Fraser and Paré's

# Diagnosis of
# Diseases
## of the
# CHEST

Fraser and Paré's

# *Diagnosis of*
# Diseases
# *of the*
# CHEST

*Fourth Edition*

*Volume III*

**R. S. Fraser, M.D.**
Professor of Pathology
McGill University Health Centre
Royal Victoria Hospital
Montreal, Quebec

**Neil Colman, M.D.**
Associate Professor of Medicine
McGill University Health Centre
Montreal General Hospital
Montreal, Quebec

**Nestor L. Müller, M.D., Ph.D.**
Professor of Radiology
University of British Columbia
Vancouver Hospital and Health
 Sciences Centre
Vancouver, British Columbia

**P. D. Paré, M.D.**
Professor of Medicine
University of British Columbia
St. Paul's Hospital
Vancouver, British Columbia

*W.B. SAUNDERS COMPANY*
**A Division of Harcourt Brace & Company**
Philadelphia   London   Toronto   Montreal   Sydney   Tokyo

**W.B. SAUNDERS COMPANY**
*A Division of Harcourt Brace & Company*

The Curtis Center
Independence Square West
Philadelphia, Pennsylvania 19106

**Library of Congress Cataloging-in-Publication Data**

Fraser and Paré's Diagnosis of diseases of the chest / Richard S. Fraser . . . [et al.].—4th ed.

p.    cm.

ISBN 0–7216–6194–7

1. Chest—Diseases—Diagnosis.    I. Fraser, Richard S.
   [DNLM: 1. Thoracic Diseases—diagnosis.    2. Diagnostic Imaging.
   WF 975D536 1999]

RC941.D52  1999    617.5′4075—dc21

DNLM/DLC                                                    98–36145

ISBN 0–7216–6194–7 (set)
ISBN 0–7216–6195–5 (vol. I)
ISBN 0–7216–6196–3 (vol. II)
ISBN 0–7216–6197–1 (vol. III)
ISBN 0–7216–6198–X (vol. IV)

FRASER AND PARÉ'S DIAGNOSIS OF DISEASES OF THE CHEST

Printed in the United States of America.

Last digit is the print number:     9    8    7    6    5    4    3    2    1

This book is dedicated to

ROBERT G. FRASER AND J. A. PETER PARÉ

who had the inspiration to recognize the importance of radiologic findings in
the diagnosis of chest disease, the dedication and perseverance to document
these and other findings in the initial editions of this book, and the grace to
teach us the value of both

and to

OUR WIVES AND CHILDREN

without whose encouragement and patience during our many hours of
reading, writing, and editing this edition would not have been completed.

# Preface to the Fourth Edition

Previous editions of this book were based on the principle that the radiograph is the "focal point" or "first step" in the diagnosis of chest disease. We agree with the fundamental importance of the radiograph in this respect; however, we feel that it is best considered as one of two "pillars" of diagnosis, the other being the clinical history. Although it is of course possible to render an opinion about the nature of a patient's illness on the basis of only one of these pillars, this is fraught with potential error and should be avoided in most cases. Instead, it is our belief that the combination of a good clinical history and high-quality posteroanterior and lateral chest radiographs provides the respiratory physician or radiologist with sufficient information to significantly limit the differential diagnosis in the vast majority of patients who have chest disease and to enable a specific (and often correct) diagnosis in many. Additional information derived from ancillary radiologic procedures, laboratory tests, pulmonary function tests, and pathologic examination enables further refinement of differential diagnosis and a confident diagnosis in almost all patients. Of these additional tests, one that has undergone significant advance in the recent past is computed tomography (CT), particularly with the advent of high-resolution (HRCT) and spiral CT. The former has enabled much clearer delineation of the location and extent of disease in the lungs, pleura, and mediastinum, and the latter has greatly improved the ability to image the airways and vessels. The current edition of this book has changed to reflect the increased availability and diagnostic accuracy of these procedures; in addition, numerous figures have been added to illustrate the various abnormalities that they can identify.

Some might argue that a knowledge of the etiology, pathogenesis, and pathologic characteristics of disease is unnecessary for the clinician or radiologist to diagnose chest disease. It is our belief, however, that a thorough understanding of the overall nature of such disease will result in improved diagnostic skill. This potential refinement may be apparent in several areas, including better appreciation of the nature of radiologic abnormalities (e.g., via a knowledge of gross pathologic findings), improved knowledge of the potential value of new diagnostic tests (e.g., via an understanding of the molecular and genetic abnormalities associated with certain diseases and with the techniques by which these are identified), and a more thorough understanding of the associations between certain diseases or disease processes (e.g., viral infection and neoplasia). For these reasons, we have included a significant amount of material that is not directly relevant to diagnosis. We recognize the limitations of this approach, particularly with respect to a consideration of disease pathogenesis—the remarkable amount of research in chest disease, especially that related to cellular and molecular mechanisms, is difficult to summarize accurately, particularly since three of us have limited involvement in fundamental research. Moreover, it is inevitable that the progress that is currently being made in this research is such that some of the material in the text will be outdated at the time it is published. Despite these limitations, we consider an understanding of the etiology and pathogenesis of chest disease to be of sufficient importance to describe them to the best of our ability.

The organization of this book is based on a fairly consistent consideration of specific diseases under the headings of epidemiology, etiology and pathogenesis, pathologic characteristics, radiologic manifestations, clinical manifestations, laboratory findings (including pulmonary function tests), and prognosis and natural history. As with previous editions, a discussion of treatment has been omitted because of the rapidity with which therapeutic strategies may change and the implications that this may have. The scope of the book is such that it is meant primarily for specialists in chest disease, including pneumologists, thoracic surgeons, chest radiologists, and pathologists whose interest lies in this field. However, we believe that residents in training for these specialties will also find the text useful.

What will our readers find that is different from previous editions? Allusion has already been made to the extensive expansion of the discussion of HRCT and the addition of numerous new illustrations. Many new pathologic illustrations, both gross and microscopic, have also been included in an attempt to better explain the anatomic basis of disease. In addition to extensive updating of the material in previous editions, new sections have been written on CT of the normal lung, pulmonary transplantation, the effects on the chest of human immunodeficiency virus (HIV) infection, and pulmonary hemorrhage syndromes. The discussion of pulmonary neoplasia has been reorganized to conform more closely to the latest World Health Organization Classification of Lung Tumors. The Tables of Differential Diagnosis have been simplified to include primarily those diseases that are likely to be encountered by most pulmonary physicians; along with an increase in the number of illustrative examples, it is hoped that this version will provide a more simple and practical guide to differential diagnosis of the commonly enountered radiographic patterns of chest disease.

To make the text more accessible to the reader, the 21 chapters of the previous three editions have been expanded to 79. The subdivision is somewhat arbitrary and has necessitated repetition of material in some areas; for example, the inclusion of a chapter on chest disease in HIV infection necessarily involves a discussion of pulmonary infections and neoplasms that are also included in other, more comprehensive chapters on these subjects. As much as possible, we have tried to limit discussion of a particular topic to one place in the text; nevertheless, we have sometimes repeated material in order to minimize the necessity for the reader to refer to other sections of the book. We have also grouped chapters into larger categories based on anatomic location or presumed etiology and pathogenesis of disease; such grouping is again somewhat arbitrary, but hopefully will provide the reader easier access to appropriate information.

The reference list of the previous editions has been culled in an attempt to include those articles that are most relevant to the points we have chosen to emphasize; however, numerous reports published before 1990 have been retained. As might be expected, many references to articles published in the 1990s have also been added in an attempt to bring the text as up to date as possible. The resulting reference list contains a somewhat daunting total of approximately 31,000 citations! The inclusion of a list such as this might be questioned in light of the relatively easy availability of personal computers and electronic reference archives. However, we feel it is useful to have such references accessible to those who wish quick access to literature sources in book form. In addition, and perhaps more important in a book compiled by only four authors, we wish to provide a "factual" basis for our assertions as much as possible. As will be appreciated by those who publish in medical journals, it is inevitable that there are errors in our reference list, sometimes with respect to omission of an author or the spelling of his or her name and sometimes with respect to inappropriate attribution of statements or to omission of a key article. We apologize for these errors in advance and ask for our readers' understanding and the feedback to correct them. (Correspondence may be sent to [DDC@pathology.lan.mcgill.ca].)

The last edition of this book included a quotation from Ecclesiastes concerning the passage of time. We would also like to offer a quote of general philosophic interest, although one that is perhaps more directly related to the subject matter of this book. It derives from Maimonides, the great twelfth century scholar and physician:

> *Do not consider a thing as proof because you find it written in books: . . . there are fools who accept a thing as (such), because it is in writing.*

What we offer in the following pages are a concept of disease of the chest and an approach to its diagnosis based on the combined experience and knowledge of reported observations of four individuals. As in our everyday practice, we have attempted to be as open-minded to new ideas and as unbiased in our selection of material as possible. Despite this, such bias is to some extent inevitable and errors of commission or omission must be present. We do not, of course, advocate the unequivocal acceptance of Maimonides' aphorism; however, we trust that our readers will take his words to heart and consider the following pages and indeed the entire subject of chest disease with a questioning and open mind.

RSF

NLM

NC

PDP

# Acknowledgments

The production of a book such as *Fraser and Paré's Diagnosis of Diseases of the Chest* is a huge task, and we have been fortunate in having the support and encouragement of many colleagues and friends in our endeavor. The availability and efficiency of modern computers have meant that much writing and editing have been performed directly by us; nevertheless, we could not have accomplished our task without secretarial help from Laura Fiorita, Stella Totilo, and Andrea Sanders at the McGill University Health Centre (MUHC); Catherine Goyette and Tamara Eigendorf at St. Paul's Hospital and the University of British Columbia; and Jenny Silver at the Vancouver Hospital and Health Sciences Centre. The diligence with which these individuals carried out their tasks shows in the final product and is deeply appreciated.

The majority of the case histories and radiologic illustrations reproduced in the text are derived from patients of staff members of the MUHC (particularly the Royal Victoria Hospital, the Montreal General Hospital, and the Montreal Chest Hospital Institute) and the Vancouver Hospital and Health Sciences Centre. Almost all illustrations of pathology are related to patients from the MUHC. We are indebted to our colleagues who cared for these patients, not only for their generosity in permitting us to publish the illustrations of various diseases but also for the benefit of their experience and guidance over the years. A number of these colleagues deserve particular mention for their comments and help on selected topics; these include Drs. Richard Menzies and John Kosiuk at the MUHC; Drs. Pearce Wilcox, John Fleetham, Brad Munt, and Hugh Chaun and Ms. Elisabeth Baile at the University of British Columbia; and Drs. A. Jean Buckley, John Aldrich, John Mayo, and Daniel Worsley at the Vancouver Hospital and Health Sciences Centre.

The photographic work throughout these volumes was the accomplishment of many individuals. Illustrations from former editions were provided by members of the Department of Visual Aids of the Royal Victoria Hospital; Susie Gray at the Department of Radiology, University of Alabama; Joseph Donohue, Anthony Graham, and Michael Paré of Montreal; and Sally Osborne at St. Paul's Hospital, Vancouver. Those involved in the production of new illustrations for this edition include Marcus Arts and Helmut Bernhard at the Montreal Neurological Institute Photography Department; Diane Minshall and Stuart Greene at St. Paul's Hospital, University of British Columbia; and Janis Franklin and Michael Robertson at the Vancouver Hospital Sciences Centre.

Throughout our writing and editing, we received support and cooperation from several individuals at W.B. Saunders, notably our Chief Editor, Lisette Bralow, our developmental editors Janice Gaillard and Melissa Messersmith, and our copy editors Sue Reilly and Lee Ann Draud, all of whom helped us overcome a number of the obstacles we encountered at various times. Finally, we acknowledge and thank our wives and children, without whose patience and encouragement this book would not have been completed.

RSF
NLM
NC
PDP

# Contents

## VOLUME ONE

## VOLUME TWO

# V O L U M E   T H R E E

# V O L U M E   F O U R

# VII
## IMMUNOLOGIC LUNG DISEASE

# Connective Tissue Diseases

The autoimmune connective tissue diseases comprise a group of disorders whose common denominator is damage to components of connective tissue at a variety of sites in the body. Specific diseases include systemic lupus erythematosus, rheumatoid disease, progressive systemic sclerosis, dermatomyositis and polymyositis, ankylosing spondylitis, Sjögren's syndrome, mixed connective tissue disease, and relapsing polychondritis. The manifestations of respiratory system involvement vary in type and severity among these disease entities, but in each, such involvement can be a cause of mortality and considerable morbidity. These diseases are often a source of great diagnostic challenge. At the end of the day, definitive diagnosis is often possible using the information derived from clinical, laboratory, radiologic, and pathologic studies. However, at presentation, full clinical expression of any of the disorders may be absent, and the placing of patients in particular diagnostic "pigeon holes" may be difficult. Although it might reasonably be argued that the vasculitides are part of the connective tissue disease group (and in fact, several of the entities discussed within it occasionally manifest this process), for purposes of discussion we have grouped them separately (Chapter 40, *see* page 1489). In addition, although ankylosing spondylitis is usually considered to be a connective tissue disease,[1] this abnormality is discussed in Chapter 78 (disorders of the chest wall, *see* page 3022).

## SYSTEMIC LUPUS ERYTHEMATOSUS

Systemic lupus erythematosus (SLE) is a multisystem autoimmune disorder for which several groups of diagnostic criteria have been proposed (Table 39–1).[2] Patients are considered to have the disease if four criteria are met sequentially or simultaneously during any period of observation. However, there are many patients who demonstrate only some of the features of classic SLE without ever evolving to the full-fledged syndrome.[2] Patients with such "overlap" syndromes or "lupus-like" disorders tend to have a good prognosis, even with conservative management.

Pulmonary involvement in SLE was first appreciated by Osler when he described a woman who had bilateral lung consolidation, hemoptysis, skin rash, anemia, and nephritis.[3] Overall, about 50% to 60% of patients have pleuropulmonary involvement at some time in their clinical course.[4] In a series of 1000 European patients studied prospectively, 3% had lung involvement and 17% pleural involvement at the onset of the disease;[5] over the period of observation a further 7% developed lung disease and 36% pleural disease.

### Epidemiology

The incidence and prevalence of SLE vary geographically, as well as with race, age, and sex. For example, the overall prevalence of the disease in Birmingham, England, is approximately 25 per 100,000 population,[6] the rate for men being 4 in 100,000 and for women 45 in 100,000 (the higher prevalence in women is a characteristic of other

## Table 39–1. CLINICAL FEATURES OF CLASSIC SYSTEMIC LUPUS ERYTHEMATOSUS

| | |
|---|---|
| Rash | Serositis |
| Discoid lupus | Renal disorder |
| Photosensitivity | Neurologic disorder |
| Oral ulcers | Hematologic disorder |
| Arthritis | Immunologic disorder |

From Panush RS, Greer JM, Morshedian KK: What is lupus? What is not lupus? Rheum Dis Clin North Am 19:223, 1993.

studies as well[7, 8]). In this study, higher rates were seen in African Caribbeans (207 per 100,000) and Asians (49 per 100,000) than in whites (20 per 100,000). A marked excess of SLE in African American women compared with whites has also been described in San Francisco and New York.[9] These figures contrast with those of studies from Africa that generally show a low prevalence of the disease in the black population,[10] and specifically a lower prevalence in South African blacks than in whites. Marked differences have also been reported in the prevalence of SLE among Chinese living in different parts of the world;[10] for example, Chinese in Malaysia have a higher prevalence than the native Malay population,[11] whereas in San Francisco there is no such excess.[9] It is unclear to what extent these differences in prevalence are related to genetic heterogeneity among populations in different parts of the world or to environmental influences.

The mean age at diagnosis in the Birmingham study cited previously was approximately 41 years (range, 11 to 83 years).[6] In contrast with earlier studies showing a younger age predominance,[9, 12] older age at diagnosis is a consistent finding in European women, having been noted in studies from Sweden, Iceland, and England.[10] In a study from the Midlands of England,[7] for example, the highest prevalence was seen in women between the ages of 40 to 49 (10.5 per 100,000) and 50 to 59 years (18.4 per 100,000).

### Serology

The screening test most commonly used in patients suspected of having SLE is a search for antinuclear antibodies (ANA). The sensitivity of the test varies from laboratory to laboratory, depending on the cut-off points used for positivity.[13] The specificity depends on the clinical setting in which it is used; it is probably wise to avoid using it as a definitive diagnostic tool in patients who have vague complaints or symptoms.[14] Most authorities agree that about 5% to 10% of patients who satisfy the diagnostic criteria for SLE are ANA negative,[15] although some patients who initially have a negative test result subsequently test positive.[16, 17]

Four patterns of antinuclear staining have been described: (1) *speckled*, the most frequent pattern, is associated with sera containing antibodies to such well-defined nuclear antigens as ribonucleoprotein (nRNP) and Sm (a soluble non-nucleic glycoprotein macromolecule), two of the major antigens present in saline-soluble extractable nuclear antigen (ENA); (2) *rim*, a pattern that is highly specific for patients who have SLE and is associated with antibodies in the serum against native deoxyribonucleic acid (nDNA Ab); (3) *nucleolar*, which is present in 50% of patients who have progressive systemic sclerosis (PSS) but seldom in those with SLE; and (4) *homogeneous*, the pattern seen in patients who have antibodies against nucleoprotein. Several patterns of ANA staining may be seen in an individual patient. ANA-negative patients who have SLE have antibodies that are directed preferentially against macromolecules located predominantly, if not solely, in the cytoplasm; these are not detected by the ANA test.

ANA production seems to be antigen driven and T cell dependent.[18] These autoantibodies are not generated randomly, because only a small proportion of available nuclear proteins is involved in the autoimmune reaction; moreover, some ANAs serve as markers of specific disease subsets. Many of the common autoantigens in SLE are constituents of large macromolecular complexes of proteins and nucleic acids.[18] Linked sets of autoantibodies to the individual components of the complex tend to be produced together, a phenomenon that could be explained by the processing of intact antigenic particles by antigen-presenting cells, followed by presentation of component peptide fragments to T lymphocytes.

Antibodies to double-stranded DNA (dsDNA) are highly specific for SLE, whereas antibodies to single-stranded DNA (ssDNA) are seen in a wide variety of autoimmune disorders, including SLE.[18, 19, 19a] However, most of the anti-dsDNA antibodies produced in SLE react with both ssDNA and dsDNA. The production of anti-dsDNA antibodies, often with reciprocal depression of serum complement, correlates with disease activity in many, but not all,[20] patients. The mechanism by which anti-DNA antibodies cause disease remains unclear[21] and other non-DNA-binding antibodies are under investigation with respect to pathogenesis. These include anti-Sm and RNP antibodies targeted against both the proteins and RNA of small nuclear ribonucleoprotein (snRNP) and antibodies directed against various components of the chromatin DNA–protein complex, such as the histones of nucleosomes.[18] Because some of these non-DNA autoantibodies can react with cell membranes, it is important to consider them in disease pathogenesis.[22]

Both cytoplasmic (c) and peripheral (p) antineutrophil cytoplasmic antibodies (ANCA) can also be found in SLE.[23, 24] In one study of 114 consecutive patients who had SLE in a Toronto Rheumatic Diseases clinic, 10% had c-ANCA and 25% p-ANCA;[23] however, no association was found between the presence of these antibodies and disease activity or expression.

A variety of investigators have attempted to identify relationships between pulmonary disease and specific autoantibodies, with somewhat conflicting results. The most clear association is that of antiphospholipid antibodies with thrombocytopenia and thromboembolic disease, including both venous thrombosis and pulmonary thromboembolism. Although some workers have reported an association between the presence of anti-Ro and lung disease in SLE,[25, 26] others have not.[27] A weak association between anti-U1-RNP and pulmonary fibrosis has been documented in a study from the Netherlands;[28] antibodies against the eukaryotic ribosomal protein L7 (found in approximately one third of patients who have SLE) also seem to correlate with the presence of lung fibrosis. Interestingly, the latter antibody has been found in about 40% of patients who have progressive systemic sclerosis, in which it appears to have no correlation with lung fibrosis.[29]

While it is worthwhile noting the wide variety of autoantibodies described in patients who have SLE, it is important to recognize that the antibody pattern, and often the clinical features, tend to remain the same over time in specific individuals.[30]

### Etiology and Pathogenesis

The etiology and pathogenesis of SLE are incompletely understood and undoubtedly complex. The marked heterogeneity in clinical and laboratory abnormalities[31] suggests that a variety of genetic, environmental, and hormonal influences may initiate or modulate the abnormal immunologic reactions found in the disease.

### Genetic Factors

There is considerable evidence that genetic factors play an important role in both disease susceptibility and expression. Such evidence comes from epidemiologic studies of the incidence and prevalence of disease in related individuals, experimental investigations in lupus-prone mice, and studies of major histocompatibility haplotypes. The role of many genes has been examined, especially those encoding elements of the immune system.[30, 30a] Associations with major histocompatibility haplotypes, as well as with deficiencies of early components of the complement system, are well established. There is also increasing evidence for participation of genes regulating T-cell receptors, immunoglobulins, cytokines,[30, 30b] and even angiotensin-converting enzyme.[30c]

Estimates of the concordance of SLE among monozygotic twins vary from 15%[32] to 30%.[31] In one investigation of 728 first-degree relatives of 102 patients who had SLE, approximately 10% of the patients had a relative with the disease.[33] The overall prevalence of SLE among these relatives was 1.4%, a value much larger than that of the general population, in which it has been estimated to be only 0.2% to 0.3%.[30]

Many investigators have examined the relationship between SLE or SLE subtypes and specific genotypes of the major histocompatibility gene complex (human leukocyte antigens [HLA]). Since the class II MHC molecule is involved in antigen-specific T-cell responses involving helper T cells and the class I molecule is related to activation of antigen-specific cytotoxic T cells, an association between the disease and these molecules has some biologic plausibility. Normally, T cells do not respond to a self-antigen bound within an MHC molecule; however, in SLE, certain antigens are able to initiate and perpetuate autoimmune responses.[30]

Early workers identified a strong association between SLE and HLA-DR3 and HLA-DR2, particularly in patients who have subacute cutaneous lupus;[34] in some studies, 100% of such patients had DR3 and B8 antigens (the latter possibly being coinherited with DR3).[35] A Swiss study in Caucasian patients who had SLE revealed the complete absence of DRw15/3 and DRw15/7 heterozygotes;[36] the authors hypothesized that the presence of these alleles might be linked ultimately to the formation of a molecule that confers resistance to SLE. A study from Northern India found a significant increase in the prevalence of HLA-DR4 in patients (38%) compared with controls (18%).[37] Haplotype B8-DR3 was also found frequently in this patient group. A Canadian study underlines the importance of ethnicity in examining these associations. Canadians of Anglo-Saxon origin had a higher prevalence of the HLA-B8, DR3, C4A null haplotype, whereas DQ6 was associated with SLE in French Canadians.[38] Despite these findings, it is evident that the disease has no HLA associations at all in some racial groups.[30]

Several groups have shown that particular HLA alleles may be more closely associated with certain autoantibodies than with SLE itself. For example anti-Ro and anti-La antibodies are strongly associated with the presence of DR2 and DR3 and with heterozygosity for the HLA-DQ alleles DQw1 and DQw2.[30] The application of PCR and oligonucleotide probe technology has allowed the determination of HLA variants at the DNA level. The results of such studies have shown that there may be shared sequences among the different HLA alleles that are associated with disease susceptibility.[30]

Genetically determined complement deficiency is also strongly associated with the development of SLE, although this explains only a minority of cases in most populations. In one investigation of 81 people who had SLE from 14 families, there was a strong association between C4A deletion and disease,[39] confirming results described earlier in which the C4A gene deletion was associated with subacute cutaneous lupus and Sjögren's syndrome.[40] The mechanism by which complement deficiency may be involved in the development of SLE is unclear; however, it may be important in the clearing of immune complexes, and its dysfunction could allow for the deposition of such complexes in tissue. Although a deficiency early in the complement cascade may be suggested by particular features of SLE, lung involvement is not a characteristic feature of such deficiency.

### Environmental Factors

A variety of environmental factors have been implicated in the pathogenesis of SLE, the most extensively investigated being light, microorganisms, and drugs.

**Light.** One to two thirds of patients who have SLE develop a skin rash on exposure to light. In addition, both sunlight and the ultraviolet B radiation emitted by cool, white fluorescent lamps may induce exacerbations of systemic disease.[31] The mechanisms underlying these reactions are unclear. However, there is evidence that ultraviolet light may increase the expression of SLE-related antigens such as Ro, La, and RNP at the plasma membrane.[31] It may also induce the release of cytokines in the epidermis and dermis, which in turn may initiate an inflammatory reaction directed against keratinocytes.[41]

**Infection.** A number of groups have shown elevated antibody titers to certain viruses in the serum of patients who have SLE.[42-46] In addition, ultrastructural investigations have shown so-called tubuloreticular structures (TRS) within endothelial cells of glomeruli, skin, and lung;[47] although these do not represent virus material, they are commonly seen in infections such as viral pneumonia, as well as in SLE and other presumed autoimmune disorders.[47] TRS can be induced experimentally in lymphoblasts by interferon,[48] and it has thus been postulated that viral antigen may initiate the formation of TRS by inducing interferon production by sensitized lymphocytes. Supporting this hypothesis are studies that have documented interferon levels directly proportional to disease activity in the serum of patients who have active SLE as well as patients who have other autoimmune disease.[47, 49]

The precise virus or viruses that may be involved in these reactions have not been identified. In one case-control study in which 195 patients who had SLE were compared with 143 sex- and age-matched controls, a history of shingles was found to be strongly associated with a risk for the disease, implicating herpes zoster.[50] Endogenous retroviruses mediate lupus in some murine models[29, 51] and there is con-

siderable homology in the nucleotide sequences of the circulating DNA strands found in patients who have SLE and portions of human immunodeficiency virus-1 (HIV-1).[52] If these circulating nucleic acids act as antigens, then the potential for retroviruses in the etiology of SLE becomes apparent.

Patients who have SLE and who are receiving immunosuppressive therapy seem especially prone to the development of *Salmonella* infection;[53] in fact, several patients have been described in whom the first presentation of SLE was concurrent with *Salmonella* bacteremia.[54] Although this association is more likely to be related to a specific defect in host defense, the possibility that salmonellosis may occasionally induce SLE has not been excluded.[54]

Heat shock proteins of infecting organisms are similar in structure to those produced by humans in response to a variety of infections and other stresses. Some investigators have speculated that antibodies produced against these bacterial proteins may cross-react with those of humans and have a pathogenetic role in a variety of connective tissue diseases.[55]

**Drugs.** It is well recognized that SLE can be induced by certain drugs, including hydralazine; procainamide; isoniazid; phenytoin and other anticonvulsants; quinidine; methyldopa; chlorpromazine; sulfasalazine; and the beta-adrenoreceptor blocking agents, acebutolol, labetalol, pindolol, and propranolol.[56-65] Disease related to these agents is typically devoid of serious manifestations, such as nephritis and cerebritis.[62]

In addition to these drugs, there is also convincing evidence of an association between SLE and long-standing treatment with penicillamine.[66] This drug is associated with a wide range of immunologic disorders, including myasthenia gravis, an immune-complex pulmonary-renal hemorrhagic syndrome, obliterative bronchiolitis, pemphigus, polymyositis, and membranous glomerulonephritis.[66] Interestingly, SLE associated with penicillamine shows clinical and laboratory features that are somewhat different from those seen with other drugs that induce the SLE syndrome; in addition to having elevated levels of ANA, affected patients are more likely to develop glomerulonephritis and neurologic disorders, and to have hypocomplementemia and antibodies to dsDNA.

Although the precise pathogenesis of drug-related disease remains obscure, certain clinical, epidemiologic, and laboratory features suggest that it is more than a simple unveiling of a latent predisposition to idiopathic SLE. Patients who acquire drug-induced SLE are almost invariably "slow acetylators" of the responsible medication; the few affected patients who are "fast acetylators" have often received large doses of the drug.[67] Acetylation takes place in the liver through the enzyme *N*-acetyltransferase. The process is genetically determined, rapid-acetylating patients probably having an autosomal dominant gene, whereas slow-acetylating patients are homozygotes for the allele coding for slow acetylation.[68] In addition to the inherited control of acetylation, patients who develop drug-induced SLE are commonly found to carry the HLA-DR4 locus.

The genetic control of susceptibility to the drug-provoked variant of SLE was demonstrated in one study of 26 patients who had hydralazine-induced SLE, 25 of whom were slow acetylators.[68] In contrast with control groups of rapid acetylators and patients who had hypertension who were receiving the drug but did not show HLA-DR4, all slow-acetylating women who had HLA-DR4 developed the disease; men who developed SLE were receiving higher daily doses of the drug and were slow acetylators with HLA-DR4. Additional evidence implicating acetylation in the pathogenesis of the disease lies in the demonstration that acetylprocainamide in generally accepted therapeutic dosages can be given with impunity to patients who have procainamide-induced SLE.[69, 70]

It has also been suggested that drugs causing SLE may be transformed to reactive metabolites as a result of oxidation by activated phagocytic cells.[71, 72] The action of these metabolites on the surface of monocytes responsible for inducing an immune response could then be the initiating process in the abnormal drug reaction. Antigen-specific CD4 cells may become autoreactive after treatment with DNA methylation inhibitors, a mechanism that also may be important in some cases of drug-induced disease.[31]

**Miscellaneous Environmental Factors.** A variety of other potential environmental influences on the development of SLE have been described. The recognition that a cluster of four workers involved in the production of scouring powder that had a high silica content had connective tissue disease led to the examination of 50 workers in the same plant:[73] 32 of these workers had symptoms of a systemic disease. Among them were 3 who had SLE and 5 who had an overlap syndrome. In a case-control epidemiologic study from Japan, an age-adjusted odds ratio of 2.3 was found for SLE among current smokers compared with a control group of health examination participants from public health centers.[74] In another Japanese study, frequent ingestion of meat was associated with a relative risk of SLE of 3.4 compared with rare ingestion of meat.[75] Although extensively studied, silicone breast implants have not been convincingly shown to be associated with the development of SLE.[76, 77]

### Endocrine Factors

Several observations support the hypothesis that there is an endocrine component in the pathogenesis of SLE. As indicated previously, epidemiologic studies have documented a pronounced susceptibility of women for the disease. Moreover, an increased risk for the development of SLE has been shown in postmenopausal woman who receive estrogen replacement therapy, the risk increasing proportionately with duration of therapy.[78] (Despite this, the use of oral contraceptives and postmenopausal hormone replacement therapy has not been associated with deterioration in patients who have established SLE.[31]) In a study of the genetic and endocrine features of 16 men who had SLE, a higher-than-expected incidence of hyperestrogenemia and hypoandrogenemia was found.[79] Experiments on castrated male mice, in which the incidence of SLE-like disease is higher, also suggest an important hormonal effect.[34]

### Immune Factors

As previously discussed, the production of autoantibodies to cellular macromolecules is an important immunologic disturbance in patients who have SLE. However, it is not certain to what extent these antibodies are pathogenic and to what extent they simply reflect the consequences of tissue damage.[31] If the former, they could theoretically mediate tissue injury by either an immune-complex mediated inflammatory response or by antibody-mediated cellular damage.[31] That antibodies are indeed pathogenetic is supported by the observation that B-cell activation is directed against a defined and limited range of cellular antigens, and by animal models of SLE that are characterized by B-cell hyperactivity.[31] It is notable that a higher ratio of helper (CD4) to suppressor (CD8) lymphocytes in the peripheral blood has been associated with disease activity in general, and lung involvement in particular.[26]

It is unclear whether SLE is related to excessive T-cell help or defective T-cell suppression;[31] however, interleukin-6, a lymphokine that may be involved in an autocrine pathway for B-cell activation, is elevated in the sera of patients who have SLE.[80] In addition, tumor necrosis factor-alpha (TNF-alpha) release is inhibited from the peripheral blood monocytes of patients who have SLE;[81] correction of this deficit by the administration of recombinant TNF-alpha inhibits the abnormal B-cell proliferation.

In contrast with findings in the blood, bronchoalveolar lavage (BAL) fluid from patients who have SLE reveals increased levels of activated CD8 cells and natural killer cells independent of changes in peripheral lymphocyte distribution and general disease activity. Activation of these cells can be associated with the production of $O_2$ radicals, which can cause tissue damage on their release.[82] BAL mononuclear cells have also been shown to have enhanced production of transforming growth factor-beta, which is an important mitogen for fibroblasts.[83] Both these functions could account, in part, for lung damage in patients who have SLE.

### *Pathologic Characteristics*

At autopsy, pathologic changes in the lungs and pleura are common in patients who have SLE.[3, 84–86] However, because of the frequent involvement of other organs and tissues, it is not always clear in an individual patient which of these changes is related to a direct effect of SLE and which to an effect of therapy or of complicating disease in the lungs or other site. In many instances, it is probably the latter that is important.[84] Pathologic findings that have been proposed as being caused by SLE itself, at least in some patients, include pleuritis and pleural fibrosis (with or without effusion), interstitial pneumonitis and fibrosis, vasculitis, pulmonary arterial hypertension,[87] pulmonary hemorrhage,[88] lymphocytic interstitial pneumonitis,[89] and follicular bronchiolitis.[90]

Pleural fibrosis is the most common finding at autopsy, having been reported in as many as 80% to 100% of cases in some series;[85, 87, 92] acute fibrinous pleuritis is seen less frequently.[87] In patients who have pleural effusion, immune complexes have been found in the walls of the parietal pleural capillaries.[93]

Although focal parenchymal interstitial inflammation and fibrosis have been documented with reasonable frequency by some investigators,[85, 87] diffuse interstitial pneumonitis is uncommon; in one series of 120 patients, only 5 cases were identified.[84] Pathologic findings in these cases are similar to those of idiopathic pulmonary fibrosis.[95, 96] Immunopathologic studies of biopsy specimens in one study showed granular deposition of IgG, C3, and DNA in alveolar walls, and electron microscopy revealed electron-dense deposits in a similar location;[96] eluates from frozen lung tissue contained antinuclear and anti-DNA activity.

"Acute lupus pneumonitis" refers to an uncommon manifestation of SLE characterized by fever, dyspnea, hypoxemia, and patchy, diffuse radiographic opacities in the absence of infection.[97] Pathologic features in these patients are variable. Some cases show diffuse alveolar damage (intra-alveolar proteinaceous exudate, hyaline membranes, and an interstitial mononuclear inflammatory infiltrate)[92, 98] and others capillaritis and alveolar hemorrhage (Fig. 39–1; *also see* page 1513).[99–103] Immunofluorescent deposits of DNA, anti-DNA Ab, IgG, and C3 as well as subendothelial electron-dense deposits can be identified within the lungs of many patients who have acute lupus pneumonitis, with or without hemorrhage.[99, 100, 102, 103]

Some patients develop pulmonary hypertension, characterized pathologically by intimal fibrosis, medial hypertrophy, and (sometimes) plexiform lesions; in most of these, there is a history of Raynaud's phenomenon.[105, 106] The vessels of some patients who have the antiphospholipid syndrome show concentric intimal hyperplasia.[107]

### Radiologic Manifestations

Radiologic abnormalities may be seen in the lungs, pleura, and heart, alone or in combination. In one study of

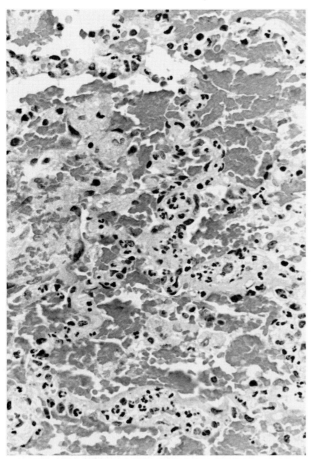

**Figure 39–1. Systemic Lupus Erythematosus—Capillaritis with Pulmonary Hemorrhage.** A magnified view of lung parenchyma shows several alveolar air spaces filled with red blood cells. The adjacent septa contain a moderate number of neutrophils, some of which appear fragmented. (×300.)

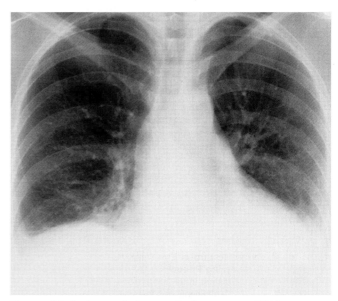

**Figure 39–2. Systemic Lupus Erythematosus (SLE).** A posteroanterior chest radiograph demonstrates small pleural effusions and decreased lung volumes. Mild enlargement of the cardiopericardial silhouette was shown at echocardiography to be due to a pericardial effusion. This constellation of findings is characteristic of SLE. The patient was a 30-year-old woman.

21 patients who had radiographic abnormalities in the thorax, the findings included pleural effusion in 13, various pulmonary parenchymal changes in 10, pericardial effusion in 5, and cardiomegaly in 5.[108] In another investigation of 275 patients, 46% had normal chest radiographs, 35% had pleural effusion or thickening, 13% had pulmonary abnormalities, and 37% had cardiomegaly or pericardial effusion.[109]

As is evident from these figures, pleural effusion is the most common thoracic manifestation of SLE.[108, 110] It is frequently bilateral; although usually small (Fig. 39–2), it may be massive.[109, 110] Such pleural involvement is frequently an early manifestation of SLE: in one series of 57 patients, pleural effusion occurred in 42;[111] in 3 of these, pleuritis appeared as an isolated first sign of SLE, and in 16 others it was associated with only minor antecedent symptoms of the disease. In 23 of the 42 cases the effusion was bilateral, either simultaneously or alternately; 13 of the 19 cases of unilateral effusion were situated on the left. The effusions may resolve completely[112] or result in mild residual pleural thickening.[109]

The radiographic abnormalities in the lungs usually are nonspecific and commonly consist of rather poorly defined patchy areas of parenchymal consolidation involving mainly the lung bases.[110, 113] In most patients—up to 70% in some series[110]—these areas are the result of infection; occasionally, they represent bronchiolitis obliterans organizing pneumonia (BOOP) (Fig. 39–3).[114] The radiographic findings in acute lupus pneumonitis consist of patchy unilateral or bilateral areas of ground-glass opacity (Fig. 39–4) or air-space consolidation, often associated with pleural effusions.[110] Occasionally, the chest radiograph is normal.[115]

Alveolar hemorrhage, whether or not accompanied by the clinical syndrome of acute lupus pneumonitis, is manifested radiologically by bilateral, patchy, ill-defined areas of consolidation involving mainly the lower lung zones.[110] In

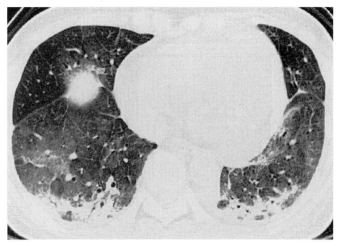

**Figure 39–3. Systemic Lupus Erythematosus (SLE): Bronchiolitis Obliterans Organizing Pneumonia.** An HRCT scan demonstrates localized areas of consolidation in the lower lobes. These have a predominantly peribronchial and subpleural distribution. Focal areas of ground-glass attenuation are also evident. The patient was a 46-year-old woman with SLE who presented with progressive shortness of breath and poorly defined areas of consolidation on the chest radiograph. The diagnosis of bronchiolitis obliterans organizing pneumonia was confirmed by lung biopsy.

patients who have severe hemorrhage, the radiographs may demonstrate extensive bilateral areas of ground-glass opacity or multifocal or confluent areas of consolidation (Fig. 39–5).[112, 116] It has been suggested that magnetic resonance (MR) imaging may show characteristic findings in these cases, consisting of intermediate signal intensity on proton density spin-echo images and low signal on T2-weighted images.[117]

Radiographic evidence of interstitial fibrosis is seen in a small percentage of patients who have SLE (Fig. 39–6); it was reported in 3 of 28 patients in one series,[118] 1 of 44 patients in a second,[119] and was not evident in any of 270 patients in a third.[109] In another investigation of the incidence of abnormalities in an outpatient SLE clinic over a 1-year period, diffuse interstitial lung disease was found in 18 patients (approximately 3% of those studied).[120]

Horizontal line shadows are seen relatively commonly in patients who have SLE. They are usually present in the lung bases, are sometimes migratory, and are probably attributable to subsegmental atelectasis. Cavitary pulmonary nodules are rare; in one study of six patients who had SLE or mixed connective tissue disease with this abnormality,[121] the lesion proved to be the result of infection or pulmonary infarction in five. Although local parenchymal changes may be fairly extensive without producing symptoms,[122] it is likely that the converse is more often the case—many patients complain of dyspnea and have considerable impairment of pulmonary function without manifesting parenchymal abnormalities on the radiograph. In some of these patients, sequential radiographs show progressive loss of lung volume,[97] a shrinkage that may be associated with an elevated diaphragm as a result of muscle weakness.[110, 123, 124]

The presence and extent of parenchymal abnormalities in patients who have SLE are frequently underestimated on the chest radiograph.[125–127] In a prospective study of 48

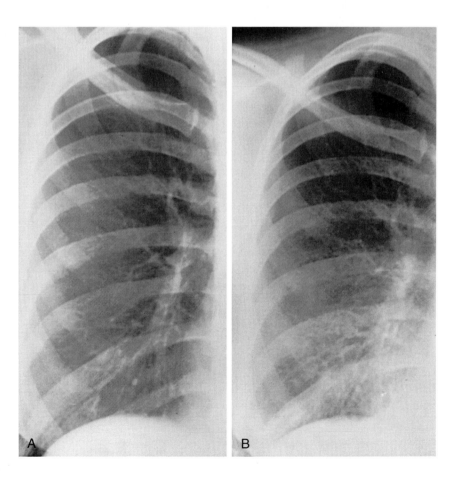

**Figure 39–4. Acute Lupus Pneumonitis.** A detail view of the right lung from a posteroanterior radiograph *(A)* is normal. Two days later, following the onset of dyspnea and cough in this patient with systemic lupus erythematosus *(B)*, the right lung shows increased opacity and poorly defined markings in the mid and lower portions of the chest. Similar features were identified in the left lung. Note that there is no recruitment of upper zone vessels to suggest that pulmonary venous hypertension was a cause for the pulmonary abnormality. The changes are consistent with acute noncardiac pulmonary edema.

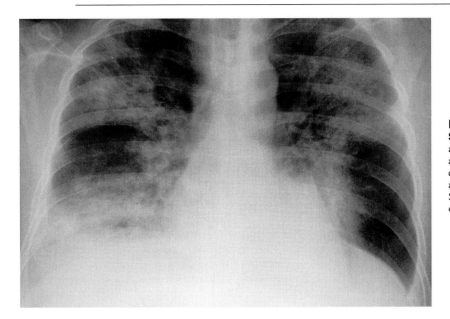

**Figure 39–5. Diffuse Pulmonary Hemorrhage in Systemic Lupus Erythematosus (SLE).** A postero-anterior chest radiograph demonstrates extensive bilateral areas of consolidation with relative sparing of the peripheral lung regions. Small bilateral pleural effusions are also evident. The patient was a 24-year-old man with SLE who presented with hemoptysis. The parenchymal opacities resolved within 72 hours.

patients who had serologically confirmed disease but no prior clinical evidence of pulmonary involvement, chest radiographs demonstrated evidence of fibrosis in 3 patients (6%) and were normal in 45 (94%).[125] Of the 45 patients who had normal radiographs, 17 (38%) had abnormal findings on HRCT. The most common abnormalities were interlobular septal thickening (33% of patients), intralobular interstitial thickening (33%), small rounded areas of consolidation (22%), and areas of ground-glass attenuation (13%). The abnormalities occurred mainly in the lower lobes in 14 patients and in the middle lobes in 3; the fibrosis involved mainly the subpleural lung regions and had an appearance

similar to that of interstitial fibrosis seen in other connective tissue disorders. The duration of SLE clinically in this group of patients ranged from 8 to 52 months.

In another prospective study, 34 patients who had SLE were assessed using chest radiography, HRCT, and pulmonary function tests.[126] The plain chest radiograph was abnormal in 8 patients (24%), pulmonary function abnormalities were present in 14 (41%), and HRCT abnormalities were identified in 24 (70%). The authors reported that 11 patients (32%) had definite evidence of interstitial lung disease, which was mild in 5 patients and moderately advanced in 6. Nine of the 11 patients who had evidence of interstitial lung

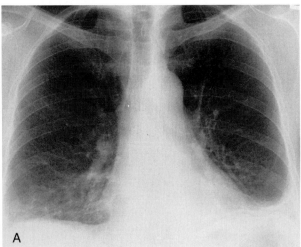

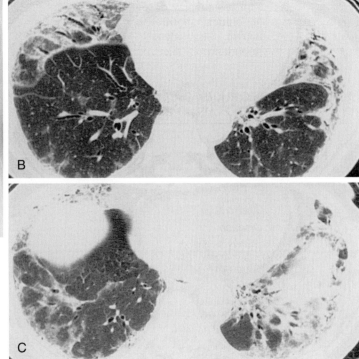

**Figure 39–6. Systemic Lupus Erythematosus (SLE): Pulmonary Fibrosis.** A posteroanterior chest radiograph *(A)* demonstrates irregular linear opacities in the lower lung zones. HRCT scans *(B and C)* demonstrate parenchymal abnormalities involving the right middle lobe, the lingula, and the lower lobes. The findings consist of areas of ground-glass attenuation as well as irregular linear opacities, distortion of lung architecture, and bronchial dilation indicative of fibrosis. The patient was a 53-year-old woman who had long-standing SLE.

disease on HRCT were asymptomatic, 7 had normal chest radiographs, and 4 had normal pulmonary function tests. Airway disease—defined as bronchial dilation or bronchial wall thickening—was observed in 12 patients (9 of whom had never smoked cigarettes).

As might be expected, the prevalence of parenchymal abnormalities is highest in patients who have long-standing SLE and chronic respiratory symptoms. In one study of 10 patients who had a mean duration of SLE of 7.5 years and who had respiratory symptoms for a mean of 2.5 years, all patients had abnormal pulmonary function tests and HRCT scans (4 had normal chest radiographs).[127] The most common abnormalities on HRCT were areas of ground-glass attenuation (seen in 8 patients), honeycombing (in 7), and pleural thickening (in 8). Two patients had airway abnormalities, consisting of bronchial dilation in one and centrilobular nodular and branching linear opacities ("tree-in-bud" appearance) in the other.

Cardiovascular changes frequently occur in association with pulmonary and pleural manifestations; increase in the size of the cardiac silhouette is generally the result of pericardial effusion, which usually is relatively small but may be massive.[109, 128] Both cardiomegaly and pulmonary edema may be caused by primary lupus myocardiopathy. The radiographic manifestations of drug-induced SLE are no different from those of the idiopathic form.[129]

### Clinical Manifestations

The clinical manifestations of pleuropulmonary involvement in SLE are numerous (Table 39–2). Even when combined with a knowledge of radiologic abnormalities, their diagnostic significance may be uncertain. On the one hand, similar signs, symptoms, and radiographic changes could be due to any one of several manifestations of SLE or to infection. On the other hand, as discussed in the section on radiology, subclinical pleuropulmonary abnormalities are common if searched for assiduously enough with HRCT or function studies. The clinical significance of these latter abnormalities is unknown. Although it is likely wrong to attribute the same importance to them that one would to

### Table 39–2. PLEUROPULMONARY DISEASE IN SYSTEMIC LUPUS ERYTHEMATOSUS

*Pleural Disease*
  Pleuritis with and without effusion

*Parenchymal Disease*
  Acute lupus pneumonitis
  Interstitial pneumonitis and fibrosis
  Pulmonary hemorrhage

*Vascular Disease*
  Pulmonary artery thrombosis
  Pulmonary thromboembolism
  Pulmonary hypertension

*Airway Disease*
  Obliterative bronchiolitis
  Bronchiolitis obliterans organizing pneumonia

*Neuromuscular Disease*
  Diaphragmatic dysfunction

clinically evident disease, close follow-up is probably advisable; for example, in one patient who had this constellation of radiologic and clinical findings, histologic abnormalities consistent with acute lupus pneumonitis were demonstrated on a transbronchial biopsy specimen.[130]

Although more than one variety of pleuropulmonary disease may occur in an individual patient, and there is some overlap in clinical manifestations, the different forms are conveniently discussed separately. The most common abnormality is pleural disease.

### Pleural Disease

Clinically detectable involvement of the pleura occurs during the course of disease in up to 70% of patients and is the presenting manifestation in 5%.[131] The subject is discussed in detail in Chapter 69 (*see* page 2753).

### Acute Lupus Pneumonitis

Symptomatic acute lupus pneumonitis is an uncommon manifestation of SLE, estimates of its incidence varying from 1% to 12%.[92, 132] Patients may present with the abrupt onset of dyspnea, fever, cough, cyanosis, pleuritic chest pain, and, occasionally, hemoptysis. Although this can be the sole and presenting manifestation of disease, it is more commonly associated with multisystem disease and serologic findings of SLE.[4] The complication appears to be particularly common in postpartum exacerbations.[1] It may resolve completely with appropriate therapy; however, chronic interstitial disease persists in some patients.[4]

The clinical manifestations and radiologic features are similar to those of pneumonia caused by bacteria and a variety of nonbacterial opportunistic microorganisms and of thromboembolic disease; the distinction among them is clearly vital to proper patient management. Practically, the diagnosis is often one of exclusion, being made after aggressive attempts at identifying an infectious or thromboembolic etiology for the radiographic abnormalities have failed.

### Diffuse Interstitial Pneumonitis and Fibrosis

Data on the prevalence and clinical features of interstitial pneumonitis and fibrosis in patients who have SLE are scanty, since the literature is derived from case reports and retrospective review.[3] Nevertheless, the complication is clearly uncommon: as indicated previously, radiographic evidence of disease has been noted in 0 to 3% of patients,[8, 109] and in one autopsy study of 120 patients, moderate or severe fibrosis was noted in only 4 individuals.[84] Although the disease resembles that of idiopathic pulmonary fibrosis in both pathologic and radiologic aspects, from clinical and functional points of view its course is usually less severe.[3] It may develop *de novo* or follow one or more episodes of acute lupus pneumonitis.[1] Patients complain of dyspnea and have bibasilar crackles on physical examination and restrictive lung function.[95]

The diagnosis is usually apparent on the basis of radiologic and clinical findings.[1] However, in some cases it may be difficult to distinguish radiographically apparent fibrotic disease from the plate shadows seen at the bases of the lungs in patients who have SLE and diaphragmatic dysfunction (*see* farther on).[133]

### Diffuse Alveolar Hemorrhage

The triad of anemia, air-space consolidation, and hemoptysis should suggest the possibility of diffuse alveolar hemorrhage. In fact, because of its prognostic implication, the diagnosis should be considered in a patient who has dyspnea and diffuse air-space opacities radiologically even in the absence of hemoptysis.[134] We and others believe that the abnormality is part of the clinicopathologic spectrum of acute lupus pneumonitis.[1] The manifestation is rare; it occurred in only 1.6% of patients in one series[134] and was responsible for 3.7% of 510 hospitalizations for complications of SLE in another.[135]

Anemia with a dropping hematocrit in the face of worsening radiologic abnormalities is characteristic. Hemoptysis may be absent, mild,[136, 137] or severe.[101, 102, 138, 139] Although the hemorrhage usually occurs in the setting of established SLE, it may be the sole and presenting manifestation;[135] in this situation, patients are usually considered to suffer from pulmonary hemosiderosis until other features of SLE become evident.[137, 140] As indicated previously, the pathologic basis of the abnormality is usually capillaritis, a complication that is most likely immune mediated.[110, 135] Many patients have concomitant lupus nephritis.[135] With cessation of bleeding, radiographic and clinical improvement is rapid; in fact, the chest radiograph may become normal within 2 to 4 days.[3] The differential diagnosis of hemoptysis in patients who have SLE includes heart failure, necrotizing infection, and thromboembolic disease. The severity of bleeding from any of these conditions may be aggravated by lupus-related thrombocytopenia.

The mortality rate of diffuse alveolar hemorrhage has generally been reported to be in excess of 50%,[99, 101, 134, 135, 138] although occasional groups have documented better results,[142, 143] possibly as a result of earlier diagnosis and aggressive management.

### Disease Associated with Antiphospholipid Antibodies

Antiphospholipid antibodies are a heterogeneous group of immunoglobulins directed against negatively charged phospholipids, protein-phospholipid complexes, or plasma proteins such as beta$_2$-glycoprotein-I.[144] They can be identified by a variety of tests, including an ELISA (which measures anticardiolipin antibodies and is the most reliable),[145] the VDRL, and a functional coagulation assay that detects the antiprothrombinase, lupus anticoagulant; each of these tests probably recognizes different, although overlapping, antibody populations.[146, 147]

Although these antibodies can be present in patients who meet standard diagnostic criteria for SLE, they are found as often in those who do not.[148] When the latter patients experience thrombotic events they are said to have the primary antiphospholipid syndrome (Hughes' syndrome).[149, 150] A number of similarities and differences in the clinical behavior and laboratory findings of these two groups of patients have been described. In a large European study, in which both groups were strictly defined, there were similar histories of venous thrombosis, pulmonary thromboembo-

lism, arterial thrombosis, thrombocytopenia, livedo reticularis, and pulmonary hypertension;[151] however, patients who had SLE demonstrated more frequent hemolytic anemia, neutropenia, and valvular heart disease than did the group that had "primary" disease. Both types of patients are at increased risk of recurremt embolic events after discontinuation of anticoagulation therapy.[94]

Patients who have SLE show different clinical manifestations related to the presence or absence of anticardiolipin antibodies. In one study of 842 patients, those in whom the antibody was of IgG type had a more significant history of thrombosis (30% vs. 9%), spontaneous fetal losses (31% vs. 17%), thrombocytopenia (30% vs. 18%), and livedo reticularis (22% vs. 10%), when compared with patients who had negative titers;[5] unfortunately, correlations with antibody level and persistence were not examined in the study. Similar risks were noted for IgM antibodies, which were less prevalent overall. These findings are in keeping with those of other reports in which a strong association between the presence of antiphospholipid antibodies in SLE and pulmonary thromboembolism, deep venous thrombosis, thrombocytopenia, recurrent fetal loss, leg ulcers, and central nervous system disease has been documented.[3, 146, 152–154] In fact, the results of a meta-analysis of 26 articles suggested that patients who have SLE and the lupus anticoagulant have a sixfold greater risk for venous thrombosis than those who do not have the antibody, while the presence of anticardiolipin antibodies doubles this risk.[155] Despite these findings, it is important to note that in *unselected* patients who have SLE, the presence of these antibodies has a low predictive value for these clinical features.[156–158]

The pathogenesis of the procoagulant effect of these antibodies is unknown. Some have speculated that they may bind to the prothrombinase complex and inhibit its activity.[146] There seems to be a particularly strong association between thrombotic events and the presence of anticardiolipin antibodies that bind the plasma protein beta$_2$-glycoprotein-I (a cofactor of anticardiolipin). Antibodies to this cofactor have also been associated with the antiphospholipid syndrome in the absence of anticardiolipin antibodies, in both patients who have SLE and those who do not.[159] Despite these observations, the explanation for a number of important clinical features remains obscure, including the reason for the episodic nature of the clotting, the mechanism of the initiating event, and the localization of thrombotic events,[160] and further investigations are necessary to clarify the inconstant relationship of the antibodies to thrombotic events.[147, 161] Patients who have SLE and antiphospholipid antibodies also have reduced free protein S levels and generate more thrombin than lupus patients who have normal free protein S levels, both factors that contribute to their thrombotic state.[162] Although endothelial injury may precede vascular occlusion, there is no histologic evidence of vasculitis.[31]

The presence of clinical manifestations related to antiphospholipid antibodies is associated with decreased survival in patients who have SLE.[163] On the other hand, some patients have transient, low-grade levels of these antibodies when their disease is active; generally, they do not have the thrombotic complications characteristic of patients who have persistent high antibody levels, particularly of the IgG type.[156, 164–166]

## Pulmonary Hypertension

Clinically important pulmonary hypertension is rare in SLE.[1] However, when sensitive techniques such as echocardiography are used to identify its presence, the prevalence in case series ranges from 4% to as high as 43%.[167–170] Clinical signs and symptoms include dyspnea on exertion, chest pain, dry cough, fatigue, ankle swelling, jugular venous distention, right ventricular heave, augmentation of the intensity of the second heart sound, and auscultation of a murmur of tricuspid insufficiency.[171] Although radiographs usually show the characteristic features of hypertension, they may be normal early in the disease process.[3]

An underlying mechanism responsible for the hypertension, such as interstitial fibrosis and thromboembolism, can be found in some patients; in others, the pathogenesis is inapparent. In the latter-named situation, the disease resembles primary pulmonary hypertension clinically, radiologically, and pathologically. Up to 75% of affected patients demonstrate Raynaud's phenomenon as part of their clinical picture, compared with only 25% of the lupus population in general.[172] The prevalence of anticardiolipin antibody is high in patients who have hypertension; however, this finding is of uncertain significance, since there is no relationship between the titer of the antibody and the severity of the hypertension,[173] and patients usually do not show any other evidence of the antiphospholipid syndrome.[174]

Antiendothelial cell antibodies have been identified in a number of patients who have SLE.[175] These antibodies induce the release of endothelin-1, a potent pulmonary artery vasoconstrictor that could play a role in vascular injury.[175] The level of these antibodies, of both the IgG and IgM type, is higher in patients who have pulmonary hypertension than in those who do not. Titers are also higher in patients who have digital vasculopathy and Raynaud's phenomenon.[176] Although these findings suggest a role for these antibodies in the pathogenesis of pulmonary hypertension, the details of the possible mechanism are unclear. Fatal pulmonary hypertension has been described in a set of identical twins who had SLE, suggesting a genetic factor in the pathogenesis in at least some cases.[177] Immunoglobulin and complement have occasionally been found in the pulmonary artery wall, suggesting that immune complex deposition may somehow be involved.[171] The high frequency of Raynaud's phenomenon and the occurrence of pulmonary hypertension, measured echocardiographically, during flares of disease, also suggest a possible vasospastic reaction.[4]

The presence of pulmonary hypertension is a poor prognostic sign, the 2-year mortality exceeding 50%.[3] In one study of 24 patients who had SLE and pulmonary hypertension (21 of whom seemed to have idiopathic disease), 13 patients died, most as a result of cor pulmonale;[174] 4 were lost to follow-up, and only 7 remained alive and accounted for at the end of the period of observation.

## Diaphragmatic Dysfunction

In 1965, a group of patients was described with a combination of SLE and dyspnea, associated with progressive elevation of the hemidiaphragms and decrease in vital capacity.[97] Although conflicting data have been published[178] and other explanations have been offered,[179] this "shrinking

lung" syndrome is generally considered to be the result of diaphragmatic weakness;[180–183] expiratory muscle function is also often impaired.[183] Patients who have the syndrome present with dyspnea on exertion and, frequently, orthopnea. Although the latter is an important clinical clue to the presence of diaphragmatic weakness, similar abnormalities can occur in patients who have chest wall pain. For example, in one investigation of 12 patients who had low lung volumes on chest radiographs and no parenchymal or pleural disease on HRCT, 9 had normal diaphragmatic strength as assessed by measurement of transdiaphragmatic pressures;[178] all had chest wall pain. The other 3 patients generated normal transdiaphragmatic pressures when the phrenic nerves were stimulated.

The pathogenesis of respiratory muscle weakness, and diaphragmatic weakness in particular, is obscure. Phrenic nerve function is intact.[183] There is little evidence for a generalized myopathy,[183] and there is no correlation between the presence of lymphocytic vasculitis in muscle biopsy specimens and respiratory muscle function. There is a single autopsy report of diffuse diaphragmatic fibrosis in one affected patient.[184] Associated pleural disease is also unlikely to explain the functional abnormalities, as diffuse pleural thickening in other disorders is not associated with major reductions in transdiaphragmatic pressure.[183] Despite the severity of the abnormalities found in these patients, the clinical course is relatively stable,[180, 181] and some patients have improved with therapy.[182, 185, 186]

## Bronchiolitis

Several cases of obliterative bronchiolitis similar to that seen in rheumatoid disease have been described in patients who have SLE.[187–189] Affected patients have air-flow obstruction on lung function testing and no parenchymal changes on chest radiography. Bronchiolitis obliterans with organizing pneumonia (BOOP) has also been described in some patients.[190–194] The latter present with subacute respiratory illness, restrictive lung function, and radiologic changes similar to those of idiopathic BOOP (*see* page 2344).[195] The disorder must be distinguished from acute lupus pneumonitis, diffuse pulmonary hemorrhage, lung infarction, and pneumonia. Open lung biopsy constitutes the gold standard for diagnosis, but transbronchial biopsy may also be useful.[191, 192]

## Miscellaneous Abnormalities

Although rare, hypopharyngeal or laryngeal involvement by SLE can occur and cause acute, life-threatening upper airway obstruction.[1] Involvement of the cricoarytenoid joint as well as inflammation and edema of supraglottic structures has been described.[1] In one series of 22 patients who had normal chest radiographs and who were admitted to the hospital for an acute exacerbation of SLE, 6 had unexplained elevation of the alveolar-arterial oxygen gradient when arterial blood gas analysis was performed;[196] this reverted to normal when steroids were given to treat other active disease. The authors hypothesized that the elevation was the result of intrapulmonary leukoagglutination; however, occult interstitial disease had not been excluded by HRCT.

Other pulmonary abnormalities described in association

with SLE include "pseudolymphoma" (presenting as lung nodules),[197] amyloidosis,[3, 198] and lymphocytic interstitial pneumonia (presenting as nodular, focal, or diffuse disease).[199, 200] Nasal signs and symptoms are minor but seem to be common when looked for;[201] in one series of 36 patients, 21 had nonspecific nasal symptoms and 12 had evidence of chronic inflammatory changes in the nose.

### Drug-Induced Lupus

The clinical manifestations of drug-induced lupus do not appear until months or years after the initiation of therapy. In most cases, the onset is insidious and is heralded by prolonged discomfort in the joints.[59, 202] Additional relatively common manifestations include pleuritis, pericarditis, fever, and skin rashes. Pulmonary involvement is unusual;[203, 204] for example, clinical and radiographic evidence of pulmonary disease was found in only 3 of 44 patients in one series.[205] However, results of bronchoalveolar lavage in one patient indicate that alveolitis may be present in asymptomatic individuals.[206]

The diagnosis should be considered in any patient on medication who develops suspicious symptoms; it is strengthened by the finding of a positive blood test for ANA, and confirmed by the disappearance of symptoms and signs with cessation of drug therapy. Although clinical manifestations disappear within days to weeks, serologic abnormalities may continue for months.[58, 70, 207, 208]

### *Pulmonary Function Tests*

A characteristic feature of pulmonary function in SLE (seen also in progressive systemic sclerosis) is a severity of impairment out of proportion to the rather mild changes usually apparent clinically and radiographically.[181, 209, 210] Evidence of impaired function can be found in patients who have normal chest radiographs in whom there is no history of previous pulmonary or pleural disease;[211] however, function is typically more severely impaired in patients who have such a history.

The most common abnormality is an isolated reduction in diffusing capacity.[211, 212] Many asymptomatic patients also have abnormalities of small airway function.[211] Although it has been questioned whether these are more frequent than those in the normal population,[212] the progression of air-flow obstruction unrelated to smoking in patients who have SLE suggests that the changes are real.[213] Dyspnea is common in patients who have SLE and correlates strongly with the maximal uptake of oxygen during exercise.[214] As discussed earlier, dyspnea that is unexplained by radiographic evidence of pulmonary or pleural disease may be related to impaired diaphragmatic function;[180, 181, 215, 216] weakness of both expiratory and inspiratory muscles of breathing, unrelated to steroid therapy, has also been described.[180] Dyspnea may also be associated with increased respiratory drive and an increased ventilatory response to $CO_2$ rebreathing.[217]

Most commonly, routine pulmonary function studies reveal a decrease in lung volumes. Diffusing capacity and arterial oxygen saturation are also usually reduced, with low or normal $P_{CO_2}$, compensated respiratory alkalosis, and reduced lung compliance.[95, 209, 210] Confirmation of suspected pulmonary arterial hypertension may require catheterization

or echocardiography; the original report of the use of measurement of $V_D/V_T$ as a means of detecting this manifestation of autoimmune disease[218] has not been borne out.[219] Pulmonary function studies have been reported to remain abnormal after acute lupus pneumonitis has undergone complete radiographic resolution[92] and after clinical remission has occurred following withdrawal of the drug in procainamide-induced disease.[220]

### *Prognosis and Natural History*

Most patients who have SLE follow a chronic course punctuated by acute exacerbations; a minority present with fulminating disease, sometimes rapidly fatal as a result of renal failure or superimposed infection. When it does ensue, death typically occurs after many years from renal failure, central nervous system involvement, infection, or myocardial infarction.[221–223, 223a] There is also evidence that women who have SLE are at increased risk for the development of malignancy.[91]

The reported 10-year survival rates range from 60%[221] to 90%.[9, 217, 224] Improvement in survival statistics in relatively recent series may be related to better therapy, although it is perhaps more likely the result of earlier diagnosis.[225] The prognosis is worse for men and for patients who have renal involvement at the onset of disease, particularly those who have the nephrotic syndrome. Patients younger than 16 years of age who have no evidence of renal disease do well.[224] Older patients have been variously described as doing well[225] or as having increased mortality.[226] Socioeconomic status was linked to increased mortality in one American study;[226] once correction was made for such status, there was no association of mortality with race. The amount of circulating DNA antibody and DNA–anti-DNA complexes correlate with both the activity and severity of disease.[227, 228]

Although a number of subtle immunologic defects predisposing to infection have been demonstrated in patients who have SLE,[3] serious infection is primarily associated with the use of corticosteroids and other immunosuppressive drugs.[229] Bacterial pneumonia is more common in patients who have active SLE.[230] In addition to immunosuppression, risk factors for bacterial infection include renal failure, pulmonary edema, and respiratory muscle weakness. Tuberculosis, often presenting atypically with miliary or localized extrapulmonary disease, is an important complication in patients from areas with a high prevalence of the infection.[231, 232] A number of opportunistic pathogens have also been described, including *Nocardia, Pneumocystis carinii, Cryptococcus, Aspergillus,* and cytomegalovirus.[1, 230] In addition to morbidity, pulmonary infection is also an important cause of mortality, being responsible for 15% of deaths in one autopsy series;[84] generalized sepsis was responsible for a further 28% of deaths.

## HYPOCOMPLEMENTEMIC URTICARIAL VASCULITIS

The term *hypocomplementemic urticarial vasculitis* (HUV) is used to refer to a syndrome characterized by persistent urticaria, leukocytoclastic vasculitis, and hypocomplementemia. A variety of other presumed immunologically mediated manifestations may also be present, including arthritis and arthralgias, glomerulonephritis, episcleritis, uveitis, and central nervous system abnormalities.[233–235] Patients have low serum Clq levels, associated with the presence of an antibody to this complement component.[236, 237] The antibody is not seen in other diseases except for SLE, in which its prevalence is much less (35%) than in HUV.[237] This observation, as well as the paucity of serum autoantibodies typical of SLE and the characteristic cutaneous findings, suggest that HUV is an entity distinct from SLE.[233, 234] The pathogenesis of the disease is believed to be related to immune complex deposition. Description of the disease in a set of identical twins suggests that genetic influences may be important.[238]

Obstructive lung disease, sometimes reversible,[233, 239] has been described in a number of patients with HUV. For example, in one series of 18 patients, 11 had dyspnea and moderate to severe air-flow obstruction on lung function testing; 6 died of respiratory insufficiency.[236] Although almost all affected patients have been smokers, the severity of the associated lung disease has been out of proportion to what might be expected with the degree of cigarette smoking, suggesting that the obstructive disease is directly related to the presence of HUV.[233–235] Despite the documentation of normal or elevated levels of alpha$_1$-antitrypsin in most patients,[234] it has been suggested that panacinar emphysema is present in some patients.[233–235] Pulmonary vasculitis has not been documented.

# RHEUMATOID DISEASE

The frequency with which rheumatoid arthritis is associated with extra-articular manifestations—76% of cases in one series of 127 patients[240]—clearly justifies the concept of rheumatoid disease (RD) as a systemic process. In contrast with the female sex predominance characteristic of rheumatoid arthritis (female to male, two or three to one[241]), extra-articular manifestations of rheumatoid disease are more common in men. In the series just cited, these manifestations were present in patients who had the most severe joint involvement and included subcutaneous nodules, pulmonary fibrosis, digital vasculitis, skin ulceration, lymph node enlargement, neuropathy, splenomegaly, episcleritis, and pericarditis.[240]

Although pleuropulmonary and joint involvement are intimately related,[242–244] the prevalence of lung disease in a reported series of patients who have RD varies considerably. At least part of this variation depends on the criteria for diagnosis. For example, interstitial lung disease is seen in 1% to 5% of patients who have RD when the diagnosis is based on chest radiographic findings.[245–247] However, as many as 40% of patients have a reduction in diffusing capacity in keeping with early fibrosis.[248] Evidence of fibrosis can also be detected at a relatively early stage on HRCT; for example, in one series of 38 asymptomatic patients, 11 (29%) had abnormal scans (abnormalities were also detected in 27 of 39 patients who had chest symptoms).[249] In another series of 36 patients who had RD of recent onset, 5 (14%) had clinically significant interstitial lung disease and 16 (44%) had abnormalities on HRCT, pulmonary function studies, BAL analysis, and [99m]Tc-DTPA nuclear scans that

were compatible with interstitial disease but judged to be clinically unimportant.[250] The significance of these changes remains to be determined by long-term outcome studies.

The majority of patients who have pleuropulmonary disease have clinical evidence of arthritis, and in about 70% to 80% the sheep cell agglutination or latex fixation tests are positive for rheumatoid factor.[241] Occasionally, arthritis is not clinically evident when a pleuropulmonary abnormality becomes manifest; in such circumstances, the diagnosis may be suggested on the basis of positive serology or may not be suspected until the arthritis becomes evident.[251–253]

The pleuropulmonary manifestations of rheumatoid disease are listed in Table 39–3. Although these abnormalities may be present in any combination, each is sufficiently distinctive clinically, pathologically, and radiologically to warrant separate consideration.[242–244] Sclerosing mediastinitis and pericarditis occur occasionally, the latter usually in association with extensive joint involvement and subcutaneous nodules.[254, 255]

## Pathogenesis

Rheumatoid disease is a systemic abnormality of unknown etiology that is characterized principally by chronic inflammation and destruction of joints.[256] The pathogenesis is complicated and incompletely understood, and may include a combination of inflammatory, immunologic, hormonal, and genetic factors. A variety of cells, including macrophages, T and B lymphocytes, synoviocytes, and endothelial cells, have been implicated in the development of the disease.[257] T- and B-cell activation with cytokine release culminates in joint destruction. Although the events that initiate this process are unknown, a variety of infectious agents have been considered.[258]

## Table 39–3. PLEUROPULMONARY MANIFESTATIONS OF RHEUMATOID DISEASE

**Parenchymal Disease**
  Interstitial pneumonitis and fibrosis
  Upper lobe fibrobullous disease
  Rheumatoid nodule
  Caplan's syndrome

**Pleural Disease**
  Pleural effusion
  Pneumothorax

**Airway Disease**
  Obliterative bronchiolitis
  Bronchiolitis obliterans with organizing pneumonia
  Follicular bronchiolitis
  Bronchiectasis
  Upper airway disease

**Vascular Disease**
  Pulmonary hypertension
  Pulmonary arteritis
  Hyperviscosity syndrome

**Secondary Abnormalities**
  Drug reactions
  Infection
  Malignancy

Several lines of study indicate an important role for cell-mediated immunity in the pathogenesis of the disease. Some investigators have suggested that activation of circulating T lymphocytes makes them susceptible to endothelial binding and transmigration.[259] Activated T lymphocytes demonstrate increased avidity of their adhesion receptors both for extracellular matrix proteins in the joint and for a number of cellular adhesion molecules, a process that may trigger a mitogenic response in the synovial cells and the secretion of tissue-damaging proteases.[260] T lymphocyte-independent dysregulation of the synovial cell cycle, prompting excessive growth, may also be important.[261]

Among the proinflammatory cytokines locally released in this chronic inflammatory process, tumor necrosis factor-alpha (TNF-alpha), produced mainly by activated macrophages,[262] seems to play an especially important role.[263, 264] Its effects are amplified by its ability to induce the release of other cytokines, such as interleukin-1 and granulocyte-macrophage colony-stimulating factor.[265]

As with other connective tissue diseases, serologic abnormalities are common in RD and presumably reflect an underlying derangement of immunologic function. The presence of rheumatoid factor (RF) (anti-IgG immunoglobulin) is the most common. Since these antibodies are also found in other autoimmune and infectious diseases as well as in normal individuals, their precise contribution to the pathogenesis of RD is unclear.[266] Nevertheless, most patients who have RD have high titers of RF, and about 15% to 30% have ANAs.[241] Although low titers of ANA and rheumatoid factors are found in approximately 5% of normal individuals, in 20% to 30% of asbestos workers who have interstitial fibrosis,[267] and in a number of patients who have idiopathic pulmonary fibrosis,[268] high titers are almost invariably associated with RD. In contrast with synovitis, the extra-articular manifestations of rheumatoid disease, and particularly some pleuropulmonary lesions, seem to develop as a result of dysfunction of humoral immunity. For example, in rheumatoid pleural and pericardial fluids, immune complex–like activity is virtually always present, levels of RF are high, and complement is low.[269]

As in idiopathic pulmonary fibrosis, activated macrophages in lung affected by RD synthesize and secrete fibroblast growth factors and neutrophil chemotactic factors.[270] Patients who have RA without evident pulmonary involvement also have abnormalities in BAL fluid, the major finding being an increase in activated helper T cells.[271] Some have speculated that these activated lymphocytes may produce IgM locally followed by the formation of immune complexes that may be directly cytolytic or cause damage indirectly by neutrophil recruitment.[272] This hypothesis is supported by the observation that IgM and rheumatoid factor may be found in pulmonary arterioles and alveolar walls and in the parenchyma adjacent to cavitated rheumatoid lung nodules.[269, 273] In fact, patients who have pulmonary disease have a higher level of BAL immune complexes compared with those who do not have lung disease.[274] To complicate matters, some patients have a neutrophilic alveolitis, and their BAL fluid shows a reduction in the CD4+/CD8+ lymphocyte ratio.[244] There is a strong correlation between the degree of such BAL neutrophilia and the severity of pulmonary function abnormalities, suggesting that neutrophilia is more likely to be present in more advanced fibrotic disease.[275]

Similar findings have been documented for BAL eosinophilia and the level of BAL histamine.[276] There is an increased elaboration of TNF-alpha by alveolar macrophages in patients who have RA, both with and without interstitial lung disease.

Both hormonal and genetic factors have also been implicated in the pathogenesis of RD. Several observations suggest that there may be an important influence of sex hormones. For example, despite RD being more common in women, its peak incidence is at the time of menopause. In addition, premenopausal women do better than postmenopausal woman who have the disease, oral contraceptive pills may be protective, and pregnancy has been associated with dramatic improvement.[277] A number of associations with specific HLA haplotype have been described for RD, that with HLA-B40 being the most notable.[278, 279] In one investigation, the relative risk for lung involvement as opposed to other extra-articular manifestations was approximately 40 in patients who had this haplotype.[278]

## Parenchymal Disease

### Diffuse Interstitial Pneumonitis and Fibrosis

Interstitial pneumonitis in RD is similar both pathologically and radiographically to the interstitial pneumonitis that occurs in association with a variety of other etiologies as well as with idiopathic pulmonary fibrosis. Although its precise prevalence depends on the method of diagnosis—clinical, radiologic, functional, or histologic—it is probably the most common form of pulmonary involvement in RD.[280]

#### Pathologic Characteristics

Histologic changes in the early stages of the disease consist of an interstitial infiltrate of lymphocytes, histiocytes, and plasma cells (Fig. 39–7),[281, 282] the last-named often more frequent than in idiopathic pulmonary fibrosis.[283] Nodular aggregates of lymphocytes, sometimes with germinal centers, may be prominent in both the parenchymal interstitium[284] and in interstitial tissue adjacent to bronchioles and interlobular septa (follicular bronchiolitis; see farther on).[285] Alveolar air spaces may be unaffected but often contain an increased number of macrophages.

With progression of the disease, the infiltrate decreases in severity and is replaced by fibrous tissue, which in the advanced stage results in an appearance of "honeycomb" lung (Fig. 39–7). These changes are entirely nonspecific and cannot in themselves lead to a diagnosis of rheumatoid disease; occasionally, necrobiotic nodules or the nodules of Caplan's syndrome are associated with the pneumonitis,[281, 286] suggesting the rheumatoid etiology. Large amounts of IgM and lesser quantities of IgG have been found within alveolar walls and small vessels in some immunofluorescent studies.[284]

#### Radiologic Manifestations

The prevalence of radiographic evidence of pulmonary fibrosis in patients who have rheumatoid disease ranges from

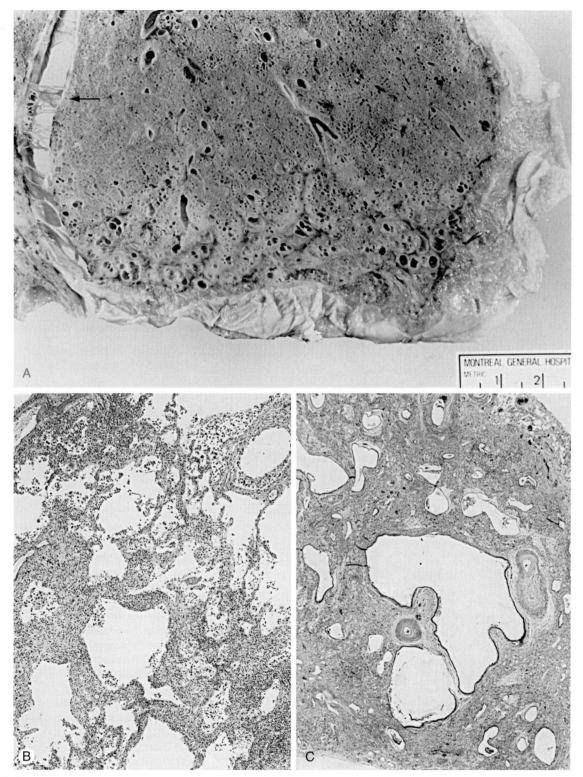

**Figure 39–7. Interstitial Fibrosis in Rheumatoid Disease.** The base of a lower lobe in a patient with long-standing rheumatoid disease *(A)* shows diffuse pleural fibrosis and interpleural adhesions within the fissure *(arrow)*. The lung parenchyma shows interstitial thickening, which is most severe in the basal subpleural region, where early honeycombing is evident. A section from a transition area between normal and affected lung *(B)* shows moderately severe interstitial inflammation, composed predominantly of lymphocytes. A section from the most basal region *(C)* reveals replacement of normal parenchyma by fibrous tissue and multiple variably sized cystic spaces. *(B, ×40; C, ×20.)*

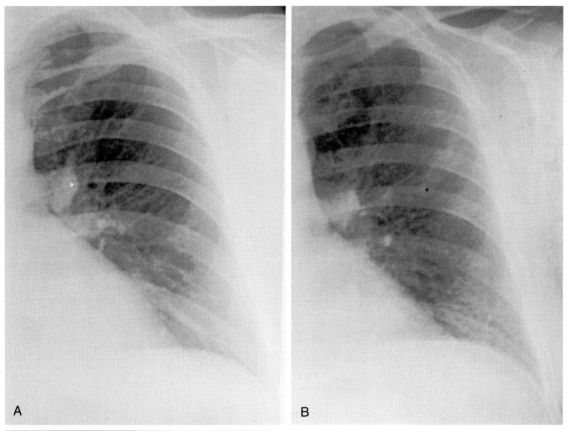

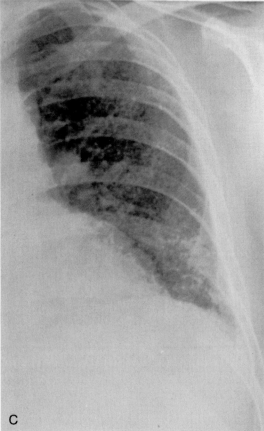

**Figure 39–8. Early Radiographic Features of Rheumatoid Pulmonary Disease.** Illustrated are sequential detail views of the left lung from posteroanterior chest radiographs. In *A*, the lung is normal. Two years later *(B)*, a faint reticulonodular pattern has developed at the base of the left lung and slight elevation of the hemidiaphragm has occurred, reflecting loss of lung volume. Two years later *(C)*, the reticulonodular pattern has become coarser and has progressed to involve the whole lung; the hemidiaphragm has undergone further elevation and has lost its sharp definition as a result of contiguous parenchymal disease. Similar findings were present in the right lung. The patient was a 48-year-old man who had long-standing rheumatoid arthritis.

about 2% to 10% in different series.[287, 288] We believe that the most representative data come from a study in which the chest radiographs of 309 patients who had RD were compared with those of sex- and age-matched controls;[289] in this study, a reticulonodular pattern consistent with fibrosis was seen in 4.5% of patients who had RD as compared with 0.3% of the controls.

The pattern and distribution of fibrosis on both the chest radiograph and HRCT are indistinguishable from those of idiopathic pulmonary fibrosis.[112, 290, 291] In the early stage, the radiographic appearance consists of irregular linear opacities causing a fine reticular or reticulonodular pattern (Fig. 39–8).[112, 292] The abnormality usually involves mainly the lower lung zones,[292] although it occasionally affects the mid-lung zones predominantly.[287] With progression of disease, the reticular or reticulonodular pattern becomes more coarse and diffuse, and honeycombing may be seen.[292] Follow-up may demonstrate progressive loss of lung volume.

Similar to the radiograph, the predominant abnormality on HRCT consists of a reticular pattern caused by a combination of intralobular lines and irregular thickening of interlobular septa (Fig. 39–9).[112, 291] These are present mainly in the subpleural parenchyma and the lower lung zones.[291] Although irregular linear opacities representing fibrosis can be seen on HRCT at any level, honeycombing is usually most marked near the diaphragm.[291, 293]

In one review of the CT findings in 77 patients, 8 (10%) demonstrated features of pulmonary fibrosis (small irregular linear opacities with associated architectural distortion and honeycombing).[294] Seven also had areas of ground-glass attenuation and 5 had pleural thickening or effusion. Honeycombing was seen exclusively in the peripheral lung in 5 patients and involved both the central and peripheral lung in 3 patients. Follow-up of 4 patients over a 4-year period demonstrated progression of honeycombing from the peripheral to the central parts of both lungs and from the lung bases towards the apices.[294] In three patients, the areas of ground-glass attenuation were replaced by honeycombing.

### Clinical Manifestations

Interstitial pneumonitis associated with RD is most frequent in sero-positive men between 50 and 60 years of age.[244] The complication has been reported to occur more commonly in patients with a positive lupus erythematosus (LE) cell test. Most (albeit not all[245]) investigators have found its frequency to be much greater in the presence of subcutaneous nodules.[296–298]

The most common symptom is dyspnea on effort,[297, 299] sometimes associated with cough and pleuritic pain. Finger clubbing may be present, not uncommonly associated with cor pulmonale,[297, 300] and may antedate the onset of respira-

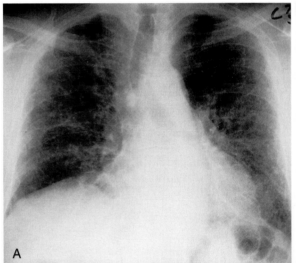

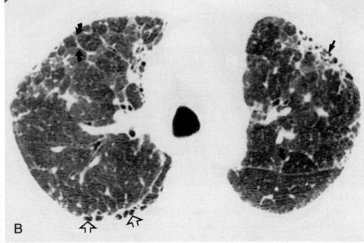

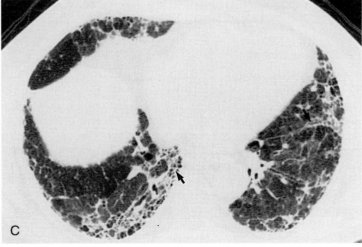

**Figure 39–9. Rheumatoid Disease: Interstitial Pneumonitis and Fibrosis.** A posteroanterior chest radiograph *(A)* demonstrates a diffuse reticulonodular pattern associated with a decrease in lung volumes. HRCT scans *(B and C)* demonstrate a reticular pattern involving mainly the peripheral lung. The reticular pattern is due to a combination of intralobular linear opacities *(straight arrows)* and thickening of the interlobular septa *(curved arrows)*. "Honeycombing" is evident, particularly in the right lower lobe *(open arrows)*. No nodules are evident on the CT scan. (The nodularity on the radiograph is due to linear opacities seen end-on.) The patient was a 73-year-old man who had long-standing rheumatoid disease.

tory symptoms.[301] Crackles may be audible on auscultation of the chest.[302] Anemia and slight lymphocytosis develop in some advanced cases. Pulmonary function tests typically show a restrictive ventilatory defect.[303] The diffusing capacity also is commonly reduced,[296, 300] even in patients who have normal chest radiographs.

The natural history of interstitial fibrosis in RD is not well defined.[242] The prognosis undoubtedly depends to some extent on how the disease is identified (e.g., by HRCT scanning in an asymptomatic individual or by chest radiography in a symptomatic patient). In general, it appears that the disease is more benign than idiopathic pulmonary fibrosis.[242] Nevertheless, although it remains stable or progresses very slowly in some patients, in others it progresses rapidly and leads to death from respiratory insufficiency.[244] In one study of 49 patients who required hospitalization for lung disease in the setting of rheumatoid arthritis, the median survival was 3.5 years and the 5-year survival only 39%.[302]

### Upper Lobe Fibrobullous Disease

Although rare, the number of reports of fibrosis confined to the upper lobes and associated with bullae or cavities is sufficient to justify inclusion of this form of parenchymal abnormality as a separate manifestation of rheumatoid disease.[251, 304–306] The pathogenic basis of this unusual variety is unclear. Search for acid-fast organisms has produced negative results. Chest radiographs reveal patchy upper lobe fibrosis and cystic spaces consistent with either cavities or bullae, the pattern closely resembling that seen in patients who have advanced ankylosing spondylitis (Fig. 39–10).[251, 305] In one patient, the upper lobe opacity was associated with obliterative bronchiolitis. In two others, pathologic examination of the lungs at autopsy revealed numerous cavitated necrobiotic nodules whose presence had not been suspected radiographically or clinically.[307]

### Rheumatoid Nodules

A rheumatoid (necrobiotic) nodule is a well-circumscribed, tumor-like mass found most commonly in the subcutaneous tissues and less often in the peritoneum, dura, sclera, and visceral organs.[308] It is a relatively rare manifestation of pleuropulmonary rheumatoid disease and usually is associated with advanced rheumatoid arthritis and with multiple subcutaneous rheumatoid nodules in the elbows or elsewhere.[298, 309–312]

#### Pathologic Characteristics

The pathologic features of rheumatoid nodules are the same regardless of their location in the body.[308] In the lungs, they may be solitary or multiple and are usually situated peripherally in relation to the pleura or interlobular septa;[253, 313] an endobronchial location has also been described.[314] Occasionally, nodules are found in the chest wall adjacent to the parietal pleura.[315] Grossly, the nodules are well defined and frequently contain a soft, yellowish central area. Histologically, this central portion is composed of amorphous necrotic material surrounded by a well-defined layer of palisading epithelioid histiocytes (with their long axis perpendicular to the zone of necrosis) (Fig. 39–11); the

adjacent tissue shows fibrosis and a variably intense plasma cell and lymphocyte infiltrate. Microscopic "nodules" with an identical histologic appearance can be identified occasionally.[285]

#### Radiologic Manifestations

The necrobiotic nodule represents a relatively rare cause of solitary or multiple nodules in the lungs. It has been estimated that they can be detected radiographically in approximately 2 per 1,000 patients who have rheumatoid disease.[317] As might be expected, they are seen more commonly with CT, being observed in 3 of 77 patients in one series.[294] Typically, they present as well-circumscribed nodules or masses, usually multiple, ranging from 5 mm to 7 cm in diameter, commonly situated in the periphery of the lung next to the pleura (Fig. 39–12).[294, 310] They may be very numerous, resembling metastases (Fig. 39–13), and may wax and wane in concert with the subcutaneous nodules and in proportion to the activity of underlying arthritis.[318, 319] Cavitation is common, the walls being thick and having a smooth inner lining. During remission of arthritis, the cavities may become thin walled and gradually disappear, and during exacerbations they may refill and become opacified.[309] Pleural effusion[309, 320] and spontaneous pneumothorax[309, 318, 321] may coexist.

#### Clinical Manifestations

Necrobiotic nodules are almost always asymptomatic. Rarely, they are associated with hemoptysis or cause sudden pain or dyspnea when pneumothorax results from rupture into the pleural cavity.[322] In one patient, a cavitated nodule was complicated by an aspergilloma.[323] An appreciable number of cases have been reported in patients who do not have rheumatoid factor;[252, 314, 324] in addition, it is not unusual for the abnormality to be present in the absence of symptomatic arthritis, which may or may not develop later.[252, 253, 313, 324] Histologic proof of diagnosis is often required, because pulmonary carcinoma can present in an identical clinical and radiographic fashion.[325]

### Caplan's Syndrome

Caplan's syndrome was first described in 1953 in coal miners in South Wales and is characterized radiographically by single or multiple well-defined spherical pulmonary opacities ranging from 0.5 to 5.0 cm in diameter.[326] In contrast with the slow development of progressive massive fibrosis in coal-worker's pneumoconiosis, these lesions usually develop rapidly and tend to appear in "crops." In many cases, the background of simple pneumoconiosis is slight or even absent.[327] Since the original description of the disease in coal workers, the number of pneumoconioses with which these lesions may be associated has grown to include many relating to industries in which silica or silicates are a hazard,[328, 329] such as boiler scaling;[330] the manufacture of roof tiles;[331] asbestos mining;[332–334] and exposure to aluminum powder,[335] kaolin,[336] and dolomite.[337]

The condition is uncommon; in one survey of 21,000 miners in 23 collieries only 55 cases were identified, the incidence in individual collieries ranging from approxi-

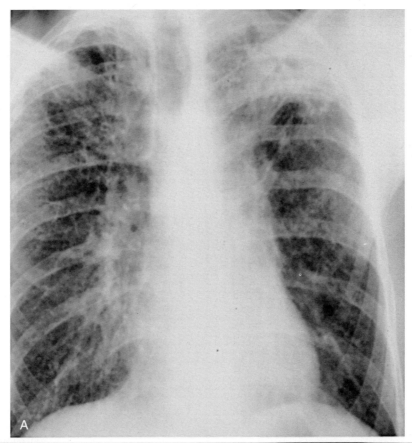

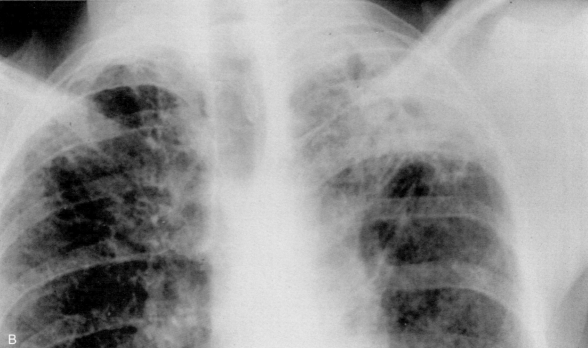

**Figure 39–10. Upper Lobe Fibrobullous Disease of Rheumatoid Origin Accompanied by Fungus Ball Formation.** A posteroanterior radiograph *(A)* and a magnified view *(B)* of both upper lungs reveal inhomogeneous consolidation in the apical portion of the left upper lobe; the left hilum is elevated. A coarse reticular pattern is present in the right upper lobe and a fine reticulation is evident elsewhere in both lungs.

*Illustration continued on following page*

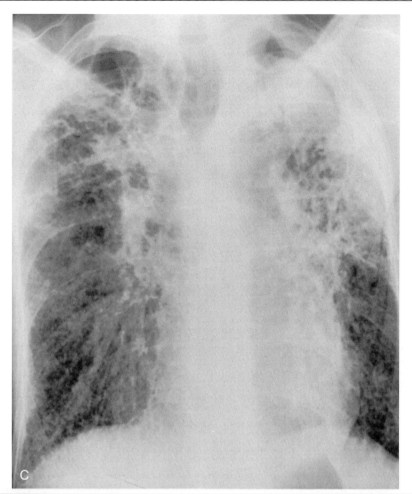

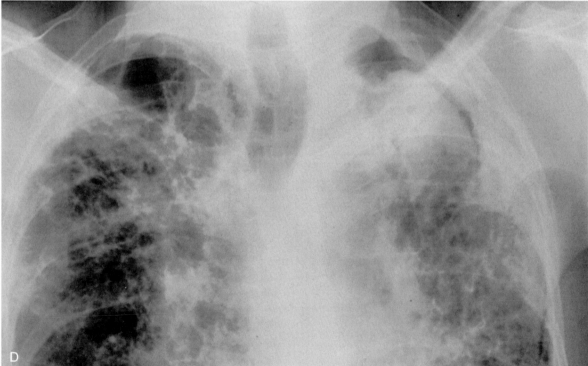

**Figure 39–10** *Continued.* Similar views obtained 6 years later *(C* and *D)* show the reticular pattern to have become much coarser throughout both lungs, particularly in the upper zones. Large bullae have developed in both apices; on the left, the largest bulla contains a homogeneous ovoid opacity consistent with a fungus ball. Cardiac size has increased. The patient was a middle-aged man with a long history of severe rheumatoid arthritis. Repeated bronchial and gastric washings were negative for acid-fast bacilli.

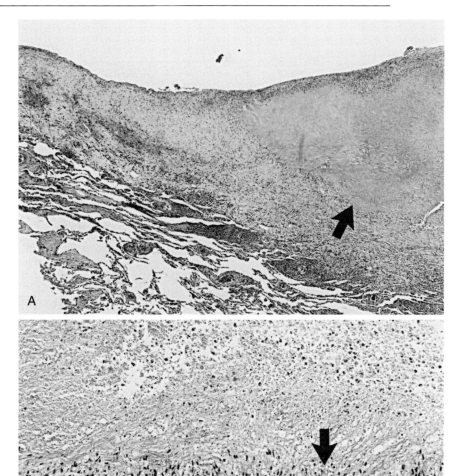

**Figure 39–11. Rheumatoid Nodule.** A section through the pleura and peripheral lung *(A)* shows fibrous tissue and chronic inflammatory cells present in a subpleural location adjacent to a focus of necrotic tissue. A magnified view *(B)* shows a layer of palisaded epithelioid histiocytes *(between arrows)* adjacent to necrotic debris. The patient had long-standing rheumatoid arthritis. The lesion was an incidental finding in a lobe removed for carcinoma. *(A, ×25; B, ×100.)* (Courtesy of Dr. S. Sahai, Reddy Memorial Hospital, Montreal, Canada.)

mately 2% to 6% of all men affected by pneumoconiosis.[338] Despite this, in individuals who suffer from both pneumoconiosis and rheumatoid arthritis, the prevalence is substantial; in one report of 26 such patients, 8 (30%) were found to have typical nodules in the lungs.[339] In another survey of 890 coal miners, the radiograph showed the characteristic opacities in 20 cases;[340] 11 (55%) of these 20 patients had clinical evidence of rheumatoid arthritis, whereas only 3% of a group of patients who had progressive massive fibrosis were so affected.

Although the pathogenesis of the nodules in Caplan's syndrome is unknown, the available evidence supports the hypothesis that the lesions represent a hypersensitivity reaction to dust particles.[341, 342] Typing of HLA-A, HLA-B, and HLA-DR antigens in 79 patients who had Caplan's syndrome revealed the overall prevalence of HLA-DR4 to be similar to that found in patients who had RD without pneumoconiosis;[343] the antigen Bw45 was present only in patients who had rheumatoid factor and was considerably more frequent (14%) than in a population of 316 individuals who had not been exposed to coal dust (1%). Patients who did not have rheumatoid factor showed an increased prevalence of HLA-A1 and HLA-B8 (59% and 52%, respectively) when compared with the group whose rheumatoid factor was positive (30% and 25%, respectively).

### Pathologic Characteristics

Grossly, the nodules of Caplan's syndrome can be solitary or multiple, the latter sometimes coalescing into large, lobulated masses.[329, 344, 345] Individual nodules are usually well defined and measure 1 to 2 cm in diameter. Characteris-

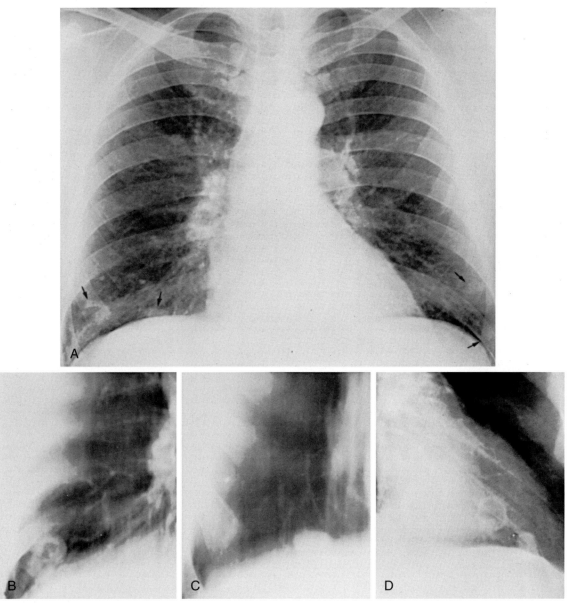

**Figure 39–12. Rheumatoid Nodules.** A posteroanterior chest radiograph *(A)* in a 41-year-old man with a 1-year history of rheumatoid arthritis demonstrates two well-circumscribed nodules in the base of the right lung and at least two in the left base *(arrows);* the more lateral of the two lesions on the right has cavitated. Tomographic sections of the right base at different levels *(B* and *C)* show at least two nodules just above the costophrenic angle (one of which is cavitated) and a third nodule of homogeneous density more posteriorly situated. A thoracotomy was performed and three nodules were removed from the right middle and lower lobes; characteristic histologic features of rheumatoid nodules were seen. Six years later, an oblique radiograph of the lower portion of the left lung *(D)* reveals two nodules, one of which presents as a ring shadow and the other as a nodule of homogeneous density.

tically, they show alternating concentric rings of light and dark areas; liquefaction necrosis and calcification may be evident. Histologically, the central portion is composed of necrotic collagen that is surrounded by a layer of macrophages and polymorphonuclear leukocytes. Some of the macrophages in this zone contain dust particles, and it is thought that when these cells die the dust remains behind, forming the characteristic darkened ring.[344] It is this pigmented ring that distinguishes the Caplan's nodule from the necrobiotic nodule of uncomplicated rheumatoid disease. Palisaded epithelioid cells similar to those of the typical rheumatoid nodule are seen in some cases. The periphery of the nodule is composed of collagen and a variably intense lymphocytic infiltrate; adjacent vessels frequently show endarteritis obliterans.

### Radiologic Manifestations

Radiographically, there is little to distinguish the nodular lesions of Caplan's syndrome from the necrobiotic nodules of rheumatoid disease unassociated with pneumoconiosis. As indicated previously, the nodules tend to develop rapidly and appear in crops. They may increase in number, remain unchanged, or calcify; cavitation may occur and may be followed by fibrosis or disappearance of the lesion.[326, 329, 346]

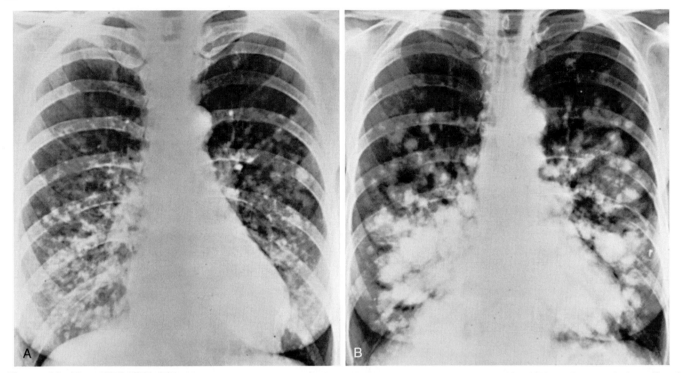

**Figure 39–13. Multiple Rheumatoid Nodules.** For many years prior to the radiograph illustrated in *A,* this middle-aged woman had manifested clinical evidence of rheumatoid arthritis. Multiple small, discrete nodules ranging from barely visible to approximately 1 cm in diameter are scattered throughout both lungs, with some mid-zonal and basal predominance. Seven years later *(B),* the nodules had increased markedly in size, some reaching a diameter of 3 cm; none showed evidence of cavitation. The patient manifested no symptoms or signs referable to her chest. Biopsy of a left-sided nodule revealed a typical rheumatoid nodule.

### Clinical Manifestations

The opacities may appear before, coincident with, or after the clinical onset of arthritis, and there is no apparent relationship between the severity of the arthritis and the extent and type of radiographic change in the lungs. As with the more common necrobiotic nodule, symptoms are usually absent.

### Pleural Disease

Pleural abnormalities are probably the most frequent manifestation of rheumatoid disease in the thorax.[1] For example, in one series of 516 patients who had rheumatoid arthritis, 108 (21%) gave a history of pleurisy and 17 (3%) had pleural effusions for which no other cause could be found;[347] these figures were in contrast to those observed in 301 controls who had degenerative joint disease, of whom only 12% gave a history of pleurisy and only one had pleural effusion.

#### *Pleuritis and Pleural Effusion*

##### Pathologic Characteristics

Needle biopsy specimens of the pleura usually show only nonspecific chronic inflammation;[348–350] rheumatoid nodules are seen rarely.[351, 352] Pleural fibrosis and adhesions are common findings at autopsy (*see* Fig. 39–7).[281] Thoracoscopic examination sometimes shows the parietal pleura to possess a "gritty" appearance caused by numerous nodules

about 0.5 mm in diameter;[353, 354] histologically, these consist of small papillae of fibrovascular tissue whose surface is lined by a layer of stratified, focally multinucleated epithelioid cells.

In some cases, cytologic examination of pleural fluid reveals clumps of acellular granular material associated with large, elongated multinucleated giant cells and a background of necrotic material (Fig. 39–14).[356–359] These abnormalities are related to rupture of pleural-based rheumatoid nodules into the pleural space and are highly suggestive of rheumatoid effusion.[354] The biochemical and other features of the fluid are discussed on page 2754.

##### Radiologic Manifestations

Pleural effusions are usually small and unilateral,[112, 360] but may be bilateral or large.[361, 362] Although they usually resolve over a period of weeks or months, they may recur or occasionally persist for many months or even years (Fig. 39–15).[349, 363, 364] Of the 25 cases in one investigation, 23 were unilateral (14 on the right and 9 on the left).[349] In the great majority of cases, the effusion is the sole radiographic abnormality apparent in the thorax; in fact, it has been suggested that the presence of associated parenchymal disease suggests a nonrheumatoid etiology.[349] Despite this, several cases have been reported in which there were underlying parenchymal rheumatoid nodules and, unexpectedly, a significant blood eosinophilia.[318, 350, 351] As with diffuse pulmonary fibrosis, pleural effusion associated with rheumatoid disease is much more likely to occur in patients who have subcutaneous nodules than in those who do not.[350, 351, 365]

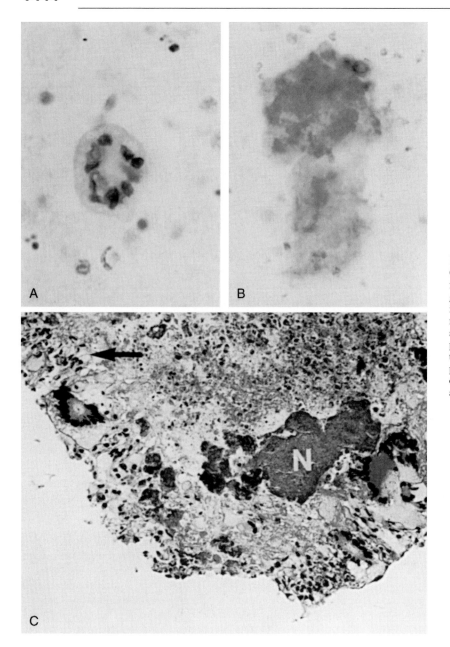

**Figure 39–14. Rheumatoid Pleural Effusion: Cytologic Appearance.** Highly magnified views of a filter preparation of pleural fluid show a multinucleated giant cell and scattered mononuclear cells *(A)* and an irregular fragment of more or less amorphous, acellular material *(B)*. Taken together, these findings are highly suggestive of a rheumatoid etiology. A section of a closed pleural biopsy specimen from the same patient *(C)* shows that the likely origin of the material seen on the filter preparation is a disrupted rheumatoid nodule composed of necrotic material (N), epithelioid histocytes *(arrow)*, and multinucleated giant cells. (*A* and *B*, Papanicolaou ×450; *C*, hematoxylin-eosin ×130.)

## Clinical Manifestations

The effusion may be entirely unsuspected because of lack of symptoms,[366] as was the case in approximately 50% of patients in one series.[349] Occasionally, it develops abruptly and is associated with pain and fever.[367] As the amount of fluid increases, so does the likelihood of dyspnea; rarely, the effusion is so massive that it is associated with respiratory failure.[368] The effusion may antedate clinical evidence of rheumatoid arthritis[348, 349, 365, 369] or may occur when joint disease is only mild;[370] in many cases, it is associated with episodic exacerbations of arthritis[349, 351] and in some with pericarditis. Effusion can be transient, persistent, or relapsing.[131] When chronic, it may lead to fibrothorax requiring decortication.[131] Distinction from infectious or malignant causes is obviously of paramount importance.[352]

### *Pneumothorax*

Pneumothorax is an uncommon complication of rheumatoid disease. It is often associated with rupture of rheuma-

toid nodules into the pleural space;[244, 371] in some patients, it is related to advanced interstitial fibrosis.

## Airway Disease

Clinically significant airway disease is uncommon in nonsmoking patients who have rheumatoid arthritis.[243] Nevertheless, about 15% of such patients have been found to have functional evidence of air-flow obstruction.[316, 372] In addition, it is important to consider the potential for the interaction between cigarette smoke and RD, which may be significant. For example, in one study of 200 unselected patients, half of whom had rheumatoid arthritis and half of whom had osteoarthritis (the age, sex, smoking, and atopic histories of the two groups being comparable), wheezing was found to be much more prevalent in the group with rheumatoid arthritis (18% vs. 4%); moreover, on function testing, this group had significantly greater air-flow obstruc-

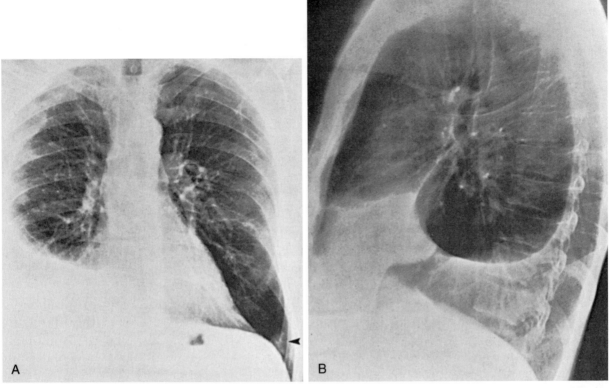

**Figure 39–15. Rheumatoid Pleural Effusion.** Posteroanterior *(A)* and lateral *(B)* radiographs reveal a moderate accumulation of fluid in the right pleural space. Apart from the solitary nodular opacity in the left costophrenic angle *(arrow)*, the nature of which was not established, the lungs are clear. The effusion showed little change in quantity during several months of observation. The patient was a 54-year-old man with rheumatoid arthritis.

tion and airway hyperresponsiveness than the control population.[373] Specific airway complications of RD include obliterative bronchiolitis, BOOP, bronchiectasis, follicular bronchitis/bronchiolitis, and bronchial inflammation and fibrosis associated with Sjögren's syndrome *(see* page 1466); upper airway obstruction, related to ankylosis of the cricoarytenoid and cricothyroid joints, and sleep apnea are additional complications.

### Obliterative Bronchiolitis

The association of obliterative bronchiolitis with RD was first reported in six women who had rheumatoid arthritis and developed rapidly progressive obstructive pulmonary disease.[374] Since this description, there have been many examples of a similar nature.[306, 375–378] Several screening surveys of patients with RD have revealed an association of bronchiolitis and obstructive pulmonary disease with the presence of HLA-DR4 antigen or symptoms of the "sicca" syndrome (or both).[379–381] There also seems to be an increased prevalence of HLA-B40 antigen in patients who have obliterative bronchiolitis, both with and without rheumatoid arthritis, while an increased prevalence of DR1 has been seen in patients who have RD-associated obliterative bronchiolitis alone.[382] In the latter group of patients, HLA-B5 and HLA-A3 have been absent, implying that expression of these antigens might in some way be protective against the development of bronchiolar disease.

At the onset of obliterative bronchiolitis, many patients have been receiving penicillamine;[374, 383–386] rarely, a history

of gold therapy is elicited.[376, 387] This association with medication may be purely coincidental, since in two reviews of 200 patients who were receiving therapy with these two drugs, not a single example of bronchiolitis was uncovered.[388, 389] Nevertheless, the complication has been reported in one patient receiving gold who did not have RD,[104] and it does seem to occur more commonly in patients taking penicillamine. Some have suggested that the use of this drug might be a marker of more aggressive disease.

Histologically, the abnormality is characterized by a variably intense inflammatory infiltrate of lymphocytes and plasma cells in and around the walls of bronchioles and (occasionally) small bronchi.[374, 375, 390] Disruption of the epithelium is seen in some cases, resulting in an intraluminal polypoid mass of inflammatory cells and fibroblasts;[375] more often, however, the fibroblastic proliferation occurs between the airway muscle and intact epithelium ("constrictive" bronchiolitis) (Fig. 39–16). In the late stages, there may be complete fibrous obliteration of airway lumina.[306, 374, 375] The surrounding parenchyma and pulmonary vasculature are typically unremarkable; in some cases, additional abnormalities related to RD (e.g., organizing pneumonia or lymphoid hyperplasia[285]) are present.

The chest radiograph is usually normal or shows only hyperinflation;[374, 391] a single case has been reported in which there was fine nodularity.[390] In one investigation of the HRCT findings in four patients, abnormalities consisted of a mosaic perfusion pattern, with some areas of lung showing decreased attenuation and vascularity and others showing increased attenuation and vascularity;[392] bronchiectasis,

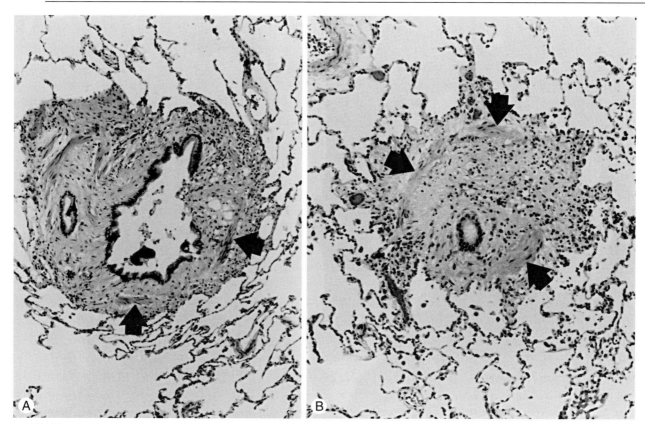

**Figure 39–16. Rheumatoid Disease: Obliterative Bronchiolitis.** Sections of two membranous bronchioles show partial *(A)* and almost complete *(B)* luminal obliteration by fibrous tissue with relatively few inflammatory cells *(arrows* indicate the muscularis mucosa). The adjacent lung parenchyma is normal. The patient was a 45-year-old woman who had long-standing rheumatoid disease.

mainly at a subsegmental level, was also noted. In another study of two patients, mosaic perfusion and bronchiectasis were also found;[391] in addition, expiratory CT showed focal areas of air trapping consistent with small airway obstruction (Fig. 39–17).

When bronchiolitis occurs in association with penicilla-mine, it is usually within 1 year of beginning therapy.[393] Most patients have shortness of breath. Frequently, this worsens at a much faster rate than that usually seen in patients who have chronic obstructive pulmonary disease (COPD);[374–376] occasionally, there is more insidious deteriora-tion.[375] Chronic cough and sputum production are usually present; curiously, most patients also have chronic sinusi-tis.[378] A mid-inspiratory squeak is often present on physical examination.[374, 390] Arthritic deformity is usually evident; however, rare cases have been described in which oblitera-tive bronchiolitis and circulating ANA and rheumatoid factor have been unassociated with evidence of joint involvement or other manifestation of connective tissue disease.[377, 394, 395] It has been speculated that the abnormal serology in these cases may be secondary to bronchiolitis rather than being indicative of a true immunopathogenesis.[394] Pulmonary func-tion tests typically show an obstructive pattern with a low diffusing capacity; a few patients have a restrictive or mixed obstructive-restrictive pattern.[244, 393]

### Bronchiolitis Obliterans with Organizing Pneumonia

Bronchiolitis obliterans organizing pneumonia (BOOP) has also been described in a number of patients who have

RD.[316, 396–398] Pathologic and radiologic findings are iden-tical to those of idiopathic BOOP (*see* page 2344). Symp-toms are nonspecific, patients typically complaining of cough and dyspnea over relatively short periods (weeks to months).[396–398] Pulmonary function studies reveal a restrictive or mixed restrictive-obstructive pattern.[316] It is important to distinguish the abnormality from interstitial pneumonitis and fibrosis, since BOOP usually improves markedly with ther-apy. In most cases, a confident diagnosis can be made on the basis of clinical and radiologic findings (including HRCT); occasionally, lung biopsy is required.

### Follicular Bronchitis/Bronchiolitis

Follicular bronchitis/bronchiolitis is a relatively uncom-mon histologic manifestation of pulmonary rheumatoid dis-ease. Pathologically, it is characterized by the presence of abundant lymphoid tissue, frequently with prominent germi-nal centers, situated in the walls of bronchioles and, to some extent, bronchi (Fig. 39–18).[399, 400] Although the alveolar interstitium may contain a similar lymphocytic infiltrate, this is often minimal; however, similar lymphoid aggregates are not uncommonly present in the pleura and intralobular septa.[285, 399] The lesion is not specific and can be found in association with other connective tissue diseases[399, 400] and a variety of other conditions.[399] A familial form associated with ANA and elevated serum immunoglobulin has also been described.[401] Although it is possible that the abnormal-ity represents active inflammation of the bronchioles (i.e., a true bronchiolitis), it is probable that most cases are in fact

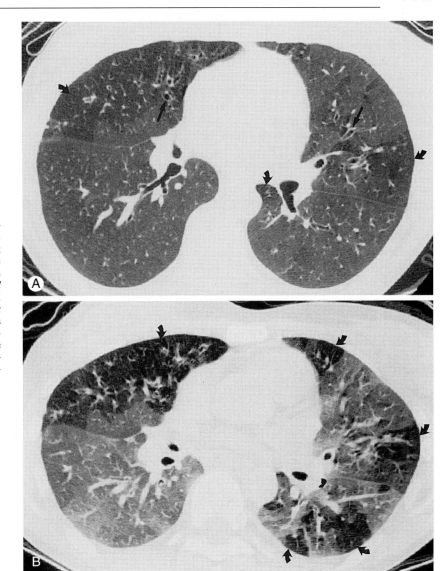

**Figure 39–17. Rheumatoid Disease: Obliterative Bronchiolitis.** An HRCT scan performed at end-inspiration *(A)* demonstrates bronchiectasis in the right middle lobe and lingula *(straight arrows)*. Note the areas of decreased attenuation and vascularity in the middle lobe, the lingula, and the left lower lobe *(curved arrows)* with slight increase in vascularity in normal lung, a pattern known as *mosaic perfusion.* Another scan performed at maximal expiration *(B)* demonstrates areas of air trapping *(arrows)*. Note the marked decrease in vascularity in the areas of air trapping. The patient was a 30-year-old woman with rheumatoid disease and a clinical diagnosis of obliterative bronchiolitis. She was not receiving penicillamine.

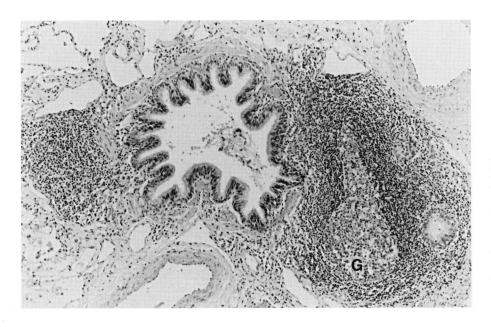

**Figure 39–18. Rheumatoid Disease— Follicular Bronchiolitis.** The wall of a membranous bronchiole contains two foci of lymphoid tissue, one with a prominent germinal center (G). The patient was a 44-year-old man with long-standing rheumatoid disease.

the result of hyperplasia of the lymphoid tissue that normally occurs in this region (*see* page 1273).

The chest radiograph characteristically shows a diffuse reticulonodular pattern.[399, 400] HRCT demonstrates nodules, mainly in a centrilobular, subpleural and peribronchial distribution;[294, 312, 402] these are usually very small but occasionally are 1 cm or more in diameter (Fig. 39–19). Other findings include bronchial wall thickening and centrilobular branching linear opacities.[312]

The most common clinical finding is progressive shortness of breath.[399, 400, 402] Cough and sputum production are usually present;[378] fever and recurrent pneumonia occur occasionally. For unknown reasons, the condition is relatively more frequent in adolescents who have juvenile rheumatoid arthritis. Some patients give a history of gold or penicillamine therapy before the onset of disease.[400] Pulmonary function studies reveal evidence of airway obstruction,[400] restriction, or combined restriction-obstruction.[316] As with BOOP it is important to distinguish follicular bronchiolitis from interstitial pneumonitis and fibrosis, since the former seems to respond favorably to therapy.[393]

### Bronchiectasis

An association between rheumatoid arthritis and bronchiectasis was first reported in 1985[403] and has been confirmed in several series.[404–406] In one of these, two groups of patients were examined, one with pulmonary fibrosis and the other with bronchiectasis;[404] surprisingly, rheumatoid arthritis was equally prevalent in both groups.

It is possible that the bronchiectasis is a predisposing condition for the development of the arthritis rather than an extra-articular manifestation of RD. Evidence in favor of this hypothesis includes the observation that it preceded the development of RA in 30 of 32 patients in one series[407] and 12 of 14 in another.[406] When bronchiectasis is recognized following the onset of arthritis, it is usually in the setting of prolonged, severe arthritis treated with systemic corticoste-

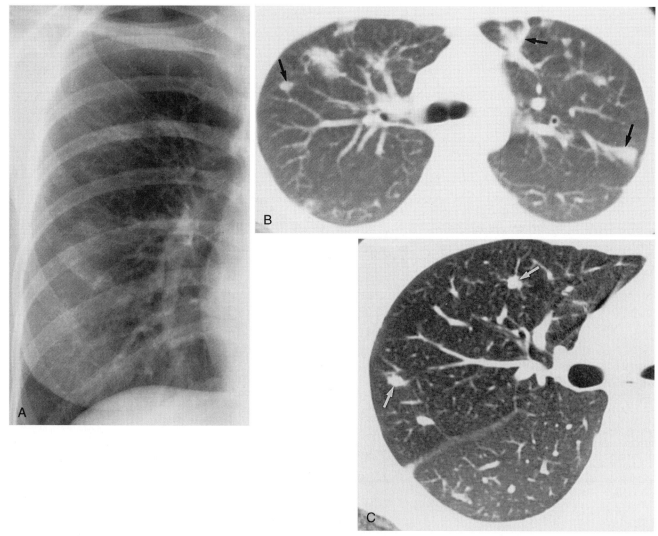

**Figure 39–19. Rheumatoid Disease: Follicular Bronchiolitis.** A view of the right lung from a posteroanterior chest radiograph *(A)* shows ill-defined nodular opacities. A similar pattern was present in the left lung. A conventional 10-mm-collimation CT scan *(B)* demonstrates focal nodular areas of consolidation in both lungs, located in a predominantly peribronchovascular distribution *(arrows)*. An HRCT scan targeted to the right lung *(C)* demonstrates sharply defined peribronchovascular nodular infiltrates in the right upper lobe *(arrows)*. The patient was a 24-year-old woman with rheumatoid disease and biopsy-proven follicular bronchiolitis.

roids.[408] In this situation, it might be the consequence of infection related to immunosuppression.

The condition may be even more common in patients who have rheumatoid arthritis than these clinically based series might suggest; for example, in one investigation of 20 nonsmoking patients who had normal chest radiographs and who underwent HRCT scanning of the chest, 5 were unexpectedly found to have bronchiectasis.[409] In another series, patients who had rheumatoid arthritis and interstitial lung disease on the chest radiograph were compared with a control group of patients with RD who had no evidence of interstitial lung disease on HRCT.[410] Bronchiectasis was seen in 6 of the patients who had interstitial lung disease; although this was likely traction bronchiectasis in 4 patients, in 2 it was believed to be the predominant finding. Four of the patients who had normal chest radiographs had bronchiectasis on HRCT scans. In a third series of 84 unselected patients who had rheumatoid arthritis, bronchiectasis or bronchiolectasis was the most common CT abnormality being observed in 30% of the entire group (Fig. 39–20);[249] only a minority of these patients (7 of 23) had evidence of honeycombing or other distortion of lung architecture.

### Upper Airway Disease

Upper airway involvement in RD can be manifested in several ways.[1, 243, 411] Evidence of inflammation of the cricoarytenoid and cricothyroid joints is common; in one series, it was identified at autopsy in 88% of patients, and by CT scan of the larynx in 45%.[411] Such disease is usually asymptomatic; however, the joints may become fixed in the adducted position, resulting in significant upper airway obstruction. This may become apparent only when viral upper respiratory tract infection or endotracheal intubation causes laryngeal edema. Less severe involvement may result in hoarseness; a change in singing or speaking voice; a sense of pain, fullness, or foreign body in the throat; pain with phonation; radiation of pain to the ear; dysphagia; or odynophagia.[411] Even asymptomatic patients have been shown to have increased translaryngeal resistance.[411]

Involvement of the temporomandibular and/or cervical vertebral joints has been associated with the development of sleep apnea.[412] Both central and obstructive patterns of apnea have been described, the authors of one study attributing the central form to inhibitory input from mechanoreceptors stimulated during upper airway collapse.[412] Other reported abnormalities of the upper airway include rheumatoid nodules of the vocal cords, dislocation of the larynx due to cervical spine deformity, laryngeal neuropathy (presumably as a result of involvement of the vasa nervorum), and ulceration of the esophagus in association with cricoarytenoid arthritis.[411]

Significant temporomandibular and cervical spine immobility may make visualization of the vocal cords and intubation difficult. Severe arthritic involvement of the larynx may necessitate preoperative tracheostomy to establish an airway safely.[243]

### Pulmonary Vascular Disease

#### Pulmonary Hypertension and Vasculitis

Pulmonary arterial hypertension in RD occurs most frequently in association with diffuse interstitial fibrosis,[413] in which case its pathogenesis and pathologic characteristics are the same as those associated with fibrosis of other etiologies.[413] Rarely, hypertension develops in the absence of parenchymal disease;[414–416] in this situation, it is often associated with Raynaud's phenomenon (Fig. 39–21).[245, 415] The pathogenesis of disease in some of these cases appears to be related to an immune complex–mediated arteritis;[1] however, this is not always present.[417] (When considering the significance of pulmonary vasculitis in cases of pulmonary hypertension, it is important to remember that it may be secondary to the hypertension rather than a primary process.[416]) As discussed farther on, there may also be a relationship with hyperviscosity syndrome. In fact, pulmonary vasculitis is rare in RD.[417–422] None was found in a series of open lung biopsies in 40 patients who had rheumatoid arthritis;[406] in

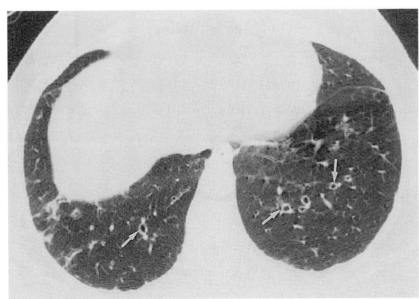

**Figure 39–20. Rheumatoid Disease: Bronchiectasis.** An HRCT scan in a 54-year-old woman with long-standing rheumatoid disease and chronic symptoms of nonproductive cough demonstrates bronchiectasis in both lower lobes *(arrows)*.

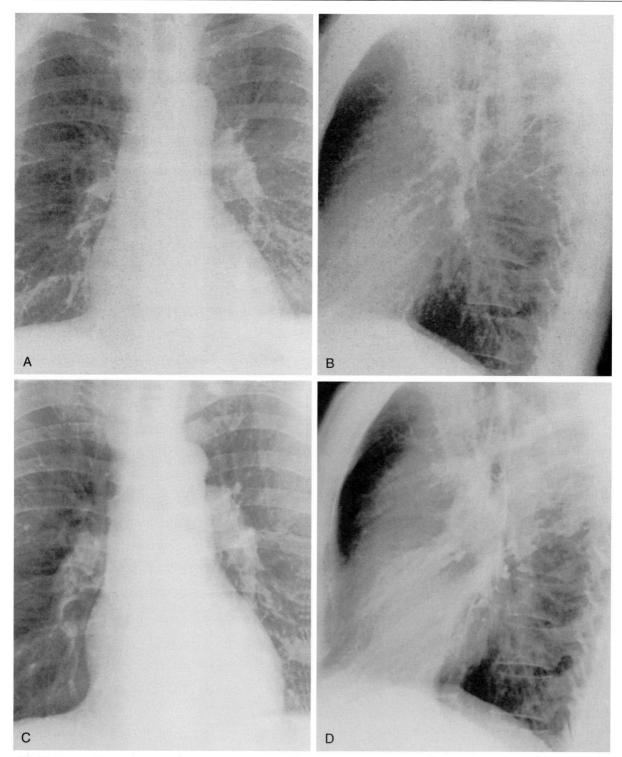

**Figure 39–21. Precapillary Pulmonary Hypertension in Rheumatoid Disease Unassociated with Interstitial Pulmonary Fibrosis.** The initial posteroanterior *(A)* and lateral *(B)* chest radiographs of this 51-year-old man are normal. Three years later *(C and D)*, there had developed enlargement of both hila compatible with pulmonary arterial dilation. Cardiac size is unchanged. Note that the lungs show no evidence of interstitial lung disease.

another review of 50 patients who had systemic rheumatoid vasculitis, pulmonary changes "consistent with vasculitis" were found in only one individual.[423] Although usually an isolated finding, vasculitis is occasionally associated with parenchymal disease.[243] In patients who have RD and systemic vasculitis indistinguishable from polyarteritis nodosa,

involvement of the bronchial arteries has been documented rarely.[424] Diffuse alveolar hemorrhage associated with the presence of antineutrophil cytoplasmic antibodies (ANCAs) has also been reported.[355, 425] However, when considering this diagnosis, it should be remembered that some investigators have detected ANCAs in as many as 12% of patients who have RD and no evidence of pulmonary or systemic vasculitis.[426]

### Hyperviscosity Syndrome

Hyperviscosity syndrome is a rare manifestation of RD that is seen when rheumatoid factor forms conglomerates sufficient in size and number to interfere with blood flow in small vessels.[427] Clinically, the condition is characterized by weakness, dyspnea, a bleeding diathesis, striking purplish-red palmar erythema, and high serum viscosity. A single case has been described of a patient who had both hyperviscosity and pulmonary hypertension;[428] the classic findings of hyperviscosity were minimal in this patient, suggesting that the diagnosis of hyperviscosity should at least be considered in patients who have RD and pulmonary hypertension.

### Miscellaneous Abnormalities

A number of other abnormalities of the respiratory system have been described in patients who have rheumatoid disease, including bronchocentric granulomatosis,[429] idiopathic hemosiderosis, and chronic eosinophilic pneumonia.[1] Whether the conditions represent additional rare manifestations of RD in the lungs, or are simply coincidental, is not clear. Diffuse interstitial amyloidosis also has been described in some patients who have had long-standing rheumatoid arthritis.[430]

Some patients who have rheumatoid arthritis have a significant reduction in chest wall compliance, probably related to involvement of the costosternal and costovertebral joints.[431] This could contribute to dyspnea in such patients. A reduction in respiratory muscle strength and an increase in respiratory drive have also been documented in patients who have RD.[432] It has been hypothesized that the weakness may be the result of corticosteroid therapy and/or rheumatoid myositis, while increased stimulation to neural afferents arising from muscle, joint, or lung receptors accounts for the increase in drive.[432]

Pulmonary disease in patients who have RD can also represent a complication of therapy. The effects of drugs used in the management of rheumatoid arthritis, including methotrexate, gold salts, and penicillamine, are discussed in greater detail in Chapter 63 (see page 2537). It is obviously important to distinguish these effects from other pulmonary manifestations of RD and from opportunistic infection or malignancy due to immunosuppression arising from treatment.

### Prognosis and Natural History

The prognosis and course of RD clearly depend to some extent on the severity and type of systemic disease. With respect to pleuropulmonary involvement, some of the abnormalities (e.g., rheumatoid nodules, pleural effusion and fibrosis, and BOOP) are not life threatening and are not directly related to decreased survival in the vast majority of patients. However, other complications (e.g., interstitial pneumonitis, obliterative bronchiolitis, and pulmonary hypertension) are frequently more serious.

In comparison with age- and sex-specific rates in the general population, a threefold increase in mortality overall has been reported in patients who have RD.[433] During the first 5 years after diagnosis, a highly significant number of deaths from circulatory, respiratory, and musculoskeletal disorders has been found;[433, 434] later, infection and amyloidosis are major causes of death.[433, 435] For example, in a Japanese series of more than 1,000 autopsies of patients who had RD, the most common causes of death were infection (27%), respiratory disease (18%), and amyloidosis (13%).[436] Pneumonia occurs more frequently in patients who have RD, and deaths due to respiratory infection exceed the expected rate by more than four times.[243] Of particular note is the increased risk for the development of opportunistic lung infection with *Pneumocystis carinii*,[437, 438] *Aspergillus* species,[439] and *Nocardia asteroides*,[440] secondary to the use of "low-dose" methotrexate therapy.

An association between pulmonary carcinoma and interstitial fibrosis has been seen in some series of patients who have RD,[242, 243] a relationship that is presumably similar to that seen with other etiologies of pulmonary fibrosis (see page 1080). A report on the incidence of malignancy in 530 patients receiving immunosuppressive agents for RA, predominantly azathioprine, over a 7-year period of follow-up, revealed 20 cancers.[441] The standardized mortality ratio (SMR) for lymphoproliferative disorders and myeloma was particularly striking (8.05), although excess pulmonary carcinoma was also noted (SMR = 3.37).

### Pleuropulmonary Disease in Juvenile Rheumatoid Arthritis

Juvenile rheumatoid arthritis is characterized by chronic synovitis and a variety of visceral abnormalities that, by definition, have their onset in individuals younger than 16 years of age. The condition has been divided into a number of clinical variants, including (1) an acute systemic form characterized by fever, rash, lymph node enlargement, hepatosplenomegaly, and a variable degree of arthritis (seen in approximately 20% of patients); and (2) polyarticular forms in which four or less joints are involved (about 50% of cases).

Clinically manifest pleuropulmonary complications are uncommon: in one series of 191 patients who had active disease, only eight (4%) were so affected;[442] a review of the literature to 1980 revealed only eight other cases.[442] Most patients have the systemic form of the illness, although abnormalities can also occur in pauciarticular and polyarticular forms. Despite these findings, one group of investigators documented frequent pulmonary function abnormalities in the absence of symptoms or radiographic findings, with significant reduction in mid-expiratory flows being found in patients who had active disease;[443] diffusing capacity was also somewhat reduced.

As with adult RD, pleuritis and pleural effusion are the most common manifestations of thoracic involvement in juvenile RA. Follicular bronchiolitis appears to be the most frequent form of pulmonary disease.[399, 442] A single case of pulmonary hypertension has been reported;[417] histocompatibility testing showed the presence of DR3 and DRw52, both of which have also been associated with idiopathic pulmonary hypertension in children and with pulmonary hypertension in patients who have progressive systemic sclerosis.

## PROGRESSIVE SYSTEMIC SCLEROSIS

Progressive systemic sclerosis (PSS, scleroderma) is a generalized disorder of connective tissue characterized by a variety of inflammatory, fibrotic, and degenerative changes often accompanied by vasculopathy. It is an uncommon condition, with an estimated incidence of only 12 cases per million population per year.[444] The majority of patients are in the fourth to sixth decades of life. There is a female predominance of approximately three to one,[445, 446] but no significant racial predominance.[446]

Although pulmonary disease is common in PSS, there is a significant disparity between the frequency of clinical, pathologic, radiologic, and functional disease. In many cases, abnormalities of pulmonary function are demonstrable when the chest radiograph is perfectly normal.[447–451] For example, in one review of 800 patients, radiographic abnormalities were present in the lungs in 25% of patients and pulmonary symptoms in 16%;[448] however, some aspects of pulmonary function were almost invariably abnormal. In an additional review of 890 patients in the University of Pittsburgh scleroderma databank, 60% had a forced vital capacity (FVC) greater than 75% predicted, 27% had moderate restrictive disease (FVC between 50% and 75% predicted), and 13% had severe restriction (FVC < 50% predicted).[452] Similar differences in the ability to identify disease occur between standard radiography and more sophisticated tests of early lung disease. For example, in one study of 16 patients whose chest radiographs were normal, 7 (44%) had abnormalities on HRCT scans and 11 (73%) had abnormalities on BAL similar to those found in patients who had obvious abnormalities on plain radiographs.[453] In another investigation in which the plain radiograph was abnormal in 42% of patients, HRCT was abnormal in 71%.[454]

The word *scleroderma* is used here as a descriptive term for the thickened and fixed skin and subcutaneous tissue over the fingers, face, and elsewhere on the body. Although characteristically found in PSS, it is in fact a clinical sign that can be found in a number of disorders of local or general distribution and of varied etiology (Table 39–4). Many of these "sclerodermas" closely resemble PSS, and some are variants that are generally accepted as having a similar pathogenesis. Examples include CREST syndrome (*see* page 1460) and mixed connective tissue disease (*see* page 1469). In addition, features of PSS are also found in patients who have symptoms and signs more indicative of other well-defined disorders; these diseases are discussed individually.

### Pathogenesis

#### Interstitial Pneumonitis and Fibrosis

In many respects, the interstitial lung disease seen in PSS resembles that of idiopathic pulmonary fibrosis. Pathologically, it is characterized by an accumulation of immune and inflammatory effector cells in the parenchymal intersti-

## Table 39–4. Diseases Associated with Sclerosis

*Diseases Associated with Generalized Sclerosis*

Scleroderma
  Acrosclerosis
  Progressive systemic sclerosis
Porphyria cutanea tarda
Scleromyxedema
Carcinoid syndrome
Primary amyloidosis
Mixed connective tissue disease
Graft-versus-host disease
CREST syndrome
Diffuse fasciitis with eosinophilia
Metastatic malignancy
  Melanoma
  Lung carcinoma
Insulin-dependent diabetes mellitus in children
Occupational exposure to silica, silicates, and vinyl chloride

*Diseases Associated with Localized Sclerosis*

Scleroderma
  Morphea
  Linear scleroderma
Lichen sclerosus et atrophicus
Carcinoma en cuirasse (metastatic carcinoma of breast)
Acro-osteolysis
Drug-induced
  Bleomycin
  Pentazocine
Trauma-induced: vibratory
  Pneumatic hammers
  Chain saws

Modified from Chanda JJ: Med Clin North Am 64:969, 1980.

tium,[455–463] associated in some patients with the subsequent development of fibrosis.[457, 459] Ultrastructural studies of material obtained at open lung biopsy suggest that endothelial and/or epithelial damage may precede the inflammation and fibrosis.[460] Although the nature of the initial insult is not known, it is likely that the ensuing reaction is related to the subsequent development of clinically evident disease; patients who have persistent evidence of alveolitis on BAL tend to show greater rates of decline in lung function than do those who have no evidence of active inflammation.[461, 464] Damage to type II pneumocytes may lead to the production of tissue factor, the primary cellular initiator of the coagulation cascade;[465] this in turn may result in local fibrin deposition, which could contribute to interstitial fibrosis via its subsequent organization.

Much of the information concerning the nature of the inflammatory reaction in the lungs of patients who have PSS has been derived from studies of cells and cell products obtained by BAL. The relative importance of each cell type to the development of fibrosis is not clear; it is likely, however, that the alveolar macrophage plays an important role. There is ample evidence that these cells are in a highly active state,[457, 458, 461] a feature manifested in BAL fluid by the presence of various cytokines (including interleukin-6), tumor necrosis factor-alpha, fibronectin, transforming growth factor-beta, and other growth factors such as insulin-like growth factor-I,[466] which are implicated in both fibroblast activation and chemotaxis.[457, 458, 461, 467–471a] In addition, there is *in vitro* evidence that these cells secrete interleukin-8, another cytokine that acts as a chemoattractant for neutrophils.[472, 473] Neutrophils in turn may release elastase, which has tissue-damaging properties; in support of this hypothesis are the results of one study in which more extensive fibrosis (as assessed by HRCT scanning) was found in patients who had BAL neutrophilia than in those who did not.[463]

Although other cells are undoubtedly involved in the pathogenesis of pulmonary disease in PSS, their precise roles are unclear. The number of lymphocytes in BAL fluid of patients who have PSS is increased by clonal expansion, suggesting a reaction to specific antigens;[456] however, there seems to be no correlation between activation of T lymphocytes and the presence or absence of pulmonary fibrosis.[457] Recruitment and activation of interstitial mast cells are also seen in PSS;[474] *in vitro* studies suggest that release of histamine and tryptase by these cells may be involved in fibroblast activation.[474] In one study, the percentage of eosinophils in BAL correlated with a ground-glass appearance of the lung on HRCT, a finding that was believed to reflect inflammation.[463] However, the relationship, if any, of this finding to the development of fibrosis remains to be determined.

A number of serologic abnormalities have been found in the blood of patients who have PSS. Some have been associated with various clinical features of disease; however, the nature and significance of this association are far from clear. Antinuclear antibodies are present in most patients who have PSS;[444] those who have the CREST variant frequently have the anticentromeric form, an antibody that is unusual in PSS and in other autoimmune connective tissue diseases.[475] A clinical subset of PSS characterized by diffuse cutaneous change, progressive pulmonary fibrosis, and poor prognosis has been associated with an antibody to an epitope of DNA, termed *topoisomerase I* (topo I, or Scl-70).[476, 477, 477a] Anti-RNA polymerase III antibodies were described in 23% of 252 consecutive patients who had PSS in one investigation;[478] the antibody seemed specific for PSS and was most closely associated with extensive cutaneous involvement, pulmonary fibrosis, and heart disease. Antihistone antibodies also correlate with the presence of severe pulmonary fibrosis in patients who have PSS.[479]

A variety of other findings in the blood of patients who have PSS might be related to disease pathogenesis. For example, affected patients have a reduction in the number of circulating T cells, particularly T-suppressor cells and natural killer cells.[480] In one study of six patients who had PSS and evidence of alveolitis, four had impaired release of interferon-gamma by peripheral lymphocytes;[481] the latter can suppress fibroblast proliferation, and its deficiency was associated with a deterioration in lung function. In another investigation, the serum concentration of procollagen type I carboxyterminal propeptide, an index of collagen synthesis, was higher in patients who had more diffuse disease; they were also more likely to have lung fibrosis and joint involvement.[482]

Endothelin-1 is a potent vasoconstrictor, derived largely from endothelial cells, that may cause tissue fibrosis by direct stimulation of fibroblasts;[483] it is therefore an attractive potential link between the vascular and fibrotic tissue changes seen in PSS. Several experimental observations support a pathogenic role for this substance. For example, macrophages of patients who have PSS show excessive endothelin-1 production *in vitro*.[484] Increased levels of endothelin-1 and increased endothein-1 receptor expression have also been demonstrated in the affected parenchyma of patients who have fibrotic lung disease.[485] Finally, higher than normal levels of circulating endothelin-1 have been found in some patients who have PSS (although the relationship between these levels and either pulmonary fibrosis or hypertension has not been consistent).[483, 486]

There is also evidence suggesting that genetic factors influence susceptibility to or expression of PSS. Familial clustering of the disease has been well described.[487, 488] However, no consistent association between HLA haplotype and PSS has been found between as opposed to within centers, perhaps reflecting differences in populations in various geographic locations. A study of connective tissue disease and autoantibodies in the families of 63 patients who had PSS in Britain revealed the presence of ANAs more often in relatives than in controls;[444] however, antibodies with a high specificity for PSS were found only in affected patients. This finding could be explained as well by environmental influences as by genetic ones. In fact, the finding of an increased frequency of ANAs in the spouses of probands suggests that environmental factors are involved in the pathogenesis of PSS; this interpretation is supported by the observation that the development of scleroderma-like disorders has been associated with exposure to a variety of environmental agents (*see* Table 39–4, page 1452).

Gastroesophageal reflux and pulmonary aspiration are common in patients who have PSS; since the severity of reflux is positively correlated with the severity of lung function impairment,[489] it is possible that recurrent aspiration contributes to or is the cause of the lung damage, in at least some patients. However, patients who have BAL evidence of alveolitis are more likely to have esophageal involvement than patients who do not have alveolitis (95% vs. 68%, respectively);[461] thus, the association of reflux with lung function impairment could also be due to their both being markers of disease severity. A third explanation is afforded by the results of another investigation in which differences in the prevalence of alveolitis were no longer apparent when cigarette smoking was taken into account—both lung function and reflux were worsened by smoking.[489]

### Pulmonary Hypertension

The pathogenesis of Raynaud's phenomenon and the pulmonary hypertension with which it can be associated in the CREST variant of PSS is poorly understood. It is likely, however, that the initial event is pure vasospasm, perhaps caused by an imbalance between thromboxane $A_2$, a potent vasoconstrictor and platelet aggregator produced largely by platelets, and prostacyclin (prostaglandin $I_2$), a vasodilator and inhibitor of platelet aggregation released from vascular endothelium.[490, 491] The results of a number of studies involving a variety of vasodilators directed not only toward relief of digital arterial spasm but also against pulmonary vasoconstriction support this hypothesis.[492–497] There is also evidence that patients who have PSS have defective endothelial cell function, manifested by absent substance-P–induced arterial vasodilation early in the course of the disease.[497a] Levels of antiendothelial cell antibodies are higher in patients with PSS who have digital infarcts or pulmonary arterial hypertension than in patients who do not have these complications.[497b] In patients who have Raynaud's phenomenon, it is presumed that recurrent episodes of vasoconstriction lead eventually to intimal fibrosis of digital vessels, with or without thrombosis, a supposition that has been supported by some pathologic studies.[498, 499]

Whether similar events occur in the pulmonary circulation is not clear. One patient who had Raynaud's phenomenon, cutaneous sclerosis, and minimal bibasilar pulmonary fibrosis complained of dyspnea occasioned by cold weather; when the patient was exposed to cold in the laboratory with a catheter in place, there was a rapid rise in pulmonary artery pressure, attesting to the presence of vasospasm in the pulmonary artery circulation.[494] However, another study of nine patients who had PSS and CREST syndrome failed to confirm this response following hand immersion in cold water.[500] Moreover, no consistent findings have been demonstrated in measurements of the diffusing capacity following

exposure to cold in patients who have Raynaud's phenomenon; some investigators have demonstrated a rise in single-breath diffusing capacity for CO on exposure,[501, 502] while others have shown a fall.[503] (Normal individuals show no change in diffusing capacity during the test.[502]) The same variability has been seen in the response of the pulmonary arteries to vasodilators in patients who have PSS, improvement in flow being seen in some patients[504] but not in others.[505] If vasospasm does lead to permanent obstruction in the pulmonary artery circulation, this might explain the variability in findings in the right-sided circulation in this disease.

### Pathologic Characteristics

Pathologic changes occur in the pleura, alveolar interstitium, bronchioles, and vasculature. Unexplained pleural effu-

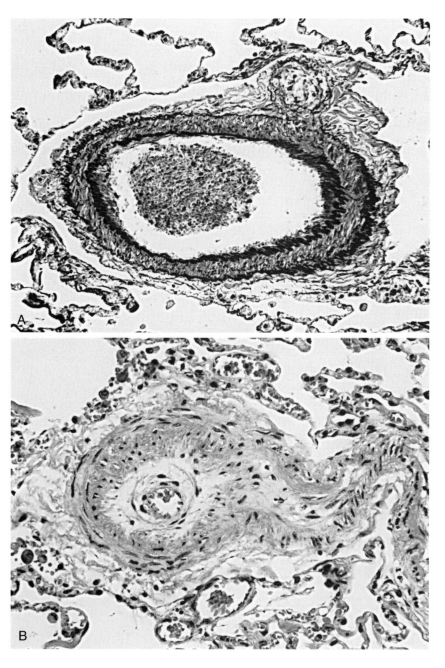

**Figure 39–22. Overlap Syndrome (Systemic Lupus Erythematosus with CREST) and Pulmonary Arterial Hypertension.** A 26-year-old woman with long-standing celiac disease presented with findings consistent with SLE according to American Rheumatological Association criteria. She subsequently developed the CREST syndrome, and evidence of pulmonary hypertension; she died 1 month later. An autopsy showed normal lung parenchyma and extensive narrowing of small pulmonary arteries and arterioles. A medium-sized muscular artery with medial muscle hypertrophy is shown in *A*. A small artery showing muscle hypertrophy and loose subendothelial connective tissue is seen in *B*. (*A*, Verhoeff–Van Gieson ×130; *B*, ×250.)

sion is infrequent, as is fibrinous pleuritis; in fact, the latter was found in one autopsy study to be no more common in patients who had PSS than in controls.[506] By contrast, pleural fibrosis is not uncommon—28% of 58 cases in the latter study[506]—and may be either local or diffuse. At autopsy, some degree of parenchymal interstitial fibrosis is frequent, although in many cases it is only focal.[507] More severely affected lungs show bilateral interstitial thickening that is most marked in the subpleural regions of the lower lobes and is grossly and microscopically similar to idiopathic pulmonary fibrosis.[508] Obliterative bronchiolitis, by itself, is not a feature of PSS, despite the frequent use of penicillamine as therapy. However, bronchiolar disease is common in the setting of severe fibrosis at autopsy.[393] Follicular bronchiolitis and bronchiolitis obliterans organizing pneumonia are seen occasionally.[509, 510]

Although pathologic evidence of pulmonary arterial hypertension is seen most often in association with diffuse interstitial fibrosis, vascular changes can also be present in areas of lung uninvolved by the latter process, and occasionally occur in the absence of interstitial disease.[507, 511] Many patients who have the latter finding probably have CREST syndrome rather than pure PSS.[512] Although some investigators have found histologic abnormalities at all levels of the arterial system,[507] others have identified predominant involvement of small muscular arteries and arterioles.[513, 514] In the latter vessels, the intima is moderately to severely thickened by loose fibroblastic connective tissue that in later stages is transformed into mature collagen (Fig. 39–22).[514] The media usually shows some degree of hypertrophy;[507] in some cases, however, it appears atrophic.[514] Arteritis, fibrinoid necrosis, and plexiform lesions are uncommon. Intimal and medial thickening can progress to virtually complete obliteration of vessel lumina with consequent pulmonary arterial hypertension and right ventricular hypertrophy.

### Radiologic Manifestations

The systemic nature of progressive systemic sclerosis can often be appreciated on the chest radiograph, which may demonstrate abnormalities involving the lungs, pleura, esophagus, and chest wall.

### The Lungs

Evidence of interstitial fibrosis has been reported to be present on the chest radiograph in 20% to 65% of patients who have PSS.[515–517] The initial radiographic abnormalities may be subtle and typically consist of a fine reticulation;[517] as the disease progresses, the reticulation tends to become coarser and easier to detect as it extends from the lung bases to involve the lower two thirds of the lungs (Fig. 39–23).[517] (As with idiopathic pulmonary fibrosis and rheumatoid disease, there is a tendency for predominant involvement of the lower lung zones, with little or no evidence of upper zone abnormality, at least in the initial stages of the disease.[516–518]) Serial radiographs over a 2- to 3-year period may show progressive and uniform loss of lung volume in addition to a worsening of the interstitial disease, a finding of considerable value in diagnosis; we have been impressed by the tendency for both PSS and idiopathic pulmonary fibrosis to show this progressive loss of volume, in contrast with other causes of diffuse interstitial fibrosis.

HRCT frequently demonstrates evidence of interstitial

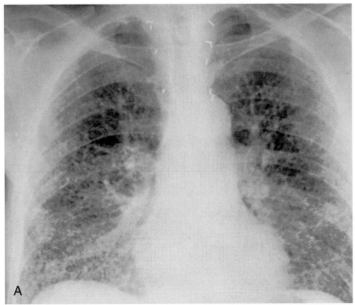
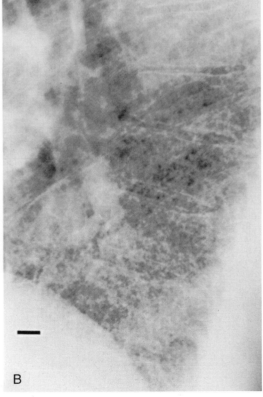

**Figure 39–23. Progressive Systemic Sclerosis (PSS): Interstitial Fibrosis.** A posteroanterior chest radiograph *(A)* and a detail view of the lower zones from a lateral projection *(B)* reveal a reticular pattern involving mainly the lower lung zones. Metallic clips in the upper mediastinum relate to prior bilateral sympathetectomy. The patient was a 45-year-old man with a long history of PSS.

pneumonitis and fibrosis in patients who have normal or questionable radiographic findings.[516, 517] For example, in one prospective study of 23 patients, a definitive reticular pattern consistent with fibrosis was seen on the chest radiograph in 9 (39%) and minimal or equivocal findings in 6 (26%); by contrast, evidence of fibrosis was seen on HRCT in 21 patients (91%).[516] Only 9 patients (39%) had dyspnea at rest or on exercise. In a second study of 18 patients who had dyspnea or restrictive lung disease as determined by pulmonary function tests, 10 (59%) had evidence of fibrosis on the chest radiograph as compared to 15 (88%) on HRCT.[518]

The HRCT findings include parenchymal and subpleural micronodules, intralobular linear opacities giving a reticular pattern, subpleural lines, areas of ground-glass attenuation, and honeycombing (Fig. 39–24).[510, 516] The abnormalities involve mainly the lower lobes and have a predominant peripheral and posterior distribution.[510] Because of this distribution, CT scans should be performed with the patient prone to detect mild abnormalities and to avoid confusing early disease with reversible gravity-induced density.[510] When the chest radiograph is normal or equivocal, nodules measuring 2 to 3 mm in diameter are commonly seen on CT, reflecting the presence of follicular bronchiolitis.[510]

The pattern of abnormality on HRCT has been shown to reflect the relative proportions of fibrosis and inflamma-tion. In one study of 12 patients, comparison was made between the CT findings and open lung biopsy specimens obtained from 20 different lobes.[519] In 13 of the lobes, HRCT demonstrated a predominant reticular pattern; in the other 7 lobes, there was an equivalent extent of reticulation and ground-glass attenuation. On histologic examination, the predominant reticular pattern was associated with a predominantly fibrotic appearance in 12 of 13 lobes; in the lobes that had an equivalent extent of reticulation and ground-glass attenuation, there was an inflammatory appearance in 4 lobes and a fibrotic appearance in 3 lobes. CT thus allowed correct discrimination between inflammatory and fibrotic histologic findings in 16 (80%) of 20 biopsy specimens. In another investigation, short-term functional improvement following therapy with corticosteroids was observed in three of seven patients who had equivalent extent of ground-glass attenuation and reticulation and in none of six patients who had predominant reticulation.[520] Despite this apparent therapeutic benefit, in a follow-up of 66 patients who had interstitial pneumonitis and fibrosis associated with PSS, the CT appearances were not predictive of 4-year survival.[520]

Patients who have interstitial pneumonitis and fibrosis associated with PSS frequently have mediastinal lymph node enlargement on CT (defined as a short-axis diameter > 10 mm). In one series of 53 patients, mediastinal lymphadenop-

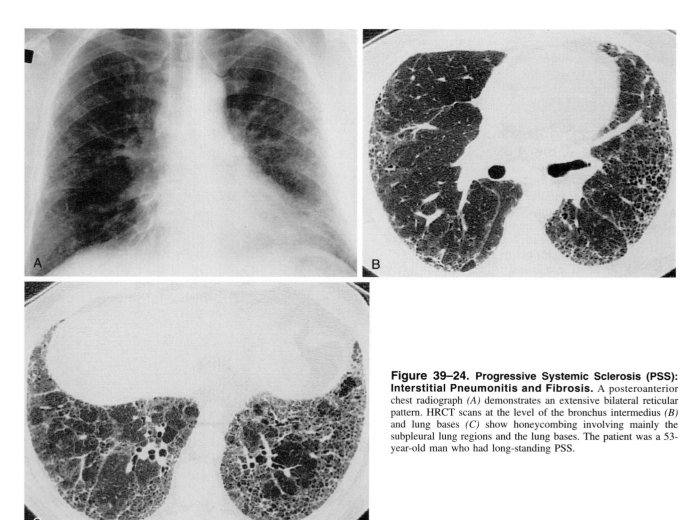

**Figure 39–24. Progressive Systemic Sclerosis (PSS): Interstitial Pneumonitis and Fibrosis.** A posteroanterior chest radiograph *(A)* demonstrates an extensive bilateral reticular pattern. HRCT scans at the level of the bronchus intermedius *(B)* and lung bases *(C)* show honeycombing involving mainly the subpleural lung regions and the lung bases. The patient was a 53-year-old man who had long-standing PSS.

athy was not seen in any of the patients who had normal parenchyma on CT, but was present in 23% of those who had mild parenchymal disease and in 42% of those who had honeycombing.[510] In another study of 25 patients who had PSS and diffuse interstitial lung disease, mediastinal adenopathy was present in 15 (60%).[521] The likelihood of lymphadenopathy appears to be related to the presence of parenchymal abnormalities rather than the specific pattern of disease seen on HRCT. In a review of the CT findings in 73 patients, lymphadenopathy was identified in 35 (48%).[522] It was present in 70% of patients who had parenchymal abnormalities regardless of whether the pattern consisted of areas of ground-glass attenuation, a linear pattern, or honeycombing. Only 6 (17%) of the 35 patients who had normal lung parenchyma on CT had lymphadenopathy.

When considering pulmonary abnormalities, it should be remembered that they may be a manifestation of secondary lung disease; for example, esophageal dysmotility may lead to aspiration pneumonia.[122, 523]

### The Pleura

Radiographic evidence of pleural effusion or thickening is less common in PSS than in other connective tissue diseases, being seen in approximately 10% to 15% of patients.[524, 525] Pleural thickening is seen more commonly on CT: in one series of 55 patients evaluated with HRCT, diffuse pleural thickening was seen in one third, all of whom also had pulmonary abnormalities.[510] Pneumothorax is rare.[516]

### The Esophagus

The esophagus is reported to be involved clinically and radiologically in about 50% of patients who have PSS;[526, 527] however, it is likely that the true frequency is even greater, since patients who have minimal involvement unaccompanied by dysphagia are unlikely to be referred for radiologic examination.[448] For example, in one study of 36 patients who underwent either manometric or barium examination of the esophagus, 33 manifested abnormal esophageal motility.[528] Although the majority of patients who have radiographic evidence of esophageal involvement complain of dysphagia, this is not invariable.[448]

The atrophy and atony of the esophagus that result in aperistalsis can lead to dilation, which may be manifested on plain radiographs as an air esophagogram (Fig. 39–25). However, for maximal sensitivity, the presence or absence of esophageal aperistalsis must be assessed by fluoroscopic study and barium swallow—preferably in the horizontal position, since in many cases the motility disturbance is not evident in the erect position. In fact, the presence of a substantial amount of gas in the esophagus on a lateral radiograph of the chest is a useful sign of PSS, especially if it is unassociated with an air-fluid level and if gas is present in the gastric fundus.[529] The latter two qualifications are important, since an esophageal air-fluid level and a gasless stomach are characteristic features of achalasia, the chief differential diagnostic possibility. The association of an air-containing esophagus with the lung changes described previously is virtually pathognomonic of PSS.[530]

### The Chest Wall

Erosion of the cortex of the superior aspects of the ribs in the posterior axillary line (superior rib notching) has been reported in approximately 15% of patients who have PSS.[448, 525] The finding is of unknown pathogenesis and is not specific, since it may also be observed in rheumatoid disease, SLE, and Sjögren's syndrome.

### *Clinical Manifestations*

The patient who has advanced PSS presents a distressing picture that is dominated by a thickened inelastic and waxy appearance of the skin, most prominent about the face and extremities. Although these abnormalities may not be the earliest manifestations,[531, 532] they are the most characteristic and are observed eventually in almost every patient.[122] The skin is frequently bronze and sometimes contains calcium deposits.[122, 526] It is not nearly as thick in CREST syndrome as in PSS. A rapid increase in skin thickness is a poor prognostic sign, especially with respect to the development of overt renal disease; however, skin thickness can wax and wane and paradoxically can show dramatic improvement after the kidneys have become involved[533] or the patient has survived a renal crisis.[534] Involvement of the skin of the thoracic wall generally does not interfere with pulmonary function; however, one patient who had severe chest wall involvement did demonstrate restriction functionally, despite an unremarkable HRCT scan of the lung and a normal diffusing capacity.[534a]

Although pulmonary symptoms are the presenting manifestation of disease in less than 1% of patients,[535] more than 60% have dyspnea at some point in the course of the disease (usually in the late stages).[536] Patients may have a slightly productive cough or hemoptysis, the latter as a result of bleeding from ectatic bronchial vessels; massive pulmonary hemorrhage is extremely rare.[537, 538] Basilar crackles are reported to occur in approximately 50% of patients.[539] When lung disease is rapidly progressive or the radiographic features are atypical, bronchiolitis obliterans organizing pneumonia should be considered.[509]

Esophageal involvement should be suspected if the patient complains of difficulty in swallowing; however, as indicated previously, esophageal dilation and disturbed motility can be detected in many patients before dysphagia becomes clinically manifest.[540] Involvement of the esophagus appears to bear no relationship to the progression or severity of visceral or cutaneous sclerosis; patients who die from their disease may manifest only mild esophageal changes, whereas those whose skin disease shows improvement may manifest progressive esophageal disease. Esophageal dysmotility causes reflux and can be complicated by esophageal candidiasis and stricture formation.[541] In addition to the symptoms and signs referable to the skin and gastrointestinal tract and to Raynaud's phenomenon, patients may have weight loss and low-grade fever.

Cardiac involvement is common and may be primary or secondary to systemic or pulmonary hypertension.[536] Sclerosis of the cardiac muscle may result in biventricular failure; however, right ventricular failure alone is more likely to be related directly to pulmonary vascular disease. Patients who have new-onset biventricular failure may also have

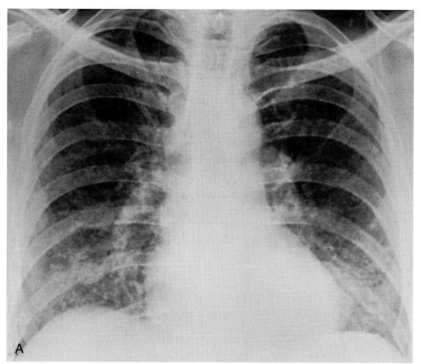

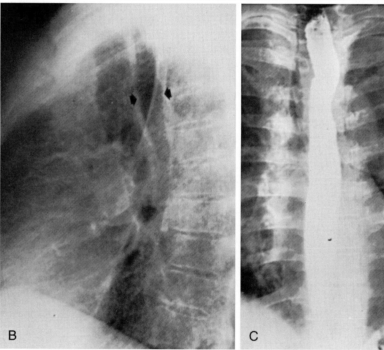

**Figure 39–25. Esophageal Distention in Progressive Systemic Sclerosis (PSS).** Posteroanterior *(A)* and lateral *(B)* radiographs of the chest reveal a fine reticular pattern throughout both lungs; the reticulation is more prominent in the bases. In lateral projection, an abnormal accumulation of gas behind the trachea *(arrows)* represents an air-distended esophagus. A radiograph of the chest following ingestion of barium *(C)* shows uniform dilation of the esophagus; fluoroscopic examination revealed aperistalsis. The patient was a 53-year-old man with PSS.

PSS-related myocarditis.[542] Although changes in the cardiac muscle are seen frequently at autopsy, clinical findings of heart failure due to myocardial fibrosis are uncommon, and an abnormal left ventricular ejection fraction is seen in only 15% of patients.[536] A prolonged PR interval or a left or a right bundle branch block may be the only manifestation of myocardial fibrosis;[448] in one investigation using Holter monitor analysis, disturbances in conduction or rhythm were identified in 26 of 46 patients, some of whom complained of palpitations or syncope.[543]

Pericardial involvement is uncommon clinically, occurring in only 7% of patients in one study;[536] this contrasts with the frequent involvement of the pericardium at autopsy or by echocardiography, in which it has been found in as many as 60% of cases.[536] Pericardial disease may be acute or chronic; large effusions may indicate the development of renal failure. Complicating tamponade or constrictive pericarditis has been described.[536]

Arthralgia, particularly of the hands, occurs in 50% to 80% of patients at some stage in the course of the disease.[544] Clinical evidence of renal involvement has been reported in approximately 25% of patients,[448] although at autopsy the kidneys are found to be affected in the great majority. Renal crisis, characterized by malignant hypertension, microangiopathic hemolytic anemia, azotemia, and hyperreninemia, is one of the most feared complications of PSS.[545] Typically, it occurs early in course of the disease in patients who have rapidly progressive cutaneous thickening.

As indicated previously, some patients who have PSS have symptoms and signs of other connective tissue diseases, placing them in a category commonly referred to as "overlap syndrome." These combinations are discussed in greater length in the section on mixed connective tissue disease (MCTD), a syndrome whose clinical and laboratory features are so consistent that it is usually considered a separate entity (*see* page 1469). In addition to this and the CREST syndrome, there exist a number of other disease processes, some of which appear to be of autoimmune pathogenesis, that closely mimic PSS (*see* Table 39–4). Examples include a PSS-like syndrome with skin, joint, and pulmonary manifestations that has been described in children who have insulin-dependent diabetes mellitus[546] and a combination of PSS and myxedema associated with circulating antithyroid antibodies.[547]

Another disease complex that some authors regard as a variant of PSS is diffuse fasciitis with eosinophilia,[548, 549] a syndrome that includes cutaneous sclerosis with sparing of the skin of the hands and feet, blood eosinophilia, increased serum levels of eosinophilic chemotactic factor, and (sometimes) polyarthritis.[549, 550] As the name implies, the inflammatory process involves predominantly fascia. Although the lungs are spared, the chest wall may be affected, resulting in restrictive lung function.[551, 552] The eosinophilia is predominantly in the blood, although some eosinophils may also be present with other mononuclear cells in the inflamed fascia; one case associated with granulomatous vasculitis has been reported.[553]

A variety of diseases associated with cutaneous sclerosis may be confused with PSS (*see* Table 39–4). Diffuse sclerosis of skin and viscera similar to PSS is an occasional accompaniment of carcinoid syndrome. A PSS-like illness has also been reported during therapy with hydroxytryptophan and carbidopa (*see* page 1752).[554] A more recent addition to the many PSS-like lesions encountered in clinical practice is chronic graft-versus-host disease;[555] this complication of bone marrow transplantation presents with features of PSS and Sjögren's syndrome, obstructive airway disease with obliterative bronchiolitis, and recurrent pulmonary infections (*see* page 1729).[556] Finally, many survivors of toxic oil syndrome in Spain have developed a clinical condition virtually identical to PSS (*see* page 2587).[557]

In many instances, these overlap syndromes are associated with Raynaud's phenomenon, which can result in further diagnostic confusion. Raynaud's phenomenon also occurs in the majority of patients who have PSS, as for example, in 22 of 27 patients in one series[448] and in 39 of 44 in another.[515] It usually precedes skin changes[517, 558] and may antedate or occur simultaneously with clinical or functional evidence of pulmonary parenchymal involvement.[558] In one series of 91 patients who initially presented with Raynaud's phenomenon, clinical findings included arthralgia or a history of arthritis in 27%, skin abnormalities in 30%, esophageal hypomotility in 14%, a lowered diffusing capacity in 23%, and renal disease in 5%;[559] none of the last three abnormalities was associated with symptoms. Twenty-six of the 91 cases could be classified as PSS or CREST syndrome,

8 as SLE, and 5 as MCTD; the remaining 52 could not be precisely categorized, although 20 had some evidence of systemic disease. In this series, both the number of different serum autoantibodies and the titer of ANAs were positively correlated with the number of affected organ systems.

A considerable contribution to the understanding of the natural history of Raynaud's phenomenon was made by the recognition that an abnormal pattern on nailfold capillary microscopy can be seen in patients who have PSS.[560] This pattern has been found to be more sensitive than the presence of ANAs, digital ulcers, or decreased esophageal motility in predicting which patients who have Raynaud's phenomenon and poorly defined connective tissue disease will subsequently develop PSS.[560] The abnormality has also been correlated with clinical and laboratory findings of pulmonary hypertension in patients who have PSS.[561]

### Pulmonary Function Tests

Pulmonary function is almost invariably disturbed in patients who have PSS, even when the chest radiograph is normal. In the presence of radiographic evidence of interstitial fibrosis, serial studies of pulmonary function may show progressive deterioration coincident with worsening of the radiographic abnormality.[451] However, although there is substantial individual variability, studies of serial pulmonary function changes in patients who have PSS and patients who have idiopathic pulmonary fibrosis have revealed a relatively indolent progression in the former compared with the latter.[562–565]

The usual functional aberrations consist of a restrictive impairment with progressively diminishing vital capacity and residual volume.[452, 566, 567] The results of some studies also indicate that obstruction may be present in the absence of a smoking history;[566, 568, 569] this obstruction is characterized by a normal (as opposed to supranormal) $FEV_1/FVC$ in association with increased residual volume.[568] However, some investigators have disputed this association.[570] Both diffusing capacity and lung compliance are almost invariably reduced,[448, 569, 571–574] the former being the most sensitive of the standard lung function studies for predicting early lung involvement.[575] The findings documented in some case reports suggest that ventilatory failure can be the result of diaphragmatic muscle dysfunction;[576, 577] reversal of muscle weakness with therapy in one patient suggests that such dysfunction may be related to inflammation rather than fibrosis.[577]

In one investigation of exercise tests in 15 patients, circulatory impairment was evident in most, with a low $O_2$ pulse and low anaerobic threshold;[578] 14 had normal spirometry or restrictive lung function, while one smoker had obstructive airways disease. Despite these changes, the limitation to exercise was not due to the abnormal lung function. In another study of 34 patients who had PSS and abnormal lung function characterized by a reduction in the diffusing capacity, incremental exercise testing revealed significant exercise impairment;[579] reductions in oxygen uptake were accompanied by a high dead-space ventilation and a widened alveolar-arterial oxygen gradient during exercise. Among 78 patients who had normal lung function, exercise testing was able to reveal subtle abnormalities; 12 (15%) of these had increased dead space–to–tidal volume ratios during exercise.

### Prognosis and Natural History

The prognosis of PSS is poor: in two early series of 236[526] and 198[580] patients, the 5-year survival rates were reported to be 49% and 67%, respectively. Similar results were found in a more recent study of 264 patients:[581] after an average of 5.2 years of follow-up, 50% were known to have died, 68% of the deaths being directly attributable to PSS. The prognosis is poorer for men and African Americans than for women and whites;[445, 526, 582] a decreased survival time has also been found in older patients after allowance has been made for the natural increase in mortality with age.[580]

The cause of death may be related to cardiovascular, pulmonary, or renal complications;[445, 580, 583] however, with better management of renal failure, pulmonary disease has emerged as the most common fatal complication.[584] Despite this, involvement of the lungs does not necessarily constitute a bad prognostic sign; in one series, the interval from the onset of clinically evident pulmonary disease to death was as long as 37 years.[539] In a follow-up study of 71 patients, a lowered diffusing capacity for CO was associated with a poor prognosis, particularly if the overall pattern was obstructive and the patient was male.[585] Despite general acceptance of an increased incidence of pulmonary carcinoma in patients who have PSS (Fig. 39–26),[586, 587] a comprehensive analysis of this relationship suggests that it may be fortuitous.[588] Systemic amyloidosis is a rare complication.[589]

## CREST SYNDROME

CREST syndrome (limited systemic sclerosis) is generally regarded as a variant of PSS. As originally described, the syndrome included the clinical findings of subcutaneous calcification, Raynaud's phenomenon, sclerodactyly, and multiple telangiectasia (CRST syndrome).[590, 591] It was subsequently realized that esophageal involvement is a common additional manifestation, thus creating a group of five abnormalities for which the word *CREST* constitutes an acronym.

The serum of patients who have CREST syndrome usually does not contain the autoantibodies seen in the other autoimmune diseases; however, there is frequently a positive reaction to the centromeric portion of dividing chromosomes. This anticentromere antibody has been found in the sera of more than 50% of patients judged on clinical grounds to have CREST syndrome, in less than 10% of those who have PSS, and rarely in patients who have other connective tissue diseases.[477, 592–594] However, when all individuals who have anticentromere antibody are considered, only a minority have CREST syndrome (e.g., 4% in one study and 16% in another).[595, 596] In patients who have CREST syndrome, the prevalence of interstitial lung disease is considerably lower in those who have anticentromere antibody in their serum than in those who do not;[592] such patients also manifest less skin and joint involvement.[597] As with PSS, analysis of the BAL fluid of patients who have CREST syndrome reveals increased numbers of neutrophils, eosinophils, and lymphocytes, indicative of an alveolitis.[598, 599] A familial occurrence of the syndrome in association with HLA haplotype DR5 has been described.[600]

The clinical manifestations in patients who have CREST syndrome have important differences in their frequency in comparison to those in patients who have PSS. For example, in one investigation of 13 patients who had CREST syndrome and 26 who had PSS, no significant differences in the age of onset of Raynaud's phenomenon, the frequency of finger ulceration, sclerodactyly, or abnormal esophageal peristalsis or dysphagia were identified;[601] however, patients who had CREST syndrome had an appreciably lower incidence of arthralgia (54%) and arthritis (15%) than did those who had PSS (88% and 65%, respectively). In CREST syndrome, skin involvement is usually limited to the distal portions of the extremities.[524, 592] Radionuclide studies of myocardial function and perfusion indicate that abnormalities of left ventricular function are relatively minor in patients who have CREST syndrome compared with those with PSS.[602]

One of the more important differences between CREST syndrome and PSS is the incidence of pulmonary hypertension. As with PSS, this complication can be secondary to parenchymal interstitial fibrosis; more often, however, it occurs as an isolated finding without evidence of other pulmonary disease. In one study of 331 patients, 30 (9%) were so affected;[512] by contrast, none of 342 patients who had PSS and no CREST features had pulmonary hypertension. In another study of 34 consecutive patients who had PSS and no clinical evidence of pulmonary hypertension (most of whom had CREST syndrome), 35% had echocardiographic evidence of pulmonary hypertension.[603] Pathologic findings in these cases are similar to those in hypertension associated with other connective tissue diseases or primary (idiopathic) pulmonary hypertension.

The prevalence of radiographic abnormalities in the chest varies in different reports. For example, in one study of nine patients, none had radiographic evidence of pulmonary interstitial disease, pleural effusion, or pleural thickening.[515] By contrast, a comparison of the chest radiographs of 88 patients who had CREST syndrome and 77 patients with PSS revealed similar abnormalities in the two groups:[524] 33% of patients who had CREST had evidence of fibrosis on the chest radiograph as compared with 40% of patients who had PSS; the pattern of pulmonary abnormalities was similar.

Patients who have CREST syndrome may show a restrictive pattern on pulmonary function testing;[592, 597] the combination of a low diffusing capacity and a relatively high vital capacity may reflect primary vascular disease.[524] In patients who have Raynaud's phenomenon, the membrane component of the diffusing capacity (Dm) correlates best with the presence of nailfold capillary abnormalities and the presence of antinuclear antibodies, findings that suggest early PSS. By contrast, the reduction in the capillary blood volume component of the diffusing capacity (Vc) is the major cause of a lower-than-normal diffusing capacity in patients who have Raynaud's phenomenon;[604] this finding suggests the presence of vascular changes in the pulmonary circulation similar to those seen in the extremities.[604]

CREST syndrome usually has a more indolent course than PSS; however, the original hypothesis that it represents a benign variant has been invalidated by the appreciation of cases of late-onset pulmonary hypertension,[605] in which the prognosis is poor. In the study of 30 patients cited previously, the 2-year survival was only 40%.[512]

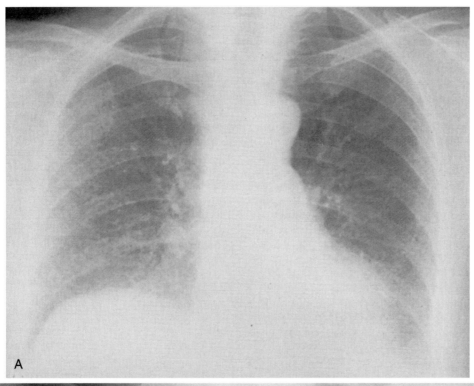

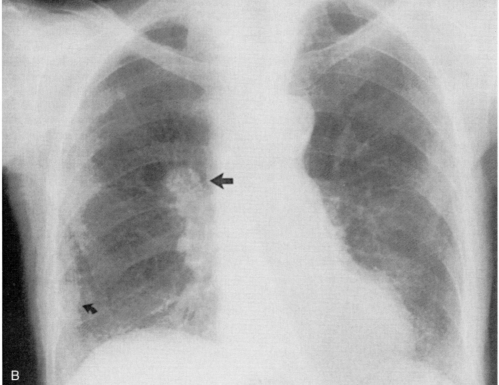

**Figure 39–26. Pulmonary Carcinoma Associated with Long-Standing Diffuse Interstitial Fibrosis Caused by Progressive Systemic Sclerosis.** A posteroanterior chest radiograph *(A)* reveals a fine reticular pattern throughout both lungs with some basal predominance. Two years later *(B),* a 1.7-cm nodular opacity *(curved arrow)* had developed in the right lower lobe, and the right hilum had increased in size as a result of lymph node enlargement *(large arrow).* At autopsy, the pulmonary lesion was a small cell carcinoma; metastases were present within hilar lymph nodes. The patient was a 56-year-old woman with typical features of PSS.

## RAYNAUD'S PHENOMENON

Raynaud's phenomenon (vasospasm of the digital arteries resulting in blanching and cyanosis) occurs most commonly as an isolated finding[492, 559] or in association with "primary" (idiopathic) pulmonary arterial hypertension.[606–610] When it occurs in association with another connective tissue disease, it is usually an early sign, antedating cutaneous sclerosis and other manifestations of generalized disease. When it occurs alone, with normal serology, capillaroscopy, and absence of any systemic features of connective tissue disease, it is more properly called *Raynaud's disease*.[611] Some patients who present with Raynaud's phenomenon are found subsequently to have more extensive disease, including minor degrees of arthralgia-arthritis, vasculopathy, or dermal thickening with or without circulating autoantibodies. While some of these patients eventually develop diagnostic criteria of a specific connective tissue disease, others do not, perhaps reflecting the existence of a connective tissue disease of which Raynaud's phenomenon is the main feature.[559, 610]

## DERMATOMYOSITIS AND POLYMYOSITIS

The terms *dermatomyositis* and *polymyositis* refer to a group of disorders characterized by weakness and, sometimes, pain in the proximal limb muscles and (occasionally) in the muscles of the neck. About 50% of patients have a characteristic heliotrope skin rash, erythema or purpura on the extensor surfaces of the extremity joints, and Gottron's papules (flat-topped violaceous papules on the dorsal aspect of the interphalangeal joints of the hand, which develop central atrophy with hypopigmentation and telangiectasia), which enable the distinction of dermatomyositis from polymyositis.[612] In a minority of cases, there is associated neoplastic disease. Five diagnostic criteria have been defined to distinguish these diseases from the muscular dystrophies:[613, 614] (1) symmetric weakness of the limb girdle muscles and anterior neck flexors progressing over weeks or months, with or without dysphagia or respiratory muscle involvement; (2) biopsy evidence of muscle necrosis and regeneration; (3) elevation of serum skeletal muscle enzyme levels, particularly creatine phosphokinase and aldolase and, to a lesser extent, aspartate and alanine transaminase, and lactate dehydrogenase; (4) electromyographic changes; and (5) skin involvement as described earlier.

Although the clinical picture differs considerably from case to case, the common denominator is muscular weakness. The thorax is commonly affected at some point in the disease, generally in one or more of three forms: (1) hypoventilation and respiratory failure as a result of direct involvement of the respiratory muscles; (2) interstitial pneumonitis indistinguishable from that seen in other connective tissue diseases; and (3) aspiration pneumonia secondary to pharyngeal muscle weakness.

The disease is worldwide in distribution and occurs twice as often in women as in men. Its incidence shows two peaks, the first during the first decade and the second in the fifth and sixth decades.[613, 615–617] Despite this, dermatomyositis/polymyositis (DM/PM) is an uncommon cause of connective tissue disease in children, accounting for only 5% of cases among 4,585 children referred to rheumatology centers in southern New England.[618] The estimated disease prevalence in this region was 0.4 per 100,000 children at risk. The overall incidence is approximately 5 to 10 cases per million population, with a more recent increase in incidence, particularly in black women.[619, 620]

DM/PM has been classified into five groups according to the predominance of skin or muscle involvement and the presence of other diseases:[613, 614] primary idiopathic polymyositis; primary idiopathic dermatomyositis; dermatomyositis or polymyositis associated with neoplasia; dermatomyositis or polymyositis developing in childhood and associated with vasculitis; and dermatomyositis or polymyositis associated with other connective tissue diseases. This classification is based solely on clinical findings; studies aimed at distinguishing the groups on the basis of serum enzyme levels,[615] electromyographic patterns, and the ultrastructure of muscle fibers have not proven useful.[621–623] However, attempts to classify patients according to type of autoantibody might prove more fruitful (*see* farther on).[624, 625]

### Etiology and Pathogenesis

The differential diagnosis of myositis is broad.[620] A wide variety of microorganisms can cause acute myositis, and the resulting disease must be distinguished from DM/PM.[626] The possibility that some of these organisms are also implicated in the pathogenesis of the "idiopathic" form of disease by the initiation of immune mechanisms has also been considered. In many patients who have dermatomyositis, electron-microscopic examination has shown intracytoplasmic, paramyxovirus-like tubular structures within endothelial cells in the vicinity of active dermal and muscle inflammation.[627, 628] (In lung specimens that have been examined by electron microscopy, these inclusions have not been identified.[629]) Although it has been speculated that a virus might be involved in the genesis of these structures, similar inclusions have been identified in other connective tissue and neoplastic diseases;[628, 630] in addition, serologic and cultural investigations generally have not yielded evidence of viral infection[627] and attempts to isolate a viral genome by polymerase chain reaction testing of muscle tissue have not been successful.[626]

There have also been reports of an association between polymyositis and HIV infection in patients with and without acquired immunodeficiency syndrome. Pathologically, this resembles the idiopathic form of polymyositis, and the virus itself does not directly invade the muscle.[626] Infection with human T-cell leukemia virus (HTLV-1) has also been associated with polymyositis in areas endemic for the organism, notably Japan and Jamaica.[626] The onset of myositis associated with certain antibodies is seasonally clustered in the United States; for example, patients who have anti Jo-1 antibody syndrome (*see* farther on) tend to develop their first muscular weakness in the spring.[620] Taken together, all these observations suggest that viral infection might in some way initiate an immune response directed toward muscle tissue.

Patients who have dermatomyositis and polymyositis have a high frequency of antibodies to nuclear and cytoplasmic antigens,[631] some of which show strong associations with specific clinical features. For example, a group of myositis-associated autoantibodies, the antisynthetases, are strongly linked to the development of interstitial lung disease, patients having these antibodies accounting for about 80% of all patients with DM/PM who have this complication.[624, 631, 632] These antibodies are directed against the aminoacyl-tRNA synthetases, cytoplasmic enzymes that catalyze the binding of amino acids to the appropriate tRNA for incorporation into polypeptide chains. A distinct synthetase is present for each amino acid. The most common, anti-Jo-1, is found in about 20% of patients who have DM/PM;[633] others have been labeled anti-PL-7, anti-PL-12, anti-EJ, and anti-OJ.[631, 634–636] HLA-DR3 is more common in whites who have anti-Jo-1 than in other patients who have myositis, and DRw52 is present in almost all patients who have these antibodies,[624, 631] suggesting that a genetic predisposition is required for their development.

Each of these antibodies has been associated with an antisynthetase syndrome, which, when compared with DM/PM in patients without such antibodies, has a high frequency of interstitial lung disease (50% to 100% vs. 10%), arthritis (60% to 100% vs. 30%), Raynaud's phenomenon (60% vs. 93%), fever during active disease (87% vs. 23%), flaring of disease during treatment withdrawal (60% vs. 20%), and hyperkeratotic lines on the hands with scaling and fissuring ("mechanic's hands," 71%).[631] Because some features of other connective diseases (e.g., sclerodactyly, Raynaud's phenomenon, and sicca syndrome) may occur, this disorder can be confused with PSS or mixed connective tissue disease. When polymyositis or dermatomyositis is associated with malignancy, these antibodies are usually absent.[620]

It is generally considered unlikely that antisynthetase antibodies are pathogenetic. Observations in favor of this hypothesis include the finding that disease may be suppressed by treatment, despite the presence of high antibody titers, and that the responsible antigens are present in every cell, whereas the disease is organ specific. Despite these arguments, muscle disease is rare in the absence of these antibodies, and if they are an epiphenomenon, they are presumably closely associated with pathogenetic mechanisms.[631]

There are several lines of evidence suggesting that a cell-mediated immune reaction is important in the pathogenesis of DM/PM.[620] Histologic examination of affected muscle shows a predominantly lymphocytic infiltrate; CD8 + cytotoxic T cells predominate and are directed at an unknown antigen. Studies have shown an increased number of activated T cells in peripheral blood, increased migration of mononuclear cells to muscle, and an increased proliferative response of monocytes to autologous muscle *in vitro*. The presence of myositis-specific antibodies, as discussed earlier, also suggests a role for helper T cells in disease pathogenesis. Vascular injury in DM is prominent and is characterized by loss of muscle capillaries and ischemic muscle damage, processes that appear to be mediated by local complement activation in small muscle vessels.[631, 637, 638] Deposition of immunoglobulin has also been found in muscle blood vessels in some studies, particularly in children who have dermatomyositis.[620]

It has been proposed that in response to an initial undefined injury, muscle antigen is presented by intramuscular macrophages to T cells.[637, 639] Following their activation and proliferation, these cells release cytokines that lead to further recruitment of mononuclear cells and up-regulation of MHC antigens and adhesion molecules on the surface of muscle cells. These allow the muscle cells to serve as antigen presenters to T cells and, in turn, to further recruit more mononuclear cells.[637, 639] Activation of B cells by helper T cells results in the production of autoantibodies that are the consequence rather than the cause of muscle injury. Instead, destruction of muscle is the result of direct T-cell-mediated cytotoxicity or cytokine production.[637]

### Pathologic Characteristics

Histologic examination of muscle biopsy specimens from patients who have polymyositis reveals both degenerative and regenerative changes, often with a variation in cross-sectional diameter of adjacent fibers; phagocytosis of necrotic muscle may be seen (Fig. 39–27). A mononuclear infiltrate, often most prominent in a perivascular location, and interstitial fibrosis provide evidence of the inflammatory nature of the disease. Electron-microscopic studies have shown disorganization and loss of myofibrils, swelling of mitochondria, distortion and clumping of Z bands, and dilation of endoplasmic reticulum with clumping of myofilaments.[622, 623]

Pathologic findings of interstitial lung disease are indistinguishable from those of interstitial pneumonitis associated with other connective tissue diseases.[629, 640–642] Bronchiolitis obliterans organizing pneumonia is seen in some cases.[642] In contrast with DM/PM of childhood in which necrotizing vasculitis may be widespread,[613] histologic evidence of vascular involvement is rare in adult disease.[629, 644] Severe plexogenic pulmonary arteriopathy was found in one patient at autopsy.[645]

### Radiologic Manifestations

The frequency of parenchymal abnormalities evident on the chest radiograph has ranged from 0 to 9% in different series.[617, 629, 646] The most representative figure is probably that derived from a Mayo Clinic study in which 213 patients had the diagnosis established by a combination of muscle biopsy, electromyography, and detection of enzyme abnormalities; in this investigation, only 10 (5%) showed radiographic evidence of interstitial pulmonary disease.[617]

The radiographic findings of interstitial fibrosis in patients who have DM/PM are indistinguishable from those of idiopathic pulmonary fibrosis and consist of a symmetrical, predominantly basal, reticular or reticulonodular pattern.[617, 647] This pattern can become diffuse over time and progress to honeycombing.[647, 648] Some patients develop relatively acute abnormalities over a 2- to 3-week period.[617, 649] In these individuals, the chest radiograph usually demonstrates bilateral areas of consolidation superimposed on a reticulonodular pattern, an abnormality related to either diffuse alveolar damage[642, 649] or bronchiolitis obliterans organizing pneumonia (BOOP).[649, 651, 652] On HRCT, the consolidation may have a predominantly peribronchoarterial or subpleural distribution (Fig. 39–28).[651, 653] BOOP may also present with bilateral interstitial or nodular infiltrates.[642]

In one investigation of 25 patients, 23 had parenchymal abnormalities on HRCT, including linear opacities (92%), ground-glass attenuation (92%), air-space consolidation

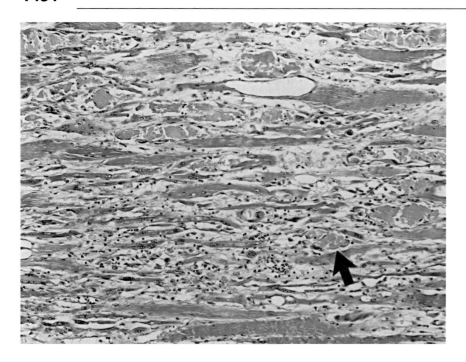

**Figure 39–27. Polymyositis with Systemic Lupus Erythematosus (SLE).** The section is from the diaphragm of a 22-year-old man with SLE admitted for progressive weakness. A serum creatinine phosphokinase level was markedly elevated. Interstitial inflammation and numerous degenerated muscle fibers, some undergoing phagocytosis *(arrow)*, are evident. (×100.)

(52%), small nodules (28%), and honeycombing (16%).[653] The linear opacities involved mainly the peripheral portions of the middle and lower lung zones, similar to the distribution of interstitial pneumonitis and fibrosis in other connective tissue diseases. In the majority of cases, the consolidation involved the middle and lower lung zones and was shown histologically to represent BOOP; in two cases, it was diffuse and was shown at autopsy to be related to diffuse alveolar damage.[653] In another study of 19 patients,

all had bilateral areas of ground-glass attenuation and patchy areas of consolidation involving mainly the lower lung zones;[653a] a predominantly subpleural distribution was present in 16 patients (84%). Other common findings included interlobular septal thickening, subpleural lines, and irregular peribronchoarterial thickening. Bronchial or bronchiolar dilation (traction bronchiectasis or bronchiolectasis) was seen in 7 patients; none had honeycombing. HRCT scans performed during mean follow-up of 2 years after treatment with corti-

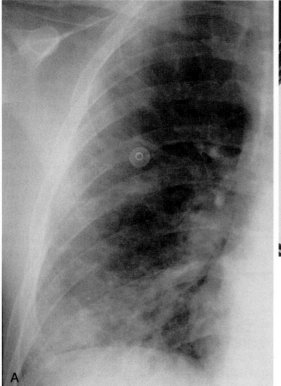

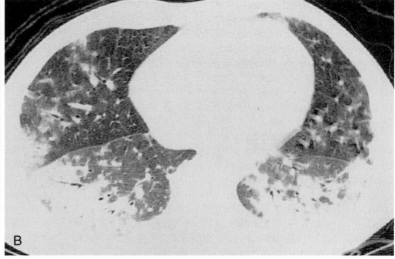

**Figure 39–28. Polymyositis: Bronchiolitis Obliterans Organizing Pneumonia (BOOP).** A view of the right lung from a posteroanterior chest radiograph *(A)* demonstrates areas of consolidation. Similar findings were present in the left lung. An HRCT scan through the lower lung zones *(B)* demonstrates that the consolidation involves mainly the peripheral lung regions. The patient was a 27-year-old man who presented with fever, cough, progressive shortness of breath, and muscle weakness. The diagnoses of BOOP and polymyositis were both proven by biopsy.

costeroids and/or immunosuppressants showed marked improvement in all but 1 patient.

When polymyositis involves the respiratory muscles, particularly the diaphragm, diaphragmatic elevation and small-volume lungs are apparent, often in conjunction with basal linear opacities.[654] When pharyngeal muscle paralysis is present, unilateral or bilateral segmental pneumonia may result from aspiration of food and oral secretions; in fact, such aspiration pneumonia has been reported in 15% to 20% of patients.[649]

### Clinical Manifestations

Patients usually present with symmetric weakness of the neck[655] and proximal limb muscles that progresses rapidly over weeks or months rather than years, as is characteristic of the muscular dystrophies. In some patients, muscle destruction is extremely rapid and is associated with diffuse, profound weakness and pain, tenderness, and swelling of affected areas.[613] In patients whose disease tends to be more chronic, muscle weakness is often ascribed incorrectly to a catabolic protein-losing condition[656] or to concomitant steroid therapy.[640] Sometimes, manifestations of other connective tissue diseases overshadow those of muscle weakness, and the latter may be overlooked. Symptoms and signs of these disorders range from relatively localized vascular or visceral disease, such as Raynaud's phenomenon, hypomotility of the distal esophagus and small bowel, or cardiac arrhythmias,[613] to full-blown connective tissue diseases, such as SLE.

A minority of patients have symptoms and signs referable to the respiratory system. Those related to respiratory muscle weakness are probably the most common; in one study of 89 patients, 6 had myositis sufficient to cause respiratory embarrassment.[615] If severe enough, such disease can result in extreme dyspnea, cyanosis, ineffective cough,[657] and, rarely, respiratory failure. Interstitial pneumonitis and fibrosis also may cause dyspnea, which is occasionally the major presenting symptom.[644] More often, extensive disease is unassociated with symptoms and is discovered on a screening chest radiograph.[617] Rare patients have been described who had dyspnea as a result of capillaritis and diffuse alveolar hemorrhage.[658] Clinical evidence of pulmonary hypertension is rare.

Patients who have pharyngeal weakness may have drooling, dyspnea, ineffective cough, and an inability to lie flat; in this situation, aspiration or infection is common. Other patients present with only minor skin involvement and Raynaud's phenomenon; in this group, esophageal and/or pharyngeal dysfunction frequently lead to dysphagia and aspiration pneumonia.[659] In one review of the clinical and autopsy records of 65 patients who had DM/PM and associated pulmonary disease, a history of dyspnea was found in 31, cough in 23, and chest pain in 6.[660] Dysphagia was present in a similar proportion of patients with and without pneumonia. Interstitial lung disease was noted at autopsy in 27 patients. Bronchopneumonia was identified in 35 patients and pulmonary vasculitis in 5, all the latter having associated interstitial lung disease.

The incidence of coexistent carcinoma probably is not nearly as great as is often assumed,[613] and exhaustive investigation for associated malignancy is seldom warranted in the absence of suspicious signs and symptoms of cancer. Only about 5% to 15% of patients have been reported to have malignancy in various series,[615, 616, 661] although these figures generally exceed the expected frequency in control populations.[662, 663] This excess risk of carcinoma tapers rapidly with time. In one series of 539 patients who had DM in which there was a sixfold increase in carcinoma within 1 year of the diagnosis, no excess cancers were found after the second year of follow-up.[664] Carcinomas can be found in a wide variety of sites, including the stomach, prostate, pancreas, lung, lymphatic and hematopoietic systems, and ovary.[615, 664]

### Laboratory Findings and Pulmonary Function Tests

Measurement of serum creatine phosphokinase is useful in establishing the diagnosis of DM/PM, particularly in eliminating the possibility of muscular dystrophy. However, values may be within normal limits, even in patients who have active myositis and muscle atrophy resulting from severe long-standing disease.[655, 665] Enzyme levels usually decrease 3 to 4 weeks before muscle strength improves and increase 5 to 6 weeks before clinical relapse.[666] Muscle biopsies have been reported to be normal in 10% to 50% of cases;[615, 666] in one series, positive electromyographic changes were observed in 56 of the 61 patients in whom this procedure was performed.[615]

Pulmonary function tests show no abnormality in most patients; in those in whom diffuse interstitial fibrosis has developed, findings are identical to those of PSS.[659, 667, 668] When the diaphragm is paralyzed in the absence of other muscle involvement,[669] the vital capacity is decreased, flow rates and transdiaphragmatic pressure are reduced, and hypoxemia develops, with or without a rise in $P_{CO_2}$. Such ventilatory failure may be reversible.[669, 670] In some patients who do not have cardiorespiratory symptoms, muscle weakness masks significant underlying cardiopulmonary disease; in one such series of 11 patients, 7 had echocardiographic evidence of pulmonary hypertension that was associated with abnormalities of exercise performance.[671]

### Prognosis and Natural History

In one study of 124 patients followed over 2½ years, the overall mortality from the time of first hospitalization was 36%, death usually being caused by aspiration pneumonia.[672] The 5-year mortality rate in one series of 182 patients who had DM followed in Japan was 27%, the most common causes of death being malignancy and interstitial lung disease.[673] The prognosis is considerably better in children than in adults. In patients who have chronic active disease associated with muscle atrophy, the prognosis appears to be particularly poor; in one study of 6 such patients, only 2 survived 1 year.

## SJÖGREN'S SYNDROME

In 1933, Sjögren described a clinical triad of keratoconjunctivitis sicca, xerostomia, and recurrent swelling of the parotid gland that has come to bear his name.[674] By its most stringent definition, the abnormality is now considered to be an autoimmune process associated with destruction of salivary and lacrimal gland tissues. Patients who have compatible symptoms but who do not have autoantibodies or evidence of glandular disease on biopsy can be said to have the sicca (dry mouth) syndrome.[675]

Although Sjögren's syndrome (SS) may be seen in the absence of other connective tissue disease (primary Sjögren's syndrome), such disease is frequently present; for example, in one study of 171 patients, rheumatoid arthritis or another connective tissue disorder coexisted in 100 (59%).[676] Sicca syndrome itself represented primary SS in less than half the cases, the remainder being patients who had other connective tissue diseases that manifested sicca components.[676] Clinical features of sicca syndrome are present to some extent in many patients who have autoimmune diseases; if not readily apparent, they can usually be detected by assessment of exocrine gland histology or function. Employing a variety of techniques, different investigators have found defective glandular function in patients who have rheumatoid disease,[676] PSS,[677, 678] SLE,[679, 680] primary biliary cirrhosis,[681] Hashimoto's thyroiditis, pernicious anemia, and primary hypothyroidism.[680] SS shows a remarkable female sex predominance (90%);[682–685] the mean age in one series of 171 patients was 57 years.[682]

Patients who have SS frequently have pleuropulmonary abnormalities; some of these appear to be a reflection of another underlying connective tissue disease, whereas others are probably specific for the syndrome. These disorders include lymphocytic interstitial pneumonitis, pleuritis with or without effusion, and tracheobronchial gland inflammation.[686–690]

### Etiology and Pathogenesis

Evidence for an autoimmune pathogenesis of SS is quite strong. Primary SS is characterized by autoantibodies to small nuclear/cytoplasmic particles.[643] These anti-Ro and anti-La antibodies (SSA and SSB) are present in more than 90% of patients and are associated with an increased frequency of purpura, hypergammaglobulinemia, severe salivary gland dysfunction, lymphopenia, and leukopenia.[691] There has been much speculation that this antibody response is directed toward salivary gland cells that have been altered by a virus.[691] Implicated organisms include Epstein-Barr virus, hepatitis C virus, human herpesvirus-6, and retroviruses.[692–696] It has been postulated that viral infection of salivary epithelial cells up-regulates expression of HLA-D/DR as well as a variety of molecules that promote lymphocyte adhesion.[697] This results in the epithelial cells acting as antigen-presenting cells to CD4+ T cells, which in turn stimulate B lymphocytes to form autoantibody to the presented antigen.[695] The latter may undergo clonal expansion, which may be related to the markedly elevated risk of developing lymphoma in the salivary glands and cervical lymph nodes.[698] Activated T cells are the predominant cell in the exocrine gland infiltrate,[699, 700] and cytokines produced in the salivary glands are similar to those produced by helper T lymphocytes.[693] Epithelial cells themselves may act as sources of the proinflammatory cytokines, interleukin-1, and interleukin-6.[701]

Genetic factors are also likely to be important in the pathogenesis of SS. There is a high prevalence of HLA-B8, HLA-DR3, and HLA-DRw52 in white and African American, but not Japanese,[702] populations with primary SS and anti-Ro, anti-La antibodies.[643] Familial aggregation of the disorder and its association with other autoimmune diseases also suggest a role for genetic factors.[703]

Patients who have primary SS frequently develop lymphocytic alveolitis, whose intensity is linked to the intensity of the associated pulmonary, but not systemic, disease.[704] Despite this, alveolar macrophage activation has not been documented in BAL samples from such patients.[705]

### Pathologic Characteristics

Pathologic findings in the trachea and bronchi in some patients include atrophy of mucous glands associated with a lymphoplasmacytic cellular infiltrate.[706, 707] These abnormalities are believed to be analogous to salivary gland involvement and to be responsible for chronic cough. Despite this, morphometric measurements in some studies have shown an increase in mucous gland and goblet cell size and number.[708] Fibrosis and mononuclear cell infiltration of small airways has also been reported in patients who manifest evidence of obstructive airway disease.[709]

Pulmonary parenchymal disease may take several forms, the most common of which is a diffuse, usually bilateral, interstitial infiltrate of lymphocytes and plasma cells associated with a variable number of histiocytes and multinucleated giant cells (lymphoid interstitial pneumonitis).[710–712] This infiltrate is usually most dense in relation to bronchioles and their accompanying vessels, but can extend into the alveolar interstitium itself. Fibrosis may occur and is prominent in some cases.[712–714] Occasionally, the disease presents as a mass lesion ("pseudolymphoma").[715] The pathologic differentiation of malignant from benign infiltrates in both localized and diffuse forms of disease may be difficult (*see* pages 1269 and 1271).

Occasional cases of SS and pulmonary amyloidosis have also been reported;[711, 716–718] one unusual example was associated with bullae whose pathogenesis was believed to be related to partial obstruction of small airways by an inflammatory cell infiltrate.[719] Systemic necrotizing vasculitis affecting either small or large vessels has also been identified in some patients;[720] however, involvement of the pulmonary vasculature has not been documented. Bronchiolitis obliterans organizing pneumonia,[393] follicular bronchiolitis,[393] and plexogenic pulmonary arteriopathy[721] have been described rarely.

### Radiologic Manifestations

The frequency of abnormalities on the chest radiograph varies considerably in different series. For example, in one study of 42 patients, 14 (33%) showed a reticulonodular pattern (Fig. 39–29)[684] and in another review of 343 patients, pulmonary involvement was demonstrated in 31 (9%);[721] however, in a third study of 171 patients, only 3 (1.7%) showed radiographic abnormalities consistent with fibrosis.[682]

The reticulonodular pattern seen in SS usually has a basal predominance.[722] Lung biopsy in a small number of patients has shown that this pattern may be caused by lymphoid interstitial pneumonia, interstitial fibrosis, or, less commonly, frank lymphoma.[722–724] The HRCT findings were

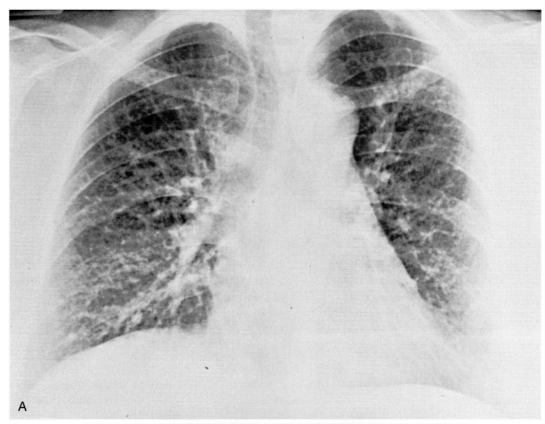

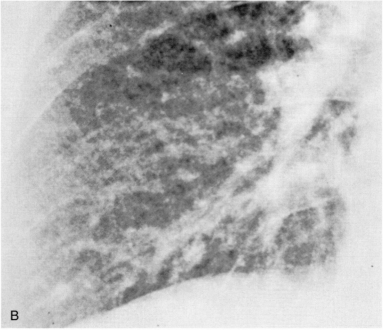

**Figure 39–29. Sjögren's Syndrome.** This 45-year-old woman presented with keratoconjunctivitis sicca, xerostomia, and recurrent swelling of the parotid glands. A posteroanterior chest radiograph *(A)* reveals a diffuse, coarse reticular pattern throughout both lungs, seen to better advantage in the magnified view of the right lower zone *(B)*. Note also the enlargement of the left lobe of the thyroid.

assessed in a prospective study of 50 patients in whom the onset of SS had occurred a mean of 12 years (range 2 to 37 years) prior to the scans;[725] 37 (74%) of the 50 patients had no respiratory symptoms at the time of the scan. Abnormalities were detected in 17 patients (34%) on HRCT compared with 7 (14%) on chest radiographs. The most common

findings consisted of bronchiolectasis and poorly defined centrilobular nodular or branching linear opacities (seen in 11 patients), areas of ground-glass attenuation (in 7), and honeycombing (in 4). The latter was bilateral and asymmetric and present almost exclusively in the periphery of the lower lobes.

A characteristic pattern of extensive areas of ground-glass attenuation with scattered thin-walled cysts has been reported in some patients with lymphoid interstitial pneumonitis (Fig. 39–30).[726–728] Similar findings have been described in lymphoid interstitial pneumonia not associated with Sjögren's syndrome.[726, 729] An open lung biopsy specimen in one patient demonstrated interstitial and peribronchiolar lympho-plasmacytic infiltrates associated with overinflation of the secondary pulmonary lobule.[727] Another pattern that may be seen with lymphoid interstitial pneumonia consists of interlobular septal thickening and nodular thickening of the bronchovascular bundles, an appearance that cannot be distinguished from lymphoma. In one series, the HRCT findings consisted of thin-walled cysts ranging from 2 to 15 mm in diameter and multiple irregular, solid soft tissue nodules, the majority of which lie adjacent to the cysts.[728] Other findings described in patients who have SS include parenchymal consolidation as a result of bronchopneumonia,[684] a focal mass due to focal lymphoid hyperplasia (pseudolymphoma),[715] and pleural effusion.[724]

### Clinical Manifestations

The chief symptoms of SS are a gritty or burning sensation of the eyes; dryness of the mouth, nose, and skin; and (sometimes) dyspareunia.[730] The lack of saliva can result in dental caries and decreased taste perception. Involvement of the nasal and nasopharyngeal mucosa may lead to diminished olfactory acuity and to obstruction of the eustachian tubes, with resultant chronic otitis media and deafness.[730–733] Nasal crusting is common and is often associated with epistaxis. Xerostomia and keratoconjunctivitis are usually not associated with enlargement of salivary and lacrimal glands; in one series, for example, the latter was identified in only 6 of 71 patients who had sicca syndrome and in 1 of 94 who had SS and rheumatoid disease.[676] When it does occur, lacrimal and submandibular salivary gland enlargement is usually bilateral; by contrast, parotid gland enlargement is unilateral in most patients.[676] Enlargement of one or more parotid or submandibular glands has been described in 25% to 50% of patients.[685] Involvement of the larynx may result in hoarseness and cough.

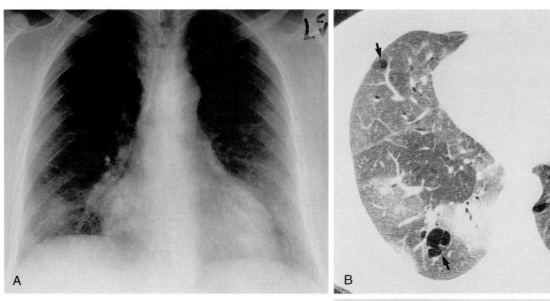

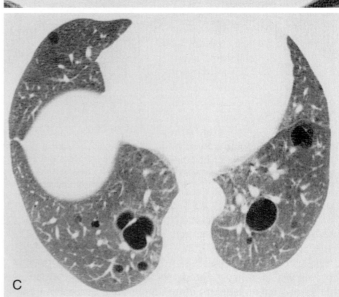

**Figure 39–30. Sjögren's Syndrome: Lymphoid Interstitial Pneumonitis (LIP).** A posteroanterior chest radiograph *(A)* in a 50-year-old woman with long-standing Sjögren's syndrome demonstrates poorly defined, hazy, increased opacity in both lungs and focal areas of consolidation in the right lower lobe. An HRCT scan *(B)* through the lower lung zones demonstrates extensive areas of ground-glass attenuation in both lungs and focal area of consolidation in the right lower lobe. Small cystic spaces *(arrows)* are present in both lungs. The diagnosis of LIP was proven by lung biopsy. An HRCT scan 6 months later *(C)* demonstrates almost complete resolution of the parenchymal infiltrates. However, the cysts have become more conspicuous. They are presumably related to partial obstruction of small airways. The patient was a lifelong nonsmoker.

Although it is seldom a severe problem, clinically evident pulmonary involvement has been reported in approximately 10% to 45% of patients who have primary SS.[712, 718, 734, 734a] Cough due to tracheobronchial gland inflammation and atrophy is relatively frequent.[688] Such disease may be associated with manifestations of atelectasis, bronchitis, bronchiectasis, and recurrent bronchopneumonia.[1] Lymphocytic infiltration and fibrosis of the pulmonary interstitium may be associated with dyspnea; in some patients, crackles may also be heard at the lung bases. In one HRCT investigation of 16 patients who had dyspnea, 6 had evidence of parenchymal fibrosis,[735] 5 others had peribronchial thickening, and 3 had pleural thickening. Peribronchial disease may be associated with dyspnea when there is hyperinflation and obstructive lung function[736] or airway hyperresponsiveness.[737] An association between SS and pulmonary lymphangioleiomyomatosis has also been described in a single patient.[738] Pleuritis is relatively uncommon in primary SS, but is seen more often in the secondary form.[688]

Other symptoms seen at some time in the course of primary SS include polyarthralgia (approximately 95%), Raynaud's phenomenon (80%), and hypothyroidism (15%).[689] Dysphagia may be caused by cricopharyngeal webs.[733] Cranial and peripheral neuropathy has been reported,[739] in association with antineuronal antibodies.[740] Renal tubular acidosis is found in some patients and has been ascribed to hyperglobulinemia; however, characteristic histologic changes of SS may be present in the kidney in the absence of hyperglobulinemia.[741] A single patient has been reported in whom periodic paralysis was presumably caused by renal tubular acidosis.[742] Purpura hyperglobulinemia and thrombocytopenic purpura are rare manifestations.[676, 682, 743]

Approximately one half to two thirds of patients who have SS manifest symptoms and signs of an associated connective tissue disease.[676, 684] In the early stages, it may be difficult to distinguish such patients from those who have primary SS.[744]

### Laboratory Findings and Pulmonary Function Tests

Although the diagnosis of SS is usually based on characteristic clinical manifestations, it may be substantiated by tests of glandular secretory function, by biopsy of minor salivary glands, and by the detection of various serum antibodies. The former include Schirmer's test for the measurement of tear formation, and slit-lamp examination of the eyes after instillation of a drop of rose bengal dye into the conjunctival sac for identification of superficial corneal scarring due to inadequate lacrimal gland secretion. Salivary gland function may also be assessed by scintillation scanning or radionuclide excretion studies. Lysozyme concentration has been shown to be reduced in both tears[685] and saliva.[745]

Although a variety of autoantibodies, including rheumatoid factor and ANA, may be found in patients who have primary SS, they occur much more commonly in SS associated with other connective tissue diseases.[680] Antibodies to native DNA are not present.[680] Measurement of antibodies to the extractable nuclear antigens SSA and SSB and to gamma globulin shows considerable sensitivity for SS. A high percentage of patients who have SS have immune complexes, usually related to IgG.[680] A low-molecular-weight protein constituent of cell membrane known as beta$_2$-microglobulin is also present in high concentration in both saliva and sera; levels are even higher when renal or lymphoproliferative complications are present.[746]

Significant abnormalities of lung function are found in about 25% of patients who have primary SS.[734] As might be expected in a disease that can involve the pulmonary interstitium, bronchi, or both, pulmonary function test results may be restrictive, obstructive, or mixed in pattern.[747–750] Airway dysfunction is not associated with loss of elastic recoil.[751] Airway hyperresponsiveness appears to be common, being described in 60% in one series of 15 patients from Japan,[752] a result similar to that of an earlier report from Sweden.[737]

### Prognosis and Natural History

The course and prognosis of lung disease in primary SS is poorly described; however, it may progress relatively rapidly, and abnormalities of lung function may become more prevalent with time in patients followed prospectively.[734] Patients who have SS, both primary and secondary, are at increased risk for the development of non-Hodgkin's lymphoma, sometimes primary in the lung.[680, 753] Those who develop this complication generally manifest a severe sicca syndrome and parotid swelling and have an increased likelihood of lymph node enlargement, splenomegaly, leukopenia, vasculitis, neuropathy, Raynaud's phenomenon, purpura, and hyperglobulinemia; gammopathy may be monoclonal and is usually related to IgM.[680, 730]

## OVERLAP SYNDROMES AND MIXED CONNECTIVE TISSUE DISEASE

Many patients who have connective tissue disease show features of more than one specific entity, in which case they are commonly referred to as having *overlap syndromes* or *unclassified (undifferentiated) connective tissue disease*.[754, 754a] Such syndromes include those with features of rheumatoid arthritis and SLE, Sjögren's syndrome and SLE, dermatomyositis and SLE,[755] and, occasionally, even more complex combinations (e.g., dermatomyositis, rheumatoid disease, Sjögren's syndrome, Hashimoto's thyroiditis, and SLE[756]). These overlap syndromes form a significant proportion of all connective tissue diseases. For example, in one series of 73 patients said to have had PSS, 20 were noted to have symptoms and signs that overlapped with other autoimmune diseases and to have clinical and radiographic features that differed from PSS and from CREST syndrome;[575] this overlap group showed a marked female predominance (9:1) and had significantly more pleuropulmonary disease. Approximately half of these patients were diagnosed and accepted as having PSS for a number of years before the features of other connective tissue diseases became apparent. In another review of 84 patients initially felt to have an overlap syndrome, 33 developed findings that permitted diagnosis of a specific connective tissue disease over a 5-year period.[754a]

One form of overlap disease merits more detailed discussion. In 1972, Sharp and associates[757] described a symptom complex that included features of SLE, PSS, and polymyositis that they and others[758, 759] were prepared to accept as a distinct entity. Patients who had this mixed connective tissue disease (MCTD) typically had high serum titers of antibody to extractable nuclear antigen (anti-nRNP Ab), a feature that has become the hallmark of the syndrome.[755] Despite this, there is some debate about whether the presence of anti-nRNP distinguishes patients who have MCTD from those who have other connective tissue overlap syndromes. In one study of 27 patients who had overlap syndromes followed prospectively, 17 were positive for anti-nRNP and 10 were not;[755] no clear distinction could be made between the two groups, leading the investigators to conclude that MCTD was not distinct from overlap syndromes in general. In keeping with these conclusions, clinically acceptable cases of MCTD account for only 5% to 10% of patients who have anti-nRNP Ab; moreover in some patients who manifest the clinical criteria of MCTD, the results of this antibody determination are negative. By contrast, the results of one long-term study showed a correlation between the presence and level of anti-nRNP Ab and the state of disease activity;[754] in patients whose disease became inactive, the autoantibody disappeared, whereas most of those who progressed to a fatal outcome continued to have high titers.

Initially, MCTD was considered to be a relatively benign form of connective tissue disease that responded readily to corticosteroid therapy. However, it is now clear that patients may develop the more ominous features of other connective tissue diseases that do not respond to corticosteroid therapy; for example, it has been estimated that central nervous system involvement occurs in 30% to 50% of patients, and membranous glomerulonephritis develops in some.[241] Fatal diffuse interstitial lung disease, diffuse alveolar hemorrhage, and pulmonary arterial hypertension have also been described.[355, 754, 760, 760a] Less severe pulmonary disease probably develops in 15% to 20% of patients.[761, 762]

Pathologic characteristics of pulmonary changes in MCTD have been infrequently described. Fibrous pleural adhesions were noted in one case,[763] and there have been several reports of interstitial pneumonitis and fibrosis.[760, 764] Immunofluorescent and electron-microscopic studies in these cases have shown no evidence of immune complex deposition.[760] In three cases of pulmonary hypertension unassociated with parenchymal disease, histologic features included plexogenic pulmonary arteriopathy in two[760, 765] and recurrent small vessel thromboemboli in one.[763] IgG was identified in the pulmonary arterial walls in one of these cases.[760]

The radiologic manifestations of MCTD include findings seen in patients who have SLE, progressive systemic sclerosis, and polymyositis.[766] The frequency of pulmonary abnormalities varies considerably in different series. For example, in a retrospective study of 81 patients from the Mayo Clinic, an interstitial pattern was seen on the chest radiograph in 19% of cases;[767] on the other hand, careful prospective study of 34 patients demonstrated interstitial infiltrates in 85% of cases.[768] The infiltrates consisted of irregular linear opacities giving a reticular pattern and involving mainly the lung bases.[768] With progression of disease, the fibrosis gradually extends superiorly; in the late stage, honeycombing may be identified.[766, 768] HRCT essentially corroborates the radiographic findings and shows a predominantly subpleural distribution of fibrosis, similar to that seen in the interstitial fibrosis associated with other connective tissue diseases.[766] Other radiographic abnormalities include areas of parenchymal consolidation that may be

related to aspiration pneumonia[766, 767] or diffuse pulmonary hemorrhage (Fig. 39–31).[769, 770]

Pleural effusion has been reported in 5% of patients;[767] in one case, it consisted of an exudate containing 95% neutrophils.[771] Pericardial effusion and evidence of congestive heart failure secondary to myocarditis may also be seen.[766] Mediastinal lymphadenopathy has been reported in two patients.[772, 773]

The course of MCTD is variable. An evaluation of the original 25 patients reported by Sharp and coworkers[757] showed that the arthritis, serositis, fever, and myositis responded to corticosteroids and became less severe with time.[774] However, the clinical picture more closely resembled PSS, and the skin and esophageal lesions did not respond to therapy. On the other hand, a prospective analysis of another group of 34 patients in whom a diagnosis of MCTD was eventually made and who were followed for a mean duration of more than 6 years indicated that some patients who presented with rather limited disease and were diagnosed as having SLE or PSS may progress to a clinical picture more compatible with MCTD.[754] Conversely, in another investigation of 46 patients initially believed to have MCTD and followed prospectively, 12 were found to "differentiate" into SLE and 13 into PSS (11 had died and 7 were lost to follow-up);[775] this suggested that MCTD may be an intermediate step in the progression to a more distinct connective tissue disease in many patients. The outcome was linked to specific HLA haplotypes, suggesting it was genetically determined.

## RHEUMATIC PNEUMONITIS

In 1937, Masson and associates[776] described morphologic changes in the lungs of patients who had died of rheumatic fever that they considered specific for this condition and that they termed *rheumatic pneumonitis*. Although it is likely that most such cases are analogous to the localized or diffuse alveolar damage that can complicate other insults such as uremia, shock, and radiation,[777] the findings in occasional patients suggest that true "primary" rheumatic pneumonitis may occur.[778–780]

In all of these conditions, the histologic picture is that of diffuse alveolar damage, with pulmonary congestion, intraalveolar proteinaceous exudate, and hyaline membranes. Organization of the exudate can lead to significant air-space fibrosis.[781] Vasculitis has occasionally been described in smaller branches of the pulmonary arteries.[777] When these pathologic changes are present in the lungs in association with rheumatic fever, the disease is usually very severe and is accompanied by extensive cardiac involvement.[782, 783] The radiographic pattern is generally one of pulmonary edema, progressing from relatively mild interstitial edema through all stages to severe air-space involvement. Hemoptysis occurs in approximately one third of cases, and dyspnea may be severe.

## RELAPSING POLYCHONDRITIS

Relapsing polychondritis is an unusual systemic disorder characterized principally by widespread inflammation

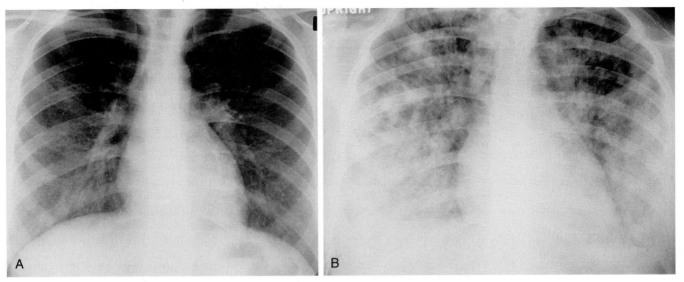

**Figure 39–31. Diffuse Pulmonary Hemorrhage in Mixed Connective Tissue Disease.** A 17-year-old woman presented with hemoptysis. A posteroanterior (PA) chest radiograph *(A)* demonstrates poorly defined areas of increased opacity in the right lung and left lower lobe. The patient was shown to have mixed connective tissue disease. The clinical and radiographic findings resolved following treatment with corticosteroids. Six months later, the patient presented with a recurrent episode of hemoptysis. A PA chest radiograph at this time *(B)* shows extensive bilateral consolidation. The radiographic findings cleared within 72 hours following treatment with corticosteroids.

and destruction of cartilage in a variety of sites throughout the body; involvement of the eye, ear, and systemic vessels is also occasionally seen. The condition is uncommon: in one comprehensive review of the literature in 1976, only 136 cases were identified.[784] There is no sex predominance, and the disease occurs at all ages, with a peak incidence between 40 and 60 years.[784]

### Etiology and Pathogenesis

The etiology and pathogenesis of relapsing polychondritis are unknown. An associated autoimmune disorder has been found in 20% to 25% of cases,[784, 785] suggesting that the disease may have an immunologic basis. Anticartilage antibodies have been detected in some patients,[786–788] and it has been shown that exposure of peripheral blood lymphocytes to cartilage antigen *in vitro* results in increased blastogenesis[789] and the production of macrophage migration-inhibiting factor.[790] In two patients, granular deposits of C3 and immunoglobulin were identified at the chondrofibrous junction of ear cartilage.[785] In another, low levels of complement were found in the subcutaneous fluid overlying affected ear cartilage;[791] however, simultaneous measurement of serum complement showed a normal level, suggesting that the complement system was activated locally. Although some of these findings may reflect simply the normal immune response to cartilage damage, the sum of evidence suggests that abnormal immunity is important at some point in the disease. This hypothesis has been strengthened by the observation that the antibodies to collagen seen in relapsing polychondritis are directed toward minor matrix collagens and therefore unlikely to be nonspecific responses to tissue injury.[792, 793]

As with many other connective tissue diseases, there is evidence for genetic factors in the pathogenesis of relapsing polychondritis. A relatively strong association with HLA-DR4 has been described in patients who have the disease;

for example, in one investigation this was identified in 56% of patients and in only 25% of controls.[794] Hydralazine, a drug also responsible for an SLE-like syndrome, has been reported to have induced the disease in a woman who was a slow acetylator and was HLA-DR4 positive.[795]

### Pathologic Characteristics

Relapsing polychondritis affects cartilage in many anatomic sites, including the ribs, tracheobronchial tree, ear lobes, nose, and axial and peripheral joints.[784, 786, 796, 797] The gross appearance of the trachea and major bronchi at autopsy has been described infrequently; however, severe narrowing has been observed in a few cases.[788, 789, 799] Microscopically, affected cartilage shows fragmentation, loss of the normal basophilic staining, and replacement by fibrous tissue. In clinically active disease, an inflammatory infiltrate composed of lymphocytes, plasma cells, and occasional neutrophils is often present at the fibrous-cartilaginous interface.[785, 798] Histochemical studies show a variable loss of glycosaminoglycans from the cartilage matrix,[788, 798] and electron-microscopic examination has revealed degeneration of chondrocytes as well as elastic and collagen fibers.[800–802]

### Radiologic Manifestations

The most common radiographic manifestation in the chest is tracheal stenosis.[786] Less commonly, there is narrowing of the major[786, 803] or segmental bronchi (Fig. 39–32).[804] Bilateral upper lobe opacities were noted radiographically in one patient who was found at autopsy to have obstructive pneumonitis and extensive airway obliteration in the same anatomic distribution.[805] The tracheal narrowing usually measures only a few centimeters in length,[805] although diffuse tracheal stenosis may occur.[806] Thickening of the tracheal or bronchial wall can also be seen on CT, in association with narrowing of the lumen (Fig. 39–33).[807–809]

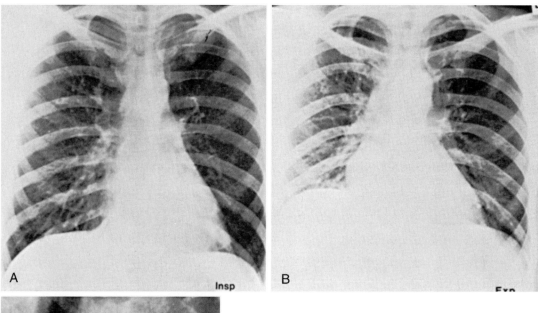

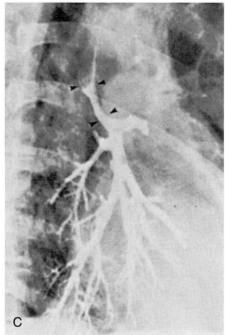

**Figure 39–32. Bronchial Narrowing in Relapsing Polychondritis.** Posteroanterior chest radiographs at inspiration *(A)* and expiration *(B)* in a 25-year-old man with relapsing polychondritis demonstrate a moderate degree of oligemia of the left lung. The volume of the left lung on inspiration is roughly normal, although it shows a severe degree of air trapping on expiration *(B)*. A left bronchogram *(C)* demonstrates a severe degree of narrowing of the whole length of the left main bronchus *(arrowheads);* the lower lobe bronchi were otherwise normal. This bronchial narrowing resulted from chondritis affecting the cartilage rings of this airway. Some years later, the patient died in respiratory insufficiency when a similar process affected the major bronchi of the right lung. (Courtesy of Dr. John Henderson, Ottawa General Hospital.)

Occasionally, bronchiectasis is evident, presumably secondary to recurrent pneumonia.[804] The extent and degree of tracheal and bronchial stenosis are best assessed using spiral CT with thin-collimation (3-mm) and multiplanar or three-dimensional reconstructions.[810, 810a]

### Clinical Manifestations

As the name indicates, the disease is typically relapsing and remitting and usually has a prolonged course. The most common clinical manifestations in one series of 23 patients were swelling and redness of the ears (in 88%) and arthralgia (in 81%).[784] Nasal chondritis is also frequent and may result in a saddle deformity. Such deformity and audiovestibular damage can mimic that seen in Wegener's granulomatosis and Cogan's syndrome, respectively.[811] Cutaneous manifestations are the presenting feature in more than 50% of patients,

and usually consist of erythema, swelling, and pain as a reflection of involvement of the underlying cartilage; direct involvement of the skin can be manifested as vasculitis and can resemble erythema nodosum.[812]

Respiratory tract involvement is not uncommon. Involvement of the larynx and trachea was present in 13 (56%) patients in the series cited previously;[784] in 14%, it was responsible for the presenting signs and symptoms of the disease. Symptoms of respiratory tract disease include dyspnea, cough, hoarseness, stridor, wheezing, and tenderness over the laryngotracheal cartilages.[813] Airway obstruction can occur as a consequence of encroachment of the airway by acutely inflamed mucosa, by scarring later in the course of disease, or by dynamic collapse of the airway secondary to cartilage dissolution.[1] Such airway involvement may occur even in the absence of previous nasal or auricular pathology.[1]

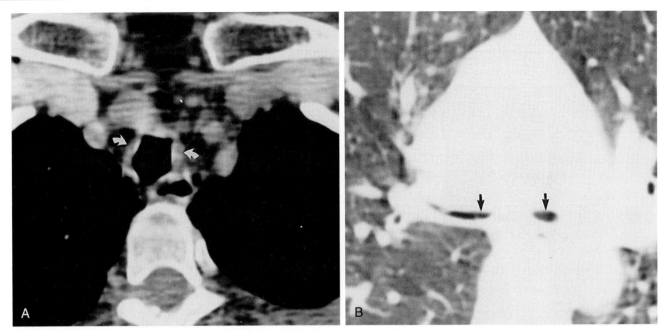

**Figure 39–33. Relapsing Polychondritis.** An HRCT scan *(A)* demonstrates mild thickening of the cartilaginous portion of the tracheal wall *(arrows)*. A scan at the level of the main bronchi photographed at lung windows *(B)* demonstrates narrowing of the lumen of both the right and left main bronchi *(arrows)*. The patient was a 51-year-old woman who presented with a 6-month history of sore throat, hoarseness, and dry cough. The diagnosis was proven by tracheal biopsy. (From Müller et al: Can Assoc Radiol J 40:213, 1989.)

Many other clinical manifestations can be seen, related to episcleritis, iritis, ear involvement (usually hearing impairment), cataracts, heart failure or arrhythmia (secondary to myocarditis), and aortic valvular insufficiency.[786, 797, 814, 815] Twenty-nine of 129 patients followed at the Mayo Clinic had evidence of coexistent glomerulonephritis,[816] most likely on the basis of immune complex–mediated glomerular injury.[817] One case has been reported of acute glomerulonephritis associated with diffuse alveolar hemorrhage.[818] Chondrolysis of the joints can lead to severe arthritis.

The diagnosis is made on the basis of recurrent inflammation of two or more cartilaginous sites, most commonly the ears and nose.[818] Laboratory findings include anemia and abnormalities of liver function. During acute exacerbations, acid mucopolysaccharides may be recovered from the urine and presumably are derived from affected cartilage.[786] Pulmonary function studies in patients who have airway involvement demonstrate signs of intrathoracic or extrathoracic upper airway obstruction on flow-volume curves, the appearance of the curve depending on the site of obstruction.[813]

The prognosis of patients who have evidence of airway obstruction is poor; 13 of 62 in one series died despite attempts at therapy.[813] In another review of 112 patients, the most frequent causes of death were infection, systemic vasculitis, and malignancy;[819] only 10% of the deaths could be attributed to airway involvement by chondritis. The 5- and 10-year probabilities of survival after diagnosis were 74% and 55%, respectively.

## PULMONARY INVOLVEMENT IN INFLAMMATORY BOWEL DISEASE

Although idiopathic inflammatory bowel disease (IBD; Crohn's disease and ulcerative colitis) is generally not considered to be in the spectrum of the connective tissue diseases, it may well be immunologically mediated and is thus included in this chapter. Clinically apparent respiratory involvement in these disorders is rare; in one early report of the association, only three cases were identified in a series of 1,400 patients followed for more than 40 years.[820] In fact, most of the descriptions of an association between pleuropulmonary disease and IBD are culled from individual case reports; these reports were summarized and 33 new patients were added in a 1993 review.[821]

In contrast with clinically evident pulmonary disease, subclinical abnormalities appear to be relatively common, an observation that strengthens the hypothesis that the association between involvement of the two organ systems is not coincidental. For example, in two studies of patients who had Crohn's disease of varying activity, but who were asymptomatic from a pulmonary point of view and who had normal chest radiographs, evidence of lymphocytic alveolitis was seen in BAL fluid;[822, 823] most patients were not receiving anti-inflammatory drugs at the time of bronchoscopy. In another investigation of 26 children who had Crohn's disease and normal chest radiographs, a significant reduction in the diffusing capacity was identified when their bowel disease was active compared with when it was quiescent.[824] In another investigation, 54 patients who had Crohn's disease, 21 who had ulcerative colitis, and 43 healthy controls underwent pulmonary function testing; abnormalities were found in 54%, 38%, and 7%, respectively.[825] Obstructive disorders were more frequent in patients who had ulcerative colitis, whereas restriction with reduction in diffusing capacity was seen in the patients who had Crohn's disease. These results were not entirely confirmed in another study in which the reduction in vital capacity of 29 adult patients who had Crohn's disease was attributed to intercurrent medical disease;[826] the hemoglobin-corrected transfer factor for CO was

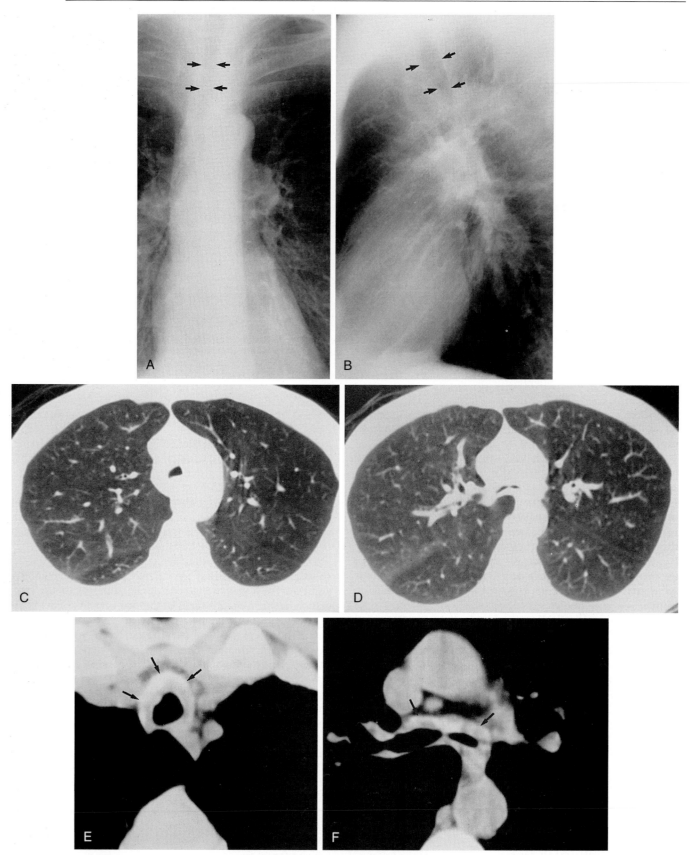

**Figure 39–34. Ulcerative Tracheobronchitis Associated with Ulcerative Colitis.** A 50-year-old man with ulcerative colitis presented with progressive shortness of breath and stridor. Views from posteroanterior *(A)* and lateral *(B)* chest radiographs demonstrate diffuse narrowing of the tracheal lumen *(arrows)*. The degree of tracheal narrowing and the presence of bilateral bronchial narrowing are better seen on the CT scans photographed on lung windows *(C* and *D)*. Soft tissue windows demonstrate marked thickening of the wall of the trachea *(E)* and the right and left main bronchi *(F) (arrows)*. The diagnosis of ulcerative tracheobronchitis was proven by biopsy.

reduced in these patients compared with the control group. Evidence of small airway dysfunction was described by another group in 30 patients who had IBD (12 with Crohn's disease and 18 with ulcerative colitis);[826a] a decrease in diffusing capacity was also found when the bowel disease was clinically active. Increases in the functional residual capacity and residual volume have also been noted in groups of patients who had IBD.[826–828]

Airway complications are probably the most common manifestations of pleuropulmonary disease in patients who have IBD, especially ulcerative colitis.[821] Chronic bronchitis and bronchiectasis have been seen in a number of such patients in the absence of a smoking history;[828a, b] ulcerative tracheobronchitis (Fig. 39–34),[829] BOOP,[830, 831] obliterative bronchiolitis, and diffuse panbronchiolitis[832, 833] have also been described. Subglottic stenosis has also been a manifestation of both ulcerative colitis and Crohn's disease.

The radiographic and HRCT findings were described in seven patients with ulcerative colitis who presented with cough and recurrent respiratory infections.[834] The chest radiographs were normal in two patients and showed evidence of bronchial wall thickening in three and bronchiectasis in two. HRCT findings included bronchiectasis in six patients and centrilobular nodularity suggestive of peripheral airway disease in four. Three patients had narrowing of the major bronchi, in one associated with narrowing of the distal trachea. Bronchial biopsy in six patients demonstrated acute and chronic inflammation of the mucosa and submucosa associated with peribronchial fibrosis.

In many patients who have chronic bronchitis and bronchiectasis, the severity of pulmonary symptoms parallels the severity of the bowel disease. For unknown reasons, disease in the lungs may flare dramatically following bowel resection. In contrast with the usual disappointing response to inhaled and systemic corticosteroids in patients who have bronchiectasis or chronic bronchitis, many patients who have IBD improve with such therapy or with lavage of steroids directly onto the bronchial mucosa. Although disease may occur at any level of the airways, it typically does not progress to involve other sites.[821]

In addition to BOOP, a variety of parenchymal lung diseases have been associated with IBD. Eosinophilia with lung infiltrates has been described most commonly in patients taking sulfasalazine and other anti-inflammatory medication (*see* page 2557); however, some patients have not given this history,[821] raising the possibility that the reaction may be an intrinsic manifestation of IBD. Nonspecific interstitial pneumonitis and fibrosis have also been described in occasional patients,[835, 836] only some of whom were taking medication known to cause lung disease.[821] Rare pulmonary abnormalities described in patients who have IBD include cavitating lung nodules with and without associated pyoderma gangrenosum,[821] nodular amyloidosis,[837] focal granulomatous lung disease ("metastatic" Crohn's disease),[838, 839] sarcoidosis,[821] chronic eosinophilic pneumonia,[840] pulmonary vasculitis,[841] and colobronchial[842] and esophagopulmonary[843] fistulas. Although some of these abnormalities undoubtedly represent complications of the bowel disease, others are probably coincidental associations.

Pleural disease can also occur in patients who have IBD. One group reported 41 patients who had serositis (32 with ulcerative colitis and 9 with Crohn's disease), usually pericarditis but on occasion pleuritis;[821] approximately half were not taking anti-inflammatory medication for their bowel disease at the time of presentation. Serositis may be recurrent, and parallel exacerbations of disease were noted in many patients; symptoms included chest pain and rarely, pericardial tamponade.

## PULMONARY INVOLVEMENT IN PRIMARY BILIARY CIRRHOSIS

Pulmonary disease has been described occasionally in patients who have primary biliary cirrhosis (PBC), most often in association with Sjögren's syndrome.[681, 844–846] Although it is possible that the latter condition is in fact responsible for the pulmonary abnormalities, the documentation of alveolitis on BAL in patients who have PBC without Sjögren's syndrome suggests a pathogenetic role of PBC itself.[845] Reported pulmonary complications include bronchiolitis, BOOP, diffuse alveolar hemorrhage, and interstitial pneumonitis.[847, 848]

# REFERENCES

1. Wiedemann HP, Matthay RA: Pulmonary manifestations of the collagen vascular diseases. Clin Chest Med 10:677, 1989.
2. Panush RS, Greer JM, Morshedian KK: What is lupus? What is not lupus? Rheum Dis Clin North Am 19:223, 1993.
3. Orens JB, Martinez FJ, Lynch JP III: Pleuropulmonary manifestations of systemic lupus erythematosus. Rheum Dis Clin North Am 20:159, 1994.
4. Quismorio FP: Clinical and pathologic features of lung involvement in systemic lupus erythematosus. Semin Respir Med 9:297, 1988.
5. Cervera R, Khamashta MA, Font J, et al: Systemic lupus erythematosus: Clinical and immunologic patterns of disease expression in a cohort of 1,000 patients. Medicine (Baltimore) 72:113, 1993.
6. Hopkinson ND, Doherty M, Powell RJ: Clinical features and race-specific incidence/prevalence rates of systemic lupus erythematosus in a geographically complete cohort of patients. Ann Rheum Dis 53:675, 1994.
7. Hopkinson ND, Doherty M, Powell RJ: The prevalence and incidence of systemic lupus erythematosus in Nottingham, UK. Br J Rheum 32:110, 1993.
8. Johnson AE, Goron C, Palmer RG, et al: The prevalence and incidence of systemic lupus erythematosus in Birmingham, England: Relationship to ethnicity and country of birth. Arthritis Rheum 38:551, 1995.
9. Fessel WJ: Systemic lupus erythematosus in the community. Arch Intern Med 134:1027, 1974.
10. Hopkinson N: Epidemiology of systemic lupus erythematosus. Ann Rheum Dis 51:1291, 1992.
11. Frank A: Apparent predisposition to systemic lupus erythematosus in Chinese patients in West Malaysia. Ann Rheum Dis 39:266, 1980.
12. Siegel M, Lee SL: The epidemiology of systemic lupus erythematosus. Semin Arthritis Rheum 3:1, 1973.
13. Dawkins RL, Peter JB: Laboratory tests in clinical immunology: A critique. Am J Med 68:3, 1980.
14. Thomas C, Robinson JA: The antinuclear antibody test: When is a positive result clinically relevant? Postgrad Med 94:55, 1993.
15. Synkowski DR, Mogavero HS Jr, Provost TT: Lupus erythematosus: Laboratory testing and clinical subsets in the evaluation of patients. Med Clin North Am 64:921, 1980.
16. Maddison PJ, Provost TT, Reichlin M: Serological findings in patients with "ANA-negative" systemic lupus erythematosus. Medicine (Baltimore) 60:87, 1981.
17. Ferreiro JE, Reiter WM, Saldana MJ: Systemic lupus erythematosus presenting as chronic serositis with no demonstrable antinuclear antibodies. Am J Med 76:1100, 1984.
18. Reeves WH, Satoh M, Wang J, et al: Antibodies to DNA, DNA-binding proteins, and histones. Rheum Dis Clin North Am 20:1, 1994.
19. Pisetsky DS: Anti-DNA antibodies in systemic lupus erythematosus. Rheum Dis Clin North Am 18:437, 1992.
19a. Hahn BH: Antibodies to DNA. N Engl J Med 338:1359, 1998.
20. Vlachoyiannopoulos PG, Karassa FB, Karakostas KX, et al: Systemic lupus erythematosus in Greece: Clinical features, evolution, and outcome—a descriptive analysis of 292 patients. Lupus 2:303, 1993.
21. Rahman MAA, Isenberg DA: Autoantibodies in systemic lupus erythematosus. Curr Opin Rheumatol 6:468, 1994.
22. Jacob L, Viard JP: Anti-DNA antibodies and their relationships with anti-histone and anti-nucleosome specificities. Eur J Med 1:425, 1992.
23. Pauzner R, Urowitz M, Gladman D, et al: Antineutrophil cytoplasmic antibodies in systemic lupus erythematosus. J Rheum 21:1670, 1994.
24. Merkel PA, Polisson RP, Chang Y, et al: Prevalence of antineutrophil cytoplasmic antibodies in a large inception cohort of patients with connective tissue disease. Ann Intern Med 126:866, 1997.
25. Hedgpeth T, Boulware DW: Interstitial pneumonitis in antinuclear antibody–negative systemic lupus erythematosus: A new clinical manifestation and possible association with anti-Ro (SS-A) antibodies. Arthritis Rheum 31:545, 1988.
26. Smolen JS, Morimoto C, Steinberg AD, et al: Systemic lupus erythematosus: Delineations of subpopulations by clinical, serologic, and T-cell subset analysis. Am J Med Sci 289:139, 1985.
27. Mittenburg AM, Roos A, Slegtenhorst L, et al: IgA anti-ds DNA antibodies in systemic lupus erythematosus: Occurrence, incidence, and association with clinical and laboratory variables of disease activity. J Rheum 20:53, 1993.
28. Groen H, Ter Brog EJ, Postma DS et al: Pulmonary function in systemic lupus erythematosus is related to distinct clinical, serologic, and nailfold capillary patterns. Am J Med 93:619, 1992.
29. Neu E, von Mikecz AH, Hemmerich PH, et al: Autoantibodies against eukaryotic protein L7 in patients suffering form systemic lupus erythematosus and progressive systemic sclerosis: Frequency and correlation with clinical, serological, and genetic parameters. The SLE Study Group. Clin Exp Immunol 100:198, 1995.
30. Arnett FC, Reveille JD: Genetics of systemic lupus erythematosus. Rheum Dis Clin North Am 18:865, 1992.
30a. Martin-Villa JM, Martinez-Laso J, Moreno-Pelayo MA, et al: Differential contribution of HLA-DR, DQ, and TAP2 alleles to systemic lupus erythematosus susceptibility in Spanish patients: Role of TAP2*01 alleles in Ro autoantibody production. Ann Rheum Dis 57:214, 1998.
30b. Manger K, Repp R, Spriewald BM, et al: Fcgamma receptor IIa polymorphism in Caucasian patients with systemic lupus erythematosus: Association with clinical symptoms. Arthritis Rheum 41:1181, 1998.
30c. Tassiulas IO, Aksentijevich I, Salmon JE, et al: Angiotensin I converting enzyme gene polymorphisms in systemic lupus erythematosus: Decreased prevalence of DD genotype in African American patients. Clin Nephrol 50:8, 1998.
31. Systemic lupus erythematosus: Emerging concepts: I. Dermatologic and joint disease, the antiphospholipid antibody syndrome, pregnancy, and hormonal therapy: Morbidity and mortality, and pathogenesis. Ann Intern Med 123:42, 1995.
32. Jarvinen P, Aho K: Twin studies in rheumatic diseases. Semin Arthritis Rheum 24:19, 1994.
33. Yeh HM, Chen JR, Tsai JJ, et al: Prevalence of familial systemic lupus erythematosus in Taiwan. Kaohsiung J Med Sci 9:664, 1993.
34. Steinberg AD, Raveché ES, Laskin CA, et al: Systemic lupus erythematosus: Insights from animal models. Ann Intern Med 100:714, 1984.
35. Decker JL, Steinberg AD, Reinertsen JL, et al: Systemic lupus erythematosus: Evolving concepts. Ann Intern Med 91:587, 1979.
36. Reinharz D, Tiercy JM, Mach B, et al: Absence of DRw15/3 and of DRw15/7 heterozygotes in Caucasian patients with systemic lupus erythematosus. Tissue Antigens 37:10, 1991.
37. Mehra NK, Pande I, Taneja V, et al: Major histocompatibility complex genes and susceptibility to systemic lupus erythematosus in northern India. Lupus 2:313, 1993.
38. Goldstein R, Sengar DP: Comparative studies of the major histocompatibility complex in French Canadian and non–French Canadian Caucasians with systemic lupus erythematosus. Arthritis Rheum 36:1121, 1993.
39. Huang DF, Siminovitch KA, Liu XY, et al: Population and family studies of three disease-related polymorphic genes in systemic lupus erythematosus. J Clin Invest 95:1766, 1995.
40. Petri M, Watson R, Winkelstein JA, et al: Clinical expression of systemic erythematosus in patients with C4A deficiency. Medicine (Baltimore) 72:236, 1993.
41. Hess EV, Farhey Y: Epidemiology, genetics, etiology, and environmental relationships of systemic lupus erythematosus. Curr Opin Rheumatol 6:474, 1994.
42. Wallace SL, Diamond H, Kaplan D: Recent advances in rheumatoid diseases: The connective tissue diseases other than rheumatoid arthritis—1970 and 1971. Ann Intern Med 77:455, 1972.
43. Block SR, Christian CL: The pathogenesis of systemic lupus erythematosus. Am J Med 59:453, 1975.
44. Phillips PE, Christian CL: Myxovirus antibody increases in human connective tissue disease. Science 168:892, 1970.
45. Hollinger FB, Sharp JT, Lidsky MD, et al: Antibodies to viral antigens in systemic lupus erythematosus. Arthritis Rheum 14:1, 1971.
46. Goodman JR, Sylvester RA, Talal N, et al: Virus-like structures in lymphocytes of patients with systemic and discoid lupus erythematosus. Ann Intern Med 79:396, 1973.
47. Hammar SP, Winterbaur RH, Bockus D, et al: Endothelial cell damage and tubuloreticular structures in interstitial lung disease associated with collagen vascular disease and viral pneumonia. Am Rev Respir Dis 127:77, 1983.
48. Rich S: Human lupus inclusions and interferon. Science 213:772, 1981.
49. Hooks JJ, Moutsopoulos HM, Geis SA, et al: Immune interferon in the circulation of patients with auto-immune disease. N Engl J Med 301:5, 1979.
50. Strom BL, Reidenberg MM, West S, et al: Shingles, allergies, family medical history, oral contraceptives, and other potential risk factors for systemic lupus erythematosus. Am J Epidemiol 140:632, 1994.
51. Kalden JR, Gay S: Retroviruses and autoimmune rheumatic diseases. Clin Exp Immunol 98:1, 1994.
52. Kalden JR, Winkler TH, Herrmann M, et al: Pathogenesis of SLE: Immunopathology in man. Rheumatol Int 11:95, 1991.
53. Shahram F, Akbarian M, Davatchi F: Salmonella infection in systemic lupus erythematosus. Lupus 2:55, 1993.
54. Li EK, Cohen MG, Ho AK, et al: Salmonella bacteraemia occurring concurrently with the first presentation of systemic lupus erythematosus. Br J Rheum 32:66, 1993.
55. Schultz DR, Arnold PI: Head shock (stress) proteins and autoimmunity in rheumatic diseases. Semin Arthritis Rheum 22:357, 1993.
56. Dupont A, Six R: Lupus-like syndrome induced by methyldopa. BMJ 285:693, 1982.
57. Harrington TM, Davis DE: Systemic lupus-like syndrome induced by methyldopa therapy. Chest 79:696, 1981.
58. McCracken M, Benson EA, Hickling P: Systemic lupus erythematosus induced by aminoglutethimide. BMJ 281:1254, 1980.
59. Hughes GRV: Hypotensive agents, beta-blockers, and drug-induced lupus. BMJ 284:1358, 1982.
60. Record NB Jr: Acebutolol-induced pleuropulmonary lupus syndrome. Ann Intern Med 95:326, 1981.
61. West SG, McMahon M, Protanova JP: Quinidine-induced lupus erythematosus. Ann Intern Med 100:840, 1984.
62. Price EJ, Venables PJ: Drug-induced lupus. Drug Safety 12:283, 1995.
63. Laversuch CJ, Collins DA, Charles PJ, et al: Sulphasalazine-induced autoimmune abnormalities in patients with rheumatic disease. Br J Rheum 344:435, 1995.
64. Sato-Matsumura KC, Koizumi H, Matsumura T, et al: Lupus erythematosus–like syndrome induced by thiamazole and propylthiouracil. J Dermatol 21:501, 1994.
65. Drory VE, Korczyn AD: Hypersensitivity vasculitis and systemic lupus erythematosus induced by anticonvulsants. Clin Neuropharmacol 16:19, 1993.

66. Chalmers A, Thompson D, Stein HE, et al: Systemic lupus erythematosus during penicillamine therapy for rheumatoid arthritis. Ann Intern Med 97:659, 1982.

67. Harland SJ, Facchini V, Timbrell JA: Hydralazine-induced lupus erythematosus–like syndrome in a patient of the rapid acetylator phenotype. BMJ 281:273, 1980.

68. Batchelor JR, Welsh KI, Tinoco RM, et al: Hydralazine-induced systemic lupus erythematosus: Influence of HLA-DR and sex on susceptibility. Lancet 1:1107, 1980.

69. Kluger J, Drayer DE, Reidenberg MM, et al: Acetylprocainamide therapy in patients with previous procainamide-induced lupus syndrome. Ann Intern Med 95:326, 1981.

70. Stec GP, Lertora JJL, Atkinson AJ Jr, et al: Remission of procainamide-induced lupus erythematosus with *N*-acetylprocainamide therapy. Ann Intern Med 90:799, 1979.

71. Rubin RI: Autoantibody specificity in drug-induced lupus and neutrophil-mediated metabolism of lupus-inducing drugs. Clin Biochem 25:223, 1992.

72. Uetrecht J: Metabolism of drugs by activated leukocytes: Implications for drug-induced lupus and other drug hypersensitivity reactions. Adv Exp Med Biol 283:1221, 1991.

73. Sanchez-Roman J, Wichman I, Salaberri J, et al: Multiple clinical and biological autoimmune manifestations in 50 workers after occupational exposure to silica. Ann Rheum Dis 52:534, 1993.

74. Nagata C, Fujita S, Iwata H, et al: Systemic lupus erythematosus: A case-control epidemiologic study in Japan. Int J Dermatol 34:333, 1995.

75. Minami Y, Sasaki T, Komatsu S, et al: Female systemic lupus erythematosus in Miyagi Prefecture, Japan: A case-control study of dietary and reproductive factors. Tohoku J Exp Med 169:245, 1993.

76. Hirmand H, Latrenta GS, Hoffman LA: Autoimmune disease and silicone breast implants. Oncology 7:17, 1993.

77. Sanchez-Guerrero J, Colditz GA, Elizabeth PH, et al: Silicone breast implants and the risk of connective-tissue diseases and symptoms. N Engl J Med 332:1666, 1995.

78. Sanchez-Guerrero J, Liang MH, Karlson EW, et al: Postmenopausal estrogen therapy and the risk for developing systemic lupus erythematosus. Ann Intern Med 122:430, 1995.

79. Inman RD, Jovanovic L, Markenson JA, et al: Systemic lupus erythematosus in men: Genetic and endocrine features. Arch Intern Med 142:1813, 1982.

80. Tsokos GC: Lymphocytes, cytokines, inflammations, and immune trafficking. Curr Opin Rheumatol 6:461, 1994.

81. Mitamura K, Kang H, Tomita Y, et al: Impaired tumour necrosis factor-alpha (TNF-alpha) production and abnormal B-cell response to TNF-alpha in patients with systemic lupus erythematosus (SLE). Clin Exp Immunol 85:386, 1991.

82. Groen H, Aslander M, Bootsma H, et al: Bronchoalveolar lavage cell analysis and lung function impairment in patients with systemic lupus erythematosus (SLE). Clin Exp Immunol 94:127, 1993.

83. Deguchi Y: Spontaneous increase of transforming growth factor-beta production by bronchoalveolar mononuclear cells of patients with systemic autoimmune diseases affecting the lung. Ann Rheum Dis 51:362, 1992.

84. Haupt HM, Moore GW, Hutchins GM: The lung in systemic lupus erythematosus: Analysis of the pathologic changes in 120 patients. Am J Med 71:791, 1981.

85. Gross M, Esterly JR, Earle RH: Pulmonary alterations in systemic lupus erythematosus. Am Rev Respir Dis 105:572, 1972.

86. Klemperer P, Pollack AD, Baehr G: Pathology of disseminated lupus erythematosus. Arch Pathol 32:569, 1941.

87. Miller LR, Greenberg SD, McLarty JW: Lupus lung. Chest 88:265, 1985.

88. Byrd RB, Trunk G: Systemic lupus erythematosus presenting as pulmonary hemosiderosis. Chest 64:128, 1973.

89. Matthay RA, Schwarz MI, Petty TL, et al: Pulmonary manifestations of systemic lupus erythematosus: Review of twelve cases of acute lupus pneumonitis. Medicine (Baltimore) 54:397, 1974.

90. Pertschuk LP, Moccia LF, Rosen Y, et al: Acute pulmonary complications in systemic lupus erythematosus: Immunofluorescence and light microscopic study. Am J Clin Pathol 68:553, 1977.

91. Ramsey-Goldman R, Mattai SA, Schilling E, et al: Increased risk of malignancy in patients with systemic lupus erythematosus. J Invest Med 46:217, 1998.

92. Matthay RA, Schwartz MI, Petty TL, et al: Pulmonary manifestations of systemic lupus erythematosus: Review of twelve cases of acute lupus pneumonitis. Medicine (Baltimore) 54:397, 1975.

93. Schocket AL, Lain D, Kohler PF, et al: Immune complex vasculitis as a cause of ascites and pleural effusions in systemic lupus erythematosus. J Rheumatol 5:33, 1978.

94. Schulman S, Svenungsson E, Granqvist S, et al: Anticardiolipin antibodies predict early recurrence of thromboembolism following anticoagulant therapy. Am J Med 104:332, 1998.

95. Eisenberg H, Dubois EL, Sherwin RP, et al: Diffuse interstitial lung disease in systemic lupus erythematosus. Ann Intern Med 79:37, 1973.

96. Inque T, Kanayama Y, Ohe A, et al: Immunopathologic studies of pneumonitis in systemic lupus erythematosus. Ann Intern Med 91:30, 1979.

97. Hoffbrand BI, Beck ER: "Unexplained" dyspnoea and shrinking lungs in systemic lupus erythematosus. BMJ 1:1273, 1965.

98. Harvey AM, Shulman LE, Tumulty PA, et al: Systemic lupus erythematosus: Review of the literature and clinical analysis of 138 cases. Medicine (Baltimore) 33:291, 1954.

99. Churg A, Franklin W, Chan KL, et al: Pulmonary hemorrhage and immune-complex deposition in the lung: Complications in a patient with systemic lupus erythematosus. Arch Pathol Lab Med 104:388, 1980.

100. Rodriquez-Iturbe B, Garcia R, Rubio L, et al: Immunohistologic findings in the lung in systemic lupus erythematosus. Arch Pathol Lab Med 101:201, 1977.

101. Marino CT, Pertschuk LP: Pulmonary hemorrhage in systemic lupus erythematosus. Arch Intern Med 141:201, 1981.

102. Eagen JW, Memoli VA, Roberts JL, et al: Pulmonary hemorrhage in systemic lupus erythematosus. Medicine (Baltimore) 57:545, 1978.

103. Myers JL, Katzenstein A-LA: Microangiitis in lupus-induced pulmonary hemorrhage. Am J Clin Pathol 85:552, 1986.

104. Schwartzman KJ, Bowie DM, Yeadon C, et al: Constrictive bronchiolitis obliterans following gold therapy. Eur Respir J 8:2191, 1995.

105. Nair SS, Askari AL, Popelka CG, et al: Pulmonary hypertension and systemic lupus erythematosus. Arch Intern Med 140:109, 1980.

106. Editorial: Pulmonary hypertension and systemic lupus erythematosus. J Rheumatol 13:1, 1986.

107. Hughson MD, McCarty GA, Brumback RA: Spectrum of vascular pathology affecting patients with the antiphospholipid syndrome. Hum Pathol 26:716, 1995.

108. Garland LH, Sisson MA: Roentgen findings in the "collagen" diseases. Am J Roentgenol 71:581, 1954.

109. Bulgrin JG, Dubois EL, Jacobson G: Chest roentgenographic changes in systemic lupus erythematosus. Radiology 74:42, 1960.

110. Wiedemann HP, Matthay RA: Pulmonary manifestations of systemic lupus erythematosus. J Thorac Imaging 7(2):1, 1992.

111. Belli N, Coppola G: Lesions induced by an antilung serum. Ann Ist Forlanini 20:45, 1960.

112. Gamsu G: Radiographic manifestations of thoracic involvement by collagen vascular diseases. J Thorac Imaging 7:1, 1992.

113. Gould DM, Daves ML: A review of roentgen findings in systemic lupus erythematosus (SLE). Am J Med Sci 235:596, 1958.

114. Gammon RB, Bridges TA, Al-Nezir H, et al: Bronchiolitis obliterans organizing pneumonia associated with systemic lupus erythematosus. Chest 102:1171, 1992.

115. Susanto I, Peters JI: Acute lupus pneumonitis with normal chest radiograph. Chest 111:1781, 1997.

116. Onomura K, Nakata H, Tanaka Y, Tsuda T: Pulmonary hemorrhage in patients with systemic lupus erythematosus. J Thorac Imaging 6:57, 1991.

117. Hsu BY, Edwards DK, Drambert MA: Pulmonary hemorrhage complicating systemic lupus erythematosus: Role of MR imaging in diagnosis. Am J Roentgenol 158:519, 1992.

118. Huang CT, Hennigar GR, Lyons HA: Pulmonary dysfunction in systemic lupus erythematosus. N Engl J Med 272:288, 1965.

119. Gross M, Esterly JR, Earle RH: Pulmonary alterations in systemic lupus erythematosus. Am Rev Respir Dis 105:572, 1972.

120. Eisenberg H, Dubois EL, Sherwin RP, et al: Diffuse interstitial lung disease in systemic lupus erythematosus. Ann Intern Med 79:37, 1973.

121. Webb WR, Gamsu G: Cavitary pulmonary nodules with systemic lupus erythematosus: Differential diagnosis. Am J Roentgenol 136:27, 1981.

122. Divertie MB: Lung involvement in the connective-tissue disorders. Med Clin North Am 48:1015, 1964.

123. Martens J, Demedts M, Vanmeenen MT, Dequeker J: Respiratory muscle dysfunction in systemic lupus erythematosus. Chest 84:170, 1983.

124. Thompson PJ, Dhillon DP, Ledingham J, Turner-Warwick M: Shrinking lungs, diaphragmatic dysfunction, and systemic lupus erythematosus. Am Rev Respir Dis 132:926, 1985.

125. Bankier AA, Kiener HP, Wiesmayr MN, et al: Discrete lung involvement in systemic lupus erythematosus: CT assessment. Radiology 196:835, 1995.

126. Fenlon HM, Doran M, Sant SM, Breatnach E: High-resolution chest CT in systemic lupus erythematosus. Am J Roentgenol 166:301, 1996.

127. Ooi GC, Ngan H, Peh WCG, et al: Systemic lupus erythematosus patients with respiratory symptoms: The value of HRCT. Clin Radiol 52:775, 1997.

128. Taylor TL, Ostrum H: The roentgen evaluation of systemic lupus erythematosus. Am J Roentgenol 82:95, 1959.

129. Auerbach RC, Snyder NE, Bragg DG: The chest roentgenographic manifestations of pronestyl-induced lupus erythematosus. Radiology 109:287, 1973.

130. Susanto I, Peters JI: Acute lupus pneumonitis with normal chest radiograph. Chest 111:1781, 1997.

131. Joseph JJ, Sahn SA: Connective tissue disease and the pleura. Chest 104:262, 1993.

132. Levin DC: Proper interpretation of pulmonary roentgen changes in systemic lupus erythematosus. Am J Roentgenol 111:510, 1971.

133. Weinrib L, Sharma OP, Quismorio Jr FP: A long-term study of interstitial lung disease in systemic lupus erythematosus. Semin Arthritis Rheum 20:48, 1990.

134. Abud-Mendoza C, Diaz-Jouanen E, Alarcon-Sergovia D: Fatal pulmonary hemorrhage in systemic lupus erythematosus: Occurrence without hemoptysis. J Rheumatol 12:558, 1985.

135. Zamora MR, Warner ML, Tuder R, et al: Diffuse alveolar hemorrhage and systemic lupus erythematosus: Clinical presentation, histology, survival, and outcome. Medicine (Baltimore) 76:192, 1997.

136. Gamsu G, Webb WR: Pulmonary hemorrhage in systemic lupus erythematosus. J Can Assoc Radiol 29:66, 1978.

137. Kuhn C: Systemic lupus erythematosus in a patient with ultrastructural lesions of the pulmonary capillaries previously reported in the review as due to idiopathic pulmonary hemosiderosis. Am Rev Respir Dis 106:931, 1972.

138. Mintz G, Galindo LF, Fernandez-Diez J, et al: Acute massive pulmonary hemorrhage in systemic lupus erythematosus. J Rheumatol 5:39, 1978.

139. Ramirez RE, Glasier C, Kirks D, et al: Pulmonary hemorrhage associated with systemic lupus erythematosus in children. Radiology 152:409, 1984.

140. Byrd RB, Trunk G: Systemic lupus erythematosus presenting as pulmonary hemosiderosis. Chest 68:128, 1975.

141. McColl GJ, Buchanan RR: Familial CREST syndrome. J Rheumatol 21:754, 1994.

142. Schwab EP, Schumacher Jr HR, Freudunlich B, et al: Pulmonary alveolar hemorrhage in systemic lupus erythematosus. Semin Arthritis Rheum 23:8, 1993.

143. Onomura K, Nakaa H, Tanaka Y, et al: Pulmonary hemorrhage in patients with systemic lupus erythematosus. J Thorac Imaging 6:57, 1991.

144. Finazzi G, Brancaccio V, Moia M, et al: Natural history and risk factors for thrombosis in 360 patients with antiphospholipid antibodies: A four-year prospective study from the Italian registry. Am J Med 100:530, 1996.

145. Lockshin MD: Lupus and antiphospholipid antibody syndrome: Either, neither, or both. Am J Med 96:1, 1994.

146. Viard JP, Amoura Z, Bach JF: Association of anti-$\beta_2$ glycoprotein I antibodies with lupus-type circulating anticoagulant and thrombosis in systemic lupus erythematosus. Am J Med 93:181, 1992.

147. Matsuda J, Saitoh N, Gohchi K, et al: Detection of beta$_2$-glycoprotein-I–dependent antiphospholipid antibodies and anti-beta$_2$-glycoprotein-I antibody in patients with systemic lupus erythematosus and in patients with syphilis. Int Arch Allergy Immunol 103:239, 1994.

148. Pilling J, Cutaia M: The antiphospholipid syndrome. Chest 112:1451, 1997.

149. Asherson RA, Khamashta MA, Ordi-Ros J, et al: The "primary" antiphospholipid syndrome: Major clinical and serological features. Medicine (Baltimore) 68:366, 1989.

150. Wilson WA, Gharavi AE: Hughes syndrome: Perspectives on thrombosis and antiphospholipid antibody. Am J Med 101:574, 1996.

151. Vianna JL, Khamashta MA, Ordi-Ros J, et al: Comparison of the primary and secondary antiphospholipid syndrome: Am J Med 96:3, 1994.

152. Toubi E, Khamashta MA, Panarra A, et al: Association of antiphospholipid antibodies with central nervous system disease in systemic lupus erythematosus. Am J Med 99:397, 1995.

153. Pines A, Kaplinsky N, Olchovsky D, et al: Pleuro-pulmonary manifestations of systemic lupus erythematosus: Clinical features of its subgroups. Chest 88:129, 1985.

154. Alarcon-Segovia D, Deleze M, Oria CV, et al: Antiphospholipid antibodies and the antiphospholipid syndrome in systemic lupus erythematosus: A prospective analysis of 500 consecutive patients. Medicine (Baltimore) 68:353, 1989.

155. Wahl DG, Guillemin F, de Maistre E, et al: Risk for venous thrombosis related to antiphospholipid antibodies in systemic lupus erthematosus—a meta-analysis. Lupus 6:467, 1997.

156. Sachse C, Luthke K, Hartung K, et al: Significance of antibodies to cardiolipin in unselected patients with systemic lupus erythematosus: Clinical and laboratory associations. The SLE Study Group. Rheumatol Int 15:23, 1995.

157. Sammaritano LR, Gharavi AE: Antiphospholipid antibody syndrome. Clin Lab Med 12:41, 1992.

158. Merkel PA, Chang Y, Pierangeli SS, et al: The prevalence and clinical associations of anticardiolipin antibodies in a large inception cohort of patients with connective tissue diseases. Am J Med 101:576, 1996.

159. Cabral AR, Amigo MC, Cabiedes J, et al: The antiphospholipid/cofactor syndromes: A primary variant with antibodies to $\beta_2$-glycoprotein-I but no antibodies detectable in standard antiphospholipid assays. Am J Med 101:472, 1996.

160. Lockshin MD: Antiphospholipid antibody: Future developments. Lupus 3:309, 1994.

161. Hanly JG, Hong C, James H, et al: Requirement of beta$_2$-glycoprotein-I as cofactor in the binding for IgM and IgA anticardiolipin antibodies. J Rheumatol 22:1091, 1995.

162. Ginsberg JS, Demers C, Brill-Edwards P, et al: Acquired free protein S deficiency is associated with antiphospholipid antibodies and increased thrombin generation in patients with systemic lupus erythematosus. Am J Med 98:379, 1995.

163. Gulko PS, Reveille JD, Koopman WJ, et al: Anticardiolipin antibodies in systemic lupus erythematosus: Clinical correlates, HLA associations, and impact on survival. J Rheumatol 20:1684, 1993.

164. Escalante A, Brey RL, Mitchell BD, et al: Accuracy of anticardiolipin antibodies in identifying a history of thrombosis among patients with systemic lupus erythematosus. Am J Med 98:559, 1995.

165. Out HJ, van Vliet M, de Groot PG, et al: Prospective study of fluctuations of lupus anticoagulant activity and anticardiolipin antibody titre in patients with systemic lupus erythematosus. Ann Rheum Dis 51:353, 1992.

166. Ishii Y, Nagasawa K, Mayumi T, et al: Clinical importance of persistence of anticardiolipin antibodies in systemic lupus erythematosus. Ann Rheum Dis 49:387, 1990.

167. Winslow TM, Ossipov MA, Fazio GP, et al: Five-year follow-up study of the prevalence and progression of pulmonary hypertension in systemic lupus erythematosus. Am Heart J 129:510, 1995.

168. Simonson JS, Schiller NB, Petri M, et al: Pulmonary hypertension in systemic lupus erythematosus. J Rheumatol 16:918, 1989.

169. Ansari A, Larson PH, Bates HD: Vascular manifestations of systemic lupus erythematosus. Angiology 37:423, 1986.

170. Badui E, Garcia-Rubi D, Robles E, et al: Cardiovascular manifestations in systemic lupus erythematosus: Prospective study of 100 patients. Angiology 36:431, 1985.

171. Quismorio Jr FP, Sharma O, Koss M, et al: Immunopathologic and clinical studies in pulmonary hypertension associated with systemic lupus erythematosus. Semin Arthritis Rheum 13:349, 1984.

172. Boumpas DT, Austin HA III, Fessler BJ, et al: Systemic lupus erythematosus: Emerging concepts: I. Renal, neuropsychiatric, cardiovascular, pulmonary, and hematologic disease. Ann Intern Med 122:940, 1995.

173. Miyata M, Suzuki K, Sakuma F, et al: Anticardiolipin antibodies are associated with pulmonary hypertension in patients with mixed connective tissue disease or systemic lupus erythematosus. Int Arch Allergy Immunol 100:351, 1993.

174. Asherson RA, Higenbottam TW, Dinh Xuan AT, et al: Pulmonary hypertension in a lupus clinic: Experience with twenty-four patients. J Rheumatol 17:1292, 1990.

175. Yoshio T, Masuyama J, Mimori A, et al: Endothelin-1 release from cultured endothelial cells induced by sera from patients with systemic lupus erythematosus. Ann Rheum Dis 54:361, 1995.

176. Yoshio T, Masuyama J, Sumiya M, et al: Antiendothelial cell antibodies and their relation to pulmonary hypertension in systemic lupus erythematosus. J Rheumatol 21:2058, 1994.

177. Wilson L, Tomita T, Braniecki M: Fatal pulmonary hypertension in identical twins with systemic lupus erythematosus. Hum Pathol 22:295, 1991.

178. Laroche CM, Mulvey DA, Hawkins PN, et al: Diaphragm strength in the shrinking lung syndrome of systemic lupus erythematosus. Q J Med 71:429, 1989.

179. Laroche CM: The diaphragm in SLE [letter]. Chest 94:1115, 1988.

180. Martens J, Demedts M, Vanmeenen MT, et al: Respiratory muscle dysfunction in systemic lupus erythematosus. Chest 84:170, 1983.

181. Gibson GJ, Edmonds JP, Hughes GRV: Diaphragm function and lung involvement in systemic lupus erythematosus. Am J Med 63:926, 1977.

182. Thompson PJ, Dhisslon DP, Ledingham J, et al: Shrinking lungs, diaphragmatic dysfunction, and systemic lupus erythematosus. Am Rev Respir Dis 132:926, 1985.

183. Wilcox PG, Stein HB, Clarke SD, et al: Phrenic nerve function in patients with diaphragmatic weakness and systemic lupus erythematosus. Chest 93:352, 1988.

184. Rubin LA, Urowitz MB: Shrinking lung syndrome in SLE: A clinical pathologic study. J Rheumatol 10:973, 1983.

185. Walz-Leblanc BA, Urowitz MB, Gladman DD, et al: The "shrinking lungs syndrome" in systemic lupus erythematosus—improvement with corticosteroid therapy. J Rheumatol 19:1970, 1992.

186. Elkayam O, Segal R, Capsi D, et al: Restrictive lung disease due to diaphragmatic dysfunction in systemic lupus erythematosus: Two case reports. Clin Exp Rheumatol 10:267, 1992.

187. Kallenbach J, Zwi S, Goldman HI: Airway obstruction in a case of disseminated lupus erythematosus. Thorax 33:814, 1978.

188. Venizelos PC, Al-Bazzaz F: Pulmonary function abnormalities in systemic lupus erythematosus responsive to glucocorticoid therapy. Chest 79:702, 1981.

189. Kinney WW, Angelillo VA: Bronchiolitis in systemic lupus erythematosus. Chest 82:646, 1982.

190. Gammon RB, Bridges TA, Al-Nezir H, et al: Bronchiolitis obliterans organizing pneumonia associated with systemic lupus erythematosus. Chest 102:1171, 1992.

191. Azzam ZS, Bentur L, Rubin AHE, et al: Bronchiolitis obliterans organizing pneumonia. Chest 104:1899, 1993.

192. Nakamura K, Hirakata M, Fujii T, et al: Three cases with systemic rheumatic disease who developed pulmonary lesions suggestive of bronchiolitis obliterans organizing pneumonia. Ryumachi 35:9, 1995.

193. Mana F, Mets T, Vincken W, et al: The association of bronchiolitis obliterans organizing pneumonia, systemic lupus erythematosus, and Hunner's cystitis. Chest 104:642, 1993.

194. Nakamura K, Akizuki M, Ichikawa Y, et al: Occurrence of bronchiolitis obliterans organizing pneumonia (BOOP) in a flare-up stage of systemic lupus erythematosus (SLE). Ryumachi 33:156, 1993.

195. Epler GR, Colby TV, Carrington CB, et al: Bronchiolitis obliterans organizing pneumonia. N Engl J Med 312:152, 1985.

196. Abramson SB, Dobro J, Eberle MA, et al: Acute reversible hypoxemia in systemic lupus erythematosus. Ann Intern Med 114:941, 1991.

197. Yum MN, Ziegler JR, Walker PD, et al: Pseudolymphoma of the lung in a patient with systemic lupus erythematosus. Am J Med 66:172, 1979.

198. Marenco JL, Sanchez-Burson J, Ruiz Campos J: Pulmonary amyloidosis and unusual lung involvement in SLE. Clin Rheumatol 13:525, 1994.

199. Yood RA, Steigman DM, Gill LR: Lymphocytic interstitial pneumonitis in a patient with systemic lupus erythematosus. Lupus 4:161, 1995.

200. Nishizaka Y, Oda Y: A case of systemic lupus erythematosus associated with Sjögren's syndrome diagnosed by lung localization. Jpn J Thorac Dis 30:689, 1992.

201. Robson AK, Burge SM, Millard PR: Nasal mucosal involvement in lupus erythematosus. Clin Otolaryngol 17:341, 1992.

202. Skaer TL: Medication-induced systemic lupus erythematosus. Clin Ther 14:496, 1992.

203. Mansilla-Tinoco R, Harland SJ, Ryan PJ, et al: Hydralazine antinuclear antibodies and the lupus syndrome. BMJ 284:936, 1982.

204. Kaplan AI, Zakher F, Sabin S: Drug-induced lupus erythematosus with *in vivo* lupus erythematosus cells in pleural fluid. Chest 73:875, 1978.

205. Perry HM Jr: Late toxicity of hydralazine resembling systemic lupus erythematosus or rheumatoid arthritis. Am J Med 54:58, 1973.

206. Goldberg SK, Lipshutz JB, Ricketts RM, et al: Procainamide-induced lupus lung disease characterized by neutrophil alveolitis. Am J Med 76:146, 1984.

207. Freestone S, Ramsay IE: Transient monoclonal gammopathy in hydralazine-induced lupus erythematosus. BMJ 285:1536, 1982.

208. Bass BH: Hydralazine lung. Thorax 36:695, 1981.

209. Huang CT, Hennigar GR, Lyons HA: Pulmonary dysfunction in systemic lupus erythematosus. N Engl J Med 272:288, 1965.

210. Gold WM, Jennings DB: Pulmonary function in patients with lupus erythematosus. Am Rev Respir Dis 93:556, 1966.
211. Bankier AA, Kiener HP, Wiesmayr MN, et al: Discrete lung involvement in systemic lupus erythematosus: CT assessment. Radiology 196:835, 1995.
212. Andonopoulos AP, Constantopoulos SH, Galanopoulou V, et al: Pulmonary function of nonsmoking patients with systemic lupus erythematosus. Chest 94:312, 1988.
213. Eichacker PQ, Pinsker KM, Epstein A, et al: Serial pulmonary function testing in patients with systemic lupus erythematosus. Chest 94:129, 1988.
214. Hellman DB, Kirsch CM, Whiting-O'Keefe Q, et al: Dyspnea in ambulatory patients with SLE: Prevalence, severity, and correlation with incremental exercise testing. J Rheumatol 22:455, 1995.
215. Jacobelli S, Moreno R, Massardo L, et al: Inspiratory muscle dysfunction and unexplained dyspnea in systemic lupus erythematosus. Arthritis Rheum 28:781, 1985.
216. de Jongste JC, Neijens HJ, Duiverman EJ, et al: Respiratory tract disease in systemic lupus erythematosus. Arch Dis Child 61:478, 1986.
217. Scano G, Goti P, Duranti R, et al: Control of breathing in a subset of patients with systemic lupus erythematosus. Chest 108:759, 1995.
218. Nadel JA, Gold WM, Burgess JH: Early diagnosis of chronic pulmonary vascular obstruction: Value of pulmonary function tests. Am J Med 44:16, 1968.
219. Mohsenifar Z, Tashkin DP, Levy SE, et al: Lack of sensitivity of measurements of VD/VT at rest and during exercise in detection of hemodynamically significant pulmonary vascular abnormalities in collagen vascular disease. Am Rev Respir Dis 123:508, 1981.
220. Byrd RB, Schanzer B: Pulmonary sequelae in procainamide lupus-like syndrome. Dis Chest 55:170, 1969.
221. Estes D, Christian CL: The natural history of systemic lupus erythematosus by prospective analysis. Medicine (Baltimore) 50:85, 1971.
222. Urowitz MB, Bookman AAM, Koehler BE, et al: The bimodal mortality pattern of systemic lupus erythematosus. Am J Med 60:221, 1976.
223. Mody GM, Parag KB, Nathoo BC, et al: High mortality with systemic lupus erythematosus in hospitalised African blacks. Br J Rheumatol 33:1151, 1994.
223a. Blanco FJ, Gomez-Reino JJ, de la Mata J, et al: Survival analysis of 306 European Spanish patients with systemic lupus erythematosus. Lupus 7:159, 1998.
224. Wallace DJ, Podell T, Weiner J, et al: Systemic lupus erythematosus—survival patterns: Experience with 609 patients. JAMA 245:934, 1981.
225. Baker SB, Rovira JR, Campion EW, et al: Late-onset systemic lupus erythematosus. Am J Med 66:727, 1979.
226. Ward MM, Pyun E, Studenski S: Long-term survival in systemic lupus erythematosus: Patient characteristics associated with poorer outcomes. Arthritis Rheum 38:274, 1995.
227. Bardana EJ, Harbeck RJ, Hoffman AA, et al: The prognostic and therapeutic implications of DNA: Anti-DNA immune complexes in systemic lupus erythematosus (SLE). Am J Med 59:515, 1975.
228. Morrow WJW, Isenberg DA, Todd-Pokropek A, et al: Useful laboratory measurements in the management of systemic lupus erythematosus. Q J Med 51:125, 1982.
229. Hellmann DB, Petri M, Whiting-O'Keefe Q: Fatal infections in systemic lupus erythematosus: The role of opportunistic organisms. Medicine (Baltimore) 66:341, 1987.
230. Nived O, Sturfelt G, Wollheim F: Systemic lupus erythematosus and infection: A controlled and prospective study including an epidemiological group. Q J Med 55:271, 1985.
231. Feng PH, Tan TH: Tuberculosis in patients with systemic lupus erythematosus. Ann Rheum Dis 41:11, 1982.
232. Victorio-Navarra ST, EE D, Arroyo CG, et al: Tuberculosis among Filipino patients with systemic lupus erythematosus. Semin Arthritis Rheum 26:628, 1996.
233. Zeiss CR, Burch FX, Marder RJ, et al: A hypocomplementemic vasculitic urticarial syndrome: Report of four new cases and definition of the disease. Am J Med 68:867, 1980.
234. Schwartz HR, McDuffie FC, Black LF, et al: Hypocomplementemic urticarial vasculitis: Association with chronic obstructive pulmonary disease. Mayo Clin Proc 57:231, 1982.
235. Fortson JS, Zone JJ, Hammond ME, et al: Hypocomplementemic urticarial vasculitis responsive to dapsone. J Am Acad Dermatol 15:1137, 1986.
236. Wisnieski JJ, Baer AN, Christensen J, et al: Hypocomplementemic urticarial vasculitis syndrome: Clinical and serologic findings in 18 patients. Medicine (Baltimore) 74:24, 1995.
237. Wisnieski JJ, Jones SM: IgG autoantibody to the collagen-like region of the Clq in hypocomplementemic urticarial vasculitis syndrome, systemic lupus erythematosus, and six other musculoskeletal or rheumatic diseases. J Rheumatol 19:884, 1992.
238. Wisnieski JJ, Emancipator SN, Korman NJ, et al: Hypocomplementemic urticarial vasculitis syndrome in identical twins. Arthritis Rheum 37:1105, 1994.
239. Estrada Rodriguez JL, Lopes Serrano C, Belchi Hernandez J, et al: Hypocomplementemic urticarial vasculitis syndrome, asthma, and anaphylactic reaction with ampicillin. J Investig Allergol Clin Immunol 1:69, 1991.
240. Gordon DA, Stein JL, Broder I: The extra-articular features of rheumatoid arthritis: A systemic analysis of 127 cases. Am J Med 54:445, 1973.
241. Kohler PF, Vaughan J: The autoimmune diseases. JAMA 248:2646, 1982.
242. Helmers R, Galvin J, Hunninghake GW: Pulmonary manifestations associated with rheumatoid arthritis. Chest 100:235, 1991.
243. Baydur A, Mongan ES: Thoracic manifestations in rheumatoid arthritis. Semin Respir Med 9:305, 1988.
244. Anaya JM, Diethelm L, Ortiz LA, et al: Pulmonary involvement in rheumatoid arthritis. Semin Arthritis Rheum 24:242, 1995.
245. Walker WC, Wright V: Pulmonary lesions and rheumatoid arthritis. Medicine (Baltimore) 47:501, 1968.
246. Jurik AG, Davidsen D, Graudal H: Prevalence of pulmonary involvement in rheumatoid arthritis and its relationship to some characteristics of the patients: A radiological and clinical study. J Rheumatol 11:217, 1982.
247. Hyland RH, Gordon DA, Broder I, et al: A systematic controlled study of pulmonary abnormalities in rheumatoid arthritis. J Rheumatol 10:395, 1983.
248. Roschmann RA, Rothenberg RJ: Pulmonary fibrosis in rheumatoid arthritis: A review of clinical features and therapy. Semin Arthritis Rheum 16:174, 1987.
249. Remy-Jardin M, Remy J, Cortet B, et al: Lung changes in rheumatoid arthritis: CT findings. Radiology 193:375, 1994.
250. Gabbay E, Tarala R, Will R, et al: Interstitial lung disease in recent-onset rheumatoid arthritis. Am J Respir Crit Care Med 156:528, 1997.
251. Petrie GR, Bloomfield P, Grant IWB, et al: Upper lobe fibrosis and cavitation in rheumatoid disease. Br J Dis Chest 74:263, 1980.
252. Eraut D, Evans J, Caplin M: Pulmonary necrobiotic nodules without rheumatoid arthritis. Br J Dis Chest 72:301, 1978.
253. Nusslein HG, Rodl W, Giedel J, et al: Multiple peripheral pulmonary nodules preceding rheumatoid arthritis. Rheumatology 7:89, 1987.
254. Mole TM, Glover J, Sheppard MN: Sclerosing mediastinitis: A report on 18 cases. Thorax 50:280, 1995.
255. Jurik AG, Graudal H: Pericarditis in rheumatoid arthritis: A clinical and radiological study. Rheumatol Int 6:37, 1986.
256. Sakkas LI, Chen PF, Platsoucas CD: T-cell antigen receptors in rheumatoid arthritis. Immunol Res 13:117, 1994.
257. Panayi GS: The pathogenesis of rheumatoid arthritis: From molecules to the whole patient. Br J Rheumatol 32:533, 1993.
258. Small P: Rheumatoid arthritis—an infectious disease? Ann Allergy 60:377, 1988.
259. Ziff M: Role of endothelium in the pathogenesis of rheumatoid synovitis. Int J Tissue React 15:135, 1993.
260. Postigo AA, Garcia-Vicuna R, Laffon A, et al: The role of adhesion molecules in the pathogenesis of rheumatoid arthritis. Autoimmunity 16:69, 1993.
261. Muller-Ladner U: T-cell–independent cellular pathways of rheumatoid joint destruction. Curr Opin Rheumatol 7:222, 1995.
262. Das UN: Interaction(s) between essential fatty acids, eicosanoids, cytokines, growth factors, and free radicals: Relevance to new therapeutic strategies in rheumatoid arthritis and other collagen vascular diseases. Prostaglandins Leukot Essent Fatty Acids 44:201, 1991.
263. Feldmann M, Brennan FM, Elliot M, et al: TNF-alpha as a therapeutic target in rheumatoid arthritis. Circ Shock 43:179, 1994.
264. Feldmann M, Brennan FM, Williams RO, et al: Evaluation of the role of cytokines in autoimmune disease: The importance of TNF-alpha in rheumatoid arthritis. Prog Growth Factor Res 4:247, 1992.
265. Brennan FM, Feldmann M: Cytokines in autoimmunity. Curr Opin Immunol 4:754, 1992.
266. Kalsi J, Isenberg D: Rheumatoid factor. Primary or secondary event in the pathogenesis of RA. Int Arch Allergy Immunol 102:209, 1993.
267. Turner-Warwick M, Parkes WR: Circulating rheumatoid and antinuclear factors in asbestos workers. BMJ 3:492, 1970.
268. Turner-Warwick M, Doniach D: Auto-antibody studies in interstitial pulmonary fibrosis. BMJ 1:886, 1965.
269. Kanok JM, Steinberg P, Cassidy JT, et al: Serum IgE levels in patients with selective IgA deficiency. Ann Allergy 41:220, 1978.
270. Wells AU, Hansell DM, du Bois RM: Interstitial lung disease in the collagen vascular diseases. Semin Respir Med 14:33, 1993.
271. Kolarz G, Scherak O, Popp W, et al: Bronchoalveolar lavage in rheumatoid arthritis. Br J Rheumatol 32:556, 1993.
272. Kelly CA: Rheumatoid arthritis: Other rheumatoid lung problems. Baillieres Clin Rheumatol 7:17, 1993.
273. DeHoratius RJ, Abruzzo JL, Williams RC Jr: Immunofluorescent and immunologic studies of rheumatoid lung. Arch Intern Med 129:441, 1972.
274. Gosset P, Perez T, Lassalle P, et al: Increased TNF-alpha secretion by alveolar macrophages from patients with rheumatoid arthritis. Am Rev Respir Dis 143:593, 1991.
275. Garcia JGN, James HL, Zinkgraf S, et al: Lower respiratory tract abnormalities in rheumatoid interstitial lung disease. Am Rev Respir Dis 136:811, 1987.
276. Casale TB, Little MM, Furst D, et al: Elevated BAL fluid histamine levels and parenchymal pulmonary disease in rheumatoid arthritis. Chest 96:1016, 1989.
277. Da Silva JA, Hall GM: The effects of gender and sex hormones on outcome in rheumatoid arthritis. Baillieres Clin Rheumatol 6:196, 1992.
278. Charles PJ, Sweatman MC, Markwicj JR, et al: HLA-B40—a marker for susceptibility to lung disease in rheumatoid arthritis. Dis Markers 9:97, 1991.
279. Hakala M, Ruuska P, Hameenkorpi R, et al: Diffuse interstitial lung disease in rheumatoid arthritis: Views on immunological and HLA findings. Scand J Rheumatol 15:368, 1986.
280. Scherak O, Popp W, Kolarz G, et al: Bronchoalveolar lavage and lung biopsy in rheumatoid arthritis: In vivo effects of disease modifying antirheumatic drugs. J Rheumatol 20:944, 1993.
281. Scadding JG: The lungs in rheumatoid arthritis. Proc R Soc Med 62:227, 1969.
282. Hakala M, Pääkkö P, Huhti E, et al: Open lung biopsy of patients with rheumatoid arthritis. Clin Rheumatol 9:452, 1990.

283. Nozawa Y: Histopathological findings of the lung in collagen disease, especially on their differential diagnosis. Acta Pathol Jpn 22:843, 1972.

284. DeHoratius RJ, Abruzzo JL, Williams RC Jr: Immunofluorescent and immunologic studies of rheumatoid lung. Arch Intern Med 129:441, 1972.

285. Yousem SA, Colby TV, Carrington CB: Lung biopsy in rheumatoid arthritis. Am Rev Respir Dis 131:770, 1985.

286. Cruickshank B: Interstitial pneumonia and its consequences in rheumatoid disease. Br J Dis Chest 53:226, 1959.

287. Walker WC, Wright V: Rheumatoid pleuritis. Ann Rheum Dis 26:467, 1967.

288. Frank ST, Weg JG, Harkleroad LE, Fitch RF: Pulmonary dysfunction in rheumatoid disease. Chest 63:27, 1973.

289. Jurik AG, Davidsen D, Graudal H: Prevalence of pulmonary involvement in rheumatoid arthritis and its relationship to some characteristics of the patients—a radiological and clinical study. Scand J Rheumatol 11:217, 1982.

290. Turner-Warwick M, Burrows B, Johnson A: Cryptogenic fibrosing alveolitis: clinical features and their influence on survival. Thorax 35:171, 1980.

291. Staples CA, Müller NL, Vedal S, et al: Usual interstitial pneumonia: correlation of CT with clinical, functional, and radiologic findings. Radiology 162:377, 1987.

292. Locke CB: Rheumatoid lung. Clin Radiol 14:43, 1963.

293. Steinberg DL, Webb WR: CT appearances of rheumatoid lung disease. J Comput Assist Tomogr 8:881, 1984.

294. Remy-Jardin M, Remy J, Cortet B, et al: Lung changes in rheumatoid arthritis: CT findings. Radiology 193:375, 1994.

295. Popper MS, Bogdonoff ML, Hughes RL: Interstitial rheumatoid lung disease: A reassessment and review of the literature. Chest 62:243, 1972.

296. Cudkowicz L, Madoff IM, Abelmann WH: Rheumatoid lung disease: A case report which includes respiratory function studies and a lung biopsy. Br J Dis Chest 55:35, 1961.

297. Patterson CD, Harville WE, Pierce JA: Rheumatoid lung disease. Ann Intern Med 62:685, 1965.

298. Robertson JL, Brinkman GL: Nodular rheumatoid lung disease. Am J Med 31:483, 1961.

299. Brannan HM, Good CA, Divertie MB, et al: Pulmonary disease associated with rheumatoid arthritis. JAMA 189:914, 1964.

300. Lee FI, Brain AT: Chronic diffuse interstitial pulmonary fibrosis and rheumatoid arthritis. Lancet 2:693, 1962.

301. Sievers K, Aho K, Hurri L, et al: Studies of rheumatoid pulmonary disease: A comparison of roentgenological findings among patients with high rheumatoid factor titers and with completely negative reactions. Acta Tubercul Scand 45:21, 1964.

302. Hakala M: Poor prognosis in patients with rheumatoid arthritis hospitalized for interstitial lung fibrosis. Chest 93:114, 1988.

303. Ognibene AJ: Systemic "rheumatoid disease" with interstitial pulmonary fibrosis: A report of two cases. Arch Intern Med 105:762, 1960.

304. Petty TL, Wilkins M: The five manifestations of rheumatoid lung. Dis Chest 49:75, 1966.

305. Strohl KP, Feldman NT, Ingram RH Jr: Apical fibrobullous disease with rheumatoid arthritis. Chest 75:739, 1979.

306. McCann BG, Hart GJ, Stokes TC, et al: Obliterative bronchiolitis and upper-zone pulmonary consolidation in rheumatoid arthritis. Thorax 38:73, 1983.

307. Yue CC, Park CH, Kushner I: Apical fibrocavitary lesions of the lung in rheumatoid arthritis: Report of two cases and review of the literature. Am J Med 81:741, 1986.

308. Ellman P, Cudkowicz L, Elwood JS: Widespread serous membrane involvement by rheumatoid nodules. J Clin Pathol 7:239, 1954.

309. Burrows FGO: Pulmonary nodules in rheumatoid disease: A report of two cases. Br J Radiol 40:256, 1967.

310. Sienewicz DJ, Martin JR, Moore S, et al: Rheumatoid nodules in the lung. J Can Assoc Radiol 13:73, 1962.

311. Dumas LW, Gregory RL, Ozer FL: Case of rheumatoid lung with cavity formation. BMJ 1:383, 1963.

312. Hayakawa H, Sato A, Imokawa S, et al: Bronchiolar disease in rheumatoid arthritis. Am J Respir Crit Care Med 154:1531, 1996.

313. Walters MN, Ojeda VJ: Pleuropulmonary necrobiotic rheumatoid nodules: A review and clinicopathological study of six patients. Med J Aust 144:648, 1986.

314. Johnson TS, White P, Weiss ST, et al: Endobronchial necrobiotic nodule antedating rheumatoid arthritis. Chest 82:199, 1982.

315. Tserkezoglou A, Metakidis S, Papastamatiou-Tsimara H, et al: Solitary rheumatoid nodule of the pleura and rheumatoid pleural effusion. Thorax 33:769, 1978.

316. Perez T, Remy-Jardin M, Cortet B: Airways involvement in rheumatoid arthritis: Clinical, functional, and HRCT findings. Am J Respir Crit Care Med 157:1658, 1998.

317. Shannon TM, Gale ME: Noncardiac manifestations of rheumatoid arthritis in the thorax. J Thorac Imaging 7:19, 1992.

318. Portner MM, Gracie WA Jr: Rheumatoid lung disease with cavitary nodules, pneumothorax, and eosinophilia. N Engl J Med 275:697, 1966.

319. Morgan WKC, Wolfel DA: The lungs and pleura in rheumatoid arthritis. Am J Roentgenol 98:334, 1966.

320. Stengel BF, Watson RA, Darling RJ: Pulmonary rheumatoid nodule with cavitation and chronic lipid effusion. JAMA 198:1263, 1966.

321. Rubin EH, Gordon M, Thelmo WL: Nodular pleuropulmonary rheumatoid disease: Report of two cases and review of the literature. Am J Med 42:567, 1967.

322. Jones JS: An account of pleural effusions, pulmonary nodules, and cavities attributable to rheumatoid disease. Br J Dis Chest 72:39, 1978.

323. McConnochie K, O'Sullivan M, Khalil JF, et al: *Aspergillus* colonization of pulmonary rheumatoid nodule. Respir Med 83:157, 1989.

324. Burke GW, Carrington CB, Grinnan R: Pulmonary nodules and rheumatoid factor in the absence of arthritis. Chest 72:538, 1977.

325. Jolles H, Moseley PL, Peterson MW: Nodular pulmonary opacities in patients with rheumatoid arthritis. Chest 96:1022, 1989.

326. Caplan A: Certain unusual radiological appearances in the chest of coal miners suffering from rheumatoid arthritis. Thorax 8:29, 1953.

327. Constantinidis K: Pneumoconiosis and rheumatoid arthritis: Caplan's syndrome. Br J Clin Pract 31:25, 1977.

328. Chatgidakis CB, Theron CP: Rheumatoid pneumoconiosis (Caplan's syndrome): A discussion of the disease and a report of a case in a European Witwatersrand gold miner. Arch Environ Health 2:397, 1961.

329. Caplan A, Cowen EDH, Gough J: Rheumatoid pneumoconiosis in a foundry worker. Thorax 13:181, 1958.

330. Campbell JA: A case of Caplan's syndrome in a boiler-scaler. Thorax 13:177, 1958.

331. Hayes DS, Posner E: A case of Caplan's syndrome in a roof tile maker. Tubercle 41:143, 1960.

332. Rickards AG, Barrett GM: Rheumatoid lung changes associated with asbestosis. Thorax 13:185, 1958.

333. Morgan WKC: Rheumatoid pneumoconiosis in association with abestosis. Thorax 19:433, 1964.

334. Greaves IA: Rheumatoid "pneumoconiosis" (Caplan's syndrome) in an asbestos worker: A 17 years' follow-up. Thorax 34:404, 1979.

335. Jordan JW: Pulmonary fibrosis in a worker using an aluminum powder. Br J Industr Med 18:21, 1961.

336. Wells IP, Bhatt RC, Flanagan M: Kaolinosis: A radiological review. Clin Radiol 36:579, 1985.

337. Anttila S, Sutinen S, Paakko P: Rheumatoid pneumoconiosis in a dolomite worker: A light and electron microscopic and x-ray microanalytical study. Br J Dis Chest 78:195, 1984.

338. Lindars DC, Davies D: Rheumatoid pneumoconiosis: A study in colliery populations in the East Midlands coal field. Thorax 22:525, 1967.

339. Fritze E, Dickmans H: Pneumoconiosis causing a round infiltrate. Radiologe 2:270, 1964.

340. Miall WE, Caplan A, Cochrane AL, et al: An epidemiological study of rheumatoid arthritis associated with characteristic chest x-ray appearances in coal workers. BMJ 2:1231, 1953.

341. Dines DE: Pulmonary disease of vascular origin. Dis Chest 54:3, 1968.

342. Benedek TG: Rheumatoid pneumoconiosis: Documentation of onset and pathogenic considerations. Am J Med 55:515, 1973.

343. Darke C, Wagner MMF, Nuki G, et al: HLA-A, -B, and -DR antigens and properdin factor B allotypes in Caplan's syndrome. Br J Dis Chest 77:235, 1983.

344. Gough J, Rivers D, Seal RME: Pathological studies of modified pneumoconiosis in coal miners with rheumatoid arthritis (Caplan's syndrome). Thorax 10:9, 1955.

345. Hurd ER: Extraarticular manifestations of rheumatoid arthritis. Semin Arthritis Rheum 8:151, 1979.

346. Ramirez-R J, Lopez-Majano V, Schultze G: Caplan's syndrome: A clinicopathologic study. Am J Med 37:643, 1964.

347. Walker WC, Wright V: Rheumatoid pleuritis. Ann Rheum Dis 26:467, 1967.

348. Ward R: Pleural effusion and rheumatoid disease. Lancet 2:1336, 1961.

349. Carr DT, Mayne JG: Pleurisy with effusion in rheumatoid arthritis, with reference to the low concentration of glucose in pleural fluid. Am Rev Respir Dis 85:345, 1962.

350. Mays EE: Rheumatoid pleuritis: Observations in eight cases and suggestions for making the diagnosis in patients without the "typical findings." Dis Chest 53:202, 1968.

351. Campbell GD, Ferrington E: Rheumatoid pleuritis with effusion. Dis Chest 53:521, 1968.

352. Berger HW, Seckler SG: Pleural and pericardial effusions in rheumatoid disease. Ann Intern Med 64:1291, 1966.

353. Faurschou P, Francis D, Faarup P: Thoracoscopic, histological, and clinical findings in nine cases of rheumatoid pleural effusion. Thorax 40:371, 1985.

354. Aru A, Engel U, Francis D: Characteristic and specific histological findings in rheumatoid pleurisy. Acta Pathol Microbiol Immunol Scand 94:57, 1986.

355. Schwarz MI, Zamora MR, Hodges TN, et al: Isolated pulmonary capillaritis and diffuse alveolar hemorrhage in rheumatoid arthritis and mixed connective tissue disease. Chest 113:1609, 1998.

356. Nosanchuk JS, Naylor B: A unique cytologic picture in pleural fluid from patients with rheumatoid arthritis. Am J Clin Pathol 50:330, 1968.

357. Becker SN: Cytodiagnosis of rheumatoid pleural effusion. Cleve Clin Q 50:445, 1983.

358. Pettersson T, Soderblom T, Nyberg P, et al: Pleural fluid soluble interleukin-2 receptor in rheumatoid arthritis and systemic lupus erythematosus. J Rheumatol 21:1820, 1994.

359. Montes S, Guasrda LA: Cytology of pleural effusions in rheumatoid arthritis. Diagn Cytopathol 4:71, 1988.

360. Martel W, Abell MR, Mikkelsne WM, et al: Pulmonary and pleural lesions in rheumatoid disease. Radiology 90:641, 1968.

361. Brennan SR, Daly JJ: Large pleural effusions in rheumatoid arthritis. Br J Dis Chest 73:133, 1979.

362. Pritkin JD, Jensen WA, Yenokida GG, et al: Respiratory failure due to a massive rheumatoid effusion. J Rheumatol 17:673, 1990.

363. Lee PR, Sox HC, North FS, et al: Pleurisy with effusion in rheumatoid arthritis. Arch Intern Med 104:634, 1959.

364. Faurschou P, Francis D, Faarup P: Thoracoscopic, histologic, and clinical findings in nine cases of rheumatoid pleural effusion. Thorax 40:371, 1985.

365. Leading article: Pleurisy and rheumatoid arthritis. BMJ 2:1, 1968.
366. Locke CB: Rheumatoid lung. Clin Radiol 14:43, 1963.
367. Torrington KG: Rapid appearance of rheumatoid pleural effusion. Chest 73:409, 1978.
368. Pritikin JD, Jensen WA, Yenokida GG, et al: Respiratory failure due to a massive rheumatoid pleural effusion. J Rheumatol 17:673, 1990.
369. Grossman LA, Kaplan HJ, Ownby FD, et al: Acute pericarditis: With subsequent clinical rheumatoid arthritis. Arch Intern Med 109:665, 1962.
370. Schools GS, Mikkelsen WM: Rheumatoid pleuritis. Arthritis Rheum 5:369, 1962.
371. Adelman HM, Dupont EL, Flannery MT, et al: Case report: Recurrent pneumothorax in a patient with rheumatoid arthritis. Am J Med Sci 308:171, 1994.
372. Vergnenegre A, Pugnere N, Antonini MT, et al: Airway obstruction and rheumatoid arthritis. Eur Respir J 10:1072, 1997.
373. Hassan WU, Keaney NP, Holland CD, et al: Bronchial reactivity and airflow obstruction in rheumatoid arthritis. Ann Rheum Dis 53:511, 1994.
374. Geddes DM, Corrin B, Brewerton DA, et al: Progressive airway obliteration in adults and its association with rheumatoid disease. Q J Med 46:427, 1977.
375. Begin R, Masse S, Cantin A, et al: Airway disease in a subset of nonsmoking rheumatoid patients: Characterization of the disease and evidence for an autoimmune pathogenesis. Am J Med 72:743, 1982.
376. Lahdensuo A, Mattila J, Vilppula A: Bronchiolitis in rheumatoid arthritis. Chest 85:705, 1984.
377. Jacobs P, Bonnyns M, Depierreux M, et al: Rapidly fatal bronchiolitis obliterans with circulating antinuclear and rheumatoid factors. Eur J Resp Dis 65:384, 1984.
378. Hayakawa H, Sato A, Imokawa S, et al: Bronchiolar disease in rheumatoid arthritis. Am J Respir Crit Care Med 154:1531, 1996.
379. Hakala M, Paakko P, Sutinen S, et al: Association of bronchiolitis with connective tissue disorders. Ann Rheum Dis 45:656, 1986.
380. Scott TE, Wise RA, Hochberg MC, et al: HLA-DR4 and pulmonary dysfunction in rheumatoid arthritis. Am J Med 82:765, 1987.
381. Radoux V, Menard HA, Begin R, et al: Airway disease in rheumatoid arthritis patients: One element of a general exocrine dysfunction. Arthritis Rheum 30:249, 1987.
382. Sweatman MC, Markwick JR, Charles PJ, et al: Histocompatibility antigens in adult obliterative bronchiolitis with or without rheumatoid arthritis. Dis Markers 4:19, 1986.
383. Murphy KC, Atkins CJ, Offer RC, et al: Obliterative bronchiolitis in two rheumatoid arthritis patients treated with penicillamine. Arthritis Rheum 24:557, 1981.
384. Lyle WH: D-Penicillamine and fatal obliterative bronchiolitis. Lancet 1:105, 1977.
385. Epler GR, Snider GC, Gainsler EH, et al: Bronchiolitis and bronchitis in connective tissue disease, a possible relationship to the use of penicillamine. JAMA 242:528, 1979.
386. Stein HC, Patternson AC, Offer RC, et al: Adverse effects of D-penicillamine in rheumatoid arthritis. Ann Intern Med 92:24, 1980.
387. Holness L, Tenenbaum J, Cooter NBE, et al: Fatal bronchiolitis obliterans associated with chrysotherapy. Ann Rheum Dis 42:593, 1983.
388. Halla JT, Cassady J, Hardin JG: Sequential gold and penicillamine therapy in rheumatoid arthritis: Comparative study of effectiveness and toxicity and review of the literature. Am J Med 72:423, 1982.
389. Cooke NT, Bamji AN: Gold and pulmonary function in rheumatoid arthritis. Br J Rheumatol 22:18, 1983.
390. Herzog CA, Miller RR, Hoidal JR: Case reports: Bronchiolitis and rheumatoid arthritis. Am Rev Respir Dis 124:636, 1981.
391. Aquino SL, Webb RW, Golden J: Bronchiolitis obliterans associated with rheumatoid arthritis: Findings on HRCT and dynamic expiratory CT. J Comput Assist Tomogr 18:555, 1994.
392. Padley SPG, Adler BD, Hansell DM, Müller NL: Bronchiolitis obliterans: High-resolution CT findings and correlation with pulmonary function tests. Clin Radiol 47:236, 1993.
393. Wells AU, du Bois RM: Bronchiolitis in association with connective tissue disorders. Clin Chest Med 14:655, 1993.
394. Jacobs P, Bonnyns M, Depierreux M, et al: Rapidly fatal bronchiolitis obliterans with circulating antinuclear and rheumatoid factors. Eur J Resp Dis 65:384, 1984.
395. Schwarz MI, Lynch DA, Tuder R: Bronchiolitis obliterans—the lone manifestation of rheumatoid arthritis? Eur Respir J 7:817, 1994.
396. Rees JH, Woodhead MA, Sheppard MN, et al: Rheumatoid arthritis and cryptogenic organising pneumonitis. Respir Med 85:243, 1991.
397. van Thiel RJ, van der Burg S, Groote AD, et al: Bronchiolitis obliterans organizing pneumonia and rheumatoid arthritis. Eur Respir J 4:905, 1991.
398. Ippolito JA, Palmer L, Spector S, et al: Bronchiolitis obliterans organizing pneumonia and rheumatoid arthritis. Semin Arthritis Rheum 23:70, 1993.
399. Yousem SA, Colby TV, Carrington CB: Follicular bronchitis/bronchiolitis. Hum Pathol 16:700, 1985.
400. Fortoul TI, Cano-Valle F, Oliva E, et al: Follicular bronchiolitis in association with connective tissue diseases. Lung 163:305, 1985.
401. Franchi LM, Chin TW, Nussbaum E, et al: Familial pulmonary nodular lymphoid hyperplasia. J Pediatr 121:89, 1992.
402. Kinoshita M, Higashi T, Tanaka C, et al: Follicular bronchiolitis associated with rheumatoid arthritis. Int Med 31:674, 1992.
403. Bamji A, Cooke N: Rheumatoid arthritis and chronic bronchial suppuration. Scand J Rheum 14:15, 1985.
404. Solanki T, Neville E: Bronchiectasis and rheumatoid disease: Is there an association? Br J Rheumatol 31:691, 1992.
405. Bate AS, Sidebottom D, Cooper RG, et al: DNA variants of alpha₁-antitrypsin in rheumatoid arthritis with and without pulmonary complications. Dis Markers 8:317, 1990.
406. Despaux J, Polio JC, Toussirot E, et al: Rheumatoid arthritis and bronchiectasis: A retrospective study of 14 cases. Rev Rhum Engl Ed 63:801, 1996.
407. McMahon MJ, Swinson DR, Shettar S, et al: Bronchiectasis and rheumatoid arthritis: A clinical study. Ann Rheum Dis 52:776, 1993.
408. Shadick NA, Fanta CH, Weinblatt ME, et al: Bronchiectasis: A late feature of severe rheumatoid arthritis. Medicine (Baltimore) 73:161, 1994.
409. Hassan WU, Keaney NP, Holland CD, et al: High-resolution computed tomography of the lung in lifelong non-smoking patients with rheumatoid arthritis. Ann Rheum Dis 54:308, 1995.
410. McDonagh J, Greaves M, Wright AR, et al: High-resolution computed tomography of the lungs in patients with rheumatoid arthritis and interstitial lung disease. Br J Rheumatol 33:118, 1994.
411. Blosser S, Wigley FM, Wise RA: Increase in translaryngeal resistance during phonation in rheumatoid arthritis. Chest 102:387, 1992.
412. Oyama T, Okuda Y, Oyama H, et al: Sleep apnea syndrome in rheumatoid arthritis (RA) patients complicated with cervical and temporomandibular lesions. Ryumachi 35:3, 1995.
413. Heath D, Gillund TD, Kay JM, et al: Pulmonary vascular disease in honeycomb lung. J Pathol Bacteriol 95:423, 1968.
414. Jordan JD, Snyder CH: Rheumatoid disease of the lung and cor pulmonale: Observations in a child. Am J Dis Child 108:174, 1964.
415. Gardner DL, Duthie JJR, MacLeod J, et al: Pulmonary hypertension in rheumatoid disease: Report of a case with intimal sclerosis of the pulmonary and digital arteries. Scot Med J 2:183, 1957.
416. Kay JM, Banik S: Unexplained pulmonary hypertension with pulmonary arteritis in rheumatoid disease. Br J Dis Chest 71:63, 1977.
417. Padeh S, Laxer RM, Silver MM, et al: Primary pulmonary hypertension in a patient with systemic-onset juvenile arthritis. Arthritis Rheum 34:1575, 1991.
418. Baydur A, Mongan ES, Slager UT: Acute respiratory failure and pulmonary arteritis without parenchymal involvement: Demonstration in a patient with rheumatoid arthritis. Chest 75:518, 1979.
419. Armstrong JG, Steele RH: Localised pulmonary arteritis in rheumatoid disease. Thorax 37:313, 1982.
420. Morikawa J, Kitamura K, Habuchi Y, et al: Pulmonary hypertension in a patient with rheumatoid arthritis. Chest 93:876, 1988.
421. Young ID, Ford SE, Ford PM: The association of pulmonary hypertension with rheumatoid arthritis. J Rheumatol 16:1266, 1989.
422. Balagopal VP, da Costa P, Greenstone MA: Fatal pulmonary hypertension and rheumatoid vasculitis. Eur Respir J 8:331, 1995.
423. Scott DGI, Bacon PA, Tribe CR: Systemic rheumatoid vasculitis: A clinical and laboratory study of 50 cases. Medicine (Baltimore) 60:288, 1981.
424. Sokoloff L, Bunim JJ: Vascular lesions in rheumatoid arthritis. J Chronic Dis 5:668, 1957.
425. Torralbo A, Herrero JA, Portoles J, et al: Alveolar hemorrhage associated with antineutrophil cytoplasmic antibodies in rheumatoid arthritis. Chest 105:1590, 1994.
426. Cambridge G, Williams M, Leaker B, et al: Anti-myeloperoxidase antibodies in patients with rheumatoid arthritis: Prevalence, clinical correlates, and IgG subclass. Ann Rheum Dis 53:24, 1994.
427. Jasin HE, LoSpalluto J, Ziff M: Rheumatoid hyperviscosity syndrome. Am J Med 49:484, 1970.
428. Eaton AM, Serota H, Kernodle GW, et al: Pulmonary hypertension secondary to serum hyperviscosity in a patient with rheumatoid arthritis. Am J Med 82:1039, 1987.
429. Hellems SO, Kanner RE, Renzetti Jr AD: Bronchocentric granulomatosis associated with rheumatoid arthritis. Chest 83:831, 1983.
430. Sumiya M, Ohya N, Shinoura H, et al: Diffuse interstitial pulmonary amyloidosis in rheumatoid arthritis. J Rheumatol 23:933, 1996.
431. Bégin R, Radoux V, Cantin A, et al: Stiffness of the rib cage in a subset of rheumatoid patients. Lung 166:141, 1988.
432. Gorini M, Ginanni R, Spinelli A, et al: Inspiratory muscle strength and respiratory drive in patients with rheumatoid arthritis. Am Rev Respir Dis 142:289, 1990.
433. Prior P, Symmons DPM, Scott DL, et al: Cause of death in rheumatoid arthritis. Br J Rheumatol 23:92, 1984.
434. Mutru O, Laakso M, Isomaki H, et al: Ten-year mortality and causes of death in patients with rheumatoid arthritis. BMJ 290:1797, 1985.
435. Vandenbroucke JP, Hazevoet HM, Cats A: Survival and cause of death in rheumatoid arthritis: A 25-year prospective follow-up. J Rheumatol 11:158, 1984.
436. Toyoshima H, Kusaba T, Yamaguchi M: Cause of death in autopsied RA patients. Ryumachi 33:209, 1993.
437. Barrera P, Laan RF, van Riel PL, et al: Methotrexate-related pulmonary complications in rheumatoid arthritis. Ann Rheum Dis 53:434, 1994.
438. Wollner A, Mohle-Boetani J, Lambert RE, et al: *Pneumocystis carinii* pneumonia complicating low-dose methotrexate treatment for rheumatoid arthritis. Thorax 46:205, 1991.
439. O'Reilly S, Hartley P, Jeffers M, et al: Invasive pulmonary aspergillosis associated with low-dose methotrexate therapy for rheumatoid arthritis: A case report of treatment with itraconazole. Tubercle Lung Dis 75:153, 1994.
440. Cornelissen JJ, Bakker LJ, Van der Veen MJ, et al: *Nocardia asteroides* pneumonia complicating low-dose methotrexate treatment of refractory rheumatoid arthritis. Ann Rheum Dis 50:642, 1991.

441. Matteson EL, Hickey AR, Maguire L, et al: Occurrence of neoplasia in patients with rheumatoid arthritis enrolled in a DMARD Registry. Rheumatoid Arthritis Azathioprine Registry Steering Committee. J Rheumatol 18:809, 1991.

442. Athreya BH, Doughty RA, Bookspan M, et al: Pulmonary manifestations of juvenile rheumatoid arthritis. Clin Chest Med 1:361, 1980.

443. Pelucchi A, Lomater C, Gerloni V, et al: Lung function and diffusing capacity for carbon monoxide in patients with juvenile chronic arthritis: Effect of disease activity and low-dose methotrexate therapy. Clin Exp Rheumatol 12:675, 1994.

444. Maddison PJ, Stephens C, Briggs D, et al: Connective tissue disease and autoantibodies in the kindreds of 63 patients with systemic sclerosis. Medicine (Baltimore) 72:103, 1993.

445. Masi AT, D'Angelo WA: Epidemiology of fatal systemic sclerosis (diffuse scleroderma): A 15-year survey in Baltimore. Ann Intern Med 66:870, 1967.

446. Medsger TA Jr, Masi AT: Epidemiology of systemic sclerosis (scleroderma). Ann Intern Med 74:714, 1971.

447. Huang CT, Lyons HA: Comparison of pulmonary function in patients with systemic lupus erythematosus, scleroderma, and rheumatoid arthritis. Am Rev Respir Dis 93:865, 1966.

448. Bianchi FA, Bistue AR, Wendt VE, et al: Analysis of twenty-seven cases of progressive systemic sclerosis (including two with combined systemic lupus erythematosus) and a review of the literature. J Chron Dis 19:953, 1966.

449. Adhikari PK, Bianchi FA, Boushy SF, et al: Pulmonary function in scleroderma: Its relation to changes in the chest roentgenogram and the skin of the thorax. Am Rev Respir Dis 86:823, 1962.

450. Wilson RJ, Rodnan GP, Robin ED: An early pulmonary physiologic abnormality in progressive systemic sclerosis (diffuse scleroderma). Am J Med 36:361, 1964.

451. Miller RD, Fowler WS, Helmholz FH Jr: Scleroderma of the lungs. Proc Mayo Clin 34:66, 1959.

452. Steen VD, Conte C, Owens GR, et al: Severe restrictive lung disease in systemic sclerosis. Arthritis Rheum 37:1283, 1994.

453. Harrison NK, Glanville AR, Strickland B, et al: Pulmonary involvement in systemic sclerosis: The detection of early changes by thin-section CT scan, bronchoalveolar lavage, and Tc-DTPA clearance. Respir Med 83:403, 1989.

454. Dellafiore L, Colombo B, Del Sante M, et al: Pulmonary involvement in scleroderma assessed with high-resolution computerized tomography and functional tests. Radiol Med 87:608, 1994.

455. Frigieri L, Mormile F, Grilli N, et al: Bilateral bronchoalveolar lavage in progressive systemic sclerosis: Interlobar variability, lymphocyte subpopulations, and functional correlations. Respiration 58:132, 1991.

456. Yurovsky VV, Sutton PA, Schulze DH, et al: Expansion of selected V delta 1 + gamma delta T cells in systemic sclerosis patients. J Immunol 153:881, 1994.

457. Gudbjornsson B, Hallgren R, Nettelbladt O, et al: Phenotypic and functional activation of alveolar macrophages, T lymphocytes, and NK cells in patients with systemic sclerosis and primary Sjögren's syndrome. Ann Rheum Dis 53:574, 1994.

458. Wallaert B, Bart F, Aerts C, et al: Activated macrophages in subclinical pulmonary inflammation in collagen vascular diseases. Thorax 43:24, 1988.

459. Martinot JB, Wallaert B, Hatron PY, et al: Clinical and subclinical alveolitis in collagen vascular diseases: Contribution of alpha₂-macroglobulin levels in BAL fluid. Eur Respir J 2:437, 1989.

460. Harrison NK, Myers Ar, Corrin B, et al: Structural features of interstitial lung disease in systemic sclerosis. Am Rev Respir Dis 144:706, 1991.

461. Silver RM, Miller KS, Kinsella MB, et al: Evaluation and management of scleroderma lung disease using bronchoalveolar lavage. Am J Med 88:470, 1990.

462. Kahaleh MB: Raynaud's phenomenon and vascular disease in scleroderma. Curr Opin Rheumatol 6:621, 1994.

463. Wells AU, Hansell DM, Rubens MB, et al: Fibrosing alveolitis in systemic sclerosis. Am J Respir Crit Care Med 150:462, 1994.

464. Behr J, Vogelmeier C, Beinert T, et al: Bronchoalveolar lavage for evaluation and management of scleroderma disease of the lung. Am J Respir Crit Care Med 154:400, 1996.

465. Imokawa S, Sato A, Hayakawa H, et al: Tissue factor expression and fibrin deposition in the lungs of patients with idiopathic pulmonary fibrosis and systemic sclerosis. Am J Respir Crit Care Med 156:631, 1997.

466. Harrison NK, Cambrey AD, Myers AR, et al: Insulin-like growth factor-I is partially responsible for fibroblast proliferation induced by bronchoalveolar lavage fluid from patients with systemic sclerosis. Clin Sci 86:141, 1994.

467. Corrin B, Butcher D, McAnulty BJ, et al: Immunohistochemical localization of transforming growth factor-beta₁ in the lungs of patients with systemic sclerosis, cryptogenic fibrosing alveolitis and other lung disorders. Histopathology 24:145, 1994.

468. Deguchi Y, Kishimoto S: Spontaneous activation of transforming growth factor-beta gene transcription in bronchoalveolar mononuclear cells of individuals with systemic autoimmune diseases with lung involvement. Lupus 1:27, 1991.

469. Deguchi Y: Spontaneous increase of transforming growth factor beta production of bronchoalveolar mononuclear cells of patients with systemic autoimmune disease affecting the lung. Ann Rheum Dis 51:362, 1992.

470. Ludwicka A, Trojanowska M, Smith EA, et al: Growth and characterization of fibroblasts obtained from bronchoalveolar lavage of patients with scleroderma. J Rheumatol 19:1716, 1992.

471. Bolster MB, Ludwicka A, Sutherland SE, et al: Cytokine concentrations in bronchoalveolar lavage fluid of patients with systemic sclerosis. Arthritis Rheum 40:743, 1997.

471a. Hasegawa M, Sato S, Fujimoto M, et al: Serum levels of interleukin 6 (IL-6), oncostatin M, soluble IL-6 receptor, and soluble gp130 in patients with systemic sclerosis. J Rheumatol 25:308, 1998.

472. Crestani B, Seta N, Palazzo E, et al: Interleukin-8 and neutrophils in systemic sclerosis with lung involvement. Am J Respir Crit Care Med 150:1263, 1994.

473. Southcott AM, Jones KP, Li D, et al: Interleukin-8: Differential expression in lone fibrosing alveolitis and systemic sclerosis. Am J Respir Crit Care Med 151:1604, 1995.

474. Chanez P, Lacoste JY, Guillot B, et al: Mast cells' contribution to the fibrosing alveolitis of the scleroderma lung. Am Rev Respir Dis 147:1497, 1993.

475. Fritzler MJ, Kinsella TD: The CREST syndrome: A distinct serologic entity with anticentromere antibodies. Am J Med 69:520, 1980.

476. Kuwana M, Kaburaki J, Mimori T, et al: Autoantigenic epitopes on DNA topoisomerase I: Clinical and immunogenetic associations in systemic sclerosis. Arthritis Rheum 36:1406, 1993.

477. Spencer-Green G, Alter D, Welch HG: Test performance in systemic sclerosis: Anti-centromere and anti-Scl antibodies. Am J Med 103:242, 1997.

477a. Greidinger EL, Flaherty KT, White B, et al: African-American race and antibodies to topoisomerase I are associated with increased severity of scleroderma lung disease. Chest 114:801, 1998.

478. Okano Y, Steen VD, Medsger Jr TA: Autoantibody reactive with RNA polymerase III in systemic sclerosis. Ann Intern Med 119:1005, 1993.

479. Sato S, Ihn H, Kikuchi K, et al: Antihistone antibodies in systemic sclerosis: Association with pulmonary fibrosis. Arthritis Rheum 37:391, 1994.

480. Frieri M, Angadi C, Paolano A, et al: Altered T-cell subpopulations and lymphocytes expressing natural killer cell phenotypes in patients with progressive systemic sclerosis. J Allergy Clin Immunol 87:773, 1991.

481. Prior C, Haslam PL: In vivo levels and in vitro production of interferon-gamma in fibrosing interstitial lung diseases. Clin Exp Immunol 88:280, 1992.

482. Kikuchi K, Inh H, Sato S, et al: Serum concentration of procollagen type I carboxyterminal propeptide in systemic sclerosis. Arch Dermatol Res 286:77, 1994.

483. Morelli S, Ferri C, Polettini E, et al: Plasma endothelin-1 levels, pulmonary hypertension, and lung fibrosis in patients with systemic sclerosis. Am J Med 99:255, 1995.

484. Odoux C, Crestani B, Lebrun G, et al: Endothelin-1 secretion by alveolar macrophages in systemic sclerosis. Am J Respir Crit Care Med 156:1429, 1997.

485. Abraham DJ, Vancheeswaran R, Dashwood MR, et al: Increased levels of endothelin-1 and differential type A and B receptor expression in scleroderma-associated fibrotic lung disease. Am J Pathol 151:831, 1997.

486. Vancheeswaran R, Magoulas T, Efrat G, et al: Circulating endothelin-1 levels in systemic sclerosis subsets—a marker of fibrosis or vascular dysfunction? J Rheumatol 21:1838, 1994.

487. McGregor AR, Watson A, Yunis E, et al: Familial clustering of scleroderma spectrum disease. Am J Med 84:1023, 1988.

488. Sasaki T, Denpo K, Ono H, et al: HLA in systemic scleroderma (PSS) and familial scleroderma. J Dermatol 18:18, 1991.

489. Troshinsky MB, Kane GC, Varga J, et al: Pulmonary function and gastroesophageal reflux in systemic sclerosis. Ann Intern Med 121:6, 1994.

490. Leading article: Pathophysiology of Raynaud's phenomenon. BMJ 281:1027, 1980.

491. Kahaleh MB: Raynaud's phenomenon and vascular disease in scleroderma. Curr Opin Rheumatol 6:621, 1994.

492. Stranden E, Roald OK, Krohg K: Treatment of Raynaud's phenomenon with the 5-HT₂-receptor antagonist ketanserin. BMJ 285:1069, 1982.

493. Smith CD, McKendry RJR: Controlled trial of nifedipine in the treatment of Raynaud's phenomenon. Lancet 2:1299, 1982.

494. Naslund MJ, Pearson TA, Ritter JM: A documented episode of pulmonary vasoconstriction in systemic sclerosis. Johns Hopkins Med J 148:78, 1981.

495. Martin MFR, Tooke JE: Effects of prostaglandin E₁ on microvascular haemodynamics in progressive systemic sclerosis. BMJ 285:1688, 1982.

496. Clifford PC, Martin MFR, Sheddon EJ, et al: Treatment of vasospastic disease with prostaglandin E₁. BMJ 281:1031, 1980.

497. Miyazaki S, Miura K, Kasai Y, et al: Relief from digital vasospasm by treatment with captopril and its complete inhibition by serine proteinase inhibitors in Raynaud's phenomenon. BMJ 284:310, 1981.

497a. Cailes J, Winter S, du Bois RM, et al: Defective endothelially mediated pulmonary vasodilation in systemic sclerosis. Chest 114:178, 1998.

497b. Negi VS, Tripathy NK, Misra R, et al: Antiendothelial cell antibodies in scleroderma correlate with severe digital ischemia and pulmonary arterial hypertension. J Rheumatol 25:462, 1998.

498. Rodnan GP, Myerowitz RL, Justh GO: Morphologic changes in the digital arteries of patients with progressive systemic sclerosis (scleroderma) and Raynaud phenomenon. Medicine (Baltimore) 59:393, 1980.

499. Rawson AJ, Woske HM: A study of the etiologic factors in so-called primary pulmonary hypertension. Arch Intern Med 105:203, 1960.

500. Shuck JW, Oetgen WJ, Tesar JT: Pulmonary vascular response during Raynaud's phenomenon in progressive systemic sclerosis. Am J Med 78:221, 1985.

501. Wise RA, Wigley F, Newball HH, et al: The effect of cold exposure on diffusing capacity in patients with Raynaud phenomenon. Chest 81:695, 1982.

502. Miller MJ: Effect of the cold pressor test on diffusing capacity. Chest 84:26, 1983.

503. Vergnon JM, Barthélémy JC, Riffat J, et al: Raynaud's phenomenon of the lung. Chest 101:1312, 1992.

504. Thurm CA, Wigley FM, Dole WP, et al: Failure of vasodilator infusion to alter pulmonary diffusing capacity in systemic sclerosis. Am J Med 90:547, 1991.

505. Sfikakis PP, Kyriakidis MK, Vergos CG, et al: Cardiopulmonary hemodynamics in systemic sclerosis and response to nifedipine and captopril. Am J Med 90:541, 1991.

506. D'Angelo WA, Fries JF, Masi AT, et al: Pathologic observations in systemic sclerosis (scleroderma): A study of fifty-eight autopsy cases and fifty-eight matched controls. Am J Med 46:428, 1969.

507. Young RH, Mark GJ: Pulmonary vascular changes in scleroderma. Am J Med 64:998, 1978.

508. Harrison NK, Myers AR, Corrin B, et al: Structural features of interstitial lung disease in systemic sclerosis. Am Rev Respir Dis 144:706, 1991.

509. Bridges AJ, Hsu KC, Dias-Arias AA, et al: Bronchiolitis obliterans organizing pneumonia and scleroderma. J Rheumatol 19:1136, 1992.

510. Remy-Jardin M, Remy J, Wallaert B, Bataille D, Hatron PY: Pulmonary involvement in progressive systemic sclerosis: Sequential evaluation with CT, pulmonary function tests, and bronchoalveolar lavage. Radiology 188:499, 1993.

511. Kazemi H, Nash G: Progressive systemic sclerosis and pulmonary hypertension. N Engl J Med 286:91, 1972.

512. Stupi AM, Steen VD, Owens GR, et al: Pulmonary hypertension in the CREST syndrome variant of systemic sclerosis. Arthritis Rheum 29:515, 1986.

513. Rawson AJ, Woske HM: A study of the etiologic factors in so-called primary pulmonary hypertension. Arch Intern Med 105:233, 1960.

514. Naeye RL: Pulmonary vascular lesions in systemic scleroderma. Dis Chest 44:374, 1963.

515. Taormina VJ, Miller WT, Gefter WB, et al: Progressive systemic sclerosis subgroups: Variable pulmonary features. Am J Roentgenol 137:277, 1981.

516. Schurawitzki H, Stiglbauer R, Graninger W, et al: Interstitial lung disease in progressive systemic sclerosis: High-resolution CT versus radiography. Radiology 176:755, 1990.

517. Arroliga AC, Podell DN, Matthay RA: Pulmonary manifestations of scleroderma. J Thorac Imaging 7:30, 1992.

518. Warrick JH, Bhalla M, Schabel SI, Silver RM: High-resolution computed tomography in early scleroderma lung disease. J Rheumatol 18:1520, 1991.

519. Wells AU, Hansell DM, Corrin B, et al: High-resolution computed tomography as a predictor of lung histology in systemic sclerosis. Thorax 47:508, 1992.

520. Wells AU, Hansell DM, Rubens MB, et al: The predictive value of appearances on thin-section computed tomography in fibrosing alveolitis. Am Rev Respir Dis 148:1076, 1993.

521. Bhalla M, Silver RM, Shepard JAO, McLoud TC: Chest CT in patients with scleroderma: Prevalence of asymptomatic esophageal dilatation and mediastinal lymphadenopathy. Am J Roentgenol 161:269, 1993.

522. Wechsler RJ, Steiner RM, Spirn PW, et al: The relationship of thoracic lymphadenopathy to pulmonary interstitial disease in diffuse and limited systemic sclerosis: CT findings. Am J Roentgenol 167:101, 1996.

523. Opie LH: The pulmonary manifestations of generalised scleroderma (progressive systemic sclerosis). Dis Chest 28:665, 1955.

524. Owens GR, Fino GJ, Herbert DL, et al: Pulmonary function in progressive systemic sclerosis: Comparison of CREST syndrome variant with diffuse scleroderma. Chest 84:546, 1983.

525. McCarthy DS, Baragar FD, Dhingra S, et al: The lung in systemic sclerosis (scleroderma): A review and new information. Semin Arthritis Rheum 17:271, 1988.

526. Farmer RG, Gifford RW Jr, Hines EA Jr: Prognostic significance of Raynaud's phenomenon and other clinical characteristics of systemic sclerosis: A study of 271 cases. Circulation 21:1088, 1960.

527. Mahrer PR, Evans JA, Steinberg I: Scleroderma: Relation of pulmonary changes to esophageal disease. Ann Intern Med 40:92, 1954.

528. Taormina VJ, Miller WT, Gefter WB, et al: Progressive systemic sclerosis subgroups: Variable pulmonary features. Am J Roentgenol 137:277, 1981.

529. Martinez LO: Air in the esophagus as a sign of scleroderma (differential diagnosis with some other entities). J Can Assoc Radiol 25:234, 1974.

530. Dinsmore RE, Goodman D, Dreyfuss JR: The air esophagram: A sign of scleroderma involving the esophagus. Radiology 87:348, 1966.

531. Lomeo RM, Corenella RJ, Schabel ST, et al: Progressive systemic sclerosis sine scleroderma presenting as pulmonary interstitial fibrosis. Am J Med 87:525, 1989.

532. Ferri C, Bernini L, Gremignai G, et al: Lung involvement in systemic sclerosis since scleroderma treated by plasma exchange. Int J Artificial Organs 15:426, 1992.

533. Medsger TA Jr, Steen VD, Ziegler G, et al: The natural history of skin involvement in progressive systemic sclerosis. Arthritis Rheum 23:720, 1980.

534. Wasner C, Cooke CR, Fries JF: Successful medical treatment of scleroderma renal crisis. N Engl J Med 299:873, 1978.

534a. Aguayo SM, Richardson CL, Roman J: Severe extrapulmonary thoracic restriction caused by morphea, a form of localized scleroderma. Chest 104:1304, 1993.

535. Bettmann MA, Kantrowitz F: Rapid onset of lung involvement in progressive systemic sclerosis. Chest 75:509, 1979.

536. Owens GR, Follansbee WP: Cardiopulmonary manifestations of systemic sclerosis. Chest 91:118, 1987.

537. Kallenbach J, Prinsloo I, Zwi S: Progressive systemic sclerosis complicated by diffuse pulmonary haemorrhage. Thorax 32:767, 1977.

538. Alvarez Vega JL, Salazar Vallinas JM, Ortega Alberdi R, et al: Pulmonary haemorrhage and focal necrotizing glomerulonephritis in a case of systemic sclerosis. Clin Rheumatol 11:116, 1992.

539. Weaver AL, Divertie MB, Titus JL: Pulmonary scleroderma. Dis Chest 54:490, 1968.

540. Montesi A, Pesaresi A, Cavalli ML, et al: Oropharyngeal and esophageal function in scleroderma. Dysphagia 6:219, 1991.

541. Hendel L: Esophageal and small intestinal manifestations of progressive systemic sclerosis: A clinical and experimental study. Dan Med Bull 41:371, 1994.

542. Clemson BS, MIller WR, Luck JC, et al: Acute myocarditis in fulminant systemic sclerosis. Chest 101:872, 1992.

543. Clements PJ, Furst DE, Cabeen W, et al: The relationship of arrhythmias and conduction disturbances to other manifestations of cardiopulmonary disease in progressive systemic sclerosis (PSS). Am J Med 71:38, 1981.

544. Clark JA, Winkelmann RK, McDuffie FC, et al: Synovial tissue changes and rheumatic factor in scleroderma. Mayo Clin Proc 46:97, 1971.

545. Steen VD: Renal involvement in systemic sclerosis. Clin Dermatol 12:253, 1994.

546. Buckingham BA, Uitto J, Sandborg C, et al: Scleroderma-like changes in insulin-dependent diabetes mellitus: Clinical and biochemical studies. Diabetes Care 7:163, 1984.

547. Gordon MB, Klein I, Dekker A, et al: Thyroid disease in progressive systemic sclerosis: Increased frequency of glandular fibrosis and hypothyroidism. Ann Intern Med 95:431, 1981.

548. Solomon G, Barland P, Rifkin H: Eosinophilic fasciitis responsive to cimetidine. Ann Intern Med 97:547, 1982.

549. Kent LT, Cramer SF, Moskowitz RW, et al: Eosinophilic fasciitis: Clinical, laboratory, and microscopic consideration. Arthritis Rheum 24:677, 1981.

550. Michet CJ Jr, Doyle JA, Ginsburg WW: Eosinophilic fasciitis: Report of 15 cases. Mayo Clin Proc 56:27, 1981.

551. Sills EM: Diffuse fasciitis with eosinophilia in childhood. Johns Hopkins Med J 151:203, 1982.

552. Wood SH, Cantrell BB, Shulman LE: Eosinophilic fasciitis. Johns Hopkins Med J 148:81, 1981.

553. Lewkonia RW, Marx LH, Atkinson MH: Granulomatous vasculitis in the syndrome of diffuse fasciitis with eosinophilia. Arch Intern Med 142:73, 1982.

554. Sternberg EM, Van Woert MH, Young SN, et al: Development of a scleroderma-like illness during therapy with L-5-hydroxytryptophan and carbidopa. N Engl J Med 303:782, 1980.

555. Soubani AO, Miller KB, Hassoun PM: Pulmonary complications of bone marrow transplantation. Chest 109:1066, 1996.

556. Johnson FL, Stokes DC, Ruggiero M, et al: Chronic obstructive airways disease after bone marrow transplantation. J Pediatr 105:370, 1984.

557. James TN: The toxic oil syndrome. Clin Cardiol 17:463, 1994.

558. Hayman LD, Hunt RE: Pulmonary fibrosis in generalized scleroderma: Report of a case and review of the literature. Dis Chest 21:691, 1952.

559. Kallenberg CG, Wouda AA, The TH: Systemic involvement and immunologic findings in patients presenting with Raynaud's phenomenon. Am J Med 69:675, 1980.

560. Harper FE, Maricq HR, Turner RE, et al: A prospective study of Raynaud phenomenon and early connective tissue disease: A 5-year report. Am J Med 72:883, 1982.

561. Ohtsuka T, Hasegawa A, Nakano A, et al: Nailfold capillary abnormality and pulmonary hypertension in systemic sclerosis. Int J Dermatol 36:116, 1997.

562. Colp CR, Riker J, Williams MH Jr: Serial changes in scleroderma and idiopathic interstitial lung disease. Arch Intern Med 132:506, 1973.

563. Greenwald GI, Tashkin DP, Gong H, et al: Longitudinal changes in lung function and respiratory symptoms in progressive systemic sclerosis: Prospective study. Am J Med 83:83, 1987.

564. Abramson MJ, Barnett AJ, Littlejohn GO, et al: Lung function abnormalities and decline of spirometry in scleroderma: An overrated danger? Postgrad Med J 67:632, 1991.

565. Wells AU, Cullinan P, Hansell DM, et al: Fibrosing alveolitis associated with systemic sclerosis has a better prognosis than lone cryptogenic fibrosing alveolitis. Am J Respir Crit Care Med 149:1583, 1994.

566. Schneider PD, Wise RA, Hochberg MC, et al: Serial pulmonary function in systemic sclerosis. Am J Med 73:385, 1982.

567. Jacobsen S, Halberg P, Ullman S, et al: A longitudinal study of pulmonary function in Danish patients with systemic sclerosis. Clin Rheumatol 16:384, 1997.

568. Guttadauria M, Ellman H, Emmanuel G, et al: Pulmonary function in scleroderma. Arthritis Rheum 20:1071, 1977.

569. Blom-Bulow B, Jonson B, Brauer K: Lung function in progressive systemic sclerosis is dominated by poorly compliant lungs and stiff airways. Eur J Resp Dis 66:1, 1985.

570. Kostopoulos C, Rassidakis A, Sfikakis PP, et al: Small airways dysfunction in systemic sclerosis. Chest 102:875, 1992.

571. Catterall M, Rowell NR: Respiratory function in progressive systemic sclerosis. Thorax 18:10, 1963.

572. Sackner MA, Akgun N, Kimbel P, et al: The pathophysiology of scleroderma involving the heart and respiratory system. Ann Intern Med 60:611, 1964.

573. Hughes DTD, Lee FI: Lung function in patients with systemic sclerosis. Thorax 18:16, 1963.

574. Ritchie B: Pulmonary function in scleroderma. Thorax 19:28, 1964.

575. Scheja A, Akesson A, Wollmer P, et al: Early pulmonary disease in systemic sclerosis: A comparison between carbon monoxide transfer factor and static lung compliance. Ann Rheum Dis 52:725, 1993.

576. Iliffe GD, Pettigrew NM: Hypoventilatory respiratory failure in generalised scleroderma. BMJ 286:337, 1983.

577. Chausow AM, Kane T, Levinson D, et al: Reversible hypercapnic respiratory insufficiency in scleroderma caused by respiratory muscle weakness. Am Rev Respir Dis 130:142, 1984.

578. Sudduth CD, Strange C, Cook WR, et al: Failure of the circulatory system limits exercise performance in patients with systemic sclerosis. Am J Med 95:413, 1993.

579. Schwaiblmair M, Behr J, Fruhmann G: Cardiorespiratory responses to incremental exercise in patients with systemic sclerosis. Chest 110:1520, 1996.

580. Medsger TA Jr, Masi AT, Rodnan GP, et al: Survival with systemic sclerosis (scleroderma): Life-table analysis of clinical and demographic factors in 309 patients. Ann Intern Med 75:369, 1971.

581. Altman RD, Medsger Jr TA, Bloch Da, et al: Predictors of survival in systemic sclerosis (scleroderma). Arthritis Rheum 34:403, 1991.

582. Rodnan GP: The natural history of progressive systemic sclerosis (diffuse scleroderma). Bull Rheum Dis 13:301, 1963.

583. Bulpitt KJ, Clements PJ, Lachenbruch PA, et al: Early undifferentiated connective tissue disease: III. Outcome and prognostic indicators in early scleroderma (systemic sclerosis). Ann Intern Med 118:602, 1993.

584. Wells AU, Hansell DM, du Bois RM: Interstitial lung disease in the collagen vascular diseases. Semin Respir Med 14:33, 1993.

585. Peters-Golden M, Wise RA, Hochberg MC, et al: Carbon monoxide diffusing capacity as predictor of outcome in systemic sclerosis. Am J Med 77:1027, 1984.

586. Sarma DP, Weilbaecher TG: Systemic scleroderma and small cell carcinoma of the lung. J Surg Oncol 29:28, 1985.

587. Peters-Golden M, Wise RA, Hochberg M, et al: Incidence of lung cancer in systemic sclerosis. J Rheumatol 12:1136, 1985.

588. Talbott JH, Barrocas M: Progressive systemic sclerosis (PSS) and malignancy, pulmonary and non-pulmonary. Medicine (Baltimore) 58:182, 1979.

589. Benharroch D, Sukenik S, Sacks M: Bronchioloalveolar carcinoma and generalized amyloidosis complicating progressive systemic sclerosis. Hum Pathol 23:839, 1992.

590. Winterbauer RH: Multiple telangiectasia, Raynaud's phenomenon, sclerodactyly, and subcutaneous calcinosis: A syndrome mimicking hereditary hemorrhagic telangiectasia. Bull Johns Hopkins Hosp 114:361, 1964.

591. Thomas EWP: Calcinosis cutis and scleroderma: Thibierge-Weissenbach syndrome. Lancet 2:389, 1942.

592. Steen VD, Ziegler GL, Rodnan GP, et al: Clinical and laboratory associations of anticentromere antibody in patients with progressive systemic sclerosis. Arthritis Rheum 27:125, 1984.

593. Fritzler MJ, Kinsella TD: The CREST syndrome: A distinct serologic entity with anticentromere antibodies. Am J Med 69:520, 1980.

594. Caramaschi P, Biasi D, Manzo T, et al: Anticentromeres antibody—clinical associations: A study of 44 patients. Rheumatol Int 14:253, 1995.

595. Zuber M, Gotzen R, Filler I: Clinical correlation of anticentromere antibodies. Clin Rheumatol 13:427, 1994.

596. Chan HL, Lee YS, Hong HS, et al: Anticentromere antibodies (ACA): Clinical distribution and disease specificity. Clin Exp Dermatol 19:298, 1994.

597. Steen VD, Owens GR, Fino GJ, et al: Pulmonary involvement in systemic sclerosis (scleroderma). Arthritis Rheum 28:759, 1985.

598. Pesci A, Bertorelli G, Manganelli P, et al: Bronchoalveolar lavage analysis of interstitial lung disease in CREST syndrome. Clin Exp Rheumatol 4:121, 1986.

599. Bolster MB, Silver RM: Lung disease in systemic sclerosis (scleroderma). Baillieres Clin Rheumatol 7:79, 1993.

600. McColl GJ, Buchanan RR: Familial CREST syndrome. J Rheum 21:754, 1994.

601. Velayos EE, Masi AT, Stevens MB, et al: The "CREST" syndrome: Comparison with systemic sclerosis (scleroderma). Arch Intern Med 139:1240, 1979.

602. Follansbee WP, Curtiss EI, Medsger TA Jr, et al: Myocardial function and perfusion in the CREST syndrome variant of progressive systemic sclerosis: Exercise radionuclide evaluation and comparison with diffuse scleroderma. Am J Med 77:489, 1984.

603. Battle RW, Davitt MA, Cooper SM, et al: Prevalence of pulmonary hypertension in limited and diffuse scleroderma. Chest 110:1515, 1996.

604. Groen H, Wichers G, Ter Borg EJ, et al: Pulmonary diffusing capacity disturbances are related to nailfold capillary changes in patients with Raynaud's phenomenon with and without an underlying connective tissue disease. Am J Med 89:34, 1990.

605. Salerni R, Rodnan GP, Leon DF, et al: Pulmonary hypertension in the CREST syndrome of progressive systemic sclerosis (scleroderma). Ann Intern Med 86:394, 1977.

606. Winters WJ Jr, Joseph RR: "Primary" pulmonary hypertension and Raynaud's phenomenon: Case report and review of the literature. Arch Intern Med 114:821, 1964.

607. Smith WM, Kroop IG: Raynaud's disease in primary pulmonary hypertension. JAMA 165:1245, 1957.

608. Celoria GC, Friedell GH, Sommers SC: Raynaud's disease and primary pulmonary hypertension. Circulation 22:1055, 1960.

609. Wade G, Ball J: Unexplained pulmonary hypertension. Q J Med 26:83, 1957.

610. Rawson AJ, Woske HM: A study of the etiologic factors in so-called primary pulmonary hypertension. Arch Intern Med 105:203, 1960.

611. Planchon B, Pistorius MA, Beurrier P, et al: Primary Raynaud's phenomenon: Age of onset and pathogenesis in a prospective study of 424 patients. Angiology 45:677, 1994.

612. Tanimoto K, Nakano K, Kano S, et al: Classification criteria for polymyositis and dermatomyositis. J Rheumatol 22:668, 1995.

613. Bohan A, Peter JB: Polymyositis and dermatomyositis: I. N Engl J Med 292:344, 1975.

614. Leong KH, Boey ML: Inflammatory myopathies. Singapore Med J 33:186, 1992.

615. Rose AL, Walton JN: Polymyositis: A survey of 89 cases with particular reference to treatment and prognosis. Brain 89:747, 1966.

616. Winkelmann RK, Mulder DW, Lambert EH, et al: Course of dermatomyositis/polymyositis: Comparison of untreated and cortisone-treated patients. Mayo Clin Proc 43:545, 1968.

617. Frazier AR, Miller RD: Interstitial pneumonitis in association with polymyositis and dermatomyositis. Chest 65:403, 1974.

618. Denardo BA, Tucker LB, Miller LC, et al: Demography of a regional pediatric rheumatology patient population: Affiliated Children's Arthritis Centers of New England. J Rheumatol 21:1553, 1994.

619. Cronin ME, Plotz PH: Idiopathic inflammatory myopathies. Rheum Dis Clin North Am 16:655, 1990.

620. Plotz PH, Rider LG, Targoff IN, et al: Myositis: Immunologic contributions to understanding cause, pathogenesis, and therapy. Ann Intern Med 122:715, 1995.

621. Editorial: Classification of polymyositis. JAMA 204:1187, 1968.

622. Mintz G, González-Angulo A, Fraga A: Ultrastructure of muscle in polymyositis. Am J Med 44:216, 1968.

623. González-Angulo A, Fraga A, Mintz G, et al: Submicroscopic alterations in capillaries of skeletal muscles in polymyositis. Am J Med 45:873, 1968.

624. Love LA, Leff RL, Fraser DD, et al: A new approach to the classification of idiopathic inflammatory myopathy: Myositis-specific autoantibodies define useful homogenous patient groups. Medicine (Baltimore) 70:360, 1991.

625. Miller FW: Classification and prognosis of inflammatory muscle disease. Rheum Dis Clin North Am 20:811, 1994.

626. Ytterberg SR: The relationship of infectious agents to inflammatory myositis. Rheum Dis Clin North Am 20:995, 1994.

627. Hashimoto K, Robison L, Velayos E, et al: Dermatomyositis: Electron microscopic, immunologic, and tissue culture studies of paramyxovirus-like inclusions. Arch Dermatol 103:120, 1971.

628. Landry M, Winkelman RK: Tubular cytoplasmic inclusion in dermatomyositis. Mayo Clin Proc 47:479, 1972.

629. Salmeron G, Greenberg SD, Lidsky MD: Polymyositis and diffuse interstitial lung disease: A review of the pulmonary histopathologic findings. Arch Intern Med 141:1005, 1981.

630. Fraire AE, Smith MN, Greenberg SD, et al: Tubular structures in pulmonary endothelial cells in systemic lupus erythematosus. Am J Clin Pathol 56:244, 1971.

631. Targof IN: Immune manifestations of inflammatory muscle disease. Rheum Dis Clin North Am 20:857, 1994.

632. Grau JM, Miro O, Pedrol E, et al: Interstitial lung disease related to dermatomyositis: Comparative study with patients without lung involvement. J Rheumatol 23:1921, 1996.

633. Wasicek CA, Reichlin M, Montes M, et al: Polymyositis and interstitial lung disease in a patient with anti-Jo-1 prototype. Am J Med 76:538, 1984.

634. Targoff IN, Trieu EP, Miller W: Reaction of anti-OJ autoantibodies with components of the multi-enzyme complex of aminoacyl-tRNA synthetases in addiction to isoleucyl-tRNA synthetase. J Clin Invest 91:2556, 1993.

635. Targoff IN, Arnett FC: Clinical manifestations in patients with antibody to PL-12 antigen (alanyl-tRNA synthetase). Am J Med 88:21, 1990.

636. Targoff IN, Trieu EP, Plotz PH, et al: Antibodies to glycyl-transfer RNA synthetase in patients with myositis and interstitial lung disease. Arthritis Rheum 35:821, 1992.

637. Hohlfeld R, Goebels N, Engel AG: Cellular mechanisms in inflammatory myopathies. Baillieres Clin Neurol 2:617, 1993.

638. Dalakas MC: Clinical, immunopathologic, and therapeutic considerations of inflammatory myopathies. Clin Neuropharmacol 15:327, 1992.

639. Kalovidouris AE: Mechanisms of inflammation and histopathology in inflammatory myopathy. Rheum Dis Clin North Am 20:881, 1994.

640. Thomson PL, MacKay IR: Fibrosing alveolitis and polymyositis. Thorax 25:504, 1970.

641. Duncan PE, Griffin JP, Garcia A, et al: Fibrosing alveolitis in polymyositis: A review of histologically confirmed cases. Am J Med 57:621, 1974.

642. Tazelaar HD, Viggiano RW, Pickersgill J, et al: Interstitial lung disease in polymyositis and dermatomyositis: Clinical features and prognosis as correlated with histologic findings. Am Rev Respir Dis 141:727, 1990.

643. von Mühlen CA, Tan EM: Autoantibodies in the diagnosis of systemic rheumatic diseases. Semin Arthritis Rheum 24:323, 1995.

644. Schwarz MT, Matthay RA, Sahn SA, et al: Interstitial lung disease in polymyositis and dermatomyositis: Analysis of six cases and review of the literature. Medicine (Baltimore) 55:89, 1976.

645. Bunch TW, Tancredi RG, Lie JT: Pulmonary hypertension in polymyositis. Chest 79:105, 1981.

646. Bohan A, Peter JB, Bowman RL, et al: A computer-assisted analysis of 153 patients with polymyositis and dermatomyositis. Medicine (Baltimore) 56:255, 1977.

647. Schwarz Mi, Matthay RA, Sahn SA, Stanford RE, et al: Interstitial lung disease in polymyositis and dermatomyositis: Analysis of six cases and review of the literature. Medicine (Baltimore) 55:89, 1976.

648. Hyun BH, Diggs CI, Toone EC: Dermatomyositis with cystic fibrosis (honeycombing) of the lung. Dis Chest 42:449, 1962.

649. Schwarz MI: Pulmonary and cardiac manifestations of polymyositis-dermatomyositis. J Thorac Imaging 7:46, 1992.

650. Fudman EJ, Schnitzer TJ: Dermatomyositis without creatinine kinase elevation. Am J Med 80:329, 1986.

651. Müller NL, Miller RR: Diseases of the bronchioles: CT and histopathologic findings. Radiology 196:3, 1995.

652. Tazelaar HD, Viggiano RW, Pickersgill J, et al: Interstitial lung disease in polymyositis and dermatomyositis. Am Rev Respir Dis 141:727, 1990.

653. Ikezoe J, Johkoh T, Nohno N, et al: High-resolution CT findings of lung disease in patients with polymyositis and dermatomyositis. J Thorac Imaging 11:250, 1996.

653a. Mino M, Noma S, Taguchi Y, et al: Pulmonary involvement in polymyositis and dermatomyositis: Sequential evaluation with CT. Am J Roentgenol 169:83, 1997.

654. Schiavi EA, Roncoroni AJ, Puy RJM: Isolated bilateral diaphragmatic paresis with interstitial lung disease: An unusual presentation of dermatomyositis. Am Rev Respir Dis 129:337, 1984.

655. Ogle S: Retrospective study of polymyositis in Auckland over 10 years. NZ Med J 92:433, 1980.

656. Webb DR, Currie GD: Pulmonary fibrosis masking polymyositis. JAMA 222:1146, 1972.

657. Sano M, Suzuki M, Sato M, et al: Fatal respiratory failure due to polymyositis. Int Med 33:185, 1994.

658. Schwarz MI, Sutarik JM, Nick JA, et al: Pulmonary capillaritis and diffuse alveolar hemorrhage. Am J Respir Crit Care Med 151:2037, 1991.

659. Hepper NGG, Ferguson RH, Howard FM Jr: Three types of pulmonary involvement in polymyositis. Med Clin North Am 28:1031, 1964.

660. Lakhanpal S, Lie JT, Conn DL, et al: Pulmonary disease in polymyositis/dermatomyositis: A clinicopathological analysis of 65 autopsy cases. Ann Rheum Dis 46:23, 1987.

661. Benbassat J, Gefel D, Larholt K, et al: Prognostic factors in polymyositis/dermatomyositis: A computer-assisted analysis of ninety-two cases. Arthritis Rheum 28:249, 1985.

662. Bernard P, Bonnetblanc JM: Dermatomyositis and malignancy. J Invest Dermatol 100:128S, 1993.

663. Callen JP: Relationship of cancer to inflammatory muscle diseases: Dermatomyositis, polymyositis, and inclusion body myositis. Rheum Dis Clin North Am 20:943, 1994.

664. Chow WH, Gridley G, Mellemjaer L, et al: Cancer risk following polymyositis and dermatomyositis: A nationwide cohort study in Denmark. Cancer Causes Control 6:9, 1995.

665. Bunch TW, Worthington JW, Combs JJ, et al: Azathioprine with prednisone for polymyositis: A controlled clinical trial. Ann Intern Med 92:365, 1980.

666. Bohan A, Peter JB: Polymyositis and dermatomyositis: II. N Engl J Med 292:403, 1975.

667. Camp AV, Lane DJ, Mowat AG: Dermatomyositis with parenchymal lung involvement. BMJ 1:155, 1972.

668. Pace WR Jr, Decker JL, Martin CJ: Polymyositis: Report of two cases with pulmonary function studies suggestive of progressive systemic sclerosis. Am J Med Sci 245:322, 1963.

669. Schiavi EA, Roncoroni AJ, Puy RJM: Isolated bilateral diaphragmatic paresis with interstitial lung disease: An unusual presentation of dermatomyositis. Am Rev Respir Dis 129:337, 1984.

670. Haskard DO: Successful treatment of dermatomyositis complicated by ventilatory failure. Ann Rheum Dis 42:460, 1983.

671. Hebert CA, Byrnes TJ, Baethge BA, et al: Exercise limitation in patients with polymyositis. Chest 98:352, 1990.

672. Medsger TA Jr, Robinson H, Masi AT: Factors affecting survivorship in polymyositis: A life-table study of 124 patients. Arthritis Rheum 14:249, 1971.

673. Hidano A, Torikai S, Uemura T, et al: Malignancy and interstitial pneumonitis as fatal complications in dermatomyositis. J Derm 19:153, 1992.

674. Sjögren H: Zur Kenntnis der Keratoconjunctivitis sicca (keratitis filiformis bei Hypofunktion der Tränendrüsen). (Keratoconjunctivitis sicca [keratitis filiformis with hypofunction of the lacrimal glands].) Acta Ophthalmol 2(Suppl):1, 1933.

675. Fox RI, Saito I: Criteria for diagnosis of Sjögren's syndrome. Rheum Dis Clin North Am 20:391, 1994.

676. Whaley K, Williamson J, Chisholm DK, et al: Sjögren's syndrome: I. Sicca components. Q J Med 42:279, 1973.

677. Alarcón-Segovia D, Ibanez G, Hernóndez-Ortíz J, et al: Sjögren's syndrome in progressive systemic sclerosis (scleroderma). Am J Med 57:78, 1974.

678. Cipoletti JF, Buckingham RB, Barnes EL, et al: Sjögren's syndrome in progressive systemic sclerosis. Ann Intern Med 87:535, 1977.

679. Alarcón-Segovia D, Ibáñez G, Velásquez-Forero F, et al: Sjögren's syndrome in systemic lupus erythematosus: Clinical and subclinical manifestations. Ann Intern Med 81:577, 1974.

680. Moutsopoulos HM, Chused TM, Mann DL, et al: Sjögren's syndrome (sicca syndrome): Current issues. Ann Intern Med 92:212, 1980.

681. Alarcón-Segovia D, Díaz-Jouanen E, Fishbein E: Features of Sjögren's syndrome in primary biliary cirrhosis. Ann Intern Med 79:31, 1973.

682. Whaley K, Webb J, McEvoy BA, et al: Sjögren's syndrome: II. Clinical associations and immunological phenomena. Q J Med 42:513, 1973.

683. Talal N, Bunim JJ: The development of malignant lymphoma in the course of Sjögren's syndrome. Am J Med 36:529, 1964.

684. Silbiger ML, Peterson CC Jr: Sjögren's syndrome: Its roentgenographic features. Am J Roentgenol 100:554, 1967.

685. Shearn MA: Sjögren's syndrome. Med Clin North Am 61:271, 1977.

686. Fairfax AJ, Haslam PL, Pavia D, et al: Pulmonary disorders associated with Sjögren's syndrome. Q J Med 50:279, 1981.

687. Constantopoulos SH, Drosos AA, Maddison PJ, et al: Xerotrachea and interstitial lung disease in primary Sjögren's syndrome. Respiration 46:310, 1984.

688. Constantopoulos SH, Tsianos EV, Moutsopoulos HM: Pulmonary and gastrointestinal manifestations of Sjögren's syndrome. Rheum Dis Clin North Am 18:617, 1992.

689. Kelly CA, Foster H, Pal B, et al: Primary Sjögren's syndrome in northeast England—a longitudinal study. Br J Rheum 31:787, 1992.

690. Bardana EJ, Montanaro A: Sjögren's syndrome: A rheumatic disorder with prominent respiratory manifestations. Ann Allergy 64:3, 1990.

691. Cummings NA, Schall GL, Asofsky R, et al: Sjögren's syndrome—newer aspects of research, diagnosis, and therapy. Ann Intern Med 75:937, 1971.

692. Mariette X: Sjögren's syndrome and virus. Ann Med Interne 146:243, 1995.

693. Fox RI: Epidemiology, pathogenesis, animal models, and treatment of Sjögren's syndrome. Curr Opin Rheumatol 6:501, 1994.

694. Miyasaka N, Saito I, Haruta J: Possible involvement of Epstein-Barr virus in the pathogenesis of Sjögren's syndrome. Clin Immunol Immunopathol 72:166, 1994.

695. Moutsopoulos HM, Papadopoulos GK: Possible viral implication in the pathogenesis of Sjögren's syndrome. Eur J Med 1:219, 1992.

696. Clark DA, Lamey PJ, Jarrett RF, et al: A model to study viral and cytokine involvement in Sjögren's syndrome. Autoimmunology 18:7, 1994.

697. Aziz KE, McCluskey PJ, Montanaro A, et al: Vascular endothelium and lymphocyte adhesion molecules in minor salivary glands of patients with Sjögren's syndrome. J Clin Lab Immunol 37:39, 1992.

698. Fox RI, Kang HI: Pathogenesis of Sjögren's syndrome. Rheum Dis Clin North Am 18:517, 1992.

699. Levy Y, Dueymes M, Pennec YL, et al: IgA Sjögren's syndrome. Clin Exp Rheumatol 12:543, 1994.

700. Smith MD, Lamour A, Boylston A, et al: Selective expression of V beta families by T cells in the blood and salivary gland infiltrate of patients with primary Sjögren's syndrome. J Rheumatol 21:1832, 1994.

701. Skopoulis FN, Moutsopoulos HM: Autoimmune epitheliitis: Sjögren's syndrome. Clin Exp Rheumatol 11:S9, 1994.

702. Miyagawa S, Dohi K, Shima H, et al: Absence of HLA-B8 and HLA-DR3 in Japanese patients with Sjögren's syndrome positive for anti-SSA (R0). J Rheumatol 19:1922, 1992.

703. Reveille JD, Arnett FC: The immunogenetics of Sjögren's syndrome. Rheum Dis Clin North Am 18:539, 1992.

704. Dalavanga YA, Constantopoulos SH, Galanopoulos V, et al: Alveolitis correlates with clinical pulmonary involvement in primary Sjögren's syndrome. Chest 99:1394, 1991.

705. Gudbjornsson B, Hallgren R, Nettelbladt O, et al: Phenotypic and functional activation of alveolar macrophages, T lymphocytes, and NK cells in patients with systemic sclerosis and primary Sjögren's syndrome. Ann Rheum Dis 53:574, 1994.

706. Bucher UG, Reid L: Sjögren's syndrome: Report of a fatal case with pulmonary and renal lesions. Br J Dis Chest 53:237, 1959.

707. Ellman P, Weber FP, Goodier TEW: A contribution to the pathology of Sjögren's disease. Q J Med 77:33, 1951.

708. Andoh Y, Shimura S, Sawai T, et al: Morphometric analysis of airways in Sjögren's syndrome. Am Rev Respir Dis 148:1358, 1993.

709. Newball HH, Brahim SA: Chronic obstructive airway disease in patients with Sjögren's syndrome. Am Rev Respir Dis 115:295, 1977.

710. Liebow AA, Carrington CB: Diffuse pulmonary lymphoreticular infiltrations associated with dysproteinemia. Med Clin North Am 57:809, 1973.

711. Bonner H Jr, Ennis RS, Geellhoed GW, et al: Lymphoid infiltration and amyloidosis of lung in Sjögren's syndrome. Arch Pathol 95:42, 1973.

712. Deheinzelin D, Capelozzi VL, Kairalla RA, et al: Interstitial lung disease in primary Sjögren's syndrome. Am J Respir Crit Care Med 154:794, 1996.

713. Karlish AJ: Lung changes in Sjögren's syndrome. Proc R Soc Med 62:22, 1969.

714. Scully RF, Galdabini JJ, McNelly BU: Case records of the Massachusetts General Hospital: Weekly clinicopathological exercises. Case 28–1975. N Engl J Med 293:136, 1975.

715. Tsuzaka K, Akama H, Yamada H, et al: Pulmonary pseudolymphoma presented with a mass lesion in a patient with primary Sjögren's syndrome: Beneficial effect of intermittent intravenous cyclophosphamide. Scand J Rheumatol 22:90, 1993.

716. Motegi M, Suzuki Y, Takayanagi N, et al: A case of multiple nodular pulmonary amyloidosis associated with Sjögren's syndrome. Jpn J Thorac Dis 32:1016, 1994.

717. Wong BC, Wong KL, Ip MS, et al: Sjögren's syndrome with amyloid A presenting as multiple pulmonary nodules. J Rheumatol 21:165, 1994.

718. Strimlan CV, Rosenow III EC, Divertie MB, et al: Pulmonary manifestations of Sjögren's syndrome. Chest 70:354, 1976.

719. Kobayashi H, Matsuoka R, Kitamura S, et al: Sjögren's syndrome with multiple bullae and pulmonary nodular amyloidosis. Chest 94:438, 1988.

720. Tsokos M, Lazarou SA, Moutsopoulos HM: Vasculitis in primary Sjögren's syndrome: Histologic classification and clinical presentation. Am J Clin Pathol 88:26, 1987.

721. Strimlan CV, Rosenow EC III, Divertie MB, et al: Pulmonary manifestations of Sjögren's syndrome. Chest 70:354, 1976.

722. Tanoue LT: Pulmonary involvement in collagen vascular disease: A review of the pulmonary manifestations of the Marfan syndrome, ankylosing spondylitis, Sjögren's syndrome, and relapsing polychondritis. J Thorac Imaging 7:62, 1992.

723. Strimlan CV, Rosenow EC III, Divertie MB, et al: Pulmonary manifestations of Sjögren's syndrome. Chest 70:354, 1975.

724. Kadota JI, Kusano S, Kawakami K, et al: Usual interstitial pneumonia associated with primary Sjögren's syndrome. Chest 180:1756, 1995.

725. Franquet T, Giménez A, Monill JM, et al: Primary Sjögren's syndrome and associated lung disease: CT findings in 50 patients. Am J Roentgenol 169:655, 1997.

726. Carignan S, Staples CA, Müller NL: Intrathoracic lymphoproliferative disorders in the immunocompromised patient: CT findings. Radiology 197:53, 1995.

727. Meyer CA, Pina JS, Taillon D, et al: Inspiratory and expiratory high-resolution CT findings in a patient with Sjögren's syndrome and cystic lung disease. Am J Roentgenol 168:101, 1997.

728. Desai SR, Nicholson AG, Stewart S, et al: Benign pulmonary lymphocytic infiltration and amyloidosis: Computed tomographic and pathologic features in three cases. J Thorac Imaging 12:215, 1997.

729. Ichikawa Y, Kinoshita M, Koga T, et al: Lung cyst formation in lymphocytic interstitial pneumonia: CT features. J Comput Assist Tomogr 18:745, 1994.

730. Hughes GRV, Whaley K: Sjögren's syndrome. BMJ 4:533, 1972.

731. Powell RD, Larson AL, Henkin RI: Nasal mucous membrane biopsy in Sjögren's syndrome: A new diagnostic technique. Ann Intern Med 81:25, 1974.

732. Henkin RI, Talal N, Larson AL, et al: Abnormalities of taste and smell in Sjögren's syndrome. Ann Intern Med 76:375, 1972.

733. Doig JA, Whaley K, Dick WC, et al: Otolaryngological aspects of Sjögren's syndrome. BMJ 4:460, 1971.

734. Kelly C, Gardiner P, Pal B, et al: Lung function in primary Sjögren's syndrome. Thorax 46:180, 1991.

734a. Salaffi F, Manganelli P, Carotti M, et al: A longitudinal study of pulmonary involvement in primary Sjögren's syndrome: Relationship between alveolitis and subsequent lung changes on high-resolution computed tomography. Br J Rheumatol 37:263, 1998.

735. Gardiner P, Ward C, Allison A, et al: Pleuropulmonary abnormalities in primary Sjögren's syndrome. J Rheumatol 20:831, 1993.

736. Lahdensuo A, Korpela M: Pulmonary findings in patients with primary Sjögren's syndrome. Chest 108:316, 1995.

737. Gudbjornsson B, Hedenstrom H, Stalenheim G, et al: Bronchial hyperresponsiveness to methacholine in patients with primary Sjögren's syndrome. Ann Rheum Dis 50:36, 1991.

738. Desche P, Couderc LJ, Espardeau B: Sjögren's syndrome and pulmonary lymphangiomyomatosis. Chest 94:897, 1988.

739. Kaltreider HB, Talal N: The neuropathy of Sjögren's syndrome: Trigeminal nerve involvement. Ann Intern Med 70:751, 1969.

740. Moll JW, Markusse HM, Pijnenburg JJ, et al: Antineuronal antibodies in patients with neurologic complications of primary Sjögren's syndrome. Neurology 43:2574, 1993.

741. Shioji R, Furuyama T, Onodera S, et al: Sjögren's syndrome and renal tubular acidosis. Am J Med 48:456, 1970.

742. Raskin RJ, Tesar JT, Lawless OJ: Hypokalemic periodic paralysis in Sjögren's syndrome. Arch Intern Med 141:1671, 1981.

743. Steinberg AD, Green WT Jr, Talal N: Thrombotic thrombocytopenic purpura complicating Sjögren's syndrome. JAMA 215:757, 1971.

744. Fox RI, Howell FV, Bone RC, et al: Primary Sjögren's syndrome: Clinical and immunopathologic features. Semin Arthritis Rheum 14:77, 1984.

745. Moutsopoulos HM, Karsh J, Wolf RO, et al: Lysozyme determination in parotid saliva from patients with Sjögren's syndrome. Am J Med 69:39, 1980.

746. Michalski JP, Daniels TE, Talal N, et al: Beta₂-microglobulin and lymphocytic infiltration in Sjögren's syndrome. N Engl J Med 293:1228, 1975.

747. Segal I, Fink G, Machtey I, et al: Pulmonary function abnormalities in Sjögren's syndrome and the sicca complex. Thorax 36:286, 1981.

748. Constantopoulos SH, Papadimitriou CS, Moutsopoulos HM: Respiratory manifestations in primary Sjögren's syndrome: A clinical, functional, and histologic study. Chest 88:226, 1985.

749. Papathanasiou MP, Constantopoulos SH, Tsampoulas C, et al: Reappraisal of respiratory abnormalities in primary and secondary Sjögren's syndrome: A controlled study. Chest 90:370, 1986.

750. Martinez-Cordero E, Andrade-Ortega L, Martinez-Miranda E: Pulmonary function abnormalities in patients with primary Sjögren's syndrome. J Investig Allergol Clin Immunol 3:205, 1993.

751. Newball HH, Brahim SA: Chronic obstructive airway disease in patients with Sjögren's syndrome. Am Rev Respir Dis 115:295, 1977.

752. Ohmoto A, Kohno M, Matsuyama R: Bronchial hypersensitivity in Sjögren's syndrome. Ryumachi 34:10, 1994.

753. Kamholz S, Sher A, Barland P, et al: Sjögren's syndrome: Severe upper airways obstruction due to primary malignant tracheal lymphoma developing during successful treatment of lymphocytic interstitial pneumonitis. J Rheumatol 14:588, 1987.

754. Sullivan WD, Hurst DJ, Harmon CE, et al: A prospective evaluation emphasizing pulmonary involvement in patients with connective tissue disease. Medicine (Baltimore) 63:92, 1984.

754a. Danieli MG, Fraticelli P, Salvi A, et al: Undifferentiated connective tissue disease: Natural history and evolution into definite CTD assessed in 84 patients initially diagnosed as early UCTD. Clin Rheumatol 17:195, 1998.

755. Lazaro MA, Maldonado Cocco JA, Catoggio LJ, et al: Clinical and serologic characteristics of patients with overlap syndrome: Is mixed connective tissue disease a distinct clinical entity? Medicine (Baltimore) 68:58, 1989.

756. Tuffanelli DL, Winkelmann RK: Scleroderma and its relationship to the "collagenoses": Dermatomyositis, lupus erythematosus, rheumatoid arthritis, and Sjögren's syndrome. Am J Med Sci 243:133, 1962.

757. Sharp GC, Irvin WS, Tan EM, et al: Mixed connective tissue disease—apparently distinct rheumatic disease syndrome associated with a specific antibody to an extractable nuclear antigen (ENA). Am J Med 52:148, 1972.

758. Silver TM, Farber SJ, Bole GG, et al: Radiological features of mixed connective tissue disease and scleroderma—systemic lupus erythematosus overlap. Radiology 120:269, 1976.

759. Editorial: Mixed connective tissue disease. BMJ 4:315, 1972.

760. Wiener-Kronish JP, Solinger AM, Warnock ML, et al: Severe pulmonary involvement in mixed connective tissue disease. Am Rev Respir Dis 124:499, 1981.

760a. Horiki T, Fuyuno G, Ishii M, et al: Fatal alveolar hemorrhage in a patient with mixed connective tissue disease presenting polymyositis features. Intern Med 37:554, 1998.

761. Prakash UBS, Luthra HS, Divertie MB: Intrathoracic manifestations in mixed connective tissue disease. Mayo Clin Proc 60:813, 1985.

762. Derderian SS, Tellis CJ, Abbrecht PH, et al: Pulmonary involvement in mixed connective tissue disease. Chest 88:45, 1985.

763. Jones MB, Osterholm RK, Wilson RB, et al: Fatal pulmonary hypertension and resolving immune-complex glomerulonephritis in mixed connective tissue disease: A case report and review of the literature. Am J Med 65:855, 1978.

764. Clinicopathologic Conference: Mixed connective tissue disease. Am J Med 65:833, 1978.

765. Kobayashi H, Sano T, Ii K, et al: Mixed connective tissue disease with fatal pulmonary hypertension. Acta Pathol Jpn 32:1121, 1982.

766. Prakash UBS: Lungs in mixed connective tissue disease. J Thorac Imaging 7:55, 1992.

767. Prakash UBS, Luthra HS, Divertie MB: Intrathoracic manifestations in mixed connective tissue disease. Mayo Clin Proc 60:813, 1985.

768. Sullivan WD, Hurst DJ, Harmon CE, et al: A prospective evaluation emphasizing pulmonary involvement in patients with mixed connective tissue disease. Medicine (Baltimore) 63:92, 1984.

769. Germain MJ, Davidman M: Pulmonary hemorrhage and acute renal failure in a patient with mixed connective tissue disease. Am J Kidney Dis 3:420, 1984.

770. Müller NL, Miller RR: Diffuse pulmonary hemorrhage. Radiol Clin North Am 29:965, 1991.

771. Hoogsteden HC, van Dongen JJ, van der Kwast TH, et al: Bilateral exudative pleuritis, an unusual pulmonary onset of mixed connective tissue disease. Respiration 48:164, 1985.

772. Guit GL, Shaw PC, Ehrlich J, Kroon HM, Oudkerk M: Mediastinal lymphadenopathy and pulmonary arterial hypertension in mixed connective tissue disease. Radiology 154:305, 1985.

773. Gordonson J, Quinn M, Kaufman R, Van den Tweel JG: Mediastinal lymphadenopathy and undifferentiated connective tissue disease: Case report and review. Am J Roentgenol 131:325, 1978.

774. Nimelstein SH, Brody S, McShane D, et al: Mixed connective tissue disease: A subsequent evaluation of the original 25 patients. Medicine (Baltimore) 59:239, 1980.

775. Gendi NS, Welsh KI, Van Venrooij WJ, et al: HLA type as a predictor of mixed connective tissue disease differentiation: Ten-year clinical and immunogenetic follow-up of 46 patients. Arthritis Rheum 38:259, 1995.

776. Masson P, Riopelle J-L, Martin P: Poumon rhumatismal [Rheumatoid lung]. Ann Anat Pathol 14:359, 1937.

777. Spencer H: Pathology of the Lung: Excluding Pulmonary Tuberculosis. New York, Pergamon Press, 1962.

778. Raz I, Fisher J, Israeli A, et al: An unusual case of rheumatic pneumonia. Arch Intern Med 145:1130, 1985.

779. Tanaka H, Kobayashi H, Kano S, et al: Autopsy of a patient with rheumatic fever who initially presented with acute respiratory failure. Jpn J Thorac Dis 33:678, 1995.

780. Ephrem D: Rheumatic pneumonia in a 10-year-old Ethiopian child. East Afr Med J 67:740, 1990.

781. Grunow WA, Esterly JR: Rheumatic pneumonitis. Chest 61:298, 1972.

782. Brown G, Goldring D, Behrer MR: Rheumatic pneumonia. J Pediatr 52:598, 1958.

783. Goldring D, Behrer MR, Brown G, et al: Rheumatic pneumonitis: II. Report on the clinical and laboratory findings in twenty-three patients. J Pediatr 53:547, 1958.

784. McAdam LP, O'Hanlan MA, Bluestone R, et al: Relapsing polychondritis: Prospective study of 23 patients and a review of the literature. Medicine (Baltimore) 55:193, 1976.

785. Valenzuela R, Cooperrider PA, Gogate P, et al: Relapsing polychondritis: Immunomicroscopic findings in cartilage of ear biopsy specimens. Hum Pathol 11:19, 1980.

786. Dolan DL, Lemmon GB Jr, Teitelbaum SL: Relapsing polychondritis: Analytical literature review and studies on pathogenesis. Am J Med 41:285, 1966.

787. Hughes RAC, Berry CL, Seifert M, et al: Relapsing polychondritis: Three cases with a clinicopathological study and literature review. Q J Med 41:363, 1972.

788. Homma S, Matsumoto T, Abe H, et al: Relapsing polychondritis: Pathological and immunological findings in an autopsy case. Acta Pathol Jpn 34:1137, 1984.

789. Herman JH, Dennis MV: Immunopathologic studies in relapsing polychondritis. J Clin Invest 52:549, 1973.

790. Rajapakse DA, Bywaters EGL: Cell-mediated immunity to cartilage proteoglycan in relapsing polychondritis. Clin Exp Immunol 16:497, 1974.

791. McKenna CH, Luthra HS, Jordon RE: Hypocomplementemic ear effusion in relapsing polychondritis. Mayo Clin Proc 51:495, 1976.

792. Alsalameh S, Mollenhauer J, Scheuplein F, et al: Preferential cellular and humoral immune reactivities to native and denatured collagen types IX and XI in a patient with fatal relapsing polychondritis. J Rheumatol 20:1419, 1993.

793. Yang CL, Brinckmann J, Rui HF, et al: Autoantibodies to cartilage collagens in relapsing polychondritis. Arch Dermatol Res 285:245, 1993.

794. Lang B, Rothenfusser A, Lanchbury JS, et al: Susceptibility to relapsing polychondritis is associated with HLA-DR4. Arthritis Rheum 36:660, 1993.

795. Dahlqvist A, Lundberg E, Ostberg Y: Hydralazine-induced relapsing polychondritis-like syndrome: Report of a case with severe chronic laryngeal complications. Acta Otolaryngol 96:355, 1983.

796. Pearson CM, Kline HM, Newcomber VD: Relapsing polychondritis. N Engl J Med 263:51, 1960.

797. Hainer JW, Hamilton GW: Aortic abnormalities in relapsing polychondritis: Report of a case with dissecting aortic aneurysm. N Engl J Med 280:1166, 1969.

798. Kindblom L-G, Dalen P, Edmar G, et al: Relapsing polychondritis: A clinical, pathologic-anatomic, and histochemical study of two cases. Acta Pathol Microbiol Scand 85:656, 1977.

799. Higenbottam T, Dixon J: Chondritis associated with fatal intramural bronchial fibrosis. Thorax 34:563, 1979.

800. Hashimoto K, Arkin CR, Kang AH: Relapsing polychondritis: An ultrastructural study. Arthritis Rheum 20:91, 1977.

801. Dryll A, Lansaman J, Meyer O, et al: Relapsing polychondritis: An ultrastructural study of elastic and collagen fibres degradation revealed by tannic acid: Case report. Virchows Arch 390:109, 1981.

802. Mitchell N, Shepard N: Relapsing polychondritis: An electron-microscopic study of synovium and articular cartilage. J Bone Joint Surg 54A:1235, 1972.

803. Crockford MP, Kerr IH: Relapsing polychondritis. Clin Radiol 39:386, 1988.

804. Davis SD, Berkmen YM, King T: Peripheral bronchial involvement in relapsing polychondritis: Demonstration by thin-section CT. Am J Roentgenol 153:953, 1989.

805. Kilman WJ: Narrowing of the airway in relapsing polychondritis. Radiology 126:373, 1978.

806. Choplin RH, Wehunt WD, Theros EG: Diffuse lesions of the trachea. Semin Roentgenol 18:38, 1983.

807. Mendelson DS, Som PM, Crane R, et al: Relapsing polychondritis studied by computed tomography. Radiology 157:489, 1985.

808. Müller NL, Miller RR, Ostrow DN, Paré PD: Clinico-radiologic-pathologic conference: Diffuse thickening of the tracheal wall. Can Assoc Radiol J 40:213, 1989.

809. Im JG, Chung JW, Han SK, et al: CT manifestations of tracheobronchial involvement in relapsing polychondritis. J Comput Assist Tomogr 12:792, 1988.

810. Quint LE, Whyte RI, Kazerooni EA, et al: Stenosis of the central airways: Evaluation by helical CT with multiplanar reconstructions. Radiology 194:871, 1995.

810a. Remy-Jardin M, Remy J, Artaud D, et al: Volume rendering of the tracheobronchial tree: Clinical evaluation of bronchographic images. Radiology 208:761, 1998.

811. Hunninghake GW, Fauci AS: Pulmonary involvement in the collagen vascular diseases. Am Rev Respir Dis 119:471, 1979.

812. White JW Jr: Relapsing polychondritis. South Med J 78:448, 1985.

813. Eng J, Sabanathan S: Airway complications in relapsing polychondritis. Ann Thorac Surg 51:686, 1991.

814. Manna R, Annese V, Ghirlanda G, et al: Relapsing polychondritis with severe aortic insufficiency. Clin Rheumatol 4:474, 1985.

815. Isaak BL, Liesegang TJ, Michet CJ Jr: Ocular and systemic findings in relapsing polychondritis. Ophthalmology 93:681, 1986.

816. Chang-Miller A, Okamura M, Torres VE, et al: Renal involvement in relapsing polychondritis. Medicine (Baltimore) 66:202, 1987.

817. Ruhlen JL, Huston KA, Wood WG: Relapsing polychondritis with glomerulonephritis. JAMA 245:847, 1981.

818. Neild GH, Cameron JS, Lessot MH, et al: Relapsing polychondritis with crescentic glomerulonephritis. BMJ 1:743, 1978.

819. Michet CJ Jr, McKenna CH, Luthra HS, et al: Relapsing polychondritis: Survival and predictive role of early disease manifestations. Ann Intern Med 104:74, 1986.

820. Kraft SC, Earle RH, Roesler M, et al: Unexplained bronchopulmonary disease with inflammatory bowel disease. Arch Intern Med 136:454, 1976.

821. Camus P, Piard F, Ashcroft T, et al: The lung in inflammatory bowel disease. Medicine (Baltimore) 72:151, 1993.

822. Smiéjan JM, Cosnes J, Chollet-Martin S, et al: Sarcoid-like lymphocytosis of the lower respiratory tract in patients with active Crohn's disease. Ann Intern Med 104:17, 1986.

823. Bonniere P, Wallaert B, Cortot A, et al: Latent pulmonary involvement in Crohn's disease: Biological, functional, bronchoalveolar lavage, and scintigraphic studies. Gut 27:919, 1986.

824. Mucnk A, Murciano D, Pariente R, et al: Latent pulmonary function abnormalities in children with Crohn's disease. Eur Respir J 8:377, 1995.

825. Sommer H, Schmidt M, Gruber KD: Pulmonary functional disorders in ulcerative colitis and Crohn's disease. Deutsche Medizinische Wochenschrift 111:812, 1986.

826. Neilly JB, Maon ANH, McSharry C, et al: Pulmonary abnormalities in Crohn's disease. Respir Med 83:487, 1989.

826a. Tzanakis N, Samiou M, Bouros D, et al: Small airways function in patients with inflammatory bowel disease. Am J Respir Crit Care Med 157:382, 1998.

827. Douglas JG, McDonald CF, Leslie MJ, et al: Respiratory impairment in inflammatory bowel disease: Does it vary with disease activity? Respir Med 83:389, 1989.

828. Pasquis P, Colin R, Denis PH, et al: Transient pulmonary impairment during attacks of Crohn's disease. Respiration 41:56, 1981.

828a. Spira A, Grossman R, Balter M: Large airway disease associated with inflammatory bowel disease. Chest 113:1723, 1998.

828b. Eaton TE, Lambie N, Wells AU: Bronchiectasis following colectomy for Crohn's disease. Thorax 53:529, 1998.

829. Vasishta S, Wood JB, McGinty F: Ulcerative tracheobronchitis years after colectomy for ulcerative colitis. Chest 106:1279, 1994.

830. Swinburn CR, Jackson GJ, Cobden I, et al: Bronchiolitis obliterans organising pneumonia in a patient with ulcerative colitis. Thorax 43:735, 1988.

831. Matsumoto K, Hirano T, Kondo Y, et al: A case of bronchiolitis obliterans organizing pneumonia associated with ulcerative colitis. Jpn J Thorac Dis 31:245, 1993.

832. Wilcox P, Miller R, Miller G, et al: Airway involvement in ulcerative colitis. Chest 92:18, 1987.

833. Desai SJ, Gephardt GN, Stoller JK: Diffuse panbronchiolitis preceding ulcerative colitis. Chest 95:1342, 1989.

834. Garg K, Lynch DA, Newell JD II: Inflammatory airways disease in ulcerative colitis: CT and high-resolution CT features. J Thorac Imaging 8:159, 1993.

835. Kayer K, Probst F, Gabius HJ, et al: Are there characteristic alterations of lung tissue associated with Crohn's disease? Pathol Res Pract 186:485, 1990.

836. Shneerson JM: Steroid-responsive alveolitis associated with ulcerative colitis. Chest 101:585, 1992.

837. Beer TW, Edwards CW: Pulmonary nodules due to reactive systemic amyloidosis (AA) in Crohn's disease. Thorax 48:1287, 1993.

838. Calder CJ, Lacy D, Raafat F, et al: Crohn's disease with pulmonary involvement in a 3-year-old boy. Gut 34:1636, 1993.

839. Puntis JW, Tarlow MJ, Raafat F, et al: Crohn's disease of the lung. Arch Dis Child 65:1270, 1990.

840. Grantham JG, Meadows JA III, Gleich GJ: Chronic eosinophilic pneumonia degranulation and release of major basic protein. Am J Med 80:89, 1986.

841. Sargent D, Sessions JT, Fairman RP: Pulmonary vasculitis complicating ulcerative colitis. South Med J 78:624, 1985.

842. Domej W, Kullnig P, Petritsch W, et al: Colobronchial fistula: A rare complication of Crohn's colitis. Am Rev Respir Dis 142:1225, 1990.

843. Steel A, Dyer NH, Matthews HR: Cervical Crohn's disease with oesophagopulmonary fistula. Postgrad Med J 64:706, 1988.

844. Rodriguez-Roisin R, Pares A, Bruguera M, et al: Pulmonary involvement in primary biliary cirrhosis. Thorax 36:208, 1981.

845. Wallaert B, Bonniere P, Prin L, et al: Primary biliary cirrhosis: Subclinical inflammatory alveolitis in patients with normal chest roentgenograms. Chest 90:842, 1986.

846. Wallace JG Jr, Tong MJ, Ueki BH, et al: Pulmonary involvement in primary biliary cirrhosis. J Clin Gastroenterol 9:431, 1987.

847. Strobel ES, Bonnet RB, Werner P, et al: Bronchiolitis obliterans organising pneumonia and primary biliary cirrhosis-like lung involvement in a patient with primary biliary cirrhosis. Clin Rheumatol 17:246, 1998.

848. Komatsu T, Utsunomiya K, Oyaizu T: Goodpasture's syndrome associated with primary biliary cirrhosis. Intern Med 37:611, 1998.

# *Vasculitis*

This chapter includes a variety of conditions whose sole or predominant histologic feature is inflammation of pulmonary vessels; discussion is limited to disorders in which the inflammatory reaction is directed primarily against the vessel wall (*see* farther on) and is of proven or presumed immunologic origin. Such disease occurs in several well-characterized clinicopathologic entities, such as Wegener's granulomatosis, Churg-Strauss syndrome, microscopic poly-angiitis, Takayasu's arteritis, and Behçet's disease. Other conditions in which systemic vasculitis is prominent but in which the nature of associated pulmonary disease is poorly defined (such as polyarteritis nodosa [PAN]) are also discussed. Vasculitis associated with connective tissue diseases (such as systemic lupus erythematosus [SLE] and rheumatoid disease) and with drugs is dealt with in Chapters 39 and 63, respectively.

Although the precise cause and pathogenesis of most types of primary pulmonary vasculitis are unknown, it is widely believed by dint of clinical, serologic, and pathologic features that most are associated with some alteration of immunity. Such alteration is likely genetically determined, at least partly, and the presence, type, and extent of the vasculitic process are probably determined by a combination of the individual host response and the particular inciting antigen to which the patient is responding. Pathogenetic mechanisms may be related to several forms of immune reaction and likely involve a complex interaction between cell adhesion molecules, cytokines, cell enzymes, antibodies, and various inflammatory and immune mediator cells.[1, 2] Specific agents responsible for inducing an abnormal immune reaction are also varied; although rarely documented, the most commonly implicated are drugs and microorganisms.

Deposition of immune complexes in vessel walls has been extensively investigated and is likely to be important in several systemic vasculitides, including Henoch-Schönlein purpura, mixed cryoglobulinemia, and PAN; the occasional instances of pulmonary vasculitis in these diseases most likely have the same pathogenesis. Immune complexes can theoretically be derived from circulating preformed antigen-antibody complexes or by an *in situ* reaction of antigen and antibody in the vessel wall. In the majority of cases, specific inciting antigens are unknown; exceptions include hepatitis B and C antigen, some streptococcal proteins, and immunoglobulin (such as occurs in cryoglobulinemia).[3]

There is also evidence that non–immune complex antibody-mediated vascular disease is important in the pathogenesis of some forms of vasculitis. The most extensively investigated of such antibodies are those directed against neutrophil components (antineutrophil cytoplasmic antibodies [ANCA]) (*see* page 1492); other antibodies, such as those directed to endothelial cells themselves, may also have a role.[4, 5] Although there are several theoretical mechanisms by which the latter might cause tissue damage, including complement fixation, neutrophil recruitment, and antibody-dependent cytotoxicity,[1] whether any are operative in a particular vasculitic syndrome or whether they represent simply a secondary reaction to tissue damaged by another mechanism has not been established.

The presence of granulomatous inflammation, either in relation to vessels themselves or in the adjacent parenchyma, implies that cell-mediated immunity is also important in some pulmonary vasculitides, such as Wegener's granulomatosis, giant cell arteritis, and Takayasu's arteritis. The mechanisms involved, however, are poorly understood.[6]

Pathologic diagnosis of vasculitis is not always straightforward, and not all vasculitis documented histologically represents a primary process: a number of pulmonary conditions, particularly infections, but also sarcoidosis, emboli of injected foreign material, and thromboemboli, can result in inflammation of a vessel wall by extension of disease from the vascular lumen or adjacent lung parenchyma. These conditions are best considered secondary vasculitides and obviously have different implications than primary disease.[7] This secondary process is fairly common, and to be confident of a diagnosis of primary pulmonary vasculitis, it is essential

that appropriate cultures be performed on biopsy material and that tissue be thoroughly examined histologically to exclude an infectious or other cause, particularly when disease is relatively localized. It is also important to interpret the results of pathologic examination in the context of clinical, radiologic, and laboratory findings.

Clinical and radiologic manifestations of pulmonary vasculitis can be related to the vascular inflammation itself or to the pneumonitis that accompanies some of the disorders. During the acute stages, the effects of vasculitis include alveolar hemorrhage and vascular thrombosis, with or without parenchymal necrosis. With more prolonged disease, weakening of the vessel wall can result in aneurysm formation, whereas obliteration of the vessel lumens can cause pulmonary hypertension. Because of the frequent occurrence of concomitant extrapulmonary vasculitis and the common presence of glomerulonephritis, signs and symptoms of extrathoracic disease may overshadow the pulmonary manifestations.

Over the years, a number of classifications of systemic and pulmonary vasculitis have been proposed, reflecting to some extent the limited understanding of etiology and pathogenesis.[8, 9] The one we find most useful is based on a consideration of the size of vessel affected as proposed in the Chapel Hill Consensus Conference on the Nomenclature of Systemic Vasculitis (Table 40–1).[10] Although lympho-

---

**Table 40–1. NAMES AND DEFINITIONS OF VASCULITIDES ADOPTED BY THE CHAPEL HILL CONSENSUS CONFERENCE ON THE NOMENCLATURE OF SYSTEMIC VASCULITIS***

**LARGE VESSEL VASCULITIS**

Giant cell (temporal) arteritis — Granulomatous arteritis of the aorta and its major branches, with a predilection for the extracranial branches of the carotid artery. *Often involves the temporal artery. Usually occurs in patients older than 50 and often is associated with polymyalgia rheumatica*

Takayasu's arteritis — Granulomatous inflammation of the aorta and its major branches. *Usually occurs in patients younger than 50*

**MEDIUM-SIZED VESSEL VASCULITIS**

Polyarteritis nodosa† (classic polyarteritis nodosa) — Necrotizing inflammation of medium-sized or small arteries without glomerulonephritis or vasculitis in arterioles, capillaries, or venules

Kawasaki disease — Arteritis involving large, medium-sized, and small arteries associated with mucocutaneous lymph node syndrome. *Coronary arteries are often involved. Aorta and veins may be involved. Usually occurs in children*

**SMALL VESSEL VASCULITIS**

Wegener's granulomatosis‡ — Granulomatous inflammation involving the respiratory tract and necrotizing vasculitis affecting small to medium-sized vessels (e.g., capillaries, venules, arterioles, and arteries). *Necrotizing glomerulonephritis is common*

Churg-Strauss syndrome‡ — Eosinophil-rich and granulomatous inflammation involving the respiratory tract and necrotizing vasculitis affecting small to medium-sized vessels and associated with asthma and eosinophilia

Microscopic polyangiitis† (microscopic polyarteritis)‡ — Necrotizing vasculitis, with few or no immune deposits, affecting small vessels (i.e., capillaries, venules, or arterioles). *Necrotizing arteritis involving small and medium-sized arteries may be present. Necrotizing glomerulonephritis is common. Pulmonary capillaritis often occurs*

Henoch-Schönlein purpura — Vasculitis, with IgA-dominant immune deposits, affecting small vessels (i.e., capillaries, venules, or arterioles). *Typically involves skin, gut, and glomeruli and is associated with arthralgias or arthritis*

Essential cryoglobulinemic vasculitis — Vasculitis, with cryoglobulin immune deposits, affecting small vessels (i.e., capillaries, venules, or arterioles) and associated with cryoglobulins in serum. *Skin and glomeruli are often involved*

Cutaneous leukocytoclastic angiitis — Isolated cutaneous leukocytoclastic angiitis without systemic vasculitis or glomerulonephritis

*Large vessel refers to the aorta and the largest branches directed toward major body regions (e.g., to the extremities and the head and neck); medium-sized vessel refers to the main visceral arteries (e.g., renal, hepatic, coronary, and mesenteric arteries); small vessel refers to venules, capillaries, arterioles, and the intraparenchymal distal arterial radicals that connect with arterioles. Some small and large vessel vasculitides may involve medium-sized arteries, but large and medium-sized vessel vasculitides do not involve vessels smaller than arteries. Essential components are represented by normal type; italicized type represents usual, but not essential, components.*

†Preferred term.

‡Strongly associated with antineutrophil cytoplasmic autoantibodies.

From Jennette C, Falk RJ: Nomenclature of systemic vasculitides: Proposal of an international consensus conference. Arthritis Rheum 37:187, 1994.

matoid granulomatosis has often been classified with the pulmonary vasculitides, we consider it to represent a neoplastic process and discuss it separately (*see* page 1280). A discussion of necrotizing sarcoid granulomatosis is included in this chapter because of its prominent vascular involvement, recognizing that the disease may be better considered a secondary vasculitis. The subject of vasculitis in general and pulmonary vasculitis in particular has been the subject of a number of reviews.[8, 9, 11–13, 13a, 267]

## WEGENER'S GRANULOMATOSIS

Wegener's granulomatosis is a multisystem disease with variable clinical expression, which, in its full-blown state, is characterized pathologically by necrotizing granulomatous inflammation of the upper and lower respiratory tracts, glomerulonephritis, and necrotizing vasculitis of the lungs and a variety of systemic organs and tissues. A classification scheme developed by the American College of Rheumatology in 1990 considered four principal criteria in the diagnosis (Table 40–2):[14] (1) nasal or oral inflammation; (2) an abnormal chest radiograph; (3) an abnormal urinary sediment; and (4) granulomatous inflammation on a biopsy specimen (in the event a specimen is unavailable, hemoptysis can be substituted as the fourth criterion). Using a reference group of 722 patients with other forms of vasculitis and 85 patients considered to have Wegener's granulomatosis on the basis of more extensive criteria, the presence of two or more of these criteria was associated with a diagnostic sensitivity of approximately 88% and a specificity of 92%.[14]

Two clinical variants of Wegener's granulomatosis have been described in addition to the full-blown systemic disease. The more common is manifested primarily or solely in the respiratory tract and is thus known as *limited (nonrenal)* Wegener's granulomatosis.[15, 16] In many cases, the qualifier "limited" refers chiefly to an absence of clinical manifestations of renal and other visceral disease; concomitant

## Table 40–2. CRITERIA AND DEFINITIONS USED FOR THE CLASSIFICATION OF WEGENER'S GRANULOMATOSIS*

| CRITERION | DEFINITION |
|---|---|
| Nasal or oral inflammation | Development of painful or painless oral ulcers or purulent or bloody nasal discharge |
| Abnormal chest radiograph | Chest radiograph showing the presence of nodules, fixed infiltrates, or cavities |
| Urinary sediment | Microhematuria (>5 red blood cells per high-power field) or red cell casts in urine sediment |
| Granulomatous inflammation on biopsy | Histologic changes showing granulomatous inflammation within the wall of an artery or in the perivascular or extravascular area (artery or arteriole) |

*For purposes of classification, a patient is said to have Wegener's granulomatosis if at least 2 of these 4 criteria are present.

Modified from Leavitt RY, Fauci AS, Bloch DA, et al: The American College of Rheumatology 1990 criteria for the classification of Wegener's granulomatosis. Arthritis Rheum 33:1101, 1990.

involvement of the upper respiratory tract and skin is not uncommon,[16–18] and a number of patients with apparently limited disease have been found at autopsy or biopsy to have histologic evidence of glomerulonephritis or systemic vasculitis and granulomatous inflammation.[16, 19] (In fact, 7 of the 16 patients initially described with this form of disease showed such systemic involvement, although it was usually mild and focal in nature.[16]) Thus, from a pathogenetic point of view, it is probably appropriate to consider these cases as part of a spectrum of disease rather than as a separate entity.[15] From a practical point of view, a diagnosis of "limited" Wegener's granulomatosis should be made only after investigations have excluded the possibility of an infectious cause, especially when disease consists of a solitary pulmonary nodule. A second, less common clinical variant of Wegener's granulomatosis is characterized by prominent and sometimes prolonged involvement of the mucous membranes of the upper respiratory tract and skin.[20, 21]

### Epidemiology

Wegener's granulomatosis is a rare disease. For example, the incidence in the adult population has been estimated to be about 8.5 per 1 million annually in Norfolk, England[22] and about 1.3 per 100,000 per 5 years in the Leicester region.[23] In the United States, the prevalence has been estimated to be about 3 per 100,000.[24] The disease typically affects adults in their thirties to fifties, the mean age in three large series being 46, 41, and 56 years.[24–26] In some series, however, older individuals have constituted a significant proportion of affected individuals; for example, in one study of 51 patients, 29 (57%) were less than 60 years of age, and 22 (43%) were 60 years old or older.[27] There is evidence that the clinical features and prognosis of disease in such individuals differ from those in younger patients (*see* farther on).[27] Wegener's granulomatosis is particularly rare in children, but has been seen in an appreciable number of adolescents;[28, 29] in a review of 180 cases referred to the U.S. National Institutes of Health (NIH) over a 24-year period, 15% were in patients younger than 19 years.[25] There is no sex predominance.[25, 26] The rarity of cases developing during pregnancy indicates that it is not a risk factor (although it has been suggested that the disease might be more severe in this condition).[30, 31]

One group of investigators found evidence for a seasonal variation in the onset of symptoms, being highest (approximately 35% of patients) in the spring and lowest (14%) in the summer.[32] Others have found no evidence of such variation[24] or have found a higher incidence in the winter.[22] In one epidemiologic study from New York State, significant differences in the reported incidence of disease were found between different counties, the highest rates being in nonmetropolitan areas.[24]

### Etiology and Pathogenesis

A variety of etiologic agents and pathogenetic processes have been considered in Wegener's granulomatosis, including infectious organisms, heredity, antibodies (particularly those directed to neutrophil proteinase), antigen-antibody complex deposition, and cell-mediated immunity. As with the autoimmune connective tissue diseases, it is likely that more than one of these is involved.

### Infection

The prominent involvement of the upper and lower respiratory tracts as well as the occurrence of occasional cases predominantly limited to these sites strongly suggests that the causative agent of Wegener's granulomatosis is inhaled. Most investigation concerning the nature of such a putative agent has centered on infectious organisms, for which a number of observations suggest a possible role.[33] Clinical experience has shown that the development of relapses is preceded in some cases by evidence of bacterial or viral infection, often of the upper or lower respiratory tract.[34] Some investigators have shown such relapse to be associated with an increased likelihood of chronic nasal colonization by *Staphylococcus aureus*;[35] a possible association with lower respiratory tract infection by the same organism has also been reported.[36, 37] Evidence for a relation between systemic vasculitis (including some cases diagnosed as Wegener's granulomatosis) and chronic infection by parvovirus B19 has also been published.[38]

Several investigators have shown a beneficial response to therapy with trimethoprim-sulfamethoxazole,[39] particularly when disease is limited clinically to the upper and lower respiratory tracts[40] or after remission of disease following standard immunosuppressive therapy.[41] Although it has been suggested that this response may represent immunosuppressant or anti-inflammatory actions of the drugs,[39, 42] the possibility of a direct effect on an unrecognized microbe cannot be excluded. Despite these findings, lung cultures in cases of Wegener's granulomatosis are typically sterile, and no organisms have been identified by light or electron microscopic examination.

### Other Inhaled Substances

Inhaled substances other than microorganisms have been less investigated as possible causes of Wegener's granulomatosis. Granulomatous lesions closely resembling those of Wegener's granulomatosis have been induced in previously sensitized rabbits after inhalation of an aerosol consisting of bovine serum albumin and the T-cell mitogen concanavalin A, and it has been suggested that inhalation of naturally occurring concanavalin A or other plant lectins might thus be a pathogenetic factor.[43] A possible association with inhaled silica has also been identified;[44] in one case-control study, a nearly sevenfold risk for Wegener's granulomatosis was found in workers exposed to silica or grain dust.[45]

### Genetic Factors

In contrast to many diseases with a presumed immunopathogenesis, there is little evidence for a hereditary influence in Wegener's granulomatosis. Necrotizing granulomas and vasculitis consistent with Wegener's granulomatosis have been reported in family members,[46–48] and families with different forms of vasculitis (including Wegener's granulomatosis) have also been identified;[49] however, these situa-

tions are rare. Studies of the distribution of major histocompatibility complex (MHC) alleles have produced variable results, some showing an association between Wegener's granulomatosis and DR1,[50] DR2,[51] and DR13/DR6[52] and others no difference between the frequency of any MHC allele in control individuals and patients with Wegener's granulomatosis.[53]

An association between PiZ allele carriers and both Wegener's granulomatosis and ANCAs has been found by several groups of investigators.[54–56] For example, in one study of 105 C-ANCA–positive patients, there were 17 heterozygotes and 1 homozygote for PiZ;[57] 66 patients were considered to have Wegener's granulomatosis, of whom 15 (23%) were found to be heterozygotes. The pathogenetic significance of this association is unclear, particularly because vasculitides other than Wegener's granulomatosis have also been associated with a PiZZ genotype;[56] however, it does suggest the possibility of a genetic susceptibility for the development of the disease.

### Antineutrophil Cytoplasmic Antibodies

ANCAs react with substances in neutrophil azurophilic granules and monocyte lysosomes. Three forms can be identified by indirect immunofluorescence.[58, 59, 59a] *C-ANCA* produces cytoplasmic staining in alcohol-fixed cells and is directed predominantly to the serine proteinase, proteinase 3 (PR3). PR3 is structurally homologous to elastase, cathepsin G, and other neutrophil enzymes and has a variety of functions, including host defense and regulation of proliferation and differentiation of hematopoietic cells; its major natural inhibitor is alpha$_1$-antitrypsin (certain ANCAs also have an inhibitory action[60]). *P-ANCA* produces perinuclear staining in alcohol-fixed neutrophils and cytoplasmic staining in formalin-fixed material; it reacts predominantly with myeloperoxidase, but also with other enzymes, such as elastase, lysozyme, lactoferrin, and cathepsin D.[61] *Atypical ANCA* produce nuclear or varied cytoplasmic staining on alcohol-fixed material and are directed to a variety of antigens. In addition to immunofluorescence, ANCAs can be detected by enzyme-linked immunosorbent assay (ELISA) and radioimmunoassay.[62] In fact, it has been recommended that the presence of ANCAs be confirmed by ELISA after their detection on screening immunofluorescence.[59]

C-ANCA has been strongly associated with Wegener's granulomatosis, being seen in as many as 90% of patients with disseminated disease and, in some studies, showing a change in titer with disease activity (*see* page 1505); it is also present in many patients with microscopic polyangiitis and in some with infections (such as amebiasis, aspergillosis, bacterial endocarditis, and chromomycosis[63, 64, 441]), idiopathic necrotizing glomerulonephritis, idiopathic pulmonary hemosiderosis,[65] and nonclassifiable vasculitis.[58] P-ANCA and atypical ANCAs have also been detected in patients who have various vasculitides (particularly Churg-Strauss syndrome and microscopic polyangiitis) as well as those who have ulcerative colitis, Crohn's disease, autoimmune hepatic disease, some infections, and connective tissue disease such as rheumatoid disease and SLE.[58, 59, 61] In addition to systemic production, there is evidence that the antibodies may be elaborated locally in the respiratory tract.[66]

The high frequency of C-ANCA in Wegener's granulomatosis and its association with disease activity have suggested that they might have a pathogenic role in the development of vasculitis. A variety of experimental observations support this hypothesis.[67] In unstimulated neutrophils, PR3 is present within the azurophilic granules and thus unavailable for interaction with circulating antibodies. When neutrophils are activated—for example, by tumor necrosis factor-α or interleukin 1 (IL-1) or 8 (IL-8)—granules migrate to the cell surface where the PR3 becomes accessible.[68–70] When C-ANCA is added to such primed neutrophils *in vitro*, the latter undergo degranulation and release free radicals and potentially noxious enzymes.[69, 71] In fact, complexes of elastase and alpha₁-antitrypsin have been found to be elevated in the plasma of patients who have Wegener's granulomatosis, the levels varying with disease activity.[72] There is also evidence that the antibodies can stimulate both neutrophils and monocytes to produce cytokines that theoretically can enhance the local inflammatory reaction.[73, 74] Moreover, ANCAs from patients with clinically active disease were found in one study to induce a greater neutrophil respiratory burst than those from patients with inactive disease (the difference between the ANCAs in the two groups being a relatively greater amount of immunoglobulin G3 in those with active disease).[75] Hypothetically, therefore, an inflammatory stimulus such as an infection could lead to vasculitis by activating neutrophils in the presence of ANCAs.

PR3 has also been identified in human endothelial cells by some,[76] albeit not all,[77] investigators; as with neutrophils, stimulation by a variety of cytokines, such as tumor necrosis factor-α and IL-1, may lead to migration and expression of the enzyme on the cell surface. Cytotoxic effects have been documented in such "primed" endothelial cells incubated with C-ANCA and activated neutrophils *in vitro*.[78, 79] Antibodies to PR3 are also capable of increasing adherence of both neutrophils and T lymphocytes to cultured endothelial cells,[80, 81] and there is evidence that integrin adhesion molecules are up-regulated on leukocytes in patients with active Wegener's granulomatosis.[82] Thus, it is possible that an interaction between ANCAs and endothelial cells, either directly or indirectly via activated neutrophils or T cells, may also be involved in the development of vasculitis.

There is also evidence that ANCAs may be part of a cell-mediated immune response in Wegener's granulomatosis, possibly via PR3-mediated T-cell mitogenesis.[83] Several observations implicate such a response in the pathogenesis of the disease, including the presence of granulomatous inflammation in tissue specimens and an increase in markers of T-cell activity in the serum of patients with active disease.[84] The results of experimental studies of PR3–T cell interaction have been somewhat contradictory, however, and a definite role in pathogenesis is uncertain at the present time.[85]

Despite the attractiveness of these hypothetical mechanisms, it is clear that ANCA-mediated injury cannot be the entire explanation of the pathogenesis of Wegener's granulomatosis: not all patients have elevated ANCAs and the serum level of antibody does not always correlate with the severity of disease; moreover, some patients who have C-ANCA do not have Wegener's granulomatosis. In addition, although some experimental animal models have provided evidence of a pathogenetic role for ANCAs, conclusive proof is lacking.[67]

### Anti–Endothelial Cell Antibodies

Anti–endothelial cell antibodies are also common in a number of systemic vasculitides, including Wegener's granulomatosis.[86, 99] For example, in one investigation of 32 patients who had the latter condition, they were identified in all those considered to have clinically active disease, including some who were negative for C-ANCA;[87] moreover, the antibody level was positively correlated with disease activity. However, as indicated previously, it is not certain whether these antibodies are pathogenic or are part of the reaction to endothelial damage. In one *in vitro* study, they were shown to up-regulate several cell adhesion molecules and to induce the secretion of various cytokines, including IL-1β, IL-6, IL-8, and monocyte chemoattractant protein-1;[88] although the antibodies displayed no cytotoxic activity, it was concluded that they could play a pathogenetic role by facilitating leukocyte recruitment and adhesion to endothelial surfaces. Despite these observations, some investigators have found little evidence for a pathogenetic role in the disease.[89]

### Immune Complexes

Circulating immune complexes (including those related to PR3-ANCA)[54] have been demonstrated in some patients with active Wegener's granulomatosis;[26, 90–92] in some studies, they have been found to be associated with disease activity, and in one case, they disappeared during remission induced by immunosuppressive therapy.[90] In addition, subepithelial electron-dense deposits as well as complement and IgG have been found in renal glomeruli of some patients,[93, 94] suggesting that immune complex deposition may play a role in the pathogenesis of the glomerulonephritis. Immunohistochemical examination of pulmonary tissue for the presence of immune complex deposits has led to conflicting results: some workers have reported granular deposition of IgG and C3 in the walls of alveoli and medium-sized blood vessels,[91] others have shown IgG and IgM on alveolar walls but not within vessels,[92] and still others (the majority) have found no evidence of immune complex deposition.[93, 95, 96]

### Cell-Mediated Immunity

As indicated previously, the frequent presence of granulomatous inflammation in active lesions, in relation to both vessels and extravascular tissue, implies a cell-mediated component in the pathogenesis of Wegener's granulomatosis. As with antibody-mediated disease, several clinical and experimental observations support this hypothesis. For example, some investigators have found T lymphocytes from patients with Wegener's granulomatosis to have an increased proliferative response to purified PR3 and to nonfractionated proteins of neutrophil azurophilic granules.[97] Others have found the number of CD4+ T cells to be decreased and the number of CD8+ cells increased in patients with Wegener's granulomatosis compared with healthy individuals;[98] moreover, both CD4+ and CD8+ cell subsets showed evidence of activation in Wegener's granulomatosis. The documentation of elevated levels of serum markers of T-cell activation in many patients with active disease also suggests a cell-mediated response.[84] Despite these observations, the details of possible cell-mediated mechanisms in the pathogenesis

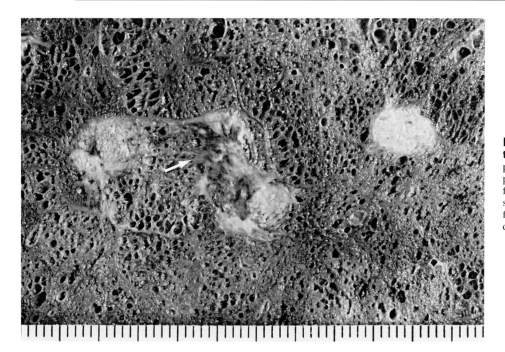

**Figure 40–1. Wegener's Granulomatosis.** Two discrete foci of necrosis, one partially bounded by interlobular septa, are present in the lung parenchyma. Treatment for Wegener's granulomatosis had been instituted 3 weeks before death, and some fibrosis, probably related to its effect, is evident in the larger lesion *(arrow).*

of Wegener's granulomatosis are unclear. Although cell-mediated immunity may be depressed in patients with advanced disease who have therapeutically induced immunosuppression,[100] delayed hypersensitivity skin reactions are positive in those tested before therapy.[101]

### Pathologic Characteristics

Pathologic features of Wegener's granulomatosis are variable, but overall quite characteristic of the disease.[16, 102–105] Grossly, pulmonary involvement is typically characterized by well-circumscribed nodules or masses ranging in diameter from 1 to 10 cm, often with central necrosis (Fig. 40–1); cavitation may be present, especially in larger masses. Occasionally, disease is manifested by a solitary nodule[106] or by focal or diffuse hemorrhagic consolidation.[103]

Microscopically, the nodules are composed of variable amounts of inflammatory and necrotic tissue, typically associated with effacement of normal lung architecture (Fig. 40–2).[104, 105, 107] The inflammatory infiltrate is composed predominantly of lymphocytes, plasma cells, and histiocytes, with lesser numbers of eosinophils, multinucleated giant cells, and polymorphonuclear leukocytes. Characteristically, the last-named tend to be aggregated in small microabscess-like clusters (Fig. 40–3*A*). As the disease progresses, these clusters become necrotic and are often bordered by a layer of macrophages or epithelioid histiocytes (Fig. 40–3*B*). With further progression, individual necrotic areas enlarge and coalesce, resulting in a characteristic serpiginous outline (Fig. 40–4). At this time, the necrotic tissue usually has a basophilic, granular appearance and is bordered by a distinct layer of epithelioid histiocytes (granulomatous inflammation). Small granulomas, usually poorly formed but sometimes well circumscribed and resembling those of sarcoidosis, also may be present in the surrounding inflammatory infiltrate. Depending on the stage of the disease and the effect of therapy, some lesions show relatively less inflammatory cell infiltrate and more fibrosis.

Additional histologic findings in the lung parenchyma include air-space filling by blood, macrophages or fibroblastic tissue, nonspecific or follicular bronchiolitis, and obstructive pneumonitis.[104] Usually, these are relatively minor in extent; occasionally, they comprise a prominent component

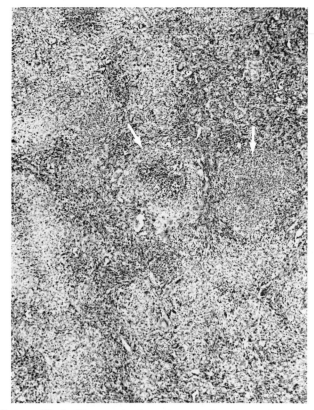

**Figure 40–2. Wegener's Granulomatosis—Parenchymal Destruction.** A section of a grossly nodular focus of consolidation shows complete effacement of lung parenchyma by a mixed inflammatory infiltrate. Multiple small foci of necrosis containing polymorphonuclear leukocytes are present *(arrows).*

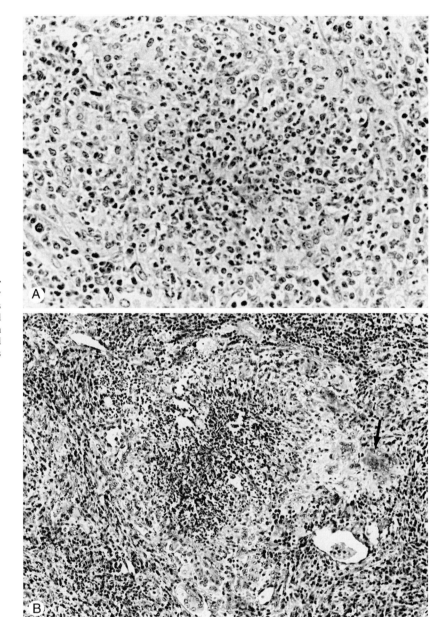

**Figure 40–3. Wegener's Granulomatosis—Pulmonary Parenchymal Inflammation.** Sections *(A, B)* show distinct aggregates of neutrophils within a polymorphous infiltrate of macrophages, lymphocytes, eosinophils, and isolated polymorphonuclear leukocytes. The aggregate in *B* is partly necrotic and bordered by a layer of epithelioid histiocytes and occasional multinucleated giant cells *(arrow)*. *(A,* ×200; *B,* ×120.)

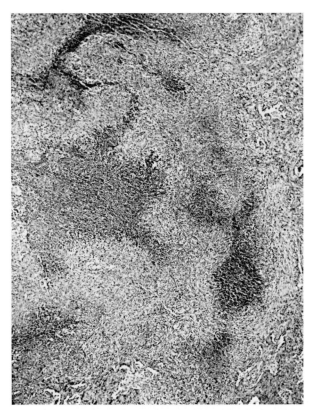

**Figure 40–4. Wegener's Granulomatosis—Parenchymal Necrosis.** A low-power view of a grossly nodular focus of consolidation shows almost complete effacement of lung parenchyma by a chronic inflammatory infiltrate containing irregularly shaped (serpiginous) foci of dark-staining necrotic material. (×40.)

of biopsy material, in which case there may be histologic confusion with other conditions, such as bronchiolitis obliterans organizing pneumonia,[108] eosinophilic pneumonia, or Churg-Strauss syndrome.[109]

Although inflammation is typically most prominent in the parenchyma, involvement of the airways is also common, either by direct extension from a parenchymal focus or independently.[102, 110] This involvement can take the form of mucosal or submucosal granulomatous inflammation (Fig. 40–5); the epithelium may be intact or superficially ulcerated, in which case there may be a polypoid mass of granulation tissue that causes airway obstruction. The subglottic trachea is a relatively common site of the latter complication.

Pulmonary arteries and veins of small to medium size show focal or extensive inflammation, manifested by one of three patterns (Fig. 40–6): (1) fibrinoid necrosis of the media; (2) infiltration of the vessel wall, often the media and sometimes all layers, by a mixed inflammatory infiltrate similar to that in the parenchyma; or (3) well-defined granulomas or aggregates of multinucleated giant cells. Thrombosis may or may not be present. To be characterized as a true vasculitis and not secondary to the parenchymal inflammation, inflamed vessels should ideally be situated in relatively normal parenchyma outside the inflammatory or necrotic zones; because they are often not observed in this location, however, their presence at the margin of the involved tissue or in foci of relatively mild inflammation is usually taken as evidence of primary vascular abnormality. Elastic tissue

stains may be useful for detecting remnants of partly destroyed vessels.

In cases characterized grossly by focal or diffuse hemorrhagic consolidation, the histologic appearance is different and is best described as capillaritis or microangiitis.[103, 107, 111–113] In these cases, the underlying lung architecture is maintained, but the alveolar air spaces are filled with red blood cells; hemosiderin-laden macrophages indicative of prior hemorrhage and foci of organizing fibrinous exudate (presumably reflecting healing alveolar wall damage) may also be seen. Alveolar septa are thickened by a variable number of polymorphonuclear leukocytes that may be focally necrotic (Fig. 40–7). Fibrin thrombi may be evident in the vascular lumen. In addition to capillaries, arterioles and venules are also often affected. The findings associated with microangiitis may be the only histologic manifestation of Wegener's granulomatosis or may be present in association with the classic parenchymal and vascular changes described previously.

As might be expected, therapy for Wegener's granulomatosis has an effect on all the histologic abnormalities just described.[114] Findings related to such therapy may be seen shortly after its institution (in some cases within 1 week)[104] and include decreased prominence of active vascular and parenchymal inflammation, parenchymal fibrosis (manifested as either focal scars or more diffuse interstitial disease) and bronchiolar fibrosis.

In the upper respiratory tract, involvement of the mucous membranes of the paranasal sinuses results in thickening in the early stages and, in some cases, eventually in destruction of bone and cartilage. The histologic appearance is similar to that seen in the lung parenchyma, although nonspecific chronic inflammation may be the only abnormality in small biopsy specimens.[116–118] Characteristically the kidneys show a focal and segmental necrotizing glomerulonephritis histologically similar to that seen in PAN and a variety of other conditions.[119] In one review of 349 cases of Wegener's granulomatosis published between 1979 and 1995, 267 (77%) were reported to have had renal involvement;[120] in renal biopsy specimens, extracapillary proliferation (crescent formation) was evident in 94 (70%), fibrinoid necrosis in 72 (54%), granuloma formation in 7 (5%), and interstitial vasculitis in 25 (19%). Vasculitis in systemic vessels is similar to that seen in the lung; the bronchial arteries are occasionally affected.[103] Rarely, disease in extrapulmonary sites is manifested as a masslike lesion resembling a neoplasm or an abscess;[121, 122] in cases in which other features of Wegener's granulomatosis are inapparent, the possibility of misdiagnosis is obvious.

### Radiologic Manifestations

In an analysis of the findings in 158 patients with Wegener's granulomatosis referred to the NIH, pulmonary parenchymal abnormalities were identified on the initial chest radiograph in 45% and eventually developed in 85%.[123] The typical pattern consists of nodules ranging in size from a few millimeters to 10 cm in diameter (Fig. 40–8);[124–126] rarely, there is a reticulonodular interstitial pattern.[127, 128] In 80% to 95% of cases, the nodules are fewer than 10.[125, 126, 136] They are bilateral in approximately 75% of cases[124] and are

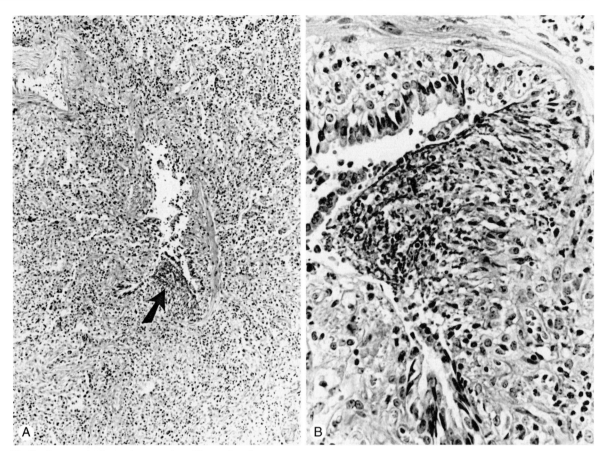

**Figure 40–5. Wegener's Granulomatosis—Airway Involvement.** A section of lung *(A)* shows severe parenchymal fibrosis and chronic inflammation associated with effacement of normal architecture. A membranous bronchiole shows focal acute inflammation and necrosis of the mucosa *(arrow,* magnified in *B).* The difference in histologic appearance of this focus of inflammation from that of the surrounding lung suggests that it is a manifestation of primary mucosal injury rather than an extension of the parenchymal disease. Typical features of Wegener's granulomatosis were present elsewhere in the biopsy specimen.

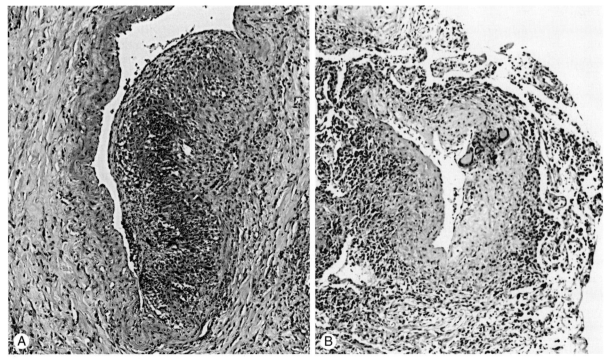

**Figure 40–6. Wegener's Granulomatosis—Vasculitis.** A section of a medium-sized pulmonary artery *(A)* shows a focus of acute inflammation and necrosis in the media identical to that of the parenchymal inflammation typical of Wegener's granulomatosis. A section of a similar size vessel from another case *(B)* shows a focus of granulomatous inflammation in the media. *(A,* ×80; *B,* ×100.)

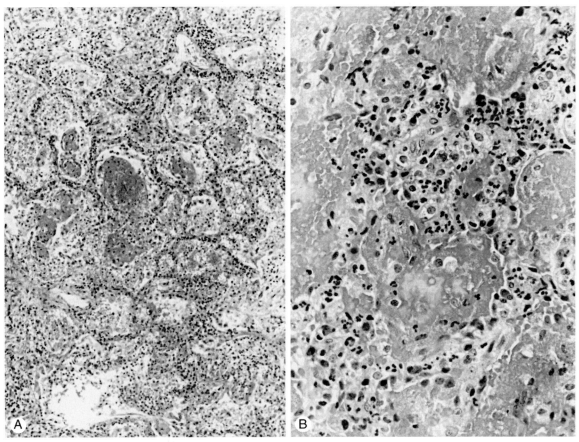

**Figure 40–7. Wegener's Granulomatosis—Capillaritis.** A section from an open-lung biopsy specimen of a patient with bilateral air-space disease *(A)* shows filling of alveolar air spaces by blood and mild-to-moderate thickening of alveolar septa. On higher magnification *(B)*, the latter can be seen to be the result of an infiltrate of polymorphonuclear leukocytes.

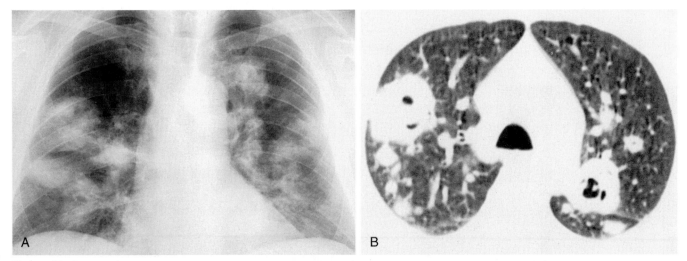

**Figure 40–8. Wegener's Granulomatosis.** A posteroanterior chest radiograph *(A)* and a CT scan at the level of the upper lobes *(B)* demonstrate multiple bilateral nodules ranging from a few millimeters to 5 cm in diameter. The larger nodules are cavitated. The patient was a 54-year-old man; open-lung biopsy showed features typical of Wegener's granulomatosis.

usually widely distributed, with no predilection for any lung zone.[124, 129, 130] With progression of disease, the nodules tend to increase in size and in number.[124] Calcification is rare (Fig. 40–9).[115, 131] Cavitation occurs eventually in approximately 50% of cases.[124, 133] The cavities are usually thick walled and tend to have an irregular, shaggy inner lining;[124, 126, 133] less commonly, they are thin walled[115, 133, 134] or contain an air-fluid level (Fig. 40–10). The cavities may become large, sometimes involving a whole lobe.[131] Rarely, individual pulmonary opacities, with or without cavitation, decrease in size or even disappear before therapy.[132]

Computed tomography may demonstrate nodules that are not apparent on radiography and is superior in demonstrating the presence of cavitation;[115, 133, 134a] in fact, cavitation is evident on CT in the majority of nodules that measure more than 2 cm.[126] As on radiography, the nodules tend to have a random distribution;[126, 134] occasionally, they are predominantly or exclusively subpleural in location[134] or have a peribronchovascular distribution.[133, 135] CT may also show "feeding vessels" leading into the nodules (Fig. 40–11), although the usefulness of this finding in differential diagnosis is questionable.[133, 135] Occasionally, a peripheral pulmonary artery is identified that is irregular and stellate in shape and larger than its corresponding bronchus *(vasculitis sign).*[133]

Acute air-space consolidation or ground-glass opacities secondary to pulmonary hemorrhage (Fig. 40–12) is the second most common radiographic finding in Wegener's granulomatosis and may occur with or without the presence of nodules (Fig. 40–13).[124, 129, 133] The areas of consolidation are quite variable in appearance, some being dense and localized,[124] some involving a whole lobe,[136, 137] and others being bilateral and patchy or confluent (Fig. 40–14).[122, 133] In one review of the radiographic findings in 77 patients with pulmonary Wegener's granulomatosis, nodules were identified on the radiograph in 69% of cases and areas of consolidation in 53%;[124] 49% of nodules and 17% of areas of consolidation had evidence of cavitation. Diffuse bilateral areas of ground-glass opacity or consolidation were seen in 8% of cases. On CT, the areas of consolidation may be random in distribution; sometimes they appear as peripheral wedge-shaped lesions abutting the pleura mimicking pulmo-

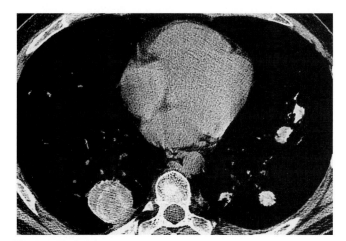

**Figure 40–9. Wegener's Granulomatosis.** HRCT scan in a 39-year-old man demonstrates several bilateral calcified lung nodules. The diagnosis of Wegener's granulomatosis was based on a combination of clinical findings and positive C-ANCA.

nary infarcts[135] or have a peribronchoarterial distribution (Fig. 40–15).[126, 133, 138] Calcification within areas of consolidation is rare.[124] Less common parenchymal abnormalities evident on CT include interlobular septal thickening, centrilobular interstitial thickening, and parenchymal bands.[134a]

Bronchial wall involvement by Wegener's granulomatosis may result in airway narrowing and lead to segmental, lobar, or total lung atelectasis.[124, 131] The bronchial abnormalities themselves or those affecting the trachea are seldom visible on the radiograph.[125, 139] For example, in one study of 51 patients who underwent bronchoscopy, 30 (59%) had tracheal or endobronchial disease, including subglottic stenosis, ulcerating tracheobronchitis, and tracheal or bronchial stenosis;[139] in none of these cases were these abnormalities evident on radiography. Tracheal and bronchial wall thickening and narrowing of the lumen, however, can usually be detected on CT.[125, 133, 134, 140] The tracheal rings may be abnormally thickened and calcified.[141] Rarely, tracheal[141a] or esophageal[141b] involvement leads to a tracheoesophageal fistula.

Pleural effusions may be unilateral or bilateral and small or large. They have been reported in as few as 3% and as many as 55% of cases in various series,[131, 133, 134, 142] the best estimate of frequency probably being about 10%.[124] Rarely, there are other pleural abnormalities, such as unilateral or bilateral pleural thickening,[131] pneumothorax, hydropneumothorax,[133, 143] or pyopneumothorax.[144]

Hilar or mediastinal lymph node enlargement, or both, has been reported on radiography or CT in 2% to 15% of cases.[124, 125, 133] The hilar lymphadenopathy may be unilateral or bilateral. Occasionally, enlarged mediastinal nodes compress the trachea or bronchi.[144a]

## Clinical Manifestations

The onset of Wegener's granulomatosis may be acute and its course fulminating,[145] but is more commonly insidious. The latter is particularly seen in patients with "limited" disease, in whom the diagnosis may not be made until many years after the onset of symptoms.[25] Although the disease may be associated initially with such nonspecific symptoms as fever, malaise, weight loss, and fatigue, the majority of patients present with complaints referable to the nose, paranasal sinuses, ear, or chest;[25] in fact, many patients initially consult an otolaryngologist or ophthalmologist. In the review of 180 patients referred to the NIH cited previously, clinical features of ear, nose, and throat; pulmonary; and ocular disease were present initially in approximately 75%, 50%, and 15%, respectively.[25] A few patients present with symptoms and signs of widespread disease.

Thoracic symptoms consist most often of cough, hemoptysis, dyspnea, and pleuritic pain.[25, 26] Cough, usually nonproductive, is the most frequent, occurring in 60 of 77 patients with pulmonary disease in one review.[26] Hemoptysis is seen in about 30% to 40% of these patients; occasionally, it is massive, the clinical presentation mimicking Goodpasture's syndrome.[93, 146, 147] Dyspnea occurs particularly with alveolar hemorrhage and, occasionally, as a result of tracheal involvement.[148, 149]

There is some evidence that clinical manifestations are different in older individuals.[27] For example, in one investigation of 67 patients, of whom 33 were older than 60 years

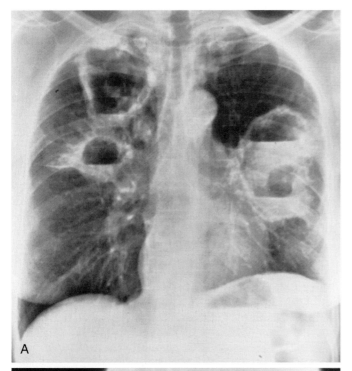

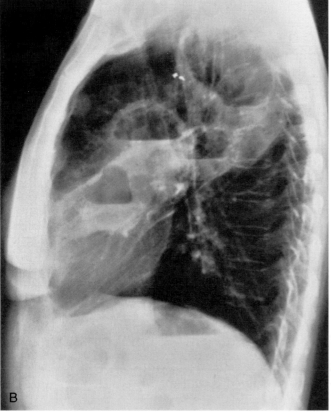

**Figure 40–10. Wegener's Granulomatosis—Cavitation.** Posteroanterior *(A)* and lateral *(B)* radiographs in a 55-year-old woman reveal multiple, large, thick-walled cavities with air-fluid levels. The left upper lung zone is oligemic, suggesting the possibility of stenosis of the left upper lobe bronchus with secondary hypoxic vasoconstriction.

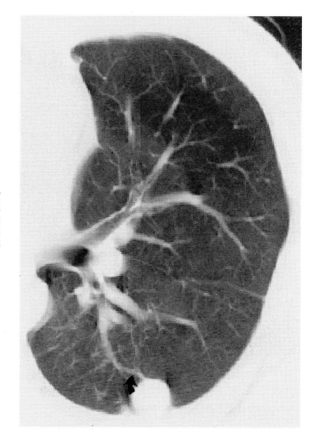

**Figure 40–11. Wegener's Granulomatosis.** A view of the left lung from a CT scan in a 42-year-old man with Wegener's granulomatosis demonstrates a 1.5-cm subpleural nodule. A vessel *(arrow)* can be seen to course into the nodule *(feeding vessel sign)*. This finding has also been described in other conditions in which pulmonary vessels are predominantly affected, such as metastatic carcinoma and septic emboli.

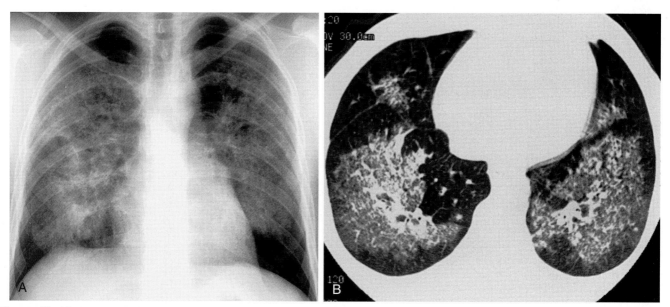

**Figure 40–12. Wegener's Granulomatosis—Air-Space Hemorrhage.** A posteroanterior chest radiograph *(A)* in a 20-year-old man shows extensive bilateral areas of consolidation with relative sparing of the lung apices and bases. Several irregular linear opacities suggestive of fibrosis are also evident. HRCT scan *(B)* demonstrates bilateral areas of ground-glass attenuation and consolidation with relative sparing of the subpleural lung regions. A few small nodular and irregular linear opacities are also evident. The patient had had recurrent episodes of pulmonary hemorrhage.

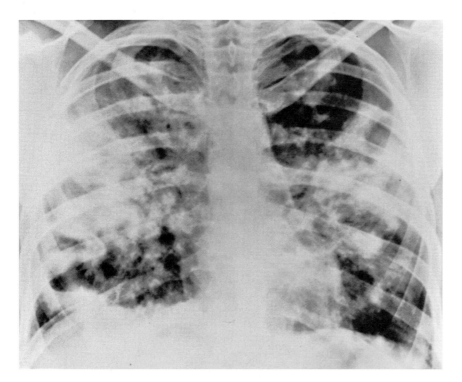

**Figure 40–13. Wegener's Granulomatosis, Limited Form.** A posteroanterior chest radiograph in a 24-year-old man demonstrates extensive bilateral air-space consolidation. Cavities are present in the right lower and left upper lobes. The patient presented with a 2-month history of increased exertional dyspnea, dry cough, malaise, and nocturnal fever. He died approximately 2 weeks later. Pathologic diagnosis at autopsy was Wegener's granulomatosis, limited form. (Courtesy of Dr. Michael Lefcoe, Victoria Hospital, London, Ontario.)

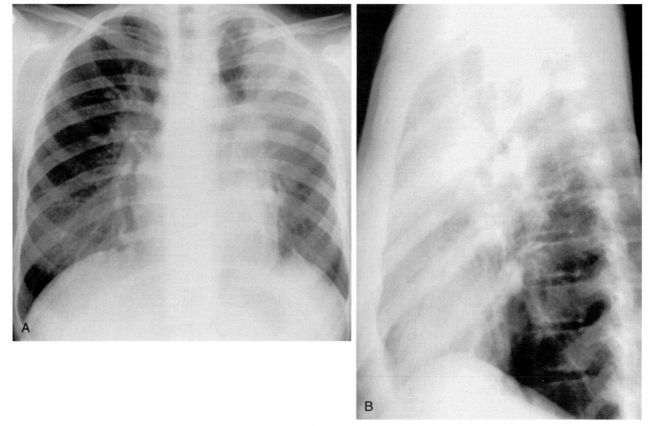

**Figure 40–14. Wegener's Granulomatosis with Nonsegmental Consolidation.** Posteroanterior *(A)* and lateral *(B)* chest radiographs reveal extensive air-space consolidation in the left upper and lower lobes; faint air bronchograms are visible in both areas. Elevation of the left main and upper lobe bronchi and a left juxtaphrenic peak indicate a mild degree of atelectasis. Open-lung biopsy revealed features typical of Wegener's granulomatosis.

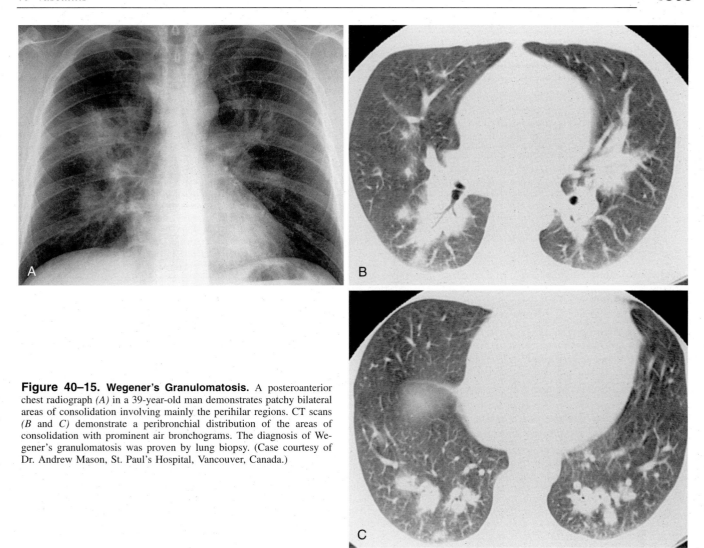

**Figure 40–15. Wegener's Granulomatosis.** A posteroanterior chest radiograph *(A)* in a 39-year-old man demonstrates patchy bilateral areas of consolidation involving mainly the perihilar regions. CT scans *(B* and *C)* demonstrate a peribronchial distribution of the areas of consolidation with prominent air bronchograms. The diagnosis of Wegener's granulomatosis was proven by lung biopsy. (Case courtesy of Dr. Andrew Mason, St. Paul's Hospital, Vancouver, Canada.)

of age, the prevalence of upper respiratory tract involvement and hemoptysis was significantly less common and that of renal insufficiency and central nervous system involvement significantly more common in the older group.[150]

Associations of Wegener's granulomatosis with immunologically mediated diseases, such as Hashimoto's thyroiditis[151] and CREST syndrome,[152] have been documented; however, the number of cases is so small that a spurious association cannot be excluded. One group of investigators found that patients with Wegener's granulomatosis had an increased likelihood of a history of an allergic disorder (predominantly skin, drug, and insect reactions) compared with healthy individuals and patients without vasculitis who were attending a general rheumatology clinic.[153]

Although virtually any organ or tissue can be affected in Wegener's granulomatosis, the most common are the lungs, upper respiratory tract (including the nose, nasal sinuses, middle ear, larynx, and subglottic trachea), kidneys, systemic vessels, joints, skin, and eyes.[101]

### Upper Respiratory Tract

The upper respiratory tract is affected at the onset of disease in about 50% to 75% of patients and at some time

during its course in almost all patients.[25] The most common manifestations are those related to sinusitis and nasal ulceration. The latter may be associated with destruction of bone and cartilage and significant nasal deformity. Manifestations of otitis, including pain and hearing loss, are also common.

Involvement of the larynx and subglottic region of the trachea is surprisingly frequent and may be manifested by hoarseness or, in severe cases, dyspnea. In one series of 189 patients with Wegener's granulomatosis followed at the NIH, subglottic stenosis was documented in 43 (23%);[154] the complication often developed in the absence of other features of active Wegener's granulomatosis. Occasionally, it is the initial manifestation of disease.[155] In a small number of patients, open surgical reconstruction is necessary;[25, 156] rarely, the process leads to a tracheoesophageal fistula[157] or is severe enough to cause airway obstruction and death.[158]

### Kidney

Although manifestations of renal disease occur in 75% to 85% of patients at some time in the course of the disease,[25, 159] only rarely are they the presenting clinical features.[160–162] Aneurysms similar to those seen in PAN have been identified by angiography in some cases.[141, 163]

## Musculoskeletal System

Musculoskeletal symptoms occur in about 30% of patients at the onset of disease. Joint involvement usually takes the form of arthralgia; arthritis, sometimes migratory and similar to rheumatoid arthritis, occurs occasionally.[164] Skeletal muscle involvement is usually manifested by myalgia; jaw claudication[165] and acute myositis[166] have been reported rarely. The former may lead to a mistaken diagnosis of giant cell arteritis.[167] Bone involvement occurs most often secondary to nasal or sinusoidal disease and is thus usually seen in the facial bones; examples arising at other sites have been reported rarely.[168]

## Central and Peripheral Nervous Systems

Neurologic manifestations are relatively uncommon at presentation, but develop in 20% to 35% of patients during the course of disease.[25, 169] In one review of 324 consecutive patients, 109 (34%) had neurologic involvement;[169] peripheral neuropathy occurred in 53, cranial neuropathy in 21, external ophthalmoplegia in 16, cerebrovascular events in 13, seizures in 10, and cerebritis in 5. Peripheral nervous system involvement is typically manifested as mononeuritis multiplex or polyneuritis. Cranial neuropathies may be related to meningeal involvement,[170, 171] and may be the only manifestation of disease for several years before there is clinical evidence of involvement elsewhere.[172] The diagnosis has been confirmed in some of these cases by measuring C-ANCA in cerebrospinal fluid.[173] Headache,[174] hydrocephalus,[175] and Horner's syndrome[176] occur occasionally. In one patient, cerebritis developed during cyclophosphamide therapy.[177]

## Eye

Ocular involvement is seen in about 10% to 15% of patients at the onset of disease and may be manifested by conjunctivitis, dacrocystitis, scleritis, proptosis (related to a retro-orbital pseudotumor), visual loss (usually as a result of optic nerve entrapment by a pseudotumor), diplopia, or pain.[178, 179]

## Heart and Large Systemic Vessels

Although evidence of myocardial involvement is not uncommon at autopsy, related clinical manifestations are infrequent.[180] They are usually the result of vascular occlusion and include conduction abnormalities and heart failure.[181–183] Valvulitis[184, 185] and congestive cardiomyopathy[185a] have been documented rarely. Pericarditis occurs in about 10% of patients; rarely, associated effusion is sufficient to result in hemodynamic compromise.[25] Clinical symptoms related to involvement of large systemic arteries are uncommon but can be associated with ischemic lesions, aneurysm formation, or rupture.[186, 187]

## Skin

Skin involvement occurs in about 10% to 15% of patients.[25, 188, 189] In one review of 244 patients, of whom 30 (14%) had skin disease, the most common manifestation was palpable purpura;[188] other findings included pyoderma-like ulcers, papules, petechiae, nodules, and bullae. Vascular occlusion may cause gangrene of the distal extremities.[190] There is evidence that the histologic pattern of skin involvement may be related to different clinical manifestations; in one study of 75 biopsy specimens from 46 patients, patients with leukocytoclastic vasculitis had more rapidly progressive and widespread disease (particularly musculoskeletal and renal) than patients without skin lesions or those whose biopsy specimens showed granulomatous inflammation;[191] the latter patients frequently had neither renal nor pulmonary manifestations of Wegener's granulomatosis.

## Miscellaneous Sites

Although *gastrointestinal* lesions are seen at autopsy in many patients,[192–194] prior signs and symptoms are uncommon. Intestinal perforation has been reported[195] and some patients have findings suggestive of idiopathic inflammatory bowel disease.[49, 192] Esophageal disease is rare.[196] Involvement of the *urogenital tract* (apart from glomerulonephritis) is relatively uncommon, but can be manifested by prostatitis, orchitis, ureteral stenosis, bladder pseudotumor, or penile ulceration.[197, 198] Distinction between Wegener's granulomatosis of the bladder and cyclophosphamide-related cystitis may be difficult.

Rarely affected tissues or organs include the *oral cavity* (manifested in some patients by swollen, erythematous ["strawberry"] gums),[199, 200] *salivary glands*,[201, 202] *pituitary* (with panhypopituitarism or diabetes insipidus),[203, 204] *retroperitoneum* (resulting in disease that resembles retroperitoneal fibrosis),[121] *breast* (not uncommonly misinterpreted clinically as carcinoma),[205, 206] and *mediastinum*.[121]

## Laboratory Findings and Diagnosis

### Hematologic and Miscellaneous Serologic Abnormalities

Laboratory findings include anemia, sometimes hemolytic in type;[207] thrombocytosis; and leukocytosis, occasionally with eosinophilia.[208] In the NIH review of 158 patients, the mean white count at presentation was $10.5 \times 10^9$/liter;[25] approximately two thirds of patients had a platelet count greater than $400 \times 10^9$/liter, and three quarters a hemoglobin less than 125 g/liter. These hematologic abnormalities tend to be less severe in patients without renal involvement.[120] As might be expected, markers of endothelial damage and coagulation disturbance, such as thrombin–antithrombin III complexes, fibrin-D-dimers, von Willebrand's factor, and thrombomodulin, are elevated in many patients. In fact, some investigators have found their levels to be closely related to disease activity.[209] The erythrocyte sedimentation rate is elevated (>70 mm/hour) in most patients. Hypercalcemia—presumably related to the presence of epithelioid histiocytes as in other granulomatous diseases—has been documented rarely.[210]

Rheumatoid factor may be detected in the serum, usually in low titers.[90, 101] Some patients have an elevated level of IgE.[91, 96, 164] Anticardiolipin antibodies are fairly common; in one investigation of 25 patients, they were detected in 10 (40%).[211] Anti–glomerular basement membrane antibodies are rarely present.[211] As discussed previously (*see* page 1492), immune complexes can be found in the serum in 15% to 20% of patients.

A number of investigators have attempted to identify markers of disease activity other than ANCA. In one study, monitoring of soluble endothelial leukocyte adhesion molecule-1, a neutrophil chemoattractant and possible marker of endothelial cell damage or activation, was shown to be useful both in diagnosis and in following disease activity.[212] Similar results have been found for other cell adhesion molecules (such as intercellular adhesion molecule-1 and vascular cell adhesion molecule-1),[213, 214] soluble serum thrombomodulin (a marker of endothelial cell injury),[215, 216] the soluble form of CD30 activation molecule,[217] and anti–endothelial cell antibodies.[87]

### Antineutrophil Cytoplasmic Antibodies

The diagnosis and management of Wegener's granulomatosis have been aided by the ability to measure serum ANCA levels. As discussed previously, most investigators have found C-ANCA in approximately 85% to 90% of patients with disseminated WG[218–220] and about 75% of those with limited disease[221] (however, *see* farther on); P-ANCA (directed to myeloperoxidase or leukocyte elastase) are found in a minority.[222, 223] The specificity of C-ANCA for Wegener's granulomatosis has been found to be relatively high by some investigators,[219, 224] although the antibody can also be seen in a variety of other conditions, including non-Wegener's granulomatosis vasculitis and some infections (e.g., amebiasis and chromomycosis[63, 64]). In one literature review, their incidence in the former group was 45% in microscopic polyangiitis, 10% in Churg-Strauss syndrome, and 5% in classic PAN.[58]

In addition to diagnosis, there is evidence that measurement of C-ANCA can be used to follow the course of disease and to guide therapy in patients with known Wegener's granulomatosis. A decrease in ANCA level has been documented in some patients during induction therapy.[225] Moreover, several groups of investigators have found relapses of disease to be preceded by an increase in the serum ANCA level[218, 224, 226] or to be associated with a persistently high ANCA level despite clinical improvement after immunosuppressive therapy.[225, 227] For example, in one investigation of 58 patients in whom the serum ANCA levels were prospectively assessed over a 24-month period, the antibodies were found to increase in 20 patients, of whom 9 were randomly assigned to receive treatment with prednisolone and cyclophosphamide;[228] the remaining 11 received no therapy until the onset of clinical disease. Nine of the latter patients relapsed (six within 3 months), whereas none of the group treated on the basis of an elevated ANCA level alone developed active disease. It has also been suggested that measurement of ANCA-related inhibition of PR3 activity may be an even more sensitive predictor of relapse.[60]

Despite these observations, it is clear that not all relapses of Wegener's granulomatosis are associated with an increase in ANCA titer and that some patients with a positive test result do not have the disease.[60, 225] For example, in one investigation of 53 patients in whom serial C-ANCA titers were obtained, a rise in titer preceded clinical exacerbation of disease in only 24% of patients.[229] Moreover, in another

study of 235 patients from a variety of "nonspecialist" centers in southwest England, investigators found an overall sensitivity and specificity of 65% and 77%;[230] false-positive tests—almost one third of which were related to C-ANCA—were identified in patients with infection, fibrotic lung disease, connective tissue disease, malignancy, and pulmonary thromboembolism. False-positive diagnoses of Wegener's granulomatosis based on clinical features and a positive C-ANCA test have also been reported in cases of ulcerative colitis, pulmonary aspergillosis, and disseminated *Mycobacterium bovis* infection.[231–233] In one review and meta-analysis of the literature to 1995, the overall sensitivity of C-ANCA testing for Wegener's granulomatosis ranged from 34% to 92% and the specificity from 88% to 100%;[234] the pooled sensitivity was 66%, and the pooled specificity was 98%. For active disease, the pooled sensitivity and specificity were 91% and 99%; for inactive disease, they were 63% and 99.5%.

On the basis of the current information, it seems reasonable to conclude that the presence of a positive test for C-ANCA is highly suggestive of vasculitis; when present in a patient with two or more clinical and radiologic criteria of Wegener's granulomatosis (as defined in the 1990 American College of Rheumatology classification, *see* page 1491),[14] a diagnosis of Wegener's granulomatosis is virtually ensured. In C-ANCA–positive patients with fewer American College of Rheumatology criteria or with atypical clinical or radiologic features, further investigation (including biopsy, if not already performed) is indicated. Similarly, patients with clinical and radiologic features of Wegener's granulomatosis and a negative ANCA test may require additional investigation. Although the significance of an increase in C-ANCA titer in a patient with known Wegener's granulomatosis in the absence of a clinical exacerbation is uncertain, he or she should at least be followed with particular care.

### Bronchoscopy

The frequency of airway abnormalities detected at bronchoscopy is high. In one study of 51 patients with biopsy-proven Wegener's granulomatosis who underwent the procedure, 30 (59%) had evidence of tracheobronchial disease, including subglottic, tracheal, or bronchial stenosis in 9 (30%), ulcerating tracheobronchitis with or without inflammatory pseudotumors in 18 (60%), and hemorrhage without an identifiable source in 2 (4%).[235] Biopsy of affected areas yields tissue that supports the diagnosis of Wegener's granulomatosis in some patients; the diagnosis has also been confirmed occasionally by transbronchial biopsy.[236]

In one study, bronchoalveolar lavage of patients with active Wegener's granulomatosis showed a marked increase in neutrophils (mean, 42% of white cells) and a mild increase in eosinophils (mean, 4%).[237] Increased levels of neutrophil-related cytokines and neutrophil products, such as IL-8, granulocyte colony-stimulating factor, and IL-1$\beta$, have also been documented in some patients.[238]

### Cytology

As might be expected, cytologic examination of specimens obtained by bronchial washing or brushing usually is not useful in diagnosis. However, the diagnosis can be suspected in material obtained by transthoracic needle aspiration on the basis of the presence of neutrophils, necrotic debris, and multinucleated giant cells.[239] The diagnosis has also been suggested on material obtained by nasal scraping.[240]

### Pulmonary Function Tests

Pulmonary function tests may show restrictive or obstructive disease. Flow/volume curves may be useful in diagnosing and following patients with tracheal or bronchial obstruction.[241, 242] Lowered values for pulmonary diffusing capacity usually do not improve with therapy, suggesting the possibility of an alveolitis attributable to either Wegener's granulomatosis itself or cyclophosphamide toxicity.[242]

### Natural History and Prognosis

Before the use of cyclophosphamide, the clinical course of Wegener's granulomatosis was generally progressive, death occurring within 6 months from uremia or, less often, from respiratory failure, coronary vasculitis, or myocarditis.[101] For example, in one series of 56 patients reported in 1958, 52 were dead within 2 years, the great majority (83%) from renal failure.[243] Combined corticosteroid and cytotoxic drug therapy, primarily with cyclophosphamide, has resulted in both clinical remissions of the disease and apparent cures, even in patients with renal involvement.[142, 244, 245] In the NIH review of 158 patients (of whom 138 were treated with combined therapy), complete remission of disease was documented in 75% of patients and marked improvement in another 15%.[25] The median time to achieve remission, however, was approximately 12 months and was as long as 6 years in some individuals. Moreover, 50% of patients with a complete remission experienced a relapse of disease after 3 months to 16 years. Similar results were found in another study of 28 patients, in whom the relapse rate was 44% and the median time to relapse was 42 months.[246] With the institution of controlled, randomized trials to evaluate both traditional and innovative forms of therapy, it is hoped that these figures may be improved.[247]

Despite the favorable impact of corticosteroid and cytotoxic drug therapy, morbidity and mortality are still substantial. For example, follow-up of 77 patients enrolled in the 1990 American College of Rheumatology vasculitis classification study revealed a significant increase in mortality compared with the general population (standard mortality ratio of 4.6 for women and 6.8 for men).[248] Other investigators have reported case fatality rates of 20% to 28%.[26] In the NIH study, 13% of patients were considered to have died of Wegener's granulomatosis or complications related to its treatment.[25] Renal failure requiring dialysis developed in 17 (11%) patients. Some degree of hearing or visual loss occurred in 33 and 8 patients, respectively. Chronic atrophic rhinitis and recurrent sinonasal infections were seen in almost 50% of individuals. Serial pulmonary function tests showed progressive deterioration in 17%, attributed to Wegener's granulomatosis, cyclophosphamide therapy, or both. Endobronchial fibrosis resulted in recurrent postobstructive pneumonia in several patients; as indicated previously (*see* page 1503), tracheal stenosis, usually subglottic, is also common.

As might be expected with prolonged treatment with cyclophosphamide and glucocorticoids, complications possibly related to these agents are also significant. In the NIH study, they included diabetes mellitus (8%), cystitis (43%), bladder cancer (2.8%), myelodysplasia (2%), cataracts (21%), infertility (16 of 28 women between 18 and 35 years), and aseptic necrosis of bone (3%).[25] Seventy-three patients experienced infections requiring hospitalization and intravenous antibiotic therapy;[25] *Pneumocystis carinii* has been found to be a particularly important opportunistic pathogen in some series.[249]

Several factors have been identified that may help predict disease outcome. As indicated previously, the prognosis in patients with the limited form of Wegener's granulomatosis is better than in those with classic disease, presumably because of the absence of significant renal involvement;[15, 16, 26, 136] in fact, prolonged, relatively symptom-free survival is possible.[250] Despite this, recurrence or progression of disease, sometimes rapid, can occur.[106, 251] In patients with disseminated disease, there is also evidence that the presence of PiZ heterozygosity is associated with a worse prognosis.[57] Some investigators have found the risk of mortality from infectious complications[150] or from uncontrolled pulmonary vasculitis[27] to be substantially higher in patients older than 60 years of age.

## CHURG-STRAUSS SYNDROME

In 1951, Churg and Strauss described a syndrome characterized clinically by asthma, fever, and blood eosinophilia and pathologically by necrotizing vasculitis and extravascular granulomatous inflammation.[252] This abnormality (Churg-Strauss syndrome, allergic granulomatosis and angiitis) has had a somewhat complicated conceptual history. At some times, it has been considered to represent a variant of Wegener's granulomatosis[253, 254] and at others part of a spectrum of disease that includes PAN (the term *overlap syndrome* sometimes being used to refer to the latter cases).[3, 253] In addition, some cases of Churg-Strauss syndrome share features with nonvasculitic conditions, such as hypereosinophilic syndrome or eosinophilic pneumonia.[255–257] Despite the fact that it is difficult to classify vasculitic disease with eosinophilia precisely in some patients, maintenance of Churg-Strauss syndrome as a disease entity is generally thought to serve a useful purpose.

Compounding these terminology and conceptual issues are the variable criteria that have been used to define Churg-Strauss syndrome. In their original report, Churg and Strauss stressed the histologic aspects of the disease as distinctive diagnostic features. It became clear, however, that not all of the histologic abnormalities were seen in every patient with the syndrome and that not every patient with the histologic changes described by Churg and Strauss had the clinical features of Churg-Strauss syndrome.[258] A group of clinical criteria were proposed in 1984 in an attempt to standardize the diagnosis, including the presence of asthma, a peak peripheral blood eosinophilia level of more than $1.5 \times 10^9$/liter, and systemic vasculitis involving two or more extrapulmonary organs.[258] This list was altered and expanded in the American College of Rheumatology vasculitis classification system proposed in 1990 to include asthma, peripheral blood eosinophilia greater than 10%, mononeuropathy or polyneuropathy, nonfixed pulmonary "infiltrates," paranasal sinus abnormality, and the presence of extravascular eosinophils (Table 40–3);[259] the presence of four or more of these criteria was found to be diagnostic of Churg-Strauss syndrome with a sensitivity of 85% and a specificity of almost 100%.

As with Wegener's granulomatosis, some patients have disease with a histologic appearance characteristic of Churg-Strauss syndrome that is localized to a single organ or tissue *(limited Churg-Strauss syndrome).*[260] The most common site of such disease is the gastrointestinal tract; the lung is rarely affected in this fashion.

### Epidemiology

Churg-Strauss syndrome is rare; only 138 cases had been documented in the English literature by 1984,[258] and in the American College of Rheumatology classification study, only 20 examples were identified among 787 cases of vasculitis.[261] The annual incidence in the Norfolk region of England has been estimated to be 2.4 per 1 million (approximately 30% that of Wegener's granulomatosis and the same as that of microscopic polyangiitis).[22]

Many patients experience the onset of allergic phenomena (asthma or rhinitis) in early adulthood; the mean age in one series of 12 patients was 25 years and in a literature review of 31 patients was 28 years.[258] Vasculitis develops most often in middle-aged adults, the mean age of onset being 38 to 48 years in different reviews.[258, 262] There is no sex predominance. Some authors have suggested that there may be an increased likelihood of the onset of disease in the spring.[256]

### Table 40–3. CRITERIA AND DEFINITIONS USED FOR THE CLASSIFICATION OF CHURG-STRAUSS SYNDROME

| CRITERION | DEFINITION |
| --- | --- |
| Asthma | History of wheezing or diffuse high-pitched wheezes on expiration |
| Eosinophilia | Eosinophilia >10% on white blood cell differential count |
| History of allergy | History of seasonal allergy (e.g., allergic rhinitis) or other documented allergies, including food, contactants, and others *except* for drug allergy |
| Mononeuropathy or polyneuropathy | Development of mononeuropathy, multiple mononeuropathies, or polyneuropathy (i.e., glove/stocking distribution) attributable to a systemic vasculitis |
| Pulmonary infiltrates, nonfixed | Migratory or transitory pulmonary infiltrates on radiographs (not including fixed infiltrates), attributable to a systemic vasculitis |
| Paranasal sinus abnormality | History of acute or chronic paranasal sinus pain or tenderness or radiographic opacification of the paranasal sinuses |
| Extravascular eosinophils | Biopsy including artery, arteriole, or venule, showing accumulations of eosinophils in extravascular areas |

Modified from Masi AT, Hunder GG, Lie JT, et al: The American College of Rheumatology 1990 criteria for the classification of Churg-Strauss syndrome (allergic granulomatosis and angiitis). Arthritis Rheum 33:1098, 1990.

### Etiology and Pathogenesis

The cause of Churg-Strauss syndrome is unknown; as with other vasculitides, more than one agent may be involved. The association with asthma, rhinitis, and an elevated level of serum IgE; the response to corticosteroids; and the pathologic findings are suggestive of a hypersensitivity reaction to an unidentified antigen or antigens. Some investigators have found an association with a history of vaccination or desensitization therapy,[263] smoking freebase cocaine,[264] *Ascaris* infestation,[265] and exposure to pigeons,[266] lending support to this hypothesis. In the majority of patients, however, a potential causative antigen has not been identified.

Although the pathogenesis of the disease is also unclear, immunologic mechanisms are implicated by several clinical and experimental observations. Circulating immune complexes have been documented in some cases.[258, 268] The presence of ANCA in the serum also suggests an immune component in pathogenesis; however, these are not present in all patients and are mostly P-ANCA (*see* farther on), for which a pathogenetic role is less clear than for C-ANCA. Flare-ups of disease have been reported during pregnancy, suggesting the possibility of a hormonal influence;[269, 270] however, these examples are so rare that a pathogenic relationship is uncertain.

### Pathologic Characteristics

The characteristic microscopic findings of Churg-Strauss syndrome consist of a combination of vasculitis, necrotizing extravascular granulomatous inflammation, and prominent tissue infiltration by eosinophils (Fig. 40–16).[271, 272] As indicated previously, however, not all three features are present in every case, and not all patients with this combination of findings have the clinical syndrome of Churg-Strauss syndrome. Thus, as in other vasculitides, definitive diagnosis requires careful consideration of clinical, radiologic, and laboratory findings as well as those found on tissue examination.

Vasculitis occurs predominantly in small-to-medium-sized arteries and veins and consists of a transmural infiltrate of lymphocytes, plasma cells, histiocytes, multinucleated giant cells, and a large number of eosinophils; the pattern is similar in both pulmonary and extrapulmonary foci. Fibrinoid necrosis of vessel walls and granulomas may be present, and a variable degree of fibrosis can be seen in older lesions. From a practical point of view, it is worth noting that vasculitis itself was not included as a diagnostic criterion in the American College of Rheumatology classification scheme, the presence of extravascular eosinophils being found to be a more sensitive and specific indicator.[259]

Extravascular granulomatous inflammation typically consists of a central focus of necrotic material, frequently with numerous admixed eosinophils, surrounded by palisaded epithelioid histiocytes and multinucleated giant cells. Although granulomas may be seen within the lung itself, they occur more commonly in extrapulmonary sites.[272] Within the pulmonary parenchyma, it is more common to see alveolar interstitial and air-space infiltration by eosinophils and macrophages in a pattern similar to eosinophilic

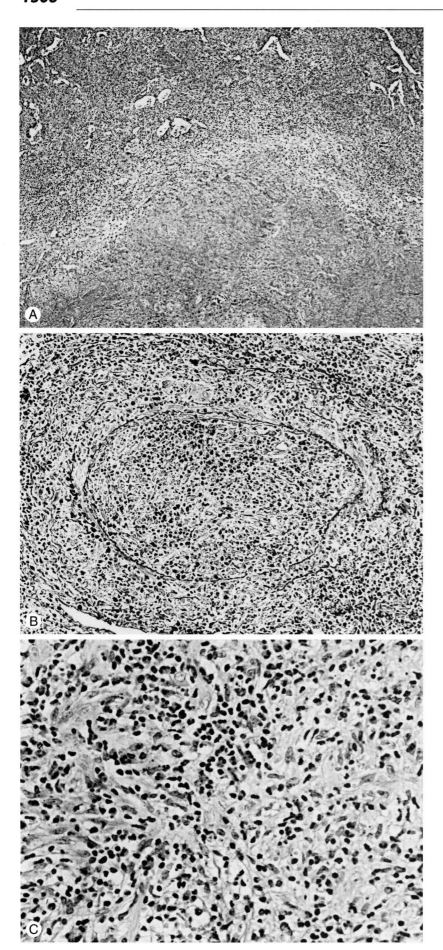

**Figure 40–16. Churg-Strauss Syndrome—Histologic Appearance.** A low-power view of lung parenchyma *(A)* shows a well-defined focus of necrosis in the lower portion, adjacent to which is an inflammatory infiltrate that obscures the lung architecture. A pulmonary artery in the latter area *(B)* shows disruption of elastic laminae and complete luminal occlusion. A high-power view of the inflammatory infiltrate *(C)* shows it to consist of a mixture of macrophages, lymphocytes, and bilobed eosinophils. (*A*, ×40; *B*, Verhoeff-Van Gieson, ×80; *C*, ×325.) (Courtesy Dr. S. Sahai.)

pneumonia.[252, 272] Histologic changes of chronic asthma (goblet cell metaplasia, basement membrane thickening, and muscle hypertrophy) are frequently evident in the walls of bronchioles and small bronchi;[272] apart from these changes, significant bronchial disease appears to be rare.[274] One case has been reported in which the major pulmonary abnormality appeared to be diffuse panbronchiolitis.[275]

### Radiologic Manifestations

The chest radiograph is abnormal in approximately 70% of patients.[276] In the majority, the abnormalities consist of transient patchy nonsegmental areas of consolidation without predilection for any lung zone.[276, 277] In 40%, these changes precede the development of clinical evidence of systemic vasculitis.[276] The areas of consolidation may be symmetric and have a nonsegmental distribution similar to that observed in chronic eosinophilic pneumonia (Fig. 40–17).[276–278] A diffuse interstitial, reticular, or reticulonodular pattern and miliary lesions may also occur, but are uncommon.[276, 277] Occasionally, the abnormalities consist of bilateral small and large nodular opacities, which may become confluent; in contrast to Wegener's granulomatosis, cavitation is rare (Fig. 40–18).[276, 279, 280] Unilateral or bilateral pleural effusions occur in approximately 30% of patients,[276] and hilar lymphadenopathy has been observed in a small number.[276, 278]

In one review of the HRCT findings at the time of diagnosis in 17 patients, the most common abnormality (seen in approximately 60%) consisted of areas of ground-glass attenuation or consolidation in either a patchy or a predominant peripheral distribution (Fig. 40–19);[280] 2 patients also had small centrilobular nodules. In another two patients, the predominant abnormality consisted of multiple nodules measuring 0.5 to 3.5 cm in diameter, several of which were cavitated. One patient had interlobular septal thickening resulting from interstitial pulmonary edema secondary to cardiac involvement, two had bronchial wall thickening or

dilation (findings commonly seen in patients with asthma), and two had normal HRCT findings. Small unilateral or bilateral pleural effusions were identified in two patients.

A single case has also been reported in which HRCT demonstrated enlarged peripheral pulmonary arteries, some of which had an irregular, stellate configuration and which correlated with the presence of vasculitis histologically.[281] In another patient, who had concurrent Churg-Strauss syndrome and giant cell arteritis, the parenchymal abnormalities on HRCT consisted of interstitial disease and small parenchymal nodules.[282]

### Clinical Manifestations

As indicated previously, patients with Churg-Strauss syndrome typically have a history of allergic phenomena—most often nasal polyposis, sinusitis, or asthma—that precedes the other components of the disease by months or years. Occasionally, asthma diminishes in severity when the clinical manifestations of vasculitis become apparent.[271] It has also been suggested that full-blown disease may be suppressed in some patients taking corticosteroids for asthma.[283] Pulmonary manifestations that develop during the vasculitic phase of disease include cough and (rarely) hemoptysis. Deep vein thrombosis, with or without pulmonary thromboembolism, occurs rarely.[284]

Churg-Strauss syndrome is a multisystem disease with predilection for involvement of the lungs, skin, gastrointestinal tract, and nervous system; the lower urinary tract, spleen, and heart are less commonly affected, and virtually any organ or tissue can be involved occasionally.[3, 252, 271] *Gastrointestinal* involvement occurs in 35% to 60% of patients,[285] manifested most often by pain and less frequently by diarrhea or bleeding; underlying pathologic conditions include cholecystitis, colonic or small bowel ulceration or perforation, and formation of a masslike lesion.[286, 287] *Neurologic* disease most often takes the form of a peripheral neuropathy,

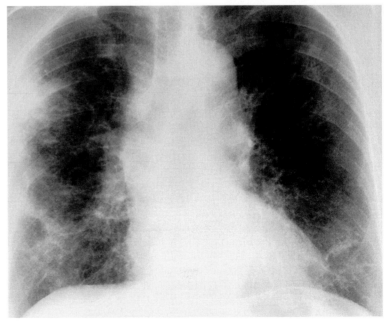

**Figure 40–17. Churg-Strauss Syndrome.** A posteroanterior chest radiograph in a 71-year-old woman demonstrates patchy bilateral areas of consolidation in a predominantly subpleural distribution. The diagnosis of Churg-Strauss syndrome was proven by open-lung biopsy.

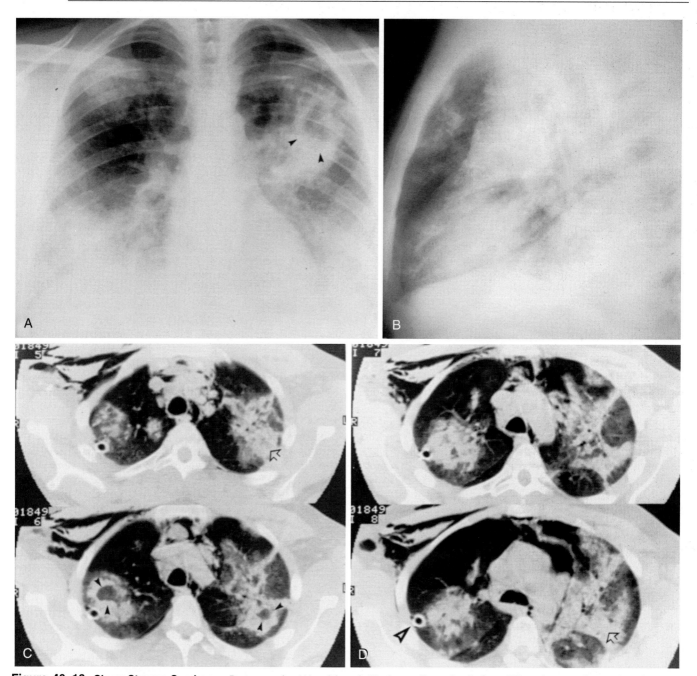

**Figure 40–18. Churg-Strauss Syndrome.** Posteroanterior *(A)* and lateral *(B)* chest radiographs disclose diffuse air-space disease throughout both lungs with moderate lower zonal predominance. The consolidation on the left contains a large central lucency *(arrowheads)*, suggesting cavitation. The consolidation involves both central and peripheral portions of the lungs. Several days later, conventional CT images through the upper lobes *(C and D)* reveal broad zones of air-space consolidation *(open arrows)*; both upper lobes contain lucencies *(small arrowheads)* consistent with cavitation. (The chest tube on the right *[large arrowheads]* was inserted for relief of a right pneumothorax; pneumomediastinum and subcutaneous emphysema are seen anteriorly.) An open-lung biopsy disclosed histologic features compatible with Churg-Strauss syndrome. The patient was a 20-year-old man with asthma, minimal cough, fever, and blood eosinophilia.

usually mononeuritis multiplex.[288] Cranial nerve disease almost always involves the optic nerve;[289] however, involvement of other nerves has also been reported.[288, 290] Cerebral infarction is rare.[288] *Cardiac* disease is also common and again may take several clinicopathologic forms, including angina; myocardial infarction; or sudden death as a result of coronary arteritis or myocarditis; and pericarditis (occasionally complicated by tamponade).[291–293] Heart failure also may be the result of hypertension secondary to renal disease.

*Skin* rash is one of the most common clinical features of Churg-Strauss syndrome. In one review of 90 patients, it was seen in 36 (40%);[294] in 5, it was the initial manifestation of disease. The most common findings reported in this review were purpura and petechiae on the lower extremities and cutaneous nodules and papules on the elbows. *Renal* disease is present in 30% to 50% of patients,[285] usually manifested by an active urinary sediment and histologic features of glomerulonephritis;[258, 271] progression to renal

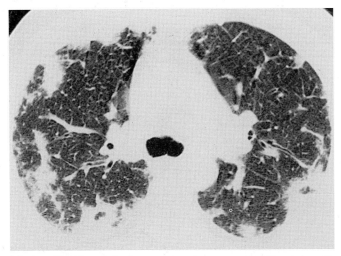

**Figure 40–19. Churg-Strauss Syndrome.** An HRCT scan in a 52-year-old man demonstrates bilateral areas of consolidation in a predominantly subpleural distribution. The diagnosis was proven by open-lung biopsy.

failure is relatively infrequent (only about 10% of patients reported by 1984).[258] Migratory *polyarthritis* occurs in a minority of cases.[271] Vasculitis of the temporal artery has been reported to mimic giant cell arteritis.[295]

### Laboratory Findings and Diagnosis

The white cell count is typically elevated as a result of eosinophilia; in one literature review of 85 cases, the mean peak count was $12.9 \times 10^9$/liter (range 1.5 to $29 \times 10^9$/liter).[258] Significant eosinophilia in blood and other fluids (such as pleural effusion) is also seen occasionally in Wegener's granulomatosis and microscopic polyangiitis.[285, 296] As might be expected, an elevated eosinophil count is also found in specimens obtained by bronchoalveolar lavage.[297, 298] In one investigation, no significant correlation was found between bronchoalveolar lavage results and clinical manifestations or pulmonary function abnormalities;[297] moreover, sequential evaluation in two patients demonstrated persistent bronchoalveolar lavage eosinophilia despite disappearance of clinical and radiologic abnormalities after corticosteroid therapy.

Hypergammaglobulinemia E is a common feature of the vasculitic phase of the disease.[258, 259] Anemia is present in the majority of patients;[258] rarely, it is related to an autoimmune hemolytic process.[299] An elevated rheumatoid factor is also seen in many patients.[258] ANCAs are present in about 75% of patients;[300–303] about three quarters of these are related to myeloperoxidase (P-ANCA) and the remainder to proteinase-3 (C-ANCA). In one study, the presence of ANCA did not appear to be associated with disease activity.[304]

### Natural History and Prognosis

In one prospective study of 82 patients followed from 1980 to 1993 and treated according to several protocols, five factors were selected to form a prognostic score: (1) increased blood creatinine; (2) proteinuria; (3) cardiomyopathy; (4) gastrointestinal tract involvement; and (5) central nervous system signs (measurements of ANCA and the presence of comorbid disease were not included in the analysis).[262] When none of the factors was present, the 5-year mortality was approximately 12%; when one was identified, it was 26%; and when three or more were present, it was 46%. The results of this study confirmed the authors' previous findings that the prognosis of Churg-Strauss syndrome is similar to that of classic PAN.[305] In another review of 45 patients (35 with classic PAN, 8 with Churg-Strauss syndrome, and 2 with overlap syndrome), the overall 5-year mortality was found to be 58%;[306] an increased risk of death was associated with cardiac or renal but not gastrointestinal disease.

## POLYARTERITIS NODOSA

PAN was one of the first forms of vasculitis to be identified and, as such, has been associated with much interest and study over the years. According to concepts that developed in the first part of the twentieth century and that persisted until the late 1980s, the disease was characterized histologically by necrotizing vasculitis that affected predominantly small-to-medium-sized muscular arteries of the systemic circulation; the lesions were typically unassociated with granulomatous inflammation, patchy in distribution, and often located at vessel branch points and associated with localized aneurysms. Renal disease, consisting principally of glomerulonephritis, was common. In addition to cases with these features, there were patients with similar clinical disease but in whom vasculitis affected predominantly small vessels *(microscopic PAN)*. Partly as a result of the identification of ANCAs and the increased experience with small vessel vasculitis in the 1980s, it has been proposed that these two forms of disease be more clearly separated. Thus, according to the participants at the International Consensus Conference on Vasculitis at Chapel Hill in 1990, the term *classic PAN* should be used to refer to cases of vasculitis involving only medium-sized or small arteries; cases characterized by inflammation of arterioles, venules, or capillaries (including those of the glomeruli) should be referred to as *microscopic polyangiitis*.[10] According to these definitions, PAN is much less common than microscopic polyangiitis.[10, 307]

Several observations can be cited in support of the distinction between these two conditions. Although pulmonary disease (usually capillaritis and parenchymal hemorrhage) is common in microscopic polyangiitis, the incidence of vasculitis in the pulmonary circulation in classic PAN is almost nonexistent.[308] Although the authors of a 1957 review of 111 cases of PAN identified 32 with lung involvement,[309] the clinical and pathologic features of these cases as well as others reported in the literature[310–312] suggest that the majority are better classified as microscopic polyangiitis, Wegener's granulomatosis, Churg-Strauss syndrome, or even simple pulmonary eosinophilia (Loeffler's syndrome). (Despite this, involvement of the bronchial arteries as part of systemic vasculitis can occur [Fig. 40–20],[313] and rare cases of apparent pulmonary artery inflammation have been reported in

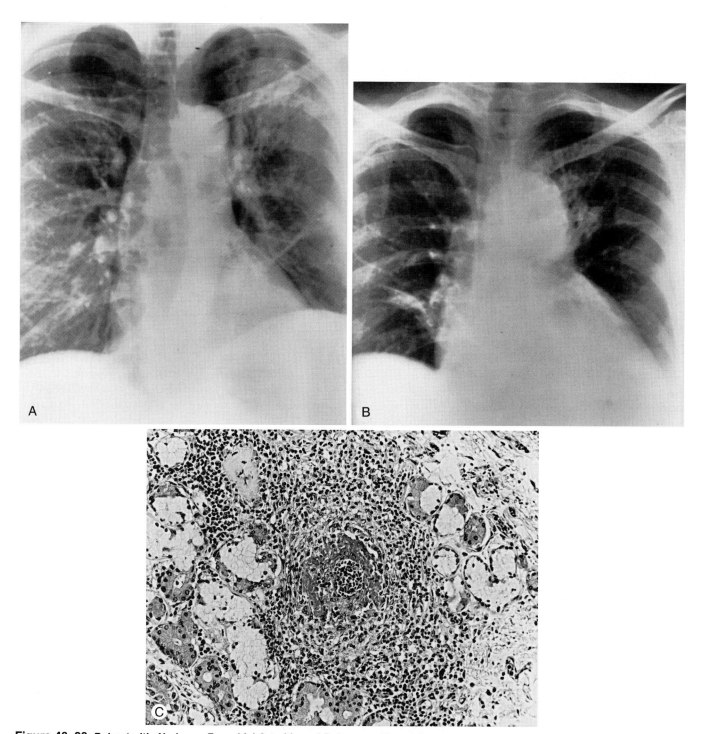

**Figure 40–20. Polyarteritis Nodosa—Bronchial Arteritis and Pulmonary Hemorrhage.** This 67-year-old woman presented with fever, malaise, and myalgias. Laboratory investigation revealed biochemical evidence of renal failure; a kidney biopsy specimen showed necrotizing glomerulonephritis. A chest radiograph at that time *(A)* showed diffuse air-space consolidation in the left upper lobe, thought to be consistent with pulmonary hemorrhage. Six days later *(B)*, there was considerable improvement. Autopsy 2 days later showed only red blood cells and scattered hemosiderin-laden macrophages in the left upper lobe parenchyma and peribronchovascular interstitial tissue. Although pulmonary arteries were normal, multiple bronchial arteries showed fibrinoid necrosis associated with an acute inflammatory infiltrate *(C)*. The upper lobe hemorrhage was presumed to be derived from rupture of one or more of these vessels followed by tracking of blood from the peribronchial interstitium into the air spaces. Crescentic glomerulonephritis and necrotizing vasculitis in several medium-sized arteries in abdominal viscera and soft tissue were also present.

classic PAN.[314, 315]) A second important difference between classic PAN and microscopic polyangiitis is the incidence of ANCA, which is virtually nil in the former and high in the latter.[303, 316]

As just indicated, it is probable that the majority of clinical symptoms and radiologic abnormalities related to the lungs are not the result of pulmonary involvement by classic PAN itself. This conclusion was supported by the results of a review of the radiographic findings in 28 patients;[317] except for 4 patients in whom parenchymal nodules and patchy consolidation were observed, all other abnormalities were readily attributable to cardiac decompensation.

## MICROSCOPIC POLYANGIITIS

As discussed in the previous section, microscopic polyangiitis can be considered as a necrotizing vasculitis that affects predominantly small vessels (arterioles, venules, and capillaries); although large vessel involvement, such as seen in classic PAN, may also be present, it is typically a minor component of the disease. Men are affected somewhat more commonly than women, and the average age of onset is about 50 years.[285]

The cause and pathogenesis of the condition are uncertain. In contrast to classic PAN, evidence of hepatitis B infection is rare,[285] and other potential inciting agents are usually not identified. Many affected patients have ANCAs, and it is possible that these antibodies are involved pathogenetically via mechanisms discussed previously (see page 1492). A number of cases have been associated with the PiZZ phenotype, suggesting the possibility of a hereditary factor.[56] Although immune complex deposition has been implicated in the pathogenesis of disease in some experimental animal models that resemble microscopic polyangiitis[318, 319] as well as in occasional patients with pulmonary capillaritis associated with other diseases such as SLE or Henoch-Schönlein purpura,[320, 321] evidence of tissue deposition of immune complexes is characteristically absent in microscopic polyangiitis. Drug ingestion (e.g., propylthiouracil)[322] and influenza vaccination[323] have been implicated in some cases.

Histologically, the lungs show intra-alveolar hemorrhage and, in more chronic cases, variable numbers of hemosiderin-laden macrophages.[324, 326] Typically, there is a patchy neutrophilic infiltrate in the alveolar septa associated with edema, necrosis, and (sometimes) fibrin thrombi (Fig. 40–21); fibroblast proliferation indicative of healing can also be seen. Arterioles and venules may be involved, but larger vessels are typically normal. Bronchial vessels are also commonly affected.[326]

From a diagnostic point of view, it is important to remember that the finding of alveolar hemorrhage and capillaritis represents a histologic reaction rather than a specific disease entity.[113, 327] In addition to microscopic polyangiitis, some patients manifest features of other vasculitides, such as Wegener's granulomatosis,[103, 111] Behçet's syndrome, or Henoch-Schönlein purpura;[321, 324] others have a connective tissue disease (usually SLE),[273, 325] antiphospholipid syndrome,[328] IgA nephropathy,[329] or drug hypersensitivity.[324] An association with Churg-Strauss syndrome,[330] hemolytic uremic syndrome,[331] hypocomplementemic urticarial vasculitis,[332] and myelodysplastic syndromes[333] has also been documented.

Radiographic features consist of patchy, bilateral airspace opacities caused by alveolar hemorrhage.[334, 335] Pleural effusion has been reported in approximately 15% of cases and pulmonary edema in 6%.[335]

Depending on the extent and nature of renal, pulmonary, and systemic vascular involvement, clinical findings can be quite variable. Renal disease is the most common and important manifestation and is present at the onset of disease in most patients. Pulmonary involvement develops in about 15% to 30% of patients and is characterized principally by hemoptysis;[285] cough, chest pain, and shortness of breath may be present.[324] One unusual case was associated with progressive obstructive lung disease.[336] In one review of the clinical features of the disorder, myalgias, arthralgias, and arthritis were found to be present in about 65% to 70% of patients; cutaneous lesions (purpura, splinter hemorrhages) in 45% to 55%; gastrointestinal symptoms (abdominal pain or bleeding) in 30% to 60%; and peripheral neuropathy in 15% to 35%.[285]

ANCAs are present in the majority of patients.[285] P-ANCA related to myeloperoxidase is most common; however, anti-PR3 C-ANCA is seen occasionally.[285, 337] Eosinophilia is present in some patients; rheumatoid factor can be detected in 40% to 50% and ANA in 20% to 30%.[285]

As in Wegener's granulomatosis, corticosteroid and cyclophosphamide therapy induce disease remission, often complete and for a prolonged period, in many patients;[338] however, relapse is not uncommon. In one study, the risk of death was higher in patients who presented with pulmonary hemorrhage, or with C-ANCA compared to P-ANCA.[339]

## TAKAYASU'S ARTERITIS

Takayasu's arteritis is an uncommon vasculitis affecting principally the aorta and its major branches; approximately 300 cases had been reported by 1996.[340] Depending on the specific sites involved, the condition has been classified into several types.[341, 342] Although the arteritis is usually confined to the systemic circulation, pulmonary artery involvement is found in an appreciable number of cases; for example, in one review of 76 autopsies, the main pulmonary artery was found to be affected in 34 and the intrapulmonary arterial branches in 21.[343] Angiographic studies have shown a wide variation in the incidence of pulmonary involvement, ranging from about 15% to 85% of patients.[344–346] A combination of findings has been proposed for diagnosis;[347–349] according to the American College of Rheumatology vasculitis classification scheme, the presence of three or more of the criteria listed in Table 40–4 is associated with sensitivity and specificity of diagnosis of approximately 90% and 98%.[348]

### Epidemiology

The disease has a marked predilection for women (approximately 90% to 95% of cases[347, 350–352]) and usually has its onset between 10 and 40 years of age. Most reports have originated in Southeast Asia; however, it has been suggested that the disease might be underdiagnosed in Europe and

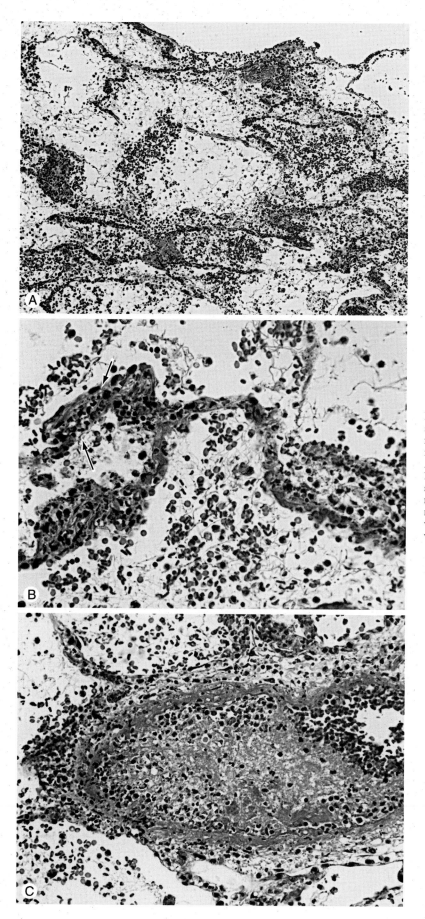

**Figure 40–21. Microscopic Polyangiitis.** A section of lung from a patient with hemoptysis and patchy, bilateral air-space opacities *(A)* shows the alveolar air spaces to contain red blood cells and fibrin. An inflammatory cellular infiltrate is located predominantly in and adjacent to the alveolar septa. A magnified view *(B)* shows intact and fragmented *(arrows)* leukocytes in the alveolar wall. A small pulmonary artery *(C)* shows inflammation and fibrinoid necrosis of the media and recent thrombosis; numerous necrotic and fragmented polymorphonuclear leukocytes (leukocytoclasis) are evident in the vessel wall at the endothelial surface. The larger pulmonary vessels were normal. *(A,* ×100; *B,* ×325; *C,* ×250.)

**Table 40–4. 1990 CRITERIA FOR THE CLASSIFICATION OF TAKAYASU'S ARTERITIS***

| CRITERION | DEFINITION |
| --- | --- |
| Age at disease onset ≤40 years | Development of symptoms or findings related to Takayasu's arteritis at age ≤40 years |
| Claudication of extremities | Development and worsening of fatigue and discomfort in muscles of one or more extremity while in use, especially the upper extremities |
| Decreased brachial artery pulse | Decreased pulsation of one or both brachial arteries |
| Blood pressure difference >10 mm Hg | Difference of >10 mm Hg in systolic blood pressure between arms |
| Bruit over subclavian arteries or aorta | Bruit audible on auscultation over one or both subclavian arteries or abdominal aorta |
| Arteriogram abnormality | Arteriographic narrowing or occlusion of the entire aorta, its primary branches, or large arteries in the proximal upper or lower extremities, not due to arteriosclerosis, fibromuscular dysplasia, or similar causes; changes usually focal or segmental |

*For purposes of classification, a patient is said to have Takayasu's arteritis if at least 3 of these 6 criteria are present.
Modified from Arend WP, Michel BA, Bloch DA, et al: The American College of Rheumatology 1990 criteria for the classification of Takayasu arteritis. Arthritis Rheum 33:1131, 1990.

North America.[353] A difference in the anatomic distribution of disease between different nationalities has been found by some investigators;[342] in a study of 80 Japanese patients and 102 Indian patients, vascular lesions tended to occur primarily in the ascending aorta, aortic arch, or its branches in the former and primarily in the abdominal aorta and renal arteries in the latter.

### Etiology and Pathogenesis

Although the etiology and pathogenesis of Takayasu's arteritis are unknown, a variety of observations strongly suggest an immunologic basis. For example, some patients have serologic abnormalities[354] or extravascular disease known to be associated with abnormal immune reactions, including glomerulonephritis; skin lesions, such as erythema nodosum, facial lupus rash, and erythema induratum; and connective tissue diseases, such as rheumatoid arthritis and polymyositis.[355, 356] In one study of 19 patients, 18 were found to have anti–endothelial cell antibodies (ANCA, ANA, anti-DNA antibodies, extractable nuclear antibodies, anti-Ro antibodies, and anticardiolipin antibodies were all absent);[357] however, it is not known whether these are pathogenic or secondary to vascular injury. Other investigators have also found no evidence of ANCA formation.[358] Evidence of altered cell-mediated immunity, including an increased CD4/CD8 ratio, has been documented in some patients.[359]

Other pathogenetic factors are less well established. An association has been reported with several HLA antigens (most commonly B52 and B39.2[360]), and occasional familial cases have been documented, suggesting a hereditary factor.[359] The strong association with young women also suggests a hormonal influence, a possibility supported by the observation of elevated urinary estrogens in one study.[361]

### Pathologic Characteristics

Pathologically, most changes are limited to the larger elastic vessels and consist of a patchy panarteritis. The adventitia shows fibrosis and a mixed, largely mononuclear inflammatory cell infiltrate resembling that seen in syphilis; fibrous obliteration and a perivascular mononuclear infiltrate of the vasa vasorum are also frequent.[351, 362] In histologically active lesions—which may be present in patients with clinically inactive disease[352]—the medium contains necrotizing or nonnecrotizing granulomas, either well or poorly formed; scattered multinucleated giant cells also occur in association with a nonspecific inflammatory cellular infiltrate. Older lesions show only fibrosis and disruption of the elastic laminae. Intimal fibrosis is frequent and may be present in the smaller arteries and arterioles (as was the case in one patient in whom it was considered to be responsible for pulmonary hypertension[363]). Abnormalities of arterioles and small arteries, consisting of a deficiency of the outer media accompanied by capillary proliferation, have also been described.[364] Rare cases have been found to have pathologic features of acute interstitial pneumonitis[365] or usual interstitial pneumonitis.[355]

### Radiologic Manifestations

The most common radiographic abnormalities involve the aorta and consist of contour irregularities (reported in about 10% to 75% of patients) and calcification (in 10% to 25%).[366, 367] These findings are uncommon in premenopausal women and should alert the physician to the diagnosis.[366] In one review of 49 patients, abnormalities were detected on the chest radiograph in 67%;[366] the most common consisted of a wavy or scalloped contour of the descending thoracic aorta (45%) (Fig. 40–22), ectasia of the aortic arch (18%), calcification of the wall of the aorta at the level of the aortic arch or descending aorta (18%), and cardiomegaly (16%).[366] Less common abnormalities include dilation of the ascending aorta, aneurysms of the descending aorta, oligemia distal to obstructed pulmonary arteries, and pulmonary edema.[366, 367] Rarely, occlusion of the aorta distal to the left subclavian artery results in rib notching.[366] Pulmonary arterial hypertension is a late manifestation.[368]

In one retrospective CT analysis of pulmonary parenchymal abnormalities in 25 patients, localized areas of low attenuation and decreased vascularity were identified in 11 (44%);[369] these were shown to correspond to areas of decreased vascularity distal to pulmonary arteritis on pulmonary angiography and to perfusion defects on technetium 99m–macroaggregated albumin perfusion scintigraphy. The findings were better seen on HRCT than on conventional CT. Other abnormalities seen on CT included localized subpleural irregular linear opacities (in 48% of patients) and localized areas of pleural thickening (in 36%).

Aortic and pulmonary artery abnormalities in Takayasu's arteritis may be assessed using contrast-enhanced spiral CT or magnetic resonance (MR) imaging (Fig. 40–23).[370–372]

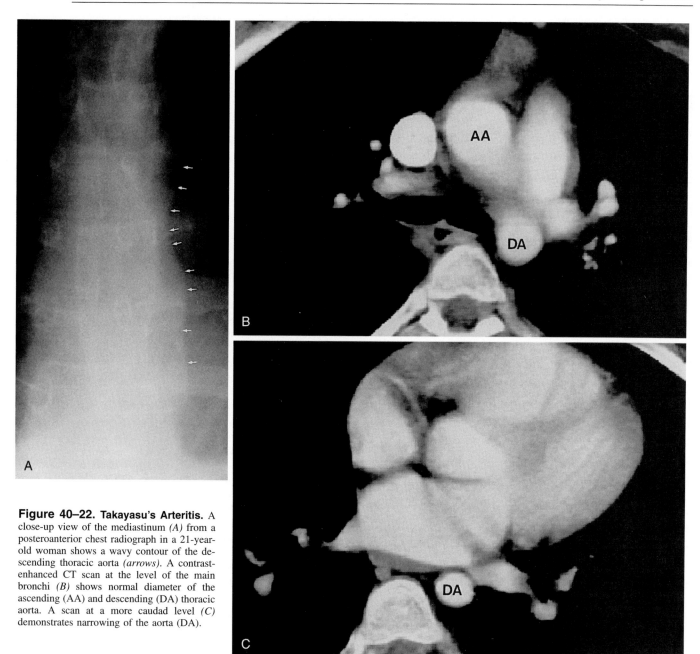

**Figure 40–22. Takayasu's Arteritis.** A close-up view of the mediastinum *(A)* from a posteroanterior chest radiograph in a 21-year-old woman shows a wavy contour of the descending thoracic aorta *(arrows)*. A contrast-enhanced CT scan at the level of the main bronchi *(B)* shows normal diameter of the ascending (AA) and descending (DA) thoracic aorta. A scan at a more caudad level *(C)* demonstrates narrowing of the aorta (DA).

In one study, contrast-enhanced spiral CT (CT angiography) was prospectively performed in 12 patients and 10 healthy adults.[370] Precontrast images revealed high attenuation of the aortic wall in 10 patients and mural calcification in the aorta in 9. Arterial-phase images demonstrated circumferential thickening of 1 to 4 mm of the aortic wall in all patients and enhancement in five; delayed-phase CT obtained 20 to 40 minutes after intravenous injection demonstrated circumferential enhancement of the aortic wall in eight. (The wall of the aorta in the 10 healthy adults was <1 mm in thickness or was imperceptible, demonstrated no calcification, and could not be visualized on the precontrast and delayed images.) In two patients, the pulmonary trunk and right and left main pulmonary arteries demonstrated variable wall thickening with both early and delayed enhancement.

The findings on MR imaging were assessed in another investigation of 77 patients using cardiac-gated spin-echo technique.[371] Aortic lesions—including stenosis, dilation, aneurysms, wall thickening, and mural thrombi—were clearly seen, particularly on sagittal images; cine MR also allowed recognition of the presence of aortic regurgitation. The most common findings were stenosis of the descending thoracic aorta (37% of cases), dilation of the ascending aorta (32% of cases), and contour irregularities of the descending thoracic aorta (22% of cases). In 54 patients (70%), MR images revealed abnormalities in the pulmonary arterial system. The most common finding consisted of "an abnormal treelike appearance" of the peripheral vessels; this was noted in 66% of cases and considered to represent occlusive changes in the arterial lumens. Less common abnormalities included dilation of the pulmonary trunk (19% of cases) and thrombi in central pulmonary arteries (3%).

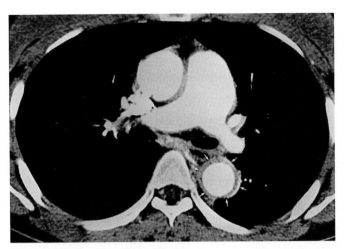

**Figure 40–23. Takayasu's Arteritis.** A contrast-enhanced CT scan in a 32-year-old woman demonstrates circumferential thickening of the wall of the descending thoracic aorta *(arrows)*, a characteristic finding in Takayasu's arteritis. (Case courtesy of Dr. Jung-Gi Im, Department of Radiology, Seoul National University Hospital, Seoul, Korea.)

Several investigators have also assessed the incidence and patterns of pulmonary artery involvement after conventional or digital pulmonary angiography.[366, 373, 374] As mentioned previously, the incidence of pulmonary involvement in the various series ranges from about 15% to 85%. The high incidence in some of the studies probably reflects a selection bias, because pulmonary angiography was not performed routinely.[366] Based on findings on CT[369] and MR imaging,[371] we believe that pulmonary artery involvement probably occurs in about 50% to 70% of cases. The frequency of such involvement shows a positive correlation with the degree of brachiocephalic vessel disease but not with extent or severity of aortic disease.[371] Rarely, pulmonary artery disease is the initial manifestation of Takayasu's arteritis.[375] The most common abnormalities consist of stenosis or occlusion of segmental or subsegmental branches, usually of an upper lobe; less often, they involve the middle lobe, lingula, or lower lobe segmental or subsegmental vessels. The abnormalities tend to progress over time.[371]

Scintigraphy may demonstrate decreased perfusion distal to narrowed or occluded pulmonary arteries.[366] In one case, radionuclide imaging showed complete obstruction of the right pulmonary artery and compromised perfusion in the left upper and lower lobes;[376] ventilation was normal. In another study of 57 patients in which technetium 99m–macroaggregated albumin was used, the relationship between inflammatory activity—determined on the basis of the physical findings and laboratory data (the erythrocyte sedimentation rate and level of C-reactive protein)—and pulmonary arterial changes was assessed;[377] the incidence of scintigraphic abnormality in the patients with active inflammation (7 of 21 patients, 33%) was lower than that in the patients with chronic disease (22 of 32, 69%). The lower incidence of scintigraphic abnormality in the former patients suggested to the authors that no stenotic or occlusive changes had yet been produced in the pulmonary artery.

### Clinical Manifestations

Systemic vasculitis and fibrosis result in both nonspecific constitutional symptoms and a variety of specific symptoms.[352] The former include fever, myalgias, arthralgias, and weight loss and are typically present for months to years before the more specific features of the disease become manifest. The latter are usually related to vascular stenosis and include angina pectoris, headache, syncope, impaired vision, and claudication in upper or lower extremities. A bruit, most often heard over the carotid artery, is common.[352] Localized pain over the affected arteries may be present. Arterial pulses may be diminished or, in severe cases, absent altogether; a difference in systolic blood pressure may be evident between the two arms. In long-standing disease with renal artery involvement, systemic hypertension may also be seen.

Clinical evidence of pulmonary involvement almost always occurs in patients with systemic findings; rarely, it is the first manifestation of the disease.[378] Many patients are asymptomatic despite the presence of clinical signs or radiologic abnormalities indicative of pulmonary disease.[350] Chest pain and hemoptysis occur occasionally.[378] In some cases, a midsystolic murmur in the pulmonic area is suggestive of pulmonary artery involvement, particularly when an early systolic click is absent. Laboratory findings include an elevated erythrocyte sedimentation rate and anemia.[359]

In a study of 60 patients followed at the NIH over a 6-month to 20-year period, only 2 patients died (one of suicide and the other suddenly during clinical remission; an autopsy was not performed).[352] Serious morbidity (i.e., permanent disability as a result of inability to perform daily functions) was found in about 50%, and a further 25% had episodes of temporary disability during periods of active disease.

## GIANT CELL ARTERITIS

Giant cell (temporal) arteritis is one of the most common systemic vasculitides.[261] The larger vessels of the head and neck are most frequently affected; necrotizing and nonnecrotizing granulomatous inflammation of both large elastic and medium-sized muscular pulmonary arteries has been documented rarely (Fig. 40–24).[379, 380] The cause and pathogenesis are unknown; however, in a retrospective, case-control study of 100 patients with giant cell arteritis and 100 with hip fractures, evidence of definite, probable, or possible infection before or during the illness was three times more likely in the former than the latter, suggesting to the authors that infection might induce the vasculitis.[381] The abnormality usually affects individuals older than age 50.

Symptoms usually consist of headache, jaw claudication, polymyalgia rheumatica, and loss of vision; tenderness in the region of the temporal artery or scalp is not uncommon. The erythrocyte sedimentation rate is typically elevated. In one review of 146 patients, symptoms and signs of upper respiratory tract involvement, including sore throat, hoarseness, and a choking sensation, were present in 6 (4%) as the initial manifestation and 13 (9%) at some point in the disease.[382] In another review of 39 patients, evidence of pleuropulmonary involvement was found in 5 (17%).[383] One patient has been reported who apparently had pulmonary infarction.[384] Another patient was found to have a bilateral reticular interstitial pattern on the chest radiograph;[385] transbronchial biopsy demonstrated ill-defined granulomas within the bronchial wall and alveolar interstitium. Pleural effusion

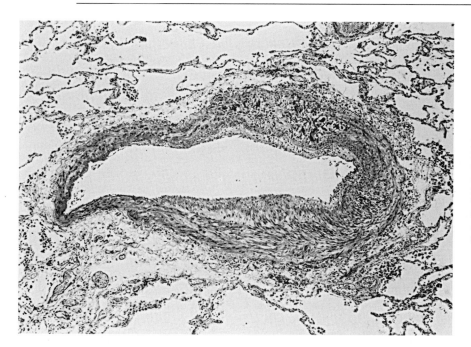

**Figure 40–24. Giant Cell Arteritis.** A 74-year-old woman was admitted to the hospital for investigation of frontal headaches. She developed signs of brain stem and cerebral infarcts and died soon thereafter. Autopsy confirmed the cerebral findings and showed granulomatous vasculitis involving the temporal arteries as well as the aorta and elastic and large muscular pulmonary arteries. A section from one of the latter shows well-defined granulomas within the media. (×60.)

has been documented in some patients;[383, 386] histologic features have been those of nonspecific pleuritis.[386]

From a diagnostic point of view, it is important to remember that not all patients with histologically evident giant cell vasculitis have the clinical syndrome of giant cell arteritis; moreover, not all those with clinical features suggestive of the disease ultimately prove to have it. For example, some patients have been described with clinically typical, biopsy-proven giant cell (temporal) arteritis who also had radiographically demonstrable pulmonary nodules;[387, 388] however, the observation that inflammation of the temporal artery can occur in Wegener's granulomatosis[167] suggests that these cases may represent variants of the latter disease. Other patients have been described who have clinical but not histologic features of giant cell (temporal) arteritis and who have ultimately been diagnosed to have Churg-Strauss syndrome.[389] Finally, patients have also been reported who have giant cell arteritis either limited to the pulmonary vessels,[390, 391] or involving pulmonary vessels and the aorta[392] or small, noncranial systemic vessels *(disseminated visceral giant cell arteritis)*;[393, 394] the fundamental nature of disease in all these individuals is unclear.

## BEHÇET'S DISEASE

Behçet's disease is an uncommon systemic disorder characterized principally by recurrent aphthous stomatitis, genital ulcers, skin lesions, and uveitis; in addition, a wide variety of other organs and tissues may be involved, including the kidneys, joints, central nervous system, gastrointestinal tract, pericardium, and lung.[395] Men are affected more often than women, and the age of onset is usually between 20 and 30 years. The incidence is highest in the Middle East and Japan.[396] Pulmonary involvement is infrequent. For example, in one retrospective autopsy review of 170 patients, pulmonary thrombosis was identified only once.[396] In another review of 72 patients, 7 were found to have evidence of

pulmonary vascular involvement.[397] Approximately 90 cases had been reported by 1989.[397] It has been proposed that some, if not all, cases of Hughes-Stovin syndrome—thrombosis of pulmonary arteries and systemic veins associated with headache, fever, cough, papilledema, and hemoptysis—are in reality examples of Behçet's disease.[398]

Although the cause is unknown, there has been speculation that it may be a virus.[398] Several investigators have also noted the precipitation of attacks by a variety of foods, especially walnuts.[399, 400] An increased frequency of HLA-B5 has been reported,[401] suggesting a hereditary factor in pathogenesis. The basic pathogenic abnormality is believed to be vasculitis, possibly on the basis of immune complex deposition.[398] Focal segmental glomerulonephritis has been documented in some cases[395, 402] and has been associated with subendothelial electron dense deposits and immunofluorescent evidence of IgG and C3 deposition. In addition, several investigators have found circulating immune complexes whose levels have shown some correlation with disease activity.[403, 404] Autoantibodies against oral mucosa and lymphocyte sensitization to mucosal antigens have been demonstrated;[402] however, it is not certain whether these are pathogenic or represent a response to tissue injury. The presence of C-ANCA has also been documented in some cases,[405] raising the possibility of neutrophil-mediated toxicity *(see page 1492).*

The principal histologic abnormality in the lungs is transmural inflammation (predominantly lymphocytes, plasma cells, and polymorphonuclear leukocytes) of virtually any pulmonary vessel.[397, 398, 406] The inflammatory process can extend into adjacent airways, with bronchial artery erosion and secondary hemoptysis. The same clinical finding can occur with involvement of the pulmonary vessels. Although histologic features of recent vascular necrosis are uncommonly seen, elastic tissue stains often demonstrate medial destruction of muscular and elastic arteries, sometimes severe enough to be associated with aneurysmal dilation. Recent or organized thrombi and parenchymal infarcts may be present and may be related to either local vasculitis and thrombosis or thromboembolism secondary to systemic thrombophlebitis.[406] Immunofluorescent studies of one lung biopsy specimen showed granular deposition of IgG, C3, and C4 in the walls of small veins, in the same location where an inflammatory cellular infiltrate was seen on light microscopic examination.[400]

Pulmonary artery aneurysms are manifested radiographically by round perihilar opacities or the rapid development of unilateral hilar enlargement (Fig. 40–25).[407–409] The aneurysms may be single or multiple, and unilateral or bilateral; they usually measure from 1 to 3 cm in diameter.[407–410] Although they may have sharply defined margins, the latter

are more commonly poorly defined as a result of surrounding hemorrhage.[407] The presence, size, and location of the aneurysms can be assessed with CT, MR, or angiography (Fig. 40–26);[407–409, 411] both CT and MR may also demonstrate thrombosed pulmonary artery aneurysms that are not seen at angiography.[407, 412] When considering pulmonary angiography in patients with Behçet's disease, it should be remembered that insertion of a venous catheter may lead to venous thrombosis or to propagation of an existing thrombus,[407, 413] complications that may result in significant deterioration.[409, 414]

Thrombotic occlusion of the pulmonary vasculature most commonly involves the right interlobar artery followed

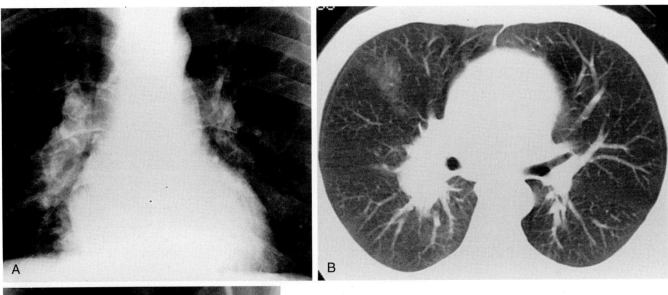

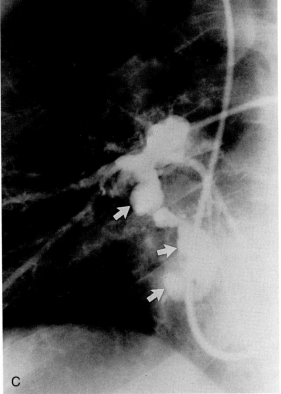

**Figure 40–25. Behçet's Disease.** A 28-year-old patient with Behçet's disease presented with massive hemoptysis. A view from a posteroanterior chest radiograph *(A)* demonstrates prominence of the inferior aspect of the right hilum. A CT scan *(B)* shows prominence of the right hilum and localized areas of ground-glass attenuation in the right middle lobe secondary to pulmonary hemorrhage. A selective right pulmonary angiogram *(C)* demonstrates irregular aneurysm formation involving the right interlobar, right lower lobe, and right posterior basal segmental pulmonary arteries *(arrows)*. The hemoptysis resolved after occlusion of the right interlobar pulmonary artery with coils. (Case courtesy of Professor Martine Remy-Jardin, Universitaire de Lille, Lille, France.)

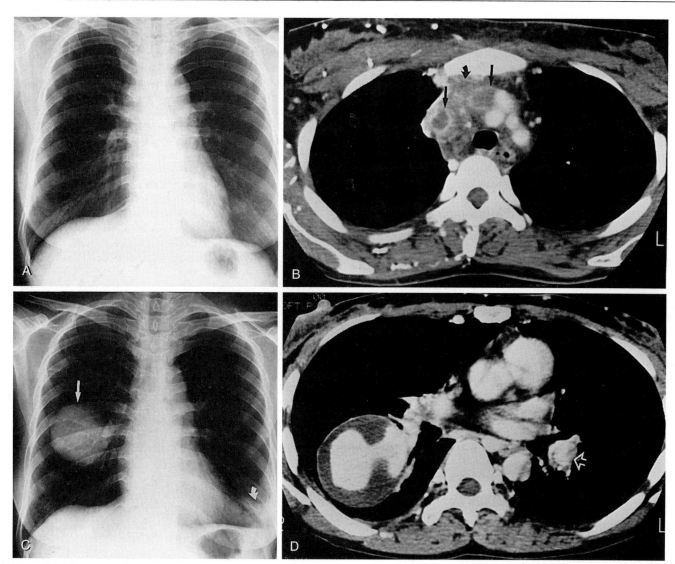

**Figure 40–26. Behçet's Disease.** A posteroanterior chest radiograph *(A)* in a 37-year-old woman with Behçet's disease shows widening of the right upper mediastinum. A contrast-enhanced CT scan *(B)* demonstrates thrombosis of the right and left brachiocephalic veins *(straight arrows)* and increased attenuation of the mediastinal fat *(curved arrow)*, suggestive of edema. Also note collateral veins in the mediastinum and chest wall. A posteroanterior chest radiograph obtained 6 months later *(C)* shows a round, well-defined mass in the right lower lobe *(straight arrow)* and localized consolidation in the left lower lobe *(curved arrow)*. The upper mediastinum appears normal. A contrast-enhanced CT scan *(D)* obtained at the same time as *C* shows a large aneurysm of the right pulmonary artery with enhancement of the patent lumen and a circumferential thrombus. Also note dilated left descending pulmonary artery *(arrowhead)*. (A to D from Ahn JM, lm JG, Ryoo JW, et al: Thoracic manifestations of Behçet syndrome: Radiographic and CT findings in nine patients. Radiology 194:199, 1995. Case courtesy of Dr. Jung-Gi Im, Department of Radiology, Seoul National University Hospital, Seoul, Korea.)

in decreasing order by lobar and segmental arteries.[412] Such occlusion may result in localized areas of consolidation as a result of pulmonary infarction (rarely associated with cavitation),[410] areas of oligemia,[410] and areas of atelectasis.[407] Lung scintigraphy shows ventilation-perfusion mismatch or a combination of matched and mismatched perfusion defects.[409, 415] Pulmonary hemorrhage as a result of vasculitis or pulmonary artery rupture can also result in focal, multifocal, or diffuse air-space consolidation.[407, 409, 410]

Thrombosis of the superior vena cava or brachiocephalic veins may be manifested by mediastinal widening on the chest radiograph *(see* Fig. 40–26).[408] CT scans in five patients with such widening showed it to be secondary to thrombosis or narrowing of the superior vena cava leading to collateral circulation and mediastinal edema.[408] Mediastinal widening may also result from aortic aneurysm formation.[407]

Unilateral or bilateral pleural effusions may occur, usually as a result of pulmonary infarction.[377, 410] Rarely, an effusion represents hemothorax resulting from rupture of a pulmonary artery,[416] chylothorax secondary to thrombosis of the superior vena cava and brachiocephalic vein,[417] or vasculitis of the pleura itself.[407] A case of hydropneumothorax secondary to rupture of a cavitated infarct into the pleural space has also been described.[410]

Clinically, Behçet's disease is characterized by exacerbations and remissions of uveitis and oral and genital ulcers. Other findings include skin lesions (particularly erythema nodosum); arthritis; thrombophlebitis; neurologic syndromes; and, less frequently, colitis, epididymitis, orchitis, and systemic arterial thrombosis and aneurysms.[402] Pulmonary disease is usually manifested several years after the onset of systemic disease;[418] however, it may be the initial feature.[419] Clinical findings include dyspnea, cough, chest pain, and hemoptysis.[397] The last-named is the most common and serious, sometimes being massive and leading to death.[406, 418, 420] In fact, in one series of 72 patients, 15 of the 16 who died did so as a result of pulmonary hemorrhage, usually within 2 years after the onset of pulmonary disease.[397] Clinical features of superior vena caval obstruction occur occasionally.[421] Obstructive airway disease, sometimes responsive to bronchodilator therapy, has been noted by a number of investigators;[422–424] others have found evidence of restrictive lung disease, usually mild.[397] A patient with sleep apnea hypothesized to be secondary to palatal involvement has also been reported.[425]

## MIXED CRYOGLOBULINEMIA

Mixed cryoglobulinemia is an uncommon disease characterized by purpura, arthralgia, glomerulonephritis, and the presence in the serum of globulins that precipitate on exposure to cold temperatures (cryoglobulins). These proteins can be present in a variety of lymphoproliferative, infectious, and connective tissue disorders; there is evidence that many cases are related to hepatitis C infection.[426, 427] In most cases, the globulins are composed of complexes of IgM directed against IgG (hence the qualifier *mixed*). Most manifestations of disease are believed to result from tissue deposition of these immune complexes followed by an inflammatory response.

Pulmonary involvement has been described in a number of clinicopathologic reports[428–430] and in one series of 23 patients whose lung function was studied.[431] Several pathologic abnormalities have been identified, the most common being capillaritis and intra-alveolar hemorrhage.[429, 430] Pathologic examination of lung tissue from one patient who manifested dyspnea and severe hypoxemia showed extensive occlusion of small arteries, arterioles, and capillaries by granular eosinophilic material, unassociated with significant inflammatory reaction;[429] the material was identified by electron microscopic and immunochemical studies as aggregates of IgM and IgG, and the authors proposed that cryoglobulin precipitation in the vascular lumens resulted in capillary block and consequent hypoxemia. A case of bronchiolitis obliterans organizing pneumonia has also been reported.[440]

In one series of 23 patients, radiographic evidence of diffuse interstitial lung disease was present in 18;[431] symptoms related to the chest were unusual, one patient presenting with hemoptysis, another with pleural pain, and a third with a clinical picture of asthma. Pulmonary function tests indicated small airway obstruction and an increase in the alveolar-arterial gradient for oxygen. A case complicated by adult respiratory distress syndrome has also been reported in which the initial chest radiograph demonstrated left upper lobe consolidation that progressed within 4 days to have a panlobar distribution.[432]

## HENOCH-SCHÖNLEIN PURPURA

Henoch-Schönlein purpura is a distinctive vasculitic syndrome characterized by purpura, abdominal pain, gastrointestinal hemorrhage, arthritis or arthralgia, and glomerulonephritis. The disease appears most often during childhood or adolescence but can occur at any age.[433] Although many patients give a history of antecedent infection or drug ingestion, no specific agent has been proven to be etiologic. Circulating and tissue-related immune complexes, most often containing IgA, have been identified in a number of cases, and it has been speculated that the disease results from activation of complement by IgA via the alternate pathway.[253] IgA-related ANCAs that did not interact with either PR3 or myeloperoxidase were identified in 11 of 14 adult patients in one investigation;[434] however, their pathogenetic role, if any, is unclear. Some patients have been found to have alpha$_1$-antitrypsin deficiency.[435]

Involvement of the respiratory tract is rare; in one review of 77 adult patients with the condition, only 4 had evidence of pulmonary disease (none of whom underwent biopsy).[433] The occasional cases examined pathologically have shown capillaritis and intra-alveolar hemorrhage.[436–438] Immunohistochemical study in one case showed IgA deposition along alveolar septa.[437]

Radiographic manifestations are typically those of bilateral air-space disease, reflecting intra-alveolar hemorrhage; the pattern is predominantly interstitial in some cases.[439] Clinically, the disease is characterized by episodes of resolution and relapse, typically ending with spontaneous remission.[253] The combination of arthritis, abdominal pain (with or without melena), palpable purpura, and nephritis should suggest the diagnosis. Pulmonary involvement is characterized by hemoptysis.[433, 436, 437, 444] The prognosis is usually good, although severe renal involvement or gastrointestinal or pulmonary hemorrhage may result in death.[443]

## NECROTIZING SARCOID GRANULOMATOSIS

Necrotizing sarcoid granulomatosis is an uncommon disorder that usually is recognized only after histologic examination of excised lung tissue. It was first defined pathologically as a mass of confluent granulomas associated with a variable amount of necrosis and prominent, focally destructive vasculitis.[444] It is because of the latter that a discussion of the disease is included within the chapter on pulmonary vasculitides. Despite the presence of vascular inflammation, however, it is not clear whether or not this is the primary process in the disorder, and it is possible that a clearer elucidation of etiology and pathogenesis might result in a more appropriate classification.[445] Only about 100 cases had been reported by 1996.[446] Most patients are middle-aged adults, an average age of 49 years being found in three series.[447–449] A distinct female predominance has been found by several groups of investigators.[447–450]

As indicated, the cause and pathogenesis of necrotizing sarcoid granulomatosis are unknown, and it is not certain if the histologic findings represent a disease entity per se or simply an unusual reaction to several unknown agents. The vascular involvement, granulomatous inflammation, and apparently good response to corticosteroid therapy have suggested a hypersensitivity reaction. In one immunofluorescent study, a strong reaction was found to *Aspergillus fumigatus* within the necrotic material;[447] apart from this isolated observation, however, there have been no clues as to the identity of a possible antigen. Nonnecrotizing vasculitis is common

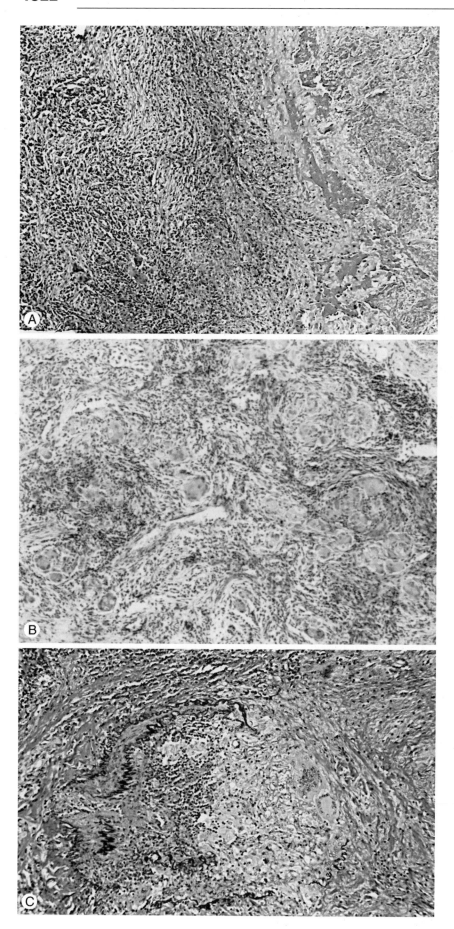

**Figure 40–27. Histoplasmosis Simulating Necrotizing Sarcoid Granulomatosis.** A 33-year-old woman presented with fever and malaise. Radiographs showed a well-defined nodular opacity in the right upper lobe. A low-power view of the excised nodule *(A)* shows necrosis on the right and a chronic inflammatory infiltrate on the left. A magnified view of the parenchymal inflammation *(B)* shows it to consist of several nonnecrotizing granulomas amid a background of lymphocytes, fibroblasts, and isolated multinucleated giant cells. A pulmonary artery adjacent to the focus of parenchymal inflammation *(C)* shows destruction of elastic laminae and obliteration of the lumen by a granulomatous inflammatory infiltrate. Because of the necrosis, granulomas, and vasculitis, the biopsy specimen was initially interpreted as necrotizing sarcoid granulomatosis (a limited form of Wegener's granulomatosis might also have been considered). Silver stains showed numerous organisms consistent with *Histoplasma capsulatum* within the necrotic areas. (*A,* ×40; *B,* ×100; *C,* Verhoeff Van Gieson, ×130.)

in otherwise classic sarcoidosis (although usually less marked in extent and severity than in necrotizing sarcoid granulomatosis).[451] This finding, in addition to the occasional documentation of granulomatous inflammation in hilar lymph nodes and other extrapulmonary sites,[447, 448, 450, 452, 453] suggests that necrotizing sarcoid granulomatosis might be a variant of classic sarcoidosis, possibly representing the histologic counterpart of the nodular form of the disease observed radiologically.[448, 454]

Culture and thorough examination of tissue with special stains must always be performed to exclude the possibility of infection; we and others[448] have observed cases simulating necrotizing sarcoid granulomatosis in which the aforementioned procedures have provided proof of an infectious cause (Fig. 40–27). In fact, because of the similarity of the histologic pattern to that of known infections, it is possible that some reported cases of necrotizing sarcoid granulomatosis represent infection by an unidentified organism.

The most striking histologic feature is the presence of confluent parenchymal granulomas admixed with a chronic inflammatory infiltrate of histiocytes, multinucleated giant cells, lymphocytes, and fibroblasts.[444, 447, 448] Necrosis may be seen within individual granulomas, but is more often evident as an area of coagulative or granular necrosis within the confluent granulomatous mass itself; in one patient, the necrosis was described as being suppurative in nature.[455] Vasculitis affects small-to-medium-sized arteries and veins and can take several forms, including the presence of granulomas in part or all of the vessel wall, abundant medial giant cells in a pattern similar to temporal arteritis, or a transmural lymphohistiocytic infiltrate. Granulomatous inflammation of smaller airways may lead to luminal obliteration and obstructive pneumonitis. Involvement of the pleura can also occur and is sometimes prominent.[450] Although regional lymph nodes occasionally show small foci of nonnecrotizing granulomas, an appearance similar to classic sarcoidosis has been noted only occasionally.[448]

The radiologic pattern in the majority of patients is that of multiple well-defined nodules (Fig. 40–28).[448, 455, 456] Most commonly, they measure 5 to 10 mm in diameter; however,

a miliary pattern and nodules as large as 4 cm in diameter may be seen.[448, 455, 456] On HRCT, the nodules have a predominantly peribronchoarterial and subpleural distribution, similar to that of sarcoidosis.[457] The nodules may increase in size and number over time or, occasionally, resolve;[448] cavitation occurs rarely.[115, 447]

Other radiologic manifestations include a solitary nodule or mass,[448, 457] bilateral areas of consolidation (Fig. 40–29), and, less commonly, a bilateral interstitial reticular pattern.[448, 455, 457] On HRCT, the areas of consolidation may have a predominantly peribronchoarterial[457] or subpleural distribution.[458] Hilar lymph node enlargement was not a feature in the original report of 11 cases,[444] but was noted in 1 of 13 patients in one series[447] and in 6 of 12 in another.[448] Pleural effusion may occur,[447] but is uncommon.

Patients may be asymptomatic or present with cough, fever, sweats, malaise, dyspnea, hemoptysis, or pleuritic pain.[450] A localized wheeze was found in one patient who had endobronchial involvement.[450] Extrapulmonary findings are usually absent, although uveitis and hypothalamic insufficiency have been reported.[446, 448] One patient has been reported who presented with recurrent headaches and transient right hemipareses as a result of a retro-orbital mass (shown to be composed of a necrotizing granulomatous inflammatory infiltrate) 12 years before the appearance of a similar inflammatory mass in the lung.[453] In one investigation of six patients, a restrictive pattern of pulmonary function was found in four and an obstructive-restrictive pattern in one.[450]

The course of necrotizing sarcoid granulomatosis is typically benign. Radiologic evidence of disease diminishes with corticosteroid therapy or, occasionally, spontaneously. Relapse has occurred in some patients after cessation of therapy.[447]

## MISCELLANEOUS PULMONARY VASCULITIDES

In addition to the disease entities described previously, there exist a number of cases associated with pulmonary

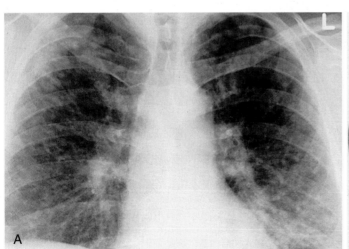
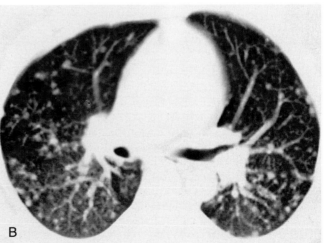

**Figure 40–28. Necrotizing Sarcoid Granulomatosis.** A view of the chest from a posteroanterior radiograph *(A)* in a 41-year-old man demonstrates numerous bilateral small nodular opacities. A conventional CT scan *(B)* demonstrates the majority of the nodules to be closely associated with pulmonary vessels. Subpleural nodules are also evident. The diagnosis of necrotizing sarcoid granulomatosis was proven by open-lung biopsy.

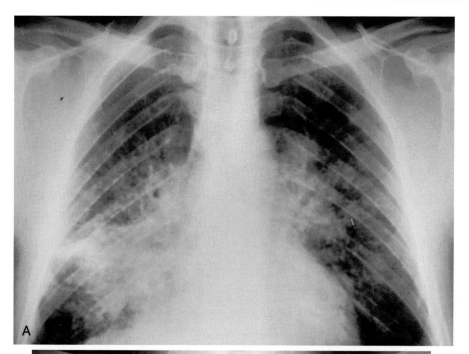

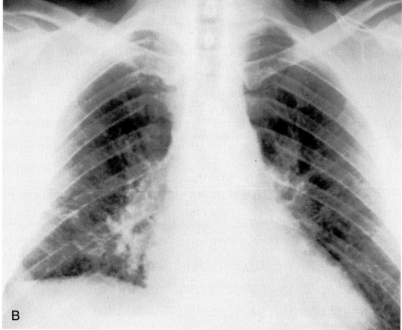

**Figure 40–29. Necrotizing Sarcoid Granulomatosis.** A posteroanterior chest radiograph *(A)* of a 50-year-old man reveals bilateral areas of consolidation and small nodular opacities that predominantly affect the perihilar parenchyma bilaterally. Mediastinal lymph nodes are not enlarged; hilar nodes cannot be evaluated because of contiguous parenchymal consolidation. An open-lung biopsy disclosed isolated and confluent nonnecrotizing granulomas and a granulomatous vasculitis that completely enveloped partly occluded and recanalizing arteries. A posteroanterior chest radiograph 4 months later *(B)* after the institution of corticosteroid therapy reveals remarkable clearing of the parenchymal disease.

vasculitis that defy precise clinicopathologic classification. Some of these may represent variants of the better-characterized vasculitides and have been described by the term *polyangiitis overlap syndrome* by some authors.[3] These and other workers have listed combinations of diseases, such as Takayasu's arteritis and PAN, Churg-Strauss syndrome and PAN, giant cell arteritis and Wegener's granulomatosis, and so on. Coexistent Wegener's granulomatosis and anti–glomerular basement membrane disease has also been described.[459] Because of their varied and atypical manifestations, it is clear that these variants can cause considerable diagnostic difficulty. The possibility of pulmonary vasculitis should not be discounted, however, simply because of a lack of clinicopathologic features enabling precise classification.

Several other rare forms of pulmonary vasculitis have also been reported that have no apparent relationship with any of the vasculitides discussed previously. These include the following:

1. A familial disorder characterized by onset in adolescence, polyarthritis and nonnecrotizing granulomatous arteritis, and apparent inheritance in a dominant fashion;[460] autopsy of one patient showed involvement of the lungs, although there had been no pulmonary symptoms.

2. Another apparently hereditary disorder characterized by severe episodic attacks of pulmonary hypertension, peripheral eosinophilia, and pulmonary arteritis with massive eosinophil infiltration.[461]

3. One case in which multiple aneurysms and histologi-

cally nonspecific vasculitis involved chiefly large and medium-sized pulmonary and systemic arteries; the only pulmonary complaint was asthma, which had an onset 5 years before symptoms of arteritis.[462]

4. Occasional cases in which granulomatous inflammation appears to be limited to the pulmonary vasculature;[463] whether these represent a *forme fruste* of Takayasu's disease or a completely different entity is uncertain.

5. One case of generalized visceral and lymph node as well as vascular granulomatous inflammation.[464]

# REFERENCES

1. Sneller MC, Fauci AS: Pathogenesis of vasculitis syndromes. Med Clin North Am 81:221, 1997.
2. Sundy JS, Haynes BF: Pathogenic mechanisms of vessel damage in vasculitis syndromes. Rheum Dis Clin North Am 21:861, 1995.
3. Leavitt RY, Fauci AS: Pulmonary vasculitis. Am Rev Respir Dis 134:149, 1986.
4. Brasile L, Kremer JM, Clarke JL, et al: Identification of an autoantibody to vascular endothelial cell-specific antigens in patients with systemic vasculitis. Am J Med 87:74, 1989.
5. Ferraro G, Meroni PL, Tincani A, et al: Anti-endothelial cell antibodies in patients with Wegener's granulomatosis and micropolyarteritis. Clin Exp Immunol 79:47, 1990.
6. Rasmussen N, Petersen J: Cellular immune responses and pathogenesis in C-ANCA positive vasculitides. J Autoimmun 6:227, 1993.
7. Ulbright TM, Katzenstein A-LA: Solitary necrotizing granulomas of the lung: Differentiating features and etiology. Am J Surg Pathol 4:13, 1980.
8. Lie JT: Nomenclature and classification of vasculitis: Plus ca change, plus c'est la meme chose. Arthritis Rheum 37:181, 1994.
9. Jennette JC, Falk RJ: Small-vessel vasculitis. N Engl J Med 337:1512, 1997.
10. Jennette JC, Falk RJ, Andrassy K, et al: Nomenclature of systemic vasculitides. Proposal of an International Consensus Conference. Arthritis Rheum 37:187, 1994.
11. Travis WD, Fleming MV: Vasculitis of the lung. Pathology 4:23, 1996.
12. Ciaccia A, Ferrari M, Facchini FM, et al: Pulmonary vasculitis: Classification, clinical features, and management. Clin Rev Allergy Immunol 15:73, 1997.
13. Savage CO, Harper L, Adu D: Primary systemic vasculitis. Lancet 349:553, 1997.
13a. Burns A: Pulmonary vasculitis. Br J Hosp Med 58:389, 1997.
14. Leavitt RY, Fauci AS, Bloch DA, et al: The American College of Rheumatology 1990 criteria for the classification of Wegener's granulomatosis. Arthritis Rheum 33:1101, 1990.
15. Luqmani RA, Bacon PA, Beaman M, et al: Classical versus nonrenal Wegener's granulomatosis. QJM 87:161, 1994.
16. Carrington CB, Liebow AA: Limited forms of angiitis and granulomatosis of Wegener's type. Am J Med 41:497, 1966.
17. Cassan SM, Coles DT, Harrison EG Jr: The concept of limited forms of Wegener's granulomatosis. Am J Med 49:366, 1970.
18. Israel HL, Patchefsky AS: Wegener's granulomatosis of lung: Diagnosis and treatment, experience with 12 cases. Ann Intern Med 74:881, 1971.
19. Wolff SM, Fauci AS, Horn RG, et al: Wegener's granulomatosis. Ann Intern Med 81:513, 1974.
20. Fienberg R: The protracted superficial phenomenon in pathergic (Wegener's) granulomatosis. Hum Pathol 12:458, 1981.
21. Kihiczak D, Nychay SG, Schwartz RA, et al: Protracted superficial Wegener's granulomatosis. J Am Acad Dermatol 30:863, 1994.
22. Watts RA, Carruthers DM, Scott DG: Epidemiology of systemic vasculitis: Changing incidence or definition? Semin Arthritis Rheum 25:28, 1995.
23. Andrews M, Edmunds M, Campbell A, et al: Systemic vasculitis in the 1980s: Is there an increasing incidence of Wegener's granulomatosis and microscopic polyarteritis? J R Coll Physicians Lond 24:284, 1990.
24. Cotch MF, Hoffman GS, Yerg DE, et al: The epidemiology of Wegener's granulomatosis: Estimates of the five-year period prevalence, annual mortality, and geographic disease distribution from population-based data sources. Arthritis Rheum 39:87, 1996.
25. Hoffman GS, Kerr GS, Leavitt RS, et al: Wegener granulomatosis: An analysis of 158 patients. Ann Intern Med 116:488, 1992.
26. Cordier JF, Valeyre D, Guillevin L, et al: Pulmonary Wegener's granulomatosis: A clinical and imaging study of 77 cases. Chest 97:906, 1990.
27. Vassallo M, Shepherd RJ, Iqbal P, et al: Age-related variations in presentation and outcome in Wegener's granulomatosis. J R Coll Physicians Lond 31:396, 1997.
28. Neumann G, Benz-Bohm G, Rister M: Wegener's granulomatosis in childhood: Review of the literature and case report. Pediatr Radiol 14:267, 1984.
29. Hall SL, Miller LC, Duggan E, et al: Wegener's granulomatosis in pediatric patients. J Pediatr 106:739, 1985.
30. Habib A, MacKay K, Abrons HL: Wegener's granulomatosis complicating pregnancy: Presentation of two patients and review of the literature. Clin Nephrol 46:332, 1996.
31. Luisiri P, Lance NJ, Curran JJ: Wegener's granulomatosis in pregnancy. Arthritis Rheum 40:1354, 1997.
32. Raynauld JP, Bloch DA, Fries JF: Seasonal variation in the onset of Wegener's granulomatosis, PAN and giant cell arteritis. J Rheumatol 20:1524, 1993.
33. George J, Levy Y, Kallenberg CG, et al: Infections and Wegener's granulomatosis—a cause and effect relationship? QJM 90:367, 1997.
34. Pinching AJ, Rees AJ, Pussell BA, et al: Relapses in Wegener's granulomatosis: The role of infection. BMJ 281:836, 1980.
35. Stegeman CA, Tervaert JW, Sluiter WJ, et al: Association of chronic nasal carriage of Staphylococcus aureus and higher relapse rates in Wegener granulomatosis. Ann Intern Med 120:12, 1994.
36. van Putten JW, van Haren EH, Lammers JW: Association between Wegener's granulomatosis and Staphylococcus aureus infection? Eur Respir J 9:1955, 1996.
37. Valenti S, Vignolo C, Benevolo E, et al: Mixed infection by Staphylococcus and Candida, and Wegener's granulomatosis. Monaldi Arch Chest Dis 51:387, 1996.
38. Finkel TH, Torok TJ, Ferguson PJ, et al: Chronic parvovirus B19 infection and systemic necrotising vasculitis: Opportunistic infection or aetiological agent? Lancet 343:1255, 1994.
39. DeRemee RA, McDonald TJ, Weiland LH: Wegener's granulomatosis: Observations on treatment with antimicrobial agents. Mayo Clin Proc 60:27, 1985.
40. Reinhold-Keller E, De Groot K, Rudert H, et al: Response to trimethoprim/sulfamethoxazole in Wegener's granulomatosis depends on the phase of disease. QJM 89:15, 1996.
41. Stegeman CA, Cohen Tervaert JW, de Jong PE, et al: Trimethoprim-sulfamethoxazole (co-trimoxazole) for the prevention of relapses of Wegener's granulomatosis. Dutch Co-Trimoxazole Wegener Study Group. N Engl J Med 335:16, 1996.
42. Roberts DE, Curd JG: Sulfonamides as antiinflammatory agents in the treatment of Wegener's granulomatosis. Arthritis Rheum 33:1590, 1990.
43. Willoughby WF, Barbaras JE, Wheelis R: Immunologic mechanisms in experimental interstitial pneumonitis. Chest 69(Suppl):290, 1976.
44. Neyer U, Woss E, Neuweiler J: Wegener's granulomatosis associated with silicosis. Nephrol Dial Transplant 9:559, 1994.
45. Nuyts GD, Van Vlem E, De Vos A, et al: Wegener granulomatosis is associated with exposure to silicon compounds: A case-control study. Nephrol Dial Transplant 10:1162, 1995.
46. Muniain MA, Moreno JC, Gonzalez Campora R: Wegener's granulomatosis in two sisters. Ann Rheum Dis 45:417, 1986.
47. Knudsen BB, Joergensen T, Munch-Jensen B: Wegener's granulomatosis in a family. Scand J Rheumatol 17:225, 1988.
48. Rottem M, Cotch MF, Fauci AS, et al: Familial vasculitis: Report of 2 families. J Rheumatol 21:561, 1994.
49. Wilson RH, Kerr PP, McLoughlin J, et al: Symptomatic colitis as the initial presentation of Wegener's granulomatosis. Br J Clin Pract 47:315, 1993.
50. Papiha SS, Murty GE, Ad'hia A, et al: Association of Wegener's granulomatosis with HLA antigens and other genetic markers. Ann Rheum Dis 51:246, 1992.
51. Elkon KB, Sutherland DC, Rees AJ, et al: HLA antigen frequencies in systemic vasculitis: Increase in HLA-DR2 in Wegener's granulomatosis. Arthritis Rheum 26:102, 1983.
52. Hagen EC, Stegeman CA, D'Amaro J, et al: Decreased frequency of HLA-DR13DR6 in Wegener's granulomatosis. Kidney Int 48:801, 1995.
53. Zhang L, Jayne DR, Zhao MH, et al: Distribution of MHC class II alleles in primary systemic vasculitis. Kidney Int 47:294, 1995.
54. Baslund B, Szpirt W, Eriksson S, et al: Complexes between proteinase 3, alpha 1-antitrypsin and proteinase 3 anti-neutrophil cytoplasm autoantibodies: A comparison between alpha 1-antitrypsin PiZ allele carriers and noncarriers with Wegener's granulomatosis. Eur J Clin Invest 26:786, 1996.
55. Testa A, Audrain M, Baranger T, et al: Anti-neutrophil cytoplasm antibodies and alpha-1-antitrypsin phenotype. Clin Exp Immunol 93:S16, 1993.
56. Mazodier P, Elzouki ANY, Segelmark M, et al: Systemic necrotizing vasculitides in severe alpha$_1$-antitrypsin deficiency. QJM 89:599, 1996.
57. Elzouki AN, Segelmark M, Wieslander J, et al: Strong link between the alpha 1-antitrypsin PiZ allele and Wegener's granulomatosis. J Intern Med 236:543, 1994.
58. Kallenberg CG, Brouwer E, Weening JJ, et al: Anti-neutrophil cytoplasmic antibodies: Current diagnostic and pathophysiological potential. Kidney Int 46:1, 1994.
59. Savige JA, Davies DJ, Gatenby PA: Anti-neutrophil cytoplasmic antibodies (ANCA): Their detection and significance: Report from workshops. Pathology 26:186, 1994.
59a. Baslund B, Petersen J: Antineutrophil cytoplasm autoantibodies (ANCA): The need for specific and sensitive assays. Autoimmunity 27:231, 1998.
60. Daouk GH, Palsson R, Arnaout MA: Inhibition of proteinase 3 by ANCA and its correlation with disease activity in Wegener's granulomatosis. Kidney Int 47:1528, 1995.
61. Wiik A, Stummann L, Kjeldsen L, et al: The diversity of perinuclear antineutrophil cytoplasmic antibodies (pANCA) antigens. Clin Exp Immunol 101(S):15, 1995.
62. Hagen EC, Andrassy K, Chernok E, et al: The value of indirect immunofluorescence and solid phase techniques for ANCA detection: A report on the first phase of an international cooperative study on the standardization of ANCA assays. J Immunol Methods 159:1, 1993.
63. Galperin C, Shoenfeld Y, Gilburd B, et al: Anti-neutrophil cytoplasmic antibodies in patients with chromomycosis. Clin Exp Rheumatol 14:479, 1996.
64. Pudifin DJ, Duursma J, Gathiram V, et al: Invasive amoebiasis is associated with the development of anti-neutrophil cytoplasmic antibody. Clin Exp Immunol 97:48, 1994.
65. Blanco A, Solis P, Gomez S, et al: Antineutrophil cytoplasmic antibodies (ANCA) in idiopathic pulmonary hemosiderosis. Pediatr Allergy Immunol 5:235, 1994.
66. Baltaro RJ, Hoffman GS, Sechler JMG, et al: Immunoglobulin G antineutrophil cytoplasmic antibodies are produced in the respiratory tract of patients with Wegener's granulomatosis. Am Rev Respir Dis 143:275, 1991.
67. Kallenberg CG, Brouwer E, Mulder AH, et al: ANCA—pathophysiology revisited. Clin Exp Immunol 100:1, 1995.
68. Csernok E, Ernst M, Schmitt W, et al: Activated neutrophils express proteinase 3 on their plasma membrane in vitro and in vivo. Clin Exp Immunol 95:244, 1994.
69. Falk RJ, Terrell RS, Charles LA, et al: Anti-neutrophil cytoplasmic autoantibod-

ies induce neutrophils to degranulate and produce oxygen radicals in vitro. Proc Natl Acad Sci U S A 87:4115, 1990.

70. Csernok E, Lüdemann J, Wolfgang L, et al: Ultrastructural localization of proteinase 3, the target antigen of anti-cytoplasmic antibodies circulating in Wegener's granulomatosis. Am J Pathol 137:1113, 1990.

71. Grimminger F, Hattar K, Papavassilis C, et al: Neutrophil activation by anti-proteinase 3 antibodies in Wegener's granulomatosis: Role of exogenous arachidonic acid and leukotriene B4 generation. J Exp Med 184:1567, 1996.

72. Haubitz M, Schulzeck P, Schellong S, et al: Complexed plasma elastase as an in vivo marker for leukocyte activation in antineutrophil cytoplasmic antibody-associated vasculitis. Arthritis Rheum 40:1680, 1997.

73. Brooks CJ, King WJ, Radford DJ, et al: IL-1 beta production by human polymorphonuclear leucocytes stimulated by anti-neutrophil cytoplasmic autoantibodies: Relevance to systemic vasculitis. Clin Exp Immunol 106:273, 1996.

74. Casselman BL, Kilgore KS, Miller BF, et al: Antibodies to neutrophil cytoplasmic antigens induce monocyte chemoattractant protein-1 secretion from human monocytes. J Lab Clin Med 126:495, 1995.

75. Mulder AH, Stegeman CA, Kallenberg CG: Activation of granulocytes by anti-neutrophil cytoplasmic antibodies (ANCA) in Wegener's granulomatosis: A predominant role for the IgG3 subclass of ANCA. Clin Exp Immunol 101:227, 1995.

76. Mayet WJ, Csernok E, Szymkowiak C, et al: Human endothelial cells express proteinase 3, the target antigen of anticytoplasmic antibodies in Wegener's granulomatosis. Blood 82:1221, 1993.

77. King WJ, Adu D, Daha MR, et al: Endothelial cells and renal epithelial cells do not express the Wegener's autoantigen, proteinase 3. Clin Exp Immunol 102:98, 1995.

78. Mayet WJ, Schwarting A, Meyer zum Buschenfelde KH: Cytotoxic effects of antibodies to proteinase 3 (C-ANCA) on human endothelial cells. Clin Exp Immunol 97:458, 1994.

79. Savage COS, Pottinger BE, Gaskin G, et al: Autoantibodies developing to myeloperoxidase and proteinase 3 in systemic vasculitis stimulate neutrophil cytotoxicity towards cultured endothelial cells. Am J Pathol 141:335, 1992.

80. Mayet W-J, Meyer zum Büschenfelde K-H: Antibodies to proteinase 3 increase adhesion of neutrophils to human endothelial cells. Clin Exp Immunol 94:440, 1993.

81. Mayet W-J, Schwarting A, Orth TH, et al: Antibodies to proteinase 3 increase adhesion of T-lymphocytes to human endothelial cells via VCAM-1. Arthritis Rheum 37:S220, 1994.

82. Haller H, Eichhorn J, Pieper K, et al: Circulating leukocyte integrin expression in Wegener's granulomatosis. J Am Soc Nephrol 7:40, 1996.

83. Brouwer E, Stegeman CA, Huitema MG, et al: T cell reactivity to proteinase 3 and myeloperoxidase in patients with Wegener's granulomatosis (Wegener's granulomatosis). Clin Exp Immunol 98:448, 1994.

84. Stegeman CA, Cohen Tervaert JW, Huitema MG, et al: Serum markers of T cell activation in relapses of Wegener's granulomatosis. Clin Exp Immunol 91:415, 1993.

85. Mathieson PW, Oliveira DBG: The role of cellular immunity in systemic vasculitis. Clin Exp Immunol 100:183, 1995.

86. Navarro M, Cervera R, Font J, et al: Anti-endothelial cell antibodies in systemic autoimmune diseases: Prevalence and clinical significance. Lupus 6:521, 1997.

87. Gobel U, Eichhorn J, Kettritz R, et al: Disease activity and autoantibodies to endothelial cells in patients with Wegener's granulomatosis. Am J Kidney Dis 28:186, 1996.

88. Del Papa N, Guidali L, Sironi M, et al: Anti-endothelial cell IgG antibodies from patients with Wegener's granulomatosis bind to human endothelial cells in vitro and induce adhesion molecule expression and cytokine secretion. Arthritis Rheum 39:758, 1996.

89. Varagunam M, Nwosu Z, Adu D, et al: Little evidence for anti-endothelial cell antibodies in microscopic polyarteritis and Wegener's granulomatosis. Nephrol Dial Transplant 8:113, 1993.

90. Howell SB, Epstein WV: Circulating immunoglobulin complexes in Wegener's granulomatosis. Am J Med 60:259, 1976.

91. Shasby DM, Schwarz MI, Forstot JZ, et al: Pulmonary immune complex deposition in Wegener's granulomatosis. Chest 81:3, 1982.

92. Hui AN, Ehresmann GR, Quismorio FP, et al: Wegener's granulomatosis: Electron microscopic and immunofluorescent studies. Chest 80:6, 1981.

93. Stokes TC, McCann BG, Rees RT, et al: Acute fulminating intrapulmonary haemorrhage in Wegener's granulomatosis. Thorax 37:315, 1982.

94. Horn RG, Fauci AS, Rosenthal AS, et al: Renal biopsy pathology in Wegener's granulomatosis. Am J Pathol 74:423, 1974.

95. Donald KJ, Edwards RF, McEvoy JDS: An ultrastructural study of the pathogenesis of tissue injury in limited Wegener's granulomatosis. Pathology 8:161, 1976.

96. Israel HL, Patchefsky AS, Saldana MJ: Wegener's granulomatosis, lymphomatoid granulomatosis, and benign lymphocytic angiitis and granulomatosis of lung: Recognition and treatment. Ann Intern Med 87:691, 1977.

97. Ballieux BE, van der Burg SH, Hagen EC, et al: Cell-mediated autoimmunity in patients with Wegener's granulomatosis. Clin Exp Immunol 100:186, 1995.

98. Schlesier M, Kaspar T, Gutfleisch J, et al: Activated CD4+ and CD8+ T-cell subsets in Wegener's granulomatosis. Rheumatol Int 14:213, 1995.

99. van Vollenhoven RF: Adhesion molecules, sex steroids, and the pathogenesis of vasculitis syndromes. Curr Opinion Rheumatol 7:4, 1995.

100. Shillitoe EJ, Lehner T, Lessof MH: Immunological features of Wegener's granulomatosis. Lancet 1:281, 1974.

101. Fauci AS, Wolff SM: Wegener's granulomatosis: Studies in eighteen patients and a review of the literature. Medicine 52:535, 1973.

102. Godman GC, Churg J: Wegener's granulomatosis: Pathology and review of the literature. AMA Arch Pathol 58:533, 1954.

103. Yoshikawa Y, Watanabe T: Pulmonary lesions in Wegener's granulomatosis: A clinicopathologic study of 22 autopsy cases. Hum Pathol 17:401, 1986.

104. Travis WD, Hoffman GS, Leavitt RY, et al: Surgical pathology of the lung in Wegener's granulomatosis: Review of 87 open lung biopsies from 67 patients. Am J Surg Pathol 15:315, 1991.

105. Mark EJ, Matsubara O, Tan-Liu NS, et al: The pulmonary biopsy in the early diagnosis of Wegener's (pathergic) granulomatosis: A study based on 35 open lung biopsies. Hum Pathol 19:1065, 1988.

106. Katzenstein AL, Locke WK: Solitary lung lesions in Wegener's granulomatosis: Pathologic findings and clinical significance in 25 cases. Am J Surg Pathol 19:545, 1995.

107. Gaudin PB, Askin FB, Falk RJ, et al: The pathologic spectrum of pulmonary lesions in patients with anti-neutrophil cytoplasmic autoantibodies specific for anti-proteinase 3 and anti-myeloperoxidase. Am J Clin Pathol 104:7, 1995.

108. Uner AH, Rozum-Slota B, Katzenstein AL: Bronchiolitis obliterans-organizing pneumonia (BOOP)-like variant of Wegener's granulomatosis: A clinicopathologic study of 16 cases. Am J Surg Pathol 20:794, 1996.

109. Yousem SA, Lombard CM: The eosinophilic variant of Wegener's granulomatosis. Hum Pathol 19:682, 1988.

110. Yousem SA: Bronchocentric injury in Wegener's granulomatosis: A report of five cases. Hum Pathol 22:535, 1991.

111. Travis WD, Carpenter HA, Lie JT: Diffuse pulmonary hemorrhage: An uncommon manifestation of Wegener's granulomatosis. Am J Surg Pathol 11:702, 1987.

112. Myers JL, Katzenstein AA: Wegener's granulomatosis presenting with massive pulmonary hemorrhage and capillaritis. Am J Surg Pathol 11:895, 1987.

113. Travis WD, Colby TV, Lombard C, et al: A clinicopathologic study of 34 cases of diffuse pulmonary hemorrhage with lung biopsy confirmation. Am J Surg Pathol 14:1112, 1990.

114. Mark EJ, Flieder DB, Matsubara O: Treated Wegener's granulomatosis: Distinctive pathological findings in the lungs of 20 patients and what they tell us about the natural history of the disease. Hum Pathol 28:450, 1997.

115. Frazier AA, Rosado-de-Christenson ML, Galvin JR, Fleming MV: Pulmonary angiitis and granulomatosis: Radiologic-pathologic correlation. RadioGraphics 18:687, 1998.

116. Matsubara O, Yoshimura N, Doi Y, et al: Nasal biopsy in the early diagnosis of Wegener's (pathergic) granulomatosis: Significance of palisading granuloma and leukocytoclastic vasculitis. Virchows Arch 428:13, 1996.

117. Devaney KO, Travis WD, Hoffman G, et al: Interpretation of head and neck biopsies in Wegener's granulomatosis: A pathologic study of 126 biopsies in 70 patients. Am J Surg Pathol 14:555, 1990.

118. Del Buono EA, Flint A: Diagnostic usefulness of nasal biopsy in Wegener's granulomatosis. Hum Pathol 22:107, 1991.

119. Weiss MA, Crissman JD: Renal biopsy findings in Wegener's granulomatosis: Segmental necrotizing glomerulonephritis with glomerular thrombosis. Hum Pathol 15:943, 1984.

120. Bajema IM, Hagen EC, van der Woude FJ, et al: Wegener's granulomatosis: A meta-analysis of 349 literary case reports. J Lab Clin Med 129:17, 1997.

121. Goulart RA, Mark EJ, Rosen S: Tumefactions as an extravascular manifestation of Wegener's granulomatosis. Am J Surg Pathol 19:145, 1995.

122. Boubenider SA, Akhtar M, Nyman R: Wegener's granulomatosis limited to the kidney as a masslike lesion. Nephron 68:500, 1994.

123. Hoffman GS, Kerr GS, Leavitt RY, et al: Wegener granulomatosis: An analysis of 158 patients. Ann Intern Med 116:488, 1992.

124. Cordier JF, Valeyre D, Guillevin L, et al: Pulmonary Wegener's granulomatosis: A clinical and imaging study of 77 cases. Chest 97:906, 1990.

125. Aberle DR, Gamsu G, Lynch D: Thoracic manifestations of Wegener granulomatosis: Diagnosis and course. Radiology 174:703, 1990.

126. Weir IH, Müller NL, Chiles C, et al: Wegener's granulomatosis: Findings from computed tomography of the chest in 10 patients. Can Assoc Radiol J 43:31, 1992.

127. Edwards CW: Vasculitis and granulomatosis of the respiratory tract. Thorax 37:81, 1982.

128. Wechsler RJ, Steiner RM, Israel HL, et al: Chest radiography in lymphomatoid granulomatosis: Comparison with Wegener granulomatosis. Am J Roentgenol 142:679, 1984.

129. McGregor MBB, Sandler G: Wegener's granulomatosis: A clinical and radiological survey. Br J Radiol 37:430, 1964.

130. Bischoff ME: Noninfectious necrotizing granulomatosis: The pulmonary roentgen signs. Radiology 75:752, 1960.

131. Maguire R, Fauci AS, Doppman JL, et al: Unusual radiographic features of Wegener's granulomatosis. Am J Roentgenol 130:233, 1978.

132. Hunninghake GW, Fauci AS: Pulmonary involvement in the collagen vascular diseases. Am Rev Respir Dis 119:471, 1979.

133. Papiris SA, Manoussakis MN, Drosos AA, et al: Imaging of thoracic Wegener's granulomatosis: The computed tomographic appearance. Am J Med 93:529, 1992.

134. Maskell GF, Lockwood CM, Flower CDR: Computed tomography of the lung in Wegener's granulomatosis. Clin Radiol 48:377, 1993.

134a. Reuter M, Schnabel A, Wesner F, et al: Pulmonary Wegener's granulomatosis: Correlation between high-resolution CT findings and clinical scoring of disease activity. Chest 114:500, 1998.

135. Kuhlman JE, Hruban RH, Fishman ER: Wegener granulomatosis: CT features of parenchymal lung disease. J Comput Assist Tomogr 15:948, 1991.

136. Gohel VK, Dalinka MK, Israel HL, et al: The radiological manifestations of Wegener's granulomatosis. Br J Radiol 46:427, 1973.

137. Roghair GD, Ross P: Wegener's granulomatosis: Case reports. Br J Radiol 43:216, 1970.

138. Foo SS, Weisbrod GL, Herman SJ, Chamberlain DW: Wegener granulomatosis presenting on CT with atypical bronchovasocentric distribution. J Comput Assist Tomogr 14:1004, 1990.

139. Daum TE, Specks U, Colby TV, et al: Tracheobronchial involvement in Wegener's granulomatosis. Am J Respir Crit Care Med 151:522, 1995.

140. Stein MG, Gamsu G, Webb WR, et al: Computed tomography of diffuse tracheal stenosis in Wegener granulomatosis. J Comput Assist Tomogr 10:868, 1986.

141. Baker SB, Robinson DR: Unusual renal manifestations of Wegener's granulomatosis: Report of two cases. Am J Med 64:883, 1978.

141a. Conces DJ Jr, Kesler KA, Datzman M, Tarver RD: Tracheoesophageal fistula due to Wegener's granulomatosis. J Thoracic Imaging 10:126, 1995.

141b. Kulis JC, Nequin ND: Tracheoesophageal fistula due to Wegener's granulomatosis. JAMA 191:54, 1965.

142. Pinching AJ, Lockwood CM, Pussell BA, et al: Wegener's granulomatosis: Observations on 18 patients with severe renal disease. QJM 52:435, 1983.

143. Jaspan T, Davison AM, Walker WC: Spontaneous pneumothorax in Wegener's granulomatosis. Thorax 37:774, 1982.

144. Wolffenbuttel BH, Weber RF, Kho GS: Pyopneumothorax: A rare complication of Wegener's granulomatosis. Eur J Respir Dis 67:223, 1985.

144a. Cohen MI, Gore RM, August CZ, Ossoff RH: Tracheal and bronchial stenosis associated with mediastinal adenopathy in Wegener granulomatosis: CT findings. J Comput Assist Tomogr 8:327, 1984.

145. Kjellstrand CM, Simmons RL, Uranga VM, et al: Acute fulminant Wegener granulomatosis: Therapy with immunosuppression, hemodialysis, and renal transplantation. Arch Intern Med 134:40, 1974.

146. Richards BT, Razavi M, Leftwich WB: Wegener's granulomatosis with severe hemoptysis. Am Rev Respir Dis 85:890, 1962.

147. Hensley MJ, Feldman NT, Lazarus JM, et al: Diffuse pulmonary hemorrhage and rapidly progressive renal failure: An uncommon presentation of Wegener's granulomatosis. Am J Med 66:894, 1979.

148. Arauz JC, Fonseca R: Wegener's granulomatosis appearing initially in the trachea. Ann Otol Rhinol Laryngol 91:593, 1982.

149. Hellmann D, Laing T, Petri M, et al: Wegener's granulomatosis: Isolated involvement of the trachea and larynx. Ann Rheum Dis 46:628, 1987.

150. Krafcik SS, Covin RB, Lynch JP 3rd, et al: Wegener's granulomatosis in the elderly. Chest 109:430, 1996.

151. Masor JJ, Gal AA, LiVolsi VA: Case report: Hashimoto's thyroiditis associated with Wegener's granulomatosis. Am J Med Sci 308:112, 1994.

152. Le Thi Huong D, Gatfosse M, Papo T, et al: Wegener's granulomatosis and CREST syndrome. Br J Rheumatol 33:1087, 1994.

153. Cuadrado MJ, D'Cruz D, Lloyd M, et al: Allergic disorders in systemic vasculitis: A case-controlled study. Br J Rheumatol 33:749, 1994.

154. Langford CA, Sneller MC, Hallahan CW, et al: Clinical features and therapeutic management of subglottic stenosis in patients with Wegener's granulomatosis. Arthritis Rheum 39:1754, 1996.

155. Gans R, de Vries N, Donker AJ, et al: Circulating anti-neutrophil cytoplasmic autoantibodies in subglottic stenosis: A useful aid in diagnosing vasculitis in this condition? QJM 80:565, 1991.

156. Herridge MS, Pearson FG, Downey GP: Subglottic stenosis complicating Wegener's granulomatosis: Surgical repair as a viable treatment option. J Thorac Cardiovasc Surg 111:961, 1996.

157. Conces DJ Jr, Kesler KA, Datzman M, et al: Tracheoesophageal fistula due to Wegener granulomatosis. J Thorac Imaging 10:126, 1995.

158. Matt BH: Wegener's granulomatosis, acute laryngotracheal airway obstruction and death in a 17-year-old female: Case report and review of the literature. Int J Pediatr Otorhinolaryngol 37:163, 1996.

159. Fauci AS, Balow JE, Brown R, et al: Successful renal transplantation in Wegener's granulomatosis. Am J Med 60:437, 1976.

160. van der Woude FJ, Hoorntje SJ, Weening JJ, et al: Renal involvement in Wegener's granulomatosis: Report of three unusual cases. Nephron 32:185, 1982.

161. Anderson CL, Stavrides A: Rapidly progressive renal failure as the primary manifestation of Wegener's granulomatosis. Am J Med Sci 275:109, 1978.

162. Woodworth TG, Abuelo JG, Austin HA III, et al: Severe glomerulonephritis with late emergence of classic Wegener's granulomatosis: Report of 4 cases and review of the literature. Medicine 66:181, 1987.

163. Moutsopoulos HM, Avgerinos PC, Tsampoulas CG, et al: Selective renal angiography in Wegener's granulomatosis. Ann Rheum Dis 42:192, 1983.

164. Brandwein S, Esdaile J, Danoff D, et al: Wegener's granulomatosis: Clinical features and outcome in 13 patients. Arch Intern Med 143:476, 1983.

165. Vermeulen JP, Mahowald ML: A case of Wegener's granulomatosis presenting with jaw claudication. J Rheumatol 11:707, 1984.

166. Shuhart DT, Torretti DJ, Maksimak JF, et al: Acute myositis as an unusual presentation of Wegener's granulomatosis. Arch Pediatr Adolesc Med 148:875, 1994.

167. Nishino H, DeRemee RA, Rubino FA, et al: Wegener's granulomatosis associated with vasculitis of the temporal artery: Report of five cases. Mayo Clin Proc 68:115, 1993.

168. Hennington MH, Detterbeck FC, Kahai J, et al: Wegener's granulomatosis mimicking a sternal abscess. South Med J 89:438, 1996.

169. Nishino H, Rubino FA, DeRemee RA, et al: Neurological involvement in Wegener's granulomatosis: An analysis of 324 consecutive patients at the Mayo Clinic. Ann Neurol 33:4, 1993.

170. Jinnah HA, Dixon A, Brat DJ, et al: Chronic meningitis with cranial neuropathies in Wegener's granulomatosis: Case report and review of the literature. Arthritis Rheum 40:573, 1997.

171. Hern JD, Hollis LJ, Mochloulis G, et al: Early diagnosis of Wegener's granulomatosis presenting with facial nerve palsy. J Laryngol Otol 110:459, 1996.

172. Kashiyama T, Suzuki A, Mizuguchi K: Wegener's granulomatosis with multiple cranial nerve involvements as the initial clinical manifestations. Intern Med 34:1110, 1995.

173. Spranger M, Schwab S, Meinck HM, et al: Meningeal involvement in Wegener's granulomatosis confirmed and monitored by positive circulating antineutrophil cytoplasm in cerebrospinal fluid. Neurology 48:263, 1997.

174. Makura ZG, Robson AK: Wegener's granulomatosis presenting as a temporal headache. J Laryngol Otol 110:802, 1996.

175. Koga H, Oochi N, Osato S, et al: Case report: Wegener's granulomatosis accompanied by communicating hydrocephalus. Am J Med Sci 307:278, 1994.

176. Nishino H, Rubino FA: Horner's syndrome in Wegener's granulomatosis: Report of four cases. J Neurol Neurosurg Psychiatry 56:897, 1993.

177. Kroneman OC III, Pevzner M: Failure of cyclophosphamide to prevent cerebritis in Wegener's granulomatosis. Am J Med 80:526, 1986.

178. Haynes BF, Fishman ML, Fauci AS, et al: The ocular manifestations of Wegener's granulomatosis: Fifteen years' experience and review of the literature. Am J Med 63:131, 1977.

179. Stavrou P, Deutsch J, Rene C, et al: Ocular manifestations of classical and limited Wegener's granulomatosis. QJM 86:719, 1993.

180. Goodfield NE, Bhandari S, Plant WD, et al: Cardiac involvement in Wegener's granulomatosis. Br Heart J 73:110, 1995.

181. Lawson TM, Williams BD: Silent myocardial infarction in Wegener's granulomatosis. Br J Rheumatol 35:188, 1996.

182. Allen DC, Doherty CC, O'Reilly DP: Pathology of the heart and the cardiac conduction system in Wegener's granulomatosis. Br Heart J 52:674, 1984.

183. Schiavone WA, Ahmad M, Ockner SA: Unusual cardiac complications of Wegener's granulomatosis. Chest 88:745, 1985.

184. Davenport A, Goodfellow J, Goel S, et al: Aortic valve disease in patients with Wegener's granulomatosis. Am J Kidney Dis 24:205, 1994.

185. Fox AD, Robbins SE: Aortic valvulitis complicating Wegener's granulomatosis. Thorax 49:1176, 1994.

185a. Delevaux I, Hoen B, Selton-Suty C, et al: Relapsing congestive cardiomyopathy in Wegener's granulomatosis. Mayo Clin Proc 72:848, 1997.

186. Yamasaki S, Eguchi K, Kawabe Y, et al: Wegener's granulomatosis overlapped with Takayasu arteritis. Clin Rheumatol 15:303, 1996.

187. Aoki N, Soma K, Owada T, et al: Wegener's granulomatosis complicated by arterial aneurysm. Intern Med 34:790, 1995.

188. Daoud MS, Gibson LE, DeRemee RA, et al: Cutaneous Wegener's granulomatosis: Clinical, histopathologic, and immunopathologic features of thirty patients. J Am Acad Dermatol 31:605, 1994.

189. Frances C, Du LT, Piette JC, et al: Wegener's granulomatosis: Dermatological manifestations in 75 cases with clinicopathologic correlation. Arch Dermatol 130:861, 1994.

190. Handa R, Wali JP: Wegener's granulomatosis with gangrene of toes. Scand J Rheumatol 25:103, 1996.

191. Barksdale SK, Hallahan CW, Kerr GS, et al: Cutaneous pathology in Wegener's granulomatosis. A clinicopathologic study of 75 biopsies in 46 patients. Am J Surg Pathol 19:161, 1995.

192. Sokol RJ, Farrell MK, McAdams AJ: An unusual presentation of Wegener's granulomatosis mimicking inflammatory bowel disease. Gastroenterology 87:426, 1984.

193. Oddis CV, Schoolwerth AC, Abt AB: Wegener's granulomatosis with delayed pulmonary and colonic involvement. South Med J 77:1589, 1984.

194. Haworth SJ, Pusey CD: Severe intestinal involvement in Wegener's granulomatosis. Gut 25:1296, 1984.

195. Geraghty J, Mackay IR, Smith DC: Intestinal perforation in Wegener's granulomatosis. Gut 27:450, 1986.

196. Spiera RF, Filippa DA, Bains MS, et al: Esophageal involvement in Wegener's granulomatosis. Arthritis Rheum 37:1404, 1994.

197. Davenport A, Downey SE, Goel S, et al: Wegener's granulomatosis involving the urogenital tract. Br J Urol 78:354, 1996.

198. Huong DL, Papo T, Piette JC, et al: Urogenital manifestations of Wegener granulomatosis. Medicine 74:152, 1995.

199. Eufinger H, Machtens E, Akuamoa-Boateng E: Oral manifestations of Wegener's granulomatosis. Int J Oral Maxillofac Surg 21:50, 1992.

200. Napier SS, Allen JA, Irwin CR, et al: Strawberry gums: A clinicopathological manifestation diagnostic of Wegener's granulomatosis? J Clin Pathol 46:709, 1993.

201. Ah-See KW, McLaren K, Maran AG: Wegener's granulomatosis presenting as major salivary gland enlargement. J Laryngol Otol 110:691, 1996.

202. Lustmann J, Segal N, Markitziu A: Salivary gland involvement in Wegener's granulomatosis: A case report and review of the literature. Oral Surg Oral Med Oral Pathol 77:254, 1994.

203. Roberts GA, Eren E, Sinclair H, et al: Two cases of Wegener's granulomatosis involving the pituitary. Clin Endocrinol 42:323, 1995.

204. Rosete A, Cabral AR, Kraus A, et al: Diabetes insipidus secondary to Wegener's granulomatosis: Report and review of the literature. J Rheumatol 18:761, 1991.

205. Jordan JM, Rowe WT, Allen NB: Wegener's granulomatosis involving the breast: Report of three cases and review of the literature. Am J Med 83:159, 1987.

206. Gobel U, Kettritz R, Kettritz U, et al: Wegener's granulomatosis masquerading as breast cancer. Arch Intern Med 155:205, 1995.

207. Crummy CS, Perlin E, Moquin RR: Microangiopathic hemolytic anemia in Wegener's granulomatosis. Am J Med 51:544, 1971.

208. Krupsky M, Landau Z, Lifschitz-Mercer B, et al: Wegener's granulomatosis with peripheral eosinophilia: Atypical variant of a classic disease. Chest 104:1290, 1993.

209. Hergesell O, Andrassy K, Nawroth P: Elevated levels of markers of endothelial cell damage and markers of activated coagulation in patients with systemic necrotizing vasculitis. Thromb Haemost 75:892, 1996.

210. Shaker JL, Redlin KC, Warren GV, et al: Case report: Hypercalcemia with inappropriate 1,25-dihydroxyvitamin D in Wegener's granulomatosis. Am J Med Sci 308:115, 1994.

211. Savige JA, Chang L, Wilson D, et al: Autoantibodies and target antigens in antineutrophil cytoplasmic antibody (ANCA)-associated vasculitides. Rheumatol Int 16:109, 1996.

212. Yaqoob M, West DC, McDicken I, et al: Monitoring of endothelial leucocyte adhesion molecule-1 in anti-neutrophil-cytoplasmic-antibody-positive vasculitis. Am J Nephrol 16:106, 1996.

213. Mrowka C, Sieberth HG: Circulating adhesion molecules ICAM-1, VCAM-1 and E-selectin in systemic vasculitis: Marked differences between Wegener's granulomatosis and SLE. Clin Invest 72:762, 1994.

214. Stegeman CA, Tervaert JW, Huitema MG, et al: Serum levels of soluble adhesion molecules intercellular adhesion molecule 1, vascular cell adhesion molecule 1, and E-selectin in patients with Wegener's granulomatosis: Relationship to disease activity and relevance during followup. Arthritis Rheum 37:1228, 1994.

215. Boehme MW, Schmitt WH, Youinou P, et al: Clinical relevance of elevated serum thrombomodulin and soluble E-selectin in patients with Wegener's granulomatosis and other systemic vasculitides. Am J Med 101:387, 1996.

216. Ohdama S, Matsubara O, Aoki N: Plasma thrombomodulin in Wegener's granulomatosis as an indicator of vascular injuries. Chest 106:666, 1994.

217. Wang G, Hansen H, Tatsis E, et al: High plasma levels of the soluble form of CD30 activation molecule reflect disease activity in patients with Wegener's granulomatosis. Am J Med 102:517, 1997.

218. Egner W, Chapel HM: Titration of antibodies against neutrophil cytoplasmic antigens is useful in monitoring disease activity in systemic vasculitides. Clin Exp Immunol 82:244, 1990.

219. Nölle B, Specks U, Lüdemann J, et al: Anticytoplasmic antibodies: Their immunodiagnostic value in Wegener's granulomatosis. Ann Intern Med 111:28, 1989.

220. Weber MFA, Andrassy K, Pullig O, et al: Antineutrophil cytoplasmic antibodies and antiglomerular basement membrane antibodies in Goodpasture's syndrome and in Wegener's granulomatosis. J Am Soc Nephrol 2:1227, 1992.

221. Kallenberg CGM, Mulder AHL, Cohen Tervaert JW: Anti-neutrophil cytoplasmic antibodies: A still growing class of autoantibodies in inflammatory disorders. Am J Med 93:675, 1992.

222. Cohen Tervaert JW, Mulder AHL, Stegeman CA, et al: The occurrence of autoantibodies to human leukocyte elastase in Wegener's granulomatosis and other inflammatory disorders. Ann Rheum Dis 52:115, 1993.

223. Cohen Tervaert JW, Goldschmeding R, Elema JD, et al: Association of autoantibodies to myeloperoxidase with different forms of vasculitis. Arthritis Rheum 33:1264, 1990.

224. Cohen Tervaert JW, van der Woude FJ, Fauci AS, et al: Association between active Wegener's granulomatosis and anticytoplasmic antibodies. Arch Intern Med 149:2461, 1989.

225. de'Olivera J, Gaskin G, Dash A, et al: Relationship between disease activity and anti-neutrophil cytoplasmic antibody concentration in long-term management of systemic vasculitis. Am J Kidney Dis 25:380, 1995.

226. Jayne D, Heaton A, Brownlee A, et al: Sequential antineutrophil cytoplasm antibody titres in the management of systemic vasculitis. Nephrol Dial Transplant 5:309, 1990.

227. Power WJ, Rodriguez A, Neves RA, et al: Disease relapse in patients with ocular manifestations of Wegener granulomatosis. Ophthalmology 102:154, 1995.

228. Tervaert JWC, Huitema MG, Hene RJ, et al: Prevention of relapses in Wegener's granulomatosis by treatment based on antineutrophil antibody titre. Lancet 336:709, 1990.

229. Kerr GS, Fleisher TA, Hallahan CW, et al: Limited prognostic value of changes in antineutrophil cytoplasmic antibody titers in patients with Wegener's granulomatosis. Adv Exp Med Biol 336:411, 1993.

230. Davenport A, Lock RJ, Wallington TB: Clinical relevance of testing for antineutrophil cytoplasm antibodies (ANCA) with a standard indirect immunofluorescence ANCA test in patients with upper or lower respiratory tract symptoms. Thorax 49:213, 1994.

231. Davenport A: "False postive" perinuclear and cytoplasmic anti-neutrophil cytoplasmic antibody results leading to misdiagnosis of Wegener's granulomatosis and/or microscopic polyarteritis. Clin Nephrol 37:124, 1992.

232. Salerno SM, Ormseth EJ, Roth BJ, et al: Sulfasalazine pulmonary toxicity in ulcerative colitis mimicking clinical features of Wegener's granulomatosis. Chest 110:556, 1996.

233. Cho C, Asuncion A, Tatum AH: False-positive antineutrophil cytoplasmic antibody in aspergillosis with oxalosis. Arch Pathol Lab Med 119:558, 1995.

234. Rao JK, Weinberger M, Oddone EZ, et al: The role of antineutrophil cytoplasmic antibody (c-ANCA) testing in the diagnosis of Wegener granulomatosis: A literature review and meta-analysis. Ann Intern Med 123:925, 1995.

235. Daum TE, Specks U, Colby TV, et al: Tracheobronchial involvement in Wegener's granulomatosis. Am J Respir Crit Care Med 151:522, 1995.

236. Givens CD Jr, Newman JH, McCurley TL: Diagnosis of Wegener's granulomatosis by transbronchial biopsy. Chest 88:794, 1985.

237. Hoffman GS, Sechler JMG, Gallin JI, et al: Bronchoalveolar lavage analysis in Wegener's granulomatosis: A method to study disease pathogenesis. Am Rev Respir Dis 143:401, 1991.

238. Mukae H, Matsumoto N, Ashitani J, et al: Neutrophil-related cytokines and neutrophil products in bronchoalveolar lavage fluid of a patient with ANCA negative Wegener's granulomatosis. Eur Respir J 9:1950, 1996.

239. Kaneishi NK, Howell LP, Russell LA, et al: Fine needle aspiration cytology of pulmonary Wegener's granulomatosis with biopsy correlation: A report of three cases. Acta Cytol 39:1094, 1995.

240. Granados R, Constantine NM, Cibas ES: Nasal scrape cytology in the diagnosis of Wegener's granulomatosis: A case report. Acta Cytol 38:463, 1994.

241. McDonald TJ, Neel HB III, DeRemee RA: Wegener's granulomatosis of the subglottis and the upper portion of the trachea. Ann Otol Rhinol Laryngol 91:588, 1982.

242. Rosenberg DM, Weinberger SE, Fulmer JD, et al: Functional correlates of lung involvement in Wegener's granulomatosis: Use of pulmonary function tests in staging and follow-up. Am J Med 69:387, 1980.

243. Walton EW: Giant-cell granuloma of the respiratory tract (Wegener's granulomatosis). BMJ 2:265, 1958.

244. Fischer E, Blumberg A: Prolonged anuria in Wegener's granulomatosis: Recovery of renal function. JAMA 240:1174, 1978.

245. Dahlberg PJ, Newcomer KL, Yutuc WR, et al: Renal failure in Wegener's granulomatosis: Recovery following dialysis and cyclophosphamide-prednisone therapy. Am J Med Sci 287:47, 1984.

246. Gordon M, Luqmani RA, Adu D, et al: Relapses in patients with a systemic vasculitis. QJM 86:779, 1993.

247. Jayne DR, Rasmussen N: Treatment of antineutrophil cytoplasm autoantibody-associated systemic vasculitis: Initiatives of the European Community Systemic Vasculitis Clinical Trials Study Group. Mayo Clin Proc 72:737, 1997.

248. Matteson EL, Gold KN, Bloch DA, et al: Long-term survival of patients with Wegener's granulomatosis from the American College of Rheumatology Wegener's Granulomatosis Classification Criteria Cohort. Am J Med 101:129, 1996.

249. Ognibene FP, Shelhamer JH, Hoffman GS, et al: Pneumocystis carinii pneumonia: A major complication of immunosuppressive therapy in patients with Wegener's granulomatosis. Am J Respir Crit Care Med 151:795, 1995.

250. Sheldon P: Cryptic Wegener's granulomatosis revealed after 18 years. Br J Rheumatol 33:296, 1994.

251. Odeh M, Best LA, Kerner H, et al: Localized Wegener's granulomatosis relapsing as diffuse massive intra-alveolar hemorrhage. Chest 104:955, 1993.

252. Churg J, Strauss L: Allergic granulomatosis, allergic angiitis, and periarteritis nodosa. Am J Pathol 27:277, 1951.

253. Fauci AS, Haynes BF, Katz P: The spectrum of vasculitis: Clinical, pathologic, immunologic, and therapeutic considerations. Ann Intern Med 89:660, 1978.

254. Fienberg R: Allergic granulomatosis. Am J Surg Pathol 6:189, 1982.

255. Lanham JG, Cooke S, Davies J, et al: Endomyocardial complications of the Churg-Strauss syndrome. Postgrad Med J 61:341, 1985.

256. Steinfeld S, Golstein M, De Vuyst P: Chronic eosinophilic pneumonia (CEP) as a presenting feature of Churg-Strauss syndrome (Churg-Strauss syndrome). Eur Respir J 7:2098, 1994.

257. Hueto-Perez-de-Heredia JJ, Dominguez-del-Valle FJ, Garcia E, et al: Chronic eosinophilic pneumonia as a presenting feature of Churg-Strauss syndrome. Eur Respir J 7:1006, 1994.

258. Lanham JG, Elkon KB, Pusey CD, et al: Systemic vasculitis with asthma and eosinophilia: A clinical approach to the Churg-Strauss syndrome. Medicine 63:65, 1984.

259. Masi AT, Hunder GG, Lie JT, et al: The American College of Rheumatology 1990 criteria for the classification of Churg-Strauss syndrome (allergic granulomatosis and angiitis). Arthritis Rheum 33:1094, 1990.

260. Lie JT: Limited forms of Churg-Strauss syndrome. Pathol Annu 28(Part 2):199, 1993.

261. Bloch DA, Michel BA, Hunder GG, et al: The American College of Rheumatology 1990 criteria for the classification of vasculitis: Patents and methods. Arthritis Rheum 33:1068, 1990.

262. Guillevin L, Lhote F, Gayraud M, et al: Prognostic factors in PAN and Churg-Strauss syndrome. A prospective study in 342 patients. Medicine 75:17, 1996.

263. Guillevin L, Guittard T, Bletry O, et al: Systemic necrotizing angiitis with asthma: Causes and precipitating factors in 43 cases. Lung 165:165, 1987.

264. Orriols R, Munoz X, Ferrer J, et al: Cocaine-induced Churg-Strauss vasculitis. Eur Respir J 9:175, 1996.

265. Chauhan A, Scott DGI, Neuberger J, et al: Churg-Strauss vasculitis and ascaris infection. Ann Rheum Dis 49:320, 1990.

266. Guillevin L, Amouroux J, Arbeille B, et al: Churg-Strauss angiitis: Arguments favoring the responsibility of inhaled antigens. Chest 100:1472, 1991.

267. Kallenberg CG, Heeringa P: Pathogenesis of vasculitis. Lupus 7:280, 1998.

268. Sale S, Patterson R: Recurrent Churg-Strauss vasculitis: With exophthalmus, hearing loss, nasal obstruction, amyloid deposits, hyperimmunoglobulinemia-E, and circulating immune complexes. Arch Intern Med 141:1363, 1981.

269. Lima F, Buchanan N, Froes L, et al: Pregnancy in granulomatous vasculitis. Ann Rheum Dis 54:604, 1995.

270. Connolly JO, Lanham JG, Partridge MR: Fulminant pregnancy-related Churg-Strauss syndrome. Br J Rheumatol 33:776, 1994.

271. Chumbley LC, Harrison EG Jr, DeRemee RA: Allergic granulomatosis and angiitis (Churg-Strauss syndrome) report and analysis of 30 cases. Mayo Clin Proc 52:477, 1977.

272. Koss MN, Antonovych T, Hochholzer L: Allergic granulomatosis (Churg-Strauss

syndrome) pulmonary and renal morphologic findings. Am J Surg Pathol 5:21, 1981.

273. Schwarz MI, Zamora MR, Hodges TN, et al: Isolated pulmonary capillaritis and diffuse alveolar hemorrhage in rheumatoid arthritis and mixed connective tissue disease. Chest 113:1609, 1998.

274. Alvarez-Sala R, Prados C, Armada E, et al: Congestive cardiomyopathy and endobronchial granulomas as manifestations of Churg-Strauss syndrome. Postgrad Med J 71:365, 1995.

275. Sasaki A, Hasegawa M, Nakazato Y, et al: Allergic granulomatosis and angiitis (Churg-Strauss syndrome): Report of an autopsy case in a nonasthmatic patient. Acta Pathol Jpn 38:781, 1988.

276. Lanham JG, Elkon KB, Pusey CD, et al: Systemic vasculitis with asthma and eosinophilia: A clinical approach to the Churg-Strauss syndrome. Medicine 63:65, 1984.

277. Chumbley LC, Harrison EG, DeRemee RA: Allergic granulomatosis and angiitis (Churg-Strauss syndrome): Report and analysis of 30 cases. Mayo Clin Proc 52:477, 1977.

278. Levin DC: Pulmonary abnormalities in the necrotizing vasculitides and their rapid response to steroids. Radiology 97:521, 1970.

279. Degesys GE, Mintzer RA, Vrla RF: Allergic granulomatosis: Churg-Strauss syndrome. Am J Roentgenol 135:1281, 1980.

280. Worthy SA, Müller NL, Hansell DM, Flower CDR: Churg-Strauss syndrome: The spectrum of pulmonary CT findings in 17 patients. Am J Roentgenol 170:297, 1998.

281. Buschman DL, James AW Jr, Talmadge EK: Churg-Strauss pulmonary vasculitis: High-resolution computed tomography scanning and pathologic findings. Am Rev Respir Dis 142:458, 1990.

282. Amato MSP, Barbas CSV, Delmonte VC, et al: Concurrent Churg-Strauss syndrome and temporal arteritis in a young patient with pulmonary nodules. Am Rev Respir Dis 139:1539, 1989.

283. Churg A, Brallas M, Cronin SR, et al: Formes frustes of Churg-Strauss syndrome. Chest 108:320, 1995.

284. Ames PR, Roes L, Lupoli S, et al: Thrombosis in Churg-Strauss syndrome: Beyond vasculitis? Br J Rheumatol 35:1181, 1996.

285. Lhote F, Guillevin L: Polyarteritis nodosa, microscopic polyangiitis, and Churg-Strauss syndrome: Clinical aspects and treatment. Rheum Dis Clin North Am 21:911, 1995.

286. Burke AP, Sobin LH, Virmani R: Localized vasculitis of the gastrointestinal tract. Am J Surg Pathol 19:338, 1995.

287. Guillevin L, Lhote F, Gallais V, et al: Gastrointestinal tract involvement in PAN and Churg-Strauss syndrome. Ann Med Interne 146:260, 1995.

288. Sehgal M, Swanson JW, DeRemee RA, et al: Neurologic manifestations of Churg-Strauss syndrome. Mayo Clin Proc 70:337, 1995.

289. Weinstein JM, Chui H, Lane S, et al: Churg-Strauss syndrome (allergic granulomatous angiitis): Neuro-ophthalmologic manifestations. Arch Ophthalmol 101:1217, 1983.

290. Shintani S, Tsuruoka S, Yamada M: Churg-Strauss syndrome associated with third nerve palsy and mononeuritis multiplex of the legs. Clin Neurol Neurosurg 97:172, 1995.

291. Kozak M, Gill EA, Green LS: The Churg-Strauss syndrome: A case report with angiographically documented coronary involvement and a review of the literature. Chest 107:578, 1995.

292. Drogue M, Vergnon JM, Wintzer B, et al: Prinzmetal's angina pectoris revealing aneurysm of the right coronary artery during evolution of Churg-Strauss syndrome. Chest 103:978, 1993.

293. Sharma A, De Varennes B, Sniderman AD: Churg-Strauss syndrome presenting with marked eosinophilia and pericardial effusion. Can J Cardiol 9:329, 1993.

294. Davis MD, Daoud MS, McEvoy MT, et al: Cutaneous manifestations of Churg-Strauss syndrome: A clinicopathologic correlation. J Am Acad Dermatol 37:199, 1997.

295. Nagpal S: Churg-Strauss syndrome with non-giant cell eosinophilic temporal arteritis. J Rheumatol 21:366, 1994.

296. Krupsky M, Landau Z, Lifschitz-Mercer B, et al: Wegener's granulomatosis with peripheral eosinophilia: Atypical variant of a classic disease. Chest 104:1290, 1993.

297. Wallaert B, Gosset P, Prin L, et al: Bronchoalveolar lavage in allergic granulomatosis and angiitis. Eur Respir J 6:413, 1993.

298. Olivieri D, Pesci A, Bertorelli G: Eosinophilic alveolitis in immunologic interstitial lung disorders. Lung 168:964, 1990.

299. Kojima K, Omoto E, Katayama Y, et al: Autoimmune hemolytic anemia in allergic granulomatous angiitis (Churg-Strauss syndrome). Int J Hematol 63:149, 1996.

300. Fienberg R, Mark EJ, Goodman M, et al: Correlation of antineutrophil cytoplasmic antibodies with the extrarenal histopathology of Wegener's (pathergic) granulomatosis and related forms of vasculitis. Hum Pathol 24:160, 1993.

301. Guillevin L, Visser H, Noel LH, et al: Antineutrophil cytoplasm antibodies in systemic PAN with and without hepatitis B virus infection and Churg-Strauss syndrome—62 patients. J Rheumatol 20:1345, 1993.

302. Cohen Tervaert JW, Goldschmeding R, Von Dem Borne AEGKR, et al: Antimyeloperoxidase antibodies in the Churg-Strauss Syndrome. Thorax 46:70, 1991.

303. Cohen Tervaert JW, Limburg PC, Elema JD, et al: Detection of autoantibodies against myeloid lysosomal enzymes: A useful adjunct to classification of patients with biopsy-proven necrotizing arteritis. Am J Med 91:59, 1991.

304. Cohen P, Guillevin L, Baril L, et al: Persistence of antineutrophil cytoplasmic antibodies (ANCA) in asymptomatic patients with systemic PAN or Churg-Strauss syndrome: Follow-up of 53 patients. Clin Exp Rheumatol 13:193, 1995.

305. Guillevin L, Le THD, Godeau P, et al: Clinical findings and prognosis of PAN and Churg-Strauss angiitis: A study in 165 patients. Br J Rheumatol 27:258, 1988.

306. Fortin P, Larson MG, Watters AK, et al: Prognostic factors in systemic necrotizing vasculitis of the PAN group: A review of 45 cases. J Rheumatol 22:78, 1995.

307. Watts RA, Jolliffe VA, Carruthers DM, et al: Effect of classification on the incidence of PAN and microscopic polyangiitis Arthritis Rheum 39:1208, 1997.

308. Hunninghake GW, Fauci AS: Pulmonary involvement in the collagen vascular diseases. Am Rev Respir Dis 119:471, 1979.

309. Rose GA, Spencer H: Polyarteritis nodosa. QJM 26:43, 1957.

310. Landman S, Burgener F: Pulmonary manifestations in Wegener's granulomatosis. Am J Roentgenol 122:750, 1974.

311. Rose GA: Clinical features of PAN with lung involvement. Br J Tuberc 51:113, 1957.

312. Spencer H: Pulmonary lesions in PAN. Br J Tuberc 51:123, 1957.

313. Matsumoto T, Homma S, Okada M, et al: The lung in PAN: A pathologic study of 10 cases. Hum Pathol 24:717, 1993.

314. Robinson BWS, Sterrett G: Bronchiolitis obliterans associated with PAN. Chest 102:309, 1992.

315. Nick J, Tuder R, May R, et al: Polyarteritis nodosa with pulmonary vasculitis. Am J Respir Crit Care Med 153:450, 1996.

316. Guillevin L, Lhote F, Amouroux J, et al: Antineutrophil cytoplasmic antibodies, abnormal angiograms and pathological findings in PAN and Churg-Strauss syndrome: Indications for the classification of vasculitides of the PAN group. Br J Rheumatol 35:958, 1996.

317. Garland LH, Sisson MA: Roentgen findings in the "collagen" diseases. Am J Roentgenol 71:581, 1954.

318. Scherzer H, Ward PA: Lung and dermal vascular injury produced by preformed immune complexes. Am Rev Respir Dis 117:551, 1978.

319. Bellon B, Bernaudin J-F, Mandet C, et al: Immune complex-mediated lung injury produced by horseradish peroxidase (HRP) and anti-HRP antibodies in rats. Am J Pathol 107:16, 1982.

320. Kradin RL, Kiprov D, Dickersin GR, et al: Immune complex disease with fatal pulmonary hemorrhage: Its occurrence in a patient with myasthenia gravis. Arch Pathol Lab Med 105:582, 1981.

321. Yokose T, Aida J, Ito Y, et al: A case of pulmonary hemorrhage in Henoch-Schönlein purpura accompanied by PAN in an elderly man. Respiration 60:307, 1993.

322. Ohtsuka M, Yamashita Y, Doi M, et al: Propylthiouracil-induced alveolar haemorrhage associated with antineutrophil cytoplasmic antibody. Eur Respir J 10:1405, 1997.

323. Kelsall JT, Chalmers A, Sherlock CH, et al: Microscopic polyangiitis after influenza vaccination. J Rheumatol 24:1198, 1997.

324. Mark EJ, Ramirez JR: Pulmonary capillaritis and hemorrhage in patients with systemic vasculitis. Arch Pathol Lab Med 109:413, 1985.

325. Myers JL, Katzenstein A-LA: Microangiitis in lupus-induced pulmonary hemorrhage. Am J Clin Pathol 85:552, 1986.

326. Akikusa B, Sato T, Ogawa M, et al: Necrotizing alveolar capillaritis in autopsy cases of microscopic polyangiitis: Incidence, histopathogenesis, and relationship with systemic vasculitis. Arch Pathol Lab Med 121:144, 1997.

327. Green RJ, Ruoss SJ, Kraft SA, et al: Pulmonary capillaritis and alveolar hemorrhage: Update on diagnosis and management. Chest 110:1305, 1996.

328. Gertner E, Lie JT: Pulmonary capillaritis, alveolar hemorrhage, and recurrent microvascular thrombosis in primary antiphospholipid syndrome. J Rheumatol 20:1224, 1993.

329. Lai FM, Li EKM, Suen MWM, et al: Pulmonary hemorrhage: A fatal manifestation in IgA nephropathy. Arch Pathol Lab Med 18:542, 1994.

330. Clutterbuck EJ, Pusey CD: Severe alveolar haemorrhage in Churg-Strauss syndrome. Eur J Respir Dis 71:158, 1987.

331. Green J, Brenner B, Gery R, et al: Adult hemolytic uremic syndrome associated with nonimmune deposit crescentic glomerulonephritis and alveolar hemorrhage. Am J Med Sci 296:121, 1988.

332. Martini A, Ravelli A, Albani S, et al: Hypocomplementemic urticarial vasculitis syndrome with severe systemic manifestations. J Pediatr 124:742, 1994.

333. Enright H, Miller W: Autoimmune phenomena in patients with myelodysplastic syndromes. Leuk Lymphoma 24:483, 1997.

334. Lewis EJ, Schur PH, Busch GJ, et al: Immunopathologic features of a patient with glomerulonephritis and pulmonary hemorrhage. Am J Med 54:507, 1973.

335. Haworth SJ, Savage COS, Carr D, et al: Pulmonary hemorrhage complicating Wegener's granulomatosis and microscopic polyarteritis. BMJ 290:1175, 1985.

336. Brugiere O, Raffy O, Sleiman C, et al: Progressive obstructive lung disease associated with microscopic polyangiitis. Am J Respir Crit Care Med 155:739, 1997.

337. Bosch X, Lopez-Soto A, Mirapeix E, et al: Antineutrophil cytoplasmic autoantibody-associated alveolar capillaritis in patients presenting with pulmonary hemorrhage. Arch Pathol Lab Med 118:517, 1994.

338. Nachman PH, Hogan SL, Jennette JC, et al: Treatment response and relapse in antineutrophil cytoplasmic autoantibody-associated microscopic polyangiitis and glomerulonephritis. J Am Soc Nephrol 7:33, 1996.

339. Hogan SL, Nachman PH, Wilkman AS, et al: Prognostic markers in patients with antineutrophil cytoplasmic autoantibody-associated microscopic polyangiitis and glomerulonephritis. J Am Soc Nephrol 7:23, 1996.

340. Dabague J, Reyes PA: Takayasu arteritis in Mexico: A 38-year clinical perspective through literature review. Int J Cardiol 54:S103, 1996.

341. Ueno A, Awane Y, Wakabayashi A, et al: Successfully operated obliterative

brachiocephalic arteritis (Takayasu) associated with the elongated coarctation. Jpn Heart J 8:538, 1967.

342. Hata A, Noda M, Moriwaki R, et al: Angiographic findings of Takayasu arteritis: New classification. Int J Cardiol 54:S155, 1996.

343. Nasu T: Takayasu's truncoarteritis in Japan: A statistical observation of 76 autopsy cases. Pathol Microbiol 43:140, 1975.

344. Sharma S, Kamalakar T, Rajani M, et al: The incidence and patterns of pulmonary artery involvement in Takayasu's arteritis. Clin Radiol 42:177, 1990.

345. Neng-shu H, Fan L, En-hui W, et al: Pulmonary artery involvement in aortoarteritis: An analysis of DSA. Chin Med J 103:666, 1990.

346. Yamato M, Lecky JW, Hiramatsu K, et al: Takayasu arteritis: Radiographic and angiographic findings in 59 patients. Radiology 161:329, 1986.

347. Ishikawa K: Diagnostic approach and proposed criteria for the clinical diagnosis of Takayasu's arteriopathy. J Am Coll Cardiol 12:964, 1988.

348. Arend WP, Michel BA, Bloch DA, et al: The American College of Rheumatology 1990 criteria for the classification of Takayasu arteritis. Arthritis Rheum 33:1129, 1990.

349. Sharma BK, Jain S, Suri S, et al: Diagnostic criteria for Takayasu arteritis. Int J Cardiol 54:S141, 1997.

350. Lupi HE, Sànchez TG, Horwitz S, et al: Pulmonary artery involvement in Takayasu's arteritis. Chest 67:69, 1967.

351. Nasu T: Pathology of pulseless disease: A systematic study and critical review of twenty-one autopsy cases reported in Japan. Angiology 14:225, 1963.

352. Kerr GS, Hallahan CW, Giordano J, et al: Takayasu arteritis. Ann Intern Med 120:919, 1994.

353. Sharma BK, Siveski-Iliskovic N, Singal PK: Takayasu arteritis may be underdiagnosed in North America. Can J Cardiol 11:311, 1995.

354. Lupi-Herrera E, Sanchez-Torres G, Marcushamer J, et al: Takayasu's arteritis: Clinical study of 107 cases. Am Heart J 93:94, 1977.

355. Greene NB, Baughman RP, Kim CK: Takayasu's arteritis associated with interstitial lung disease and glomerulonephritis. Chest 89:605, 1986.

356. Sharma BK, Jain S, Sagar S: Systemic manifestations of Takayasu arteritis: The expanding spectrum. Int J Cardiol 54:S149, 1996.

357. Eichhorn J, Sima D, Thiele B, et al: Anti-endothelial cell antibodies in Takayasu arteritis. Circulation 94:2396, 1996.

358. Garcia-Torres R, Noel LH, Reyes PA, et al: Absence of ANCA in Mexican patients with Takayasu's arteritis. Scand J Rheumatol 26:55, 1997.

359. Kerr GS: Takayasu's arteritis. Rheum Dis Clin North Am 21:1041, 1995.

360. Kimura A, Kitamura H, Date Y, et al: Comprehensive analysis of HLA genes in Takayasu arteritis in Japan. Int J Cardiol 54:S61, 1996.

361. Numano F, Shimamoto T: Hypersecretion of estrogen and Takayasu's disease. Am Heart J 81:591, 1971.

362. Saito Y, Hirota K, Ito I, et al: Clinical and pathological studies of five autopsied cases of aortitis syndrome: Part I. Findings of the aorta and its branches, peripheral arteries and pulmonary arteries. Jpn Heart J 13:20, 1972.

363. Ishihama Y, Iwasaki T, Onga H, et al: An autopsy case of Takayasu's arteritis with pulmonary hypertension. Jpn Circ J 37:647, 1973.

364. Rose AG, Halper J, Factor SM: Primary arteriopathy in Takayasu's disease. Arch Pathol Lab Med 108:644, 1984.

365. Kreidstein SH, Lytwyn A, Keystone EC: Takayasu arteritis with acute interstitial pneumonia and coronary vasculitis: Expanding the spectrum: Report of a case. Arthritis Rheum 36:1175, 1993.

366. Yamato M, Lecky JW, Hiramatsu K, et al: Takayasu arteritis: Radiographic and angiographic findings in 59 patients. Radiology 161:329, 1986.

367. Hachiya J: Current concept of Takayasu's arteritis. Semin Roentgenol 5:245, 1970.

368. Liu YQ, Jin BL, Ling J: Pulmonary artery involvement in aortoarteritis: An angiographic study. Cardiovasc Intervent Radiol 17:2, 1994.

369. Takahashi K, Honda M, Furuse M, et al: CT findings of pulmonary parenchyma in Takayasu arteritis. J Comput Assist Tomogr 20:742, 1996.

370. Park JH, Chung JW, Im JG, et al: Takayasu arteritis: Evaluation of mural changes in the aorta and pulmonary artery with CT angiography. Radiology 196:89, 1995.

371. Yamada I, Numano F, Suzuki S: Takayasu arteritis: Evaluation with MR imaging. Radiology 188:89, 1993.

372. Matsunaga N, Hayashi K, Sakamoto I, et al: Takayasu arteritis: Protean radiologic manifestations and diagnosis. Radiographics 17:579, 1997.

373. Yamada I, Shibuya H, Matsubara O, et al: Pulmonary artery disease in Takayasu's arteritis: Angiographic findings. Am J Roentgenol 159:263, 1992.

374. Sharma S, Kamalakar T, Rajani M, et al: The incidence and patterns of pulmonary artery involvement in Takayasu's arteritis. Clin Radiol 42:177, 1990.

375. Hayashi K, Nagasaki M, Matsunaga N, et al: Initial pulmonary artery involvement in Takayasu arteritis. Radiology 159:401, 1986.

376. Bremerich J, Müller-Brand J, Perruchoud AP: Pulmonary vessel involvement in Takayasu arteritis. Clin Nucl Med 20:848, 1995.

377. Hayashi K, Sakamoto I, Matsunaga N: Pulmonary arterial lesions in Takayasu arteritis: Relationship of inflammatory activity to scintigraphic findings and sequential changes. Ann Nucl Med 10:219, 1996.

378. Nakabayashi K, Kurata N, Nangi N, et al: Pulmonary artery involvement as first manifestation in three cases of Takayasu arteritis. Int J Cardiol 54:S177, 1996.

379. Klein RG, Hunder GG, Stanson AW, et al: Large artery involvement in giant cell (temporal) arteritis. Ann Intern Med 83:806, 1975.

380. Ladanyi M, Fraser RS: Pulmonary involvement in giant cell arteritis. Arch Pathol Lab Med 111:1178, 1987.

381. Russo MG, Waxman J, Abdoh AA, et al: Correlation between infection and the onset of the giant cell (temporal) arteritis syndrome: A trigger mechanism? Arthritis Rheum 38:374, 1995.

382. Larson TS, Hall S, Hepper NGG, et al: Respiratory tract symptoms as a clue to giant cell arteritis. Ann Intern Med 101:594, 1984.

383. Gur H, Rapman E, Ehrenfeld M, et al: Clinical manifestations of temporal arteritis: A report from Israel. J Rheumatol 23:1927, 1996.

384. de Heide LJ, Pieterman H, Hennemann G: Pulmonary infarction caused by giant-cell arteritis of the pulmonary artery. Neth J Med 46:36, 1995.

385. Karam GH, Fulmer JD: Giant cell arteritis presenting as interstitial lung disease. Chest 82:781, 1982.

386. Romero S, Vela P, Padilla I, et al: Pleural effusion as manifestation of temporal arteritis. Thorax 47:398, 1992.

387. Bradley JD, Pinals RS, Blumenfeld HB, et al: Giant cell arteritis with pulmonary nodules. Am J Med 77:135, 1984.

388. Zenone T, Souquet PJ, Bohas C, et al: Unusual manifestations of giant cell arteritis: Pulmonary nodules, cough, conjunctivitis and otitis with deafness. Eur Respir J 7:2252, 1994.

389. Lesser RS, Aledort D, Lie JT: Non-giant cell arteritis of the temporal artery presenting as the polymyalgia rheumatica-temporal arteritis syndrome. J Rheumatol 22:2177, 1995.

390. Wagenaar SSC, Westermann CJJ, Corrin B: Giant cell arteritis limited to large elastic pulmonary arteries. Thorax 36:876, 1981.

391. Okubo S, Kunieda T, Ando M, et al: Idiopathic isolated pulmonary arteritis with chronic cor pulmonale. Chest 94:665, 1988.

392. Glover MU, Muniz J, Bessone L, et al: Pulmonary artery obstruction due to giant cell arteritis. Chest 91:925, 1987.

393. Takashi M, Kamimura A, Koizumi F: Disseminated visceral giant cell arteritis. Acta Pathol Jpn 37:863, 1987.

394. Lie JT: Disseminated visceral giant cell arteritis. Am J Clin Pathol 69:299, 1978.

395. Gamble CN, Wiesner KB, Shapiro RF, et al: The immune complex pathogenesis of glomerulonephritis and pulmonary vasculitis in Behçet's disease. Am J Med 66:1031, 1979.

396. Lakhanpal S, Tani K, Lie JT, et al: Pathologic features of Behçet's syndrome: A review of Japanese autopsy registry data. Hum Pathol 16:790, 1985.

397. Raz I, Okon E, Chajek-Shaul T: Pulmonary manifestations in Behçet's syndrome. Chest 95:585, 1989.

398. Slavin RE, de Groot WJ: Pathology of the lung in Behçet's disease: Case report and review of the literature. Am J Surg Pathol 5:779, 1981.

399. Wilcox CG: Behçet's disease: A review. J Assoc Military Dermatol 9:23, 1983.

400. Petty TL, Scoggin CH, Good JT: Recurrent pneumonia in Behçet's syndrome: Roentgenographic documentation during 13 years. JAMA 238:2529, 1977.

401. Tanaka K, Kajiyama K, Imamura T, et al: Genetic and environmental factors in the development of Behçet's disease. Tohoku J Exp Med 145:205, 1985.

402. Herreman G, Beaufils H, Godeau P, et al: Behçet's syndrome and renal involvement: A histological and immunofluorescent study of 11 renal biopsies. Am J Med Sci 284:10, 1982.

403. Gupta RC, O'Duffy JD, McDuffie FC, et al: Circulating immune complexes in active Behçet's disease. Clin Exp Immunol 34:213, 1978.

404. Levinsky RF, Lehner T: Circulating soluble immune complexes in recurrent oral ulceration and Behçet's syndrome. Clin Exp Immunol 32:193, 1978.

405. Yang CW, Park IS, Kim SY, et al: Antineutrophil cytoplasmic autoantibody associated vasculitis and renal failure in Behçet disease. Nephrol Dial Transplant 8:871, 1993.

406. Efthimiou J, Johnston C, Spiro SG, et al: Pulmonary disease in Behçet's syndrome. QJM 58:259, 1986.

407. Tunaci A, Berkmen YM, Gökmen E: Thoracic involvement in Behçet's disease: Pathologic, clinical, and imaging features. Am J Roentgenol 164:51, 1995.

408. Ahn JM, Im JG, Ryoo JW, et al: Thoracic manifestations of Behçet syndrome: Radiographic and CT findings in nine patients. Radiology 194:199, 1995.

409. Erkan F, Cavdar T: Pulmonary vasculitis in Behçet's disease. Am Rev Respir Dis 146:232, 1992.

410. Grenier P, Bletry O, Cornud F, et al: Pulmonary involvement in Behçet disease. Am J Roentgenol 137:565, 1981.

411. Puckette TC, Jolles H, Proto AV: Magnetic resonance imaging confirmation of pulmonary artery aneurysm in Behçet's disease. J Thorac Imaging 9:172, 1994.

412. Numan F, Islak C, Berkmen T, et al: Behçet disease: Pulmonary arterial involvement in 15 cases. Radiology 192:465, 1994.

413. Efthimiou J, Johnston C, Spiro SG, et al: Pulmonary disease in Behçet's syndrome. QJM 58:259, 1986.

414. Raz I, Elimelech O, Chajek-Shaul T: Pulmonary manifestations in Behçet's syndrome. Chest 95:585, 1989.

415. Winer-Muram HT, Headley AS, Menke P, et al: Radiologic manifestations of thoracic vascular Behçet's disease in African-American men. J Thorac Imaging 9:176, 1994.

416. Davies JD: Behçet's syndrome with hemoptysis and pulmonary lesions. J Pathol 109:351, 1973.

417. Cöplü L, Emri S, Selçuk ZT, et al: Life threatening chylous pleural and pericardial effusion in a patient with Behçet's syndrome. Thorax 47:64, 1992.

418. Erkan F, Cavdar T: Pulmonary vasculitis in Behçet's disease. Am Rev Respir Dis 146:232, 1992.

419. Jerray M, Benzarti M, Rouatbi N: Possible Behçet's disease revealed by pulmonary aneurysms. Chest 99:1291, 1991.

420. Reza MJ, Demanes DJ: Behçet's disease: A case with hemoptysis, pseudotumor cerebri, and arteritis. J Rheumatol 5:320, 1978.

421. Cadman EC, Lundberg WB, Mitchell MS: Pulmonary manifestations in Behçet's syndrome. Arch Intern Med 136:944, 1976.

422. Ahonen AV, Stenius-Aarniala BS, Viljanen BC, et al: Obstructive lung disease in Behçet's syndrome. Scand J Respir Dis 59:44, 1978.

423. Gibson JM, O'Hara MD, Beare JM, et al: Bronchial obstruction in a patient with Behçet's disease. Eur J Respir Dis 63:356, 1982.

424. Evans WV, Jenkins RM: Pulmonary function in Behçet's syndrome. Scand J Respir Dis 60:314, 1979.

425. Sakurai N, Koike Y, Kaneoke Y, et al: Sleep apnea and palatal myoclonus in a patient with neuro-Behçet syndrome. Intern Med 32:336, 1993.

426. Agnello V, Knight G, Abel G: Interferon α2a for cryoglobulinemia associated with hepatitis C virus. N Engl J Med 331:751, 1994.

427. Sansonno D, Cornacchiulo V, Iacobelli AR, et al: Localization of hepatitis C virus antigens in liver and skin tissues of chronic C-virus infected patients with mixed cryoglobulinemia. Hepatology 21:305, 1995.

428. Cryer PE, Kissane J: Mixed cryoimmunoglobulinemia. Am J Med 61:95, 1976.

429. Chejfee G, Lichtenberg L, Lertratanakul Y, et al: Quarterly case: Respiratory insufficiency in a patient with mixed cryoglobulinemia. Ultrastruct Pathol 2:295, 1981.

430. Martinez JS, Kohler PF: Variant "Goodpasture's syndrome"? The need for immunologic criteria in rapidly progressive glomerulonephritis and hemorrhagic pneumonitis. Ann Intern Med 75:67, 1971.

431. Bombardieri S, Paoletti P, Ferri C, et al: Lung involvement in essential mixed cryoglobulinemia. Am J Med 66:748, 1979.

432. Stagg MP, Lauber J, Michalski JP: Mixed essential cryoglobulinemia and adult respiratory distress syndrome: A case report. Am J Med 87:445, 1989.

433. Cream JJ, Gumpel JM, Peachey RDG: Schönlein-Henoch purpura in the adult: A study of 77 adults with anaphylactoid or Schönlein-Henoch purpura. QJM New Series 39:461, 1970.

434. Ronda N, Esnault VL, Layward L, et al: Antineutrophil cytoplasm antibodies (ANCA) of IgA isotype in adult Henoch-Schönlein purpura. Clin Exp Immunol 95:49, 1994.

435. Elzouki AN, Sterner G, Eriksson S: Henoch-Schönlein purpura and alpha 1-antitrypsin deficiency. Nephrol Dial Transplant 10:1454, 1995.

436. Jacome AF: Pulmonary hemorrhage and death complicating anaphylactoid purpura. South Med J 60:1003, 1967.

437. Kathuria S, Cheifec G: Fatal pulmonary Henoch-Schönlein syndrome. Chest 182:654, 1982.

438. Wright WK, Krous HF, Griswold WR, et al: Pulmonary vasculitis with hemorrhage in anaphylactoid purpura. Pediatr Pulmonol 17:269, 1994.

439. Fulmer JD, Kaltreider HB: The pulmonary vasculitides. Chest 82:615, 1982.

440. Zackrison LH, Katz P: Bronchiolitis obliterans organizing pneumonia associated with essential mixed cryoglobulinemia. Arthritis Rheum 36:1627, 1993.

441. Subra JF, Michelet C, Laporte J, et al: The presence of cytoplasmic antineutrophil cytoplasmic antibodies (C-ANCA) in the course of subacute bacterial endocarditis with glomerular involvement: Coincidence or association? Clin Nephrol 49:15, 1998.

442. Shichiri M, Tsutsumi K, Yamamoto I, et al: Diffuse intrapulmonary hemorrhage and renal failure in adult Henoch-Schönlein purpura. Am J Nephrol 7:140, 1987.

443. Paller AS, Kelly K, Sethi R: Pulmonary hemorrhage: An often fatal complication of Henoch-Schönlein purpura. Pediatr Dermatol 14:299, 1997.

444. Liebow AA: Pulmonary angiitis and granulomatosis. Am Rev Respir Dis 108:1, 1973.

445. Gibbs AR, Williams WJ, Kelland D: Necrotising sarcoidal granulomatosis: A problem of identity: A study of seven cases. Sarcoidosis 4:94, 1987.

446. Le Gall F, Loeuillet L, Delaval P, et al: Necrotizing sarcoid granulomatosis with and without extrapulmonary involvement. Pathol Res Pract 192:306, 1996.

447. Koss MN, Hochholzer L, Feigin DS, et al: Necrotizing sarcoid-like granulomatosis: Clinical, pathologic, and immunopathologic findings. Hum Pathol 11:510, 1980.

448. Churg A, Carrington CB, Gupta R: Necrotizing sarcoid granulomatosis. Chest 76:706, 1979.

449. Saldana MJ: Necrotizing sarcoid granulomatosis: Clinicopathologic observations in 24 patients (abstract). Lab Invest 38:364, 1978.

450. Chittock DR, Joseph MG, Paterson NA, et al: Necrotizing sarcoid granulomatosis with pleural involvement: Clinical and radiographic features. Chest 106:672, 1994.

451. Rosen Y, Moon S, Huang C-T, et al: Granulomatous pulmonary angiitis in sarcoidosis. Arch Pathol Lab Med 101:170, 1977.

452. Singh N, Cole S, Krause PJ, et al: Necrotizing sarcoid granulomatosis with extrapulmonary involvement. Am Rev Respir Dis 124:189, 1981.

453. Dykhuizen RS, Smith CC, Kennedy MM, et al: Necrotizing sarcoid granulomatosis with extrapulmonary involvement. Eur Respir J 10:245, 1997.

454. Fisher MR, Christ ML, Bernstein JR: Necrotizing sarcoid-like granulomatosis radiologic-pathologic correlation. J Can Assoc Radiol 35:313, 1984.

455. Rolfes DB, Weiss MA, Sanders MA: Necrotizing sarcoid granulomatosis with suppurative features. Am J Clin Pathol 82:602, 1984.

456. Stephen JG, Braimbridge MV, Corrin B, et al: Necrotizing "sarcoidal" angiitis and granulomatosis of the lung. Thorax 31:356, 1976.

457. Niimi H, Hartman TE, Müller NL: Necrotizing sarcoid granulomatosis: Computed tomography and pathologic findings. J Comput Assist Tomogr 19:920, 1995.

458. Adlakha A, Kang E, Adlakha K, et al: Nonproductive cough, dyspnea, malaise, and night sweats in a 47-year-old woman. Chest 109:1385, 1996.

459. Wahls TL, Bonsib SM, Schuster VL: Coexistent Wegener's granulomatosis and anti-glomerular basement membrane disease. Hum Pathol 18:202, 1987.

460. Rotenstein D, Gibbas DL, Majmudar B, et al: Familial granulomatous arteritis with polyarthritis of juvenile onset. N Engl J Med 306:86, 1982.

461. Kawashima A, Kimura A, Katsuda S, et al: Pulmonary vasculitis with hypereosinophilia and episodic pulmonary hypertension: Report of three siblings. Pathol Int 45:66, 1995.

462. Hartley JPR, Dinnen JS, Seaton A: Pulmonary and systemic aneurysms in a case of widespread arteritis. Thorax 33:493, 1978.

463. Lie JT: Isolated pulmonary Takayasu arteritis: Clinicopathologic characteristics. Mod Pathol 9:469, 1996.

464. Shintaku M, Mase K, Ohtsuki H, et al: Generalized sarcoidlike granulomas with systemic angiitis, crescentic glomerulonephritis, and pulmonary hemorrhage: Report of an autopsy case. Arch Pathol Lab Med 113:1295, 1989.

# *Sarcoidosis*

Sarcoidosis (Boeck's sarcoid, Besnier-Boeck-Schaumann disease) is a relatively common disease of the lungs and other organs that is difficult to characterize precisely. In 1991, members of the World Association of Sarcoidosis and other Granulomatous Disorders proposed that it should be defined descriptively.[1, 2] Although their definition is cumbersome, it encompasses most of the important features of the disease and emphasizes the fact that the criteria for diagnosis are based on a combination of clinical, radiologic, and laboratory findings. According to the World Association, sarcoidosis is

a multisystem disorder of unknown cause(s). It most commonly affects young and middle-aged adults and frequently presents with bilateral hilar lymphadenopathy, pulmonary infiltration (sic), and ocular and skin lesions. Liver, spleen, lymph nodes, salivary glands, heart, nervous system, muscles, bone and other organs may also be involved. The diagnosis is established when clinico-radiological findings are supported by histologic evidence of non-caseating epithelioid cell granulomas. Granulomas of known causes and local sarcoid reactions must be excluded.

Frequently observed immunological features are depression of cutaneous delayed-type hypersensitivity and increased helper cell (CD4)/suppressor cell (CD8) ratio at the site of involvement. Circulating immune complexes along with other signs of B cell hyperactivity may also be detectable. Other markers of the disease include elevated levels of serum angiotensin converting enzyme (ACE), increased uptake of radioactive gallium, abnormal calcium metabolism and abnormal fluorescein angiography. The Kveim-Siltzbach test, when appropriate cell suspensions are available, may be of diagnostic help.

The course and prognosis may correlate with the mode of the onset and the extent of the disease. An acute onset with erythema nodosum or asymptomatic bilateral hilar lymphadenopathy usually heralds a self-limiting course, whereas an insidious onset, especially with multiple extra-pulmonary lesions, may be followed by relentless, progressive fibrosis of the lungs and other organs.

Corticosteroids relieve symptoms, suppress the formation of granulomas and normalize the serum ACE levels and the gallium uptake.

As this description indicates, sarcoidosis is a systemic disease with a variety of clinical and radiologic features that are associated histologically with granulomatous inflammation. Because other diseases, such as tuberculosis or fungal infection, extrinsic allergic alveolitis, and lymphoma, can simulate the histologic or radiologic features of the disease,[3] the diagnosis is frequently one of exclusion. Many investigators have attempted to identify the etiology of the disease and its pathogenetic mechanisms; in the 1980s and 1990s, particular emphasis has been placed on its molecular biology. However, despite an abundance of published reports, an understanding of the initiating events and pathogenesis of the disease and the reasons why it progresses in some patients and undergoes spontaneous resolution in others remain obscure.

## EPIDEMIOLOGY

Precise figures regarding the incidence of sarcoidosis are difficult to obtain, partly because many cases never come to clinical attention. For example, a comprehensive review of the world literature to 1967 revealed that approximately 50% of patients with the disease were asymptomatic when it was first recognized (25% presented with respiratory symptoms, usually dyspnea, and the remaining 25% had extrathoracic symptoms only).[4] Similarly, the authors of an autopsy study from Sweden published in 1964 concluded that there are approximately 10 times more cases of sarcoidosis than are detected during life.[5] The following statistics relating to the incidence and prevalence of sarcoidosis must be considered in the light of these observations.

There is considerable variation in the reported incidence and prevalence of sarcoidosis in different countries and continents. Although such geographic variation undoubtedly is associated predominantly with true differences in incidence, it is also likely to be related to local awareness of and interest in the disease.[6] As a generalization, the disease is more common in temperate than in tropical climates,[4, 7] many large series having been reported from Scandinavia, England, and the United States.[8–15] The prevalence in Sweden, Norway, and Finland is approximately 64, 27, and 11 per 100,000 population, respectively.[15, 16] In the United States, a reasonable estimate of the prevalence of a radiographic pattern consistent with the diagnosis is about 10 per 100,000 examinations.[4] African Americans, especially females, have a particularly high prevalence.[7, 18] In a review of newly diagnosed cases of sarcoidosis in patients belonging to a Detroit Health Maintenance organization between 1990 and 1994 and constituting about 5% of the metropolitan population in the ages studied, annual incidence rates were found to be 39.1 per 100,000 for African American women, 29.8 for African American men, 12.1 for white women, and 9.6 for white men.[19] African American women between the ages of 30 and 39 years were at the greatest risk, with an annual incidence of 107 per 100,000. A disproportionately high prevalence has also been observed in Puerto Ricans living in the United States,[20, 21] in West Indians in the United Kingdom,[22] and in inhabitants of Germany, Ireland, and the Czech Republic.[7, 23] It is less common in some other European countries, such as Spain, in which the annual incidence has been estimated to be only 1.4 per 100,000.[24]

The disease is uncommon in Southeast Asia and Japan;[17] for example, in Hokkaido, Japan, the prevalence is only 3.7 per 100,000.[15] It is especially rare in Chinese individuals; in one mass community radiographic survey of 3.6 million people in Taiwan, no cases were identified![25] In the United States, recognition of the disease in a Chinese patient has been considered to justify publication.[25, 26] Despite these observations, the disease can be seen in these individuals;[27] for example, of eight patients with sarcoidosis seen over a period of 10 years in Singapore, five were Chinese.[28] Mass radiographic surveys have also found the prevalence to be very low among the aboriginal peoples of New Zealand and Canada.[5] Although sarcoidosis has been thought to be rare in Africa,[4] a relatively recent study from Cape Town documented a prevalence of 27 per 100,000 in black South Africans and 6 per 100,000 in white South Africans.[7] Although historically believed to be uncommon in South America,[29] there is evidence that this may be related to underestimation of disease prevalence.[7]

The relative prevalence in men and women varies among series, with no sex predominance reported in some and a definite female predominance in others;[4, 8, 15, 23, 30] however, as mentioned previously, there is a clear-cut increased risk in African American women.

Although the disease may occur at any age, it is recognized most commonly in patients between the ages of 20 and 40 years.[4, 9] In one review of 1,254 patients, 50% were in this age group;[9] only 2% were younger than 10 years, and only 4% were older than 60. An 81-year-old woman in the United Kingdom has been touted as the oldest patient reported with the disease in the world.[31] Estimates of the incidence of the disease in children may be low because screening chest radiographs are less likely to be obtained in this age group.[32] The lack of screening of asymptomatic children may also be the explanation for reports in the American medical literature suggesting that sarcoidosis is more likely to be associated with symptoms in children than in adults.[33, 34] Thus, in an analysis of the clinical and radiographic characteristics of pulmonary sarcoidosis in 26 children ranging in age from 2.5 to 17 years (mean, 13 years), 25 were symptomatic at the time of diagnosis.[35] By contrast, in a study from Japan where schoolchildren had had yearly chest radiographs, 42 of 45 children with a diagnosis of sarcoidosis were asymptomatic.[32]

## ETIOLOGY AND PATHOGENESIS

The etiology of sarcoidosis is unknown. However, the observation that the lungs and mediastinal and hilar lymph nodes are the structures most often involved (in 80% to 90% of cases in large series[8, 9]) suggests that the disease is caused by some agent that enters the body via the lungs, presumably by inhalation. Support for this hypothesis is provided by the observation that alveolitis characteristic of sarcoidosis can be identified by bronchoalveolar lavage (BAL) in patients who have extrathoracic sarcoidosis and no clinical, radiographic,[38] or physiologic[39] evidence of pulmonary or mediastinal disease. As discussed farther on, both the molecular biologic and histologic findings are in keeping with an inflammatory and immunologic response to an antigenic stimulus. Potential etiologic or pathogenic factors involved in the disease include microorganisms, heredity, cigarette smoke, and immunologic reactions.

### Infection

The results of several experimental, epidemiologic, and clinical investigations suggest that sarcoidosis may be caused by a transmissible agent such as a microorganism. Granulomas have been found in the footpads or viscera of mice after the inoculation of homogenates of human sarcoid tissue.[40–42] Tadpole-shaped structures suggestive of bacteria have been identified by electron microscopy in the granulomas of some patients.[43, 44] "Tubulospherical bodies" have also been identified in leukocytes within the vitreous humor of affected patients by the same technique;[45] moreover, transmission of granulomatous uveitis has been documented in mice after inoculation of the abnormal leukocytes. A single case of possible person-to-person transmission of the disease by a bone marrow transplant has been reported.[46] Several cases of disease recurrence in transplanted lungs have also been documented;[47, 48] however, it is unclear whether this is related to spread of infection or another process. Examples of the disease have also been reported in which there has been temporal clustering in nonconsanguineous relatives (such as in-laws)[49] and in close acquaintances,[50] suggesting exposure to a single etiologic agent. An excess prevalence of the disease has been documented in nurses.[51] Despite all these observations, attempts to culture organisms from tissue specimens are invariably unrewarding. (It has been speculated that this failure might be related to the presence of organisms without cell walls, resulting in a "slow bacterial infection" phenomenon.[52, 53])

The microorganisms that have been subject to the most investigation as possible causes of sarcoidosis are *Mycobacterium tuberculosis*[52–58] and nontuberculous mycobacteria.[52,

[55, 57, 58] The polymerase chain reaction has been used in a number of studies in an attempt to identify mycobacterial DNA in sarcoid tissue. Unfortunately, the findings have been variable. In one investigation, mycobacterial DNA was found in 7 of 16 tissue samples from patients with sarcoidosis, and in only 1 of 16 samples from patients with a variety of malignancies;[56] the positive control patient had radiologic changes consistent with remote tuberculosis. In this study, *M. tuberculosis* DNA was identified in sarcoid specimens with the same frequency as 4 samples known to be infected with the organism. In another investigation of 104 patients who had undergone BAL for probable tuberculosis (62 patients), possible sarcoidosis (20 patients), or other reasons (22 patients), *M. tuberculosis* DNA was found in 50% and nontuberculous mycobacterial DNA in 20% of the patients with sarcoidosis;[52] these values were significantly different from those of the control patients. In another study of 20 patients who had sarcoidosis and 20 controls, cell wall–deficient L forms of *M. tuberculosis* were identified in the blood by culture and monoclonal antibody techniques in 19 of the patients and in none of the controls.[53] Although the results of these and other studies[36, 57, 59] suggest that mycobacteria have a role in the development of sarcoidosis, many investigators have been unable to identify mycobacterial DNA in tissue specimens of sarcoidosis using similar techniques.[55, 58, 60–62] The failure of some of the workers to use tuberculosis-positive control subjects to validate the sensitivity of the particular technique[58] weakens the argument that mycobacteria are not implicated in the disease;[63] however, other workers who have used appropriate controls[64, 65] and more sensitive techniques[64] have also failed to identify mycobacterial antigen in appropriate specimens.

Support for the hypothesis that mycobacteria are involved in the etiology of sarcoidosis also comes from analyses of peripheral T-cell subsets; although not documented by all investigators,[66] many groups have found that some patients with sarcoidosis have a proliferation of the γδ subgroup of T cells that is similar to the pattern of T-cell proliferation seen in defense against mycobacteria.[67–72] There have also been case reports of patients who have had simultaneous or sequential tuberculosis and sarcoidosis.[37] Although the weight of all the evidence appears to favor an etiologic role for *M. tuberculosis* in sarcoidosis, given the discrepancy in results between different reports, further studies are required before such a role is considered definite.

A variety of other microorganisms have also been investigated as potential etiologic agents of sarcoidosis. A possible relation between sarcoidosis and infection by *Yersinia enterocolitica* was described by one group in 1979;[73] although this organism most often infects the gastrointestinal tract, it can cause a clinical picture that is virtually identical to sarcoidosis, including the presence of erythema nodosum and acute arthritis. Reports in the Chinese literature (available in abstract form) have both implicated[74, 75] and rejected[76] *Borrelia burgdorferi* (the agent responsible for Lyme disease) as a potential cause. In one investigation of 21 patients with sarcoidosis in an endemic area for Lyme disease in Italy, no antibodies to *Borrelia* were found;[77] however, in another study from Japan a strong association was found between serologic evidence of infection with this organism and sarcoidosis.[77a] Reports from two centers in Japan also implicate the bacterium *Propionibacterium acnes* as a caus-

ative agent in Japanese patients.[78, 79] The results of all these studies require confirmation and elaboration before any particular agent is accepted as being the etiology or having a role in the pathogenesis of sarcoidosis.

Although the preferential expression of specific T cell–receptor genes in sarcoidosis could be explained by stimulation of T cells by specific infectious agents, this reaction has also been seen after stimulation by autoantigens.[80] Bacterial and mycobacterial heat-shock proteins, which are homologous with human heat-shock proteins, have a postulated role in autoimmunity related to molecular mimicry of self-proteins[80] and could theoretically be involved in the pathogenesis of sarcoidosis. In fact, alveolar macrophages from patients who have sarcoidosis express endogenous heat-shock protein that could be a target for specific T-cell clones.[80]

## Genetic Factors

As with many other diseases, genetic factors likely have a role in the pathogenesis of sarcoidosis. Conceptually, the disease may develop in genetically predisposed hosts who are exposed to antigens that trigger the characteristic granulomatous inflammatory response.[81] Genetic differences that promote susceptibility to sarcoidosis could reside in loci that influence immune regulation, T-cell function, or antigen presentation or recognition.[81]

The strongest support for a hereditary susceptibility to the disease comes from observations of familial clustering.[82] Sarcoidosis has occurred in several members of a family[83–85] and in identical twins.[8, 86, 87] In fact, the high prevalence of the disease in the Republic of Ireland has been linked to occurrence of the disease among siblings; in one study comprising 114 index patients who had biopsy-proven sarcoidosis and a total sibling pool of 534 individuals, 11 (approximately 10%) of the index patients were found to have at least one sibling who had sarcoidosis.[88] The importance of familial sarcoidosis was also investigated in a survey of 1,082 consecutive patients who had the disease;[82] a first- or second-degree relative was recognized as having had sarcoidosis in 14% of patients. The association was more common in African Americans (17%) than in whites (6%). The most frequent relationship was sibling-pairs, followed by parent-offspring. Analysis of the pattern of disease occurrence in these families strongly suggested that the risk was conferred genetically rather than by an environmental factor.

Because the pathogenesis of sarcoidosis may involve antigen recognition, processing, and presentation, there has been considerable study of the relationship of the disease and its specific manifestations with human leukocyte antigen (HLA)-related genes.[82, 89–93a, b] In whites, an association between susceptibility to sarcoidosis and class I HLA-A1 and B8 has been described, and the presence of class II antigen HLA-DR3 has been associated with a favorable prognosis;[81, 89, 92] however, such observations have not been applicable to other populations.[81] It has been suggested that more emphasis should be placed on the associations of class II antigens with the susceptibility to the disease, because these are more likely involved in macrophage/T-cell interaction.[82] In fact, alveolar macrophages of patients who have sarcoidosis have a higher density of class II molecules (DR, DQ, DP) on their surface, a feature that might account for their ability to enhance antigen presentation to lymphocytes and stimulate the local accumulation of activated helper T cells,[94] which is a characteristic finding in the disorder. It is also possible that other genes, such as those encoding the immunoglobulin heavy chain constant region[92] or an isoform of serum angiotensin converting enzyme,[95] also influence susceptibility to sarcoidosis and its clinical expression.

## Immunologic Factors

The pulmonary alveolar macrophage plays a key role in the pathogenesis of sarcoidosis. It is responsible for the processing and subsequent presentation of the putative "sarcoid antigen" to immunocompetent cells, thereby initiating the lymphocytic alveolitis that is characteristic of this disorder.[96] Although the proportion of macrophages in BAL fluid of patients with sarcoidosis is reduced compared with that of healthy individuals, their absolute number is increased.[97] This increase is the result of both local proliferation and recruitment of blood monocytes from the peripheral circulation.[98] Although their primary role is probably the initiation of T cell–mediated immune reactions that lead to granuloma formation, there is also a subset that has suppressor activity.[99, 100] The final outcome of the inflammatory reaction may well depend on the balance of activity of these functionally different cells.

The ability of pulmonary alveolar macrophages to present antigen to helper T cells is enhanced by an increase in the density of class II major histocompatibility complex molecules and other molecules involved in T-cell activation, such as CD86, on their surface;[94, 101] in fact, a threefold increase in this ability has been observed in patients with the disease.[102, 103] Activation of macrophages in sarcoidosis is characterized by clustering of lymphocytes around them (peripolesis)[104] and by the elaboration of a variety of cytokines, the cell membrane glycoprotein CD14,[105] and a number of adhesion molecules.[106–111] In aggregate, these molecules enhance the migration and activation of a variety of cells, including lymphocytes, polymorphonuclear leukocytes, and fibroblasts, which participate in the inflammatory reaction and fibrosis characteristic of the disorder.[97] Cytokines released include interleukin (IL)-1,[112–115] IL-2,[116, 117] IL-6,[114, 115, 118–120] IL-8,[118, 121] tumor necrosis factor-α (TNF-α),[112, 114, 115, 120, 122, 123] insulin-like growth factor-1,[123a] and monocyte chemotactic protein-1 (MCP-1).[121] Once macrophages are incorporated into the granulomas as epithelioid histiocytes, they secrete transforming growth factor-β₁ (TGF-β₁); this may modulate the fibrosis that accompanies granuloma evolution by its anti-inflammatory actions.[124]

Evidence of a lymphocytic alveolitis is common on analysis of BAL fluid from patients who have sarcoidosis and is principally related to an increase in CD4 helper cells;[125, 126] however, an excess of CD8 (suppressor) cells is seen rarely.[125] In general, the role of T cells seems to be twofold—antigen recognition and amplification of the local cellular immune response.[81] To this end, activated lymphocytes release a number of cytokines, including IL-1,[127] IL-2,[127–132] IL-4,[128] IL-6,[127] RANTES,[127a] macrophage inhibition factor,[133] TNF-α,[128] granulocyte-macrophage colony-stimu-

lating factor (GM-CSF),[128] and interferon gamma (IFN-γ).[127, 128, 134] The pattern of cytokine release (principally, IFN-γ and IL-2) suggest that these helper lymphocytes are predominantly of the Th-1 phenotype in areas of granuloma formation.[81, 135] It has also been suggested that abnormal IL-12 production by pulmonary macrophages could account for the granulomatous inflammation of sarcoidosis by means of its increasing the release of IFN-γ.[80] All these cytokines have a number of effects on alveolar macrophages, including chemotaxis, an increase in their expression of surface HLA class II molecules, and inhibition of migration from the lung parenchyma. Activated lymphocytes also express an increased number of IL-2 receptors on their surface, thereby enhancing the effectiveness of IL-2 as a T-cell growth factor by autocrine and paracrine mechanisms.[96] In addition to the release of cytokines, activation of lymphocytes is manifested by the expression of several surface activation markers, including CD69, HLA-DR, Leu-8, and CD25.[136]

The preferential proliferation of T-cell clones that express subsets of αβ T-cell receptors is consistent with their recent stimulation by antigen,[137–145] as the role of such cells is to recognize antigen presented in the context of its pairing with HLA class II molecules.[81] A similar response has been seen in T cells derived from tissue exposed to the Kveim reagent,[146] which presumably contains the sarcoid antigen responsible for initiation of the granulomatous inflammatory lesions of sarcoidosis.

In addition to local proliferation of lymphocytes under the influence of IL-2 and other cytokines, lymphocytes are recruited to the lung under the influence of IL-1 and IL-2.[147] The major evidence for this is the observation of a very high ratio of CD4 to CD8 lymphocytes in affected tissue, coupled with depletion of CD4 lymphocytes in the peripheral circulation.[147] The number of CD4 lymphocytes in BAL fluid, as well as their relative proportion, is influenced by the duration and extent of disease, with higher CD4 levels generally being found in patients who have early or extrapulmonary disease.[148]

Although information is incomplete, immunohistochemical analyses of sarcoid granulomas have led to a reasonable understanding of the mechanisms of their formation.[103] Macrophage markers in the center of newly formed granulomas and in areas around blood vessels suggest that they have been recently recruited from the peripheral circulation.[103] In more mature granulomas, the proliferating cells are lymphocytes of the helper/memory phenotype (CD4/CD45RO).[103, 149] Lymphocytes are compartmentalized within granulomas, with CD4 cells being found in the inner portions and CD8 cells scattered around the outer rim.[150] In animal models, CD4 cells favor the growth of granulomas whereas CD8 cells restrict their growth;[103] the degree to which a similar "balance of forces" influences the course of human sarcoid granulomas is unknown.

The precise factors that determine whether fibrosis is the outcome of the granulomatous inflammation of sarcoidosis are uncertain. In addition to activated lymphocytes and macrophages, neutrophils, eosinophils, and mast cells are found in increased numbers at sites of granuloma formation; all can theoretically participate in the development of fibrosis.[103] A number of cytokines released from lymphocytes and macrophages enhance fibrosis, including IFN-γ,[151] IL-1, IL-6, fibronectin, alveolar macrophage-derived growth factor

(AMDGF), and platelet-derived growth factor (PDGF).[152–156] Oxygen radicals, proteinases, cationic proteins, and various other substances released from activated inflammatory cells can also contribute to pulmonary injury and subsequent fibrosis.[103, 157]

Recruitment and proliferation of fibroblasts is associated with their activation and enhanced secretion of matrix components.[103] As mentioned previously, why some patients have spontaneous resolution of disease and others progressive fibrosis is not clear. An IL-1 receptor antagonist has been found within sarcoid granulomas, where it could function as an immunomodulator of inflammation.[158]

An impressive number of systemic abnormalities of both cell-mediated and humoral immunity have also been documented in patients who have sarcoidosis. However, it is uncertain to what extent these are involved in pathogenesis of disease rather than reflecting a secondary reaction to it. Cutaneous anergy is common and can be explained by peripheral T-cell lymphopenia and hyporesponsiveness of peripheral lymphocytes to antigenic stimuli.[149, 159] Examination of blood cell subsets reveals a pattern that is the reverse of that found in the lung, with an increase in the number of cells expressing suppressor-cytotoxic activity and a decrease in the CD4 helper-inducer subset.[149] B-cell hyperactivity is suggested by the finding of a polyclonal increase in circulating immunoglobulins, the presence of circulating immune complexes,[160] the presence of autoantibodies,[161] and high levels of antibodies to *Mycoplasma pneumoniae* and some viruses. Immune complexes and complement can also be found in BAL fluid.[103] These observations are most likely an epiphenomenon relating to B-cell activation in granulomatous inflammation because peripheral B lymphocytes demonstrate impaired function *in vitro*.[103, 149, 162]

In contrast to the spontaneous production of IFN-γ by lung macrophages, peripheral blood monocytes show inhibition of IFN-γ production after exposure to provocative stimuli.[163, 164] Using flow cytometry, it has been shown that leukocytes of all types demonstrate increased expression of adhesion molecules, a feature that may partly explain their eventual extravasation and aggregation in tissue granulomas.[165]

### Cigarette Smoke

Although not a uniform finding,[166] most investigators have found that sarcoidosis is more common in nonsmokers than in smokers.[167–171] Moreover, the alveolitis of patients who smoke is less intense than that of nonsmokers who have a similar stage of disease.[172] Although the mechanism by which this occurs is uncertain, there is evidence that it is related to modulation of local immune phenomena;[171, 173] for example, activated alveolar macrophages from patients who smoke have been found to release less TNF-α than those of nonsmokers.[173] Despite these observations, continued smoking after the diagnosis has been made does not favorably alter the course and prognosis of the disease.[171, 174]

### PATHOLOGIC CHARACTERISTICS

The pathologic hallmark of sarcoidosis is the granuloma, which is identical to that caused by many well-defined etiologic agents—a more or less well-circumscribed collection of epithelioid histiocytes sometimes associated with multinucleated giant cells (Fig. 41–1). The histiocytes typically have abundant lightly eosinophilic cytoplasm and oval or kidney-shaped, vesicular nuclei. Lymphocytes, plasma cells (occasionally), and neutrophils and eosinophils (rarely) can also be found within the granuloma.

Cytoplasmic inclusions are often present within the cells of the granuloma, especially the multinucleated giant cells; they include the asteroid body, the lamellated or conchoidal (Schaumann) body (Fig. 41–2),[175] and small needle-shaped or ovoid, refractile particles, many of which represent calcium oxalate.[176] It has been hypothesized that the latter particles form the nucleus on which a protein matrix, calcium salts, and iron are deposited to form the Schaumann body.[176] All these inclusions are more commonly identified in the granulomas of sarcoidosis than in granulomas of other causes;[177] however, in an individual case, they are of no diagnostic value.[176, 178] Small ovoid or spindle-shaped, yellow-brown structures termed *Hamazaki-Wesenberg bodies* are not uncommonly identified in lymph nodes affected by sarcoidosis.[179–181] Although they superficially resemble fungi (particularly because some appear to bud), they have been shown to represent ceroid within giant intracellular and extracellular liposomes.[180, 181] As with other granuloma-related structures, these unusual bodies can be seen in lymph nodes associated with many other diseases (both granulomatous and nongranulomatous) and are not specific for sarcoidosis.

Although the majority of sarcoid granulomas are non-necrotizing, necrosis has been documented in 5% to 40% of cases.[178, 182, 183] It usually occupies the central one fourth or less of the granuloma; rarely, it is more extensive (Fig. 41–3). Most often, the necrotic material is amorphous and contains degenerated, hyperchromatic nuclei; occasionally, it possesses a finely granular appearance resembling the caseous material of tuberculous or fungal infection.

Although it is probable that many granulomas resolve completely over time,[183] some undoubtedly undergo progressive fibrosis. Fibroblasts are present in considerable numbers at the periphery of more mature granulomas,[184, 185] and it appears that the fibrosis begins at this site. In this circumstance, concentric lamellae of collagen can be seen to separate the histologically "active" central portion of the granuloma from the adjacent tissue (*see* Fig. 41–1). With time, the fibrosis proceeds inward until the entire granuloma is converted into a scar (*see* Fig. 41–1). This pattern of peripheral lamellar fibrosis is characteristic of healing sarcoidosis and is evidence in favor of the diagnosis.

The finding of non-necrotizing granulomas does not constitute absolute evidence of sarcoidosis, because such lesions are by no means specific. Local or diffuse non-necrotizing granulomas can be found in the lungs and intrathoracic lymph nodes as well as many other organs in a wide variety of conditions, including infections (particularly mycobacterial and fungal),[177] extrinsic allergic alveolitis, berylliosis, neoplasms[186] (particularly pulmonary carcinoma,[187] Hodgkin's and non-Hodgkin's lymphoma, and seminoma), drugs,[188] and foreign material such as talc or aspirated food. In some cases, ancillary procedures such as culture, histochemical staining, immunohistochemical reactions, polymerase chain reaction, or polarization microscopy may clarify the etiology of the granulomatous process. How-

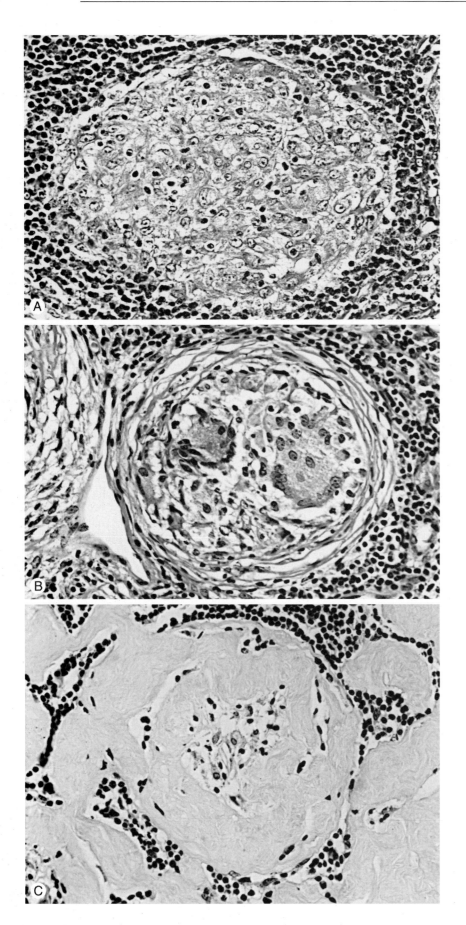

**Figure 41–1. Sarcoidosis: Granulomas.** Histologic sections show three well-circumscribed granulomas in different stages. The most active (A) shows numerous epithelioid histiocytes and scattered small mononuclear cells (probably a combination of lymphocytes and monocytes); there is no fibrosis or necrosis. A later stage (B) shows a distinct zone of collagen possessing a clear-cut lamellated appearance at the periphery; two multinucleated giant cells are evident. An even later stage (C) shows almost complete replacement of the granuloma by mature fibrous tissue. (A, B, C, ×300.)

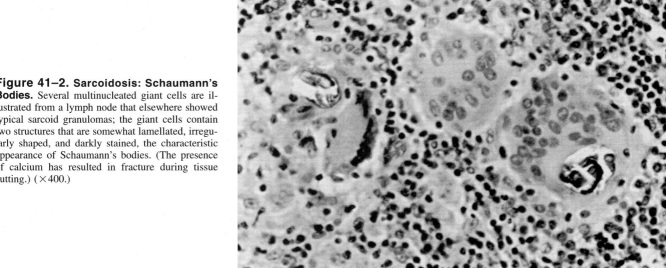

**Figure 41–2. Sarcoidosis: Schaumann's Bodies.** Several multinucleated giant cells are illustrated from a lymph node that elsewhere showed typical sarcoid granulomas; the giant cells contain two structures that are somewhat lamellated, irregularly shaped, and darkly stained, the characteristic appearance of Schaumann's bodies. (The presence of calcium has resulted in fracture during tissue cutting.) (×400.)

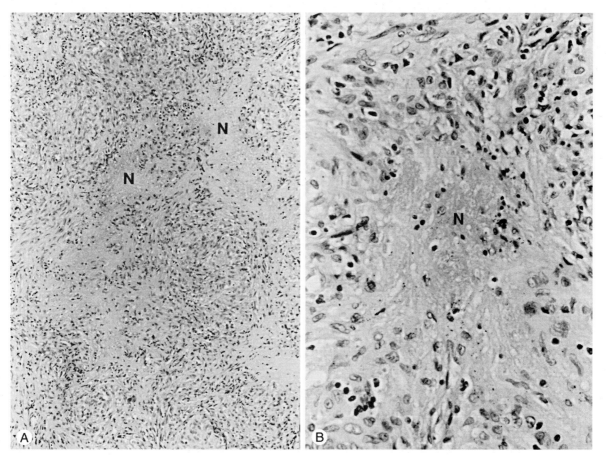

**Figure 41–3. Sarcoidosis: Necrosis.** A section from a mediastinoscopic lymph node biopsy specimen shows confluent granulomatous inflammation associated with a moderate amount of necrosis (N). Although the presence of such necrosis significantly increases the likelihood of an infectious etiology, it does not exclude a diagnosis of sarcoidosis. The patient was an asymptomatic 25-year-old woman who had mediastinal lymph node enlargement on CT and a reticulonodular pattern on the chest radiograph; culture of the excised tissue showed no growth.

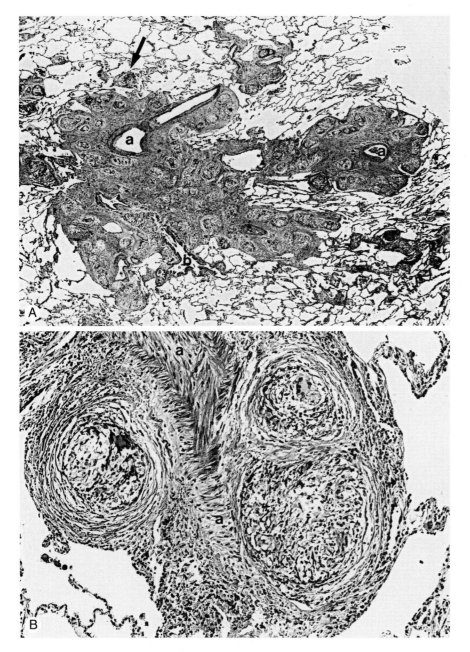

**Figure 41–4. Pulmonary Sarcoidosis.** A low magnification view of lung parenchyma *(A)* shows numerous granulomas associated with a moderate amount of collagen; both granulomas and fibrous tissue are located predominantly in the interstitium adjacent to pulmonary arteries (a) and bronchioles (b). Only an occasional granuloma appears to be located within parenchymal interstitium *(arrow).* A magnified view *(B)* shows three granulomas with a peripheral rim of lamellated fibrous tissue adjacent to a tangentially sectioned pulmonary artery (a). (*A,* ×15; *B,* ×120.)

ever, even negative results of these and other investigations do not absolutely confirm a diagnosis of sarcoidosis.

Pulmonary involvement in sarcoidosis is characteristically most prominent in the peribronchovascular, interlobular septal, and pleural interstitial tissue (Fig. 41–4). In the early stages, granulomas are typically discrete and histologically active; as the disease progresses, they often become confluent and associated with fibrosis, resulting in more or less diffuse interstitial thickening. The parenchymal interstitium may also be affected, although invariably much less so than that in peribronchovascular, septal, and pleural locations. Such disease is manifested by a mononuclear cell infiltrate (predominantly lymphocytes) in alveolar septa (Fig. 41–5);[184, 189] rarely, granuloma formation is evident (Fig. 41–6).[190–192] Ultrastructural examination of alveolar septa in patients with alveolitis has shown the presence of lymphocytes and monocytes in capillary lumina and adjacent interstitium associated with evidence of endothelial and epithelial damage;[193, 194] in many cases, such damage can be identified in alveoli that appear normal by light microscopy.[194]

Individual foci of parenchymal disease are usually minute (identifiable only on microscopy) but can conglomerate with each other and with granulomas in the peribronchovascular and septal interstitium to form relatively discrete masses several centimeters in diameter, an appearance sometimes referred to as "nodular sarcoidosis." Although evolution of disease from a stage of alveolitis to one of granuloma formation and eventually fibrosis is probably the rule in many cases, a number of studies indicate that such a process is by no means invariable.[195–198]

Granulomatous inflammation of pulmonary vessels is common in sarcoidosis (Fig. 41–7); in one study of open-lung biopsy specimens from 128 patients, it was identified in 88 (69%).[199] Vessels of all sizes and types are affected, including elastic and muscular arteries, arterioles and venules, veins, lymphatics, and bronchial vessels.[200] Although the granulomatous inflammation can be associated with disruption of the elastic laminae, necrosis of the vessel wall does not occur and thrombosis is rare. Despite these observations, significant luminal compression can occur, and it is possible that this is the mechanism of parenchymal necrosis seen in some cases. Although it is likely the vascular inflammation is secondary to extension of perivascular interstitial disease in most cases, primary vascular disease also appears to occur.[200]

In addition to their location in peribronchial connective tissue, granulomas affect the airway mucosa and are commonly seen in bronchial biopsy specimens; although probably most frequent in small airways, they can also occur in the walls of larger bronchi,[201] sometimes to such an extent as to cause airway stenosis.[202, 203] Rarely, evidence of granulomatous inflammation can be seen in sputum or bronchial wash specimens.[204]

The gross appearance of pulmonary sarcoidosis depends on the stage and severity of disease. In early, relatively mild disease in which granulomatous inflammation is most prominent in relation to peribronchovascular, interlobular, and pleural connective tissue, the appearance may resemble lymphangitic carcinomatosis. As the disease progresses, involvement of the lung parenchyma may become evident

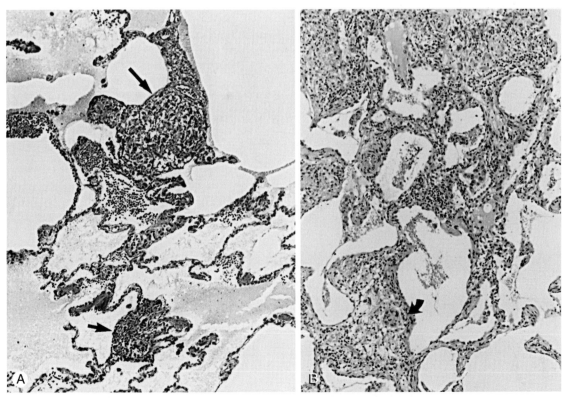

**Figure 41–5. Sarcoidosis: Interstitial Pneumonitis.** A section of lung parenchyma that elsewhere showed typical features of sarcoidosis *(A)* reveals patchy interstitial thickening by an infiltrate of mononuclear inflammatory cells. In one focus *(short arrow)*, these are predominantly lymphocytes, whereas in a second focus *(long arrow)*, the cells are larger and give the impression of early granuloma formation. A section from another biopsy specimen *(B)* shows a moderate degree of interstitial thickening with more clear-cut granuloma formation *(arrow)*. *(A,* ×100; *B,* ×140.)

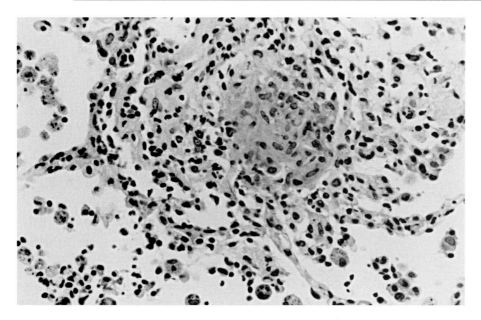

**Figure 41–6. Sarcoidosis: Alveolar Air-Space Involvement.** A highly magnified view of several alveoli shows an infiltrate of inflammatory cells (predominantly lymphocytes) in the alveolar interstitium and adjacent air spaces; a small granuloma can also be seen. Granulomatous inflammation typical of sarcoidosis was present elsewhere in this open biopsy specimen. (×450.)

as foci of nodular or interstitial fibrosis. This process is usually most severe in the upper lobes, where it can possess a honeycomb appearance similar to that of idiopathic pulmonary fibrosis (except for its presence in both subpleural and central regions) (Fig. 41–8). Sometimes, it takes the form of more or less solid areas of fibrous tissue associated with bronchiectasis. The latter can be severe enough to result in the formation of "cavities"; not infrequently, these are associated with the development of fungus balls,[205] a complication sometimes associated with fatal hemoptysis.[205, 206] Solitary or (rarely) multiple cavities unassociated with bronchiectasis can also occur (Fig. 41–9) and suffer the same complication. Fibrosis of the pleura and adjacent parenchymal interstitium is sometimes manifested by slightly elevated white plaques on the visceral pleural surface (Fig. 41–10); rarely, pleural thickening is massive.[207]

Lymph node involvement typically takes the form of more or less diffuse replacement of the node by granulomas (Fig. 41–11), often with a variable histologic appearance.[208] Initially, the granulomas are discrete and appear active; as in pulmonary disease, however, they can become confluent and undergo progressive fibrosis, eventually resulting in completely fibrotic nodes in which granulomas are difficult to recognize. Grossly, such lymph nodes are rubbery or hard and may be ill defined at their periphery.

## RADIOLOGIC MANIFESTATIONS

The radiographic changes in thoracic sarcoidosis can be usefully classified for descriptive purposes into four groups or stages:[209]

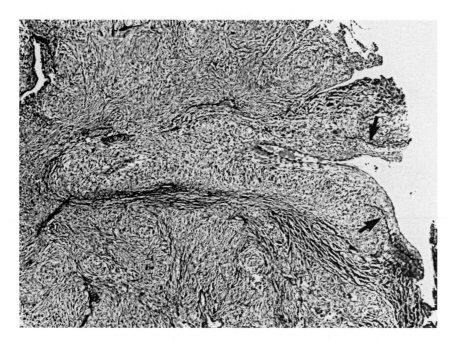

**Figure 41–7. Sarcoidosis: Vascular Involvement.** The section shows replacement of lung parenchyma by numerous granulomas associated with a moderate amount of fibrous tissue. The media of a pulmonary artery are largely replaced by more or less confluent granulomas. (Residual internal elastic lamina is indicated by *arrows.*) (Verhoeff–van Gieson, ×52.)

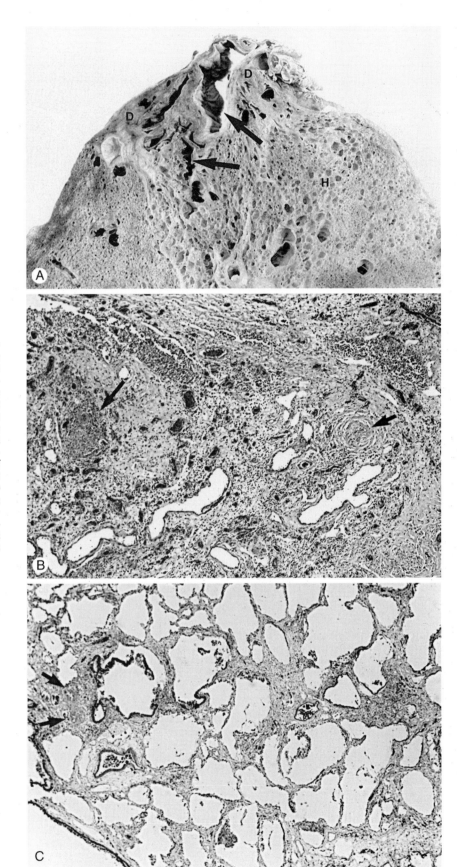

**Figure 41–8. Sarcoidosis: Interstitial Fibrosis.** A section of the apical portion of an upper lobe *(A)* from a patient with long-standing sarcoidosis shows foci of dense fibrosis in which the lung parenchyma is completely destroyed (D); extensive but less severe fibrosis with a "honeycomb" appearance (H) is also present in areas where the parenchyma is also evident. Bronchi in the region of severe fibrosis are ectatic *(arrows)*. A histologic section from the area of dense fibrosis *(B)* shows replacement of lung parenchyma by collagen and scattered aggregates of lymphocytes. The only evidence of sarcoidosis is two granulomas, one *(short arrow)* almost completely fibrosed and the other *(long arrow)* more active in appearance. A section from the area of "honeycombing" *(C)* shows less extensive fibrosis and numerous irregular cystic spaces representing dilated transitional airways. Two largely fibrosed granulomas are present *(arrows).* (*B,* ×40; *C,* ×20.)

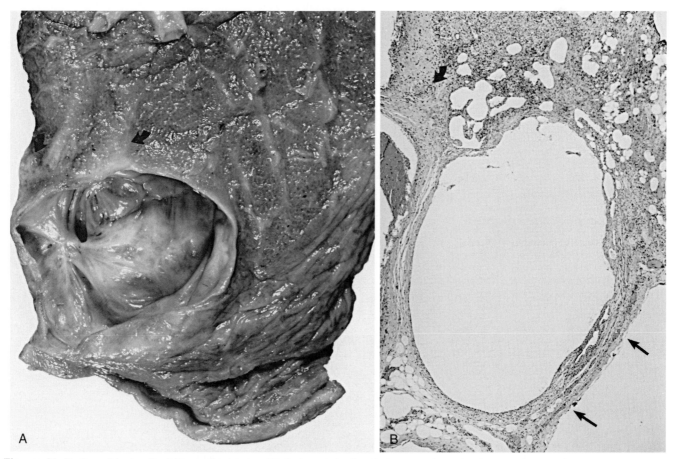

**Figure 41–9. Sarcoidosis: Cyst Formation.** A magnified view of the lingula from a patient with long-standing sarcoidosis *(A)* shows a well-circumscribed cyst approximately 2 cm in diameter. There is no bronchiectasis and only a few very small foci of parenchymal fibrosis *(arrows)*. Histologic examination of the cyst wall showed it to be composed of fibrous tissue containing scattered non-necrotizing granulomas. A section of lung from another patient *(B)* shows a subpleural cystic space, in this case lined only by fibrous tissue. The adjacent lung also shows fibrosis and occasional granulomas *(curved arrow)*. *(Straight arrows* indicate pleura.)

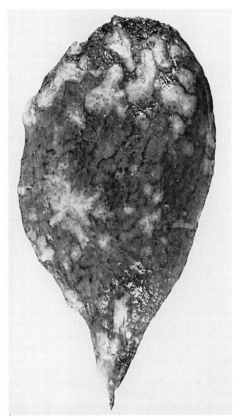

**Figure 41–10. Sarcoidosis: Pleural Fibrosis.** The costal visceral pleura of this left upper lobe shows multiple irregularly shaped plaquelike foci. Histologic examination revealed them to be composed largely of mature fibrosis tissue containing scattered granulomas in the pleura and underlying lung parenchyma. Typical features of largely inactive-appearing sarcoidosis were also evident in hilar and mediastinal lymph nodes and the more central lung regions.

Stage 0: No demonstrable abnormality
Stage 1: Hilar and mediastinal lymph node enlargement unassociated with pulmonary abnormality
Stage 2: Hilar and mediastinal lymph node enlargement associated with pulmonary abnormality
Stage 3: Diffuse pulmonary disease unassociated with node enlargement

The main utility of this staging system is in predicting outcome. In one survey of 3,676 patients from nine countries, 8% had normal chest radiographs at presentation, 51% had Stage 1 disease, 29% had Stage 2 disease, and 12% had Stage 3 disease.[210] On follow-up, 65% of patients with Stage 1 disease showed resolution of the radiographic findings, compared with 49% of patients with Stage 2 disease and only 20% with Stage 3 disease. It should be noted, however, that several other classifications of sarcoidosis have been proposed.[209, 211, 212] Furthermore, the staging system is only a means to describe the radiographic findings and patients do not necessarily progress sequentially from one stage to the next.[211] For example, both hilar and mediastinal lymphadenopathy occasionally develop after involvement of an extrathoracic site or, rarely, after development of parenchymal abnormalities.[212–216]

## Lymph Node Enlargement without Pulmonary Abnormality

On the chest radiograph, lymph node enlargement without parenchymal disease is seen at presentation in approximately 50% of patients.[210, 213, 217] The combination of bilateral hilar and right paratracheal lymph node enlargement (the "1-2-3" sign[218]) is a characteristic and common manifestation (Fig. 41–12);[213] the former is present in more than 95% of patients and the latter in about 70% with intrathoracic lymph node enlargement.[211, 219] Other common sites of lymphadenopathy include the aortopulmonary window (approximately 50% of cases) and subcarinal region (20% of cases).[211, 213, 219] Anterior mediastinal lymphadenopathy is seldom prominent, but can be identified on the radiograph in approximately 15% of cases.[211, 215] Enlargement of paravertebral nodes is uncommon in our experience, although the incidence in reported series varies greatly (e.g., in only 1 of 62 patients in one series[220] and 6 [20%] of 30 cases in another[221]).

Hilar lymph node enlargement is usually bilateral and symmetric. Unilateral enlargement is uncommon, being reported in only 3% to 5% of cases (Fig. 41–13).[222, 223] In one study of the chest radiographs of 800 patients, 38 (5%) showed unilateral node enlargement;[224] of these, erythema nodosum was present in 6 patients, a surprisingly high incidence. The authors suggested that mediastinal node enlargement may have its onset or may regress unilaterally or asymmetrically.

Occasionally, hilar and mediastinal node enlargement is sufficient to compress the major bronchi (Fig. 41–14). Such compression may lead to lobar atelectasis, most commonly involving the middle lobe.[216] Rarely, enlarged nodes cause narrowing of a central pulmonary artery, particularly the truncus anterior, and lead to decreased pulmonary perfusion.[216, 225, 226] Similarly, a few cases of superior vena caval syndrome or obstruction of the innominate vein by massively enlarged lymph nodes have been reported.[216, 227–229]

Calcification of hilar lymph nodes is apparent radiographically in approximately 5% of patients at presentation.[223, 230] In some cases, the calcification resembles the eggshell calcification of silicosis.[223] (In fact, sarcoidosis is considered to be the most common cause of circumferential or eggshell calcification in patients not exposed to silica.[216, 231]) Nodal calcification is usually a late manifestation and is almost invariably associated with advanced disease; it has also been reported after corticosteroid therapy.[232] In one study of 111 patients followed for 10 years or more, calcification of mediastinal lymph nodes was detected radiographically in more than 20%.[232]

Paratracheal node enlargement seldom occurs without concomitant enlargement of hilar nodes.[233] This bilaterally symmetric hilar and paratracheal lymph node enlargement contrasts sharply with the node enlargement of primary tuberculosis, which tends to be unilateral and less sharply demarcated.[234] The contrast is even more evident with lymphoma. For example, enlargement in Hodgkin's disease tends to occur predominantly in the anterior mediastinal and paratracheal groups; when it affects the hilar nodes, it is predominantly unilateral and asymmetric. As indicated previously, anterior mediastinal node enlargement is seldom a prominent

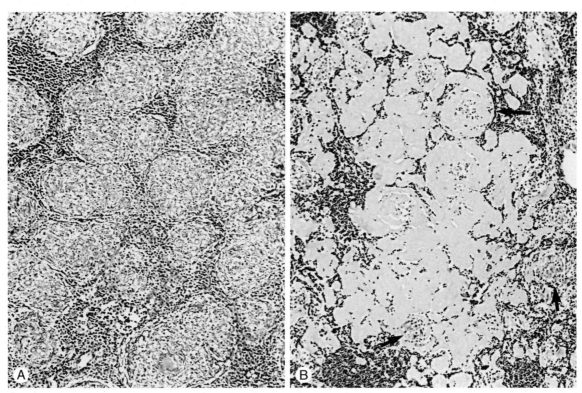

**Figure 41–11. Sarcoidosis: Lymph Node Involvement, Active and Healed.** A section of a mediastinal lymph node *(A)* shows discrete and focally confluent granulomas that virtually obliterate the normal nodal architecture. There is no necrosis. A section of a node from another patient *(B)* shows lamellae of mature collagen, focally with a nodular appearance *(long arrow)*, representing former active granulomas. Occasional small aggregates of epithelioid histiocytes can still be identified *(short arrows)*. (*A* and *B*, ×40.)

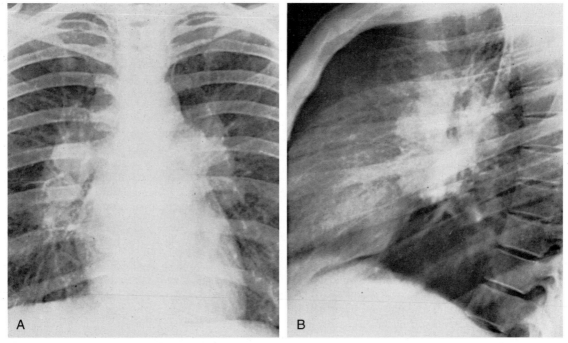

**Figure 41–12. Sarcoidosis: Lymph Node Involvement Alone.** Posteroanterior *(A)* and lateral *(B)* radiographs of a 32-year-old asymptomatic woman demonstrate marked enlargement of both hila, the lobulated contour being typical of lymph node enlargement. Nodes are also enlarged in the right paratracheal and aortopulmonary regions. The lungs are clear.

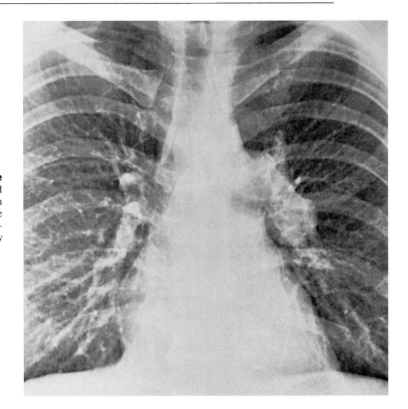

**Figure 41–13. Sarcoidosis: Unilateral Hilar Lymph Node Enlargement.** A posteroanterior radiograph of this 26-year-old asymptomatic man reveals marked enlargement of the left hilum in a configuration characteristic of enlarged lymph nodes. There is no evidence of node enlargement in the right hilum or paratracheal chain. The lungs are clear. The diagnosis was established by biopsy of a left scalene node.

feature of sarcoidosis and is characteristically associated with paratracheal and symmetric bilateral hilar lymphadenopathy.

The prevalence of lymphadenopathy and its distribution as described earlier refer to the findings on the chest radiograph. As expected, both hilar and mediastinal lymphadenopathy is seen more commonly on computed tomography than on radiography.[235, 236] Furthermore, the mediastinal lymphadenopathy can be seen on CT to involve more nodal stations than are apparent on radiography (Fig. 41–15, Table 41–1).[236, 237] CT may also demonstrate enlarged nodes in sites other than the hila and mediastinum, including internal mammary, axillary, and infradiaphragmatic regions.[237–239] Calcification of hilar and mediastinal nodes is also seen more commonly than on the radiograph (Fig. 41–16);[240, 241] in one study of 18 patients, the finding was identified on CT at presentation in 4 (22%) and on follow-up scans performed 4 to 49 months later in 8 (44%).[240]

## Table 41–1. FREQUENCY OF LYMPHADENOPATHY SEEN IN A STUDY OF 25 PATIENTS WITH SARCOIDOSIS

| NODE GROUP | RADIOGRAPH | CT |
|---|---|---|
| Hilar | 84 | 88 |
| Right paratracheal | 76 | 100 |
| Aortopulmonary window | 72 | 92 |
| Subcarinal | 12 | 64 |
| Anterior mediastinal | 12 | 48 |
| Posterior mediastinal | 0 | 16 |

Modified from Sider L, Horton ES Jr: Hilar and mediastinal adenopathy in sarcoidosis as detected by computed tomography. J Thorac Imag 5:77, 1990.

Two other investigators compared the pattern and distribution of calcified mediastinal lymph nodes in sarcoidosis and tuberculosis.[241] In the patients with sarcoidosis, the CT scans were performed within 0 to 32 years (median 3 years) of diagnosis. Nodal calcification was present in 26 of 49 (53%) patients with sarcoidosis and 13 of 28 (46%) patients with tuberculosis. In both groups, the lymphadenopathy frequently involved both the hilar and mediastinal lymph nodes. When hilar lymph node calcification was present, it was more likely to be bilateral in sarcoidosis (65% of patients) than in tuberculosis (8% of patients). The diameter of the calcified lymph nodes was larger in sarcoidosis than in tuberculosis, the mean short-axis nodal diameter being 12 mm in the former compared with 7 mm in the latter. The pattern of calcification was more commonly focal in sarcoidosis and diffuse in tuberculosis. An eggshell pattern of calcification was identified in 9% of patients with sarcoidosis and 8% of patients with tuberculosis.

It is important to appreciate that Stages 0 and 1 refer only to radiographically evident disease and not to disease determined by pathologic or physiologic examination. As in other interstitial diseases, the lungs can be involved in the absence of a demonstrable abnormality on the chest radiograph.[242–244] In fact, the chest radiograph is normal (Stage 0) in about 10% of patients who have biopsy-proven intrathoracic sarcoidosis.[210, 242] Similarly, in a study of 21 consecutive patients with Stage 1 disease who underwent open-lung biopsy, typical sarcoid granulomas were present in all;[245] however, the extent of granulomatous inflammation and fibrosis was significantly less than that seen in open-lung biopsy specimens of patients with radiographic evidence of diffuse lung involvement. The authors of the last study also cited six articles from the literature in which the results of lung biopsy of patients with Stage 1 disease were reported:

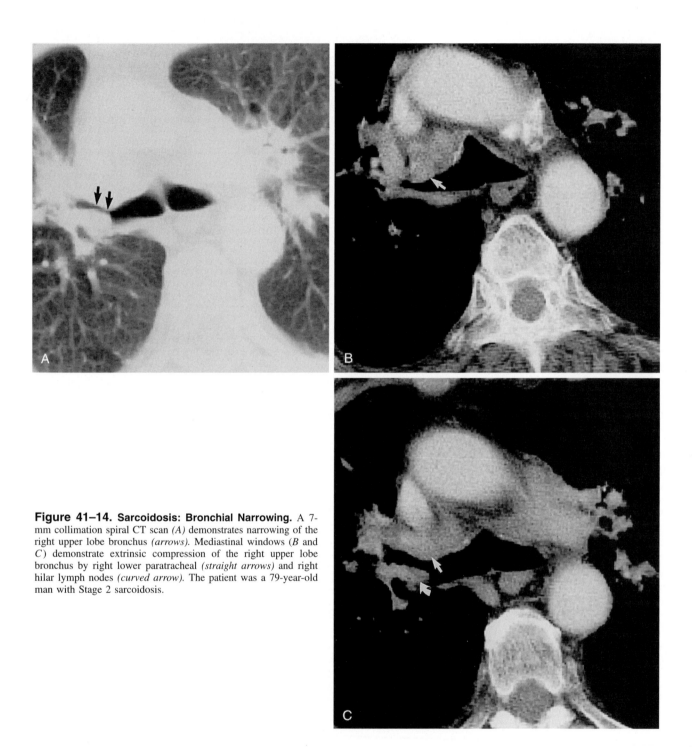

**Figure 41–14. Sarcoidosis: Bronchial Narrowing.** A 7-mm collimation spiral CT scan *(A)* demonstrates narrowing of the right upper lobe bronchus *(arrows)*. Mediastinal windows *(B* and *C)* demonstrate extrinsic compression of the right upper lobe bronchus by right lower paratracheal *(straight arrows)* and right hilar lymph nodes *(curved arrow)*. The patient was a 79-year-old man with Stage 2 sarcoidosis.

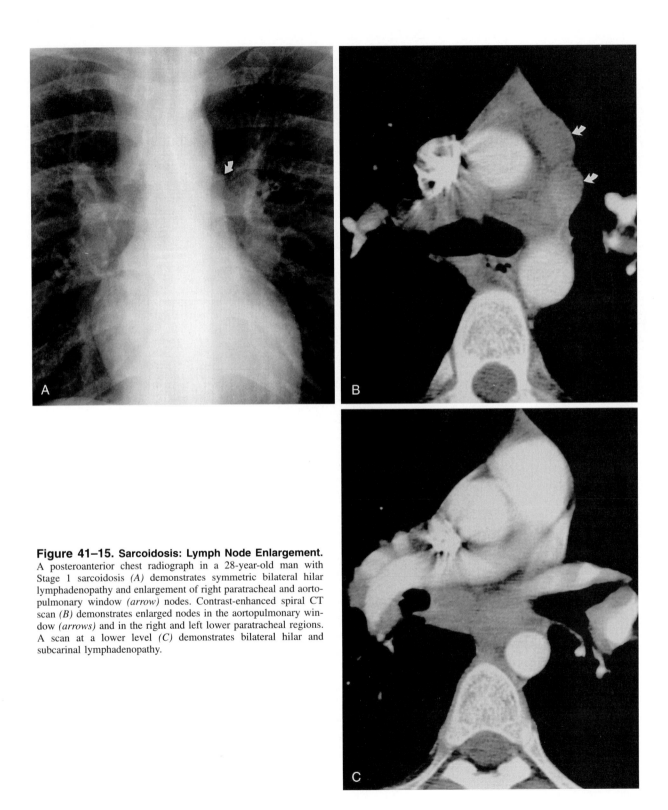

**Figure 41–15. Sarcoidosis: Lymph Node Enlargement.**
A posteroanterior chest radiograph in a 28-year-old man with Stage 1 sarcoidosis *(A)* demonstrates symmetric bilateral hilar lymphadenopathy and enlargement of right paratracheal and aortopulmonary window *(arrow)* nodes. Contrast-enhanced spiral CT scan *(B)* demonstrates enlarged nodes in the aortopulmonary window *(arrows)* and in the right and left lower paratracheal regions. A scan at a lower level *(C)* demonstrates bilateral hilar and subcarinal lymphadenopathy.

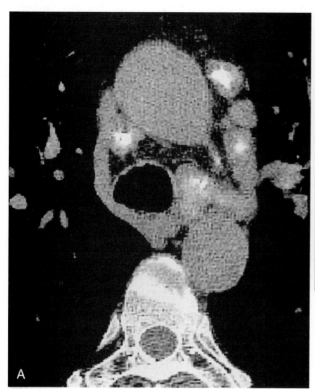
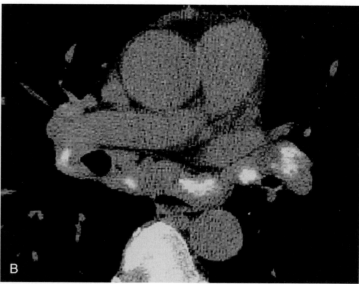

**Figure 41–16. Sarcoidosis: Calcified Lymph Nodes.** An HRCT scan *(A)* in a 59-year-old man with long-standing Stage 2 sarcoidosis demonstrates calcified aortopulmonary window and paratracheal lymph nodes. A scan at a lower level *(B)* demonstrates calcified bilateral hilar and subcarinal lymph nodes.

lung tissue containing granulomas was obtained in 50% to 100% of cases.[245] As might be expected, parenchymal abnormalities are seen more commonly on HRCT than on the radiograph.[235] For example, in one study of 44 patients, mild parenchymal abnormalities were detected on HRCT in all 6 patients with radiographic Stage 1 disease.[246]

Sixty-five per cent to 80% of patients with Stage 1 sarcoidosis eventually show complete radiographic resolution.[14, 210, 247] In one study of 308 patients, normal chest radiographs were present in 44% after 1 year of follow-up and in 82% after 5 years.[247] Occasionally, enlarged hilar and mediastinal nodes regress to normal size only to undergo enlargement once again at a later date.[248–250] On the other hand, hilar and paratracheal node enlargement can persist unchanged for 15 years or more.[251, 252] In one study of 12 patients with chronic hilar and mediastinal lymph node enlargement, 7 remained asymptomatic for a mean period of 16 years despite persistent node enlargement, 2 patients had disfiguring facial sarcoidosis for which corticosteroid therapy was administered for 18 and 27 years, and 3 developed diffuse pulmonary disease after 10 years of stable node enlargement (Fig. 41–17).[253] Tests performed on patients with node enlargement to evaluate cellular activity after a mean interval of more than 16 years included measurement of serum levels of angiotensin-converting enzyme (ACE) (elevated in 8 of 12 patients) and gallium 67 scanning (hilar uptake in all 8 patients tested). The results of these tests were similar for patients who remained well and for those who had symptomatic or progressive disease, indicating that these parameters of active granulomatous inflammation do not necessarily reflect the duration of the disease, its outcome, or the need for treatment.

### Diffuse Pulmonary Disease with or without Lymph Node Enlargement

Parenchymal disease is seen on the chest radiograph at presentation in approximately 40% of patients with sarcoidosis and occurs at some time during the course of the disease in 50% to 65%.[210, 211, 247, 254] At presentation, the pulmonary disease is associated with lymph node enlargement (Stage 2) in approximately 30% of patients; the remaining 10% have no evidence of lymph node enlargement (Stage 3).[210, 247] In one 15-year follow-up study of 308 patients, 9% with Stage 1 disease at presentation progressed to Stage 2 and an additional 2% progressed to Stage 3 apparently without passing through Stage 2.[247] In approximately 70% of 128 patients with Stage 2 disease at presentation, the radiographic findings returned to normal, in 5% they remained at Stage 2, and in 25% they progressed to Stage 3.

The parenchymal abnormalities in sarcoidosis are typically bilateral and symmetrical; although they may be diffuse, in 50% to 80% of patients they involve mainly the upper lung zones.[235, 255–257] Occasionally, disease is asymmetric, either during the stage of development or resolution;[252] sometimes, it is unilateral.[258] Although there is no question that HRCT can reveal parenchymal disease in the absence of abnormality on conventional radiographs, we have found that when radiographs display disease, the extent and profusion of opacities are little different from those revealed by HRCT.[259]

The most frequent patterns are nodular and reticulonodular; less commonly, a reticular pattern, air-space consolidation, or ground-glass opacities predominate.[254, 259, 260, 261] The pattern and extent of parenchymal abnormalities are better depicted on HRCT than on the radiograph.[235, 246, 259,]

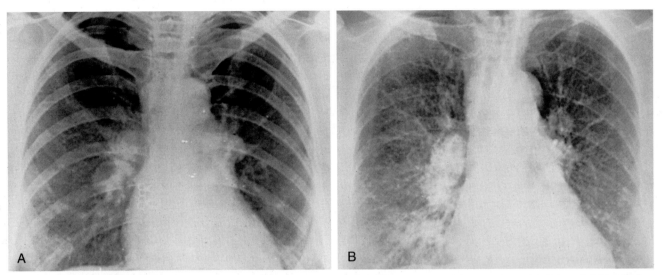

**Figure 41–17. Sarcoidosis: Lymph Node Enlargement Persisting for 13 Years.** A posteroanterior radiograph *(A)* reveals bilateral hilar and paratracheal lymph node enlargement. The lungs are clear. Thirteen years later *(B)*, the node enlargement is still evident and is accompanied by diffuse interstitial pulmonary disease. The patient was a woman who was 60 years old at the time of the second radiograph.

[261, 262] Magnetic resonance (MR) imaging is inferior to HRCT in the demonstration of parenchymal lung disease and is rarely used in assessment.[263]

**Nodular Pattern.** A nodular pattern is present on the chest radiograph in 30% to 60% of patients (Fig. 41–18).[256,

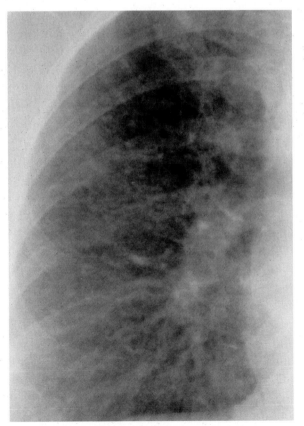

**Figure 41–18. Sarcoidosis: Nodular Pattern.** A view of the right lung from a posteroanterior chest radiograph demonstrates numerous nodules measuring approximately 3 mm in diameter, most abundant in the middle and upper lung zones. Similar findings were present in the left lung. The patient was a 37-year-old woman with Stage 2 sarcoidosis.

[260–262] The nodules usually have irregular margins and involve mainly the middle and upper lung zones. They vary in size and frequently range from 1 to 10 mm in diameter, although the majority measure less than 3 mm.

On HRCT, nodules are seen at presentation in 90% to 100% of patients with parenchymal abnormalities.[246, 255, 264] They are most numerous along the bronchoarterial and pleural interstitium and adjacent to the interlobar fissures (Fig. 41–19).[235, 246, 255] In fact, extensive nodular thickening of the bronchoarterial interstitium involving mainly the middle and upper lung zones is a characteristic feature of the disease.[255, 265] Nodules are also commonly seen along the interlobular septa and centrilobular structures.[235, 264, 265] Correlation of HRCT with pathologic findings has shown that the nodules represent a conglomeration of granulomas.[235, 266]

Uncommonly, nodules are diffuse throughout the lung parenchyma; in one study of 150 patients, a diffuse miliary pattern was observed in 2 (Fig. 41–20).[230] Nodules may also appear as dense, round, sharply marginated opacities greater than 1 cm in diameter simulating a metastatic neoplasm (Fig. 41–21).[267–269] This pattern was observed in 3 of 150 patients in one study;[217] all were African American. Rarely, nodules of this type are solitary.[270, 271] (However, a solitary nodule can be a carcinoma even in a young patient with proven sarcoidosis.[272]) Although nodules greater than 1 cm in diameter are seldom the only finding in pulmonary sarcoidosis, large nodules are frequently seen in association with smaller nodular opacities. Nodules greater than 1 cm in diameter associated with smaller nodules were observed on HRCT in 33% of 159 patients in one study;[256] three were cavitated.

**Reticulonodular Pattern.** A reticulonodular pattern is present in 25% to 50% of patients with radiographically evident parenchymal abnormalities (Fig. 41–22).[256, 259, 260, 273] The pattern may result from a combination of nodules and thickening of the interlobular septa or a combination of nodules and irregular linear opacities (reticular pattern).

**Reticular Pattern.** A reticular pattern is seen in 15% to 20% of patients (Fig. 41–23).[259, 260] It may result from thickening of interlobular septa, nonseptal (intralobular) irregular lines, traction bronchiectasis, or, less commonly, honey-

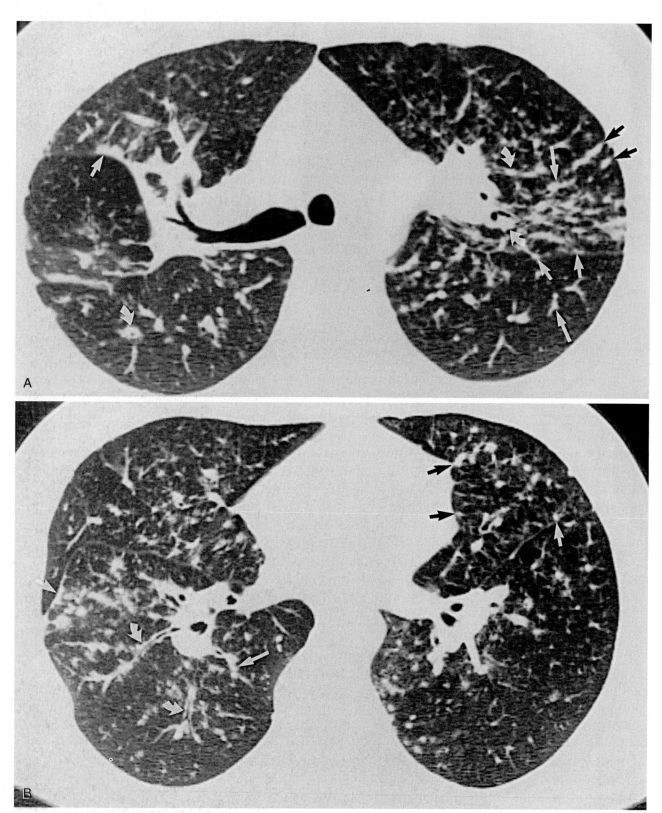

**Figure 41–19. Sarcoidosis: HRCT Appearance.** HRCT scans at the level of the right upper lobe bronchus *(A)* and the inferior pulmonary veins *(B)* demonstrate multiple small nodules. These are located mainly along the bronchi *(curved white arrows)*, pulmonary vessels *(long straight white arrows)*, subpleural lung regions, and the interlobar fissures *(short straight white arrows)*. Nodular thickening of interlobular septa is also evident *(black arrows)*. The patient was a 37-year-old man with Stage 2 sarcoidosis.

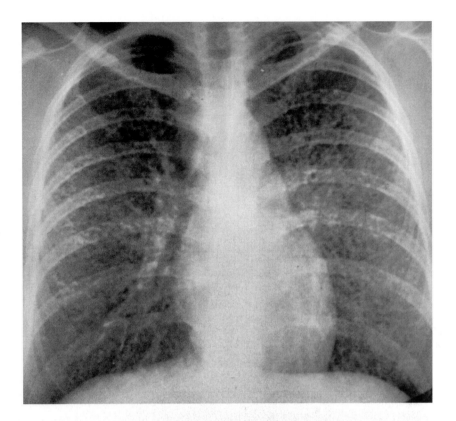

**Figure 41–20. Sarcoidosis: Diffuse Nodular Pattern.** A posteroanterior radiograph reveals a nodular pattern throughout both lungs with some midzonal predominance. There is no evidence of hilar or mediastinal lymph node enlargement. This 26-year-old woman complained of mild dyspnea on exertion. The diagnosis was made by open-lung biopsy.

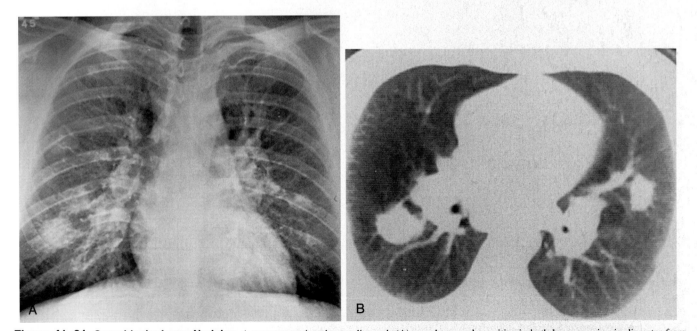

**Figure 41–21. Sarcoidosis: Large Nodules.** A posteroanterior chest radiograph *(A)* reveals several opacities in both lungs ranging in diameter from 1 to 2 cm. The opacities have ill-defined margins but are homogeneous in density. Hilar lymph node enlargement is present bilaterally, and there is also suggestive evidence of mild enlargement of paratracheal nodes. A CT scan through the lower portion of the thorax *(B)* reveals homogeneous masses in both lungs and bilateral hilar node enlargement. The resolution of the image is insufficient to permit evaluation of lung parenchyma generally.

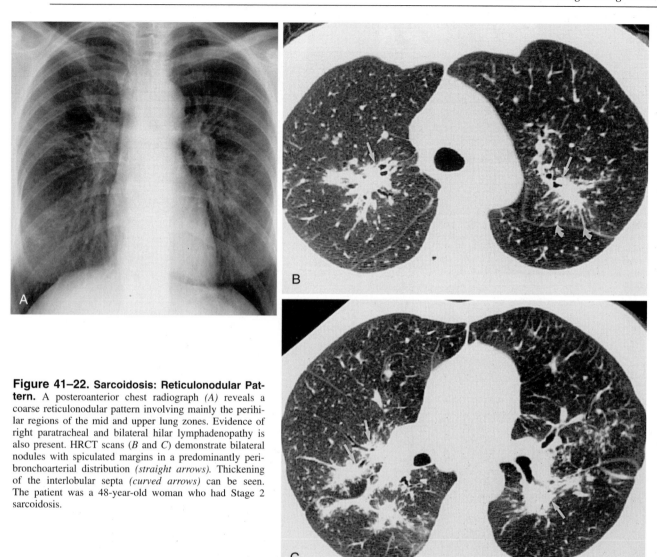

**Figure 41–22. Sarcoidosis: Reticulonodular Pattern.** A posteroanterior chest radiograph *(A)* reveals a coarse reticulonodular pattern involving mainly the perihilar regions of the mid and upper lung zones. Evidence of right paratracheal and bilateral hilar lymphadenopathy is also present. HRCT scans *(B* and *C)* demonstrate bilateral nodules with spiculated margins in a predominantly peribronchoarterial distribution *(straight arrows)*. Thickening of the interlobular septa *(curved arrows)* can be seen. The patient was a 48-year-old woman who had Stage 2 sarcoidosis.

combing (Fig. 41–24). On HRCT, smooth or nodular thickening of interlobular septa has been described in 20% to 90% of patients and nonseptal irregular lines in 20% to 70% (Fig. 41–25).[235, 256, 262–264] The interlobular septal thickening is seldom extensive and, like the nodular opacities, tends to involve mainly the central regions of the middle and upper lung zones. Irregular linear opacities are usually associated with distortion of the architecture of the secondary pulmonary lobules, indicating the presence of fibrosis; however, they are occasionally reversible.[235, 263] Fibrosis also leads to dilatation and distortion of bronchi (traction bronchiectasis), predominantly in the parahilar regions of the upper lung zones, and to honeycombing *(see* Fig. 41–24).[257, 273] The latter usually involves the subpleural lung regions of the middle and upper lung zones.[257]

**Air-Space Consolidation.** Parenchymal consolidation is the predominant finding on the chest radiograph in 10% to 20% of patients with sarcoidosis (Fig. 41–26).[217, 235, 260] The consolidation typically has a bilateral and symmetric distribution, again involving mainly the mid and upper lung zones. The appearance may resemble pulmonary edema.[209, 213] Occasionally, it has a lobar distribution;[256] rarely, it has a periph-

eral distribution resembling chronic eosinophilic pneumonia (Fig. 41–27).[274] In patients in whom the disease is largely confined to the upper lung zones, the pattern may mimic postprimary tuberculosis; in one series of 616 patients, this was identified in 54 (9%).[275]

On HRCT, the areas of consolidation may be peribronchial *(see* Fig. 41–26) or, less commonly, peripheral in distribution.[276] Air bronchograms can be seen in the majority of cases.[276] In one review of the HRCT findings in 10 patients, additional findings of small nodules, thickening of the bronchoarterial interstitium, and interlobular septa were present in all cases;[276] the areas of consolidation involved mainly the upper lung zones in four cases, the lower lung zones in one, and all lung zones in five patients.

**Ground-Glass Opacities.** Hazy areas of increased opacity without obscuration of the vascular markings (ground-glass opacities) are seldom seen on the radiograph but are commonly present on HRCT (Fig. 41–28). In one review of the chest radiographs in 1,652 patients, only 10 (0.6%) showed diffuse ground-glass abnormalities; all had associated hilar or mediastinal lymphadenopathy.[277] By contrast, areas of ground-glass attenuation have been reported on HRCT in

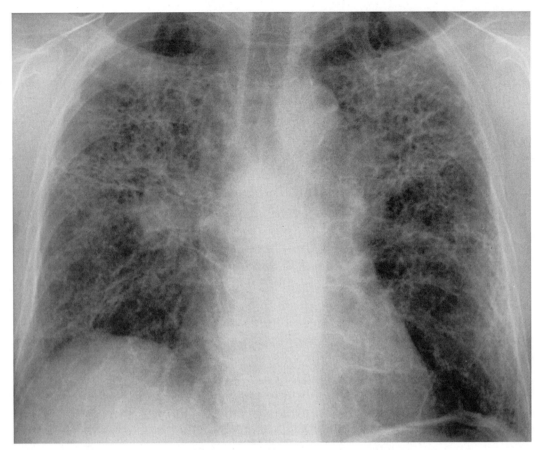

**Figure 41–23. Sarcoidosis: Reticular Pattern Associated with Fibrosis.** A posteroanterior chest radiograph in a 67-year-old woman with sarcoidosis demonstrates a coarse reticular pattern involving mainly the perihilar regions of the mid and upper lung zones.

**Figure 41–24. Sarcoidosis: Pulmonary Fibrosis.** An HRCT image at the level of the aortic arch in a 36-year-old man with sarcoidosis demonstrates fibrosis involving mainly the upper and mid lung zones. The fibrosis is associated with distortion of lung architecture and posterior displacement of ectatic upper lobe bronchi. Note thickening of interlobular septa *(straight arrows)*, a few residual centrilobular nodules *(curved arrows)*, and focal areas of ground-glass attenuation *(open arrows)*. Gallium-67 lung scan showed no uptake; the radiograph showed a reticular pattern.

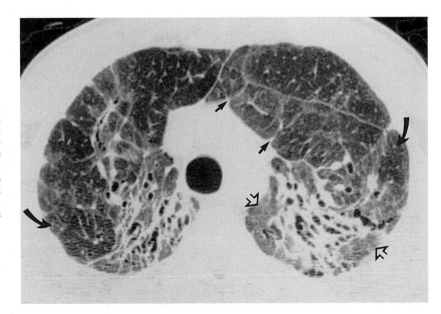

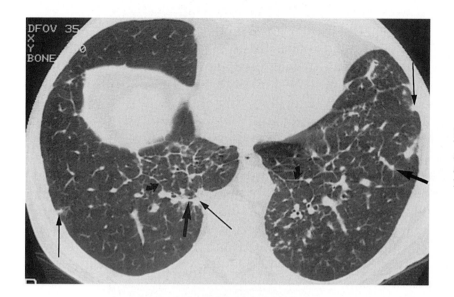

**Figure 41–25. Sarcoidosis: Interlobular Septal Thickening.** HRCT scan through the lower lung zones demonstrates smooth *(curved arrows)* and nodular *(short straight arrows)* thickening of the interlobular septa. Subpleural nodules *(long thin arrows)* are also evident.

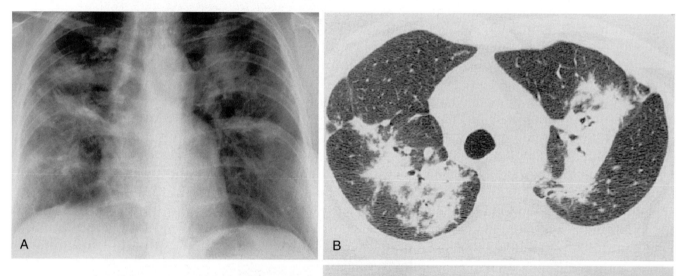

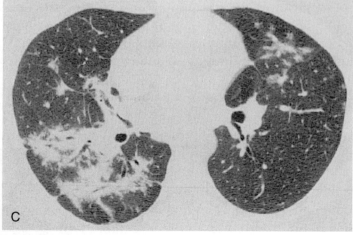

**Figure 41–26. Sarcoidosis: Air-Space Consolidation.** A posteroanterior chest radiograph *(A)* in a 39-year-old woman with Stage 2 sarcoidosis demonstrates patchy bilateral areas of consolidation. Air bronchograms can be seen, particularly on the right side. The consolidation involves mainly the perihilar regions of the mid and upper lung zones. HRCT images *(B* and *C)* demonstrate a peribronchial distribution of the areas of consolidation and clearly defined air bronchograms.

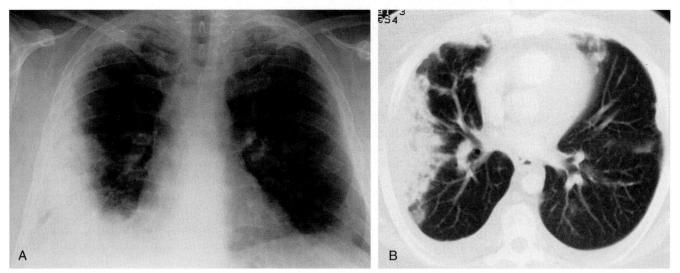

**Figure 41–27. Sarcoidosis: Subpleural Consolidation.** A posteroanterior chest radiograph *(A)* in a 34-year-old man demonstrates extensive right subpleural consolidation. A small area of consolidation is also present in the left lower lobe. A CT scan *(B)* demonstrates subpleural consolidation in the right lung and focal area of consolidation in the lingula. The patient had no hilar or mediastinal lymphadenopathy on the radiograph or CT. The diagnosis of Stage 3 sarcoidosis was proven by video-assisted thoracoscopic biopsy of the right lower lobe.

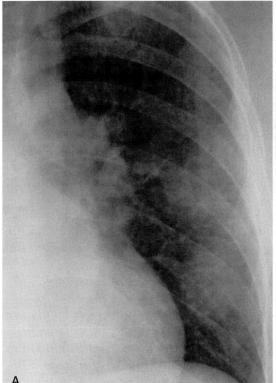

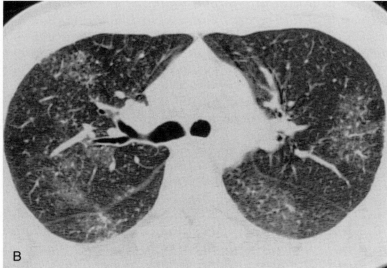

**Figure 41–28. Sarcoidosis: Ground-Glass Attenuation.** A close-up view of the left lung from a posteroanterior chest radiograph *(A)* and an HRCT scan *(B)* demonstrate patchy areas of ground-glass attenuation containing a few poorly defined nodules. The patient was a 32-year-old man who had Stage 2 sarcoidosis. The diagnosis was proven by transbronchial biopsy.

20% to 60% of patients.[256, 264, 266, 273] In the vast majority of these cases, the ground-glass attenuation is a secondary feature seen in association with small nodules; rarely, it is the predominant abnormality.[266, 278] Correlation of HRCT and pathologic findings has shown the pattern to be related to the presence of interstitial granulomatous inflammation;[266, 278, 279] occasionally, it is the result of microscopic foci of fibrosis in the parenchyma.[278]

When pulmonary disease and lymph node enlargement coexist, their radiologic appearance is no different from that of separate involvement. However, in such circumstances the two manifestations may differ greatly in their temporal relationship in different patients. Diffuse pulmonary disease usually appears when hilar node enlargement is present, although the latter may be regressing. Node enlargement may also disappear and be replaced by diffuse pulmonary involvement, either concurrently (Fig. 41–29) or several years later (Fig. 41–30), or it may remain and diffuse pulmonary involvement may be superimposed on it.

**Fibrosis.** In 50% to 70% of patients with Stage 2 disease and 20% to 40% with Stage 3, the radiologic abnormalities eventually resolve.[210, 247] Many patients with persistent radiographic abnormalities improve clinically;[280] approximately 20% develop pulmonary fibrosis.[14, 213] There are no radiographic criteria that allow distinction of reversible from irreversible disease.[213] On HRCT, nodules, consolidation, ground-glass attenuation and interlobular septal thickening may resolve, remain stable, or progress on follow-up.[240, 264, 281] Irregular linear opacities are most commonly irreversible but occasionally resolve.[240, 264] Irreversible abnormalities indicative of fibrosis on HRCT include architectural distortion, traction bronchiectasis, and honeycombing.[240, 264, 281] Except

for the demonstration of irreversible abnormalities in pulmonary fibrosis, HRCT is not helpful in predicting outcome, there being no difference in the pattern or extent of parenchymal abnormalities in patients with persistent or progressive disease and in patients who improve on follow-up.[264]

The fibrosis in sarcoidosis typically involves mainly the upper lung zones (Fig. 41–31).[209, 213] It is usually associated with upward retraction of the hila and with well-defined structural changes in the lungs, including bulla formation, traction bronchiectasis, and compensatory overinflation of the lower lobes (*see* Fig. 41–23).[282] When fibrosis and compensatory overinflation are severe, changes in the heart and pulmonary vasculature are those of pulmonary hypertension and cor pulmonale of any cause. On HRCT, the fibrosis has a characteristic peribronchovascular distribution radiating from the hila to the upper lobes (*see* Fig. 41–24).[240, 246, 257] Additional findings include irregular lines of attenuation with associated architectural distortion, central conglomeration of ectatic bronchi (Fig. 41–32), conglomerate masses, and, in approximately 40% of cases, subpleural honeycombing (Fig. 41–33).[257] Differentiation of conglomerate masses of fibrosis in sarcoidosis from those in silicosis can be readily made by the presence of air bronchograms in the former.[257]

### Other Radiologic Manifestations

Unusual manifestations of sarcoidosis have been the subject of a review in which abnormalities of bone, pleura, mediastinum, lungs, and the cardiovascular system are discussed in detail.[283] The interested reader is directed to this review for in-depth coverage of these admittedly uncommon

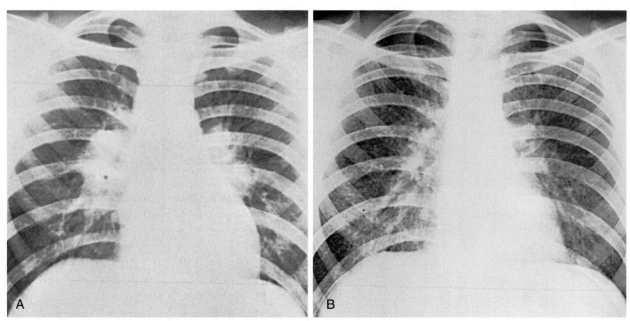

**Figure 41–29. Sarcoidosis: Lymph Node Enlargement Undergoing Rapid Resolution Followed by Pulmonary Involvement.** At the time of the radiograph illustrated in *A,* this 28-year-old man complained of recent onset of headaches, low-grade fever, fatigue, moderate exertional dyspnea, and pleuritic pain. A posteroanterior radiograph *(A)* demonstrated enlargement of the hilar and paratracheal lymph nodes, bilaterally and symmetrically; the lungs were clear. The diagnosis of sarcoidosis was established by axillary and cervical lymph node biopsy. The patient's symptoms rapidly abated over the following 2 weeks but returned 3 months later. A radiograph at this time *(B)* revealed complete disappearance of the mediastinal and hilar lymph node enlargement. However, a diffuse reticular pattern throughout both lungs was now evident. Complete radiographic resolution occurred in 3 months without treatment.

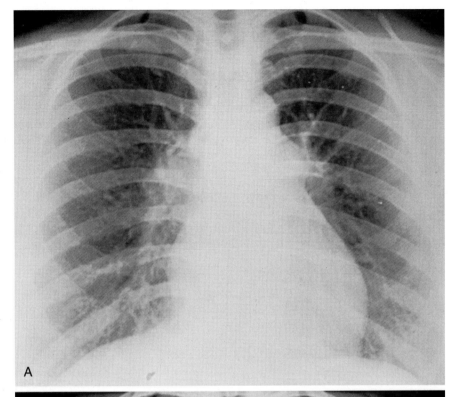

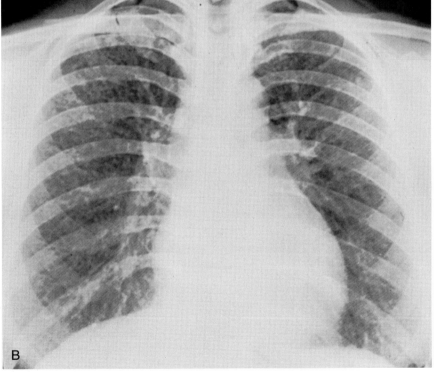

**Figure 41–30. Sarcoidosis: Lymph Node Enlargement with Clearing and Late Pulmonary Involvement.** A posteroanterior radiograph *(A)* of a 31-year-old asymptomatic woman demonstrates enlargement of the tracheobronchial and hilar lymph nodes bilaterally. The diagnosis of sarcoidosis was established by scalene node biopsy. The node enlargement disappeared over the following 4 months, and the chest radiograph returned to normal. Four years later, a posteroanterior radiograph *(B)* revealed diffuse involvement of both lungs by a coarse reticulonodular pattern compatible with a diagnosis of sarcoidosis. Although the hila are normal at this time, there is a suggestion of slight enlargement of right paratracheal nodes.

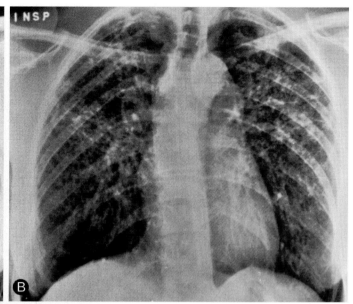

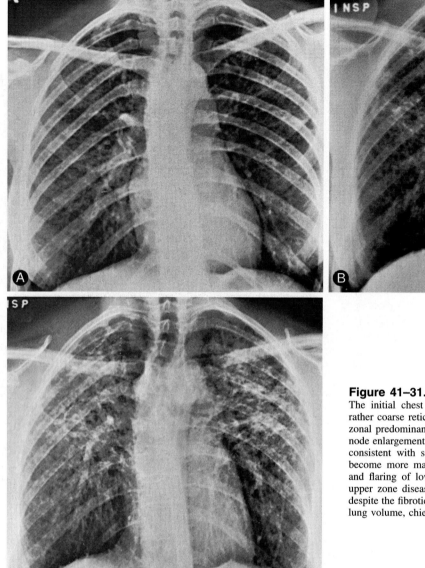

**Figure 41–31. Sarcoidosis: Progressive Pulmonary Fibrosis.** The initial chest radiograph *(A)* of this 37-year-old woman reveals a rather coarse reticular pattern throughout both lungs with definite upper-zonal predominance. There is no evidence of hilar or mediastinal lymph node enlargement. Open-lung biopsy showed non-necrotizing granulomas consistent with sarcoidosis. Three years later *(B),* the reticulation had become more marked and there had occurred an upward displacement and flaring of lower zone vessels, indicating the fibrotic nature of the upper zone disease. This was more evident 1 year later *(C).* Note that despite the fibrotic nature of the disease, there was no overall reduction in lung volume, chiefly because of overinflation of lower zone parenchyma.

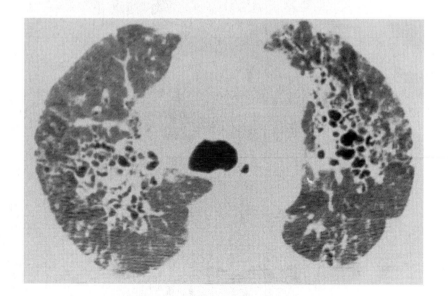

**Figure 41–32. Sarcoidosis: Pulmonary Fibrosis.** An HRCT scan at the level of the tracheal carina demonstrates central conglomeration of ectatic bronchi (traction bronchiectasis) and subpleural nodules. The patient was a 60-year-old man who had Stage 3 sarcoidosis.

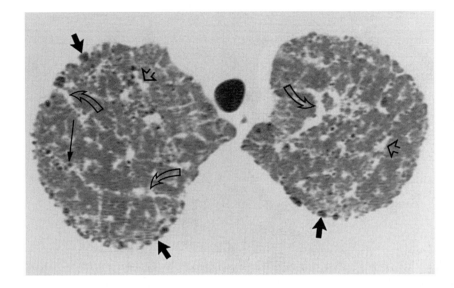

**Figure 41–33. Sarcoidosis: Honeycombing.** An HRCT scan through the upper lobes in a 30-year-old woman with Stage 3 sarcoidosis demonstrates extensive subpleural honeycombing *(short arrows)*. Honeycomb formation is also present adjacent to some of the interlobular septa *(long arrow)*; nodular thickening can be seen adjacent to other interlobular septa *(curved open arrows)* and along the vessels *(open straight arrows)*.

manifestations, and only a brief description is given here. Such atypical features appear to be particularly common in older individuals. In one study of 29 patients who presented after the age of 50 years, 17 (59%) had atypical findings, including mediastinal node enlargement alone or in combination with unilateral hilar node enlargement in 8 patients, solitary or multiple pulmonary masses in 3, and atelectasis in 3.[284]

**Cavitation.** This is a very uncommon manifestation of sarcoidosis (Fig. 41–34).[256, 283, 285–287] In one series of 1,254 cases in which the thorax was involved in 94%, cavitation was present in only 8 cases (0.6%).[9] The abnormality is more commonly apparent on HRCT than on the radiograph; for example, in one review of 159 patients, cavitated nodules

were seen in 3.[256] The cavities tend to be thin walled and are seen in association with other parenchymal abnormalities.[285, 288] They may resolve spontaneously[286] or develop superimposed infection or mycetoma formation.[237, 287, 288] The latter complication occurs in approximately 40% of cystic lesions in sarcoidosis; although most often located in foci of bronchiectasis they may also be seen in bullae or cavities (Fig. 41–35).[261, 288–290]

It is important to eliminate other causes before accepting sarcoidosis as the cause of cavitation.[285, 288] Of greatest importance in this regard are tuberculosis and fungal infection. In addition, true cavitation should be distinguished from a "multicystic" pattern caused by bullae or bronchiectasis.[267, 291]

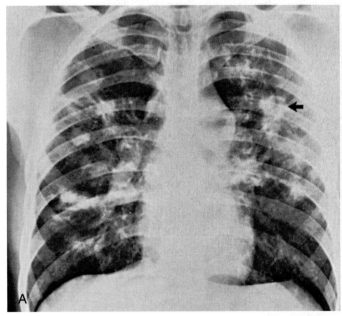
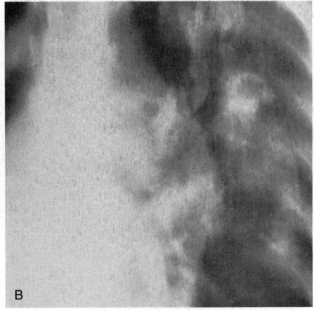

**Figure 41–34. Sarcoidosis: Large Nodules with Cavitation.** A posteroanterior radiograph *(A)* reveals a multitude of poorly defined opacities throughout both lungs, without anatomic predilection. The opacities range up to 3 cm in diameter and most are homogeneous. A single mass *(arrow)* shows a central radiolucency consistent with cavitation, visualized to better advantage on an anteroposterior tomogram *(B)*. There is bilateral hilar and paratracheal lymph node enlargement. Non-necrotizing granulomas were identified in tissue obtained by transbronchial biopsy. The patient was a 22-year-old man.

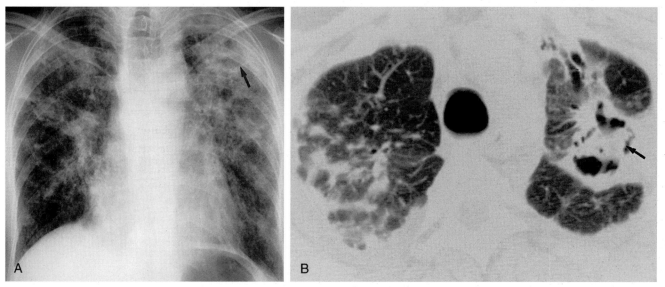

**Figure 41–35. Sarcoidosis: Fungus Ball Formation.** A posteroanterior chest radiograph *(A)* in a 61-year-old woman who had long-standing sarcoidosis shows a coarse reticulonodular pattern in the upper lobes associated with superior retraction of the hila (indicative of pulmonary fibrosis). A cavity *(arrow)* is seen in the left upper lobe. A CT scan *(B)* demonstrates a fungus ball *(arrow)* within the cavity. The patient presented with a history of weight loss and recurrent episodes of blood-streaked sputum.

**Atelectasis and Air Trapping.** This is also a rare manifestation of pulmonary sarcoidosis, being observed in only 1 of 150 cases in one series,[217] in 1 of 198 in another,[223] and in 3 of 300 in a third.[289] The atelectasis may be caused by extrinsic compression of bronchi by enlarged lymph nodes, by bronchial mucosal inflammation, or, perhaps most commonly, by a combination of the two.[283, 292] The diagnosis can be confirmed by bronchial biopsy.[293, 294] Occasionally, enlarged hilar and mediastinal nodes compress and narrow major bronchi without causing atelectasis *(see* Fig. 41–14).[295] Both endobronchial involvement and nodal compression can cause regional hypoventilation and resultant hypoxic vasoconstriction and local oligemia. Expiratory HRCT can show air trapping, most commonly at the level of the secondary pulmonary lobules.[261, 295a]

**Pleural Disease.** The reported prevalence of pleural effusion in sarcoidosis ranges from 0.7% to 7%;[217, 289, 296–299] tabulation of the findings of several studies involving 3,146 patients revealed a prevalence of 2.4%.[283] Approximately one third of cases are bilateral. In one study of 227 patients in which evidence of pleural involvement was specifically sought, pleural effusion was found in 15 (7%) and pleural thickening in 8 (3%).[299] All of the patients with effusion manifested moderately advanced pulmonary sarcoidosis, and non-necrotizing granulomas were identified on pleural biopsy in 7 of the 15 cases. Pleural effusion tended to clear in 4 to 8 weeks, but in some cases progressed to chronic pleural thickening. Several investigators have suggested that the presence of pleural effusion in association with pulmonary sarcoidosis should raise the possibility of complicating tuberculosis,[300] coincidental pneumonia, or heart failure.[9, 251, 252, 301]

Pleural thickening and fibrothorax are undoubtedly much more common in sarcoidosis than has been emphasized in the literature, having been identified often at thoracotomy and autopsy.[283] Such thickening can occur independently of effusion and may be unilateral or bilateral.[299, 302] It is usually asymptomatic but may be associated with progres-

sive dyspnea.[302] Rarely, sarcoidosis presents as a discrete pleural mass.[303]

Spontaneous pneumothorax has been estimated to occur in 1% to 2% of cases.[304, 305] Bullae tend to develop in the upper lobes in advanced fibrotic disease and have been said to rupture in approximately 5% of cases.[304] However, it is probable that in the absence of bullae, pneumothorax represents a coincidental occurrence and is of the same etiology as that which occurs spontaneously in a susceptible young male population. Bilateral pneumothorax occurs rarely.[306, 307]

**Skeletal Disease.** Radiographic evidence of bone involvement is seen in approximately 3% of patients,[283] usually in the setting of long-standing disease. The short tubular bones of the hands and feet are most commonly affected.[283, 308] Findings include cystic lesions, punched-out cortical lesions, or a lacelike trabecular pattern. Rapid progression may lead to pathologic fractures.[283] Rarely, combined osteolytic and osteoblastic changes have been described in the vertebral bodies, sternum, or ribs.[283, 309–311] In one study of untreated patients who had chronic sarcoidosis, 14 of 25 had evidence of vertebral osteoporosis;[312] possible mechanisms include osteoclastic stimulation by granulomas and production of osteoclastic-activating factor by lymphocytes.[308]

**Cardiovascular Disease.** Although abnormalities of the heart, pericardium, and pulmonary vasculature are not uncommon pathologically, they are usually of insufficient severity to cause radiographic manifestations. Enlargement of the cardiac silhouette may be the result of congestive cardiomyopathy, valvular disease, pericardial effusion, and left ventricular aneurysm.[313, 314, 314a] Such cardiac abnormalities may occur in patients with or without lymphadenopathy or evidence of pulmonary disease.[314] MR imaging can be helpful in demonstrating the presence of myocardial involvement.[314] Pulmonary hypertension and cor pulmonale, caused by a combination of obliteration of the pulmonary vascular bed and hypoxic vasoconstriction, tend to occur in the late stage of the disease but can develop earlier.[295] Obstruction of major pulmonary arteries and veins and the superior vena cava by enlarged lymph nodes is rare.[295]

**Abdominal Manifestations.** Abdominal lymphadenopathy, hepatomegaly, and splenomegaly are common radiologic findings in sarcoidosis.[238, 239, 315, 316] For example, in one investigation of 59 patients, abdominal CT scans showed extensive lymphadenopathy in 6 (10%), hepatomegaly in 5 (8%), and splenomegaly in 4 (6%) patients.[239] Nodules were seen in the spleen in 8 patients (15%) and in the liver in 3 (5%). In another review of 46 patients, lymphadenopathy was present in 20 (43%), splenomegaly or low-attenuation lesions in 24 (52%), and hepatomegaly or low-attenuation liver lesions in 7 (15%).[315] The presence of such CT abnormalities is associated with elevated serum ACE levels[239] but not with the stage of thoracic disease.[239, 315]

## CLINICAL MANIFESTATIONS

The reported prevalence of symptoms in sarcoidosis is partly dependent on the means by which the disease is diagnosed. For example, in areas in which radiographic screening is used for routine health care, more asymptomatic patients will be identified; however, if positive findings on biopsy are required for diagnosis, fewer asymptomatic patients will be found. In our and other investigators' experience,[4] symptoms occur in approximately 50% of affected individuals. However, others have found a considerably lesser prevalence; for example, in one review of 227 patients with biopsy-proven disease, only 15% were asymptomatic.[317]

Symptoms often develop insidiously and are frequently associated with multisystem involvement. Constitutional symptoms, including weight loss, fatigue, weakness, and malaise are common. Fever occurs in 15% to 20% of patients;[9] however, in one series it was reported in approximately 40%, with more than one half experiencing night sweats and one third reporting chills.[318] The acute onset of symptoms, usually with erythema nodosum, is particularly common in Scandinavian women; as many as a third of these individuals have been found to present in this fashion.[12] A predilection for erythema nodosum has also been reported in Irish women in London and Puerto Ricans in New York City.[319] The triad of bilateral hilar lymphadenopathy, erythema nodosum, and polyarticular arthritis/arthralgia (Löfgren's syndrome) has also long been recognized as an acute presentation (*see* farther on).[320] Whether coincidental or linked via common susceptibility or exposure, sarcoidosis has been described in association with a variety of connective tissue disorders, including rheumatoid arthritis, ankylosing spondylitis, systemic lupus erythematosus, and progressive systemic sclerosis;[321, 323] in fact, the prevalence of such associations may be underestimated, because symptoms caused by sarcoidosis could easily be attributed to the underlying connective tissue disease, or vice versa.

Signs and symptoms can be related to the involvement of many organs and tissues,[322] the most common being the lungs, heart, skin, and eyes.

**Lungs.** Symptoms of pulmonary involvement develop in about one third of patients[5, 8, 9] and include dry cough and shortness of breath.[3, 5, 324, 325] Hemoptysis is uncommon.[326] For example, in one series of 433 patients, it occurred in

only 25 (6%); it was mild in 19, moderate in 4, and massive in 2.[327] The complication is usually attributable to an aspergilloma in an ectatic bronchus or cystic space.[328, 329] Chest pain can be caused by excessive coughing and rarely is pleuritic in type.[330–332] Symptoms related to pleural involvement (effusion, fibrosis, or pneumothorax) are also rare;[332a] the authors of one literature review estimated that only about 2% of patients were so afflicted.[333]

Auscultatory signs of pleuropulmonary disease usually are absent in the early stages of the disease, although a few scattered crackles can be heard in some patients; with the development of pulmonary fibrosis, crackles can become more widespread. Rhonchi or wheezes may be audible in patients with endobronchial involvement;[334–339] wheezes also may be appreciated in the occasional patient who develops airway hyperresponsiveness.[340] Clubbing is rare, but may be seen in patients with bronchiectasis or pulmonary fibrosis.[342]

**Heart and Blood Vessels.** The cardiovascular system can be affected directly or indirectly. *Indirect* involvement includes pulmonary arterial hypertension and cor pulmonale secondary to extensive parenchymal fibrosis, hypoxemia, or (rarely) compression of the pulmonary arteries[341, 343, 344] or veins[345] by enlarged hilar or mediastinal lymph nodes. Such extrinsic compression can also affect the superior vena cava[346] and left innominate vein;[347] compression of the latter vessel has also been reported to cause massive left-sided pleural effusion.[347] Pulmonary hypertension is generally associated with Stage 3 disease, but can also occur in patients who have Stage 1 or 2 disease.[348–350]

*Direct* involvement of the heart can be manifested in a variety of ways, including paroxysmal arrhythmias,[351–354] left ventricular failure,[351–356] valvular abnormalities such as mitral insufficiency,[351, 353] angina-like chest pain due to small vessel involvement,[352, 357] sudden death,[351] and ventricular aneurysm.[351–355, 358] Despite this impressive list and the fact that histologic examination reveals granulomatous myocarditis in 25% to 50% of patients at autopsy,[8, 351–354, 359-361] clinical effects are recognized in only a minority.

The authors of one comprehensive autopsy study of 108 patients who had clinically evident cardiac sarcoidosis, concluded that cardiac dysfunction was caused by granulomatous infiltration in 89%.[355] Sixty of the 89 had died suddenly, and in 10 of these the sudden death was the initial manifestation of disease; 20 others had died of progressive cardiac failure, 3 from recurring pericardial effusion, and 6 from unknown causes. Of 163 cases of cardiac disease secondary to sarcoidosis studied in the United Kingdom, the age at presentation with cardiac abnormalities ranged from 18 to 77 (mean, about 45) years, with no sex predominance;[362] however, in another report of 320 autopsies in Japan, a 2 to 1 female predominance was documented.[361] In an American series, the average age of the 70 patients who died was 47 years;[362] death was sudden in 45 patients, and in 26 of these no previous diagnosis of heart disease or sarcoidosis had been made. Most patients presented with either complete or partial heart block. The time interval from the onset of cardiac symptoms to death from myocardial involvement has been reported to range from 3 months to 15 years.[363] In the series of 108 autopsies cited previously, a ventricular aneurysm was identified in 8.[355] This complication appears to be particularly common in African Americans;[364] there is also evidence that it is more likely to occur in patients who receive corticosteroids.[355]

As might be expected from the previous discussion, electrocardiographic abnormalities occur more frequently in patients with sarcoidosis than in matched controls.[351, 365, 366] In fact, the diagnosis of sarcoidosis should be considered in any young individual with unexplained arrhythmia, heart block, or congestive heart failure, even in the absence of typical radiographic features of sarcoidosis.[351, 352]

Cardiac sarcoidosis is difficult to diagnose. It is one of the few conditions that can cause a focal abnormality of wall motion on echocardiography in the absence of coronary artery disease, typically in the upper septal area with preservation of apical function (a distinctly unusual pattern to be caused by coronary artery disease).[352] Although echocardiography may be useful in diagnosis, other studies are generally required. Radionuclide imaging with thallium-201 may reveal myocardial perfusion defects;[367, 368] unlike patients who have coronary artery disease, these lesions are reversible with dipyridamole infusion.[369] Larger defects have been described using technetium-99m sestamibi and single-photon emission computed tomography, with greater sensitivity than with thallium.[370] Whether gallium-67 uptake in affected myocardium predicts corticosteroid responsiveness remains to be determined.[371] There is little experience with MR imaging.[353, 372] Although myocardial biopsy is highly specific, the procedure lacks sensitivity. In the final analysis, the diagnosis of cardiac sarcoidosis in a patient with pulmonary and systemic disease is often presumptive.[351, 353]

**Lymph Nodes.** As indicated previously, enlarged mediastinal or hilar lymph nodes may cause clinical signs and symptoms as a result of vascular compression.[343–347] Enlargement of peripheral lymph nodes is said to be clinically evident in about 75% of cases.[9] In fact, it is possible that nodal involvement occurs at some time in every case of sarcoidosis whether nodes are palpable or not; for example, lymph node biopsies from regions such as the scalene area are positive in 80% of cases, even when they are not palpable.[373, 374] Palpable lymph nodes are found most frequently in the cervical area, but they also may be felt in the axilla, epitrochlear regions, and the groin.[4]

**Eyes.** The incidence of ocular involvement varies considerably from series to series, depending at least partly on the interest of the physician or ophthalmologist in sarcoidosis as a generalized disease and partly on the sophistication of the ophthalmologic examination. If slit lamp examination is utilized, the eye can be found to be affected in about 25% of patients.[375] Acute or chronic anterior uveitis is the most frequent finding (about two thirds of patients);[375] posterior and generalized uveitis are each seen in about 15% of patients.[375] Other ocular abnormalities include conjunctivitis, scleritis, lacrimal gland enlargement (*see* farther on), choroidoretinitis, periphlebitis retinae, macular and optic nerve edema, retinal hemorrhage, and (rarely) neovascularization.[375]

In general, acute ocular disease is more commonly seen in acute sarcoid syndromes, whereas chronic problems occur in patients with chronic fibrotic pulmonary and systemic disease.[375] Ocular symptoms may constitute the presenting feature of sarcoidosis[376] and may be confused with many conditions, even an orbital tumor (in a patient with proptosis related to a retro-ocular mass of granulomatous inflammatory

tissue).[377] Likewise, choroidal granulomas can be the sole manifestation of the disease and can be confused with metastatic carcinoma.[378] Blindness developed in 3.5% of 145 patients in one early series.[9]

**Skin.** Cutaneous involvement occurs in 20% to 30% of patients;[9, 379, 380] for example, of 818 patients observed in an English sarcoidosis clinic, 251 (31%) had erythema nodosum and 147 (21%) had some other dermatologic manifestation at some time in their disease course.[381] Patients with skin disease (except for erythema nodosum) are more likely to have lymph node, hepatic, and splenic involvement than patients without cutaneous lesions.[380]

Skin lesions may be "specific" (granulomas present pathologically) or nonspecific. The most frequent nonspecific abnormality is erythema nodosum, which has been reported in 3% to 25% of cases.[382] This is a form of panniculitis that most commonly involves the shins and is characterized by the development of crops of transient, nonulcerating nodules that are usually tender, multiple, and bilateral; the lesions resolve slowly, leaving bruiselike patches without scarring.[383]

Lupus pernio ("purple lupus") consists of purplish nodules usually occurring on the face, neck, shoulders, digits, and (sometimes) the mucous membrane of the nose; it is often associated with involvement of nasal bones.[384] Large plaques resembling psoriasis may develop over the trunk or extremities. Both abnormalities are usually associated with a chronic course; for example, in one series, radiologic resolution of pulmonary disease occurred in only 22% of the patients with skin plaques and in none of those with lupus pernio.[379] Lupus pernio itself seldom, if ever, resolves completely[385, 386] and patients may be left with unsightly, telangiectatic scars.[385]

"Specific" dermal involvement is manifested most often as smooth, soft, red-brown asymptomatic papulonodular lesions; these can be found anywhere on the body and may be solitary or coalescent, deep or superficial. Papules appear in crops and are scattered over the face or grouped closely together at the nape of the neck.[381] Although they tend to occur early in acute disease, like lupus pernio they can be seen in the subacute and chronic phases, during which they tend to coalesce into pebbled, brownish or purplish smooth plaques.[381] Rare dermal manifestations of sarcoidosis include a localized scleroderma-like lesion,[381a] a rhinophyma-like lesion,[381b] and leukocytoclastic vasculitis.[381c]

Involvement of old and recent cutaneous scars by granulomatous inflammation is well recognized in patients with sarcoidosis.[4, 387] The development of non-necrotizing granulomas at the venipuncture site of six blood donors, five of whom also had bilateral hilar lymph node enlargement radiographically, also has been reported.[388]

**Liver and Spleen.** The incidence of hepatic and splenic involvement depends on whether the figures are obtained from clinical or pathologic studies. Whereas autopsy reveals granulomas at these sites in approximately two thirds of cases, the liver and spleen are palpable on physical examination in only about 20% of patients.[389] The degree of liver involvement is seldom sufficient to cause symptoms, with evidence of disease usually being derived from liver biopsy, measurement of serum liver enzymes, or hepatomegaly in patients with known sarcoidosis.

Hepatic involvement can be associated with a variety of histologic and clinical abnormalities that mimic those of other primary liver diseases.[390, 390a] Rarely, there is a picture of active liver disease with abnormalities of liver function and liver cell destruction and fibrosis on biopsy.[390] MR imaging can be useful in distinguishing this form of disease from neoplasia or other inflammatory conditions.[389] Occasionally, granulomatous inflammation is responsible for a nodular rather than a diffusely infiltrative appearance on CT of the liver and spleen. In a review of 32 patients who had this abnormality, the chest film was normal in 25%, whereas the majority had evidence of advanced pulmonary disease, high ACE levels, systemic and/or abdominal symptoms, and abdominal adenopathy.[391]

Sarcoidosis can also lead to a picture of chronic cholestasis, a complication that is most common in young black men and has a poor prognosis.[389] It may be difficult to distinguish from primary biliary cirrhosis,[392–395] especially in cases in which the latter is accompanied by lung disease; however, primary biliary cirrhosis is much more common in women, has a different appearance on liver biopsy, and is associated with antimitochondrial antibodies.[389] With or without evidence of cholestasis, some patients with chronic sarcoidosis develop portal hypertension as a result of obstruction of the portal vein radicals by foci of granulomatous inflammation.[389] Budd-Chiari syndrome has also resulted from narrowing and subsequent thrombosis of the hepatic veins secondary to granulomatous inflammation.[389, 390a]

The discovery of non-necrotizing granulomas in liver tissue obtained by biopsy carried out for reasons other than to substantiate a clinical diagnosis of sarcoidosis presents a rather perplexing problem. The cause can be identified in about 90% of cases;[389, 392, 393, 396] in addition to sarcoidosis,[397] it includes infection, primary biliary cirrhosis, neoplasms (particularly Hodgkin's disease[398, 399]), Crohn's disease, chronic active hepatitis, and drug reactions. The term *granulomatous hepatitis* has been used to describe the disease in the 10% of patients in whom these or other causes have been excluded. Such patients are usually febrile; the condition may remit spontaneously or require corticosteroid therapy.[389]

As in the liver, splenic sarcoidosis is seldom symptomatic. Occasionally, splenomegaly develops and becomes so severe as to necessitate splenectomy because of hypersplenism or because of a space-occupying effect.[8, 400] Of 32 patients with splenomegaly in one study, 7 had hypersplenism and most responded to corticosteroid therapy;[401] the spleen decreased in size in all but 1 patient, who required splenectomy.

**Gastrointestinal Tract.** Symptomatic involvement of the gastrointestinal tract is very rare.[402, 403] However, the demonstration of markedly increased intestinal permeability (associated histologically with edema and T-cell accumulation) in conjunction with evidence of active, subclinical pulmonary disease might implicate the gut in the pathogenesis of sarcoidosis.[404] A study of the incidence of humoral sensitivity to dietary proteins has revealed that about 40% of patients who have sarcoidosis show a specific sensitization to the wheat protein α-gliadin.[405] This could be related to the increase in gut permeability or could represent an altered gastrointestinal immune response. Celiac disease has also been found rarely in patients who have sarcoidosis.[406]

The esophagus can be affected by extension from contiguous mediastinal lymph nodes, sometimes with resulting dysphagia.[407, 408] One patient has been described in whom infiltration of Auerbach's plexus by granulomas resulted in achalasia.[409] An endoscopic biopsy study of 60 patients with sarcoidosis revealed the presence of granulomas in 6.[410] Cases have also been reported of abdominal sarcoidosis associated with ascites[411] and a perforated appendix.[412]

**Salivary and Lacrimal Glands.** Involvement of salivary glands is not uncommon; for example, in one study of 75 patients who underwent random biopsy of the lower lip, granulomas were found in the minor salivary gland in 44 (58%).[413] In another investigation of 537 patients, parotid gland enlargement was described in 33 (6%);[403] it was bilateral in 24. As in Sjögren's syndrome, lymphocytic infiltration of the salivary glands is associated with expression of HLA-DR antigen on the epithelial cells,[414] which also express a high level of IL-2 receptors. The combination of parotid gland involvement, uveitis, and pyrexia is called uveoparotid fever; the combination of parotid gland enlargement, uveitis, and facial nerve palsy is known as Heerfordt's syndrome. Although clinically evident parotid gland involvement may be absent in patients who have uveitis, the volume of saliva and enzyme secretion from both this gland and the submaxillary gland is often decreased.[415]

Involvement of the lacrimal glands also is probably common, although these are rarely sampled. In Scadding's classic review, the glands were palpable in only 2 of 275 cases;[4] however, such involvement may result in keratoconjunctivitis sicca and duct obstruction.[416]

**Musculoskeletal System and Joints.** Three forms of joint involvement have been described:[417] (1) migratory polyarthritis associated with erythema nodosum, fever, and hilar lymph node enlargement; (2) single or recurrent episodes of polyarticular or monoarticular arthritis; and (3) persistent arthritis. The first of these is the most frequent. It is really a polyarthralgia rather than an arthritis and tends to involve the larger joints, particularly the ankles, wrists, elbows, and knees.[308, 418, 419] In our experience, inflammation of the periarticular tissue may be prominent in such patients. Symptoms are usually self-limited and last from a few days to several months;[418, 419] occasionally, they recur or are associated with chronic myalgia and fibromyalgia.[418] Typically, patients are left free of disability.

True arthritis is uncommon and usually is seen in patients with multiple system involvement.[420] It tends to develop during the course of chronic pulmonary disease[421] and, although usually transient, can persist for as long as a year. Rarely, a patient develops a chronic arthropathy with joint deformation and destruction.[308] When joint involvement is prominent clinically, synovial biopsy is likely to reveal granulomas.[422, 423]

Among the bones, those of the hands and feet are the most commonly involved;[308] the axial skeleton is occasionally the site of cyst formation.[308, 424, 425] As indicated previously, lupus pernio may be associated with involvement of nasal bones.[308] Bone pain is very uncommon,[400] even in the rare patient with hypertrophic pulmonary osteoarthropathy. Involvement of skeletal muscle by granulomatous inflammation can give rise to weakness.[426] Rarely, syndromes of acute polymyositis or chronic myopathy have been described.[308, 427] Much more commonly, patients receiving corticosteroids develop a steroid myopathy that can clinically imitate sarcoid myopathy.[308]

**Kidney.** Clinical or functional evidence of renal disease is uncommon,[428–430] despite the fact that granulomas are found in the kidneys in 5% to 20% of autopsied patients.[431] Clinically significant disease occurs principally by two mechanisms: (1) direct involvement of the kidneys by granulomatous inflammation (interstitial nephritis); and (2) as a result of abnormal calcium metabolism, with nephrocalcinosis, urolithiasis, or hypercalcemic renal failure. The use of corticosteroids for the treatment of sarcoidosis has likely resulted in a decrease in the prevalence of renal failure by the second mechanism.[432] Given the relative rarity of renal disease in patients with sarcoidosis, coincidental pathology must be considered in the differential diagnosis.

Granulomatous interstitial nephritis is a rare cause of renal failure. However, in one survey of renal biopsies done at three general hospitals serving a population of 700,000 patients in England, four such cases were discovered.[432] These patients constituted 7% of the 58 patients who had biopsies for the diagnosis of chronic renal failure; in 2, renal biopsy results were the first sign of sarcoidosis.

Hypercalcemia occurs in up to 30% of patients who have sarcoidosis. Hypercalciuria is even more common and accounts for the increased frequency of renal stones; occasionally, these provide the first indication of the disease.[433] The pathogenesis of the hypercalcemia is at least partly related to dysregulated production of 1,25-dihydroxyvitamin $D_3$ (calcitriol) by epithelioid histiocytes within pulmonary and other granulomas.[396, 434, 433, 435] Conversion was initially believed to occur only in the kidneys; however, levels of this hormone have been shown to be elevated in the serum of patients who have sarcoidosis and hypercalcemia who are anephric[436] or who have end-stage renal disease.[437] The variation in vitamin D metabolism is seasonal, being accentuated in the summer as a result of an increase in activation of vitamin D by ultraviolet radiation.[438] Although hypercalcemia rarely leads to renal failure, it is commonly associated with interstitial calcium deposition, chronic inflammation, and interstitial fibrosis. We have seen one patient in whom intense sunbathing appeared to precipitate symptomatic hypercalcemia. It is also possible that production of parathyroid hormone–related protein by epithelioid macrophages in sarcoid granulomas may contribute to the development of hypercalcemia.[438a]

There is also evidence that calcitriol may have a role in the pathogenesis of sarcoidosis; it contributes to the proliferation and differentiation of circulating monocytes into macrophages, is able to stimulate epithelioid histiocytes in granulomas to produce ACE, and inhibits proliferation and lymphokine production of T-helper cells.[439]

Glomerular disease is rare in sarcoidosis, although it is likely that there are more cases of membranous nephropathy than can be explained by chance.[440–443] A single case of minimal change disease has also been reported.[443a] Glomerular calcinosis has also been reported.[444] Rarely, urinary tract sarcoidosis mimics other urologic disease; for example, renal sarcoidosis may be confused with a neoplasm, and retroperitoneal lymph node enlargement has been a cause of ureteric obstruction.[432] Compression of the renal artery by enlarged retroperitoneal lymph nodes has also been reported.[432, 445]

**Central and Peripheral Nervous System.** Involvement of the nervous system is evident in 5% of patients during life[446–448] and in 15% to 25% at autopsy. Abnormalities occur in the cranial and peripheral nerves, the brain, the spinal cord, and the meninges.[449–457] Among patients who have neurologic manifestations of sarcoidosis, these constitute the first clinical evidence of disease in 50% to 75% of patients. Although any cranial nerve can be affected, the second and seventh are most commonly involved, presumably as a result of extension of disease from underlying meninges[438] or from nasal lesions.[459] Unilateral or bilateral facial palsy is sometimes associated with uveoparotid fever. A case of bilateral diaphragmatic paresis secondary to phrenic nerve involvement has also been reported.[459a] Cerebral lesions can result in grand mal seizures and can simulate metastatic carcinoma.[460] Psychiatric presentations include delirium, depression, personality changes, and psychosis.[447, 461]

Even in the presence of established sarcoidosis, other explanations for central nervous system (CNS) pathology should be considered before arriving at a diagnosis of CNS involvement.[448] For example, patients who have sarcoidosis appear to be at risk for progressive multifocal leukoencephalopathy,[459, 462] a fatal disease with characteristics that can be misinterpreted as being caused by cerebral sarcoidosis. MR imaging with gadolinium enhancement is the most sensitive diagnostic test to detect CNS sarcoidosis, especially in patients who have meningeal involvement.[463]

A characteristic intracranial localization of sarcoidosis is the hypothalamus and pituitary gland.[446, 464–466] Affected patients often complain of polyuria and polydipsia, symptoms usually associated with a deficiency of antidiuretic hormone (ADH) and diabetes insipidus. It has been shown, however, that many patients with hypothalamic-pituitary sarcoidosis have adequate reserves of ADH, in which case the cause of these symptoms remains obscure.[466] In one patient, hypothalamic involvement was the cause of narcolepsy;[467] resolution occurred with cranial radiation therapy.

**Upper Respiratory Tract.** Clinically evident involvement of the upper respiratory passages is rare. The epiglottis is the most common site to be affected; its enlargement as a result of granuloma accumulation can cause significant obstruction,[468, 469] sometimes requiring tracheostomy.[470, 471] Laryngeal granulomas have been identified in 1% to 2% of patients;[472] symptoms include dyspnea, cough, and hoarseness. Stridor is evident occasionally.[505] Hoarseness can also result from the extension of disease into the recurrent laryngeal nerve from contiguous lymph nodes in the mediastinum.[473] Upper airway obstruction causing sleep apnea has also been described in one patient.[473a]

**Miscellaneous Sites.** Although clinically evident breast involvement is extremely rare, tumors caused by conglomerated granulomas have been described.[304, 474, 475] Likewise, endometrial sarcoidosis is rare.[476]

## PULMONARY FUNCTION TESTS

Pulmonary parenchymal involvement in sarcoidosis usually produces a restrictive impairment with reduction in lung volumes.[477] Although attempts have been made to show that progression of stage in sarcoidosis is linked to progressive deterioration in lung function,[478, 479] pulmonary function varies considerably among patients who manifest similar degrees of disease radiographically.[480, 481] For example, in one investigation of patients with pathologically proven pulmonary sarcoidosis and no evidence of parenchymal abnormality on plain radiographs, only 80% were found to have a normal vital capacity (VC) and 70% a normal diffusing capacity (DLCO);[482] by contrast, 35% of patients with radiographic evidence of parenchymal disease had a normal VC and almost 35% a normal DLCO.

Most (albeit not all[483]) investigators have shown an increasing prevalence of low DLCO with increasing radiographic stage.[477, 478, 484] However, within any particular stage, the results are quite variable. The DLCO can remain reduced when other function tests have improved and after symptoms have disappeared and the chest radiograph has returned to normal;[485, 486] in such cases, lung biopsy reveals interstitial granulomatous or fibrotic disease.[487] A reduction in both static and dynamic pulmonary compliance has also been described.[488–490]

Reductions in DLCO and alterations in gas exchange can be present on exercise, even in asymptomatic patients.[491–494] In those with normal spirometry, gas exchange abnormalities on exercise are much more likely in the presence of an abnormal DLCO; in one study, only one of 17 patients with a normal DLCO had abnormal gas exchange on exercise, whereas 7 of 9 patients with a reduced DLCO had this finding.[495] In the same investigation, ventilation requirements and dead space/tidal volume ratio (VD/VT) during exercise also tended to be abnormal in patients with abnormal DLCOs; however, impairment was still noted in a significant minority of patients with normal spirometry and DLCO, an observation that illustrates the sensitivity of exercise testing for the demonstration of physiologic derangement.

Abnormalities of cardiocirculatory function, such as excessive heart rate and low $O_2$ pulse, have also been found on exercise testing in patients with sarcoidosis.[349, 496, 497] These might be the result of subclinical impairment of right[349, 496] or left[497] ventricular function by cardiac sarcoidosis or, in the case of right-sided disease, changes in the lung vasculature secondary to pulmonary disease.

Although the majority of patients who have sarcoidosis and abnormal lung function have restrictive abnormalities, many manifest an obstructive deficit as well. In a small number the pattern is solely obstructive.[498] In fact, in one investigation of 123 African Americans who had sarcoidosis (about 90% of whom had never smoked), airway obstruction was present in 78 (63%);[484] in another study of 107 newly diagnosed patients (of whom 30 had never smoked) 61 (57%) had evidence of air flow obstruction.[478] In contrast to many previous studies, air flow obstruction was the most common functional abnormality, with restrictive lung volumes being noted in only 7 patients and an abnormally low DLCO in 29. Using sensitive tests of small airways dysfunction, such as dynamic compliance, measurement of upstream resistance, and ratio of closing volume to vital capacity, impairment of small airways function can be demonstrated in asymptomatic nonsmoking patients who have sarcoidosis.[478, 484, 499–504]

When clinical signs or routine function tests suggest the presence of airway obstruction, a number of mechanisms must be considered. Sarcoidosis may affect airways of all sizes, including the larynx or trachea. Evidence of small airway disease may be seen on expiratory HRCT. In one report of three patients who had sarcoidosis, expiratory HRCT scans showed patchy air trapping at the level of the secondary pulmonary lobules, consistent with small airway disease.[506] Several investigators have looked at bronchial response to methacholine in patients who have sarcoidosis, and some have found airway hyperresponsiveness.[340, 507–509a] Peak inspiratory mouth pressures may also be reduced in patients with sarcoidosis; in some cases, this has been ascribed to granulomatous inflammation of the respiratory musculature.[510]

Although radiographic findings correlate poorly with clinical and functional impairment in cross-sectional studies, serial radiographs are an accurate means of predicting functional impairment in longitudinal studies. In a study comparing sequential radiographs and pulmonary function tests in 64 patients, the authors showed that when patients were used as their own control, changes in the severity of parenchymal abnormalities on the radiograph correlated well with functional changes over time.[260] In patients whose chest radiographs improved, both the vital capacity and the DLCO improved, although the functional parameters seldom returned to normal even when the radiograph showed complete resolution of the parenchymal abnormalities.

The severity of clinical and functional impairment in patients who have sarcoidosis has been compared with the findings on HRCT in several studies.[246, 259, 264, 511] These have shown a significant but modest correlation between extent of parenchymal abnormalities on HRCT and severity of dyspnea (r = 0.6), DLCO (r = −0.5 to −0.6), and vital capacity (r = −0.4 to −0.8). In one study, patients with nodular opacities were shown to have less clinical impairment than patients who had irregular linear opacities.[259] In another investigation, no significant correlation was found between nodular opacities and functional parameters.[264] In two studies in which HRCT and radiographic findings were compared, the former were found to be superior to the latter in demonstrating the presence of parenchymal abnormalities;[246, 259] however, the radiographic and CT assessments of disease severity showed similar correlations with clinical and functional impairment.

## LABORATORY FINDINGS

A variety of laboratory techniques have been used to support a diagnosis of sarcoidosis, to clarify its pathogenesis, to assess the likelihood of response to therapy, to monitor response to treatment, and to estimate prognosis. Attempts have been made to correlate the findings of different tests with each other and with clinical features, radiographic stage, and pulmonary function abnormalities. Such tests include the measurement of differential cell counts in BAL fluid, biochemical assays of a variety of substances in BAL fluid and serum (especially serum ACE), and gallium-67 uptake by the lungs. Although innumerable reports have been published, resulting in an abundance of information, the conclusions of various authors differ in many respects and in some instances are contradictory. The most important variables accounting for these inconsistencies are the methodology employed, the patient population studied, and the activity of the disease.

**Analysis of BAL Fluid.** Information regarding the number, type, and state of activation of inflammatory and immune cells and the presence of cytokines and other mediators of inflammation and fibrosis in BAL fluid was outlined previously (*see* page 1536); the value of these measurements in estimating prognosis is discussed on page 1572.

**Gallium 67 Scanning.** This test has been used for many years to detect sites of inflammation or neoplasia, both in the lungs and elsewhere (*see* page 331).[512] The results of many (albeit not all[513]) investigations suggest that the correlation between the percentage of lymphocytes found in BAL fluid and gallium 67 scintiscans is good.[514, 515] The sensitivity of gallium 67 scintigraphy in detecting inflammatory lesions in general has been estimated to range from 80% to more than 90%. This test has been used, on occasion, to detect the presence of pulmonary disease in patients who have Stages 0 and 1 sarcoidosis.[516, 517]

When sarcoidosis is suspected, the pattern of gallium uptake may also have diagnostic importance. Provided certain technical considerations are taken into account, the findings of a "lambda" gallium distribution (well circumscribed, uniform, symmetric uptake of gallium in both the parahilar and infrahilar lymph nodes and in the right paratracheal mediastinal lymph nodes) or a "panda" image (abnormal bilateral, symmetric uptake by the lacrimal and parotid glands with or without submandibular gland uptake) *together with* bilateral symmetric hilar lymphadenopathy or bilateral symmetric pulmonary fibrosis have both been found to be highly specific for sarcoidosis (Fig. 41–36).[517] In one investigation of 162 patients who had sarcoidosis, these patterns of gallium uptake were seen in approximately 30% of the 21 patients who had Stage 0 disease, 75% of the 39 patients who had Stage 1 disease, 90% of 47 patients who had Stage 2 disease, and 70% of the 21 patients who had "Stage 4" involvement.[475] There were no false-positive diagnoses made in 167 human immunodeficiency virus (HIV)-positive patients (most of whom had acquired immunodeficiency syndrome). This investigation included many patients who had atypical radiographic features of sarcoidosis, such as unilateral hilar lymphadenopathy or asymmetric lung opacities.

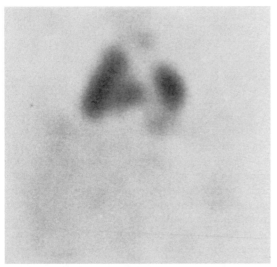

**Figure 41–36. Sarcoidosis: Lambda Pattern.** A coronal single photon emission computed tomography (SPECT) image obtained 24 hours after intravenous administration of gallium-67 citrate shows increased activity in both hila and in the right paratracheal region. (Courtesy of Dr. Daniel Worsley, Department of Radiology, Vancouver General Hospital, Vancouver, British Columbia.)

The "panda" pattern *without* parenchymal lung disease or symmetric hilar lymphadenopathy has been seen in 8% of HIV-positive patients, in patients with Sjögren's syndrome, and after irradiation of the head and neck;[517] however, it has not been described in untreated patients with lymphoma in the absence of an associated condition such as Sjögren's syndrome or previous radiation therapy.[517] In another report, bilateral hilar uptake of gallium was documented in 81 of 172 (47%) patients with sarcoidosis but in none of 21 with lymphoma.[518]

In summary, it seems reasonable to conclude that the identification of a lambda or panda pattern of gallium uptake in the appropriate clinical and radiologic context lends strong support for a diagnosis of sarcoidosis; the test may be particularly useful when radiologic features of disease, including those on HRCT scans, are atypical.

**Angiotensin-Converting Enzyme.** Measurement of ACE in the serum or in BAL fluid has been extensively investigated for its usefulness in the diagnosis of sarcoidosis. ACE normally resides within pinocytotic vesicles in pulmonary capillary endothelial cells where it converts angiotensin I into angiotensin II as the former passes through the pulmonary circulation. Although some of the ACE in sarcoidosis probably comes from this source, there is evidence that a considerable portion is derived from the granulomas themselves. Such evidence includes (1) the demonstration by immunofluorescence of ACE in sarcoid granulomas;[519] (2) ultrastructural studies suggesting that epithelioid cells possess a synthetic, rather than a phagocytic, function;[11] (3) the demonstration *in vitro* of secretion of ACE by epithelioid cells;[520] (4) the observation that ACE levels are increased in granulomatous diseases other than sarcoidosis (e.g., in talc-induced pulmonary granulomas in rabbits[521]); (5) the finding in patients with sarcoidosis of ACE activity in circulating monocytes, the precursors of epithelioid cells;[522, 523] and (6) the observation in a murine model of granulomatous inflammation that the ACE activity as assessed by the tissue level of ACE messenger RNA (mRNA) correlates with the burden of granulomatous tissue assessed histologically.[524] ACE may also have a role as a modulator of granuloma formation by means of local production of angiotensin II in granulomas,[439] because this substance is chemotactic for macrophages and may increase their activation in an autocrine fashion.[439]

The level of ACE in BAL fluid is elevated in many patients who have active sarcoidosis.[331, 525, 526] In these patients, the lavage ACE-to-albumen ratio is 10-fold higher than the same ratio in the serum,[526] indicating that the increased ACE is the result of local production rather than altered capillary permeability. In one investigation, high levels of ACE in BAL fluid were detected in all 16 patients with active disease, some of whom had normal values for ACE in their serum.[525] In a second study, levels of ACE in BAL fluid were higher in patients with Stage 2 and Stage 3 disease than in those who had Stage 1 disease.[527] However, the wide distribution of ACE levels in BAL fluid in both control patients and those with sarcoidosis,[526] as well as the lack of specificity of the finding,[527] limits the clinical usefulness of this measure. Although serum ACE levels may be reduced in drug-induced pulmonary disease and adult respiratory distress syndrome, they are often increased in a variety of diseases other than sarcoidosis.[528, 529]

Both spectrophotometric and radioimmunoassay methods have been used to measure the level of serum ACE;[523, 530–532] in general, levels are accepted as being raised when they are 2 SD above the control mean value. Mean values of serum ACE are significantly higher in healthy children and adolescents up to the age of 20 than in adults.[533–535] Men and women have similar levels, and there is no change with aging. African Americans tend to have higher levels than whites.[536]

A number of variants in the ACE gene have been described that may influence ACE levels in the normal population.[537–540] However, the variant genes do not seem to be risk factors for the development of sarcoidosis or for a modification of disease severity in patients who have sarcoidosis. In one investigation, the distribution of genotypes was found to be similar in patients with sarcoidosis and control individuals;[540] although ACE levels correlated weakly with disease severity (as assessed by radiographic stage), there was no relationship between ACE genotype and radiographic stage. However, in one study from Japan, a correlation was found between ACE genotype and the presence of airway hyper-responsiveness.[509a]

The incidence of increased serum ACE levels ranges from 33% to almost 90% in series of patients who have recent onset of clinically active sarcoidosis and are not being treated with steroids.[531–534, 536, 541–546] There is evidence that applying a different normal range for the serum ACE values for each genotype can improve the sensitivity of the test for the diagnosis of sarcoidosis.[547, 548] With few exceptions,[533, 549] normal results are found more often in Stage 1 than in Stage 2 disease; serum ACE levels were increased in 7 (39%) of 18 patients with Stage 0 in one investigation.[39, 542, 543] There are few reports in which the levels of serum ACE have been documented in patients considered on clinical grounds to have inactive sarcoidosis; however, 2 of 12 such patients in one series[543] and 11% in another[523] had elevated values.

Although measurement of serum ACE levels has some value in supporting a diagnosis of sarcoidosis, it must be remembered that false-positive results (values that are 2 SD above the control mean) occur in 1% to 6% of normal subjects[523, 531, 533, 542, 545, 550] and in patients with a variety of other diseases (Table 41–2). However, patients who have sarcoidosis are much more likely to have higher values of serum ACE than those with the conditions in this rather formidable list; moreover, the prevalence of abnormal values is generally much greater in groups of patients who have sarcoidosis than in patients with other conditions.

In summary, despite the occurrence of false-positive results in many pulmonary diseases that resemble sarcoidosis, the measurement of serum ACE levels is occasionally useful in supporting a diagnosis. Its association with disease activity and usefulness in the monitoring of disease course and response to therapy are discussed farther on (see page 1573).

**Miscellaneous Serum Abnormalities.** A variety of other biochemical abnormalities have been documented in patients who have sarcoidosis; as with alterations in ACE levels, attempts have been made to use these in diagnosis and follow-up. The serum lysozyme level is often increased and has been proposed as a useful index of disease activity.[551, 552] After an evaluation of levels of this enzyme and of serum ACE in patients with sarcoidosis,[534, 546, 553] one group of

## Table 41–2. DISEASES ASSOCIATED WITH ELEVATED SERUM ANGIOTENSIN-CONVERTING ENZYME

| DISEASE | SELECTED REFERENCES |
|---|---|
| *Infection* | |
| Tuberculosis | 533, 550 |
| *Mycobacterium intracellulare* infection | |
| Coccidioidomycosis | 544 |
| Leprosy | 536 |
| *Neoplasms* | |
| Lymphoma | 533, 536 |
| Multiple myeloma | |
| *Immunologic Disease* | |
| Extrinsic allergic alveolitis | 550 |
| Ulcerative colitis | 676 |
| Idiopathic pulmonary fibrosis | 550 |
| *Airway Disease* | |
| Chronic obstructive pulmonary disease | |
| Asthma | 530, 550 |
| *Inorganic Dust Inhalation* | |
| Silicosis | |
| Asbestosis | 534, 544 |
| Berylliosis | 536 |
| *Metabolic Disease* | |
| Hyperthyroidism | 544 |
| Amyloidosis | 523 |
| Gaucher's disease | 523, 677 |
| Diabetes mellitus | |
| *Miscellaneous Diseases* | |
| Osteoarthritis | 536 |
| Hepatitis and alcoholic cirrhosis | 678, 679 |
| Biliary cirrhosis | 523, 533 |
| Lymphangioleiomyomatosis | 523 |
| Chronic granulomatous disease of children | 680 |
| Chronic fatigue–immune dysfunction syndrome | 681 |
| Familial Mediterranean fever | 682 |

investigators concluded that lysozyme was more likely to be elevated in the early stages of the disease, particularly in patients who have erythema nodosum.[553] These investigators also found the levels of both enzymes to decrease before clinical improvement could be detected. Of some interest was the observation that serum levels of ACE and lysozyme were not related in normal subjects but showed a positive correlation when they were elevated in patients with active sarcoidosis; this suggests separate sources for these enzymes when ACE activity is normal and a common source (e.g., epithelioid histiocytes) when ACE activity is increased.[534] Like ACE, the lysozyme level can be raised in pulmonary diseases that are included in the differential diagnosis of sarcoidosis.[554]

The level of serum alkaline phosphatase has been found to be increased in 30% to 45% of patients who have sarcoidosis,[9] accompanied by an elevated urinary level of the amino acid hydroxyproline during the acute stage of the disease.[555] In one study, the level of serum $\beta_2$-microglobulin, a low-molecular-weight protein associated with the histocompatibility antigens and thought to reflect activation of immunocompetent cells (particularly lymphocytes), was found to be elevated in 63% of 132 patients with sarcoidosis at a time when only 32% had elevated values of ACE.[556]

Hypercalcemia is seen in about 10% of patients who have sarcoidosis; hypercalciuria occurs in about 30%.[557] The former is said by most, but not all,[558] investigators, to be more evident in the summer months, presumably as a result of increased exposure to sunlight.[438, 559, 560] The hypercalcemia usually can be corrected by corticosteroid therapy, thereby serving to differentiate it from the hypercalcemia of hyperparathyroidism. In fact, some patients who have sarcoidosis and whose hypercalcemia fails to respond to corticosteroid therapy have subsequently been found to have hyperparathyroidism.[561–565] Aside from the renal effects of hypercalcemia (*see* page 1566), metastatic calcification can occur in organs and tissues other than the kidney, including the eyes, lungs, stomach, blood vessels, and even ear cartilage.[566]

**Hematologic Abnormalities.** Hematologic abnormalities are common in patients with sarcoidosis. In one early review, investigators found hemoglobin values below 11 gm/dl in 22% of patients.[9] In a later study of 75 patients with active pulmonary sarcoidosis, one or more hematologic abnormalities were documented in 87%;[567] anemia was present in 21 patients (28%), in 17 of whom bone marrow examination revealed granulomas. Some patients with anemia show evidence of increased hemolysis.[568, 569]

Leukopenia and lymphocytopenia are common, with white blood cell counts below $5.0 \times 10^9$ per liter being observed in approximately 30% of patients. Eosinophilia greater than 5% is present in about one third of cases. Thrombocytopenia is rare and is associated with a poor prognosis;[9, 570] death was documented in 6 of 24 patients reported in the literature by 1980.[571]

## DIAGNOSIS AND DIFFERENTIAL DIAGNOSIS

As indicated previously, about 50% of patients are asymptomatic when first seen, the disease being discovered on a screening chest radiograph or radiograph taken for unrelated reasons that reveals bilateral symmetric hilar and paratracheal lymph node enlargement. Patients who have malignancy, especially lymphoma and (uncommonly) renal cell carcinoma,[572] can also present with similar radiographic findings, but usually in association with symptoms. Even when the hilar node enlargement is asymmetric, sarcoidosis is almost certainly the diagnosis if the patient is asymptomatic. For example, in one series of 100 patients who had bilateral hilar node enlargement, all of the 30 who were asymptomatic had sarcoidosis.[573] The syndrome of bilateral hilar lymph node enlargement, fever, arthralgia, and erythema nodosum has been accepted by most investigators as synonymous with sarcoidosis, whether or not pathologic proof is available, and with this we are in complete agreement.[574–575a] As discussed earlier, we limit the use of gallium scanning to selected patients in whom the clinical and radiologic features of disease are atypical. In patients with an interstitial pattern on the chest radiograph and no evidence of adenopathy, the identification of bilateral hilar lymphadenopathy on previous radiographs may be a diagnostic clue. The description of an individual as "asymptomatic with a normal physical examination" presumes that a careful history has been taken, including a work history to exclude exposure to beryllium or organic dusts and a social and travel history to assess for possible exposure to infectious organisms.

As discussed previously, HRCT has been shown to be superior to chest radiography in the diagnosis of sarcoidosis. The procedure may demonstrate parenchymal abnormalities in patients who have only hilar lymphadenopathy apparent on the radiograph and is superior to the radiograph in demonstrating both the pattern and extent of disease.[235, 246] In one study of 140 consecutive patients with various chronic interstitial lung diseases, chest radiographs and HRCT scans were separately read by three independent observers without knowledge of clinical and pathologic data;[256] on average, the three observers made a correct confident diagnosis of sarcoidosis based on the findings on HRCT in 66% of 53 cases compared with 30% on the radiograph. As might be expected, the diagnostic accuracy improves considerably when the HRCT analysis is combined with the radiographic findings and clinical data. For example, in a study of 208 patients who had chronic interstitial lung disease, a confident correct diagnosis of sarcoidosis was made based on the clinical findings alone in 33% of 80 patients, on a combination of clinical and radiographic findings in 52%, and on a combination of clinical, radiographic, and HRCT findings in 80%. Of the 208 cases, only one (berylliosis) was misdiagnosed as sarcoidosis and only two cases of sarcoidosis were misdiagnosed (one as extrinsic allergic alveolitis [EAA] and the other as silicosis). We therefore conclude that in the appropriate clinical context, a confident diagnosis of sarcoidosis can usually be made based on a combination of clinical, radiographic, and HRCT findings, thus precluding the need for lung biopsy.

In cases in which the diagnosis cannot be confidently made on the basis of these findings, it can usually be established by the identification of non-necrotizing granulomas on biopsy specimens. It should be remembered, however, that other granulomatous diseases, including tuberculosis, brucellosis, fungal infection, and EAA can present pathologic and clinical pictures similar to that of sarcoidosis.[576] Many of these can be excluded by the identification of microorganisms by special stains, polymerase chain reaction, and/or culture. However, EAA may be difficult to differentiate from sarcoidosis,[577] particularly with small biopsy samples as obtained by transbronchial biopsy. Careful follow-up of patients in whom a diagnosis of sarcoidosis has been made occasionally results in the identification of a specific etiology for the granulomatous inflammation.[5]

### Biopsy

In a minority of cases, the diagnosis is established pathologically after biopsy of a characteristic skin lesion, the liver, or a palpable peripheral lymph node, most often one situated in the supraclavicular region; however, diagnostic tissue is obtained in the majority of patients by transbronchial biopsy. Biopsies of bronchial mucosa alone are also useful; for example, in one series of 22 patients, biopsy specimens from this site revealed granulomas in 17.[578] In other studies, bronchial biopsy has been found to yield specimens consistent with sarcoidosis in about 50% of patients;[579, 580] in one of these studies, the yield was considerably higher in African Americans (85%) than in whites (38%).[580]

The reported yield with transbronchial biopsy varies considerably, depending on the stage of the disease, the number of biopsy specimens obtained, and the number of tissue sections examined microscopically.[581] For example, in one series an average yield of 62% for all stages of disease increased to 76% when Stage 2 was considered alone.[582] In other studies in which 4 to 10 biopsy samples have been taken from multiple areas, diagnostic specimens have been documented in 90% to 100% of patients.[317, 578, 583–586] When ocular sarcoidosis is suspected in patients who have normal chest radiographs, transbronchial biopsy has provided tissue consistent with the diagnosis in 37 of 60 procedures (62%).[587]

In patients who have Stage 1 disease, scalene node biopsy shows non-necrotizing granulomatous inflammation in approximately 80% of patients[582] and is complementary to transbronchial biopsy when results from this procedure are negative.[588] However, this procedure is seldom necessary. Mediastinoscopy yields diagnostic tissue in 95% to 100% of cases;[589] however, it should be reserved for patients in whom less invasive procedures have not provided a diagnosis or for patients in whom the initial clinical evaluation strongly suggests lymphoma.

Transthoracic needle biopsy provides a low yield in diffuse pulmonary disease but can be useful in patients who have large nodules.[590] Transbronchial needle aspiration (TBNA) performed during bronchoscopy has also been found valuable by some investigators; for example, in one study, evidence of nodal granulomatous inflammation was found in 16 of 30 patients (53%) with Stage 1 disease and in 10 of 21 (48%) with Stage 2 disease.[591] Others have been even more successful, finding TBNA to be positive in 90% of patients with Stage 1 disease.[592] Although open-lung biopsy undoubtedly produces the most satisfactory tissue specimens for diagnosis, it is associated with a higher morbidity and mortality than other biopsy procedures. Biopsy of other tissues, such as salivary glands and conjunctiva, is not indicated in most patients because of its relatively low yield.[593, 594]

When tissue confirmation is required for the diagnosis, our approach in most patients is to obtain at least four specimens by transbronchial biopsy and one or more specimens by bronchial wall biopsy (in the latter case, "blindly" if the mucosa appears normal and directed in the presence of a mucosal abnormality). One or two additional specimens are submitted for fungal and mycobacterial culture when there is any suggestion of infection or an unusual clinical presentation. The latter procedure is important; for example, in one investigation, culture of specimens from patients in whom transbronchial biopsy revealed granulomas that were negative with special stains revealed mycobacterial or fungal organisms in 10 of 92 specimens.[595]

### The Kveim Test

The Kveim test consists of the intradermal injection of 0.1 to 0.2 ml of saline suspension of a crude extract of tissue showing sarcoid-related granulomatous inflammation, usually obtained from the spleen of patients with active disease. The test site is marked and sampled 4 to 6 weeks after the injection;[596] a positive reaction is indicated by the development of non-necrotizing granulomatous inflammation.

Most investigators have found the incidence of positive reactions in patients with active sarcoidosis to range from about 70% to 85%.[597–601] Positive reactivity has been as high as 88% in patients with bilateral hilar lymph node enlargement, erythema nodosum, and arthralgia;[589] however, it is less common in other groups. For example, in one study of 74 patients who had pulmonary parenchymal disease without hilar lymph node enlargement, Kveim tests were positive in only 53%;[589] similar results were documented in a more recent report.[601]

Because the highest yield is seen in patients in whom tissue confirmation is rarely, if ever, necessary and because of concerns regarding transmission of infectious disease,[602] difficulty in validation and standardization of reagents, restricted availability,[3] and the high yield afforded by transbronchial biopsy, the Kveim test has been abandoned as a diagnostic procedure in most centers.

## PROGNOSIS AND NATURAL HISTORY

### Morbidity and Mortality

For several reasons, it is difficult to make precise statements concerning the prognosis of sarcoidosis. As discussed previously, many patients are asymptomatic and never come to medical attention; moreover, the diagnosis is recognized premortem less than half the time in patients who die of the disease.[603, 604] However, if biopsy proof and a "characteristic" clinical picture are required for inclusion in a particular series, obviously the percentage of patients with symptoms and the prognosis will be different from those in series that include patients discovered by radiographic screening. As a result, the prognosis of patients with sarcoidosis varies considerably in published reports. Prognosis also varies with patient population characteristics, such as ethnic origin and age, and with the length of follow-up after diagnosis; some patients have an early remission only to relapse subsequently, whereas others resolve completely even after a prolonged period of disease activity.

As might be expected, the prognosis is undoubtedly better in a nonreferral setting than in tertiary care institutions (from which most series originate). This point was clearly made in an analysis of the course and prognosis of 86 patients who were seen over a 10-year period in a prepaid health maintenance organization:[605] no patients died, and none developed severe disability. Among a group of 295 patients enrolled in a tertiary care institution in Japan between 1978 and 1990, 27 (9%) were considered to have severe disease.[606] Mortality was seen in this group only, with 5 patients dying during the period of observation; 8 of the 27 had had mild clinical signs and symptoms at first presentation. In a review of 254 Danish patients followed a mean of 27 years from the time of diagnosis, 33 (13%) died of sarcoidosis;[607] the likelihood of death was slightly greater in the first 20 years of observation.[608] The presence of respiratory symptoms at the time of diagnosis was an independent predictor of death, even after adjusting for age, sex, radiographic stage, and lung function at presentation.

The overall *reported* mortality rate in patients who have sarcoidosis ranges from 5% to 10%; in patients followed for many years, the percentage is probably closer to 10%.[319, 609–612] These figures very likely reflect a referred patient population with advanced disease. Estimates of mortality rates in the United States have been made by workers at the Centers for Disease Control and Prevention in Atlanta, Georgia, using the admittedly imperfect tool of death certificate reporting.[613] According to this group, the age-adjusted rates increased between 1979 and 1991 from 1.3 to 1.6 per million population in men and from 1.9 to 2.5 per million in women. Reported mortality varied by region and by race, being highest in African Americans in all regions. Among whites, the highest mortality rates were in the northern states and among African Americans the highest rates were in the mid Atlantic and northern Midwestern states. The authors of some,[609, 614, 615] but not all,[605, 610, 616] reviews have also found a poorer prognosis for African Americans. The elderly are more likely to be left with disability than the young.[617] Pregnancy and the immediate postpartum period have also been associated with an increased mortality rate.[618]

Most patients who die of sarcoidosis do so as a result of cor pulmonale secondary to pulmonary fibrosis or from cardiac arrhythmia secondary to granulomatous myocardial disease.[356, 603] Myocardial involvement can also lead to the formation of a ventricular aneurysm and fatal cardiac failure.[356] Occasionally, death results from CNS disease,[459, 462] renal failure associated with nephrocalcinosis, or hemorrhage caused by an aspergilloma.

The over-representation of cardiac sarcoidosis as a cause of death in autopsy studies suggests that cardiac involvement also worsens prognosis.[604] In a study of Japanese patients, sarcoidosis was more likely to resolve spontaneously in the absence of chronic tonsillitis, the authors postulating that disease course was modified by an immune response to persistent antigenic stimulation.[619] The presence of erythema nodosum, arthralgia, and bilateral hilar lymph node enlargement (with or without low-grade fever) at the time of initial diagnosis almost invariably indicates a favorable prognosis,[12, 14, 251, 319, 574, 575, 620, 621] although a few patients who have this constellation of findings develop chronic disease.[622, 623]

The incidence of severe disability appears to be increased in patients who have clinically evident extrathoracic involvement,[614] especially those with persistent skin lesions,[253, 386, 609, 622] bone lesions, hepatomegaly, splenomegaly, or hypercalcemia.[617, 621, 622, 624] Disability also tends to be more severe in patients who have an intermittent course that includes frequent relapses[12] and in young children.[625, 626] Although the disease has been considered to be clinically less severe in Europe than in North America,[610] one group who performed a retrospective analysis of 1,609 cases of sarcoidosis in London, New York, Paris, Los Angeles, and Tokyo failed to demonstrate significant differences.[319]

### Relationship with Neoplasia

Although the presence of both sarcoidosis and malignancy has been described in some patients, whether this combination of diseases is coincidental or the result of a pathogenetic association has been a long-standing debate.[627, 628] Non-necrotizing granulomas can be found in association with a variety of neoplasms; usually, they are localized, often in lymph nodes draining the site of malignancy.[629] Although some investigators have claimed that this establishes a pathogenetic link between sarcoidosis and malignancy,[628] this argument seems flawed,[630] principally because the presence of such localized granuloma formation does not necessarily indicate a diagnosis of sarcoidosis. In one investigation in which stringent criteria were employed for accepting a pathogenetic rather than a coincidental association between the two conditions, no evidence for such a link was found.[630] However, in another review of 131 cases of coexistent sarcoidosis and malignancy, a causal relationship was suggested by the following observations:[627] (1) there was a nonrandom distribution of tumor types; (2) sarcoidosis almost invariably preceded the onset of lymphoproliferative malignancy (arguing against a tumor-induced sarcoid tissue response); and (3) the observed incidences of pulmonary carcinoma and malignant lymphoproliferative disease were significantly higher than expected. Other investigators have also described a possible link between sarcoidosis and lymphoproliferative disorders; for example, in one study of six patients whose cancers preceded the diagnosis of sarcoidosis by a mean of 9 months, four had hematologic malignancy.[631] Despite these findings, it is possible that increased surveillance of cancer patients might account for a higher than expected incidence of sarcoidosis in such a population.

The discovery of nine cases of sarcoidosis among 1,570 patients with germ cell tumors seen at the Memorial Sloan-Kettering Cancer Center between 1980 and 1989 (a prevalence far in excess of that expected by chance),[632] in conjunction with previous reports in the literature of this association,[633–643] led one group to propose the existence of a "sarcoid-like lymphadenopathy" and testicular germ cell tumor syndrome. Similar observations have been made in other reviews.[644] Although the excess number of patients with sarcoidosis in these series might be accounted for by referral bias or increased radiologic surveillance, the importance of tissue diagnosis of malignancy when the only abnormality seen on staging is mediastinal or bilateral hilar adenopathy cannot be overstressed.[644] Bilateral hilar adenopathy as a result of metastatic spread of germ cell cancer is distinctly unusual; it was noted in only 0.8% of patients treated with chemotherapy at Memorial Sloan-Kettering.[632]

### Prognostic Factors

Most observers agree that prognosis is strongly related to the radiographic stage of disease on presentation; in general, patients with Stage 1 disease fare better than those with Stage 2 disease and patients with Stage 2 disease fare better than those with Stage 3 disease.[319, 608, 617, 645] An absence of improvement in the chest radiograph over a 1-year period is a poor prognostic sign, whereas radiographic resolution that lasts for 2 years can be regarded as a cure.[617] Clearing of the chest radiograph is usually associated with a return to normal function,[645] although some patients have a persistent diffusion defect.[646] The risk of developing abnormal pulmonary function when the initial assessment of function is normal appears small.[611] The prognosis of patients who manifest air flow obstruction on routine pulmonary function tests does not appear to differ from that of patients without obstruction.[647]

Considerable effort has been directed at identifying markers of "activity" in patients who have sarcoidosis, with the hope that such markers will allow identification of those likely to develop progressive disease. Such patients could then be treated with corticosteroids in the hope of modifying the course of disease before the development of significant fibrosis. The alternative and putatively less desirable approach would be to begin therapy after significant alteration in lung or other organ function has already occurred, with the hope of preventing further deterioration and perhaps reversing changes related to the presence of granulomatous inflammation. Unfortunately, although a number of rough correlations between test results and disease outcome have been identified, none has sufficient precision to allow for intelligent decisions regarding the timing of institution of therapy.

Although the degree of BAL lymphocytosis reflects the intensity of alveolitis, the number of lymphocytes has not proved useful as an independent marker of prognosis or as a guide to therapy.[189, 648–652] This might be expected, because the most intense lymphocytosis in BAL is seen in patients with favorable prognosis, such as those with Stage 1 disease or erythema nodosum.[172, 651] Attempts to correlate specific lymphocyte subtypes with prognosis have yielded contradictory results,[172, 651–657] possibly because of differences in methodology or in the distribution of radiographic stage in patients studied.[5] Markers of lymphocyte activation are seen more frequently in patients who have more advanced disease; however, whether evaluation of the degree of lymphocyte activation has predictive value in individual patients, with sufficient sensitivity and specificity to guide therapy, remains to be determined.

Although serial measurement of serum ACE levels appears to be a reasonable method of monitoring disease activity, with levels generally falling and rising with clinical[662] and functional[663] evidence of change, the levels may vary significantly when all other parameters of disease activity are stable,[664] and they do not always distinguish clinically progressive from inactive disease.[665] Evidence that measurement of serum ACE levels can play a role in predicting prognosis or the outcome of therapy is not good.[189] Moreover, it seems unlikely that the measurement of serum ACE levels adds to the information available from clinical, radiologic, and functional evaluation.[666]

Although gallium 67 scanning has also been found to be an indicator of disease activity,[667, 668] it has not been shown to be a predictor of prognosis in most studies. The results of one long-term investigation indicated that patients who have proven pulmonary sarcoidosis in whom a gallium scan is negative are not likely to show deterioration in their disease after a 2-year period.[669] Its high degree of interobserver variability, radiation exposure to the patient,

**Table 41–3. SARCOIDOSIS: TESTS OF ACTIVITY AND PROGNOSIS**

| TEST | SELECTED REFERENCES |
|---|---|
| *Radiology* | |
| Gallium scanning | 514, 667, 668, 683 |
| Stage according to radiographic pattern | 608 |
| *Pulmonary Function Tests* | See text |
| *Analysis of Bronchoalveolar Lavage Fluid* | |
| Lymphocyte number | 649, 652 |
| Lymphocyte subsets | 651–653, 681, 684 |
| Lymphocyte activation markers | 126, 659–661 |
| Fibroblast activation markers (fibronectin, hyaluron, vitonectin) | 557, 675 |
| Mast cell number | 672, 685 |
| IgG and IgA | 670 |
| Cytokines (TNF-$\alpha$, IL-6, IL-1$\beta$, GM-CSF) | 114, 123, 686 |
| Macrophage acid phosphatase | 687 |
| Macrophage oxygen radical production | 148 |
| D Dimer | 688 |
| Collagenase | 673 |
| *Hematologic* | |
| Platelet count | 571 |
| *Analysis of Serum Constituents* | |
| Angiotensin-converting enzyme | 664, 665 |
| Soluble interleukin-2 receptors | 116, 117, 123 |
| Procollagen III peptide | 689, 690 |
| Neopterin | 674, 691 |
| ICAM-1 | 692 |
| Antiphospholipid antibody | 693 |
| Interferon gamma | 671 |
| Progastrin-releasing peptide | 694 |
| KL-6 | 695 |
| Monocyte chemoattractant protein-1 | 698 |
| Monocyte inflammatory protein-1$\alpha$ | 698 |
| *Analysis of Tissue Samples* | |
| Presence of granulomas on bronchial biopsy specimens | 696 |
| *Miscellaneous* | |
| Respiratory epithelial permeability to Tc-DTPA | 697 |

TNF-$\alpha$, tumor necrosis factor-$\alpha$; IL, interleukin; GM-CSF, granulocyte-macrophage colony-stimulating factor; ICAM-1, intercellular adhesion molecule-1.

and cost[3] have limited its application in patients with sarcoidosis; in addition, as with the measurement of serum ACE, the procedure adds little to routine measures.[666]

Many other tests have been evaluated for their ability to detect disease activity and predict disease progression (Table 41–3). Despite the finding that some correlate with disease progression,[670–673] none has been applied to a sufficiently large population of patients in a prospective fashion to allow for intelligent decision-making regarding therapy. Moreover, results have been inconsistent in different studies[115, 674, 675] and no test has been demonstrated to be superior to standard clinical evaluation (including lung function testing and chest radiography) in guiding management.

# REFERENCES

1. Yamamoto M, Sharma OP, Hosada Y: The 1991 descriptive definition of sarcoidosis. Sarcoidosis 9(Suppl):33, 1993.
2. Nagai S: Pulmonary sarcoidosis: Pathogenesis and population differences. Intern Med 34:833, 1995.
3. Kirtland SH, Winterbauer RH: Pulmonary sarcoidosis. Semin Respir Med 14:344, 1993.
4. Scadding JG: Sarcoidosis. London, Eyre and Spottiswoode, 1967.
5. Brown JK: Pulmonary sarcoidosis: Clinical evaluation and management. Semin Respir Med 12:215, 1991.
6. Gupta SK: Sarcoidosis in India. Semin Respir Med 12:75, 1991.
7. James DG: Epidemiology of sarcoidosis. Sarcoidosis 9:79, 1992.
8. Longcope WT, Freiman DG: A study of sarcoidosis: Based on a combined investigation of 160 cases including 30 autopsies from The Johns Hopkins Hospital and Massachusetts General Hospital. Medicine 31:1, 1952.
9. Mayock RL, Bertrand P, Morrison CE, et al: Manifestations of sarcoidosis: Analysis of 145 patients, with a review of nine series selected from the literature. Am J Med 35:67, 1963.
10. Terris M, Chaves AD: An epidemiologic study of sarcoidosis. Am Rev Respir Dis 94:50, 1966.
11. Israel HL, Sones M: Sarcoidosis: Clinical observations on one hundred and sixty cases. AMA Arch Intern Med 102:766, 1958.
12. Rudberg-Roos I: The course and prognosis of sarcoidosis as observed in 296 cases. Acta Tuberc Scand 52(Suppl):1, 1962.
13. James DG: Erythema nodosum. BMJ 1:853, 1961.
14. Scadding JG: Prognosis of intrathoracic sarcoidosis in England: A review of 136 cases after five years' observation. BMJ 2:1165, 1961.
15. Pietinalho A, Hiraga Y, Hosoda Y, et al: The frequency of sarcoidosis in Finland and Hokkaido, Japan: A comparative epidemiological study. Sarcoidosis 12:61, 1995.
16. Akisada M, Tasaka A, Mikami R: Lymphography in sarcoidosis: Comparison with roentgen findings in the chest. Am J Roentgenol 93:1273, 1969.
17. Da Costa JL: Geographic epidemiology of sarcoidosis in Southeast Asia. Am Rev Respir Dis 108:1269, 1973.
18. Rybicki BA, Maliarik MJ, Popovich J Jr, et al: Epidemiology, demographics and genetics of sarcoidosis. Semin Respir Infect 13:166, 1998.
19. Rybicki BA, Major M, Popovich J Jr, et al: Racial differences in sarcoidosis incidence: A 5-year study in a health maintenance organization. Am J Epidemiol 145:234, 1997.
20. Zaki MH, Addrizzo JR, Patton JM, et al: Further exploratory studies in sarcoidosis: An epidemiologic investigation to compare the prevalence of tuberculous infection and/or disease among contacts of matched sarcoidosis and asthmatic patients. Am Rev Respir Dis 103:539, 1971.
21. Keller AZ: Anatomic sites, age attributes, and rates of sarcoidosis in U.S. veterans. Am Rev Respir Dis 107:615, 1973.
22. Honeybourne D: Ethnic differences in the clinical features of sarcoidosis in south-east London. Br J Dis Chest 74:63, 1980.
23. Kolek V: Epidemiological study on sarcoidosis in Moravia and Silesia. Sarcoidosis 11:110, 1994.
24. Mana J, Badrinas F, Morera J, et al: Sarcoidosis in Spain. Sarcoidosis 9:118, 1992.
25. Hsing CT, Han FC, Liu HC, et al: Sarcoidosis among Chinese. Am Rev Respir Dis 89:917, 1964.
26. Present DH, Siltzbach LE: Sarcoidosis among the Chinese and a review of the worldwide epidemiology of sarcoidosis. Am Rev Respir Dis 95:285, 1967.
27. Panna LN, Man CA, Guan BO: Sarcoidosis among Chinese. Chest 80:74, 1981.
28. Lee SK, Narendran K, Chiang GS: Pulmonary sarcoidosis in Singapore. Ann Acad Med Singapore 14:446, 1985.
29. Purriel P, Navarrete E: Epidemiology of sarcoidosis in Uruguay and other countries of Latin America. Am Rev Respir Dis 84:155, 1961.
30. Fazzi P, Solfanelli S, De Pede F, et al: Sarcoidosis in Tuscany: A preliminary report. Sarcoidosis 9:123, 1992.
31. Brown IG, Hamblin TJ, Mikhail JR: Oldest case of sarcoidosis in the world. BMJ 283:190, 1981.
32. Kendig EL Jr, Niitu Y: Sarcoidosis in Japanese and American children. Chest 77:514, 1980.
33. Kendig EL, Brummer DL: The prognosis of sarcoidosis in children. Chest 70:351, 1976.
34. Kendig EL Jr: Sarcoidosis. Am J Dis Child 136:11, 1982.
35. Merten DF, Kirks DR, Grossman H: Pulmonary sarcoidosis in childhood. Am J Roentgenol 135:673, 1980.
36. Vago L, Barberis M, Gori A, et al: Nested polymerase chain reaction for Mycobacterium tuberculosis IS6110 sequence on formalin-fixed paraffin-embedded tissues with granulomatous diseases for rapid diagnosis of tuberculosis. Am J Clin Pathol 109:411, 1998.
37. Wong CF, Yew WW, Wong PC, et al: A case of concomitant tuberculosis and sarcoidosis with mycobacterial DNA present in the sarcoid lesion. Chest 114:626, 1998.
38. Wallaert B, Ramon P, Fournier EC, et al: Activated alveolar macrophage and lymphocyte alveolitis in extrathoracic sarcoidosis without radiological mediastinopulmonary involvement. Ann NY Acad Sci 465:201, 1986.
39. Wallaert B, Ramon P, Fournier EC, et al: Bronchoalveolar lavage, serum angiotensin-converting enzyme and gallium-67 scanning in extrathoracic sarcoidosis. Chest 82:553, 1982.
40. Mitchell DN, Rees RJW, Goswami KKA: Transmissible agents from human sarcoid and Crohn's disease tissues. Lancet 2:761, 1976.
41. Mitchell DN, Rees RJW: The nature and physical characteristics of a transmissible agent from human sarcoid tissue. Ann NY Acad Sci 278:233, 1976.
42. Mitchell DN, Rees RJW: Further observations on the nature and physical characteristics of transmissible agents from human sarcoid and Crohn's disease tissues. In Williams WJ, Davies BH (eds): Eighth International Conference on Sarcoidosis and Other Granulomatous Disease. Cardiff, UK, Alpha Omega Publishing Ltd, 1978, p 121.
43. Wang N-S, Schraufnagel DE, Sampson MG: The tadpole-shaped structure in human non-necrotizing granulomas. Am Rev Respir Dis 123:560, 1981.
44. Dewar A, Corrin B, Turner-Warwick M: Tadpole shaped structures in a further patient with granulomatous lung disease. Thorax 39:466, 1984.
45. Wirostko E, Johnson L, Wirostko B: Sarcoidosis-associated uveitis. Parasitization of vitreous leucocytes by mollicute-like organisms. Acta Ophthalmol 67:415, 1989.
46. Heyll A, Meckenstock G, Aul C, et al: Possible transmission of sarcoidosis via allogenic bone marrow transplantation. Bone Marrow Transplant 14:161, 1994.
47. Martinez FJ, Orens JB, Deeb M, et al: Recurrence of sarcoidosis following bilateral allogeneic lung transplantation. Chest 106:1597, 1994.
48. Johnson BA, Duncan SR, Ohori NP, et al: Recurrence of sarcoidosis in pulmonary allograft recipients. Am Rev Respir Dis 148:1373, 1993.
49. Edmonstone WM, Wilson AG: Temporal clustering of familial sarcoidosis in nonconsanguineous relatives. Br J Dis Chest 78:184, 1984.
50. Stewart IC, Davidson NM: Clustering of sarcoidosis. Thorax 37:398, 1982.
51. Edmondstone WM: Sarcoidosis in nurses: Is there an association? Thorax 43:342, 1988.
52. Saboor SA, Johnson NM, McFadden J: Detection of mycobacterial DNA in sarcoidosis and tuberculosis with polymerase chain reaction. Lancet 339:1012, 1992.
53. Almenoff PL, Johnson A, Lesser M, et al: Growth of acid fast L forms in the blood of patients with sarcoidosis. Thorax 51:530, 1996.
54. Scadding JG: Sarcoidosis. London, Eyre and Spottiswoode, 1967.
55. Richter E, Greinert U, Kirsten D, et al: Assessment of mycobacterial DNA in cells and tissues of mycobacterial and sarcoid lesions. Am J Respir Crit Care Med 153:375, 1996.
56. Fidler HM, Rook GA, Johnson N, et al: Mycobacterium tuberculosis DNA in tissue affected by sarcoidosis. BMJ 306:546, 1993.
57. Mitchell IC, Turk JL, Mitchell DN: Detection of mycobacterial RRNA in sarcoidosis with liquid-phase hybridisation. Lancet 339:1015, 1992.
58. Bocart D, Lecossier D, De Lassence A, et al: A search for mycobacterial DNA in granulomatous tissue from patients with sarcoidosis using the polymerase chain reaction. Am Rev Respir Dis 145:1142, 1992.
59. Popper HH, Winter E, Hofler G: DNA of Mycobacterium tuberculosis in formalin-fixed, paraffin-embedded tissue in tuberculosis and sarcoidosis detected by polymerase chain reaction. Am J Clin Pathol 101:738, 1994.
60. Lisby G, Milman N, Jacobsen GK: Search for Mycobacterium paratuberculosis DNA in tissue from patients with sarcoidosis by enzymatic gene amplification. APMIS 101:876, 1993.
61. Gerdes J, Richter E, Rüsch-Gerdes S, et al: Mycobacterial nucleic acids in sarcoid lesions (letter). Lancet 339:1536, 1992.
62. Thakker B, Black M, Foulis AK: Mycobacterial nucleic acids in sarcoid lesions (letter). Lancet 339:1536, 1992.
63. Joyce-Brady M. Tasted great, less filling: The debate about mycobacteria and sarcoidosis. Am Rev Respir Dis 145:986, 1992.
64. Vokura M, Lecossier D, du Bois RM, et al: Absence of DNA from mycobacteria of the M. tuberculosis complex in sarcoidosis. Am J Respir Crit Care Med 156:1000, 1997.
65. Richter E, Greinert U, Kirsten D, et al: Assessment of mycobacterial DNA in cells and tissues of mycobacterial and sarcoid lesions. Am J Respir Crit Care Med 153:375, 1996.
66. Wilsher ML, Hallowes M, Birchall NM: Gamma/delta T lymphocytes in the blood of patients with sarcoidosis. Thorax 50:858, 1995.
67. Balbi B, Valle MT, Oddera S, et al: T-lymphocytes with γδ + and γδ2 + antigen receptors are present in increased proportions in a fraction of patients with tuberculosis or with sarcoidosis. Am Rev Respir Dis 148:1685, 1993.
68. Shigehara K, Shijubo N, Nakanishi F, et al: Circulating gamma-delta T-cell-receptor–positive lymphocytes. Respiration 62:84, 1995.
69. Nakata K, Sugie T, Nakano H, et al: Gamma-delta T cells in sarcoidosis: Correlation with clinical features. Am J Respir Crit Care Med 149:981, 1994.
70. Nakata K, Sugie T, Cohen H, et al: Expansion of circulating gamma delta T cells in active sarcoidosis closely correlates with defects in cellular immunity. Clin Immunol Immunopathol 74:217, 1995.
71. Raulf M, Liebers V, Steppert C, et al: Increased gamma/delta-positive T-cells in blood and bronchoalveolar lavage of patients with sarcoidosis and hypersensitivity pneumonitis. Eur Respir J 7:140, 1994.
72. Grunewald J, Shigematsu M, Nagai S, et al: T-cell receptor V gene expression in HLA-typed Japanese patients with pulmonary sarcoidosis. Am J Respir Crit Care Med 151:151, 1995.

73. Agner E, Larsen JH: *Yersinia enterocolitica* infection and sarcoidosis: A report of seven cases. Scand J Respir Dis 60:230, 1979.

74. Hua B, Li QD, Wang FM, et al: *Borrelia burgdorferi* infection may be the cause of sarcoidosis. Chin Med J (Engl) 105:560, 1992.

75. Liu HG: Spirochetes in the cheilitis granulomatosa and sarcoidosis. Chung Hua I Hsueh Tsa Chih 73:142, 1993.

76. Lian W, Luo W: *Borrelia burgdorferi* DNA in biological samples from patients with sarcoidosis during the polymerase chain reaction techniques. Chin Med Sci J 10:93, 1995.

77. Arcangeli G, Calabro S, Cisno F, et al: Determination of antibodies to *Borrelia burgdorferi* in sarcoidosis. Sarcoidosis 11:32, 1994.

77a. Ishihara M, Ohno S, Ono H, et al: Seroprevalence of anti-Borrelia antibodies among patients with confirmed sarcoidosis in a region of Japan where Lyme borreliosis is endemic. Graefes Arch Clin Exp Ophthalmol 236:280, 1998.

78. Nakata Y, Kataoka M, Kimura I: Sarcoidosis and *Propionibacterium acnes*. Nippon Rinsho 52:1492, 1994.

79. Eishi Y: Seeking a causative agent of sarcoidosis. Nippon Rinsho 52:1486, 1994.

80. Moller DR: Etiology of sarcoidosis. Clin Chest Med 18:695, 1997.

81. Newman LS, Rose CS, Maier LA: Sarcoidosis. N Engl J Med 336:1224, 1997.

82. Rybicki BA, Maliarik MJ, Major M, et al: Genetics of sarcoidosis. Clin Chest Med 18:707, 1997.

83. Huan P, Hachulla E, Delaporte E, et al: Familial sarcoidosis: 3 cases in the same family. Rev Med Interne 16:280, 1995.

84. Bamberry P, Kaur U, Bhusnurmath SR, et al: Familial idiopathic granulomatosis: Sarcoidosis and Crohn's disease in two Indian families. Thorax 46:919, 1991.

85. James DG, Williams WJ: Epidemiology. *In* Smith LH Jr (ed): Sarcoidosis and Other Granulomatous Disorders. Philadelphia, WB Saunders, 1985, pp 242–246.

86. Plummer NS, Symmers WS, Winner HI: Sarcoidosis in identical twins: With torulosis as a complication in one case. BMJ 2:599, 1957.

87. Yoshikawa T, Yamamoto M, Inaba S, et al: Sarcoidosis in identical twins. Nippon Kyobi Shikkan Gakkai Zasshi 32:610, 1994.

88. Brennan NJ, Crean P, Long JP, et al: High prevalence of familial sarcoidosis in an Irish population. Thorax 39:14, 1984.

89. Berlin M, Fogdell-Hahn A, Olerup O, et al: HLA-DR predicts the prognosis of sarcoidosis in Scandinavian patients with pulmonary sarcoidosis. Am J Respir Crit Care Med 156:1601, 1997.

90. Ina Y, Takada K, Yamamoto M, et al: HLA and sarcoidosis in the Japanese. Chest 95:1257, 1989.

91. Abe S, Yamaguchi E, Makimura S, et al: Association of HLA-DR with sarcoidosis: Correlation with clinical course. Chest 92:487, 1987.

92. Martinetti M, Tinelli C, Kolek V, et al: "The sarcoidosis map": A joint survey of clinical and immunogenetic findings in two European countries. Am J Respir Crit Care Med 152:557, 1995.

93. Pasturenzi L, Martinetti M, Cuccia M, et al: HLA class I, II and III polymorphism in Italian patients with sarcoidosis. Chest 104:1170, 1993.

93a. Maliarik MJ, Chen KM, Major ML, et al: Analysis of HLA-DPB1 polymorphisms in African-Americans with sarcoidosis. Am J Respir Crit Care Med 158:111, 1998.

93b. Schurmann M, Bein G, Kirsten D, et al: HLA-DQB1 and HLA-DPB1 genotypes in familial sarcoidosis. Respir Med 92:649, 1998.

94. Spurzem JR, Saltini C, Kirby M, et al: Expression of HLA class II genes in alveolar macrophages of patients with sarcoidosis. Am Rev Respir Dis 140:89, 1989.

95. Furuya K, Yamaguchi E, Itoh A, et al: Deletion polymorphism in the angiotensin I converting enzyme (SACE) gene as a genetic risk factor for sarcoidosis. Thorax 51:777, 1996.

96. O'Connor CM, Fitzgerald MX: Speculations on sarcoidosis. Respir Med 86:277, 1992.

97. Daniele RP: Immunology of sarcoidosis. Semin Respir Med 12:204, 1991.

98. Semenzato G: Immunology of interstitial lung diseases: Cellular events taking place in the lung of sarcoidosis, hypersensitivity pneumonitis and HIV infection. Eur Respir J 4:94, 1991.

99. Spiteri MA, Clarke SW, Poulter LW: Alveolar macrophages that suppress T-cell responses may be crucial to the pathogenetic outcome of pulmonary sarcoidosis. Eur Respir J 5:394, 1992.

100. Zissel G, Homolka J, Schlaak J, et al: Anti-inflammatory cytokine release by alveolar macrophages in pulmonary sarcoidosis. Am J Respir Crit Care Med 154:713, 1996.

101. Nicod LP, Isler P: Alveolar macrophages in sarcoidosis coexpress high levels of CD86 (B7.2), CD40, and CD30L. Am J Respir Cell Mol Biol 17:91, 1997.

102. Ina Y, Takada K, Yamamoto M, et al: Antigen-presenting capacity in patients with sarcoidosis. Chest 98:911, 1990.

103. Semenzato G, Agostini C, Chilosi M: Immunology and immunohistology. *In* James DG (ed): Sarcoidosis and Other Granulomatous Disorders. New York, Marcel Dekker, 1994.

104. Van Maarsseveen TC, De Groot J, Stam J, et al: Peripolesis in alveolar sarcoidosis. Am Rev Respir Dis 147:1259, 1993.

105. Striz I, Zheng L, Wang YM, et al: Soluble CD14 is increased in bronchoalveolar lavage of active sarcoidosis and correlates with alveolar macrophage membrane-bound CD14. Am J Respir Crit Care Med 151:544, 1995.

106. Ishii Y, Kitamura S: Elevated levels of soluble ICAM-1 in serum and BAL fluid in patients with active sarcoidosis. Chest 107:1636, 1995.

107. Melis M, Gjomarkaj M, Pace E, et al: Increased expression of leukocyte function association antigen-1 (LFA-1) and intercellular adhesion molecule-1 (ICAM-1) by alveolar macrophages of patients with pulmonary sarcoidosis. Chest 100:910, 1991.

108. Smith DL, deShazo RD: Integrins, macrophages and sarcoidosis. Chest 102:659, 1992.

109. Dalhoff K, Bohnet S, Braun J, et al: Intercellular adhesion molecule 1 (ICAM-1) in the pathogenesis of mononuclear cell alveolitis in pulmonary sarcoidosis. Thorax 48:1140, 1993.

110. Schaberg T, Rau M, Stephan H, et al: Increased number of alveolar macrophages expressing surface molecules of the CD11/CD18 family in sarcoidosis and idiopathic pulmonary fibrosis is related to the production of superoxide anions by these cells. Am Rev Respir Dis 147:1507, 1993.

111. Lynch JP 3d, Standiford TJ, Rolfe MW, et al: Neutrophilic alveolitis in idiopathic pulmonary fibrosis: The role of interleukin-8. Am Rev Respir Dis 145:1433, 1992.

112. Müller-Quernheim J, Pfeifer S, Männel D, et al: Lung-restricted activation of the alveolar macrophage/monocyte system in pulmonary sarcoidosis. Am Rev Respir Dis 145:187, 1992.

113. Yamaguchi E, Okazaki N, Tsuneta Y, et al: Interleukins in pulmonary sarcoidosis: Dissociative correlations of lung interleukins 1 and 2 with the intensity of alveolitis. Am Rev Respir Dis 138:645, 1988.

114. Steffen M, Petersen J, Oldigs M, et al: Increased secretion of tumor necrosis factor-alpha, interleukin-1-beta, and interleukin-6 by alveolar macrophages from patients with sarcoidosis. J Allergy Clin Immunol 91:939, 1993.

115. Pueringer RJ, Schwartz DA, Dayton CS, et al: The relationship between alveolar macrophage TNF, IL-1, and PGE2 release, alveolitis, and disease severity in sarcoidosis. Chest 103:832, 1993.

116. Ina Y, Takada K, Sato T, et al: Soluble interleukin 2 receptors in patients with sarcoidosis: Possible origin. Chest 102:1128, 1992.

117. Pforte A, Brunner A, Gais P, et al: Concomitant modulation of serum-soluble interleukin-2 receptor and alveolar macrophage interleukin-2 receptor in sarcoidosis. Am Rev Respir Dis 147:717, 1993.

118. Girgis RE, Basha MA, Maliarik M, et al: Cytokines in the bronchoalveolar lavage fluid of patients with active pulmonary sarcoidosis. Am J Respir Crit Care Med 152:71, 1995.

119. Sahashi K, Ina Y, Takada K, et al: Significance of interleukin 6 in patients with sarcoidosis. Chest 106:156, 1994.

120. Homolka J, Müller-Quernheim J: Increased interleukin 6 production by bronchoalveolar lavage cells in patients with active sarcoidosis. Lung 171:173, 1993.

121. Car BD, Meloni F, Luisetti M, et al: Elevated IL-8 and MCP-1 in the bronchoalveolar lavage fluid of patients with idiopathic pulmonary fibrosis and pulmonary sarcoidosis. Am J Respir Crit Care Med 149:655, 1994.

122. Zheng L, Teschler H, Guzman J, et al: Alveolar macrophage TNF-α release and BAL cell phenotypes in sarcoidosis. Am J Respir Crit Care Med 152:1061, 1995.

123. Ziegenhagen MW, Benner UK, Zizzel G, et al: Sarcoidosis: TNF-α release from alveolar macrophages and serum level of sIL-2 are prognostic markers. Am J Respir Crit Care Med 156:1586, 1997.

123a. Allen JT, Bloor CA, Knight RA, et al: Expression of insulin-like growth factor binding proteins in bronchoalveolar lavage fluid of patients with pulmonary sarcoidosis. Am J Respir Cell Mol Biol 19:250, 1998.

124. Limper AH, Colby TV, Sanders MS, et al: Immunohistochemical localization of transforming growth factor-β₁ in the nonnecrotizing granulomas of pulmonary sarcoidosis. Am J Respir Crit Care Med 149:197, 1994.

125. Agostini C, Trentin L, Zambello R, et al: CD8 alveolitis in sarcoidosis: Incidence, phenotypic characteristics and clinical features. Am J Med 95:466, 1993.

126. Ainslie GM, Poulter LW, du Bois RM: Relation between immunocytological features of bronchoalveolar lavage fluid and clinical indices in sarcoidosis. Thorax 44:501, 1989.

127. Hoshino T, Itoh K, Gouhara R, et al: Spontaneous production of various cytokines except IL-4 from CD4+ T cells in the affected organs of sarcoidosis patients. Clin Exp Immunol 102:399, 1995.

127a. Kodama N, Yamaguchi E, Hizawa N, et al: Expression of RANTES by bronchoalveolar lavage cells in nonsmoking patients with interstitial lung diseases. Am J Respir Cell Mol Biol 18:526, 1998.

128. Garlepp MJ, Rose AH, Dench JE, et al: Clonal analysis of lung and blood T cells in patients with sarcoidosis. Thorax 49:577, 1994.

129. Hunninghake GW, Bedell GN, Zavala DC, et al: Role of interleukin-2 release by lung T-cells in active pulmonary sarcoidosis. Am Rev Respir Dis 128:634, 1983.

130. Semenzato G, Agostini C, Trentin L, et al: Evidence of cells bearing interleukin-2 receptor at sites of disease activity in sarcoid patients. Clin Exp Immunol 57:331, 1984.

131. Muller-Quernheim J, Saltini C, Sondermeyer P, et al: Compartmentalized activation of the interleukin-2 gene by lung T lymphocytes in active pulmonary sarcoidosis. J Immunol 137:3475, 1986.

132. Konishi K, Moller DR, Saltini C, et al: Spontaneous expression of the interleukin-2 receptor gene and presence of functional interleukin-2 receptors on T lymphocytes in the blood of individuals with active pulmonary sarcoidosis. J Clin Invest 82:775, 1988.

133. Kataria YP, Holter JF: Immunology of sarcoidosis. Clin Chest Med 18:719, 1997.

135. Bäumer I, Zissel G, Schlaak M, et al: Th1/Th2 cell distribution in pulmonary sarcoidosis. Am J Respir Cell Mol Biol 16:171, 1997.

134. Moseley PL, Hemken C, Monick M, et al: Interferon and growth factor activity for human lung fibroblasts: Release from bronchoalveolar cells for patients with active sarcoidosis. Chest 89:657, 1986.

136. Hol BEA, Hintzen RQ, Van Lier RAW, et al: Soluble and cellular markers of T cell activation in patients with pulmonary sarcoidosis. Am Rev Respir Dis 148:643, 1993.

137. Tamura N, Moller DR, Balbi B, et al: Preferential usage of the T-cell antigen

receptor β-chain constant region cβ1 element by lung T-lymphocytes of patients with pulmonary sarcoidosis. Am Rev Respir Dis 143:635, 1991.

138. Bellocq A, Lecossier D, Pierre-Audigier C, et al: T cell receptor repertoire of T lymphocytes recovered from the lung and blood of patients with sarcoidosis. Am J Respir Crit Care 149:646, 1994.

139. Forrester JM, Wang Y, Ricalton N, et al: TCR expression of activated T cell clones in the lungs of patients with pulmonary sarcoidosis. J Immunol 153:4291, 1994.

140. Forman JD, Kelin JT, Silver RF, et al: Selective activation and accumulation of oligoclonal V beta-specific T cells in active pulmonary sarcoidosis. J Clin Invest 94:1533, 1994.

141. Jones CM, Lake RA, Wijeyekoon JB, et al: Oligoclonal V gene usage by T lymphocytes in bronchoalveolar lavage fluid from sarcoidosis patients. Am J Respir Cell Mol Biol 14:470, 1996.

142. Zissel G, Bäumer I, Fleischer B, et al: TCR Vβ families in T cell clones from sarcoid lung parenchyma, BAL, and blood. Am J Respir Crit Care Med 156:1593, 1997.

143. Jones CM, Lake RA, Wijeyekoon JB, et al: Oligoclonal V gene usage by T lymphocytes in bronchoalveolar lavage fluid from sarcoidosis patients. Am J Respir Cell Mol Biol 14:470, 1996.

144. Trentin L, Zambello R, Facco M, et al: Selection of T lymphocytes bearing limited TCR-Vβ regions in the lung of hypersensitivity pneumonitis and sarcoidosis. Am J Respir Crit Care Med 155:587, 1997.

145. Usui Y, Kohsaka H, Eishi Y, et al: Shared amino acid motifs in T-cell receptor β junctional regions of bronchoalveolar T cells in patients with pulmonary sarcoidosis. Am J Respir Crit Care Med 154:50, 1996.

146. Klein JT, Horn TD, Forman JD, et al: Selection of oligoclonal V beta-specific T cells in the intradermal response to Kveim-Siltzbach reagent in individuals with sarcoidosis. J Immunol 154:1450, 1995.

147. Thomas PD, Hunninghake GW: Current concepts of the pathogenesis of sarcoidosis. Am Rev Respir Dis 135:747, 1987.

148. Groen H, Hamstra M, Aalbers R, et al: Clinical evaluation of lymphocyte sub-populations and oxygen radical production in sarcoidosis and idiopathic pulmonary fibrosis. Respir Med 88:55, 1994.

149. Semenzato G, Ango MR, Chilosi M: Immunology of extrapulmonary sarcoid lesions. Semin Respir Med 13:380, 1992.

150. Kita S, Tsuda T, Sugisaki K, et al: Characterization of distribution of T lymphocyte subsets and activated T lymphocytes infiltrating into sarcoid lesions. Intern Med 34:847, 1995.

151. Moseley PL, Hemken C, Monick M, et al: Interferon and growth factor activity for human lung fibroblasts: Release from bronchoalveolar cells from patients with active sarcoidosis. Chest 89:657, 1986.

152. Bitterman PB, Adelberg S, Crystal RG: Mechanisms of pulmonary fibrosis: Spontaneous release of the alveolar macrophage-derived growth factor in the interstitial lung disorders. J Clin Invest 72:1801, 1983.

153. Cantin AM, Boileau R, Begin R: Increased procollagen III aminoterminal peptide-related antigens and fibroblast growth signals in the lungs of patients with idiopathic pulmonary fibrosis. Am Rev Respir Dis 137:572, 1988.

154. Yamauchi K, Martinet Y, Crystal RG: Modulation of fibronectin gene expression in human mononuclear phagocytes. J Clin Invest 80:1720, 1987.

155. Martinet Y, Rom WN, Grotendorst GR, et al: Exaggerated spontaneous release of platelet-derived growth factor by alveolar macrophages from patients with idiopathic pulmonary fibrosis. N Engl J Med 317:202, 1987.

156. Scappaticci E, Libertucci D, Bottomicca F, et al: Platelet-activating factor in bronchoalveolar lavage from patients with sarcoidosis. Am Rev Respir Dis 146:433, 1992.

157. Calhoun WJ, Salisbury SM, Chosy LW, et al: Increased alveolar macrophage chemiluminescence and airspace cell superoxide production in active pulmonary sarcoidosis. J Lab Clin Med 112:147, 1988.

158. Rolfe MW, Standiford TJ, Kunkel SL, et al: Interleukin-1 receptor antagonist expression in sarcoidosis. Am Rev Respir Dis 18:1378, 1993.

159. Lecossier D, Valeyre D, Loiseay A, et al: Antigen-induced proliferative response of lavage and blood T lymphocytes. Am Rev Respir Dis 144:861, 1991.

160. Papadopoulos KI, Hornblad Y, Liljebladh H, et al: High frequency of endocrine autoimmunity in patients with sarcoidosis. Eur J Endocrinol 134:331, 1996.

161. Schoenfeld N, Schmolke B, Schmitt M, et al: Specification and quantitation of circulating immune complexes in the serum of patients with active pulmonary sarcoidosis. Thorax 49:688, 1994.

162. Barth J, Falsafi-Amin R, Petermann W, et al: B-lymphocyte response in peripheral blood of patients with pulmonary sarcoidosis. Sarcoidosis 9:49, 1992.

163. Bertran G, Arzt E, Resnik E, et al: Inhibition of interferon gamma production by peripheral blood mononuclear leukocytes of patients with sarcoidosis: Pathogenic implications. Chest 101:996, 1992.

164. Rottoli P, Muscettola M, Grasso G, et al: Impaired interferon-gamma production by peripheral blood mononuclear cells and effects of calcitriol in pulmonary sarcoidosis. Sarcoidosis 10:108, 1993.

165. Shakoor Z, Hamblin AS: Increased CD11/CD18 expression on peripheral blood leucocytes of patients with sarcoidosis. Clin Exp Immunol 90:99, 1992.

166. Bresnitz EA, Stolley PD, Israel HL, et al: Possible risk factors for sarcoidosis: A case-control study. Ann NY Acad Sci 465:632, 1986.

167. Douglas JG, Middleton WG, Gaddie J, et al: Sarcoidosis: A disorder commoner in non-smokers? Thorax 41:787, 1986.

168. Hance AJ, Basset P, Saumon G, et al: Smoking and interstitial lung disease: The effect of cigarette smoking on the incidence of pulmonary histiocytosis X and sarcoidosis. Ann NY Acad Sci 465:643, 1986.

169. Comstock GW, Keltz H, Sencer DJ: Clay eating and sarcoidosis: A controlled study in the state of Georgia. Am Rev Respir Dis 84(Suppl):130, 1961.

170. Revsbech P: Is sarcoidosis related to exposure to pets or the housing conditions? A case-referent study. Sarcoidosis 9:101, 1992.

171. Valeyre D, Soler P, Clerici C, et al: Smoking and pulmonary sarcoidosis: Effect of cigarette smoking on prevalence, clinical manifestations, alveolitis, and evolution of the disease. Thorax 43:516, 1988.

172. Drent M, van Velzen-Blad H, Diamant M, et al: Relationship between presentation of sarcoidosis and T lymphocyte profile: A study in bronchoalveolar lavage fluid. Chest 104:795, 1993.

173. Yamaguchi E, Itoh A, Furuya K, et al: Release of tumour necrosis factor-alpha from human alveolar macrophages is decreased in smokers. Chest 103:479, 1993.

174. Strom KE, Eklund AG. Smoking does not prevent the onset of respiratory failure in sarcoidosis. Sarcoidosis 10:26, 1993.

175. Jones WW: The nature and origin of Schaumann bodies. J Pathol Bacteriol 79:193, 1960.

176. Reid JD, Andersen ME: Calcium oxalate in sarcoid granulomas: With particular reference to the small ovoid body and a note on the finding of dolomite. Am J Clin Pathol 90:545, 1988.

177. Hsu RM, Connors AF Jr, Tomashefski JF Jr: Histologic, microbiologic, and clinical correlates of the diagnosis of sarcoidosis by transbronchial biopsy. Arch Pathol Lab Med 120:364, 1996.

178. Rosen Y, Vuletin JC, Pertschuk LP, et al: Sarcoidosis: From the pathologist's vantage point. Pathol Ann 14(part 1):405, 1979.

179. Williams WJ, Williams D: "Residual bodies" in sarcoid and sarcoid-like granulomas. J Clin Pathol 20:574, 1967.

180. Sieracki JC, Fisher ER: The ceroid nature of the so-called Hamazaki-Wesenberg bodies. Am J Clin Pathol 59:248, 1973.

181. Doyle WF, Brahman HD, Burgess JH: The nature of yellow-brown bodies in peritoneal lymph nodes: Histochemical and electron microscopic evaluation of these bodies in a case of suspected sarcoidosis. Arch Pathol 96:320, 1973.

182. Ricker W, Clark M: Sarcoidosis: A clinico-pathologic review of 300 cases, including 22 autopsies. Am J Clin Pathol 19:725, 1949.

183. Mitchell DN, Scadding JG, Heard BE, et al: Sarcoidosis: Histopathological definition and clinical diagnosis. J Clin Pathol 30:395, 1977.

184. Rosen Y, Athanassiades TJ, Moon S, et al: Nongranulomatous interstitial pneumonitis in sarcoidosis: Relationship to development of epithelioid granulomas. Chest 74:122, 1978.

185. Arnoux AG, Jaubert F, Stanislas-Leguern G, et al: In vitro granuloma-like formations in bronchoalveolar cell cultures from patients with sarcoidosis. Ann NY Acad Sci 465:183, 1986.

186. Hunsaker AR, Munden RF, Pugatch RD, et al: Sarcoid-like reaction in patients with malignancy. Radiology 200:255, 1996.

187. Laurberg P: Sarcoid reactions in pulmonary neoplasms. Scand J Respir Dis 56:20, 1975.

188. Wood GM, Bolton RP, Muers MF, et al: Pleurisy and pulmonary granulomas after treatment with acebutolol. BMJ 285:936, 1982.

189. Thomas PD, Hunninghake GW: Current concepts of the pathogenesis of sarcoidosis. Am Rev Respir Dis 135:747, 1987.

190. Rosen Y, Athanassiades TJ, Moon S, et al: Nongranulomatous interstitial pneumonitis in sarcoidosis. Chest 74:122, 1978.

191. Shigematsu N, Emori K, Matsuba K, et al: Clinicopathologic characteristics of pulmonary acinar sarcoidosis. Chest 73:186, 1978.

192. Battesti JP, Saumon G, Valeyre D, et al: Pulmonary sarcoidosis with an alveolar radiographic pattern. Thorax 37:448, 1982.

193. Takemura T, Hiraga Y, Oomichi M, et al: Ultrastructural features of alveolitis in sarcoidosis. Am J Respir Crit Care Med 152:360, 1995.

194. Planes C, Valeyre D, Loiseau A, et al: Ultrastructural alterations of the air-blood barrier in sarcoidosis and hypersensitivity pneumonitis and their relation to lung histopathology. Am J Respir Crit Care Med 150:1067, 1994.

195. Keogh BA, Hunninghake GW, Line BR, et al: The alveolitis of pulmonary sarcoidosis: Evaluation of natural history and alveolitis-dependent changes in lung function. Am Rev Respir Dis 128:256, 1983.

196. Cantin A, Begin R, Rola-Pleszozynski M, et al: Heterogeneity of bronchoalveolar lavage cellularity in stage III pulmonary sarcoidosis. Chest 83:485, 1983.

197. Staton GW Jr, Check IJ, Fajman WA, et al: Analysis of homogeneity of alveolitis in pulmonary sarcoidosis by bilateral bronchoalveolar lavage, gallium-67 lung uptake, and chest radiograph. Sarcoidosis 4:8, 1987.

198. Sanguinetti CM, Montroni M, Balbi B, et al: Does activity of pulmonary sarcoidosis depend on disease duration: A correlation between bronchoalveolar lavage, scintigraphic, radiologic, and physiologic parameters and time of onset of the disease. Sarcoidosis 4:18, 1987.

199. Rosen Y, Moon S, Huang C-T, et al: Granulomatous pulmonary angiitis in sarcoidosis. Arch Pathol Lab Med 101:170, 1977.

200. Takemura T, Matsui Y, Saiki S, et al: Pulmonary vascular involvement in sarcoidosis: A report of 40 autopsy cases. Hum Pathol 23:1216, 1992.

201. Rossman MD, Daniele RP, Dauber JH: Nodular endobronchial sarcoidosis: A study comparing blood and lung lymphocytes. Chest 79:427, 1981.

202. Olsson T, Björnstad-Pettersen H, Stjernberg NL: Bronchostenosis due to sarcoidosis. Chest 75:663, 1979.

203. Hadfield JW, Page RL, Flower CDR, et al: Localized airways narrowing in sarcoidosis. Thorax 37:443, 1982.

204. Aisner SC, Gupta PK, Frost JH: Sputum cytology in pulmonary sarcoidosis. Acta Cytol 21:394, 1977.

205. Wollschlager C, Khan F: Aspergillomas complicating sarcoidosis: A prospective study in 100 patients. Chest 86:585, 1984.

206. Edelman RR, Johnson TS, Jhaveri HS, et al: Fatal hemoptysis resulting from erosion of a pulmonary artery in cavitary sarcoidosis. Am J Roentgenol 145:37, 1985.
207. Kanada DJ, Scott D, Sharma OP: Unusual presentations of pleural sarcoidosis. Br J Dis Chest 74:203, 1980.
208. van Maarsseveen AC, Veldhuizen RW, Stam J, et al: A quantitative histomorphologic analysis of lymph node granulomas in sarcoidosis in relation to radiological stage I and II. J Pathol 134:441, 1983.
209. DeRemee RA: The roentgenographic staging of sarcoidosis: Historic and contemporary perspectives. Chest 83:128, 1983.
210. James DG, Neville E, Siltzbach LE, et al: A worldwide review of sarcoidosis. Ann NY Acad Sci 278:321, 1976.
211. Chiles C, Putman CE: Pulmonary sarcoidosis. Semin Respir Med 13:345, 1992.
212. Miller BH, Rosado-de-Christenson M, McAdams HP, et al: Thoracic sarcoidosis: Radiologic-pathologic correlation. RadioGraphics 15:421, 1995.
213. Berkmen YM: Radiologic aspects of intrathoracic sarcoidosis. Semin Roentgenol 20:356, 1985.
214. Ellis K, Renthal G: Pulmonary sarcoidosis: Roentgenographic observations on course of disease. AJR 88:1070, 1962.
215. Littner MR, Schachter EN, Putman CE, et al: The clinical assessment of roentgenographically atypical pulmonary sarcoidosis. Am J Med 62:361, 1977.
216. Rockoff SD, Rohatgi PK: Unusual manifestations of thoracic sarcoidosis. AJR 144:513, 1985.
217. Kirks DR, McCormick VD, Greenspan RH: Pulmonary sarcoidosis: Roentgenologic analysis of 150 patients. Am J Roentgenol 117:777, 1973.
218. Theros EG: RPC of the month from the AFIP. Radiology 92:1557, 1969.
219. Bein ME, Putman CE, McLoud TC, et al: A reevaluation of intrathoracic lymphadenopathy in sarcoidosis. Am J Roentgenol 131:409, 1978.
220. Bein ME, Putman CE, McLoud TC, et al: A reevaluation of intrathoracic lymphadenopathy in sarcoidosis. Am J Roentgenol 131:409, 1978.
221. Schabel SI, Foote GA, McKee KA: Posterior lymphadenopathy in sarcoidosis. Radiology 129:591, 1978.
222. Kent DC: Recurrent unilateral hilar adenopathy in sarcoidosis. Am Rev Respir Dis 91:272, 1965.
223. Rabinowitz JG, Ulreich S, Soriano C: The usual unusual manifestations of sarcoidosis and the "hilar-haze"—A new diagnostic aid. Am J Roentgenol 120:821, 1974.
224. Spann RW, Rosenow EC III, DeRemee RA, et al: Unilateral hilar or paratracheal adenopathy in sarcoidosis: A study of 38 cases. Thorax 26:296, 1971.
225. Westcott JL, Graff AC Jr: Sarcoidosis, hilar adenopathy, and pulmonary artery narrowing. Radiology 108:585, 1973.
226. Faunce HF, Ramsay GC, Sy W: Protracted yet variable major pulmonary artery compression in sarcoidosis. Radiology 119:313, 1976.
227. Radke JR, Kaplan H, Conway WA: The significance of superior vena cava syndrome developing in a patient with sarcoidosis. Radiology 134:311, 1980.
228. Morgans WE, Al-Jilahawi AN, Mbatha PB: Superior vena caval obstruction caused by sarcoidosis. Thorax 35:397, 1980.
229. Javaheri S, Hales K: Sarcoidosis: Cause of innominate vein obstruction and massive pleural effusion. Lung 157:81, 1980.
230. Scadding JG: The late stages of pulmonary sarcoidosis. Postgrad Med J 46:530, 1970.
231. Gross BH, Schneider HJ, Proto AV: Eggshell calcification of lymph nodes: An update. Am J Roentgenol 135:1265, 1980.
232. Israel HL, Lenchner G, Steiner RM: Late development of mediastinal calcification in sarcoidosis. Am Rev Respir Dis 124:302, 1981.
233. Wurm K, Reindell H: On the differential roentgenological diagnosis of sarcoidosis (Boeck's disease) and lymphogranulomatosis. Radiologe 2:134, 1962.
234. Wurm K: The stages of pulmonary sarcoidosis. Ger Med Monthly 5:386, 1960.
235. Müller NL, Kullnig P, Miller RR: The CT findings of pulmonary sarcoidosis: Analysis of 25 patients. AJR 152:1179, 1989.
236. Sider L, Horton ES Jr: Hilar and mediastinal adenopathy in sarcoidosis as detected by computed tomography. J Thorac Imag 5:77, 1990.
237. Kuhlman JE, Fishman EK, Hamper UM, et al: The computed tomographic spectrum of thoracic sarcoidosis. RadioGraphics 9:449, 1989.
238. Saksouk FA, Haddad MC: Detection of mesenteric involvement in sarcoidosis using computed tomography. Br J Radiol 60:1135, 1987.
239. Warshauer DM, Dumbleton SA, Molina PL, et al: Abdominal CT findings in sarcoidosis: Radiologic and clinical correlation. Radiology 192:93, 1994.
240. Murdoch J, Müller NL: Pulmonary sarcoidosis: Changes on follow-up CT examination. AJR 159:473, 1992.
241. Gawne-Cain ML, Hansell DM: The pattern and distribution of calcified mediastinal lymph nodes in sarcoidosis and tuberculosis: A CT study. Clin Radiol 51:263, 1996.
242. Epler GR, McLoud TC, Gaensler EA, et al: Normal chest roentgenograms in chronic diffuse infiltrative lung disease. N Engl J Med 298:934, 1978.
243. Schlossberg O, Sfedu E: Disseminated sarcoidosis. Sarcoidosis 4:149, 1987.
244. Israel RH: Diagnosing sarcoidosis (letter). JAMA 241:1791, 1979.
245. Rosen Y, Amorosa JK, Moon S, et al: Occurrence of lung granulomas in patients with stage I sarcoidosis. Am J Roentgenol 129:1083, 1977.
246. Brauner MW, Grenier P, Mompoint D, et al: Pulmonary sarcoidosis: Evaluation with high-resolution CT. Radiology 172:467, 1989.
247. Hillerdal G, Nöu E, Osterman K, et al: Sarcoidosis: Epidemiology and prognosis. Am Rev Respir Dis 130:29, 1984.
248. Symmons DPM, Woods KL: Recurrent sarcoidosis. Thorax 35:879, 1980.
249. Baughman RP: Sarcoidosis: Usual and unusual manifestations (clinical conference). Chest 94:165, 1988.
250. Steiger V, Fanburg BL: Recurrence of thoracic lymphadenopathy in sarcoidosis (letter). N Engl J Med 314:1512, 1986.
251. Ellis K, Renthal G: Pulmonary sarcoidosis: Roentgenographic observations on course of disease. Am J Roentgenol 88:1070, 1962.
252. Stone DJ, Schwartz A: A long-term study of sarcoid and its modification by steroid therapy: Lung function and other factors in prognosis. Am J Med 41:528, 1966.
253. Israel HL, Sperber M, Steiner RM: Course of chronic hilar sarcoidosis in relation to markers of granulomatous activity. Invest Radiol 18:1, 1983.
254. Kirks DR, McCormick VD, Greenspan RH: Pulmonary sarcoidosis: Roentgenologic analysis of 150 patients. AJR 117:777, 1979.
255. Mathieson JR, Mayo JR, Staples CA, Müller NL: Chronic diffuse infiltrative lung disease: Comparison of diagnostic accuracy of CT and chest radiography. Radiology 171:111, 1989.
256. Grenier P, Valeyre D, Cluzel P, et al: Chronic diffuse interstitial lung disease: Diagnostic value of chest radiography and high-resolution CT. Radiology 179:123, 1991.
257. Primack SL, Hartman TE, Hansell DM, Müller NL: End-stage lung disease: CT findings in 61 patients. Radiology 189:681, 1993.
258. Mesbahi SJ, Davies P: Unilateral pulmonary changes in the chest x-ray in sarcoidosis. Clin Radiol 32:283, 1981.
259. Müller NL, Mawson JB, Mathieson JR, et al: Sarcoidosis: Correlation of extent of disease at CT with clinical, functional, and radiographic findings. Radiology 171:613, 1989.
260. McLoud TC, Epler GR, Gaensler EA, et al: A radiographic classification for sarcoidosis: Physiologic correlation. Invest Radiol 17:129, 1982.
261. Traill ZC, Maskell GF, Gleeson FV: High-resolution CT findings of pulmonary sarcoidosis. Am J Roentgenol 168:1557, 1997.
262. Grenier P, Chevret S, Beigelman C, et al: Chronic diffuse infiltrative lung disease: Determination of the diagnostic value of clinical data, chest radiography, and CT with Bayesian analysis. Radiology 191:383, 1994.
263. Müller NL, Mayo JR, Zwirewich CV: Value of MR imaging in the evaluation of chronic infiltrative lung diseases: Comparison with CT. AJR 158:1205, 1992.
264. Remy-Jardin M, Giraud F, Remy J, et al: Pulmonary sarcoidosis: Role of CT in the evaluation of disease activity and functional impairment and in prognosis assessment. Radiology 191:675, 1994.
265. Gruden JF, Webb WR: Identification and evaluation of centrilobular opacities on high-resolution CT. Semin Ultrasound CT MRI 16:435, 1995.
266. Nishimura K, Itoh H, Kitaichi M, et al: Pulmonary sarcoidosis: Correlation of CT and histopathologic findings. Radiology 189:105, 1993.
267. Felson B: Uncommon roentgen patterns of pulmonary sarcoidosis. Dis Chest 34:357, 1958.
268. Rubinstein I, Solomon A, Baum GL, et al: Pulmonary sarcoidosis presenting with unusual roentgenographic manifestations. Eur J Respir Dis 67:335, 1985.
269. Chao DC, Hassenpflug M, Sharma OP: Multiple lung masses, pneumothorax, and psychiatric symptoms in a 29-year-old African-American woman. Chest 108:871, 1995.
270. Pinsker KL: Solitary pulmonary nodule in sarcoidosis. JAMA 240:1379, 1978.
271. Rose RM, Lee RG, Costello P: Solitary nodular sarcoidosis. Clin Radiol 36:589, 1985.
272. Hasan FM, Mark EJ: A young man with a diagnosis of sarcoidosis and a pulmonary mass. N Engl J Med 306:412, 1982.
273. Lynch DA, Webb WR, Gamsu G, et al: Computed tomography in pulmonary sarcoidosis. J Comput Assist Tomogr 13:405, 1989.
274. Glazer HS, Levitt RG, Shackelford GD: Peripheral pulmonary infiltrates in sarcoidosis. Chest 86:741, 1984.
275. Teirstein AS, Siltzbach LE: Sarcoidosis of the upper lung fields simulating pulmonary tuberculosis. Chest 64:303, 1973.
276. Johkoh T, Ikezoe J, Takeuchi N, et al: CT findings in "pseudoalveolar" sarcoidosis. J Comput Assist Tomogr 16:904, 1992.
277. Tazi A, Desfemmes-Baleyte T, Soler P, et al: Pulmonary sarcoidosis with a diffuse ground glass pattern on the chest radiograph. Thorax 49:793, 1994.
278. Leung AN, Miller RR, Müller NL: Parenchymal opacification in chronic infiltrative lung diseases: CT-pathologic correlation. Radiology 188:209, 1993.
279. Nishimura K, Itoh H, Kitaichi M, et al: CT and pathological correlation of pulmonry sarcoidosis. Semin Ultrasound CT MRI 16:361, 1995.
280. Thomas PD, Hunninghake GW: Current concepts of the pathogenesis of sarcoidosis. Am Rev Respir Dis 135:747, 1987.
281. Brauner MW, Lenoir S, Grenier P, et al: Pulmonary sarcoidosis: CT assessment of lesion reversibility. Radiology 182:349, 1992.
282. Miller A: The vanishing lung syndrome associated with pulmonary sarcoidosis. Br J Dis Chest 75:209, 1981.
283. Rockoff SD, Rohatgi PK: Unusual manifestations of thoracic sarcoidosis. Am J Roentgenol 144:513, 1985.
284. Conant EF, Glickstein MF, Mahar P, et al: Pulmonary sarcoidosis in the older patient: Conventional radiographic features. Radiology 169:315, 1988.
285. Ichikawa Y, Fujimoto K, Shiraishi T, et al: Primary cavitary sarcoidosis: High-resolution CT findings. Am J Roentgenol 163:745, 1994.
286. Canessa PA, Torraca A, Lavecchia MA, et al: Primary acute pulmonary cavitation in asymptomatic sarcoidosis. Sarcoidosis 6:158, 1989.
287. Biem J, Hoffstein V: Aggressive cavitary pulmonary sarcoidosis. Am Rev Respir Dis 143:428, 1991.
288. Gorske KJ, Fleming RJ: Mycetoma formation in cavitary pulmonary sarcoidosis. Radiology 95:279, 1970.
289. Freundlich IM, Libshitz HI, Glassman LM, et al: Sarcoidosis: Typical and atypical thoracic manifestations and complications. Clin Radiol 21:376, 1970.

290. Israel HL, Ostrow A: Sarcoidosis and aspergilloma. Am J Med 47:243, 1969.

291. Felson B: Less familiar roentgen patterns of pulmonary granulomas: Sarcoidosis, histoplasmosis and noninfectious necrotizing granulomatosis (Wegener's syndrome). Am J Roentgenol 81:211, 1959.

292. Dorman RL Jr, Whitman GJ, Chew FS: Thoracic sarcoidosis. AJR 164:1368, 1995.

293. Goldenberg GJ, Greenspan RH: Middle-lobe atelectasis due to endobronchial sarcoidosis with hypercalcemia and renal impairment. N Engl J Med 262:1112, 1960.

294. Citron KM, Scadding JG: Stenosing non-caseating tuberculosis (sarcoidosis) of the bronchi. Thorax 12:10, 1957.

295. Henry DA, Kiser PE, Scheer CE, et al: Multiple imaging evaluation of sarcoidosis. RadioGraphics 6:75, 1986.

295a. Gleeson FV, Traill ZC, Hansell DM: Evidence on expiratory CT scans of small-airway obstruction in sarcoidosis. Am J Roentgenol 166:1052, 1996.

296. Sharma OP, Gordonson J: Pleural effusion in sarcoidosis: A report of six cases. Thorax 30:95, 1975.

297. Chusid EL, Siltzbach LE: Sarcoidosis of the pleura. Ann Intern Med 81:190, 1974.

298. Beekman JF, Zimmet SM, Chun BK, et al: Spectrum of pleural involvement in sarcoidosis. Arch Intern Med 136:323, 1976.

299. Wilen SB, Rabinowitz JG, Ulreich S, et al: Pleural involvement in sarcoidosis. Am J Med 57:200, 1974.

300. Knox AJ, Wardman AG, Page RL: Tuberculous pleural effusion occurring during corticosteroid treatment of sarcoidosis. Thorax 41:651, 1986.

301. Berte SJ, Pfotenhauer MA: Massive pleural effusion in sarcoidosis. Am Rev Respir Dis 86:261, 1962.

302. Lum GH, Poropatich RK: Unilateral pleural thickening. Chest 110:1348, 1996.

303. Loughney E, Higgins BG: Pleural sarcoidosis: A rare presentation. Thorax 52:200, 1997.

304. Whitcomb ME, Hawley PC, Domby WR, et al: The role of fiberoptic bronchoscopy in the diagnosis of sarcoidosis: Clinical conference in pulmonary disease from Ohio State University, Columbus. Chest 74:205, 1978.

305. Gomm SA: An unusual presentation of sarcoidosis: Spontaneous haemopneumothorax. Postgrad Med J 60:621, 1984.

306. Ross RJ, Empey DW: Bilateral spontaneous pneumothorax in sarcoidosis. Postgrad Med J 59:106, 1983.

307. Sharma SK, Pande JN, Mukhopadhay AK, et al: Bilateral recurrent spontaneous pneumothoraces in sarcoidosis. Jpn J Med 26:69, 1987.

308. Rizzato G, Montemurro L: The locomotor system. In James DG (ed): Sarcoidosis and Other Granulomatous Disorders. New York, Marcel Dekker, 1994.

309. Stump D, Spock A, Grossman H: Vertebral sarcoidosis in adolescents. Radiology 121:153, 1976.

310. Oven TJ, Sones M, Morrissey WL: Lytic lesion of the sternum: Rare manifestation of sarcoidosis. Am J Med 80:285, 1986.

311. Yaghmai I: Radiographic, angiographic and radionuclide manifestations of osseous sarcoidosis. RadioGraphics 3:375, 1983.

312. Rizzato G, Montemurro L, Fraioli P: Bone mineral content in sarcoidosis. Semin Respir Med 13:411, 1992.

313. Chiles C, Adams GW, Ravin CE: Radiographic manifestations of cardiac sarcoid. Am J Roentgenol 145:711, 1985.

314. Riedy K, Fisher MR, Belic N, et al: MR imaging of myocardial sarcoidosis. Am J Roentgenol 151:915, 1988.

314a. Mazzone P, Arroliga A: Acute dyspnea and hypoxia in a 37-year-old woman with sarcoidosis. Chest 113:830, 1998.

315. Folz SJ, Johnson CD, Swensen SJ: Abdominal manifestations of sarcoidosis in CT studies. J Comput Assist Tomogr 19:573, 1995.

316. Farman J, Ramirez G, Brunetti J, et al: Abdominal manifestations of sarcoidosis: CT appearances. Clin Imaging 19:30, 1995.

317. Thrasher DR, Briggs DD Jr: Pulmonary sarcoidosis. Clin Chest Med 3:537, 1982.

318. Nolan JP, Klatskin G: The fever of sarcoidosis. Ann Intern Med 61:455, 1964.

319. Siltzbach LE, James DG, Neville E, et al: Course and prognosis of sarcoidosis around the world. Am J Med 57:847, 1974.

320. Löfgren S, Lundbäck H: The bilateral hilar lymphoma syndrome: I. A study of the relation to age and sex in 212 cases: II. A study of the relation to tuberculosis and sarcoidosis in 212 cases. Acta Med Scand 142:259, 1952.

321. Kucera Maj RF: A possible association of rheumatoid arthritis and sarcoidosis. Chest 95:604, 1989.

322. Lynch JP III, Sharma OP, Baughman RP: Extrapulmonary sarcoidosis. Semin Respir Infect 13:229, 1998.

323. Enzenauer RJ, West SG: Sarcoidosis in autoimmune disease. Semin Arthritis Rheum 22:1, 1992.

324. Kataria YP, Shaw RA, Campbell PB: Sarcoidosis: An overview: II. Clin Notes Respir Dis 20:3, 1982.

325. Blackmon GM, Raghu G: Pulmonary sarcoidosis: A mimic of respiratory infection. Semin Respir Infect 10:176, 1995.

326. Rubinstein I, Baum GL, Hiss Y, et al: Hemoptysis in sarcoidosis. Eur J Respir Dis 66:302, 1985.

327. Chang JC, Driver AG, Townsend CA, et al: Hemoptysis in sarcoidosis. Sarcoidosis 4:49, 1987.

328. Israel HL, Lenchner GS, Atkinson GW: Sarcoidosis and aspergilloma: The role of surgery. Chest 82:430, 1982.

329. Johns CJ: Management of hemoptysis with pulmonary fungus ball in sarcoidosis. Chest 82:400, 1982.

330. Gardiner IT, Uff JS: Acute pleurisy in sarcoidosis. Thorax 33:124, 1978.

331. Kanada DJ, Scott D, Sharma OP: Unusual presentations of pleural sarcoidosis. Br J Dis Chest 74:203, 1980.

332. Liss HP: Pleuropericarditis in sarcoidosis. South Med J 79:258, 1986.

332a. Froudarakis ME, Bouros D, Voloudaki A, et al: Pneumothorax as a first manifestation of sarcoidosis. Chest 112:278, 1997.

333. Soskel NT, Sharma OP: Pleural involvement in sarcoidosis: Case presentation and detailed review of the literature. Semin Respir Med 13:492, 1992.

334. Benatar SR, Clark TJH: Pulmonary function in a case of endobronchial sarcoidosis. Am Rev Respir Dis 110:490, 1974.

335. Olsson T, Bjornstad-Pettersen H, Stjernberg NL: Bronchostenosis due to sarcoidosis: A cause of atelectasis and airway obstruction simulating pulmonary neoplasm and chronic obstructive pulmonary disease. Chest 75:663, 1979.

336. Hadfield JW, Page RL, Flower CDR, et al: Localised airway narrowing in sarcoidosis. Thorax 37:443, 1982.

337. Stjernberg N, Thunell M: Pulmonary function in patients with endobronchial sarcoidosis. Acta Med Scand 215:121, 1984.

338. Fouty BW, Pomeranz M, Thigpen TP, et al: Dilatation of bronchial stenoses due to sarcoidosis using flexible fiberoptic bronchoscope. Chest 106:677, 1994.

339. Udwadia ZF, Pilling JR, Jenkins PF, et al: Bronchoscopic and bronchographic findings in 12 patients with sarcoidosis and severe progressive airways obstruction. Thorax 45:272, 1990.

340. Bechtel JT, Starr T III, Dantzker DR, et al: Airway hyperreactivity in patients with sarcoidosis. Am Rev Respir Dis 1241:759, 1981.

341. Damuth TE, Bower JS, Cho K, et al: Major pulmonary artery stenosis causing pulmonary hypertension in sarcoidosis. Chest 78:888, 1980.

342. Shah A, Bhagat R: Digital clubbing in sarcoidosis. Indian J Chest Dis Allied Sci 34:217, 1992.

343. Martin JM, Dowling GP: Sudden death associated with compression of pulmonary arteries in sarcoidosis. Can Med Assoc J 133:423, 1985.

344. Khan MM, Gill DS, McConkey B: Myopathy and external pulmonary compression caused by sarcoidosis. Thorax 36:703, 1981.

345. Hoffstein V, Ranganathan N, Mullen JB: Sarcoidosis simulating pulmonary veno-occlusive disease. Am Rev Respir Dis 134:809, 1986.

346. Morgans WE, Al-Jilahawi AN, Mbatha PB: Superior vena caval obstruction caused by sarcoidosis. Thorax 35:397, 1980.

347. Javaheri S, Hales CA: Sarcoidosis: A cause of innominate vein obstruction and massive pleural effusion. Lung 157:81, 1980.

348. Thunell M, Bjerle P, Olofsson BO, et al: Cardiopulmonary function in sarcoidosis. Acta Med Scand 215:215, 1984.

349. Baughman RP, Gerson M, Bosken CH: Right and left ventricular function at rest and with exercise in patients with sarcoidosis. Chest 85:301, 1984.

350. Guskowski J, Hawrykiewicz I, Zych D, et al: Pulmonary haemodynamics at rest and during exercise in patients with sarcoidosis. Respiration 46:26, 1984.

351. Fleming HA: Cardiac sarcoidosis. In James DG (ed): Sarcoidosis and Other Granulomatous Disorders. New York, Marcel Dekker, 1994.

352. Oakley CM: Cardiac sarcoidosis. Thorax 44:371, 1989.

353. Sharma OP, Maheshwari A, Tahker K: Myocardial sarcoidosis. Chest 103:253, 1993.

354. Sharma OP: Myocardial sarcoidosis: A wolf in sheep's clothing. Chest 106:988, 1994.

355. Roberts WC, McAllister HA Jr, Ferrans VJ: Sarcoidosis of the heart: A clinicopathologic study of 35 necropsy patients (group I) and review of 78 previously described necropsy patients (Group II). Am J Med 63:86, 1977.

356. Virmani R, Bures JC, Roberts WC: Cardiac sarcoidosis: Major cause of sudden death in young individuals. Chest 77:423, 1980.

356a. Yazaki Y, Isobe M, Hiramitsu S, et al: Comparison of clinical features and prognosis of cardiac sarcoidosis and idiopathic dilated cardiomyopathy. Am J Cardiol 82:537, 1998.

357. Wait JL, Movahed A: Anginal chest pain in sarcoidosis. Thorax 44:391, 1989.

358. Ahmed SS, Rozefort R, Taclob LT, et al: Development of ventricular aneurysm in cardiac sarcoidosis. Angiology 28:323, 1977.

359. Editorial: Myocardial sarcoidosis. Lancet 2:1351, 1972.

360. Silverman KJ, Hutchins GM, Buckley BH: Cardiac sarcoid: A clinicopathologic study of 84 unselected patients with systemic sarcoidosis. Circulation 58:1204, 1978.

361. Iwai K, Tachibana T, Takemura T, et al: Pathological studies on sarcoidosis autopsy: I. Epidemiological features of 320 cases in Japan. Acta Pathol Jpn 43:372, 1993.

362. Fleming HA: Sarcoid heart disease: A review and an appeal. Thorax 35:641, 1980.

363. Botti RE, Young FE: Myocardial sarcoid, complete heart block and aortic stenosis. Ann Intern Med 51:811, 1959.

364. Chun SK, Andy JJ, Jilly P, et al: Ventricular aneurysm in sarcoidosis. Chest 68:392, 1975.

365. Thunell M, Bjerle P, Stjernberg N: ECG abnormalities in patients with sarcoidosis. Acta Med Scand 213:115, 1983.

366. Suzuki T, Kanda T, Kubota S, et al: Holter monitoring as a noninvasive indicator of cardiac involvement in sarcoidosis. Chest 106:1021, 1994.

367. Kinney EL, Jackson GL, Reeves WC, et al: Thallium-scan myocardial defects and echocardiographic abnormalities in patients with sarcoidosis without clinical cardiac dysfunction. Am J Med 68:497, 1980.

368. Kinney EL, Jackson GL, Reeves WC, et al: Thallium-scan myocardial defects and echocardiographic abnormalities in patients with sarcoidosis without clinical cardiac dysfunction: An analysis of 44 patients. Am J Med 68:497, 1980.

369. Tellier P, Paycha F, Antony I, et al: Reversibility by dipyridamole of thallium-201 myocardial scan defects in patients with sarcoidosis. Am J Med 85:189, 1988.

370. Le Guludec D, Menad F, Faraggi M, et al: Myocardial sarcoidosis: Clinical value of technetium-99m sestamibi tomoscintigraphy. Chest 106:1675, 1994.
371. Okayama K, Kurata C, Tawarahara K, et al: Diagnostic and prognostic value of myocardial scintigraphy with thallium-201 and gallium-67 in cardiac sarcoidosis. Chest 107:330, 1995.
372. Dupuis JM, Victor J, Furber A, et al: Value of magnetic resonance imaging in cardiac sarcoidosis: Apropos of a case. Arch Mal Coeur Vaiss 87:105, 1994.
373. Lillington GA, Jamplis RW: Scalene node biopsy. Ann Intern Med 59:101, 1963.
374. Editorial: "Diagnosis" of sarcoidosis. N Engl J Med 267:103, 1962.
375. James DG, Angi MR: Ocular sarcoidosis. In James DG (ed): Sarcoidosis and Other Granulomatous Disorders. New York, Marcel Dekker, 1994.
376. Shah S, Cole MD, Nicholls A: Ocular and renal sarcoidosis. J R Soc Med 88:597, 1995.
377. Faller M, Purohit A, Kennel N, et al: Systemic sarcoidosis initially presenting as an orbital tumour. Eur Respir J 8:474, 1995.
378. Campo RV, Aaberg TM: Choroidal granuloma in sarcoidosis. Am J Ophthalmol 97:419, 1984.
379. Sharma OP: Cutaneous sarcoidosis: Clinical features and management. Chest 61:320, 1972.
380. Olive KE, Kataria YP: Cutaneous manifestations of sarcoidosis: Relationships to other organ system involvement, abnormal laboratory measurements, and disease course. Arch Intern Med 145:1811, 1985.
381. James DG, Epstein WL: Cutaneous sarcoidosis. In James DG (ed): Sarcoidosis and Other Granulomatous Disorders. New York, Marcel Dekker, 1994.
381a. Burov EA, Kantor GR, Isaac M: Morpheaform sarcoidosis: report of three cases. J Am Acad Dermatol 39:345, 1998.
381b. Goldenberg JD, Kotler HS, Shamsai R, et al: Sarcoidosis of the external nose mimicking rhinophyma. Case report and review of the literature. Ann Otol Rhinol Laryngol 107:514, 1998.
381c. Garcia-Porrua C, Gonzalez-Gay MA, Garcia-Pais MJ, et al: Cutaneous vasculitis: an unusual presentation of sarcoidosis in adulthood (review). Scand J Rheumatol 27:80, 1998.
382. Sheffield EA: Pathology of sarcoidosis. Clin Chest Med 18:741, 1997.
383. Dorland's Illustrated Medical Dictionary, 28th ed. Philadelphia, WB Saunders, 1994.
384. Spiteri MA, Matthey F, Gordon T, et al: Lupus pernio: A clinicoradiological study of thirty-five cases. Br J Dermatol 112:315, 1985.
385. Veien NK, Stahl D, Brodthagen H: Cutaneous sarcoidosis in Caucasians. J Am Acad Dermatol 16(3 Pt 1):534, 1987.
386. Hanno R, Callen JP: Sarcoidosis: A disorder with prominent cutaneous features and their interrelationship with systemic disease. Med Clin North Am 64:847, 1980.
387. James DG: Dermatological aspects of sarcoidosis. Q J Med 28:109, 1959.
388. Hancock BW: Cutaneous sarcoidosis in blood donation venipuncture sites. BMJ 4:706, 1972.
389. Sherlock S: The liver in sarcoidosis. In James DG (ed): Sarcoidosis and Other Granulomatous Disorders. New York, Marcel Dekker, 1994.
390. Devaney K, Goodman ZD, Epstein MS, et al: Hepatic sarcoidosis: Clinicopathologic features in 100 patients. Am J Surg Pathol 17:1272, 1993.
390a. Ishak KG: Sarcoidosis of the liver and bile ducts (review). Mayo Clin Proc 73:467, 1998.
391. Warshauer DM, Molina PL, Hamman SM, et al: Nodular sarcoidosis of the liver and spleen: Analysis of 32 cases. Radiology 195:757, 1995.
392. Cunningham D, Mills PR, Quigley EMM, et al: Hepatic granulomas: Experience over a 10-year period in the west of Scotland. Q J Med 51:162, 1982.
393. Scheuer PJ: Hepatic granulomas. BMJ 285:833, 1982.
394. Rudzki C, Ishak KG, Zimmerman HJ: Chronic intrahepatic cholestasis of sarcoidosis. Am J Med 59:373, 1975.
395. Keeffe EB: Sarcoidosis and primary biliary cirrhosis. Am J Med 83:977, 1987.
396. McCluggage WG, Sloan JM: Hepatic granulomas in Northern Ireland: A thirteen-year review. Histopathology 25:219, 1994.
397. Maddrey WC, Johns CJ, Boitnott JK, et al: Sarcoidosis and chronic hepatic disease: A clinical and pathologic study of 20 patients. Medicine 49:375, 1970.
398. Kadin ME, Donaldson SS, Dorfman RF: Isolated granulomas in Hodgkin's disease. N Engl J Med 283:859, 1970.
399. Bagley CM, Roth JA, Thomas LB, et al: Liver biopsy in Hodgkin's disease. Ann Intern Med 76:219, 1972.
400. Joseph RR, Cohen RV: Sarcoidosis: An exercise in differential diagnosis. Dis Chest 52:458, 1967.
401. Kataria YP, Whitcomb ME: Splenomegaly in sarcoidosis. Arch Intern Med 140:35, 1980.
402. Sprague R, Harper P, McClain S, et al: Disseminated gastrointestinal sarcoidosis: Case report and review of the literature. Gastroenterology 87:421, 1984.
403. James DG: Alimentary tract. In James DG (ed): Sarcoidosis and Other Granulomatous Disorders. New York, Marcel Dekker, 1994.
404. Wallaert B, Colombel JF, Adenis A, et al: Increased intestinal permeability in active pulmonary sarcoidosis. Am Rev Respir Dis 145:1440, 1992.
405. McCormick PA, Feighery C, Dolan C, et al: Altered gastrointestinal immune response in sarcoidosis. Gut 29:1628, 1988.
406. Douglas JG, Gillon J, Logan RF, et al: Sarcoidosis and coeliac disease: An association? Lancet 2:13, 1984.
407. Cook DM, Dines DE, Dycus DS: Sarcoidosis: Report of a case presenting as dysphagia. Chest 57:84, 1970.
408. Davies RJ: Dysphagia, abdominal pain, and sarcoid granulomata. BMJ 3:564, 1972.
409. Dufresne CR, Jeyasingham K, Baker RR: Achalasia of the cardia associated with pulmonary sarcoidosis. Surgery 94:32, 1983.
410. Palmer ED: Note on silent sarcoidosis of the gastric mucosa. J Lab Clin Med 52:231, 1958.
411. Papowitz AJ, Li JKH: Abdominal sarcoidosis with ascites. Chest 59:692, 1971.
412. Munt PW: Sarcoidosis of the appendix presenting as appendiceal perforation and abscess. Chest 66:295, 1974.
413. Nessan VJ, Jacoway JR: Biopsy of minor salivary glands in the diagnosis of sarcoidosis. N Engl J Med 301:922, 1979.
414. Giotaki HA, Zioga CP, Ioachim-Velogianni EE: Monoclonal antibodies to epithelioid cells in lip biopsy in sarcoidosis. Sarcoidosis 9:35, 1992.
415. Bhoola KD, McNicol MW, Oliver S, et al: Changes in salivary enzymes in patients with sarcoidosis. N Engl J Med 281:877, 1969.
416. Fisher OE, Burton GG, Bryan WF: Sarcoidosis involving the lacrimal sac. Am Rev Respir Dis 103:708, 1971.
417. Kaplan H: Sarcoid arthritis: A review. Arch Intern Med 112:924, 1963.
418. Gran JT, Bohmer E: Acute sarcoid arthritis: A favourable outcome? A retrospective survey of 49 patients with review of the literature. Scand J Rheumatol 25:70, 1996.
419. Glennas A, Kvien TK, Melby K, et al: Acute sarcoid arthritis: Occurrence, seasonal onset, clinical features and outcomes. Br J Rheumatol 34:45, 1995.
420. Grigor RR, Hughes GRV: Chronic sarcoid arthritis. Br Med J 2:1044, 1976.
421. Perruquet JL, Harrington TM, Davis DE, et al: Sarcoid arthritis in a North American Caucasian population. J Rheumatol 11:521, 1984.
422. Sokoloff L, Bunim JJ: Clinical and pathological studies of joint involvement in sarcoidosis. N Engl J Med 260:841, 1959.
423. Halevy J, Segal I, Pitlik S, et al: Unusual clinical presentation of acute sarcoidosis. Respiration 40:237, 1981.
424. Marymount JV, Murphy DA: Sarcoidosis of the axial skeleton. Clin Nucl Med 19:1060, 1994.
425. Mana J, Segarra MI, Casas R, et al: Multiple atypical bone involvement in sarcoidosis. J Rheumatol 20:394, 1993.
426. Talbot PS: Sarcoid myopathy. BMJ 4:465, 1967.
427. Ost D, Yeldandi A, Cugell D: Acute sarcoid myositis with respiratory muscle involvement: Case report and review of the literature. Chest 107:879, 1995.
428. King BP, Esparza AR, Kahn SI, et al: Sarcoid granulomatous nephritis occurring as isolated renal failure. Arch Intern Med 136:241, 1976.
429. Bear RA, Handelsman S, Lang A, et al: Clinical and pathological features of six cases of sarcoidosis presenting with renal failure. Can Med Assoc J 121:1367, 1979.
430. van Dorp WT, Jie K, Lobatto S, et al: Renal failure due to granulomatous interstitial nephritis after pulmonary sarcoidosis. Nephrol Dial Transplant 2:573, 1987.
431. King BP, Esparza AR, Kahn SI, et al: Sarcoid granulomatous nephritis occurring as isolated renal failure. Arch Intern Med 136:241, 1976.
432. Hoffbrand BI: The kidney in sarcoidosis. In James DG (ed): Sarcoidosis and Other Granulomatous Disorders. New York, Marcel Dekker, 1994.
433. Rizzato G, Fraiolo P, Montemurro L: Nephrolithiasis as a presenting feature of chronic sarcoidosis. Thorax 50:555, 1995.
434. Sharma OP: Vitamin D, calcium and sarcoidosis. Chest 109:535, 1996.
435. Hamada K, Nagai S, Tsutsumi T, et al: Ionized calcium and 1,25-dihydroxyvitamin D concentration in serum of patients with sarcoidosis. Eur Respir J 11:1015, 1998.
436. Barbour GL, Coburn JW, Slatopolsky E, et al: Hypercalcemia in an anephric patient with sarcoidosis: Evidence for extrarenal generation of 1,25-dihydroxyvitamin D. N Engl J Med 305:440, 1981.
437. Maesaka JK, Batuman V, Pablo NC, et al: Elevated 1,25-dihydroxyvitamin D levels: Occurrence with sarcoidosis with end-stage renal disease. Arch Intern Med 142:1206, 1982.
438. Bonnema SJ, Moller J, Marving J, et al: Sarcoidosis causes abnormal seasonal variation in 1,25-dihydroxycholecalciferol. J Intern Med 239:393, 1996.
438a. Zeimer HJ, Greenaway TM, Slavin J, et al: Parathyroid-hormone-related protein in sarcoidosis. Am J Pathol 152:17, 1998.
439. Costabel U, Teschler H: Biochemical changes in sarcoidosis. Clin Chest Med 18:827, 1997
440. Taylor RG, Fisher C, Hoffbrand BI: Sarcoidosis and membranous glomerulonephritis: A significant association. Br Med J 284:1297, 1982.
441. Taylor TK, Senekjian HO, Knight TF, et al: Membranous nephropathy with epithelial crescents in a patient with pulmonary sarcoidosis. Arch Intern Med 139:1183, 1979.
442. Molle D, Baumelou A, Beaufils H, et al: Membranoproliferative glomerulonephritis associated with pulmonary sarcoidosis. Am J Nephrol 6:386, 1986.
443. Vidal F, Oliver JA, Campanya E, et al: Sarcoidosis presenting as multiple pulmonary nodules and nephrotic syndrome. Postgrad Med J 62:1147, 1986.
443a. North-Coombes JD, Healy GF, Cochrane J: Sarcoid-associated minimal change disease: A case report. J South Carolina Med Assoc 94:351, 1998.
444. Trillo A, Orozco R, Jindal K: Glomerular calcinosis in sarcoidosis. Arch Pathol Lab Med 116:1221, 1992.
445. Godin M, Fillastre J-P, Ducastelle T, et al: Sarcoidosis: Retroperitoneal fibrosis, renal arterial involvement and unilateral focal glomerulosclerosis. Arch Intern Med 140:1240, 1980.
446. Delaney P: Neurologic manifestations in sarcoidosis. Review of the literature, with a report of 23 cases. Ann Intern Med 87:336, 1977.
447. Stoudemire A, Linfors E, Houpt JL: Central nervous system sarcoidosis. Gen Hosp Psychiatry 5:129, 1983.

448. Oksanen VE: Neurosarcoidosis. *In* James DG (ed): Sarcoidosis and Other Granulomatous Disorders. New York, Marcel Dekker, 1994.

449. Pascuzzi RM, Shapiro SA, Rau AN, et al: Sarcoid myelopathy. J Neuroimaging 6:61, 1996.

450. O'Reilly BJ, Burrows EH: VIIIth cranial nerve involvement in sarcoidosis. J Laryngol Otol 109:1089, 1995.

451. Westlake WH, Heath JD, Spalton DJ: Sarcoidosis involving the optic nerve and hypothalamus. Arch Opthalmol 113:669, 1995.

452. Stubgen JP: Neurosarcoidosis presenting as a retroclival mass. Surg Neurol 43:85, 1995.

453. Rieger J, Hosten N: Spinal cord sarcoidosis. Neuroradiology 36:627, 1994.

454. Boucher RM, Grace J, Java DJ Jr: Sarcoidosis presenting as multiple cranial neuropathies and a parotid mass. Otolaryngol Head Neck Surg 111:652, 1994.

455. Graf M, Wakhloo A, Schmidtke K, et al: Sarcoidosis of the spinal cord and medulla oblongata: A pathological and neuroradiological case report. Clin Neuropathol 13:19, 1994.

456. Fried ED, Landau AJ, Sher JH, et al: Spinal cord sarcoidosis: A case report and review of the literature. J Assoc Acad Minor Phys 4:132, 1993.

457. Godwin JE, Sahn SA: Sarcoidosis presenting as progressive ascending lower extremity weakness and asymptomatic meningitis with hypoglycorrhachia. Chest 97:1263, 1990.

458. Grizzanti JN, Knapp AB, Schecter AJ, et al: Treatment of sarcoid meningitis with radiotherapy. Am J Med 73:605, 1982.

459. Delaney P: Neurologic manifestations in sarcoidosis: Review of the literature, with a report of 23 cases. Ann Intern Med 87:336, 1977.

459a. Robinson LR, Brownsberger R, Raghu G: Respiratory failure and hypoventilation secondary to neurosarcoidosis. Am J Respir Crit Care Med 157:1316, 1998.

460. Karnik AS: Nodular cerebral sarcoidosis simulating metastatic carcinoma. Arch Intern Med 142:385, 1982.

461. O'Brien GM, Baughman RP, Broderick JP, et al: Paranoid psychosis due to neurosarcoidosis. Sarcoidosis 11:34, 1994.

462. Rosenbloom MA, Uphoff DF: The association of progressive multifocal leukoencephalopathy and sarcoidosis. Chest 83:572, 1983.

463. Sharma OP: Neurosarcoidosis. Chest 112:220, 1997.

464. Cariski AT: Isolated CNS sarcoidosis. JAMA 245:62, 1981.

465. Ismail F, Miller JL, Kahn SE, et al: Hypothalamic-pituitary sarcoidosis: A case report. S Afr Med J 67:139, 1985.

466. Stuart CA, Neelon FA, Lebovitz HE: Disordered control of thirst in hypothalamic-pituitary sarcoidosis. N Engl J Med 303:1078, 1980.

467. Rubinstein I, Gray TA, Moldofsky H, et al: Neurosarcoidosis associated with hypersomnolence treated with corticosteroids and brain irradiation. Chest 94:205, 1988.

468. Bower JS, Belen JE, Weg JG, et al: Manifestations and treatment of laryngeal sarcoidosis. Am Rev Respir Dis 122:325, 1980.

469. Fogel TD, Weissberg JB, Dobular K, et al: Radiotherapy in sarcoidosis of the larynx: Case report and review of the literature. Laryngoscope 94:1223, 1984.

470. Di Benedetto R, Lefrak S: Systematic sarcoidosis with severe involvement of the upper respiratory tract. Am Rev Respir Dis 102:801, 1970.

471. Carasso B: Sarcoidosis of the larynx causing airway obstruction. Chest 65:693, 1974.

472. Firooz03 H, Young R, Lee T: Sarcoidosis of the larynx. Radiology 95:425, 1970.

473. Chijimatsu Y, Tajima J, Washizaki M, et al: Hoarseness as an initial manifestation of sarcoidosis. Chest 78:779, 1980.

473a. Shah RN, Mills PR, George PJ, et al: Upper airways sarcoidosis presenting as obstructive sleep apnoea. Thorax 53:232, 1998.

474. Rigden B: Sarcoid lesion in breast after probable sarcoidosis in lung. BMJ 2:1533, 1978.

475. Kosuda T, Tanaka I, Irie H, et al: Breast sarcoidosis: 2 case reports and a review of 19. Nippon Rinsho 52:1608, 1994.

476. Murphy O, Hogan J, Bredin CP: Endometrial and pulmonary sarcoidosis. Ir J Med Sci 161:14, 1992.

477. Badr AI, Sharma OP: Pulmonary function. *In* James DG (ed): Sarcoidosis and Other Granulomatous Disorders. New York, Marcel Dekker, 1994.

478. Harrison BDW, Shaylor JM, Stokes TC, et al: Airflow limitation in sarcoidosis—a study of pulmonary function in 107 patients with newly diagnosed disease. Respir Med 85:59, 1991.

479. Miller A, Chuang M, Teirstein AS, et al: Pulmonary function in stage I and II pulmonary sarcoidosis. Ann NY Acad Sci 278:292, 1976.

480. Colp C, Park SS, Williams MH Jr: Pulmonary function follow-up of 120 patients with sarcoidosis. Ann NY Acad Sci 278:301, 1976.

481. Keogh BA, Crystal RG: Pulmonary function testing in interstitial pulmonary disease: What does it tell us? Chest 78:856, 1980.

482. Winterbauer RH, Hutchinson JF: Use of pulmonary function tests in the management of sarcoidosis. Chest 78:640, 1980.

483. Dujic Z, Tocilj J, Eterovic D: Increase of lung transfer factor in early sarcoidosis. Respir Med 89:9, 1995.

484. Sharma OP, Johnson R: Airway obstruction in sarcoidosis: A study of 123 nonsmoking black American patients with sarcoidosis. Chest 94:343, 1988.

485. Boushy SF, Kurtzman RS, Martin ND, et al: The course of pulmonary function in sarcoidosis. Ann Intern Med 62:939, 1965.

486. Pulmonary function in sarcoidosis (lead article). BMJ 1:710, 1967.

487. Young RC Jr, Carr C, Shelton TG, et al: Sarcoidosis: Relationship between changes in lung structure and function. Am Rev Respir Dis 95:224, 1967.

488. Snider GL, Doctor L: The mechanics of ventilation in sarcoidosis. Am Rev Respir Dis 89:897, 1964.

489. Sellers RD, Siebens AA: The effects of sarcoidosis on pulmonary function with particular reference to changes in pulmonary compliance. Am Rev Respir Dis 91:660, 1965.

490. Brådvik I, Wollmer P, Blom-Bülow, et al: Lung mechanics and gas exchange during exercise in pulmonary sarcoidosis. Chest 99:572, 1991.

491. Ingram CG, Reid PC, Johnston RN: Exercise testing in pulmonary sarcoidosis. Thorax 37:129, 1982.

492. Matthews JI, Hooper RG: Exercise testing in pulmonary sarcoidosis. Chest 83:75, 1983.

493. Athos L, Mohler JG, Sharma OM: Exercise testing in the physiologic assessment of sarcoidosis. Ann NY Acad Sci 465:491, 1986.

494. Demeter SL: Gas exchange across abnormal interstitial tissue in pulmonary sarcoidosis: Results of therapy. Angiology 38:256, 1987.

495. Miller A, Brown LK, Sloane MF, et al: Cardiorespiratory responses to incremental exercise in sarcoidosis patients with normal spirometry. Chest 107:323, 1995.

496. Sietsema KE, Kraft M, Ginzton L, et al: Abnormal oxygen uptake responses to exercise in patients with mild pulmonary sarcoidosis. Chest 102:838, 1992.

497. Gibbons WJ, Levy RD, Nava S et al: Subclinical cardiac dysfunction in sarcoidosis. Chest 100:44, 1991.

498. Dines DE, Stubbs SE, McDougall JC: Obstructive disease of the airways associated with stage I sarcoidosis. Mayo Clin Proc 53:788, 1978.

499. Renzi GD, Renzi PM, Lopez-Majano V, et al: Airway function in sarcoidosis: Effect of short-term steroid therapy. Respiration 42:98, 1981.

500. Radwan L, Grebska E, Koziorowski A: Small airways function in pulmonary sarcoidosis. Scand J Respir Dis 59:37, 1978.

501. Angyropoulou PK, Patakas DA, Louridas GE: Airway function in stage I and stage II pulmonary sarcoidosis. Respiration 46:17, 1984.

502. Scano G, Monechi GC, Stendardi L, et al: Functional evaluation in stage I pulmonary sarcoidosis. Respiration 49:195, 1986.

503. Coates R, Neville E: The development of airways obstruction in sarcoidosis among smokers and non-smokers. Sarcoidosis 10:115, 1993.

504. Remy-Jardin M, Giraud F, Remy J, et al: Pulmonary sarcoidosis role of CT in the evaluation of disease activity and functional impairment and in prognosis assessment. Radiology 191:675, 1994.

505. Brandstetter RD, Messina MS, Sprince NL, et al: Tracheal stenosis due to sarcoidosis. Chest 80:656, 1981.

506. Gleeson FV, Traill ZC, Hansell DM: Evidence on expiratory CT scans of small-airway obstruction in sarcoidosis. AJR 166:1052, 1996.

507. Manresa Presas F, Romero Colomer P, Rodriguez Sanchon B: Bronchial hyperreactivity in fresh stage I sarcoidosis. Ann NY Acad Sci 465:523, 1986.

508. Marcias S, Ledda MA, Perra R, et al: Aspecific bronchial hyperreactivity in pulmonary sarcoidosis. Sarcoidosis 11:118, 1994.

509. Boulet LP, Milot J, La Forge J, et al: Lymphocytic alveolitis and airway responsiveness in recently diagnosed sarcoidosis. Sarcoidosis 9:43, 1992.

509a. Niimi T, Tomita H, Sato S, et al: Bronchial responsiveness and angiotensin-converting enzyme gene polymorphism in sarcoidosis patients. Chest 114:495, 1998.

510. Baydur A, Pandya K, Sharma OP, et al: Control of ventilation, respiratory muscle strength, and granulomatous involvement of skeletal muscles in patients with sarcoidosis. Chest 103:396, 1993.

511. Bergin CJ, Bell DY, Coblentz CL, et al: Sarcoidosis: Correlation of pulmonary parenchymal pattern at CT with results of pulmonary function tests. Radiology 171:619, 1989.

512. Ebright JR, Soin JS, Manoli RS: The gallium scan: Problems and misuse in examination of patients with suspected infection. Arch Intern Med 142:246, 1982.

513. Myslivecek M, Husak V, Kolek V, et al: Absolute quantitation of gallium-67 citrate accumulation in the lungs and its importance for the evaluation of disease activity in pulmonary sarcoidosis. Eur J Nucl Med 19:1016, 1992.

514. Okada M, Takahashi H, Nukiwa T, et al: Correlative analysis of longitudinal changes in bronchoalveolar lavage, 67 gallium scanning, serum angiotensin-converting enzyme activity, chest x-ray, and pulmonary function tests in pulmonary sarcoidosis. Jpn J Med 26:360, 1987.

515. Line BR, Hunninghake GW, Keogh BA, et al: Gallium-67 scanning to stage the alveolitis of sarcoidosis: Correlation with clinical studies, pulmonary function studies and bronchoalveolar lavage. Am Rev Respir Dis 123:440, 1981.

516. Klech H, Kohn H, Kummer F, et al: Assessment of activity in sarcoidosis: Sensitivity and specificity of 67 gallium scintigraphy, serum ACE levels, chest roentgenography, and blood lymphocyte populations. Chest 82:732, 1982.

517. Sulavik SB, Spencer RP, Palestro CJ, et al: Specificity and sensitivity of distinctive chest radiographic and/or GA images in the noninvasive diagnosis of sarcoidosis. Chest 103:403, 1993.

518. Israel HL, Albertine KH, Park CH, et al: Whole-body gallium 67 scans: Role in diagnosis of sarcoidosis. Am Rev Respir Dis 144:1182, 1991.

519. Pertschuk LP, Silverstein E, Friedland J: Immunohistologic diagnosis of sarcoidosis. Am J Clin Pathol 75:350, 1981.

520. Okabe T, Suzuki A, Ishikawa H, et al: Cells originating from sarcoid granulomas in vitro. Am Rev Respir Dis 124:608, 1981.

521. Horowitz J, Kueppers F, Rosen S: Angiotensin-converting enzyme concentrations in rabbits with talc-induced pulmonary granulomas. Am Rev Respir Dis 124:306, 1981.

523. Rohrbach MS, DeRemee RA: Pulmonary sarcoidosis and serum angiotensin-converting enzyme. Mayo Clin Proc 57:64, 1982.

524. Gilbert S, Steinbrech DS, Landas SK, et al: Amounts of angiotensin-converting enzyme mRNA reflect the burden of granulomas in granulomatous lung disease. Am Rev Respir Dis 148:483, 1993.

525. Perrin-Fayolle M, Pacheco Y, Harf R, et al: Angiotensin-converting enzyme in bronchoalveolar lavage fluid in pulmonary sarcoidosis. Thorax 36:790, 1981.

526. Allen RK, Pierce RJ, Barter CE: Angiotensin-converting enzyme in bronchoalveolar lavage fluid in sarcoidosis. Sarcoidosis 9:54, 1992.

527. Specks U, Martin WJ II, Rohrbach MS: Bronchoalveolar lavage fluid angiotensin-converting enzyme in interstitial lung diseases. Am Rev Respir Dis 141:117, 1990.

528. Lieberman J: Elevation of serum angiotensin-converting-enzyme (ACE) level in sarcoidosis. J Med 59:365, 1975.

529. Fanburg BL, Schoenberger MD, Bachus B, et al: Elevated serum angiotensin-I converting enzyme in sarcoidosis. Am Rev Respir Dis 114:525, 1976.

530. Sandron D, LeCossier D, Moreau F, et al: Angiotensin-converting enzyme in sarcoidosis and other pulmonary diseases: A comparison of two methods of determination. Lung 157:31, 1979.

531. Rohatgi PK, Ryan JW: Simple radioassay for measuring serum activity of angiotensin-converting enzyme in sarcoidosis. Chest 78:69, 1980.

532. Brice EAW, Friedlander W, Bateman ED, et al: Serum angiotensin-converting enzyme activity, concentration, and specific activity in granulomatous interstitial lung disease, tuberculosis, and COPD. Chest 107:706, 1995.

533. Studdy P, Bird R, James DG: Serum angiotensin-converting enzyme (SACE) in sarcoidosis and other granulomatous disorders. Lancet 2:1331, 1978.

534. Gronhagen-Riska C: Angiotensin-converting enzyme: I. Activity and correlations with serum lysozyme in sarcoidosis, other chest or lymph node diseases and healthy persons. Scand J Respir Dis 60:83, 1979.

535. Glatt A: Angiotensin-converting enzyme in sarcoidosis (letter). Mayo Clin Proc 58:140, 1983.

536. Lieberman J, Nosal A, Schlessner LA, et al: Serum angiotensin-converting enzyme for diagnosis and therapeutic evaluation of sarcoidosis. Am Rev Respir Dis 120:329, 1979.

537. Furuya K, Yamaguchi E, Kawakami Y: Angiotensin-converting enzyme (ACE) polymorphism and serum ACE activities in sarcoidosis. Nippon Rinsho 52:1561, 1994.

538. Tiret L, Rigat B, Visvikis S, et al: Evidence, from combined segregation and linkage analysis, that a variant of the angiotensin I-converting enzyme (ACE) gene controls plasma ACE levels. Am J Hum Genet 51:197, 1992.

539. Rigat B, Hubert C, Corvol P, et al: PCR detection of the insertion/deletion polymorphism of the human angiotensin converting enzyme gene (DCP1) (dipeptidyl carboxypeptidase). Nucl Acid Res 20:1433, 1992.

540. Arbustini E, Grasso M, Leo G, et al: Polymorphism of angiotensin-converting enzyme gene in sarcoidosis. Am J Respir Crit Care Med 153:851, 1996.

541. Rossman MD, Dauber JH, Cardillo ME, et al: Pulmonary sarcoidosis: Correlation of serum angiotensin-converting enzyme with blood and bronchoalveolar lymphocytes. Am Rev Respir Dis 125:366, 1982.

542. Bhigjee AI, Pillay NL, Omar MAK, et al: Serum angiotensin-converting in sarcoidosis. S Afr Med J 58:615, 1980.

543. Allen R, Mendelsohn FAO, Csicsmann J, et al: A clinical evaluation of serum angiotensin-converting enzyme in sarcoidosis. Aust NZ J Med 10:496, 1980.

544. Rohatgi PK: Serum angiotensin-converting enzyme in pulmonary disease (review). Lung 160:287, 1982.

545. Rohatgi PK, Ryan JW, Lindeman P: Value of serial measurement of serum angiotensin-converting enzyme in the management of sarcoidosis. Am J Med 70:44, 1981.

546. Gronhagen-Riska C, Selroos O, Wagar G, et al: Angiotensin-converting enzyme: II. Serum activity in early and newly diagnosed sarcoidosis. Scand J Respir Dis 60:94, 1979.

547. Tomita H, Yasutaka I, Sugiura Y, et al: Polymorphism in the angiotensin-converting enzyme (ACE) gene and sarcoidosis. Am J Respir Crit Care Med 156:255, 1997.

548. Sharma P, Smith I, Maguire G, et al: Clinical value of ACE genotyping in diagnosis of sarcoidosis. Lancet 349:1602, 1997.

549. Bunting PS, Szalai JP, Katic M: Diagnostic aspects of angiotensin-converting enzyme in pulmonary sarcoidosis. Clin Biochem 20:213, 1987.

550. Baur X, Fruhmann G, Dahlheim H: Follow-up of angiotensin-converting enzyme in serum of patients with sarcoidosis. Respiration 41:133, 1981.

551. Pascual RS, Gee JBL, Finch SC: Usefulness of serum lysozyme measurement in diagnosis and evaluation of sarcoidosis. N Engl J Med 289:1074, 1973.

552. Zorn SK, Stevens CA, Schachter EN, et al: The angiotensin-converting enzyme in pulmonary sarcoidosis and the relative diagnostic value of serum lysozyme. Lung 157:87, 1980.

553. Gronhagen-Riska C, Selroos O: Angiotensin-converting enzyme: IV. Changes in serum activity and in lysozyme concentrations as indicators of the course of untreated sarcoidosis. Scand J Respir Dis 60:337, 1979.

554. Turton CWG, Grundy E, Firth G, et al: Value of measuring serum angiotensin-I converting enzyme and serum lysozyme in the management of sarcoidosis. Thorax 34:57, 1979.

555. Massaro D, Handler AE, Katz S, et al: Excretion of hydroxyproline in patients with sarcoidosis. Am Rev Respir Dis 93:929, 1966.

556. Parrish RW, Williams JD, Davies BH: Serum beta-2-microglobulin and angiotensin-converting enzyme activity in sarcoidosis. Thorax 37:936, 1982.

557. Sharma OP: Vitamin D, calcium, and sarcoidosis. Chest 109:535, 1996.

558. Goldstein RA, Israel HL, Becker KL, et al: The infrequency of hypercalcemia in sarcoidosis. Am J Med 51:21, 1971.

559. Papapoulos SE, Clemens TL, Fraher LJ, et al: 1,25-dihydroxycholecalciferol in the pathogenesis of the hypercalcaemia of sarcoidosis. Lancet 1:627, 1979.

560. Taylor RL, Lynch HJ Jr, Wysor WG Jr: Seasonal influence of sunlight on the hypercalcemia of sarcoidosis. Am J Med 34:221, 1963.

561. Rømer FK: Renal manifestations and abnormal calcium metabolism in sarcoidosis. Q J Med 49:233, 1980.

562. Lief PD, Bogartz LJ, Koerner SK, et al: Sarcoidosis and primary hyperparathyroidism: An unusual association. Am J Med 47:825, 1969.

563. Burr JM, Farrell JJ, Hills AG: Sarcoidosis and hyperparathyroidism with hypercalcemia: Special usefulness of the cortisone test. N Engl J Med 261:1271, 1959.

564. Dent CE, Watson L: Hyperparathyroidism and sarcoidosis. BMJ 1:646, 1966.

565. Robinson RG, Kerwin DM, Tsou E: Parathyroid adenoma with coexistent sarcoid granulomas: A hypercalcemic patient. Arch Intern Med 140:1547, 1980.

566. Batson JM: Calcification of the ear cartilage associated with the hypercalcemia of sarcoidosis: Report of a case. N Engl J Med 265:876, 1961.

567. Lower EE, Smith JT, Martelo OJ, et al: The anemia of sarcoidosis. Sarcoidosis 5:51, 1988.

568. West WO: Acquired hemolytic anemia secondary to Boeck's sarcoid: Report of a case and review of the literature. N Engl J Med 261:688, 1959.

569. Kondo H, Sakai S, Sakai Y: Autoimmune haemolytic anaemia, Sjögren's syndrome and idiopathic thrombocytopenic purpura in a patient with sarcoidosis. Acta Haematol 89:209, 1993.

570. Semple P d'A: Thrombocytopenia, hemolytic anaemia, and sarcoidosis. BMJ 4:440, 1975.

571. Knodel AR, Beekman JF: Severe thrombocytopenia and sarcoidosis. JAMA 243:258, 1980.

572. Bogaerts Y, Van Der Straeten M, Tasson J, et al: Sarcoidosis or malignancy: A diagnostic dilemma. Eur J Respir Dis 64:541, 1983.

573. Winterbauer RH, Belic N, Moores KD: A clinical interpretation of bilateral hilar adenopathy. Ann Intern Med 78:65, 1973.

574. Meyer A, Raugel M, Jullien JL, et al: Nontuberculous mediastinal adenopathies with erythema nodosum (Löfgren's syndrome): Four new case reports. Rev Tuberc (Paris) 23:357, 1959.

575. Rajasuriya K, Nagaratnam N, Somasunderam M: Syndrome of erythema nodosum, bilateral hilar enlargement and polyarthritis. Br J Dis Chest 53:314, 1959.

575a. Reich JM, Brouns MC, O'Connor EA, et al: Mediastinoscopy in patients with presumptive stage I sarcoidosis: a risk/benefit, cost/benefit analysis. Chest 113:147, 1998.

576. Bacharach T, Zalis EG: Sarcoid syndrome associated with coccidioidomycosis. Am Rev Respir Dis 88:248, 1963.

577. Cohen SH, Fink JN, Garancis JC, et al: Sarcoidosis in hypersensitivity pneumonitis. Chest 72:588, 1977.

578. Mitchell DM, Mitchell DN, Collins JV, et al: Transbronchial lung biopsy through fibreoptic bronchoscope in diagnosis of sarcoidosis. BMJ 280:679, 1980.

579. Bjermer L, Thunell M, Rosenhall L, et al: Endobronchial biopsy positive sarcoidosis: Relation to bronchoalveolar lavage and course of disease. Respir Med 85:229, 1991.

580. Torrington KG, Shorr AF, Parker JW: Endobronchial disease and racial differences in pulmonary sarcoidosis. Chest 111:619, 1997.

581. Takayama K, Nagata N, Miyagawa Y, et al: The usefulness of step sectioning of transbronchial lung biopsy specimen in diagnosing sarcoidosis. Chest 102:1441, 1992.

582. Stjernberg N, Thunell M, Lundgren R: Comparison of flexible fiberoptic bronchoscopy and scalene lymph node biopsy in the diagnosis of sarcoidosis. Endoscopy 15:300, 1983.

583. Mitchell DM, Mitchell DN, Collins JV, et al: Transbronchial lung biopsy through fibreoptic bronchoscope in diagnosis of sarcoidosis. Br J Dis Chest 74:320, 1980.

584. Roethe RA, Fuller PB, Byrd RB, et al: Transbronchoscopic lung biopsy in sarcoidosis: Optimal number and sites for diagnosis. Chest 77:400, 1980.

585. Pinsker KL, Kamholz SL: Diagnosis of sarcoidosis by transbronchial lung biopsy. Chest 79:123, 1981.

586. Gilman MJ, Wang KP: Transbronchial lung biopsy in sarcoidosis: An approach to determine the optimal number of biopsies. Am Rev Respir Dis 122:721, 1980.

587. Ohara K, Okubo A, Kamata K, et al: Transbronchial lung biopsy in the diagnosis of suspected ocular sarcoidosis. Arch Opthalmol 111:642, 1993.

588. Ohmichi M, Yamada G, Hiraga Y: Transbronchial lung biopsy (TBLB) and scalene node biopsy in sarcoidosis. Nippon Rinsho 52:1539, 1994.

589. Mikhail JR, Mitchell DN, Drury RAB, et al: A comparison of the value of mediastinal lymph node biopsy and the Kveim test in sarcoidosis. Am Rev Respir Dis 104:544, 1971.

590. Vernon SE: Nodular pulmonary sarcoidosis: Diagnosis with fine needle aspiration biopsy. Acta Cytol 29:473, 1985.

591. Morales CF, Patefield AJ, Strollo PJ Jr, et al: Flexible transbronchial needle aspiration in the diagnosis of sarcoidosis. Chest 106:709, 1994.

592. Wang KP, Fuenning C, Johns CJ, et al: Flexible transbronchial needle aspiration for the diagnosis of sarcoidosis. Ann Otol Rhinol Laryngol 98:298, 1989.

593. Nessan VJ, Jacoway JR: Biopsy of minor salivary glands in the diagnosis of sarcoidosis. N Engl J Med 301:922, 1979.

594. Solomon DA, Horn BR, Byrd RB, et al: The diagnosis of sarcoidosis by conjunctival biopsy. Chest 74:271, 1978.

595. Hsu RM, Connors AF Jr, Tomashefski JF Jr: Histologic, microbiologic, and clinical correlates of the diagnosis of sarcoidosis by transbronchial biopsy. Arch Pathol Lab Med 120:364, 1996.

596. James DG, Sharma OP, Bradstreet P: The Kveim-Siltzbach test: Report of a new British antigen. Lancet 2:1274, 1967.

597. Anderson R, James DG, Peters PM, et al: The Kveim test in sarcoidosis. Lancet 2:650, 1963.

598. Hirsch JG, Cohn ZA, Morse SI, et al: Evaluation of the Kveim reaction as a diagnostic test for sarcoidosis. N Engl J Med 265:827, 1961.

599. American Thoracic Society: Brummer DI, chairman; Chaves AD, Cugell DW, et al: The Kveim test. A statement by the committee on therapy. Am Rev Respir Dis 103:435, 1971.

600. Siltzbach LE: The Kveim test in sarcoidosis: A study of 750 patients. JAMA 178:476, 1961.

601. Mana J, Pujol R, Salazar A, et al: The Kveim-Siltzbach test in sarcoidosis. Med Clin 104:645, 1995.

602. Wigley RD: Moratorium on Kveim tests (letters to the editor). Lancet 341:1284, 1993.

603. Perry A, Vuitch F: Causes of death in patients with sarcoidosis: A morphologic study of 38 autopsies with clinicopathologic correlations. Arch Pathol Lab Med 119:167, 1995.

604. Sugie T, Hashimoto N, Iwai K: Clinical and autopsy studies on prognosis of sarcoidosis. Nippon Rinsho 52:1567, 1994.

605. Reich JM, Johnson RE: Course and prognosis of sarcoidosis in a nonreferral setting: Analysis of 86 patients observed for 10 years. Am J Med 78:61, 1985.

606. Takada K, Ina Y, Noda M, et al: The clinical course and prognosis of patients with severe, moderate or mild sarcoidosis. J Clin Epidemiol 46:359, 1993.

607. Vestbo J, Viskum K: Respiratory symptoms at presentation and long-term vital prognosis in patients with pulmonary sarcoidosis. Sarcoidosis 11:123, 1994.

608. Viskum K, Vestbo J: Vital prognosis in intrathoracic sarcoidosis with special reference to pulmonary function and radiological stage. Eur Respir J 6:349, 1993.

609. Sones M, Israel HL: Course and prognosis of sarcoidosis. Am J Med 29:84, 1960.

610. Israel HL: Prognosis of sarcoidosis. Ann Intern Med 73:1038, 1970.

611. McLoud TC, Epler GR, Gaensler EA, et al: A radiographic classification for sarcoidosis: Physiologic correlation. Invest Radiol 17:129, 1982.

612. O'Brien LE, Forsman PJ, Wiltse HE: Early onset sarcoidosis with pulmonary function abnormalities. Chest 65:472, 1974.

613. Gideon NM, Mannino DM: Sarcoidosis mortality in the United States 1979–1991: An analysis of multiple-cause mortality data. Am J Med 100:423, 1996.

614. Israel HL, Karlin P, Menduke H, et al: Factors affecting outcome of sarcoidosis: Influence of race, extrathoracic involvement, and initial radiologic lung lesions. Ann NY Acad Sci 465:609, 1986.

615. Johns CJ, Schonfeld SA, Scott PP, et al: Longitudinal study of chronic sarcoidosis with low-dose maintenance corticosteroid therapy: Outcome and complications. Ann NY Acad Sci 465:702, 1986.

616. Young RC Jr, Titus-Dillon PY, Schneider ML, et al: Sarcoidosis in Washington, D.C.: Clinical observations in 105 black patients. Arch Intern Med 125:102, 1970.

617. Editorial: Management of pulmonary sarcoidosis. Lancet 1:890, 1982.

618. Haynes de Regt R: Sarcoidosis and pregnancy. Obstet Gynecol 70(3 Pt 1):369, 1987.

619. Ikeda T, Hayashi S, Kamikawaji N, et al: Adverse effect of chronic tonsillitis on clinical course of sarcoidosis in relation to HLA distribution. Chest 101:758, 1992.

620. Glennas A, Kvien TK, Melby K, et al: Acute sarcoid arthritis: Occurrence, seasonal onset, clinical features and outcome. Br J Rheumatol 34:45, 1995.

621. Mana J, Salazar A, Manresa F: Clinical factors predicting persistence of activity in sarcoidosis: A multivariate analysis of 193 cases. Respiration 61:219, 1994.

622. Neville E, Walker AN, James DG: Prognostic factors predicting the outcome of sarcoidosis: An analysis of 818 patients. Q J Med 52:525, 1983.

623. Gran JT, Bohmer E: Acute sarcoid arthritis: A favourable outcome? A retrospective survey of 49 patients with review of the literature. Scand J Rheumatol 25:70, 1996.

624. Salazar A, Mana J, Corbella X, et al: Splenomegaly in sarcoidosis: A report of 16 cases. Sarcoidosis 12:131, 1995.

625. Siltzbach LE, Greenberg GM: Childhood sarcoidosis—a study of 18 patients. N Engl J Med 279:1239, 1968.

626. Kendig EL, Brummer DL: The prognosis of sarcoidosis in children. Chest 70:351, 1976.

627. Brincker H: Coexistence of sarcoidosis and malignant disease: Causality or coincidence. Sarcoidosis 7:80, 1990.

628. Brincker H, Wilbek E: The incidence of malignant tumours in patients with respiratory sarcoidosis. Br J Cancer 29:247, 1974.

629. Romer FK: Sarcoidosis and cancer. *In* James DG (ed): Sarcoidosis and Other Granulomatous Disorders. New York, Marcel Dekker, 1994.

630. Reich JM, Mullooly JP, Johnson RE: Linkage-analysis of malignancy-associated sarcoidosis. Chest 107:605, 1995.

631. Suen JS, Forse MS, Hyland RH, et al: The malignancy-sarcoidosis syndrome. Chest 98:1300, 1990.

632. Toner GC, Bosl GJ: Sarcoidosis, "sarcoid-like lymphadenopathy" and testicular germ cell tumours. Am J Med 89:651, 1990.

633. Biglino A, Cariti G, Musset M, et al: Pulmonary sarcoidosis associated with Leydig cell testicular neoplasm. Chest 94:428, 1988.

634. Gefter WB, Glick JH, Epstein DM, et al: Sarcoidosis: A cause of intrathoracic lymphadenopathy after treatment of testicular carcinoma. Am J Roentgenol 139:820, 1982.

635. Geller RA, Kuremsky DA, Copeland JS, et al: Sarcoidosis and testicular neoplasm: An unusual association. J Urol 118:487, 1977.

636. Trump DL, Ettinger DS, Feldman MJ, et al: Sarcoidosis and sarcoid-like lesions: Their occurrence after cytotoxic and radiation therapy of testis cancer. Arch Intern Med 141:37, 1981.

637. Gefter WB, Glick JH, Epstein DM, et al: Sarcoidosis: A cause of intrathoracic lymphadenopathy after treatment of testicular carcinoma. Am J Roentgenol 139:820, 1982.

638. O'Connell M, Powell S, Horwich A: Sarcoid-like lymphadenopathy in malignant teratoma. Postgrad Med J 59:108, 1983.

639. Colebunders R, Bultinck J, Servais J, et al: A patient with testis seminoma, sarcoidosis, and neutropenic enterocolitis. Hum Pathol 15:394, 1984.

640. Blacher EJ, Maynard JF: Seminoma and sarcoidosis: An unusual association. Urology 26:288, 1985.

641. Fossa SD, Abeler V, Marton PF, et al: Sarcoid reaction of hilar and paratracheal lymph nodes in patients treated for testicular cancer. Cancer 56:2212, 1985.

642. Urbanski SJ, Alison RE, Jewett MAS, et al: Association of germ cell tumours of the testis and intrathoracic sarcoid-like lesions. Can Med Assoc J 137:416, 1987.

643. Heffner JE, Milam MG: Sarcoid-like hilar and mediastinal lymphadenopathy in a patient with metastatic testicular cancer. Cancer 60:1545, 1987.

644. Leatham EW, Eeles R, Sheppard M, et al: The association of germ cell tumours of the testis with sarcoid-like processes. Clin Oncol (R Coll Radiol) 4:89, 1992.

644a. Rayson D, Burch PA, Richardson RL: Sarcoidosis and testicular carcinoma. Cancer 83:337, 1998.

645. Huhti E, Poukkula A, Lilja M: Prognosis for sarcoidosis in a defined geographical area. Br J Dis Chest 81:381, 1987.

646. Johnston RN: Pulmonary sarcoidosis after ten to twenty years. Scott Med J 31:72, 1986.

647. Meier-Sydow J, Rust MG, Kappos A, et al: The long-term course of airflow obstruction in obstructive variants of the fibrotic stage of sarcoidosis and of idiopathic pulmonary fibrosis. Ann NY Acad Sci 465:515, 1986.

648. Bjermer L, Rosenhall L, Angstrom T, et al: Predictive value of bronchoalveolar lavage cell analysis in sarcoidosis. Thorax 43:284, 1988.

649. Laviolette M, La Forge J, Tennina S, et al: Prognostic value of bronchoalveolar lavage lymphocyte count in recently diagnosed pulmonary sarcoidosis. Chest 100:380, 1991.

650. Foley NM, Coral AP, Tung K, et al: Bronchoalveolar lavage cell counts as a predictor of short term outcome in pulmonary sarcoidosis. Thorax 44:732, 1989.

651. Ward K, O'Connor C, Odlum C, et al: Prognostic value of bronchoalveolar lavage in sarcoidosis: The critical influence of disease presentation. Thorax 44:6, 1989.

652. Verstraeten A, Demedts M, Verwilghen J, et al: Predictive value of bronchoalveolar lavage in pulmonary sarcoidosis. Chest 98:560, 1990.

653. Gerli R, Darwish S, Broccucci L, et al: Helper inducer T cells in the lungs of sarcoidosis patients: Analysis of the pathogenic and clinical significance. Chest 95:811, 1989.

654. Israel-Biet D, Venet A, Chretien J: Persistent high alveolar lymphocytosis as a predictive criterion of chronic pulmonary sarcoidosis. Ann NY Acad Sci 465:395, 1986.

655. Buchalter S, App W, Jackson L, et al: Bronchoalveolar lavage cell analysis in sarcoidosis: A comparison of lymphocyte counts and clinical course. Ann NY Acad Sci 465:678, 1986.

656. Baughman RP, Fernandez M, Bosken CH, et al: Comparison of gallium-67 scanning, bronchoalveolar lavage, and serum angiotensin-converting enzyme levels in pulmonary sarcoidosis: Predicting response to therapy. Am Rev Respir Dis 129:676, 1984.

657. Rust M, Bergmann L, Kuhn T, et al: Prognostic value of chest radiograph, serum angiotensin-converting enzyme and T helper cell count in blood and in bronchoalveolar lavage of patients with pulmonary sarcoidosis. Respiration 48:231, 1985.

658. Costabel U, Bross KJ, Guzman J, et al: Predictive value of bronchoalveolar T cell subsets for the course of pulmonary sarcoidosis. Ann NY Acad Sci 465:418, 1986.

659. Schoenfeld N, Schmitt M, Remy N, et al: Activation of bronchoalveolar lavage T lymphocytes and clinical, function and radiological features in sarcoidosis. Sarcoidosis 12:135, 1995.

660. Xaubet A, Agusti C, Roca J, et al: BAL lymphocyte activation antigens and diffusing capacity are related in mild to moderate pulmonary sarcoidosis. Eur Respir J 6:715, 1993.

661. Mukae H, Kohno S, Morikawa T, et al: Two-color analysis of lymphocyte subsets of bronchoalveolar lavage fluid and peripheral blood in Japanese patients with sarcoidosis. Chest 105:1474, 1994.

662. Ueda E, Kawabe T, Tachibana T, et al: Serum angiotensin-converting enzyme activity as an indicator of prognosis in sarcoidosis. Am Rev Respir Dis 121:667, 1980.

663. Weaver LJ, Solliday NH, Celic L, et al: Serial observations of angiotensin-converting enzyme and pulmonary function in sarcoidosis. Arch Intern Med 141:931, 1981.

664. Selroos O, Gronhagen-Riska C: Angiotensin converting enzyme: III. Changes in serum level as an indicator of disease activity in untreated sarcoidosis. Scand J Respir Dis 60:328, 1979.

665. Straub JP, van Kamp GJ, van Maarsseveen TC, et al: Biochemical parameters in BAL of sarcoidosis. Sarcoidosis 12:51, 1995.

666. Turner-Warwick M, McAllister W, Lawrence R, et al: Corticosteroid treatment in pulmonary sarcoidosis: Do serial lavage lymphocyte counts, serum angiotensin-converting enzyme measurements, and gallium-67 scans help management? Thorax 41:903, 1986.

667. Rohatgi PK, Bates HR, Noss RW: Computer-assisted sequential quantitative analysis of gallium scans in pulmonary sarcoidosis. Eur J Respir Dis 66:248, 1985.

668. Niden AH, Mishkin FS, Salem F, et al: Prognostic significance of gallium lung scans in sarcoidosis. Ann NY Acad Sci 465:435, 1986.

669. Baughman RP, Shipley R, Eisentrout CE: Predictive value of gallium scan,

angiotensin-converting enzyme level, and bronchoalveolar lavage in two-year follow-up of pulmonary sarcoidosis. Lung 165:371, 1987.

670. Vandenplas O, Depelchin S, Delaunois L, et al: Bronchoalveolar lavage immunoglobulin A and G and antiproteases correlate with changes in diffusion indices during the natural course of pulmonary sarcoidosis. Eur Respir J 7:1856, 1994.

671. Prior C, Haslam PL: Increased levels of serum interferon-gamma in pulmonary sarcoidosis and relationship with response to corticosteroid therapy. Am Rev Respir Dis 143:53, 1991.

672. Bjermer L, Eklund A, Blaschke E: Bronchoalveolar lavage fibronectin in patients with sarcoidosis: Correlation to hyaluronan and disease activity. Eur Respir J 4:965, 1991.

673. Ward K, O'Connor CM, Odlum C, et al: Pulmonary disease progress in sarcoid patients with and without bronchoalveolar lavage collagenase. Am Rev Respir Dis 142:636, 1990.

674. Homolka J, Lorenz J, Zuchold HD, et al: Evaluation of soluble CD 14 and neopterin as serum parameters of the inflammatory activity of pulmonary sarcoidosis. Clin Invest 70:909, 1992.

675. Eklund AG, Sigurdardottir O, Öhrn M: Vitronectin and its relationship to other extracellular matrix components in bronchoalveolar lavage fluid in sarcoidosis. Am Rev Respir Dis 145:646, 1992.

676. Letizia C, D'Ambrosio C, Agostini D, et al: Serum angiotensin converting enzyme activity in Crohn's disease and ulcerative colitis. Ital J Gastroenterol 25:23, 1993.

677. Silverstein E, Pertschuk LP, Friedland J: Immunofluorescent detection of angiotensin-converting enzyme (ACE) in Gaucher cells. Am J Med 69:408, 1980.

678. Matsuki K, Sakata T: Angiotensin-converting enzyme in diseases of the liver. Am J Med 73:549, 1982.

679. Borowsky SA, Lieberman J, Strome S, et al: Elevation of serum angiotensin-converting enzyme level: Occurrence in alcoholic liver disease. Arch Intern Med 142:893, 1982.

680. Rømer FK, Faber V, Koch C, et al: Serum-angiotensin-enzyme in chronic granulomatous disease (letter). Lancet 1:1237, 1979.

681. Lieberman J, Bell DS: Serum angiotensin-converting enzyme as a marker for the chronic fatigue-immune dysfunction syndrome: A comparison to serum angiotensin-converting enzyme in sarcoidosis. Am J Med 95:407, 1993.

682. Lindsay M, Sharma OP: Familial Mediterranean fever: Another cause of raised serum angiotensin converting enzyme; another abortive attempt at masquerading as sarcoidosis. Sarcoidosis 10:132, 1993.

683. Lawrence EC, Brouseau KP, Berger MB, et al: Elevated concentrations of soluble interleukin-2 receptors in serum samples bronchoalveolar lavage fluids in active sarcoidosis. Am Rev Respir Dis 137:759, 1988.

684. Suzuki K, Tamura N, Iwase A, et al: Prognostic value of Ia + T lymphocytes in bronchoalveolar lavage fluid in pulmonary sarcoidosis. Am J Respir Crit Care Med 154:707, 1996.

685. Bjermer L, Engstrom-Laurent A, Thunell M, et al: Hyaluronic acid in bronchoalveolar lavage fluid in patients with sarcoidosis: Relationship to lavage mast cells. Thorax 42:933, 1987.

686. Itoh A, Yamaguchi E, Furuya K, et al: Correlation of GM-CSF mRNA in bronchoalveolar fluid with indices of clinical activity in sarcoidosis. Thorax 48:1230, 1993.

687. Capelli A, Lusuardi M, Carli S, et al: Acid phosphatase (EC 3.1.3.2) activity in alveolar macrophages from patients with active sarcoidosis. Chest 99:546, 1991.

688. Perez RL, Duncan A, Hunler RL, et al: Elevated d dimer in the lungs and blood of patients with sarcoidosis. Chest 103:1100, 1993.

689. Luisetti M, Bulgheroni A, Bacchella L, et al: Elevated serum procollagen III aminopeptide levels in sarcoidosis. Chest 98:1414, 1990.

690. Poole A, Myllyla R, Davies BH: Activities of enzymes of collagen biosynthesis and levels of type III procollagen in peptide in the serum of patients with sarcoidosis. Life Sci 45:319, 1989.

691. Lacronique J, Auzeby A, Valeyre D, et al: Urinary neopterin in pulmonary sarcoidosis: Relationship to clinical and biologic assessment of the disease. Am Rev Respir Dis 139:1474, 1989.

692. Ishii Y, Kitamura S: Elevated levels of soluble ICAM-1 in serum and BAL fluid in patients with active sarcoidosis. Chest 107:1636, 1995.

693. Ina Y, Takada K, Yamamoto M, et al: Antiphospholipid antibodies: A prognostic factor in sarcoidosis? Chest 105:1179, 1994.

694. Shijubo N, Yamaguchi K, Hirasawa M, et al: Progastrin-releasing peptide(31-98) in idiopathic pulmonary fibrosis and sarcoidosis. Am J Respir Crit Care Med 154:1694, 1996.

695. Kobayashi J, Kitamura S, et al: Serum KL-6 for the evaluation of active pneumonitis in pulmonary sarcoidosis. Chest 109:1276, 1996.

696. Bjermer L, Thunell M, Rosehall L, et al: Endobronchial biopsy positive sarcoidosis: Relation to bronchoalveolar lavage and course of disease. Respir Med 85:229, 1991.

697. Chinet T, Dusser D, Labrune S, et al: Lung function declines in patients with pulmonary sarcoidosis and increased respiratory epithelial permeability to Tc-DTPA. Am Rev Respir Dis 141:445, 1990.

698. Hashimoto S, Nakayama T, Gon Y, et al: Correlation of plasma monocyte chemoattractant protein-1 (MCP-1) and monocyte inflammatory protein-1 alpha (MIP-1 alpha) levels with disease activity and clinical course of sarcoidosis. Clin Exp Immunol 111:604, 1998.

# CHAPTER 42

# Interstitial Pneumonitis and Fibrosis

A discussion of inflammatory disease of the pulmonary interstitium can be confusing partly because of the multiplicity of terms by which the abnormality has been known. In addition to the purely descriptive *interstitial pneumonitis and fibrosis*, the disorder has been labeled *idiopathic pulmonary fibrosis, cryptogenic fibrosing alveolitis, Hamman-Rich disease, diffuse interstitial fibrosis, idiopathic interstitial fibrosis, honeycomb lung, usual interstitial pneumonitis, desquamative interstitial pneumonitis, Osler-Charcot disease, diffuse pulmonary alveolar fibrosis,* and *interstitial pneumonia.*[1] Specific comments about some of these terms is warranted, particularly with respect to the distinction between usual and desquamative interstitial pneumonitis.

An important contribution to the understanding and nosology of interstitial lung disease was made by Liebow and Carrington in 1969 when they grouped various abnormalities into five categories on the basis of their histologic features:[2]

1. Classic or usual interstitial pneumonia (UIP), characterized by thickening of alveolar interstitium by fibrous tissue and mononuclear inflammatory cells, typically with variable severity from one area of lung to another

2. Desquamative interstitial pneumonia (DIP), in which there is a striking accumulation of macrophages in the alveolar air spaces associated with relatively mild but uniform interstitial thickening by mononuclear inflammatory cells and a variable, but usually small, amount of connective tissue

3. A diffuse lesion similar to UIP but with superimposed bronchiolitis obliterans (originally termed "BIP," this reaction is more commonly known today as *bronchiolitis obliterans organizing pneumonia* [BOOP, cryptogenic organizing pneumonia])

4. Lymphoid interstitial pneumonia (LIP), in which there is marked infiltration of parenchymal interstitium by lymphocytes, plasma cells, or both in a pattern that is sometimes difficult to distinguish from lymphoma

5. Giant cell interstitial pneumonia (GIP), consisting of an interstitial infiltrate of mononuclear cells associated with large numbers of multinucleated giant cells in the interstitium and adjacent air spaces

Each of these histologic patterns can be regarded as a tissue reaction to a variety of etiologic agents rather than as a manifestation of a specific disease.[3-7] For example, in addition to cases in which no etiology is apparent, BOOP can be seen in some connective tissue diseases and after infection or aspiration of gastric contents. The pattern of GIP can be seen with infection by several viruses (particularly measles virus) and with exposure to hard-metal dust (tungsten carbide and cobalt). LIP can be seen in patients who have dysproteinemia, autoimmune disease such as Sjögren's syndrome, or the acquired immunodeficiency syndrome.[8] These three forms of interstitial pulmonary disease comprise fairly distinct clinicopathologic entities and are discussed elsewhere in this text.

In contrast to LIP, GIP, and BOOP, there has been some debate concerning the distinctiveness of UIP and DIP from each other. Carrington and Liebow[2] suggested that the different histologic and radiographic features of the two abnormalities and the relatively favorable response of DIP to corticosteroid therapy implied that they have a different etiology and pathogenesis and should be considered separate entities. Other investigators, however, have documented considerable histologic overlap among patients with interstitial pneumonitis and fibrosis and have suggested that the patterns of DIP and UIP represent different stages of one disease process.[9] This interpretation is supported by reports of occasional patients in whom an initial biopsy shows a pattern of DIP and in whom subsequent biopsy or autopsy specimens show only diffuse pulmonary fibrosis.[10, 11] A variety of investigators—particularly in Great Britain—have supported this unifying concept and suggest that the two reactions should be referred to by a single term (most commonly, *cryptogenic fibrosing alveolitis*).[5, 9, 10, 12, 13] Although there is some merit in this viewpoint, we believe that the pathologic and radiologic differences between UIP and DIP and their distinctively different courses are such that the two are better considered separately, recognizing that definitive statements concerning a common etiology and pathogenesis cannot be made at this time. Of all patients with interstitial pneumonitis of unknown etiology, about 5% have a histologic pattern of DIP;[13a] most of the remainder have UIP.

Although the term *cryptogenic fibrosing alveolitis* better describes the inflammatory and fibrotic nature of both UIP and DIP, the designation idiopathic pulmonary fibrosis (IPF) has found widespread acceptance in North America[14–19] and is used throughout this text to refer to UIP. As its name implies, IPF is unassociated with other conditions known to be complicated by interstitial pneumonitis and fibrosis, such as connective tissue disease, extrinsic allergic alveolitis, exposure to occupational inorganic dusts (pneumoconiosis), or drug intake. In addition to IPF and DIP, there are two other clinicopathologic abnormalities with prominent parenchymal interstitial involvement—acute interstitial pneumonitis and nonspecific interstitial pneumonitis—that deserve to be considered separately.

# IDIOPATHIC PULMONARY FIBROSIS

## Epidemiology

Only limited data are available on the incidence and prevalence of IPF in the general population; moreover, differences in terminology, diagnostic criteria, and means of case identification make these data difficult to interpret. Early estimates of prevalence ranged from 3 to 5 per 100,000 in the United States to 6 per 100,000 in Nottingham, England.[16] The results of a more recent investigation from Bernalillo County, New Mexico suggest that the disease may be much more common, at least in this area of the world.[20] In this study, all patients 18 years of age and older referred for evaluation of interstitial lung disease during a 2-year period were identified by examination of physician referrals, hospital discharge diagnoses, pathology reports, and death certificates. The prevalence of preclinical or undiagnosed cases of IPF was estimated by reviewing lung specimens from 510 autopsies. (The study is flawed by its necessary dependence on physician diagnosis—thereby including patients with widely varying diagnostic criteria—and by its separation of the diagnoses of "IPF," "pulmonary fibrosis," and "interstitial pneumonitis." Review of hospital admissions has shown that many patients classified as having pulmonary fibrosis in fact have IPF;[21] therefore, in this respect, the number of cases of IPF may have been underestimated.)

IPF alone accounted for 23% of the prevalent cases and 31% of the incident cases of interstitial lung disease. The prevalence of IPF was 20 per 100,000 for males and 14 per 100,000 for females, values that are much greater than previous estimates. Surprisingly, there were almost as many incident cases of IPF as there were prevalent cases; as an explanation, the authors hypothesized that patients with the disease did not survive long enough to accrue in the population. Both incident and prevalent cases showed a small male predominance, a finding that is consistent with that of other reviews.[22] Although the diagnosis was made in all age groups examined, both the incidence and prevalence increased markedly with age; among men and women older than 75 years, the latter was 2.5 per 1,000 and the former 1.6 per 1,000 per year.

The finding of three cases of unsuspected interstitial lung disease (one considered to be IPF) among the 510 autopsies suggests that there may also be a substantial number of undiagnosed cases in the population.[20] As a result, the authors suggested that the 4,851 deaths attributed to IPF in the United States in 1988 likely represent a gross underestimate. This speculation is supported by the fact that examination of death certificates has been shown to be an inaccurate method of identifying this diagnosis, even in patients who have had well-recognized disease.[20, 22] In an analysis of close to 27 million deaths occurring in the United States between 1979 and 1991 in which death certificates were used to identify cases, the age-adjusted mortality rate for pulmonary fibrosis in 1991 was 50.9 per million in men and 27.2 per million in women.[23] Deaths were more common in older individuals and in whites compared with African Americans.

## Etiology and Pathogenesis

By definition, the etiology of IPF is unknown; however, evidence has accumulated in support of a role for several possible agents. Pathogenetic factors that have been most extensively studied include inherited susceptibility to disease and immunologically mediated inflammation and fibrosis in response to viral infection or other pulmonary injury.[17]

### Viral Infection

Limited information is available concerning the potential role of viruses in the initiation of lung injury in IPF. Although the diagnosis of the condition often coincides with recognition of a viral-type syndrome,[24–26] it is rare to document a specific viral infection that evolves into pathologically proven interstitial fibrosis.[27–29] The results of several serologic and immunohistochemical investigations also suggest that viruses may be involved in the ongoing pathogenesis of the disease, possibly in association with latent infection.[25] For example, in one study of 13 patients, specific immunoglobulins for Epstein-Barr virus (EBV) were found in the serum of 10.[31] Although it is conceivable that this finding reflects a nonspecific depression of cell-mediated immunity, one group of investigators found evidence of EBV replication within epithelial cells of the lower respiratory tract in 14 of 20 (70%) patients who had IPF, compared with only 9% of controls.[32]

In a study of 66 patients from Japan, a much higher prevalence of antibodies to hepatitis C virus was found among patients who had IPF (29%) than among age-matched controls (4%).[33] Similar results were demonstrated in a study of 60 Italian patients;[34] however, the prevalence of antibody to hepatitis C was also elevated in patients who had lung disease other than IPF. In another serologic investigation of 62 patients from the United Kingdom, no difference in the prevalence of antibodies to this virus was found between patients who had IPF and the general population.[35] Finally, in a study in which a polymerase chain reaction was used to identify adenovirus genome in lung tissue of patients who had fibrotic lung disease, evidence for the presence of the genome was largely confined to patients who had been treated with systemic corticosteroids,[26] suggesting that the presence of the virus was the result of reactivation or new infection induced by the therapy.

Although it is not possible to be certain, the results of these studies suggest that viral infection has a limited, if any, role in the pathogenesis of IPF.

### Other Environmental Factors

That environmental factors might be more important than usually recognized in the etiology of IPF is suggested by an epidemiologic study of 1,311 Japanese patients who had an autopsy diagnosis of IPF;[36] in this group, the rate of IPF was more than two times higher in workers exposed to dust or organic solvents than in unexposed individuals. The observation that solvents are also associated with the development of pulmonary fibrosis in animals and with the development of progressive systemic sclerosis in humans supports the possibility of an etiologic role for these agents in IPF.[37] One group identified occupational exposure to a number of dusts to be associated with an increased risk for the development of IPF, including metal dust (odds ratio, 10.97), wood dust (odds ratio, 2.94), work with cattle (odds ratio, 10.89), and home heating with wood (odds ratio, 12.55).[38] The same investigators subsequently performed a more extensive case-control study in which lifetime occupational exposures of patients who had IPF were determined by questionnaire and compared with those of controls matched for age, sex, and community.[39] After adjustment for smoking, the relative risk for IPF was again found to be increased significantly in patients who had had wood or metal dust exposure; moreover, a relation was documented between the intensity of exposure and the likelihood of disease.

Cigarette smoking also appears to increase the risk of developing IPF. In one investigation of 248 patients who smoked and 491 controls, in which conditional logistic regression analysis was used, the odds ratio for IPF in patients who had ever smoked was 1.6; however, in patients who smoked one to two packages of cigarettes per day, it was 2.3.[40] In another study of 141 patients who had IPF and a group of matched control subjects, the risk for developing IPF was increased in those taking antidepressants, even after controlling for cigarette smoking.[30]

The mechanism by which any of these inhaled substances might initiate or modify the development of IPF is unknown; however, such studies provide tantalizing clues that lung fibrosis may not always be "idiopathic."[41]

### Genetic Factors

An inherited susceptibility to IPF has been implicated by the results of several studies. For example, there is evidence that some patients with IPF have an inherited abnormality of immune function. An example of such an association in one family consisted of IPF, hypocalciuric hypercalcemia, and defective granulocyte function; all three disorders were inherited in an autosomal dominant pattern.[42–44]

A familial form of IPF (designated *familial fibrocystic pulmonary dysplasia* by some authors) that possesses pathologic and radiographic characteristics identical to those of the nonfamilial form has also been described (Fig. 42–1).[45–49] In one review of the literature in 1983, 73 definite cases were identified in 19 families;[50] additional examples have been described since.[51] Family members of these patients also have evidence of alveolitis on analysis of bronchoalveolar lavage (BAL) fluid.[52] Transmission of this familial abnormality appears to depend on a simple mendelian autosomal dominant trait with reduced penetrance.

The finding of clear-cut genetic susceptibility to disease in some patients suggests that as yet unidentified genetic factors may be important in the pathogenesis of nonfamilial IPF. Studies of the relationship between HLA histocompatibility loci and the presence of IPF have not yielded consistent results. An increased incidence of HLA-B15,[53] HLA-B8,[54] HLA-B12,[53] HLA-Dr2,[50] and Dw6[53] has been found by some workers; however, others have not confirmed these results.[53, 55] One group of investigators found an increase in S and Z Pi alleles in patients who had IPF as compared with controls;[56] an association of homozygous $\alpha_1$-antitrypsin deficiency and IPF has also been reported in a family cluster.[57] A chromosome 14 gene that encodes for immunoglobulin allotypes has also been linked to the development of pulmonary fibrosis in another family cluster.[49]

### Immunologic Factors

Whether IPF should be considered an "autoimmune" disease has been a subject of considerable conjecture. Many patients who have interstitial pneumonitis and fibrosis have clinical and serologic evidence of autoimmunity.[58–62] In some of these patients, the diagnosis of a specific connective tissue disorder, such as rheumatoid disease, progressive systemic sclerosis, dermatomyositis or polymyositis, Sjögren's syndrome, or mixed connective tissue disease, can be made on the basis of clinical findings and the presence of specific autoantibodies in the blood.[63] The number of such cases among patients with interstitial pneumonitis is considerable; for example, in one series of 220 such patients (none of whom had a history of exposure to known external fibrogenic agents), 30% were found to have a specific connective tissue disease.[64]

IPF is also occasionally associated with abnormalities in a tissue or organ that are not usually included under the umbrella of connective tissue disorders but in which an abnormality of immune function is implicated. Such abnormalities include digital vasculitis,[65] myasthenia gravis,[66] celiac disease,[67] chronic active hepatitis,[68–71] renal tubular acidosis,[72] hemolytic anemia,[73, 74] immunoglobulin A (IgA) nephropathy,[75] antiphospholipid antibody syndrome,[76] and thrombocytopenic purpura.[77] The observation that patients with IPF have a higher prevalence of atopy than controls also suggests a relationship between immunologic dysfunction and the pathogenesis of the lung disease.[78]

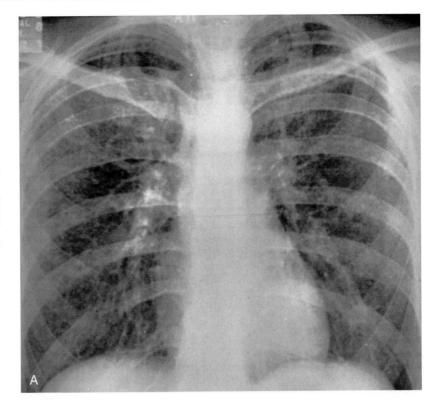

**Figure 42–1. Idiopathic Pulmonary Fibrosis (IPF) in Three Family Members.** The posteroanterior radiograph illustrated in *A* is of a young female member of the family; it reveals a rather fine reticular pattern throughout both lungs, with a vague, hazy opacity in upper lung zones bilaterally.

*Illustration continued on following page*

Serologic abnormalities are also commonly documented in patients who have IPF and no clinical evidence of extrapulmonary disease.[79] For example, it has been estimated that about one third of patients who have IPF have antinuclear antibodies and one third rheumatoid factor, usually in low titers; a few have both.[80] Immune complexes, both circulating and bound to lung tissue, have been found in a minority of patients who have IPF;[81–83] their presence appears to be associated with a more active (cellular) phase of disease.[63, 79, 84–86]

The results of some pathologic and experimental animal studies also provide evidence for an immunologic pathogenesis of IPF.[87, 88] For example, the intratracheal instillation of hapten to previously immunized hamsters has been found to result in interstitial fibrosis;[89] by contrast, mice that are unable to mount a delayed-type hypersensitivity response to the hapten do not develop a fibrogenic response after exposure.[90] In humans, IgG and C3 have been found in a granular pattern lining alveolar cells in some cases of IPF with an "active" (inflammatory) appearance, although only rarely in patients who have predominant fibrosis.[79] In one small series of 11 patients who had IPF, immunofluorescent study of transbronchial biopsy specimens revealed immunoglobulin and complement deposition.[91] Immune complexes have also been identified in the BAL fluid,[91, 92] and have been found by some investigators to be associated with disease progression.[91] Because these complexes can activate alveolar macrophages and are chemotactic for neutrophils through complement activation, their presence might initiate the inflammatory events in the lung that precede the fibrotic remodeling of lung tissue, at least in some patients.

Attempts to discover a putative antigen to which pathogenic antibodies may be directed have yielded several candidates. Antibodies to native collagen were found in 13 of 16 patients (81%) who had IPF in one investigation;[93] antibodies to proteins in alveolar epithelial cells have been found by other workers.[94, 95] However, whether these antibodies are pathogenetic or simply an epiphenomenon remains to be determined.

### Cellular Mechanisms of Disease

More is known about the mechanisms of disease pathogenesis in IPF than is known about the etiology.[95a] Damage to both epithelial and endothelial cells appears to be closely related to the development and progression of fibrosis.[96] The latter is characterized by a proliferation of myofibroblasts and the deposition of collagen and proteoglycans.[97, 98] Although some collagen is probably laid down directly in the alveolar interstitium, there is substantial evidence that the air space is a more important site of fibrogenesis, the collagen so formed subsequently being incorporated into the interstitial connective tissue (Fig. 42–2).[99–102]

Fibrosis is preceded by an inflammatory reaction in which pulmonary alveolar macrophages and lymphocytes appear to play critical roles. No single cell or cell product can explain all the events leading to fibrosis, and it is likely that a complex interaction between the epithelial, endothelial, inflammatory, and fibroblastic cells determines the rapidity and severity of its development.[96, 97, 103–106]

Ultrastructural studies in IPF have shown both epithelial and endothelial damage in the earliest stage of disease.[103] Evidence of such damage can also be seen with light microscopy as type II cell hyperplasia and (occasionally) a proteinaceous exudate within alveolar air spaces. Epithelial injury may have a variety of effects. For example, because normal

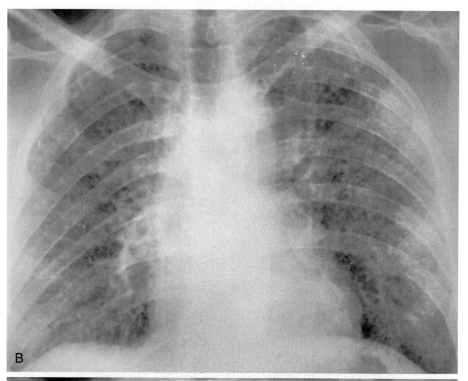

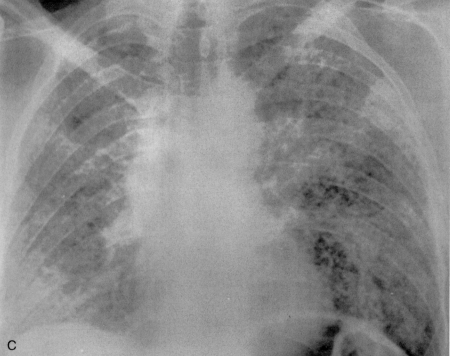

**Figure 42–1** *Continued.* Parts *B* and *C* are from a male member whose initial radiograph *(B)* reveals a coarse reticular pattern without anatomic predominance; 1 year later *(C)*, lung volume had reduced, and the reticular opacities had worsened.

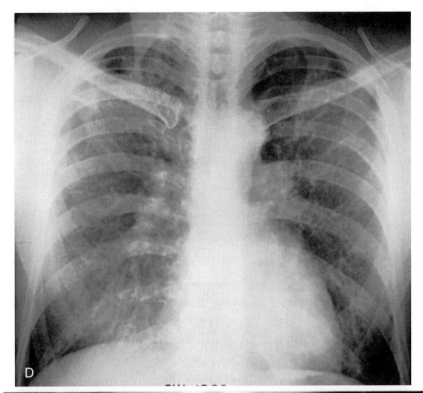

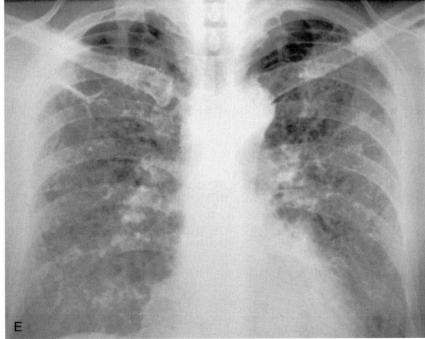

**Figure 42–1** *Continued.* Parts *D* and *E* are from another male member of the family whose initial radiograph *(D)* reveals a rather fine reticular pattern throughout both lungs similar to the changes observed in *A*; 5 years later *(E)*, the lungs had lost some volume and the reticular pattern had worsened considerably. Open-lung biopsies of the two male members of the family revealed classic changes of IPF.

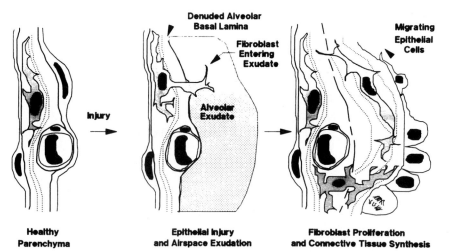

**Figure 42–2. Idiopathic Pulmonary Fibrosis.** The illustration shows a diagrammatic representation of a normal alveolus *(left)* and one that has experienced epithelial and endothelial injury *(middle)*. In the latter, a myofibroblast can be seen extending into an air-space exudate. Somewhat later *(right)*, the exudate is replaced by connective tissue produced by the fibroblasts and is covered by a layer of alveolar epithelial cells that migrate over its surface. (From Kuhn C III, Boldt J, King TE: An immunohistochemical study of architectural remodeling and connective tissue synthesis in pulmonary fibrosis. Am Rev Respir Dis 140:1693, 1989.)

alveolar epithelial cells can suppress clonal lymphocyte expansion in the alveolar air space,[103] an absence of or alteration to these cells may be related to the proliferation of lymphocytes characteristic of the alveolitis in IPF. Epithelial cells also produce inhibitors of fibroblast proliferation, such as prostaglandin $E_2$,[103] and a loss or decrease in the number of these cells would theoretically favor a shift towards fibroblast activation. Finally, there is evidence that epithelial cells are a source of endothelin-1,[107, 108] other profibrotic and proinflammatory cytokines,[96, 109, 110] and tissue factor (which favors fibrin deposition in the lungs).[111] In fact, BAL fluid from patients who have IPF reflects a procoagulant environment in the alveolar air space.[111a]

Endothelial cell damage may also be important in the pathogenesis of IPF. Theoretically, it may lead to deposition of collagen in the interstitium through the activating and attractant effects of thrombin on fibroblasts.[103] In addition, increased vascular permeability may be associated with an increase in interstitial or air-space fluid and proteins,[112] which may then undergo organization. Vascular endothelium also expresses adhesion molecules for inflammatory cells that favor their recruitment to the alveoli.[103, 113]

BAL fluid and interstitial tissue from most patients who have IPF contain excess neutrophils, eosinophils, macrophages, and (sometimes) lymphocytes.[114, 114a] All may play a role in the pathogenesis of epithelial and endothelial cell injury and interstitial fibrosis. Macrophages in particular appear to be important in the inflammatory reaction.[104] They probably increase in number by a combination of recruitment of blood monocytes and local proliferation of interstitial macrophages.[17, 115] When activated, they secrete a number of fibroblast growth factors (including fibronectin, platelet-derived growth factor, transforming growth factor β, and insulin-like growth factor),[116, 116a] inhibitors of antifibrotic cytokines,[117] IL-13 (which can inhibit the production of proinflammatory cytokines produced by macrophages),[117a] and neutrophil chemotactic factors, such as interleukin-8 (IL-8).[110, 114, 118–121a] Macrophages also secrete a variety of other cytokines, such as IL-1 and tumor necrosis factor-α (TNF-α), that are involved in the regulation of other inflammatory cells.[104, 122, 123] With neutrophils[124–126] and eosinophils,[127, 128] macrophages produce oxidants that may directly damage epithelial and endothelial cells.[17, 112, 129–131a] In addi-

tion to oxidants, neutrophils release proteases and collagenases that can degrade the connective tissue matrix,[103, 131b] thereby promoting further tissue damage. Both BAL fluid and serum also contain high concentrations of gastrin-releasing peptide, a substance that can stimulate the release of profibrotic cytokines from alveolar macrophages.[132]

Lymphocytes also undoubtedly have an important role in the pathogenesis of IPF. An influx of activated T lymphocytes, perhaps mediated by chemoattractant cytokines released by damaged epithelial cells, precedes the development of fibrosis in some models of fibrotic lung disease. Such lymphocytes enhance the release of fibrogenic and proinflammatory cytokines from pulmonary macrophages;[97, 133, 134] they may also interact directly with fibroblasts through the release of fibroblast-activating cytokines.[97] An increased number of fibroblasts with inherently augmented proliferative activity are also present in the fibrous tissue of patients with IPF.[135]

Pulmonary mast cells are increased in number in IPF; because they make direct contact with fibroblasts and are able to secrete a variety of proinflammatory and profibrotic cytokines, they may also have a role in fibrosis.[97, 136] However, they are particularly evident in the fibrotic rather than the inflammatory stage of disease, and their pathogenic role is unclear.

The cells that produce collagen in IPF have features of both fibroblastic and muscle differentiation (myofibroblasts).[137] They can frequently be identified by light microscopy in small subepithelial clusters associated with loose connective tissue. The latter has been shown to contain a significant amount of the proteoglycan versican, which has been hypothesized to have an important role in the development of mature collagen.[98] Interestingly, myofibroblasts appear to be more than just target cells in patients who have IPF; there is evidence that they are capable of producing a variety of cytokines that can modulate the behavior of other inflammatory cells, as well as mediators that have autocrine function.[97, 103] There is also evidence for an imbalance of certain cytokines, such that angiogenesis is favored in patients who have IPF; the observation that angiogenesis is related to deposition of extracellular matrix suggests that it may also have a role in pathogenesis.[138]

## Pathologic Characteristics

Pathologically, IPF is characterized by a variable degree of interstitial abnormality, areas of normal and markedly diseased lung being present in different regions of the same lobe and even in a single lobule (Fig. 42–3). In early disease, alveolar septa are slightly thickened by an infiltrate of inflammatory cells (Fig. 42–4); lymphocytes are usually the most numerous, but plasma cells, mast cells,[139] histiocytes, eosinophils, and polymorphonuclear leukocytes can be encountered in lesser numbers. In more advanced disease (*see* Fig. 42–4), the interstitial thickening is greater and is usually associated with some degree of fibrosis. Most often, this consists of mature collagen; however, foci of loose connective tissue indicative of fibrogenesis are common (Fig. 42–5). Such active fibrosis can be also be seen in alveolar air spaces and the lumens of transitional airways (Fig. 42–6);[99, 140] however, if this is present in more than an occasional focus, a diagnosis of BOOP should be entertained. (With this is mind, it should be noted that it is sometimes difficult to say with certainty if fibroblastic tissue is within an air space, the interstitium, or both.[140])

In the most severely affected areas, interstitial thickening is so marked that alveoli are reduced to small slits (*see* Fig. 42–4) or are completely obliterated; at this stage, fibrous tissue is usually more abundant than the inflammatory cell infiltrate. Such fibrosis is often associated with dilation of transitional airways (traction bronchiolectasis, Fig. 42–7), representing the histologic counterpart of grossly evident honeycomb lung (*see* farther on). Additional abnormalities that can be seen in the areas of severe fibrosis include an increase in elastic tissue, smooth muscle hyperplasia (Fig. 42–8), and epithelial metaplasia (Fig. 42–9), the latter usually of squamous or columnar mucus-secreting cells. Dystrophic calcification and osseous metaplasia occur occasionally.[141, 142]

In contrast to normal alveoli that are lined mostly by type I epithelial cells, the walls of alveoli in IPF are commonly lined predominantly by cuboidal cells (Fig. 42–10); although many of these represent hyperplastic type II cells, some do not show ultrastructural features of type II cell differentiation and appear to be derived directly from bronchiolar epithelium.[143] There is evidence that type II cells are more prominent in the least fibrotic areas and bronchiolar cells in the most fibrotic.[143, 144] Prominent nucleoli or eosinophilic inclusions resembling Mallory hyaline can be seen within the nucleus or cytoplasm, respectively, of these hyperplastic cells and should not be confused with viral inclusions (Fig. 42–11).[145, 146] Langerhans' cells are also present in increased numbers adjacent to the hyperplastic type II cells.[147] Neuroendocrine cells have been found to be sparse during the active (inflammatory) stage of disease and to be even fewer as fibrosis increases.[148]

Although IPF is predominantly an interstitial process, pathologic abnormalities can also be seen in the air spaces and vessels. A common finding is the presence of an increased number of intra-alveolar macrophages; in contrast to desquamative interstitial pneumonitis,[149] these usually vary greatly in number from alveolus to alveolus and overall are not numerous. Occasional multinucleated giant cells can be seen, both in the air spaces and the interstitium; however, well-formed granulomas do not occur. The cystic spaces of honeycomb lung frequently contain mucus derived from metaplastic epithelial cells (*see* Fig. 42–9); the mucus often contains polymorphonuclear leukocytes, which should not be considered evidence of infection. Pulmonary arteries usually show some degree of intimal fibrosis and medial muscular hyperplasia, especially in the regions of more marked interstitial fibrosis. Although such changes may be related to generalized pulmonary hypertension, in most cases they probably reflect a reaction to local interstitial disease.

Grossly, the early stage of IPF consists of only a slight coarseness of the normal parenchyma, typically most severe in the subpleural region and in the basal and posterior

*Text continued on page 1599*

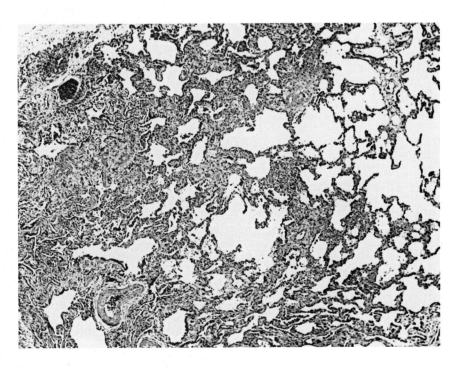

**Figure 42–3. Idiopathic Pulmonary Fibrosis: Variable Severity.** A low-magnification view of lung parenchyma shows interstitial thickening of variable severity; some alveolar septa are almost normal, whereas others show moderate or marked thickening. (×35.)

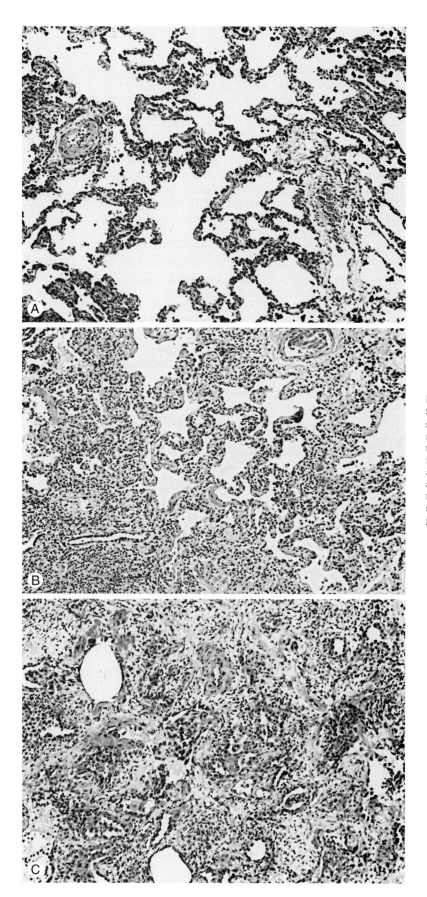

**Figure 42–4. Idiopathic Pulmonary Fibrosis: Varying Severity.** Three sections demonstrate increasing degrees of severity of pathologic abnormality. An early stage *(A)* shows mild interstitial thickening, caused predominantly by an infiltrate of lymphocytes. More advanced disease *(B)* is characterized by moderate thickening of the interstitium; although there are still abundant lymphocytes, these are now associated with appreciable fibrous tissue. Still more severe disease *(C)* is manifested by a marked reduction in the size of alveolar air spaces and a great increase in the amount of interstitial collagen. *(A, B,* and *C,* ×80.)

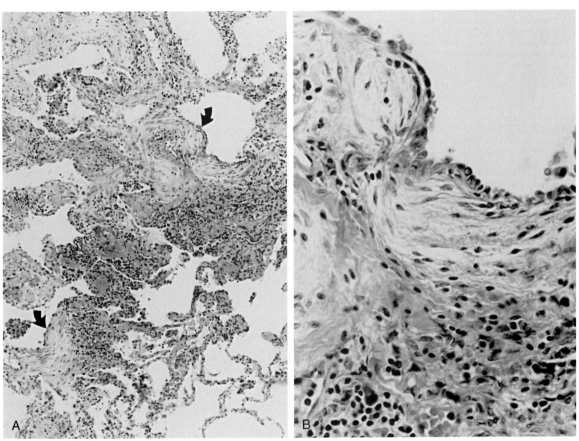

**Figure 42–5. Idiopathic Pulmonary Fibrosis: Active Fibrosis.** Sections show variably severe interstitial thickening by a combination of mononuclear inflammatory cells and collagen. In several areas (*arrows* and magnified view *[B]*), the connective tissue has a loose appearance indicative of active fibrogenesis.

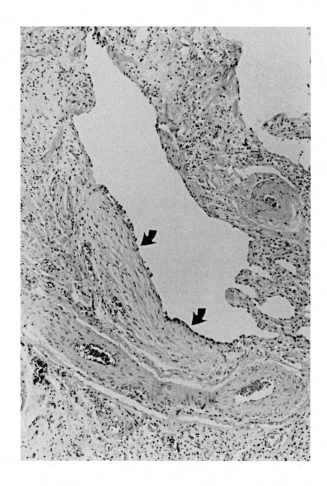

**Figure 42–6. Idiopathic Pulmonary Fibrosis (IPF): Bronchiolar Involvement.** A longitudinal section of a small membranous bronchiole shows a focus of fibroblastic tissue between the epithelium and the adjacent pulmonary artery *(arrows)*. This was the only focus of airway fibrosis identified in the biopsy, which was otherwise typical of IPF.

**Figure 42–7. Early "Honeycomb" Change.** The majority of the lung parenchyma in this autopsy specimen has been replaced by fibrous tissue and a moderate number of lymphocytes. The irregularly shaped cystic spaces—corresponding to the cells of the "honeycomb" that were seen grossly—are mostly dilated airways (small membranous and respiratory bronchioles and alveolar ducts). (×35.)

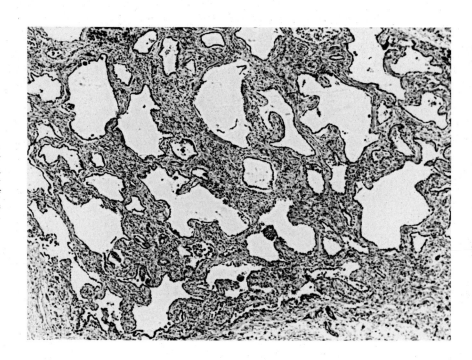

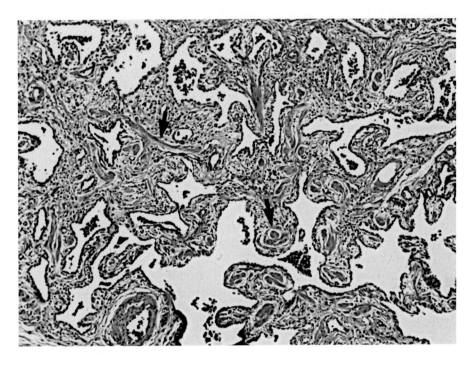

**Figure 42–8. Idiopathic Pulmonary Fibrosis: Muscular Hyperplasia.** The section shows a focus of lung with advanced interstitial fibrosis, associated with numerous haphazardly arranged bands of hyperplastic smooth muscle *(arrows)*. (×60.)

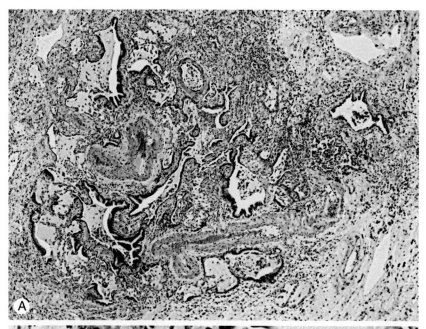

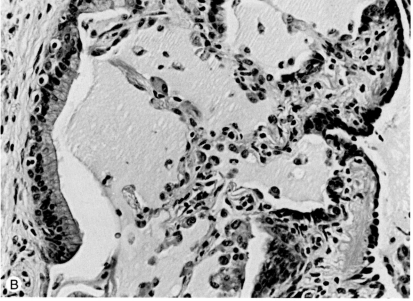

**Figure 42–9. Idiopathic Pulmonary Fibrosis: Epithelial Metaplasia.** Sections show several irregularly shaped cystic spaces lined by tall columnar cells seen to better advantage at higher magnification *(B)*. Mucus is present in several of the adjacent air spaces, representing secretion from the metaplastic epithelium. *(A, ×40; B, ×250.)*

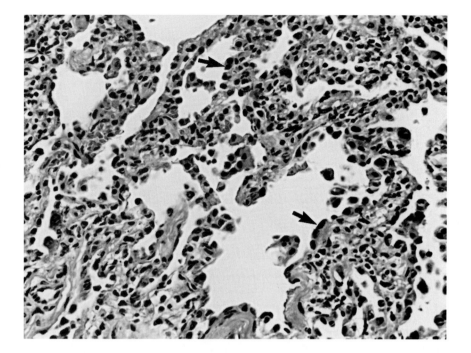

**Figure 42–10. Idiopathic Pulmonary Fibrosis: Type II Cell Hyperplasia.** The section shows mild to moderate interstitial thickening caused by a combination of fibrosis and an infiltrate of mononuclear inflammatory cells; occasional macrophages are present in adjacent air spaces, and there is prominent type II cell hyperplasia *(arrows)*. (×250.)

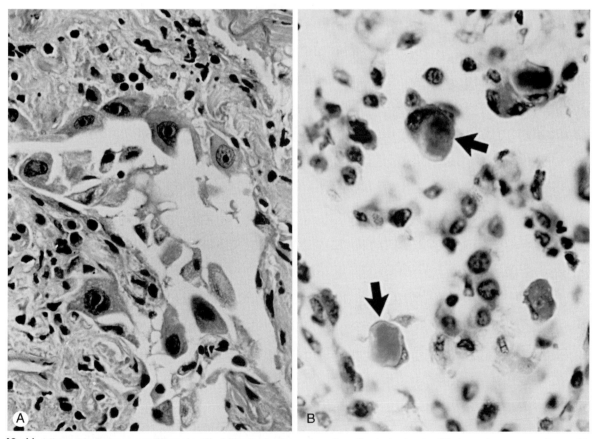

**Figure 42–11. Idiopathic Pulmonary Fibrosis: Viral-like Inclusions.** A section of a single alveolus *(A)* shows the presence of several hyperplastic type II cells with abundant cytoplasm and prominent central nucleoli, resembling cells infected by cytomegalovirus. A section from another patient *(B)* shows several intra-alveolar cells containing prominent cytoplasmic inclusions that correspond to accumulations of cytoplasmic filaments similar to those of Mallory hyaline seen in hepatocytes in alcohol toxicity. *(A,* ×320; *B,* ×600.)

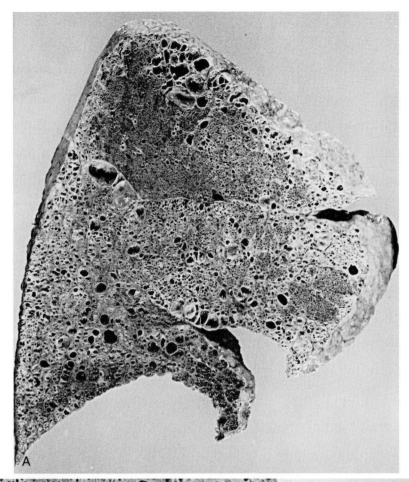

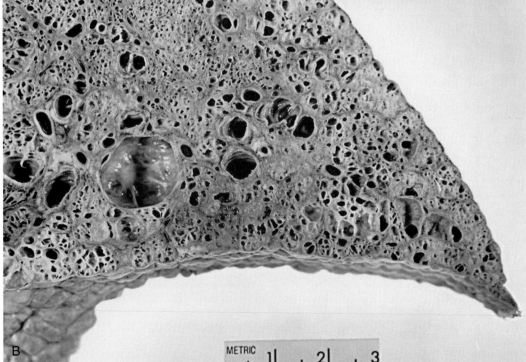

**Figure 42–12. Idiopathic Pulmonary Fibrosis: Advanced Stage.** A sagittal section of a right lung *(A)* shows advanced interstitial fibrosis with extensive "honeycomb" change. Note the relative sparing of the central portion of the upper lobe. A magnified view of the basal aspect of another slice of lower lobe from the same patient *(B)* shows severe interstitial fibrosis with virtually no remaining normal parenchyma.

portions of the lower lobes. As disease progresses, clear-cut areas of fibrosis alternating with small cystic spaces 1 to 2 mm in diameter become evident. Eventually, large portions of a lobe can be affected, resulting in innumerable 5- to 10-mm cystic spaces separated by a variable amount of fibrous tissue (honeycomb lung, Fig. 42–12). Again, these changes are usually most prominent in the lower lobes, particularly the subpleural region; the central portion of all lobes is relatively spared. The pleural surface of such a lung typically has a coarse, nodular appearance that is caused by outward bulging of the ectatic transitional airways and retraction of the adjacent fibrotic parenchyma (Fig. 42–13).

Abnormalities of the large airways can also be seen in IPF. Bronchiectasis is probably the most common; for example, in one autopsy study of 12 patients with advanced disease, it was identified in 9.[150] The observation that the ectasia is largely confined to areas of pronounced interstitial fibrosis (Fig. 42–14) suggests that its cause is retraction of the adjacent fibrous tissue (traction bronchiectasis). In another study of the proximal bronchi in patients with IPF, glandular and muscle hypertrophy were identified in all 9.[151]

Ultrastructural features of IPF have been described by several groups of investigators.[143, 144, 152–154] Basically, they consist of endothelial and epithelial damage and repair associated with multilamination of the alveolar septal basement membrane and an increase in collagen and elastic fibers in the interstitium; an increased number of myofibroblasts is also commonly seen.[153]

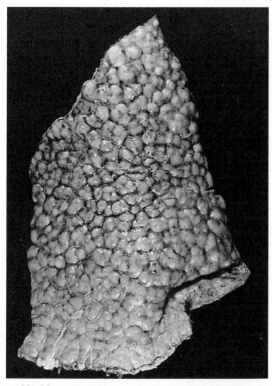

**Figure 42–13. Idiopathic Pulmonary Fibrosis: Pleural Nodularity.** The costal pleural surface of this lower lobe shows numerous nodules approximately 0.5 to 1.0 cm in diameter. The nodules correspond to dilated airways ("honeycomb cysts") bulging outward between foci of parenchymal fibrosis.

## Radiologic Manifestations

### Radiographic Findings

The most common radiographic finding of IPF, described in about 80% of patients with biopsy-proven disease, consists of bilateral irregular linear opacities causing a reticular pattern (Fig. 42–15).[155–157] Although these opacities may be diffuse throughout both lungs, in 50% to 80% of cases, they involve predominantly or exclusively the lower lung zones;[156–158] in 60%, a predominant peripheral distribution is apparent.[158] Cystic changes related to honeycombing can be identified in 30% to 70% of patients.[155, 158, 159] Basal areas of ground-glass opacity are present in about 30% and diffuse ground-glass opacity in 10% to 15% (Fig. 42–16).[155, 158] Less common abnormalities include small nodular opacities (seen in about 10% of patients) and a combination of irregular linear and nodular opacities (reticulonodular pattern, in 20%).[156]

In patients with mild disease, the findings usually consist of symmetric, basal, small to medium-sized irregular linear (reticular pattern) or ground-glass opacities.[155, 160] As the disease progresses, the abnormalities become more diffuse and assume a coarser reticular or reticulonodular pattern associated with progressive loss of volume. "End-stage" disease is characterized by the presence of cysts measuring up to 1 cm in diameter.[160] Radiographic evidence of pleural disease is uncommon; in one study of 95 patients, effusions were observed in 4%, pneumothorax in 7%, and diffuse pleural thickening in 6%.[161]

Decreased lung volumes are evident radiographically at presentation in 50% to 60% of cases.[155, 158] We have been impressed by the striking loss of lung volume apparent on serial radiograph studies over a period of several years (Fig. 42–17) and consider that a diffuse or predominantly basal reticular pattern accompanied by progressive elevation of the diaphragm—signs that occur much less frequently in other forms of diffuse interstitial fibrosis—strongly suggests the diagnosis of either IPF or progressive systemic sclerosis.[162]

The accuracy of chest radiography in the diagnosis of IPF has been assessed in several studies.[158, 163, 164] In one investigation of 118 consecutive patients with various chronic interstitial or air-space diseases, radiographs were independently reviewed by three observers without knowledge of clinical or pathologic data.[163] A confident diagnosis of IPF was made on the basis of the radiographic findings in 30% of cases; this diagnosis was correct in 87% of cases. In another study of 86 patients with various chronic interstitial lung diseases (of which 24 were IPF) and 14 control subjects, a correct diagnosis of IPF was suggested as a first-choice diagnosis in 17 of 24 (69%).[164] The diagnostic value of chest radiography when combined with clinical information was evaluated in another study of 208 patients with various chronic interstitial lung diseases;[158] the diagnosis of IPF was made with a high degree of confidence in 47% of patients with IPF based on clinical data alone and in 79% of patients based on a combination of clinical and radiographic findings. Although theses studies confirm that the radiographic findings in IPF are often sufficient to suggest the diagnosis, the chest radiograph is normal in about 10% to 15% of patients.[155, 165]

*Text continued on page 1604*

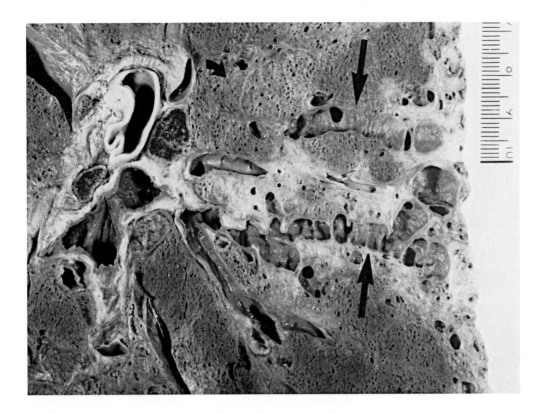

**Figure 42–14. Idiopathic Pulmonary Fibrosis: Traction Bronchiectasis.** A magnified view of the midportion of an upper lobe shows patchy fibrosis, most marked in the parenchyma adjacent to the pleura and one bronchus; it is relatively mild elsewhere *(curved arrow)*. Two bronchi show a mild to moderate degree of cylindrical bronchiectasis *(straight arrows)*.

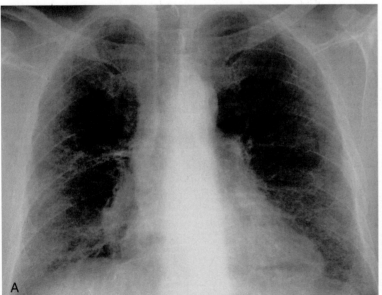

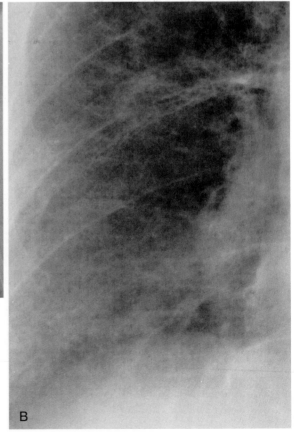

**Figure 42–15. Idiopathic Pulmonary Fibrosis.** A posteroanterior chest radiograph *(A)* reveals irregular linear opacities (reticular pattern) involving predominantly the peripheral regions of the lower lung zones. A magnified view of the right lower lung *(B)* demonstrates the reticular pattern to better advantage. The patient was a 71-year-old man with recently diagnosed idiopathic pulmonary fibrosis.

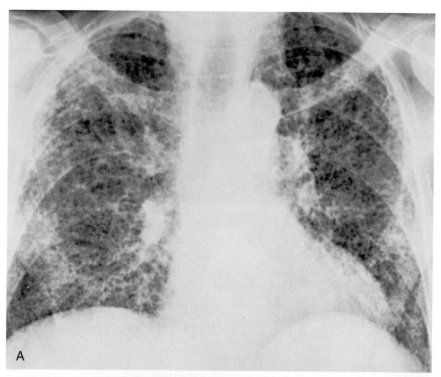

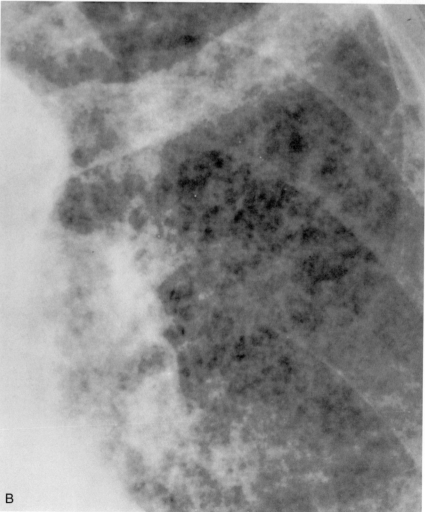

**Figure 42–16. Advanced Idiopathic Pulmonary Fibrosis with Honeycombing.** A postero-anterior radiograph *(A)* and a magnified view of the left mid lung *(B)* reveal a coarse reticular pattern without anatomic predominance. Honeycomb changes are present in several areas and are seen to good advantage in *B*.

*Illustration continued on following page*

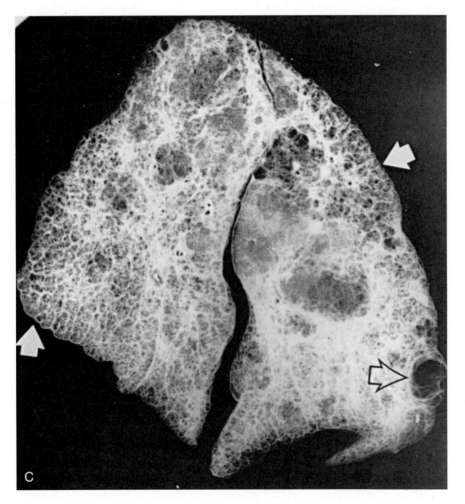

**Figure 42–16** *Continued.* A radiograph of a 1-cm-thick slice of left lung removed at autopsy *(C)* shows honeycombing *(solid arrows)* and a large subpleural bulla in the lower lobe *(open arrow).* The honeycombing is most severe in the periphery.

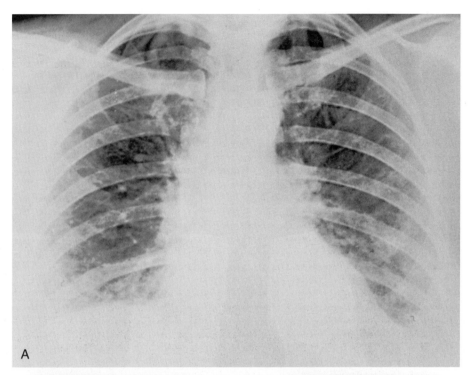

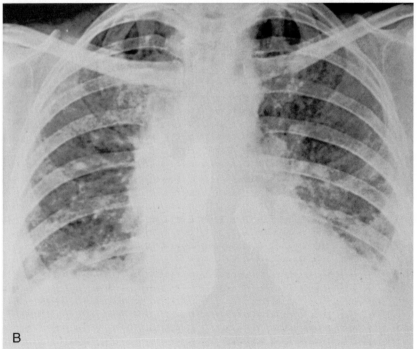

**Figure 42–17. Idiopathic Pulmonary Fibrosis (IPF).** The radiograph illustrated in *A* reveals a reticular pattern superimposed on a hazy, ground-glass opacity. Seven years later, a radiograph *(B)* reveals a more extensive reticular pattern and considerable reduction in the size of the thorax due to progressive fibrosis.

### Computed Tomography Findings

IPF is characterized on CT scans by the presence of fine or coarse irregular lines of attenuation (reticular pattern) involving predominantly the subpleural lung regions and the lower lung zones (Fig. 42–18).[166–168] A patchy distribution is apparent in most cases, with areas that have a reticular pattern intermingled with areas of normal lung (Fig. 42–19).[166, 169] The irregular lines of attenuation are usually associated with irregular pleural, vascular, and bronchial interfaces, evidence of architectural distortion, and dilation of bronchi and bronchioles (traction bronchiectasis and bronchiolectasis).[168, 170] Air-containing cysts measuring 2 to 20 mm in diameter (honeycombing) are seen in 80% to 90% of patients at presentation (*see* Fig. 42–19).[159, 171] These findings are much better appreciated on HRCT than on conventional 7 to 10-mm collimation scans.[166]

A crescentic, predominantly subpleural distribution of the reticular pattern of fibrosis is evident on HRCT in about 80% to 95% of patients;[163, 166, 168] in about 70% of patients the fibrosis is most severe in the lower lung zones, in about 20% all zones are involved to a similar degree, and in as many as 10%, mainly the upper lung zones are affected.[163, 172] Serial HRCT scans show an increase in the extent of the reticular pattern and evidence of honeycombing in virtually all cases (Fig. 42–20).[171, 173, 174] The progression of honeycombing is significantly faster in patients who have extensive areas of ground-glass attenuation on HRCT or marked disease activity on open-lung biopsy specimens.[174a] Cystic spaces related to honeycombing have been shown to decrease in size on HRCT scans performed after forced expiration.[175, 176] Rarely, fine linear or small nodular foci of calcification may be seen within areas of fibrosis as a result of ossification.[177] The subpleural predominance of reticulation or honeycombing is the most characteristic feature of IPF on HRCT; lack of this feature should suggest an alternative diagnosis.

Areas of ground-glass attenuation have been described on HRCT in 65% to 100% of patients (Fig. 42–21).[168, 174, 178] In one study of 12 patients in whom the presence of ground-

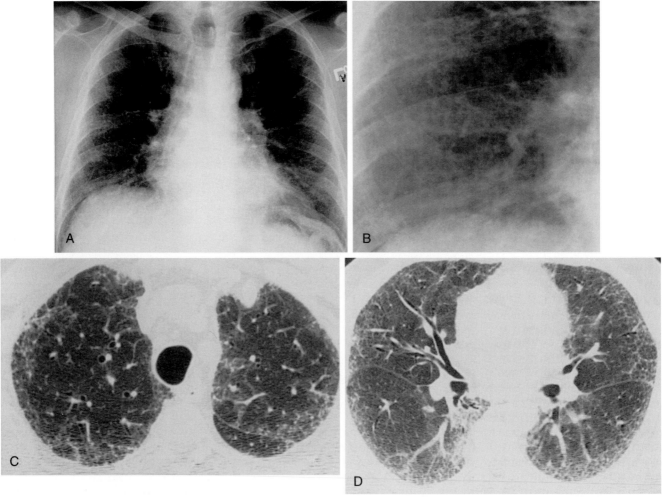

**Figure 42–18. Idiopathic Pulmonary Fibrosis.** A posteroanterior chest radiograph *(A)* reveals a fine bilateral reticular pattern and associated loss of lung volume. The reticular pattern is better appreciated on the magnified view of the right lower lung *(B)*. An HRCT scan through the lung apices *(C)* shows irregular lines of attenuation involving predominantly the subpleural lung regions. HRCT at the level of the right middle lobe bronchus *(D)* demonstrates more extensive parenchymal involvement. The predominant subpleural distribution, however, is still apparent. The reticular pattern on CT is due to irregular thickening of interlobular septa and the presence of intralobular lines. Areas of ground-glass attenuation are present, also involving mainly the subpleural lung regions. The patient was a 66-year-old man.

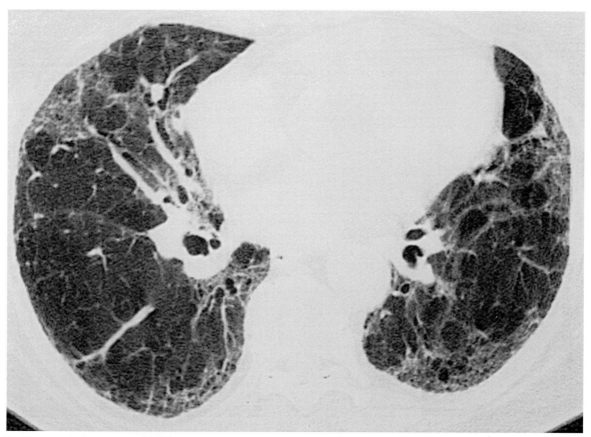

**Figure 42–19. Idiopathic Pulmonary Fibrosis.** HRCT demonstrates a characteristic variegated pattern of idiopathic pulmonary fibrosis, the findings consisting of areas with irregular lines, honeycombing, and ground-glass attenuation intermingled with areas of normal lung. The parenchymal abnormalities have a patchy but predominantly subpleural distribution. The patient was an 80-year-old woman.

glass attenuation on CT scans was compared with pathologic measures of disease activity, 7 patients were categorized histologically as having mild disease activity and 5 as having moderate to marked activity;[179] CT scans demonstrated areas of ground-glass attenuation in all 5 patients with marked disease activity (sensitivity, 100%) and in 2 of 7 with mild activity (specificity, 70%).[179] In another investigation of 14 patients, 12 (86%) with IPF who had areas of ground-glass attenuation on HRCT had marked inflammation on biopsy.[180]

Mediastinal lymph node enlargement is evident on CT in 70% to 90% of patients.[181, 182] The enlargement is usually mild, with nodes measuring between 10 and 15 mm in short-axis diameter and involving only one or two nodal stations (most commonly the right lower paratracheal region).[181] As a result, the node enlargement is typically not apparent on the radiograph. There is evidence that the prevalence of lymph node enlargement is lower in patients receiving corticosteroid therapy. In one investigation, enlarged mediastinal nodes were seen on HRCT in 3 of 22 patients (14%) who had received oral corticosteroids up to 2 months before the date of the CT examination and in 23 of 32 (71%) of patients who had not taken corticosteroids for at least 6 months before the HRCT scan.[182a]

The diagnostic accuracy of HRCT in the diagnosis of IPF has also been assessed in a number of studies.[158, 163, 183] In one, the accuracy of CT was compared with that of chest radiography in the prediction of specific diagnoses in 34 patients with IPF and 84 patients with other chronic intersti-

tial diseases.[163] The radiographs and CT scans were independently assessed by three observers without knowledge of clinical or pathologic data. A confident diagnosis of IPF was made on CT in 73% of patients; this diagnosis was correct 95% of the time. By comparison, a confident diagnosis was made in only 30% of chest radiographs (the diagnosis being correct in 87% of cases).

In another study of 41 patients with IPF and 45 with various other diffuse lung diseases, two independent observers correctly and confidently discriminated between the two groups with an accuracy of 88% on HRCT and 76% on chest radiography.[183] The false-negative rate for IPF decreased from 29% on chest radiography to 11% on HRCT, and the false-positive rate from 19% to 13%.[183] In a third series of 134 patients with various acute and chronic lung diseases, CT images and chest radiographs were reviewed separately and in random order by 20 physicians who were provided only information on patient age and sex;[184] a correct first-choice diagnosis of IPF was made on CT in 77% of cases and on the chest radiograph in 71%. In a fourth investigation of 85 patients (including 18 who had IPF and who underwent biopsy), CT scan images were reviewed by two radiologists who reached a decision by consensus.[184a] The correct diagnosis of IPF was made as a first choice diagnosis in 16 of 18 (89%) patients; the diagnosis was correct in all 12 patients in whom a first choice diagnosis of IPF was made with a high degree of confidence. The variable diagnostic accuracy of CT and chest radiography in these

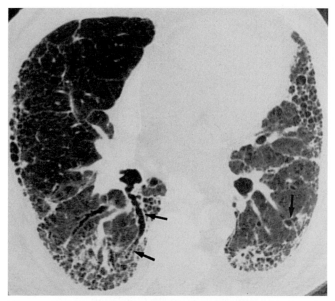

**Figure 42–20. Idiopathic Pulmonary Fibrosis with Traction Bronchiectasis.** An HRCT scan reveals bilateral honeycombing involving predominantly the subpleural lung regions. Bronchial dilation (traction bronchiectasis) *(arrows)* is evident within the areas of fibrosis, particularly in the right lower lobe. The patient was an 81-year-old man.

studies may be related, at least in part, to different patient populations.

The diagnostic accuracy based on the HRCT findings increases with severity of disease. In one study, the scans of 61 consecutive patients with end-stage lung disease (defined by the presence of honeycombing, extensive cystic change, or conglomerate fibrosis) were independently assessed by two observers without knowledge of clinical or pathologic

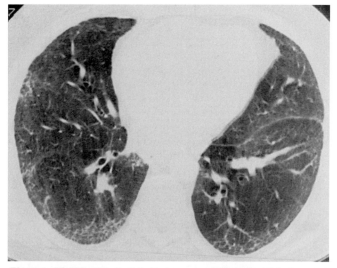

**Figure 42–21. Idiopathic Pulmonary Fibrosis with Ground-Glass Attenuation.** An HRCT scan demonstrates bilateral areas of ground-glass attenuation in a patchy distribution. Irregular thickening of interlobular septa and intralobular lines giving a fine reticular pattern are also evident, particularly in the subpleural regions of the lower lobes. Lung biopsy demonstrated a pattern of usual interstitial pneumonia with predominant inflammation and relatively mild fibrosis. The patient was a 61-year-old man.

data;[178] a correct first-choice diagnosis of IPF was made in 23 of the 26 cases (88%); when the observers were confident in their first choice diagnosis (based on the presence of predominantly subpleural and lower lung zone honeycombing), they made a correct diagnosis in all cases. (The diagnosis of IPF in these patients was established by biopsy specimens taken from relatively uninvolved areas or before the development of end-stage disease.)

Although HRCT is superior to chest radiography in the assessment of pattern and extent of parenchymal abnormalities in IPF (Fig. 42–22), a normal HRCT does not rule out the diagnosis.[165] The sensitivity of chest radiography and HRCT was assessed in a prospective study of 25 patients with dyspnea and suspected interstitial lung disease.[165] Abnormal scans compatible with interstitial lung disease were present in 22 of 25 patients (88%) with biopsy-proven IPF and abnormal radiographs in 21 of 25 (84%); the three patients with normal CT scans had less severe disease based on clinical findings, physiologic scores, gas-exchange abnormalities, and pathologic scoring of open-lung biopsy specimens. This percentage of false-negative HRCT scans in patients with IPF reported in this study seems high to us.

### Other Radiologic Techniques

Other imaging modalities, including magnetic resonance (MR) imaging[185, 186] and positron emission tomography,[187, 188] have a limited, if any, role in the diagnosis of IPF. In one study of 25 patients who had chronic lung disease (including 6 who had IPF) in which MR imaging was compared with HRCT, the former was found to be inferior in the anatomic assessment of the lung parenchyma and in the demonstration of interstitial abnormalities, particularly the presence and extent of fibrosis.[185] Similar results were obtained in another study of 10 patients.[189] In addition, although active alveolitis may result in increased signal intensity on MR imaging,[185, 186, 190] a similar increase may be seen in patients with fibrosis alone.[186]

Administration of conventional contrast medium increases the MR signal intensity of areas of honeycombing but does not influence the detection of ground-glass opacities.[189] The results of an experimental study in rats have suggested a potential role for the use of a macromolecular MR imaging contrast agent (polylysine-gadopentate dimeglumine) in differentiating alveolitis from fibrosis.[191] In this study, pulmonary injury was induced by the instillation of 200 μg of cadmium chloride in the left bronchus. Animals imaged 3 hours later (exudative phase or early alveolitis) demonstrated gradually increasing contrast enhancement on MR imaging, indicating a leak of paramagnetic macromolecules from the intravascular into the extravascular spaces. Animals imaged 8 days later (fibrotic stage) demonstrated constant lung enhancement. The enhancement during the fibrotic stage was lower than that during the exudative phase, indicating a decrease in plasma volume in the fibrotic lung.[191]

### Clinical Manifestations

Symptoms include progressive dyspnea, nonproductive cough, weight loss, and fatigue.[15, 80] Clubbing is common,[192] and its presence can antedate symptoms and other signs of

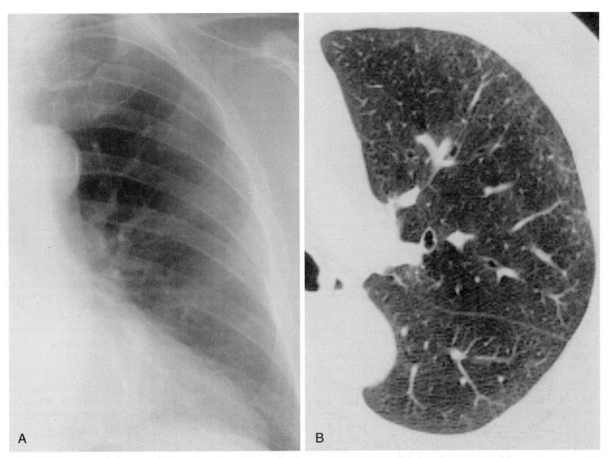

**Figure 42–22. Idiopathic Pulmonary Fibrosis: Comparison of Chest Radiography and High-Resolution CT.** A view of the left lung from a posteroanterior chest radiograph *(A)* shows questionable parenchymal abnormalities. The radiograph as well as several other radiographs obtained in this patient over a 2-year period were interpreted by several radiologists as being normal. A view of the left lung *(B)* from an HRCT scan performed during the same period reveals irregular lines and areas of ground-glass attenuation in the subpleural lung regions. The diagnosis of idiopathic pulmonary fibrosis was made prospectively based on the HRCT findings and was confirmed by open-lung biopsy. The patient was a 72-year-old man.

pulmonary disease.[193, 194] Arthralgia and myalgia have been described in patients with early disease.[195]

In the early stages, examination of the chest can be within normal limits; however, diffuse crackles, predominantly over the lung bases, are frequently heard as disease becomes more severe.[196] These have been termed *Velcro rales* because of their resemblance to the sound produced by tearing apart mated strips of Velcro adhesive.[197] Although such inspiratory crackles are characteristic of IPF, occasional expiratory crackles may also be heard, particularly when disease is advanced.[198] When an occupational history fails to reveal asbestos exposure, the combination of fine crackles, clubbing of the fingers, and dyspnea strongly suggests the diagnosis of IPF. Cyanosis and signs of pulmonary hypertension and cor pulmonale are late manifestations.

Other infrequent clinical findings include impotence (presumably caused by suppression of the hypothalamic-pituitary-testicular axis by hypoxia),[199] orthodeoxia (arterial oxygen desaturation accentuated by the upright position),[200, 201] and hyponatremia associated with the syndrome of inappropriate secretion of antidiuretic hormone.[202]

### Pulmonary Function Tests

Patients who have IPF characteristically develop restrictive derangements of lung function with low diffusing capac-

ity.[203–206] Although some authors disagree,[207] volume adjustment of diffusing capacity does not appear to be useful in IPF because there is no correlation of the severity of disease with the adjusted $D_{CO}$.[208] Most patients show normal or even increased expiratory flow rates when related to absolute lung volume; however, a minority manifest a reduction in maximum midexpiratory flow rate and $FEV_1$ relative to the reduction in vital capacity,[209] likely reflecting the effects of cigarette smoking.[210, 211] Indices of air-flow obstruction correlate closely with the presence of emphysema as determined by HRCT.[212] In the absence of emphysema, there is no relation between smoking history and functional deficits. Vital capacity, diffusing capacity,[213] gas transfer, and pulmonary hemodynamics[214, 215] appear to be more severely affected than in other interstitial lung diseases.[216] The physiologic response to the deterioration in vital capacity is to assume an increasingly rapid and shallow respiratory pattern,[203] a finding linked to reduced lung compliance.[217] These changes in ventilatory pattern do not persist during sleep, suggesting that they are dependent on cortical perception of respiratory system afferents.[218] Hypoxemia is common at rest and is caused chiefly by $\dot{V}/\dot{Q}$ inequality;[207, 219, 220] however, about 20% of this hypoxemia can be attributed to a diffusion defect.[207, 209, 219]

A number of abnormalities have been described in the exercise performance of patients who have IPF. Patients typically have a rapid, shallow breathing pattern with total ventilation being excessive for each workload,[221] a finding that is partly related to increased dead-space ventilation and partly to hyperventilation. At the same time, maximum ventilatory capacity is reduced compared with normal.[221] Patients who have IPF may also develop or have worsened arterial hypoxemia during exercise, largely as a result of diffusion impairment;[207] this could impair tissue oxygen delivery and exercise performance.

Abnormal cardiac performance with reduction in stroke volume, increase in heart rate, and elevation in pulmonary artery pressure during exercise may also limit maximum exercise tolerance.[221] In one study in which an attempt was made to determine which of these factors is most important in limiting exercise performance, excess dead space was added to the exercise circuitry, thereby selectively stressing the respiratory system.[221] Exercise performance deteriorated in a significant fashion, with decreases in exercise time, maximal workload, and maximum oxygen uptake at end exercise. There were no changes in end-exercise tidal volume or respiratory frequency, and cardiac performance was not altered. These findings suggest that exercise limitation is predominantly the result of respiratory abnormalities.

Attempts to correlate pathologic findings with particular lung function derangements have also been made. In one study, a decrease in vital capacity and diffusing capacity correlated with increasing severity of fibrosis.[209] In another, severity of disease (both inflammation and fibrosis) as determined by HRCT correlated best with diffusing capacity and oxygen desaturation on exercise.[212] However, other investigators have found these functional measurements to be poor indicators of the relative amounts of fibrous tissue and inflammatory cells.[222, 223] The finding of stability of the diffusing capacity in the face of deteriorating lung volumes in one group of patients followed for a 3-year period has provided support for these observations.[224]

### Natural History and Prognosis

In most patients with IPF, deterioration is gradual and inexorable with increasing shortness of breath often accompanied by the development of cor pulmonale. Most succumb to respiratory failure, frequently precipitated by infection;[225, 226] about 20% die from cardiac disease.[225] The overall mean survival is probably less than 5 years.[64, 226–228a–c] (Although patients have been reported to live as long as 15 years after diagnosis,[229, 230] we suspect that many of these would now be considered to have nonspecific interstitial pneumonitis [*see* farther on].) A few patients have an acute, severe exacerbation of disease after a period of relative stability;[231] pathologic examination of the lungs of these individuals often shows diffuse alveolar damage. As discussed farther on (*see* page 1619), whether this process represents an accelerated phase of IPF or a superimposed complication is not clear. When there is clinical deterioration, progression of IPF must be distinguished from complications of the disease itself, such as pneumothorax, pulmonary carcinoma, thromboembolism, and infection, and of its therapy, such as steroid-related myopathy, hypokalemia, and uncontrolled diabetes.[232] Given the age of patients usually affected, independent abnormalities, such as ischemic heart

disease with left ventricular failure, also explain increasing breathlessness in some patients.

The incidence of pulmonary carcinoma is increased in patients with IPF, reflecting the association between parenchymal scarring regardless of etiology and pulmonary neoplasia that is discussed in Chapter 31 (*see* page 1080). It has been suggested that the neoplastic proliferation may be related to epithelial metaplasia and hyperplasia of either bronchiolar or alveolar epithelium, processes that commonly exist in IPF.[233–235] Adenocarcinoma is the most frequent histologic type, although squamous cell carcinoma and large cell carcinoma have also been reported.[236–238] The radiographic manifestations of pulmonary carcinoma associated with IPF include a nodule or mass superimposed on linear and cystic opacities.[239] In one study of 32 patients, the carcinoma was located in the lower lobes in 21 (66%) and in the lung periphery, where the most advanced fibrosis was located, in 21.[240] The CT findings consisted of an ill-defined focal consolidation-like mass in 17 patients (53%), a nodule in 12 (38%), massive lymphadenopathy in 2 (6%), and diffuse air-space consolidation in 1 (3%). Clubbing appears to be an almost invariable clinical finding in patients who have this complication.[64, 241–243]

Many attempts have been made to identify specific clinical, functional, laboratory, radiologic, and pathologic features that predict prognosis and response to treatment in IPF. Conventional wisdom holds that a favorable response to therapy improves survival and, in fact, there is little doubt that patients who respond to therapy live longer than patients who do not.[204] However, those who respond to therapy also have disease profiles that independently favor longer survival.[243a] Therefore, at least some and perhaps a great deal of the difference in survival between responders and nonresponders has to do with the state of the patient before therapy was given. Given these relationships among disease severity, response to therapy, and prognosis, the need for appropriately designed therapeutic trials in well-defined patient populations is apparent.

### Clinical Criteria

There appears to be general agreement that the prognosis is better in patients who have a shorter duration of symptoms before presentation,[243–247] who have dyspnea of only mild to moderate severity,[64] or who are younger (with the exception of infants).[6] A poorer prognosis is seen in men, in patients who have severe dyspnea when first seen, in smokers, and in patients reporting mucus hypersecretion[248, 249] or receiving immunosuppressive therapy.[228, 250]

### Pulmonary Function and Laboratory Test Criteria

Survival is worse in patients who have more restrictive lung function.[205, 251, 252] Whether arterial hypoxemia independently predicts poor prognosis has not been clarified because studies on this question have yielded conflicting results.[64, 252] Not surprisingly, the absence of right-axis deviation on the electrocardiogram is associated with more prolonged survival.[64] Although patients who have IPF have higher than normal serum levels of markers of enhanced cell-mediated immunity, such as soluble CD8 and IL-2 receptors, these do not correlate with clinical indicators of disease activity or with outcome in the short to medium term.[253] Similarly, although the presence of immune complexes in serum and in lung biopsy specimens appears to correlate with less severe disease, this finding is not associated with an increased length of survival or response to corticosteroids.[85, 86] Although the finding of an elevated total plasma lactate dehydrogenase level is not specific for IPF, the level of this enzyme appears to reflect disease activity.[254] However, as with the other blood tests, the level likely has no independent prognostic value in an individual patient after considering the clinical, functional, and radiographic findings.

## Bronchoalveolar Lavage Criteria

Abnormalities in BAL fluid have been extensively studied for their predictive ability. Recognizing that the airways, particularly those of smokers, can contain an abundance of neutrophils,[255–257] and that a proper technique for alveolar sampling is important in the interpretation of results, several investigators have established that an increased percentage of neutrophils, eosinophils, or both are related to a poor clinical response to therapy.[246, 251, 258–261] On the other hand, a high BAL fluid lymphocyte count has been associated with a favorable response to therapy and better prognosis.[250, 251, 255, 261, 262, 262a]

Patients who have IPF have a lower proportion of phosphatidylglycerol and a higher proportion of phosphatidylinositol in BAL fluid than do healthy volunteers;[263] moreover, the severity of these alterations correlates with the degree of pulmonary fibrosis.[263] In addition, surfactant protein A levels in BAL fluid of patients who have IPF are lower than those in controls, and there is a good correlation between levels of this glycoprotein in BAL and survival.[264] In one study, the survival of patients above the median level was more than twice that of patients below the median;[264] however, the measurement of surfactant protein A did not improve on predictions of survival based on traditional clinical and functional parameters. In another investigation, the level of CYFRA 21-1, a cytokeratin fragment, was increased in patients who had IPF;[264a] moreover, its level correlated with the level of inflammatory cells in BAL fluid and decreased with response to therapy. Poorer survival has also been correlated with the finding of augmented release of prostaglandin $E_2$ from cultured alveolar macrophages.[251]

## Pathologic Criteria

A number of pathologic findings have been described that may be useful in defining prognosis or identifying patients who are likely to respond to therapy. Patients whose lung biopsy specimens show more cellularity, as opposed to more fibrosis, usually[6, 149, 227, 265] but not always[2, 266, 267] have a more favorable prognosis. Despite this, estimates of the degree of cellularity in biopsy specimens do not appear to be a reliable predictor of response to therapy;[85, 243, 244, 268] by contrast, there is evidence that the severity of fibrosis is an indicator of the likelihood of a lack of response.[227, 244] A semiquantitative grading system based on histologic abnormalities has been proposed as a means of assessing more accurately the extent and severity of disease.[140, 269] The expression of tenascin, an extracellular matrix glycoprotein that is particularly prominent beneath metaplastic bronchiolar-type epithelium, was associated with a shortened survival in one study of 28 patients.[270]

## Radiologic Criteria

The pattern and extent of parenchymal abnormality and the degree of volume loss correlate with the severity of functional impairment, length of survival, and overall prognosis of patients with IPF.[173, 271, 272, 272a] In one investigation of the radiographic, clinical, and functional findings in 26 patients, the lungs were divided into six zones (upper, middle, and lower lung zones of the right and left lung), each of which was graded for severity of disease according to the International Labor Office Grading System.[173] The extent and severity of parenchymal abnormalities (profusion score) correlated with the severity of dyspnea (r = 0.54) and with the impairment in gas transfer as assessed by the carbon monoxide diffusion capacity (r = −0.53).[173] Follow-up chest radiographs obtained 6 weeks to 53 months later (mean, 25 months) showed an increase in the profusion of the irregular linear opacities. The change in the average profusion score between initial and follow-up radiographs correlated with the interval decrease in total-lung capacity (r = 0.69), residual volume (r = 0.76), and interval increase in the severity of dyspnea (r = 0.65).

Reticular changes and honeycombing on HRCT in patients with IPF reflect the presence of irreversible interstitial fibrosis,[166, 168, 169, 273, 274] whereas areas of ground-glass attenuation usually reflect the presence of active pneumonitis.[179, 180, 273, 274] Based on the assumption that patients with such active disease are more likely to respond to immunosuppressive and anti-inflammatory therapy, it is reasonable to postulate that patients with predominantly ground-glass attenuation would be more likely to respond to treatment than those with predominantly reticulation or honeycombing.[179]

Several groups of investigators have addressed this issue. In one study of 19 patients with IPF, areas of ground-glass attenuation on HRCT were quantified subjectively by two independent observers;[275] the extent of attenuation showed a significant correlation with improvement in carbon monoxide diffusing capacity and forced vital capacity after corticosteroid treatment. In another study of 76 patients, CT scans were categorized as showing a predominantly ground-glass, mixed, or predominantly reticular pattern;[276] favorable response to treatment and 4-year survival in previously untreated patients were most common in patients with the ground-glass pattern, least common in those with reticulation, and intermediate in those with a mixed pattern. Despite these findings, only 8 of the 76 patients (11%) had a predominant pattern of ground-glass attenuation, and 18 (24%) had an equivalent distribution of areas of ground-glass attenuation and reticulation; thus, most patients had predominant reticulation and would not be expected to respond to corticosteroid treatment. Furthermore, in both studies, the investigators failed to distinguish patients with IPF from those who had DIP or nonspecific interstitial pneumonitis.

The prognostic significance of areas of ground-glass attenuation on HRCT in patients with IPF compared with those with DIP was assessed in a retrospective study of 23 patients (12 with IPF and 11 with DIP) who had both initial and follow-up HRCT scans (median interval, 10 months).[174] Eleven patients with IPF and 11 with DIP received treatment (mostly corticosteroids alone) between the initial and follow-up scans. On the initial scans, all 12 patients with IPF had areas of ground-glass attenuation and reticulation; 10 had honeycombing. All 11 patients with DIP had areas of ground-glass attenuation, 5 had reticulation, and 1 had honeycombing. Nine of the 12 patients (75%) with IPF showed an increase in the extent of ground-glass attenuation or progression to reticulation or honeycombing on follow-up, as compared with only two (18%) with DIP. Thus, although areas of ground-glass attenuation reflect the presence of active inflammation, in most patients with UIP, they progress to fibrosis despite treatment (Fig. 42–23).[171, 173, 174] Given the fact that so few patients who had IPF improved with therapy, the study did not have sufficient power to determine whether any particular CT abnormality had a favorable prognostic value. In one prospective investigation of 38 patients (37 of whom had IPF and one DIP), the patients who responded to a 3-month trial of high-dose corticosteroid therapy had a greater extent of ground-glass attenuation than the nonresponders;[243a] long-term survival was greatest in patients who had the lowest extent of fibrosis on pretreatment HRCT. In this study, the HRCT findings were superior to the histopathologic features in predicting mortality.

Most patients with IPF show slowly progressive deterioration. Some, however, have an accelerated course characterized by an exacerbation of dyspnea, decrease in arterial oxygen tension ($PaO_2$) of more than 10 mm Hg, and new diffuse opacities on chest radiographs over a 1-month period, in the absence of infection and left heart failure.[277, 278] In one study in which the CT findings were assessed in 17 patients who had such accelerated disease, areas of ground-glass attenuation or consolidation were identified in all cases;[278] the areas were predominantly peripheral in 6 patients, multifocal in 6, and diffuse in 5. All patients received high-dose intravenous corticosteroid therapy; despite this treatment, 1 of 6 (17%) patients with peripheral opacification, 3

of 6 (50%) with multifocal opacification, and all 5 (100%) with diffuse opacification died within a mean of 34 days (range, 12 days to 3 months).[278] The authors concluded that the pattern of distribution of parenchymal opacification on CT may be helpful in predicting prognosis and response to treatment.

It has been suggested that technetium-99m–DTPA clearance, which may reflect pulmonary inflammation, correlates with disease activity and subsequent functional and radiologic evolution.[188, 279] In one small study in which positron emission tomography scanning was employed, vascular permeability was also found to be related to disease activity.[280] Although some investigators have found evidence that a relatively low gallium scan index might predict stability of disease,[281] others have found no relation between gallium scan results and clinical course.[282]

### Summary

In summary, there is no single finding or group of findings on BAL fluid analysis, laboratory testing, or histologic or radiologic examination that allows the clinician to distinguish with *certainty* which patient will respond to therapy and which will not.[247, 262] However, it seems reasonable to conclude that therapy should be more seriously considered in patients who are more likely to have a better prognosis and who have clinical features associated with an increased likelihood of response to that therapy. Thus, younger patients with less advanced disease probably warrant a therapeutic trial, whereas older patients who have advanced fibrotic disease are unlikely to benefit from aggressive intervention.

### Diagnosis

When clinical findings and the radiographic pattern suggest interstitial lung disease, the diagnostic possibilities

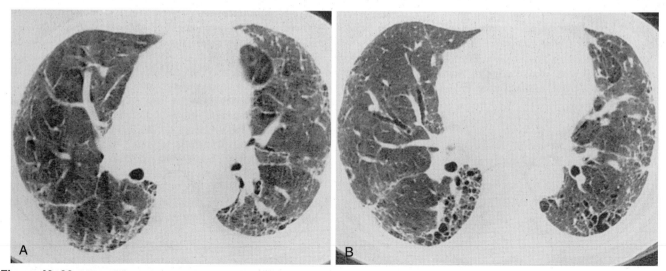

**Figure 42–23. Idiopathic Pulmonary Fibrosis: Progression Despite Treatment.** An HRCT scan *(A)* demonstrates irregular linear opacities and areas of ground-glass attenuation involving mainly the subpleural lung regions. A scan performed 1 year later at approximately the same level *(B)* reveals that the areas of ground-glass attenuation and irregular linear opacities in the posteromedial aspect of the right lower lobe have progressed to a state of honeycombing. Progression of honeycombing is also evident in the left lower lobe. The remaining areas of the lungs show relatively little change. The patient was a 69-year-old woman who was treated with corticosteroids in the interval between the two scans. (From Terriff BA, Kwan SY, Chan-Yeung M, Müller NL: Fibrosing alveolitis: Chest radiography and CT as predictors of clinical and functional impairment at follow-up in 26 patients. Radiology 184:445, 1992, with permission.)

are numerous. Although the combination of clubbing, slowly progressive worsening of dyspnea, serial reduction in pulmonary function, and radiographic evidence of progressive loss of lung volume strongly suggest the diagnosis of IPF, in most cases this is a diagnosis of exclusion. Nevertheless, it is unusual for a lung biopsy specimen to reveal a different diagnosis when a careful history, physical examination, and laboratory and radiologic investigations (including HRCT[283, 284]) have reasonably excluded other diagnostic possibilities. Connective tissue diseases, such as rheumatoid disease, progressive systemic sclerosis, Sjögren's syndrome, and dermatomyositis or polymyositis, are usually readily recognized by their clinical manifestations and specific autoantibodies. However, error may arise during the early stages of polymyositis, when muscle weakness may be overlooked or ascribed to nonspecific manifestations of the pulmonary disability or to corticosteroid therapy.[285, 286]

The diagnosis of pneumoconiosis or a drug reaction usually requires little more than an appropriate clinical history regarding occupation and medication. Similarly, a history of exposure to birds, moldy hay, or other organic dusts should raise the possibility of extrinsic allergic alveolitis. The diagnosis of IPF is virtually eliminated when diffuse interstitial lung disease is associated with hilar and paratracheal lymph node enlargement on the plain radiograph, the combination of the two strongly suggesting a diagnosis of sarcoidosis. However, as discussed previously, mediastinal lymph node enlargement is not uncommon on CT in IPF and should not be used as evidence against the presence of this disease.

The clinical findings associated with other interstitial pneumonitides, such as neurofibromatosis, Hermansky-Pudlak syndrome, dyskeratosis congenita,[287] tuberous sclerosis, and lymphangioleiomyomatosis, are also usually sufficiently characteristic to distinguish them from IPF. Pulmonary Langerhans' cell histiocytosis usually presents radiographically with normal or increased lung volume and characteristically affects the upper lung zones more than the lower.

Open-lung biopsy and thoracoscopic biopsy are the only procedures that yield sufficient tissue to confirm a diagnosis of IPF.[288] However, although transbronchial biopsy does not allow the distinction of IPF from many other conditions,[5, 289] it is a valuable procedure for the diagnosis of sarcoidosis and lymphangitic carcinoma, with which it might be confused radiographically. Whether tissue confirmation of IPF is routinely required is controversial. Because no investigations have been carried out that have specifically addressed this issue, it is not surprising to find a variety of approaches in common practice. In one study of 109 American pulmonary physicians, 22 of 23 respondents reported that they routinely obtain tissue in the evaluation of patients with interstitial lung disease (although most use transbronchial biopsy).[290] By contrast, most British pulmonary specialists are content to make the diagnosis of IPF on the basis of clinical and radiologic features alone.[291] In our view and that of others,[14] when the clinical, laboratory, and radiologic features (including those of HRCT scans) are typical of IPF, biopsy is not indicated, particularly when a treatment decision will not depend on the findings of the biopsy. In other words, the cost-effectiveness and risks of biopsy have to be weighed against the benefits.[14]

## DESQUAMATIVE INTERSTITIAL PNEUMONITIS

As discussed previously (*see* page 1584), there has been some debate concerning the distinction of IPF from DIP: some authors believe that they should be considered separate entities and others that they represent different stages of one disease process. In our view, the pathologic and radiologic differences between the two conditions, as well as their different courses and responses to therapy, are such that the two are better considered separately.

The etiology and pathogenesis of DIP are unknown. The evidence for a viral cause is even less than that described for IPF. Although intranuclear inclusion bodies have been reported pathologically,[149, 195, 292] they likely represent the products of nuclear degeneration rather than structures of viral origin. As with IPF, immunologic factors have been implicated in disease pathogenesis; for example, the intravenous administration of Freund's adjuvant to rabbits can result in a pattern similar to that of DIP.[293] The histologic pattern of DIP has been seen in association with nitrofurantoin therapy,[294] leukemia,[295] and a variety of inhaled particulates.[296–298] DIP also bears some resemblance to smoking-related respiratory bronchiolitis (*see* page 2348);[301] in fact, some investigators believe that the latter may be an early manifestation of DIP.[7]

Unlike the variable histologic appearance characteristic of IPF, the pattern of DIP is distinctly uniform, all portions of lung on a tissue section appearing more or less similar (Fig. 42–24). The alveolar interstitium is usually mildly to moderately thickened by an infiltrate of mononuclear inflammatory cells (predominantly lymphocytes) and a small amount of collagen; lymphoid nodules are sometimes present, and type II cell hyperplasia is extensive. Alveolar air spaces are characteristically filled with numerous mononuclear cells, originally believed to be desquamated type II cells, but now known to consist predominantly of alveolar macrophages. These cells may contain small amounts of iron or other material. Occasionally, oval or rounded lamellated periodic acid–Schiff–positive structures can be identified that resemble Schaumann's bodies in sarcoidosis (Fig. 42–25);[299] the precise nature or significance of these structures, sometimes termed *blue bodies*, is unclear.

The histologic pattern of DIP can be seen focally in some cases of IPF as well as in a variety of other conditions, such as tuberculosis, Langerhans' cell histiocytosis, and rheumatoid nodules (Fig. 42–26).[300] Thus, a definitive diagnosis of DIP based solely on a small amount of tissue, such as obtained by transbronchial biopsy, should not be made.

The characteristic radiographic pattern of DIP consists of symmetric bilateral ground-glass opacification, which can be diffuse but usually involves mainly the lower lung zones (Fig. 42–27).[292, 302] In patients with fibrosis, irregular linear opacities can be seen, again predominantly in the lower lung zones (Fig. 42–28).[227, 303] Hilar lymph node enlargement has been reported in a small number of cases (*see* Fig. 42–28);[149, 304, 305] pleural effusion is rare.[292] The chest radiograph has been reported to be normal in 3% to 22% of patients with biopsy-proven disease.[165, 227, 292, 303]

The predominant abnormality on HRCT is the presence of bilateral areas of ground-glass attenuation.[306, 307] In one review of 22 patients, this involved the middle and lower lung zones in all patients and the upper lung zones in 18

*Text continued on page 1616*

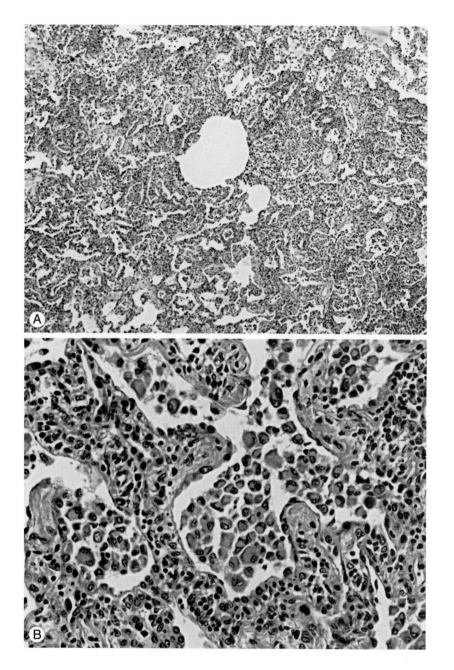

**Figure 42–24. Desquamative Interstitial Pneumonitis.** A low-magnification view of lung parenchyma *(A)* shows moderately severe, fairly uniform disease affecting all the tissue. At higher power *(B)*, interstitial thickening can be seen to be caused by a combination of mononuclear inflammatory cells (predominantly lymphocytes) and a small amount of fibrous tissue; the adjacent air spaces contain numerous macrophages. *(A, ×40; B, ×250.)* (Courtesy of Dr. Claude Auger, Jean Talon Hospital, Montreal.)

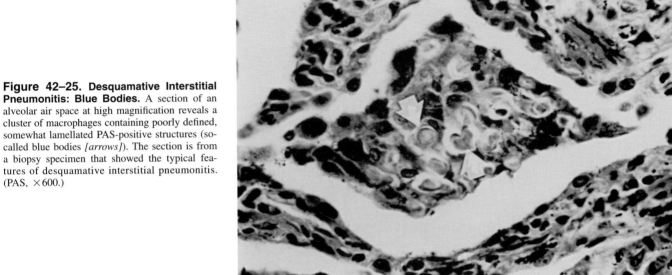

**Figure 42–25. Desquamative Interstitial Pneumonitis: Blue Bodies.** A section of an alveolar air space at high magnification reveals a cluster of macrophages containing poorly defined, somewhat lamellated PAS-positive structures (so-called blue bodies *[arrows]*). The section is from a biopsy specimen that showed the typical features of desquamative interstitial pneumonitis. (PAS, ×600.)

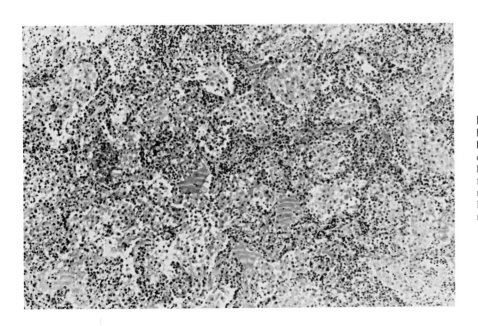

**Figure 42–26. Desquamative Interstitial Pneumonitis (DIP)–like Reaction in Langerhans' Cell Histiocytosis.** A section taken adjacent to a focus of parenchymal Langerhans' cell histiocytosis shows a moderate degree of fairly uniform interstitial pneumonitis and the presence of numerous intra-alveolar macrophages. Such a DIP-like pattern can be seen focally in several pulmonary diseases.

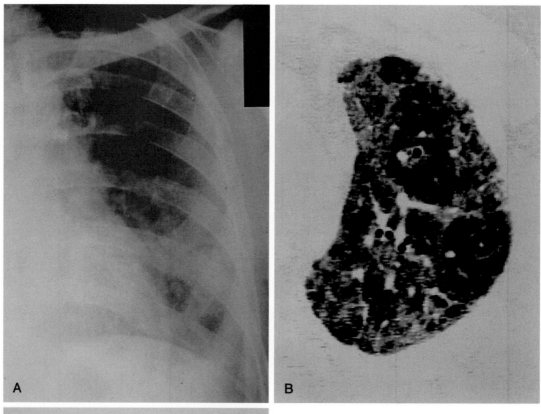

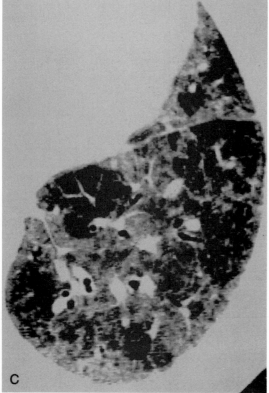

**Figure 42–27. Desquamative Interstitial Pneumonitis.** A view of the left lung from an anteroposterior chest radiograph *(A)* reveals ground-glass opacification throughout all lung zones. Views of the left lung from HRCT scans *(B* and *C)* essentially confirm the radiographic findings. The patient was a 53-year-old man with biopsy proven desquamative interstitial pneumonitis.

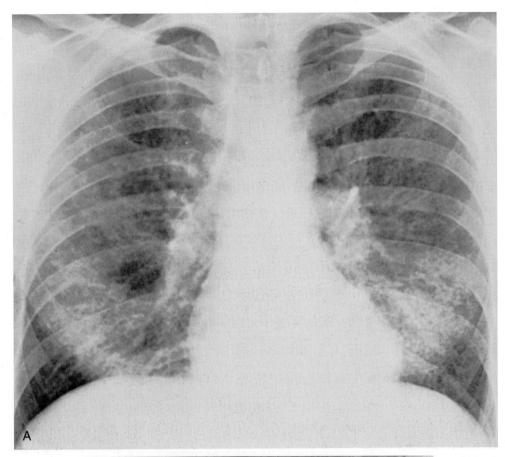

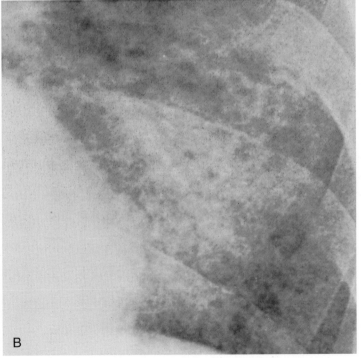

**Figure 42–28. Desquamative Interstitial Pneumonitis.** This 35-year-old policeman noted the onset of dyspnea 6 months previously while wrestling a suspect; the dyspnea had become progressively worse up to the time of hospital admission. A posteroanterior radiograph *(A)* and a magnified view of the lower portion of the left lung *(B)* reveal diffuse bilateral ground-glass opacities and lower lung zone reticular pattern. Hilar lymph nodes appear slightly enlarged.

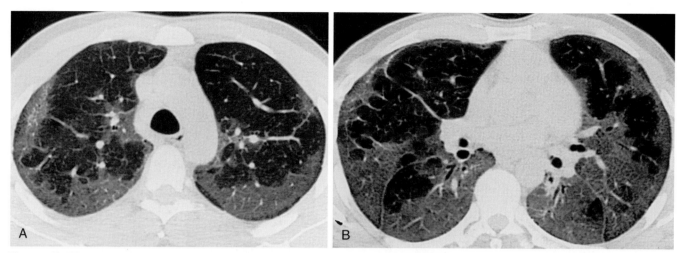

**Figure 42–29. Desquamative Interstitial Pneumonitis.** An HRCT scan at the level of the aortic arch *(A)* demonstrates areas of ground-glass attenuation that have a predominantly subpleural distribution. Another scan at the level of the superior segmental bronchi *(B)* demonstrates more extensive disease; however, the subpleural predominance is still apparent. The patient was a 39-year-old man who had biopsy proven desquamative interstitial pneumonitis. (Courtesy of Dr. David Hansell, Royal Brompton Hospital.) (From Hartman TE, Primack SL, Swensen SJ, et al: Desquamative interstitial pneumonia: Thin-section CT findings in 22 patients. Radiology 187:787, 1993, with permission.)

(82%).[307] The distribution was predominantly peripheral in 13 patients (59%) (Fig. 42–29), patchy and bilateral in 5 (23%), and diffuse in 4 (18%). Irregular lines of attenuation (reticular pattern) suggestive of fibrosis were seen in 11 patients (50%), and cystic changes (honeycombing) in 7 (32%). The fibrosis was most marked in the lower lung zones in 11 patients, middle lung zones in 1 patient, and upper lung zones in 1 patient. Mild honeycombing was seen in the 7 of the 22 patients and was present almost exclusively in the lung bases. In a second investigation of 8 patients who had DIP, all showed areas of ground-glass attenuation involving the middle and lower lung zones, predominantly in the lung periphery;[307a] less common findings included a mild reticular pattern in 5 patients, architectural distortion in 3, and traction bronchiectasis in 1. Although small cystic changes were seen in areas with ground-glass attenuation,

these were considered to represent traction bronchiolectasis rather than areas of honeycombing.

The natural history of areas of ground-glass attenuation was assessed in a follow-up study of 11 patients.[174] On initial CT scans, all 11 patients had areas of ground-glass attenuation involving about 50% of the lung parenchyma, 5 patients had irregular linear opacities involving about 5% of the lung parenchyma, and 1 patient had mild honeycombing. Follow-up HRCT scans performed after a median interval of 10 months and after treatment (predominantly corticosteroids alone) demonstrated a decrease in the extent of parenchymal abnormalities in 6 patients, no change in 3, and a slight increase in the extent of abnormalities in 2 patients. The improvement on the follow-up CT was related to a decrease in the extent of areas of ground-glass attenuation (Fig. 42–30). The two patients with progression of disease showed an

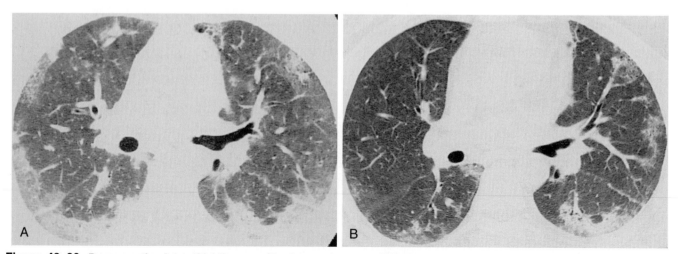

**Figure 42–30. Desquamative Interstitial Pneumonitis: Improvement on Follow-up.** An HRCT scan at presentation *(A)* reveals extensive bilateral areas of ground-glass attenuation involving predominantly the subpleural lung regions. A few irregular linear opacities are present in the subpleural regions, consistent with mild fibrosis. A scan 18 months later *(B)* demonstrates marked improvement in the areas of ground-glass attenuation. Mild residual fibrosis is present, particularly in the subpleural regions of the left lung. (Courtesy of Dr. Georgeann McGuinness, New York University Medical Center, New York.)

increase in the extent of irregular lines or the development of mild honeycombing.[174] In another follow-up investigation of eight patients, all showed initial decrease in extent of ground-glass attenuation with treatment; however, the extent of ground-glass attenuation subsequently increased in 3 patients despite treatment.[307a]

Dyspnea on exertion is seen in most patients; for example, in two series, it was the initial complaint in 38 of 44 patients (86%).[292, 308] Rarely, disease is discovered following the performance of a "routine" chest radiograph.[308] Cough has been reported in about half of patients; fever, diaphoresis, weight loss, weakness, myalgia, chest pain, and fatigue are seen in a minority. Bibasilar crackles have been described in about half of patients; clubbing is somewhat less prevalent. When disease is advanced, cyanosis can be noted.

Pulmonary function studies may be normal[292] but usually show evidence of a restrictive defect.[308] Associated airflow obstruction may be noted in patients who are smokers.[308] Gas-exchange defects are the rule.

Most patients who are treated with corticosteroids demonstrate both subjective and objective improvement in the short term;[308] 3 of 26 patients in one series had a complete remission.[308] However, progression of disease despite continued therapy has occurred frequently,[308] and only about half of patients demonstrate persistent improvement 1 year after initiation of therapy.[227, 308] In one study of 40 patients who were followed for 1 to 22 years, mortality was 28%, and mean survival was 12.2 years.[227]

## NONSPECIFIC INTERSTITIAL PNEUMONITIS

Nonspecific interstitial pneumonitis (NIP) is a form of interstitial lung disease that resembles IPF but that appears to be associated with a significantly different course and outcome.[309] The abnormality differs pathologically from IPF by its uniform appearance: as discussed previously, IPF typically shows a combination of active inflammation and fibrogenesis associated with changes of more long-standing injury, such as mature fibrous tissue and cyst formation; by contrast NIP, is characterized by an appearance that suggests a single initiating event (Fig. 42–31).

The predominant radiographic manifestations of NIP consist of areas of ground-glass opacification or consolidation involving mainly the middle and lower lung zones (Fig. 42–32).[310] Other manifestations include a reticular pattern[309] or a combination of interstitial and air-space patterns.[309–311] Reticular opacities may be seen superimposed on the areas of ground-glass opacification. In one review of the findings in seven patients, areas of parenchymal opacification were seen in five, a combination of opacification and reticulation in one, and a normal chest radiograph in one.[310] CT demonstrated abnormalities in all seven cases, the most common finding being bilateral, patchy areas of ground-glass attenuation without zonal or peripheral predominance (*see* Fig. 42–32).[310] Areas of consolidation were present in five patients; they involved mainly the lower lung zones but showed no peripheral or central predominance. Irregular linear opaci-

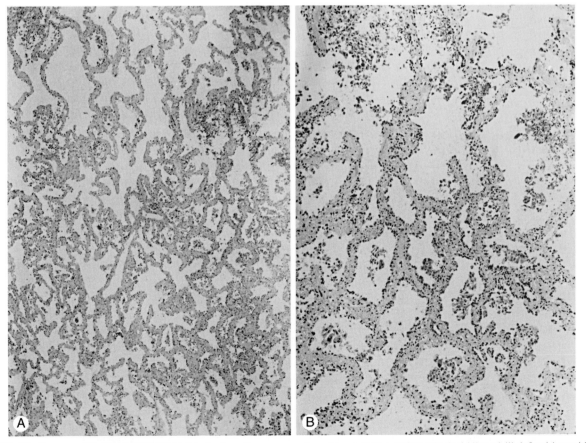

**Figure 42–31. Nonspecific Interstitial Fibrosis.** Sections from an open-lung biopsy from a patient who had bilateral ill-defined interstitial disease show thickening of the alveolar interstitium by mature collagen with few inflammatory cells; air spaces contain a mild increase in the number of alveolar macrophages. The uniform appearance of the fibrosis is distinctly different from that of idiopathic pulmonary fibrosis (compare with Figure 42–3).

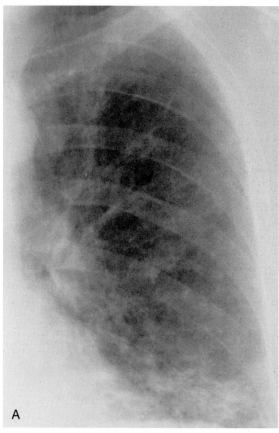

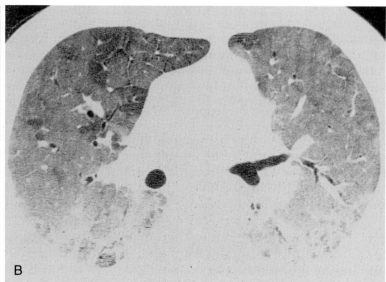

**Figure 42–32. Nonspecific Interstitial Pneumonitis.** A view of the left lung from a posteroanterior chest radiograph *(A)* reveals diffuse ground-glass opacification of the left lung and focal areas of consolidation and irregular linear opacities in the left lower lung zone. Similar findings were present in the right lung. An HRCT scan *(B)* demonstrates extensive bilateral areas of ground-glass attenuation. Small focal areas of consolidation are present in the dependent lung regions. The patient was a 44-year-old man who had biopsy proven nonspecific interstitial pneumonitis.

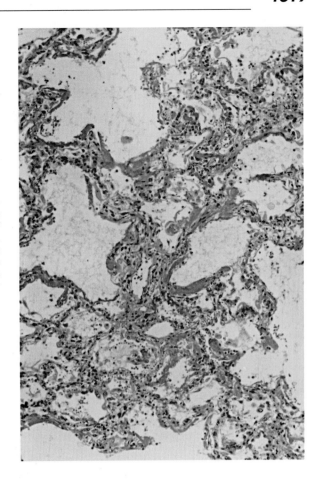

**Figure 42–33. Idiopathic Pulmonary Fibrosis with Superimposed Diffuse Alveolar Damage.** The section is from an autopsy specimen of a patient who had a 3-year history of idiopathic pulmonary fibrosis diagnosed on the basis of radiologic and clinical findings. Two weeks before his death, his chronic dyspnea rapidly worsened and became associated with air-space consolidation on the chest radiograph; both findings progressed until his death. The section shows an exudate of proteinaceous material in alveolar air spaces and prominent hyaline membranes lining alveolar ducts. The alveolar interstitium is mildly to moderately thickened by mature fibrous tissue and occasional lymphocytes.

ties were identified in two patients.[310] Similar findings have been illustrated by other investigators.[160, 170] Although these results suggest a relatively uniform pattern of abnormalities on HRCT, a variety of patterns was identified in another investigation of 27 patients who had NIP;[311a] the predominant abnormalities consisted of areas of ground-glass attenuation in 48% of patients, a reticular pattern in 22%, air-space consolidation in 19%, nodules in 7%, and honeycombing in 4%. In this study—which included 129 patients who had various forms of interstitial pneumonitis—a correct first choice diagnosis was made by two independent observers in 71% of 35 patients who had IPF, 79% of 24 patients who had BOOP, 63% of 23 patients who had DIP, 65% of 20 patients who had acute interstitial pneumonitis, and only 9% of 27 patients who had NIP. Other abnormalities that may occasionally be seen on CT include architectural distortion, traction bronchiectasis, and mediastinal lymph node enlargement.[160, 310]

This form of interstitial lung disease accounts for about 5% to 15% of patients who were historically included in series of patients who had IPF.[206, 312] Symptoms do not differ from those associated with IPF but are likely to be less severe and considerably more indolent in progression. Some patients have been reported who have influenza-like symptoms associated with mild dyspnea.[313] In one study of seven such patients, the mean duration of symptoms before diagnosis was 4 months.[313]

Survival in patients who have NIP is substantially better than that in patients who have IPF.[13a, 206, 313a] In one study,

almost 80% of 14 patients who had NIP were alive 10 years after diagnosis, compared with less than 10% of 63 patients who had IPF.[206] In another investigation of 48 patients considered to have NIP, only 5 (11%) had died in the follow-up period, and almost 50% recovered completely, figures much better than those for IPF.[309]

## ACUTE INTERSTITIAL PNEUMONITIS

In 1935, Hamman and Rich described an acute (fulminating) variety of interstitial fibrosis characterized by rapid progression of signs and symptoms leading to death in less than a year.[314] Review of the histologic descriptions of some of their patients and more recent studies of patients with similar clinical disease have shown the underlying pathologic abnormality in these cases to be diffuse alveolar damage (DAD).[315–317] About 25% to 30% of patients have an exudative pattern (air-space proteinaceous exudate, interstitial edema and (usually) mild inflammation, and hyaline membranes) and the remainder a proliferative (fibroblastic) pattern. Presumably because of the latter appearance, the abnormality was termed *diffuse interstitial fibrosis* by Hamman and Rich; subsequent authors have instead preferred the designation *acute interstitial pneumonitis*.[315, 316] In fact, a more appropriate clinical description might be the adult respiratory distress syndrome (ARDS). Whatever the terminology, it is conceivable that this abnormality may represent simply a particularly severe form of IPF; this hypothesis is

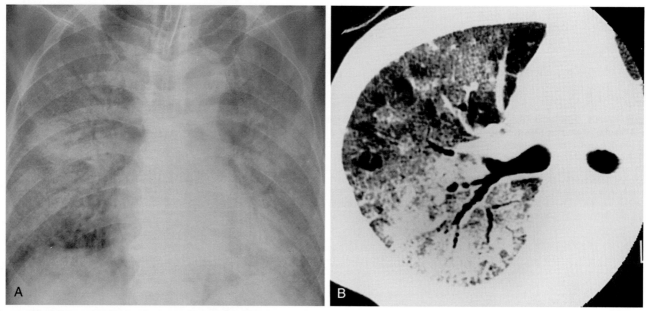

**Figure 42–34. Acute Interstitial Pneumonitis.** A posteroanterior chest radiograph *(A)* shows extensive bilateral consolidation with air bronchograms. A view of the right lung from an HRCT scan *(B)* demonstrates air-space consolidation with air bronchograms posteriorly and areas of ground-glass attenuation in the anterior aspects of the right upper lobe. The patient was a 69-year-old man who presented with symptoms of acute respiratory failure and had pathologically proven acute interstitial pneumonitis. (From Primack SL, Hartman TE, Ikezoe J, et al: Acute interstitial pneumonia: Radiographic and CT findings in nine patients. Radiology 188:817, 1993, with permission.)

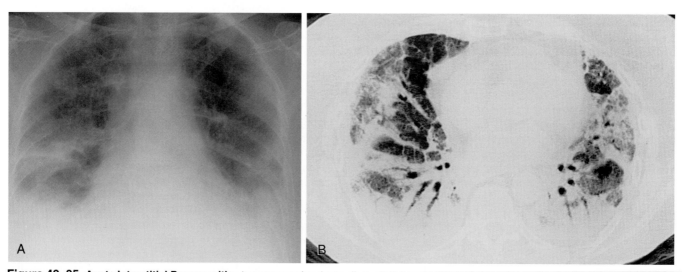

**Figure 42–35. Acute Interstitial Pneumonitis.** A posteroanterior chest radiograph *(A)* reveals bilateral areas of consolidation involving predominantly the lower lung zones. A CT scan *(B)* demonstrates areas of consolidation with air bronchograms in the dependent portions of the lower lobes and areas of ground-glass attenuation in the middle lobe and lingula. The patient was an 83-year-old woman in whom the diagnosis of acute interstitial pneumonitis was proven at autopsy. (From Primack SL, Hartman TE, Ikezoe J, et al: Acute interstitial pneumonia: Radiographic and CT findings in nine patients. Radiology 188:817, 1993, with permission.)

supported by the observation that some patients with otherwise typical IPF undergo a phase of rapidly progressive disease characterized radiologically by ARDS and pathologically by DAD (Fig. 42–33).[231] Despite these arguments, we believe that the features of most cases of *de novo* acute interstitial pneumonitis are so different from those of the usual case of IPF that they should be considered separately.

The radiologic manifestations of acute interstitial pneumonitis are similar to those of ARDS.[160, 170, 318] The main finding on the chest radiograph consists of bilateral air-space consolidation (Fig. 42–34).[318] In one study of nine patients, this finding was present in all; it was diffuse in five patients, involved mainly the upper lung zones in two, and involved mainly the lower lung zones in two (Fig. 42–35).[318] CT usually demonstrates extensive bilateral areas of ground-glass attenuation, which may be diffuse or have a patchy distribution with focal areas of sparing, resulting in a geographic appearance.[160, 170, 318] In the study cited previously, bilateral ground-glass attenuation was present in all nine cases and air-space consolidation in six.[318] As in ARDS, an anteroposterior gradient in the ground-glass attenuation or consolidation is present because of a considerable increase in attenuation in the dependent lung regions (Fig. 42–35). Additional findings seen in a small number of cases include smooth interlobular septal thickening, honeycombing, and small pleural effusions.[160, 318]

Patients may complain of an influenza-like illness and fever.[231] Dyspnea is rapidly progressive over a period of weeks. In one study of nine patients, eight died within 3 months of presentation.[318]

# REFERENCES

1. King TE, Cherniack RM, Schwarz MI: Idiopathic pulmonary fibrosis and other interstitial lung diseases of unknown etiology. *In* Murray JF, Nadel JA, (eds): Textbook of Respiratory Medicine. Vol. 2. Philadelphia, WB Saunders, 1994, p 1827.
2. Liebow AA, Carrington CB: The interstitial pneumonias. *In* Simon M, Potchen EJ, LeMay M (eds): Frontiers of Pulmonary Radiology. New York, Grune & Stratton, 1969, p 102.
3. Bhagwat AG, Wentworth P, Conen PE: Observations on the relationship of desquamative interstitial pneumonia and pulmonary alveolar proteinosis in childhood: A pathologic and experimental study. Chest 58:326, 1970.
4. Bedrossian CW, Kuhn C 3d, Luna MA, et al: Desquamative interstitial pneumonia-like reaction accompanying pulmonary lesions. Chest 72:166, 1977.
5. Henderson DW: The morphogenesis and classification of diffuse interstitial lung diseases: A clinicopathological approach, based on tissue reaction patterns. Aust N Z J Med 14(Suppl):735, 1984.
6. Stilwell PC, Norris DG, O'Connell EJ, et al: Desquamative interstitial pneumonitis in children. Chest 77:165, 1980.
7. Katzenstein AA, Myers JL: State of the art. Idiopathic pulmonary fibrosis. Am J Respir Crit Care Med 157:1301, 1998.
8. Müller NL: Chronic interstitial pneumonias. Semin Respir Med 13:309, 1992.
9. Scadding JG, Hinson KFW: Diffuse fibrosing alveolitis (diffuse interstitial fibrosis of the lungs). Thorax 22:291, 1967.
10. Patchefsky AS, Israel HL, Hoch WS, et al: Desquamative interstitial pneumonia: Relationship to interstitial fibrosis. Thorax 28:680, 1973.
11. McCann BG, Brewer DB: A case of desquamative interstitial pneumonia progressing to "honeycomb lung." J Pathol 112:199, 1974.
12. Crystal RG, Fulmer JD, Roberts WC, et al: Idiopathic pulmonary fibrosis. Ann Intern Med 85:769, 1976.
13. Fromm GB, Dunn LJ, Harris JO: Desquamative interstitial pneumonitis: Characterization of free intra-alveolar cells. Chest 77:552, 1980.
13a. Bjoraker JA, Ryu JH, Edwin MK, et al: Prognostic significance of histopathologic subsets in idiopathic pulmonary fibrosis. Am J Respir Crit Care Med 157:199, 1998.
14. du Bois RM: Idiopathic pulmonary fibrosis. Annu Rev Med 44:441, 1993.
15. Tierney LM Jr: Idiopathic pulmonary fibrosis. Semin Respir Med 12:229, 1991.
16. Coultas DB: Epidemiology of idiopathic pulmonary fibrosis. Semin Respir Med 14:181, 1993.
17. Cherniack RM, Crystal RG, Kalica AR: Current concepts in idiopathic pulmonary fibrosis: a road map for the future. Am Rev Respir Dis 143:680, 1991.
18. Marinelli WA: Idiopathic pulmonary fibrosis: Progress and challenge. Chest 108:297, 1995.
19. DePaso WJ, Winterbauer RH: Intersitial lung disease. Dis Mon 37:61, 1991.
20. Coultas DB, Zumwalt RE, Black WC, et al: The epidemiology of interstitial lung diseases. J Respir Crit Care Med 50:967, 1994.
21. Johnston IDA, Bleasdale C, Hind CRK, et al: Accuracy of diagnostic coding of hospital admissions for cryptogenic fibrosing alveolitis. Thorax 46:589, 1991.
22. Johnston I, Britton J, Kinnear W, et al: Rising mortality from cryptogenic fibrosing alveolitis. Br Med J 301:1017, 1990.
23. Mannino DM, Etzel RA, Parrish RG: Pulmonary fibrosis deaths in the United States, 1979–1991. Am J Respir Crit Care Med 153:1548, 1996.
24. Campbell EJ, Harris B, Avioli LV: Idiopathic pulmonary fibrosis. Arch Intern Med 141:771, 1981.
25. Geist LJ, Hunninghake GW: Potential role of viruses in the pathogenesis of pulmonary fibrosis. Chest 103:119, 1993.
26. Kuwano K, Nomoto Y, Kunitake R, et al: Detection of adenovirus E1A DNA in pulmonary fibrosis using nested polymerase chain reaction. Eur Respir J 10:1433, 1997.
27. Pinsker KL, Schneyer B, Becker N, et al: Usual interstitial pneumonia following Texas A2 influenza infection. Chest 80:123, 1981.
28. Kawai T, Fujiwara T, Aoyama Y, et al: Diffuse interstitial fibrosing pneumonitis and adenovirus infection. Chest 69:692, 1976.
29. Yonemaru M, Ustumi K, Kasuga I, et al: A case of pulmonary fibrosis associated with CMV inclusion body. Nippon Kyobu Shikkan Gakkai Zasshi 32:184, 1994.
30. Hubbard R, Venn A, Smith C, et al: Exposure to commonly prescribed drugs and the etiology of cryptogenic fibrosing alveolitis: A case-control study. Am J Respir Crit Care Med 157:743, 1998.
31. Vergnon JM, Vincent M, de The G, et al: Cryptogenic fibrosing alveolitis and Epstein-Barr virus: An association? Lancet 2:768, 1984.
32. Egan JJ, Stewart JP, Hasleton PS, et al: Epstein-Barr virus replication within pulmonary epithelial cells in cryptogenic fibrosing alveolitis. Thorax 50:1234, 1995.
33. Ueda T, Ohta K, Suzuki N, et al: Idiopathic pulmonary fibrosis and high prevalence of serum antibodies to hepatitis C virus. Am Rev Respir Dis 146:266, 1992.
34. Meliconi R, Andreone P, Fasano L, et al: Incidence of hepatitis C virus infection in Italian patients with idiopathic pulmonary fibrosis. Thorax 51:315, 1996.
35. Irving WL, Day S, Johnston IDA: Idiopathic pulmonary fibrosis and hepatitis C virus infection. Am Rev Respir Dis 148:1683, 1993.
36. Iwai K, Mori T, Yamada N, et al: Idiopathic pulmonary fibrosis. Am J Respir Crit Care Med 150:670, 1994.
37. Billings CG, Howard P: Hypothesis: Exposure to solvents may cause fibrosing alveolitis. Eur Respir J 7:1172, 1994.
38. Scott J, Johnston I, Britton J: What causes cryptogenic fibrosing alveolitis? A case-control study of environmental exposure to dust. Br Med J 301:1015, 1990.
39. Hubbard R, Lewis S, Richards K, et al: Occupational exposure to metal or wood dust and aetiology of cryptogenic fibrosing alveolitis. Lancet 347:284, 1996.
40. Baumgartner KB, Samet JM, Stidley CA, et al: Cigarette smoking: A risk factor for idiopathic pulmonary fibrosis. Am J Respir Crit Care Med 155:242, 1997.
41. Kennedy S, Chan-Yeung M: Taking cryptogenic out of fibrosing alveolitis. Lancet 347:276, 1996.
42. Auwerx J, Demedts M, Bouillon R, et al: Coexistence of hypocalciuric hypercalcaemia and interstitial lung disease in a family: A cross-sectional study. Eur J Clin Invest 15:6, 1985.
43. Demedts M, Auwerx J, Goddeeris P, et al: The inherited association of interstitial lung disease, hypocalciuric hypercalcemia, and defective granulocyte function. Am Rev Respir Dis 131:470, 1985.
44. Auwerx J, Boogaerts M, Ceuppens JL, et al: Defective host defense mechanisms in a family with hypocalciuric hypercalcaemia and coexisting interstitial lung disease. Clin Exp Immunol 62:57, 1985.
45. Solliday NH, Williams JA, Gaensler EA, et al: Familial chronic interstitial pneumonia. Am Rev Respir Dis 108:193, 1973.
46. Koch B: Familial fibrocystic pulmonary dysplasia: Observations in one family. Can Med Assoc J 92:801, 1965.
47. Hughes EW: Familial interstitial pulmonary fibrosis. Thorax 19:515, 1964.
48. Young WA: Familial fibrocystic pulmonary dysplasia: A new case in a known affected family. Can Med Assoc J 94:1059, 1966.
49. Musk AW, Zilko PJ, Manners P, et al: Genetic studies in familial fibrosing alveolitis: Possible linkage with immunoglobulin allotypes (Gm). Chest 89:206, 1986.
50. Libby DM, Gibofsky A, Fotino M, et al: Immunogenetic and clinical findings in idiopathic pulmonary fibrosis: Association with the B-cell alloantigen HLA-DR2. Am Rev Respir Dis 127:618, 1983.
51. Stinson JC, Tomkin GH: Familial cryptogenic fibrosing alveolitis: A case report. Ir J Med Sci 161:42, 1992.
52. Bitterman PB, Rennard SI, Keogh BA, et al: Familial idiopathic pulmonary fibrosis: Evidence of lung inflammation in unaffected family members. N Engl J Med 314:1343, 1986.
53. Raghu G, Hert R: Interstitial lung diseases: Genetic predisposition and inherited interstitial lung diseases. Semin Respir Med 14:323, 1993.
54. Turton CWG, Morris LM, Lawler SD, et al: HLA in cryptogenic fibrosing alveolitis (letter). Lancet 1:507, 1978.
55. Fulmer JD, Sposovska MS, von Gal ER: Distribution of HLA antigens in idiopathic pulmonary fibrosis. Am Rev Respir Dis 118:141, 1978.
56. Geddes DM, Webley M, Brewerton DA, et al: Alpha-1 anti-trypsin phenotypes in fibrosing alveolitis and rheumatoid arthritis. Lancet 2:1049, 1977.
57. Kim H, Lepler L, Daniels A, et al: Alpha-1 antitrypsin deficiency and idiopathic pulmonary fibrosis in a family. South Med J 89:1008, 1996.
58. Stack BHR, Grant IWB, Irvine WJ, et al: Idiopathic diffuse interstitial lung disease: A review of 42 cases. Am Rev Respir Dis 92:939, 1965.
59. Bonanni PP, Frymoyer JW, Jacox RJ: A family study of idiopathic pulmonary fibrosis: A possible dysproteinemic and genetically determined disease. Am J Med 39:411, 1965.
60. Moore FH, Hamlin JW, Lindsay S: Progressive diffuse interstitial fibrosis of the lungs (Hamman-Rich syndrome): Report of a case of seven years' duration. AMA Arch Intern Med 100:651, 1957.
61. MacKay IR, Ritchie B: Diffuse fibrosing alveolitis (diffuse interstitial fibrosis of the lungs): Two cases with autoimmune features. Thorax 20:200, 1965.
62. Read J: The pathogenesis of the Hamman-Rich syndrome: A review from the standpoint of possible allergic etiology. Am Rev Tuberc 78:353, 1958.
63. Chapman JR, Charles PJ, Venables PJW, et al: Definition and clinical relevance of antibodies to nuclear ribonucleoprotein and other nuclear antigens in patients with cryptogenic fibrosing alveolitis. Am Rev Respir Dis 130:439, 1984.
64. Turner-Warwick M, Burrows B, Johnson A: Cryptogenic fibrosing alveolitis: Clinical features and their influence on survival. Thorax 35:171, 1980.
65. Hodson ME, Haslam PL, Spiro SG, et al: Digital vasculitis in patients with cryptogenic fibrosing alveolitis. Br J Dis Chest 78:140, 1984.
66. McFadden RG, Craig ID, Paterson NAM: Interstitial pneumonitis in myasthenia gravis. Br J Dis Chest 78:187, 1984.
67. Smith MJL, Benson MK, Strickland ID: Coeliac disease and diffuse interstitial lung disease. Lancet 1:473, 1971.
68. Scadding JG: Chronic diffuse interstitial fibrosis of the lungs. Br Med J 1:443, 1960.
69. Turner-Warwick M: Fibrosing alveolitis and chronic liver disease. Q J Med 37:133, 1968.
70. Golding PL, Smith M, Williams R: Multisystem involvement in chronic liver disease: Studies on the incidence and pathogenesis. Am J Med 55:772, 1973.
71. Capron JP, Marti R, Rey JL, et al: Fibrosing alveolitis and hepatitis B surface antigen-associated chronic active hepatitis in a patient with immunoglobulin A deficiency. Am J Med 66:874, 1979.
72. Mason AMS, McIllmurray MB, Golding PL, et al: Fibrosing alveolitis associated with renal tubular acidosis. Br Med J 4:596, 1970.
73. Williams AJ, Marsh J, Stableforth DE: Cryptogenic fibrosing alveolitis, chronic active hepatitis, and autoimmune haemolytic anaemia in the same patient. Br J Dis Chest 79:200, 1985.

74. Scadding JW: Fibrosing alveolitis with autoimmune haemolytic anaemia: Two case reports. Thorax 32:134, 1977.

75. Endo Y, Hara M: Glomerular IgA deposition in pulmonary diseases. Kidney Int 29:557, 1986.

76. Kelion AD, Cockcroft JR, Ritter JM: Antiphospholipid syndrome in a patient with rapidly progressive fibrosing alveolitis. Postgrad J 71:233, 1995.

77. May JJ, Schwarz MI, Dreisin RB: Idiopathic thrombocytopenic purpura occurring with interstitial pneumonitis. Ann Intern Med 90:199, 1979.

78. Marsh P, Johnston I, Britton J: Atopy as a risk factor for cryptogenic fibrosing alveolitis. Respir Med 88:369, 1994.

79. Schwarz MI, Dreisin RB, Pratt DS, et al: Immunofluorescent patterns in the idiopathic interstitial pneumonias. J Lab Clin Med 91:929, 1978.

80. Scadding JG: Diffuse pulmonary alveolar fibrosis. Thorax 29:271, 1974.

81. Nagaya H, Buckley EC III, Sieker HO: Positive antinuclear factor in patients with unexplained pulmonary fibrosis. Ann Intern Med 70:1135, 1969.

82. Nagaya H, Sieker HO: Pathogenic mechanisms of interstitial pulmonary fibrosis in patients with serum antinuclear factor: A histologic and clinical correlation. Am J Med 52:51, 1972.

83. Nagaya H, Elmore M, Ford CD: Idiopathic interstitial pulmonary fibrosis: An immune complex disease. Am Rev Respir Dis 107:826, 1973.

84. Holgate ST, Haslam P, Turner-Warwick M: The significance of antinuclear and DNA antibodies in cryptogenic fibrosing alveolitis. Thorax 38:67, 1983.

85. Gelb AF, Dreisen RB, Epstein JD, et al: Immune complexes, gallium lung scans, and bronchoalveolar lavage in idiopathic interstitial pneumonitis-fibrosis. Chest 84:148, 1983.

86. Martinet Y, Haslam PL, Turner-Warwick M: Clinical significance of circulating immune complexes in "lone" cryptogenic fibrosing alveolitis and those with associated connective tissue disorders. Clin Allergy 14:491, 1984.

87. Fan K, D'Orsogna DE: Diffuse pulmonary interstitial fibrosis: Evidence of humoral antibody mediated pathogenesis. Chest 85:150, 1984.

88. Campbell DA, Poulter LW, Janossy G, et al: Immunohistological analysis of lung tissue from patients with cryptogenic fibrosing alveolitis suggesting local expression of immune hypersensitivity. Thorax 40:405, 1985.

89. Stein-Streilein J, Lipscomb MF, Fisch H, et al: Pulmonary interstitial fibrosis induced in hapten-immune hamsters. Am Rev Respir Dis 136:119, 1987.

90. Kimura R, Hu H, Stein-Streilein J: Immunological tolerance to hapten prevents subsequent induction of hapten-immune pulmonary interstitial fibrosis. Cell Immunol 145:351, 1992

91. Meliconi R, Senaldi G, Sturani C, et al: Complement activation products in idiopathic pulmonary fibrosis: Relevance of fragment Ba to disease severity. Clin Immunol Immunopathol 57:64, 1990.

92. Dall'Aglio, Pesci A, Bertorelli G, et al: Study of immune complexes in bronchoalveolar lavage fluids. Respiration 54:36, 1988.

93. Nakos G, Adams A, Andriopoulos N: Antibodies to collagen in patients with idiopathic pulmonary fibrosis. Chest 103:1051, 1993.

94. Wallace WA, Schofield JA, Lamb D, et al: Localization of a pulmonary autoantigen in cryptogenic fibrosing alveolitis. Thorax 49:1139, 1994.

95. Wallace WA, Roberts SN, Caldwell H, et al: Circulating antibodies to lung protein(s) in patients with cryptogenic fibrosing alveolitis. Thorax 49:218, 1994.

95a. Ward PA, Hunninghake GW: Lung inflammation and fibrosis. Am J Respir Crit Care Med 157:S123, 1998.

96. Rochester CL, Elias JA: Cytokines and cytokine networking in the pathogenesis of interstitial and fibrotic lung disorders. Semin Respir Med 14:389, 1993.

97. Kumar RK, Lykke AWJ: Messages and handshakes: Cellular interactions in pulmonary fibrosis. Pathology 18:1995.

98. Bensadoun ES, Burke AK, Hogg JA, et al: Proteoglycan deposition in pulmonary fibrosis. Am J Respir Crit Care Med 154:1819, 1996.

99. Basset F, Ferrans VJ, Takemura T, et al: Intraluminal fibrosis in interstitial lung disorders. Am J Pathol 122:443, 1986.

100. Fukuda Y, Basset F, Ferrans VJ, et al: Significance of early intra-alveolar fibrotic lesions and integrin expression in lung biopsy specimens from patients with idiopathic pulmonary fibrosis. Hum Pathol 26:53, 1995.

101. Burkhardt A: Alveolitis and collapse in the pathogenesis of pulmonary fibrosis. Am Rev Respir Dis 140:513, 1989.

102. Kuhn III C, Boldt J, King TE: An immunohistochemical study of architectural remodeling and connective tissue synthesis in pulmonary fibrosis. Am Rev Respir Dis 140:1693, 1989.

103. Sheppard MN, Harrison NK: New perspectives on basic mechanisms in lung disease—1. Thorax 47:1064, 1992.

104. Shaw RJ: The role of lung macrophages at the interface between chronic inflammation and fibrosis. Respir Med 85:267, 1991.

105. Gauldie J, Jordana M, Cox G: Cytokines and pulmonary fibrosis. Thorax 48:931, 1993.

106. Elias JA, Freundlich B, Kern JA, et al: Cytokine networks in the regulation of inflammation and fibrosis in the lung. Chest 97:1439, 1990.

107. Giaid A, Michel RP, Stewart DJ, et al: Expression of endothelin-1 in lungs of patients with cryptogenic fibrosing alveolitis. Lancet 341:1550, 1993.

108. Saleh D, Furukawa K, Tsao M-S, et al: Elevated expression of endothelin-1 and endothelin-converting enzyme-1 in idiopathic pulmonary fibrosis: Possible involvement of proinflammatory cytokines. Am J Respir Cell Mol Biol 16:187, 1997.

109. Iyonaga K, Takeya M, Saita N, et al: Monocyte chemoattractant protein-1 in idiopathic pulmonary fibrosis and other interstitial lung diseases. Hum Pathol 25:455, 1994.

110. Car BD, Meloni F, Luisetti M, et al: Elevated IL-8 and MCP-1 in the bronchoalveolar lavage fluid of patients with idiopathic pulmonary fibrosis and pulmonary sarcoidosis. Am J Respir Crit Care Med 149:655, 1994.

111. Imokawa S, Sato A, Hayakawa H, et al: Tissue factor expression and fibrin deposition in the lungs of patients with idiopathic pulmonary fibrosis and systemic sclerosis. Am J Respir Crit Care Med 156:631, 1997.

111a. Kobayashi H, Gabazza EC, Taguchi O, et al: Protein C anticoagulant system in patients with interstitial lung disease. Am J Respir Crit Care Med 157:1850, 1998.

112. Strausz J, Müller-Quernheim J, Steppling H, et al: Oxygen radical production by alveolar inflammatory cells in idiopathic pulmonary fibrosis. Am Rev Respir Dis 141:124, 1990.

113. Nakao A, Hasegawa Y, Tsuchiya Y, et al: Expression of cell adhesion molecules in the lungs of patients with idiopathic pulmonary fibrosis. Chest 108:233, 1995.

114. du Bois RM: Advances in our understanding of the pathogenesis of fibrotic lung disease. Respir Med 84:185, 1990.

114a. Wells AU, Hansell DM, Haslam PL, et al: Bronchoalveolar lavage cellularity: Lone cryptogenic fibrosing alveolitis compared with the fibrosing alveolitis of systemic sclerosis. Am J Respir Crit Care Med 157:1474, 1998.

115. Pforte A, Gerth C, Voss A: Proliferating alveolar macrophages in BAL and lung function changes in interstitial lung disease. Eur Respir J 6:951, 1993.

116. Aston C, Jagirdar J, Lee TC, et al: Enhanced insulin-like growth factor molecules in idiopathic pulmonary fibrosis. Am J Respir Crit Care Med 151:1597, 1995.

116a. Coker RK, Laurent GJ: Pulmonary fibrosis: Cytokines in the balance. Eur Respir J 11:1218, 1998.

117. Smith DR, Kunkel SL, Standiford TJ, et al: Increased interleukin-1 receptor antagonist in idiopathic pulmonary fibrosis. Am J Respir Crit Car Med 151:1965, 1995.

117a. Hancock A, Armstrong L, Gama R, et al: Production of interleukin 13 by alveolar macrophages from normal and fibrotic lung. Am J Respir Cell Mol Biol 18:60, 1998.

118. Southcott AM, Jones KP, Li D, et al: Interleukin-8: Differential expression in lone fibrosing alveolitis and systemic sclerosis. Am J Respir Crit Care Med 151:1604, 1995.

119. Lynch III JP, Standiford TJ, Rolfe MW, et al: Neutrophilic alveolitis in idiopathic pulmonary fibrosis. Am Rev Respir Dis 145:1433, 1992.

120. Ozaki T, Hayashi H, Tani K, et al: Neutrophil chemotactic factors in the respiratory tract of patients with chronic airway diseases or idiopathic pulmonary fibrosis. Am Rev Respir Dis 145:85, 1992.

121. Nakamura H, Fujishima S, Waki Y, et al: Priming of alveolar macrophages for interleukin-8 production in patients with idiopathic pulmonary fibrosis. Am J Respir Crit Care Med 152:1579, 1995.

121a. Ziegenhagen MW, Zabel P, Zissel G, et al: Serum level of interleukin 8 is elevated in idiopathic pulmonary fibrosis and indicates disease activity. Am J Respir Crit Care Med 157:762, 1998.

122. Elias JA, Gustilo K, Freundlich B: Human alveolar macrophage and blood monocyte inhibition of fibroblast proliferation. Am Rev Respir Dis 138:1595, 1988.

123. Weissler JC, Mendelson C, Moya F, et al: Effect of interstitial lung disease macrophages on T-cell signal transduction. Am J Respir Crit Care Med 149:191, 1994.

124. Maier K, Leuschel L, Costabel U: Increased levels of oxidized methionine residues in bronchoalveolar lavage fluid proteins from patients with idiopathic pulmonary fibrosis. Am J Respir Crit Care Med 143:271, 1991.

125. Behr J, Maier K, Krombach F, et al: Pathogenetic significance of reactive oxygen species in diffuse fibrosing alveolitis. Am Rev Respir Dis 144:146, 1991.

126. Obayashi Y, Yamadori I, Fujita J, et al: The role of neutrophils in the pathogenesis of idiopathic pulmonary fibrosis. Chest 112:1338, 1997.

127. Hällgren R, Bjermer L, Lundgren R, et al: The eosinophil component of the alveolitis in idiopathic pulmonary fibrosis: Signs of eosinophil activation in the lung are related to impaired pulmonary function. Am Rev Respir Dis 139:373, 1989.

128. Fujimoto K, Kubo K, Yamaguchi S, et al: Eosinophil activation in patients with pulmonary fibrosis. Chest 108:48, 1995.

129. Kiemle-Kallee J, Krelpe H, Radzun HJ, et al: Alveolar macrophages in idiopathic pulmonary fibrosis display a more monocyte-like immunophenotype and an increased release of free oxygen radicals. Eur Respir J 4:400, 1991.

130. Schaberg T, Rau M, Stephan H, et al: Increased number of alveolar macrophages expressing surface molecules of the CD11/CD18 family in sarcoidosis and idiopathic pulmonary fibrosis is related to the production of superoxide anions by these cells. Am Rev Respir Dis 147:1507, 1993.

131. Saleh D, Barnes PJ, Giaid A: Increased production of the potent oxidant peroxynitrite in the lungs of patients with idiopathic pulmonary fibrosis. Am J Respir Crit Care Med 155:1763, 1997.

131a. Behr J, Maier K, Degenkolb B, et al: Antioxidative and clinical effects of high-dose *N*-acetylcysteine in fibrosing alveolitis. Am J Respir Crit Care Med 156:1897, 1997.

131b. Yamanouchi H, Fujita J, Hojo S, et al: Neutrophil elastase: Alpha-1-proteinase inhibitor complex in serum and bronchoalveolar lavage fluid in patients with pulmonary fibrosis. Eur Respir J 11:120, 1998.

132. Shijubo N, Yamaguchi K, Hirasawa M, et al: Progastrin-releasing peptide (31-98) in idiopathic pulmonary fibrosis and sarcoidosis. Am J Respir Crit Care Med 154:1694, 1996.

133. Shaw RJ, Benedict SH, Clark RAF, et al: Pathogenesis of pulmonary fibrosis in interstitial lung disease. Am Rev Respir Dis 143:167, 1991.

134. Emura M, Nagai S, Takeuchi M, et al: In vitro production of B cell growth

factor and B cell differentiation factor by peripheral blood mononuclear cells and bronchoalveolar lavage T lymphocytes from patients with idiopathic pulmonary fibrosis. Clin Exp Immunol 82:133, 1990.

135. Jordana M, Schulman J, McSharry C, et al: Heterogeneous proliferative characteristics of human adult lung fibroblast lines and clonally derived fibroblasts from control and fibrotic lung. Am Rev Respir Dis 137:579, 1988.
136. Inoue Y, King TE Jr, Tinkle SS, et al: Human mast cell basic fibroblast growth factor in pulmonary fibrotic disorders. Am J Pathol 149:2037, 1996.
137. Khun C, McDonald JA: The roles of the myofibroblast in idiopathic pulmonary fibrosis: Ultrastructural and immunohistochemical features of sites of active extracellular matrix synthesis. Am J Pathol 138:1257, 1991.
138. Keane MP, Arenberg DA, Lynch JP 3rd, et al: The CXC chemokines, IL-8 and IL-10, regulate angiogenic activity in idiopathic pulmonary fibrosis. J Immunol 159:1437, 1997.
139. Kawanami O, Ferrans VJ, Fulmer JD, et al: Ultrastructure of pulmonary mast cells in patients with fibrotic lung disorders. Lab Invest 40:717, 1979.
140. Cherniack RM, Colby TV, Flint A, et al: Quantitative assessment of lung pathology in idiopathic pulmonary fibrosis. Am Rev Respir Dis 144:892, 1991.
141. Mendeloff J: Disseminated nodular pulmonary ossification in the Hamman-Rich lung. Am Rev Respir Dis 103:269, 1971.
142. Genereux GP: The end-stage lung. Radiology 116:279, 1975.
143. Kawanami O, Ferrans VJ, Crystal RG: Structure of alveolar epithelial cells in patients with fibrotic lung disorders. Lab Invest 46:39, 1982.
144. Sutinen S, Rainio P, Sutinen S, et al: Ultrastructure of terminal respiratory epithelium and prognosis in chronic interstitial pneumonia. Eur J Respir Dis 61:325, 1980.
145. Shimizu S, Kobayashi H, Watanabe H, et al: Mallory body-like structures in the lung. Acta Pathol Jpn 36(1):105, 1986.
146. Nonomura A, Kono N, Ohta G: Pulmonary cytoplasmic hyalin resembling Mallory's alcoholic hyalin in the liver. Acta Pathol Jpn 36(6):869, 1986.
147. Kawanami O, Basset F, Ferrans VJ, et al: Pulmonary Langerhans' cells in patients with fibrotic lung disorders. Lab Invest 44:227, 1981.
148. Wilson NJE, Gosney JR, Mayall F: Endocrine cells in diffuse pulmonary fibrosis. Thorax 48:1252, 1993.
149. Gaensler EA, Goff AM, Prowse CM: Desquamative interstitial pneumonia. N Engl J Med 274:113, 1966.
150. Westcott JL, Cole SR: Traction bronchiectasis in end-stage pulmonary fibrosis. Radiology 161:665, 1986.
151. Edwards CW, Carlile A: The larger bronchi in cryptogenic fibrosing alveolitis: A morphometric study. Thorax 37:828, 1982.
152. Coalson JJ: The ultrastructure of human fibrosing alveolitis. Virchows Arch (Pathol Anat) 395:181, 1982.
153. Adler KB, Craighead JE, Vallyathan NV, et al: Actin-containing cells in human pulmonary fibrosis. Am J Pathol 102:427, 1981.
154. Kawanami O, Matsuda K, Yoneyama H, et al: Endothelial fenestration of the alveolar capillaries in interstitial fibrotic lung diseases. Acta Pathol Jpn 42:177, 1992.
155. Carrington CB, Gaensler EA, Coutu RE, et al: Natural history and treated course of usual and desquamative interstitial pneumonia. N Engl J Med 298:801, 1978.
156. McLoud TC, Carrington CB, Gaensler EA: Diffuse infiltrative lung disease: A new scheme for description. Radiology 149:353, 1983.
157. Müller NL, Guerry-Force ML, Staples CA, et al: Differential diagnosis of bronchiolitis obliterans with organizing pneumonia and usual interstitial pneumonia: Clinical, functional, and radiologic findings. Radiology 162:151, 1987.
158. Grenier P, Chevret S, Beigelman C, et al: Chronic diffuse infiltrative lung disease: determination of the diagnostic value of clinical data, chest radiography, and CT and Bayesian analysis. Radiology 191:383, 1994.
159. Staples CA, Müller NL, Vedal S, et al: Usual interstitial pneumonia: correlation of CT with clinical, functional and radiological findings. Radiology 162:377, 1987.
160. McAdams HP, Rosado-de-Christenson ML, Wehunt WD, et al: The alphabet soup revisited: The chronic interstitial pneumonias in the 1990's. RadioGraphics 1996;16,1009
161. Picado C, Gomez de Almeida R, Xaubet A, et al: Spontaneous pneumothorax in cryptogenic fibrosing alveolitis. Respiration 48:77, 1985.
162. Feigin DS: New perspectives on interstitial lung disease. Radiol Clin North Am 21:683, 1983.
163. Mathieson JR, Mayo JR, Staples CA, Müller NL: Chronic diffuse infiltrative lung disease: Comparison of diagnostic accuracy of CT and chest radiography. Radiology 171:111, 1989.
164. Padley SPG, Hansell DM, Flower CDR, et al: Comparative accuracy of high resolution computed tomography and chest radiography in the diagnosis of chronic diffuse infiltrative lung disease. Clin Radiol 44:222, 1991.
165. Orens JB, Kazerooni DA, Martinez FJ, et al: The sensitivity of high-resolution CT in detecting idiopathic pulmonary fibrosis proved by open lung biopsy: A prospective study. Chest 108:109, 1995.
166. Müller NL, Miller RR, Webb WR: Fibrosing alveolitis: CT-pathologic correlation. Radiology 160:585, 1986.
167. Strickland B, Strickland NH: The value of high definition, narrow section computed tomography in fibrosing alveolitis. Clin Radiol 39:589, 1988.
168. Nishimura K, Kitaichi M, Izumi T, et al: Usual interstitial pneumonia: Histologic correlation with high-resolution CT. Radiology 182:342, 1992.
169. Müller NL, Miller RR: State of the art: Computed tomography of chronic diffuse infiltrative lung disease: Part 1. Am Rev Respir Dis 142:1206, 1990.
170. Müller NL, Colby TV: Idiopathic interstitial pneumonias: High-resolution CT and histologic findings. RadioGraphics 17:1016, 1997.

171. Akira M, Sakatani M, Ueda E: Idiopathic pulmonary fibrosis: Progression of honeycombing at thin-section CT. Radiology 189:687, 1993.
172. Wells AU, Rubens MB, du Bois RM, et al: Serial CT in fibrosing alveolitis: Prognostic significance of the initial pattern. Am J Roentgenol 161:1159, 1993.
173. Terriff BA, Kwan SY, Chan-Yeung M, et al: Fibrosing alveolitis: Chest radiography and CT as predictors of clinical and functional impairment at follow-up in 26 patients. Radiology 184:445, 1992.
174. Hartman TE, Primack SL, Kang EY, et al: Disease progression in usual interstitial pneumonia compared with desquamative interstitial pneumonia: Assessment with serial CT. Chest 110:378, 1996.
174a. Lee JS, Gong G, Song K-S, et al: Usual interstitial pneumonia: Relationship between disease activity and the progression of honeycombing at thin-section computed tomography. J Thorac Imaging 13:199, 1998.
175. Aquino SL, Webb WR, Zaloudek CJ, et al: Lung cysts associated with honeycombing: Change in size on expiratory CT scans. Am J Roentgenol 162:583, 1994.
176. Worthy SA, Brown MJ, Müller NL: Cystic air spaces in the lung: Change in size on expiratory high-resolution CT in 23 patients. Clin Radiol 53:515, 1998.
177. Gevenois PA, Abehsera M, Knoop C, et al: Disseminated pulmonary ossification in end-stage pulmonary fibrosis: CT demonstration. Am J Roentgenol 162:1303, 1994.
178. Primack SL, Hartman TE, Hansell DM, Müller NL: End-stage lung disease: CT findings in 61 patients. Radiology 189:681, 1993.
179. Müller NL, Staples CA, Miller RR, et al: Disease activity in idiopathic pulmonary fibrosis: CT and pathologic correlation. Radiology 165:731, 1987.
180. Leung AN, Miller RR, Müller NL: Parenchymal opacification in chronic infiltrative lung diseases: CT-pathologic correlation. Radiology 188:209, 1993.
181. Niimi H, Kang EY, Kwong JS, Müller NL: CT of chronic infiltrative lung disease: Prevalence of mediastinal lymphadenopathy. J Comput Assist Tomogr 20:305, 1996.
182. Bergin C, Castellino RA: Mediastinal lymph node enlargement on CT scans in patients with usual interstitial pneumonitis. Am J Roentgenol 154:251, 1990.
182a. Franquet T, Gimenez A, Alegret X, et al: Mediastinal lymphadenopathy in cryptogenic fibrosing alveolitis: The effect of steroid therapy on the prevalence of nodal enlargement. Clin Radiol 53:435, 1998.
183. Tung KT, Wells AU, Rubens MB, et al: Accuracy of the typical computed tomographic appearances of fibrosing alveolitis. Thorax 48:334, 1993.
184. Nishimura K, Izumi T, Kitaichi M, et al: The diagnostic accuracy of high-resolution computed tomography in diffuse infiltrative lung diseases. Chest 104:1149, 1993.
184a. Swensen SJ, Aughenbaugh GL, Myers JL: Diffuse lung disease: Diagnostic accuracy of CT in patients undergoing surgical biopsy of the lung. Radiology 205:229, 1997.
185. Müller NL, Mayo JR, Zwirewich CV: Value of MR imaging in the evaluation of chronic infiltrative lung diseases: Comparison with CT. Am J Roentgenol 158:1205, 1992.
186. Primack SL, Mayo JR, Hartman TE, et al: MRI of infiltrative lung disease: Comparison with pathologic findings. J Comput Assist Tomogr 18:233, 1994.
187. Wollmer P, Rhodes CG, Hughes JM: Regional extravascular density and fractional blood volume of the lung in interstitial disease. Thorax 39:286, 1984.
188. Pantin CF, Valind SO, Sweatman M, et al: Measures of the inflammatory response in cryptogenic fibrosing alveolitis. Am Rev Respir Dis 138:1234, 1988.
189. King MA, Bergin CJ, Ghadishah E, et al: Detecting pulmonary abnormalities on magnetic resonance images in patients with usual interstitial pneumonitis: Effect of varying window settings and gadopentetate dimeglumine. Acad Radiol 3:300, 1996.
190. McFadden RG, Carr TJ, Wood TE: Proton magnetic resonance imaging to stage activity of interstitial lung disease. Chest 92:31, 1987.
191. Berthezène Y, Vexler V, Kuwatsuru R, et al: Differentiation of alveolitis and pulmonary fibrosis with a macromolecular MR imaging contrast agent. Radiology 185:97, 1992.
192. Johnston ID, Prescott RJ, Chalmers JC, et al: British Thoracic Society study of cryptogenic fibrosing alveolitis: Current presentation and initial management. Fibrosing alveolitis subcommittee of the research committee of the British Thoracic Society. Thorax 52:38, 1997.
193. Stinson JC, Tomkin GH: Familial cryptogenic fibrosing alveolitis: A case report. Ir J Med Sci 161:42, 1992.
194. Kanematsu T, Kitaichi M, Nishimura K, et al: Clubbing of the fingers and smooth-muscle proliferation in fibrotic changes in the lung of patients with idiopathic pulmonary fibrosis. Chest 105:339, 1994.
195. Patchefsky AS, Banner M, Freundlich IM: Desquamative interstitial pneumonia: Significance of intranuclear viral-like inclusion bodies. Ann Intern Med 74:322, 1971.
196. Baughman RP, Shipley RT, Loudon RG, et al: Crackles in interstitial lung disease: Comparison of sarcoidosis and fibrosing alveolitis. Chest 100:96, 1991.
197. DeRemee RA, Harrison EG Jr, Andersen HA: The concept of classic interstitial pneumonitis-fibrosis (CIP-F) as a clinicopathologic syndrome. Chest 61:213, 1972.
198. Walshaw MJ, Nisar M, Pearson MG, et al: Expiratory lung crackles in patients with fibrosing alveolitis. Chest 97:407, 1990
199. Semple P d'a, Beastall GH, Brown TM, et al: Sex hormone suppression and sexual impotence in hypoxic pulmonary fibrosis. Thorax 39:46, 1984.
200. Tenholder MF, Russell MD, Knight E, et al: Orthodeoxia: A new finding in interstitial fibrosis. Am Rev Respir Dis 136:170, 1987.
201. Bourke SJ, Munro NC, White JE, et al: Platypnoea-orthodeoxia in cryptogenic fibrosing alveolitis. Respir Med 89:387, 1995.

202. Snell NJC, Coysh HL: Persistent hyponatremia complicating fibrosing alveolitis. Thorax 33:820, 1978.
203. Javaheri S, Sicilian L: Lung function, breathing pattern, and gas exchange in interstitial lung disease. Thorax 47:93, 1992.
204. Hanson D, Winterbauer RH, Kirtland SH, et al: Changes in pulmonary function test results after 1 year of therapy as predictors of survival in patients with idiopathic pulmonary fibrosis. Chest 108:305, 1995.
205. Agusti C, Xaubet A, Agusti Ag, et al: Clinical and functional assessment of patients with idiopathic pulmonary fibrosis: Results of a 3 year follow-up. Eur Respir J 7:643, 1994.
206. Bjoraker JA, Ryu JH, Edwin MK, et al: Prognostic significance of histopathologic subsets in idiopathic pulmonary fibrosis. Am J Respir Crit Care Med 157:199, 1998.
207. Agusti AGN, Roca J, Gea J, et al: Mechanisms of gas-exchange impairment in idiopathic pulmonary fibrosis. Am Rev Respir Dis 143:219, 1991.
208. Kaneengiser LC, Rapoport DM, Epstein H, et al: Volume adjustment of mechanics and diffusion in interstitial lung disease. Chest 96:1036, 1989.
209. Pande JN: Interrelationship between lung volume, expiratory flow, and lung transfer factor in fibrosing alveolitis. Thorax 36:858, 1981.
210. Schwartz DA, Merchant RK, Helmers RA, et al: The influence of cigarette smoking on lung function in patients with idiopathic pulmonary fibrosis. Am Rev Respir Dis 144:504, 1991.
211. Cherniack RM, Colby TV, Flint A, et al: Correlation of structure and function in idiopathic pulmonary fibrosis. Am J Respir Crit Care Med 151:1180, 1995.
212. Wells AU, King AD, Rubens MB, et al: Lone cryptogenic fibrosing alveolitis: A functional-morphologic correlation based on extent of disease on thin-section computed tomography. Am J Respir Crit Care Med 155:1367, 1997.
213. Epler GR, Saber FA, Gaensler EA: Determination of severe impairment (disability) in interstitial lung disease. Am Rev Respir Dis 121:647, 1980.
214. Weitzenblum E, Ehrart M, Rasaholinjanahary J, et al: Pulmonary hemodynamics in idiopathic pulmonary fibrosis and other interstitial pulmonary diseases. Respiration 44:118, 1983.
215. Zapletal A, Houstek J, Samanek M, et al: Lung function in children and adolescents with idiopathic interstitial pulmonary fibrosis. Pediatr Pulmonol 1:154, 1985.
216. Agusti C, Xaubet A, Roca J, et al: Interstitial pulmonary fibrosis with and without associated collagen vascular disease: Results of a two year follow up. Thorax 47:1035, 1992.
217. Hanley ME, King Jr TE, Schwarz MI, et al: The impact of smoking on mechanical properties of the lungs in idiopathic pulmonary fibrosis and sarcoidosis. Am Rev Respir Dis 144:1102, 1991.
218. Shea SA, Winning AJ, Mckenzie E, et al: Does the abnormal pattern of breathing in patients with interstitial lung disease persist in deep non-rapid eye movement sleep? Am Rev Respir Dis 139:653, 1989.
219. Cassan SM, Divertie MB, Brown AL, Jr: Fine structural morphometry on biopsy specimens of human lung. 2. Diffuse idiopathic pulmonary fibrosis. Chest 65:275, 1974.
220. Wagner PD, Dantzker DR, Dueck R, et al: Distribution of ventilation-perfusion ratios in patients with interstitial lung disease. Chest 69:256, 1976.
221. Marciniuk DD, Watts RE, Gallagher CG: Dead space loading and exercise limitation in patients with interstitial lung disease. Chest 105:183, 1994.
222. Chinet T, Jaubert F, Dusser D, et al: Effects of inflammation and fibrosis on pulmonary function in diffuse lung fibrosis. Thorax 45:675, 1990.
223. Fulmer JD, Roberts WC, von Gal ER, et al: Morphologic-physiologic correlates of the severity of fibrosis and degree of cellularity in idiopathic pulmonary fibrosis. J Clin Invest 63:665, 1979.
224. Agusti C, Xaubet A, Agusti AG, et al: Clinical and functional assessment of patients with idiopathic pulmonary fibrosis: Results of a 3 year follow-up. Eur Respir J 7:643, 1994.
225. Stack BHR, Choo-Kang YFJ, Heard BE: The prognosis of cryptogenic fibrosing alveolitis. Thorax 27:535, 1972.
226. Louw SJ, Bateman ED, Benatar SR: Cryptogenic fibrosing alveolitis: Clinical spectrum and treatment. S Afr Med J 65:195, 1984.
227. Carrington CB, Gaensler EA, Coutu RE, et al: Natural history and treated course of usual and desquamative interstitial pneumonia. N Engl J Med 298:801, 1978.
228. Schwartz DA, Van Fossen DS, Davis CS, et al: Determinants of progression in idiopathic pulmonary fibrosis. Am J Respir Crit Care Med 149:444, 1994.
228a. Selman M, Carrillo G, Salas J, et al: Colchicine, D-penicillamine, and prednisone in the treatment of idiopathic pulmonary fibrosis: A controlled clinical trial. Chest 114:507, 1998.
228b. Hubbard R, Johnston I, Britton J: Survival in patients with cryptogenic fibrosing alveolitis: A population-based cohort study. Chest 113:396, 1998.
228c. Mapel DW, Hunt WC, Utton R, et al: Idiopathic pulmonary fibrosis: Survival in population based and hospital based cohorts. Thorax 53:469, 1998.
229. Carabasi RJ: Diffuse interstitial pulmonary fibrosis (Hamman-Rich syndrome): Report of three cases. Am Rev Tuberc 78:610, 1958.
230. Muschenheim C: Some observations on the Hamman-Rich disease. Am J Med Sci 241:279, 1961.
231. Kondoh Y, Taniguchi H, Kawabata Y, et al: Acute exacerbation in idiopathic pulmonary fibrosis: Analysis of clinical and pathologic findings in three cases. Chest 103:1808, 1993.
232. Panos RJ, Mortenson RL, Niccoli SA, et al: Clinical deterioration in patients with idiopathic pulmonary fibrosis: Causes and assessment. Am J Med 88:396, 1990.
233. Haddad R, Massaro D: Idiopathic diffuse interstitial pulmonary fibrosis (fibrosing alveolitis), atypical epithelial proliferation and lung cancer. Am J Med 45:211, 1968.

234. Meyer EC, Liebow AA: Relationship of interstitial pneumonia, honeycombing and atypical epithelial proliferation to cancer of the lung. Cancer 18:322, 1965.
235. Scadding JG: Chronic diffuse interstitial fibrosis of the lungs. Br Med J 1:443, 1960.
236. Lutwyche VU: Another presentation of fibrosing alveolitis and alveolar cell carcinoma. Chest 70:292, 1976.
237. Nagai A, Chiyotani A, Nakadate T, et al: Lung cancer in patients with idiopathic pulmonary fibrosis. Tohoku J Exp Med 167:231, 1992.
238. Mizushima Y, Kobayashi M: Clinical characteristics of synchronous multiple lung cancer associated with idiopathic pulmonary fibrosis: A review of Japanese cases. Chest 108:1272, 1995.
239. Haddad R. Massaro D: Idiopathic diffuse interstitial pulmonary fibrosis (fibrosing alveolitis), atypical epithelial proliferation and lung cancer. Am J Med 45:211, 1968.
240. Lee HJ, Im JG, Ahn JM, et al: Lung cancer in patients with idiopathic pulmonary fibrosis: CT findings. 20:979, 1996.
241. Beaumont F, Jansen HM, Elema JD, et al: Simultaneous occurrence of pulmonary interstitial fibrosis and alveolar cell carcinoma in one family. Thorax 36:252, 1981.
242. Turner-Warwick M, Lebowitz M, Burrows B, et al: Cryptogenic fibrosing alveolitis and lung cancer. Thorax 35:496, 1980.
243. Tukiainen P, Taskinen E, Holsti P, et al: Prognosis of cryptogenic fibrosing alveolitis. Thorax 38:349, 1983.
243a. Gay SE, Kazerooni EA, Toews GB, et al: Idiopathic pulmonary fibrosis: Predicting response to therapy and survival. Am J Respir Crit Care Med 157:1063, 1998.
244. Winterbauer RH, Hammar SP, Hallman KO, et al: Diffuse interstitial pneumonitis: Clinicopathologic correlations in 20 patients treated with prednisone/azathioprine. Am J Med 65:661, 1978.
245. Turner-Warwick M, Burrows B, Johnson A: Cryptogenic fibrosing alveolitis: Response to corticosteroid treatment and its effect on survival. Thorax 35:593, 1980.
246. Rudd RM, Haslam PL, Turner-Warwick M: Cryptogenic fibrosing alveolitis: Relationships of pulmonary physiology and bronchoalveolar lavage to response to treatment and prognosis. Am Rev Respir Dis 124:1, 1981.
247. van Oortegem K, Wallaert B, Marquette CH, et al: Determinants of response to immunosuppressive therapy in idiopathic pulmonary fibrosis. Eur Respir J 7:1950, 1994.
248. Honda Ym Kuroki Y, Shijubo N, et al: Aberrant appearance of lung surfactant protein A in sera of patients with idiopathic pulmonary fibrosis and its clinical significance: Respiration 62:64, 1995.
249. Watters LC, King TE, Schwarz MI, et al: A clinical, radiographic, and physiologic scoring system for the longitudinal assessment of patients with idiopathic pulmonary fibrosis. Am Rev Respir Dis 133:97, 1986.
250. de Cremoux H, Bernaudin JF, Laurent P, et al: Interactions between cigarette smoking and the natural history of idiopathic pulmonary fibrosis. Chest 98:71, 1990.
251. Schwartz DA, Helmers RA, Galvin JR, et al: Determinants of survival in idiopathic pulmonary fibrosis. Am J Respir Crit Care Med 149:450, 1994.
252. Erbes R, Schaberg T, Loddenkemper R: Lung function tests in patients with idiopathic pulmonary fibrosis. Chest 111:51, 1997.
253. Meliconi R, Lalli E, Borzi RM, et al: Idiopathic pulmonary fibrosis: Can cell mediated immunity markers predict clinical outcome? Thorax 45:536, 1990.
254. Matuskewicz SP, Williamson IJ, Sime PJ, et al: Plasma lactate dehydrogenase: A marker of disease activity in cryptogenic fibrosing alveolitis and extrinsic allergic alveolitis. Eur Respir J 6:1282, 1993.
255. Haslam PL, Turton CWG, Heard B, et al: Bronchoalveolar lavage in pulmonary fibrosis: Comparison of cells obtained with lung biopsy and clinical features. Thorax 35:9, 1980.
256. Yasuoka S, Nakayama T, Kawano T, et al: Comparison of cell profiles of bronchial and bronchoalveolar lavage fluids between normal subjects and patients with idiopathic pulmonary fibrosis. Tohoku J Exp Med 146:33, 1985.
257. Watters LC, King TE, Cherniack RM, et al: Bronchoalveolar lavage fluid neutrophils increase after corticosteroid therapy in smokers with idiopathic pulmonary fibrosis. Am Rev Respir Dis 133:104, 1986.
258. Haslam PL, Turton CWG, Lukoszek A, et al: Bronchoalveolar lavage fluid cell counts in cryptogenic fibrosing alveolitis and their relation to therapy. Thorax 35:328, 1980.
259. Strumpf IJ, Feld MK, Cornelius MJ, et al: Safety of fiberoptic bronchoalveolar lavage in evaluation of interstitial lung disease. Chest 80:268, 1981.
260. Peterson MW, Monick M, Hunninghake GW: Prognostic role of eosinophils in pulmonary fibrosis. Chest 92:51, 1987.
261. Watters LC, Schwarz MI, Cherniack RM, et al: Idiopathic pulmonary fibrosis: Pretreatment bronchoalveolar lavage cellular constituents and their relationships with lung histopathology and clinical response to therapy. Am Rev Respir Dis 135:696, 1987.
262. Turner-Warwick M, Haslam PL: The value of serial bronchoalveolar lavage in assessing the clinical progress of patients with cryptogenic fibrosing alveolitis. Am Rev Respir Dis 135:26, 1987.
262a. Fireman E, Vardinon N, Burke M, et al: Predictive value of response to treatment of T-lymphocyte subpopulations in idiopathic pulmonary fibrosis. Eur Respir J 11:706, 1998.
263. Robinson PC, Watters LC, King TE, et al: Idiopathic pulmonary fibrosis: Abnormalities in bronchoalveolar lavage fluid phospholipids. Am Rev Respir Dis 137:585, 1988.

264. McCormack FX, King Jr TE, Bucher BL, et al: Surfactant protein A predicts survival in idiopathic pulmonary fibrosis. Am J Respir Crit Care Med 152:751, 1995.

264a. Kanazawa H, Yoshikawa T, Yamade M, et al: CYFRA 21-1, a cytokeratin subunit 19 fragment, in bronchoalveolar lavage fluid from patients with interstitial lung disease. Clin Sci 94:531, 1998.

265. Davis GS, Brody AR, Landis JN, et al: Quantitation of inflammatory activity in interstitial pneumonitis by bronchofiberscopic pulmonary lavage. Chest 69:265, 1976.

266. Patchefsky AS, Israel HL, Hoch WS, et al: Desquamative interstitial pneumonia: Relationship to interstitial fibrosis. Thorax 28:680, 1973.

267. Gaensler EA, Carrington CB, Coutu RE: Chronic interstitial pneumonias. Clin Notes Respir Dis 10:3, 1972.

268. Bateman ED, Turner-Warwick M, Haslam PL, et al: Cryptogenic fibrosing alveolitis: Prediction of fibrogenic activity from immunohistochemical studies of collagen types in lung biopsy specimens. Thorax 38:93, 1983.

269. Hyde DM, King TE Jr, McDermott T, et al: Idiopathic pulmonary fibrosis: Quantitative assessment of lung pathology. Comparison of a semiquantitative and a morphometric histopathologic scoring system. Am Rev Respir Dis 146:1042, 1992.

270. Kaarteenaho-Wiik R, Tani T, Sormunen R, et al: Tenascin immunoreactivity as a prognostic marker in usual interstitial pneumonitis. Am J Respir Crit Care Med 154:511, 1996.

271. Schwartz DA, Helmers RA, Galvin JR, et al: Determinants of survival in idiopathic pulmonary fibrosis. Am J Respir Crit Care Med 149:450, 1994.

272. Schwartz DA, Van Fossen DS, Davis CS, et al: Determinants of progression in idiopathic pulmonary fibrosis. Am J Respir Crit Care Med 149:444, 1994.

272a. Xaubet A, Agusti C, Luburich P, et al: Pulmonary function tests and CT scan in the management of idiopathic pulmonary fibrosis. Am J Respir Crit Care Med 158:431, 1998.

273. Hansell DM, Wells AU: State of the art. CT evaluation of fibrosing alveolitis: applications and insights. J Thorac Imaging 11:231, 1996.

274. Kazerooni EA, Martinez FJ, Flint A, et al: Thin-section CT obtained at 10-mm increments versus limited three-level thin-section CT for idiopathic pulmonary fibrosis: correlation with pathologic scoring. Am J Roentgenol 169:977, 1997.

275. Lee JS, Im JG, Ahn JM, et al: Fibrosing alveolitis: Prognostic implication of ground-glass attenuation at high-resolution CT. Radiology 184:451, 1992.

276. Wells AU, Hansell DM, Rubens MB, et al: The predictive value of appearances on thin-section computed tomography in fibrosing alveolitis. Am Rev Respir Dis 148:1076, 1993.

277. Kondoh Y, Taniguchi H, Kawabata Y, et al: Acute exacerbation in idiopathic pulmonary fibrosis: Analysis of clinical and pathologic findings in three cases. Chest 103:1808, 1993.

278. Akira M, Hamada H, Sakatani M, et al: CT findings during phase of accelerated deterioration in patients with idiopathic pulmonary fibrosis. Am J Roentgenol 168:79, 1997.

279. Wells AU, Hansell DM, Harrison NK, et al: Clearance of inhaled Tc-DTPA predicts the clinical course of fibrosing alveolitis. Eur Respir J 6:797, 1993.

280. Kaplan JD, Trulock EP, Anderson DJ, et al: Pulmonary vascular permeability in interstitial lung disease. Am Rev Respir Dis 145:1495, 1992.

281. Vanderstappen M, Mornex JF, Lahneche B, et al: Gallium-67 scanning in the staging of cryptogenic fibrosing alveolitis and hypersensitivity pneumonitis. Eur Respir J 1:517, 1988.

282. Fujishima S, Kanazawa M, Yamasawa F, et al: Clinical significance of gallium-67 scintigraphy in assessing pulmonary lesions of sarcoidosis and idiopathic pulmonary fibrosis. Nippon Kyobu Shikkan Gakkai Zasshi 30:435, 1992.

283. Nishimura K, Izumi T, Kitaichi M, et al: The diagnostic accuracy of high resolution computer tomography in diffuse infiltrative lung diseases. Chest 104:1149, 1993.

284. Tung KT, Wells AU, Rubens MB, et al: Accuracy of the typical computer tomographic appearances of fibrosing alveolitis. Thorax 48:334, 1993.

285. Webb DR, Currie GD: Pulmonary fibrosis masking polymyositis. JAMA 222:1146, 1972.

286. Thompson PL, Mackay IR: Fibrosing alveolitis and polymyositis. Thorax 25:504, 1970.

287. Imokawa S, Sato A, Toyoshima M, et al: Dyskeratosis congenita showing usual interstitial pneumonia. Int Med 33:226, 1994.

288. Bensard DD, McIntyre RC, Waring BJ, et al: Comparison of video thoracoscopic lung biopsy to open lung biopsy in the diagnosis of interstitial lung disease. Chest 103:765, 1993.

289. Chuang MT, Raskin J, Krellenstein DJ, et al: Bronchoscopy in diffuse lung disease: Evaluation by open lung biopsy in nondiagnostic transbronchial lung biopsy. Ann Otol Rhinol Laryngol 96:654, 1987.

290. Smith CM, Moser KM: Management for interstitial lung disease. State of the art. Chest 95:676, 1989.

291. Costabel U: Management of idiopathic pulmonary fibrosis: Academic postulate and clinical practice. Eur Respir J 6:770, 1993.

292. Liebow AA, Steer A, Billingsley J: Desquamative interstitial pneumonia. Am J Med 39:369, 1965.

293. Deodhar SD, Bhagwat AG: Desquamative interstitial pneumonia-like syndrome in rabbits. Arch Pathol 84:54, 1967.

294. Bone RC, Wolfe J, Sobonya RE, et al: Desquamative interstitial pneumonia following long-term nitrofurantoin therapy. Am J Med 60:697, 1976.

295. Goldstein JD, Godleski JJ, Herman PG: Desquamative interstitial pneumonitis associated with monomyelocytic leukemia. Chest 81:321, 1982.

296. Abraham JL, Hertzberg MA: Inorganic particulates associated with desquamative interstitial pneumonia. Chest 80:67S, 1981.

297. Herbert A, Sterling G, Abraham J, et al: Desquamative interstitial pneumonia in an aluminum welder. Hum Pathol 13:694, 1982.

298. Lougheed MD, Roos JO, Waddell WR, et al: Desquamative interstitial pneumonitis and diffuse alveolar damage in textile workers. Chest 108:1196, 1995.

299. Gardiner IT, Uff JS: "Blue bodies" in a case of cryptogenic fibrosing alveolitis (desquamative type): An ultra-structural study. Thorax 33:806, 1978.

300. Bedrossian CWM, Kuhn C III, Luna MA, et al: Desquamative interstitial pneumonia-like reaction accompanying pulmonary lesions. Chest 72:166, 1977.

301. Yousem SA, Colby TV, Gaensler EA: Respiratory bronchiolitis-associated interstitial lung disease and its relationship to desquamative interstitial pneumonia. Mayo Clin Proc 64:1373, 1989.

302. Gaensler EA, Goff AM, Prowse CM: Desquamative interstitial pneumonia. N Engl J Med 274:113, 1966.

303. Feigin DS, Friedman PJ: Chest radiography in desquamative interstitial pneumonitis: A review of 37 patients. Am J Roentgenol 134:91, 1980.

304. Schneider RM, Nevius DB, Brown HZ: Desquamative interstitial pneumonia in a four-year-old child. N Engl J Med 277:1056, 1967.

305. Cruz E, Rodriguez J, Lisboa C, et al: Desquamative alveolar disease (desquamative interstitial pneumonia): Case report. Thorax 24:186, 1969.

306. Vedal S, Welsh EV, Miller RR, et al: Desquamative interstitial pneumonia: Computed tomographic findings before and after treatment with corticosteroids. Chest 93:215, 1988.

307. Hartman TE, Primack SL, Swensen SJ, et al: Desquamative interstitial pneumonia: Thin-section CT findings in 22 patients. Radiology 187:787, 1993.

308. Tubbs RR, Benjamin SP, Reich NE, et al: Desquamative interstitial pneumonitis. Chest 72:159, 1977.

307a. Akira M, Yamamoto S, Hara H, et al: Serial computed tomographic evaluation in desquamative interstitial pneumonia. Thorax 52:333, 1997.

309. Katzenstein A-LA, Fiorelli RF: Nonspecific interstitial pneumonia/fibrosis: Histologic features and clinical significance. Am J Surg Pathol 18:136, 1994.

310. Park JS, Lee KS, Kim JS, et al: Nonspecific interstitial pneumonia with fibrosis: Radiographic and CT findings in seven patients. Radiology 195:645, 1995.

311. Katoh T, Andoh T, Mikawa K, et al: Computed tomographic findings in nonspecific interstitial pneumonia/fibrosis. Respirology 3:69, 1998.

311a. Johkoh T, Müller NL, Cartier Y, et al: Idiopathic interstitial pneumonias: Diagnostic accuracy of thin-section CT in 129 patients. Radiology 1999; in press.

312. Chan-Yeung M, Müller N: Cryptogenic fibrosing alveolitis. Lancet 350:651, 1997.

313. Park CS, Jeon JW, Park SW, et al: Nonspecific interstitial pneumonia/fibrosis: Clinical manifestations, histologic and radiologic features. Korean J Intern Med 11:122, 1996.

313a. Cottin V, Donsbeck A, Revel D, et al: Nonspecific interstitial pneumonia. Am J Respir Crit Care Med 158:1286, 1998.

314. Hamman L, Rich AR: Fulminating diffuse interstitial fibrosis of the lungs. Trans Am Clin Climatol Assoc 51:154, 1935.

315. Olson J, Colby TV, Elliot CG: Hamman-Rich syndrome revisited. Mayo Clin Proc 65:1538, 1990.

316. Katzenstein A-LA, Myers JL, Mazur MT: Acute interstitial pneumonia: A clinicopathologic, ultrastructural, and cell kinetic study. Am J Surg Pathol 10(4):256, 1986.

317. Porte A, Stoeckel ME, Mantz JM, et al: Acute interstitial pulmonary fibrosis: Comparative light and electron microscopic study of 19 cases. Pathogenic and therapeutic implications. Intensive Care Med 4:181, 1978.

318. Primack SL, Hartman TE, Ikezoe J, et al: Acute interstitial pneumonia: Radiographic and CT findings in nine patients. Radiology 188:817, 1993.

# CHAPTER 43

# *Langerhans' Cell Histiocytosis*

Langerhans' cell histiocytosis (Langerhans' cell granulomatosis, eosinophilic granuloma, histiocytosis X) is an uncommon disease characterized pathologically by a proliferation of specialized histiocytes known as Langerhans' cells.[1, 2] The disorder has been recognized for many years under the rubric "histiocytosis X" as a group of diseases with similar morphologic but different clinical features.[3] Although it is not always possible to fit patients into specific categories,[4] three variants traditionally have been identified.

*Letterer-Siwe disease* occurs in infants and children and is characterized by widespread dissemination and a fulminant, often fatal, course; the structures most commonly affected are the liver, spleen, lymph nodes, lungs, and bones.[5] *Hand-Schüller-Christian disease* consists of a triad of osteolytic skull lesions, exophthalmos, and diabetes insipidus and is considered by some to be a variant of multifocal eosinophilic granuloma.[5] This form of disease characteristically becomes manifest during childhood or adolescence and progresses much more slowly than Letterer-Siwe disease, most affected persons living into adult life; occasionally, it appears in adulthood.[6] *Eosinophilic granuloma* is characteristically a disease of adults that is most often localized to the lungs or bones. It occurs most frequently in whites and has been described rarely in African Americans.[7, 8] Although it was originally thought to be more common in men,[9] authors of some relatively recent reports have described a significant number of cases in women,[10, 11] and the sex distribution is currently believed to be equal.[1, 12] It is possible that this change in incidence reflects the close association of the disease with smoking (*see* farther on).[13]

As the term *histiocytosis X* implies, the cell of origin of these disorders was initially uncertain. However, following the ultrastructural observation that the histiocytes characteristic of the disorder contain Birbeck granules (intracytoplasmic structures also seen in epidermal Langerhans' cells[2]), as well as extensive immunohistochemical analyses indicating immunologic similarity with these same cells,[14, 15] it is now accepted that the proliferating cell is in fact an activated Langerhans' cell. The normal Langerhans' cell is best known as an antigen-processing and presenting cell that resides in the epidermis; however, similar cells also occur in epithelia elsewhere in the body, including the pulmonary airways (*see* page 11).[16] As a result of these observations, the disease process has come to be known as *Langerhans' cell histiocytosis* (LCH). The particular variety with which we are concerned in the following discussion is pulmonary Langerhans' cell histiocytosis (PLCH).

## ETIOLOGY AND PATHOGENESIS

The etiology and pathogenesis of PLCH are unclear. Potential etiologic agents that have been considered include viruses and tobacco smoke. The former have been suggested by the observation that occasional lesions appear to follow infection by Epstein-Barr virus or papillomavirus[17] and by the demonstration of human herpesvirus 6 DNA in the histiocytes of approximately 50% of 30 patients in one study.[18] However, the results of ultrastructural investigations[19] and other molecular biologic studies[20] have provided no confirmatory evidence of viral infection.

The evidence implicating tobacco smoke in the etiology of PLCH is more substantial. Clinically, there is a very strong association of the disorder with cigarette smoking,[13] with as many as 100% of patients in some series admitting the habit.[21] Histologically, the earliest lesions have a peribronchiolar location, a distribution identical to that of smoke-induced small airway disease.[21] Cigarette smokers also have an increased population of Langerhans' cells in bronchoalveolar lavage (BAL) fluid compared with that in normal nonsmokers.[22] Finally, peripheral blood lymphocytes exposed to tobacco glycoprotein (a potent immunostimulator isolated from cigarette smoke) show a decreased T cell proliferative response with reduced production of interleukin-2 (IL-2) in patients who have PLCH compared with the response in smoking control patients.[23] Taken together, these observations suggest that an abnormal response to cigarette smoke may be important in the pathogenesis of PLCH; however, the precise mechanisms by which this may occur are unclear.

The fundamental nature of the histiocytic proliferation in PLCH is also uncertain. Some (albeit not all[24]) investigators have found evidence that the proliferation is clonal in nature,[25–27] suggesting that it is neoplastic. This hypothesis is supported by investigations in which a variable degree of cellular atypia has been found in the histiocytes and a relatively rapid clinical course, such as that seen in malignant neoplasms, has been documented.[28] Despite these observations, the demonstration that the Langerhans' cells in pulmonary nodules have a low proliferation rate[28a] and the presence of a benign clinical course in the vast majority of patients (including those in whom the disease undergoes spontaneous remission) argue strongly against a neoplastic process; instead, most workers regard the proliferation as an abnormal inflammatory-immunologic reaction.[29]

A variety of investigations have been undertaken to better define the nature of the factors underlying such a reaction. As indicated previously, the histiocytic cells seen in LCH share morphologic and immunohistochemical features with the Langerhans cell of the skin.[2] Despite this, there are important differences between the two. LCH cells are defective in antigen presentation and have a distribution in the body quite different from that of normal Langerhans' cells.[2] Unlike normal cells, those from patients with PLCH have a greatly increased number of Birbeck granules, stain more positively for CD1a, and express a variety of antigens (such as CD1c, CD4, CD24, and CD32[30, 31]) and leukocyte (CD54 and CD58) and other adhesion molecules.[29, 32] These various CD antigens are known to be related to activation of Langerhans' cells *in vitro*, suggesting that the histiocytic cells of LCH are activated Langerhans' cells. Increases in tissue and circulating immune complexes have also been found in a number of patients who have active, as opposed to fibrotic, disease;[33] because these are known to have a stimulatory effect on Langerhans' cells, it is possible that they play a role in activation.[1] LCH histiocytes can proliferate locally,[32, 34] a phenomenon possibly related to the presence of granulocyte-macrophage colony-stimulating factor.[35-37]

The mechanism of tissue damage in PLCH is uncertain but probably involves an interaction between LCH histiocytes and other inflammatory-immune cells, particularly the lymphocyte and the alveolar macrophage. One group of investigators has shown the presence of close contact between the abnormal Langerhans' cells and CD4[+] T lymphocytes.[30] A possible role for local lymphocyte activation is also supported by the observation that immunoglobulins are increased in the BAL fluid of affected patients.[38] Moreover, the results of one immunohistochemical study of Langerhans' cells in four patients with active disease suggested that these cells are capable of inducing an *in-situ* T cell lymphocyte response.[39] Pulmonary alveolar macrophage activation also may play a role in disease pathogenesis. In common with other fibrotic lung diseases, platelet-derived growth factor produced by alveolar macrophages may be important in inducing fibroblast replication and collagen production.[40] In addition, alveolar macrophages elaborate greatly increased amounts of plasminogen activator, a protease that has been associated with tissue damage.[41]

The pathogenesis of the fibrosis in PLCH probably shares features with other chronic interstitial pulmonary diseases. One analysis of biopsy material showed that fibrosis appears to be preceded by detachment of epithelial lining cells and migration of Langerhans' cells, inflammatory cells, and myofibroblasts into the adjacent air space.[42] Active inflammatory lesions have been shown to contain abundant transforming growth factor-beta$_1$, a cytokine that promotes fibrosis,[43] suggesting a role for this agent in fibrogenesis.

The reason for the predominance of fibrosis in the upper lobes is not clear.

## PATHOLOGIC CHARACTERISTICS

Grossly, the lungs in the early or active stage of PLCH show multiple nodules, most measuring 1 to 10 mm in diameter. With time, the relatively discrete nodular lesions become confluent, resulting in irregularly shaped areas of fibrosis containing cysts of variable size. In long-standing disease, the appearance is similar to that of advanced idiopathic pulmonary fibrosis (IPF), with the presence of bands of fibrous tissue and multiple cysts of variable size (Fig. 43–1). The major distinguishing features between the two are that PLCH tends to be more severe in the upper lobes and to affect peripheral and central regions more evenly.[10, 11, 44]

Abnormalities in the early stage of disease are located predominantly in the interstitial connective tissue of small membranous and proximal respiratory bronchioles and consist mainly of a cellular infiltrate (Fig. 43–2).[11, 21, 45] In more advanced disease, this infiltrate typically extends into the

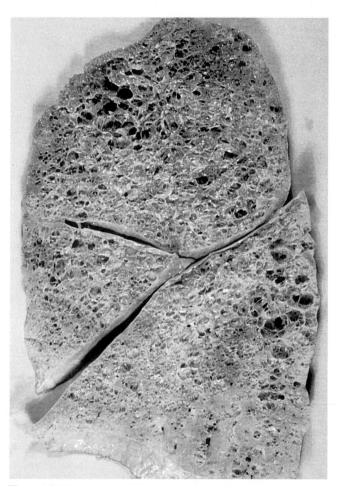

**Figure 43–1. Langerhans' Cell Histiocytosis.** A sagittal slice of the right lung in its midportion shows innumerable cystic spaces, the majority measuring about 0.5 to 1 cm in diameter. They are present in both central and peripheral regions and are more evident in the upper lobe and superior portions of the lower and middle lobes.

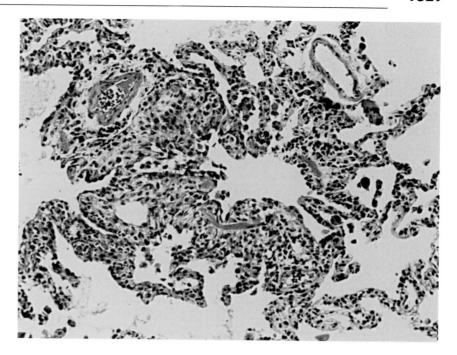

**Figure 43–2. Langerhans' Cell Histiocytosis: Early Bronchiolar Involvement.** The wall of this respiratory bronchiole is moderately thickened by an infiltrate of histiocytes and occasional eosinophils; there is no fibrosis. (×170.)

adjacent alveolar interstitium, and the central portion of the lesion undergoes fibrosis, resulting in a characteristic stellate shape (Fig. 43–3). For reasons that are not clear, some affected bronchioles appear to dilate (Fig. 43–4), resulting in the cysts that are seen in both gross specimens and

radiologic images. It is also possible that some cysts originate by cavitation of the cellular nodules.

Although a stellate appearance of the infiltrate is characteristic of the early lesions of PLCH, other morphologic patterns are commonly evident. Relatively well-circum-

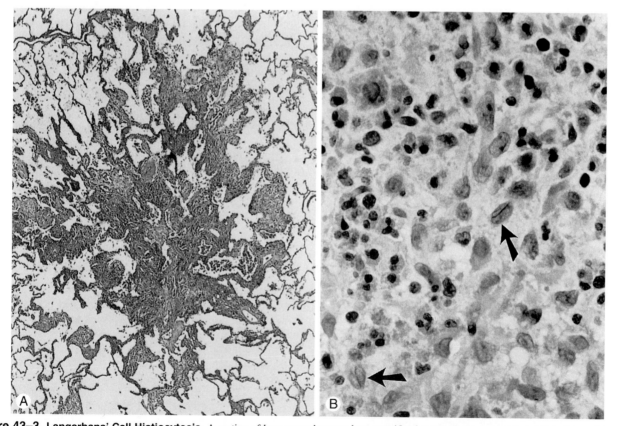

**Figure 43–3. Langerhans' Cell Histiocytosis.** A section of lung parenchyma at low magnification *(A)* shows a somewhat stellate focus of interstitial thickening caused by a cellular infiltrate and mild fibrosis. A magnified view of the infiltrate *(B)* shows it to be composed of scattered, bilobed eosinophils and numerous histiocytes with irregularly shaped, vesicular nuclei that are focally grooved *(arrows). (A,* ×32; *B,* ×400.)

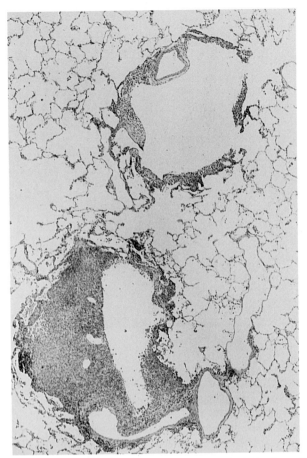

**Figure 43–4. Langerhans' Cell Histiocytosis: Early Lesions.** Two foci of disease are evident, each centered on a bronchiole. The one on the bottom is probably related to a membranous bronchiole and that on the top to a proximal respiratory bronchiole. The latter is mildly dilated and its wall slightly thickened by a cellular infiltrate; the former shows more marked, eccentric thickening as a result of a more pronounced cellular infiltrate. (×40.)

scribed, somewhat nodular cellular infiltrates without a stellate pattern can be seen, frequently adjacent to an airway. In addition, plugs of fibroblastic tissue can be present in the alveolar air spaces and the lumens of transitional airways; rarely, these are extensive enough to simulate the pattern of bronchiolitis obliterans–organizing pneumonia.[21] With progression, individual foci of disease coalesce, the fibrous tissue becomes more prominent, and an increasing amount of lung is destroyed (Fig. 43–5). In advanced disease, the lung may consist almost entirely of fibrous tissue and cystic spaces, with only scattered Langerhans' cells and few or no eosinophils. At this stage, diagnosis may be difficult, particularly in small biopsy specimens.[46]

The cellular portion of the stellate and nodular lesions consists of several types of inflammatory cells, the proportion varying from area to area. As might be expected, Langerhans' cells are frequently abundant. They are characterized by vesicular, often grooved nuclei and a moderate amount of pale, eosinophilic cytoplasm that is occasionally vacuolated (*see* Fig. 43–3B); cytologic atypia, sometimes marked, is seen occasionally.[28] Admixed among these cells are fairly numerous eosinophils and lesser numbers of neutrophils, plasma cells, lymphocytes, and multinucleated giant

cells. Despite the designation *eosinophilic granuloma*, true granuloma formation does not occur. Necrosis is very uncommon.

Alveolar macrophages are commonly increased in number at the periphery of foci of active disease; in some cases, they may be so numerous as to simulate desquamative interstitial pneumonitis.[10] The condition can also be confused with large cell lymphoma and eosinophilic pneumonia.[47] In these cases, identification of Langerhans' cells by immunohistochemical or ultrastructural means can be helpful. It is well established that these cells show a positive reaction for protein S-100,[48–50] in contrast to alveolar macrophages that typically produce a negative result. However, not all cells stain for this antigen, and a negative reaction does not exclude the diagnosis.[14] A positive reaction for CD1a is more specific and can be performed on either fresh frozen or formalin-fixed tissue.[14] Positive reactions for LN2, LN3, and vimentin and negative ones for lysozyme, leukocyte common antigen, and Leu-M1 are also characteristic.[15, 28]

Electron microscopic investigation can also be useful in selected cases. Ultrastructural studies have shown that the Langerhans cell possesses scattered surface microvilli and a moderate amount of cytoplasm that is usually rich in lysosomes and phagosomes (Fig. 43–6).[51, 52] In addition, the cytoplasm contains characteristic Birbeck granules, consisting of two parallel unit membranes separated by a thin stripe of granular or striated material (*see* Fig. 43–6); the bodies can appear to be free in the cytoplasm or attached to the plasma membrane and are sometimes expanded at one end in a form resembling a tennis racquet.

## RADIOLOGIC MANIFESTATIONS

Pulmonary involvement is characteristically bilaterally symmetric and diffuse throughout the upper and midlung zones with sparing of the costophrenic angles.[7, 9, 10] Early on, the radiographic appearance consists of a nodular pattern, with individual lesions ranging from 1 to 10 mm in diameter (Fig. 43–7); these are presumed to be predominantly cellular with minimal fibrosis,[53] and they may regress or even completely resolve.[54–57] Although cavitated nodules are only occasionally seen on the radiograph during this stage,[58] they can be identified on high-resolution computed tomography (HRCT) in approximately 10% of cases.[59, 60] In two instances, the early phase of the disease was manifested radiographically by fluffy alveolar consolidation in a butterfly distribution, strongly suggestive of pulmonary edema.[61]

In more advanced disease, the pattern may become reticulonodular (Fig. 43–8). Although this stage is usually considered to be irreversible, one patient has been described in whom the radiographic abnormalities resolved completely within 3 years following smoking cessation.[61a] The end stage of disease is characterized by a very coarse reticular pattern that, in the upper-lung zones particularly, often assumes a cystic appearance that is characteristic of honeycombing (Fig. 43–9). Usually, the cysts are about 1 cm in diameter, but they may measure up to 3 cm, especially in the lung periphery. A honeycomb pattern in the midlung and upper-lung zones is highly suggestive of PLCH; in fact, it is probable that the term *honeycomb lung* was coined originally

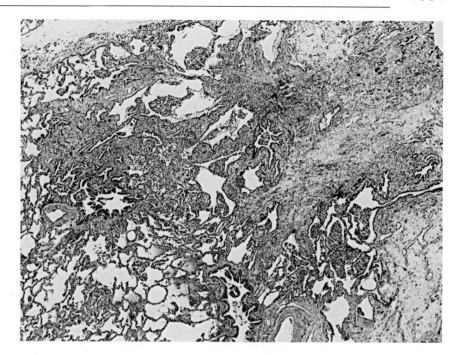

**Figure 43–5. Langerhans' Cell Histiocytosis: Interstitial Fibrosis.** The section shows lung parenchyma with a focus of active disease on the left. On the right, the lung parenchyma is almost entirely destroyed and replaced by mature fibrous tissue (F). (×25.)

to designate the severe disorganization of lung architecture that is seen in this disease.[62]

Several investigators have reviewed the computed tomography (CT) findings in PLCH.[59, 60, 63–65] The most common abnormalities on HRCT are cysts (present in approximately 80% of patients) and nodules (present in 60% to 80%). Less common findings, seen in approximately 10% of cases each, include cavitated nodules, reticulation, and areas of ground-glass attenuation.

As might be expected, the incidence of these findings depends on the stage of disease. In patients who have recent symptoms, the predominant abnormality consists of small nodules, which may vary from a few in number to a myriad (Fig. 43–10).[59, 60] The majority measure 1 to 5 mm in diameter, although larger nodules are seen in approximately 30% of cases. The nodules tend to have a centrilobular distribution corresponding to the peribronchiolar distribution of the cellular infiltrate seen histologically.[60] Their margins may be smooth or irregular. Follow-up CT scans demonstrate that cavitation of small nodules may occur within a few weeks of the initial CT scan and that larger nodules may be replaced by cysts;[59, 60] occasionally, small nodules disappear.

With progression of disease, cysts become a more prominent feature. They range from a few millimeters to several centimeters in diameter and may be round, oval, or bizarre in shape.[59, 64] The reticular and reticulonodular opacities that are frequently identified on the chest radiograph are relatively uncommon on CT,[59, 60, 64] many of the opacities probably representing cysts (Fig. 43–11).[59] In many cases, the pulmonary parenchyma between the cysts appears remarkably normal on CT.[59] With progression of disease, there is evidence of fibrosis and, eventually, extensive honeycombing (Fig. 43–12).[65] Regardless of the stage of disease, the abnormalities are most severe in the upper- and midlung zone; the lung bases are relatively spared.[59, 65–67]

The pattern and distribution of abnormalities on HRCT are usually characteristic enough to allow a confident diagnosis.[65, 66, 66a] In one study of 140 consecutive patients with chronic infiltrative lung disease, the superiority of HRCT over chest radiography in the assessment of pattern and distribution of abnormalities was the greatest for PLCH.[65] In another investigation of 61 patients with end-stage lung disease from a variety of causes, the correct first choice diagnosis of PLCH was made correctly by two independent blinded observers in eight out of eight cases.[66] The presence of nodules and cysts throughout the midlung and upper-lung zones with relative sparing of the lung bases is virtually diagnostic. In patients with only nodules, differential diagnosis is more difficult, because the pattern may resemble that of sarcoidosis, tuberculosis, or metastatic cancer. In patients who exhibit only cystic changes, the findings can be distinguished easily from those in IPF because the latter typically show most severe involvement in the subpleural lung regions and the lower-lung zones.[66] In a woman, cystic changes similar to those in PLCH may be seen in lymphangioleiomyomatosis and tuberous sclerosis;[68, 69] however, the cysts in these conditions are present diffusely throughout the lungs, without sparing of the lung bases, and nodules are rarely seen.[68, 69]

In our experience, the progressive loss of lung volume that is so characteristic of IPF is seldom seen in PLCH, perhaps because the development of cysts counteracts the retraction exerted by the fibrous tissue. The tendency for the lungs to maintain normal volume has been observed by others also; for example, in one study of 50 patients who had PLCH, none was considered to have a decrease in lung volume, and some were actually felt to show evidence of overinflation.[9] In another review of 100 patients, 60 were considered to have lung volumes within the normal range, 31 to be overinflated, and only 9 to have lung volumes below normal.[10]

Hilar and mediastinal node enlargement and pleural effusion are rare in adults,[70–73] although the former is relatively common in children.[71, 74] Spontaneous pneumothorax is a relatively common complication; in two series comprising 150 patients, it developed in 18 (12%).[9, 10] It may be the

*Text continued on page 1636*

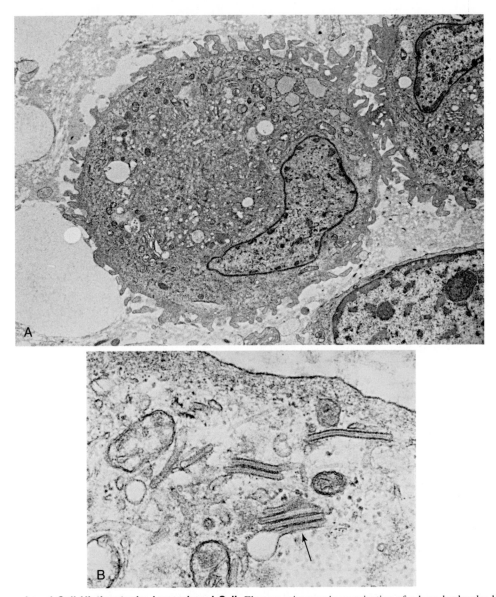

**Figure 43–6. Langerhans' Cell Histiocytosis: Langerhans' Cell.** Electron microscopic examination of a bronchoalveolar lavage fluid specimen from a patient with Langerhans' cell histiocytosis *(A)* shows a cell that superficially resembles an alveolar macrophage; however, several small tubular structures *(arrows)* can barely be discerned in the peripheral cytoplasm. At higher magnification *(B)*, the tubules can be seen to be composed of parallel membranous structures separated by finely granular material; one of these structures *(arrow)* shows a terminal expansion, resulting in a "tennis racquet" appearance. *(A, ×7000; B, ×50,650.)*

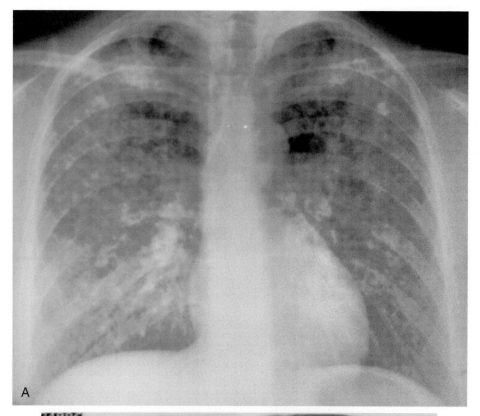

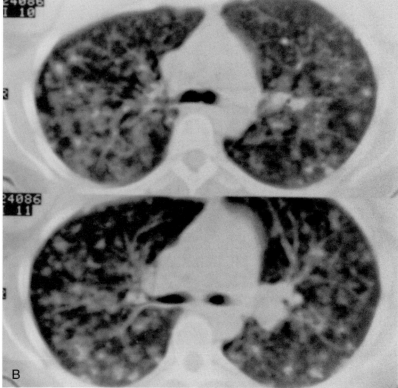

**Figure 43–7. Langerhans' Cell Histiocytosis: Active Stage.** A posteroanterior radiograph *(A)* reveals extensive bilateral pulmonary disease with sparing of the costophrenic sulci. The pattern consists of poorly defined small nodular and ground-glass opacities. Conventional 10-mm collimation CT scans through the midportion of both lungs and just below the level of the tracheal carina *(B)* reveal a multitude of poorly defined nodular opacities ranging from 3 to 10 mm in diameter. This 38-year-old man complained of increased dyspnea on effort.

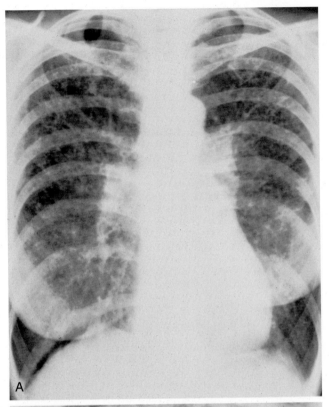

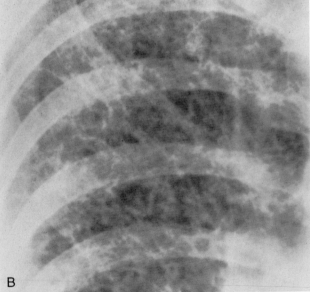

**Figure 43–8. Langerhans' Cell Histiocytosis.** For many years, this 57-year-old woman had had a chronic cough that produced small amounts of whitish-green sputum. During the last 3 to 4 years she had experienced increasing shortness of breath on exertion, to a point that she could climb only one flight of stairs before stopping. A posteroanterior radiograph *(A)* and a magnified view of the upper portion of the right lung *(B)* reveal a rather coarse reticular pattern that is more prominent in the upper than in the lower lung zones. A honeycomb pattern is suggested in the upper zones. Note sparing of the costophrenic sulci. Lung volume appears slightly increased; there are no other findings of note.

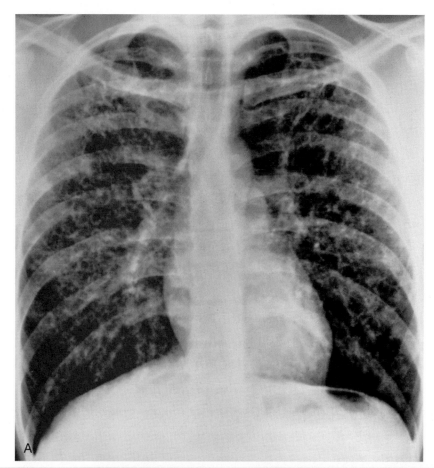

**Figure 43–9. Langerhans' Cell Histiocytosis.** A posteroanterior radiograph *(A)* and a detail view of the midportion of the right lung *(B)* reveal a rather coarse reticulonodular pattern throughout both lungs with some upper-zonal predominance. In several areas, there are ring shadows measuring 7 to 10 mm in diameter and characterized by a central radiolucency surrounded by a wall of variable thickness. This honeycomb pattern is well demonstrated in the magnified view *(arrows)*.

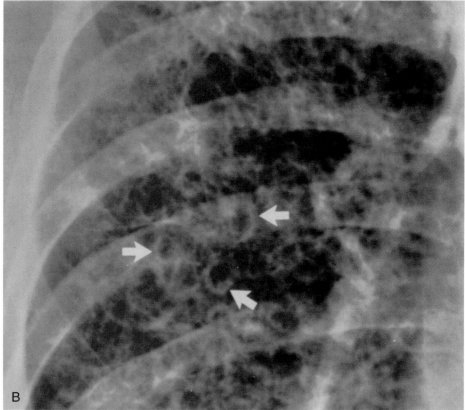

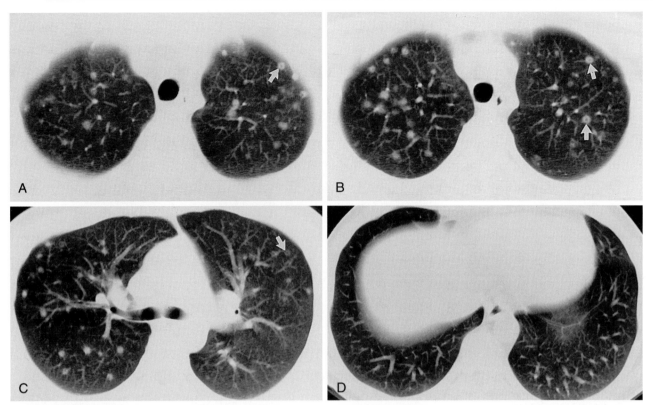

**Figure 43–10. Pulmonary Langerhans' Cell Histiocytosis: Cavitated Nodules.** A 30-year-old man presented with a pathologic fracture of the right first rib. The chest radiograph showed poorly defined small nodular opacities. A conventional 10-mm collimation CT scan demonstrates multiple bilateral nodules measuring 3 to 7 mm in diameter. Central lucencies can be seen in several of the nodules near the lung apices *(A)* and *(B)*, suggesting cavitation *(arrows)*. Similar findings are present at the level of the right upper lobe bronchus *(C)*. No nodules were identified in the lung bases *(D)*. Diagnosis of Langerhans' cell histiocytosis was proved by biopsy of the right first rib.

first manifestation of the disease[9] and occasionally occurs in the absence of radiographic abnormalities in the lungs.[71] Concomitant involvement of bones and lungs can occur[70, 75–78] but is uncommon in adults, appearing in only 5 of 100 patients in one series.[10]

## CLINICAL MANIFESTATIONS

PLCH is seen predominantly in young adults, the median age in one series being 33 years.[21] When first discovered, 20% to 25% of patients are asymptomatic,[10] the disease being identified on a screening chest radiograph. In symptomatic patients, the average duration of symptoms before presentation is about 6 months. Somewhat less than one third of patients have only nonspecific constitutional symptoms such as fatigue, weight loss, and fever.[10] Respiratory symptoms are present in the remaining two thirds and usually consist of dry cough and dyspnea. Hemoptysis is uncommon, occurring in only 6 of 100 patients in one study.[10] Chest pain can be caused by either a pneumothorax or (rarely) an osteolytic rib lesion. Physical findings are of little help in diagnosis; occasionally, crackles are heard over the lungs, or there is local tenderness over a bony lesion.[79] Finger clubbing is extremely rare.[11]

In contrast to the pediatric form of LCH (Letterer-Siwe disease), in which multiple organs are involved, disease in adults is generally confined to the lungs or bones.[10, 11] As indicated previously, concomitant involvement of the two

sites is uncommon.[10] Disease outside the lung and bones is even rarer; however, involvement of eye,[80, 81] skin,[82] colon,[83] pituitary,[20] mediastinal lymph nodes,[84] heart,[81] and brain[85] has been described. The association of diffuse lung disease with diabetes insipidus should strongly suggest the diagnosis, although this combination occasionally occurs in histoplasmosis and sarcoidosis.

## PULMONARY FUNCTION TESTS

Even in the presence of radiographic abnormalities, lung function is within the normal predicted range in many patients, in sharp contrast to those who have IPF.[86] The earliest abnormality is a reduction in the diffusing capacity.[87] In more advanced disease, pulmonary function studies show both restrictive[88] and obstructive patterns,[10] the former being manifested by decreased vital capacity, normal residual volume, and normal flow rates. In one follow-up study of 18 patients, airflow limitation appeared to increase with progression of the disease.[44] Exercise impairment is common.[88] Indices reflecting pulmonary vascular function (diffusing capacity, baseline $V_D/V_T$, and exercise $V_D/V_T$) are abnormal; there is a strong correlation between the severity of these derangements and overall exercise performance.

## DIAGNOSIS

In a young, asymptomatic adult with classic radiologic abnormalities, the diagnosis can usually be made with con-

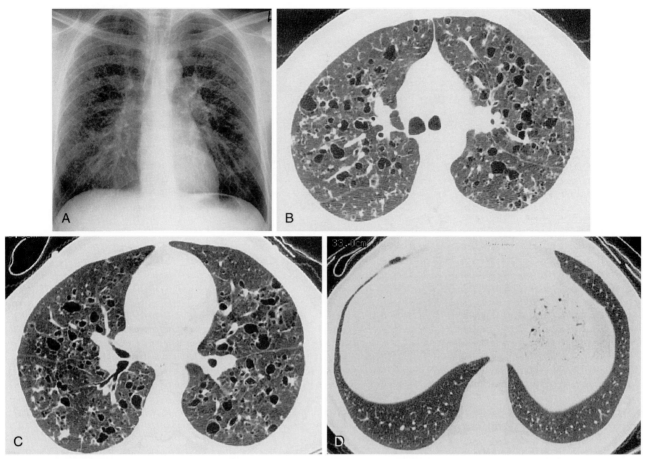

**Figure 43–11. Pulmonary Langerhans' Cell Histiocytosis.** A 30-year-old man presented with mild shortness of breath. A posteroanterior chest radiograph *(A)* shows a coarse reticular pattern as well as several cysts. Although the abnormalities are relatively diffuse in both upper and middle lung zones, there is sparing of the costophrenic sulci. High-resolution CT scan at the level of the main bronchi *(B)* demonstrates numerous bilateral cystic lesions of various sizes. Note relatively normal intervening lung parenchyma. The apparent reticular opacities on the radiograph are shown on CT to be due to cysts, there being little evidence of additional fibrosis. Note that the visualized bronchi are normal in diameter and that these do not communicate with the cysts. High-resolution CT scan at the level of the right middle lobe bronchus *(C)* demonstrates numerous bilateral cysts. Also note a few irregularly marginated small nodules. High-resolution CT scan through the lung bases *(D)* shows only a few localized cysts.

fidence without ancillary studies. Occasionally, atypical features necessitate histologic or cytologic confirmation. Langerhans' cells can be identified in specimens obtained by BAL,[44, 89, 90] a procedure that has been used for diagnosis. However, they can also be seen in cases of pulmonary fibrosis of other etiology, and it has been advocated that a differential count of greater than 3%[91] or 5%[92] must be documented for positive diagnosis. The diagnosis of PLCH is usually evident from the histologic appearance in open or thoracoscopic lung biopsy specimens. With smaller tissue fragments, however, interpretation may be difficult; for example, in two studies of transbronchial biopsy specimens, the diagnosis was considered definite in only 6 of 22 patients.[21, 93]

## PROGNOSIS AND NATURAL HISTORY

The prognosis of PLCH is generally good, particularly in patients whose disease is confined to the lungs.[94] Follow-up data in one series of 37 patients revealed that 13 improved (4 returned to normal), 11 stabilized, and 13 worsened (5 of whom died).[9] In another series of 60 patients, 16 were

initially asymptomatic and remained so, 28 had remission of symptoms (17 complete and 11 partial), 11 remained stable but symptomatic, 4 showed progression with increasing disability, and only 1 died.[10] Relapse of the disease—sometimes years after initial radiologic remission—occurs in some patients.[94a] The prognosis is worse in older patients with disseminated disease, in patients who have functional indices of airflow obstruction (lower $FEV_1$/FVC ratio and higher RV/TLC ratio),[95] and in patients who have radiographic evidence of honeycombing, especially if it is associated with repeated episodes of pneumothorax.[11] Although the morphologic appearance of the Langerhans cell is generally an imperfect predictor of clinical severity, there appears to be a subgroup of patients (mostly men) who have cytologically atypical Langerhans' cells and who experience an aggressive clinical course with extensive and unusual organ involvement.[28] Although the effects of smoking cessation on outcome are poorly documented, it seems prudent to strongly advocate this for all patients, given the close association of smoking with disease.

The results of a number of investigations suggest that LCH may be complicated by malignancy. Although the association with pulmonary carcinoma is confounded by the

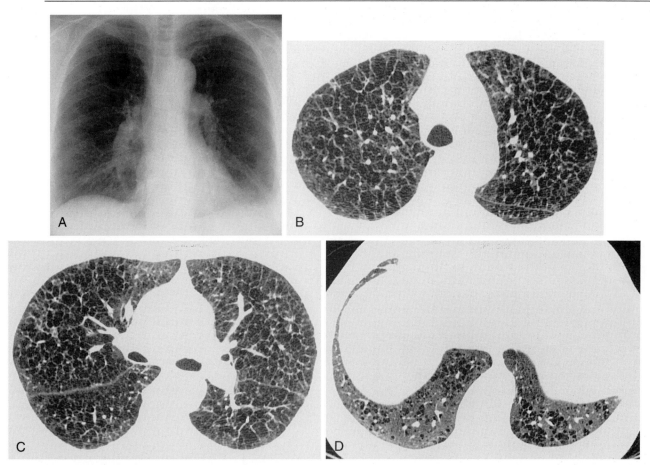

**Figure 43–12. Pulmonary Langerhans' Cell Histiocytosis: End-Stage Lung.** A 56-year-old woman with long-standing histiocytosis and severe shortness of breath was referred for lung transplant. A posteroanterior chest radiograph *(A)* shows enlarged central pulmonary arteries consistent with pulmonary arterial hypertension. However, there is only minimal evidence of parenchymal disease with a few linear opacities bilaterally. The blunting of the left costophrenic sulcus is related to previous lung biopsy. High-resolution CT scans *(B and C)* through the upper and middle lung zones demonstrate thin-walled cysts throughout both lungs. Localized areas of ground-glass attenuation are present anteriorly in focal areas of relatively spared lung. High-resolution CT through the lung bases *(D)* shows relative sparing. The areas of ground-glass attenuation are due to blood flow redistribution away from areas of abnormal lung. Pathologic specimen of the right lung is illustrated in Figure 43–1.

smoking history of most patients,[96, 97] the number of reports of other types of cancer suggests more than a spurious association. For example, in one series of 21 patients who had PLCH, 9 had malignant tumors (3 pulmonary carcinoma, 1 pulmonary carcinoid tumor, 2 lymphoma, and 5 extrapulmonary carcinoma [two patients had two neoplasms]).[96] In one review of the literature, 21 patients were identified who had a history of both PLCH and Hodgkin's disease.[98] A

review of a Dutch registry of children with a spectrum of LCH revealed 27 patients with neoplasia; 4 had lymphoma, 10 had other solid tumors, and 13 had leukemia.[82] In all of these cases, the malignancy may precede, follow, or occur simultaneously with the discovery of LCH. When malignancies are associated with PLCH, it is important to remember that the nodules of LCH can imitate metastases radiologically.

# REFERENCES

1. Schwarz MI: Interstitial lung disease associated with bronchiolitis, eosinophilic granuloma, and other unique entities. Sem Respir Med 14:375, 1993.
2. Chu T, Jaffe R: The normal Langerhans' cell and the LCH cell. Br J Cancer 23:4, 1994.
3. Lichtenstein L: Histiocytosis X: Integration of eosinophilic granuloma of bone. "Letterer-Siwe disease" and "Schüller-Christian disease" as related manifestations of a single nosologic entity. Arch Pathol 56:84, 1953.
4. Enriquez P, Dahlin DC, Hayles AB, et al: Histiocytosis X: A clinical study. Mayo Clin Proc 42:88, 1967.
5. Groopman JE, Golde DW: The histiocytic disorders: A pathophysiologic analysis. Ann Intern Med 94:95, 1981.
6. Kaufman A, Bukberg PR, Werlin S, et al: Multifocal eosinophilic granuloma ("Hand-Schüller-Christian disease"). Report illustrating H-S-C chronicity and diagnostic challenge. Am J Med 60:541, 1976.
7. Dunmore LA Jr, El-Khoury SA: Eosinophilic granuloma of the lung. A report of three cases in Negro patients. Am Rev Respir Dis 90:789, 1964.
8. Morley TF, Silverstein SD, Giudice JC, et al: Multifocal eosinophilic granuloma. Respiration 54:89, 1988.
9. Lacronique J, Roth C, Battesti J-P, et al: Chest radiological features of pulmonary histiocytosis X: A report based on 50 adult cases. Thorax 37:104, 1982.
10. Friedman PJ, Liebow AA, Sokoloff J: Eosinophilic granuloma of lung: Clinical aspects of primary pulmonary histiocytosis in the adult. Medicine 60:385, 1981.
11. Colby TV, Lombard C: Histiocytosis X in the lung. Hum Pathol 14:847, 1983.
12. Malpas JS, Norton AJ: Langerhans' cell histiocytosis in the adult. Med Pediatr Oncol 27:540, 1996.
13. Hance AJ, Basset F, Saumon G, et al: Smoking and interstitial lung disease. The effect of cigarette smoking on the incidence of pulmonary histiocytosis X and sarcoidosis. Ann N Y Acad Sci 465:643, 1986.
14. Emile JF, Wechsler J, Brousse N, et al: Langerhans' cell histiocytosis. Definitive diagnosis with the use of monoclonal antibody 010 on routinely paraffin-embedded samples. Am J Surg Pathol 19:636, 1995.
15. Azumi N, Sheibani K, Swartz WG, et al: Antigenic phenotype of Langerhans' cell histiocytosis: An immunohistochemical study demonstrating the value of LN-2, LN-3, and vimentin. Hum Pathol 19:1376, 1988.
16. Hance AJ: Pulmonary immune cells in health and disease: Dendritic cells and Langerhans' cells. Eur Respir J 6:1213, 1993.
17. McClain K, Weiss RA: Viruses and Langerhans' cell histiocytosis: Is there a link? Br J Cancer 23:S34, 1994.
18. Leahy MA, Krejci SM, Friednash M, et al: Human herpesvirus 6 is present in lesions of Langerhans' cell histiocytosis. J Invest Dermatol 101:642, 1993.
19. Mierau GW, Wills EJ, Steele PO: Ultrastructural studies in Langerhans' cell histiocytosis: A search for evidence of viral etiology. Pediatr Pathol 14:895, 1994.
20. McClain K, Jin H, Gresik V, et al: Langerhans' cell histiocytosis: Lack of a viral etiology. Am J Hematol 47:16, 1994.
21. Travis WD, Borok Z, Roum JH, et al: Pulmonary Langerhans' cell granulomatosis (histiocytosis X). A clinicopathologic study of 48 cases. Am J Surg Pathol 17:971, 1993.
22. Casolaro MA, Bernaudin JF, Saltini C, et al: Accumulation of Langerhans' cells on the epithelial surface of the lower respiratory tract in normal subjects in association with cigarette smoking. Am Rev Respir Dis 137:406, 1988.
23. Youkeles LH, Grizzanti JN, Liao Z, et al: Decreased tobacco-glycoprotein-induced lymphocyte proliferation in vitro in pulmonary eosinophilic granuloma. Am J Respir Crit Care Med 151:145, 1995.
24. Yu RC, Chu AC: Lack of T-cell receptor gene rearrangements in cells involved in Langerhans' cell histiocytosis. Cancer 75:1162, 1995.
25. Yu RC, Chu C, Buluwela L, et al: Clonal proliferation of Langerhans' cells in Langerhans' cell histiocytosis. Lancet 343:767, 1994.
26. Willman CL: Detection of clonal histiocytes in Langerhans' cell histiocytosis: Biology and clinical significance. Br J Cancer 23:S29, 1994.
27. Willman CL, Busque L, Griffith BB, et al: Langerhans'-cell histiocytosis (histiocytosis X)—a clonal proliferative disease. N Engl J Med 331:154, 1994.
28. Ben-Ezra J, Bailey A, Azumi N, et al: Malignant histiocytosis X. A distinct clinicopathologic entity. Cancer 68:1050, 1991.
28a. Brabencova E, Tazi A, Lorenzato M, et al: Langerhans cells in Langerhans cell granulomatosis are not actively proliferating. Am J Pathol 152:1143, 1998.
29. de Graaf JH, Tamminga RY, Kamps WA, et al: Langerhans' cell histiocytosis: Expression of leukocyte cellular adhesion molecules suggests abnormal homing and differentiation. Am J Pathol 144:466, 1994.
30. Tzi A, Bonay M, Grandsaigne M, et al: Surface phenotype of Langerhans' cells and lymphocytes in granulomatous lesions from patients with pulmonary histiocytosis X. Am Rev Respir Dis 147:1531, 1993.
31. Emile JF, Fraitag S, Leborgne M, et al: Langerhans' cells histiocytosis cells are activated Langerhans' cells. J Pathol 174:71, 1994.
32. Ruco LP, Stoppacciaro A, Vitolo D, et al: Expression of adhesion molecules in Langerhans' cell histiocytosis. Histopathology 23:29, 1993.
33. King TE Jr, Schwarz MI, Dreisin RE, et al: Circulating immune complexes in pulmonary eosinophilic granuloma. Ann Intern Med 91:397, 1979.
34. Hage C, Willman CL, Favara BE, et al: Langerhans' cell histiocytosis (histiocytosis X): Immunophenotype and growth fraction. Hum Pathol 24:840, 1993.
35. Emile JF, Peuchmaur M, Fraitag S, et al: Immunohistochemical detection of granulocyte/macrophage colony-stimulating factor in Langerhans' cell histiocytosis. Histopathology 23:327, 1993.
36. Barth J, Kreipe H, Radzun HJ, et al: Increased expression of growth factor genes for macrophages and fibroblasts in bronchoalveolar lavage cells of a patient with pulmonary histiocytosis X. Thorax 46:835, 1991.
37. Tazi A, Bonay M, Bergeron A: Role of granulocyte-macrophage colony stimulating factor (GM-CSF) in the pathogenesis of adult pulmonary histiocytosis X. Thorax 51:611, 1996.
38. Weinberger SE, Kelman JA, Elson NA, et al: Bronchoalveolar lavage in interstitial lung disease. Ann Intern Med 89:459, 1978.
39. Colasante A, Poletti V, Rosini S, et al: Langerhans' cells in Langerhans' cell histiocytosis and peripheral adenocarcinomas of the lung. Am Rev Respir Dis 148:752, 1993.
40. Uebelhoer M, Bewig B, Kreipe H, et al: Modulation of fibroblast activity in histiocytosis X by platelet-derived growth factor. Chest 107:701, 1995.
41. Robinson BW: Production of plasminogen activator by alveolar macrophages in normal subjects and patients with interstitial lung disease. Thorax 43:508, 1988.
42. Fukuda Y, Basset F, Soler P, et al: Intraluminal fibrosis and elastic fiber degradation lead to lung remodelling in pulmonary Langerhans' cell granulomatosis (histiocytosis X). Am J Pathol 137:415, 1990.
43. Asakura S, Colby TV, Limper AH: Tissue localization of transforming growth factor-beta$_1$ in pulmonary eosinophilic granuloma. Am J Respir Crit Care Med 154:1525, 1996.
44. Basset F, Corrin B, Spencer H, et al: Pulmonary histiocytosis X. Am Rev Respir Dis 118:811, 1978.
45. Knudson RJ, Badger TL, Gaensler EA: Eosinophilic granuloma of the lung. Med Thorac 23:248, 1966.
46. Powers MA, Askin FB, Cresson DH: Pulmonary eosinophilic granuloma. 25-year follow-up. Am Rev Respir Dis 129:503, 1984.
47. Pomeranz SJ, Proto AV: Histiocytosis X. Unusual-confusing features of eosinophilic granuloma. Chest 89:88, 1986.
48. Flint A, Lloyd RV, Colby TV, et al: Pulmonary histiocytosis X. Immunoperoxidase staining for HLA-DR antigen and S100 protein. Arch Pathol Lab Med 110:930, 1986.
49. Soler P, Chollet S, Jacque C, et al: Immunocytochemical characterization of pulmonary histiocytosis X cells in lung biopsies. Am J Pathol 118:439, 1985.
50. Webber D, Tron V, Askin F, et al: S-100 staining in the diagnosis of eosinophilic granuloma of lung. Am J Clin Pathol 84:447, 1985.
51. Akhtar M, Ali MA, Sabbah R: Ultrastructure of histiocytosis X. A study of 9 cases with review of the literature. King Faisal Specialist Hosp Med J 4:137, 1984.
52. Ide F, Iwase T, Saito I, et al: Immunohistochemical and ultrastructural analysis of the proliferating cells in histiocytosis X. Cancer 53:917, 1984.
53. Arnett NL, Schulz DM: Primary pulmonary eosinophilic granuloma. Radiology 69:224, 1957.
54. Williams AW, Dunnington WG, Berte SJ: Pulmonary eosinophilic granuloma: A clinical and pathologic discussion. Ann Intern Med 54:30, 1961.
55. Bickers JN, Buechner HA, Ekman PJ: Pulmonary eosinophilic granuloma. Its natural history and prognosis. Am Rev Respir Dis 85:211, 1962.
56. Thompson J, Buechner RHA, Fishman R: Eosinophilic granuloma of the lung. Ann Intern Med 48:1134, 1958.
57. Kittredge RD, Geller A, Finby N: The reticuloendothelioses in the lung. Am J Roentgenol 100:588, 1967.
58. Clark RL, Margulies SI, Mulholland JH: Histiocytosis X. A fatal case with unusual pulmonary manifestations. Radiology 95:631, 1970.
59. Moore ADA, Godwin JD, Müller NL, et al: Pulmonary histiocytosis X: Comparison of radiographic and CT findings. Radiology 172:249, 1989.
60. Brauner MW, Grenier P, Mouelhi MM, et al: Pulmonary histiocytosis X: Evaluation with high-resolution CT. Radiology 172:255, 1989.
61. Weber WN, Margolin FR, Nielsen SL: Pulmonary histiocytosis X. A review of 18 patients with reports of 6 cases. Am J Roentgenol 107:280, 1969.
61a. Von Essen S, West W, Sitorius M, et al: Complete resolution of roentgenographic changes in a patient with pulmonary histiocytosis X. Chest 98:765, 1990.
62. McLetchie NGB, Reynolds DP: Histiocytic reticulosis and honeycomb lungs. Can Med Assoc J 71:44, 1954.
63. Giron J, Tawil A, Trussard V, et al: Contribution of high-resolution x-ray computed tomography to the diagnosis of pulmonary histiocytosis X: Apropos of 12 cases. Ann Radiol 33:31, 1990.
64. Kulwiec EL, Lynch DA, Aguayo SM, et al: Imaging of pulmonary histiocytosis X. Radiographics 12:515, 1992.
65. Grenier P, Valeyre D, Cluzel P, et al: Chronic diffuse interstitial lung disease: Diagnostic value of chest radiography and high-resolution CT. Radiology 179:123, 1991.
66. Primack SL, Hartman TE, Hansell DM, et al: End-stage lung disease: CT findings in 61 patients. Radiology 189:681, 1993.
66a. Bonelli FS, Hartman TE, Swensen SJ, et al: Accuracy of high-resolution CT in diagnosing lung diseases. Am J Roentgenol 170:1507, 1998.
67. Müller NL, Miller RR: Computed tomography of chronic diffuse infiltrative lung disease. Part 2. Am Rev Respir Dis 142:1440, 1990.
68. Müller NL, Chiles C, Kullnig P: Pulmonary lymphangiomyomatosis: Correlation of CT with radiographic and functional findings. Radiology 175:335, 1990.
69. Lenoir S, Grenier P, Brauner MW, et al: Pulmonary lymphangiomyomatosis and tuberous sclerosis: Comparison of radiographic and thin-section CT findings. Radiology 175:329, 1990.

70. Takahashi M, Martel W, Oberman HA: The variable roentgenographic appearance of idiopathic histiocytosis. Clin Radiol 17:48, 1966.

71. Carlson RA, Hattery RR, O'Connell EJ, et al: Pulmonary involvement by histiocytosis X in the pediatric age group. Mayo Clin Proc 51:542, 1976.

72. Tittel PW, Winkler CF: Chronic recurrent pleural effusion in adult histiocytosis X. Br J Radiol 54:68, 1981.

73. Guardia J, Pedreira J-D, Esteban R, et al: Early pleural effusion in histiocytosis X. Arch Intern Med 139:934, 1979.

74. Matlin AH, Young LW, Klemperer MR: Pleural effusion in two children with histiocytosis X. Chest 61:33, 1972.

75. Favara BE, McCarthy RC, Mierau GW: Histiocytosis X. Hum Pathol 14:663, 1983.

76. Konno K, Hayashi I, Oka S: Eosinophilic granuloma (histiocytosis X) involving anterior chest wall and lung. Am Rev Respir Dis 100:391, 1969.

77. Meier B, Rhyner K, Medici TC, et al: Eosinophilic granuloma of the skeleton with involvement of the lung: A report of three cases. Eur J Respir Dis 64:551, 1983.

78. Langer A, Fettes I: Multifocal eosinophilic granuloma with a pituitary stalk lesion. West J Med 142:829, 1985.

79. Bank A, Christensen C: Unusual manifestation of Langerhans' cell histiocytosis. Acta Med Scand 223:479, 1988.

80. Yamada G, Morita Y, Yokokawa K, et al: A case of pulmonary eosinophilic granuloma with involvement of the ocular fundus. Jpn J Thorac Dis 30:1365, 1992.

81. MacCumber MW, Hoffman PN, Wand GS, et al: Ophthalmic involvement in aggressive histiocytosis X. Ophthalmology 97:22, 1990.

82. Egeler RM, Neglia JP, Arico M, et al: Acute leukemia in association with Langerhans' cell histiocytosis. Med Pediatr Oncol 23:81, 1994.

83. Rioux M, Trottier F, Rodrigue J: Colonic bull's-eye lesions in histiocytosis X. Can Assoc Radiol J 45:476, 1994.

84. Mogul M, Hartman G, Donaldson S, et al: Langerhans' cell histiocytosis presenting with the superior vena cava syndrome: A case report. Med Pediatr Oncol 21:456, 1993.

85. Usami I, Yamakoshi M, Kuroki H, et al: A case of eosinophilic granuloma associated with a brain lesion. Jpn J Thorac Dis 31:271, 1993.

86. Bates DV: Respiratory Function in Disease. 3rd ed. Philadelphia, WB Saunders, 1989.

87. Schonfeld N, Frank W, Wenig S, et al: Clinical and radiologic features, lung function and therapeutic results in pulmonary histiocytosis X. Respiration 60:38, 1993.

88. Crausman RS, Jennings CA, Tuder RM, et al: Pulmonary histiocytosis X: Pulmonary function and exercise physiology. Am J Respir Crit Care Med 153:426, 1996.

89. Verea-Hernando H, Fontan-Bueso J, Martin-Egana MT, et al: Langerhans' cells in bronchoalveolar lavage in the late stages of pulmonary histiocytosis X. Chest 81:130, 1982.

90. Basset F, Soler P, Jaurand MC, et al: Ultrastructural examination of bronchoalveolar lavage for diagnosis of pulmonary histiocytosis X: Preliminary report on 4 cases. Thorax 32:303, 1977.

91. Xaubet A, Agusti C, Picado C, et al: Bronchoalveolar lavage analysis with anti-T6 monoclonal antibody in the evaluation of diffuse lung diseases. Respiration 56:161, 1989.

92. Auerswald U, Barth J, Magnussen H: Value of CD-1–positive cells in bronchoalveolar lavage fluid for the diagnosis of pulmonary histiocytosis X. Lung 169:305, 1991.

93. Housini I, Tomashefski JF Jr, Cohen A, et al: Transbronchial biopsy in patients with pulmonary eosinophilic granuloma. Comparison with findings on open lung biopsy. Arch Pathol Lab Med 118:523, 1994.

94. Greenberger JS, Crocker AC, Vawter G, et al: Results of treatment of 127 patients with systemic histiocytosis (Letterer-Siwe's syndrome, Schüller-Christian syndrome and multifocal eosinophilic granuloma). Medicine 60:311, 1981.

94a. Tazi A, Montcelly L, Bergeron A, et al: Relapsing nodular lesions in the course of adult pulmonary Langerhans cell histiocytosis. Am J Respir Crit Care Med 157:2007, 1998.

95. Delobbe A, Durieu J, Duhamel A: Determinants of survival pulmonary Langerhans' cell granulomatosis (histiocytosis X). Eur Respir J 9:2002, 1996.

96. Tomashefski JF, Khiyami A, Kleinerman J: Neoplasms associated with pulmonary eosinophilic granuloma. Arch Pathol Lab Med 115:499, 1991.

97. Sadoun D, Vaylet F, Valeyre D, et al: Bronchogenic carcinoma in patients with pulmonary histiocytosis X. Chest 101:1610, 1992.

98. Shin MS, Buchalter SE, Ho KJ: Langerhans' cell histiocytosis associated with Hodgkin's disease: A case report. J Nat Med Assoc 86:65, 1994.

# CHAPTER 44

# The Pulmonary Manifestations of Human Immunodeficiency Virus Infection

## GENERAL EPIDEMIOLOGIC FEATURES

Since it was first described in 1981, the acquired immunodeficiency syndrome (AIDS) has become a pandemic associated with significant morbidity and mortality.[1] By the end of 1995, after considering reporting delays, underdiagnosis, and incomplete reporting, an estimated 6,000,000 cases of AIDS had occurred in adults and children, of whom 5,000,000 had died.[1] In urban centers in the sub-Saharan region of Africa, western Europe, and North America, AIDS has become the leading cause of death for both men and women between 15 and 49 years of age; in sub-Saharan Africa, it is the leading cause of potential healthy life years lost.[1] By the year 2000, the World Health Organization has estimated that about 26,000,000 people will be infected with the causative virus (human immunodeficiency virus [HIV]);[1] more than 90% of these will be living in "developing" countries, and more than 10,000,000 children younger than 10 years of age will be orphaned as the result of AIDS-related deaths.

From 1981 through 1996, 573,800 cases of AIDS in people aged 13 years or older were reported to the Centers for Disease Control and Prevention by state and local health departments in the United States.[2] In 1993, there was a large increase in the number of reported cases as a result of a refined case surveillance definition of disease that included recurrent bacterial pneumonia, tuberculosis, and a CD4+ count of less than 200/mm³.[2] Although the number of cases reported in 1996 was substantially higher than that in 1992, there was a decline from 1994 through 1996;[2, 3] in fact, 1996 was the first calendar year in which the overall incidence of AIDS decreased in the United States[3] (Fig. 44–1). Despite this, the incidence of AIDS is still increasing in some groups,[4] particularly in African-American men (19% in-

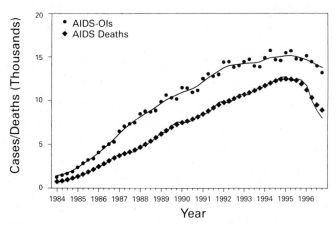

**Figure 44–1.** Estimated incidence of AIDS-opportunistic illnesses (AIDS-OIs) and estimated number of deaths among persons aged ≥13 years with AIDS (AIDS deaths), adjusted for delays in reporting, by quarter year of diagnosis/death—United States, 1984–1996.

crease in 1996 compared with 1995), Hispanic-American men (13% increase), and African-American women who have had heterosexual contact with HIV-infected men (12% increase).[3] With 42% of incident cases in 1996, the proportion of cases of AIDS in African-American patients now exceeds that in non-Hispanic whites, whereas women now account for about 20% of adults reported to have the disease.[3] The highest overall rates have been reported from Washington, D.C. (232 per 100,000 population in 1996), New York, New Jersey, Florida, and California;[5] the lowest rates (fewer than 10 cases per 100,000 population) are found in the Midwest.

The two most important risk factors for HIV infection are sexual contact with an infected person and intravenous drug use. About 45% of cases of AIDS in the United States in 1996 occurred in male homosexuals, 5% in male homosexual intravenous drug users, 30% in intravenous drug users, and 18% in patients who had heterosexual contact with an infected person.[3] Hemophiliac patients and other transfusion recipients accounted for 3.6% of cases from 1981 to 1987 and for 1.6% of cases in 1994.[6] Strikingly, the cumulative incidence of AIDS cases acquired heterosexually is 11-fold higher in African-American women than in white women and 7-fold higher in African-American men than in white men.[7] Most cases of such heterosexual transmission in the United States are related to contact of infected intravenous drug users with their partners.[2] In fact, among women, more cases of AIDS are currently the result of heterosexual transmission from an infected contact than any other single cause, including exposure to HIV by personal intravenous drug abuse.[3, 8] Although the overall proportion of cases in male homosexuals is decreasing,[6] recent increases in gonococcal infection rates among homosexual men in some American cities[9] could presage an increase in HIV infection (in part because an increase in gonorrhea rate is associated with reversion to high-risk behaviors for HIV infection).[10]

Of special interest to health care workers is the risk of developing HIV infection after inadvertent percutaneous exposure to contaminated blood. Among nurses performing procedures and emergency department physicians, the overall risk for HIV infection has been estimated to range from 1 in 3,800 to 1 in 187,000 in areas of high and low seroprevalence for HIV, respectively.[11] Among health care workers

who have accidental skin puncture by an HIV-contaminated source, the average risk is about 0.3%. Logistic regression analysis of 33 cases and 665 controls in one study showed that significant risk factors for seroconversion were deep injury, injury with a device that was visibly contaminated with the patient's blood, injury involving a needle that had been placed in the patient's artery or vein, and exposure to blood from a patient who died of AIDS within 2 months of the injury.[12]

An improved survival of patients who have AIDS has led to an increase in its prevalence, despite the modest decline in incidence. The prevalence of AIDS in the United States has been estimated to be 225,470 cases among people 13 years of age or older in 1996,[3] representing an increase of more than 65% since 1993[2] and 11% since 1995.[3] About 80% of the increase occurred in men;[3] by risk/exposure category, homosexual men accounted for the largest number of prevalent cases (48%), followed by intravenous drug users (34%, 18% of whom were also homosexual men) and people infected through heterosexual contact (15%).[3] The largest proportionate increase from 1995 to 1996 was in infection acquired through heterosexual contact (25%), whereas the largest absolute increase occurred among male homosexuals (9,890).[3] Transmission of HIV by intravenous drug use has been a significant determinant of the extent of the AIDS epidemic; needle-born infection, infection of a sexual partner, and perinatal transmission have all been important in this regard.[6, 13]

As indicated previously, AIDS is an important cause of death in young people in the United States; it is a leading cause in those aged 25 to 44 years (Fig. 44–2)[6] and is now ranked seventh for children aged 1 to 4 years.[1] Despite this, the overall death rate in patients who have the disease declined 23% in 1996 compared with 1995 (*see* Fig. 44–1).[3, 14] This striking decrease occurred in men and women, in all racial and ethnic groups and in all risk/exposure categories. It reflects the impact of newer antiretroviral therapies and prevention of opportunistic infection by prophylactic regimens.[3] However, the estimated number of cases of HIV infection and AIDS combined is about 2.5

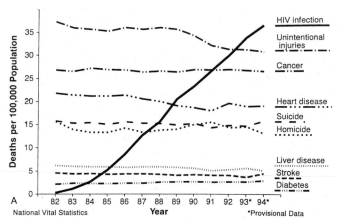

**Figure 44–2.** Death rates from leading causes of death among persons aged 25–44 years, by year, in the United States, 1982–1994. Rates are based on national vital statistics for underlying causes of death, using final mortality data for 1982 to 1992 and provisional data (based on a 10% sample of death certificates) for 1993 and 1994. (Courtesy of Richard M. Selik, M.D., Centers for Disease Control and Prevention, Atlanta, GA.)

times that of AIDS cases alone.[3] In the absence of effective therapy, AIDS develops about 10 years after the initial HIV infection; as a consequence, focusing on AIDS incidence and prevalence alone reflects rates of infection that have occurred a decade earlier.[15]

In the "developing" world, heterosexual transmission of disease has been the dominant mode of infection, resulting in a proportionately greater burden of disease among women and children than has been seen in the United States. In fact, by the year 2000, it is estimated that the number of new infections in women will equal those in men worldwide.[1] The highest incidence rates are seen in women between the ages of 15 and 25 years.[1] The spread of infection in "developing" countries has been rampant, and its full impact has yet to be felt;[6] for example, it has been estimated that AIDS will double or triple the adult mortality rates in the sub-Saharan region of Africa from levels that were already eight times higher than those in "developed" countries.[1] In fact, AIDS is already the leading cause of death in Abidjan and Kinshasa and in the rural communities of Uganda and Tanzania.[1] In countries such as Uganda, in which almost 10% of the total population of 19,000,000 is believed to be infected with HIV, AIDS will inevitably become the predominant health problem of the entire population.[1] In Kigali, Rwanda, the HIV seroprevalence was an astounding 32% among a representative sample of nearly 1,500 childbearing women attending pediatric and prenatal clinics in the city's sole community hospital.[16]

Although HIV infection was noted much later in Asia than in the rest of the world, more than 4 million people in this region were estimated to be infected in 1996.[1] The disease was initially noted in intravenous drug users in Thailand, Myanmar, and India. In the first of these countries, the seroprevalence increased from 1.2% to 45% in this population between 1988 and 1991.[1] At the same time, HIV infection was noted in 30% to 65% of female prostitutes in various cities of Thailand and India;[1] spread of the virus occurred rapidly from those individuals to their clientele. As a result of these factors, the seroprevalence of HIV has soared; for example, various investigators in India reported it to have increased from 0% to 70% among intravenous drug users and from 1.4% to 40% among patients attending clinics for sexually transmitted disease between 1986 and 1994.[17] As in Africa, infection has also been spread by long-distance truck drivers and migrant workers,[17] and infection in commercial blood donors has contaminated the blood supply.[18] Ninety per cent of infected individuals in "developing" countries are between 15 and 45 years of age and are poor. The male-to-female ratio is 5 to 1; most affected women are prostitutes.

From the beginning of the AIDS epidemic, pulmonary disease has been a major cause of morbidity and mortality, particularly in "developed" countries. In fact, the first cases described in 1981 were in homosexual men who had *Pneumocystis carinii* pneumonia (PCP).[19, 20] In one study of 1,067 patients whose clinical course was reviewed at the first National Heart Lung and Blood Institute (NHLBI) workshop on the disease, 441 had suffered a pulmonary complication, of which PCP was by far the most common.[21] At the time of the second NHLBI workshop in 1986, bacterial pneumonia and tuberculosis had also been recognized as important complications;[22, 23] this recognition was reinforced with the

expansion of the surveillance definition of AIDS in 1993 to include these two infections.[24]

A review of the medical records of more than 18,000 HIV-infected patients who received care in 10 American cities confirmed a clear association between the degree of immunosuppression, as reflected in the blood CD4+ lymphocyte count, and the risk of developing particular respiratory disorders.[25] Common respiratory tract illnesses, such as bronchitis, sinusitis, and pharyngitis, were seen with all CD4+ T lymphocyte counts, although at a greater frequency than that seen in a seronegative population.[24] With lower counts, pulmonary infections occurred with increasing frequency. About 80% of cases of bacterial pneumonia and pulmonary tuberculosis were associated with a CD4+ count of less than 400 cells/$\mu$l. With counts of less than 300 cells/$\mu$l, bacterial pneumonia was often recurrent and infection by nontuberculous mycobacteria was seen; counts of less than 200 cells/$\mu$l were often associated with PCP, disseminated tuberculosis, or Kaposi's sarcoma (KS). Patients who had the most severe degree of immunosuppression (counts of less than 100 cells/$\mu$l) tended to develop disseminated infection caused by *Mycobacterium avium–intracellulare*, cytomegalovirus (CMV), and various fungi. Similar observations have been made in the Pulmonary Complications of HIV Infection Study, in which a cohort of 1,353 HIV-infected patients was followed prospectively for a 5-year period.[26]

As the previous discussion indicates, the most common and important pulmonary complications of AIDS are infections, of which bacteria, *P. carinii*, *Mycobacterium tuberculosis,* and CMV are the most frequent causes. Neoplasms—predominantly lymphoma and KS—are less frequent but also of major import. Additional, relatively uncommon complications are seen in some patients (Table 44–1). Many of these abnormalities are also discussed in other chapters, to which the reader may refer for additional information.

## PULMONARY INFECTION

Many organisms have been found to cause pulmonary disease in patients who are HIV positive. Although some—such as *M. tuberculosis, P. carinii,* and CMV—are also seen in other immunodeficient patients, they tend to be particularly prevalent in the AIDS population; moreover, HIV-infected patients often have higher organism loads. A number of unusual organisms, such as *Rhodococcus* and cryptosporidia, are also seen almost exclusively in the setting of HIV infection. Simultaneous infection by more than one organism is relatively common, particularly in patients who have advanced disease;[27] there is evidence that the incidence of such multiple infections has increased since the beginning of the AIDS epidemic.[27] Nonetheless, the clinical manifestations of pulmonary infection caused by these organisms may differ from those in other hosts, even patients who have other forms of immunodeficiency.

### Nontuberculous Bacteria

Bacterial pneumonia is more frequent in HIV-positive patients than in seronegative controls, the risk being highest

### Table 44–1. PULMONARY MANIFESTATIONS OF ACQUIRED IMMUNODEFICIENCY SYNDROME

| CONDITION | SELECTED REFERENCES | CONDITION | SELECTED REFERENCES |
|---|---|---|---|
| *Infections* | | *Neoplasia* | |
| **Bacteria** | | Kaposi's sarcoma | 477, 478 |
| *Streptococcus pneumoniae* | 32 | Non-Hodgkin's lymphoma | 526, 565 |
| *Haemophilus influenzae* | 30, 35 | Hodgkin's disease | 478, 545, 597 |
| *Staphylococcus aureus* | 38 | Pulmonary carcinoma | 544 |
| *Legionella* species | 39, 40 | Smooth muscle neoplasms | 596 |
| *Pseudomonas aeruginosa* | 29, 41, 42 | *Miscellaneous Conditions* | |
| *Rhodococcus equi* | 30, 45 | | |
| *Nocardia* species | 29 | Nonspecific interstitial pneumonitis | 553 |
| *Streptococcus agalactiae* | 30 | Lymphocytic interstitial pneumonitis | 569 |
| Enterobacteriaceae | 30 | Lymphocytic alveolitis | 570 |
| *Moraxella catarrhalis* | 28 | "Primary" pulmonary hypertension | 576 |
| *Treponema pallidum* | 581 | Pulmonary alveolar proteinosis | 578, 580 |
| *Pasteurella multocida* | 582 | Diffuse alveolar hemorrhage | 608 |
| *Salmonella* species | 583 | Respiratory muscle dysfunction | 598 |
| *Mycobacterium tuberculosis* | 78 | Sarcoidosis | 599, 600 |
| *Mycobacterium avium–intracellulare* complex | 169, 182 | Bronchiolitis obliterans organizing pneumonia | 601 |
| *Mycobacterium kansasii* | 188 | Drug reaction | 602 |
| *Mycobacterium gordonae* | 584, 585 | Emphysema-like changes | 603, 604 |
| *Mycobacterium xenopi* | 586, 587 | Lymphocytic bronchiolitis | 605 |
| *Mycobacterium celatum* | 187, 588 | Bronchiectasis | 606 |
| *Mycobacterium haemophilum* | 75 | Pulmonary edema secondary to AIDS-related cardiac disease | 609 |
| *Mycobacterium simiae* | 187, 589 | | |
| *Mycobacterium fortuitum* | 187 | | |
| *Mycobacterium genavense* | 187, 590 | | |
| **Fungi** | | | |
| *Pneumocystis carinii* | 200–202 | | |
| *Cryptococcus* species | 192 | | |
| *Histoplasma capsulatum* | 413 | | |
| *Coccidioides immitis* | 420 | | |
| *Blastomyces dermatitidis* | 422 | | |
| *Aspergillus* species | 401 | | |
| *Sporothrix schenckii* | 591 | | |
| *Paracoccidioides brasiliensis* | 401, 401a | | |
| *Mucorales* species | 401 | | |
| *Penicillium marneffei* | 592 | | |
| **Viruses** | | | |
| Primary human immunodeficiency virus pneumonia | 442 | | |
| Cytomegalovirus | 593 | | |
| Adenovirus | 436 | | |
| Varicella | 593a | | |
| Vaccine-associated measles virus | 607 | | |
| **Parasites** | | | |
| *Toxoplasma* species | 463 | | |
| *Strongyloides stercoralis* | 369, 468 | | |
| Cryptosporidia | 471 | | |
| Microsporidia | 594 | | |
| Platyhelminths | 595 | | |

among those whose CD4 lymphocyte counts are lower than 200/μl.[28] For example, in a multicenter, prospective study of 1,130 HIV-positive and 167 HIV-negative adults followed for up to 64 months, the rate of bacterial pneumonia was 5.5 per 100 person-years in the former group and only 0.9 per 100 person-years in the latter.[28] Among those who had CD4 lymphocyte counts below 200 cells/μl, the rate was 10.8 per 100 person-years, compared with 2.3 for infected individuals who had counts greater than 500 cells/μl. The impact of this increased risk is substantial: in many centers, bacterial pneumonia is the most common cause of infection requiring hospitalization in patients who have AIDS.[29] Intravenous drug users are at particular risk; in this population, pneumonia rates are more than double those of other patients

who have HIV infection, after controlling for baseline CD4 lymphocyte count.[28] As might be expected, bacterial pneumonia is also the most common pulmonary abnormality at autopsy.[28a]

In addition to a low CD4[+] count, a number of immune deficits have been described in HIV-infected individuals that contribute to the increased risk of bacterial infection.[29–31] B-cell dysfunction, manifested by poor immunization and infection-related antibody response, is prominent.[29, 30] Defects in chemotaxis, phagocytosis, and intracellular killing by monocytes/macrophages and neutrophils are important in explaining susceptibility to certain organisms, such as *Staphylococcus aureus* and encapsulated bacteria.[29, 30] Deficits in local defense, such as depression of specific immunoglobulin A (IgA) at mucosal surfaces, may also contribute to infection risk.[29, 31] In late-stage disease, granulocytopenia related to medication use is not uncommon and is an additional factor accounting for the increased susceptibility to infection by these agents.[30]

Although the clinical and radiologic features of bacterial pneumonia in HIV-infected patients are similar to those in the normal host (see Chapter 26),[30, 31a, 31b] some remarks concerning infections caused by specific organisms are appropriate.

### Streptococcus pneumoniae

*Streptococcus pneumoniae* is the leading cause of bacterial respiratory disease associated with bacteremia among HIV-infected adults.[32] In San Francisco, the rate of pneumococcal bacteremia in patients who have AIDS is more than 100 times that in age-matched populations (9.4 per 1,000 per year, compared with 0.07).[32] In one study of HIV-infected prostitutes in Nairobi, the risk of developing pneumococcal pneumonia with bacteremia was about 18 times that in non–HIV-infected controls (79 of 587, compared with 1 of 132 over a 3-year period of observation);[33] the incidence in these individuals was 42.5 per 1,000 person-years. Recurrent bacteremic pneumococcal pneumonia is also common in this group. In one review, this developed in 20 of 156 patients (13%), compared with 12 of 180 controls (7%);[32] in another study of Kenyan female prostitutes, the recurrence rate was 264 per 1,000 person-years.[33] The organism is also the most common cause of nonbacteremic bacterial pneumonia in HIV-infected patients.[28, 34, 35] The mortality caused by *S. pneumoniae* was 19% (4 of 21 patients), compared with 4% (3 of 69 patients) in one study;[35] however, others have reported a much more favorable prognosis.[29, 33]

### Haemophilus influenzae

*Haemophilus influenzae* is also a relatively common cause of bacterial pneumonia in HIV-infected individuals.[30, 35] For example, in one study of 79 such patients who had bacterial pneumonia and from whom causative organisms were successfully cultured, 12 (15%) had this organism.[28] In another study of 51 patients who had *H. influenzae* pneumonia requiring hospitalization in New York City, more than half were HIV positive.[36] The incidence of *H. influenzae* pneumonia among HIV-infected men 20 to 49 years of age has been estimated at 23 to 41 per 100,000.[29] As with other bacterial pneumonias, the risk of infection increases with increasing immunosuppression.[37]

### Staphylococcus aureus

With some exceptions,[28, 28a] *S. aureus* has not been reported to be a common cause of pneumonia in HIV-infected patients.[29] Although the organism is frequently recovered from the respiratory tract secretions of these patients when they have lung disease, it is pathogenic in only a minority of cases. For example, in one investigation of 129 consecutive patients who had respiratory tract disease, the organism was recovered from 30 (23%);[38] however, it was thought to be responsible for pneumonia in only 8 (of whom 3 died).

### Legionella Species

*Legionella* species organisms are also infrequent causes of pneumonia.[30] For example, in one series of 237 HIV-infected patients who developed bacterial pneumonia, *Legionella pneumophila* was identified in only 1 patient.[28] In another study, *Legionella* species infection accounted for eight infections among seven patients who had advanced HIV infection (representing only about 2% of the patient population under investigation);[39] the median CD4 lymphocyte count for these patients was 83/μl; half of the infections were nosocomial in origin. Although *L. pneumophila* is the most common species identified, other species are occasionally responsible.[40] Concomitant infection with *P. carinii* or mycobacteria is common.[29]

### Pseudomonas aeruginosa

Except at autopsy,[28a] *Pseudomonas aeruginosa* is another uncommon cause of acute bacterial pneumonia in HIV-infected patients.[29, 41] A number of risk factors have been described, including steroid use, myelosuppressive therapy, neutropenia, and indwelling central venous catheters.[29] Although usually nosocomial in origin and relatively acute in onset, infection may be indolent.[42] In a retrospective review of 1,852 adults followed at a university-based outpatient AIDS clinic, 16 individuals were identified who had *Pseudomonas* species lung infection;[42] all had CD4 lymphocyte counts of 25/ml or less. In 12 of these patients, the infection was indolent and appeared to be acquired, resembling that seen in cystic fibrosis. This form of disease occurred in the absence of other recognized risk factors and was initially associated with a low mortality rate; however, the relapse rate was high, and the median survival was only 4.5 months.

### Rhodococcus equi

*R. equi (Corynebacterium equi)* is a common pulmonary pathogen in foals and is being increasingly recognized in humans. Infection is most frequent in immunocompromised individuals, particularly in patients who have AIDS;[43, 44] in fact, the identification of the organism should prompt consideration of concomitant HIV infection.[30] Interestingly, immunosuppression appears to be associated with localization of disease to the lungs; in one review of 72 patients, 52 of 62 (84%) who were immunocompromised had pulmonary disease, as opposed to only 3 of 10 (30%) of those who were immunocompetent.[44] The organism is a normal inhabitant of soil, and it is believed that infection occurs from this site by inhalation. Risk factors for infection include exposure to farm dust or horses or cohabitation with an infected individual.[45]

The organism is a facultative intracellular aerobic bacterium that may be coccoid or have a long, curved, clubbed shape.[43, 44] It is gram positive and variably acid fast and is considered to be intermediate between fast-growing nontuberculous *Mycobacterium* and *Nocardia* species. In the lungs, it is commonly present in alveolar macrophages, within which it appears to be able to survive and replicate;[46] in fact, virulence of different strains is partly dependent on this ability. Initial attachment to the macrophage surface requires complement and is mediated by leukocyte complement receptor.[47] There is evidence from a number of experimental investigations that pathogenicity is also related to bacterial infection by specific plasmids.[48, 49] As might be expected, adequate T cell function, particularly by CD8+ cells, is an important host factor in determining bacterial clearance.[50]

Pathologic findings typically consist of an ill-defined area of consolidation, sometimes with a central cavity. Microscopically, affected lung is usually destroyed and replaced by an inflammatory infiltrate composed of neutrophils and numerous macrophages[51, 52] (Fig. 44–3). The latter have abundant, foamy, or granular cytoplasm that typically contains numerous gram-positive bacilli. A substantial number of cases also have intracytoplasmic Michaelis-Gutmann bodies, characteristic of malakoplakia (*see* page 724).[52–55] Occasionally, the macrophages blend imperceptibly with a population of spindle-shaped cells organized in fascicles, simulating a mesenchymal neoplasm (*see* Fig. 44–3).

Radiologic manifestations usually consist of a round opacity or area of consolidation limited to one lobe, most commonly an upper lobe.[54] Several opacities may coalesce and undergo cavitation with a fluid level.[56, 57] Pleural effusion is present in about 20% of patients. In most cases, the abnormality persists for more than 1 month despite antibiotic therapy.

Pulmonary disease is usually insidious in onset and characterized by fever, malaise, productive cough, and pleuritic chest pain.[29, 43] Some patients have evidence of extrathoracic involvement at the time of presentation, most often affecting the eye, subcutaneous tissue, central nervous system (CNS), and lymph nodes. Pericardial involvement may be complicated by tamponade.[58] Necrotizing mediastinitis may also be seen.

The organism can frequently be isolated from the blood.[43] It is easily cultured on nonselective media but can

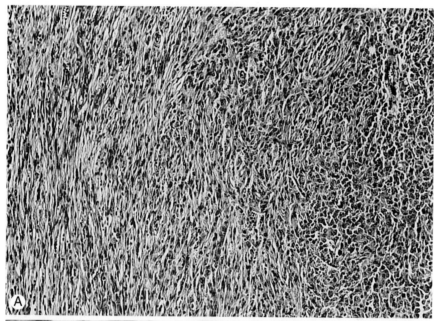

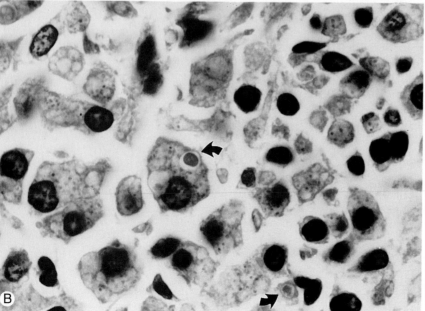

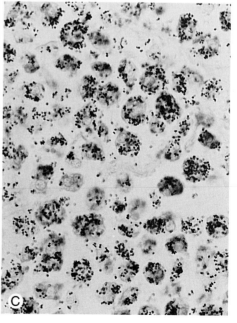

**Figure 44–3. Rhodococcosis.** A section from an ill-defined upper lobe nodule in a patient with AIDS *(A)* shows numerous oval histiocyte-like cells on the right and spindle cells on the left. A magnified view of the histiocytes *(B)* shows them to have coarsely vacuolated cytoplasm containing scattered small dots that represent bacteria. Several Michaelis-Gutmann bodies suggestive of malakoplakia are evident *(arrows)*. Gram stain *(C)* reveals numerous intracytoplasmic bacteria. *(A,* ×100; *B,* ×1300; *C,* ×600.)

be mistaken for contaminating diphtheroids.[29] Because it may be acid fast, it also can be misinterpreted as a species of *Mycobacterium*, particularly in the setting of a cavitated upper lobe mass. The bacterium has been identified cytologically in specimens derived by bronchoalveolar lavage (BAL), bronchial brushing, and transthoracic needle aspiration[59–61] and in tissue obtained from biopsy of an endobronchial mass.[62]

Rhodococcal infection is a serious disease in immunocompromised patients; in one review of six patients who had AIDS, it was considered to be fatal in four.[44] Chronic disease is not uncommon; in the four patients who died in this series, the times to death were 4, 9, 14, and 21 months.[44]

### *Bartonella henselae* and *Bartonella quintana*

*Bartonella (Rochalimaea) henselae* and *Bartonella quintana* are the causative agents of bacillary angiomatosis, a reactive vasoproliferative lesion that occurs almost exclusively in patients who have AIDS.[63–65] The organisms are fastidious gram-negative bacilli that can be seen to have a characteristic trilaminar wall on electron microscopy.[63–65] The mode of transmission is not known; however, because *B. henselae* is the most common cause of cat-scratch disease,[63, 66] it is likely that it involves animal or insect vectors.

The foci of vascular proliferation may affect many tissues, including the skin, bone, brain, and a variety of viscera.[63–67] Intrathoracic manifestations include polypoid endobronchial lesions, pulmonary parenchymal nodules or masses, mediastinal lymph node enlargement, and pleural effusions.[65, 68–71] The typical skin lesions bleed easily and are polypoid, well-circumscribed, tender, and erythematous.[64–67]

However, some are violaceous in color and less well defined, resembling KS; in fact, in one series of nine patients, they were initially misdiagnosed as KS in six.[65] Histologic features are those of a proliferation of capillary-like vessels associated with plump endothelial cells.[72] Neutrophils and clumps of eosinophilic or amphophilic material formed by aggregated bacilli may be seen in the interstitial tissue between the vessels. Spindle cells are present in some cases and may make the distinction from KS difficult.[73] Organisms can be identified by Warthin-Starry stain or immunohistochemical analysis.

In a review of the radiologic findings in nine patients, eight had lung nodules measuring between 1 mm and 1.5 cm in diameter.[65] The nodules had smooth margins and either well- or ill-defined borders; they had a propensity to be located adjacent to vascular structures.[65] One patient presented with a 6-cm peripheral mass that invaded the adjacent chest wall and showed marked enhancement after intravenous administration of contrast[70] (Fig. 44–4). Most patients have hilar or mediastinal lymph node enlargement;[65] evidence of intra-abdominal lymph node involvement is also common. The enlarged nodes show marked enhancement after intravenous administration of contrast.[65] Pleural effusions are often large. Less common findings include enhancing soft tissue masses in the skin and low-attenuation lesions in the liver or spleen.[65]

Symptoms include fever, chills, night sweats, weight loss, anemia, and (occasionally) hemoptysis or chest pain.[65, 67, 69, 70] Lymphadenopathy in the axilla, neck, or groin is common.[65] Patients usually respond rapidly to appropriate antibiotic therapy; however, if untreated, they may die of overwhelming infection.[65]

**Figure 44–4. Bacillary Angiomatosis.** A 26-year-old woman who had AIDS presented with chest pain, low-grade fever, and weight loss. The chest radiograph demonstrated a mass in the right lung. A CT scan *(A)* shows a peripheral right lower lobe mass that is invading the chest wall. A scan taken after intravenous administration of contrast *(B)* demonstrates marked heterogeneous enhancement of the mass. Histologic assessment showed features of bacillary angiomatosis. (From Coche E, Beigelman C, Lucidarme O, et al: Thoracic bacillary angiomatosis in a patient with AIDS. Am J Roentgenol 165:56, 1995. Courtesy of Dr. Philippe Grenier, Hôpital Pitie-Salpétrière, Paris, France.)

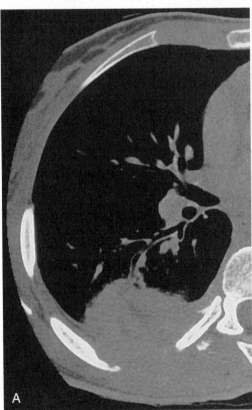
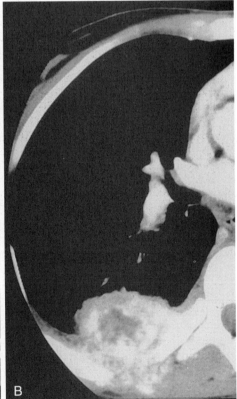

### Nocardia asteroides

The clinical presentation of lung infection related to *Nocardia asteroides* is similar to that of *R. equi*. The duration of symptoms has varied from 1 to 6 months before diagnosis. Although infection is frequently disseminated, the disease presents radiographically in the lung as lobar or multilobar areas of air-space opacification in more than half of affected patients.[29] The upper lobes are most commonly affected, and areas of cavitation are typical. Unusual radiologic manifestations include solitary masses, a reticulonodular pattern, and pleural effusion.[74] Culture of the organism from sputum or BAL fluid is definitive for the diagnosis; however, the organism may take up to 4 weeks to grow. Identification of typical slender branching filaments on Gram stain of sputum or BAL fluid should also suggest the diagnosis.

## Mycobacteria

### Mycobacterium tuberculosis

For a variety of reasons, *M. tuberculosis* can be considered the most important "opportunistic" organism in patients infected with HIV. HIV infection is a major factor in the increasing prevalence and incidence of tuberculosis worldwide.[75] Tuberculosis is the only HIV-related infection that is transmissible to the normal host; it is also both preventable and curable.[75] Patients who are infected with both HIV and *M. tuberculosis* are at high risk of developing active tuberculosis. In some HIV-infected groups, such as those in sub-Saharan Africa,[76] the prevalence of tuberculous infection is high; as a result, tuberculosis control measures in many countries are being overwhelmed.[75] Finally, there is evidence that tuberculosis accelerates the course of HIV disease.[75]

#### Epidemiology

Until 1984, the incidence of tuberculosis in the United States had been declining.[77] Between 1985 and 1991, however, about 39,000 more cases were estimated to occur than would have been expected had historical rates of decline continued unabated.[77] A number of observations supported the hypothesis that this unexpected increase in tuberculosis was at least partly related to the increase in HIV infection that was being observed at the same time.[78] For example, areas of the United States that had the largest increase in tuberculosis incidence had parallel increases in AIDS prevalence; moreover, groups that had the highest prevalence of AIDS also had the highest increase in incidence of tuberculosis. Extrapulmonary tuberculosis, which commonly develops in patients who have AIDS, had shown a much larger increase in incidence than had pulmonary tuberculosis. The incidence of tuberculosis in patients who had AIDS was also found to be about 500 times that of the normal population; in addition, there was evidence that 8% *per year* of HIV-infected people who had positive tuberculin skin test results developed tuberculosis.[79] An examination of AIDS and tuberculosis registries of the Centers for Disease Control and Prevention in Atlanta, Georgia, showed that the percentage of tuberculosis cases that matched with an AIDS case increased steadily from 1981 to 1990 (from 0.1% to 9.5%).[80] On the basis of these observations, it was estimated that at least 30% of excess tuberculosis cases in the United States could be accounted for by coexisting HIV infection.

Worldwide, a high and increasing prevalence of HIV infection has been found in patients who have tuberculosis. Figures have been particularly concerning in the sub-Saharan region of Africa.[81, 82] For example, the prevalence of HIV seropositivity among more than 400 patients hospitalized for tuberculosis in Kinshasa, Democratic Republic of Congo, between 1985 and 1987 was about 40%.[83] Among 158 patients who had new-onset thoracic tuberculosis in Burundi in the early 1990s, 105 (66%) were HIV positive.[84] In one study of 59 consecutive patients who had pulmonary tuberculosis over a 17-month period in a single department of internal medicine in Rwanda, 48 (81%) were HIV positive.[85] In another investigation of 237 patients hospitalized for acute respiratory illness and studied prospectively in Tanzania, tuberculosis was diagnosed in 182;[86] more than half were HIV seropositive.

Although the prevalence of HIV infection in patients who have tuberculosis in "developed" countries is less than in the sub-Saharan region, it is still impressive. For example, in one investigation of 500 patients who had pulmonary tuberculosis in Los Angeles, 25% of the men and 4% of the women who were tested proved to be HIV seropositive.[87] Although the prevalence of seropositivity was much higher in those patients who had obvious risk factors for HIV infection (46% of men and 12% of women), HIV was detected unexpectedly in about 7% of patients who were not thought to be at risk for infection by the virus. In another study of 183 patients who required hospitalization for tuberculosis (because of serious illness, doubtful compliance with medical advice, or homelessness) and who had no previous history of HIV infection, 33 (18%) were discovered to be coinfected with HIV.[88]

Tuberculosis has also been found to be a frequent complication of HIV infection, especially in populations in which the prevalence of infection with *M. tuberculosis* is high. For example, in an investigation of 249 HIV-positive women in Kinshasa who were followed prospectively for 32 months, 19 (almost 8%) developed tuberculosis (3.1 cases per 100 person-years), compared with 0.3% (0.12 cases per 100 person-years) of seronegative control patients.[89] In another prospective study of 460 HIV-positive and 998 HIV-negative Rwandan women, the rate ratio for development of tuberculosis in the HIV-positive group was 22.[90] In Haiti, the odds ratio for developing tuberculosis was about 16 times greater for HIV-positive patients 20 to 39 years old than for HIV-negative controls.[91] It has been estimated that 30% to 60% of adults living in "developing" countries are infected with *M. tuberculosis;*[76] the implications of infection with HIV in this context are obvious.

A similar magnitude of increased risk for the development of tuberculosis in HIV-positive patients has been described in the United States, despite the fact that tuberculosis is less prevalent.[27, 79, 92, 93] In 1995, the annual incidence of tuberculosis in the United States was 8.7 per 100,000 persons.[92] By contrast, in a study of 1,130 HIV-positive patients followed prospectively for a median of 53 months, 31 developed tuberculosis (0.7 cases per 100 person-years, a relative risk almost 100 times that of the general population);[92] the incidence was higher in the eastern United States and in patients who had more severe immunosuppression and who tested positive for purified protein derivative (PPD) at entry into the study.

The risk of developing tuberculosis in HIV-positive patients is partly confounded by other risk factors for tuberculosis, which are also more common in seropositive patients, such as homelessness, drug abuse, and incarceration in prison.[94–97] In one study, the rates of infection with *M. tuberculosis*, as manifested by a positive PPD test result, were similar in 217 HIV-positive drug users enrolled in a methadone maintenance program in New York City and 303 HIV-negative addicts.[79] However, tuberculosis developed in 8 of the seropositive subjects and in none of those who were seronegative during the period of observation. The risk of developing active disease was largely confined to individuals who were PPD positive at entry into the study (rate ratio, 24). Similar results were reported in intravenous drug users in San Francisco, where the risk of developing tuberculosis was more than 10 times greater in HIV-seropositive addicts who had a positive PPD test result than in those who were PPD negative at the beginning of the observation period.[98]

Although the results of the New York study cited previously showed that most of the new cases of tuberculosis appeared to be the result of reactivation of latent infection,[79] new infection has been important in some populations.[99, 100] For example, using DNA fingerprinting of *M. tuberculosis* isolates, more than one third of the incident cases of tuberculosis in San Francisco and New York have been found to be related to recently transmitted infection;[99, 100] the phenomenon was noted in both HIV-seronegative patients and in patients who had AIDS. Nosocomial transmission of tuberculosis,[101–106] including outbreaks of multidrug-resistant organisms,[101, 102, 105, 106] has also been well described in HIV-infected patients; the use of aerosolized pentamidine has been related to such infection.[101–105]

### Pathogenesis

Because the development of tuberculosis after infection by *M. tuberculosis* is largely dependent on a CD4 lymphocyte–mediated increase in the ability of macrophages to phagocytose and kill the organisms (*see* page 804),[78] it is not surprising that HIV infection is associated with an increased prevalence of the disease. In addition to progressive depletion and dysfunction of CD4 lymphocytes derived from both the peripheral blood and the lungs of HIV-infected patients who have tuberculosis,[107] HIV infection is associated with a number of defects in macrophage function.[78] Depletion of CD4 cells may also impair defense against mycobacteria by a reduction in activation of cytolytic CD8 lymphocytes and by a blunted antibody response of B lymphocytes.[108] As a result of these effects, patients who have HIV infection are at high risk for both primary infection after exposure to mycobacteria and reactivation or progression of disease, once infected.[78]

There is also some evidence that tuberculosis leads to progression of HIV infection. The disease results in activation of T cells and macrophages, which contain the virus. This leads to the production of tumor necrosis factor-α (TNF-α), a cytokine that induces expression of HIV in latently infected cells.[109] Lysis of macrophages infected with mycobacteria may also disseminate virus to uninfected cells.[108] In one study of BAL fluid specimens obtained from segments of lung involved with active tuberculosis and from segments of relatively normal lung, HIV levels in the former were higher than those in the latter and exceeded levels found in plasma, indicating local viral production;[110] the levels declined with treatment of the mycobacterial infection.

### Radiologic Manifestations

The patterns of abnormality seen in patients who have AIDS differ from the ones seen in those who do not,[111–114] the former having a greater prevalence of lymph node enlargement, lower lobe disease, and extensive parenchymal involvement and a lower prevalence of cavitation[115–118] (Fig. 44–5). For example, in one investigation of 67 HIV-seropositive and 158 HIV-seronegative patients who had smear or culture-positive pulmonary tuberculosis, parenchymal opacities were seen in 56 of the 67 (83%) HIV-positive patients, cavitation in 40 (60%), and pleural effusion in 6 (9%);[117] lymphadenopathy was evident in 46% of patients in whom the hila were not obscured by confluent parenchymal opacities (13 of 28). Of the 158 HIV-negative patients, parenchymal opacities were seen in 156 (99%), cavitation in 136 (87%), and pleural effusion in 19 (12%); lymphadenopathy was evident in 16% of patients in whom the hila were not obscured by confluent parenchymal disease (11 of 70). The chest radiograph was normal in 5 of 67 (7%) HIV-positive patients and in only 1 (0.6%) of 158 HIV-negative patients.

In a second investigation of 67 HIV-positive and 31 HIV-negative patients who had cultures positive for *M. tuberculosis*, findings seen more commonly in the former patients included mediastinal lymphadenopathy (60% versus 23%) and an atypical distribution of parenchymal opacities (55% versus 10%);[113] less common findings included parenchymal opacities characteristic of reactivation tuberculosis (30% versus 77%) and cavitation (18% versus 52%). There was no significant difference in the prevalence of pleural effusion (30% versus 23%) or normal radiographs (3% versus 10%).

As the findings of these studies suggest, there is considerable variation in the reported frequency of the chest radiographic manifestations of tuberculosis in HIV-positive patients. Hilar or mediastinal lymph node enlargement has been reported in 20% to 60% of patients,[117–119] cavitary disease in 0% to 40%,[117–121] atypical distribution (middle or lower lobe predominance) or atypical pattern (diffuse reticulation or miliary nodules) in 40% to 60%,[113, 117–119, 122] and pleural effusion in 10% to 40%.[113, 117–119] Normal radiographs have been documented in 3% to 15% of cases.[113, 123–127] The prevalence of the various abnormalities is influenced by the country of origin of the patient and by the degree of immunosuppression. For example, cavitation is seen less commonly in patients from the United States than in patients from North and Central Africa.[117, 119, 121, 128] In patients who have relatively normal immune status (greater than 200 CD4 cells/μl), the appearance is generally similar to that seen in postprimary tuberculosis in the normal host (Fig. 44–6); markedly immunosuppressed patients, on the other hand, tend to have a pattern similar to that of primary tuberculosis in the normal host or disseminated disease[115–117, 125, 126] (Fig. 44–7). For example, in one investigation of 97 HIV-positive patients, hilar or mediastinal lymph node enlargement was evident on the chest radiograph in 20 of 58 (34%) patients

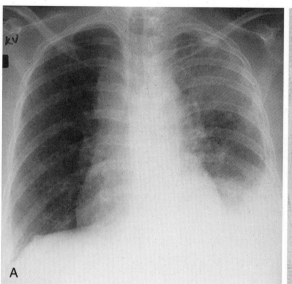

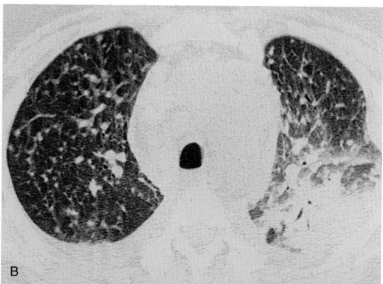

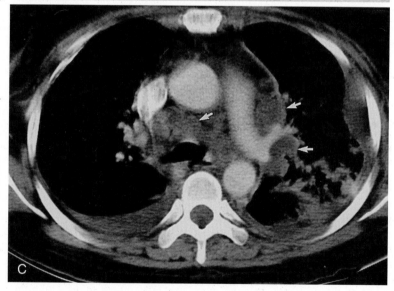

**Figure 44–5. Pulmonary Tuberculosis.** An anteroposterior chest radiograph *(A)* in a 43-year-old man with AIDS demonstrates air-space consolidation in the left upper lobe, miliary nodules, mediastinal lymphadenopathy, and bilateral pleural effusions. An HRCT scan *(B)* demonstrates a focal area of consolidation in the left upper lobe and miliary nodules. A scan following intravenous administration of contrast *(C)* demonstrates extensive left hilar and mediastinal lymphadenopathy *(arrows)* and small bilateral pleural effusions. The enlarged lymph nodes have low attenuation, a common finding in patients who have AIDS and tuberculosis.

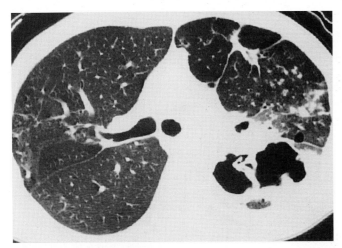

**Figure 44–6. Tuberculosis.** An HRCT scan in a 39-year-old patient with AIDS demonstrates a large cavity in the superior segment of the left lower lobe, localized areas of scarring in the left upper lobe, and focal centrilobular nodules in the left upper and right upper lobes. The findings are characteristic of reactivation tuberculosis with endobronchial spread.

who had CD4 cell counts lower than 200 cells/$\mu$l, compared with 4 of 29 (14%) whose counts were greater than 200 cells/$\mu$l.[116] Patients who have lower cell counts are also more likely to have normal chest radiographs; in one investigation, 10 (21%) of 48 patients who had fewer than 200 CD4 cells/$\mu$l had this finding, compared with only 1 of 20 (5%) patients who had more than 200 CD4 cells/$\mu$l.[125]

The CT findings have been described in several reports.[111, 113, 129–131] The most common abnormality consists of enlarged hilar and mediastinal lymph nodes, typically associated with low attenuation[114, 129, 130] (Fig. 44–8). In one review of 25 patients, extensive node enlargement was present in 23 (92%) and focal hilar lymphadenopathy in 2.[130] In 20 of the 25 (80%), the enlarged nodes had low attenuation; in 5 of these, the periphery showed marked enhancement after intravenous administration of contrast. In another investigation of 29 HIV-positive and 47 HIV-negative patients, the most common abnormalities in the former patients included lymphadenopathy (in 22 [76%]), nodules less than 1 cm in diameter (in 20 [69%]), dense consolidation (in 11 [38%]), and pleural effusion (in 7 [24%]);[131] lymphadenopathy was seen more commonly in HIV-positive than in HIV-negative patients (76% versus 55%). Findings seen less commonly in HIV-positive patients included cavitation (24% versus 49%), 1- to 3-cm-diameter nodules (14% versus 47%), and bronchial wall thickening (14% versus 45%). A linear correlation between the CD4 cell count and the number of lobes involved ($r = 0.84$) and between the CD4 cell count and the number of nodules ($r = 0.97$) was seen in the HIV-positive patients. Those who had more than 200 CD4 cells/$\mu$l were more likely to have cavitation than patients who had lower counts (50% versus 13%) and less likely to have lymphadenopathy (33% versus 70%). Two patients, both with CD4 cell counts of less than 20 cells/$\mu$l, had normal CT scans.

### Clinical Manifestations

The clinical features of tuberculosis in patients who have AIDS vary with the degree of immunosuppression.[75] When immune function is relatively preserved, the manifes-

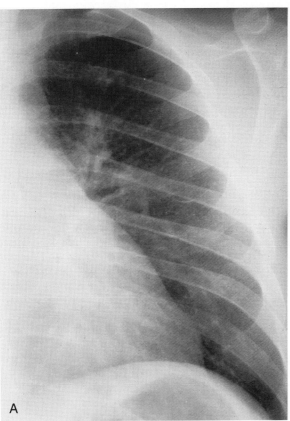

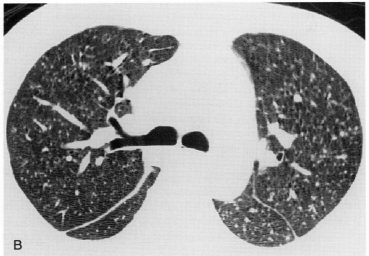

B

**Figure 44–7. Miliary Tuberculosis.** A view of the left lung from a posteroanterior chest radiograph *(A)* in a 35-year-old patient with AIDS shows miliary nodules. An HRCT scan *(B)* shows numerous nodules in a random distribution throughout both lungs; a small right pleural effusion is also evident.

A

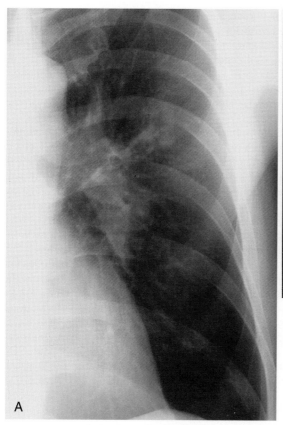

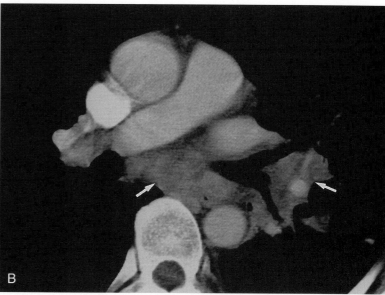

**Figure 44–8. Tuberculosis.** A view of the left lung from a posteroanterior chest radiograph *(A)* in a 45-year-old patient with AIDS demonstrates poorly defined opacities in the left upper lobe and enlargement of the left hilum. A contrast-enhanced CT scan *(B)* demonstrates nonenhancing low-attenuation left hilar and subcarinal lymph nodes *(arrows)*. The diagnosis of tuberculosis was confirmed by sputum culture.

tations tend to be the same as those in patients who are not HIV positive.[75] However, in patients in whom CD4 counts are depressed, the likelihood of atypical features is increased. Extrapulmonary tuberculosis is significantly more common in patients who are infected with HIV than in seronegative patients and is seen in more than 50% at some point in the course of the disease; moreover, it is the sole manifestation of the disease in about one quarter.[132] In one study, extrapulmonary disease was found in 30 of 43 (70%) patients who had CD4 counts of less than 100 cells/$\mu$l and in only 5 of 18 (28%) patients whose CD4 count was higher than 300 cells/$\mu$l.[133] Lymph node involvement, including radiographic evidence of mediastinal adenopathy, is particularly common.[126, 133] Gastrointestinal symptoms, disseminated disease (greater than one noncontiguous extrapulmonary site or a positive culture from blood, bone marrow, or liver biopsy), and miliary disease are also significantly more common in HIV-infected than in seronegative patients.[77, 135] Other unusual clinical manifestations of tuberculosis in HIV-infected patients are abscesses, intra-abdominal lymph node enlargement, and an adult respiratory distress syndrome–like picture.[77, 136, 137]

Coexisting HIV infection also alters the clinical features of tuberculous pleuritis. In one series of 112 patients from Tanzania who had this form of disease, of whom 65 (58%) were HIV positive, disseminated tuberculosis was found more often in HIV-positive than in HIV-negative individuals (30% versus 10%).[138] Dyspnea, fever, fatigue, night sweats, diarrhea, severe tachypnea, hepatomegaly, splenomegaly, and lymphadenopathy were all significantly more common in HIV-positive than in HIV-negative patients. Tuberculosis is

an uncommon cause of pleural effusion in patients with AIDS in North America; however, it is more common as a manifestation of tuberculosis in HIV-infected than in HIV-negative patients.[139] In one study, it was responsible for 5 of 58 (8%) effusions;[140] a large effusion was characteristic of tuberculosis. The complication may be associated with substantial weight loss and lower lobe consolidation.[139] Compared with HIV-negative patients who have pleural tuberculosis, disease in seropositive patients is more often associated with evidence of a greater burden of microorganisms; thus, organisms are more likely to be demonstrated in specimens of pleural tissue and in sputum.[141]

### Diagnosis

Significant obstacles hinder a rapid diagnosis of tuberculosis in patients who are HIV positive. The symptoms are nonspecific, the radiographic manifestations are often atypical, and infection is frequently extrapulmonary. Therefore, a high index of suspicion is the first diagnostic step, especially in patients who are at increased risk for developing the disease. These include intravenous drug abusers, the homeless, prisoners, and immigrants from areas where tuberculosis is endemic, patients in whom the tuberculin skin test is positive, and individuals who have had recent exposure to a person with active disease.[136, 142, 143] Even when radiographic and clinical manifestations are typical, the inability to obtain adequate material for culture and smear is a common cause of failure to make the diagnosis.[144]

**Tuberculin Skin Testing.** Tuberculin skin testing is of only modest value in the diagnosis. As discussed previously, there is no doubt that seropositive PPD reactors are at high risk for developing active disease. However, the prevalence of tuberculin reactivity varies directly with the absolute CD4 lymphocyte count, whereas the prevalence of anergy to a common battery of skin test antigens varies inversely.[145] Therefore, skin test negativity in patients who have advanced degrees of immunosuppression has poor negative predictive value for the presence of infection. Overall, only about 40% to 55% of HIV-infected patients who have tuberculosis show a positive PPD reaction.[146] As a result of these observations, it has been recommended that a cutaneous induration of 5 mm be considered positive in patients who are HIV seropositive.[75] However, some investigators have found evidence that this practice may be inappropriate;[147] in a study of 444 patients, seropositive drug users were somewhat less likely to be PPD positive (24 of 160 [15%]) than seronegative drug users (68 of 284 [24%]); the median induration size was the same *among reactors* in both groups.

Whether anergic HIV-infected patients are also at high risk for developing tuberculosis is another matter. In one study, the incidence of active tuberculosis was 10.4 per 100 patient-years in PPD-positive patients infected with HIV and 12.4 per 100 person-years in anergic patients;[148] these results were not significantly different. Among the anergic patients, the risk seemed to be confined to those known to be at high risk for developing the disease, that is, in intravenous drug abusers rather than homosexual men. Anergy was seldom noted when the CD4 lymphocyte count was greater than 500 cells/μl,[148] suggesting that a negative test result in such patients is likely to be a true negative. In a second study of 68 anergic HIV-positive drug addicts, 5 (7.6%, or 6.6 cases per 100 person-years) developed active tuberculosis during a 31-month period of observation.[149] This rate was similar to that observed among HIV-positive, tuberculin-positive drug addicts; by contrast, no cases of active tuberculosis were seen among 52 anergic, seronegative addicts.

Two-stage tuberculin skin testing has also been examined in HIV-infected patients;[150, 151] its value is likely to depend on the prevalence of tuberculosis in the population tested. In a study of 709 HIV-seropositive patients from Richmond, Virginia, only 18 (2.7%) demonstrated a booster effect (defined as an increase in induration from less than 5-mm diameter to one greater than 5-mm diameter on sequential PPD testing).[150] By contrast, 17 of 59 (29%) Ugandan HIV-seropositive patients had a boosted response;[151] when examined by multiple logistic regression, such responses were independently associated with a CD4 count between 200 and 500 cells/μl and with better nutritional status.

**Bacteriology.** The prevalence of positive sputum smears and culture is about the same in HIV-infected and uninfected patients who have pulmonary tuberculosis.[152] Overall, about 60% to 70% of such patients have a positive smear.[152, 153] Even in the setting of a high prevalence of *M. avium–intracellulare* infection, the finding of a positive sputum smear for acid-fast organisms has diagnostic value;[154] in one study, the positive predictive value for tuberculosis of a positive smear was 92% for expectorated sputum, 71% for induced sputum, and 71% for BAL specimens.[154]

When it cannot be produced, sputum induction with aerosolized saline and bronchoscopy with lavage can be of value.[136] Occasionally, specimens obtained by transbronchial or bronchial biopsy[136, 155] or transbronchial needle aspiration[155a] are diagnostic. Care should be taken to avoid nosocomial transmission of infection during the performance of these examinations.[156] Obviously, specimens from other sites in patients suspected of having tuberculosis should also be examined for mycobacteria by smear and culture;[75] infection may be identified in affected lymph nodes by aspiration in about 65% to 90% of patients[78] as well as in specimens of bone marrow, urine, and blood.[75]

### Prognosis and Natural History

Tuberculosis is an important cause of death among patients who have AIDS.[157] Although most patients in whom the infection is recognized and treated by effective drug therapy do well,[157] the disease may be recognized only at autopsy or may progress as a result of noncompliance with therapy or resistance of the organism to drugs.[157–160]

In an investigation of 132 patients in San Francisco who had AIDS and tuberculosis between 1981 and 1988 (before the inclusion of pulmonary tuberculosis as an AIDS-defining illness), the latter was recognized only at death in 7 patients.[157] The median survival of the 125 treated patients after the diagnosis of tuberculosis was 16 months. Tuberculosis was considered to be a major contributor to death in 5 of the 7 untreated patients and in 8 of the 125 treated patients. Most of the attributable deaths occurred within 1 month of initiation of therapy. In another study from Kenya, the mortality within 6 months of initiation of antituberculous therapy among HIV-infected patients was higher than that in seronegative patients (rate ratio, 3.8).[161] Although most of the excess mortality occurred after the first month of therapy and was not the result of tuberculosis, there was also an increased mortality of HIV-positive patients who received suboptimal therapy compared with HIV-negative patients. In a third investigation from the Democratic Republic of Congo, the mortality in 170 HIV-seropositive patients who had tuberculosis was compared with that in an identically treated group of 597 HIV-seronegative patients;[162] 1 year after the diagnosis of tuberculosis, more than 30% of the former patients had died, compared with only 4% of the latter. Although partly related to other manifestations of AIDS, the relapse rate of tuberculosis among HIV-positive patients was almost three-fold that among the HIV-negative patients.

Although the high mortality rate of patients who have AIDS and tuberculosis is in large part directly related to their degree of immunosuppression,[163] there is evidence that infection with *M. tuberculosis* adversely affects the course of HIV infection. In a retrospective cohort study conducted at four American medical centers, 106 HIV-seropositive patients who had active tuberculosis were compared with 106 seropositive patients who did not.[164] Active tuberculosis was associated with an increased risk of death (odds ratio > 2.0) after controlling for age, intravenous drug use, previous opportunistic infection, baseline CD4 count, and antiretroviral therapy. This reduced survival was seen even after excluding from the analysis patients who had early death due to tuberculosis. Although the development of tuberculosis may be a better indicator of more advanced immunosuppression among HIV-infected patients than is the CD4 lymphocyte count, the data are also consistent with the hypothesis that tuberculosis accelerates the clinical course of HIV infection.

HIV infection has also been associated with a high prevalence of multidrug-resistant (MDR) tuberculosis.[158] In some studies in the New York City area, such infection has been found in almost 20% of HIV-infected patients and 5% of seronegative patients.[158] This phenomenon is likely related to a more rapid progression to active disease among HIV-infected patients after infection with MDR organisms,[165, 166] which are prevalent in their milieu. MDR tuberculosis is difficult to treat, and mortality is high. For example, in one study of 171 treated patients who had the disease (most were not infected with HIV), 63 (37%) died, most from tuberculosis.[159] In another group of 62 HIV-infected patients who developed tuberculosis resistant to two or more standard antituberculous drugs, almost all died (median survival, 2.1 months);[167] this compares with a median survival of 14.6 months among 55 HIV-infected patients who had been treated for drug-sensitive tuberculosis.

### *Mycobacterium avium–intracellulare* Complex

Disseminated infection by organisms of the *M. avium–intracellulare* complex (MAC) is the most common systemic bacterial infection in patients who have AIDS, occurring in up to 50% of affected individuals.[75, 168] In the absence of prophylactic therapy, the incidence of bacteremia is approximately 20% at 1 year and 40% at 2 years following a

diagnosis of AIDS.[134] Most patients have an advanced degree of immunosuppression, with CD4 lymphocyte counts of less than 50 cells/$\mu$l.[75] Clinical findings are nonspecific. Persistent fever and fatigue are the most common symptoms; night sweats, anorexia, chronic abdominal pain, and diarrhea are present occasionally.[75, 169] Patients are often cachectic, and hepatosplenomegaly with lymphadenopathy may be seen. Anemia may be severe and is the most common laboratory abnormality.[75, 169]

The histologic reaction to the MAC organisms is unusual in that granulomatous inflammation and necrosis are typically absent; the usual finding is that of aggregates of macrophages "stuffed" with organisms[170–172] (Fig. 44–9). This reaction is seen most often in lymph nodes, which may be significantly enlarged as a result of the accumulation of the macrophages. It can also be seen in the lung parenchyma, in some cases associated with fibrosis (Fig. 44–10). The organism is somewhat smaller than most other mycobacteria and may be more difficult to recognize on smears; organisms within macrophages stain with periodic acid–Schiff as well as with acid-fast stains.[173] They can be identified more precisely by immunofluorescent or polymerase chain reaction (PCR) techniques.[174]

The radiographic and CT findings resemble those of tuberculosis and include focal areas of air-space consolidation, nodules, and mediastinal lymph node enlargement[175–179]

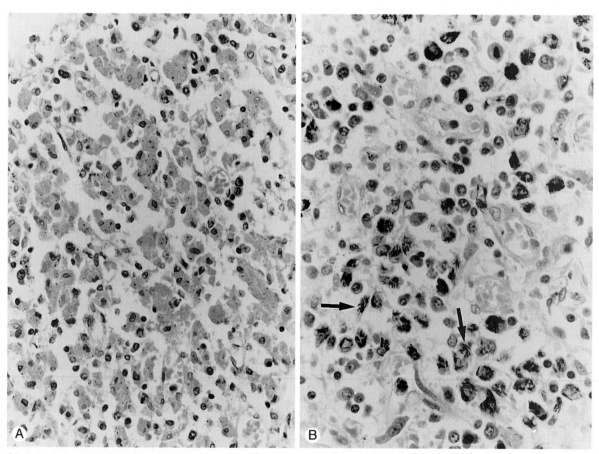

**Figure 44–9.** *Mycobacterium avium–intracellulare* **Complex: Lymph Node Infection.** A magnified view of a mediastinal lymph node that measured 2 cm in its long axis *(A)* shows effacement of normal nodal structure by a population of macrophages with abundant cytoplasm. A Ziehl-Neelsen stain *(B)* shows these cells to contain numerous acid-fast bacilli *(black* in this illustration); the organisms are so abundant that their elongated nature can only be appreciated in occasional cells *(arrows)*.

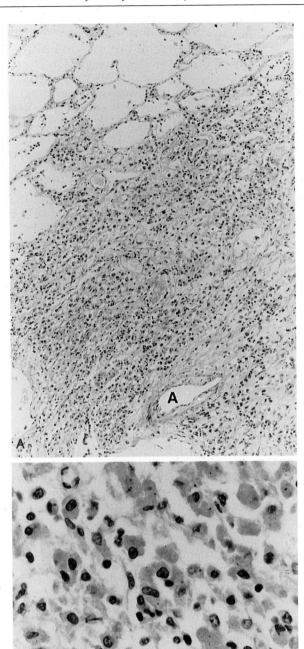

**Figure 44–10.** *Mycobacterium–intracellulare* Complex: Pulmonary Fibrosis. A section through an ill-defined area of parenchymal consolidation shows expansion of the interstitial tissue next to a small vessel *(A)*; some of the adjacent alveolar septa are also involved. The infiltrate is composed of macrophages, lymphocytes, and loose fibrous tissue; the macrophages are focally aggregated and have an appearance typical of *M. avium–intracellulare* infection *(B)*.

(Fig. 44–11). One group studied 53 patients who had AIDS and culture-proven pulmonary disease (29 with *M. tuberculosis*, 20 with MAC, and 4 with other nontuberculous species);[178] only patients who were free of concurrent infection and whose symptoms improved after appropriate mycobacterial therapy alone were included. The most common abnor-

malities were small nodules (usually centrilobular, in 15 patients), areas of ground-glass attenuation (in 11), and enlarged mediastinal lymph nodes (in 10). Compared with patients who had tuberculosis, patients who had nontuberculous infection were more likely to have extensive disease or bilateral involvement and less likely to have lymphadenopathy (43% versus 76%). MAC has also been reported as a cause of endobronchial obstruction.[180, 181]

Organisms may be cultured from respiratory tract secretions in patients who have disseminated infection[182] or before the onset of bacteremia.[183] Despite this, radiographically evident pulmonary disease is uncommon;[134, 169] for example, in a study of 48 patients in whom the organism was isolated from respiratory tract specimens, only 2 had lung disease attributed to the organism.[184] Most patients who have abnormal chest radiograph results and positive cultures of sputum or BAL fluid have other explanations for the radiographic findings.[184]

The diagnosis of MAC pulmonary disease is made by culture of respiratory tract secretions in the setting of a compatible radiographic picture for which no other cause can be demonstrated. Such a diagnosis should be followed by a search for evidence of systemic infection.[185] As mentioned previously, a positive acid-fast smear of sputum has a high positive predictive value (92%) for tuberculosis, even in populations in which MAC is more prevalent than *M. tuberculosis*.[154, 186]

### Other Nontuberculous Mycobacteria

Of the many medically significant mycobacterial species other than *M. avium–intracellulare* or *M. tuberculosis*, more than half have caused disease in HIV-infected patients[187] (*see* Table 44–1). Both colonization and infection are more common in the HIV-infected population than in uninfected patients.[187] Although some of the organisms also cause systemic illness or focal disease outside the lung, many have been identified only in the lung.

*Mycobacterium kansasii* can cause pulmonary disease in HIV-infected patients who have advanced degrees of immunosuppression.[188–190] In one investigation of 19 patients, 14 had disease confined to the lungs;[188] 3 had both pulmonary and extrapulmonary disease, and 2 had extrapulmonary infection exclusively. All patients had a CD4 count of less than 200 cells/μl (mean, 49 cells/μl). In another series of 49 HIV-infected patients from whom the organism was isolated, 17 had disseminated disease, and 29 had positive sputum smears;[190] only 1 patient was thought to have colonization without infection. Radiographically, patients had upper lobe interstitial or air-space opacities, diffuse interstitial disease, or thin-walled cavitary lesions.[187, 188] Most patients had fever and cough of at least 2 weeks' duration before diagnosis; sputum production, chest pain, hemoptysis, and night sweats were also evident.[188] Although concurrent infection was found in more than half of the patients, including PCP in 6, the clinical and radiographic presentation of patients who had combined infection did not differ from that of patients who had isolated *M. kansasii* infection. In another study of the radiographic findings in 16 patients who had AIDS and culture-proven *M. kansasii* pulmonary infection, 12 (75%) had areas of consolidation, 3 (19%) had cavitation, 4 (25%) had lymphadenopathy, and 2 (12%) had pleural effusion.[191]

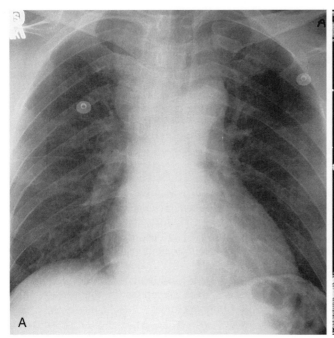
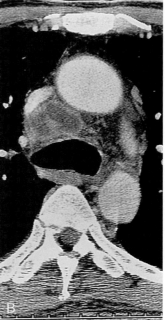

**Figure 44–11.** *Mycobacterium avium–intercellulare.* An anteroposterior chest radiograph *(A)* in a 47-year-old patient with AIDS demonstrates widening of the right superior mediastinum. A contrast-enhanced CT scan *(B)* demonstrates an enlarged right paratracheal lymph node. The enlarged node has central low attenuation and rim enhancement. The patient had culture-proven disseminated *M. avium–intracellulare* complex. (From Kang EY, Staples CA, McGuinness G, et al: Detection and differential diagnosis of pulmonary infections and tumors in patients with AIDS: Value of chest radiography versus CT. Am J Roentgenol 166:15, 1996.)

### Fungi

By far the most important fungus to cause pulmonary disease in patients who are HIV positive is *P. carinii*; however, other organisms account for a significant number of AIDS-defining illnesses,[192, 193] and a variety of additional fungi are occasional causes of infection (*see* Table 44–1). Despite this rather extensive list, with the exception of PCP, pulmonary fungal infections are distinctly uncommon in HIV-infected patients outside geographic areas in which a given fungus is endemic.[194, 195] However, the clinician must be alert to the possibility of fungal pneumonia in patients who have resided in or traveled through such endemic areas.

### *Pneumocystis carinii*

#### Epidemiology

Since the first descriptions of profound immunodeficiency occurring in previously healthy homosexual men in 1981,[196, 197] the histories of AIDS and PCP have been closely associated. From the early 1980s to the early 1990s, the infection had been documented in more than 100,000 Americans, most of whom were also infected with HIV.[198] During this time, PCP occurred in 75% of patients who had AIDS[199] and constituted the most common AIDS-defining diagnosis and the most common cause of life-threatening illness.[200–202]

Coinciding with the increased use of primary and secondary prophylaxis against PCP and of effective antiretroviral therapy in the late 1980s, the incidence of PCP began to decline.[199, 203] For example, among patients in Australia, the cumulative risk of developing PCP in the 2 years after the diagnosis of AIDS was 70% between 1983 and 1987 and 48% between 1991 and 1994.[168] Similarly, about half of infections requiring hospitalization in Toronto early in the AIDS era were caused by *P. carinii*, whereas after management evolved, the figure was only 29%.[204] Among 1,182 HIV-seropositive patients followed prospectively for a 52-month period beginning in 1988 as part of the Pulmonary Complications of HIV Infection Study, only 145 (12%) developed PCP.[205] In fact, the incidence of any of these major opportunistic infections associated with AIDS (PCP, CMV retinitis, and MAC infection) decreased from 21.9 per 100 person-years in 1994 to 3.7 per 100 person-years in 1997;[18] this improvement is largely attributable to the effectiveness of intensive antiretroviral therapy.

Despite the decrease in its incidence, PCP is still an important infection: it is the AIDS-defining illness in 25% of all patients infected with HIV[206] and has been the first opportunistic infection in about 15% of HIV-infected individuals who have received prophylaxis and 45% of those who have not.[199] In two series from the United States, 25% of those admitted to the hospital with the infection died.[207, 208] Infection with *P. carinii* is also a common harbinger of death from AIDS-related illness in the United States; for example, in one investigation of 6,692 patients infected with HIV who were followed from 1990 to 1994, almost 25% of the patients had PCP in the 6 months before death.[209] In other areas of the world, such as Africa, in which the prevalence of tuberculosis in patients who have AIDS is higher, the relative importance of PCP is less; for example, in one series of 53 HIV-seropositive patients who underwent autopsy, PCP accounted for only 9% of the deaths.[210] In another study of 222 seropositive patients admitted to the hospital in Burundi with respiratory tract illness, only 11 (5%) had PCP.[211]

A number of risk factors for PCP have been identified in HIV-seropositive patients. The most important is the degree of immunosuppression, as indicated by the CD4 lymphocyte count.[205, 212, 213] In the Pulmonary Complications of HIV Infection Study, 79% of the 145 patients who developed PCP had CD4 counts of less than 100 cells/μl, and 95% had counts of less than 200 cells/μl.[205] In another review of 1,665 HIV-seropositive patients who were followed prospectively for a 4-year period in the Multi-Center AIDS Cohort Study, the relative risk of developing PCP in the absence of prophylaxis over the initial 6 months was 4.9 in patients whose CD4 count was less than 200 cells/μl compared with those who had higher counts.[205, 213] PCP can also occur during the profound, albeit transient, lymphopenia that can characterize primary HIV infection.[214]

The use of antibiotic prophylaxis substantially affects the risk of developing PCP among HIV-infected patients who have low CD4 lymphocyte counts.[205, 213] For example, in the Pulmonary Complications of HIV Infection Study, the risk within 6 months in patients whose CD4 count was less than 200 cells/μl was ninefold higher in those not receiving prophylaxis, compared to those who received this therapy.[205] For reasons that are unclear, African Americans have less than one third the risk of developing PCP than do white Americans.[205] The presence of constitutional signs and symptoms is associated with an increased risk of developing PCP in patients who have CD4 counts both above[205, 212] and below[213] 200 cells/μl.

## Pathogenesis

The general pathogenetic features of PCP have been discussed previously (*see* page 910); it is worthwhile to discuss briefly the mechanisms by which HIV infection alters host defense against the organism. As already indicated, cell-mediated immune responses mediated by CD4 lymphocytes constitute the primary defense against *P. carinii*.[206] The increased risk of developing PCP with diminishing CD4 counts in human patients as well as in murine models of immunodeficiency and immune reconstitution is clear evidence of this effect.[206]

Alveolar macrophages also have an important role in defense.[215] These cells bind and phagocytose the organisms and subsequently release a variety of inflammatory substances, including reactive oxidants, eicosanoid metabolites, and cytokines;[215] of these, TNF-α appears to play a key role.[216] Immunocompetent mice administered a TNF-α inhibitor gene demonstrate impaired clearance of *P. carinii*;[216] when these animals are made immunodeficient by CD4 depletion, such a regimen leads to more severe and chronic infection. The mechanisms by which TNF-α mediates these effects are unclear, although there is evidence that an increased amount may enhance inflammation and edema.[215] However, the cytokine cannot be detected in cell-free BAL fluid from all immunosuppressed patients who have PCP,[215] and its precise role in human infection is unclear. There is also evidence that alveolar lymphocytes of patients infected with *P. carinii* elaborate greatly increased quantities of HIV compared with HIV-seropositive patients who are not infected;[217] this increase in viral load may be related to the effects of TNF-α.[218]

With the relative failure of immune mechanisms to control the infection, an acute inflammatory reaction associated with neutrophil and eosinophil infiltration may be prominent.[219] Although HIV-infected patients who develop PCP have, on the average, better oxygenation and less BAL neutrophilia than do seronegative patients who have PCP,[220] an increased number of neutrophils in BAL fluid correlates with poorer oxygenation and poorer patient survival.[220] Some investigators have found evidence that the acute inflammatory reaction in the lungs correlates with the number of organisms,[221] whereas others have not.[220]

Humoral immunity has been shown to be a component of host defense in murine models of *P. carinii* infection, and an antibody response has also been documented in human studies.[206] It is possible that antigenic variation in major surface glycoproteins of the organism may allow some strains to escape from humoral host defense.[206] There is also evidence that *P. carinii* is toxic to alveolar epithelial cells at points of adherence and that it inhibits their replication,[219] effects that may contribute to the development of alveolar edema[198] and abnormal surfactant function.[222]

## Pathologic Characteristics

Gross specimens of lung affected by PCP may have an appearance resembling confluent bronchopneumonia (Fig. 44–12) or more extensive consolidation simulating acute airspace pneumonia. Disease typically involves several lobes on both the right and left sides; occasionally, it is limited predominantly to one lobe in either a diffuse or nodular fashion[223–225] (Fig. 44–13), most often in patients who have been treated prophylactically. An endobronchial mass has been described rarely.[226]

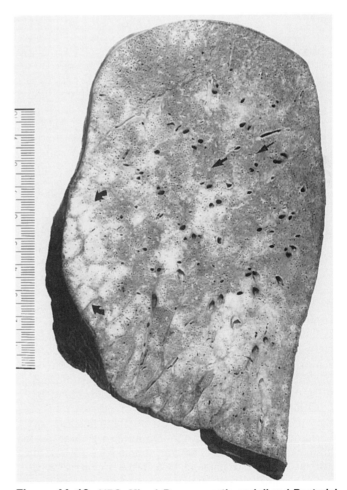

**Figure 44–12. AIDS: Mixed *Pneumocystis carinii* and Bacterial Pneumonia.** A slice of an upper lobe shows multiple foci of consolidation, some minute and relatively evenly spaced (*straight arrows*), consistent with bronchopneumonia, and others involving entire lobules (*curved arrows*). Microscopically, the latter were associated with the presence of *P. carinii* and the former with an unidentified bacterium.

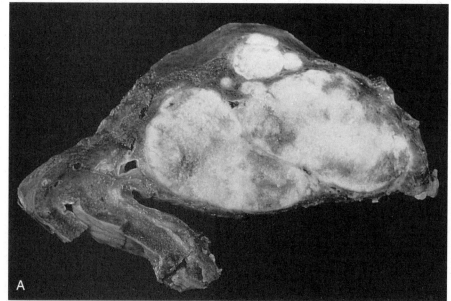

**Figure 44–13. AIDS: Localized (Nodular)** *Pneumocystis carinii* **Infection.** A resected specimen *(A)* shows a multilobulated focus of consolidation associated with several smaller satellite nodules, suggestive of tuberculous or fungal infection. A section of the nodule *(B* and *C)* shows abundant macrophages surrounding finely vacuolated proteinaceous material, which (on Grocott stain) was seen to contain numerous cysts of *Pneumocystis carinii.* The patient had been treated prophylactically with pentamidine. *(A* and *B* from Thurlbeck WM, Churg AM [eds]: Pathology of the Lung, 2nd ed. New York, Thieme Medical Publishers, 1995.)

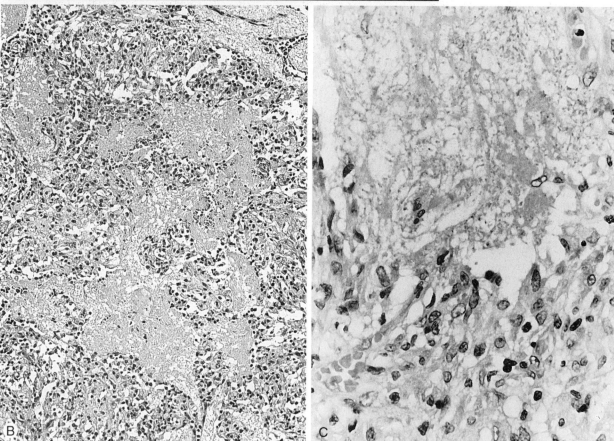

There is considerable variation in the type and severity of histologic findings.[227] The typical case is characterized by alveolar interstitial inflammation, proliferation of type II alveolar epithelial cells, and a finely vacuolated eosinophilic "exudate" within alveolar air spaces[228] (Fig. 44–14). The latter consists of cysts and trophozoites admixed with host-derived material, including surfactant, fibrin, immunoglobulins, and adhesive matrix proteins, such as fibronectin and vitronectin.[229, 230] The amount of intra-alveolar exudate may

be very large, particularly in patients who die with active disease (Fig. 44–15). The alveolar interstitium usually contains lymphocytes and plasma cells; however, in patients who have very low CD4 counts, these may be few in number or absent altogether, the only abnormality being the presence of intra-alveolar cysts (Fig. 44–16). The various histochemical and immunohistochemical techniques that can be used to identify the organisms are discussed in Chapter 28 (*see* page 912).

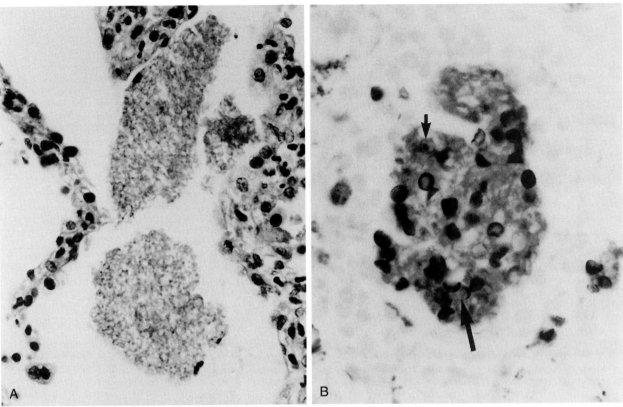

**Figure 44–14.** *Pneumocystis carinii* **Pneumonia.** A magnified view of a transbronchial biopsy specimen *(A)* from a 42-year-old man with AIDS shows mild interstitial thickening due to edema and a mononuclear inflammatory cell infiltrate; two clusters of finely vacuolated proteinaceous material are present within alveolar air spaces. A silver stain of one of these clusters *(B)* shows it to contain multiple round *(short arrow)* or sickle-shaped *(long arrow)* cysts. (*A*, ×440; *B*, Grocott silver methenamine, ×1000.)

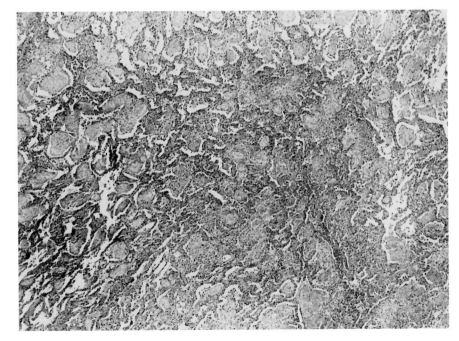

**Figure 44–15. AIDS:** *Pneumocystis carinii* **Pneumonia.** The section shows consolidation of virtually all alveolar air spaces by proteinaceous material that contained numerous *P. carinii* cysts on Grocott stain. The alveolar septa are mildly thickened by a mononuclear inflammatory cell infiltrate. (×40.)

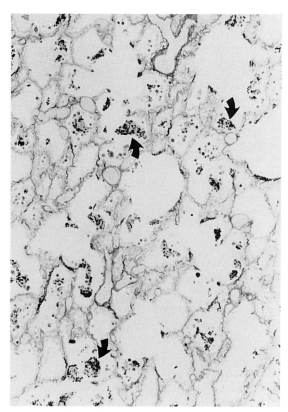

**Figure 44–16. AIDS:** *Pneumocystis carinii* **Infection with Minimal Inflammatory Reaction.** This Grocott stained section shows scattered clusters of *P. carinii* cysts within alveolar airspaces *(arrows)*. The adjacent alveolar walls contain virtually no inflammatory cells. (×80.)

Other histologic findings that may be seen either alone or in association with the typical features include diffuse alveolar damage,[231, 232] granulomatous inflammation (Fig. 44–17) (in which organisms may be few in number and difficult to identify in BAL fluid[233]),[234–236] bronchiolitis obliterans with organizing pneumonia,[227] vascular invasion (Fig. 44–18) (sometimes with vasculitis),[237] parenchymal calcification (*see* Fig. 44–17) (usually associated with prior treatment), necrosis, and cyst formation.[238–240] Pathologic findings in the latter complication are variable: some cases consist of blebs and others of parenchymal cystlike spaces lined by either a thin layer of fibrous tissue or by lung parenchyma consolidated by the foamy exudate of typical *Pneumocystis* species infection.[240] (When considering the diagnosis of parenchymal cystic spaces, it is important to remember that they are occasionally caused by organisms other than *P. carinii* [Fig. 44–19]). There is evidence that the pathogenesis of at least some of the PCP-related cystic spaces is related to tissue invasion by trophozoites followed by necrosis.[241] All these atypical pathologic manifestations are more common in patients who have received prophylactic therapy for *P. carinii* infection.

Although organisms often disappear quickly in tissue sections after therapy in patients who have PCP in the absence of AIDS, such clearing is frequently less rapid and may be absent altogether in patients who are HIV positive.[242, 243] When they are identified in this circumstance, cysts often show morphologic evidence of degeneration.[231]

### Radiologic Manifestations

The reported prevalence of normal radiographs in patients who have proven PCP has ranged from 0% to 39%;[244–248] however, it is generally accepted that the most appropriate estimate is about 10%.[247, 249] The most common radiographic manifestation consists of bilateral and symmetric ground-glass, finely granular or reticular opacities[244–247, 249, 250] (Fig. 44–20). The abnormalities can be diffuse, but often have a perihilar, lower zone predominance;[246, 247, 249, 250] less commonly, there is an upper zone predominance (Fig. 44–21). If left untreated, the opacities usually progress to predominantly perihilar or diffuse air-space consolidation[244] (Fig. 44–22).

The development of air-filled cysts or pneumatoceles (Fig. 44–23) has been reported in about 5% to 35% of patients.[246, 251–253] The cysts can be seen anywhere in the lungs, although they are more common in the upper lobes. They range from 1 to 10 cm in diameter and generally have walls 1 mm or less in thickness.[251–253] They are usually spherical. In one study of 34 patients, the cysts varied from 1 to 5 cm in diameter and were most commonly seen in the upper lung zones;[253] they were multiple in 32 of the 34 patients. Follow-up of the patients who survived the acute episode of pneumonia showed that most cysts completely resolved over a period of 5 days to 1 year (average, 5 months); a small number showed no significant change in the size. Although most pneumatoceles seen in patients who have AIDS are the result of PCP, they may also result from other causes, such as anaerobic bacterial infection (Fig. 44–24).

Pneumothorax occurs in about 5% to 10% of patients.[246, 249, 250, 254–260] Factors associated with the complication include the presence of cysts on the chest radiograph,[228, 257] a history of cigarette smoking,[258] and the use of aerosolized pentamidine.[228, 260] In one investigation, pneumothorax developed in 12 (35%) of the 34 patients who had radiographically evident cysts compared with only 2 (7%) of those who did not.[253] The pneumothorax may be unilateral or bilateral[261–264] (Fig. 44–25) and may be recurrent.[255] Pneumomediastinum occurs occasionally, either by itself or in association with pneumothorax.[246, 254]

Additional radiographic abnormalities seen in a small percentage of patients include focal parenchymal consolidation,[245, 246, 249, 250] single or multiple nodules[265–268] (Fig. 44–26), miliary nodules,[249, 269] cavitation,[245, 250, 265, 266, 270] hilar or mediastinal lymph node enlargement,[246, 249, 268, 271] lymph node and visceral calcification,[249, 272, 273] and pleural effusion.[245, 249, 250, 268]

The characteristic HRCT findings of PCP consist of symmetric bilateral areas of ground-glass attenuation[177, 274–277] (Fig. 44–27). As with radiographs, the abnormalities can be diffuse; however, they often involve mainly the perihilar regions or have a patchy distribution with intervening areas of normal parenchyma that are frequently sharply marginated by the interlobular septa[274, 275] (Fig. 44–28). Other common findings include cyst formation (Fig. 44–29), small nodules, irregular linear opacities (Fig. 44–30), and interlobular septal thickening.

In one series of 24 patients, areas of ground-glass attenuation were present on the HRCT scan in 22 (92%), consolidation in 9 (38%), cyst formation in 8 (33%), small

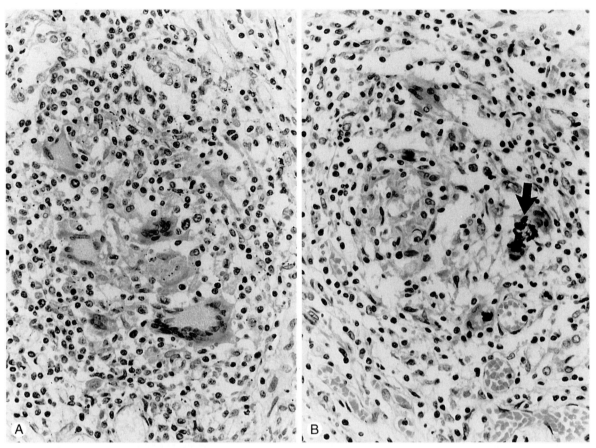

**Figure 44–17.** *Pneumocystis carinii* **Pneumonia: Granulomatous Inflammatory Reaction.** The sections are from an autopsy of a patient who had been diagnosed to have *P. carinii* pneumonia 2 months before death, for which he received standard therapy. In *A,* mononuclear cells surround a loosely formed granuloma consisting largely of multinucleated giant cells. A second poorly formed granuloma *(B)* is associated with focal calcification *(arrow).*

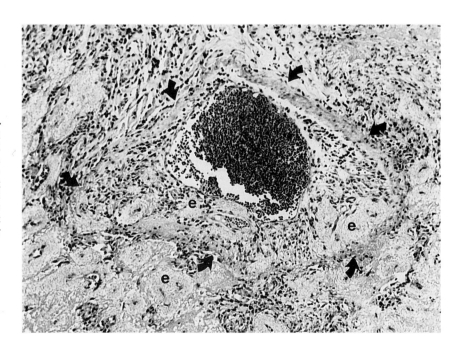

**Figure 44–18. AIDS and** *Pneumocystis cari-nii* **Infection: Vascular Infiltration.** A magnified view of a pulmonary artery from a grossly ill-defined area of consolidation shows the presence of abundant, somewhat foamy exudate (e) characteristic of *P. carinii* infection. The material is located in the lung parenchyma adjacent to the vessel and in the arterial intima *(arrows* indicate the media, which is partially destroyed in its lower and left portions). Abundant organisms were identified in the exudate using silver stain.

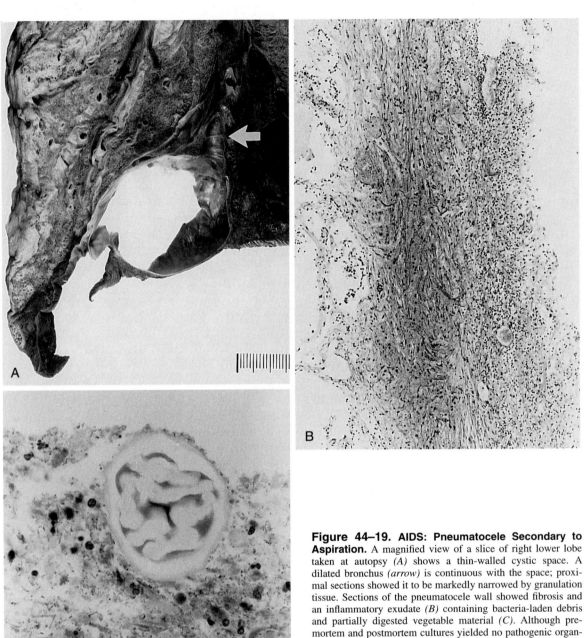

**Figure 44–19. AIDS: Pneumatocele Secondary to Aspiration.** A magnified view of a slice of right lower lobe taken at autopsy *(A)* shows a thin-walled cystic space. A dilated bronchus *(arrow)* is continuous with the space; proximal sections showed it to be markedly narrowed by granulation tissue. Sections of the pneumatocele wall showed fibrosis and an inflammatory exudate *(B)* containing bacteria-laden debris and partially digested vegetable material *(C)*. Although premortem and postmortem cultures yielded no pathogenic organisms, the cause of the pneumatocele was presumed to be aspiration and anaerobic bacterial infection. (Radiographs of the patient are shown in Fig. 44–24.)

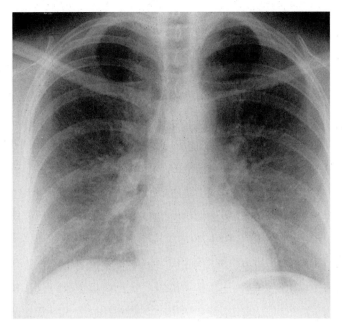

**Figure 44–20.** *Pneumocystis carinii* **Pneumonia (PCP).** A posteroanterior chest radiograph in a 41-year-old woman who had AIDS and proven PCP demonstrates bilateral symmetric ground-glass opacities involving mainly the middle and lower lung zones.

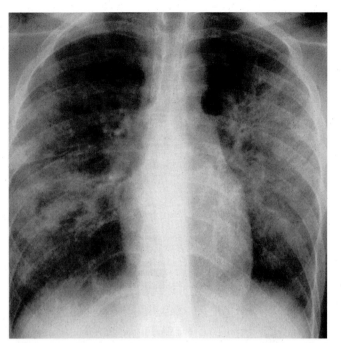

**Figure 44–22.** *Pneumocystis carinii* **Pneumonia (PCP).** A posteroanterior chest radiograph in a 31-year-old patient who had AIDS and PCP demonstrates bilateral areas of air-space consolidation involving mainly the middle lung zones.

nodules in 6 (25%), irregular linear opacities in 4 (17%), interlobular septal thickening in 4 (17%), lymph node enlargement in 6 (25%), pleural effusion in 4 (17%), and pneumothorax in 4 (17%).[177] In a second series of 39 patients, areas of ground-glass attenuation were present in 86%, cyst formation in 38%, a reticular interstitial pattern in 18%, and small nodules in 18%.[275] The prevalence of these

findings is somewhat related to the stage of disease;[114, 249] the initial abnormalities usually consist of areas of ground-glass attenuation that progress to consolidation, whereas irregular linear opacities (reticulation) and interlobular septal thickening are seen most commonly in patients who have subacute or resolving disease.[114, 249]

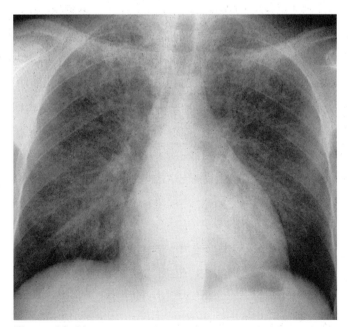

**Figure 44–21.** *Pneumocystis carinii* **Pneumonia (PCP) with Upper Lobe Distribution.** A chest radiograph demonstrates bilateral ground-glass opacities and ill-defined nodules involving mainly the upper lobes. The patient was a 26-year-old man with AIDS. The diagnosis of PCP was confirmed by bronchoalveolar lavage.

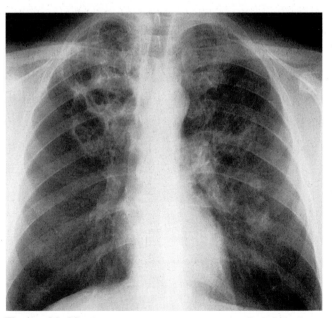

**Figure 44–23.** *Pneumocystis carinii* **Pneumonia (PCP): Pneumatoceles.** A posteroanterior chest radiograph in a 53-year-old patient with AIDS demonstrates numerous cystic lesions involving mainly the right upper lobe. The pneumatoceles had not been present on a chest radiograph performed 3 months previously.

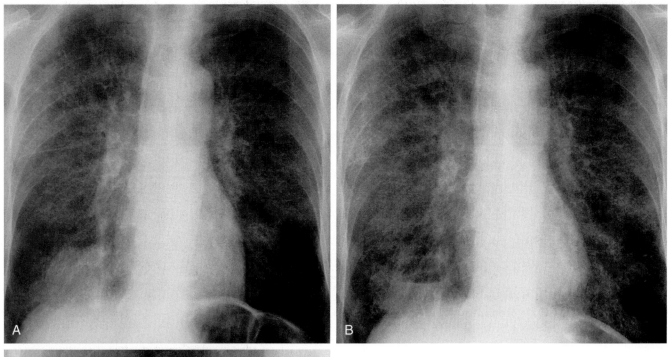

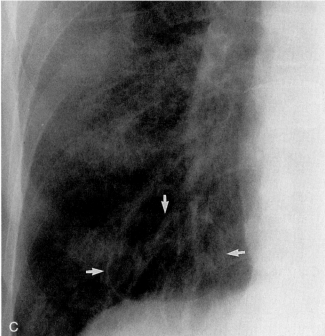

**Figure 44–24. Pneumatocele Due to Aspiration.** A posteroanterior chest radiograph *(A)* in a patient with AIDS and *Pneumocystis carinii* pneumonia (PCP) demonstrates bilateral ground-glass opacities and a fine reticulonodular pattern. A focal area of consolidation is present in the right lower lobe. A posteroanterior chest radiograph taken 1 week later *(B)* demonstrates an air-fluid level within the right lower lobe consolidation. A view of the right lower lung from a posteroanterior chest radiograph performed 3 weeks later *(C)* demonstrates a thin-walled cyst *(arrows)*. This was presumed to represent a pneumatocele secondary to anaerobic bacterial infection, superimposed on PCP. (The specimen is illustrated in Fig. 44–19.)

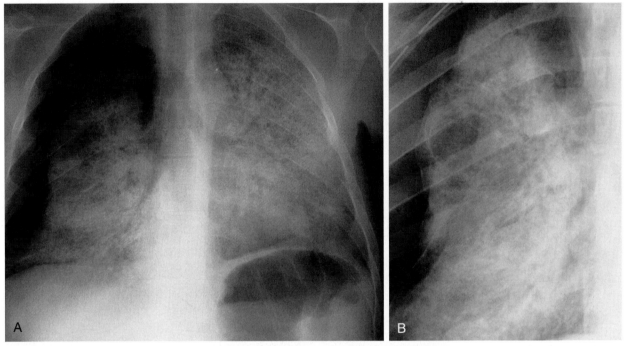

**Figure 44–25.** *Pneumocystis carinii* **Pneumonia (PCP) with Cystic Lesions and Pneumothorax.** A 31-year-old patient with AIDS presented with acute-onset shortness of breath. An anteroposterior chest radiograph *(A)* demonstrates a large right pneumothorax, extensive areas of consolidation in both lungs, and cysts. The cystic lesions are better seen on the magnified view of the right lung *(B)* from the anteroposterior radiograph performed after insertion of a chest tube. PCP was confirmed by bronchoalveolar lavage.

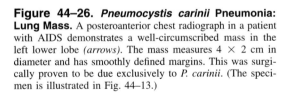

**Figure 44–26.** *Pneumocystis carinii* **Pneumonia: Lung Mass.** A posteroanterior chest radiograph in a patient with AIDS demonstrates a well-circumscribed mass in the left lower lobe *(arrows)*. The mass measures 4 × 2 cm in diameter and has smoothly defined margins. This was surgically proven to be due exclusively to *P. carinii*. (The specimen is illustrated in Fig. 44–13.)

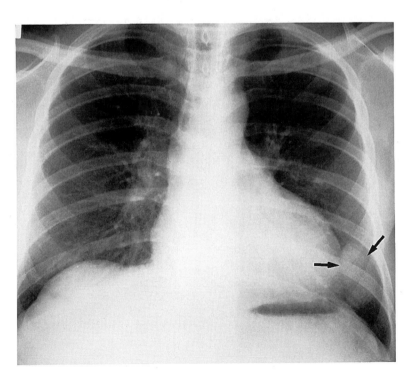

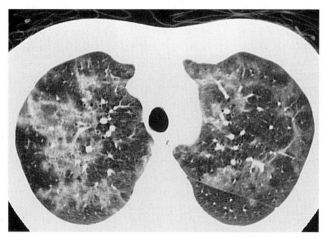

**Figure 44–27.** *Pneumocystis carinii* **Pneumonia (PCP).** An HRCT scan in a 35-year-old man with proven PCP demonstrates bilateral areas of ground-glass attenuation. (Courtesy of Dr. Andrew Mason, Department of Radiology, St. Paul's Hospital, Vancouver, BC.)

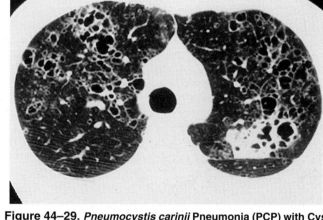

**Figure 44–29.** *Pneumocystis carinii* **Pneumonia (PCP) with Cystic Changes.** An HRCT scan through the upper lobes in a 30-year-old patient with AIDS and proven PCP demonstrates numerous irregularly shaped cysts in a random distribution. Focal areas of ground-glass attenuation and consolidation are also evident.

Most patients who have AIDS and PCP have characteristic radiographic findings, therefore obviating the need for CT.[278] However, the latter can be helpful in the assessment of patients with symptomatic disease who have normal or nonspecific radiographic findings.[279–281] As might be expected, HRCT may demonstrate parenchymal abnormalities in patients who have normal radiographs.[279–281] For example, in one investigation of 13 such patients who had a high clinical index of suspicion for PCP, all four patients who had patchy areas of ground-glass attenuation on HRCT had *P. carinii* identified in BAL fluid specimens;[280] the BAL fluid in the 9 patients who had normal HRCT scans was negative. In a second prospective investigation of 51 patients who had a high clinical pretest probability of PCP and normal, equivocal, or nonspecific chest radiographic findings, HRCT showed parenchymal abnormalities in all 6 patients who had PCP proven by BAL (sensitivity, 100%)

and was falsely positive in 5 of 45 patients with negative BAL (specificity, 89%).[281]

HRCT is also superior to chest radiography in differentiating PCP from other pulmonary infections and tumors in patients who have AIDS.[279] For example, in one review of the radiographs and HRCT scans from 139 HIV-positive patients (including 106 who had proven thoracic complications and 33 who had no evidence of active intrathoracic disease), 90% were correctly identified by two observers as having intrathoracic abnormalities on the radiograph compared with 96% on CT.[279] Among the patients who had no complications, 73% were correctly identified at radiography and 86% at CT. A confident first-choice diagnosis was made in 47% of CT interpretations (correct in 87%) compared with 34% on the radiograph (correct in 67%). A correct diagnosis of PCP was made in 87% of 19 cases. The diagnosis of PCP in these cases was based on the presence of areas of ground-glass attenuation. The value of this finding was

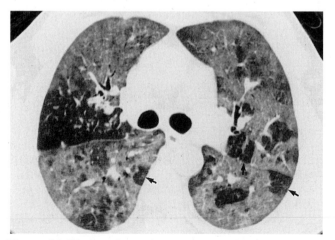

**Figure 44–28.** *Pneumocystis carinii* **Pneumonia.** An HRCT scan in a 46-year-old man with AIDS demonstrates bilateral areas of ground-glass attenuation with a mosaic pattern. Note the sharp demarcation between normal and abnormal lung parenchyma, several of the areas of spared lung parenchyma having a size and configuration that corresponds to that of secondary pulmonary lobules *(arrows).*

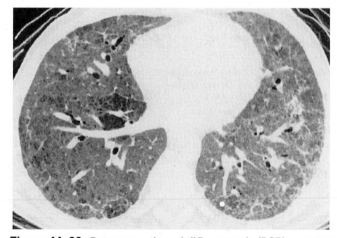

**Figure 44–30.** *Pneumocystis carinii* **Pneumonia (PCP).** An HRCT scan in a 42-year-old patient with AIDS and proven PCP demonstrates extensive bilateral areas of ground-glass attenuation. Focal areas of normal lung parenchyma, areas of decreased attenuation, and irregular linear opacities involving mainly the subpleural lung regions are also evident.

also assessed in another study that included 102 patients who had AIDS and proven thoracic complications and 20 HIV-positive patients without active intrathoracic disease.[177] A correct first-choice diagnosis of PCP was made based on HRCT in 29 (83%) of 35 patients; the diagnosis was made with a high degree of confidence in 25. Although ground-glass attenuation in patients who have AIDS can be the result of several other abnormalities, such as CMV pneumonia or lymphocytic interstitial pneumonitis (LIP), in most cases, it is a manifestation of PCP.

Scintigraphy plays a limited role in the diagnosis of PCP.[114, 247] Although gallium-67 citrate scintigraphy has a relatively high sensitivity (80% to 95%), its specificity is low (50% to 75%).[282–286] Furthermore, the procedure requires 48 to 72 hours after intravenous injection for the blood pool to clear the chest and thus allow optimal imaging.[286] Other parenchymal abnormalities that can increase pulmonary gallium uptake in patients who have AIDS include tuberculosis, MAC infection, CMV pneumonia, lymphoma, and nonspecific inflammation.[282, 283, 286]

## Clinical Manifestations

The clinical features of PCP are nonspecific. Patients commonly complain of fever, nonproductive cough, and progressive dyspnea on exertion.[201] Sputum production has been noted in less than 25% of patients.[287] Hemoptysis is rare.[288] The patient's temperature may be as high as 39° to 40° C.[206] Less common manifestations include weight loss, chest pain, night sweats, chills, fatigue, and malaise.[206] Wheezing may be a feature of infection in patients who have underlying asthma.[289] The constellation of productive cough, shaking chills, and pleuritic chest pain is unusual and should suggest another diagnosis.[201, 290] About 5% of patients do not have symptoms.[206, 291]

There are important differences in clinical presentation between patients who have AIDS and patients who have other causes of immunosuppression. In the former group, the infection tends to have a more indolent onset with relative preservation of gas exchange.[287] However, the rate of progression of the infection varies widely; some patients have fulminant disease with respiratory failure within days of onset of symptoms,[201, 206, 292] whereas others have relatively insidious disease associated with low-grade symptoms.[201] An extreme example of the latter form was reported in three patients who had chronic fibrosing disease associated with clinical stability over 4 to 24 months.[293]

The physical examination contributes little to the diagnosis.[201] Tachypnea is common;[206] cyanosis and respiratory distress can be seen with advanced diseased.[294] Examination usually reveals that the lungs are normal, although crackles and wheezes are apparent on auscultation in some patients.[201] Clubbing and hypertrophic osteoarthropathy are seen rarely;[295] in our experience, they may be associated with underlying bronchiectasis as a result of previous infection, including PCP. The finding of abnormalities such as oral candidiasis or KS may provide an important indicator of underlying HIV infection in patients in whom the diagnosis was not suspected previously.[201]

The physician should also be alert to the possibility of extrapulmonary *P. carinii* infection. A number of examples have been documented in untreated patients and in patients

who have received prophylaxis for PCP with aerosolized pentamidine only.[296] Virtually every organ system has been involved, including the heart, thyroid, bone marrow, brain, lymph nodes, gastrointestinal tract, and eye.[28a, 296, 297] Cutaneous infection can mimic KS;[298] other manifestations include otitis media and externa,[296, 299] sinusitis,[201] and splenomegaly.[296, 297]

## Laboratory Findings

Although a number of biochemical abnormalities occur in patients who have PCP, they unfortunately lack specificity.[206] Anemia, lymphopenia, and hypoalbuminemia are common.[206] The serum angiotensin-converting enzyme level may be elevated;[300] however, the degree of overlap between levels in normal individuals and in patients who have PCP and the lack of specificity of an elevated level precludes use in diagnosis.[206] Serum lactate dehydrogenase (LDH) is also commonly elevated;[301–304] however, this is also a nonspecific finding,[304] the degree of elevation reflecting the severity of pneumonia of any cause. When disease is minimal or the chest radiograph is normal, the value of LDH may also be normal.[206, 305] Despite these observations, the sensitivity of an elevated level of LDH for the diagnosis of PCP among patients with *symptomatic* disease is high; for example, in one study in which the receiver-operator curves were described, the sensitivity of the serum LDH was 0.94 at a cut-off value of 220 IU/liter.[304] Pleural effusion is exudative;[306] cytologic analysis of the fluid typically reveals the organism.[263, 306–308]

## Pulmonary Function Tests

PCP causes restrictive changes in lung function characterized by a reduction in lung volumes. This is associated with a low diffusing capacity, hypoxemia, and deterioration in gas exchange with exercise.[206, 309] After recovery from pneumonia, lung volumes return to normal, and the diffusion capacity improves without returning to normal.[310, 311] Each of these tests has a high sensitivity but low specificity for the diagnosis of PCP when applied to patients who have lung disease. The measurement of diffusing capacity and the determination of arterial oxygen desaturation with exercise have been especially evaluated as diagnostic tools.[312–318]

Applying a threshold of a 5% reduction in arterial oxygen saturation with exercise as abnormal, the value of exercise testing was determined in one group of 90 HIV-infected patients, of whom 53 were ultimately shown to have PCP;[312] 21 of the 77 available chest radiographs were normal. The sensitivity of a reduced oxygen saturation for the diagnosis of PCP was 100% and the specificity 36%; most important, the negative predictive value was 100%. Measurements of the diffusing capacity and resting arterial blood gas analysis had no diagnostic value. In another study in which an arterial oxygen desaturation of 3% with exercise was considered abnormal, the sensitivity of the test for PCP was 77% and the specificity 91%.[316] In a third investigation of 318 patients who were investigated for suspected PCP, the diagnosis was confirmed in 154;[319] 118 had other chest disease, and in the remainder, no diagnosis was determined. Only 13 of the patients who had PCP were able to complete a full 10-minute exercise test without developing desaturation; the odds ratio for PCP when arterial oxygen desaturation was present was 5.43.

The value of single or serial measurements of the diffusing capacity also lies in its high negative predictive value. In one study of 118 patients who developed a respiratory illness while being followed, 78 had PCP;[313] the diffusion capacity was less than 70% in 72, giving a sensitivity of 92% and a negative predictive value of 98% when compared with the entire group. The specificity of a low diffusion capacity for the diagnosis of PCP is poor in HIV-infected patients, in part because those who have no history of lung disease or who have recovered from previous infection frequently have a low diffusion capacity.[320] For example, in one group of 1,171 HIV-infected patients in whom the diffusing capacity was followed serially, a fall in diffusion capacity of 20% in the absence of signs, symptoms, and radiographic abnormalities was documented in 64 (6%);[317] none of these patients was found to have pulmonary infection.

PCP can precipitate asthma in some patients.[321] In one investigation of 37 patients who had PCP and in whom peak expiratory flow was measured before and after administration of a bronchodilator, the initial values were low in 84% of the patients;[321] more than half of these patients showed an increase of more than 15% in peak expiratory flow after administration of a bronchodilator. By contrast, in a control group of HIV-infected patients who did not have PCP, only 3% had improvement in lung function after bronchodilator administration. Comparison of methacholine responsiveness in another group of 25 HIV-infected drug addicts and a control group of 25 HIV-seronegative addicts showed no differences; less than 20% of these individuals had airway hyper-responsiveness.[322] In a smaller study of HIV-infected patients, seven who had recovered from PCP had bronchial hyper-responsiveness, whereas HIV-infected controls who were asymptomatic did not.[323]

### Diagnosis

The best strategy for the diagnosis of PCP, as determined by both outcome criteria and the cost-effectiveness of resource utilization, has not been determined. Whether diagnosis can be based on clinical criteria alone or whether definitive diagnosis by analysis of lung secretions or tissue is always required is a matter of debate (*see* later).[319, 324–327] A number of methods for establishing a secure diagnosis of PCP have been developed.

**Induced Sputum Analysis.** Induced sputum analysis is a simple procedure that has been widely used for the diagnosis of PCP.[328] By careful attention to technique, the use of liquefied sputum samples,[329] and immunofluorescent examination with monoclonal antibodies,[330–332] the sensitivity of the procedure has been as high as 92%.[330] However, many investigators have reported less favorable results.[333–338] In a 1996 review, the overall sensitivity of the test was found to be 67% (279 of 415 patients tested).[328] The sensitivity is not altered in patients who have undergone aerosolized pentamidine prophylaxis[339, 340] or who have recurrent disease.[336]

Despite the potential benefits of induced sputum analysis, there are many limitations to the test. Not all patients are able to produce sputum after nebulized saline inhalation,[305] and the technique must be avoided in those who are too dyspneic, nauseated, or uncooperative.[328] Experienced personnel must perform the collection, preparation, and analysis of the specimens to maximize the results.[305] The use of monoclonal antibodies adds time and expense to the procedure.[305] Similarly, although the use of PCR has been found to improve the sensitivity of the test,[336, 337, 341, 342] its application is limited by lack of standardization, cost, and time required to obtain the results.[342] Furthermore, induced sputum induction is unlikely to be cost-effective in institutions in which the overall prevalence of PCP is low or in which the pretest probability of PCP is low in any individual patient.[305, 338, 343, 344] Because its negative predictive value is less than 50%,[305] induced sputum analysis should be followed by bronchoscopy and BAL when a definitive diagnosis is required.

**Bronchoalveolar Lavage.** Fiberoptic bronchoscopy with BAL is the procedure of choice for the diagnosis of PCP in patients who have AIDS. In the absence of prolonged empiric therapy before bronchoscopy,[345] its sensitivity for diagnosis is greater than 95%, a level that effectively negates the need for transbronchial or open-lung biopsy in most patients.[346–348] (The subject of the means by which lavage fluid is examined [i.e., histochemistry, immunofluorescence, or PCR] is considered in Chapter 28 [*see* page 916].) The yield of BAL is improved by performing the lavage at the site of greatest disease radiographically.[332, 349, 350] "Blind" BAL has also been performed in intubated patients with some success; in one study of 30 such patients, the diagnosis was confirmed in 22 (73% sensitivity rate).[351]

**Empiric Therapy.** When the clinical presentation suggests a high probability of PCP, some authorities advocate empiric therapy in the absence of a definitive diagnosis to avoid the potential complications and costs of invasive investigation.[319, 325, 327] Using a decision tree with branches based on published data and expert opinion, one group compared the outcome based on the results of bronchoscopy to initial empiric therapy followed by investigation of those not responding to treatment within five days.[327] Patients in the latter group met the Centers for Disease Control and Prevention criteria for the diagnosis of presumptive PCP—an HIV-seropositive patient who presents with dyspnea and nonproductive cough of moderate severity, in the absence of the use of prophylaxis for *P. carinii* and of a previous history of PCP; the physical examination reveals crackles, laboratory testing shows moderate hypoxemia, and the chest radiograph reveals diffuse interstitial disease. Based on the assumption that at least 72% of patients who met these criteria had PCP, the authors concluded that there was no advantage to early bronchoscopy (i.e., the 1-month survival for both strategies would be the same). Whether this conclusion is applicable in any particular site depends to a large extent on the prevalence of PCP in the patient population.

Another group of 318 patients who had suspected PCP was studied to determine whether simple clinical information could accurately predict the presence or absence of PCP.[319] The diagnosis was proved by invasive means in 154 of the patients; 118 had other chest disease, and no definite diagnosis was made in 46. An algorithm was developed that was associated with a positive predictive value for confirmed PCP of 95% and that also identified patients who had a very small chance of having the disease (negative predictive value, 85%). The algorithm was based on clinical findings of fever, cough, and dyspnea occurring in a patient who had not received prophylaxis and had not had a previous episode of PCP; the chest radiograph showed interstitial disease, and arterial oxygen desaturation during exercise was demonstrated. When all of these features were present, the specificity for PCP and the positive predictive value were 100%; however, the sensitivity of this constellation of findings was only 21%. For patients with symptoms who had not received prophylaxis but had arterial oxygen desaturation during exercise, the specificity was 97% and positive predictive value 95%; the corresponding sensitivity was 46%. In the absence of typical symptoms and with the prior use of PCP prophylaxis, PCP was considered unlikely. Using this algorithm, invasive investigation could have been avoided in 59% of patients. In seven patients, the treatment of PCP would have been delayed, whereas four patients who had other diseases (two who had tuberculosis and two who had bacterial pneumonia) would have been treated initially with therapy directed at PCP.

In another study of 73 HIV-seropositive men referred for investigation because of respiratory problems, empiric therapy was initiated when the clinical picture was considered highly suggestive of PCP;[325] for the purposes of the study, all patients also had bronchoscopy and lavage to confirm the diagnosis. Adopting the empiric approach would have led to correct treatment in 43 of 45 patients and would have saved 44 of the 45 bronchoscopy procedures performed in the group of patients in whom the diagnosis of PCP was considered highly likely.

Despite the findings of these studies, not all investigators have agreed on using an empiric approach. For example, one group found empiric therapy for PCP to be a strong predictor of in-hospital mortality, after adjustment for severity of illness;[352] they attributed this finding to a failure to initiate treatment expeditiously when patients had diseases other than PCP. In our own setting, in which the prevalence of PCP is high in patients who have typical clinical and radiographic features and the prevalence of tuberculosis is relatively low, we frequently make an empiric diagnosis of PCP. However, when the severity of illness is such that the patient might not survive an error in judgment, we proceed to immediate invasive investigation.

## Prognosis and Natural History

In the early days of the AIDS epidemic, the mortality rate related to PCP was high, with about 25% or more patients dying during the first episode.[353] The 30-day mortality rate of 3,981 patients who required admission to a Veterans Affairs medical center in the United States with a first episode of PCP in the years 1987 to 1991 was 19%.[354] Currently, the early survival of patients who have a first episode of PCP is greater than 85%.[353] This improvement in survival coincided with the availability of antiretroviral therapy and the prophylactic use of drugs against *P. carinii*, which may modulate the severity of "breakthrough" disease.[355–357] Improved survival may also be related to increased awareness of early symptoms and better treatment of the pneumonia.[355, 358]

The long-term survival of patients who have PCP remains poor, largely as a result of the progressive nature of the underlying illness and its attendant immunosuppression. Slightly more than half of patients survive 1 year after the first diagnosis of PCP,[195] whereas only about 40% remain alive after 2 years.[355] In a study of patients who had received ventilatory support for PCP, 80% were alive 1 year after discharge from the hospital and only 6% were alive after 4 years.[359]

There are a large number of predictors of survival in patients who have PCP. Many are indicators of disease severity and have been combined into a variety of scoring systems, which can be used to estimate survival on admission to the hospital and to guide resource use.[360–362]

Several demographic and historical features are related to both short- and long-term prognosis. Older age has been associated with a poor outcome in a number of studies.[356, 363–365] This is likely the result of a number of factors, including increased severity of disease at presentation, failure to recognize underlying HIV infection on admission (and thereby failure to consider the diagnosis of PCP in a timely fashion), delay in initiation of therapy,[363] and non–HIV-related comorbidity.[366] Skill in care may also influence patient survival. In one large study, it appeared that the 30-day mortality rate was better when the patient was admitted to a hospital with more experience in dealing with PCP;[354] the results of a longitudinal analysis suggested that there was a learning curve for appropriate management of these patients. In a retrospective chart review of a cohort of 2,174 patients who had been hospitalized for PCP, several factors were found to influence survival after correction for initial disease severity, including the intensity and timing of medical care.[367] Survival was adversely influenced by the lack of private medical insurance (which influenced the availability of antiretroviral therapy[331]) and by the type of hospital to which the patient was admitted—the prognosis was worse in patients admitted to a Veterans Affairs hospital. The long-term survival after diagnosis of PCP is also worse in intravenous drug users, at least partly because of their failure to use antiretroviral therapy.[368]

Several clinical parameters reflect the severity of pneumonia and are predictive of both mortality and the need for admission to an intensive care unit. In a multivariate analysis of mortality risk in patients admitted to an intensive care unit for complications of HIV infection (including 174 patients who had respiratory failure), in-hospital death was significantly associated with functional status, time since AIDS diagnosis, HIV disease stage, a simplified acute physiology score, and the need for and duration of mechanical ventilation.[369] A PCP severity scoring system that incorporated clinical factors such as performance status, respiratory rate, severity of fever, and degree of dyspnea was also able to predict survival and improvement in another study of 78 patients.[360]

A number of laboratory abnormalities have also been found to have predictive value in patients who develop PCP. Some—such as serum albumin,[365, 370] body mass index,[361] and serum hemoglobin[370, 371]—reflect the nutritional status and degree of debilitation of the patient. Others—such as the alveolar-arterial oxygen gradient,[361, 362, 372–374] arterial $P_{O_2}$,[360, 375] and serum LDH[362, 365, 373, 374, 376]—reflect the severity of pneumonia. The CD4 lymphocyte count, which is a direct indication of the degree of immunosuppression and a reflection of the stage of HIV infection, also has important prognostic import.[361, 371, 377] For example, in a study of patients who received mechanical ventilation for PCP, the mortality rate of patients who had a CD4 count greater than 100 cells/µl was 25% (1 of 4), whereas all 20 patients whose CD4 count was less than 10 cells/µl died.[377] Certain abnormalities of BAL fluid, such as neutrophilia,[362, 373, 378, 379] an increased level of interleukin-8,[380] eosinophilia,[362] and an increased protein content,[378] are also strong predictors of in-hospital mortality and morbidity. A decreased density of cysts within the typical foamy alveolar exudate was found by one group of investigators to be associated with a poorer prognosis;[381] the authors speculated that the basis for this might be a relative increase in the number of free trophozoites.

Some patients who have clinical and radiographic improvement after therapy for PCP have persistence of organisms in lung tissue as revealed by either BAL or transbronchial biopsy.[372, 382–384] For example, in one study of 56 patients who had follow-up bronchoscopy with BAL 21 days after the initiation of therapy for PCP, 32 responded to therapy and 24 did not;[382] both failure of therapy and early recurrence of PCP among responders were associated with a failure to clear organisms from the BAL after completion of a course of therapy. Although some patients who have delayed clearance of *P. carinii* from BAL fluid specimens appear to have responded adequately to therapy,[384, 385] persistence of organisms constitutes a risk for early relapse and impaired survival.[372]

As might be expected, the finding of additional pulmonary pathogens, including bacteria, *M. tuberculosis*, fungi, and parasites, may also worsen the prognosis of patients who have PCP.[206] Although the results of early studies suggested that concomitant CMV infection was also associated with poor outcome,[206] those of subsequent ones have not concurred.[386] In an investigation of 111 patients who had a first diagnosis of PCP, the outcome among the 57 patients in whom CMV was not isolated was the same as that in the 54 in whom it was.[386] However, there is evidence that some patients who have combined infection with *P. carinii* and CMV may be adversely affected by the use of corticosteroids for the management of PCP.[387–389] One group found that such patients had twice the mortality within 3 months of bronchoscopy than did CMV-negative subjects;[388] this difference in mortality could not be explained by severity of pneumonia at the time of bronchoscopy or by baseline CD4 lymphocyte count. In another study of 65 patients hospitalized for the treatment of PCP, 45 were also CMV positive on BAL.[387] Ten patients died; all had concurrent CMV infection. All 20 patients who were CMV negative on BAL survived. Although these observations might be explained by the hypothesis that patients who have coinfection are more immunocompromised, they are also consistent with the conclusion that coinfection of PCP and CMV worsens the outcome of corticosteroid-treated patients.

Although the frequency of acute respiratory failure after PCP appears to be decreasing, the mortality associated with such episodes is increasing. In one review of 456 episodes of PCP, the incidence of acute respiratory failure declined from 21% between 1981 and 1987 to 9% between 1987 and 1991;[390] however, the case fatality rate among mechanically ventilated patients increased from 50% to 89% during the same period. Patients requiring mechanical ventilation despite the prior use of appropriate antibiotics and systemic corticosteroids have a very poor prognosis. This phenomenon has come to be known as the "third era" of respiratory failure and PCP.[391] (The "first era" refers to the time before the use of corticosteroids, during which the outcome of patients who required mechanical ventilation was dismal;[392, 393] the "second era" refers to the time during which patients were treated with corticosteroids, about half of whom survived.[392, 394–396]) Not surprisingly, failure to respond to therapy is a marker of high mortality in patients who develop PCP and respiratory failure.[393, 397, 398]

### *Cryptococcus* Species

Cryptococcosis, usually caused by *Cryptococcus neoformans*, is the most common systemic fungal infection in HIV-infected patients.[192] It is seen in about 10% of patients who have AIDS,[399, 400] usually when the CD4 count is less than 200 cells/µl.[401] Although CNS disease dominates the clinical picture, the lungs are not uncommonly affected. For example, in one study of 31 HIV-infected patients who developed cryptococcal infection, 12 had cryptococcal pneumonia;[402] 11 patients also had evidence of extrapulmonary disease.

Most cases of pneumonia are clinically silent and discovered serendipitously during the course of investigation of CNS or systemic complaints.[193] In one investigation of 106 patients who had AIDS and cryptococcal infection, cryptococcal pneumonia was the presenting illness in only 4.[403] Of the patients who had disseminated infection in this study, one third complained of cough and dyspnea;[403] however, many of these had concomitant infection with *P. carinii*, which presumably accounted for the symptoms. In another series of 48 patients who had disseminated cryptococcosis, the organism was first isolated from the lung in 12.[404]

Pulmonary signs and symptoms are nonspecific. Fever, cough, dyspnea, sputum production, and pleuritic chest pain have all been described.[404, 405] Hemoptysis is uncommon.[404] Tachypnea may be noted, and crackles may be heard on auscultation of the chest.[402]

The most common radiologic manifestations consist of a reticular or reticulonodular interstitial pattern (seen in about 50% to 60% of patients) or discrete nodules (seen in 30%).[114, 406–408] The latter tend to occur early in the course of AIDS and in patients who have less severe immunosuppression.[114, 408] Less common manifestations include ground-glass opacities, air-space consolidation, miliary nodules (Fig. 44–31), lymphadenopathy, and pleural effusions.[114, 406, 408]

Culture and smear of expectorated sputum are positive in less than 25% of patients who have cryptococcal pneumonia.[192] Bronchoscopy is usually required to confirm the diagnosis and exclude coexisting infection, such as PCP.[403] Culture of BAL fluid obtained by bronchoscopy is a sensitive test.[402, 404, 409] In three studies of 25 patients who underwent the procedure, it was positive in 21;[402, 404, 409] smears of BAL fluid revealed the organism in 9 of 11 patients.[409] Some workers have found the detection of cryptococcal antigen in BAL fluid in a titer exceeding or equal to 1:8 to be an even better test. In a prospective series of 220 immunocompromised patients who underwent bronchoscopy for fever and pulmonary symptoms (of whom 188 had AIDS and 8 had cryptococcal pneumonia), the sensitivity and specificity for the diagnosis of the pneumonia were 100% and 98%, respectively;[410] the corresponding positive and negative predictive values were 67% and 100%.

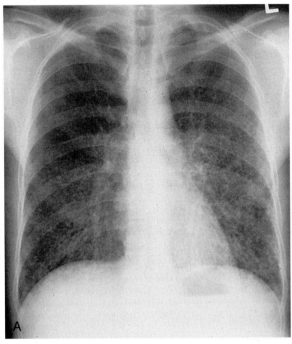
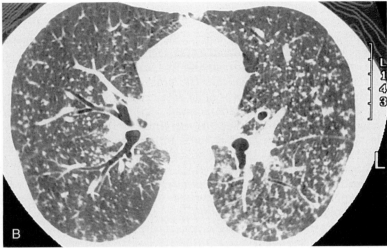

**Figure 44–31. Disseminated Cryptococcosis.** A posteroanterior chest radiograph *(A)* and an HRCT scan *(B)* in a 37-year-old patient with AIDS and disseminated cryptococcosis demonstrate miliary nodules. (From Kang EY, Staples CA, McGuinness G, et al: Detection and differential diagnosis of pulmonary infections and tumors in patients with AIDS: Value of chest radiography versus CT. Am J Roentgenol 166:15, 1996.)

The prognosis of patients who have AIDS and develop cryptococcal infection is poor; less than half survive 1 year despite long-term therapy with antifungal agents.[195]

### Histoplasma capsulatum

In the United States, histoplasmosis occurs in about 2% of patients who have AIDS, a prevalence that increases to 5% in endemic areas.[114] About 75% of these patients have disseminated disease and are markedly immunosuppressed, typically having CD4 counts of less than 100 cells/$\mu$l.[114, 411, 412] In some reviews, the incidence has been remarkably high; for example, in one series from Indianapolis, it was reported in 27% of HIV-infected patients during a local epidemic.[413] Although the findings of this study imply that new infection is involved in the development of the disease in some cases, the observation that patients can also develop the disease in areas in which the organism is not endemic indicates that reactivation of latent infection is involved in some cases.[414]

The radiologic manifestations of disseminated histoplasmosis are nonspecific. More than half of affected individuals have radiographic evidence of pulmonary involvement at the time of diagnosis.[414–416] For example, in one review of 27 patients, the chest radiograph was abnormal in 23 (85%);[412] findings included diffuse nodular opacities 3 mm or less in diameter in 9 patients (39%), nodules greater than 3 mm in diameter in 1, small linear or irregular opacities in 7 (30%), and focal or patchy areas of consolidation in 7 (30%). Small pleural effusions were present in 5 patients and hilar or paratracheal lymphadenopathy in 1. The radiographic and HRCT findings of miliary histoplasmosis are similar to those of miliary tuberculosis.[412, 417]

The systemic and pulmonary symptoms of disseminated histoplasmosis in patients who have AIDS are also nonspecific. Fever, weight loss, diarrhea, lymphadenopathy, and hepatosplenomegaly are the most common manifestations.[192] Cough and dyspnea are seen in patients who have lung involvement.

The diagnosis of disseminated histoplasmosis is usually made by detecting *Histoplasma* polysaccharide antigen (HPA) in the blood or urine or by the identification of the organism on smear or culture from the blood or bone marrow.[192] Because of the high frequency of concurrent pulmonary infection,[413] the diagnosis of pulmonary histoplasmosis in the setting of disseminated disease should not be assumed in patients who have radiographic abnormalities. BAL fluid often reveals the organisms on smear and culture in patients who have pulmonary involvement.[192] Testing for the presence of HPA in BAL fluid has the advantage of providing more rapid results; in one study of 27 patients who had pulmonary histoplasmosis, HPA was detected in 19 (70%).[418]

Although antifungal therapy can induce clinical remission, relapse is common, even with maintenance therapy.[419] In one series of 52 patients who had disseminated disease, 16 died before institution of effective follow-up, and 4 were lost to follow-up;[416] only 7 of the remaining 32 were alive and had improved after therapy; the others had died or experienced relapse of systemic fungal infection.

### Coccidioides immitis

Coccidioidomycosis is common among HIV-infected patients who live in areas endemic for the infection. In one study from Arizona, the cumulative incidence of active disease among 170 patients followed prospectively was 25% by 41 months.[420] Risk factors included a CD4 lymphocyte count of less than 250 cells/$\mu$l and a diagnosis of AIDS at entry into the study; evidence of prior infection did not appear to predict the development of disease. In a review of 77 HIV-seropositive patients who developed coccidioidomycosis, 20 had focal and 31 diffuse pulmonary disease;[421]

20 patients developed systemic disease, and 6 developed subclinical infection, as indicated by serologic findings.

Presenting symptoms are nonspecific and include fever, weight loss, cough, and fatigue.[201] The identification of an abnormal chest radiograph result usually triggers investigation that leads to the diagnosis. The usual manifestations consist of focal or diffuse areas of air-space consolidation;[421] less common findings include nodules, cavitation, hilar lymph node enlargement, and pleural effusion. Definitive diagnosis of disease requires culture of the organism from tissue or fluid samples or its identification in cytologic or histologic specimens.[193] Sputum, BAL fluid, and bronchial and transbronchial biopsy specimens all have a high diagnostic yield.[193, 401] Bronchoscopy may reveal the presence of mucosal ulceration.[401] Serologic testing has a high sensitivity overall but may fail to show infection in patients who have advanced immunosuppression.[193] High mortality rates are seen in patients who have low CD4 counts and in those who have diffuse lung involvement.[421]

### Blastomyces dermatitidis

Blastomycosis has been recognized uncommonly as an opportunistic infection in HIV-infected patients, fewer than 60 patients having been described by 1997.[422] Almost all have a history of residence in an area in which the organism is endemic. Most have CD4 lymphocyte counts of less than 200 cells/μl and a history of prior or concomitant opportunistic infection.[422] About half have focal lung disease; the remainder have disseminated infection.[423]

The chest radiograph may show focal consolidation, diffuse interstitial or miliary changes and (rarely) bilateral nodules, cavitary disease, or pleural effusion.[422] Symptoms of pulmonary involvement are nonspecific and consist of cough, sputum production, and dyspnea; pleuritic chest pain has been described occasionally.[401, 423] Culture of the organism from BAL fluid, skin, or cerebrospinal fluid has provided

a definitive diagnosis in most patients;[423] occasionally, it has been based on the cytologic or histologic identification of the organisms in specimens of sputum, BAL fluid, or tissue.[422] Serologic testing has no value in diagnosis.

About 30% to 35% of patients follow a rapidly fatal course, with death occurring within 3 weeks as a result of overwhelming lung disease with or without systemic dissemination.[422] Infection of the CNS has proved uniformly fatal.

### Aspergillus Species

Invasive pulmonary aspergillosis is uncommon in patients who have AIDS, occurring in only about 0.1% to 0.5%.[401] However, most cases have been described after 1990, making this organism an emerging pathogen in this clinical context.[424, 425] Most patients who develop pulmonary aspergillosis have neutropenia and a history of broad-spectrum antibiotic and glucocorticoid use.[401, 426–429] In the absence of these factors, patients who develop invasive lung disease usually have advanced HIV infection, generally with a CD4 lymphocyte count of less than 50 cells/μl.[424] Some have had particularly heavy aspergillus exposure through smoking marijuana.[426] The lung is the sole site of infection in somewhat more than half of patients who have pulmonary aspergillosis; in the others, systemic spread is evident.[429]

As in other patients, pulmonary aspergillosis in patients who have AIDS is manifested in several ways that can be broadly categorized as saprophytic, allergic, or invasive. The latter is probably the most common and may present as upper lobe cavitary disease, which may resemble chronic necrotizing aspergillosis[427, 430] (Fig. 44–32) or which may be characterized by one or two large cavities without surrounding infiltration[401, 430] (Fig. 44–33). Such cavitary disease was described in 13 of 33 patients in one series[424] and in 5 of 13 in another.[426] Symptoms consist of fever, cough, chest pain, and dyspnea;[427] they tend to be insidious in onset and

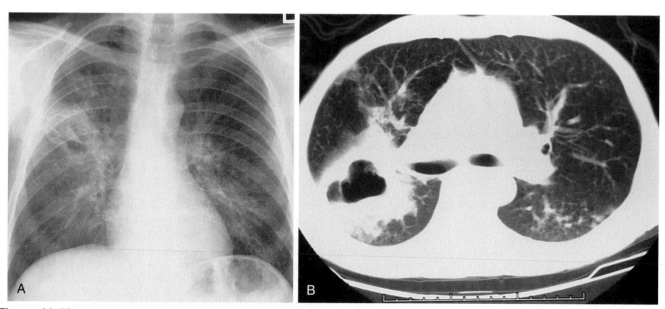

**Figure 44–32. Angioinvasive Aspergillosis.** A posteroanterior chest radiograph *(A)* in a 42-year-old patient with AIDS demonstrates a poorly defined irregular, thick-walled cavity in the right upper lobe and patchy areas of consolidation. A conventional CT scan *(B)* shows a well-defined, irregular, thick-walled cavity in the posterior segment of the right upper lobe and patchy surrounding consolidation. Pathologically proven angioinvasive aspergillosis.

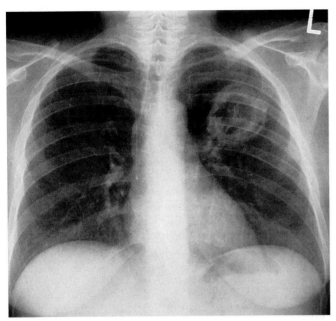

**Figure 44–33. Angioinvasive Aspergillosis.** A posteroanterior chest radiograph shows a thick-walled cavity in the left upper lobe with an intracavitary mass. The patient was a 36-year-old woman with AIDS. At bronchoscopy, she was also found to have pseudomembranous tracheobronchial aspergillosis. (Courtesy of Dr. Catherine Staples.)

progression.[426] Occasionally, there is complicating pneumothorax;[401] fatal hemoptysis is not uncommon.[427]

Bilateral air-space or interstitial opacities are seen in about half of patients.[424] These may have a nodular or reticular appearance radiographically, similar to that of PCP.[401] Focal alveolar or interstitial opacities have been seen in a minority of individuals, as in 9 of 36 patients in one review.[427] Such disease may remain relatively stable over several months or disseminate to the lungs bilaterally or systemically.[427] Necrotizing tracheobronchial aspergillosis is characterized by mucosal pseudomembranes both bronchoscopically and pathologically;[424, 427, 431] patients may have wheezing and dyspnea, and chest radiographs may be normal or show ill-defined opacities. CT may demonstrate nodular thickening of the tracheal or bronchial wall.[114] Associated lung disease may be the result of airway obstruction or spread of *Aspergillus* infection.[427]

Allergic aspergillosis is relatively uncommon in patients who have AIDS; however, all of the typical clinical and radiologic features may be seen.[426, 427] Aspergilloma formation has also been described in some patients.[432, 432a] In one investigation of 10 such individuals, 7 had previous tuberculosis and 3 previous PCP.[432] All aspergillomas developed in the upper lobes and presented as an intracavitary mass with a crescent sign or a filling defect in a cavitary infiltrate. The disease is usually relatively innocuous; however, it may be complicated by troublesome and, sometimes, life-threatening hemoptysis. Rarely, local or bilateral invasive disease ensues; for example, in the previously cited study of 10 patients, follow-up in 8 showed that 1 had improved, 3 had remained stable, and 4 (all of whom had CD4 cell counts of less than 100 cells/μl) had progressed despite therapy.[432]

Definitive diagnosis of *Aspergillus* infection requires culture of the organism from a normally sterile site or pathologic demonstration of tissue invasion. Most often, these are done by needle aspiration of lung or transbronchial biopsy;[426–428] when the airways are involved, bronchial biopsy may also reveal tissue invasion.[427] The identification of the organism in sputum or BAL fluid has little diagnostic importance by itself. For example, in one series of 972 patients who had AIDS and who were observed over a 10-year period in one institution, the organisms were isolated from respiratory sites before death in 45;[433] only 4 had invasive pulmonary aspergillosis at autopsy. Despite these and other observations, in the setting of a compatible clinical and radiologic picture and in the absence of identification of other causes, the possibility of invasive aspergillosis should be seriously considered.[401] Repeated isolation of the organism strengthens the likelihood that infection is present.[193] Despite its lack of specificity for invasive disease, BAL fluid culture appears to be a sensitive test: growth of *Aspergillus* organisms was demonstrated from BAL fluid in all 28 patients in one series;[424] no other organism was found in 27 of these patients.

More than half of patients who have invasive aspergillosis die from the infection,[427] usually as a result of massive hemoptysis, extensive lung disease with respiratory failure, or systemic dissemination.[424, 427] Because the infection occurs in the setting of advanced immunosuppression, the long-term survival of patients is limited whether or not the initial infection is eradicated. In one series of 33 patients, 31 died during the follow-up period;[424] the mean interval between diagnosis and death was 8 weeks (range, 3 days to 13 months), and only 6 patients had become culture negative with therapy.

### Viruses

The clinical significance of the identification of a viral organism in the lung is often uncertain in HIV-infected patients. Nevertheless, it is clear that a number of viruses can cause pulmonary disease,[434] the most commonly implicated being CMV and HIV itself. Other viruses are recovered from BAL fluid less often. Sometimes, they are the only pathogen isolated, suggesting that they are truly the cause of the underlying pulmonary disease.[435] The specific virus recovered in the latter cases tends to follow trends in the community and, with few exceptions, is associated with self-limited illness;[435] the major exception is the occurrence of fatal and disseminated adenovirus infection, which has been described in a review of several case reports.[436]

### Pulmonary Human Immunodeficiency Virus Infection

HIV can be found in the lungs of patients who are asymptomatic as well as in those who have pulmonary disease.[434, 437–441] It can be detected by PCR in cells in BAL fluid in most HIV-seropositive patients;[442] infection of macrophages, lymphocytes, and fibroblasts also has been identified in tissue samples. Although the significance of these findings is unclear, a number of respiratory disorders occur in the absence of apparent opportunistic infection or neoplasm, and it is conceivable that the virus is directly responsible for some of them.[442]

HIV-infected patients frequently have reductions in diffusing capacity and evidence of a lymphocytic alveolitis in the absence of clinical or radiologic findings of pulmonary disease.[443–445] These abnormalities have been associated with an increase in pulmonary alveolar permeability as assessed by 99m Tc–diethylenetriamine penta-acetate (DTPA) scanning, implying injury to the alveolar epithelium.[445] The lymphocytosis comprises an increase in both cytotoxic and suppressor T lymphocytes[442] and may be induced by cytokine release from infected pulmonary macrophages.[446] As is discussed farther on (*see* page 1685), lymphocytic infiltration of pulmonary tissue is the predominant histologic abnormality in patients who have LIP and nonspecific interstitial pneumonitis (NSIP). It is possible that all these abnormalities are manifestations of the same process and represent a reaction to HIV infection.[442]

### Cytomegalovirus

CMV can frequently be detected on culture of BAL fluid obtained from patients infected with HIV.[447–451] However, this finding is seldom associated with significant morbidity or mortality, and it is likely that the organism is not pathogenic in most cases. For example, in one study of 46 HIV-infected patients who had pulmonary symptoms, the virus was detected in the BAL fluid of 33 (72%);[447] only 1 of these patients subsequently developed clinically significant CMV infection. Moreover, the patients did not have evidence of cytopathic change in specimens obtained by transbronchial biopsy. In another investigation of 114 HIV-infected patients who had pneumonia, CMV pneumonitis was present pathologically in only 2;[448] 1 of these patients had concurrent PCP. It does not appear to make a difference whether the organism is detected by culture or by the presence of typical cellular inclusions in cytologic specimens.[449–451] In one study of 36 patients who had a positive CMV culture associated with cytopathic change on cytologic examination, 38 who had a positive culture only, and 40 patients who had no evidence of CMV by BAL, the 6-month mortality rate was the same in both CMV-positive patient groups, albeit increased compared with the patients who had no CMV in their BAL fluid.[452] The hypothesis that CMV lacks a pathogenic effect in many cases is corroborated by the histologic observation that numerous infected cells may be present in the lung in the absence of evidence of tissue damage or inflammatory reaction (Fig. 44–34).

Despite the previous observations, there is no doubt that CMV can cause pulmonary damage and disseminated infection in some patients. For example, in one review of 54 autopsies performed on patients who had AIDS, 39 (72%) had histologic evidence of CMV infection, of whom 31 (80%) had pneumonitis;[453] CMV was the only organism identified in 2 of these patients, both of whom had severe lung disease. In a second study of 75 autopsies, histologic evidence of CMV pneumonia was identified in 81%;[454] CMV was thought to have caused significant disease in 21 patients, and 5 were considered to have died as a direct result of the pneumonia. In another study of 85 episodes of pneumonia occurring in 68 HIV-infected patients, CMV was identified as the only infectious agent in 9 episodes, 2 of which were severe.[455]

The most common histologic manifestation of CMV-induced pulmonary damage is pneumonitis, characterized by a mixed neutrophilic and mononuclear inflammatory cell infiltrate in alveolar septa and adjacent air spaces (Fig. 44–35). Typical nuclear and cytoplasmic inclusions are usually easily identifiable; to be confident of the diagnosis, these should be seen in cells intimately admixed with the inflamed tissue. Rare manifestations of CMV infection in patients who have AIDS include multiple pulmonary nodules (some of which have decreased in size following antiviral therapy),[456] upper airway obstruction related to necrotizing tracheitis,[457] necrotizing bronchiolitis,[458] and diffuse alveolar hemorrhage associated with disseminated infection, viremia, and pathologic evidence of pulmonary vasculitis.[459]

The most common radiographic findings consist of bilateral ground-glass opacities or areas of consolidation.[460, 461] Less common manifestations include reticular opacities, discrete nodules or masses, and rarely, miliary nodules.[461, 462] Similar findings have been described on CT[461] (Fig. 44–36). As is evident from the previous discussion, the manifestations of pulmonary CMV infection range from simple colonization to subclinical pneumonia to clinically evident disease that may be sufficiently severe to cause respiratory failure and death.[434] Fever, dyspnea, and dry cough are common findings in patients who have pneumonitis.

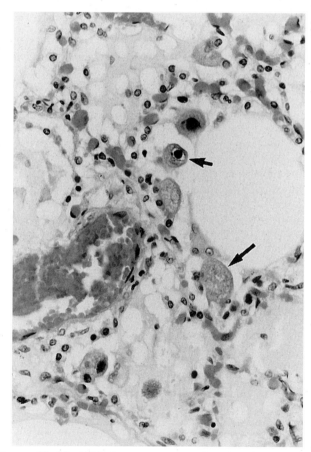

**Figure 44–34. AIDS: Cytomegalovirus (CMV) Pulmonary Infection.** The section shows alveolar air-space edema and septal capillary congestion; there is no evidence of a cellular inflammatory reaction. The edema was also present in alveoli unassociated with the virus and was thought to be secondary to left heart failure. Several enlarged cells containing intranuclear (*short arrow*) and intracytoplasmic (*long arrow*) inclusions characteristic of CMV are evident. The absence of tissue necrosis and inflammatory reaction suggests that the virus is exerting little, if any, effect on lung structure or function.

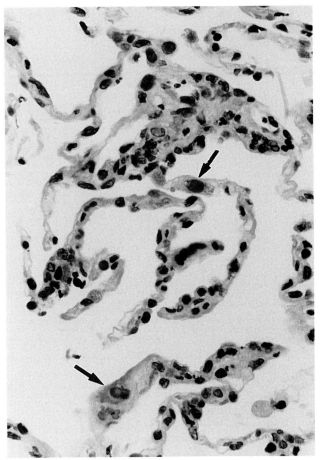

**Figure 44–35. AIDS: Cytomegalovirus (CMV) Pneumonitis.** A magnified view of a transbronchial biopsy specimen shows mild to moderate alveolar interstitial thickening by lymphocytes and occasional neutrophils. Two enlarged cells with ill-defined nuclear inclusions of CMV are evident *(arrows)*. (The presence of the organism was confirmed immunohistochemically). The intimate association of the virus and inflammatory cells suggests virus-induced tissue damage.

The diagnosis of pulmonary CMV infection is made most often by culture or by the identification of viral inclusions in cells in BAL fluid or sputum.[434] However, as indicated previously, most such cases are either unassociated with radiologic or clinical evidence of disease or have concurrent disease caused by other organisms or pathologic processes, making it difficult to determine the precise contribution of CMV to the clinical picture.[434] The diagnosis of CMV-induced disease usually requires the demonstration of tissue damage or an inflammatory reaction in biopsy specimens. The addition of CMV-specific DNA probes and monoclonal antibodies may increase the utility of cytologic examination in this respect; in one study, the finding of more than 0.5% of positive cells using monoclonal antibodies correlated with clinical features and histologic evidence of CMV pneumonia.[434] The finding of a negative culture of CMV from BAL fluid has a high negative predictive value for CMV pneumonitis.[463]

## Parasites

### *Toxoplasma gondii*

Although it has been estimated that about half of the world's population is infected with *Toxoplasma gondii*,[464]

clinically evident disease is uncommon, and the organism is usually maintained in an inactive state in the normal host. With the profound immunosuppression that accompanies HIV infection, 3% to 40% of patients who have AIDS have developed CNS toxoplasmosis, depending on the series.[464] Pulmonary involvement may occur in association with such CNS disease, as part of disseminated infection, or (rarely) as the sole site of clinical illness.[434] Overall, only about 0.5% of patients who have AIDS have developed *T. gondii* pneumonia;[464] in most cases, it is believed to be the result of reactivation of previously acquired infection.

Pulmonary infection typically develops in patients who have severe immunosuppression; for example, in one series of 13 patients, the mean CD4 lymphocyte count was 32 cells/μl.[465] Signs and symptoms are nonspecific, consisting of fever, cough, and dyspnea. The principal radiographic manifestation is a fine reticulonodular or ground-glass pattern, which resembles that seen in patients who have PCP;[465–466b] occasionally, there is diffuse nodular disease.[434] The diagnosis can be established in most cases by the identification of organisms in specimens of BAL fluid stained with methenamine silver.[434, 465, 467]

### *Strongyloides stercoralis*

HIV-infected patients are at risk for systemic dissemination of *S. stercoralis* after infestation;[468, 469] however, this complication is rare. The diagnosis should be considered in a patient who has a severe febrile illness associated with gastrointestinal and pulmonary symptoms.[434, 469] Recent travel to an endemic area is a helpful clue; however, the disease has been reported up to 40 years after primary infection and in the absence of a history of travel to an endemic area.[468] Coexisting parasitemia and meningitis are common and should prompt a search for the larvae.[434] Radiographic manifestations include a diffuse fine nodular or reticulonodular pattern and air-space consolidation.[468, 470] Examination of BAL fluid and stool shows numerous larvae.[468, 469] Eosinophilia is characteristically absent.[434] Most patients who develop diffuse pneumonia have died despite the institution of therapy.[468]

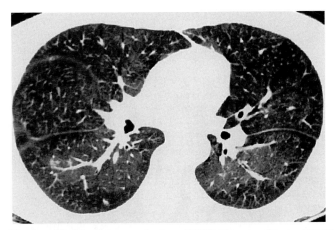

**Figure 44–36. Cytomegalovirus (CMV) Pneumonia.** An HRCT scan in a 38-year-old woman with AIDS demonstrates bilateral areas of ground-glass attenuation with relative sparing of the subpleural lung regions. Repeated bronchoalveolar lavages showed large numbers of CMV organisms and no other organisms.

### Cryptosporidia

Although patients who have AIDS are commonly infected with *Cryptosporidium* species, extraintestinal spread is uncommon.[471] Pulmonary involvement probably occurs most often by aspiration of organisms from the intestine; however, it has also been suggested that it may develop by inhalation or by hematogenous spread of infected blood monocytes.[471] The organisms can be identified on the ciliated border of the tracheobronchial mucosa (Fig. 44–37) or within the submucosal glands; in one patient, they were present within an alveolar exudate.[473, 474] Most patients have a picture of chronic bronchitis; however, many have had concurrent infection with other pathogens, and the precise contribution of the parasite to the pulmonary disease has not always been clear.[471] Radiographic abnormalities have been seen only in patients infected with other pathogens.[471]

## PULMONARY NEOPLASIA

About 25% of patients who have AIDS develop a malignant neoplasm at some point in the course of the disease.[475] In one cohort of 1,073 asymptomatic HIV-infected individuals from 6 American states followed from 1988 to 1994, the total cancer incidence was 3.99 per 100 person-years.[472] As opportunistic infections are better controlled,[476] these are likely to become even more common. Three cancers—Kaposi's sarcoma (KS), non-Hodgkin's lymphoma, and cervical carcinoma—are indicator conditions for the diagnosis of AIDS.[475] Several other neoplasms, including pulmonary carcinoma, may also be increased in frequency in patients who have HIV infection (*see* Table 44–1, page 1644).

### Kaposi's Sarcoma

KS occurs in about 15% to 20% of HIV-infected male homosexuals and in 1% to 3% of other HIV-infected patients.[475] Since the beginning of the AIDS epidemic, the incidence of the tumor as an AIDS-defining illness has progressively declined;[477] whether more intense antiretroviral therapy will alter the incidence further remains to be determined. The neoplasm is more common in patients whose immune function is worse.

KS has been identified as the cause of pulmonary disease in about one third of patients who have extrapulmonary KS.[478] About half of patients who die and have cutaneous KS have evidence of pulmonary involvement at autopsy.[478] In some autopsy series, the most commonly affected site has been the lung.[28a] Although pulmonary KS usually follows the appearance of cutaneous tumors, occasionally it is seen in the absence of skin involvement.[478]

### Etiology and Pathogenesis

The fundamental nature of KS has been debated, and there has been speculation that it may represent either a hyperplastic or a neoplastic process;[479] most evidence suggests that the latter is more likely to be correct. The disease undoubtedly behaves like a malignant neoplasm in immunosuppressed patients. In addition, one group of investigators was able to demonstrate the concordance of the methylation patterns of an X-linked androgen-receptor gene in multiple lesions from a group of women who had AIDS, providing strong evidence that the lesions were monoclonal in origin.[479] If this is correct, each KS lesion presumably arises from a monoclonal population of circulating progenitor cells that implant and proliferate in multiple sites.[479] In fact, circulating spindle cells resembling those of KS can be cultured from the blood of patients who have KS or who are at high risk for developing it.[480]

Despite the observations suggesting the potential for autonomous (neoplastic) growth of KS lesions, there is no doubt that a variety of normal inflammatory mediators have potent effects on the cells they contain. For example, KS-like tumors can be induced in nude mice injected with cells from human tumors;[481] these cells are able to recruit and induce the proliferation of mouse cells by secreting cytokines that have autocrine and paracrine growth effects, in-

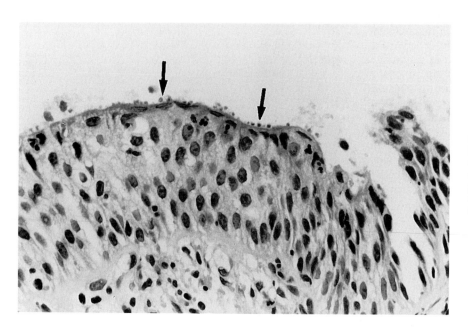

**Figure 44–37.** *Cryptosporidium* **Species: Bronchial Infection.** A magnified view of a bronchial biopsy specimen shows squamous metaplasia and mild chronic inflammation in the lamina propria. A number of round cryptosporidia are evident on the epithelial surface *(arrows)*. The patient had a history of recent onset of cough.

cluding a potent angiogenic factor. The HIV Tat protein interacts synergistically with one of these cytokines, basic fibroblast growth factor, to promote growth of the lesions.[482] It is possible that the same fibroblast growth factor interacts with vascular endothelial growth factor to induce the proliferation of vessels that is characteristic of early lesions.[483] There is also experimental evidence that corticosteroid stimulates the proliferation of KS cells through the modulation of glucocorticoid receptor expression.[484] Cytoplasmic levels of the proto-oncogene Bcl-2, a substance that inhibits apoptosis, are elevated in KS lesions;[485] it has been speculated that the combination of up-regulation of this protein and the stimulatory action of inflammatory and angiogenic cytokines and the HIV-1 Tat protein may be responsible for the progression of the lesions.[485] One group showed that cells derived from higher-grade lesions had fewer exogenous growth factor requirements, suggesting a greater capacity for autonomous growth of more "poorly differentiated" tumors.[486]

The occurrence of KS in clusters of patients and the importance of immunosuppression in its development are consistent with an infectious etiology. The most likely candidate is human herpesvirus 8 (KS-associated herpesvirus [KSHV]),[487] which has been detected in about 80% to 100% of KS lesions obtained from patients who have AIDS.[488–491] Although such a finding does not by itself establish a causal link between the virus and the tumor—for example, it is also consistent with preferential colonization of KS lesions by the organism[488]—a number of observations provide strong evidence that the organism is truly pathogenic. One group of investigators found evidence for the virus by PCR in 30 of 33 ejaculates (91%), but seldom in blood or tissue such as normal skin;[492] this suggests that the virus can be transmitted sexually and could explain the strong association of KS with male homosexuals who have AIDS. In one prospective study of 400 HIV-positive men in San Francisco, the prevalence of KSHV infection was temporally and independently associated with the development of KS, after controlling for CD4 count and the number of homosexual partners.[493]

Serum antibodies to KSHV also have been found to correlate with the presence of KS.[494] For example, in one high-risk population, the positive and negative predictive values of the presence of these antibodies for KS were 82% and 75%, respectively.[494] In another study, serologic evidence of infection was found in 32 of 40 patients (80%) who had KS, but in only 7 of 40 HIV-infected male homosexuals (18%) who did not;[495] no antibodies were detected among 122 blood donors, 22 patients infected with Epstein-Barr virus (EBV), and 20 HIV-infected hemophiliacs. In the latter investigation, examination of serial blood samples showed evidence of seroconversion before the development of KS in 21 of the 40 homosexual men (52%); the median time between seroconversion and the appearance of the tumor was 33 months. The antigen detected in this study was thought to be latent because its synthesis was neither enhanced by phorbol esters nor inhibited by antiviral drugs; the authors speculated that KSHV might be a transforming virus by which latently expressed proteins induce tumorigenesis.

Additional observations supporting a pathogenic link between KSHV and KS include the following: (1) the ability to propagate the virus from KS skin lesions,[496] (2) the finding of a close association between the virus and tumor cells *in vitro*,[496] (3) the presence of viral DNA in significantly greater amounts in tumorous than in nontumorous tissue,[491] (4) the identification of viral DNA in apparently early lesions in a significant number of cases,[496a] and (5) the association of seroconversion to the virus with the development of a febrile illness and lymph node enlargement clinically and foci of nodal KS histologically.[496b]

Despite these observations in support of an etiologic association between the virus and the tumor, it remains to be determined whether KS is related to transformation of normal cells by the virus or whether the tumor results from an immune-mediated inflammatory and angiogenic response to virus-infected cells.[496, 497]

### Pathologic Characteristics

Grossly, pulmonary lesions are typically most prominent in the pleural or bronchovascular interstitium. This may result in an appearance similar to lymphangitic carcinomatosis, except that involved regions are red or purplish rather than white and are usually larger (Fig. 44–38). Expansion of tumor outside the bronchovascular interstitium may result in nodules or, occasionally, ill-defined areas of parenchymal "consolidation" (Fig. 44–39). When present in airway mucosa, the lesions commonly appear as purplish, plaquelike elevations;[498] rarely, there is significant airway stenosis.[499] Involvement of lymph nodes is not uncommon and may result in their enlargement. Localized tumors may also be seen in the thoracic duct (*see* page 2769).

Histologically, the lesions are composed of cytologically atypical spindle cells between which are variable numbers of small, slitlike vascular spaces containing hemosiderin-laden macrophages and red blood cells (*see* Fig. 44–38). Corresponding to the gross appearance, lesions are often located in the peribronchovascular interstitium; involvement of the parenchymal interstitium occurs occasionally.[500]

### Radiologic Manifestations

The characteristic radiographic finding consists of bilateral, symmetric, poorly defined nodular or linear opacities (Fig. 44–40). Although sometimes diffuse, they often have a predominantly perihilar distribution.[501–505] The nodules measure 0.5 to 3 cm in diameter and have a tendency to coalesce.[501, 502, 504] Bronchovascular bundles may show thickening, which often progresses to perihilar consolidation[505] (Fig. 44–41). Other radiographic findings include thickening of the interlobular septa (Kerley B lines), pleural effusions (in 30% to 70% of patients),[501–503, 505] and hilar or mediastinal lymph node enlargement (in 5% to 15%).[503–506] In 5% to 15% of patients who have pulmonary parenchymal involvement at autopsy or endoscopy, the radiograph is normal.[501, 503, 505]

The characteristic HRCT findings consist of irregularly shaped, spiculated or poorly defined nodules in a predominantly perihilar and peribronchoarterial distribution[177, 503, 507, 508, 508a] (Fig. 44–42). Other common abnormalities include bronchial wall thickening (Fig. 4–43), interlobular septal thickening, focal areas of ground-glass attenuation or airspace consolidation, and pleural effusion. The areas of ground-glass attenuation may be the result of hemor-

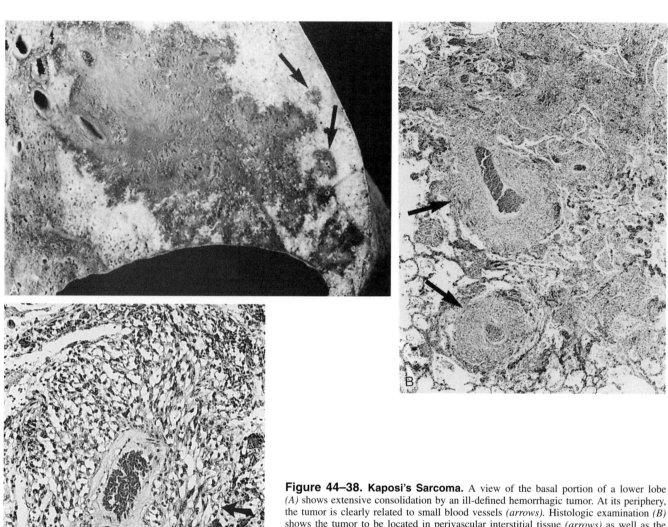

**Figure 44–38. Kaposi's Sarcoma.** A view of the basal portion of a lower lobe *(A)* shows extensive consolidation by an ill-defined hemorrhagic tumor. At its periphery, the tumor is clearly related to small blood vessels *(arrows)*. Histologic examination *(B)* shows the tumor to be located in perivascular interstitial tissue *(arrows)* as well as the adjacent lung parenchyma. A magnified view *(C)* shows typical spindle-shaped cells at lower right *(arrows)*. The lack of spindle cell appearance elsewhere is the result of the tumor being cut in cross section. *(B, ×25; C, ×150).*

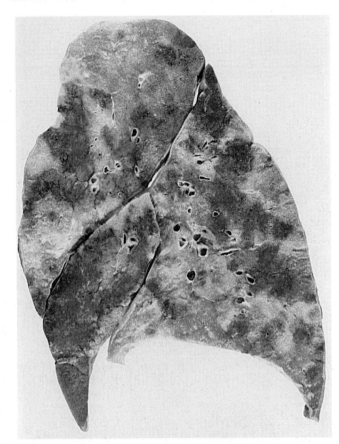

**Figure 44–39. Kaposi's Sarcoma.** A slice of right lung shows multiple foci of hemorrhagic consolidation without specific anatomic localization. The middle lobe is almost completely involved.

rhage[278, 508b] but should raise the possibility of concomitant PCP (Fig. 44–44). In one review of the findings in 26 patients who had KS, nodules were seen on CT in 22 (85%), peribronchoarterial thickening in 21 (81%), hilar or mediastinal lymphadenopathy in 13 (50%), interlobular septal thickening in 10 (38%), consolidation in 9 (35%), ground-glass attenuation in 6 (23%), and pleural effusion in 9 (35%).[177] Less common findings include a parenchymal mass; cavitation; involvement of the sternum, ribs, or thoracic spine; and pericardial effusion.[177, 507] There is considerable variation in the reported prevalence of lymphadenopathy evident on CT, ranging from about 15% to 50%.[114, 177, 503, 507, 508]

The characteristic appearance of KS on CT of the chest allows a confident radiologic diagnosis in most cases. For example, in one investigation of 102 patients who underwent the procedure, a correct first-choice diagnosis of KS was made in 26 (83%) of 32 patients who had the disease.[177] However, although CT permits accurate assessment of the presence, pattern, and distribution of parenchymal abnormalities in KS, it is poorly sensitive in the detection of endobronchial lesions.[114] Tumors large enough to cause atelectasis or stridor may be identified as intraluminal soft tissue lesions,[114, 503] but smaller lesions are seldom seen.

Magnetic resonance (MR) imaging and scintigraphy have limited, if any, role in the assessment of KS. On MR imaging, pulmonary parenchymal lesions have high signal intensity on T1-weighted images and decreased signal intensity on T2-weighted images.[509] There is a marked increase in signal intensity on T1-weighted images after intravenous administration of gadolinium.[509] Gallium 67 citrate scintigraphy is almost always negative.[114, 510] However, both cutaneous and pulmonary lesions show increased uptake of thallium 201 chloride.[511, 512] Increased uptake of thallium 201 but not gallium is also seen in pulmonary lymphoma and pulmonary carcinoma;[513] however, pulmonary infections often show increased uptake on gallium 67 scintigraphy but no uptake on thallium 201 scintigraphy.[513] Sequential thallium and gallium scans can therefore be used to help distinguish KS from pulmonary infection and lymphoma. Despite this capability, the combination of studies is costly and results in considerable delay in establishing the diagnosis and therefore is seldom used in clinical practice.

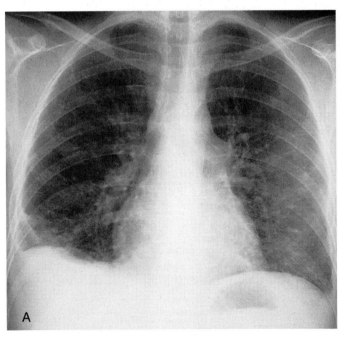

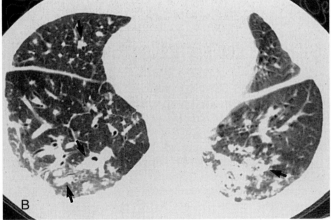

**Figure 44–40. Kaposi's Sarcoma.** An anteroposterior chest radiograph *(A)* shows bilateral, symmetric, poorly defined nodular and linear opacities and small bilateral pleural effusions. An HRCT scan *(B)* demonstrates nodular thickening of the bronchoarterial bundles *(arrows)*, interlobular septal thickening, and small bilateral pleural effusions. (From Kang EY, Staples CA, McGuinness G, et al: Detection and differential diagnosis of pulmonary infections and tumors in patients with AIDS: Value of chest radiography versus CT. Am J Roentgenol 166:15, 1996.)

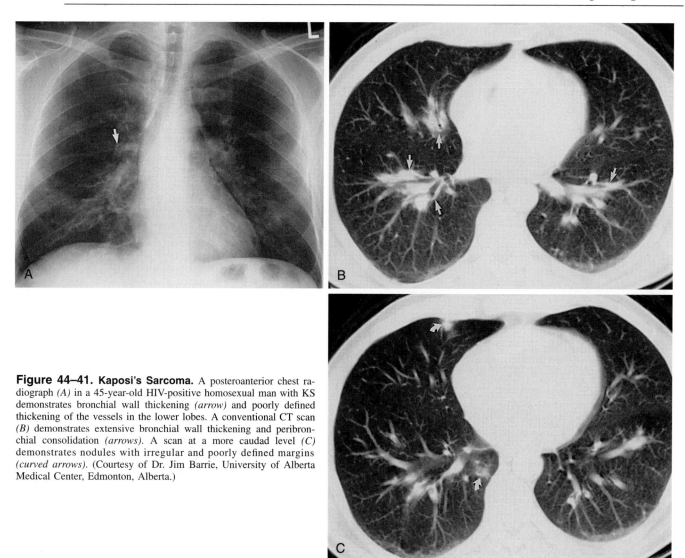

**Figure 44–41. Kaposi's Sarcoma.** A posteroanterior chest radiograph *(A)* in a 45-year-old HIV-positive homosexual man with KS demonstrates bronchial wall thickening *(arrow)* and poorly defined thickening of the vessels in the lower lobes. A conventional CT scan *(B)* demonstrates extensive bronchial wall thickening and peribronchial consolidation *(arrows)*. A scan at a more caudad level *(C)* demonstrates nodules with irregular and poorly defined margins *(curved arrows)*. (Courtesy of Dr. Jim Barrie, University of Alberta Medical Center, Edmonton, Alberta.)

### Clinical Manifestations

Most patients who have pulmonary KS have symptoms.[475] Dyspnea and cough are reported most commonly;[506] occasionally, blood streaking of sputum, fever, and chest pain are present.[478] These symptoms do not help distinguish KS from opportunistic infection, which commonly accompanies it;[515] however, the presence of blood streaking should strongly suggest endobronchial involvement in a patient who has cutaneous KS.[478] Although progression of disease is often relatively indolent, respiratory failure occurring over a period of days has been reported.[516] Pericardial tamponade as a result of KS was the cause of marked respiratory embarrassment in one patient.[517]

Examination of the lungs is often unremarkable. Findings of pleural effusion are sometimes present.[515] Occasionally, a focal wheeze related to an endobronchial obstructing lesion can be appreciated on auscultation;[475] crackles have also been reported in some patients.[478] Lesions of the larynx and upper trachea may cause hoarseness and stridor.[475, 518]

### Diagnosis

The bronchoscopic appearance of the lesions is unique and consists of violaceous or bright-red, irregularly shaped, flat or slightly raised plaques, most often located at the carinae of segmental and large subsegmental bronchi. The identification of such lesions is sufficient to make the diagnosis in most cases, and biopsy confirmation is not necessary. In fact, the histologic diagnosis of KS on small bronchial biopsy specimens can be difficult, particularly in early lesions.[475] The presence of airway lesions at bronchoscopy is almost always associated with the presence of KS in the more distal lung parenchyma (although the latter can be present in the absence of endobronchial disease).[514, 519] In one study of 168 patients in whom the diagnosis of pulmonary KS was made bronchoscopically,[514] 26 (16%) had the disease in the absence of skin lesions. In another study of 39 patients who had cutaneous KS, 19 had disease visible bronchoscopically;[519] 4 of these patients did not have radiographic abnormalities. In the absence of endobronchial le-

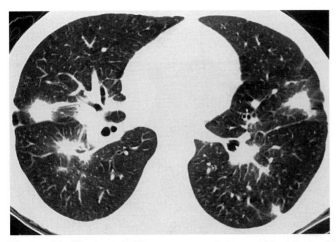

**Figure 44–42. Kaposi's Sarcoma.** An HRCT scan in a 34-year-old man with AIDS and KS demonstrates bilateral nodules with spiculated margins and peribronchial thickening. (Courtesy of Dr. Andrew Mason, Department of Radiology, St. Paul's Hospital, Vancouver, BC.)

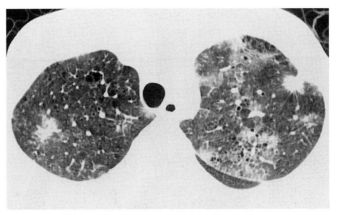

**Figure 44–44. Kaposi's Sarcoma and *Pneumocystis carinii* Pneumonia (PCP).** An HRCT scan demonstrates bilateral nodules with spiculated margins and extensive areas of ground-glass attenuation. The patient was shown to have both Kaposi's sarcoma and PCP. (Courtesy of Dr. Andrew Mason, Department of Radiology, St. Paul's Hospital, Vancouver, BC.)

sions, the diagnosis is usually based on the radiologic findings.[475]

The documentation of herpesvirus 8 DNA in tissue samples by PCR may be useful in confirming the diagnosis, particularly in specimens that are small or contain a lesion that is in an early stage.[489, 490, 496a] However, it must be remembered that viral DNA can also be identified in nontumerous tissue (particularly in patients who have KS, but also in a small number of those who do not).[491] In a limited study, the detection of human herpesvirus 8 in BAL fluid was also found to be highly sensitive and specific for the diagnosis of pulmonary KS and was positive in several patients who did not have endobronchial disease.[520] However, further studies are necessary to validate these findings before the test can be considered routine. Detection of the virus might also prove useful in the diagnosis of effusion resulting from pleural KS. Effusions are exudative and se-

rous or serosanguineous.[521] The finding of such an effusion in a patient who has AIDS and cutaneous KS is highly suggestive of such pleural involvement.[521]

Laboratory findings are nonspecific. Lung function testing usually shows a low diffusion capacity; restrictive lung function can be seen in patients who have extensive pulmonary involvement.[522]

### Prognosis

The tumor can regress in some patients who have been given intensive antiretroviral therapy.[514] Nevertheless, the prognosis of patients who have pulmonary KS is poor, the median survival varying between 2 and 10 months.[475] Poor prognostic factors are the presence of pleural effusion, severe breathlessness, a CD4 lymphocyte count of less than 100 cells/$\mu$l, absence of cutaneous KS, previous opportunistic infection, low white blood cell count or hemoglobin, and the absence of radiologic response to treatment.[475]

### Non-Hodgkin's Lymphoma

Non-Hodgkin's lymphoma develops in about 5% to 10% of HIV-infected patients, an incidence that is more than 60-fold higher than that expected in the general population.[523] Pulmonary involvement has been recognized clinically in about 1% to 15% of affected patients.[524] Some investigators have found it to be the most common form of malignancy in patients who have AIDS and hemophilia.[525] Thoracic involvement is usually recognized during the staging of lymphoma identified in an extrathoracic site; occasionally, the lung is the presenting or sole site of disease.[475] At autopsy, the lung is the most common site of extranodal disease; for example, in one study of 28 autopsies, pulmonary involvement was noted in 20 (71%).[524] Plasma cell dyscrasias, including myeloma, are relatively uncommon.[525a]

In the setting of HIV-infection, non-Hodgkin's lymphoma is generally high grade, widely disseminated, and extranodal at presentation;[526] about 20% of cases present in the CNS.[527] Approximately one third are classified histologically as small noncleaved cell (Burkitt's lymphoma–like), a

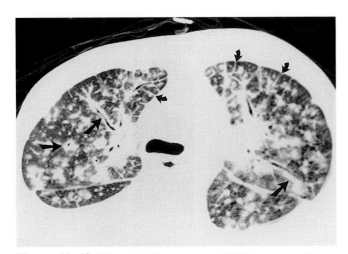

**Figure 44–43. Kaposi's Sarcoma.** An HRCT scan in a 28-year-old man with AIDS demonstrates extensive bilateral thickening of the bronchoarterial bundles *(straight arrows)*, irregularly marginated nodules, and thickening of the interlobular septa *(curved arrows)*. (From Worthy S, Kang EY, Müller NL: Acute lung disease in the immunocompromised host: Differential diagnosis at high-resolution CT. Semin Ultrasound CT MRI 16:353, 1995.)

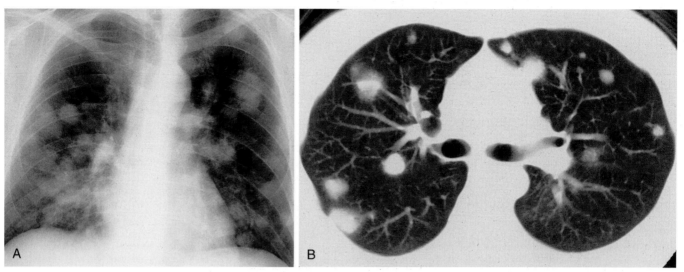

**Figure 44–45. Non-Hodgkin's Lymphoma.** A posteroanterior chest radiograph *(A)* in a 41-year-old man with AIDS demonstrates numerous bilateral nodules of varying size. A CT scan *(B)* shows that the nodules have smooth or slightly irregular margins and are distributed randomly throughout both lungs. There was no evidence of lymph node enlargement on the radiograph or CT.

rare tumor type in the United States before the AIDS era;[475] by 1985, such a tumor had become an AIDS-defining illness in the setting of HIV infection.[475] Most of the remaining cases are classified as diffuse large cell (immunoblastic) lymphoma. The molecular genetic profile of the large and small categories is different: the Burkitt's lymphoma–like type shows the presence of c-*myc* gene rearrangement and the absence of Bcl-6 gene rearrangement in almost all cases, the presence of p53 gene mutations in two thirds, and evidence of EBV infection in one third;[527] by contrast, almost all large cell lymphomas contain EBV, 25% display c-*myc* gene rearrangements, 20% show Bcl-6 gene rearrangements, and few exhibit p53 gene mutations. These observations suggest that different pathogenetic mechanisms may underlie the development of the two tumors.[527]

Almost all tumors show evidence of B-cell differentiation.[528] Occasional cases of T-cell lymphoma have also been described;[528] some of these have presented in the lung as a mass lesion that has shown relatively indolent growth.[529] Rare examples of Ki-1 anaplastic large cell lymphoma, angiotrophic large cell lymphoma, low grade B-cell lymphoma (Maltoma), and Sézary's syndrome have been reported.[530] The lung parenchyma, airways, pleura, and lymph nodes can be involved with tumor in all these histologic subtypes;[475] pathologic characteristics are similar to those of non-Hodgkin's lymphoma unassociated with AIDS. An additional very rare form of lymphoma that has been associated with herpesvirus 8 infection presents as serous effusions in the pleura, pericardium, or peritoneum ("primary effusion lymphoma").[475, 487, 531]

The most common radiologic findings of intrathoracic non-Hodgkin's lymphoma in AIDS consist of single or multiple pulmonary nodules and pleural effusions[114, 532–536] (Fig. 44–45). The nodules are usually well circumscribed and range from 0.5 to 5 cm in diameter[114, 532–534] (Fig. 44–46). On CT, they may have smooth or spiculated margins (Fig. 44–47) and often have air bronchograms (Fig. 44–48). Other common manifestations include reticular or reticulonodular opacities and bilateral areas of consolidation.[114, 532, 534] Both

the nodules and the masslike areas of consolidation may cavitate.[534, 535] Pleural effusions have been reported in 25% to 75% of patients[532, 534, 535, 537] and usually are seen in association with parenchymal abnormalities; occasionally, they are the only finding.[532, 538] Abnormalities described in a small number of patients include tracheal irregularity or polypoid endobronchial tumors,[114, 539, 540] extrathoracic masses spreading into the mediastinum,[535] and rib destruction.[114] The prevalence of lymphadenopathy has ranged from 0%[533, 535] to

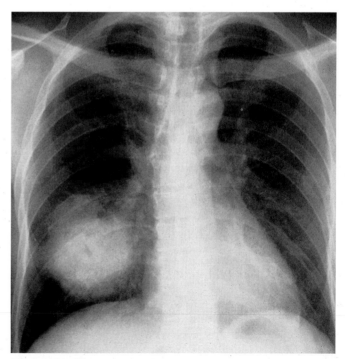

**Figure 44–46. Non-Hodgkin's Lymphoma.** A posteroanterior chest radiograph in a 38-year-old man with AIDS demonstrates an inhomogeneous 5-cm-diameter right lower lobe mass and adjacent poorly defined areas of consolidation.

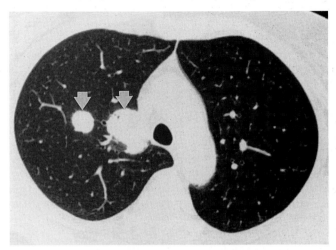

**Figure 44–47. Non-Hodgkin's Lymphoma.** An HRCT scan in a 56-year-old woman with AIDS demonstrates two nodules in the apical segment of the right upper lobe *(arrows)*. The nodules have slightly spiculated margins. Localized bubble-like lucencies related to patent airways can be seen in the larger nodule. (From Worthy S, Kang EY, Müller NL: Acute lung disease in the immunocompromised host: Differential diagnosis at high-resolution CT. Semin Ultrasound CT MRI 16:353, 1995.)

55%[537] in various studies; a reasonable overall estimate is 30%.[532, 534]

Most patients who have non-Hodgkin's lymphoma affecting the lungs have signs and symptoms.[524] In one series of 38 such patients, the most common symptoms were cough (71%), dyspnea (63%), and pleuritic chest pain (26%);[141] hemoptysis and orthopnea occurred infrequently. The physical findings were also nonspecific. Three quarters of patients were tachypneic. The nature of the other findings varies with the particular manifestation of disease in the lung; for example, dullness to percussion and diminished breath

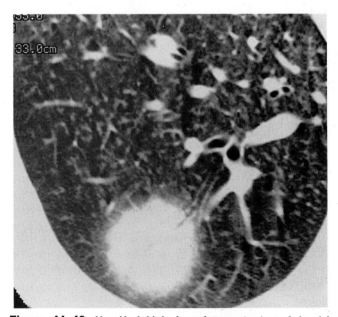

**Figure 44–48. Non-Hodgkin's Lymphoma.** A view of the right lower lobe from an HRCT scan in a patient with AIDS and non-Hodgkin's lymphoma demonstrates a nodule with an air bronchogram. (From Mason AC, Müller NL: The role of computed tomography in the diagnosis and management of human immunodeficiency virus (HIV)–related pulmonary diseases. Semin Ultrasound CT MRI 19:154, 1998.)

sounds may be present in association with pleural effusion.[524] Comorbid pulmonary disease is common; in the last-cited series, it was identified either before or after death in more than half of patients.[524]

Most patients have an advanced degree of immunosuppression; for example, the mean CD4 count in the series of 38 patients cited previously was only 67 cells/$\mu$l.[524] An elevated LDH level, high sedimentation rate, hematologic abnormalities, and abnormal gas exchange are present in 90% or more of patients;[524] however, none of these findings is useful in distinguishing lymphoma from other causes of pulmonary disease. Effusions are exudative with elevated white and red blood cell counts; in the absence of infection, the glucose is low in almost half of patients.[524] In one study of 13 patients, pulmonary function studies showed restriction in 31% and mixed restriction and obstruction in 8%;[524] the examination was normal in 69%.

Procedures that were useful in obtaining material for diagnosis of lymphoma in the largest series of cases included transbronchial biopsy (successful in 58%), thoracentesis (75%), and open-lung biopsy (75%).[524] Mediastinoscopy was diagnostic in only 1 of 3 patients, and transthoracic needle aspiration yielded diagnostic material in only 2 of 9 attempts.[524] When definitive diagnosis is required, more than one procedure may be required.[523]

The overall prognosis of patients who have non-Hodgkin's lymphoma in the setting of AIDS is poor; median survival from the time of diagnosis is generally between 4 and 6 months.[475] Bone marrow involvement and poor performance status are associated with a poor outcome.[528] Pulmonary disease is rarely the direct cause of mortality.[475]

**Pulmonary Carcinoma**

Initial reports in which pulmonary carcinoma was found to occur at a young age and to behave in an aggressive fashion in a number of patients who were HIV seropositive raised the possibility of a pathogenic association between the two conditions.[541–543] The results of extensive epidemiologic surveys subsequently confirmed the link between HIV infection and an increased risk for the development of pulmonary carcinoma.[544–546] For example, in a review of an HIV and AIDS data file that included 26,181 cases, 36 cases of primary pulmonary carcinoma were identified;[544] the observed-to-expected ratio (standard incidence ratio) compared with that of the U.S. population was 6.5. This was probably an underestimate of the risk, because it was likely that not all cases of pulmonary carcinoma in the AIDS population had been identified and that some patients in the general population were infected with HIV.[544] Although the results of this study were not corrected for the amount of cigarettes smoked, a strong and statistically significant risk for pulmonary carcinoma persisted even after assuming that all patients in the HIV-infected cohort were smokers. The biologic mechanism for this increased risk remains to be determined; however, some investigators have found evidence of increased genomic instability in tumors derived from HIV-infected patients compared with those from HIV-indeterminate individuals.[546a] The clinical and radiologic manifestations of pulmonary carcinoma in patients who have AIDS are similar to those in HIV-negative individuals.[547–551a]

## MISCELLANEOUS PULMONARY ABNORMALITIES

In addition to infection and malignancy, HIV infection has been associated with a variety of other pulmonary abnormalities (*see* Table 44–1). Their relative rarity in the general population compared with patients who are HIV seropositive suggests that some of these, such as pulmonary hypertension and LIP, are complications of the infection. However, it is possible that some of the other associations (e.g., with sarcoidosis) are spurious.

### Nonspecific Interstitial Pneumonitis

NSIP is a relatively common abnormality in HIV-positive patients that is characterized histologically by a mild to moderate infiltrate of lymphocytes and occasional plasma cells in the peribronchiolar, perivascular, and interlobular septal interstitial tissue[552] (Fig. 44–49); in contrast to LIP (*see* farther on), involvement of the alveolar interstitium is relatively mild or absent altogether. By definition, the cause of the inflammation cannot be detected and the diagnosis is made after infection and malignancy have been excluded as causes of radiologic abnormalities. Despite the frequency of the latter two complications, NSIP is likely the most common pulmonary abnormality identified in seropositive patients. For example, in one study of 24 HIV-infected patients who did not have symptoms but who had a nonpulmonary defining illness for AIDS or a CD4 lymphocyte count of less than 200 cells/μl, extensive pulmonary investigation was performed with the aim of determining the prevalence of occult PCP.[553] All patients had a normal chest radiograph and no history of previous *Pneumocystis* infection or prophylactic therapy. Gas exchange and lung function were within normal limits. Although transbronchial biopsy and BAL detected no organisms, 11 of 23 specimens showed chronic, nonspecific interstitial inflammation of the pulmonary parenchyma.

In a second study of 110 HIV-seropositive patients who were investigated because of the new appearance of any combination of pulmonary signs, symptoms, and radiographic abnormalities, NSIP was identified in 41 (38%) and was seen in association with 48 of 152 (32%) episodes of clinical pneumonitis.[554] Of these 41 patients, more than half had normal chest radiographs; 13 had no previous pulmonary history, whereas 28 had concurrent KS, previous experimental therapies that could have conceivably been a cause of interstitial pneumonia (such as interferon-α, interleukin-2, or suramin), or a history of previous PCP or drug abuse.[554] Similar results were seen in a group of 351 HIV-seropositive patients who underwent investigation because of suspected PCP.[555] Of the 67 who did not have the infection, 16 (24%) had NSIP on histologic examination; this was the most common diagnosis made in this group of patients.

The radiologic findings usually consist of a fine reticular or reticulonodular pattern or ground-glass opacities in the perihilar regions or distributed diffusely throughout both lungs.[556, 557] The appearance resembles that of PCP. In one

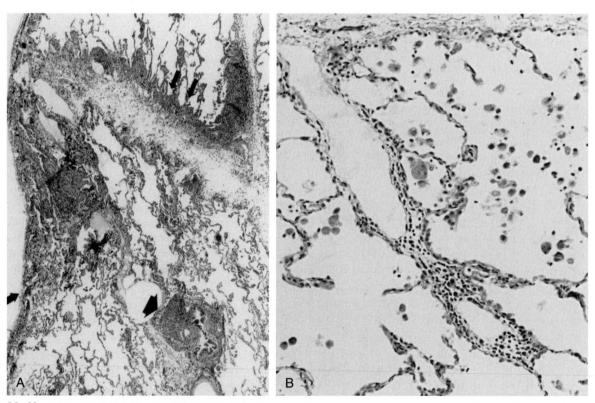

**Figure 44–49. AIDS: Nonspecific Interstitial Pneumonitis.** A section from an open-lung biopsy *(A)* shows a lymphoid infiltrate present predominantly in the interstitial tissue adjacent to a bronchiole *(large arrow)*, interlobular septum *(double arrows)*, and pleura *(thin arrow)*. Note the almost complete absence of parenchymal interstitial infiltration. Another section shows a mild lymphocytic infiltrate limited to the tissue adjacent to a small lymphatic vessel. *(A, ×42; B, ×188)*. (From Travis WD, Fox CH, Devaney KO, et al: Lymphoid pneumonitis in 50 adult patients infected with the human immunodeficiency virus. Hum Pathol 23:529, 1992.)

series of 36 patients diagnosed by transbronchial or open-lung biopsy, 16 (44%) had normal chest radiographs.[556]

The clinical presentation of patients who have NSIP is diverse but in general terms is indistinguishable from that associated with opportunistic infection.[554, 555] Most patients have fever, cough, and dyspnea that is usually mild. Mild to moderate deficits in gas exchange are common.[554] Patients tend to present earlier in their clinical course than those who have *Pneumocystis* pneumonia; immunosuppression is less advanced, weight is higher, and the serum albumin and LDH levels are closer to normal.[555]

Although subsequent episodes of NSIP occur in some patients, resolution or stabilization is the rule, even in the absence of therapy.[554, 555] The main diagnostic consideration is to distinguish it from opportunistic infection or any other pathologic process. Whether NSIP causes significant lung damage in the long term, has any prognostic significance, or predisposes to other lung disease is not known.

### Lymphocytic Interstitial Pneumonitis

LIP is a lymphoproliferative disorder characterized histologically by infiltration of the pulmonary parenchyma by cytologically mature lymphocytes and plasma cells (*see* page 1271).[558, 559] Although rare in HIV infected adults,[478] it is relatively common in children,[560, 561] in whom it is an AIDS-defining disease.[562]

The pathogenesis is unknown. In some studies, it has been associated with high titers of EBV antibodies, suggesting that it may represent a manifestation of infection by this virus;[563] however, some investigators have failed to find evidence of EBV in tissue specimens examined by *in situ*

hybridization.[552] As indicated previously, it is also possible that the reaction is a direct effect of HIV infection. The detection of the virus in some biopsy specimens by *in situ* hybridization and the results of experimental studies in sheep infected with ovine lentivirus (an organism related to HIV) support this hypothesis.[552, 564]

The observations that LIP and NSIP may both be a direct result of HIV infection and that there is some histologic overlap between the two have led to speculation that the two abnormalities may represent a spectrum of disease rather than separate entities;[558] however, differences in their presentation and course and the lack of progression of NSIP to LIP in some follow-up studies suggest that they should be considered distinct clinically.[552]

Histologically, LIP is characterized by a more or less diffuse infiltrate of mononuclear cells, usually predominantly T lymphocytes[234, 552] (Fig. 44–50). Although involvement of interstitial tissue adjacent to small vessels and airways is common, the infiltrate is most prominent in the alveolar interstitium. Focal nodular accumulations of lymphoid cells, some of which may have germinal centers, can be seen. Cytologically, the cells appear mature and show minimal nuclear atypia. The diagnosis of a reactive process is supported by the presence of polyclonality on immunohistochemical or molecular analysis, one or both of which should be performed to exclude lymphoma.

Radiographic findings consist of fine or coarse reticular or reticulonodular opacities,[566] multiple nodules measuring 2 to 5 mm in diameter,[31a] or poorly defined, hazy (ground-glass) opacities (Fig. 44–51). Occasionally, areas of consolidation may be seen superimposed on a background reticulonodular pattern.[566] HRCT scanning demonstrates areas of ground-glass attenuation[534] or ill-defined 2- to 4-mm nodules,

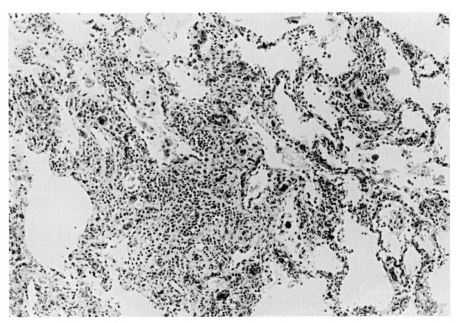

**Figure 44–50. AIDS: Lymphocytic Interstitial Pneumonitis.** A section of lung shows a moderately severe mononuclear inflammatory cell infiltrate composed predominantly of lymphocytes in the peribronchiolar and alveolar interstitium.

frequently in a peribronchial distribution.[567] Cysts similar to those seen in PCP have been seen in some patients.[534] The abnormalities may resemble those of other lymphoproliferative disorders; for example, in one series of five adult patients who had LIP, the HRCT findings (ill-defined 2- to 4-mm nodules) were similar to those in three patients who had an "atypical lymphoproliferative disorder" and one who had mucosa-associated lymphoma (maltoma).[567]

Patients present with the insidious onset of dyspnea, usually accompanied by cough and fever.[558, 559, 568] Auscultation may be normal or reveal crackles.[558] The abnormality is often associated with a CD8 lymphocytosis, diffuse hypergammaglobulinemia, a Sjögren's syndrome–like disorder, and lymphocytic infiltration of peripheral lymph nodes, liver, kidneys, bone marrow, and nasopharynx.[478, 558, 569] An HLA-DR5 haplotype is common in such patients, especially African Americans.[569] Pulmonary function studies have revealed restriction and a low diffusing capacity.[558] Gas exchange may be impaired.[558]

Lung biopsy is required for definitive diagnosis. The finding of a lymphocytic alveolitis on analysis of BAL fluid is insufficient because of its lack of specificity. For example, in one investigation of 154 HIV-infected patients who developed pulmonary infection or neoplasia, lymphocytic alveolitis was found in 78%;[570] the abnormality was also observed in 72% of 122 patients who had no radiographic or clinical evidence of pulmonary disease. In the 37 patients whose BAL lymphocytes were typed, 40% to 93% were CD8 in type. Diffuse reticular interstitial opacification was seen on radiographs in 36% of patients. These findings and symptoms of cough and dyspnea were associated with a lower blood CD4 count than that in patients who were asymptomatic and who had normal radiographs. Pulmonary function studies revealed abnormal gas exchange in 85% of the 33

patients tested;[570] however, in 5 patients who had significant radiographic abnormalities, function studies were completely normal. Open-lung biopsy performed in 4 patients who did not have tumor or opportunistic infection showed a diffuse lymphocytic infiltrate within the lymphatic channels with sparing of the alveolar septa, distinguishing the abnormality from LIP; bronchiolitis was also observed in 3 patients. As expected, the infiltrating lymphocytes were CD8 in type. The precise nature of BAL-documented lymphocytic alveolitis and its relation to NSIP and LIP is unclear; however, it is possible that it represents a cytokine-driven host response to infection in the lung with HIV.[571]

Transbronchial biopsy is the procedure of choice for the diagnosis of LIP;[478] however, open-lung biopsy may be required,[552] especially when ancillary clinical features of the disease are absent. The clinical course is variable. Some patients have had very mild disease, which has resolved spontaneously, whereas others have developed respiratory failure.[478, 558]

### Human Immunodeficiency Virus–Associated "Primary" Pulmonary Hypertension

Pulmonary hypertension unassociated with a clear-cut cause has been described in a number of patients who have AIDS (*see* page 1914).[572–576] Although direct involvement of the pulmonary vascular endothelium by HIV has not been described,[575] the improvement in pulmonary vascular resistance in some patients after antiretroviral therapy suggests a direct role of the virus in its pathogenesis.[576] Plexiform lesions have been identified on histologic examination in about 85% of cases;[574, 577] recurrent thromboembolism and veno-occlusive disease are uncommon causes.[574]

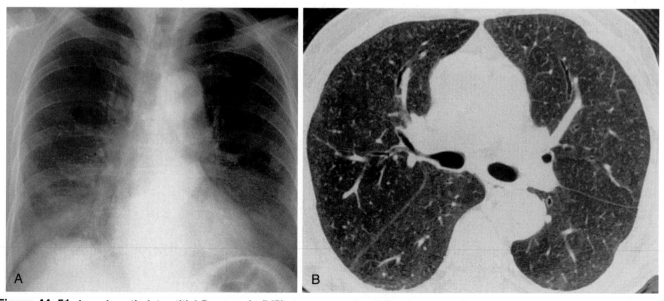

**Figure 44–51. Lymphocytic Interstitial Pneumonia (LIP).** A posteroanterior chest radiograph *(A)* in a 74-year-old man with AIDS demonstrates extensive bilateral hazy increase in opacity of both lungs. An HRCT scan *(B)* demonstrates diffuse ground-glass attenuation and poorly defined small nodules. The diagnosis of LIP was confirmed at open-lung biopsy.

## Pulmonary Alveolar Proteinosis

Both primary (idiopathic)[578] and secondary[579, 580] pulmonary alveolar proteinosis have been described in patients who have AIDS. There is evidence that the secondary form may be more common than is generally recognized in the setting of PCP. In one study of 26 patients who had this infection, lipoproteinaceous material similar to that seen in alveolar proteinosis but different from the typical foamy exudate of PCP was found in nine cases on electron and light microscopy examination of BAL fluid samples;[580] no such material could be found in control samples obtained from patients who did not have PCP.

# REFERENCES

1. Quinn TC: Global burden of the HIV pandemic. Lancet 348:99, 1996.
2. Anonymous: Update: Trends in AIDS incidence, deaths and prevalence—United States, 1996. JAMA 277:874, 1997.
3. Anonymous: Update: Trends in AIDS incidence—United States, 1996. MMWR 46:861, 1997.
4. Ward JW, Duchin JS: The epidemiology of HIV and AIDS in the United States. AIDS Clin Rev 1, 1997–98.
5. Anonymous: AIDS Rates. MMWR 46:333, 1997.
6. Gourevitch MN: The epidemiology of HIV and AIDS: Current trends. Med Clin North Am 80:1223, 1996.
7. Grinstead OA, Peterson JL, Faigeles B, et al: Antibody testing and condom use among heterosexual African Americans at risk for HIV infection: The National AIDS Behaviourial Surveys. Am J Public Health 87:85, 1997.
8. Cu-Uvin S, Flanigan TP, Rich JD, et al: Human immunodeficiency virus infection and acquired immunodeficiency syndrome among North American women. Am J Med 101:316, 1996.
9. Anonymous: Gonorrhea among men who have sex with men: Selected sexually transmitted diseases clinics, 1993–1996. MMWR 46:889, 1997.
10. Petridou E, Dafni U, Freeman J, et al: Routinely reported sexually transmitted diseases presage the evolution of the AIDS epidemic. Epidemiology 8:449, 1997.
11. Marcus R, Culver DH, Bell DM, et al: Risk of human immunodeficiency virus infection among emergency department workers. Am J Med 94:363, 1993.
12. Cardo DM, Culver DH, Ciesielski CA, et al: A case-control study of HIV seroconversion in health care workers after percutaneous exposure. N Engl J Med 337:1485, 1997.
13. Hamers FF, Batter V, Downs AM, et al: The HIV epidemic associated with injecting drug use in Europe: Geographic and time trends. AIDS 11:1365, 1997.
14. Palella FJ Jr, Delaney KM, Moorman AC, et al: Declining morbidity and mortality among patients with advanced human immunodeficiency virus infection. N Engl J Med 338:853, 1998.
15. Ware JH, Antman EM: National HIV case reporting for the United States: A defining moment in the history of the epidemic. N Engl J Med 337:1162, 1997.
16. Allen S, Lindan C, Serufilira A, et al: Human immunodeficiency virus infection in urban Rwanda. JAMA 266:1657, 1991.
17. Pais P: HIV and India: Looking into the abyss. Trop Med Int Health 1:295, 1996.
18. Bollinger RC, Tripathy SP, Quinn TC: The human immunodeficiency virus epidemic in India: Current magnitude and future projections. Medicine 74:97, 1995.
19. Gottlieb MS, Schroff R, Schanker HM, et al: *Pneumocystis carinii* pneumonia and mucosal candidiasis in previously healthy homosexual men: Evidence of a new acquired cellular immunodeficiency. N Engl J Med 305:1425, 1981.
20. Curran JW: Epidemiologic aspects of the current outbreak of Kaposi's sarcoma and opportunistic infections. N Engl J Med 306:248, 1982.
21. Hopewell PC, Luce JM: Pulmonary involvement in the acquired immunodeficiency syndrome. Chest 87:104, 1985.
22. Murray JF, Garay SM, Hopewell PC, et al: Pulmonary complications of the acquired immunodeficiency syndrome: An update. Am Rev Respir Dis 135:504, 1987.
23. Rankin JA, Collman R, Daniele RP: Acquired immune deficiency syndrome and the lung. Chest 94:155, 1988.
24. Rosen MJ: Overview of pulmonary complications. Clin Chest Med 4:621, 1996.
25. Hanson DL, Chu SY, Farizo KM, et al: Distribution of CD4+ T lymphocytes at diagnosis of acquired immunodeficiency syndrome-defining and other human immunodeficiency virus-related illnesses. Arch Intern Med 155:1537, 1995.
26. Wallace JM, Hansen NI, Lavange L, et al: Respiratory disease trends in the pulmonary complications of HIV infection study cohort. Am J Respir Crit Care Med 155:72, 1997.
27. Sehonanda A, Choi YJ, Blum S: Changing patterns of autopsy findings among persons with acquired immunodeficiency syndrome in an inner-city population: A 12-year retrospective study. Arch Pathol Lab Med 120:459, 1996.
28. Hirschtick RE, Glassroth J, Jordan MC, et al: Bacterial pneumonia in persons infected with the human immunodeficiency virus. N Engl J Med 333:845, 1995.
28a. Afessa B, Green W, Chiao J, et al: Pulmonary complications of HIV infection. Autopsy findings. Chest 113:1225, 1998.
29. Daley CL: Bacterial pneumonia in HIV-infected patients. Semin Respir Infect 8:104, 1993.
30. Noskin GA, Glassroth J: Bacterial pneumonia associated with HIV-1 infection. Clin Chest Med 17:713, 1996.
31. Davis L, Beck JM, Shellito J: Update: HIV infection and pulmonary host defenses. Semin Respir Infect 8:75, 1993.
31a. Richards PJ, Armstrong P, Parkin JM, et al: Chest imaging in AIDS. Clin Radiol 53:554, 1998.
31b. Amin Z, Miller RF, Shaw PJ: Lobar or segmental consolidation on chest radiographs of patients with HIV infection. Clin Radiol 52:541, 1997.
32. Janoff EN, Breiman RF, Daley CL, et al: Pneumococcal disease during HIV infection: Epidemiologic, clinical and immunologic perspectives. Ann Intern Med 117:314, 1992.
33. Gilks CF, Ojoo SA, Ojoo JC, et al: Invasive pneumococcal disease in a cohort study of predominantly HIV-1 infected female sex-workers in Nairobi, Kenya. Lancet 347:718, 1996.
34. Miller RF, Foley NM, Kessel D, et al: Community acquired lobar pneumonia in patients with HIV infection and AIDS. Thorax 49:367, 1994.
35. Falco V, Fernandez de Sevilla T, Alegre J, et al: Bacterial pneumonia in HIV-infected patients: A prospective study of 68 episodes. Eur Respir J 7:235, 1994.
36. Schlamm HT, Yancovitz SR: *Haemophilus influenzae* pneumonia in young adults with AIDS, ARC or risk of AIDS. Am J Med 86:11, 1989.
37. Steinhart R, Reingold AL, Taylor F, et al: Invasive *Haemophilus influenzae* infections in men with HIV infection. JAMA 268:3350, 1992.
38. Levine SJ, White DA, Fels AOS: The incidence and significance of *Staphylococcus aureus* in respiratory cultures from patients infected with the human immunodeficiency virus. Am Rev Respir Dis 141:89, 1990.
39. Blatt SP, Dolan MJ, Hendrix CW, et al: Legionnaire's disease in human immunodeficiency virus-infected patients: Eight cases and review. Clin Infect Dis 18:227, 1994.
40. Johnson KM, Huseby JS: Lung abscess caused by *Legionella micdadei*. Chest 111:252, 1997.
41. Mitchell DM, Miller RF: New developments in the pulmonary diseases affecting HIV infected individuals. Thorax 50:293, 1995.
42. Baron AD, Hillander H: *Pseudomonas aeruginosa* bronchopulmonary infection in late human immunodeficiency virus disease. Am Rev Respir Dis 148:992, 1993.
43. Scott MA, Graham BS, Verrall R, et al: *Rhodococcus equi:* An increasingly recognized opportunistic pathogen. Report of 12 cases and review of 65 cases in the literature. Am J Clin Pathol 103:649, 1995.
44. Verville TD, Huycke MM, Greenfield RA, et al: *Rhodococcus equi* infections of humans: 12 cases and a review of the literature. Medicine 73:119, 1994.
45. Arlotti M, Zoboli G, Moscatelli GL, et al: *Rhodococcus equi* infection in HIV-positive subjects: A retrospective analysis of 24 cases. Scand J Infect Dis 28:463, 1996.
46. Hondalus MK, Mosser DM: Survival and replication of *Rhodococcus equi* in macrophages. Infect Immun 62:4167, 1994.
47. Hondalus MK, Diamond MS, Rosenthal LA, et al: The intracellular bacterium *Rhodococcus equi* requires Mac-1 to bind to mammalian cells. Infect Immunol 61:2919, 1993.
48. Takai S, Sasaki Y, Ikeda T, et al: Virulence of *Rhodococcus equi* isolates from patients with and without AIDS. J Clin Microbiol 32:457, 1994.
49. Nordmann P, Keller M, Espinasse F, et al: Correlation between antibiotic resistance, phage-like particle presence, and virulence in *Rhodococcus equi* human isolates. J Clin Microbiol 32:377, 1994.
50. Nordmann P, Ronco E, Nauciel C: Role of T-lymphocyte subsets in *Rhodococcus equi* infection. Infect Immunol 60:2748, 1992.
51. Samies JH, Hathaway BN, Echols RM, et al: Lung abscess due to *Corynebacterium equi:* Report of the first case in a patient with acquired immune deficiency syndrome. Am J Med 80:685, 1986.
52. Kwon KY, Colby TV: Rhodococcus equi pneumonia and pulmonary malakoplakia in acquired immunodeficiency syndrome. Pathologic features. Arch Pathol Lab Med 118:744, 1994.
53. De Peralta-Venturina MN, Clubb FJ, Kielhofner MA: Pulmonary malacoplakia associated with *Rhodococcus equi* infection in a patient with acquired immunodeficiency syndrome. Am J Clin Pathol 102:459, 1994.
54. Scannell KA, Portoni EJ, Finkle HI, et al: Pulmonary malacoplakia and *Rhodococcus equi* infection in a patient with AIDS. Chest 97:1000, 1990.
55. Yuoh G, Hove MG, Wen J, et al: Pulmonary malacoplakia in acquired immunodeficiency syndrome: An ultrastructural study of morphogenesis of Michaelis-Gutmann bodies. Mod Pathol 9:476, 1996.
56. MacGregor JH, Samuelson WM, Sane DC, et al: Opportunistic lung infection caused by *Rhodococcus (Corynebacterium) equi.* Radiology 160:83, 1986.
57. Van Etta LL, Filce GA, Ferguson RM, et al: *Corynebacterium equi:* A review of 12 cases of human infection. Rev Infect Dis 5:1012, 1983.
58. Legras A, Lemmens B, Dequin PF, et al: Tamponade due to *Rhodococcus equi* in acquired immunodeficiency syndrome. Chest 106:1278, 1994.
59. Lachman MF: Cytologic appearance of *Rhodococcus equi* in bronchoalveolar lavage specimens: A case report. Acta Cytol 39:111, 1995.
60. van Hoeven KH, Dookhan DB, Petersen RO: Cytologic features of pulmonary malakoplakia related to *Rhodococcus equi* in an immunocompromised host. Diagn Cytopathol 15:325, 1996.
61. Sughayer M, Ali SZ, Erozan YS, et al: Pulmonary malacoplakia associated with *Rhodococcus equi* infection in an AIDS patient: Report of a case with diagnosis by fine needle aspiration. Acta Cytol 41:507, 1997.
62. Shapiro JM, Romney BM, Weiden MD, et al: *Rhodococcus equi* endobronchial mass with lung abscess in a patient with AIDS. Thorax 47:62, 1992.
63. Slater LN, Welch DF, Hensel D, et al: A newly recognized fastidious gram-negative pathogen as a cause of fever and bacteremia. N Engl J Med 323:1587, 1990.
64. Adal KA, Cockerell CJ, Petri WA: Cat scratch disease, bacillary angiomatosis, and other infections due to *Rochalimaea*. N Engl J Med 330:1509, 1994.
65. Moore EH, Russell LA, Klein JS, et al: Bacillary angiomatosis in patients with AIDS: Multiorgan imaging findings. Radiology 197:67, 1995.
66. Koehler JE, LeBoit PE, Egbert BM, et al: Cutaneous vascular lesions and disseminated cat-scratch disease in patients with the acquired immunodeficiency syndrome (AIDS) and AIDS-related complex. Ann Intern Med 109:449, 1988.
67. LeBoit PE, Berger TG, Egbert BM, et al: Bacillary angiomatosis: The histopathology and differential diagnosis of a pseudoneoplastic infection in patients with human immunodeficiency virus disease. Am J Surg Pathol 13:909, 1989.

68. Slater LN, Kyung-Whan M: Polypoid endobronchial lesions: A manifestation of bacillary angiomatosis. Chest 102:972, 1992.
69. Foltzer MA, Guiney WB, Wager GC, et al: Bronchopulmonary bacillary angiomatosis. Chest 104:973, 1993.
70. Coche E, Beigelman C, Lucidarme O, et al: Thoracic bacillary angiomatosis in a patient with AIDS. Am J Roentgenol 165:56, 1995.
71. Foltzer MA, Guiney WB Jr, Wager GC, et al: Bronchopulmonary bacillary angiomatosis. Chest 104:973, 1993.
72. Tsang WY, Chan JK: Bacillary angiomatosis: A "new" disease with a broadening clinicopathologic spectrum. Histol Histopathol 7:143, 1992.
73. Kostianovsky M, Greco MA: Angiogenic process in bacillary angiomatosis. Ultrastruct Pathol 18:349, 1994.
74. Kramer MR, Uttamchandani RB: The radiographic appearance of pulmonary nocardiosis associated with AIDS. Chest 98:382, 1990.
75. Chin DP, Hopewell PC: Mycobacterial complications of HIV infection. Clin Chest Med 17:697, 1996.
76. World Health Organization: Statement on AIDS and Tuberculosis. Geneva, March 1989.
77. Haas DW, Des Prez RM: Tuberculosis and acquired immunodeficiency syndrome: A historical perspective on recent developments. Am J Med 96:439, 1994.
78. Barnes PF, Bloch AB, Davidson PT, et al: Tuberculosis in patients with human immunodeficiency virus infection. N Engl J Med 324:1644, 1991.
79. Selwyn PA, Hartel D, Lewis VA, et al: A prospective study of the risk of tuberculosis among intravenous drug users with human immunodeficiency virus infection. N Engl J Med 320:545, 1989.
80. Burwen DR, Bloch AB, Griffin LD, et al: National trends in the concurrence of tuberculosis and acquired immunodeficiency syndrome. Arch Intern Med 155:1281, 1995.
81. De Cock KM, Soro B, Coulibaly IM, et al: Tuberculosis and HIV infection in sub-Saharan Africa. JAMA 268:1581, 1992.
82. Eriki PP, Okwera A, Aisu T, et al: The influence of human immunodeficiency virus infection on tuberculosis in Kampala, Uganda. Am Rev Respir Dis 143:185, 1991.
83. Colebunders RL, Ryser RW, Nzilambi N, et al: HIV infection in patients with tuberculosis in Kinshasa, Zaire. Am Rev Respir Dis 139:1082, 1989.
84. Milka-Cabanne N, Braunder M, Kamanfu G, et al: Radiographic abnormalities in tuberculosis and risk of coexisting human immunodeficiency virus infection: Methods and preliminary results from Bujumbura, Burundi. Am J Respir Crit Care Med 152:794, 1995.
85. Batungwanayo J, Taelman H, Dhote R, et al: Pulmonary tuberculosis in Kigali, Rwanda: Impact of human immunodeficiency virus infection on clinical and radiographic presentation. Am Rev Respir Dis 146:53, 1992.
86. Daley CL, Mugusi F, Chen LL, et al: Pulmonary complications of HIV infection in Dar es Salaam, Tanzania. Am J Respir Crit Care Med 154:105, 1996.
87. Asch SM, London AS, Barnes PF, et al: Testing for human immunodeficiency virus infection among tuberculosis patients in Los Angeles. Am J Respir Crit Care Med 155:378, 1997.
88. Barnes PF, Silva C, Otaya M: Testing for human immunodeficiency virus infection in patients with tuberculosis. Am J Respir Crit Car Med 153:1448, 1996.
89. Braun MM, Badi N, Ryder RW, et al: A retrospective cohort study of the risk of tuberculosis among women of childbearing age with HIV infection in Zaire. Am Rev Respir Dis 143:501, 1991.
90. Allen S, Batungwanayo J, Kerlikowske K, et al: Two-year incidence of tuberculosis in cohorts of HIV-infected and uninfected urban Rwandan women. Am Rev Respir Dis 146:1439, 1992.
91. Long R, Scalcini M, Manfreda J, et al: Impact of human immunodeficiency virus type 1 on tuberculosis in rural Haiti. Am Rev Respir Dis 143:69, 1991.
92. Markowitz N, Hansen NI, Hopewell PC, et al: Incidence of tuberculosis in the United States among HIV-infected persons. Ann Intern Med 126:123, 1997.
93. Heckbert SR, Elarth A, Nolan CM: The impact of human immunodeficiency virus infection on tuberculosis in young men in Seattle-King County, Washington. Chest 102:433, 1992.
94. Friedman LN, Williams MT, Singh TP, et al: Tuberculosis, AIDS and death among substance abusers on welfare in New York City. N Engl J Med 334:828, 1996.
95. Brudney K, Dobkin J: Resurgent tuberculosis in New York City: Human immunodeficiency virus, homelessness and the decline of tuberculosis control programs. Am Rev Respir Dis 144:745, 1991.
96. Gelman BB, Wolf DA, Olano JP, et al: Incarceration and the acquired immunodeficiency syndrome: Autopsy results in Texas prison inmates. Hum Pathol 27:1282, 1996.
97. Lyon R, Haque AK, Asmuth DM, et al: Changing patterns of infections in patients with AIDS: A study of 279 autopsies of prison inmates and nonincarcerated patients at a university hospital in eastern Texas, 1984–1993. Clin Infect Dis 23:241, 1996.
98. Daley CL, Hahn JA, Moss AR, et al: Incidence of tuberculosis in injection drug users in San Francisco. Am J Respir Crit Care Med 157:19, 1998.
99. Small PM, Hopewell PC, Singh SP, et al: The epidemiology of tuberculosis in San Francisco: A population-based study using conventional and molecular methods. N Engl J Med 330:1703, 1994.
100. Alland D, Kalkut GE, Moss AR, et al: Transmission of tuberculosis in New York City: An analysis by DNA fingerprinting and conventional epidemiologic methods. N Engl J Med 330:1710, 1994.
101. Fischl MA, Uttamchandani RB, Daikos GL, et al: An outbreak of tuberculosis caused by multiple-drug-resistant tubercle bacilli among patients with HIV infection. Ann Intern Med 117:177, 1992.
102. Beck-Sagué C, Dooley SW, Hutton MD, et al: Hospital outbreak of multidrug-resistant mycobacterium tuberculosis infections: Factors in transmission to staff and HIV-infected patients. JAMA 268:1280, 1992.
103. Di Perri G, Cruciani M, Danzi MC, et al: Nosocomial epidemic active tuberculosis among HIV-infected patients. Lancet 2:1502, 1989.
104. Dooley SW, Villarino ME, Lawrence M, et al: Nosocomial transmission of tuberculosis in a hospital unit for HIV-infected patients. JAMA 267:2632, 1992.
105. Edlin BR, Tokars JI, Grieco MH, et al: An outbreak of multidrug-resistant tuberculosis among hospitalized patients with the acquired immunodeficiency syndrome. N Engl J Med 326:1514, 1992.
106. Pearson ML, Jereb JA, Frieden TR, et al: Nosocomial transmission of multidrug-resistant mycobacterium tuberculosis. Ann Intern Med 117:191, 1992.
107. Law KF, Jagirdar J, Weiden MD, et al: Tuberculosis in HIV-positive patients: Cellular response and immune activation in the lung. Am J Respir Crit Care Med 153:1377, 1996.
108. Hill AR: Mycobacterial infections in AIDS. Can J Infect Dis 2:19, 1991.
109. Wallis RS, Vjecha M, Amir-Tahmasseb M, et al: Influence of tuberculosis on human immunodeficiency virus (HIV-1): Enhanced cytokine expression and elevated beta 2-microglobulin in HIV-1-associated tuberculosis. J Infect Dis 167:43, 1993.
110. Nakata K, Rom WN, Honda Y, et al: Mycobacterium tuberculosis enhances human immunodeficiency virus-1 replication in the lung. Am J Respir Crit Care Med 155:996, 1997.
111. Leung AN, Brauner MW, Gamsu G, et al: Pulmonary tuberculosis: Comparison of CT findings in HIV-seropositive and HIV-seronegative patients. Radiology 198:687, 1996.
112. Greenberg SD, Frager D, Suster B, et al: Active pulmonary tuberculosis in patients with AIDS: Spectrum of radiographic findings (including a normal appearance). Radiology 193:115, 1994.
113. Haramati LB, Jenny-Avital ER, Alterman DD: Effect of HIV status on chest radiographic and CT findings in patients with tuberculosis. Clin Radiol 52:31, 1997.
114. McGuinness G: Changing trends in the pulmonary manifestations of AIDS. Radiol Clin North Am 35:1029, 1997.
115. Goodman PC: Tuberculosis and AIDS. Radiol Clin North Am 33:707, 1995.
116. Jones BE, Young SMM, Antoniskis D, et al: Relationship of the manifestations of tuberculosis to CD4 cell counts in patients with human immunodeficiency virus infection. Am Rev Respir Dis 148:1292, 1993.
117. Long R, Maycher B, Scalcini M, et al: The chest roentgenogram in pulmonary tuberculosis patients seropositive for human immunodeficiency virus type 1. Chest 99:123, 1991.
118. Harries AD: Tuberculosis in human immunodeficiency virus infection in developing countries. Lancet 335:387, 1990.
119. Saks AM, Posner R: Tuberculosis in HIV positive patients in South Africa: A comparative radiological study with HIV negative patients. Clin Radiol 46:387, 1992.
120. Louie E, Rice LB, Holzman RS: Tuberculosis in non-Haitian patients with acquired immunodeficiency syndrome. Chest 90:542, 1986.
121. Rieder HL, Cauthen GM, Bloch AB, et al: Tuberculosis and acquired immunodeficiency syndrome: Florida. Arch Intern Med 149:1268, 1989.
122. Chaisson RE, Schecter GF, Theuer CP, et al: Tuberculosis in patients with the acquired immunodeficiency syndrome. Am Rev Respir Dis 136:570, 1987.
123. Pitchenik AE, Rubinson HA: The radiographic appearance of tuberculosis in patients with the acquired immunodeficiency syndrome (AIDS) and pre-AIDS. Am Rev Respir Dis 131:393, 1985.
124. Kramer F, Modilevesky T, Waliany AR, et al: Delayed diagnosis of tuberculosis in patients with human immunodeficiency syndrome. Am J Med 89:451, 1990.
125. Greenberg SD, Frager D, Suster B, et al: Active pulmonary tuberculosis in patients with AIDS: Spectrum of radiographic findings (including a normal appearance). Radiology 193:115, 1994.
126. Keiper MD, Beumont M, Elshami A, et al: CD4 T lymphocyte count and the radiographic presentation of pulmonary tuberculosis: A study of the relationship between these factors in patients with human immunodeficiency virus infection. Chest 107:74, 1995.
127. Lessnau KD, Gorla M, Talavera W: Radiographic findings in HIV-positive patients with sensitive and resistant tuberculosis. Chest 106:687, 1994.
128. Colebunders RL, Ryder RW, Nzilambi N, et al: HIV infection in patients with tuberculosis in Kinshasa, Zaire. Am Rev Respir Dis 139:1082, 1989.
129. Perich J, Ayuso MC, Vilana R, et al: Disseminated lymphatic tuberculosis in acquired immunodeficiency syndrome: Computed tomography findings. Can Assoc Radiol J 41:353, 1990.
130. Pastores SM, Naidich DP, Aranda CP, et al: Intrathoracic adenopathy associated with pulmonary tuberculosis in patients with human immunodeficiency virus infection. Chest 103:1433, 1993.
131. Laissy JP, Cadi M, Boudiaf ZE, et al: Pulmonary tuberculosis: Computed tomography and high-resolution computed tomography patterns in patients who are either HIV-negative or HIV-seropositive. J Thorac Imaging 13:58, 1998.
132. Chaisson RE, Schecter GF, Theuer CP, et al: Tuberculosis in patients with the acquired immunodeficiency syndrome: Clinical features, response to therapy, and survival. Am Rev Respir Dis 136:570, 1987.
133. Jones BE, Young SMM, Antoniskis D, et al: Relationship of the manifestations of tuberculosis to CD4 cell counts in patients with human immunodeficiency virus infection. Am Rev Respir Dis 148:1292, 1993.

134. Hocqueloux L, Lesprit P, Herrmann J-L, et al: Pulmonary *Mycobacterium avium* complex disease without dissemination in HIV-infected patients. Chest 113:542, 1998.

135. Shafer RW, Goldberg R, Sierra M, et al: Frequency of *Mycobacterium tuberculosis* bacteremia in patients with tuberculosis in an area endemic for AIDS. Am Rev Respir Dis 140:1611, 1989.

136. Fertel D, Pitchenik AE: Tuberculosis in acquired immune deficiency syndrome. Semin Respir Infect 4:198, 1989.

137. Farrar DJ, Flanigan TP, Gordon NM, et al: Tuberculous brain abscess in a patient with HIV infection: Case report and review. Am J Med 102:297, 1997.

138. Richter C, Perenboom R, Mtoni I, et al: Clinical features of HIV-seropositive and HIV-seronegative patients with tuberculosis pleural effusion in Dar es Salaam, Tanzania. Chest 106:1471, 1994.

139. Frye MD, Pozik CJ, Sahn SA: Tuberculous pleurisy is more common in AIDS than in non-AIDS patients with tuberculosis. Chest 112:393, 1997.

140. Joseph J, Strange C, Sahn SA: Pleural effusions in hospitalized patients with AIDS. Ann Intern Med 118:856, 1993.

141. Relkin F, Aranda CP, Garay SM, et al: Pleural tuberculosis and HIV infection. Chest 105:1338, 1994.

142. Layton MC, Cantwell MF, Dorsinville GJ, et al: Tuberculosis screening among homeless persons with AIDS living in single-room-occupancy hotels. Am J Public Health 85:1556, 1995.

143. Martin Sanchez V, Alvarez-Guisasola F, Cayla JA, et al: Predictive factors of *Mycobacterium tuberculosis* infection and pulmonary tuberculosis in prisoners. Int J Epidemiol 24:630, 1995.

144. Kramer F, Modilevsky T, Waliany AR, et al: Delayed diagnosis of tuberculosis in patients with human immunodeficiency virus infection. Am J Med 89:451, 1990.

145. Markowitz N, Hansen NI, Wilcosky TC, et al: Tuberculin and anergy testing in HIV-seropositive and HIV-seronegative persons. Ann Intern Med 119:185, 1993.

146. Ellner JJ: Tuberculosis in the time of AIDS: The facts and the message. Chest 98:1051, 1990.

147. Gourevitch MN, Hartel D, Schoenbaum EE, et al: Lack of association of induration size with HIV infection among drug users reacting to Tuberculin. Am J Respir Crit Care Med 154:1029, 1996.

148. Moreno S, Baraia-Etxaburu J, Bouza E, et al: Risk for developing tuberculosis among anergic patients infected with HIV. Ann Intern Med 119:194, 1993.

149. Selwyn PA, Sckell BM, Alcabes P, et al: High risk of active tuberculosis in HIV-infected drug users with cutaneous anergy. JAMA 268:504, 1992.

150. Webster CT, Gordin FM, Matts JP, et al: Two-stage tuberculin skin testing in individuals with human immunodeficiency virus infection. Am J Respir Crit Care Med 151:805, 1995.

151. Hecker MT, Johnson JL, Whalen CC, et al: Two-step tuberculin skin testing in HIV-infected persons in Uganda. Am J Respir Crit Care Med 155:81, 1997.

152. Smith RL, Yew K, Berkowitz KA, et al: Factors affecting the yield of acid-fast sputum smears in patients with HIV and tuberculosis. Chest 106:684, 1994.

153. Finch D, Beatty CD: The utility of a single sputum specimen in the diagnosis of tuberculosis: Comparison between HIV-infected and non-HIV-infected patients. Chest 111:1174, 1997.

154. Yajko DM, Nasson PS, Sanders CA, et al: High predictive value of the acid-fast smear for *Mycobacterium tuberculosis* despite the high prevalence of *Mycobacterium avium* complex in respiratory specimens. Clin Infect Dis 19:334, 1994.

155. Wasser LS, Whaw GW, Talavera W: Endobronchial tuberculosis in the acquired immunodeficiency syndrome. Chest 94:1240, 1988.

155a. Harkin TJ, Ciotoli C, Addrizzo-Harris DJ, et al: Transbronchial needle aspiration (TBNA) in patients infected with HIV. Am J Respir Crit Care Med 157:1913, 1998.

156. FitzGerald JM, Grzybowski S, Allen EA: The impact of human immunodeficiency virus infection on tuberculosis and its control. Chest 100:191, 1991.

157. Small PM, Schecter GF, Goodman PC, et al: Treatment of tuberculosis in patients with advanced human immunodeficiency virus infection. N Engl J Med 324:289, 1991.

158. Gordin FM, Nelson ET, Matts JP, et al: The impact of human immunodeficiency virus infection on drug-resistant tuberculosis. Am J Respir Crit Car Med 154:1478, 1996.

159. Goble M, Iseman MD, Madsen LA, et al: Treatment of 171 patients with pulmonary tuberculosis resistant to isoniazid and rifampin. N Engl J Med 328:527, 1993.

160. Frieden TR, Sterling T, Pablos-Mendez A, et al: The emergency of drug-resistant tuberculosis in New York City. N Engl J Med 328:521, 1993.

161. Nunn P, Brindle R, Carpenter L, et al: Cohort study of human immunodeficiency virus infection in patents with tuberculosis in Nairobi, Kenya: Analysis of early (6-month) mortality. Am Rev Respir Dis 146:849, 1992.

162. Perriëns JH, Colebunders RL, Karahunga C, et al: Increased mortality and tuberculosis treatment failure rate among human immunodeficiency virus (HIV) seropositive compared with HIV seronegative patients with pulmonary tuberculosis treated with "standard" chemotherapy in Kinshasa, Zaire. Am Rev Respir Dis 144:750, 1991.

163. Whalen C, Okwera A, Johnson J, et al: Predictors of survival in human immunodeficiency virus-infected patients with pulmonary tuberculosis. Am J Respir Crit Care Med 153:1977, 1996.

164. Whalen C, Horsburgh CR, Hom D, et al: Accelerated course of human immunodeficiency virus infection after tuberculosis. Am J Respir Crit Care Med 151:129, 1995.

165. Small PM, Shafer RW, Hopewell PC, et al: Exogenous reinfection with multidrug-resistant *Mycobacterium tuberculosis* in patients with advanced HIV infection. N Engl J Med 328:1137, 1993.

166. Daley CL, Small PM, Schecter GF, et al: An outbreak of tuberculosis with accelerated progression among persons infected with the human immunodeficiency virus: An analysis using restriction-fragment-length polymorphisms. N Engl J Med 326:231, 1992.

167. Fischl MA, Daikos GL, Uttamchandani RB, et al: Clinical presentation and outcome of patients with HIV infection and tuberculosis caused by multiple-drug-resistant bacilli. Ann Intern Med 117:184, 1992.

168. Dore GJ, Hoy JF, Mallal SA, et al: Trends in incidence of AIDS illnesses in Australia from 1983 to 1994: The Australian AIDS cohort. J Acquir Immune Defic Syndr Hum Retrovirol 16:39, 1997.

169. Horsburgh CR: *Mycobacterium avium* complex infection in the acquired immunodeficiency syndrome. N Engl J Med 324:1332, 1991.

170. Niedt GW, Schinella RA: Acquired immunodeficiency syndrome. Arch Pathol Lab Med 109:727, 1985.

171. Farhi DC, Mason UG III, Horsburgh CR: Pathologic findings in disseminated *Mycobacterium avium–intracellulare* infection. Am J Clin Pathol 85:67, 1986.

172. Chester AC, Winn WC: Unusual and Newly Recognized Patterns of Nontuberculous Mycobacterial Infection with Emphasis on the Immunocompromised Host. *In* Sommers SC, Rosen PP, Fechner RE (eds): Pathology Annual. Part I. Vol 21. Norwalk, CT, Appleton-Century-Crofts, 1986.

173. Pappolla MA, Mehta VT: PAS reaction stains phagocytosed atypical mycobacteria in paraffin sections. Arch Pathol Lab Med 108:372, 1984.

174. Cook SM, Bartos RE, Pierson CL, et al: Detection and characterization of atypical mycobacteria by the polymerase chain reaction. Diag Mol Pathol 3:53, 1994.

175. Marinelli DL, Albelda SM, Williams TM, et al: Non-tuberculous mycobacterial infection in AIDS: Clinical, pathologic and radiographic features. Radiology 160:77, 1986.

176. Goodman PC: Mycobacterial disease in AIDS. J Thorac Imaging 6:22, 1991.

177. Hartman TE, Primack SL, Müller NL, et al: Diagnosis of thoracic complications in AIDS: Accuracy of CT. Am J Roentgenol 162:547, 1994.

178. Laissy JP, Cadi M, Cinqualbre A, et al: *Mycobacterium tuberculosis* versus nontuberculous mycobacterial infection of the lung in AIDS patients: CT and HRCT patterns. J Comput Assist Tomogr 21:312, 1997.

179. Hocqueloux L, Lesprit P, Herrmann JL, et al: Pulmonary *Mycobacterium avium* complex disease without dissemination in HIV-infected patients. Chest 113:542, 1998.

180. Mehle ME, Adamo JP, Mehta AC, et al: Endobronchial *Mycobacterium avium–intracellulare* infection in a patient with AIDS. Chest 96:119, 1989.

181. Packer SJ, Cesario T, Williams JH: *Mycobacterium avium* complex infection presenting as endobronchial lesions in immunosuppressed patients. Ann Intern Med 109:389, 1988.

182. Nassos PS, Yajko DM, Sanders CA, et al: Prevalence of *Mycobacterium avium* complex in respiratory specimens from AIDS and non-AIDS patients in a San Francisco Hospital. Am Rev Respir Dis 143:66, 1991.

183. Chin DP, Hopewell PC, Yajko DM, et al: *Mycobacterium avium* complex in the respiratory or gastrointestinal tract and the risk of *M. avium* complex bacteremia in patients with human immunodeficiency virus infection. J Infect Dis 169:289, 1994.

184. Rigsby MO, Curtis AM: Pulmonary disease from nontuberculous mycobacteria in patients with human immunodeficiency virus. Chest 106:913, 1994.

185. Chin DP: *Mycobacterium avium* complex and other nontuberculous mycobacterial infections in patients with HIV. Semin Respir Infect 8:124, 1993.

186. Salzman SH, Schindel ML, Aranda CP, et al: The role of bronchoscopy in the diagnosis of pulmonary tuberculosis in patients at risk for HIV infection. Chest 102:143, 1992.

187. Benator DA, Gordin FM: Nontuberculous mycobacteria in patients with human immunodeficiency virus infection. Semin Respir Infect 11:285, 1996.

188. Levine B, Chaisson RE: *Mycobacterium kansasii*: A cause of treatable pulmonary disease associated with advanced human immunodeficiency virus (HIV) infection. Ann Intern Med 114:861, 1991.

189. Bamberger DM, Driks MR, Gupta MR, et al: *Mycobacterium kansasii* among patients infected with human immunodeficiency virus in Kansas City. Kansas City AIDS Research Consortium. Clin Infect Dis 18:395, 1994.

190. Witzig RS, Fazal BA, Mera RM, et al: Clinical manifestations and implications of coinfection with *Mycobacterium kansasii* and human immunodeficiency virus type 1. Clin Infect Dis 21:77, 1995.

191. Fishman JE, Schwartz DA, Sais GJ. *Mycobacterium kansasii* pulmonary infection in patients with AIDS: Spectrum of chest radiographic findings. Radiology 204:171, 1997.

192. American Thoracic Scoeity: Fungal infection in HIV-infected persons. Am J Respir Crit Care Med 152:816, 1995.

193. Stansell JD: Pulmonary fungal infections in HIV-infected persons. Semin Respir Infect 8:116, 1993.

194. Wallace JM, Rao AV, Glassroth J, et al: Respiratory illness in persons with human immunodeficiency virus infection. Am Rev Respir Dis 148:1523, 1993.

195. Moore RD, Chaisson RE: Natural history of opportunistic disease in an HIV-infected urban clinical cohort. Ann Intern Med 124:633, 1996.

196. Masu H, Michelis MA, Greene JB, et al: An outbreak of community-acquired pneumocystis carinii pneumonia: Initial manifestation of cellular immune dysfunction. N Engl J Med 305:1431, 1981.

197. Gottlieb MS, Schroff R, Schanker HM, et al: *Pneumocystis carinii* pneumonia and mucosal candidiasis in previously healthy homosexual men. N Engl J Med 305:1425, 1981.

198. Safrin S: *Pneumocystis carinii* pneumonia in patients with the acquired immunodeficiency syndrome. Semin Respir Infect 8:96, 1993.

199. Hoover DR, Saah AJ, Bacellar H, et al: Clinical manifestations of AIDS in the era of *Pneumocystis* prophylaxis. N Engl J Med 329:1922, 1993.
200. Buckley RM, Braffman MN, Stern JJ: Opportunistic infections in the acquired immunodeficiency syndrome. Semin Oncol 17:335, 1990.
201. Murray JF, Mills J: Pulmonary infectious complications of human immunodeficiency virus infection. Am Rev Respir Dis 141:1582, 1990.
202. Anonymous: AIDS surveillance in Canada. Can Med Assoc J 142:552, 1990.
203. Delmas MC, Schwoebel V, Heisterkamp SH, et al: Recent trends in *Pneumocystis carinii* pneumonia as AIDS-defining disease in nine European countries: Coordinators for AIDS Surveillance. J Acquir Immune Defic Syndr Hum Retrovirol 9:74, 1995.
204. Chien SM, Rawji M, Mintz S, et al: Changes in hospital admissions pattern in patients with human immunodeficiency virus infection in the era of *Pneumocystis carinii* prophylaxis. Chest 102:1035, 1992.
205. Stansell JD, Osmond DH, Charlebois E, et al: Predictors of *Pneumocystis carinii* pneumonia in HIV-infected persons. Am J Respir Crit Care Med 155:60, 1997.
206. Levine SJ. *Pneumocystis carinii*. Clin Chest Med 17:665, 1996.
207. Curtis JR, Ullman M, Collier AC, et al: Variations in medical care for HIV-related *Pneumocystis carinii* pneumonia: A comparison of process and outcome at two hospitals. Chest 112:398, 1997.
208. Curtis JR, Greenberg DL, Hudson LD, et al: Changing use of intensive care for HIV-infected patients with *Pneumocystis carinii* pneumonia. Am J Respir Crit Care Med 150:1305, 1994.
209. Chan IS, Neaton JD, Saravolatz LD, et al: Frequencies of opportunistic diseases prior to death among HIV-infected persons: Community programs for clinical research on AIDS. AIDS 9:1145, 1995.
210. Abouya YL, Beamel A, Lucas S, et al: *Pneumocystis carinii* pneumonia: An uncommon cause of death in African patients with acquired immunodeficiency syndrome. Am Rev Respir Dis 145:617, 1992.
211. Amanfu G, Mlika-Cabanne N, Girard PM, et al: Pulmonary complications of human immunodeficiency virus infection in Bujumbura, Burundi. Am Rev Respir Dis 147:658, 1993.
212. Phair J, Múnoz A, Detels R, et al: The risk of *Pneumocystis carinii* pneumonia among men infected with human immunodeficiency virus type 1. N Engl J Med 322:161, 1990.
213. Lundgren JD, Barton SE, Lazzarin A, et al: Factors associated with the development of *Pneumocystis carinii* pneumonia in 5,025 European patients with AIDS. Clin Infect Dis 21:106, 1995.
214. Vento S, Di Perri G, Garofano T, et al: *Pneumocystis carinii* pneumonia during primary HIV-1 infection. Lancet 342:24, 1993.
215. Limper AH: Tumor necrosis factor α-mediated host defense against pneumocystis carinii. Am J Respir Cell Mol Biol 16:110, 1997.
216. Kolls JK, Lei D, Vazquez C, et al: Exacerbation of murine *Pneumocystis carinii* infection by adenoviral-mediated gene transfer of a TNF inhibitor. Am J Respir Cell Mol Biol 16:112, 1997.
217. Israël-Biet D, Cadranel J, Even P: Human immunodeficiency virus production by alveolar lymphocytes is increased during *Pneumocystis carinii* pneumonia. Am Rev Respir Dis 148:1308, 1993.
218. Agostini C, Trentin L, Zambello R, et al: HIV-1 and the lung: Infectivity, pathogenic mechanisms, and cellular immune responses taking place in the lower respiratory tract. Am Rev Respir Dis 147:1038, 1993.
219. Limper AH: Parasitic adherence and host responses in the development of *Pneumocystis carinii* pneumonia. Semin Respir Infect 6:19, 1991.
220. Limper AH, Offord KP, Smith TF, et al: *Pneumocystis carinii* pneumonia: Differences in lung parasite number and inflammation in patients with and without AIDS. Am Rev Respir Dis 140:1204, 1989.
221. Vestbo J, Nielson TL, Junge J, et al: Amount of *Pneumocystis carinii* and degree of acute lung inflammation in HIV-associated *P carinii* pneumonia. Chest 104:109, 1993.
222. Hoffman AGD, Lawrence MG, Ognibene FP, et al: Reduction of pulmonary surfactant in patients with human immunodeficiency virus infection and *Pneumocystis carinii* pneumonia. Chest 102:1730, 1992.
223. Burke BA, Good RA: *Pneumocystis carinii* infection. Medicine 52:23, 1973.
224. Barrio JL, Suarez M, Rodriquez JL, et al: *Pneumocystis carinii* pneumonia presenting as cavitating and non-cavitating pulmonary nodules in patients with the acquired immunodeficiency syndrome. Am Rev Respir Dis 134:1094, 1986.
225. Albrecht H, Stellbrink HJ, Fenske S, et al: A novel variety of atypical *Pneumocystis carinii* infection after long-term prophylactic pentamidine inhalation in an AIDS patient: Large lower lobe pneumocystoma. Clin Invest 71:310, 1993.
226. Gagliardi AJ, Stover DE, Zaman MK: Endobronchial *Pneumocystis carinii* infection in a patient with the acquired immune deficiency syndrome. Chest 91:463, 1987.
227. Foley NM, Griffiths MH, Miller RF: Histologically atypical *Pneumocystis carinii* pneumonia. Thorax 48:996, 1993.
228. Watts JC, Chandler FW: Evolving concepts of infection by *Pneumocystis carinii*. *In* Rosen PP, Fechner RE (eds): Pathology Annual. Part 1. Vol 26. Norwalk, CT, Appleton & Lange, 1991, pp 93.
229. Bedrossian CWM: Ultrastructure of *Pneumocystis carinii*: A review of internal and surface characteristics. Semin Diagn Pathol 6:212, 1989.
230. Limper AH, Thomas CF Jr, Anders RA, et al: Interactions of parasite and host epithelial cell cycle regulation during *Pneumocystis carinii* pneumonia. J Lab Clin Med 130:132, 1997.
231. Saldana MJ, Mones JM, Martinez GR: The pathology of treated *Pneumocystis carinii* pneumonia. Semin Diagn Pathol 6:300, 1989.
232. Nash G, Fligiel S: Pathologic features of the lungs in the acquired immunodeficiency syndrome (AIDS): An autopsy study of seventeen homosexual males. Am J Clin Pathol 81:6, 1984.
233. Wakefield AE, Miller RF, Guiver LA, et al: Granulomatous *Pneumocystis carinii* pneumonia: DNA amplification studies on bronchoscopic alveolar lavage samples. J Clin Pathol 47:664, 1994.
234. Saldana MJ, Mones JM: Pulmonary pathology in AIDS: Atypical *Pneumocystis carinii* infection and lymphoid interstitial pneumonia. Thorax 49:S46, 1994.
235. Flannery MT, Quiroz E, Grundy LS, et al: *Pneumocystis carinii* pneumonia with an atypical granulomatous response. South Med J 89:409, 1996.
236. Kadakia J, Kiyabu M, Sharma OP, et al: Granulomatous response to *Pneumocystis carinii* in patients infected with HIV. Sarcoidosis 10:44, 1993.
237. Liu YC, Tomashefski JF Jr, Tomford JW, et al: Necrotizing *Pneumocystis carinii* vasculitis associated with lung necrosis and cavitation in a patient with acquired immunodeficiency syndrome. Arch Pathol Lab Med 113:494, 1989.
238. Travis WD, Pittaluga S, Lipschik GY, et al: Atypical pathologic manifestations of *Pneumocystis carinii* pneumonia in the acquired immune deficiency syndrome: Review of 123 lung biopsies from 76 patients with emphasis on cysts, vascular invasion, vasculitis and granulomas. Am J Surg Pathol 14:615, 1990.
239. Feuerstein IM, Archer A, Pluda JM, et al: Thin-walled cavities, cysts, and pneumothorax in *Pneumocystis carinii* pneumonia: Further observations with histopathologic correlation. Radiology 174:697, 1990.
240. Murry CE, Schmidt RA: Tissue invasion by *Pneumocystis carinii*: A possible cause of cavitary pneumonia and pneumothorax. Hum Pathol 23:1380, 1992.
241. Murry CE, Schmidt RA: Tissue invasion by *Pneumocystis carinii*: A possible cause of cavitary pneumonia and pneumothorax. Hum Pathol 23:1380, 1992.
242. Shelhamer JH, Ognibene FP, Macher AM, et al: Persistence of *Pneumocystis carinii* in lung tissue of acquired immunodeficiency syndrome patients treated for *Pneumocystis* pneumonia. Am Rev Respir Dis 130:1161, 1984.
243. DeLorenzo LJ, Maguire GP, Wormser GP, et al: Persistence of *Pneumocystis carinii* pneumonia in the acquired immunodeficiency syndrome. Chest 88:79, 1985.
244. Gamsu G, Hecht ST, Birnberg FA, et al: *Pneumocystis carinii* pneumonia in homosexual men. Am J Roentgenol 139:647, 1982.
245. Suster B, Akerman M, Orenstein M, et al: Pulmonary manifestations of AIDS: review of 106 episodes. Radiology 161:87, 1986.
246. DeLorenzo LJ, Huang CT, Maguire GP, et al: Roentgenographic patterns of *Pneumocystis carinii* pneumonia in 104 patients with AIDS. Chest 91:323, 1987.
247. Kuhlman JE: Pneumocystic infections: The radiologist's perspective. Radiology 198:623, 1996.
248. Opravil M, Marinceck B, Fuchs WA, et al: Shortcomings of chest radiography in detecting *Pneumocystis carinii* pneumonia. J Acquir Immune Defic Syndr Hum Retrovirol 7:39, 1994.
249. Naidich DP, McGuinness G: Pulmonary manifestations of AIDS: CT and radiographic correlations. Radiol Clin North Am 29:999, 1991.
250. Goodman PC: *Pneumocystis carinii* pneumonia. J Thorac Imaging 6:16, 1991.
251. Sandhu JS, Goodman PC: Pulmonary cysts associated with *Pneumocystis carinii* pneumonia in patients with AIDS. Radiology 173:33, 1989.
252. Gurney JW, Bates FT: Pulmonary cystic disease: Comparison of *Pneumocystis carinii* pneumatoceles and bullous emphysema due to intravenous drug abuse. Radiology 173:27, 1989.
253. Chow C, Templeton PA, White CS: Lung cysts associated with *Pneumocystis carinii* pneumonia: Radiographic characteristics, natural history, and complications. Am J Roentgenol 161:527, 1993.
254. Takahashi T, Hoshino Y, Nakamura T, et al: Mediastinal emphysema with *Pneumocystis carinii* pneumonia in AIDS. Am J Roentgenol 169:1465, 1997.
255. Beers MF, Sohn M, Swartz M: Recurrent pneumothorax in AIDS patients with *Pneumocystis* pneumonia: A clinicopathologic report of three cases and review of the literature. Chest 98:266, 1990.
256. Pastores SM, Garay SM, Naidich DP, et al: Review: Pneumothorax in patients with AIDS-related *Pneumocystis carinii* pneumonia. Am J Med Sci 312:229, 1996.
257. McClellan MD, Miller SB, Parsons PE, et al: Pneumothorax with *Pneumocystis carinii* pneumonia in AIDS: Incidence and clinical characteristics. Chest 100:1224, 1991.
258. Metersky ML, Colt HG, Olson LK, et al: AIDS-related spontaneous pneumothorax: Risk factors and treatment. Chest 108:946, 1995.
259. Tumbarello M, Tacconelli E, Pirronti T, et al: Pneumothorax in HIV-infected patients: Role of *Pneumocystis carinii* pneumonia and pulmonary tuberculosis. Eur Respir J 10:1332, 1997.
260. Sepkowitz KA, Telzak EE, Gold JW, et al: Pneumothorax in AIDS. Ann Intern Med 114:455, 1991.
261. Coker RJ, Moss F, Peters B, et al: Pneumothorax in patients with AIDS. Respir Med 87:43, 1993.
262. Bevan JS, Dooshi M, Grocutt M, et al: Bilateral spontaneous pneumothoraces complicating AIDS-related *Pneumocystis carinii* pneumonia. Respir Med 83:245, 1989.
263. Mariuz P, Raviglione MC, Gould IA, et al: Pleural *Pneumocystis carinii* infection. Chest 99:774, 1991.
264. Alkhuja S, Badhey K, Miller A: Simultaneous bilateral pneumothorax in an HIV-infected patient. Chest 112:1417, 1997.
265. Barrio JL, Suarez M, Rodriguez JL, et al: Case report: *Pneumocystis carinii* pneumonia presenting as cavitating and noncavitating solitary pulmonary nodules in patient with the acquired immunodeficiency syndrome. Am Rev Resp Dis 134:1094, 1986.
266. Klein JS, Warnock M, Webb WR, et al: Cavitating and noncavitating granulomas

in AIDS patients with *Pneumocystis* pneumonitis. Am J Roentgenol 152:753, 1989.

267. Bleiweiss IJ, Jagirdar JS, Klein MJ, et al: Granulomatous *Pneumocystis carinii* pneumonia in three patients with the acquired immune deficiency syndrome. Chest 94:580, 1988.

268. Eagar GM, Friedland JA, Sagel SS: Tumefactive *Pneumocystis carinii* infection in AIDS: Report of three cases. Am J Roentgenol 160:1197, 1993.

269. Wasser LS, Brown E, Talavera W: Miliary PCP in AIDS. Chest 96:693, 1989.

270. Chechani V, Zaman MK, Finch PJP: Chronic cavitary *Pneumocystis carinii* pneumonia in a patient with AIDS. Chest 95:1347, 1989.

271. Mayor B, Schnyder P, Giron J, et al: Mediastinal and hilar lymphadenopathy due to *Pneumocystis carinii* infection in AIDS patients: CT features. J Comput Assist Tomogr 18:408, 1994.

272. Radin DR, Baker EL, Klatt EC, et al: Visceral and nodal calcification in patients with AIDS-related *Pneumocystis carinii* infection. Am J Roentgenol 154:27, 1990.

273. Groskin SA, Massi AF, Randall PA. Calcified hilar and mediastinal lymph nodes in an AIDS patient with *Pneumocystis carinii* infection. Radiology 175:345, 1990.

274. Bergin CJ, Wirth RL, Berry GJ, et al: *Pneumocystis carinii* pneumonia: CT and HRCT observations. J Comput Assist Tomogr 14:756, 1990.

275. Kuhlman JE, Kavuru M, Fishman EK, et al: *Pneumocystis carinii* pneumonia: Spectrum of parenchymal CT findings. Radiology 175:711, 1990.

276. Moskovic E, Miller R, Pearson M: High resolution computed tomography of *Pneumocystis carinii* pneumonia in AIDS. Clin Radiol 42:239, 1990.

277. Sider L, Gabriel H, Curry DR, et al: Pattern recognition of the pulmonary manifestations of AIDS on CT scans. Radiographics 13:771, 1993.

278. Mason AC, Müller NL: The role of computed tomography in the diagnosis and management of human immunodeficiency virus (HIV)–related pulmonary diseases. Semin Ultrasound CT MRI 19:154, 1998.

279. Kang EY, Staples CA, McGuinness G, et al: Detection and differential diagnosis of pulmonary infections and tumors in patients with AIDS: Value of chest radiography versus CT. Am J Roentgenol 166:15, 1996.

280. Richards PJ, Riddell L, Reznek RH, et al: High resolution computed tomography in HIV patients with suspected *Pneumocystis carinii* pneumonia and a normal chest radiograph. Clin Radiol 51:689, 1996.

281. Gruden JF, Huang L, Turner J, et al: High-resolution CT in the evaluation of clinically suspected *Pneumocystis carinii* pneumonia in AIDS patients with normal, equivocal, or nonspecific radiographic findings. Am J Roentgenol 169:967, 1997.

282. Woolfenden JM, Carrasquillo JA, Larson SM: Acquired immunodeficiency syndrome: Ga-67 citrate imaging. Radiology 162:383, 1987.

283. Kramer EL, Sanger JJ, Garay SM, et al: Gallium-67 chest scan patterns in HIV seropositive patients: Diagnostic implications. Radiology 170:671, 1989.

284. O'Doherty MJ, Nunan TO: Nuclear medicine and AIDS. Nucl Med Commun 14:830, 1993.

285. Goldenberg DM, Sharkey RM, Udem S, et al: Immunoscintigraphy of *Pneumocystis carinii* pneumonia in AIDS patients. J Nucl Med 35:1028, 1994.

286. Kramer EL, Divgi CR: Pulmonary applications of nuclear medicine. Clin Chest Med 12:55, 1991.

287. Kovacs JA, Hiemenz JW, Macher AM, et al: *Pneumocystis carinii* pneumonia: A comparison between patients with the acquired immunodeficiency syndrome and patients with other immunodeficiencies. Ann Intern Med 100:663, 1984.

288. Ascarenhas DAN, Vasudevan VP, Vaidya KP: *Pneumocystis carinii* pneumonia: Rare causes of hemoptysis. Chest 99:251, 1991.

289. Schnipper S, Small CB, Lehach J, et al: *Pneumocystis carinii* pneumonia presenting as asthma: Increased bronchial hyperresponsiveness in *Pneumocystis carinii* pneumonia. Ann Allergy 70:141, 1993.

290. Peruzzi WT, Shapiro BA, Noskin GA, et al: Concurrent bacterial lung infection in patients with AIDS, PCP, and respiratory failure. Chest 101:1399, 1992.

291. Balestra DJ, Hennigam SH, Ross GS: Clinical prediction of *Pneumocystis* pneumonia. Arch Intern Med 152:623, 1992.

292. Torres A, El-Ebiary M, Marrades R, et al: Aetiology and prognostic factors of patients with AIDS presenting life-threatening acute respiratory failure. Eur Respir J 8:1922, 1995.

293. Wasserman K, Pothoff G, Kim E, et al: Chronic *Pneumocystis carinii* pneumonia in AIDS. Chest 104:667, 1993.

294. Gill MJ, Read R: *Pneumocystis carinii:* A review of an important opportunistic pathogen in AIDS. Can J Infect Dis 2:12, 1991.

295. Gunnarsson G, Karchmer AW: Hypertrophic osteoarthropathy associated with *Pneumocystis carinii* pneumonia and human immunodeficiency virus infection. Clin Infect Dis 22:590, 1996.

296. Northfelt DW, Clement MJ, Safrin S: Extrapulmonary pneumocytosis: Clinical features in human immunodeficiency virus infection. Medicine 69:392, 1990.

297. Lione MC, Mariuz P, Sugar J, et al: Extrapulmonary *Pneumocystis* infection. Ann Intern Med 111:339, 1991.

298. Litwin MA, Williams CM: Cutaneous *Pneumocystis carinii* infection mimicking Kaposi sarcoma. Ann Intern Med 117:48, 1992.

299. Gherman CR, Ward RR, Bassis ML: *Pneumocystis carinii* otitis media and mastoiditis as the initial manifestation of the acquired immunodeficiency syndrome. Am J Med 85:250, 1988.

300. Singer F, Talavera W, Zumoff B: Elevated levels of angiotensin-converting enzyme in *Pneumocystis carinii* pneumonia. Chest 95:803, 1989.

301. Boldt MJ, Bai TR: Utility of lactate dehydrogenase vs radiographic severity in the differential diagnosis of *Pneumocystis carinii* pneumonia. Chest 111:1187, 1997.

302. Kagawa FT, Kirsch CM, Yenokida GG, et al: Serum lactate dehydrogenase activity in patients with AIDS and *Pneumocystis carinii* pneumonia: An adjunct to diagnosis. Chest 94:1031, 1988.

303. Zaman MK, White DA: Serum lactate dehydrogenase levels and *Pneumocystis carinii* pneumonia: Diagnostic and prognostic significance. Am Rev Respir Dis 137:796, 1988.

304. Quist J, HIll AR: Serum lactate dehydrogenase (LDH) in *Pneumocystis carinii* pneumonia, tuberculosis and bacterial pneumonia. Chest 108:415, 1995.

305. Kroe DM, Kirsch CM, Jensen WA: Diagnostic strategies for *Pneumocystis carinii* pneumonia. Semin Respir Infect 12:70, 1997.

306. Horowitz ML, Schiff M, Samuels J, et al: *Pneumocystis carinii* pleural effusion: Pathogenesis and pleural fluid analysis. Am Rev Respir Dis 148:232, 1993.

307. Schaumberg TH, Schnapp LM, Taylor KG, et al: Diagnosis of *Pneumocystis carinii* infection in HIV-seropositive patients by identification of *P carinii* in pleural fluid. Chest 103:1890, 1993.

308. Balachandran I, Jones DB, Humphrey DM: A case of *Pneumocystis carinii* in pleural fluid with cytologic, histologic and ultrastructural documentation. Acta Cytol 34:486, 1990.

309. Mitchell DM, Clarke JR: The lung in HIV infection: Can pulmonary function testing help? Monaldi Arch Chest Dis 51:214, 1996.

310. Nelsing S, Jensen BN, Backer V: Persistent reduction in lung function after *Pneumocystis carinii* pneumonia in AIDS patients. Scand J Infect Dis 27:351, 1995.

311. Mitchell DM, Fleming J, Pinching AJ, et al: Pulmonary function in human immunodeficiency virus infection: A prospective 18-month study of serial lung function in 474 patients. Am Rev Respir Dis 146:745, 1992.

312. Stover DE, Greeno RA, Gagliardi AJ: The use of a simple exercise test for the diagnosis of *Pneumocystis carinii* pneumonia in patients with AIDS. Am Rev Respir Dis 139:1343, 1989.

313. Mitchell DM, Fleming J, Harris JRW, et al: Serial pulmonary function tests in the diagnosis of *P. carinii* pneumonia. Eur Respir J 6:823, 1993.

314. Smith DE, McLuckie A, Wyatt HJ, et al: Severe exercise hypoxaemia with normal or near normal x-rays: A feature of *Pneumocystis carinii* infection. Lancet 2(8619):1049, 1988.

315. Chouaid C, Housset B, Lebeau B: Cost-analysis of four diagnostic strategies for *Pneumocystis carinii* pneumonia in HIV-infected subjects. Eur Respir J 8:1554, 1995.

316. Sauleda J, Gea J, Aran X, et al: Simplified exercise test for the initial differential diagnosis of *Pneumocystis carinii* pneumonia in HIV antibody positive patients. Thorax 49:112, 1994.

317. Kvale PA, Rosen MJ, Hopewell PC, et al: A decline in the pulmonary diffusing capacity does not indicate opportunistic lung disease in asymptomatic persons infected with the human immunodeficiency virus. Pulmonary complications of HIV Infection Study Group. Am Rev Respir Dis 148:390, 1993.

318. Chouaid C, Maillard D, Housset B, et al: Cost effectiveness of noninvasive oxygen saturation measurement during exercise for the diagnosis of *Pneumocystis carinii* pneumonia. Am Rev Respir Dis 147:1360, 1993.

319. Smith DE, Forbes A, Davies S, et al: Diagnosis of *Pneumocystis carinii* pneumonia in HIV antibody positive patients by simple outpatient assessments. Thorax 47:1005, 1992.

320. Pothjoff G, Wassermann K, Ostmann H: Impairment of exercise capacity in various groups of HIV-infected patients. Respiration 61:80, 1994.

321. Schnipper S, Small CB, Lehach J, et al: *Pneumocystis carinii* pneumonia presenting as asthma: Increased bronchial hyperresponsiveness in *Pneumocystis carinii* pneumonia. Ann Allergy 70:141, 1993.

322. Moscato G, Maserati R, Marraccini P, et al: Bronchial reactivity to methacholine in HIV-infected individuals without AIDS. Chest 103:796, 1993.

323. Ong EL, Hanley SP, Mandal BK: Bronchial responsiveness in AIDS patients with *Pneumocystis carinii* pneumonia. AIDS 6:1331, 1992.

324. Kaner RJ, Stover DE: In search of shortcuts: Definitive and indirect tests in the diagnosis of *Pneumocystis carinii* pneumonia in AIDS. Am Rev Respir Dis 139:1324, 1989.

325. Miller RF, Millar AB, Weller IVD, et al: Empirical treatment without bronchoscopy for *Pneumocystis carinii* pneumonia in the acquired immunodeficiency syndrome. Thorax 44:559, 1989.

326. Glassroth J: Empiric diagnosis of *Pneumocystis carinii* pneumonia: Questions of accuracy and equity. Am J Respir Crit Care Med 152:1433, 1995.

327. Tu JV, Biem HJ, Detsky AS: Bronchoscopy versus empirical therapy in HIV-infected patients with presumptive *Pneumocystis carinii* pneumonia: A decision analysis. Am Rev Respir Dis 148:370, 1993.

328. Vander Els NJ, Stover DE: Approach to the patient with pulmonary disease. Clin Chest Med 17:767, 1996.

329. Zaman MK, Wooten OJ, Suprahmanya B, et al: Rapid noninvasive diagnosis of *Pneumocystis carinii* from induced liquefied sputum. Ann Intern Med 109:7, 1988.

330. Kovacs JA, Ng VL, Masur H, et al: Diagnosis of *Pneumocystis carinii* pneumonia: Improved detection in sputum with use of monoclonal antibodies. N Engl J Med 318:590, 1988.

331. Rocha P, Awe RJ, Guy ES, et al: A rapid and inexpensive method for processing induced sputum for detection of *Pneumocystis carinii*. Am J Clin Pathol 105:52, 1996.

332. Levine SJ, Kennedy D, Shelhamer JH, et al: Diagnosis of *Pneumocystis carinii* pneumonia by multiple lobe, site-directed bronchoalveolar lavage with immuno-fluorescent monoclonal antibody staining in human immunodeficiency virus-infected patients receiving aerosolized pentamidine chemoprophylaxis. Am Rev Respir Dis 148:838, 1992.

333. Bigby TD, Margolskee D, Curtis JL, et al: The usefulness of induced sputum in the diagnosis of *Pneumocystis carinii* pneumonia in patients with the acquired immunodeficiency syndrome. Am Rev Respir Dis 133:515, 1986.

334. Fortun J, Navas E, Marti-Belda P, et al: *Pneumocystis carinii* pneumonia in HIV-infected patients: Diagnostic yield of induced sputum and immunofluorescent stain with monoclonal antibodies. Eur Respir J 5:665, 1992.

335. Bustamante EA, Levy H: Sputum induction compared with bronchoalveolar lavage by Ballard catheter to diagnose *Pneumocystis carinii* pneumonia. Chest 105:816, 1994.

336. Kirsch CM, Jensen WA, Kagawa FT, et al: Analysis of induced sputum for the diagnosis of recurrent *Pneumocystis carinii* pneumonia. Chest 102:1152, 1992.

337. Pitchenik AE, Ganjei P, Torres A, et al: Sputum examination for the diagnosis of *Pneumocystis carinii* pneumonia in the acquired immunodeficiency syndrome. Am Rev Respir Dis 133:226, 1986.

338. Chouaid C, Housset B, Poirot JL, et al: Cost effectiveness of the induced sputum technique for the diagnosis of *Pneumocystis carinii* pneumonia (PCP) in HIV-infected patients. Eur Respir J 6:248, 1993.

339. Metersky ML, Catanzaro A: Diagnostic approach to *Pneumocystis carinii* pneumonia in the setting of prophylactic aerosolized pentamidine. Chest 100:1345, 1991.

340. Fahy JV, Chin DP, Schnapp LM, et al: Effect of aerosolized pentamidine prophylaxis on the clinical severity and diagnosis of *Pneumocystis carinii* pneumonia. Am Rev Respir Dis 146:844, 1992.

341. Leibovitz E, Pollack H, Moore T, et al: Comparison of PCR and standard cytological staining for detection of *Pneumocystis carinii* from respiratory specimens from patients with or at high risk for infection by human immunodeficiency virus. J Clin Microbiol 33:3004, 1995.

342. Chouaid C, Roux P, Lavard I, et al: Use of the polymerase chain reaction technique on induced-sputum samples for the diagnosis of *Pneumocystis carinii* pneumonia in HIV-infected patients: A clinical and cost-analysis study. Am J Clin Pathol 104:72, 1995.

343. Wehner JH, Jensen WA, Kirsch CM, et al: Controlled utilization of induced sputum analysis in the diagnosis of *Pneumocystis carinii* pneumonia. Chest 105:1770, 1994.

344. Glenny RW, Pierson DJ: Cost reduction in diagnosing *Pneumocystis carinii* pneumonia: Sputum induction versus bronchoalveolar lavage as the initial diagnostic procedure. Am Rev Respir Dis 145:1425, 1992.

345. De Gracia J, Miravittles M, Mayordomo C, et al: Empiric treatments impair the diagnostic yield of BAL in HIV-positive patients. Chest 111:1180, 1997.

346. Golden JA, Hollander H, Stulbarg MS, et al: Bronchoalveolar lavage as the exclusive diagnostic modality for *Pneumocystis carinii* pneumonia: A prospective study among patients with acquired immunodeficiency syndrome. Chest 90:18, 1986.

347. Huang L, Hecht FM, Stansell JD, et al: Suspected *Pneumocystis carinii* pneumonia with a negative induced sputum examination: Is early bronchoscopy useful? Am J Respir Crit Care Med 151:1866, 1995.

348. Savoia D, Millesimo M, Cassetta I, et al: Detection of *Pneumocystis carinii* by DNA amplification in human immunodeficiency virus-positive patients. Diagn Microbiol Infect Dis 29:61, 1997.

349. Baughman RP, Dohn MN, Shipley R, et al: Increased *Pneumocystis carinii* recovery from the upper lobes in *Pneumonocystis* pneumonia: The effect of aerosol pentamidine prophylaxis. Chest 103:426, 1993.

350. Read CA, Cerrone F, Busseniers AE, et al: Differential lobe lavage for diagnosis of acute *Pneumocystis carinii* pneumonia in patients receiving prophylactic aerosolized pentamidine therapy. Chest 103:1520, 1993.

351. Minutoli R, Eden E, Brachfeld C: Bronchoalveolar lavage via a modified stomach tube in intubated patients with the acquired immunodeficiency syndrome and diffuse pneumonia. Thorax 45:771, 1990.

352. Bennett CL, Horner RD, Weinstein RA, et al: Empirically treated *Pneumocystis carinii* pneumonia in Los Angeles, Chicago and Miami. J Infect Dis 172:312, 1995.

353. Dohn MN, Baughman RP, Vigdorth EM, et al: Equal survival rates for first, second, and third episodes of *Pneumocystis carinii* pneumonia in patients with acquired immunodeficiency syndrome. Arch Intern Med 152:2465, 1992.

354. Bennett CL, Adams J, Bennett RL, et al: The learning curve for AIDS-related *Pneumocystis carinii* pneumonia: Experience from 3,981 cases in Veterans Affairs hospitals 1987–1991. J Acquir Immune Defic Syndr Hum Retroviral 8:373, 1995.

355. Colford JM Jr, Segal M, Tabnak F, et al: Temporal trends and factors associated with survival after *Pneumocystis carinii* pneumonia in California, 1983–1992. Am J Epidemiol 146:115, 1997.

356. Lundgren JD, Barton SE, Katlama C, et al: Changes in survival over time after a first episode of *Pneumocystis carinii* pneumonia for European patients with acquired immunodeficiency syndrome. Multicentre Study Group on AIDS in Europe. Arch Intern Med 155:822, 1995.

357. Mallal SA, Martinez OP, French MA, et al: Severity and outcome of *Pneumocystis carinii* pneumonia (PCP) in patients of known and unknown HIS status. J Acquir Immune Defic Syndr Hum Retroviral 7:148, 1994.

358. Beck EJ, French PD, Helbert MH, et al: Improved outcome of *Pneumocystis carinii* pneumonia in AIDS patients: A multifactorial treatment effect. Int J STD AIDS 3:182, 1992.

359. Franklin C, Friedman Y, Wong T, et al: Improving long-term prognosis for survivors and mechanical ventilation in patients with AIDS with PCP and acute respiratory failure. Five-year follow-up of intensive care unit discharge. Arch Intern Med 155:91, 1995.

360. Vanhems P, Toma E: Evaluation of a prognostic score: *Pneumocystis carinii* pneumonia in HIV-infected patients. Chest 107:107, 1995.

361. Bennett CL, Weinstein RA, Shapiro MF, et al: A rapid preadmission method for predicting inpatients course of disease for patients with HIV-related *Pneumocystis carinii* pneumonia. Am J Respir Crit Care Med 150:1503, 1994.

362. Speich R, Opravil M, Weber R, et al: Prospective evaluation of a prognostic score for *Pneumocystis carinii* pneumonia in HIV-infected patients. Chest 102:1045, 1992.

363. Keitz SA, Bastian LA, Bennett CL, et al: AIDS-related *Pneumocystis carinii* pneumonia in older patients. J Gen Intern Med 11:591, 1996.

364. Fernandez P, Torres A, Miro JM, et al: Prognostic factors influencing the outcome in *Pneumocystis carinii* pneumonia in patients with AIDS. Thorax 50:668, 1995.

365. Benson CA, Spear J, Hines D, et al: Combined APACHE II score and serum lactate dehydrogenase as predictors of in-hospital mortality caused by first episode *Pneumocystis carinii* pneumonia in patients with acquired immunodeficiency syndrome. Am Rev Respir Dis 144:319, 1991.

366. Skiest DJ, Rubinstien E, Carley N, et al: The importance of comorbidity in HIV-infected patients over 55: A retrospective case-control study. Am J Med 101:605, 1995.

367. Horner RD, Bennett CL, Achenbach C, et al: Predictors of resource utilization for hospitalized patients with *Pneumocystis carinii* pneumonia (PCP): A summary of effects from the multi-city study of quality of PCP care. J Acquir Immun Defic Syndr Hum Retroviral 12:3679, 1996.

368. Laing R, Brettle R, Leen C, et al: Features and outcome of *Pneumocystis carinii* pneumonia according to risk category for HIV infection. Scan J Infect Dis 29:57, 1997.

369. Casalino E, Mendoza-Sassi G, Wolff M, et al: Predictors of short- and long-term survival in HIV-infected patients admitted to the ICU. Chest 113:421, 1998.

370. Bauer T, Ewig S, Hasper E, et al: Predicting in-hospital outcome in HIV-associated *Pneumocystis carinii* pneumonia. Infection 23:272, 1995.

371. Beck EJ, French PD, Helbert MH, et al: Empirically treated *Pneumocystis carinii* pneumonia in London, 1983–1989. Int J STD AIDS 3:285, 1992.

372. Brenner M, Ognibene FP, Lack EE, et al: Prognostic factors and life expectancy of patients with acquired immunodeficiency syndrome and *Pneumocystis carinii* pneumonia. Am Rev Respir Dis 136:1199, 1987.

373. Speich R, Opravil M, Weber R, et al: Prospective evaluation of a prognostic score for *Pneumocystis carinii* pneumonia in HIV-infected patients. Chest 102:1045, 1992.

374. Garay SM, Greene J: Prognostic indicators in the initial presentation of *Pneumocystis carinii* pneumonia. Chest 95:769, 1989.

375. Antinori A, Maiuro G, Pallavicini F, et al: Prognostic factors of early fatal outcome long-term survival in patient with *Pneumocystis carinii* pneumonia and acquired immunodeficiency syndrome. Eur J Epidemiol 9:183, 1993.

376. Montaner JSG, Hawley PH, Ronco JJ, et al: Multisystem organ failure predicts mortality of ICU patients with acute respiratory failure secondary to AIDS-related PCP. Chest 102:1823, 1992.

377. Kumar SD, Krieger BP: CD4 lymphocyte counts and mortality in AIDS patients requiring mechanical ventilator support due to *Pneumocystis carinii* pneumonia. Chest 113:430, 1998.

378. Sadaghdar H, Huang ZB, Eden E: Correlation of bronchoalveolar lavage findings to severity of *Pneumocystis carinii* pneumonia in AIDS: Evidence for the development of high-permeability pulmonary edema. Chest 102:63, 1992.

379. Mason GR, Hashimoto CH, Dickman PS, et al: Prognostic implications of bronchoalveolar lavage neutrophilia in patients with *Pneumocystis carinii* pneumonia and AIDS. Am Rev Respir Dis 139:1336, 1989.

380. Benfield TL, Vestbo J, Junge J, et al: Prognostic value of interleukin-8 in AIDS-associated *Pneumocystis carinii* pneumonia. Am J Respir Crit Care Med 151:1058, 1995.

381. Blumenfeld W, Miller CN, Chew KL, et al: Correlation of *Pneumocystis carinii* cyst density with mortality in patients with acquired immunodeficiency syndrome and pneumocystis pneumonia. Hum Pathol 23:612, 1992.

382. Colangelo G, Baughman RP, Dohn MN, et al: Follow-up bronchoalveolar lavage in AIDS patients with *Pneumocystis carinii* pneumonia. Am Rev Respir Dis 143:1067, 1991.

383. DeLorenzo LJ, Maguire GP, Wormser GP, et al: Persistence of *Pneumocystis carinii* pneumonia in the acquired immunodeficiency syndrome: Evaluation of therapy by follow-up trans-bronchial lung biopsy. Chest 88:79, 1985.

384. Shelhamer JH, Ognibene FP, Macher AM, et al: Persistence of *Pneumocystis carinii* in lung tissue of acquired immunodeficiency syndrome patients treated for pneumocystis pneumonia. Am Rev Respir Dis 130:1161, 1984.

385. Epstein LJ, Meyer RD, Antonson S, et al: Persistence of *Pneumocystis carinii* in patients with AIDS receiving chemoprophylaxis. Am J Respir Crit Care Med 150:1456, 1994.

386. Jacobson MA, Mills J, Rush J, et al: Morbidity and mortality of patients with AIDS and first-episode *Pneumocystis carinii* pneumonia unaffected by concomitant pulmonary cytomegalovirus infection. Am Rev Respir Dis 144:6, 1991.

387. Hyland M, Chan M, Hyland RH, et al: Associating poor outcome with the presence of cytomegalovirus in bronchoalveolar lavage from HIV patients with *Pneumocystis carinii* pneumonia. Chest 107:595, 1995.

388. Jensen AMB, Lundgren JD, Benfield T, et al: Does cytomegalovirus predict a poor prognosis in *Pneumocystis carinii* pneumonia treated with corticosteroids? A note for caution. Chest 108:411, 1995.

389. Hayner CE, Baughman RP, Linnemann CC Jr, et al: The relationship between cytomegalovirus retrieved by bronchoalveolar lavage and mortality in patients with HIV. Chest 107:735, 1995.

390. Hawley PH, Ronco JJ, Guillemi SA, et al: Decreasing frequency but worsening mortality of acute respiratory failure secondary to AIDS-related *Pneumocystis carinii* pneumonia. Chest 106:1456, 1994.

391. Wachter RM, Luce JM: Respiratory failure from severe *Pneumocystis carinii* pneumonia. Chest 106:1313, 1994.

392. Wachter RM, Russi MB, Bloch DA, et al: *Pneumocystis carinii* pneumonia and respiratory failure in AIDS: Improved outcomes and increased use of intensive care units. Am Rev Respir Dis 143:251, 1991.

393. Wachter RM, Luce JM, Safrin S, et al: Cost and outcome of intensive care for patients with AIDS, *Pneumocystis carinii* pneumonia and severe respiratory failure. JAMA 273:230, 1995.

394. Friedman Y, Franklin C, Freels S, et al: Long-term survival of patients with AIDS, *Pneumocystis carinii* pneumonia, and respiratory failure. JAMA 266:89, 1991.

395. Bozzette SA, Feigal D, Chiu J, et al: Length of stay and survival after intensive care for severe *Pneumocystis carinii* pneumonia: A prospective study. Chest 101:1404, 1992.

396. Efferen LS, Nadarajah D, Palat DS: Survival following mechanical ventilation for *Pneumocystis carinii* pneumonia in patients with the acquired immunodeficiency syndrome: A different perspective. Am J Med 87:401, 1989.

397. Staikowsky F, Lafon B, Guidet B, et al: Mechanical ventilation for *Pneumocystis carinii* pneumonia in patients with the acquired immunodeficiency syndrome: Is the prognosis really improved? Chest 104:756, 1993.

398. De Palo VA, Millstein BH, Mayo PH, et al: Outcome of intensive care in patients with HIV infection. Chest 107:506, 1995.

399. Zuger A, Louie E, Holzman RS, et al: Cryptococcal disease in patients with the acquired immunodeficiency syndrome: Diagnostic features and outcome of treatment. Ann Intern Med 104:234, 1986.

400. Eng RHK, Bishburg E, Smith SM, et al: Cryptococcal infections in patients with acquired immune deficiency syndrome. Am J Med 81:19, 1986.

401. Davies SF, Sarosi GA: Fungal pulmonary complications. Clin Chest Med 17:725, 1996.

401a. Nogueira SA, Caiuby MJ, Vasconcelos V, et al: Paracoccidioidomycosis and tuberculosis in AIDS patients: Report of two cases in Brazil. Int J Infect Dis 2:168, 1998.

402. Cameron ML, Bartlett JA, Gallis HA, et al: Manifestations of pulmonary cryptococcosis in patients with acquired immunodeficiency syndrome. Rev Infect Dis 13:64, 1991.

403. Chuck SL, Sande MA: Infections with *Cryptococcus neoformans* in the acquired immunodeficiency syndrome. N Engl J Med 321:794, 1989.

404. Chechani V, Kamholz SL: Pulmonary manifestations of disseminated cryptococcosis in patients with AIDS. Chest 98:1060, 1990.

405. Wasser L, Talavera W: Pulmonary cryptococcosis in AIDS. Chest 92:692, 1987.

406. Miller WT Jr, Edelman JM, Miller WT: Cryptococcal pulmonary infection in patients with AIDS: Radiographic appearance. Radiology 175:725, 1990.

407. Sider L, Westcott MA: Pulmonary manifestations of cryptococcosis in patients with AIDS: CT features. J Thorac Imaging 9:78, 1994.

408. Friedman EP, Miller RF, Severn A, et al: Cryptococcal pneumonia in patients with the acquired immunodeficiency syndrome. Clin Radiol 50:756, 1995.

409. Malabonga VM, Basti J, Kamholz SL: Utility of bronchoscopic sampling techniques for cryptococcal disease in AIDS. Chest 99:370, 1991.

410. Baughman RP, Rhodes JC, Dohn MN, et al: Detection of cryptococcal antigen in bronchoalveolar lavage fluid: A prospective study of diagnostic utility. Am Rev Respir Dis 145:1226, 1992.

411. Kirchner JT: Opportunistic fungal infections in patients with HIV disease. Postgrad Med 99:209, 1996.

412. Conces DJ Jr, Stockberger SM, Tarver RD, et al: Disseminated histoplasmosis in AIDS: Findings on chest radiographs. Am J Roentgenol 160:15, 1993.

413. Wheat LJ, Connolly-Stringfield PA, Baker RL, et al: Disseminated histoplasmosis in the acquired immunodeficiency syndrome: Clinical findings, diagnosis and treatment, and review of the literature. Medicine 69:361, 1990.

414. Salzman SH, Smith RL, Aranda CP: Histoplasmosis in patients at risk for the acquired immunodeficiency syndrome in a nonendemic setting. Chest 93:916, 1988.

415. Sarosi GA, Johnson PC: Progressive disseminated histoplasmosis in the acquired immunodeficiency syndrome: A model for disseminated disease. Semin Respir Infect 5:146, 1990.

416. Johnson PC, Khadori N, Najjar A, et al: Progressive disseminated histoplasmosis in patients with acquired immunodeficiency syndrome. Am J Med 85:152, 1988.

417. McGuinness G, Naidich DP, Jagirdar J, et al: High resolution CT findings in miliary lung disease. J Comput Assist Tomogr 16:384, 1992.

418. Wheat LJ, Connolly-Stringfield P, Williams B, et al: Diagnosis of histoplasmosis in patients with the acquired immunodeficiency syndrome by detection of *Histoplasma capsulatum* polysaccharide antigen in bronchoalveolar lavage fluid. Am Rev Respir Dis 145:1421, 1991.

419. Wheat LJ, Connolly-Stringfield P, Blair B, et al: Histoplasmosis relapse in patients with AIDS: Detection using *Histoplasma capsulatum* variety capsulatum antigen levels. Ann Intern Med 115:937, 1991.

420. Ampel NM, Dols CL, Galgiani JN: Coccidioidomycosis during human immunodeficiency virus infection: Results of a prospective study in a coccidioidal endemic area. Am J Med 94:235, 1993.

421. Fish DG, Ampel NM, Galgiani JN, et al: Coccidioidomycosis during human immunodeficiency virus infection: A review of 77 patients. Medicine 69:384, 1990.

422. Pappas PG: Blastomycosis in the immunocompromised patient. Semin Respir Infect 12:243, 1997.

423. Pappas PG, Pottage JC, Powderly WG, et al: Blastomycosis in patients with the acquired immunodeficiency syndrome. Ann Intern Med 116:847, 1992.

424. Lortholary O, Meyohas MC, Dupont B, et al: Invasive aspergillosis in patients with acquired immunodeficiency syndrome: Report of 33 cases. Am J Med 95:177, 1993.

425. Nash G, Irvine R, Kerschmann RL, et al: Pulmonary aspergillosis in acquired immune deficiency syndrome: Autopsy study of emerging pulmonary complication of human immunodeficiency virus infection. Hum Pathol 28:1268, 1997.

426. Denning DW, Follansbee SE, Scolaro M, et al: Pulmonary aspergillosis in the acquired immunodeficiency syndrome. N Engl J Med 324:654, 1991.

427. Miller WT Jr, Sais GJ, Frank I, et al: Pulmonary aspergillosis in patients with AIDS: Clinical and radiographic correlations. Chest 105:37, 1994.

428. Klapholz A, Salomon N, Perlman DC, et al: Aspergillosis in the acquired immunodeficiency syndrome. Chest 100:1614, 1991.

429. Minamoto GY, Barlam TF, Vander Els NJ: Invasive aspergillosis in patients with AIDS. Clin Infect Dis 14:66, 1992.

430. Staples CA, Kang EY, Wright JL, et al: Invasive pulmonary aspergillosis in AIDS: Radiographic, CT, and pathologic findings. Radiology 196:409, 1995.

431. Pervez NK, Kleinerman J, Kattan M, et al: Pseudomembranous necrotizing bronchial aspergillosis: A variant of invasive aspergillosis in a patient with hemophilia and acquired immune deficiency syndrome. Am Rev Respir Dis 131:961, 1985.

432. Addrizzo-Harris DJ, Harkin TJ, McGuinness G, et al: Pulmonary aspergilloma and AIDS: A comparison of HIV-infected and HIV-negative individuals. Chest 111:612, 1997.

432a. Torrents C, Alvarez-Castells A, de Vera PV, et al: Case report. Post-*Pneumocystis* aspergilloma in AIDS: CT features. J Comput Assist Tomogr 15:304, 1991.

433. Pursell KJ, Telzak EE, Armstrong D: *Aspergillus* species colonization and invasive disease in patients with AIDS. Clin Infect Dis 14:141, 1992.

434. Wallace JM: Viruses and other miscellaneous organisms. Clin Chest Med 17:745, 1996.

435. Connolly MG Jr, Baughman RP, Dohn MN, et al: Recovery of viruses other than cytomegalovirus from bronchoalveolar lavage fluid. Chest 105:1775, 1994.

436. King JC Jr: Community respiratory viruses in individuals with human immunodeficiency virus infection. Am J Med 102:19, 1997.

437. Rose RM, Krivine A, Pinkston P, et al: Frequent identification of HIV-1 DNA in bronchoalveolar lavage cells obtained from individuals with the acquired immunodeficiency syndrome. Am Rev Respir Dis 143:850, 1991.

438. Dean NC, Golden JA, Evans LA, et al: Human immunodeficiency virus recovery from bronchoalveolar lavage fluid in patients with AIDS. Chest 93:1176, 1988.

439. Linnemann CC Jr, Baughman RP, Frame PT, et al: Recovery of human immunodeficiency virus and detection of p24 antigen in bronchoalveolar lavage fluid from adult patients with AIDS. Chest 96:64, 1989.

440. Semenzato G, de Rossi A, Agostini C: Human retroviruses and their aetiological link to pulmonary diseases. Eur Respir J 6:925, 1993.

441. Johnson MAJ JE, Anders MAJ GT, Hawkes MAJ CE, et al: Bronchoalveolar lavage findings in patients seropositive for the human immunodeficiency virus (HIV). Chest 97:1066, 1990.

442. Mayaud CM, Cadranel J: HIV in the lung: Guilty or not guilty? Thorax 48:1191, 1993.

443. Nieman RB, Fleming J, Coker RJ, et al: Reduced carbon monoxide transfer factor (Tlco) in human immunodeficiency virus type I (HIV-I) infection as a predictor for faster progression to AIDS. Thorax 48:481, 1993.

444. French PD, Cunningham DA, Fleming J, et al: Low carbon monoxide transfer factor (TlCO) in HIV-infected patients without lung disease. Respir Med 86:253, 1992.

445. Meignan M, Guillon JM, Denis M, et al: Increased lung epithelial permeability in HIV-infected patients with isolated cytotoxic T-lymphocytic alveolitis. Am Rev Respir Dis 141:1241, 1990.

446. Dennis M, Ghadirian E: Alveolar macrophages from subjects infected with HIV-1 express macrophage inflammatory protein-1 alpha (MIP-1 alpha): Contribution to the CD8+ alveolitis. Clin Experim Immunol 96:187, 1994.

447. Mann M, Shelhamer JH, Masur H, et al: Lack of clinical utility of bronchoalveolar lavage cultures for cytomegalovirus in HIV infection. Am J Respir Crit Care Med 155:1723, 1997.

448. De La Hoz RE, Hayashi S, Cook D, et al: Investigation of the role of the cytomegalovirus as a respiratory pathogen in HIV-infected patients. Can Respir J 3:235, 1996.

449. Millar AB, Patou G, Miller RF, et al: Cytomegalovirus in the lungs of patients with AIDS: Respiratory pathogen or passenger? Am Rev Respir Dis 141:1474, 1990.

450. Miles PR, Baughman RP, Linnemann CC Jr, et al: Cytomegalovirus in the bronchoalveolar lavage fluid of patients with AIDS. Chest 97:1072, 1990.

451. Baughman RP: Cytomegalovirus: The monster in the closet? Am J Respir Crit Care Med 156:1, 1997.

452. Hayner CE, Baughman RP, Linnemann CC Jr, et al: The relationship between cytomegalovirus retrieved by bronchoalveolar lavage and mortality in patients with HIV. Chest 107:735, 1995.

453. Wallace JM, Hannah J: Cytomegalovirus pneumonitis in patients with AIDS: Findings in an autopsy series. Chest 92:198, 1987.

454. McKenzie R, Travis WD, Dolan SA, et al: The causes of death in patients with human immunodeficiency virus infection: A clinical and pathologic study with emphasis on the role of pulmonary diseases. Medicine 70:326, 1991.

455. Squire SB, Lipman MCI, Bagdades EK, et al: Severe cytomegalovirus pneumonitis in HIV infected patients with higher than average CD4 counts. Thorax 47:301, 1992.

456. Northfelt DW, Sollitto RA, Miller TR, et al: Cytomegalovirus pneumonitis: An unusual cause of pulmonary nodules in a patient with AIDS. Chest 103:1918, 1993.
457. Imoto EM, Stein RM, Shellito JE, et al: Central airway obstruction due to cytomegalovirus-induced necrotizing tracheitis in a patient with AIDS. Am Rev Respir Dis 142:884, 1990.
458. Vasudevan VP, Mascarenhas DAN, Klapper P, et al: Cytomegalovirus necrotizing bronchiolitis with HIV infection. Chest 97:483, 1990.
459. Herry I, Cadranel J, Antoine M, et al: Cytomegalovirus-induced alveolar hemorrhage in patients with AIDS: A new clinical entity? Clin Infect Dis 22:616, 1996.
460. Waxman AB, Goldie SJ, Brett-Smith H, et al: Cytomegalovirus as a primary pulmonary pathogen in AIDS. Chest 111:128, 1997.
461. McGuinness G, Scholes JV, Garay SM, et al: Cytomegalovirus pneumonitis: Spectrum of parenchymal CT findings with pathologic correlation in 21 AIDS patients. Radiology 192:451, 1994.
462. Vasudevan VP, Mascarenhs DAN, Klapper P, et al: Cytomegalovirus necrotizing bronchiolitis with HIV infection. Chest 94:483, 1990.
463. Uberti-Foppa C, Lillo F, Terreni MR, et al: Cytomegalovirus pneumonia in AIDS patients: Value of cytomegalovirus culture from BAL fluid and correlation with lung disease. Chest 113:919, 1998.
464. Campagna AC: Pulmonary toxoplasmosis. Semin Respir Infect 12:98, 1997.
465. Oksenhendler E, Cadranel J, Sarfati C, et al: *Toxoplasma gondii* pneumonia in patients with the acquired immunodeficiency syndrome. Am J Med 88:18, 1990.
466. Bergin C, Murphy M, Lyons D, et al: *Toxoplasma* pneumonitis: fatal presentation of disseminated toxoplasmosis in a patient with AIDS. Eur Respir J 5:1018, 1992.
466a. Goodman PC, Schnapp LM: Pulmonary toxoplasmosis in AIDS. Radiology 184:791, 1992.
466b. Rottenberg GT, Miszkiel K, Shaw P, et al: Fulminant *Toxoplasma gondii* pneumonia in a patient with AIDS. Clin Radiol 54:472, 1997.
467. Bonilla CA, Rosa UW: *Toxoplasma gondii* pneumonia in patients with the acquired immunodeficiency syndrome: Diagnosis by bronchoalveolar lavage. South Med J 87:659, 1994.
468. Lessnau KD, Can S, Talavera W: Disseminated *Strongyloides stercoralis* in human immunodeficiency virus-infected patients: Treatment failure and a review of the literature. Chest 104:119, 1993.
469. Celedon JC, Mathur-Wagh U, Fox J, et al: Systemic strongyloidiasis in patients infected with the human immunodeficiency virus: A report of 3 cases and review of the literature. Medicine 73:256, 1994.
470. Makris AN, Sher S, Bertoli C, et al: Pulmonary *Strongyloidiasis*: An unusual opportunistic pneumonia in a patient with AIDS. Am J Roentgenol 161:545, 1993.
471. Kemper CA: Pulmonary disease in selected protozoal infections. Semin Respir Infect 12:113, 1997.
472. Johnson CC, Wilcosky T, Kvale P, et al: Cancer incidence among an HIV infected cohort. Pulmonary complications of HIV infection Study Group. Am J Epidemiol 146:470, 1997.
473. Clavel A, Arnal AC, Sanchez EC, et al: Respiratory cryptosporidiosis: Case series and review of the literature. Infection 24:341, 1996.
474. Mohri H, Fujita H, Asakura Y, et al: Case report: Inhalation therapy of paromomycin is effective for respiratory infection and hypoxia by cryptosporidium with AIDS. Am J Med Sci 309:60, 1995.
475. White DA: Pulmonary complications of HIV-associated malignancies. Clin Chest Med 17:755, 1996.
476. Palella FJ, Delaney KM, Moorman AC, et al: Declining morbidity and mortality among patients with advanced human immunodeficiency virus infection. N Engl J Med 338:853, 1998.
477. Lifson AR, Darrow WW, Hessol NA, et al: Kaposi's sarcoma in a cohort of homosexual and bisexual men: Epidemiology and analysis for cofactors. Am J Epidemiol 131:221, 1990.
478. White DA, Matthay RA: Noninfectious pulmonary complications of infection with the human immunodeficiency virus. Am Rev Respir Dis 140:1763, 1989.
479. Rabkin CS, Janz S, Lash A, et al: Monoclonal origin of multicentric Kaposi's sarcoma lesions. N Engl J Med 336:988, 1997.
480. Browning PJ, Sechler JM, Kaplan M, et al: Identification and culture of Kaposi's sarcoma-like spindle cells from the peripheral blood of human immunodeficiency virus-1-infected individuals and normal controls. Blood 84:2711, 1994.
481. Ensoli B, Nakamura S, Salahuddin SZ, et al: AIDS-Kaposi's sarcoma-derived cells express cytokines with autocrine and paracrine growth effects. Science 243:223, 1989.
482. Ensoli B, Gendelman R, Markham P, et al: Synergy between basic fibroblast growth factor and HIV-1 Tat protein in induction of Kaposi's sarcoma. Nature 371:674, 1994.
483. Nakamura S, Murakami-Mori K, Rao N, et al: Vascular endothelial growth factor is a potent angiogenic factor in AIDS-associated Kaposi's sarcoma-derived spindle cells. J Immunol 158:4992, 1997.
484. Guo WX, Antakly T: AIDS-related Kaposi's sarcoma: Evidence for direct stimulatory effect of glucocorticoid on cell proliferation. Am J Pathol 146:727, 1995.
485. Morris CB, Gendelman R, Marrogi AJ, et al: Immunohistochemical detection of Bcl-2 in AIDS-associated and classical Kaposi's sarcoma. Am J Pathol 148:1055, 1996.
486. Bailer RT, Lazo A, Ng-Bautista CL, et al: Correlation between AIDS-related Kaposi sarcoma histological grade and in vitro behavior: Reduced exogenous growth factor requirements for isolates from high grade lesions. Lymphology 28:126, 1995.
487. Cesarman E, Knowles DM: Kaposi's sarcoma-associated herpesvirus: A lymphotropic human herpesvirus associated with Kaposi's sarcoma, primary effusion lymphoma, and multicentric Castleman's disease. Semin Diagn Pathol 14:54, 1997.
488. Chang Y, Cesarman E, Pessin M, et al: Identification of herpesvirus-like DNA sequences in AIDS-associated Kaposi's sarcoma. Science 266:1865, 1994.
489. Maiorana A, Luppi M, Barozzi P, et al: Detection of human herpes virus type 8 DNA sequences as a valuable aid in the differential diagnosis of Kaposi's sarcoma. Mod Pathol 10:182, 1997.
490. Jin Y-T, Tsai S-T, Yan J-J, et al: Detection of Kaposi's sarcoma-associated herpesvirus-like DNA sequence in vascular lesions: A reliable diagnostic marker for Kaposi's sarcoma. Am J Clin Pathol 105:360, 1996.
491. Cathomas G, Stalder A, McGandy CE, et al: Distribution of human herpesvirus 8 DNA in tumorous and nontumorous tissue of patients with acquired immunodeficiency syndrome with and without Kaposi's sarcoma. Mod Pathol 11:415, 1998.
492. Monini P, De Lellis L, Fabris M, et al: Kaposi's sarcoma-associated herpesvirus DNA sequences in prostate tissue and human semen. N Engl J Med 334:1168, 1996.
493. Martin JN, Ganem DE, Osmond DH, et al: Sexual transmission and the natural history of human herpesvirus 8 infection. N Engl J Med 338:948, 1998.
494. Miller G, Rigsby MO, Heston L, et al: Antibodies to butyrate-inducible antigens of Kaposi's sarcoma-associated herpesvirus in patients with HIV-1 infection. N Engl J Med 334:1292, 1996.
495. Gao SJ, Kinglsey L, Hoover DR, et al: Seroconversion to antibodies against Kaposi's sarcoma-associated herpesvirus-related latent nuclear antigens before the development of Kaposi's sarcoma. N Engl J Med 335:233, 1996.
496. Foreman KE, Friborg J Jr, Kong WP, et al: Propagation of a human herpesvirus from AIDS-associated Kaposi's sarcoma. N Engl J Med 336:163, 1997.
496a. O'Leary JJ, Kennedy MM, McGee JO'D: Kaposi's sarcoma–associated herpes virus (KSHV/HHV 8): Epidemiology, molecular biology and tissue distribution. J Clin Pathol 50:4, 1997.
496b. Oksenhendler E, Cazals-Hatem D, Schultz TF, et al: Transient angiolymphoid hyperplasia and Kaposi's sarcoma after primary infection with human herpesvirus 8 in a patient with human immunodeficiency virus infection. N Engl J Med 338:1585, 1998.
497. Fuster V, Vorchheimer DA: Propagating Kaposi's sarcoma-associated herpesvirus. N Engl J Med 336:214, 1997.
498. Fouret PJ, Touboul JL, Mayaud CM, et al: Pulmonary Kaposi's sarcoma in patients with acquired immune deficiency syndrome: A clinicopathological study. Thorax 42:262, 1987.
499. Chin R Jr, Jones DF, Pegram PS, et al: Complete endobronchial occlusion by Kaposi's sarcoma in the absence of cutaneous involvement. Chest 105:1581, 1994.
500. Nash G, Fligiel S: Kaposi's sarcoma presenting as pulmonary disease in the acquired immunodeficiency syndrome: Diagnosis by lung biopsy. Hum Pathol 15:999, 1984.
501. Davis SD, Henschke CI, Chamides BK, et al: Intrathoracic Kaposi sarcoma in AIDS patients: Radiographic-pathologic correlation. Radiology 163:495, 1987.
502. Sivit CJ, Schwartz AM, Rockoff SD: Kaposi's sarcoma of the lung in AIDS: Radiologic-pathologic analysis. Am J Roentgenol 148:25, 1987.
503. Naidich DP, Tarras M, Garay SM, et al: Kaposi's sarcoma: CT-radiographic correlation. Chest 96:723, 1989.
504. Goodman PC: Kaposi's sarcoma. J Thorac Imaging 6:43, 1991.
505. Gruden JF, Huang L, Webb WR, et al: AIDS-related Kaposi sarcoma of the lung: Radiographic findings and staging system with bronchoscopic correlation. Radiology 195:545, 1995.
506. Huang L, Schnapp LN, Gruden JF, et al: Presentation of AIDS-related pulmonary Kaposi's sarcoma diagnosed by bronchoscopy. Am J Respir Crit Care Med 153:1385, 1996.
507. Wolff SD, Kuhlman JE, Fishman EK: Thoracic Kaposi sarcoma in AIDS: CT findings. J Comput Assist Tomogr 17:60, 1993.
508. Khalil AM, Carette MF, Cadranel JL, et al: Intrathoracic Kaposi's sarcoma: CT findings. Chest 108:1622, 1995.
508a. Traill ZC, Miller RF, Shaw PJ: CT appearances of intrathoracic Kaposi's sarcoma in patients with AIDS. Br J Radiol 69:1104, 1996.
508b. Primack SL, Hartman TE, Lee KS, et al: Pulmonary nodules and the CT halo sign. Radiology 190:513, 1994.
509. Khalil AM, Carette MF, Cadranel JL, et al: Magnetic resonance imaging findings in pulmonary Kaposi's sarcoma: A series of 10 cases. Eur Respir J 7:1285, 1994.
510. Kramer EL, Sanger JJ, Garay SM, et al: Gallium-67 scans of the chest in patients with acquired immunodeficiency syndrome. J Nucl Med 28:1107, 1987.
511. Lee VW, Rosen MP, Baum A, et al: AIDS-related Kaposi's sarcoma: Finding on thallium-201 scintigraphy. Am J Roentgenol 151:1233, 1988.
512. Lee VW, Chen H, Panageas E, et al: Subcutaneous Kaposi's sarcoma: Thallium scan demonstration. Clin Nucl Med 15:569, 1990.
513. Lee VW, Fuller JD, O'Brien MJ, et al: Pulmonary Kaposi sarcoma in patients with AIDS: Scintigraphic diagnosis with sequential thallium and gallium scanning. Radiology 180:409, 1991.
514. Aboulafia DM: Regression of acquired immunodeficiency syndrome–related pulmonary Kaposi's sarcoma after highly active antiretroviral therapy. Mayo Clin Proc 73:439, 1998.
515. O'Brien RF: Pulmonary and pleural Kaposi's sarcoma in the acquired immune deficiency syndrome. Semin Respir Med 10:12, 1989.
516. Sadaghdar H, Eden E: Pulmonary Kaposi's sarcoma presenting as fulminant respiratory failure. Chest 100:858, 1991.
517. Stotka JL, Good CB, Downer WR, et al: Pericardial effusion and tamponade due

to Kaposi's sarcoma in acquired immunodeficiency syndrome. Chest 95:1359, 1989.

518. Irwin DH, Kaplan LD: Pulmonary manifestations of acquired immunodeficiency syndrome-associated malignancies. Semin Respir Infect 8:139, 1993.

519. Mitchell DM, McCarty M, Fleming J, et al: Bronchopulmonary Kaposi's sarcoma in patients with AIDS. Thorac 47:726, 1992.

520. Tamm M, Reichenberger F, McGandy CE, et al: Diagnosis of pulmonary Kaposi's sarcoma by detection of human herpes virus 8 in bronchoalveolar lavage. Am J Respir Crit Care Med 157:458, 1998.

521. O'Brien RF, Cohn DL: Serosanguineous pleural effusions in AIDS-associated Kaposi's sarcoma. Chest 96:460, 1989.

522. Miller RD, Tomlinson MC, Cottroll CP, et al: Bronchopulmonary Kaposi's sarcoma in patients with AIDS. Thorax 47:721, 1992.

523. Lynch JW Jr: AIDS-related non-Hodgkin's lymphoma: Useful techniques for diagnosis. Chest 110:585, 1996.

524. Eisner MD, Kaplan LD, Herndier B, et al: The pulmonary manifestations of AIDs-related non-Hodgkin's lymphoma. Chest 110:729, 1996.

525. Ragni MV, Belle SH, Jaffe RA, et al: Acquired immunodeficiency syndrome-associated non-Hodgkin's lymphomas and other malignancies in patients with hemophilia. Blood 81:1889, 1993.

525a. Fiorino AS, Atac B: Paraproteinemia, plasmacytoma, myeloma and HIV infection. Leukemia 11:2150, 1997.

526. Raphael BG, Knowles DM: Acquired immunodeficiency syndrome-associated non-Hodgkin's lymphoma. Semin Oncol 17:361, 1990.

527. Knowles DM: Molecular pathology of acquired immunodeficiency syndrome-related non-Hodgkin's lymphoma. Semin Diagn Pathol 14:67, 1997.

528. Kaplan LD, Abrams DI, Feigal E, et al: AIDs-associated non-Hodgkin's lymphoma in San Francisco. JAMA 261:719, 1989.

529. Kohler CA, Gonzales-Ayala E, Rowley E, et al: Primary pulmonary T-cell lymphoma associated with AIDS: The syndrome of the indolent pulmonary mass lesion. Am J Med 99:324, 1995.

530. Sandler AS, Kaplan L: AIDS lymphoma. Curr Opin Oncol 8:377, 1996.

531. Gaidano G, Pastore C, Gloghini A, et al: Human herpesvirus type-8 (HHV-8) in haematopoietic neoplasia. Leuk Lymphoma 24:257, 1997.

532. Sider L, Weiss AJ, Smith MD, et al: Varied appearance of AIDS-related lymphoma in the chest. Radiology 171:629, 1989.

533. Polish LB, Cohn DL, Ryder JW, et al: Pulmonary non-Hodgkin's lymphoma in AIDS. Chest 96:1321, 1989.

534. Carignan S, Staples CA, Müller NL: Intrathoracic lymphoproliferative disorders in the immunocompromised patient: CT findings. Radiology 197:53, 1995.

535. Blunt DM, Padley SPG: Radiographic manifestations of AIDS related lymphoma in the thorax. Clin Radiol 50:607, 1995.

536. Collins J, Müller NL, Leung AN, et al: Epstein Barr virus driven lymphoproliferative disorders of the lung: CT and histologic findings. Radiology 208:749, 1998.

537. Eisner MD, Kaplan LD, Herndier B, et al: The pulmonary manifestations of AIDS-related non-Hodgkin's lymphoma. Chest 110:729, 1996.

538. Morassut S, Vaccher E, Balestreri L, et al: HIV-associated human herpesvirus 8—positive primary lymphomatous effusions: Radiologic findings in six patients. Radiology 205:459, 1997.

539. McGuinness G, Gruden JF, Bhalla M, et al: AIDS-related airway disease. Am J Roentgenol 168:67, 1997.

540. Mason AC, White CS: CT appearance of endobronchial non-Hodgkin lymphoma. J Comput Assist Tomogr 18:559, 1994.

541. Alshafie MT, Donaldson B, Oluwole SF: Human immunodeficiency virus and lung cancer. Br J Surg 84:1068, 1997.

542. Mady BJ: Poorly differentiated non-small cell carcinoma of the lung in acquired immunodeficiency syndrome. Respiration 62:232, 1995.

543. Karp J, Profeta G, Marantz PR, et al: Lung cancer in patients with immunodeficiency syndrome. Chest 103:410, 1993.

544. Parker MS, Leveno DM, Campbell TJ, et al: AIDS-related bronchogenic carcinoma: Fact or fiction? Chest 113:154, 1998.

545. Gabutti G, Vercelli M, De Rosa MG, et al: AIDS related neoplasms in Genoa, Italy. Eur J Epidemiol 11:609, 1995.

546. Barchielli A, Buiatti E, Galanti C, et al: Linkage between AIDS surveillance system and population-based cancer registry data in Italy: A pilot study in Florence, 1985–1990. Tumori 81:169, 1995.

546a. Wistuba II, Behrens C, Milchgrub S, et al: Comparison of molecular changes in lung cancers in HIV-positive and HIV-indeterminate subjects. JAMA 279:1554, 1998.

547. Braun MA, Killam DA, Remick SC, et al: Lung cancer in patients seropositive for human immunodeficiency virus. Radiology 175:341, 1990.

548. Karp J, Profeta G, Marantz PR, et al: Lung cancer in patients with immunodeficiency syndrome. Chest 103:410, 1993.

549. White CS, Haramati LB, Elder KH, et al: Carcinoma of the lung in HIV-positive patients: Findings on chest radiographs and CT scans. Am J Roentgenol 164:593, 1995.

550. Fishman JE, Schwartz DS, Sais GJ, et al: Bronchogenic carcinoma in HIV-positive patients: Findings on chest radiographs and CT scans. Am J Roentgenol 164:57, 1995.

551. Gruden JF, Webb WR, Yao DC, et al: Bronchogenic carcinoma in 13 patients infected with the human immunodeficiency virus (HIV): Clinical and radiographic findings. J Thorac Imaging 10:99, 1995.

551a. Schreiner SR, Kirkpatrick BD, Askin FB: Pseudomesotheliomatous adenocarcinoma of the lung in a patient with HIV infection. Chest 113:839, 1998.

552. Travis WD, Fox CH, Devaney KO, et al: Lymphoid pneumonitis in 50 adult

patients infected with the human immunodeficiency virus: Lymphocytic interstitial pneumonitis versus nonspecific interstitial pneumonitis. Hum Pathol 23:529, 1992.

553. Ognibene FP, Masur H, Rogers P, et al: Nonspecific interstitial pneumonitis without evidence of *Pneumocystis carinii* in asymptomatic patients infected with human immunodeficiency virus (HIV). Ann Intern Med 109:874, 1988.

554. Suffredini AF, Ognibene FP, Lack EE, et al: Nonspecific interstitial pneumonitis: A common cause of pulmonary disease in the acquired immunodeficiency syndrome. Ann Intern Med 107:7, 1987.

555. Sattler F, Nichols L, Hirano L, et al: Nonspecific interstitial pneumonitis mimicking *Pneumocystis carinii* pneumonia. Am J Respir Crit Care Med 156:912, 1997.

556. Simmons JT, Suffredini AF, Lack EE, et al: Nonspecific interstitial pneumonitis in patients with AIDS: Radiologic features. Am J Roentgenol 149:265, 1987.

557. Griffiths MH, Miller RF, Semple SJG: Interstitial pneumonitis in patients infected with the human immunodeficiency virus. Thorax 50:1141, 1995.

558. Schneider RF: Lymphocytic interstitial pneumonitis and nonspecific interstitial pneumonitis. Clin Chest Med 17:763, 1996.

559. Morris JC, Rosen MJ, Marchevsky A, et al: Lymphocytic interstitial pneumonia in patients at risk for the acquired immune deficiency syndrome. Chest 91:63, 1987.

560. Sharland M, Gibb DM, Holland F: Respiratory morbidity from lymphocytic interstitial pneumonitis (LIP) in vertically acquired HIV infection. Arch Dis Child 76:334, 1997.

561. Marks MJ, Haney PJ, McDermott MP, et al: Thoracic disease in children with AIDS. Radiographics 16:1349, 1996.

562. Centers for Disease Control and Prevention: Revision of case definitions of acquired immunodeficiency syndrome for national reporting—United States. MMWR 34:373, 1985.

563. Kramer MR, Saldana MJ, Ramos M, et al: High titers of Epstein-Barr virus antibodies in adult patients with lymphocytic interstitial pneumonia associated with AIDS. Respir Med 86:49, 1992.

564. DeMartini JC, Brodie SJ, de la Concha-Bermejillo A, et al: Pathogenesis of lymphoid interstitial pneumonia in natural and experimental ovine lentivirus infection. Clin Infect Dis 17:S236, 1993.

565. Haque AK, Myers JL, Hudnall SD, et al: Pulmonary lymphomatoid granulomatosis in acquired immunodeficiency syndrome: Lesions with Epstein-Barr virus infection. Mod Pathol 11:347, 1998.

566. Oldham SAA, Castillo M, Jacobson FL, et al: HIV-associated lymphocytic interstitial pneumonia: Radiologic manifestations and pathologic correlation. Radiology 170:83, 1989.

567. McGuinness G, Soles JV, Jagirdar JS, et al: Unusual lymphoproliferative disorders in nine adults with HIV or AIDS: CT and pathologic findings. Radiology 197:59, 1995.

568. Grieco MH, Chinoy-Acharya P: Lymphocytic interstitial pneumonia associated with the acquired immune deficiency syndrome. Am Rev Respir Dis 131:952, 1985.

569. Itescu S, Brancato LJ, Buxbaum J, et al: A diffuse infiltrative CD8 lymphocytosis syndrome in human immunodeficiency virus (HIV) infection: A host immune response associated with HLA-DR5. Ann Intern Med 112:3, 1990.

570. Guillon JM, Autran B, Denis M, et al: Human immunodeficiency virus-related lymphocytic alveolitis. Chest 94:1264, 1988.

571. Agostini C, Semenzato G: Immunologic effects of HIV in the lung. Clin Chest Med 17:633, 1996.

572. Polos PG, Wolfe D, Harley RA, et al: Pulmonary hypertension and human immunodeficiency virus infection: Two reports and a review of the literature. Chest 101:474, 1992.

573. Opravil M, Pechere M, Speich R, et al: HIV-associated primary pulmonary hypertension. A case control study. Am J Respir Crit Care Med 155:990, 1997.

574. Mesa RA, Edell ES, Dunn WF, et al: Human immunodeficiency virus infection and pulmonary hypertension: Two new cases and a review of 86 reported cases. Mayo Clin Proc 73:37, 1998.

575. Mette SA, Palevsky HI, Pietra GG, et al: Primary pulmonary hypertension in association with human immunodeficiency virus infection: A possible viral etiology for some forms of hypertensive pulmonary arteriopathy. Am Rev Respir Dis 145:1196, 1992.

576. Opravil M, Pechère M, Speich R, et al: HIV-associated primary pulmonary hypertension: A case control study. Am J Respir Crit Care Med 155:990, 1997.

577. Cool CD, Kennedy D, Voelkel NF, et al: Pathogenesis and evolution of plexiform lesions in pulmonary hypertension associated with scleroderma and human immunodeficiency virus infection. Human Pathol 28:434, 1997.

578. Liu AT, Miedzinski LJ, Vallieres E, et al: Pulmonary alveolar proteinosis in an AIDS patient without concurrent pulmonary infection. Can Respir J 2:183, 1995.

579. Ruben FL, Talamo TS: Secondary pulmonary alveolar proteinosis occurring in two patients with acquired immune deficiency syndrome. Am J Med 80:1187, 1986.

580. Nhieu JT, Vojtek AM, Bernaudin JF, et al: Pulmonary alveolar proteinosis associated with *Pneumocystis carinii:* Ultrastructural identification in bronchoalveolar lavage in AIDS and immunocompromised non-AIDS patients. Chest 98:801, 1990.

581. Dooley DP, Tomski S: Syphilitic pneumonitis in an HIV-infected patient. Chest 105:629, 1994.

582. Drabick JJ, Gasser RA, Saunders NB, et al: *Pasteurella multocida* pneumonia in a man with AIDS and nontraumatic feline exposure. Chest 103:7, 1993.

583. Casado JL, Navas E, Frutos B, et al: *Salmonella* lung involvement in patients with HIV infection. Chest 112:1197, 1997.

584. Barber TW, Craven DE, Farber HW: *Mycobacterium gordonae*: A possible opportunistic respiratory tract pathogen in patients with advanced human immunodeficiency virus, type 1 infection. Chest 100:716, 1991.
585. Lessnau KD, Milanese S, Talavera W: *Mycobacterium gordonae*: A treatable disease in HIV-positive patients. Chest 104:1779, 1993.
586. El-Helou P, Rachlis A, Fong I, et al: *Mycobacterium xenopi* infection in patients with human immunodeficiency virus infection. Clin Infect Dis 25:206, 1997.
587. Eng RHK, Forrester C, Smith SM, et al: *Mycobacterium xenopi* infection in a patient with acquired immunodeficiency syndrome. Chest 86:145, 1984.
588. Zurawski CA, Cage GD, Rimland D, et al: Pneumonia and bacteremia due to *Mycobacterium celatum* masquerading as *Mycobacterium xenopi* in patients with AIDS: An underdiagnosed problem? Clin Infect Dis 24:140, 1997.
589. Wald A, Coyle MB, Carlson LC, et al: Infection with a fastidious *Mycobacterium* resembling *Mycobacterium simiae* in seven patients with AIDS. Ann Intern Med 117:586, 1992.
590. Hirschel B, Chang HR, Mach N, et al: Fatal infection with a novel, unidentified *Mycobacterium* in a man with the acquired immunodeficiency syndrome. N Engl J Med 323:109, 1990.
591. Heller HM, Fuhrer J: Disseminated sporotrichosis in patients with AIDS: Case report and review of the literature. AIDS 5:1243, 1991.
592. Piehl MR, Kaplan RL, Habr MH: Disseminated penicilliosis in a patient with acquired immunodeficiency syndrome. Arch Pathol Lab Med 112:1262, 1988.
593. Waxman AB, Goldie SJ, Brett-Smith H, et al: Cytomegalovirus as a primary pulmonary pathogen in AIDS. Chest 111:128, 1997.
593a. Fraisse P, Faller M, Rey D, et al: Recurrent varicella pneumonia complicating an endogenous reactivation of chickenpox in an HIV-infected adult patient. Eur Respir J 11:776, 1998.
594. Weber R, Kuster H, Keller R, et al: Pulmonary and intestinal microsporidiosis in a patient with the acquired immunodeficiency syndrome. Am Rev Respir Dis 146:1603, 1992.
595. Stark P, Relman DA, Santamaria-Fries M, et al: Radiologic features of a fatal platyhelminth (tapeworm) infection in an AIDS patient. Am J Roentgenol 170:136, 1998.
596. McClain KL, Leach CT, Jenson HB, et al: Association of Epstein-Barr virus with leiomyosarcomas in young people with AIDS. N Engl J Med 332:12, 1995.
597. Hessol NA, Katz MH, Liu JY, et al: Increased incidence of Hodgkin's disease in homosexual men with HIV infection. Ann Intern Med 117:309, 1992.
598. Schulz L, Nagaraja HN, Rague N, et al: Respiratory muscle dysfunction associated with human immunodeficiency virus infection. Am J Respir Crit Care Med 155:1080, 1997.
599. Newman TG, Minkowitz S, Hanna A, et al: Coexistent sarcoidosis and HIV infection: A comparison of bronchoalveolar and peripheral blood lymphocytes. Chest 102:1899, 1992.
600. Lowery WS, Whitlock WL, Dietrich RA, et al: Sarcoidosis complicated by HIV infection: Three case reports and a review of the literature. Am Rev Respir Dis 142:887, 1990.
601. Allen JN, Wewers MD: HIV-associated bronchiolitis obliterans organizing pneumonia. Chest 96:197, 1989.
602. Silverstri RC, Jensen WA, Zibrak JD, et al: Pulmonary infiltrates and hypoxemia in patients with the acquired immunodeficiency syndrome re-exposed to trimethoprim-sulfamethoxazole. Am Rev Respir Dis 136:1003, 1987.
603. Diaz PT, Clanton TL, Pacht ER: Emphysema-like pulmonary disease associated with human immunodeficiency virus infection. Ann Intern Med 116:124, 1992.
604. Guillemi SA, Staples CA, Hogg JC, et al: Unexpected lung lesions in high resolution computed tomography (HRCT) among patients with advanced HIV disease. Eur Respir J 9:33, 1996.
605. Ettensohn DB, Mayer KH, Kessimian N, et al: Lymphocytic bronchiolitis associated with HIV infection. Chest 93:201, 1988.
606. Huang L, Stansell JD: AIDS and the lung. Med Clin North Am 80:775, 1996.
607. Angel JB, Walpita P, Lerch RA, et al: Vaccine-associated measles pneumonitis in an adult with AIDS. Ann Intern Med 129:104, 1998.
608. Koziel H, Haley KM, Nasser I, et al: Pulmonary hemorrhage—an uncommon cause of pulmonary infiltrates in patients with AIDS. Chest 106:1891, 1994.
609. Michaels AD, Lederman RJ, MacGregor JS, et al: Cardiovascular involvement in AIDS. Curr Probl Cardiol 22:109, 1997.

# Transplantation

Largely as a result of an increased understanding of immunologic mechanisms and the development of powerful immunosuppressive drugs, transplantation has become an important form of therapy for many diseases. It has been estimated that more than 20,000 allogenic organ transplantations were performed in the United States in 1990;

although this figure has undoubtedly increased since that time, it is likely that many more could have been carried out were it not for limitations of cost and donor availability. In addition, more than 15,000 autologous and allogenic bone marrow transplantations (BMTs) are performed yearly worldwide. These procedures have resulted in improved quality and length of life in many patients; however, they are frequently accompanied by profound side effects. As might be expected, the necessity of preventing graft rejection by chemotherapeutic immunosuppression is associated with a significant risk of infection, often severe and caused by opportunistic organisms. In fact, it is likely that such infection is the most important complication of the procedure.[1-4] In addition, a variety of noninfectious pulmonary complications are seen in many patients, particularly those undergoing lung, heart-lung, and BMT.

## LUNG AND HEART-LUNG TRANSPLANTATION

Since the mid-1980s, lung and heart-lung transplantation have passed from the status of experimental procedures to standard therapy for a variety of otherwise fatal pulmonary conditions (Table 45–1). Thousands of operations have been performed, and new lung transplantation centers continue to develop; for example, in the 1996 annual report of the Registry of the International Society for Heart and Lung Transplantation, information had been recorded on about 1,950 heart-lung, 3,200 single-lung and 1,850 bilateral or double-lung transplantations from more than 120 centers.[5] Greater application of the procedures has been limited principally by donor availability, whereas long-term success has been constrained by the frequent development of obliterative bronchiolitis (OB).

### Technique and Patient Selection

#### Operative Procedures

Current options for lung transplantation include single-lung transplantation, double-lung transplantation (usually using a bilateral sequential single-lung procedure), heart-lung transplantation,[6-8] and lobar transplantation from living-related donors.[9] The precise indications for the selection of a particular procedure are well established in some, but not all, circumstances. For example, double-lung transplantation is necessary in patients who have septic lung disease such

## Table 45–1. LUNG DISEASES TREATED BY TRANSPLANTATION

### INTERSTITIAL LUNG DISEASE

Idiopathic pulmonary fibrosis
Drug-induced lung disease
Sarcoidosis
Langerhans' cell histiocytosis
Pneumoconiosis
Lymphangioleiomyomatosis
Lung disease as part of a systemic illness (selected cases)

### OBSTRUCTIVE LUNG DISEASE

*Nonsuppurative*

Emphysema
Obliterative bronchiolitis

*Suppurative*

Cystic fibrosis
Bronchiectasis

### VASCULAR DISEASE

Primary pulmonary hypertension
Secondary pulmonary hypertension (including chronic thromboembolic pulmonary hypertension)

### MISCELLANEOUS LUNG DISEASE

Alveolar microlithiasis

---

as diffuse bronchiectasis or cystic fibrosis because of the possibility of infection in the transplanted lung or elsewhere if the residual lung were left in place.[6–10] There is also clear-cut indication for heart-lung transplantation in patients who have Eisenmenger's complex without correctable cardiac defects, pulmonary disease with unrelated heart disease, and chronic thromboembolic pulmonary hypertension when thromboendarterectomy is not feasible.[6, 8]

Bilateral sequential single-lung transplantation has become the procedure of choice for double-lung transplantation in North America.[11, 12] In this procedure, a bilateral thoraco-sternotomy ("clamshell") incision is employed to provide exposure of both hemithoraces. Two lungs are then transplanted sequentially, each by separate vascular and bronchial anastomoses.[9] This operation is preferred by many surgeons for several reasons. One is related to the necessity for anticoagulation during cardiopulmonary bypass, a procedure that may significantly aggravate the bleeding that occurs during dissection of pleural adhesions; this complication is particularly likely to be seen in patients who have cystic fibrosis because of the extensive adhesions that often develop during the course of this disease. Although cardiopulmonary bypass can be avoided in most patients receiving sequential transplants, it is required in those undergoing either heart-lung or *en bloc* double-lung transplantation (the procedure first developed for double-lung transplantation). A second reason for sequential lung transplantation is the potential availability of the donor heart for transplantation to another patient (the "domino procedure"),[13, 14] although many such hearts appear to have been wasted.[9] The limited experience available with the use of living-related donor bilateral lobar transplantation in patients who have cystic fibrosis has been reviewed;[9] ethical and technical issues aside, this operation will likely be available to very few patients.

Single-lung transplantation is suitable for most patients requiring lung transplantation and is preferred whenever possible because it increases the pool of donor organs and decreases the waiting time that would otherwise be required for procuring two healthy lungs for double-lung transplantation.[7] As discussed farther on, post-transplantation exercise performance is similar in patients who have received double-lung and single-lung transplants.[6, 15, 16] However, whether the increased lung reserve in patients who have received a double-lung transplant will be associated with longer survival or better tolerance of OB remains to be determined.

The best procedure for patients who have primary pulmonary hypertension is uncertain. However, single-lung transplantation has been performed successfully in such patients even in the presence of right ventricular failure.[17, 18, 18a] In the latter situation, "unloading" the right ventricle allows significant functional cardiac recovery; the threshold below which this function cannot recover is unknown.[12] Disadvantages of the procedure in these patients are initial hemodynamic instability and severe gas exchange problems during subsequent rejection (most ventilation shifting to the native lung while the transplanted lung receives most of the perfusion).[6] Whether the relative availability of single lungs and the ease of the surgery compensate for these effects has not been clarified; however, survival does not appear to be affected by the type of procedure undertaken.[18a]

It was initially thought that single-lung transplantation would not be feasible in patients who have emphysema because of compression of the transplanted lung by the highly compliant and hyperinflated native lung or because of unacceptable ventilation-perfusion imbalance between the two lungs.[6, 19] However, these concerns have proved to be largely unfounded, and emphysema is now among the more common indications for single-lung transplantation.[7, 20, 21] In the setting of chronic obstructive pulmonary disease (COPD), double-lung transplantation is now confined largely to patients who have giant bullae, in whom concern about mediastinal shift and compression of the transplanted lung is still relevant, and to younger patients who are better able to tolerate the surgery and who might benefit from the greater pulmonary reserve afforded by the two lungs.[7, 22] When single-lung transplantation is performed in a patient who has emphysema, the side that has the better function, as assessed by quantitative ventilation-perfusion scanning, is conserved (assuming the absence of significant pleural adhesions from previous thoracotomy or pleurodesis on that side).[7]

### Patient Selection

Selection criteria for lung transplant recipients have been established on the basis of a combination of common sense and bitter experience.[7–9, 23–25a] General recommendations are outlined in Table 45–2; however, these criteria have varied over time and in different centers, and several comments are in order. As might be expected, the prediction of patient survival in the absence of transplantation is an imperfect art.[26] In fact, the decision to list a patient for transplantation may have as much to do with the patient's perception of the current quality of life as with the physician's estimate of the quantity of life remaining.[26a] The ability to participate in a preoperative rehabilitation program may help to optimize the patient's condition before trans-

## Table 45–2. SELECTION CRITERIA FOR LUNG TRANSPLANT RECIPIENTS

1. Age younger than 65 years for single-lung transplantation and 60 years for double-lung transplantation
2. End-stage lung disease with life expectancy of less than 12 to 18 months
3. Absence of other significant medical disease (including human immunodeficiency virus seropositivity)
4. Acceptable nutritional status (both marked obesity and marked malnutrition are relative contraindications)
5. Ambulatory with rehabilitation potential
6. Good psychological profile with demonstrated compliance with medical regimens, abstinence from cigarette smoking or other drug abuse for at least 6 months, and good emotional and logistical support system
7. Absence of multiresistant organisms on sputum culture
8. Absence of previous major thoracic surgery
9. Adequate financial resources for both transplantation and postoperative care

plantation and serves as an indicator of motivation and compliance with medical regimens.

With improving results and greater experience, age limitation has been progressively liberalized,[7–9] and many centers now accept patients up to 65 years of age for single-lung transplantation.[12] The presence of other significant medical problems is generally considered a contraindication to transplantation.[27] However, a good outcome has been described in patients who have cystic fibrosis and diabetes mellitus[28] and in a very few carefully selected patients who have systemic disease, such as progressive systemic sclerosis or systemic lupus erythematosus;[29] double-lung transplantation has even been performed successfully in a patient who had bilateral bronchioloalveolar carcinoma.[30] Osteoporosis is common in patients awaiting transplantation,[31, 32] and the procedure is usually followed by deterioration in bone mineral density as a result of the corticosteroids used for immunosuppression.[31] As a result, severe osteoporosis is a contraindication; in addition, measures to reverse or stabilize pre-existing mild or moderate osteoporosis should be employed in both the pre- and post-transplant period.

Preoperative colonization or infection by antibiotic-resistant organisms (particularly *Burkholderia cepacia*) in patients who have cystic fibrosis has had dramatic adverse consequences following lung or heart-lung transplantation. In one series of 15 such patients, 7 died, the median survival being only 28 days;[33] all deaths were the direct or indirect result of infection by the organism, whereas 14 of the 15 patients had a clinical infection attributable to the organism. As a result of this and other experience,[34] most (albeit not all[35]) authorities consider the presence of *B. cepacia* and other pan-resistant organisms to be a contraindication to transplantation. By contrast, the presence of airway colonization by *Aspergillus* species in patients who have cystic fibrosis does not appear to be complicated by invasive infection in the post-transplantation period.[9]

Ventilator dependence has generally precluded transplantation; however, the procedure can be performed successfully in this situation when patients are previously evaluated and when no additional contraindications, such as pneumonia, arise before obtaining a donor organ.[36] Although some investigators have reported success even in the absence of these provisos,[37] registry data have confirmed that ventila-

tor-dependent patients have a much higher mortality rate after transplantation than nonventilated patients.[12] Similar findings have been reported in patients undergoing retransplantation;[37a] in fact, it has been recommended that nonambulatory, ventilated patients should not be considered for retransplantation with the same priority as other patients.[37a]

Extensive pleural fibrosis has been considered a relative contraindication to lung transplantation because of the frequent presence of hyperplastic blood vessels within the adhesions. As indicated previously, dissection of such adhesions may result in excessive bleeding during cardiopulmonary bypass.[38] These concerns have resulted in a modification of the management of pneumothorax in patients who have cystic fibrosis; in some centers, pleurodesis is reserved for patients who have air leak refractory to chest tube drainage, whereas thoracoscopic blebectomy is performed with or without focal apical pleurodesis.[38, 39] However, single-lung transplantation may allow surgery on the side unaffected by pleural disease or previous dissection,[40] and the avoidance of cardiopulmonary bypass may be possible by using the bilateral sequential single-lung transplantation technique.

The use of systemic corticosteroids initially constituted a contraindication to transplantation because of fears of inadequate healing of the bronchial anastomosis. However, advances in surgical technique have reduced the frequency of postoperative bronchial dehiscence, and it is now apparent that the preoperative use of low-dose corticosteroids does not have an adverse impact on anastomotic healing.[41]

### Complications

#### *Reperfusion Edema*

Noncardiogenic pulmonary edema commonly occurs in the transplanted lung shortly after its reimplantation (reperfusion injury, the "pulmonary reimplantation response").[6, 42, 43] The pathogenesis of the complication is incompletely understood and is likely multifactorial. Potentially important factors include alveolar endothelial and epithelial damage, surfactant deficit, and abnormalities of coagulation factors. The development of pulmonary edema is also favored by the severing of pulmonary lymphatics, which necessarily occurs during transplantation, and by iatrogenic fluid overload that may occur both before and after transplantation.[44]

The severity of the increase in pulmonary vascular permeability is closely related to the time interval between excision of the donor lung and its implantation in the recipient (ischemic time).[42] The ischemia and subsequent reperfusion lead to endothelial damage,[45–48] which appears to be mediated largely by neutrophil sequestration and activation.[45, 49–51] Resident macrophages may be the source of cytokines which initiate these events.[52] Endothelial damage may ultimately be related to the effects of oxygen free radicals derived from activated neutrophils or from the endothelium itself.[53] In animal models, lipid peroxidation induced by free radicals results in an increase in endothelial permeability and edema formation that is reduced or prevented by administration of a variety of free radical scavengers.[54, 55] Moreover, the use of agents that prevent free radical formation results in the preservation of lung function during reperfusion.[56]

Coagulation factors may also be important in early reperfusion injury. In a dog model of lung transplantation, administration of $C_1$-esterase inhibitor, the main inhibitor of the blood coagulation contact system, prevented early pulmonary dysfunction;[57] the decrease in lung coagulation contact factors was associated with a reduction in complement activation, expression of leukocyte adhesion molecules, and inflammatory cell infiltration. The results of experiments in a number of animal models of reperfusion injury also implicate abnormal surfactant production and function in the gas-exchange impairment seen in the immediate post-transplantation period.[46, 58–61a] In these models, surfactant function is altered by ischemia of the donor lung;[60–62] this effect can be partly reversed by administration of exogenous surfactant[58, 59] and perhaps prevented by storage of the graft at higher lung volumes.[63] The results of an experimental study in dogs suggest an important role for endothelin-1;[63a] in this study, dogs that were given an endothelin-1–receptor antagonist had significantly improved survival and marked reduction in post-transplantation edema. Biophysical factors, such as maintenance of vascular distention during ischemic time, also may influence the severity of reperfusion injury.[63b]

Pathologic features of reperfusion injury are those of air-space and alveolar septal edema and congestion;[64] in severe cases, the appearance is that of diffuse alveolar damage (Fig. 45–1).[7, 46] Plugs of fibroblastic tissue representing organization of the air-space exudate may be identified several weeks after transplantation in severe cases (*see* Fig. 45–1).[65]

The radiologic findings of reperfusion injury are nonspecific and are similar to those in patients who have left ventricular failure, fluid overload, and acute rejection. They range from a subtle perihilar haze to patchy or confluent airspace consolidation involving mainly the middle and lower lung zones (Fig. 45–2).[66–69] Interstitial abnormalities, including peribronchial and perivascular thickening and a reticular pattern, are seen in most patients.

The spectrum of radiographic findings and the time course of reperfusion injury have been assessed in several studies. In one review of 105 consecutive patients who underwent lung transplantation, radiographic abnormalities were identified on the first postoperative chest radiograph in 141 of 148 (95%) transplanted lungs and by day 3 in 144 (97%).[67] In most cases, the abnormalities consisted predominantly of a perihilar haze or mild interstitial thickening. They were usually maximal in the first 3 days and decreased gradually thereafter; most patients had normal radiographs or only mild residual interstitial abnormalities by day 10. In another investigation of 45 patients (20 who had undergone single-lung transplantation and 25 double-lung transplantation), reperfusion edema was evident on the chest radiograph on day 1 in 39 (87%) and by day 3 in 44 (98%).[70] The

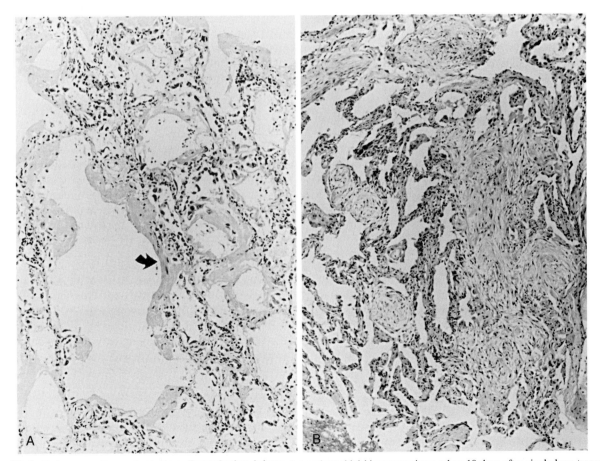

**Figure 45–1. Pulmonary Transplantation: Reperfusion Injury.** A transbronchial biopsy specimen taken 10 days after single-lung transplantation *(A)* shows air spaces partly filled with proteinaceous material, focally appearing as a hyaline membrane *(arrow)*. A follow-up biopsy about 4 weeks later *(B)* shows many air spaces filled with fibroblastic tissue, representing organization of the proteinaceous material seen in *A*. A prolonged ischemic time had occurred in the pretransplantation period.

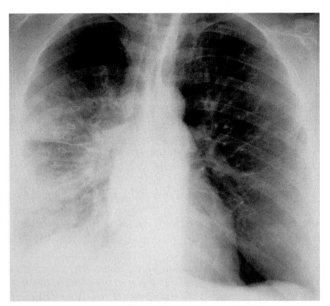

**Figure 45–2. Pulmonary Transplantation: Reperfusion Injury.** An anteroposterior chest radiograph demonstrates ground-glass opacities and poorly defined areas of consolidation in the right lung. A small right pleural effusion is also present. The patient was a 50-year-old woman with the clinical diagnosis of reperfusion edema 3 days after single right lung transplantation for emphysema.

edema was asymmetric in 9 (36%) of the patients who had undergone double-lung transplantation. There was poor correlation between the severity of radiographic findings and the alveolar-arterial oxygen gradient. A poor correlation between the extent of radiographic abnormalities and the oxygenation efficiency of the transplanted lung has also been shown by another group of investigators.[70a]

The edema usually begins immediately after transplantation, worsens over the first 48 hours, and peaks in severity between the second and fourth postoperative day.[6] Although most patients develop concomitant radiographic opacities, clinically important pulmonary dysfunction occurs in only about 15% to 35%;[12] however, in about 5% to 10% of patients, reperfusion injury is severe and may be associated with graft failure.[7] Such primary graft failure must be distinguished from other causes of air-space edema in the early post-transplantation period, such as thrombosis of the pulmonary vein and myocardial dysfunction.[71]

There is evidence that the time course of the development of edema is different in patients who have received heart-lung transplants. In one review of the radiographic findings in 20 patients who underwent heart-lung transplantation, an interstitial pattern, with or without associated air-space consolidation, was seen on the first postoperative day in all cases;[72] the abnormalities improved over the next few days but gradually increased during the second week. In another report of 10 patients who underwent heart-lung transplantation, the parenchymal abnormalities peaked on day 11 and then gradually resolved.[73]

The importance of reperfusion injury may extend beyond the initial disturbances in pulmonary function: in some animal models, there is evidence that severe reperfusion injury enhances immunogenicity of the graft by augmenting major histocompatibility complex (MHC) expression, a pro-

cess that could lead to an increased risk of subsequent rejection.[50, 74, 75]

### Hyperacute Rejection

Hyperacute rejection typically occurs within minutes of re-establishment of pulmonary perfusion and is caused by preformed alloantibodies that bind to the donor organ and activate complement.[76] The abnormality has rarely been described in lung transplant recipients.[77] It results in diffuse alveolar damage, a neutrophilic infiltrate, and positive immunoglobulin G (IgG) fluorescence in alveolar spaces and septa.[77] Screening of recipient blood for anti-HLA antibodies formed as a result of prior exposure to alloantigens through pregnancy, blood transfusion, or previous transplantation[76] and ensuring ABO compatibility has virtually eliminated this as a cause of early graft dysfunction.[12]

### Acute Rejection

Acute rejection is an almost invariable complication of lung transplantation and an important cause of morbidity;[76, 78] for example, in one investigation of 69 patients who had single-lung, double-lung, or heart-lung transplantations and who survived at least 5 days, all had at least one episode of rejection.[79] Although the reaction may be seen as early as 3 days after transplantation, it is usually first manifested after 1 to 2 weeks.[76] Its frequency diminishes with time from transplantation;[80] 60% of all cases occur during the first 3 postoperative months,[76] and rejection after 4 years is uncommon.[80] The fortunate minority of patients who do not develop clinical evidence of rejection during the first 4 months after transplantation generally continue to be free of the complication.[81]

#### Pathogenesis

Acute rejection is predominantly a cell-mediated immune response that results from the activation and proliferation of effector T cells directed against the HLA complex (MHC) of donor cells.[76, 78, 82, 82a] It is presumed that donor MHC molecules trigger reactions in recipient T lymphocytes analogous to those that would be induced by MHC–foreign antigen complexes.[76] In fact, expression of MHC gene products on various targets, including pulmonary epithelial, endothelial, and dendritic cells and alveolar macrophages, has been shown to trigger the proliferation of alloreactive cells.[78] Moreover, the risk of acute rejection has been strongly associated with HLA-DR mismatches.[82b] T-helper lymphocytes are stimulated by donor class II molecules (HLA-DP, DQ, DR) on antigen-presenting cells, such as macrophages; the lymphocytes secrete cytokines, which induce MHC expression, enhance T-lymphocyte response, and thereby both initiate and amplify the cellular inflammatory reaction.[12, 76] Recipient cytolytic (CD8+) T lymphocytes recognize donor class I MHC molecules and, after differentiation under the influence of cytokines secreted from T-helper lymphocytes, directly lyse graft endothelial and parenchymal cells.[76]

The role of humoral immunity in acute rejection is uncertain; however, biopsy specimens are striking for their absence of B lymphocytes and antibody deposition, suggesting that it is likely to be unimportant.[83]

## Pathologic Characteristics

The histologic features of acute lung rejection have been described by several groups of investigators;[84–88] although they overlap somewhat with changes seen in other conditions (e.g., infection),[84] they are sufficiently characteristic to enable confident diagnosis in most cases. As might be expected, the abnormalities vary with the severity of rejection, and grading systems reflecting such variation have been devised (Table 45–3).[85, 89] Minimal and mild rejection are seen most often;[90] severe rejection is rare.

The principal histologic finding is a mononuclear inflammatory cell infiltrate that, in the lower grades, is located predominantly in the interstitial tissue surrounding venules, arterioles, and small veins and arteries (Fig. 45–3). In more severe disease, the infiltrate extends throughout the vessel wall to involve the endothelium ("endotheliitis") and into the adjacent alveolar interstitium (Fig. 45–4). Air spaces are usually unaffected except in severe disease, in which alveolar septal necrosis may be accompanied by hemorrhage, a proteinaceous exudate, and hyaline membranes.

The inflammatory cells that infiltrate the vessel walls are predominantly mononuclear in the lower grades. As disease becomes more severe, greater numbers of eosinophils and neutrophils may be encountered; occasionally, these are prominent.[91] The mononuclear cells consist of small round or plasmacytoid lymphocytes and larger cells that have enlarged nuclei ("transformed" or "activated" lymphocytes). Plasma cells are typically absent or few in number. Follow-up biopsies in patients who have been treated for acute rejection often show perivascular fibrosis with the presence of scattered hemosiderin-laden macrophages and lymphocytes (Fig. 45–5).

Vessels are usually affected in a patchy fashion, and examination of multiple levels and biopsy fragments may be necessary to identify the abnormality. It has been suggested that a minimum of five fragments be obtained,[85] although very mild rejection may be missed even when this amount of tissue is examined. In one experimental study in which excised, transplanted dog lungs were extensively sampled after a standard series of transbronchial biopsies, five biopsy

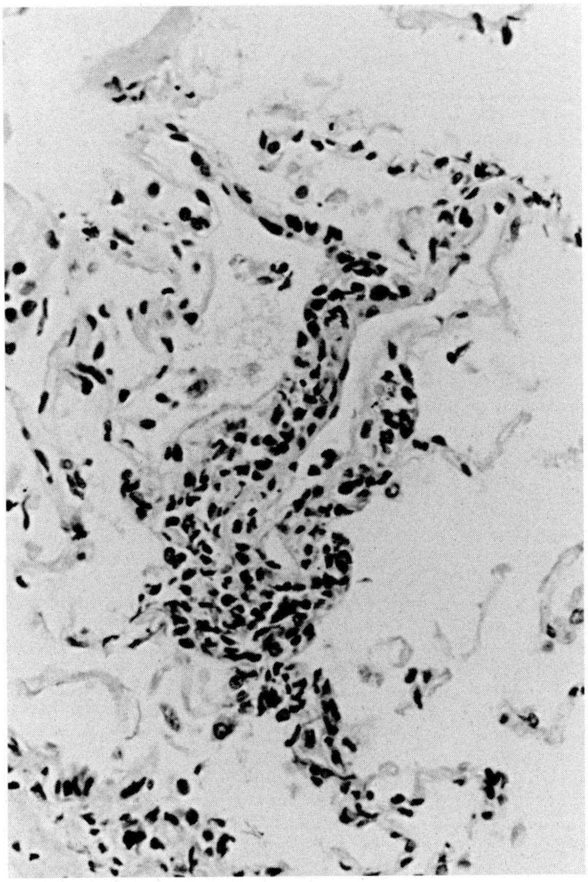

**Figure 45–3. Pulmonary Transplantation: Mild Acute Rejection.** A magnified view of a transbronchial biopsy specimen shows the wall of a small vessel to contain an infiltrate of mononuclear inflammatory cells, most with small nuclei; adjacent alveolar septa are essentially normal. Similar infiltrates were present in relation to several other pulmonary vessels.

fragments were associated with a sensitivity for the diagnosis of mild rejection of about 90%;[92] three fragments were sufficient for moderate to severe disease.

In addition to the characteristic vascular changes, bronchiolar inflammation is often seen in biopsy specimens from patients who have acute rejection. This usually takes the form of a mononuclear cell infiltrate in the mucosa (including the epithelium). It has been speculated that such inflammation may be a precursor of OB or of the lymphocytic bronchiolitis and bronchitis seen in some patients who do not have classic features of vascular rejection.[93]

## Table 45–3. REVISED WORKING FORMULATION FOR CLASSIFICATION AND GRADING OF LUNG ALLOGRAFT REJECTION—1995

Acute rejection
  Grade 0—None
  Grade 1—Minimal
  Grade 2—Mild     } with/without  { Airway inflammation—
  Grade 3—Moderate                   lymphocytic
  Grade 4—Severe                     bronchitis and
Chronic airway                       bronchiolitis
  rejection—bronchiolitis
  obliterans
  a. Active
  b. Inactive
Chronic vascular rejection—
  accelerated graft vascular
  sclerosis

Adapted from Yousem S: A perspective on the revised working formulation for the grading of lung allograft rejection. Transplant Proc 28:477, 1996. Reprinted by permission of Appleton & Lange, Inc.

## Radiologic Manifestations

The radiographic abnormalities in patients who have acute lung rejection include a fine reticular interstitial pattern, interlobular septal thickening, ground-glass opacities, patchy or confluent air-space consolidation, and new or increasing pleural effusions (Fig. 45–6).[66, 69, 94–97] The reported prevalence of these abnormalities varies considerably among studies. This variability is likely related to several factors, including different patient populations, different criteria used to diagnose acute rejection, and inconsistent terminology used to describe the parenchymal findings. The radiograph

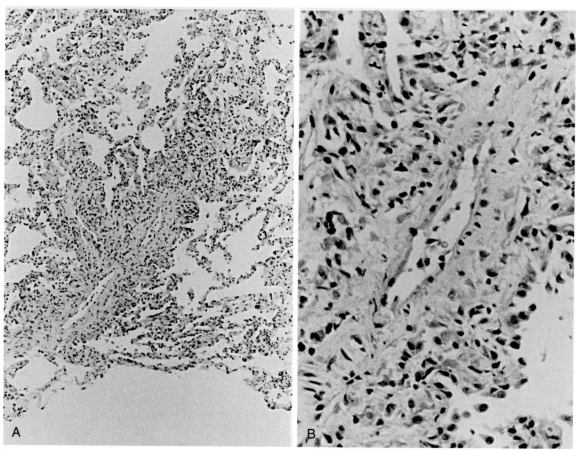

**Figure 45–4. Pulmonary Transplantation: Moderate Acute Rejection.** The wall of a small pulmonary artery *(A)* shows moderate thickening by edema and an infiltrate of inflammatory cells, some of which extend into the adjacent alveolar septa. A magnified view *(B)* shows some of the inflammatory cells to have enlarged, somewhat irregularly shaped nuclei ("transformed lymphocytes"); occasional cells are intimately associated with the endothelium ("endotheliitis") *(arrow)*. Although not easily identified in this illustration, scattered eosinophils are also present.

has been reported to show parenchymal abnormalities in 50% to 100% of patients who have clinical or biopsy-proven diagnosis of acute rejection.[67, 68, 94–96] In one investigation of 25 episodes of acute rejection in 12 patients, all of whom had symptoms, the diagnosis was confirmed by transbronchial biopsy in all cases;[96] the most common abnormalities consisted of interlobular septal thickening (seen in 19 episodes [76%]), new or increasing pleural effusion (in 17 [68%]), peribronchial cuffing (in 11 [44%]), and air-space consolidation (in 11 [44%]).

The frequency with which parenchymal abnormalities are seen is also influenced by the time at which the rejection is manifested. In one study of 45 episodes of acute rejection in 20 patients, 23 occurring within the first month after transplantation and 22 after the first month, the diagnosis of rejection was based on transbronchial biopsy in 33 episodes and on clinical findings in 12; all patients had symptoms.[95] Radiographic abnormalities were detected in 22 of 45 (49%) episodes; radiographs were abnormal in 17 of 23 (74%) episodes occurring during the first month but in only 5 of 22 episodes (23%) occurring later than the first month after transplantation.[95] The parenchymal abnormalities consisted mainly of poorly defined perihilar nodular opacities (air-space nodules), which sometimes coalesced and progressed to frank consolidation involving mainly the perihilar regions and lower lung zones.

Pleural effusions are common in association with parenchymal abnormalities in acute rejection and are occasionally the only radiographic manifestation. In one study, the radiographic findings in 22 episodes of acute rejection included a combination of parenchymal abnormalities and pleural effusion in 15 (68%) cases, pulmonary changes alone in 4 (18%), and pleural effusion alone in 3 (14%).[95] In another investigation, the chest radiographic findings were correlated with the results of transbronchial biopsies in 16 heart-lung transplant recipients who underwent 83 bronchoscopic examinations.[96] The combination of interlobular septal thickening and new or increasing pleural effusions without a concomitant increase in cardiac size or vascular pedicle width or evidence of vascular redistribution was reported to indicate acute rejection with a sensitivity of 68% (17 of 25 episodes) and a specificity of 90% (excluding the diagnosis in 52 of 58 episodes that had nonspecific or normal biopsy findings, or pulmonary infection). Although the results of this study suggest a high degree of accuracy in distinguishing acute rejection from infection, other investigators have found a lower diagnostic accuracy for acute rejection or for the distinction of rejection from infection.[67, 95]

The HRCT findings of acute lung rejection were reviewed in a study of 32 patients who had undergone single-lung, double-lung, or heart-lung transplantation.[98] A total of 190 transbronchial biopsy specimens and concurrent HRCT

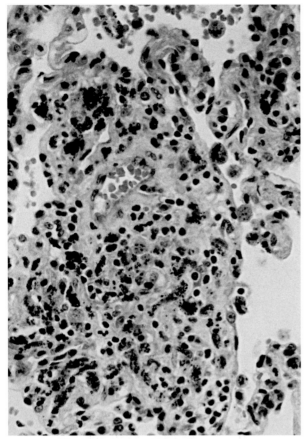

**Figure 45–5. Pulmonary Transplantation: Remote Rejection.** A magnified view of a transbronchial biopsy specimen shows marked thickening of the perivascular interstitial tissue as a result of fibrosis and an inflammatory infiltrate of lymphocytes and macrophages that contain finely granular black material (representing hemosiderin). The patient had experienced several episodes of acute rejection but was clinically well at the time of this follow-up biopsy (performed about 10 months after transplantation).

month, the HRCT findings do not allow a distinction among acute rejection, reperfusion injury, and fluid overload.

### Clinical Manifestations

Acute pulmonary rejection is associated with a nonspecific clinical picture characterized by cough, dyspnea, fever, tachypnea, and crackles on auscultation of the chest.[8, 44] These findings may be associated with arterial hypoxemia, an abnormal chest radiograph, and a reduction in perfusion to the affected lung as assessed by perfusion scintigraphy.[24] Unfortunately, infection, fluid overload, and reperfusion edema may produce similar signs and symptoms,[8, 76] and a diagnosis of rejection often depends on transbronchial biopsy.

The use of surveillance transbronchial biopsies (biopsies done in patients who have neither clinical nor radiographic abnormalities) in the post-transplantation period has led to the appreciation that some episodes of rejection are clinically silent; for example, in one study of 355 procedures performed on 161 lung transplant recipients, 50 (14%) revealed at least grade 2 rejection;[99] similar results have been reported from other centers.[81, 100–102] Most of these "silent" rejection episodes occur in the first 6 months after transplantation:[99] in one investigation, only 10 of 102 surveillance biopsies performed 2 years after transplantation revealed acute rejection, and no rejection was found in the 15 biopsies performed four years or more after transplantation.[80] There is little evidence that management based on the results of surveillance biopsies improves prognosis and outcome.[103]

When infection has been reasonably excluded by negative results on microbiologic and pathologic examination, and the clinical and radiographic picture is typical of acute rejection, a diagnosis may sometimes be inferred from a favorable response to high-dose intravenous corticosteroids.[6, 7]

### Pulmonary Function Tests

Changes in pulmonary function and their usefulness in the diagnosis of acute rejection have been evaluated in a number of studies.[104–109] A persistent decline in $FEV_1$ and FVC usually signals the development of a complication of transplantation. For example, in one investigation of 34 heart-lung transplant recipients in which histologic findings in transbronchial biopsy material were used as the gold standard, a decrease in lung function had an 84% specificity for recognizing an acute abnormality (either infection or rejection).[105] Most investigators consider a 10% fall in $FEV_1$ or FVC to be significant;[106, 107, 109] however, some accept a 5% decrease in $FEV_1$ as an indication of deterioration because this magnitude of change exceeds the coefficient of variation for repeated measurements of $FEV_1$ both in heart-lung transplant recipients and in normal volunteers.[105] As would be expected, the acceptance of a smaller deterioration in lung function as significant increases the sensitivity of the test for the detection of disease, while sacrificing specificity. Changes in lung function are more difficult to interpret in single-lung than in double-lung transplant recipients because function in the former can be influenced by disease in both the graft and the native lung.[107]

It has been an almost uniform observation that measure-

scans were obtained. Forty of the biopsy specimens (21%) showed histologic evidence of acute rejection, 111 (58%) were normal, and 39 (21%) were inconclusive. The most common abnormality seen in patients who had acute rejection was localized or widespread areas of ground-glass attenuation. This finding was identified in 26 of 40 cases (65%) diagnosed as acute rejection, compared with 5 of 11 (45%) with biopsy findings suggestive but not diagnostic of rejection, 7 of 28 (25%) with nonspecific biopsy findings, and 10 of 111 (9%) with normal biopsies. It was more likely to be present in patients who had higher grades of rejection on transbronchial biopsy specimens. Septal lines were identified in 11 cases (27%) of acute rejection, 1 of 11 (9%) with biopsy findings suggestive of rejection, 4 of 28 (14%) with nonspecific biopsy findings, and 7 of 111 (6%) with normal biopsies (Fig. 45–7). Less common abnormalities seen in acute rejection included recent or increased size of pleural effusions, basal consolidation, and peribronchial cuffing, each seen in 10 patients (25%). Although these three findings were also seen in association with reperfusion injury, in this situation, they were usually limited to the lower lung zones. The investigators concluded that in the first postoperative

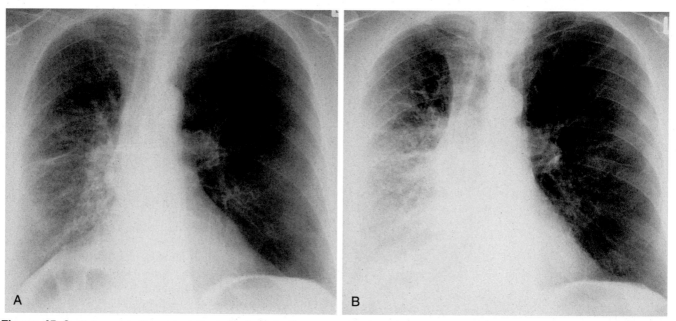

**Figure 45–6. Pulmonary Transplantation: Acute Rejection.** A 62-year-old woman underwent right lung transplantation for emphysema. A posteroanterior chest radiograph performed 6 days later *(A)* demonstrates mild interstitial thickening involving mainly the right perihilar region and right lower lobe. A radiograph 2 days later *(B)* shows an increase in the parenchymal abnormalities associated with the development of septal lines, and ground-glass opacities throughout the right middle and lower lung zones, and focal areas of consolidation. The diagnosis of acute rejection was confirmed by transbronchial biopsy.

ments of FEV$_1$ and FVC cannot distinguish between rejection and infection.[104, 105, 107] There is some evidence that the sensitivity of deterioration of lung function for the detection of rejection may be better in the first 3 postoperative months (about 85%) than subsequently (75%) in heart-lung transplant recipients;[105] similar findings may hold true for double-lung transplant recipients. Using functional criteria in single-lung transplant recipients, the overall sensitivity of lung function changes in the detection of rejection has been found to vary from about 40% to 85%.[107] The best results have been found for small changes in FVC in patients who have underlying pulmonary fibrosis, whereas the worst have been

associated with small changes in FEV$_1$ in patients who have COPD.

The significance of normal histologic findings on transbronchial biopsy specimens from patients who have deteriorating lung function is uncertain. However, it is clear that not all these patients are free of infection or rejection. Using clinical criteria as the basis for the diagnosis of rejection, one group of investigators found transbronchial biopsy to have a sensitivity of only 72%.[100] (Clinical criteria felt to indicate rejection in this study included a temperature rise of more than 0.5° C above baseline, a decrease in Pao$_2$ of more than 10 mm Hg below baseline, radiographic changes,

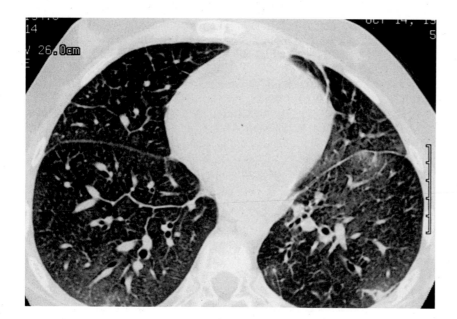

**Figure 45–7. Pulmonary Transplantation: Acute Rejection.** An HRCT scan performed 10 days after double-lung transplantation demonstrates interlobular septal thickening and patchy areas of ground-glass attenuation. The diagnosis of acute rejection was confirmed by transbronchial biopsy.

a decline in spirometric indices of more than 10% to 15% below baseline, exclusion of infection, and a favorable response to treatment with methylprednisolone.)

## Bronchoalveolar Lavage

Because serious complications of transbronchial biopsy can occur in lung transplant recipients,[76, 81] the value of bronchoalveolar lavage (BAL) has been investigated to identify findings that are both sensitive and specific for rejection. Because the procedure is useful in the identification of pathogens and is invariably performed in patients undergoing bronchoscopy for diagnosis of complications of transplantation in any event,[110–112] its use in the diagnosis of rejection would not increase the complexity of bronchoscopy. Unfortunately, although some findings are characteristic of infection or rejection, they lack sufficiently high sensitivity and specificity to permit clinical use.

BAL neutrophilia may be seen in both infection and acute or chronic rejection.[113] Similarly, although markers of eosinophil and fibroblast activation have been found in the BAL fluid of patients who have acute rejection, values overlap with those found in patients who do not have rejection.[114] T-helper lymphocytes implicated in acute rejection induce the production of $IgG_2$, and the BAL ratio of $IgG_2$ to $IgG_1$ was elevated in acute rejection in one small study;[115] although the sensitivity was about 90%, appreciation of the test's technical limitations, the small number of patients involved, and a specificity of only 80% have prevented its wider application. An elevation of the serum interleukin-2 (IL-2) receptor level, a marker of T-lymphocyte activation, has been documented in both rejection and infection;[82] it is possible that the differential analysis of BAL IL-2 receptor levels from both the transplanted and native lungs in patients who undergo single-lung transplantation will prove useful in identifying rejection.[116]

Other markers of BAL fluid abnormality, such as lymphocytosis[10] and elevated IL-4 levels,[117] lack sensitivity for the diagnosis of acute rejection, even if they appear to distinguish infection from rejection. In addition, findings identified by some investigators, such as an increase in $CD8^+$ cells during rejection,[118] have not been conclusively replicated by others.[119] In one study, the level of exhaled nitric oxide was found to be elevated in patients who had acute rejection compared with that in normal individuals and in transplant patients who had obliterative bronchiolitis;[119a] however, these results were not replicated in another investigation.[119b]

### Obliterative Bronchiolitis

Progressive airflow obstruction as a result of OB has been reported in up to 70% of patients after lung transplantation.[44, 78, 120, 121] As many as 55% of affected individuals die directly from the complication, making it the major cause of late graft failure.[76, 120, 122–125a] The complication has occurred after heart-lung, double-lung, and single-lung transplantation.[125]

### Pathogenesis

Although the precise pathogenesis of OB is uncertain, the bulk of evidence points to an immunologically mediated airway injury. In fact, most authorities use the terms *posttransplantation obliterative bronchiolitis* or *obliterative bronchiolitis syndrome* (the latter to refer to patients who have pulmonary dysfunction in the absence of histologic evidence of OB and other apparent reasons for airflow obstruction)[125–127] interchangeably with chronic rejection.[24, 76, 120, 123, 128] Numerous clinical and experimental observations support this hypothesis, including the following:

1. There is a strong association between the frequency, severity, and persistence of acute rejection and the risk of OB.[78, 122, 129, 130]

2. Identical pathologic changes are seen in the lungs of bone marrow transplant recipients who have graft-versus-host disease (GVHD) and of patients who have immunologically mediated connective tissue disease such as rheumatoid disease.

3. The prevalence of OB has been reduced by augmented immunosuppression in the post-transplantation period,[131, 132] and established OB may respond favorably to increased immunosuppression.[121, 129, 133, 134]

4. There are a higher number of T and B lymphocytes in the peribronchiolar tissue and bronchiolar lumen in patients who have OB than in those of controls.[83, 135, 136]

5. Analysis of the T-cell antigen receptor β-chain variable gene of both peripheral blood[137] and BAL fluid[138] lymphocytes in some patients who have OB has revealed clonal or oligoclonal populations, suggesting that their expansion has been the result of a response to a limited number of alloantigens.

6. Using a number of other assays, lymphocytes obtained by both BAL[139, 140] and bronchial biopsy[141] have shown donor-antigen–specific reactivity in patients who have OB.

7. The bronchial epithelium of patients who have OB has increased expression of class II MHC antigens, compared with patients who have normal histologic findings,[142] thereby providing both an inducement and a target for immune response by the recipient. In addition, rejection of other solid organ transplants is associated with injury to cells of epithelial origin.[143]

8. The presence of serum anti-HLA antibodies has been associated with a higher risk of development of OB, suggesting a role for humoral immunity.[141]

9. Some patients who have lymphocytic hyporeactivity to donor antigens have failed to develop OB.[144]

10. Bronchiolar lesions similar to those of human OB have been found in an experimental model involving heterotopic transplantation of mouse airways into subcutaneous tissue.[145]

It is probable that adhesion molecules, such as E-selectin, play an important role in regulating the events of graft rejection.[146, 147] Such molecules influence the movement of lymphocytes into the allograft and their binding to antigen-expressing donor cells; they also augment T-cell activation.[147]

Although not all investigators agree,[148] it is likely that the development of cytomegalovirus (CMV) pneumonia imposes a significant risk for the subsequent development of OB.[129, 149] For example, in one study of 118 patients, the 56 who had a history of biopsy-proven CMV pneumonia had a 74% actuarial risk of developing OB within 2 years of transplantation;[149] by contrast, the 62 patients who never developed the complication had a risk of only 22%. In addition, the use of antiviral agents for the prophylaxis of CMV pneumonia has been reported to both decrease the incidence of CMV pneumonia and delay its onset.[150, 151] This has been accompanied by a reduction in the incidence of OB and a delay in its onset. The mechanism by which CMV infection might act to cause or facilitate the development of OB is uncertain; however, pneumonia has been associated with an increase in the number and activity of antigen-presenting cells in the graft,[152–154] enhancement of donor-specific alloreactivity, and an increased expression of class II MHC antigens on endothelial and epithelial cells.[78, 125, 127, 143]

Additional factors may also be important in the pathogenesis of OB. For example, some investigators have hypothesized that the primary injury is to the lung vasculature, with OB resulting directly or indirectly from ischemic damage to the airway.[127] The development of OB coincides with the usual clustering of viral respiratory illnesses in the first quarter of the year;[155] this observation, along with the finding that histologically identified organizing pneumonia during the first year after transplantation predisposes to OB,[156] suggests that infectious organisms other than or in addition to CMV could play a role in pathogenesis. The finding that patients who have had primary pulmonary hypertension are more likely to develop OB than patients who have had other underlying pretransplant disease remains unexplained.[157]

### Pathologic Characteristics

Histologically, OB is typically manifested by an eccentric or, more often, concentric increase in the connective tissue between the muscularis mucosa and the epithelium of membranous and proximal respiratory bronchioles (Fig. 45–8).[158–160] Plugs of fibroblastic tissue within the bronchiolar lumen (i.e., internal to the epithelium) are unusual and should suggest the possibility of another etiology, particularly infection.[159] In the early stage, the abnormal connective tissue appears active, being composed of fibroblasts separated by a loose-appearing stroma. Although a mononuclear inflammatory cellular infiltrate is often present in both peribronchiolar interstitial tissue and the fibroblastic tissue itself, it is typically mild in severity. The airway epithelium may be normal but more commonly is flattened or shows squamous metaplasia.

In more advanced disease, the fibrous tissue is typically mature in appearance and may completely occlude the airway lumen (Fig. 45–9). Use of an elastic tissue stain to delineate the residual bronchiolar elastic lamina may be helpful in localizing a focus of fibrosis to an airway, particu-

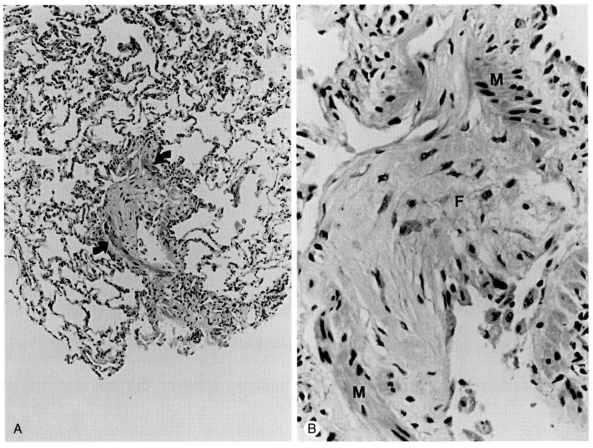

**Figure 45–8. Post-transplantation Obliterative Bronchiolitis: Early Stage.** A portion of a transbronchial biopsy specimen *(A)* shows mild interstitial pneumonitis and a small bronchiole, the lumen of which is partially occluded by fibrous tissue situated between the muscularis mucosae *(arrows)* and the epithelium. A magnified view *(B)* shows the fibrous tissue (F) to contain active-appearing fibroblasts. Note the paucity of inflammatory cells. M, muscularis mucosae.

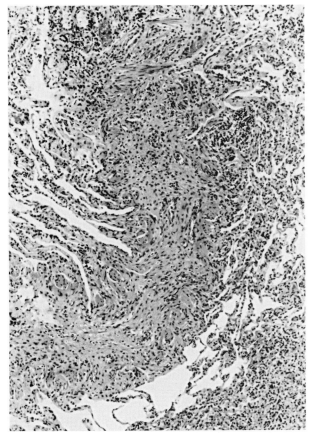

**Figure 45–9. Post-transplantation Obliterative Bronchiolitis: Late Stage.** A section from an excised donor lung about 2 years after transplantation shows a membranous bronchiole, the lumen of which is completely occluded by mature fibrous tissue containing scattered mononuclear inflammatory cells.

larly in small or distorted biopsy specimens. OB may be subdivided into active and inactive forms depending on the presence or absence of an inflammatory infiltrate (*see* Table 45–3).[89]

### Radiologic Manifestations

The radiographic findings of OB after lung transplantation include decreased peripheral vascular markings, decreased or increased lung volumes, and, less commonly, bronchial dilation.[161–163] The last-named is considered present when the internal diameter of the bronchus is greater than that of the adjacent pulmonary artery, and is seen most commonly on HRCT (Fig. 45–10);[163] for example, in one study of seven patients who had OB syndrome, two had bronchial dilation evident on the radiograph and six on HRCT.[163] The dilation involved mainly the segmental and subsegmental branches of the lower lobes. Lower lobe bronchial dilation was not seen in any of nine otherwise healthy heart-lung transplant recipients who were used as controls.

In another investigation in which the HRCT findings in 15 patients who had biopsy-proven OB after lung transplantation were compared with those in 18 control subjects, 13 patients (87%) had one or more abnormalities seen on HRCT.[164] These included bronchial dilation in 12 (80%), bronchial wall thickening in 4 (27%), and mosaic perfusion

in 6 (40%). Findings present in the control subjects included bronchial dilation in 4 (22%) and mosaic perfusion in 4 (22%). Bronchial wall thickening was not seen in any of the control subjects. Five of the patients who had OB and 16 of the control subjects also underwent expiratory HRCT scans: air trapping was seen in 4 (80%) of the former and in only 1 (6%) of the latter. The combination of bronchial dilation on the inspiratory HRCT scans and air trapping on expiratory scans was not seen in any of the control subjects.[164] In another investigation of 21 lung transplant recipients (including 11 who had biopsy-proven OB and 10 who had no histologic or functional evidence of airway disease), bronchial dilation was present on inspiratory HRCT in 4 of the 11 (36%) patients who had OB and 2 of the 10 (20%) who did not;[164a] mosaic attenuation was present in 7 (64%) of the OB patients compared with 1 of 10 (10%) of the others. On expiratory HRCT, air trapping was present in 10 of 11 patients who had OB compared with only 2 of 10 who did not. The results of these two investigations suggest that air trapping on expiratory HRCT is the most sensitive and accurate radiologic indicator of OB.[164, 164a]

The value of repeated HRCT scans in the long-term follow-up of patients who have lung transplants was assessed in a study of 13 consecutive patients.[165] A total of 140 scans were performed during a mean observation period of 26 months. OB syndrome developed in 8 patients, on average within 12 months of transplantation; histologic confirmation of OB was available in 5 patients. The first chronic changes identifiable on HRCT were a decrease in lung volume, a decrease in the peripheral vascular markings, and interlobular septal thickening, findings that appeared between 7 and 11 months after transplantation. The mean interval for the appearance of bronchial dilation was 12 months. Areas of decreased attenuation and mosaic perfusion were identified on average 16 and 21 months after transplantation, respectively. The investigators concluded that diminution of peripheral vascular markings, thickening of septal lines, and volume reduction usually precede the establishment of the diagnosis of OB, whereas decreased attenuation and mosaic perfusion are usually a late manifestation. In one study of two autopsy lungs from patients who had clinical and pathologic evidence of chronic rejection, the OB was associated with striking bronchiectasis and peribronchial fibrosis, both pathologically and on HRCT.[166]

### Clinical Manifestations

Although OB has developed as early as 2 months and as late as 4 years after transplantation, the mean time between transplantation and its recognition has been reported to vary between 6 and 12 months.[44, 76] The clinical course is variable; in some patients, the disease has an insidious onset and indolent progress, whereas in others, both the onset and course are rapid.[167] Some patients are asymptomatic, and the disease is detected by the discovery of abnormalities of surveillance lung function and lung histology.[44] Symptoms are nonspecific and include malaise, dry cough, and shortness of breath on exertion.[44] As lung function deteriorates, dyspnea worsens.[6] Wheezing and chest tightness have been found to be common by some investigators;[143] both symptoms respond poorly to bronchodilator medication.[143] Sputum

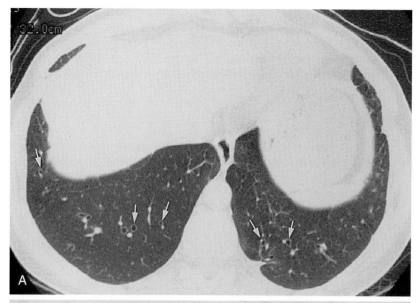

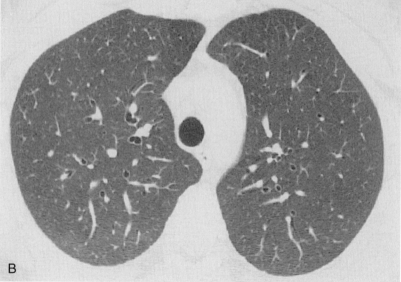

**Figure 45–10. Pulmonary Transplantation: Obliterative Bronchiolitis.** An HRCT scan *(A)* demonstrates bronchial dilation *(arrows)* and reduced vascularity throughout the basal segments of the lower lobes. The latter is best appreciated by comparison with the normal vascularity in the upper lobes *(B)*. The patient was a 24-year-old woman who had biopsy-proven obliterative bronchiolitis 18 months after double-lung transplantation.

production may occur with secondary infection but is otherwise typically absent.

There are few physical signs in early OB. Late inspiratory wheezes (squeaks) have been attributed to late opening of small airways secondary to accumulation of excess mucus and altered elastic properties of the bronchiolar wall.[125] The presence of basilar inspiratory crackles has also been described.[143] Diminished breath sounds, prolonged expiration, cyanosis, and signs of cor pulmonale accompany advanced disease.[125]

### Diagnosis

In clinical practice, the diagnosis of OB is usually based on a combination of clinical, radiologic, and functional findings. Despite this, bronchoscopy and transbronchial biopsy are useful diagnostic procedures. They permit the exclusion of abnormalities that may be confused clinically with OB, such as anastomotic stenosis, infection, and acute

rejection, and may yield tissue fragments that have diagnostic changes. Although the sensitivity of the procedure for OB is poor in most reports,[123, 168–170] varying from about 15%[168] to 40%,[123, 171] the values in some centers, such as Stanford and Pittsburgh, have been as high as 70%.[121, 145] (In these studies, the gold standard for the diagnosis has usually been the clinical and physiologic behavior of the patient; occasionally, autopsy confirmation has been obtained.[168]) As might be expected, the sensitivity appears to be greater when more and larger biopsy fragments are available for examination.[171] Bronchiolar fibrosis is occasionally seen after conditions other than chronic rejection, such as viral infection; however, the presence of a pattern of concentric submucosal fibrous tissue is highly suggestive of OB.[171] Although often associated with OB, chronic bronchial inflammation and fibrosis is not by itself an indicator of bronchiolar disease.[171] In one study, the finding of BAL neutrophilia and elevated IL-8 enabled distinction between patients who had OB and both healthy post-transplant patients and patients who had acute rejection;[172] clearly, infection had been excluded by other means in such patients. Similar results have been found by a second group of investigators.[172a]

Alteration in lung function is the most common manner by which the diagnosis of OB is made,[123] the most characteristic feature being a decline in the $FEV_1$.[7, 123, 173] A working formulation for clinical staging of graft dysfunction based on the ratio of the current $FEV_1$ to the best post-transplantation study has been generally adopted. According to this formulation, mild OB is present in patients who have a decline in $FEV_1$ to 66% to 80% of baseline, moderate OB is present in those who have values between 51% and 65% of baseline, and severe OB is present in those who have a decrease to 50% or less of baseline.[7] Although most patients have an obstructive pattern of lung dysfunction characterized by a reduction in the $FEV_1$-to-FVC ratio,[143, 174] in some there is a restrictive defect only.[143] Some investigators have also found that all patients develop an associated restrictive element of lung dysfunction with progression of OB.[143]

Although measurement of $FEV_1$ is the most widely used pulmonary function test in the diagnosis of OB, a 20%[167] to 30%[175] reduction in the $FEF_{25-75\%}$ and a decrease in flow at 50% of $FVC$[176] appear to be more sensitive measures. In one retrospective study of 94 patients (49 of whom developed OB), the bronchodilator response at low lung volumes (defined as a 25% increase in FEF at 50% vital capacity or a 30% increase in FEF at 25% vital capacity) was found to predict the development of OB with a sensitivity of 51%, a specificity of 87%, and a positive predictive value of 81%.[177]

The key to interpretation of serial lung function in the post-transplant patient is the definition of a "significant change."[143] Although criteria vary somewhat depending on the laboratory and the particular patient group, it appears that the post-transplant population behaves much like the normal population in this respect.[143] Thus, a decrease in $FEV_1$ greater than 10% in heart-lung and double-lung recipients and greater than 13% in single-lung recipients during week-to-week testing should be considered clinically significant.[143, 178] Although heart-lung and double-lung transplant recipients show more variability in lung function in the absence of infection or rejection in the first year after transplantation than at later periods, this is principally the result of improvement in function;[178] in the absence of other abnormality, such as anastomotic stenosis or infection, decreasing values of $FEV_1$ are likely secondary to OB.

### Bronchiolitis Obliterans Organizing Pneumonia

As with idiopathic bronchiolitis obliterans organizing pneumonia (BOOP) in the nontransplantation setting, this abnormality appears to represent a nonspecific reaction to epithelial injury and likely has several etiologies in patients who undergo lung transplantation. Although most often associated with mild acute rejection,[179, 180] BOOP has also been seen in the context of infection, usually CMV pneumonia;[179, 180] rarely, it occurs as an isolated finding.[179, 180] It has both followed and preceded the development of OB.[179]

Pathologic and radiologic features of transplantation-associated BOOP are no different from those of idiopathic BOOP in the nontransplant population. The clinical manifes-

tations are nonspecific. It is obviously important to identify an underlying process, whether infection or rejection, and treat it appropriately. To date, no particular prognostic importance has been attached to the development of BOOP in lung transplant patients; however, in one study of 25 patients (12 who had OB and 13 who did not), the coexistence of BOOP and acute pulmonary rejection in the first year after transplantation was strongly associated with the subsequent development of OB.[156]

### Post-transplantation Lymphoproliferative Disorder

Several histologic patterns of lymphocyte proliferation—known collectively as the post-transplantation lymphoproliferative disorder (PTLD)—can occur after bone marrow or solid organ transplantation.[12, 181] The classification and precise nature of these abnormalities has been the subject of some debate.[182] Classically, they have been regarded to be of four types: (1) a clearly benign, nonspecific hyperplastic proliferation; (2) a polymorphic proliferation of benign-appearing lymphocytes; (3) a polymorphic proliferation of cytologically atypical lymphocytes associated with necrosis and tissue invasion; and (4) a monomorphic, cytologically atypical proliferation resembling immunoblastic lymphoma (Fig. 45–11).[181, 183] Unfortunately, unlike similar lymphoid proliferations in the nontransplantation population, these morphologic patterns do not reliably predict clinical behavior in transplant recipients.

More recently, the results of a variety of clinical, morphologic, and molecular studies have suggested to some authorities that PTLDs can best be considered in three categories:[181] (1) *plasmacytic hyperplasia*, a process that most commonly arises in the oropharynx or lymph nodes, is nearly always polyclonal, usually shows evidence of multiple Epstein-Barr virus (EBV) infectious events on viral genotype analysis, and lacks oncogene or tumor suppressor gene alterations; (2) *polymorphic lymphoproliferative disorders*, abnormalities that may arise in lymph nodes or extranodal sites, are nearly always monoclonal on immunoglobulin gene rearrangement study, usually contain a single form of EBV, and lack oncogene or tumor-suppressor gene alterations; and (3) *malignant lymphoma* or *multiple myeloma*, both of which typically appear with widely disseminated disease, are monoclonal based on immunoglobulin gene rearrangements, contain a single form of EBV, and contain alterations of one or more oncogenes or tumor-suppressor genes (e.g., c-myc, ras, and p53). The use of these categories holds some promise with respect to prediction of clinical behavior.[184] However, a variety of additional morphologic and immunophenotypic forms of proliferation have also been described,[182] and it is unlikely that this classification scheme is the final one.

Most cases of PTLD have been associated with EBV-infected B cells,[183, 185] and it is likely that such infection is an essential step in the development of many lesions. Patients who are seronegative before transplantation are much more likely to develop PTLD than those who are EBV positive.[186, 187] For example, in one series of 389 consecutive solid organ transplant recipients, those who were seronegative had an incidence rate ratio (expressed per 100 person-years) of 76 for any form of lymphoproliferative disorder and 145 for fatal forms, compared with seropositive recipients.[187] In another series of 75 patients who had undergone

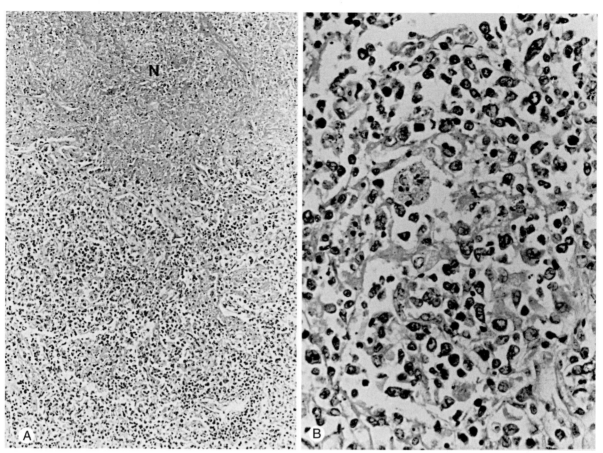

**Figure 45–11. Post-transplantation Lymphoproliferative Disorder.** Sections from a poorly demarcated pulmonary tumor show necrosis (N), destruction of lung parenchyma, and large, cytologically atypical lymphoid cells (magnified in *B*). The tumor was multifocal and present only in the lung. The patient was a 35-year-old man who received a double-lung transplant about 1.5 years before the development of the tumor.

lung transplantation, 5 of 15 (33%) seronegative recipients developed PTLD, compared with only 1 of 60 seropositive patients;[186] after excluding patients who remained seronegative after transplantation, 42% of patients who developed primary EBV infection after transplantation developed PTLD. The risk in patients who undergo lung transplantation is greater than that in patients who undergo heart, kidney, or liver transplantation; although the explanation for this is uncertain, it may be related to the higher number of EBV-positive lymphocytes in the transplanted lung or to augmented immunosuppression associated with the higher doses of cyclosporin used in the lung transplant recipients.[186] Of both theoretical interest and practical importance is the observation that multiple foci of lymphoid proliferation in the same patient may be clonally distinct, suggesting that they represent multiple primary lymphoid proliferations rather than metastases of the same lesion.[188]

Although EBV infection thus appears to be important in the development of PTLD, it is clear that therapeutic immunosuppression is also essential. The precise mechanism of the interaction between these two factors is uncertain; however, it is likely to be the result of a combination of factors, including EBV-induced B-cell proliferation; inhibition of cytotoxic T cells by cyclosporine A; cyclosporin- and EBV-related inhibition of apoptosis; and the activation of oncogenes, such as c-*myc*, or inactivation of tumor-suppressor genes.[181] Interestingly, in contrast to PTLD arising

in bone marrow transplant recipients, most cases that develop in solid organ transplant recipients appear to originate in the recipient's lymphocytes.[189, 190]

The most common radiologic findings consist of single or multiple pulmonary nodules (Fig. 45–12) and hilar or mediastinal lymphadenopathy (Fig. 45–13).[191–193a] In one investigation of 28 patients, nodules were identified on the radiograph or CT scan in 16 (57%).[192] They were relatively well circumscribed, measured between 0.3 and 5 cm in diameter, and were usually multiple and distributed randomly throughout the lungs. Patchy, predominantly peribronchial air-space consolidation associated with air bronchograms was seen in three patients, two of whom also had lung nodules. Mediastinal and hilar lymphadenopathy was seen in 17 (61%) of 28 patients (Fig. 45–14), thymic involvement in 2, pericardial thickening or effusion in 2, and pleural effusion in 4. In another investigation of four patients, all had nodules on HRCT, two had hilar and mediastinal lymphadenopathy, and one had pleural effusion.[193] In three of the four patients, a halo of ground-glass attenuation was seen surrounding the nodules; pathologic correlation in one of these showed the halo to be related to infiltration of the adjacent lung by a less dense infiltrate of lymphoid cells.[194] In a third study of 17 patients, 15 (88%) had multiple nodules on CT, 6 (35%) had interlobular septal thickening, 5 (29%) had areas of ground-glass attenuation, 4 (23%) had areas of air-space consolidation, and 5 had hilar or mediasti-

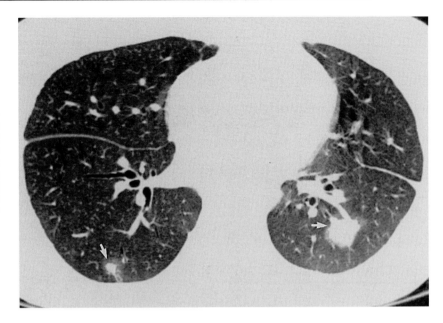

**Figure 45–12. Post-transplantation Lymphoproliferative Disorder.** An HRCT scan demonstrates bilateral nodules *(arrows)* surrounded by a poorly defined halo of ground-glass attenuation. Thickening of the left interlobar fissure as a result of a small pleural effusion is also evident. The diagnosis of post-transplantation lymphoproliferative disorder was confirmed by open-lung biopsy. The patient was a 52-year-old woman who had undergone double-lung transplantation 3 months previously.

nal lymphadenopathy.[194a] The nodules most commonly had a predominantly subpleural or peribronchovascular distribution.

The reported prevalence of PTLD in lung transplant recipients has varied from about 5% to 20%;[12, 195] most cases present in the first year after transplantation.[12] Most patients who have polymorphic, benign-appearing lesions histologically have clinically unsuspected disease.[195] On the other hand, monomorphic proliferations most commonly present in the allograft as focal or multifocal nodules or masses.[186] Localized disease in organs other than the lung, as well as disseminated disease, has also been described.[12] Ulcerative bronchitis was the presenting feature in two patients.[196]

The diagnosis can be made on specimens obtained by fine-needle aspiration;[197] however, core-needle or open-lung biopsy specimens are sometimes necessary. Regression of PTLD has followed a reduction in the intensity of maintenance immunosuppression; death may be the result of subsequent chronic rejection or nonresponsive lymphoma.[12] The 1- and 2-year actuarial survival rates after PTLD in lung transplant recipients are about 50% and 20%, respectively.[12] In one follow-up study of 26 patients who had PTLD, the prognosis was related to the initial radiographic findings.[193a] Eight (89%) of 9 patients who had solitary nodules at presentation were alive 1 year after diagnosis, compared with 6 (35%) of 17 patients who had other presentations (including multiple nodules, multifocal areas of air-space consolidation, or hilar or mediastinal lymph node enlargement).[193a]

### Infection

Pulmonary infection is the most common cause of morbidity and mortality in lung transplant recipients.[7, 12, 198–200] The average number of episodes of infection per year is almost 3;[201] such episodes account for about half of the deaths occurring during the initial hospitalization and for up to three quarters of those thereafter.[44, 199, 201] Possibly because the lung is in direct and constant contact with the environment, the infection rate is substantially higher in lung transplant recipients than in other organ recipients.[201]

Although infection is most often caused by organisms first contacted in the post-transplantation period, it may also be transmitted from the donor organ[7, 202, 203] or from foci of pretransplantation colonization in the proximal airway or sinuses of the recipient.[204] In addition to the marked immunosuppression imposed on patients to prevent rejection,[205] patients are prone to pulmonary infection because of impaired mucociliary clearance,[206, 207] the development of anastomotic stenosis or dehiscence,[208] the transection of pulmonary lymphatics, and the depression of the cough reflex as a result of lung denervation.[12] The handling, ischemia, preservation, and reimplantation of the donor lung also likely impair its defense against infection in the immediate post-transplantation period.[44]

Pathologic manifestations of infection in post-transplant patients are similar to those seen in other individuals. However, the effects of immunosuppressive therapy can clearly modify the normal inflammatory reaction. In addition, because these patients are followed very closely and transbronchial biopsy is often performed early in the course of disease or, sometimes, in apparently healthy patients for surveillance purposes, histologic abnormalities may be very subtle (*see* Fig. 45–20, page 1721). The presence of a neutrophil-rich inflammatory infiltrate in the pulmonary parenchyma should suggest the possibility of infection. However, such a reaction is not always related to this etiology. In one investigation of 13 transbronchial biopsy specimens in which the histologic abnormality was identified, an infectious (usually bacterial) cause was found in only 6;[208a] because of an association of the noninfectious cases with $\alpha_1$-antitrypsin deficiency and cigarette smoking, the authors speculated that other injurious factors might be involved in causing the reaction.

As might be expected, the spectrum of organisms responsible for complicating infection includes a variety of bacteria, viruses, fungi, and *Mycoplasma* species.[212, 217]

### Bacteria

Bacteria are the most common cause of infection in heart-lung and lung transplant recipients.[12, 201, 208] As in the

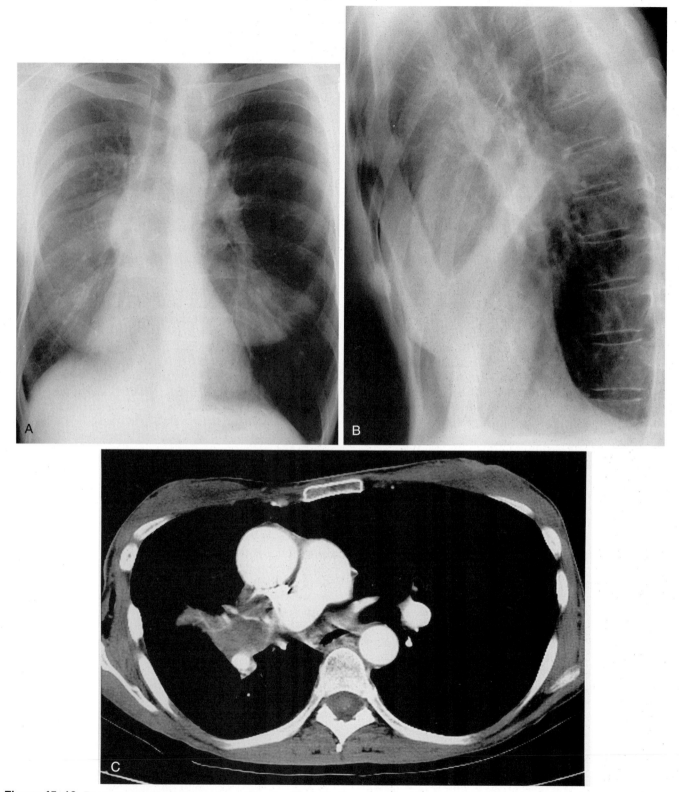

**Figure 45–13. Post-transplantation Lymphoproliferative Disorder.** Posteroanterior *(A)* and lateral *(B)* chest radiographs demonstrate enlargement of the right hilum and associated right middle lobe atelectasis. A contrast-enhanced CT scan *(C)* demonstrates right hilar lymph node enlargement associated with extrinsic compression of the right middle lobe bronchus and right middle lobe atelectasis. The patient was a 51-year-old woman who had undergone single right lung transplantation 6 months previously. (Courtesy of Dr. Ann Leung, Stanford University School of Medicine, Stanford, CA.)

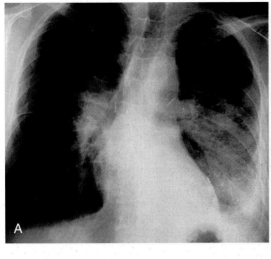

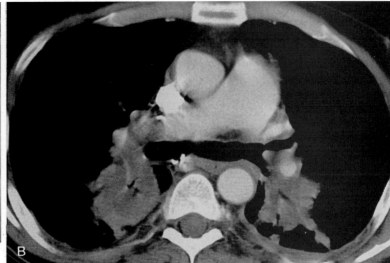

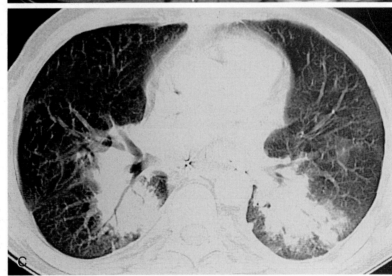

**Figure 45–14. Post-transplantation Lymphoproliferative Disorder.** An anteroposterior chest radiograph *(A)* shows enlargement of the hila, a focal convexity in the aortopulmonary window indicative of lymphadenopathy, areas of consolidation in the perihilar regions and left lower lobe, and a small left pleural effusion. A contrast-enhanced spiral CT scan photographed using mediastinal windows *(B)* confirms the presence of hilar lymphadenopathy, areas of consolidation, and a small left pleural effusion. A CT scan at a more caudad level photographed using lung windows *(C)* demonstrates a predominantly peribronchial distribution of the areas of consolidation with associated air bronchograms. The patient was a 37-year-old man who developed post-transplantation lymphoproliferative disorder 5 weeks after double-lung transplantation. The diagnosis was confirmed by open-lung biopsy.

nontransplant population, they usually cause either pneumonia or bronchitis. Although the risk of bacterial pneumonia is highest in the first 3 months after transplantation and is especially great in the first month, there remains a uniform and persistent risk over time. The incidence in the first 2 weeks after transplantation has been dramatically reduced by the use of prophylactic antibiotics tailored to culture results from the sputum of both the recipient and donor;[12, 44, 198] using this strategy, the incidence of such infections in this time period has been reported to be as low as 9%.[198]

Patients who have OB are particularly prone to bacterial lung infection, possibly because of the frequent presence of bronchiectasis.[12, 201, 209] Other specific risk factors have not been identified. Although the overall incidence of bacterial pneumonia in patients who have cystic fibrosis is not higher than that in other lung transplant recipients,[209] prior infection with multiresistant organisms, such as *B. cepacia*, is a particularly important, and often fatal, complication.[204, 209]

Gram-negative organisms, especially *Pseudomonas aeruginosa*, are the most common etiologic agents (Fig. 45–15).[44, 201, 204, 210, 211] Gram-positive species, including methicillin-resistant *Staphylococcus aureus*, are next in impor-

tance.[44, 201] Other organisms, such as *Actinomyces* species[213] and *Mycobacterium* species,[214, 215] are identified less often. Tuberculosis may develop as a primary infection, as reactivation of latent disease,[216] or after transmission of the organism from the donor.[202, 218]

The clinical presentation of bacterial pneumonia in the setting of lung transplantation may be somewhat atypical. Denervation of the lung may lead to blunting of cough, and tachypnea may not be as prominent. Fever may be suppressed as a result of corticosteroids and the white blood cell count response to infection may be blunted by the use of azathioprine.[201] The approach to patients who have suspected bacterial pneumonia is discussed in detail in Chapter 25.[6] Although infection by bacterial organisms is associated with a fair degree of morbidity, the mortality is low;[204, 210] for example, in one series of 29 patients, only 1 died.[210] Of 32 bacterial infections reported in a second series, only 2 (6%) were fatal;[204] both were caused by *Pseudomonas* species.

Bacteria may also cause acute bronchitis in lung transplant recipients,[136, 204] as in 8 of 32 bacterial infections (25%) in one series.[204] Of 49 patients who had histologic evidence

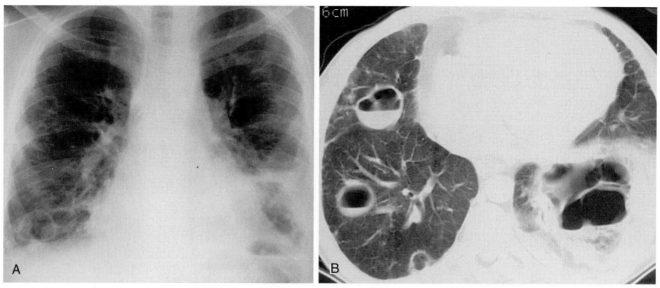

**Figure 45–15. Pulmonary Transplantation: Lung Abscesses.** A posteroanterior chest radiograph *(A)* and a conventional CT scan *(B)* demonstrate cystic lesions with air-fluid levels in the right middle lobe and in both lower lobes. Cultures grew *Pseudomonas, Enterococcus,* and *Peptostreptococcus* species. The patient was a 19-year-old man who had undergone double-lung transplantation for cystic fibrosis 18 months previously. (Courtesy of Dr. Ann Leung, Stanford University School of Medicine, Stanford, CA.)

of acute bronchitis or bronchiolitis in another review, bacterial infection explained the pathologic findings in 15 (31%).[136]

### Viruses

CMV is the second most common cause of infection in lung transplant recipients,[12, 219] and pneumonia is the most common manifestation of CMV infection. More than half of adults in the United States have serologic evidence of previous infection by CMV.[12] The organism can thus be transmitted from the lung harvested from a CMV-seropositive donor or from the transfusion of blood products from a CMV-seropositive individual; disease may also result by reactivation of latent infection in a seropositive recipient.

Because CMV is so common in the general population, it is necessary to make a careful distinction between infection and disease. The former can be defined as the identification of the organism in material obtained from any body site by culture, or cytologic, immunohistochemical, or molecular examination in the absence of symptoms and histologic changes associated with CMV.[198] CMV disease can be considered to be present if the organism is identified in material obtained from any body site by the same techniques in the presence of histologic evidence of tissue damage.

The risk and consequences of CMV infection and disease are dependent on the serologic status of both the recipient and the donor. As might be expected, the risk of infection is lowest in seronegative recipients who have received organs from seronegative donors. When seropositive blood products are also avoided in such patients, infection occurs in only about 15%. However, in these and other patients who develop primary infection, clinical disease occurs in most and is associated with a high case fatality rate (about 20% to 25%).[12] By contrast, despite the high prevalence of infection in patients who are donor positive and recipient positive or donor negative and recipient positive, disease

develops in less than one third, and the case fatality rate is lower.[12]

Because CMV-specific immune responses, especially those of antigen-specific T cells, appear to be essential for limiting primary infection and preventing disease,[220] it is undoubtedly immunosuppression that is behind the high frequency of CMV infection in these patients. Paradoxically, the results of some animal experiments of viral infection suggest that certain subsets of T-helper cells may actually enhance the toxicity of infection by lysis of infected epithelial cells or by augmenting inflammation through cytokine production.[220] The precise role of each of these mechanisms in the pathogenesis of CMV infection after lung transplantation has not been clarified. As indicated previously (*see* page 1707), it is also possible that CMV plays a role in the pathogenesis of OB.

Pathologic features of CMV infection in biopsy specimens taken from patients who have undergone lung transplantation are similar to those from other immunosuppressed patients. It is worth noting, however, that perivascular inflammation similar to that seen in acute rejection may be seen.[221] The use of antiviral agents such as ganciclovir can also result in smaller, apparently degenerated nuclear inclusions that can be overlooked unless there is a high index of suspicion and examination of several tissue levels.

Nonspecific signs and symptoms, such as fever, malaise, myalgia, arthralgia, anorexia, and fatigue are common,[222] and may occur without evident involvement of specific organ systems. Pulmonary signs and symptoms are similar to those of acute rejection. Hepatitis, colitis, retinitis, and gastroenteritis are other manifestations; their presence provides a clue to the diagnosis of pulmonary disease.[12, 222]

One of the major problems confronting the transplantation physician is distinguishing infection, particularly by CMV, from acute rejection. The timing of disease onset may be helpful in this regard. It is rare to see CMV infection within the first 2 weeks after transplantation, the mean time to the onset of symptomatic infection in the absence of prophylaxis being about 55 days after transplantation.[198] As indicated previously, definitive diagnosis of CMV pneumonia requires the histologic demonstration of tissue damage associated with evidence of CMV infection (viral inclusion bodies on histologic or cytologic examination, or positive immunohistochemical or polymerase chain reaction results).[223, 224] A *presumptive* diagnosis can be made if a culture of BAL fluid is positive for CMV, the clinical and radiologic picture is compatible with the infection, and other causes of disease have been reasonably excluded.[12] CMV infection is usually documented by the shell-vial culture technique, which allows identification of the organism in 24 to 48 hours.[12] The sensitivity and negative predictive value of the technique are extremely high; however, its specificity for the diagnosis of pneumonia is low.[223] Cytologic examination of cells in BAL fluid for viral inclusions has a low sensitivity (about 20%) but high specificity (98%) for the diagnosis of CMV pneumonia.[44] When tissue is required, transbronchial biopsy is the procedure of choice; open-lung biopsy is seldom required.[44] The sensitivity of transbronchial biopsy for the diagnosis of CMV pneumonia is difficult to determine, because of the lack of a suitable gold standard.

A variety of other viruses, including herpes simplex virus, adenovirus, influenza virus, the paramyxoviruses, respiratory syncytial virus, and parainfluenza virus, also cause pneumonia in lung transplant recipients, albeit less commonly than CMV.[12, 198, 225, 225a, b] Experimentally, the airway damage caused by parainfluenza virus appears to have a synergistic role with chronic rejection in the development of OB.[12] The association of EBV infection with the development of post-transplantation lymphoproliferative disorders is discussed elsewhere (*see* page 1711); the virus has also been implicated in the pathogenesis of smooth muscle neoplasms in the liver and, possibly, diffuse smooth muscle proliferation in the lung.[226]

### Fungi

The finding of a positive fungal culture is common in the post-transplantation period; for example, in one study of 73 heart-lung and lung transplant recipients, this was documented at some point in various sites in 59 (81%).[227] Such isolates range in importance from incidental findings in symptom-free patients to findings associated with rapidly progressive and fatal disease. Overall, invasive fungal infection, of which aspergillosis is the most common, accounts for about 10% to 15% of pulmonary infections.[198, 201, 204, 228] Disease may result from reactivation of latent infection or from recent exposure to a new environmental source, including the donor lung itself.[227]

The finding of *Aspergillus* or *Candida* species in lung specimens usually represents colonization.[6, 7, 44, 198, 229, 229a] However, both organisms can cause serious morbidity and death,[12, 198, 201, 204, 219, 230] and some have argued that all patients who have fungi isolated from BAL fluid should be treated.[198] In one series of 118 transplant recipients, 8 had pulmonary aspergillus infection (the diagnosis in most being established at autopsy);[198] although all 8 had a positive premortem culture, so did 41 patients who had a specimen submitted to the laboratory but who did not have aspergillus infection. In another study of 151 transplant recipients, aspergillus was

isolated from the airways in 69 (46%);[229] invasive disease occurred in 5 of these patients, in whom cultures were positive in only 1 at the time of tissue invasion. All of the invasive infections proved to be fatal. Patients who grew the organism in the airways in the first 6 months after transplantation had 11 times more risk of developing invasive aspergillosis than patients who did not; however, the positive predictive value was only 16%. Whether monitoring of antibodies to aspergillus will be helpful in distinguishing colonization from infection in patients who have a positive culture, but no clinical evidence of infection, remains to be determined.[231]

Pulmonary disease caused by *Aspergillus* species, predominantly *A. fumigatus*, may take any form seen in nontransplantation patients, including tracheobronchitis, bronchopneumonia, bronchocentric granulomatosis, angioinvasive disease (Fig. 45–16), allergic bronchopulmonary aspergillosis, acute eosinophilic pneumonia, fungus ball, and empyema;[12, 91, 230, 232–234] disseminated disease also occurs in some cases. The site of lung disease is usually the allograft; however, the native lung has been involved in some single-lung recipients.[12, 233, 235] In some cases, the infection begins by colonization of necrotic tissue at the bronchial anastomosis (Fig. 45–17). Although colonies that develop in this way may remain localized to the necrotic bronchial wall at this site, they may also extend through the wall into the mediastinum or pleural space, or distally along the airways, where they may cause pseudomembranous bronchitis or bronchopneumonia.[230] Definitive diagnosis of pneumonia or disseminated infection requires biopsy demonstration of tissue invasion; however, a presumptive diagnosis is reasonable when the organism is identified in a BAL specimen and the clinical picture is consistent.[12]

Although pneumonitis caused by *Candida* species is distinctly uncommon,[44] other thoracic manifestations of infection by the organism are not infrequent. These include wound infection, mediastinitis, and aneurysm of the aortic anastomosis after heart-lung transplantation.[12] Thrush due to *Candida* species is seen commonly in the upper respiratory tract after transplantation; occasionally, the infection extends to cause esophagitis or tracheobronchitis.[201] We have seen one patient who had extensive mucoid impaction in whom repeated cultures from BAL grew only *Candida* species (Fig. 45–18).

*Pneumocystis carinii* pneumonia (PCP) has been virtually eliminated in lung-transplant recipients by the use of antibiotic prophylaxis (Fig. 45–19);[12] when it does occur, it is almost always associated with noncompliance with prescribed medication.[198] The prevalence is now 2%, a figure that contrasts strikingly with the very high prevalence seen before the use of prophylaxis.[236] Many of these infections were subclinical and detected during routine surveillance bronchoscopies of symptom-free patients.[236] When pneumonia occurs, diagnosis can usually be made by bronchoscopy with BAL and transbronchial biopsy. With respect to the latter, organisms may be fewer than in other immunosuppressed patients (particularly in those undergoing surveillance biopsies), sometimes appearing as single cysts or very small aggregates of cysts rather than the usual clusters within an abundant foamy "exudate" (Fig. 45–20). In addition, the histologic reaction may be atypical (e.g., granulomatous inflammation) or manifested by a perivascular infiltrate simi-

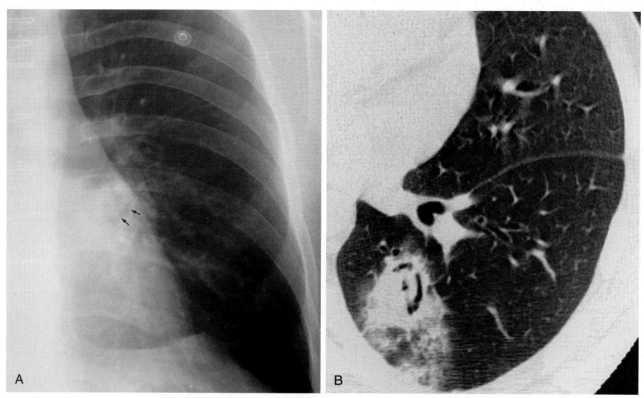

**Figure 45–16. Pulmonary Transplantation: Angioinvasive Aspergillosis.** A view of the left lower chest from an anteroposterior radiograph *(A)* demonstrates a rounded opacity containing an air crescent *(arrows)* in the lower lobe. The air crescent sign is better visualized on the CT scan *(B)*. The cavitated nodule with air crescent sign and the associated wedge-shaped area of increased opacity are characteristic of angioinvasive aspergillosis. The patient was a 36-year-old man who had undergone heart-lung transplantation 3 months previously. (Courtesy of Dr. Ann Leung, Stanford University School of Medicine, Stanford, CA.)

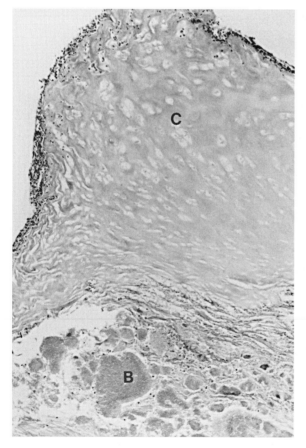

**Figure 45–17. Pulmonary Transplantation: Bronchial Anastomosis Site.** A section through the anastomotic site of a single (right) lung transplant shows necrotic cartilage (C) surrounded by a small number of neutrophils. Colonies of bacteria and fungi (B) are present in the underlying tissue. The biopsy sample was taken about 2 weeks after transplantation.

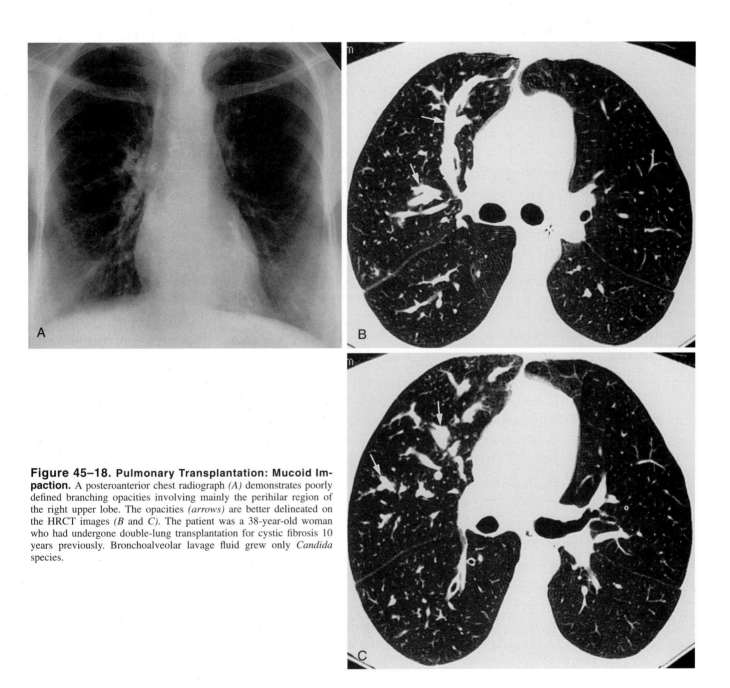

**Figure 45–18. Pulmonary Transplantation: Mucoid Impaction.** A posteroanterior chest radiograph *(A)* demonstrates poorly defined branching opacities involving mainly the perihilar region of the right upper lobe. The opacities *(arrows)* are better delineated on the HRCT images *(B and C)*. The patient was a 38-year-old woman who had undergone double-lung transplantation for cystic fibrosis 10 years previously. Bronchoalveolar lavage fluid grew only *Candida* species.

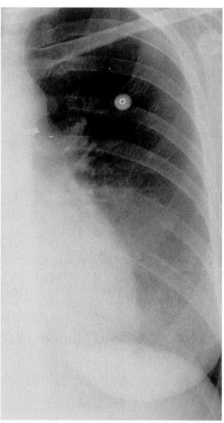

**Figure 45–19. Pulmonary Transplantation: *Pneumocystis carinii* Pneumonia.** A view of the left hemithorax demonstrates ground-glass opacities involving mainly the left lower lobe. The patient was a 29-year-old woman who developed *Pneumocystis carinii* pneumonia 4 months after heart-lung transplantation. (Courtesy of Dr. Ann Leung, Stanford University School of Medicine, Stanford, CA.)

lar to that seen in acute rejection.[221] The sensitivity of sputum analysis in the diagnosis of PCP pneumonia has not been evaluated in this setting.[44]

Other fungal organisms that have occasionally been described to cause pulmonary infection in lung transplant recipients include *Cryptococcus* species, *Coccidioides immitis*,[12] and *Scedosporium prolificans*.[237]

### Recurrence of the Primary Disease

Recurrence of the primary disease in the lung allograft has been described for sarcoidosis,[238–242] lymphangioleiomyomatosis,[243–245] diffuse panbronchiolitis,[246] alveolar proteinosis,[247] Langerhans' cell histiocytosis,[247a, b] desquamative interstitial pneumonitis,[247c, d] and giant cell pneumonitis in the absence of exposure to cobalt in the post-transplantation period.[248] Further reports of disease recurrence are to be expected,[12] given the brief history of lung transplantation relative to the lengthy history of pretransplantation morbidity.

The chest radiograph and HRCT may be normal, may show nonspecific abnormalities, or may demonstrate findings suggestive of recurrent disease. For example, in two patients who developed recurrent sarcoidosis in the lung allograft, one had normal radiologic findings and the other diffuse miliary nodules on the chest radiograph and HRCT scans.[241]

In another patient who had recurrent alveolar proteinosis, the presence of parenchymal disease 3 years after double-lung transplantation was first suggested by the presence of poorly defined, small, rounded air-space opacities on the chest radiograph.[247]

### Pleural Complications

Pleural effusion is virtually inevitable after lung transplantation.[38, 250] In one study of nine single-lung transplant recipients, ipsilateral effusion developed in all nine immediately after transplantation and continued for up to 9 days.[250] Initially, the fluid was a sanguineous exudate with predominant neutrophilia; in the following days, the lactate dehydrogenase level, cellularity, and protein content decreased markedly. By day 7, neutrophils had declined from 90% of the total cell count to 50%.

Effusions are generally small to moderate in size, but may be massive.[38] Their pathogenesis likely reflects a combination of the trauma of the surgery, increased pulmonary capillary permeability, and the disruption of lymphatic flow in the lung allograft;[38] postoperative positive fluid balance may also be a factor in some patients. As discussed previously, new or increasing pleural fluid may be a sign of acute rejection; in one investigation, the presence of these radiographic findings as well as septal lines predicted acute rejection with a sensitivity of 68% and a specificity of 90%.[38]

Other causes of pleural effusion in the post-transplantation period include parapneumonic effusion and empyema. The former was noted in 4 of 91 double-lung transplant recipients in one series;[251] all cases resolved spontaneously. Empyema occurred in 7 of the 91 patients, of whom 3 died. None of the 53 single-lung transplant recipients developed parapneumonic effusion or empyema. The risk of empyema is significantly increased in patients with cystic fibrosis who are infected with *B. cepacia* or other antibiotic-resistant organisms.[251–253] Other unusual causes of pleural effusion include chylothorax and hemothorax (the latter sometimes secondary to bleeding from a bronchial artery).[251]

Persistent or recurrent pneumothorax is also seen in some patients.[251] In one study of 138 patients who had single- and double-lung transplantation, it developed in 14 (10%);[251] in 6, it occurred after transbronchial biopsy. Other iatrogenic causes of recurrent pneumothorax include transthoracic needle aspiration, thoracentesis, and placement of a central venous catheter.[254] Pneumothorax may also develop as a consequence of other complications of transplantation, such as invasive fungal infection, or occur in the native lung as a result of the underlying disease.[38]

When pneumothorax complicates heart-lung transplantation, it is frequently bilateral because of persistent communications between the exposed left and right pleural cavities.[254] Similar communication may also follow sequential double-lung transplantation procedures using the clamshell incision approach, as a result of disruption of the anterior pleural reflections (Fig. 45–21).[38] This phenomenon clearly has important clinical and therapeutic implications. In one investigation of bilateral pneumothorax in 15 patients, causes included transthoracic needle biopsy, bronchoscopic biopsy, placement of a central venous catheter, and thoracentesis;[254] no cause was identified in 2 patients. Simultaneous bilateral pneumothoraces occurred in 6 patients (40%); 10

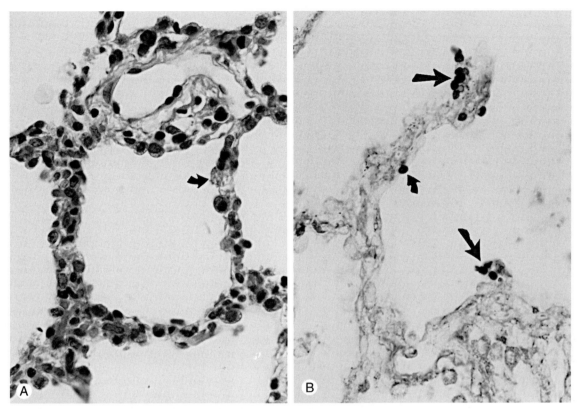

**Figure 45–20. Pulmonary Transplantation: Early _Pneumocystis carinii_ Pneumonia.** A highly magnified view of several alveoli _(A)_ shows mild interstitial thickening by an infiltrate of lymphocytes. The air spaces are unremarkable. A Grocott stain of a different region of the same transbronchial biopsy specimen _(B)_ shows occasional single cysts _(short arrow)_ and clusters of cysts _(large arrows)_ characteristic of _P. carinii_ pneumonia on the surface of the alveolar septa. In retrospect, a single focus suggestive of the organism can be seen on the hematoxylin and eosin stained section _(arrow)_. The patient had experienced a mild decrease in FEV$_1$; the chest radiograph showed no evidence of acute disease.

episodes of unilateral pneumothorax occurred in 9 patients (60%). Because the gas can preferentially accumulate in the retrosternal region, a lateral radiograph may be required to determine the size of the pneumothorax.[97, 256]

### Bronchial Complications

The two main complications related to the anastomosis are dehiscence and stenosis. The former usually occurs in the first few months after transplantation and is sometimes related to infection at the anastomotic site. With current surgical and management techniques, it is rare.[257–259] In fact, the prevalence of both complications and the associated morbidity and mortality are less now than in the early period of lung transplantation.[7] In one review of 86 anastomoses performed in 70 patients, no anastomotic leaks were identified, and only 7 anastomoses in 5 patients (7%) became stenotic.[257] In another investigation of 229 patients, complications developed in only 5 of 126 (4%) anastomoses performed in the last third of transplant recipients, compared with about 13% of anastomoses in the authors' earlier experience.[258]

Chest radiographs are of limited value in the diagnosis of bronchial dehiscence or stenosis; however, both conditions can usually be recognized on CT.[97, 249, 260–262] In one study of 23 patients who had single-lung or bilateral lung transplantation, CT scans were obtained for the evaluation of suspected or known dehiscence.[260] (The CT technique consisted of 10-mm collimation scans performed through the chest and additional 2- to 4-mm thick sections at the level of the anastomoses.) Twenty-one bronchial dehiscences were identified bronchoscopically in 17 patients; a bronchial defect was identified on CT in all 21 (sensitivity, 100%) and in 1 of 18 bronchoscopically proven intact anastomoses (specificity, 94%). The size of the bronchial defects seen on CT ranged from 0.1 to 1.5 cm, with most measuring 0.5 cm or less (Fig. 45–22). Although evidence of extraluminal air was identified in all 21 bronchoscopically proven dehiscences, it was also present in 5 (28%) of 18 intact anastomoses. In 4 of these 5, the CT scans were performed 7 to 12 days after transplantation, and the extraluminal gas represented residual gas from the time of surgery; in the other patient, air was believed to have been introduced iatrogenically at bronchoscopy in an attempt to identify a subsegmental bronchus.[260] Pneumothorax was present in association with 9 (43%) of 21 bronchial dehiscences and 6 (33%) of intact anastomoses.

Normal postoperative changes may be misinterpreted as dehiscence on conventional CT images in patients who have undergone telescoping bronchial anastomoses.[263] One of these changes is separation of the invaginated bronchial cuff and the recipient bronchus, which can result in an endoluminal flap. The gap between the flap and the wall of the recipient bronchus can simulate a bronchial wall defect, and air dissecting between the two can simulate extraluminal air. These flaps or linear air collections are seen only along

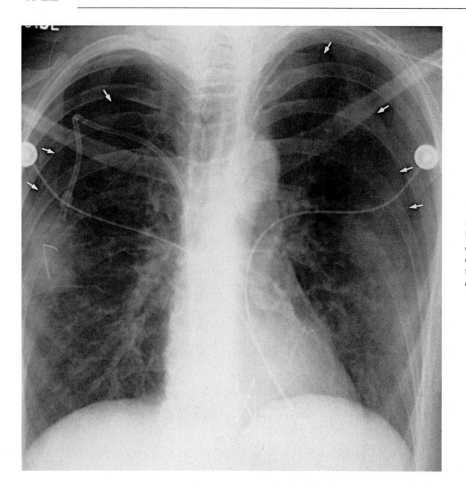

**Figure 45–21. Pulmonary Transplantation: Bilateral Pneumothoraces.** An anteroposterior chest radiograph in a 30-year-old woman shows bilateral pneumothoraces *(arrows)* that developed after transbronchial biopsy of the right lung 3 months after double-lung transplantation.

the anterior margin of the normal anastomosis, because the posterior margin of the anastomosis is sutured end to end; thus, any defect or flap along the posterior wall should suggest dehiscence. Another feature of the normal telescoping anastomosis that can be misinterpreted as dehiscence on transverse images is a small anastomotic diverticulum. This is seen as a smoothly marginated, spherical air collection at

the inferior and medial aspect of the anastomosis. Distinction of this and other normal features of telescoping anastomosis from true dehiscences can be most readily made on oblique coronal multiplanar reconstructions.[263]

CT also allows evaluation of the presence and extent of bronchial stenosis (Fig. 45–23).[66, 68, 262] Optimal assessment of bronchial caliber requires that the bronchus be in

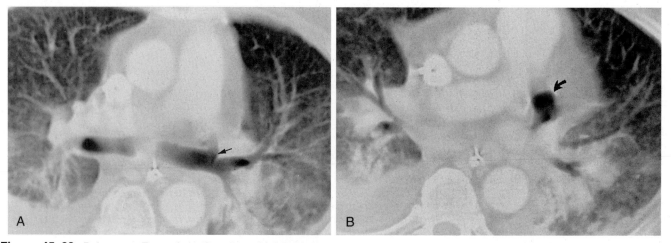

**Figure 45–22. Pulmonary Transplantation: Bronchial Dehiscence.** A CT scan *(A)* demonstrates left bronchial dehiscence *(straight arrow)*. Another scan at a more caudad level *(B)* demonstrates focal intrapericardial air collection *(curved arrow)*. The patient developed left bronchial dehiscence 8 weeks after bilateral lung transplantation for idiopathic pulmonary fibrosis. (Courtesy of Dr. Jannette Collins, University of Wisconsin-Madison Medical School, Madison, WI.)

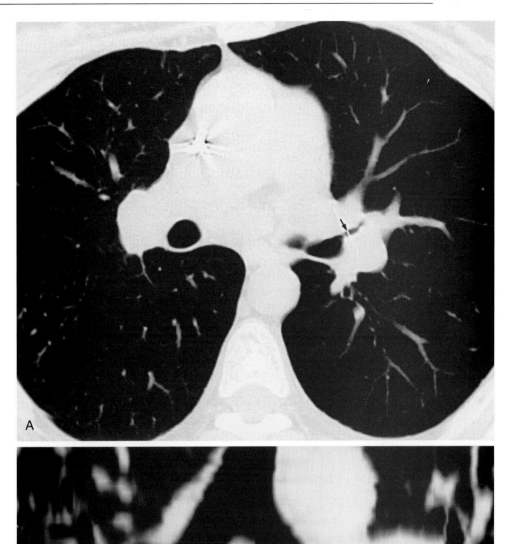

**Figure 45–23. Pulmonary Transplantation: Bronchial Stenosis.** A CT scan *(A)* demonstrates severe stenosis of the left upper lobe bronchus *(arrow)*. Coronal reconstruction *(B)* confirms the presence of stenosis in this airway and also demonstrates mild focal stenosis of the distal left main bronchus. The patient was a 31-year-old woman who had undergone double-lung transplantation for cystic fibrosis 4 months earlier. (Courtesy of Dr. Ann Leung, Stanford University School of Medicine, Stanford, CA.)

the same horizontal level as the CT image[68] or that spiral CT be performed and multiplanar reconstructions obtained.[262] In one investigation of 27 patients in whom spiral CT was performed using 3-mm collimation from a level about 2 cm above the tracheal carina, interpretation of the conventional transverse CT images for the 54 bronchial anastomoses revealed 1 mild stenosis, 1 severe stenosis, 10 anastomoses with a shelf (a common finding of no clinical significance), and 42 normal anastomoses.[262] Multiplanar reconstructions showed mild stenosis in 2 patients who had normal findings on the conventional transverse images. All 4 patients who had evidence of stenosis on multiplanar reconstructions had the findings confirmed at bronchoscopy; however, bronchoscopy demonstrated mild stenosis in 3 patients who had normal findings on CT.[262]

Patients who have anastomotic stenosis develop wheezing, breathlessness, or stridor and, in most cases, have deteriorating lung function.[264] Flow-volume loops may be useful in monitoring the patency of the anastomosis and in evaluating the functional response to stent insertion.[265] The diagnosis has been confirmed an average of about 60 days after transplantation (range, 3 to 245 days).[264] Although most stenoses can be managed successfully with stent insertion, fatal pulmonary infection occasionally ensues.[264]

Bronchiectasis is seen in some patients who have long-term transplants, particularly in those who develop OB.[158] The pathogenesis is uncertain and may be related to one or a combination of several processes, including recurrent infection, loss of normal bronchial blood flow, and chronic rejection. Chronic bronchial inflammation without ectasia is also a common finding and may also represent chronic rejection;[265a] in fact, fibrous occlusion of small bronchi identical to that in bronchioles can be seen in some patients who have OB. Smooth muscle tumors arising in the airway wall and causing severe air flow obstruction have been described in one patient.[265b]

### Pulmonary Vascular Complications

Complications related to the vascular anastomosis are uncommon.[266–268] In one review of 109 consecutive patients, 5 had postoperative pulmonary arterial or venous obstruction;[266] 2 of the 5 died before treatment, and all died between 5 and 630 days postoperatively. Lobar torsion has been reported rarely (Fig. 45–24).[255] The vascular anastomosis can be assessed radiologically using transesophageal echocardiography, CT, or angiography.[269, 270] In one investigation of 18 patients, transesophageal echocardiography allowed assessment of all right pulmonary artery anastomoses and all right and left pulmonary vein anastomoses;[269] however, none of the left pulmonary artery anastomoses could be visualized. In one case, a severe stenosis of the pulmonary vein was associated with graft dysfunction that necessitated early reoperation. Decreased perfusion in the affected lung can also be identified using technetium-99m–labeled albumin scintigraphy.[270]

Nonanastomotic pulmonary vascular abnormalities are much more common than those related to the anastomoses. They tend to be associated with the development of OB and may represent a vascular component of chronic rejection.[271] The histologic abnormalities are patchy and consist predominantly of intimal thickening by loose connective tissue containing myofibroblast-like cells.[158, 160, 271] The process affects principally large elastic and muscular arteries, arterioles, and small veins. In the first of these, accumulation of lipid-laden macrophages and cholesterol crystals may result in a resemblance to atherosclerotic plaques. Despite the rather dramatic degree of luminal narrowing in some cases, clinical effects generally appear to be slight, and arterial pressure may be within normal limits.[271] However, there is evidence that the complication occurs earlier and is associated with a bad prognosis in younger patients.[272]

As in other postoperative patients, lung transplant recipients may develop deep venous thrombosis and pulmonary thromboembolism; these complications were documented in 14 (12%) of 116 patients in one series and were considered to contribute to the death of 3 of them.[273]

### Pulmonary Function Tests

Pulmonary function improves markedly in patients after lung transplantation.[6, 7, 12, 274, 275] $FEV_1$ and FVC increase significantly, except in patients who have pulmonary hypertension whose spirometric indices are intact before the procedure.[7] After single-lung transplantation, maximal ventilatory function is usually reached within 3 months because most of the improved function is related to the allograft.[12] Analysis of the flow-volume loops of patients who received single-lung transplants for COPD may reveal a two-compartment pattern, with high initial flow derived from the allograft and terminal low flow from the native obstructed lung.[276] An early expiratory plateau has been attributed to the development of a "choke point" downstream from the anastomosis in the native proximal bronchus.[276] However, even single-lung transplant recipients generally do not have expiratory flow limitation at rest, a finding that accounts for the dramatic relief of dyspnea afforded by the surgery.[277] Patients who have fibrotic lung disease may take considerably longer to achieve maximum improvement, a delay that has been attributed to remodeling of the thoracic cavity to accommodate the larger transplanted lung.[7] As might be expected, double-lung transplant recipients have significantly better lung function than single-lung recipients; in fact, they are able to attain nearly normal function.[7, 12, 22, 275, 278–280]

When single-lung transplantation is performed for the treatment of COPD, the transplanted lung is significantly restricted and accounts for only one third of TLC.[281] The mechanism of this restriction is thought to be low transpulmonary pressure generation.[281] Although restriction in lung volumes may also be seen immediately after heart-lung transplantation, TLC ultimately returns to the recipient's preoperative value.[282] Somewhat larger donor lungs appear to adapt to the configuration of the recipient's chest wall, and it appears that it is the recipient's chest wall configuration that is the major determinant of postoperative lung volume, at least in transplantations performed for COPD.[283] Diffusion capacity is about 75% predicted after double-lung transplantation and 60% predicted after a single-lung procedure.[7] Oxygenation returns to normal in most patients; in previously hypercarbic patients, the average time to normalization of the arterial $PCO_2$ after transplantation is about 15 days.[44]

Exercise capacity is reduced in single-lung, heart-lung, and double-lung transplant recipients. Maximal oxygen uptake is about half normal, and the anaerobic threshold is reduced.[15, 16, 284–288] There are no gas-exchange abnormalities during exercise of sufficient severity to explain exercise limitation,[284, 285] and the ventilatory response to exercise (in the absence of threshold loading[289]) is normal in all respects despite lung denervation.[290] The maximal heart rate attained during exercise is well below the predicted maximum; that is, heart rate reserve is adequate.[12, 15, 16, 284, 285] Cardiac output has been normal when measured invasively;[290] however, $O_2$ pulse is low at peak exercise and increases linearly with heart rate without reaching a plateau.[284, 285, 288] This suggests that cardiac factors do not explain exercise limitation and that such limitation is located in the skeletal muscles.[284] In this respect, sustained defects in skeletal muscle oxidative capacity have been noted on phosphorus-31 magnetic resonance spectroscopy in lung transplant recipients;[291] the pathogenesis of these changes is uncertain.

Despite afferent and efferent denervation of lung after transplantation, control of breathing is not significantly altered.[12] The ventilatory response to hypercapnia may be transiently blunted in patients who were hypercarbic before surgery but returns to normal by 3 weeks after transplantation.[292] In one study of 12 heart-lung transplant recipients, the hypercarbic ventilatory response was indistinguishable from that in a group of control subjects;[293] however, $P_{0.1}$ (the mouth pressure 100 msec after airway occlusion) was increased, in all likelihood reflecting a compensatory response to abnormal respiratory system mechanics. The breathing pattern in transplant recipients is slow and deep, a

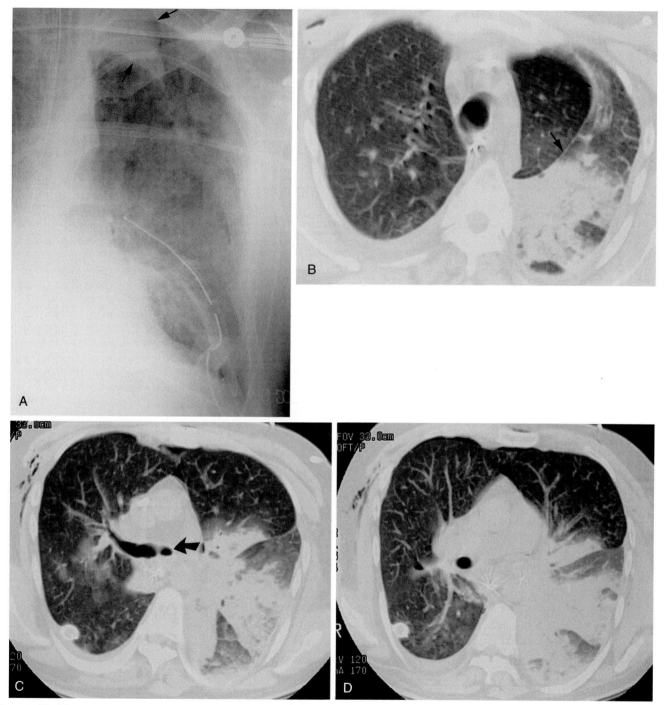

**Figure 45–24. Pulmonary Transplantation: Lobar Torsion.** A 39-year-old man underwent bilateral lung transplantation for emphysema. A view of the left lung *(A)* from a posteroanterior chest radiograph performed 3 days later demonstrates a triangular opacity in the left upper lung zone *(arrows)*. A CT scan at the level of the great vessels *(B)* shows a displaced major fissure *(arrows)*. CT scans at more caudad levels *(C* and *D)* demonstrate abrupt cut-off of the left main bronchus *(curved arrow)*, abnormal orientation and displacement of the major fissure, and consolidation of the torqued, posteriorly displaced left upper lobe. At surgery, infarction of the left upper lobe was confirmed. (Courtesy of Dr. Jannette Collins, University of Wisconsin-Madison Medical School, Madison, WI. From Collins J, Love RB: Pulmonary torsion: Complication of lung transplantation. Clin Pulmon Med 3:297, 1996.)

finding consistent with the absence of vagally mediated inflation inhibition.[293, 294] Although patients who have heart-lung transplants have a normal ability to detect added external resistive loads,[295] the intensity of sensation relative to the inspiratory resistive load is blunted compared with non-transplantation controls.[296] No significant sleep-disordered breathing has been described in heart-lung transplant recipients.[297]

The prevalence of airway hyper-responsiveness to methacholine or histamine has been found to be increased in most,[298–300] but not all,[301] studies of lung and heart-lung transplant recipients. Hyper-reactivity has been attributed to denervation hypersensitivity of muscarinic receptors.[299, 300] By contrast, the cough response to nebulized distilled water distributed by aerosol to the central airways is virtually abolished.[302]

## Prognosis

The overall 1- and 3-year survival rates are about 70% and 55%, respectively.[12] Two phases can be seen on analysis of registry data—an early decline followed by a slow attrition.[12] Higher perioperative mortality has been associated with patients who have primary pulmonary hypertension, idiopathic pulmonary fibrosis, and cystic fibrosis when compared with patients who have COPD. Both early and late survival of patients older than 60 years is somewhat less than that of younger patients.[12] Patients undergoing retransplantation[303] or on mechanical ventilation also have a higher perioperative mortality rate. Infection and graft failure are the major causes of perioperative mortality, whereas infection and OB are primarily responsible for late death.[304]

Although some patients remain ill as a result of transplant-related complications, prospective evaluation of the quality of life in some cohorts of heart-lung transplant patients has revealed a highly significant improvement in physical, social, and emotional health in surviving patients.[305, 305a] Nevertheless, only about 40% of transplantation survivors report feeling able to return to work,[305b] and only about 10% actually return to full-time employment.[306]

In a review of 230 patients who underwent retransplantation at 47 centers from 1985 to 1996, overall survival rates were 47%, 40%, and 33% at 1, 2, and 3 years, respectively.[37a] The best functional results were found in patients from more experienced centers, who were not ventilated at the time of retransplantation, and who underwent retransplantation more than 2 years after their first transplant.

## BONE MARROW TRANSPLANTATION

BMT is now standard therapy for aplastic anemia, acute and chronic leukemia, and some forms of lymphoma. It has also been used in patients with hemoglobinopathies, immunodeficiency disorders, myelodysplastic syndrome, multiple myeloma, and some solid tumors.[307] The procedure is uncommon, but not rare; more than 15,000 autologous and allogenic transplantations are performed yearly worldwide.

Pulmonary disease accounts for a substantial part of the morbidity and mortality of the procedure: more than 30% of transplantation-related deaths are related to respiratory

disorders, and pulmonary complications occur in 40% to 60% of recipients.[307, 308] These complications are classified as early or late according to whether they occur during or after the first 100 days of transplantation.[308] Specific complications are also related to the type and duration of immunologic defects produced by the underlying disease and the therapy given to the patient, the nature of the conditioning regimes employed in the pretransplantation period, and the development of graft-versus-host disease (GVHD).[307] Although recipients of syngeneic (identical twin) and autologous transplants are subject to fewer complications than patients who have allogenic grafts, the incidence of disease is nevertheless significant. The effects of stem cell transfusion are similar to those of autologous BMT.[307]

## Complications

### Pulmonary Edema

Pulmonary edema develops commonly after both allogenic and autologous BMT. For example, in one retrospective review of 55 patients, radiographic evidence of the complication was found in 29 (53%);[309] it was accompanied by hepatic dysfunction in 28, renal dysfunction in 22, and central nervous system abnormalities in 17, suggesting that the edema may be one manifestation of a systemic process. In fact, the pathogenesis is likely multifactorial. Hydrostatic forces related to fluid overload or to cardiotoxicity of immunosuppressive agents, such as doxorubicin, favor the development of edema.[307] Increased capillary permeability may also occur secondary to sepsis or to toxicity from the conditioning regimen, which may include total-body irradiation and high-dose cyclophosphamide.[307, 308]

The onset of edema is rapid and usually occurs in the second or third week after transplantation;[307] it develops earlier in patients who have allogenic transplants than in those who have autologous ones.[307] Clinical manifestations are nonspecific and include dyspnea, weight gain, and crackles on physical examination.[307] Radiographic findings are similar to those of pulmonary edema associated with fluid overload and include enlarged pulmonary vessels, interstitial thickening with peribronchial cuffing and septal lines, and, commonly, small pleural effusions.[310, 311] HRCT also frequently demonstrates areas of ground-glass attenuation involving mainly the dependent lung regions.[311] A variable degree of hypoxemia may be present.

### Diffuse Alveolar Hemorrhage

Pulmonary hemorrhage is an important complication of BMT. In one review of 141 consecutive patients who had autologous transplants, it occurred in 29 (21%);[312] 23 (79%) died, compared with death in only 14 of 112 patients (13%) who did not have hemorrhage. The complication has also been described occasionally in patients after allogenic marrow transplantation.[313] Risk factors include age older than 40 years, a primary diagnosis of solid malignancy, high fever, severe mucositis, white blood cell recovery, and renal insufficiency.[312]

Evidence of infection or other potential etiology is only occasionally noted during clinical assessment.[314, 315] However, in an autopsy study of 47 patients who died after autologous BMT,[316] 10 of the 11 patients who had diffuse alveolar hemorrhage had some other abnormality identified pathologically—7 had diffuse alveolar damage, 2 had bacterial pneumonia, 1 had invasive aspergillosis, and 2 had herpes pneumonia. Diffuse alveolar damage has also been found in a high proportion of autopsies by other investigators,[312] suggesting that it may be related to the development of the hemorrhage; however, the nature of this potential relationship is unclear.

Diffuse alveolar hemorrhage is characterized clinically by progressive dyspnea, cough, and hypoxemia;[312] hemoptysis is rare.[307] Symptoms develop about 12 days after transplantation (range, 7 to 40 days).[312] The characteristic radiographic and HRCT findings consist of bilateral or, less commonly, unilateral ground-glass opacities and patchy or confluent air-space consolidation (Fig. 45–25).[311, 317] These abnormalities tend to involve mainly the perihilar region and lower lung zones.[317] In one investigation of 39 patients in whom the diagnosis was confirmed by BAL, radiographic abnormalities were seen on average at 11 days (range, 0 to 31 days) after transplantation and preceded the BAL diagnosis by an average of 3 days (range, 0 to 24 days).[317] The radiographic findings progressed rapidly, and the most severe abnormalities were present an average of 6 days after initial presentation. Twenty-seven patients had bilateral abnormalities, 10 had unilateral abnormalities, and 2 had normal chest radiographs (Fig. 45–26).[317]

Although some investigators have found successive aliquots of BAL fluid to contain increasing amounts of blood,[318] this finding is neither sensitive nor specific for the diagnosis.[316] Systemic corticosteroids likely moderate the effects of the hemorrhage and appear to improve survival;[319, 320] clearly, excluding infection in such patients is mandatory.

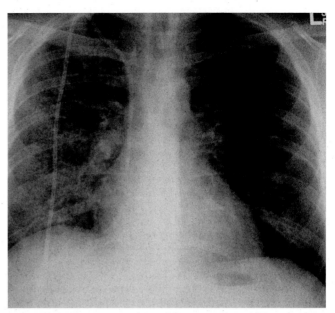

**Figure 45–26. Bone Marrow Transplantation: Diffuse Alveolar Hemorrhage.** A posteroanterior chest radiograph shows poorly defined areas of consolidation and small nodular opacities involving mainly the right lung. The patient was a 27-year-old man who developed diffuse pulmonary hemorrhage 2 weeks after bone marrow transplantation.

### Idiopathic Pneumonia Syndrome

Idiopathic pneumonia syndrome (IPS, interstitial pneumonitis, idiopathic pneumonia) has been defined as diffuse lung injury occurring after bone marrow transplantation for which an infectious etiology is not identified.[307] Interstitial pneumonitis of all etiologies accounts for about 40% of transplantation-related deaths; of these, half are noninfectious and meet the definition of IPS.[321, 322] The complication develops in about 10% of patients who have BMT.[321] The median time of onset after transplantation has been reported to be between 12 and 49 days;[323] an early peak occurs in the first 14 days and is followed by a lower but consistent incidence in the following 80 days. Most pneumonia occurring in the first 28 days after transplantation is idiopathic; after this period, the rate of IPS is about 20%.[321]

The pathogenesis of IPS is not known and may be multifactorial. The observations that acute GVHD confers a striking risk for the development of IPS (RR = 5),[323] that some patients treated with corticosteroids or cyclosporin appear to improve, that the severity of the complication can be modulated by the use of intravenous immunoglobulin prophylaxis for GVHD, and that similar disease in experimental animals is associated with an influx of CD8$^+$ T cells in the acute phase and CD4$^+$ T cells chronically[323a] suggest an immunologic component.[307, 321] However, the abnormality occurs with equal frequency in patients who have syngeneic and allogenic transplants, suggesting that it is not directly related to GVHD. There is evidence that the cumulative toxicity of radiation therapy or chemotherapy used in the conditioning regimen may be important in pathogenesis.[308] It is also possible that unrecognized infectious organisms are responsible for at least some cases of IPS. For example, in one study of 15 patients who had "idiopathic interstitial pneumonitis," herpesvirus-6 genome was found in high con-

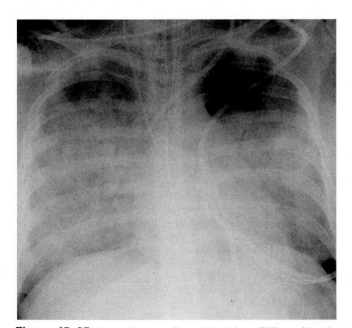

**Figure 45–25. Bone Marrow Transplantation: Diffuse Alveolar Hemorrhage.** An anteroposterior chest radiograph demonstrates extensive bilateral consolidation with air bronchograms. The patient was a 27-year-old woman who developed diffuse alveolar hemorrhage 2 weeks after bone marrow transplantation.

centrations in the lung tissue of 6 patients;[324] the finding correlated with changes in serologic titers in those patients. Risk factors for developing IPS include poor performance status before transplantation, high-dose total-body irradiation, older age, the use of methotrexate in the pretransplantation regimen, and the presence of GVHD.[307, 323, 325]

The radiologic findings of IPS are nonspecific, consisting of bilateral interstitial thickening occasionally associated with ground-glass opacities and poorly defined small nodular opacities.[311, 326, 327] The clinical manifestations are varied: radiographic changes may be associated with a complete lack of symptoms or with acute and severe respiratory distress.[321] Characteristically, patients complain of dyspnea and nonproductive cough. Crackles may be heard on auscultation. The demonstration of hypoxemia and restrictive lung function complete the totally nonspecific character of this disorder. The diagnosis is one of exclusion, particularly of infection.

The mortality rate is high, approaching 80% in some series.[308] However, less than one third of patients die of progressive respiratory failure as a direct result of IPS,[328] complicating infection being a more common cause of death.

### Obliterative Bronchiolitis

Obstructive airway disease caused by OB has also been identified as a complication of BMT.[329–333] The abnormality is uncommon; it was found in only 4 of 113 patients (3.5%) in one series[330] and in 9 of 179 (5%) in another.[333] With few exceptions,[334, 335] it follows allogenic transplantation. It may develop at any time after the third month after BMT;[307] the median interval between transplantation and diagnosis is about 260 days.[333]

Histologic features are identical to those of OB after lung transplantation, consisting most often of mild bronchiolitis and a proliferation of fibroblastic tissue between the

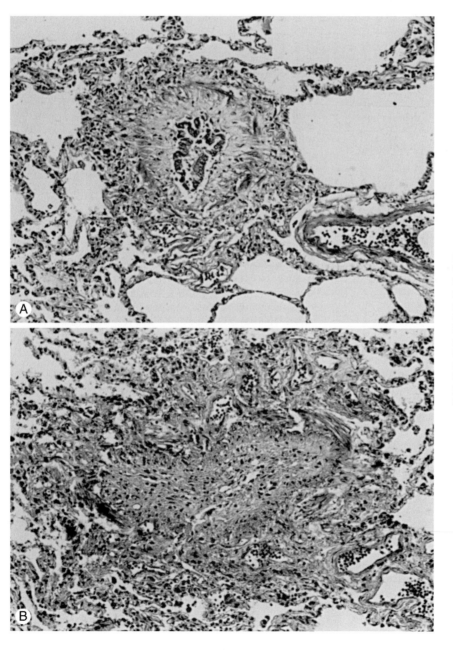

**Figure 45–27. Bone Marrow Transplantation: Obliterative Bronchiolitis.** The patient was a 37-year-old woman with acute myelogenous leukemia who had a partially matched bone marrow transplant. Six months later, she was admitted to the hospital with evidence of chronic graft-versus-host disease in skin and liver and a 1-month history of dry, nonproductive cough and increasing dyspnea. Respiratory distress increased, and she died. At autopsy, many small bronchioles showed partial *(A)* or complete *(B)* luminal obliteration by fibroblastic tissue with mild peribronchiolar lymphocytic inflammation. The parenchyma was normal. *(A* and *B,* ×150.)

epithelium and muscularis mucosae (Fig. 45–27).[330, 336, 337] Parenchymal interstitial disease is typically absent or minimal, and lymphocytic bronchitis may or may not be present.[338] Whether these cases are pathogenetically similar to cases of lymphocytic bronchitis (*see* farther on) or represent another disease process has not been established. Most patients have evidence of chronic GVHD elsewhere in the body, and it has been suggested that the bronchiolitis may represent a primary manifestation of this process in the lungs.[337, 339–341] However, the variability of BAL findings in OB (at times lymphocyte predominant [characteristic of GVHD] and at times neutrophil predominant)[342] and its demonstration in the absence of GVHD in some patients[332] suggest that the pathogenesis is more complicated and, perhaps, multifactorial.

Radiographs may be normal or may show evidence of hyperinflation. The characteristic HRCT findings consist of dilation of the segmental and subsegmental bronchi and localized areas of decreased attenuation and perfusion.[311, 327, 327a] HRCT scans performed at end-expiration may demonstrate air trapping (Fig. 45–28).[311] Recurrent pneumothorax and pneumomediastinum have been described in several patients.[338]

Initial symptoms may be attributed to an upper respiratory tract infection; eventually cough, which is progressively productive, as well as wheezing and exertional dyspnea develop.[307, 332, 333] In some patients, the abnormality is discovered because of an asymptomatic deterioration in lung function.[307] Findings of chronic GVHD, such as scleroderma, dryness of the eyes and mouth, dysphagia, serositis, and hepatic disease, are often present. Elevated levels of rheumatoid factor have been noted in some patients.[330]

Pulmonary function studies show an obstructive pattern; occasionally, restrictive lung function has also been documented.[307] The diffusing capacity may be normal or reduced.[307, 330, 333, 336] The rate of progression is variable; in one series of 35 patients, 21 deteriorated rapidly, whereas 14 had either slowly progressive or reversible disease.[332] The poorest prognosis was found among those patients who had the onset of OB within 150 days of transplantation and whose FEV$_1$ had decreased by at least 30% in the first 6 months after transplantation.

### Graft-Versus-Host Disease

GVHD is the result of recognition of recipient tissue as foreign by donor T lymphocytes.[307] The complication may be acute or chronic, the former occurring in about two thirds of patients and the latter in the remainder.[308] The lungs are frequently abnormal in patients who have chronic GVHD; findings in acute GVHD are minimal.[307] Whether the observed abnormalities are directly related to the effect of GVHD or represent the result of other processes may be difficult to ascertain. Patients who have chronic GVHD frequently have concomitant pulmonary infection by bacteria and opportunistic organisms and may develop a sicca syndrome accompanied by chronic bronchitis.[307] Some patients who have apparent IPS have a CD8+ lymphocytic alveolitis with fibrosis, as in 7 of 65 long-term survivors of BMT in one series.[343] All 7 suffered from chronic GVHD; in contrast to most patients who have IPS, the response to immunosuppressive therapy was favorable. IPS and OB can also be seen in patients who have chronic GVHD; however, both disorders can be seen in patients who do not have GVHD, making the relationship to the latter somewhat uncertain.

### Lymphocytic Bronchitis

Chronic bronchitis, characterized by a lymphocytic infiltrate in the bronchial epithelium and submucosa associated with focal epithelial necrosis, is not uncommon in patients who have undergone allogenic BMT; for example, in one investigation of 59 such patients, it was identified in 15 (25%).[344] Because the incidence and severity of these histologic changes were appreciably greater in patients who had more severe grades of GVHD, the authors of the latter study speculated that the bronchitis represented a manifestation of this process. Further, they suggested that the higher incidence of bronchopneumonia in these patients may have been caused by lymphocyte-mediated destruction of the bronchial

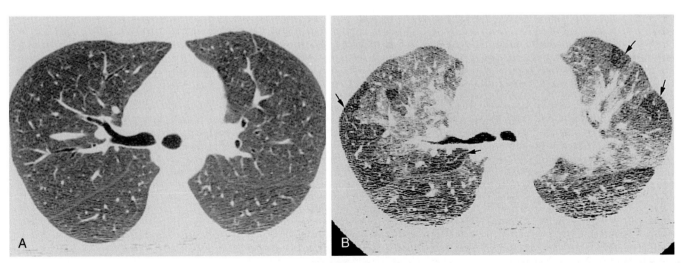

**Figure 45–28. Bone Marrow Transplantation: Obliterative Bronchiolitis.** An HRCT scan at end-inspiration *(A)* is normal whereas one performed at end-expiration *(B)* demonstrates localized areas of air trapping *(arrows)*. The patient was a 32-year-old woman who presented with dyspnea 18 months after transplantation.

epithelium. Although lymphocytic infiltration of bronchial walls has also been documented by other investigators,[345, 346] most have failed to find an association in either human autopsy material or experimental animals between the presence of inflammation and either GVHD or bronchopneumonia.[307, 308, 345] In addition, the incidence of the inflammatory infiltrate is similar in autografted and allogenically grafted dogs, implying that immunologic mechanisms may not be pathogenetically important.[345] Clinical findings include a dry, nonproductive cough, often associated with evidence of GVHD in skin, liver, and intestine.[344]

### Infection

Specific infections in patients who have BMT tend to occur at particular times, corresponding to specific defects in host defense.[347] Most diffuse radiographic infiltrates are noninfectious in origin; focal disease may be due to bacteria or fungi. Defects in humoral and cell-mediated immunity are present between 1 and 6 months after transplantation, during which time opportunistic infection is common. CMV pneumonia is a common cause of diffuse lung disease during this period (*see* farther on). After 6 months, immune function gradually returns to normal. However, GVHD may develop at this time and lead to persistent defects in cell-mediated immunity and poor antigen-specific responses; patients who have this complication are at risk of infection by opportunistic organisms and encapsulated bacteria.[347]

Confident diagnosis of bacterial pneumonia in the early post-transplantation period may be difficult as a result of the use of prophylactic antibiotics and empiric broad-spectrum antibiotics at the onset of clinical evidence of infection.[307] Nevertheless, it has been estimated that the incidence of the complication during this time is between 15% and 50%.[307, 348] Gram-negative organisms are the most common agents; gram-positive organisms such as *Streptococcus pneumoniae* and *S. aureus* are occasionally identified.[325] A focal outbreak of *Legionella* pneumonia has also been described.[325] Late bacterial pneumonia is predominantly caused by gram-positive organisms, especially *S. pneumoniae*.[325, 349, 350] Infrequent causes of bacterial pneumonia include *Mycobacterium tuberculosis*,[351, 351a] nontuberculous mycobacterial species,[352] anaerobic bacteria, and species of *Nocardia* and *Actinomyces*.[347]

*Aspergillus* is the most common fungus associated with pneumonia after BMT, having been identified as the cause of up to 36% of all nosocomial pneumonias in this setting.[347] Most cases occur within 30 days of transplantation and are associated with granulocytopenia and the use of broad-spectrum antibiotics and corticosteroids.[307] Clinical features include fever, dyspnea, and cough; hemoptysis, pleuritic pain, and sinusitis are additional symptoms that should lead to serious consideration of the diagnosis.[325] The mortality is very high, approaching 85%.[307, 308]

The incidence of PCP following BMT has been strikingly reduced by the use of prophylactic antibiotics.[307] The median time to onset of disease is 2 months after transplantation. However, patients who have chronic GVHD remain at significant risk more than 6 months after transplantation if prophylactic therapy is not maintained.[354] The yield of positive diagnosis by BAL is substantially less than that in patients who have AIDS, and transbronchial biopsy increases

the diagnostic sensitivity of bronchoscopy in this setting.[307] The onset and progression of disease are usually rapid.[325] Fungal species other than *Aspergillus* or *Pneumocystis* are only occasionally the cause of pneumonia in patients who have undergone BMT.[347, 355, 356]

CMV pneumonia occurs in 10% to 40% of BMT recipients, most often 6 to 12 weeks after the procedure.[307] It accounts for about half of all episodes of diffuse interstitial pneumonia in patients who have allogenic transplants, is much less common in those who have autologous transplants, and is seen rarely in those who have syngeneic transplants.[357] Infection may result from reactivation of latent infection in CMV antibody–positive recipients, from transfusion of CMV-positive blood products to CMV antibody–negative recipients, or from the graft itself.[307] Other risk factors include older age, conditioning regimens that include total-body irradiation, the presence of CMV viremia and excretion, T-cell depletion for GVHD prophylaxis, pretransplantation restrictive lung function, and the presence of moderate to severe GVHD.[358–363] Diffuse interstitial opacities are noted radiographically.[307] Clinical signs and symptoms are nonspecific, and include fever, nonproductive cough, dyspnea, and hypoxemia. As in patients who have lung transplants, the distinction between CMV disease and simple infection (colonization) may be difficult (*see* page 1716). The prognosis has been improved by the use of effective antiviral therapy, and it is likely that many episodes of pneumonia have been prevented by the institution of aggressive prophylaxis in patients at increased risk.[363a, 363b]

Herpes simplex pneumonia may follow gingivostomatitis in the early post-transplantation period. The complication presumably occurs by aspiration of organisms from the oral cavity and may result in focal or multifocal pulmonary opacities on chest radiographs. Diffuse pulmonary disease may also be secondary to herpes simplex viremia.[307] The diagnosis requires identification of the organism in lung tissue, because the finding of the virus in the upper airway or in BAL fluid is not specific for pneumonia.[325]

Sporadic cases of interstitial pneumonia in patients who have BMT have also been caused by parainfluenza virus, respiratory syncytial virus, adenovirus, influenza, and herpesvirus-6.[308, 364–366a] Occasionally, respiratory syncytial virus and parainfluenza virus have caused isolated outbreaks of nosocomial pneumonia.[347, 367] Upper respiratory tract involvement is frequently seen with these viruses, in contrast to CMV, which rarely causes disease at this site.[308] As discussed previously, it is possible that herpesvirus-6 is responsible for some cases of "idiopathic" interstitial pneumonitis.[324]

Parasitic or protozoal infection is relatively rare in patients who have BMT; *Toxoplasma gondii* has involved the lungs during the course of disseminated disease in patients who have received allogenic transplants.[368] Occasional cases of pneumonia caused by *Mycoplasma* or *Chlamydia* species have also been reported.[347, 353]

The radiographic manifestations of pneumonia in BMT recipients are no different from those in other hosts.[369, 370] CT can provide additional information that either changes patient management or more clearly establishes the pattern and extent of pulmonary disease (Fig. 45–29).[370–372] In one investigation in which conventional radiographs and HRCT scans were performed in 33 symptomatic episodes seen in 33 patients, 14 chest radiographs were interpreted as normal

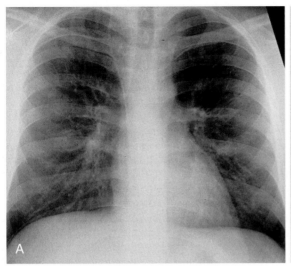

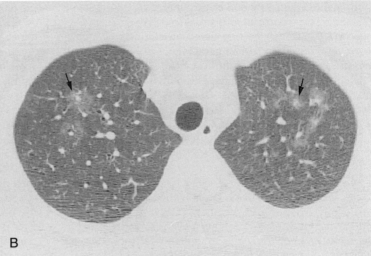

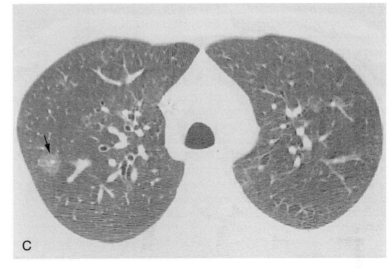

**Figure 45–29. Bone Marrow Transplantation: Angioinvasive Aspergillosis.** An anteroposterior chest radiograph *(A)* in a 19-year-old man 3 weeks after bone marrow transplantation shows questionable parenchymal opacities. HRCT scans *(B and C)* demonstrate small nodules with surrounding halos of ground-glass attenuation *(arrows).* These findings are most suggestive of angioinvasive aspergillosis. The diagnosis was confirmed by open-lung biopsy.

and 22 as demonstrating nonspecific changes;[370] however, none of the radiographic findings was considered helpful in providing sufficient information for further management. In 2 of 14 episodes (14%) in patients who had normal chest radiographs and in 9 of 22 episodes (41%) in patients who had nonspecific radiographic findings, abnormalities seen on CT resulted in a change in clinical management that included performing bronchoscopy, increasing or changing antibiotic coverage, starting white blood cell transfusions, performing biopsy, or a combination of these. In an investigation of 18 patients in whom CT scans were retrospectively reviewed after 21 episodes of intrathoracic complications, CT demonstrated diagnostically relevant findings that were not apparent at radiography in 12 of 21 cases (57%), including a ground-glass pattern in early pneumonia.[371]

In another investigation, the usefulness of HRCT was assessed prospectively in the early detection of pneumonia in 87 neutropenic patients who had 146 episodes of fever that persisted for more than 2 days despite empiric antibiotic therapy.[372] Chest radiographs and HRCT scans were normal in 56 (38%) of 146 episodes, both were abnormal in 20 (14%), and chest radiographs were normal while HRCT scans were abnormal in 70 (46%). Microorganisms were detected in 11 of 20 (55%) patients who had abnormal

radiographs and CT scans and in 30 of 70 (43%) patients in whom the HRCT scans demonstrated parenchymal abnormalities but the radiographs were normal. In 22 (31%) of these 70 episodes, abnormalities later became apparent on the radiograph. The median interval (delay) until an opacity became apparent on the chest radiograph in these patients was 5 days (range, 1 to 22 days).

The findings in these studies suggest that HRCT should be performed in bone marrow transplant recipients who have persistent fever and no evidence of pneumonia on the chest radiograph. However, similar to the chest radiograph, the HRCT findings in the various infectious complications after BMT are relatively nonspecific.[311] The main exception is the presence of a halo of ground-glass attenuation surrounding pulmonary nodules, a finding that is suggestive of invasive aspergillosis *(see* Fig. 45–29).[311, 373, 374] Uncommonly, hemorrhagic nodules are caused by other organisms, such as *Candida* species, CMV, and herpes simplex.[375]

### Pleural Disease

Pleural effusion is not uncommon after BMT; in one series of 57 patients, it developed in 9 (16%).[376] It is usually seen in association with a well-defined clinical setting, such as pulmonary edema, fluid overload, infection, noninfectious pneumonia, recurrence of neoplasm, or veno-occlusive disease.[38, 309, 377] Occasionally, patients present with large and recurrent sterile effusions; in one review of 7 such patients, the effusions were found to occur in patients who had received autologous BMT and who suffered from acute or chronic GVHD, mostly in association with systemic CMV infection.[377]

Pneumothorax sometimes accompanies severe airflow obstruction caused by OB.[38]

### Miscellaneous Complications

A number of vascular complications have been described after BMT. Some patients have developed pulmonary veno-occlusive disease;[378–380] the diagnosis is suggested by the triad of pulmonary edema, pulmonary hypertension, and normal left ventricular function. Embolization of bone and fat fragments during infusion of donor bone marrow may cause transient hypoxemia.[307] Acute respiratory distress as the result of thromboembolism has also been reported occasionally.[381]

Pulmonary alveolar proteinosis has been diagnosed in about 5% of patients who have hematologic malignancies and pulmonary symptoms.[382] It may resolve after BMT when complete remission is achieved; it has also developed after BMT in a few patients.[382] Rarely, patients have been described with the clinical and radiologic picture of BOOP.[308, 383]

Patients are at substantially increased risk of the development of secondary malignancies after BMT,[384–387] in which situation the lungs can be the site of either primary or metastatic disease.[387a] The risk is cumulative with time. In one review of 19,229 patients reported from 235 transplantation centers, 10-year survivors of BMT had a risk of developing a second (nonhematologic) malignancy that was 8.3 times that expected.[384] Hematologic malignancies, especially EBV-related B-cell lymphoproliferative disorders, are also common after BMT (Fig. 45–30).[385] In a review of 2,150 patients, the estimated actuarial incidence of any post-BMT malignancy was 9.9% (±2.3%) at 13 years, representing a standardized incidence ratio of 11.6.[385]

### Pulmonary Function Tests

Given the frequency with which patients who have BMT develop pulmonary complications, it is not surprising that lung function is often abnormal. As discussed previously, patients who develop OB typically have evidence of airway obstruction. When groups of BMT patients are followed with lung function testing prospectively after transplantation, a significant number also develop restrictive lung function with a deterioration in the diffusing capacity.[389–395] For example, in one investigation of 906 patients who had pulmonary function testing 3 months after transplantation, 34% had restrictive ventilatory defects (TLC < 80% predicted).[389] Changes may be noted even in asymptomatic patients.[392, 393] In the absence of GVHD, infection, relapse of the primary disease, and a high radiation dose during pretransplantation conditioning, these changes are transient, and lung function recovers with time.[392–395] The pathogenesis

of these functional changes in the absence of an identified cause is unclear; however, toxicity as a result of the pretransplantation conditioning regime, muscle weakness, and sequelae of intercurrent infection has been hypothesized.[307]

It is somewhat surprising that both preoperative[363, 396] and postoperative[389] abnormalities of lung function have prognostic significance in patients who have BMT. For example, in a statistical analysis of 1297 patients who had pulmonary function testing before transplantation, abnormalities in TLC, Dlco, and gas exchange were found to be significantly associated with death (although the risk was less important than that associated with other risk factors, such as relapse status and HLA mismatch).[396] Although respiratory failure was more common in patients who had abnormalities in pulmonary function before transplantation, this did not account entirely for the described increase in mortality. The risk remained statistically significant even after considering potential confounders, such as age, active malignancy at the time of transplantation, and the primary disease. The most likely explanation for the association of these functional abnormalities with outcome is the prior use of cytotoxic chemotherapy; however, the mechanism by which this affects long-term survival after transplantation is uncertain. Decreases in TLC and Dlco seem to be associated with the development of hepatic veno-occlusive disease;[388] this may account for some of the relationship between survival and lung function.

Abnormalities of pulmonary function in the post-transplantation period are also predictive of nonrelapse mortality.[389] For example, in one investigation, the presence of restrictive lung function or a fall in TLC of 15% compared with the pretransplantation period was associated with a doubling of the risk of nonrelapse mortality.[389] Death was the result of respiratory failure in these patients. These findings suggest that pulmonary function should be monitored in the post-transplantation period to appreciate early changes associated with serious lung pathology, such as interstitial pneumonia syndrome. However, whether earlier recognition of disease in these patients will alter outcome remains to be determined.

## LIVER TRANSPLANTATION

The lung is frequently diseased in patients in whom liver transplantation is anticipated as well as in those patients who have undergone the procedure.[396a] The respiratory complications of liver disease, the complications of abdominal surgery, and the infections that follow immunosuppressive medication are all discussed in the appropriate areas of this text. However, there are several complications of liver transplantation and concerns unique to liver transplantation that are briefly discussed in the following sections.

### Pulmonary Calcification

Metastatic pulmonary calcification is an uncommon cause of pulmonary disease in patients who have undergone liver transplantation; for example, in one series of 77 such patients, it was seen on the radiograph in 4 (5%).[397] The importance of the abnormality is related principally to the

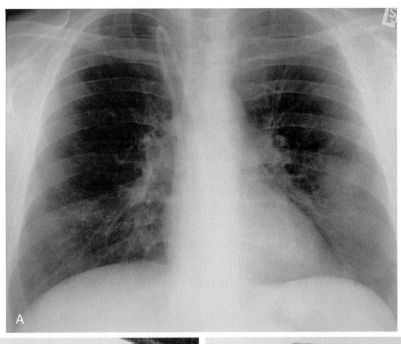

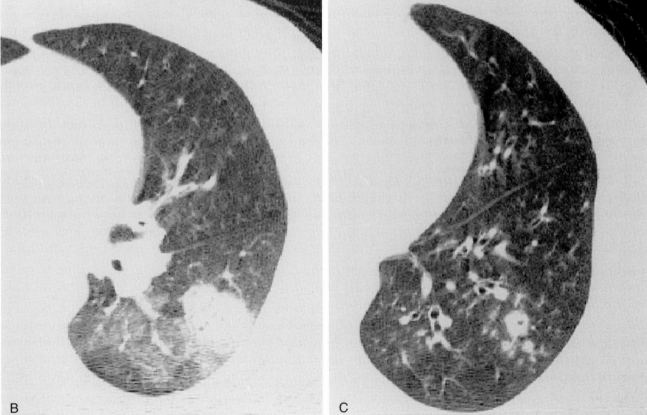

**Figure 45–30. Bone Marrow Transplantation: Post-transplantation Lymphoproliferative Disorder.** A posteroanterior chest radiograph *(A)* in a 30-year-old man shows poorly defined opacities in the left lower lobe. Views of the left lung from HRCT scans *(B* and *C)* demonstrate small nodules, focal consolidation, and areas of ground-glass attenuation. The diagnosis of post-transplantation lymphoproliferative disorder was proven at autopsy.

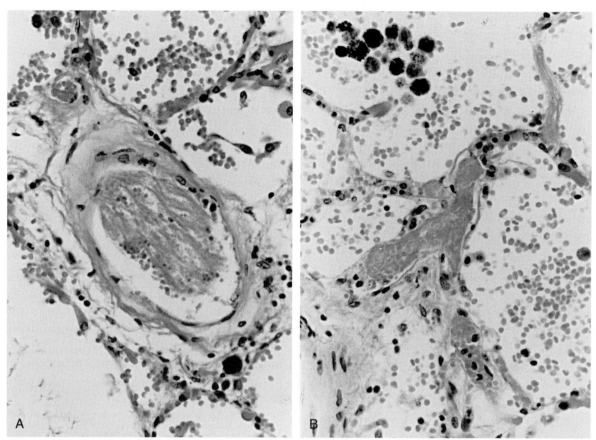

**Figure 45–31. Liver Transplantation: Microvascular Pulmonary Thrombosis.** Magnified views of lung parenchyma show complete occlusion of a small artery *(A)* and an arteriole *(B)* by fibrin-platelet thrombus. Many other vessels of similar size were affected. The patient was a 65-year-old man who became hypotensive and developed cardiac arrythmia shortly before the end of a liver transplantation procedure.

ease with which it can be confused radiographically with other complications, such as edema or infection.

Although the pathogenesis of the calcification has not been fully clarified, several risk factors have been identified. Patients typically have had postoperative renal failure and have received large volumes of blood, plasma, and elemental calcium.[398] The use of citrate-containing blood products may indirectly cause secondary hyperparathyroidism,[398] which may be aggravated by the administration of exogenous calcium.[397]

Patients usually do not have symptoms; however, dyspnea and nonproductive cough occur occasionally, and respiratory failure has been described.[399] The diagnosis can be confirmed by the use of technetium-99m phosphate scans, which show increased uptake in the lungs; CT scanning and transbronchial biopsy are specific for the diagnosis.[399]

### Pulmonary Thrombosis

Massive pulmonary platelet aggregation is a common cause of early death in patients who have undergone liver transplantation (Fig. 45–31).[400] In one autopsy study of all deaths occurring within 10 days of hepatic surgery over a 3.5-year period (including 6 liver transplantations and 13 other operations), all patients who had undergone transplantation had extensive occlusion of the pulmonary vasculature by platelet aggregates; similar findings were seen in only three of the nontransplantation patients. The latter had

conditions, such as disseminated intravascular coagulation, known to be associated with this pathologic finding; however, no cause was apparent in the liver transplant patients. Grossly, the lungs were described as having an unusual rubbery consistency.[400] Similar findings have been reported in 10 children who died suddenly after liver transplantation;[401] in 7, an elevation of pulmonary artery pressures before death suggested the presence of acute obstruction of the pulmonary vasculature.

### Hypoxemia and Liver Transplantation

Hypoxemia is common in patients who have cirrhosis;[402] the presence of severe hypoxemia in patients who have chronic liver disease and no intrinsic lung disease is termed *hepatopulmonary syndrome.*[404, 405] The pathogenesis is related to several factors. Pulmonary vascular dilation as a result of poor vascular tone and impaired hypoxic pressor response contributes to ventilation-perfusion mismatching. As cirrhosis progresses, shunt and some degree of diffusion limitation (presumably resulting from marked pulmonary capillary dilation) also become evident.[398, 402] The recognition that liver transplantation can reverse even severe preoperative hypoxemia underscores the functional nature of this disorder.[403] However, in one study, patients who had a preoperative $Po_2$ of less than 50 mm Hg had a mortality rate of 30%, compared with only 4% in those whose $Po_2$ was greater than 50 mm Hg.[403]

# REFERENCES

1. Lumbreras C, Fernandez I, Velosa J, et al: Infectious complications following pancreatic transplantation: Incidence, microbiological and clinical characteristics, and outcome. Clin Infect Dis 20:514, 1995.
2. Afessa B, Gay PC, Plevak DJ, et al: Pulmonary complications of orthotopic liver transplantation. Mayo Clin Proceed 68:427, 1993.
3. Patel R, Roberts GD, Keating MR, et al: Infections due to nontuberculous mycobacteria in kidney, heart, and liver transplant recipients. Clin Infect Dis 19:263, 1994.
4. Singh N, Gayowski T, Wagener M, et al: Pulmonary infections in liver transplant recipients receiving tacrolimus: Changing pattern of microbial etiologies. Transplantation 61:396, 1996.
5. Hosenpud JD: Registry report. J Heart Lung Transplant 15:S7, 1996.
6. Judson MA: Clinical aspects of lung transplantation. Clin Chest Med 14:335, 1993.
7. Davis RD, Pasque M: Pulmonary transplantation. Ann Surg 221:14, 1995.
8. Jenkinson SG, Levine SM: Lung transplantation. Disease-a-Month 40:1, 1994.
9. Kotloff RM, Zuckerman JB: Lung transplantation for cystic fibrosis. Chest 109:787, 1996.
10. Egan TM: Lung transplantation in cystic fibrosis. Semin Respir Infect 7:227, 1992.
11. Kaiser LR, Pasque MK, Trulock EP, et al: Bilateral sequential lung transplantation: The procedure of choice for double-lung replacement. Ann Thorac Surg 52:438, 1991.
12. Trulock EP: Lung transplantation. Am J Respir Crit Care Med 155:789, 1997
13. Yacoub MH, Banner NR, Khaghani A, et al: Heart-lung transplantation for cystic fibrosis and subsequent domino heart transplantation. J Heart Transplant 9:459, 1990.
14. Smith JA, Roberts M, McNeil K, et al: Excellent outcome of cardiac transplantation using domino donor hearts. Eur J Cardiothorac Surg 10:628, 1996.
15. Williams TJ, Patterson GA, McClean PA, et al: Maximal exercise testing in single and double lung transplant recipients. Am Rev Respir Dis 145:101, 1992.
16. Miyoshi S, Trulock EP, Schaefers HJ, et al: Cardiopulmoanry exercise testing after single and double lung transplantation. Chest 97:1130, 1990.
17. Girard C, Mornex JF, Gamondes JP, et al: Single lung transplantation for primary pulmonary hypertension without cardiopulmonary bypass. Chest 102:967, 1992.
18. Levine SM, Gibbons WJ, Bryan CL, et al: Single lung transplantation for primary pulmonary hypertension. Chest 98:1107, 1990.
18a. Gammie JS, Cheul LJ, Pham SM, et al: Cardiopulmonary bypass is associated with early allograft dysfunction but not death after double-lung transplantation. J Thorac Cardiovasc Surg 115:990, 1998.
19. Trulock EP, Egan TM, Kouchoukos NT, et al: Single lung transplantation for severe chronic obstructive pulmonary disease. Chest 96:738, 1989.
20. Bhatnagar NK: Single lung transplantation for emphysematous disease. Respir Med 87:489, 1993.
21. Kaiser LR, Cooper JD, Trulock EP, et al: The evolution of single lung transplantation for emphysema. J Thorac Cardiovasc Surg 102:333, 1991.
22. Sundaresan RS, Shiraishi Y, Trulock EP, et al: Single or bilateral lung transplantation for emphysema? J Thorac Cardiovasc Surg 112:1485, 1996.
23. Mannes GPM, de Boer WJ, van der Bij W, et al: Three hundred patients referred for lung transplantation. Chest 109:408, 1996.
24. Report of the ATS workshop on lung transplantation. Lung transplantation. Am Rev Respir Dis 147:772, 1993.
25. Egan TM, Trulock EP, Boychuk J, et al: Analysis of referrals for lung transplantation. Chest 99:867, 1991.
25a. American Thoracic Society: International guidelines for the selection of lung transplant candidates. Am J Respir Crit Care Med 158:335, 1998.
26. Edelman JD, Kotloff RM: Lung transplantation—a disease-specific approach. Clin Chest Med 18:627, 1997.
26a. Hosenpud JD, Bennett LE, Keck BM, et al: Effect of diagnosis on survival benefit of lung transplantation for end-stage lung disease. Lancet 351(9095):24, 1998.
27. Marshall SE, Kramer MR, Lewiston N, et al: Selection and evaluation of recipients for heart-lung and lung transplantation. Chest 98:1488, 1990.
28. Madden BP, Hodson ME, Tsang V, et al: Intermediate-term results of heart-lung transplantation for cystic fibrosis. Lancet 339:1583, 1992.
29. Levine SM, Anzueto A, Peters JI, et al: Single lung transplantation in patients with systemic disease. Chest 105:837, 1994.
30. Etienne B, Bertocchi M, Gamondes J-P, et al: Successful double-lung transplantation for bronchioloalveolar carcinoma. Chest 112:1423, 1997.
31. Aris RM, Neuringer IP, Weiner MA, et al: Severe osteoporosis before and after lung transplantation. Chest 109:1176, 1996.
32. Shane E, Silverberg SJ, Donovan D, et al: Osteoporosis in lung transplantation candidates with end-stage pulmonary disease. Am J Med 101:262: 1996.
33. Snell GI, de Hoyos A, Krajden M, et al: *Pseudomonas cepacia* in lung transplant recipients with cystic fibrosis. Chest 103:466, 1993.
34. Aris RM, Gilligan PH, Neuringer IP, et al: The effects of panresistant bacteria in cystic fibrosis patients on lung transplant outcomes. Am J Respir Crit Care Med 155:1699, 1997.
35. Kanj SS, Tapson V, Davis RD, et al: Infections in patients with cystic fibrosis following lung transplantation. Chest 112:924, 1997.
36. Low DE, Trulock EP, Kaiser LR, et al: Lung transplantation of ventilator-dependent patients. Chest 101:8, 1992.
37. Flume PA, Egan TM, Westerman JH, et al: Lung transplantation for mechanically ventilated patients. J Heart Lung Transplant 13:15, 1994.
37a. Novick RJ, Stitt LW, Al-Kattan K, et al: Pulmonary retransplantation: Predictors of graft function and survival in 230 patients. Ann Thorac Surg 65:227, 1998.
38. Judson MA, Sahn SA: The pleural space and organ transplantation. Am J Respir Crit Care Med 153:1153, 1996.
39. Noyes BE, Orenstein DM: Treatment of pneumothorax in cystic fibrosis in the era of lung transplantation. Chest 101:1187, 1992.
40. Dusmet M, Winton TL, Kesten S, et al: Previous intrapleural procedures do not adversely affect lung transplantation. J Heart Lung Transplant 15:249, 1996.
41. Schäfers HJ, Wagner TOF, Demertzis S, et al: Preoperative corticosteroids: A contraindication to lung transplantation? Chest 102:1522, 1992.
42. Kaplan JD, Trulock EP, Cooper JD, et al: Pulmonary vascular permeability after lung transplantation. Am Rev Respir Dis 145:954, 1992.
43. Anderson DC, Glazer HS, Semenkovich JW, et al: Lung transplant edema: Chest radiography after lung transplantation—the first 10 days. Radiology 195:275, 1995.
44. Ettinger NA, Trulock EP: Pulmonary considerations of organ transplantation. Am Rev Respir Dis 144:433, 1991.
45. Bacha EA, Herve P, Murakami S, et al: Lasting beneficial effect of short-term inhaled nitric oxide on graft function after lung transplantation. Paris-Sud University Lung Transplantation Group. J Thorac Cardiovasc Surg 112:590, 1996.
46. Novick RJ, Gehman KE, Ali IS, et al: Lung preservation: The importance of endothelial and alveolar type II cell integrity. Ann Thorac Surg 62:302, 1996.
47. Buchanan SA, Mauny MC, DeLima NF, et al: Enhanced isolated lung function after ischemia with anti-intercellular adhesion molecule antibody. J Thorac Cardiovasc Surg 111:941, 1996.
48. Chapelier A, Reignier J, Mazmanian M, et al: Amelioration of reperfusion injury by pentoxifylline after lung transplantation. The University Paris-Sud Lung Transplant Group. J Heart Lung Transplant 14:676, 1995.
49. Chapelier A, Reignier J, Mazmanian M, et al: Pentoxifylline and lung ischemia-reperfusion injury: Application to lung transplantation. Universite Paris-Sud Lung Transplant Group. J Cardiovasc Pharmacol 25:130, 1995.
50. Serrick C, La Franchesca S, Giaid A, et al: Cytokine interleukin-2 tumour necrosis factor-α and interferon-γ release after ischemia-reperfusion injury in a novel lung autograft animal model. Am J Respir Crit Care Med 152:277, 1995.
51. Binns OA, DeLima NF, Buchanan SA, et al: Neutrophil endopeptidase inhibitor improves pulmonary function during reperfusion after eighteen-hour preservation. J Thorac Cardiovasc Surg 112:607, 1996.
52. Palace GP, Del Vecchio PJ, Horgan MJ, et al: Release of tumour necrosis factor after pulmonary artery occlusion and reperfusion. Am Rev Respir Dis 147:143, 1993.
53. Unruh HW: Lung preservation and lung injury. Chest Surg Clin North Am 5:91, 1995.
54. Nezu K, Kushibe K, Tojo T, et al: Protection against lipid peroxidation induced during preservation of lungs for transplantation. J Heart Lung Transplant 13:998, 1994.
55. Qayumi AK, Jamieson WR, Poostizadeh A, et al: Comparison of new ion chelating agents in the prevention of ischemia/reperfusion injury: A swine model of heart-lung transplantation. J Invest Surg 5:115, 1992.
56. Takeuchi K, Suzuki S, Kako N, et al: A prostacyclin analogue reduces free radical generation in heart-lung transplantation. Ann Thorac Surg 54:327, 1992.
57. Salvatierra A, Velasco F, Rodriguez M, et al: C₁-esterase inhibitor prevents early pulmonary dysfunction after lung transplantation in the dog. Am J Respir Crit Care Med 155:1147, 1997.
58. Novick RJ, MacDonald J, Veldhuizen RA, et al: Evaluation of surfactant treatment strategies after prolonged graft storage in lung transplantation. Am J Respir Crit Care Med 154:98, 1996.
59. Erasmus ME, Petersen AH, Hofstede G, et al: Surfactant treatment before reperfusion improves the immediate function of lung transplants in rats. Am J Respir Crit Care Med 153:665, 1996.
60. Andrade RS, Solien EE, Wangensteen OD, et al: Surfactant dysfunction in lung preservation. Transplantation 60:536, 1995.
61. Erasmus ME, Petersen AH, Oetomo SB, et al: The function of surfactant is impaired during the reimplantation response in rat lung transplants. J Heart Lung Transplant 13:791, 1994.
61a. Hohlfeld JM, Tiryaki E, Hamm H, et al: Pulmonary surfactant activity is impaired in lung transplant recipients. Am J Respir Crit Care Med 158:706, 1998.
62. Veldhuizen RA, Lee J, Sandler D, et al: Alterations in pulmonary surfactant composition and activity after experimental lung transplantation. Am Rev Respir Dis 148:208, 1993.
63. Puskas JD, Hirai T, Christie N, et al: Reliable thirty-hour lung preservation by donor lung hyperinflation. J Thorac Cardiovasc Surg 104:1075, 1992.
63a. Shennib H, Lee AG, Kuang JQ, et al: Efficacy of administering an endothelin-receptor antagonist (SB209670) in ameliorating ischemia-reperfusion injury in lung allografts. Am J Respir Crit Care Med 157:1975, 1998.
63b. Schütte H, Hermle G, Seeger W, et al: Vascular distention and continued ventilation are protective in lung ischemia/reperfusion. Am J Respir Crit Care Med 157:171, 1998.
64. Zenati M, Yousem SA, Dowling RD, et al: Primary graft failure following pulmonary transplantation. Transplantation 50:165, 1990.

65. Yousem SA, Duncan SR, Griffith BP: Interstitial and airspace granulation tissue reactions in lung transplant recipients. Am J Surg Pathol 16:877, 1992.

66. Herman SJ, Rappaport DC, Weisbrod GL, et al: Single-lung transplantation: Imaging features. Radiology 170:89, 1989.

67. Anderson DC, Glazer HS, Semenkovich JW, et al: Lung transplant edema: chest radiography after lung transplantation: The first 10 days. Radiology 195:275, 1995.

68. Herman SJ: Radiologic assessment after lung transplantation. Radiol Clin North Am 32:663, 1994.

69. Garg K, Zamora MR, Tuder R, et al: Lung transplantation: indications, donor and recipient selection, and imaging of complications. RadioGraphics 16:355, 1996.

70. Kundu S, Herman SJ, Winton TL: Reperfusion edema after lung transplantation: Radiographic manifestations. Radiology 206:75, 1998.

70a. Ablett MJ, Grainger AJ, Keir MJ, et al: The correlation of the radiologic extent of lung transplantation edema with pulmonary oxygenation. Am J Roentgenol 171:587, 1998.

71. Sarsam MA, Yonan NA, Beton D, et al: Early pulmonary vein thrombosis after single lung transplantation. J Heart Lung Transplant 12:17, 1993.

72. Harjula ALJ, Baldwin JC, Silverman NE, et al: Implantation response following clinical heart-lung transplantation. J Cardiovasc Surg 31:1, 1990.

73. Chiles C, Guthaner DF, Jamieson SW, et al: Heart-lung transplantation: The postoperative chest radiograph. Radiology 154:299, 1985.

74. Waddell TK, Gorczynski RM, DeCampos KN, et al: Major histocompatibility complex expression and lung ischemia-reperfusion in rats. Ann Thorac Surg 62:866, 1996.

75. Adoumie R, Serrick C, Giaid A, et al: Early cellular events in the lung allograft. Ann Thorac Surg 54:1071, 1992.

76. Trulock EP: Management of lung transplant rejection. Chest 103:1566, 1993.

77. Frost AE, Jammal CT, Cagle PT: Hyperacute rejection following lung transplantation. Chest 110:559, 1996.

78. Keenan RJ, Zeevi A: Immunologic consequences of transplantation. Chest Surg Clin North Am 5:107, 1995.

79. Griffith BP, Hardesty RL, Armitage JM, et al: Acute rejection of lung allografts with various immunosuppressive protocols. Ann Thorac Surg 54:846, 1992.

80. Kesten S, Chamberlain D, Maurer J: Yield of surveillance transbronchial biopsies performed beyond two years after lung transplantation. J Heart Lung Transplant 15:384, 1996.

81. Baz MA, Layish DT, Govert JA, et al: Diagnostic yield of bronchoscopies after isolated lung transplantation. Chest 110:84, 1996.

82. Lawrence EC, Holland VA, Young JB, et al: Dynamic changes in soluble interleukin-2 receptor levels after lung or heart-lung transplantation. Am Rev Respir Dis 140:789, 1989.

82a. Sayegh MH, Turka LA: The role of T-cell activation pathway in transplant rejection. N Engl J Med 338:1813, 1998.

82b. Schulman LL, Weinberg AD, McGregor C, et al: Mismatches at the HLA-DR and HLA-B loci are risk factors for acute rejection after lung transplantation. Am J Respir Crit Care Med 157:1833, 1998.

83. Winter JB, Clelland C, Gouw AS, et al: Distinct phenotypes of infiltrating cells during acute and chronic lung rejection in human heart-lung transplants. Transplantation 59:63, 1995.

84. Nakhleh RE, Bolman RM III, Henke CA, et al: Lung transplant pathology: A comparative study of pulmonary acute rejection and cytomegaloviral infection. Am J Surg Pathol 15:1197, 1991.

85. Yousem SA, Berry GJ, Brunt EM, et al: A working formulation for the standardization of nomenclature in the diagnosis of heart and lung rejection: Lung rejection study group. J Heart Lung Transplant 9:593, 1990.

86. Clelland C, Higenbottam T, Otulana B, et al: Histologic prognostic indicators for the lung allografts of heart-lung transplants. J Heart Transplant 9:177, 1990.

87. Cagle PT, Truong LD, Holland VA, et al: Lung biopsy evaluation of acute rejection versus opportunistic infection in lung transplant patients. Transplantation 47:713, 1989.

88. Marboe CC: Pathology of lung transplantation. Pathology 4:73, 1996.

89. Yousem SA, Berry G, Cagle, PT, et al: Revision of the 1990 working formulation for the classification of pulmonary allograft rejection: Lung rejection study group. J Heart Lung Transplant 15:1, 1996.

90. Husain AN, Siddiqui MT, Montoya A, et al: Post-lung transplant biopsies: An 8-year Loyola experience. Mod Pathol 9:126, 1996.

91. Yousem SA: Graft eosinophilia in lung transplantation. Hum Pathol 23:1172, 1992.

92. Tazelaar HD, Nilsson FN, Rinaldi M, et al: The sensitivity of transbronchial biopsy for the diagnosis of acute lung rejection. J Thorac Cardiovasc Surg 105:674, 1993.

93. Yousem SA: Lymphocytic bronchitis/bronchiolitis in lung allograft recipients. Am J Surg Pathol 17:491, 1993.

94. Herman SJ, Weisbrod GL, Weisbrod L, et al: Chest radiographic findings after bilateral lung transplantation. Am J Roentgenol 153:1181, 1989.

95. Millet B, Higenbottam TW, Flower CDR, et al: The radiographic appearances of infection and acute rejection of the lung after heart-lung transplantation. Am Rev Respir Dis 140:62, 1989.

96. Bergin CJ, Castellino RA, Blank N, et al: Acute lung rejection after heart-lung transplantation: Correlation of findings on chest radiographs with lung biopsy results. Am J Roentgenol 155:23, 1990.

97. Erasmus JJ, McAdams HP, Tapson VF, et al: Radiologic issues in lung transplantation for end-stage pulmonary disease. Am J Roentgenol 169:69, 1997.

98. Loubeyre P, Revel D, Delignette A, et al: High-resolution computed tomographic findings associated with histologically diagnosed acute lung rejection in heart-lung transplant recipients. Chest 107:132, 1995.

99. Guillinger RA, Paradis IL, Dauber JH, et al: The importance of bronchoscopy with transbronchial biopsy and bronchoalveolar lavage in the management of lung transplant recipients. Am J Respir Crit Care Med 152:2037, 1995.

100. Trulock EP, Ettinger NA, Brunt EM, et al: The role of transbronchial lung biopsy in the treatment of lung transplant recipients. Chest 102:1049, 1992.

101. De Hoyos A, Chamberlain D, Schwartzman R, et al: Prospective assessment of a standardized pathologic grading system for acute rejection in lung transplantation. Chest 103:1813, 1993.

102. Boehler A, Vogt P, Zollinger A, et al: Prospective study of the value of transbronchial lung biopsy after lung transplantation. Eur Respir J 9:658, 1996.

103. Tamm M, Sharples LD, Higenbottam TW, et al: Bronchiolitis obliterans syndrome in heart-lung transplantation. Am J Respir Crit Care Med 155:1705, 1997.

104. Starnes VA, Theodore J, Oyer PE, et al: Evaluation of heart-lung transplant recipients with prospective, serial transbronchial biopsies and pulmonary function studies. J Thorac Cardiovasc Surg 98:683, 1989.

105. Otulana BA, Higenbottam T, Scott J, et al: Lung function associated with histologically diagnosed acute lung rejection and pulmonary infection in heart-lung transplant patients. Am Rev Respir Dis 142:329, 1990.

106. Otulana BA, Higenbottam T, Ferrari L, et al: The use of home spirometry in detecting acute lung rejection and infection following heart-lung transplantation. Chest 97:353, 1990.

107. Becker FS, Martinez FJ, Brunsting LA, et al: Limitations of spirometry in detecting rejection after single-lung transplantation. Am J Respir Crit Care Med 150:159, 1994.

108. Hoeper MM, Hamm M, Schäfers HJ, et al: Evaluation of lung function during pulmonary rejection and infection in heart-lung transplant patients. Chest 102:864, 1992.

109. Bjortuft O, Johansen B, Boe J, et al: Daily home spirometry facilitates early detection of rejection in single lung transplant recipients with emphysema. Eur Respir J 6:705, 1993.

110. Girgis RE, Reichenspurner H, Robbins RC, et al: The utility of annual surveillance bronchoscopy in heart-lung transplant recipients. Transplantation 60:1458, 1995.

111. Paradis IL, Duncan SR, Dauber JH, et al: Distinguishing between infection, rejection and the adult respiratory distress syndrome after human lung transplantation. J Heart Lung Transplant 11:232, 1992.

112. Chan CC, Abi-Saleh WJ, Arroliga AC, et al: Diagnostic yield and therapeutic impact of flexible bronchoscopy in lung transplant recipients. J Heart Lung Transplant 15:196, 1996.

113. Clelland C, Higenbottam T, Stewart S, et al: Bronchoalveolar lavage and transbronchial lung biopsy during acute rejection and infection in heart-lung transplant patients. Am Rev Respir Dis 147:1386, 1993.

114. Riise GC, Scherstén H, Nilsson F, et al: Activation of eosinophils and fibroblasts assessed by eosinophil cationic protein and hyalurinan in BAL. Chest 110:89, 1996.

115. Wilkes DS, Heidler KM, Niemeier M, et al: Increased bronchoalveolar IgG2/IgG1 ratio is a marker for human lung allograft rejection. J Investig Med 42:652, 1994.

116. Ross DJ, Yeh AY, Nathan SD, et al: Differential soluble interleukin-2R levels in bilateral bronchoalveolar lavage after single lung transplantation. J Heart Lung Transplant 13:972, 1994.

117. Whitehead BF, Stoehr C, Wu CJ, et al: Cytokine gene expression in human lung transplant recipients. Transplantation 56:956, 1993.

118. Crim C, Keller CA, Dunphy CH, et al: Flow cytometric analysis of lung lymphocytes in lung transplant recipients. Am J Respir Crit Care Med 153:1041, 1996.

119. Whitehead BF, Stoehr C, Finkle C, et al: Analysis of bronchoalveolar lavage from human lung transplant recipients by flow cytometry. Respir Med 89:27, 1995.

119a. Silkoff PE, Caramori M, Tremblay L, et al: Exhaled nitric oxide in human lung transplantation. A noninvasive marker of acute rejection. Am J Respir Crit Care Med 157:1822, 1998.

119b. Fisher AJ, Gabbay E, Small T, et al: Cross sectional study of exhaled nitric oxide levels following lung transplantation. Thorax 53:454, 1998.

120. Dauber JH: Posttransplant bronchiolitis obliterans syndrome: Where have we been and where are we going? Chest 109:857, 1996.

121. Reichenspurner H, Girgis RE, Robbins RC, et al: Stanford experience with obliterative bronchiolitis after lung and heart-lung transplantation. Ann Thorac Surg 62:1467, 1996.

122. Keller CA, Cagle PT, Brown RW, et al: Bronchiolitis obliterans in recipients of single, double and heart-lung transplantation. Chest 107:973, 1995.

123. Sundaresan S, Trulock EP, Mohanakumar T, et al: Prevalence and outcome of bronchiolitis obliterans syndrome after lung transplantation. Washington University Lung Transplant Group. Ann Thorac Surg 60:1341, 1995.

124. Sarris GE, Smith JA, Shumway NE, et al: Long-term results of combined heart-lung transplantation: The Stanford experience. J Heart Lung Transplant 13:940, 1994.

125. Reichenspurner H, Girgis RE, Robbins RC, et al: Obliterative bronchiolitis after lung and heart-lung transplantation. Ann Thorac Surg 60:1845, 1995.

125a. Boehler A, Kesten S, Weder W, et al: Bronchiolitis obliterans after lung transplantation. Chest 114:1411, 1998.

126. Cooper JD, Billingham M, Egan T, et al: A working formulation for the standardization of nomenclature and for clinical staging of chronic dysfunction in lung allografts. International Society for Heart and Lung Transplantation. J Heart Lung Transplant 12:713, 1993.

127. Paradis I, Yousem S, Griffith B: Airway obstruction and bronchiolitis obliterans after lung transplantation. Clin Chest Med 14:751, 1993.
128. Wahlers T, Haverich A, Schäfers HJ, et al: Chronic rejection following lung transplantation: Incidence, time pattern and consequences. Eur J Cardiothorac Surg 7:319, 1993.
129. Bando K, Paradis IL, Similo S, et al: Obliterative bronchiolitis after lung and heart-lung transplantation: An analysis of risk factors and management. J Thorac Cardiovasc Surg 110:4, 1995.
130. Higenbottam T, Otulana BA, Wallwork J: Transplantation of the lung. Eur Respir J 3:594, 1990.
131. Ross DJ, Jordan SC, Nathan SD, et al: Delayed development of obliterative bronchiolitis syndrome with OKT3 after unilateral lung transplantation. Chest 109:870, 1996.
132. Glanville AR, Baldwin JC, Burke CM, et al: Obliterative bronchiolitis after heart-lung transplantation: Apparent arrest by augmented immunosuppression. Ann Intern Med 107:300, 1987.
133. Snell GI, Esmore DS, Williams TJ: Cytolytic therapy for the bronchiolitis obliterans syndrome complicating lung transplantation. Chest 109:874, 1996.
134. Ross DJ, Lewis MI, Kramer M, et al: FK506 "rescue" immunosuppression for obliterative bronchiolitis after lung transplantation. Chest 112:1175, 1997.
135. Milne DS, Gascoigne AD, Wilkes J, et al: MHC class II and ICAM-1 expression and lymphocyte subsets in transbronchial biopsies from lung transplant recipients. Transplantation 57:1762, 1994.
136. Ohori NP, Iacono AT, Grgurich WF, et al: Significance of acute bronchitis/bronchiolitis in the lung transplant recipient. Am J Surg Pathol 18:1192, 1994.
137. Duncan SR, Valentine V, Roglic M, et al: T cell receptor biases and clonal proliferations among lung transplant recipients with obliterative bronchiolitis. J Clin Invest 97:2642, 1996.
138. DeBruyne LA, Lynch JP 3rd, Baker LA, et al: Restricted V beta usage by T cells infiltrating rejecting human lung allografts. J Immunol 156:3493, 1996.
139. Reinsmoen NL, Bolman RM, Savik K, et al: Are multiple immunopathogenetic events occurring during the development of obliterative bronchiolitis and acute rejection? Transplantation 55:1040, 1993.
140. Reinsmoen NL, Bolman RM, Savik K, et al: Differentiation of class I- and class II-directed donor-specific alloreactivity in bronchoalveolar lavage lymphocytes from lung transplant recipients. Transplantation 53:181, 1992.
141. Schulman LL, Ho EK, Reed EF, et al: Immunologic monitoring in lung allograft recipients. Transplantation 61:252, 1996.
142. Hasegawa S, Ockner DM, Ritter JH, et al: Expression of class II major histocompatibility complex antigens (HLA-DR) and lymphocyte subset immunotyping in chronic pulmonary transplant rejection. Arch Pathol Lab Med 119:432, 1995.
143. Kramer MR: Bronchiolitis obliterans following heart-lung and lung transplantation. Respir Med 88:9, 1994.
144. Reinsmoen NL, Bolman RM, Savik K, et al: Improved long-term graft outcome in lung transplant recipients who have donor antigen-specific hyporeactivity. J Heart Lung Transplant 13:30, 1994.
145. Hertz MI, Jessurun J, King MB, et al: Reproduction of the obliterative bronchiolitis lesion after heterotopic transplantation of mouse airways. Am J Pathol 142:1945, 1993.
146. Edelman JD, Kotloff RM: Lung transplantation: A disease-specific approach. Clin Chest Med 18:627, 1997.
147. Shreeniwas R, Schulman LL, Narasimhan M, et al: Adhesion molecules (E-selectin and ICAM-1) in pulmonary allograft rejection. Chest 110:1143, 1996.
148. Ettinger NA, Bailey TC, Trulock EP, et al: Cytomegalovirus infection and pneumonitis. Am Rev Respir Dis 147:1017, 1993.
149. Duncan SR, Paradis IL, Yousem SA, et al: Sequelae of cytomegalovirus pulmonary infections in lung allograft recipients. Am Rev Respir Dis 146:1419, 1992.
150. Soghikian MV, Valentine VG, Berry GJ, et al: Impact of ganciclovir prophylaxis on heart-lung and lung transplant recipients. J Heart Lung Transplant 15:881, 1996.
151. Duncan SR, Grgurich WF, Iacono AT, et al: A comparison of ganciclovir and acyclovir to prevent cytomegalovirus after lung transplantation. Am J Respir Crit Care Med 150:146, 1994.
152. Magnan A, Mege JL, Reynaud M, et al: Monitoring of alveolar macrophage production of tumour necrosis factor-alpha and interleukin-6 in lung transplant recipients. Am J Respir Crit Care Med 150:684, 1994.
153. Magnan A, Mege JL, Escallier JC, et al: Balance between alveolar macrophages IL-6 and TGF-β in lung transplant recipients. Am J Respir Crit Care Med 153:1431, 1996.
154. Zeevi A, Uknis ME, Spichty KJ, et al: Proliferation of cytomegalovirus-primed lymphocytes in bronchoalveolar lavages form lung transplant patients. Transplantation 54:635, 1992.
155. Hohlfeld J, Niedermeyer J, Hamm H, et al: Seasonal onset of bronchiolitis obliterans syndrome in lung transplant recipients. J Heart Lung Transplant 15:888, 1996.
156. Milne DS, Gascoigne AD, Ashcroft T, et al: Organizing pneumonia following pulmonary transplantation and the development of obliterative bronchiolitis. Transplantation 57:1757, 1994.
157. Kshettry VR, Kroshus TJ, Savik K, et al: Primary pulmonary hypertension as a risk factor for the development of obliterative bronchiolitis in lung allograft recipients. Chest 110:704, 1996.
158. Yousem SA, Burke CM, Billingham ME: Pathologic pulmonary alterations in long-term human heart-lung transplantation. Hum Pathol 16:911, 1985.
159. Abernathy EC, Hruban RH, Baumgartner WA, et al: The two forms of bronchiolitis obliterans in heart-lung transplant recipients. Hum Pathol 22:1102, 1991.
160. Tazelaar HD, Yousem SA: The pathology of combined heart-lung transplantation: An autopsy study. Hum Pathol 19:1403, 1988.
161. Skeens JL, Fuhrman CR, Yousem SA: Bronchiolitis obliterans in heart-lung transplantation patients: Radiologic findings in 11 patients. Am J Roentgenol 153:253, 1989.
162. Morrish WF, Herman SJ, Weisbrod GL, et al: Bronchiolitis obliterans after lung transplantation: Findings at chest radiography and high-resolution CT. Radiology 179:487, 1991.
163. Lentz D, Bergin CJ, Berry GJ, et al: Diagnosis of bronchiolitis obliterans in heart-lung transplantation patients: Importance of bronchial dilatation on CT. Am J Roentgenol 159:463, 1992.
164. Worthy SA, Park CS, Kim JS, Müller NL: Bronchiolitis obliterans after lung transplantation: High-resolution CT findings in 15 patients. Am J Roentgenol 169:673, 1997.
164a. Leung AN, Fisher K, Valentine V, et al: Bronchiolitis obliterans after lung transplantation: Detection using expiratory HRCT. Chest 113:365, 1998.
165. Ikonen T, Kivisaari L, Taskinen E, et al: High-resolution CT in long-term follow-up after lung transplantation. Chest 111:370, 1997.
166. Hruban RH, Ren H, Kuhlman JE, et al: Inflation-fixed lungs: Pathologic-radiologic (CT) correlation of lung transplantation. J Comput Assist Tomogr 14:329, 1990.
167. Nathan SD, Ross DJ, Belman MJ, et al: Bronchiolitis obliterans in single-lung transplant recipients. Chest 107:967, 1995.
168. Kramer MR, Stoehr C, Whang JL, et al: The diagnosis of obliterative bronchiolitis after heart-lung and lung transplantation: Low yield of transbronchial lung biopsy. J Heart Lung Transplant 12:675, 1993.
169. Chamberlain D, Maurer J, Chaparro C, et al: Evaluation of transbronchial lung biopsy specimens in the diagnosis of bronchiolitis obliterans after lung transplantation. J Heart Lung Transplant 13:963, 1994.
170. Pomerance A, Madden B, Burke MM, et al: Transbronchial biopsy in heart and lung transplantation: Clinicopathologic correlations. J Heart Lung Transplant 14:761, 1995.
171. Cagle PT, Brown RW, Frost A, et al: Diagnosis of chronic lung transplant rejection by transbronchial biopsy. Mod Pathol 8:137, 1995.
172. DiGiovine B, Lynch JP 3rd, Martinez FJ, et al: Bronchoalveolar lavage neutrophils is associated with obliterative bronchiolitis after lung transplantation: Role of IL-8. J Immunol 157:4194, 1996.
172a. Ward C, Snell GI, Zheng L, et al: Endobronchial biopsy and bronchoalveolar lavage in stable lung transplant recipients and chronic rejection. Am J Respir Crit Care Med 158:84, 1998.
173. Bjortuft O, Geiran OR, Fjeld J, et al: Single lung transplantation for chronic obstructive pulmonary disease: Pulmonary function and impact of bronchiolitis obliterans syndrome. Respir Med 90:553, 1996.
174. Philit F, Wiesendanger T, Archimbaud E, et al: Post-transplant obstructive lung disease ("bronchiolitis obliterans"): A clinical comparative study of bone marrow and lung transplant patients. Eur Respir J 8:551, 1995.
175. Patterson GM, Wilson S, Whang JL, et al: Physiologic definitions of obliterative bronchiolitis in heart-lung and double lung transplantation: A comparison of the forced expiratory flow between 25% and 75% of the forced vital capacity and forced expiratory volume in one second. J Heart Lung Transplant 15:175, 1996.
176. Valentine VG, Robbins RC, Berry GJ, et al: Actuarial survival of heart-lung and bilateral sequential lung transplant recipients with obliterative bronchiolitis. J Heart Lung Transplant 15:371, 1996
177. Rajagopalan N, Maurer J, Kesten S: Bronchodilator response at low lung volumes predicts bronchiolitis obliterans in lung transplant recipients. Chest 109:405, 1996.
178. Martinez JAB, Paradis IL, Dauber JH, et al: Spirometry values in stable lung transplant recipients. Am J Respir Crit Care Med 155:285, 1997.
179. Siddiqui MT, Garrity ER, Husain AN: Bronchiolitis obliterans organizing pneumonia-like reactions: A nonspecific response or an atypical form of rejection or infection in lung allograft recipients? Hum Pathol 27:714, 1996.
180. Chaparro C, Chamberlain D, Maurer J, et al: Bronchiolitis obliterans organizing pneumonia (BOOP) in lung transplant recipients. Chest 110:1150, 1996.
181. Chadburn A, Cesarman E, Knowles DM: Molecular pathology of posttransplantation lymphoproliferative disorders. Semin Diagn Pathol 14:15, 1997.
182. Swerdlow SH: Classification of the posttransplant lymphoproliferative disorders: From the past to the present. Semin Diagn Pathol 14:2, 1997.
183. Mentzer SJ, Longtine J, Fingeroth J, et al: Immunoblastic lymphoma of donor origin in the allograft after lung transplantation. Transplantation 61:1720, 1996.
184. Knowles DM, Cesarman E, Chadburn A, et al: Correlative morphologic and molecular genetic analysis demonstrates three distinct categories of posttransplantation lymphoproliferative disorders. Blood 85:552, 1995.
184a. Chadburn A, Chen JM, Hsu DT, et al: The morphologic and molecular genetic categories of posttransplantation lymphoproliferative disorders are clinically relevant. Cancer 82:1978, 1998.
185. Schenkein DP, Schwartz RS: Neoplasms and transplantation: Trading swords for plowshares. N Engl J Med 336:949, 1997.
186. Aris RM, Maia DM, Neuringer IP, et al: Post-transplantation lymphoproliferative disorder in the Epstein-Barr virus-naïve lung transplant recipient. Am J Respir Crit Care Med 154:1712, 1996.
187. Walker RC, Paya CV, Marshall WF, et al: Pretransplantation seronegative Epstein-Barr virus status is the primary risk factor for posttransplantation lymphoproliferative disorder in adult heart, lung and other solid organ transplantations. J Heart Lung Transplant 14:214, 1995.
188. Chadburn A, Cesarman E, Liu YF, et al: Molecular genetic analysis demonstrates

that multiple posttransplantation lymphoproliferative disorders occurring in one anatomic site in a single patient represent distinct primary lymphoid neoplasms. Cancer 75:2747, 1995.

189. Chadburn A, Suciu-Foca N, Cesarman E, et al: Posttransplantation lymphoproliferative disorders arising in solid organ transplant recipients are usually of recipient origin. Am J Pathol 147:1862, 1995.

190. Weissmann DJ, Ferry JA, Harris NL, et al: Posttransplantation lymphoproliferative disorders in solid organ recipients are predominantly aggressive tumors of host origin. Am J Clin Pathol 103:748, 1995.

191. Harris KM, Schwartz ML, Slasky BS, et al: Posttransplantation cyclosporine-induced lymphoproliferative disorders: Clinical and radiologic manifestations. Radiology 162:697, 1987.

192. Dodd GD III, Ledesma-Medina J, Baron RL, et al: Posttransplant lymphoproliferative disorder: Intrathoracic manifestations. Radiology 184:65, 1992.

193. Carignan S, Staples CA, Müller NL: Intrathoracic lymphoproliferative disorders in the immunocompromised patient: CT findings. Radiology 197:53, 1995.

193a. Pickhardt PJ, Siegel MJ, Anderson DC, et al: Chest radiography as a predictor of outcome in post-transplantation lymphoproliferative disorder in lung allograft recipients. Am J Roentgenol 171:375, 1998.

194. Brown MJ, Miller RR, Müller NL: Acute lung disease in the immunocompromised host: CT and pathologic examination findings. Radiology 190:247, 1994.

194a. Collins J, Müller NL, Leung AN, et al: Epstein-Barr-virus–associated lymphoproliferative disease of the lung: CT and histologic findings. Radiology 208:749, 1998.

195. Montone KT, Litzky LA, Wurster A, et al: Analysis of Epstein-Barr virus-associated posttransplantation lymphoproliferative disorder after lung transplantation. Surgery 119:544, 1996.

196. Egan JJ, Hasleton PS, Yonan N, et al: Necrotic, ulcerative bronchitis, the presenting feature of lymphoproliferative disease following heart-lung transplantation. Thorax 50:205, 1995.

197. Gattuso P, Castelli MJ, Peng Y, et al: Posttransplant lymphoproliferative disorders: A fine-needle aspiration biopsy study. Diagn Cytopathol 16:392, 1997.

198. Paradis IL, Williams P: Infection after lung transplantation. Semin Respir Infect 8:207, 1993.

199. Husain AN, Siddiqui MT, Reddy VB, et al: Postmortem findings in lung transplant recipients. Mod Pathol 9:752, 1996.

200. de Hoyos AL, Patterson GA, Maurer JR, et al: Pulmonary transplantation: Early and late results. The Toronto Lung Transplant Group. J Thorac Cardiovasc Surg 103:295, 1992.

201. Kramer MR, Marshall SE, Starnes VA, et al: Infectious complications in heart-lung transplantation. Arch Intern Med 153:2010, 1993.

202. Ridgeway AL, Warner GS, Phillips P, et al: Transmission of *Mycobacterium tuberculosis* to recipients of single lung transplants from the same donor. Am J Respir Crit Care Med 153:1166, 1996.

203. Low DE, Kaiser LR, Haydock DA, et al: The donor lung: Infectious and pathologic factors affecting outcome in lung transplantation. J Thorac Cardiovasc Surg 106:614, 1993.

204. Maurer JR, Tullis E, Grossman RF, et al: Infectious complications following isolated lung transplantation. Chest 101:1056, 1992.

205. Mermel LA, Maki DG: Bacterial pneumonia in solid organ transplantation. Semin Respir Infect 5:10, 1990.

206. Herve P, Silbert D, Cerrina J, et al: Impairment of bronchial mucociliary clearance in long-term survivors of heart-lung and double-lung transplantation. Chest 103:59, 1993.

207. Marelli D, Paul AM, Nguyen DM, et al: The reversibility of impaired mucociliary function after lung transplantation. J Thorac Cardiovasc Surg 102:908, 1991.

208. Horvath J, Dummer S, Loyd J, et al: Infection in the transplanted and native lung after single lung transplantation. Chest 104:681, 1993.

208a. McDonald JW, Keller CA, Ramos RR, et al: Mixed (neutrophil-rich) interstitial pneumonitis in biopsy specimens of lung allografts. A clinicopathologic evaluation. Chest 113:117, 1998.

209. Flume PA, Egan TM, Paradowski LJ, et al: Infectious complications of lung transplantation: Impact of cystic fibrosis. Am J Respir Crit Care Med 149:1601, 1994.

210. Deusch E, End A, Grimm M, et al: Early bacterial infections in lung transplant recipients. Chest 104:1412, 1993.

211. Bangsborg JM, Uldum S, Jensen JS, et al: Nosocomial legionellosis in three heart-lung transplant patients: Case reports and environmental observations. Eur J Clin Microbiol Infect Dis 14:99, 1995.

212. Lyon GM, Alspaugh JA, Meredith FT, et al: *Mycoplasma hominis* pneumonia complicating bilateral lung transplantation: Case report and review of the literature. Chest 112:1428, 1997.

213. Bassiri AG, Girgis RE, Theodore J: *Actinomyces odontolyticus* thoracopulmonary infections: Two cases in lung and heart-lung transplant recipients and a review of the literature. Chest 109:1109, 1996.

214. Trulock EP, Bolman RM, Genton R: Pulmonary disease caused by *Mycobacterium chelonae* in a heart-lung transplant recipient with obliterative bronchiolitis. Am Rev Respir Dis 140:802, 1989.

215. Miller RA, Lanza LA, Kline JN, et al: *Mycobacterium tuberculosis* in lung transplant recipients. Am J Respir Crit Care Med 152:374, 1995.

216. Dromer C, Nashef SA, Velly JF, et al: Tuberculosis in transplanted lungs. J Heart Lung Transplant 12:924, 1993.

217. Gass R, Fisher J, Badesch D, et al: Donor-to-host transmission of *Mycoplasma hominis* in lung allograft recipients. Clin Infect Dis 22:567, 1996.

218. Schulman LL, Scully B, McGregor CC, et al: Pulmonary tuberculosis after lung transplantation. Chest 111:1459, 1997.

219. Shreeniwas R, Schulman LL, Berkmen YM, et al: Opportunistic bronchopulmonary infections after lung transplantation: Clinical and radiographic findings. Radiology 200:349, 1996.

220. Riddell SR: Pathogenesis of cytomegalovirus pneumonia in immunocompromised hosts. Semin Respir Infect 10:199, 1995.

221. Tazelaar HD: Perivascular inflammation in pulmonary infections: Implications for the diagnosis of lung rejection. J Heart Lung Transplant 10:437, 1991.

222. Anderson DJ, Jordan MC: Viral pneumonia in recipients of solid organ transplants. Semin Respir Infect 5:38, 1990.

223. Solans EP, Garrity ER Jr, McCabe M, et al: Early diagnosis of cytomegalovirus pneumonitis in lung transplant patients. Arch Pathol Lab Med 119:33, 1995.

224. Buffone GJ, Frost A, Samo T, et al: The diagnosis of CMV pneumonitis in lung and heart/lung transplant patients by PCR compared with traditional laboratory criteria. Transplantation 56:342, 1993.

225. Ohori NP, Michaels MG, Jaffe R, et al: Adenovirus pneumonia in lung transplant recipients. Hum Pathol 26:1073, 1995.

225a. Bridges ND, Spray TL, Collinis MH, et al: Adenovirus infection in the lung results in graft failure after lung transplantation. J Thorac Cardiovasc Surg 116:617, 1998.

225b. Palmer SM Jr, Henshaw NG, Howell DN, et al: Community respiratory viral infection in adult lung transplant recipients. Chest 113:944, 1998.

226. Flint A, Lynch JP 3rd, Martinez FJ, et al: Pulmonary smooth muscle proliferation occurring after lung transplantation. Chest 112:283, 1997.

227. Kanj SS, Welty-Wolf K, Madden J, et al: Fungal infections in lung and heart-lung transplant recipients: Report of 9 cases and review of the literature. Medicine 75:142, 1996.

228. Yeldani V, Laghi F, McCabe MA, et al: *Aspergillus* and lung transplantation. J Heart Lung Transplant 14:883, 1995.

229. Cahill BC, Hibbs JR, Savik K, et al: *Aspergillus* airway colonization and invasive disease after lung transplantation. Chest 112:1160, 1997.

229a. Nunley DR, Ohori P, Grgurich WF, et al: Pulmonary aspergillosis in cystic fibrosis lung transplant recipients. Chest 114:1321, 1998.

230. Kramer MR, Denning DW, Marshall SE, et al: Ulcerative tracheobronchitis after lung transplantation. Am Rev Respir Dis 144:552, 1991.

231. Tomee JFC, Mannes GPM, van der Bij W, et al: Serodiagnosis and monitoring of aspergillus infections after lung transplantation. Ann Intern Med 125:197, 1996.

232. Egan JJ, Yonan N, Carroll KB, et al: Allergic bronchopulmonary aspergillosis in lung allograft recipients. Eur Respir J 9:169, 1996.

233. Westney GE, Kesten S, De Hoyos A, et al: *Aspergillus* infection in single and double lung transplant recipients. Transplantation 61:915, 1996.

234. Tazelaar HD, Baird AM, Mill M, et al: Bronchocentric mycosis occurring in transplant recipients. Chest 96:92, 1989.

235. McDougall JC, Vigneswaran WT, Peters SG, et al: Fungal infection of the contralateral native lung after single-lung transplantation. Ann Thorac Surg 56:176, 1993.

236. Gryzan S, Paradis IL, Zeevi A, et al: Unexpectedly high incidence of *Pneumocystis carinii* infection after heart-lung transplantation. Am Rev Respir Dis 137:1268, 1988.

237. Rabodonirina M, Paulus S, Thevenet F, et al: Disseminated *Scedosporium prolificans (S. inflatum)* infection after single-lung transplantation. Clin Infect Dis 21:1067, 1995.

238. Martel S, Carre PC, Carrera G, et al: Tumour necrosis factor-alpha gene expression by alveolar macrophages in human lung allograft recipient with recurrence of sarcoidosis. Toulouse Lung Transplantation Group. Eur Respir J 9:1087, 1996.

239. Muller C, Briegel J, Haller M, et al: Sarcoidosis recurrence following lung transplantation. Transplantation 61:1117, 1996.

240. Martinez FJ, Orens JB, Deeb M, et al: Recurrence of sarcoidosis following bilateral allogeneic lung transplantation. Chest 106:1597, 1994.

241. Kazerooni EA, Jackson C, Cascade PN: Sarcoidosis: Recurrence of primary disease in transplanted lungs. Radiology 192:461, 1994.

242. Johnson BA, Duncan SR, Ohori NP, et al: Recurrence of sarcoidosis in pulmonary allograft recipients. Am Rev Respir Dis 148:1373, 1993.

243. Nine JS, Yousem SA, Paradis IL, et al: Lymphangioleiomyomatosis: recurrence after lung transplantation. J Heart Lung Transplant 13:714, 1994.

244. O'Brien JD, Lium JH, Parosa JF, et al: Lymphangiomyomatosis recurrence in the allograft after single-lung transplantation. Am J Respir Crit Care Med 151:2033, 1995.

245. Etienne B, Bertocchi M, Gamondes J-P, et al: Relapsing pulmonary Langerhans cell histiocytosis after lung transplantation. Am J Respir Crit Care Med 157:288, 1998.

246. Baz MA, Kussin PS, Van Trigt P, et al: Recurrence of diffuse panbronchiolitis after lung transplantation. Am J Respir Crit Care Med 151:895, 1995.

247. Parker LA, Novotny DB: Recurrent alveolar proteinosis following double lung transplantation. Chest 111:1457, 1997.

247a. Gabbay E, Dark JH, Ashcroft T, et al: Recurrence of Langerhans' cell granulomatosis following lung transplantation. Thorax 53:326, 1998.

247b. Habib SB, Congleton J, Carr D, et al: Recurrence of recipient Langerhans' cell histiocytosis following bilateral lung transplantation. Thorax 53:323, 1998.

247c. King MB, Jessrun J, Hertz MI: Recurrence of desquamative interstitial pneumonia after lung transplantation. Am J Respir Crit Care Med 156:2003, 1997.

247d. Verleden GM, Sels F, Van Raemdonck D, et al: Possible recurrence of desquamative interstitial pneumonitis in a single lung transplant recipient. Eur Respir J 11:971, 1998.

248. Frost AE, Keller CA, Brown RW, et al: Giant cell interstitial pneumonitis: Disease recurrence in the transplanted lung. Am Rev Respir Dis 148:1401, 1993.

249. Collins J, Kuhlman JE, Love RB: Acute, life-threatening complications of lung transplantation. Radiographics 18:21, 1998.

250. Judson MA, Handy JR, Sahn SA: Pleural effusions following lung transplantation: Time course, characteristics, and clinical implications. Chest 109:1190, 1996.

251. Herridge MS, de Hoyos AL, Chaparro C, et al: Pleural complications in lung transplant recipients. J Thorac Cardiovasc Surg 110:22, 1995.

252. Khan SU, Gordon SM, Stillwell PC, et al: Empyema and bloodstream infection caused by *Burkholderia gladioli* in a patient with cystic fibrosis after lung transplantation. Pediatr Infect Dis J 15:637, 1996.

253. Noyes BE, Michaels MG, Kurland G, et al: *Pseudomonas cepacia* empyema necessitatis after lung transplantation in two patients with cystic fibrosis. Chest 105:1888, 1994.

254. Paranjpe DV, Wittich GR, Hamid LW, et al: Frequency and management of pneumothoraces in heart-lung transplant recipients. Radiology 190:255, 1994.

255. Collins J, Love RB: Pulmonary torsion: Complication of lung transplantation. Clin Pulm Med 3:297, 1996.

256. De Hoyos A, Maurer JR: Complications following lung transplantation. Semin Thorac Cardiovasc Surg 4:132, 1992.

257. Anderson MB, Kriett JM, Harrell J, et al: Techniques for bronchial anastomosis. J Heart Lung Transplant 14:1090, 1995.

258. Date H, Trulock EP, Arcidi JM, et al: Improved airway healing after lung transplantation: An analysis of 348 bronchial anastomoses. J Thorac Cardiovasc Surg 110:1424, 1995.

259. Colquhoun IW, Gascoigne AD, Au J, et al: Airway complications after pulmonary transplantation. Ann Thorac Surg 57:141, 1994.

260. Semenkovich JW, Glazer HS, Anderson DC, et al: Bronchial dehiscence in lung transplantation: CT evaluation. Radiology 194:205, 1995.

261. Schlueter FJ, Semenkovich JW, Glazer HS, et al: Bronchial dehiscence after lung transplantation: Correlation of CT findings with clinical outcome. Radiology 199:849, 1996.

262. Quint L, Whyte R, Kazerooni E, et al: Stenosis of the central airways: Evaluation by using helical CT with multiplanar reconstructions. Radiology 194:871, 1995.

263. McAdams HP, Murray JG, Erasmus JJ, et al: Telescoping bronchial anastomoses for unilateral or bilateral sequential lung transplantation: CT appearance. Radiology 203:202, 1997.

264. Higgins R, McNeil K, Dennis C, et al: Airway stenoses after lung transplantation: Management with expanding metal stents. J Heart Lung Transplant 13:774, 1994.

265. Anzueto A, Levine SM, Tillis WP, et al: Use of the flow-volume loop in the diagnosis of bronchial stenosis after single lung transplantation. Chest 105:934, 1994.

265a. Yousem SA, Paradis IL, Dauber JA, et al: Large airway inflammation in heart-lung transplant recipients—its significance and prognostic implications. Transplantation 49:654, 1990.

265b. Flint A, Lynch JP, Martinez FJ, et al: Pulmonary smooth muscle proliferation occurring after lung transplantation. Chest 112:283, 1997.

266. Clark SC, Levine AJ, Hasan A, et al: Vascular complications of lung transplantation. Ann Thorac Surg 61:1079, 1996.

267. Sarsam MA, Yonan NA, Beton D, et al: Early pulmonary vein thrombosis after single lung transplantation. J Heart Lung Transplant 12:17, 1993.

268. Malden ES, Kaiser LR, Gutierrez FR: Pulmonary vein obstruction following single lung transplantation. Chest 102:645, 1992.

269. Michel-Cherqui M, Brusset A, Liu N, et al: Intraoperative transesophageal echocardiographic assessment of vascular anastomoses in lung transplantation: A report on 18 cases. Chest 111:1229, 1997.

270. Gaubert JY, Moulin G, Thomas P, et al: Anastomotic stenosis of the left pulmonary artery after lung transplantation: Treatment by percutaneous placement of an endoprosthesis. Am J Roentgenol 161:947, 1993.

271. Yousem SA, Paradis IL, Dauber JH, et al: Pulmonary arteriosclerosis in long-term human heart-lung transplant recipients. Transplantation 47:564, 1989.

272. Badizadegan K, Perez-Atayde AR: Pathology of lung allografts in children and young adults. Hum Pathol 28:704, 1997.

273. Kroshus TJ, Kshettry VR, Hertz MI, et al: Deep venous thrombosis and pulmonary embolism after lung transplantation. J Thorac Cardiovasc Surg 110:540, 1995.

274. de Hoyos AL, Patterson GA, Maurer JR, et al: Pulmonary transplantation: Early and late results. J Thorac Cardiovasc Surg 103:295, 1992.

275. Dromer C, Velly JF, Jougon J, et al: Long term functional results after bilateral lung transplantation. Ann Thorac Surg 56:68, 1993.

276. Herlihy JP, Venegas JG, Systrom DM, et al: Expiratory flow pattern following single-lung transplantation in emphysema. Am J Respir Crit Care Med 150:1684, 1994.

277. Murciano D, Pichot MH, Boczkowski J, et al: Expiratory flow limitation in COPD patients after single lung transplantation. Am J Respir Crit Care Med 155:1036, 1997.

278. al-Kattan K, Tadjkarimi S, Cox A, et al: Evaluation of the long-term results of single lung versus heart-lung transplantation for emphysema. J Heart Lung Transplant 14:824, 1995.

279. Briffa NP, Dennis C, Higenbottam T, et al: Single lung transplantation for end stage emphysema. Thorax 50:562, 1995.

280. Levine SM, Anzueto A, Peters JI, et al: Medium term functional results of single-lung transplantation for endstage obstructive lung disease. Am J Respir Crit Care Med 150:398, 1994.

281. Cheriyan AF, Garrity ER Jr, Pifarre R, et al: Reduced transplant lung volumes after single lung transplantation for chronic obstructive pulmonary disease. Am J Respir Crit Care Med 151:851, 1995.

282. Lloyd KS, Barnard P, Holland VA, et al: Pulmonary function after heart-lung transplantation using larger donor organs. Am Rev Respir Dis 142:1026, 1990.

283. Brunsting LA, Lupinetti FM, Cascade PN, et al: Pulmonary function in single lung transplantation for chronic obstructive pulmonary disease. J Thorac Cardiovasc Surg 107:1337, 1994.

284. Howard DK, Iademarco EJ, Trulock EP: The role of cardiopulmonary exercise testing in lung and heart-lung transplantation. Clin Chest Med 15:405, 1994.

285. Orens JB, Becker FS, Lynch JP III, et al: Cardiopulmonary exercise testing following allogeneic lung transplantation for different underlying disease states. Chest 107:144, 1995.

286. Gibbons WJ, Levine SM, Bryan CL, et al: Cardiopulmonary exercise responses after single lung transplantation for severe obstructive lung disease. Chest 100:106, 1991.

287. Ambrosino N, Bruschi C, Callegari G, et al: Time course of exercise capacity, skeletal and respiratory muscle performance after heart-lung transplantation. Eur Respir J 9:1508, 1996.

288. Levy RD, Ernst P, Levine SM, et al: Exercise performance after lung transplantation. J Heart Lung Transplant 12:27, 1993.

289. Pellegrino R, Rodarte JR, Frost AE, et al: Breathing by double-lung recipients during exercise. Am J Respir Crit Care Med 157:106, 1998.

290. Ross DJ, Waters PF, Mohsenifar Z, et al: Hemodynamic responses to exercise after lung transplantation. Chest 103:46, 1993.

291. Evans AB, Al-Himyary AJ, Hrovat MI, et al: Abnormal skeletal muscle oxidative capacity after lung transplantation by P-MRS. Am J Respir Crit Care Med 155:615, 1997.

292. Trachiotis GD, Knight SR, Hann M, et al: Respiratory responses to $CO_2$ rebreathing in lung transplant recipients. Ann Thorac Surg 58:1709, 1994.

293. Duncan SR, Kagawa FT, Starnes VA, et al: Hypercarbic ventilatory responses of human heart-lung transplant recipients. Am Rev Respir Dis 144:126, 1991.

294. Mattila IP, Sovijarvi A, Malmberg P, et al: Altered regulation of breathing after bilateral lung transplantation. Eur J Cardiothorac Surg 9:237, 1995.

295. Tapper DP, Duncan SR, Kraft S, et al: Detection of inspiratory resistive loads by heart-lung transplant recipients. Am Rev Respir Dis 145:458, 1992.

296. Peiffer C, Silbert D, Cerrina J, et al: Respiratory sensation related to resistive loads in lung transplant recipients. Am J Respir Crit Care Med 154:924, 1996.

297. Sanders MH, Costantino JP, Owens GR, et al: Breathing during wakefulness and sleep after human heart-lung transplantation. Am Rev Respir Dis 140:45, 1989.

298. Maurer JR, McLean PA, Cooper JD, et al: Airway hyperreactivity in patients undergoing lung and heart-lung transplantation. Am Rev Respir Dis 139:1038, 1989.

299. Glanville AR, Theodore J, Baldwin JC, et al: Bronchial responsiveness after human heart-lung transplantation. Chest 97:1360, 1990.

300. Higenbottam T, Jackson M, Rashdi T, et al: Lung rejection and bronchial hyperresponsiveness to methacholine and ultrasonically nebulized distilled water in heart-lung transplantation patients. Am Rev Respir Dis 140:52, 1989.

301. Herve P, Picard N, Ladurie MLR, et al: Lack of bronchial hyperresponsiveness to methacholine and to isocapnic dry air hyperventilation in heart/lung and double-lung transplant recipients with normal lung histology. Am Rev Respir Dis 145:1503, 1992.

302. Higenbottam T, Jackson M, Woolman P, et al: The cough response to ultrasonically nebulized distilled water in heart/lung transplantation patients. Am Rev Respir Dis 140:58, 1989.

303. Novick RJ, Stitt L, Schafers HJ, et al: Pulmonary retransplantation: Does the indication for operation influence postoperative lung function? J Thorac Cardiovasc Surg 112:1504, 1996.

304. Husain AN, Siddiqui MT, Reddy VB, et al: Postmortem findings in lung transplant recipients. Mod Pathol 9:752, 1996.

305. Caine N, Sharples LD, Dennis C, et al: Measurement of health-related quality of life before and after heart-lung transplantation. J Heart Lung Transplant 15:1047, 1996.

305a. TenVergert EM, Essink-Bot M-L, Geertsma A, et al: The effect of lung transplantation on health-related quality of life. Chest 113:358, 1998.

305b. Paris W, Diercks M, Bright J, et al: Return to work after lung transplantation. J Heart Lung Transplant 17:430, 1998.

306. Schulman LL: Quality of life after lung transplantation. Chest 108:1489, 1995.

307. Soubani AO, Miller KB, Hassoun PM: Pulmonary complications of bone marrow transplantation. Chest 109:1066, 1996.

308. Breuer R, Lossos IS, Berkman N, et al: Pulmonary complications of bone marrow transplantation. Respir Med 87:571, 1993.

309. Cahill RA, Spitzer TR, Mazumder A: Marrow engraftment and clinical manifestations of capillary leak syndrome. Bone Marrow Transplant 18:177, 1996.

310. Dickout WJ, Chan CK, Hyland RH, et al: Prevention of acute pulmonary edema after bone marrow transplantation. Chest 92:303, 1987.

311. Worthy SA, Flint JD, Müller NL: Pulmonary complications after bone marrow transplantation: High-resolution CT and pathologic findings. Radiographics 17:1359, 1997.

312. Robins RA, Linder J, Stahl MG, et al: Diffuse alveolar hemorrhage in autologous bone marrow transplant recipients. Am J Med 87:511, 1989.

313. Schmidt-Wolf I, Schwerdtfeger R, Schwella N, et al: Diffuse pulmonary alveolar hemorrhage after allogeneic bone marrow transplantation. Ann Hematol 67:139, 1993.

314. Srivastava A, Gottlieb D, Bradstock KF: Diffuse alveolar haemorrhage associated with microangiopathy after allogeneic bone marrow transplantation. Bone Marrow Transplant 15:863, 1995.

315. Kane JR, Shenep JL, Krance RA, et al: Diffuse alveolar hemorrhage associated

with *Mycoplasma hominis* respiratory tract infections in a bone marrow transplant recipient. Chest 105:1891, 1994.

316. Agusti C, Ramirez J, Picado C, et al: Diffuse alveolar hemorrhage in allogeneic bone marrow transplantation. Am J Respir Crit Care Med 151:1006, 1995.

317. Witte RJ, Gurney JW, Robbins RA, et al: Diffuse pulmonary alveolar hemorrhage after bone marrow transplantation: Radiographic findings in 39 patients. Am J Roentgenol 157:461, 1991.

318. Corso S, Vukelja SJ, Wiener D, et al: Diffuse alveolar hemorrhage following autologous bone marrow infusion. Bone Marrow Transplant 12:301, 1993.

319. Metcalf JP, Rennard SI, Reed EC, et al: Corticosteroids as adjunctive therapy for diffuse alveolar hemorrhage associated with bone marrow transplantation. Am J Med 96:327, 1994.

320. Chao NJ, Duncan SR, Long GD, et al: Corticosteroid therapy for diffuse alveolar hemorrhage in autologous bone marrow transplant recipients. Ann Intern Med 114:145, 1991.

321. Clark JG, Hansen JA, Hertz MI, et al: Idiopathic pneumonia syndrome after bone marrow transplantation. Am Rev Respir Dis 147:1601, 1993.

322. Wingard JR, Mellits ED, Sostrin MB, et al: Interstitial pneumonitis after allogeneic bone marrow transplantation. Medicine 67:175, 1988

323. Crawford SW, Longton G, Storb R: Acute graft-versus-host disease and the risks for idiopathic pneumonia after marrow transplantation for severe aplastic anemia. Bone Marrow Transplant 12:225, 1993.

323a. Shankar G, Bryson S, Jennings CD, et al: Idiopathic pneumonia syndrome in mice after allogeneic bone marrow transplantation. Am J Respir Cell Mol Biol 18:235, 1998.

324. Cone RW, Hackman RC, Huang MLW, et al: Human herpesvirus 6 in lung tissue from patients with pneumonitis after bone marrow transplantation. N Engl J Med 329:156, 1993.

325. Ettinger NA, Trulock EP: Pulmonary considerations of organ transplantation. Am Rev Respir Dis 144:213, 1991.

326. Clark JG, Hansen JA, Hertz MI, et al: Idiopathic pneumonia syndrome after bone marrow transplantation. Am Rev Respir Dis 147:1601, 1993.

327. Gollub MJ, Bach AM: Imaging of complications after bone marrow transplantation. Postgrad Radiol 15:255, 1995.

327a. Padley SPG, Adler BD, Hansell DM, et al: Bronchiolitis obliterans: High resolution CT findings and correlation with pulmonary function tests. Clin Radiol 47:236, 1993.

328. Crawford SW, Hackman RC: Clinical course of idiopathic pneumonia after bone marrow transplantation. Am Rev Respir Dis 147:1393, 1993.

329. Wyatt SE, Nunn P, Hows JM, et al: Airways obstruction associated with graft-versus-host disease after bone marrow transplantation. Thorax 39:887, 1984.

330. Ralph DD, Springmeyer SC, Sullivan KM, et al: Rapidly progressive air-flow obstruction in marrow transplant recipients: Possible association between obliterative bronchiolitis and chronic graft-versus-host disease. Am Rev Respir Dis 129:641, 1984.

331. Link H, Reinhard U, Blaurock M, et al: Lung function changes after allogenic bone marrow transplantation. Thorax 41:508, 1986.

332. Clark JG, Crawford SW, Madtes DK, et al: Obstructive lung disease after allogeneic marrow transplantation. Ann Intern Med 111:368, 1989.

333. Philit F, Wiesendanger T, Archimbaud E, et al: Post-transplant obstructive lung disease ("bronchiolitis obliterans"): A clinical comparative study of bone marrow and lung transplant patients. Eur Respir J 8:551, 1995.

334. Paz HL, Crilley P, Patchefsky A, et al: Bronchiolitis obliterans after autologous bone marrow transplantation. Chest 101:775, 1992.

335. Ostrow D, Buskard N, Hill RS, et al: Bronchiolitis obliterans complicating bone marrow transplantation. Chest 87:826, 1985.

336. Wyatt SE, Nunn P, Hows JM, et al: Airways obstruction associated with graft versus host disease after bone marrow transplantation. Thorax 39:887, 1984.

337. Urbanski SJ, Kossakowska JC, Chan CK, et al: Idiopathic small airways pathology in patients with graft-versus-host disease following allogeneic bone marrow transplantation. Am J Surg Pathol 11:965, 1987.

338. Krowka MJ, Rosenow EC, Hoagland HC: Pulmonary complications of bone marrow transplantation. Chest 87:237, 1985.

339. Han CK, Hyland RH, Hutcheon MA, et al: Small-airways disease in recipients of allogeneic bone marrow transplants: An analysis of 11 cases and a review of the literature. Medicine 66:327, 1987.

340. Clark JG, Schwartz DA, Flournoy N, et al: Risk factors for airflow obstruction in recipients of bone marrow transplants. Ann Intern Med 107:648, 1987.

341. Rosenberg ME, Vercellotti GM, Snover DC, et al: Bronchiolitis obliterans after bone marrow transplantation. Am J Hematol 18:325, 1985.

342. St. John RC, Gadek JE, Tutschka PJ, et al: Analysis of airflow obstruction by bronchoalveolar lavage following bone marrow transplantation. Chest 98:600, 1990.

343. Leblond V, Zouabi H, Sutton L, et al: Late CD8+ lymphocytic alveolitis after allogeneic bone marrow transplantation and chronic graft-versus-host disease. Am J Respir Crit Care Med 150:1056, 1994.

344. Beschorner WE, Saral R, Hutchins GM, et al: Lymphocytic bronchitis associated with graft-versus-host disease in recipients of bone-marrow transplants. N Engl J Med 299:1030, 1978.

345. O'Brien KD, Hackman RC, Sale GE, et al: Lymphocytic bronchitis unrelated to acute graft-versus-host disease in canine marrow graft recipients. Transplantation 37:233, 1984.

346. Shulman HM, Sullivan KM, Weiden PL, et al: Chronic graft-versus-host syndrome in man: A long-term clinicopathologic study of 20 Seattle patients. Am J Med 69:204, 1980.

347. Crawford SW: Bone marrow transplantation and related infections. Semin Respir Infect 8:183, 1993.

348. Lossos IS, Breuer R, Or R, et al: Bacterial pneumonia in recipients of bone marrow transplantation: A five-year prospective study. Transplantation 60:672, 1995.

349. Rege K, Mehta J, Treleaven J, et al: Fatal pneumococcal infections following allogeneic bone marrow transplant. Bone Marrow Transplant 14:903, 1994.

350. Hoyle C, Goldman JM: Life-threatening infections occurring more than 3 months after BMT. 18 UK Bone Marrow Transplant Teams. Bone Marrow Transplant 14:247, 1994.

351. Martino R, Martinez C, Brunet S, et al: Tuberculosis in bone marrow transplant recipients: Report of two cases and review of the literature. Bone Marrow Transplant 18:809, 1996.

351a. Ip MS, Yuen KY, Woo PC, et al: Risk factors for pulmonary tuberculosis in bone marrow transplant recipients. Am J Respir Crit Care Med 158:1173, 1998.

352. Peters EJ, Morice R: Miliary pulmonary infection caused by *Mycobacterium terrae* in an autologous bone marrow transplant patient. Chest 100:1449, 1991.

353. Kane JR, Shenep JL, Krance RA, et al: Diffuse alveolar hemorrhage associated with *Mycoplasma hominis* respiratory tract infection in a bone marrow transplant recipient. Chest 105:1891, 1994.

354. Lyytikainen O, Ruutu T, Volin L, et al: Late onset *Pneumocystis carinii* pneumonia following allogeneic bone marrow transplantation. Bone Marrow Transplant 17:1057, 1996.

355. Garcia-Arata MI, Otero MJ, Zomeno M, et al: *Scedosporium asiospermum* pneumonia after autologous bone marrow transplantation. Eur J Clin Microbiol Infect Dis 15:600, 1996.

356. Piliero PJ, Deresiewicz RL: Pulmonary zygomycosis after allogeneic bone marrow transplantation. South Med J 88:1149, 1995.

357. Cunningham I: Pulmonary infections after bone marrow transplant. Semin Respir Infect 7:132, 1992.

358. Nagler A, Elishoov H, Kapelushnik Y, et al: Cytomegalovirus pneumonia prior to engraftment following T-cell depleted bone marrow transplantation. Med Oncol 11:127, 1994.

359. Slavin MA, Golley TA, Bowden RA: Prediction of cytomegalovirus pneumonia after marrow transplantation from cellular characteristics and cytomegalovirus culture of bronchoalveolar lavage fluid. Transplantation 58:915, 1994.

360. Foot AB, Caul EO, Roome AP, et al: Cytomegalovirus pneumonitis and bone marrow transplantation: Identification of a specific high risk group. J Clin Pathol 46:415, 1993.

361. Enright H, Haake R, Weisdorf D, et al: Cytomegalovirus pneumonia after bone marrow transplantation: Risk factors and response to therapy. Transplantation 55:1339, 1993.

362. Rubie H, Attal M, Campardou AM, et al: Risk factors for cytomegalovirus infection in BMT recipients transfused exclusively with seronegative blood products. Bone Marrow Transplant 11:209, 1993.

363. Horak DA, Schmidt GM, Zaia JA, et al: Pretransplant pulmonary function predicts cytomegalovirus-associated interstitial pneumonia following bone marrow transplantation. Chest 102:1484, 1992.

363a. Ettinger NA, Trulock EP: Pulmonary considerations of organ transplantation. Am Rev Respir Dis 144:213, 1991.

363b. Ljungman P: Cytomegalovirus pneumonia: presentation, diagnosis and treatment. Semin Respir Infect 10:209, 1995.

364. Wendt CH, Weisdorf DJ, Jordan MC, et al: Parainfluenza virus respiratory infection after bone marrow transplantation. N Engl J Med 326:921, 1992.

365. Whimbey E, Elting LS, Couch RB, et al: Influenza A virus infections among hospitalized adult bone marrow transplant recipients. Bone Marrow Transplant 13:437, 1994.

366. Whimbey E, Vartivarian SE, Champlin RE, et al: Parainfluenza virus infection in adult bone marrow transplant recipients. Eur J Clin Microbiol Infect Dis 12:699, 1993.

366a. Matsuse T, Matsui H, Shu CY, et al: Adenovirus pulmonary infections identified by PCR and in situ hybridization in bone marrow transplant recipients. J Clin Pathol 47:973, 1994.

367. Hertz MI, Englund JA, Snover D, et al: Respiratory syncytial virus-induced acute lung injury in adult patients with bone marrow transplants: a clinical approach and review of the literature. Medicine 68:269, 1989.

368. Slavin MA, Meyers JD, Remington JS, et al: *Toxoplasma gondii* infection in marrow transplant recipients: A 20 year experience. Bone Marrow Transplant 13:549, 1994.

369. Wise RH Jr, Shin MS, Gockerman JP, et al: Pneumonia in bone marrow transplant patients. Am J Roentgenol 143:707, 1984.

370. Barloon TJ, Galvin JR, Mori M, et al: High-resolution ultrafast chest CT in the clinical management of febrile bone marrow transplant patients with normal or nonspecific chest roentgenograms. Chest 99:928, 1991.

371. Graham NJ, Müller NL, Miller RR, et al: Intrathoracic complications following allogeneic bone marrow transplantation: CT findings. Radiology 181:153, 1991.

372. Heussel CP, Kauczor HU, Heussel G, et al: Early detection of pneumonia in febrile neutropenic patients: Use of thin-section CT. Am J Roentgenol 169:1247, 1997.

373. Kuhlman JE, Fishman EK, Siegelman SS: Invasive pulmonary aspergillosis in acute leukemia: Characteristic findings on CT, the CT halo sign, and the role of CT in early diagnosis. Radiology 157:611, 1985.

374. Kuhlman JE, Fishman EK, Burch PA, et al: Invasive pulmonary aspergillosis in acute leukemia: The contribution of CT to early diagnosis and aggressive management. Chest 92:95, 1987.

375. Primack SL, Hartman TE, Lee KS, Müller NL: Pulmonary nodules and the CT halo sign. Radiology 190:513, 1994.

376. Noble PW: The pulmonary complications of bone marrow transplantation in adults. West J Med 150:443, 1989.

377. Seber A, Khan SP, Kersey JH: Unexplained effusions: Association with allogeneic bone marrow transplantation and acute or chronic graft-versus-host disease. Bone Marrow Transplant 17:207, 1996.

378. Salzman D, Adkins DR, Craig F, et al: Malignancy-associated pulmonary veno-occlusive disease: Report of a case following autologous bone marrow transplantation and review. Bone Marrow Transplant 18:755, 1996.

379. Williams LM, Fussell S, Veith RW, et al: Pulmonary veno-occlusive disease in an adult following bone marrow transplantation. Chest 109:1388, 1996.

380. Kuga T, Kohda KM, Hirayama Y, et al: Pulmonary veno-occlusive disease accompanied by microangiopathic hemolytic anemia 1 year after a second bone marrow transplantation for acute lymphoblastic leukemia. Int J Hematol 64:143, 1996.

381. Uderzo C, Marraro G, Riva A, et al: Pulmonary thromboembolism in leukaemic children undergoing bone marrow transplantation. Bone Marrow Transplant 11:201, 1993.

382. Cordonnier C, Fleury-Feith JM, Escudier E, et al: Secondary alveolar proteinosis is a reversible cause of respiratory failure in leukemia patients. Am J Respir Crit Care Med 149:788, 1994.

383. Mathew P, Bozeman P, Krance RA, et al: Bronchiolitis obliterans organizing pneumonia (BOOP) in children after allogeneic bone marrow transplantation. Bone Marrow Transplant 13:221, 1994.

384. Curtis RE, Rowlings PA, Deeg HJ, et al: Solid cancers after bone marrow transplantation. N Engl J Med 336:897, 1997.

385. Bhatia S, Ramsay NK, Steinbuch M, et al: Malignant neoplasms following bone marrow transplantation. Blood 87:3633, 1996.

386. Witherspoon RP, Deeg HJ, Storb R: Secondary malignancies after marrow transplantation for leukemia or aplastic anemia. Transplant Sci 4:33, 1994.

387. Lowsky R, Lipton J, Fyles G, et al: Secondary malignancies after bone marrow transplantation in adults. J Clin Oncol 12:2187, 1994.

387a. Sánchez J, Serrano J, Gómez P, et al: Bronchial mucoepidermoid carcinoma after allogeneic bone marrow transplantation. J Clin Pathol 50:969, 1997.

388. Matute-Bello G, McDonald GD, Hinds MS, et al: Association of pulmonary function testing abnormalities and severe veno-occlusive disease of the liver after marrow transplantation. Bone Marrow Transplant 21:1125, 1998.

389. Crawford SW, Pepe M, Lin D, et al: Abnormalities of pulmonary function tests after marrow transplantation predict nonrelapse mortality. Am J Respir Crit Care Med 152:690, 1995.

390. Sutedja TG, Apperley JF, Hughes JMB, et al: Pulmonary function after bone marrow transplantation for chronic myeloid leukaemia. Thorax 43:163, 1988.

391. Prince DS, Wingard JR, Saral R, et al: Longitudinal changes in pulmonary function following bone marrow transplantation. Chest 96:301, 1989.

392. Gore EM, Lawton CA, Ash RC, et al: Pulmonary function changes in long-term survivors of bone marrow transplantation. Int J Radiat Oncol Biol Phys 36:67, 1996.

393. Lung MB, Kongerud J, Brinch L, et al: Decreased lung function in one year survivors of allogeneic bone marrow transplantation conditioned with high-dose busulphan and cyclophosphamide. Eur Respir J 8:1269, 1995.

394. Carlson K, Backlung L, Smedmyr B, et al: Pulmonary function and complications subsequent to autologous bone marrow transplantation. Bone Marrow Transplant 14:805, 1994.

395. Badier M, Guillot C, Delpierre S, et al: Pulmonary function changes 100 days and one year after bone marrow transplantation. Bone Marrow Transplant 12:457, 1993.

396. Crawford SW, Fisher L: Predictive value of pulmonary function tests before marrow transplantation. Chest 101:1257, 1992.

396a. Torbenson M, Wang J, Nichols L, et al: Causes of death in autopsied liver transplantation patients. Mod Pathol 11:37, 1998.

397. Lisbon E, Wechsler RJ, Steiner RM: Pulmonary calcinosis following orthotopic liver transplantation. J Thorac Imaging 8:305, 1993.

398. Ettinger NA, Trulock EP: Pulmonary complications of organ transplantation. Am Rev Respir Dis 143:1386, 1991.

399. O'Brien JD, Ettinger NA: Pulmonary complications of liver transplantation. Clin Chest Med 17:99, 1996.

400. Sankey EA, Crow J, Mallett SV, et al: Pulmonary platelet aggregates: possible cause of sudden perioperative death in adults undergoing liver transplantation. J Clin Pathol 46:222, 1993.

401. Gosseye S, van Obbergh L, Weynand B, et al: Platelet aggregates in small lung vessels and death during liver transplantation. Lancet 338:532, 1991.

402. Agusti AG, Roca J, Rodriquez-Roisin R: Mechanisms of gas exchange impairment in patients with liver cirrhosis. Clin Chest Med 17:49, 1996.

403. Krowka MJ, Porayko MK, Plevak DJ, et al: Hepatopulmonary syndrome with progressive hypoxemia as an indication for liver transplantation: Case reports and literature review. Mayo Clin Proc 72:44, 1997.

404. Whyte MK, Hughes JM, Peters AM, et al: Analysis of intrapulmonary right to left shunt in the hepatopulmonary syndrome. J Hepatol 29:85, 1998.

405. Herve P, Lebrec D, Brenot F, et al: Pulmonary vascular disorders in portal hypertension. Eur Respir J 11:1153, 1998.

CHAPTER *46*

# *Eosinophilic Lung Disease*

The term *eosinophilic lung disease* encompasses a group of diverse disorders characterized pathologically by the accumulation of abundant eosinophils in alveolar air spaces and interstitial tissue. Peripheral blood eosinophilia is frequently prominent, and the eosinophil is believed to play a major role in the pathogenesis. Several classifications of these disorders have been proposed.[1-4] The most convenient divides them into groups with and without etiologies (Table 46–1); those of unknown origin are defined and distinguished from one another largely by their clinical features.

## EOSINOPHIL FUNCTION

The molecular biology, function, and role of the eosinophil in disease have been reviewed, and only a brief outline is presented here.[5-8a] The damaging effects of the eosinophil are determined by the cell's recruitment, activation, degranulation, and interaction with other inflammatory and immune cells; transgenic mice that experience massive accumulation of eosinophils that have not undergone these reactions remain healthy.[7]

The mechanisms by which eosinophils accumulate in disease include activation of adhesion pathways, selective chemoattractance, and cytokine-induced prolongation of survival.[7] For example, eosinophils are capable of selective binding to vascular cell adhesion molecule-1 on endothelial cells. This reinforces the effects of a number of chemoattrac-

tant cytokines to which eosinophils respond, including interleukin (IL)-5 (potentially derived from T lymphocytes, mast cells, and [in an autocrine fashion] eosinophils themselves),[9] IL-8,[10] platelet-activating factor (PAF),[11] and RANTES (derived from T lymphocytes and platelets). The life span of tissue eosinophils may be extended by systemic and local cytokines such as IL-5 and granulocyte-macrophage colony-stimulating factor (GM-CSF).[5]

A number of substances stimulate eosinophil function, including lipids such as leukotriene $B_4$; cytokines such as IL-5, IL-2, and GM-CSF; immunoglobulins; and tachykinins such as substance P.[5] Regulatory cytokines may be derived from T lymphocytes, mast cells, macrophages, epithelial cells, platelets, or eosinophils themselves. Following activation, eosinophils in bronchoalveolar lavage (BAL) fluid may differ functionally from those derived from the peripheral blood.[12-14]

Eosinophils contain a number of preformed mediators and enzymes within cytoplasmic granules; additional mediators also may be synthesized following appropriate stimulation. The most abundant preformed substance is major basic protein, a cationic protein highly toxic to helminths and host cells. Other preformed agents include eosinophilic cationic protein, eosinophil-derived neurotoxin, and peroxidase. Eosinophils can also synthesize inflammatory lipid mediators such as prostaglandins, a variety of oxygen radicals (including superoxide anion and hydrogen peroxide), several proinflammatory cytokines (including IL-3 and GM-CSF), and neuropeptides such as vasoactive intestinal polypeptide and substance P.

Eosinophils have a variety of interactions with other inflammatory cells, which are important in explaining the pathogenesis of the diseases in which the cell is implicated. Mast cell and basophil-derived mediators facilitate eosinophil function, and mast cells and eosinophils may interact to improve host defense.[5] Eosinophil products such as peroxidase enhance the toxic properties of neutrophils and macrophages; moreover, eosinophils may activate neutrophils through release of granular proteins. The interaction of endothelial cells with eosinophils is important in their extravascular migration and is mediated by a number of factors (e.g., tumor necrosis factor α).[14a] Eosinophil products may also activate platelets and certain platelet products, such as PAF and RANTES, which favor eosinophil migration in allergic asthma.[5] Lymphocytes produce cytokines, such as IL-2, which are powerful chemoattractants for eosinophils, as well as others that promote eosinophil longevity, activation, re-

**Table 46–1. EOSINOPHILIC LUNG DISEASE**

| CLASSIFICATION | DISEASE OR SPECIFIC AGENT | SELECTED REFERENCES | CLASSIFICATION | DISEASE OR SPECIFIC AGENT | SELECTED REFERENCES |
|---|---|---|---|---|---|
| *Idiopathic Eosinophilic Lung Disease* | Simple pulmonary eosinophilia | 16, 137 | Parasites | Ascariasis | 165 |
| | Acute eosinophilic pneumonia | 27, 34 | | Paragonimiasis | 166 |
| | Chronic eosinophilic pneumonia | 22, 43 | | Strongyloidiasis | 4 |
| | Hypereosinophilic syndrome | 83 | | Tropical eosinophilia | 122 |
| | | | | Pulmonary larva migrans | 167, 168 |
| *Eosinophilic Lung Disease of Specific Etiology* | | | | Schistosomiasis | 129 |
| | | | | Ancylostomiasis | 169 |
| Drugs | Aminosalicylic acid | 138 | | *Opisthorchis sinensis* | 4 |
| | Nonsteroidal anti-inflammatory agents | 139–141 | | Opisthorchiasis | 4 |
| | Inhaled beclomethasone dipropionate | 4 | Fungi | Allergic bronchopulmonary aspergillosis | *See* page 927 |
| | Bicalutamide | 65 | | Allergic bronchopulmonary disease caused by other fungi | 170, 171 |
| | Bleomycin | 142–144 | | | |
| | Captopril | 145, 146 | | Invasive aspergillosis | 172 |
| | Carbamazepine | 147 | | *Trichosporon terrestre* | 131 |
| | Chlorpromazine | 4 | | Coccidioidomycosis | 130 |
| | Cocaine | 109, 110 | Bacteria | Tuberculosis | 173 |
| | Cromolyn sodium | 148 | | Nontuberculous mycobacterial infection | 174 |
| | Ethambutol | 149 | | Brucellosis | 134 |
| | Gold | 150, 151 | Viruses | Respiratory syncytial virus | 175 |
| | Heroin | 111 | Connective tissue disease and vasculidites | Rheumatoid disease | 132, 133 |
| | Hydrochlorothiazide | 152 | | Wegener's granulomatosis | 136 |
| | Imipramine | 153 | | Churg-Strauss granulomatosis | *See* page 1506 |
| | Interleukin-2 and -3 | 4 | | Polyarteritis nodosa and related vasculidites | 134, 135 |
| | L-tryptophan | 110, 113 | | | |
| | Mecamylamine | 154 | Inhalation of toxic material | Fumes from synthetic rubber plant | 176 |
| | Methotrexate | 155 | | | |
| | Methylphenidate | 4 | | Scotchguard (trichloroethane) | 177 |
| | Minocycline | 157, 158 | | Nickel dust | 178 |
| | Nitrofurantoin | 159 | Miscellaneous abnormalities | Scorpion sting | 179 |
| | Para-aminosalicylic acid | 160 | | Eosinophilic enteritis | 180 |
| | Penicillin | 102 | | Inflammatory bowel disease | 181 |
| | Phenytoin | 161 | | Following bone marrow transplantation | 182 |
| | Procarbazine | 162 | | Angioimmunoblastic lymphadenopathy | 183 |
| | Pyrimethamine | 4 | | | |
| | Sulfonamides | 103 | | | |
| | Trazodone | 163 | | | |
| | Trimipramine | 164 | | | |

cruitment, and function. Eosinophils also may release mitogens promoting fibroblast function.[5]

The eosinophil mediates its effector function through nonoxidative, oxidative, and humoral mechanisms.[6] Several of the preformed granular basic proteins are directly cytotoxic; moreover, subtoxic concentrations of the same substances may stimulate other inflammatory cells. Some of these products have also been shown to augment airway hyper-responsiveness in primate models.[6]

## IDIOPATHIC EOSINOPHILIC LUNG DISEASE

### Simple Pulmonary Eosinophilia

Simple pulmonary eosinophilia (Loeffler's syndrome) is an uncommon pulmonary disorder characterized by local nonsegmental areas of parenchymal consolidation, usually transient, on chest radiographs and blood eosinophilia. Some include in this syndrome conditions that occur in association with a number of etiologic agents, particularly parasites;[15] however, it seems more reasonable to confine the use of the term to cases in which the etiology is unknown (up to one third of cases[16]), while categorizing cases with known causes as specific forms of eosinophilic lung disease. The documentation of seasonal variation in the prevalence of this disorder, as well as its association with atopy, suggest that unrecog-

nized environmental antigens may be responsible in some cases.[4]

### *Pathologic Characteristics*

Because of its benign and transient nature, the pathologic features of the parenchymal consolidation have rarely been documented. In the few cases in which biopsy findings have been reported, there has been interstitial and alveolar edema admixed with a large number of eosinophilic leukocytes.[16, 17] In a description of the ultrastructural features in one patient, the alveolar and capillary basement membranes were intact and devoid of immune deposits.[18]

### *Radiologic Manifestations*

The radiographic findings characteristically consist of transitory and migratory areas of parenchymal consolidation. These may be single or multiple and are usually homogeneous in density with ill-defined margins and a nonsegmental distribution in the lung periphery (Fig. 46–1).[19, 20] The peripheral distribution is particularly well seen on CT scans (Fig. 46–2). Although the transient and shifting nature of the consolidation is a characteristic feature, the term *fleeting* perhaps exaggerates the rapidity with which change may occur; we have seen several cases in which very little change was seen over a period of several days (*see* Fig. 46–1). Despite this, even a slight decrease in the size of one area

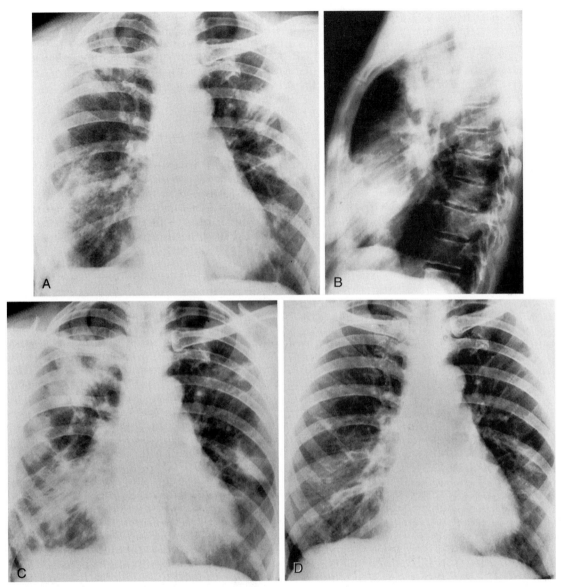

**Figure 46–1. Simple Pulmonary Eosinophilia.** Posteroanterior *(A)* and lateral *(B)* radiographs in a 61-year-old woman demonstrate bilateral areas of consolidation occupying no precise segmental distribution; note particularly the broad shadow of increased density along the lower axillary zone of the right lung. At this time her total white blood cell count was 11,000 per ml with 1,700 (15%) eosinophils. One week later *(C)*, the anatomic distribution of the areas of consolidation had changed considerably, being more extensive in the right upper and both lower lobes and less extensive in the left upper lobe; at this time the total white blood cell count was 14,000 per ml with 20% eosinophils. A diagnosis of simple pulmonary eosinophilia was made; treatment resulted in prompt remission of symptoms. One week later, the white blood cell count had returned to a normal level, the eosinophilia had disappeared, and the radiographic abnormalities had completely resolved *(D)*.

of parenchymal consolidation over a 24-hour period, if associated with a new area of consolidation, should suggest the diagnosis. To our knowledge cavitation, pleural effusion, lymph node enlargement, or cardiomegaly have not been described; however, pericardial effusion has been reported in some cases.[21]

The radiologic differential diagnosis includes the various entities in which a specific etiologic agent can be implicated, including drug- and parasite-induced eosinophilic lung disease.[22] It is also important to differentiate simple pulmonary eosinophilia from the more serious chronic eosinophilic pneumonia,[23] whose radiologic manifestations are very similar although more protracted *(see* farther on). It is also probable that some cases of mucoid impaction have been

misdiagnosed as simple pulmonary eosinophilia;[24] the distinction should be apparent in the majority of cases by the strictly segmental distribution of mucoid impaction compared with the nonsegmental and peripheral nature of involvement in simple pulmonary eosinophilia.

### Clinical Manifestations

Patients typically have few or no symptoms, the diagnosis often being suspected initially by the finding of characteristic opacities on the chest radiograph. A background of asthma and atopy is common.[24] A total white blood cell count of more than 20,000 per mm[3] is common, an increase in eosinophils being responsible for most of the elevation.

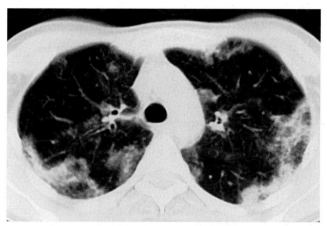

**Figure 46–2. Simple Pulmonary Eosinophilia.** A CT scan (10 mm collimation) shows bilateral areas of ground-glass attenuation and parenchymal consolidation in a characteristic peripheral distribution. The patient was a 21-year-old man.

When pulmonary parenchymal involvement is extensive, results of function tests usually indicate restrictive impairment, arterial oxygen desaturation, and a decrease in diffusing capacity.[25]

Symptoms and signs, if present, usually resolve spontaneously within 1 month.[4] A careful search should be performed for possible underlying causes of illness, such as parasites or drugs.

**Acute Eosinophilic Pneumonia**

Acute eosinophilic pneumonia is an acute febrile illness associated with hypoxemic respiratory failure, sometimes to the point of requiring mechanical ventilation, that was first described in 1989.[26, 27] Since that time, a number of isolated case reports have been published that have added to the clinical description of this disorder.[28–34] There appears to be no gender predominance, and patients of all ages have been affected.[29]

The pathogenesis of the disease is unknown. However, some workers have speculated that it may represent a hypersensitivity reaction to an unrecognized antigen.[27] In keeping with this hypothesis is the observation of an allergic diathesis in 10 of 13 patients in one series.[28] For unknown reasons and of unclear significance is the observation in one study of a significant difference in the expression of surface adhesion molecules on eosinophils in BAL fluid compared with those in peripheral blood.[35] In another study of two patients, levels of IL-5 and IL-1 receptor antagonist were high in BAL fluid when disease was active but fell with resolution of symptoms.[36] Lymphocytes (predominantly CD4⁺) and neutrophils are also increased in BAL fluid, suggesting that they may have a role in disease pathogenesis.[36a] Histologic examination of biopsies from affected patients shows diffuse alveolar damage (either acute or organizing) associated with a large number of interstitial and air-space eosinophils.[36b]

Both radiographically and on CT, the findings are similar to those of pulmonary edema. The earliest radiographic manifestation consists of reticular opacities, frequently with Kerley B lines (Fig. 46–3).[37] This progresses rapidly over a few hours or days to bilateral interstitial and air-space opacities involving mainly the lower lung zones.[37–39] Small bilateral pleural effusions are seen at some point in the course of the disease in the vast majority of patients.[40, 41] CT scans demonstrate bilateral areas of ground-glass attenuation, smooth interlobular septal thickening, small pleural effusions, and, occasionally, localized areas of consolidation or small nodules (Fig. 46–4).[39–41] In contrast to chronic eosinophilic pneumonia, a peripheral distribution is seldom seen.[37, 39]

Patients typically present with breathlessness, myalgias, and pleuritic chest pain. Physical examination reveals respiratory distress, fever, and bibasilar or diffuse crackles on auscultation of the chest.[4] Wheezing has been noted in patients in whom there is an associated bronchiolitis.[32] Peripheral eosinophilia is usually absent, although a marked elevation of BAL eosinophils—up to 80% in some patients[31]—is characteristic and is important in establishing diagnosis.[26–28, 30] Pulmonary function studies in patients who have eosinophilic infiltration of small airways show a low diffusing capacity and evidence of small airways dysfunction.[32]

Typically, there is a rapid response to corticosteroid therapy, although some patients have improved spontaneously. Unlike chronic eosinophilic pneumonia, relapse is not a feature. After therapy, lung function returns to normal.[26] It is important to distinguish the disease from drug reactions and fungal or parasitic infection, which can have similar clinical and laboratory manifestations. It is also important to keep in mind that patients who have fulminant respiratory failure may have an easily reversible cause of their disease.

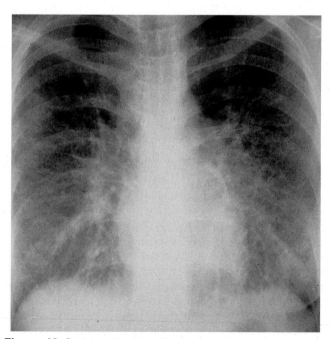

**Figure 46–3. Acute Eosinophilic Pneumonia.** A chest radiograph shows extensive bilateral interstitial changes with septal (Kerley) lines; blurring of the bronchovascular bundles is also evident. The appearance is similar to that of interstitial pulmonary edema. The patient was a 19-year-old Japanese woman. The diagnosis was proven by bronchoalveolar lavage, which demonstrated a large number of eosinophils. (Courtesy of Dr. Hiroshi Niimi, St. Marianna University School of Medicine, Yokohama, Japan.)

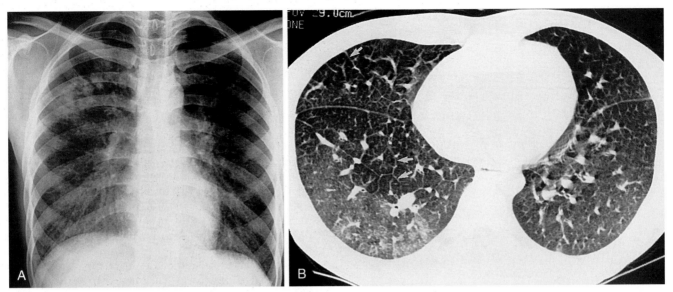

**Figure 46–4. Acute Eosinophilic Pneumonia.** A chest radiograph *(A)* reveals poorly defined asymmetric bilateral opacification, most marked in the right upper lobe. A high-resolution CT scan performed 2 days later *(B)* shows asymmetric bilateral areas of ground-glass attenuation. Mild interlobular septal thickening *(arrows)* is evident in the right lung. Transbronchial biopsy demonstrated numerous eosinophils and mononuclear cells in the alveolar spaces and alveolar walls. The patient was a 25-year-old man. (From Cheon JE, Lee KS, Jung GS, et al: Acute eosinophilic pneumonia: Radiographic and CT findings in six patients. Am J Roentgenol 167:1195, 1996. Courtesy of Dr. Kyung Soo Lee, Samsung Medical Center, Seoul, South Korea.)

## Chronic Eosinophilic Pneumonia

Although the term *chronic eosinophilic pneumonia* (CEP) was used originally in 1960,[42] a report by Carrington in 1969 is generally accepted as highlighting the clinical features that distinguish this disorder from other eosinophilic lung diseases.[23] A 1988 review summarized the literature to that date,[43] and a number of more recent series have supplemented this information.[28, 44-46] The chronicity, the severity of symptoms, and (at times) the radiologic appearance distinguish the condition from simple pulmonary eosinophilia. Women are affected twice as frequently as men; the peak incidence occurs between the ages of 30 and 39.[43]

The etiology is usually unknown, although occasional cases have been associated with *Aspergillus* infection,[47] rheumatoid disease,[48] and immune complex vasculitis in the skin.[49] The pathogenesis of the disease is also unclear; however, the frequent association with atopy and the high levels of circulating immunoglobulin (Ig) E reported during peak disease activity that return to normal during remissions, with or without treatment, suggest that it is a reagin-mediated hypersensitivity pneumonitis.[50, 51] Elaboration of cytokines such as IL-5, IL-6, IL-10,[52] and RANTES[53] in areas of affected lung seems to be important in pathogenesis, as does the presence in BAL fluid of activated helper lymphocytes.[54] Some workers have speculated that tissue damage may be related to the release of eosinophil granules, possibly in response to locally deposited immune complexes[55] or locally secreted IgA.[56] Evidence supporting this hypothesis includes the finding of high levels of eosinophilic cationic protein[57] and activated eosinophils[13, 58] in the BAL fluid of affected patients and the presence of a high level of circulating immune complexes[59] and complement activation[60] during flare-ups of disease.

There are several differences between the eosinophils obtained by BAL and those in the peripheral blood in pa-

tients who have CEP, including an increase in size[61] and the expression of surface CD69[62] and human leukocyte antigen (HLA)-DR[63] in the BAL population; the significance of these findings is not clear.

### Pathologic Characteristics

The predominant histologic finding is filling of alveolar air spaces by an inflammatory infiltrate containing a high proportion of eosinophils (Fig. 46–5).[23, 49, 55, 64] Although necrosis of lung parenchyma is unusual, aggregates of necrotic eosinophils surrounded by a rim of palisaded histiocytes ("eosinophilic microabscesses") are often present. Charcot-Leyden crystals can be seen free in the air spaces and in macrophages. The interstitium usually contains a similar, albeit less pronounced, inflammatory infiltrate and may show fibroblast proliferation and a mild increase in collagen.[23] Well-formed, nonnecrotizing granulomas are occasionally present.[23] Pulmonary vessels frequently contain scattered eosinophils and other inflammatory cells in their adventitia and, occasionally, media; however, true vasculitis (with evidence of necrosis or thrombosis) is not a feature. Airway epithelium may be ulcerated and associated with obliterative bronchiolitis,[23, 55] a finding possibly related to the development of obstructive airway disease in some cases.[55]

### Radiologic Manifestations

The radiographic pattern is identical to that of simple pulmonary eosinophilia (Loeffler's syndrome), consisting of bilateral, nonsegmental homogeneous consolidation in the lung periphery (Fig. 46–6).[43] This has led some observers to apply the designation "reversed pulmonary edema pattern" to emphasize the contrast with the perihilar or central distribution of pulmonary edema.[23, 66-68] Compared with the transitory and migratory character of the areas of consolidation in

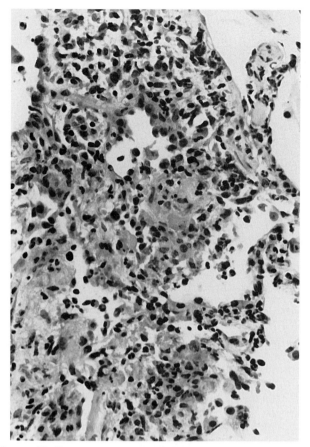

**Figure 46–5. Chronic Eosinophilic Pneumonia.** A magnified view of lung parenchyma shows numerous inflammatory cells (eosinophils, macrophages, and occasional neutrophils) in the alveolar interstitium and air spaces.

simple eosinophilic pneumonia, the lesions of CEP tend to persist unchanged for many days or even weeks unless corticosteroid therapy is instituted.

Although the reversed pulmonary edema pattern of consolidation, particularly if it affects mainly the upper lobes, is highly suggestive of CEP, it is not a universal finding. A review of the radiographic manifestations of 119 patients described in the literature by 1988 revealed that consolidation involved mainly the outer two thirds of the lungs in 74 (62%);[43] it was limited to the lung periphery in 30 cases (25%). Uncommon findings included evidence of cavitation (described in 5 of 119 cases), pleural effusion in 2, a nodular pattern in 3, and atelectasis in 2.

On CT, the peripheral distribution of the consolidation can be identified in virtually all cases (Fig. 46–7). In one review of the findings in six patients, chest radiographs and CT scans demonstrated bilateral consolidation involving mainly the upper and middle lung zones.[69] The peripheral distribution of the consolidation was apparent on the radiograph in only one of the six patients but was evident on CT in all. In another study of 17 patients, a peripheral distribution of consolidation was evident on the radiograph in 11 patients and on CT in 16.[70] Ground-glass attenuation may also be seen, usually in association with areas of consolidation but occasionally as an isolated finding.[70] Mediastinal lymph node enlargement has been reported in a small number of cases on CT[69, 71] and rarely on the radiograph.[71]

With treatment, improvement often occurs initially in the most peripheral areas of consolidation.[72] As the lesions clear, they may form bandlike opacities parallel to the pleura (Fig. 46–8).[70]

### Clinical Manifestations and Laboratory Findings

Atopy is present in about 50% of patients, asthma being the most common manifestation;[23, 28, 43] most patients are otherwise well before the onset of symptoms. In our experience and that of others,[23] there appears to be an unusual association with therapeutic desensitization to a variety of antigens. When disease develops, it is usually manifested by high fever, malaise, weight loss, cough, and dyspnea;[4, 23, 43] hemoptysis, chest pain, and myalgia occur rarely.[4] The onset of disease is frequently insidious; patients have disease for an average of 7.7 months before diagnosis.[43]

Laboratory investigation reveals blood eosinophilia in most patients, although its absence does not exclude the diagnosis when clinical and radiographic findings are compatible.[23, 43] Thrombocytosis has been described in one instance[73] as has a high carcinoembryonic antigen level in the blood.[74] Pulmonary function tests usually show a restrictive pattern with reduced diffusing capacity and impaired gas exchange, accompanied in some cases by severe hypoxemia during the acute phase.[43, 55, 75] Following remission, an obstructive ventilatory defect is a common finding. For example, in one study of 19 patients this was observed in 10;[76] eight of the remaining patients had normal lung function.

In our opinion and that of others,[77] the diagnosis can almost always be made on clinical and radiologic grounds alone without resorting to invasive procedures before institution of therapy. However, it has been confirmed by open biopsy and (occasionally) by needle biopsy[78] or fine-needle aspiration.[79] The presence of numerous eosinophils in BAL fluid also supports the diagnosis.[80, 81]

The response to corticosteroid therapy is characteristically dramatic, with rapid radiographic resolution and clear-cut clinical improvement within 24 hours.[23, 43] Most patients are completely well within 2 weeks,[43] although residual pulmonary fibrosis has been described.[82] Despite the obvious amelioration of symptoms and signs, many patients require therapy for months or even years; similarly, exacerbations are common when corticosteroids are reduced or stopped.[43, 44, 72]

### Hypereosinophilic Syndrome

Hypereosinophilic syndrome (HES, eosinophilic leukemia, disseminated eosinophilic collagen disease, Loeffler's fibroblastic parietal endocarditis) consists of prolonged blood eosinophilia associated with tissue infiltration by eosinophils and multiorgan disease. In one series of 50 patients reported from the National Institutes of Health in the United States, 35 (70%) noted the onset of disease between the ages of 20 and 50 years (mean, 33 years).[83] Although the sex incidence was not revealed in this series, other researchers have noted a male predominance.[84, 85]

Three criteria have been established for the diagnosis of idiopathic HES:[83] (1) persistent eosinophilia of 1,500 per mm³ for at least 6 months, or death before 6 months in

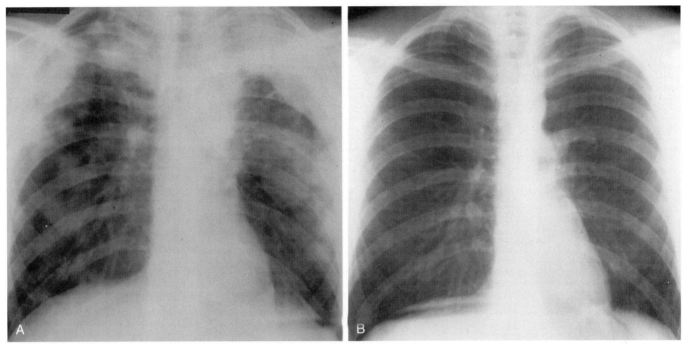

**Figure 46–6. Chronic Eosinophilic Pneumonia.** A posteroanterior chest radiograph *(A)* reveals bilateral air-space consolidation, predominantly upper lobe in distribution; note the highly characteristic peripheral (cortical) distribution of the disease *(B).* Following treatment with corticosteroids, the chest radiograph was normal. The patient was a middle-aged woman who presented with wheezing, cough, nocturnal fever, and blood eosinophilia.

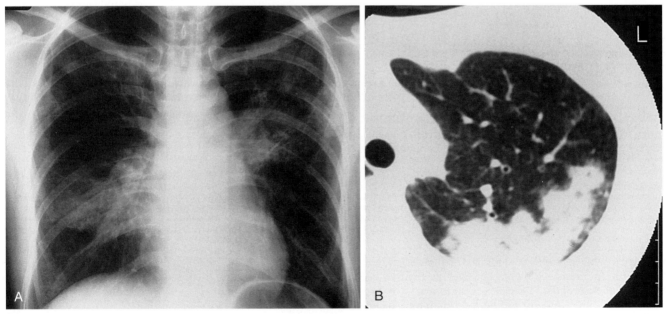

**Figure 46–7. Chronic Eosinophilic Pneumonia.** A posteroanterior chest radiograph *(A)* demonstrates bilateral perihilar and upper lobe consolidation. A peripheral predominance is not readily apparent on the radiograph. A conventional 10-mm collimation CT scan targeted to the left upper lobe *(B)* clearly demonstrates the peripheral distribution of the consolidation. The patient was a 42-year-old woman. (Courtesy of Dr. Hiroshi Niimi, St. Marianna University School of Medicine, Yokohama, Japan.)

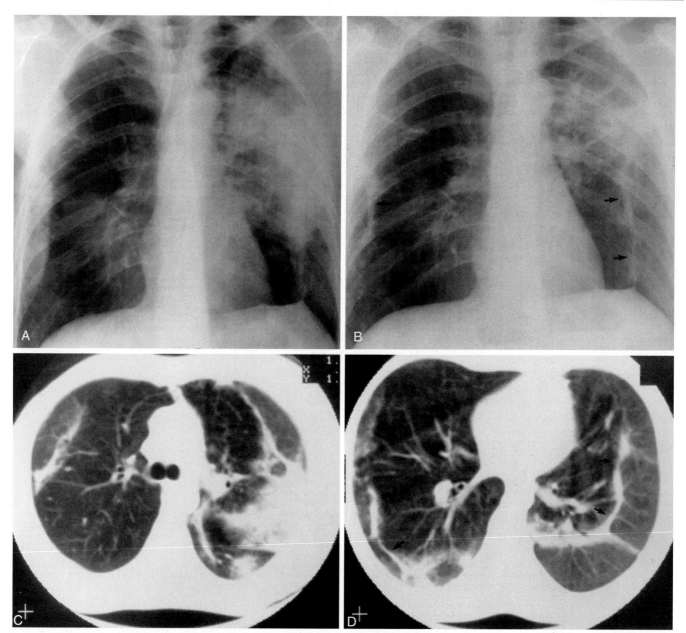

**Figure 46–8. Chronic Eosinophilic Pneumonia with Development of Vertical Linear Opacities During Resolution.** A posteroanterior chest radiograph *(A)* reveals peripherally located subpleural consolidation in both lungs, more marked on the left. Five days after institution of corticosteroid therapy *(B)*, considerable clearing of the consolidation had occurred; however, prominent bilateral vertical linear opacities *(arrows)* have appeared, sharply demarcating normal lung medially from abnormal lung laterally. CT scans through the upper and lower lobes *(C and D)* show thick, planar bands or stripes *(arrows)* that extend circumferentially around the lungs in the upper and lower lobes. The curvilinear opacities on the right are situated near the corticomedullary junction, whereas those on the left are somewhat more centrally located. Note that the lines separate normal medial lung from the peripheral shell of partially consolidated parenchyma. These opacities presumably represent the last vestiges of consolidation as clearing proceeds from peripheral to central regions. The patient was a 51-year-old woman who had cough, fever, and blood eosinophilia.

individuals with appropriate signs and symptoms; (2) lack of evidence for parasitic, allergic, or other recognized cause of eosinophilia; and (3) signs and symptoms of organ involvement, either directly related to eosinophilia or unexplained in the given clinical setting.

The cause is usually unknown; rarely, the syndrome occurs in a patient with an underlying disease such as eosinophilic leukemia.[83, 86] It is likely that the idiopathic form represents a heterogeneous group of disorders. In some patients, there is evidence of a disturbance of immunologic activity. For example, in the series of 50 patients cited

earlier, circulating immune complexes and elevated levels of IgE were found in approximately one third and a mild decrease in circulating T cells was found in a few.[83] Despite these findings, the increase in blood and tissue eosinophilia may be lymphocyte dependent, because abnormal clonal proliferation of T-helper lymphocytes has been described in patients who have the disorder.[4] The skin manifestations and the presence of bronchospasm in some patients also suggest an allergic pathogenesis.[83, 87, 88] As discussed previously, there is abundant experimental evidence indicating that the granular contents of eosinophils, particularly major basic protein and cationic protein, have potential tissue-damaging effects; the level of major basic protein has been found to be elevated in the serum of patients who have HES.[89]

Pathologic features of pulmonary disease have rarely been documented. Histologic examination in one case showed infiltration and cuffing of the small pulmonary arteries by eosinophils;[87] associated luminal obliteration can lead to parenchymal infarction. The presence of asthma is associated with bronchial changes characteristic of this disorder. Substantial pulmonary fibrosis may be found, usually in patients who also have HES-related heart disease.[83]

Initially, chest radiographs may reveal transient hazy opacities or areas of consolidation (Fig. 46–9) that can resolve spontaneously; sometimes these are associated with bronchospasm. CT may demonstrate focal parenchymal abnormalities even in patients who have normal radiographs (Fig. 46–10). When other organs are involved, an interstitial pattern has been described, presumably caused by perivascular eosinophilic infiltration or fibrosis.[37, 83, 87] Cardiac decompensation is eventually manifested by cardiomegaly, pulmonary edema, and pleural effusion.[90] Occasionally, pleural effusions are seen in patients without heart failure, possibly as a result of pulmonary thromboemboli.[91] Spontaneous pneumothorax has been reported.[92]

Initial symptoms are nonspecific, and the diagnosis is often considered only when leukocytosis and eosinophilia are detected. The major cause of morbidity and mortality is cardiac disease; the supportive structures of the atrioventricular valves are particularly prone to fibrosis, resulting in mitral and occasionally tricuspid insufficiency.[83, 91] Pulmonary arterial hypertension occasionally occurs in the absence of primary heart disease. Cough and dyspnea may reflect either pulmonary or cardiac involvement (or both).

Neurologic manifestations occur in two thirds of patients, as global central nervous system abnormalities (behavioral or cognitive), meningitis,[93] peripheral neuropathies,[94] or focal deficits resulting from embolization of cardiac mural thrombi.[83] Also present in many cases are dermatographism, angioedema of the skin, and hepatosplenomegaly caused by either eosinophilic infiltration or congestive heart failure.[90] HES has been reported to precede by 3 to 12 months or to occur concurrently with acute leukemia, usually lymphatic in type.[83, 92, 95]

There are no specific laboratory tests to confirm the diagnosis. A persistent peripheral leukocytosis and eosinophilia, a hypercellular bone marrow with eosinophilia of 25% to 75%, and evidence of multiorgan involvement should arouse suspicion. Anemia and thrombocytopenia are seen in some patients.[83] One group has reported that the circulating level of soluble IL-2 receptors correlates with disease activity and severity, a finding that underscores the apparent lymphocyte dependence of the eosinophilia.[96, 97] When the lung is affected by eosinophil tissue infiltration, BAL eosinophilia may be marked.[98, 99]

HES must be differentiated from all other causes of peripheral eosinophilia, including rheumatoid disease (which has been said to closely mimic idiopathic HES in some cases).[100] The importance of early recognition of the syndrome lies in the strong evidence that the prognosis is significantly improved if treatment is instituted promptly.[89, 101]

## EOSINOPHILIC LUNG DISEASE OF SPECIFIC ETIOLOGY

### Drugs

Drugs are an important cause of eosinophilic lung disease (*see* page 2537).[4] More than memorizing a lengthy and growing list of responsible medications, it is important for

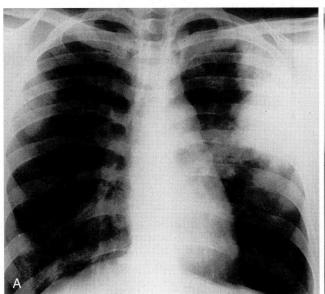 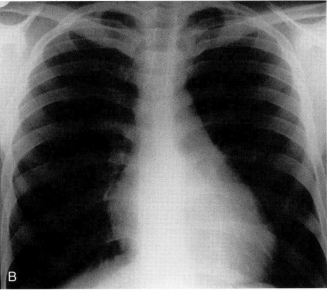

**Figure 46–9. Hypereosinophilic Syndrome.** A posteroanterior chest radiograph *(A)* shows asymmetric bilateral areas of consolidation involving predominantly the peripheral regions of the upper lobes. The patient was a 20-year-old man who had recently developed asthma and had marked eosinophilia. The parenchymal abnormalities resolved following treatment with corticosteroids; however, the patient subsequently developed myocarditis. A follow-up chest radiograph *(B)* demonstrates mild enlargement of the cardiac silhouette. The lungs are clear. (Courtesy of Dr. Christopher Flower, Addenbrooke's Hospital, Cambridge, England.)

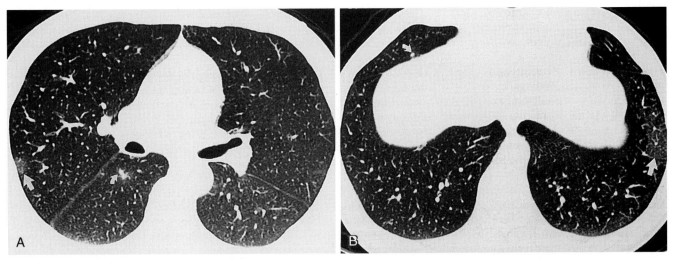

**Figure 46–10. Hypereosinophilic Syndrome.** High-resolution CT scans *(A* and *B)* demonstrate focal areas of ground-glass attenuation in the upper and lower lobes *(straight arrows)* and a few small nodules *(curved arrows)*. The chest radiograph was normal. The patient presented with a chief complaint of progressive cough. He had had peripheral eosinophilia for more than 6 months. On the current admission, bone marrow biopsy demonstrated 43% eosinophils. Abdominal ultrasound demonstrated hypoechoic lesions in the liver, biopsy of which showed eosinophil infiltration. Eosinophils were also increased in number in bronchoalveolar lavage fluid. (Courtesy of Dr. Eun-Young Kang, Korea University Guro Hospital, Seoul, Korea.)

the clinician to consider the reaction in any patient who presents with pulmonary opacities on the radiograph and blood or BAL eosinophilia and who has a history of drug exposure by any route. Reactions range from those similar to simple pulmonary eosinophilia to those resembling acute eosinophilic pneumonia. Implicated drugs include antibiotics,[102–104] nonsteroidal anti-inflammatory agents,[105, 106] drugs used for inflammatory bowel disease,[107, 108] and inhaled nontherapeutic drugs such as cocaine[109, 110] or heroin.[111]

An epidemic of a peculiar disorder, the eosinophilia-myalgia syndrome, deserves particular mention. This abnormality was first recognized in the late 1980s and has been shown to be caused by contaminants of a particular preparation of L-tryptophan.[112] Affected patients developed peripheral blood eosinophilia associated with an acute multisystemic illness that included scleroderma-like skin changes and severe myalgias. Pulmonary manifestations were common and included pneumonitis,[113] respiratory failure secondary to inflammation of respiratory muscles,[114] pleural effusion,[115] and pulmonary hypertension.[116, 117] Pulmonary function testing revealed a low diffusing capacity, with restriction due to parenchymal lung disease or myositis-associated chest wall weakness.[118, 119]

### Parasitic Infestation

Parasitic infestation is a common cause of eosinophilic lung infiltration and peripheral blood eosinophilia in "developing" countries. However, with increasing immigration to "developed" countries from these areas and with ever-increasing foreign travel, physicians should be familiar with the manifestations of these infections. All infestations are caused by metazoans, by far the majority from roundworms (nemathelminths). These diseases are described in greater detail in Chapter 30 *(see* page 1033), and only their salient features will be reviewed here.

One of the most commonly implicated parasites is *Ascaris lumbricoides.*[120] Pulmonary disease is caused by the third-stage larvae in their passage through the lungs; the response is allergic in type and invariably gives rise to blood eosinophilia. Radiographically, patchy areas of homogeneous consolidation are evident, in many cases transient and without clear-cut segmental distribution, a pattern characteristic of simple pulmonary eosinophilia. Leukocytosis of 20,000 to 25,000 per ml is common, with an eosinophilia of 30% to 70%; larvae may be found in the sputum or in gastric aspirates when pulmonary disease is active;[121] later, ova may be found in the stool.

The larval stage of *Strongyloides stercoralis* causes pulmonary disease during its migration through the lungs from pulmonary capillaries into alveolar air spaces. Because the life cycle can be perpetuated in humans indefinitely, the syndrome may be seen decades after the initial infection.[4] A mild to moderate leukocytosis, with eosinophilia, develops in the peripheral blood. In patients with hyperinfection there may be diffuse lung infiltrates, sepsis syndrome, and respiratory failure; peripheral blood eosinophilia may or may not be present.[4]

The nematodes *Ancylostoma duodenale* and Necator americanus exist in filariform larval stage in soil and infect humans by penetrating the skin. The larvae reach the pulmonary capillaries by way of the systemic veins, then migrate into the alveoli, and finally enter the esophagus and small intestine via the bronchi and trachea. Pulmonary disease appears to be less common than in *Strongyloides* infestation; however, severe infection may give rise to transient cough and hemoptysis, as well as radiographic evidence of nonsegmental homogeneous consolidation. The dog hookworm *Ancylostoma braziliense* causes a skin rash ("creeping eruption") that is associated with asymptomatic lung infiltrates of several weeks duration in about 50% of cases.[4]

Tropical eosinophilia results from infestation by several nematodes, the most common of which is *Wuchereria bancrofti.* Humans are infected from the bite of a mosquito, which introduces filariform larvae into the skin; mature worms develop and discharge microfilariae. The clinical presentation is one of asthma, frequently preceded by symptoms of fever, fatigue, weight loss, and anorexia.[122] The chest radiograph often shows a diffuse reticulonodular pattern, with hilar lymph node enlargement in some cases; ill-defined opacities or normal findings are seen occasionally.[121] Rarely, there is unilateral or bilateral nonsegmental consolidation.[123] HRCT is superior to radiography in demonstrating the pattern and extent of parenchymal abnormalities as well as the presence of mediastinal lymphadenopathy;[124] however, there is no correlation between the severity of parenchymal abnormalities on CT and pulmonary function or absolute eosinophil count.[124] The clinical manifestations are believed to be the result of the vigorous immune response directed against the microfilaria; this response is seen in only some hosts, in particular those of Indian origin, suggesting a genetic predisposition to the disease.[122] Leukocytosis is usually severe—60,000 white blood cells per ml is not unusual—with eosinophilia, sometimes as high as 60%. The eosinophils often show marked vacuolization,[125] a finding also described in patients with asthma.[126] High levels of filarial-specific IgE and IgG antibodies have been found in both blood and BAL fluid of affected patients; the observation that their levels parallel clinical activity of the disease suggests that they have a role in disease pathogenesis.[122] Pulmonary function studies may show air-flow obstruction and reduced diffusing capacity.[127] Some patients do not show complete resolution with therapy and may develop chronic restrictive interstitial disease associated with persistent eosinophilic alveolitis.[121, 128]

Pulmonary larva migrans results from infestation by larvae of the dog or cat roundworm *Toxocara canis* or *Toxocara cati.*[128a] It occurs predominantly in children who swallow soil containing eggs passed in the feces of dogs and cats; its association with pica makes some institutionalized individuals at special risk.[4] Radiographically, the chest shows local or diffuse, patchy, ill-defined opacities. Leukocytosis of 40,000 white blood cells per ml or more is common, usually with eosinophilia of at least 30%. Enzyme-linked immunosorbent assay testing is useful in confirming the diagnosis, and BAL eosinophilia may be noted.[127]

Schistosomiasis is the only parasite-induced eosino-philic lung disease caused by flatworm (platyhelminth) infestation. In the early stage of the infestation in some cases, metacercariae incite a local tissue reaction during their passage through the pulmonary capillaries, resulting in a picture of simple eosinophilic pneumonia.[129] The flukes *Opisthorchis sinensis* and *Opisthorchis viverrini* are also frequent causes of blood eosinophilia and pulmonary infiltrates in Asia.[4]

### Fungal Infection

The major fungal disease associated with pulmonary eosinophilia is allergic bronchopulmonary aspergillosis (*see* page 927); uncommonly, a variety of other mycotic organisms cause a similar hypersensitivity reaction. Coccidioidomycosis is also occasionally associated with significant eosinophilia.[130] The authors of one case report have suggested that inhalation of the fungus *Trichosporon terrestre,* which was found in the house dust of the affected patient, might cause acute eosinophilic pneumonia.[131]

### Connective Tissue Disease and Vasculitis

These diseases are characterized by their multisystemic nature and, in the majority of instances, immunopathogenesis. The most common of these that are associated with blood or tissue eosinophilia, or both, are allergic granulomatosis (Churg-Strauss syndrome, *see* page 1506) and rheumatoid disease.[132, 133] Occasionally, other conditions—including a variety of polyarteritis-like syndromes,[134, 135] giant cell arteritis,[6] and Wegener's granulomatosis[136]—are also complicated by significant eosinophilia.

### Miscellaneous Disorders

A number of other pulmonary disorders have been associated with peripheral or BAL eosinophilia (*see* Table 46–1). Although most are probably spurious associations, it is possible that some (e.g., viral bronchiolitis) may be pathogenetically related. Confusion may occur with many of the diseases discussed elsewhere in this chapter.

# REFERENCES

1. Crofton JW, Livingstone JL, Oswald NC, et al: Pulmonary eosinophilia. Thorax 7:1, 1952.
2. Citro LA, Gordon ME, Miller WT: Eosinophilic lung disease (or how to slice PIE). Am J Roentgenol 117:787, 1973.
3. Enright T, Chua S, Lim DT: Pulmonary eosinophilic syndromes. Ann Allergy 62:277, 1989.
4. Allen JN, Davis WB: Eosinophilic lung diseases. Am J Respir Crit Care Med 150:1423, 1994.
5. Kroegel C, Virchow JC, Luttmann W, et al: Pulmonary immune cells in health and disease: The eosinophil leucocyte (Part I). Eur Respir J 7:519, 1994.
6. Kroegel C, Warner JA, Virchow JC, et al: Pulmonary immune cells in health and disease: The eosinophil leucocyte (Part II). Eur Respir J 7:743, 1994.
7. Walker C, Braun RK, Boer C, et al: Cytokine control of eosinophils in pulmonary diseases. J Allergy Clin Immunol 6:1262, 1994.
8. Flier JS, Underhill LH: The immunobiology of eosinophils. N Engl J Med 324:1110, 1991.
8a. Rothenberg ME: Eosinophilia. N Engl J Med 338:1592, 1998.
9. Walker C, Bauer W, Braun RK, et al: Activated T cells and cytokines in bronchoalveolar lavages from patients with various lung diseases associated with eosinophilia. Am J Respir Crit Care Med 150:1038, 1994.
10. Erger RA, Casale TB: Interleukin-8 is a potent mediator of eosinophil chemotaxis through endothelium and epithelium. Am J Physiol 268:117, 1995.
11. Casale TB, Erger RA, Little MM: Platelet-activating factor–induced human eosinophil transendothelial migration: Evidence for a dynamic role of the endothelium. Am J Respir Cell Mol Biol 8:77, 1993.
12. Nishikawa K, Morii T, Ako H, et al: *In vivo* expression of CD69 on lung eosinophils in eosinophilic pneumonia: CD69 as a possible activation marker for eosinophils. J Allergy Clin Immunol 90:169, 1992.
13. Beninato W, Derdak S, Dixon PF, et al: Pulmonary eosinophils express HLA-DR in chronic eosinophilic pneumonia. J Allergy Clin Immunol 92:442, 993.
14. Morii T, Nishikawa K, Ako H, et al: Expression of activation antigen, CD69, on human local eosinophils. Jpn J Allergol 43:557, 1994.
14a. Erger RA, Casale TB: Tumor necrosis factor alpha is necessary for granulocyte-macrophage colony-stimulating-factor–induced eosinophil transendothelial migration. Int Arch Allergy Immunol 115:24, 1998.
15. Löffler W: Zur differential-diagnose der lungeninfiltrierungan. II. Über flüchtige succedan-infiltrate (mit eosinophilie). Beitr Klin Tuberk 79:368, 1932.
16. Ford RM: Transient pulmonary eosinophilia and asthma. A review of 20 cases occurring in 5,702 asthma sufferers. Am Rev Respir Dis 93:797, 1966.
17. Baggenstoss AH, Bayley EC, Lindberg DON: Löffler's syndrome. Report of a case with pathologic examination of the lungs. Proc Mayo Clin 21:457, 1946.
18. Bedrossian CWM, Greenberg SD, Williams LJ Jr: Ultrastructure of the lung in Löffler's pneumonia. Am J Med 58:438, 1975.
19. Peirce CB, Crutchlow EF, Henderson AT, et al: Transient focal pulmonary edema. Am Rev Tuberc 52:1, 1945.
20. Hennell H, Sussman ML: The roentgen features of eosinophilic infiltrations in the lungs. Radiology 44:328, 1945.
21. Hall JW III, Kozak M, Spink WW: Pulmonary infiltrates, pericarditis and eosinophilia. A unique case of the pulmonary infiltration and eosinophilia syndrome. Am J Med 36:135, 1964.
22. Israel HL, Diamond P: Recurrent pulmonary infiltration and pleural effusion due to nitrofurantoin sensitivity. N Engl J Med 266:1024, 1962.
23. Carrington CB, Addington WW, Goff AM, et al: Chronic eosinophilic pneumonia. N Engl J Med 280:787, 1969.
24. Chapman BJ, Capewell S, Gibson R, et al: Pulmonary eosinophilia with and without allergic bronchopulmonary aspergillosis. Thorax 44:919, 1989.
25. Morrissey JF, Gibbs GM: Pulmonary infiltration with eosinophilia occurring postpartum. Arch Intern Med 107:95, 1961.
26. Allen JN, Pacht ER, Gadek JE, et al: Acute eosinophilic pneumonia as a reversible cause of noninfectious respiratory failure. N Engl J Med 321:569, 1989.
27. Badesch DB, King TE Jr, Schwarz MI: Acute eosinophilic pneumonia: A hypersensitivity phenomenon? Am Rev Respir Dis 139:249, 1989.
28. Hayakawa H, Sato A, Toyoshima M, et al: A clinical study of idiopathic eosinophilic pneumonia. Chest 105:462, 1994.
29. Buchheit J, Eid N, Rodgers G, et al: Acute eosinophilic pneumonia with respiratory failure: A new syndrome. Am Rev Respir Dis 145:716, 1992.
30. Ogawa H, Nakamura H, Takayanagi N, et al: A case report and literature review of acute eosinophilic pneumonia. Jpn J Thoracic Dis 29:746, 1991.
31. Arakawa H, Nakajima Y, Kurihara Y, et al: Acute eosinophilic pneumonia: A report of two cases. Nippon Acta Radiologica 53:911, 1993.
32. Ogawa H, Fujimura M, Matsuda T, et al: Transient wheeze. Eosinophilic bronchobronchiolitis in acute eosinophilic pneumonia. Chest 104:493, 1993.
33. Tazelaar HD, Linz LJ, Colby TV, et al: Acute eosinophilic pneumonia: Histopathologic findings in nine patients. Am J Respir Crit Care Med 155:296, 1997.
34. Pope-Harman AL, Davis WB, Allen ED, et al: Acute eosinophilic pneumonia. A summary of 15 cases and review of the literature. Medicine (Baltimore) 75:334, 1996.
35. Okubo Y, Hossain M, Kai R, et al: Adhesion molecules on eosinophils in acute eosinophilic pneumonia. Am J Respir Crit Care Med 151:1259, 1995.
36. Allen JN, Liao Z, Wewers MD, et al: Detection of IL-5 and IL-1 receptor antagonist in bronchoalveolar lavage fluid in acute eosinophilic pneumonia. J Allergy Clin Immunol 97:1366, 1996.
36a. Fujimura M, Yasui M, Shinagawa S, et al: Bronchoalveolar lavage cell findings in three types of eosinophilic pneumonia: Acute, chronic and drug-induced eosinophilic pneumonia. Respir Med 92:743, 1998.
36b. Tazellaar HD, Linz LJ, Colby TV, et al: Acute eosinophilic pneumonia: Histopathologic findings in nine patients. Am J Respir Crit Care Med 155:296, 1997.
37. Allen JN, Davis WB: Eosinophilic lung diseases. Am J Respir Crit Care Med 150:1423, 1994.
38. Allen JN, Pacht ER, Gadek JE, et al: Acute eosinophilic pneumonia as a reversible cause of noninfectious respiratory failure. N Engl J Med 321:569, 1989.
39. Hayakawa H, Sato A, Toyoshima M, et al: A clinical study of idiopathic eosinophilic pneumonia. Chest 105:1462, 1994.
40. Cheon JE, Lee KS, Jung GS, et al: Acute eosinophilic pneumonia: Radiographic and CT findings in six patients. Am J Roentgenol 167:1195, 1996.
41. King MA, Pope-Harman AL, Allen JN, et al: Acute eosinophilic pneumonia: Radiologic and clinical features. Radiology 203:715, 1997.
42. Christoforidis AJ, Molnar W: Eosinophilic pneumonia: Report of two cases with pulmonary biopsy. JAMA 173:157, 1960.
43. Jederlinic PJ, Sicilian L, Gaensler EA: Chronic eosinophilic pneumonia: A report of 19 cases and a review of the literature. Medicine 67:154, 1988.
44. Naughton M, Fahy J, Fitzgerald MX: Chronic eosinophilic pneumonia. Chest 103:162, 1993.
45. Capewell S, Chapman BJ, Alexander F, et al: Pulmonary eosinophilia with systemic features: Therapy and prognosis. Respir Med 86:485, 1992.
46. Umeki S, Soejima R: Acute and chronic eosinophilic pneumonia: Clinical evaluation and the criteria. Intern Med 31:847, 1992.
47. Warnock ML, Fennessy J, Rippon J: Chronic eosinophilic pneumonia. A manifestation of allergic aspergillosis. Am J Clin Pathol 62:73, 1976.
48. Cooney TP: Interrelationship of chronic eosinophilic pneumonia, bronchiolitis obliterans and rheumatoid disease: A hypothesis. J Clin Pathol 34:129, 1981.
49. Chan NH, Boyko WJ, Schellenberg RR, et al: A case of eosinophilic pneumonia. Unusual immune complex vasculitis in the skin. Chest 82:113, 1982.
50. McEvoy JDS, Donald KJ, Edwards RL: Immunoglobulin levels and electron microscopy in eosinophilic pneumonia. Am J Med 64:529, 1978.
51. Turner-Warwick M, Assem ESK, Lockwood M: Cryptogenic pulmonary eosinophilia. Clin Allergy 6:135, 1976.
52. Kita H, Sur S, Hunt LW, et al: Cytokine production at the site of disease in chronic eosinophilic pneumonia. Am J Respir Crit Care Med 153:1437, 1996.
53. Kurashima K, Mukaida N, Fujimura M, et al: A specific elevation of RANTES in bronchoalveolar lavage fluids of patients with chronic eosinophilic pneumonia. Lab Invest 76:67, 1997.
54. Mukae H, Kadota J, Kohno S, et al: Increase of activated T-cells in BAL fluid of Japanese patients with bronchiolitis obliterans organizing pneumonia and chronic eosinophilic pneumonia. Chest 108:123, 1995.
55. Fox B, Seed WA: Chronic eosinophilic pneumonia. Thorax 35:570, 1980.
56. Boomars KA, van Velzen-Blad H, Mulder PG, et al: Eosinophil cationic protein and immunoglobulin levels in bronchoalveolar lavage fluid from patients with chronic eosinophilic pneumonia. Eur Respir J 9:2488, 1996.
57. Shijubo N, Shigehara K, Hirasawa M, et al: Eosinophilic cationic protein in chronic eosinophilic pneumonia and eosinophilic granuloma. Chest 106:1481, 1994.
58. Kroegel C, Matthys H, Costabel U, et al: Morphology and density features of eosinophil leukocytes in eosinophilic pneumonia. Clin Invest 70:447, 1992.
59. Demedts M, De Man F: Circulating immune complexes in chronic eosinophilic pneumonia. Acta Clin Belg 46:75, 1991.
60. Abe M, Gouya T, Tanaka K, et al: Evaluation of complement in patients with eosinophilic pneumonia. Intern Med 31:717, 1992.
61. Kroegel C, Matthys H, Costabel U: Morphology and density features of eosinophil leukocytes in eosinophilic pneumonia. A case report. Clin Invest 70:447, 1992.
62. Nishikawa K, Morii T, Ako H, et al: *In vivo* expression of CD69 on lung eosinophils in eosinophilic pneumonia: CD69 as a possible activation marker for eosinophils. J Allergy Clin Immunol 90:169, 1992.
63. Beninati W, Derdak S, Dixon PF, et al: Pulmonary eosinophils express HLA-DR in chronic eosinophilic pneumonia. J Allergy Clin Immunol 92:442, 1993.
64. Libby DM, Murphy TF, Edwards A, et al: Chronic eosinophilic pneumonia: An unusual cause of acute respiratory failure. Am Rev Respir Dis 122:497, 1980.
65. Wong PW, Macris N, DiFabrizio L, et al: Eosinophilic lung disease induced by bicalutamide: A case report and review of the medical literature. Chest 113:548, 1998.
66. Weinberg AN, Nash G: Recurrent bilateral pulmonary infiltrates with eosinophilia. N Engl J Med 286:1205, 1972.
67. Acetao JN: Fluctuating, peripheral pulmonary infiltrates. Chest 61:89, 1972.
68. Gaensler EA, Carrington CB: Peripheral opacities in chronic eosinophilic pneumonia: The photographic negative of pulmonary edema. Am J Roentgenol 128:1, 1977.
69. Mayo JR, Müller NL, Road J, et al: Chronic eosinophilic pneumonia: CT findings in six cases. Am J Roentgenol 153:727, 1989.
70. Ebara H, Ikezoe J, Johkoh T, et al: Chronic eosinophilic pneumonia: Evolution of chest radiograms and CT features. J Comput Assist Tomogr 18:737, 1994.

71. Zaki I, Wears R, Parnell A, et al: Case report: Mediastinal lymphadenopathy in eosinophilic pneumonia. Clin Radiol 48:61, 1993.

72. Pearson DJ, Rosenow EC III: Chronic eosinophilic pneumonia (Carrington's). A follow-up study. Mayo Clin Proc 53:73, 1978.

73. Brezis M, Lafair J: Thrombocytosis in chronic eosinophilic pneumonia. Chest 76:231, 1979.

74. Ashitani J, Sakamoto A, Maki H, et al: A case of eosinophilic pneumonia with elevated levels of carcino-embryonic antigen. Jpn J Thoracic Dis 32:1194, 1994.

75. Rogers RM, Christiansen JR, Coalson JJ, et al: Eosinophilic pneumonia. Physiologic response to steroid therapy and observations on light and electron microscopic findings. Chest 68:665, 1975.

76. Durieu J, Wallaert B, Tonnel AB: Long-term follow-up of pulmonary function in chronic eosinophilic pneumonia. Eur Respir J 10:286, 1997.

77. Douglas NJ, Goetzl EJ: Pulmonary eosinophilia and eosinophilic granuloma. In Murray JF, Nadel JA (eds): Textbook of Respiratory Medicine. 2nd ed. Philadelphia, WB Saunders, 1994, p 1923.

78. Perrault JL, Janis M, Wolinsky H: Resolution of chronic eosinophilic pneumonia with corticoid therapy. Demonstration by needle biopsy. Ann Intern Med 74:951, 1971.

79. Ramzy I, Geraghty R, Lefcoe MS, et al: Chronic eosinophilic pneumonia. Diagnosis by fine needle aspiration. Acta Cytol 22:366, 1978.

80. Lieske TR, Sunderrajan EV, Bassamonte PM: Bronchoalveolar lavage and technetium-99m glucoheptonate imaging in chronic eosinophilic pneumonia. Chest 85:282, 1984.

81. Dejaegher P, Dervaux L, Dubois P, et al: Eosinophilic pneumonia without radiographic pulmonary infiltrates. Chest 84:637, 1983.

82. Yoshida K, Shijubo N, Koba H, et al: Chronic eosinophilic pneumonia progressing to lung fibrosis. Eur Respir J 7:1541, 1994.

83. Fauci AS, Harley JB, Roberts WC, et al: The idiopathic hypereosinophilic syndrome. Ann Intern Med 97:78, 1982.

84. Clinicopathologic Conference: Hypereosinophilic syndrome with pulmonary hypertension. Am J Med 60:239, 1976.

85. Clinicopathologic Conference: Disseminated eosinophilic collagen disease. Am J Med 56:221, 1974.

86. Benevenisti DS, Ultmann JE: Eosinophilic leukemia: Report of five cases and review of literature. Ann Intern Med 71:731, 1969.

87. Hill R, Wang NS, Berry G: Hypereosinophilic syndrome with pulmonary vascular involvement. Angiology 35:238, 1984.

88. Bush RK, Geller M, Busse WW, et al: Response to corticosteroids in the hypereosinophilic syndrome: Association with increased serum IgE levels. Arch Intern Med 138:1244, 1978.

89. Butterfield JH, Gleich GJ: Interferon-alpha treatment of six patients with the hypereosinophilic syndrome. Ann Intern Med 121:648, 1994.

90. Epstein DM, Taormina V, Gefter WB, et al: The hypereosinophilic syndrome. Radiology 140:59, 1981.

91. Chusid MJ, Dale DC, West BC, et al: The hypereosinophilic syndrome: Analysis of fourteen cases with review of the literature. Medicine 54:1, 1975.

92. Geltner D, Friedman G, Naparstek E, et al: Acute lymphoblastic leukemia: Its occurrence with "hypereosinophilic syndrome" and bilateral spontaneous pneumothorax. Arch Intern Med 138:292, 1978.

93. Weingarten JS, O'Sheal SF, Margolis WS: Eosinophilic meningitis and the hypereosinophilic syndrome: Case report and review of the literature. Am J Med 78:674, 1985.

94. Purdie GH, Kotasek D, Rischbieth RH: The hypereosinophilic syndrome. Clin Exp Neurol 19:60, 1983.

95. Troxell ML, Mills GM, Allen RC: The hypereosinophilic syndrome in acute lymphocytic leukemia. Cancer 54:1058, 1984.

96. Prin L, Plumas J, Gruart V, et al: Elevated serum levels of soluble interleukin-2 receptor: A marker of disease activity in the hypereosinophilic syndrome. Blood 78:2626, 1991.

97. Plumas J, Gruart V, Capron M, et al: The interleukin 2 receptor in the hypereosinophilic syndrome. Leuk Lymphoma 8:449, 1992.

98. Slabbynck H, Impens N, Naegels S, et al: Idiopathic hypereosinophilic syndrome–related pulmonary involvement diagnosed by bronchoalveolar lavage. Chest 101:1178, 1992.

99. Winn RE, Kollef MH, Meyer JI: Pulmonary involvement in the hypereosinophilic syndrome. Chest 105:656, 1994.

100. Brogadir SP, Goldwein MI, Schumacher HR: A hypereosinophilic syndrome mimicking rheumatoid arthritis. Am J Med 69:799, 1980.

101. Parrillo JE, Fauci AS, Wolff SM: Hypereosinophilic syndrome: Dramatic response to therapeutic intervention. Trans Assoc Am Physicians 90:135, 1977.

102. Reichlin S, Loveless MH, Kane EG: Loeffler's syndrome following penicillin therapy. Ann Intern Med 38:113, 1953.

103. Fiengenberg DS, Weiss H, Kirshman H: Migratory pneumonia with eosinophilia associated with sulfonamide administration. Arch Intern Med 120:85, 1967.

104. Ho D, Tashkin DP, Bein ME, et al: Pulmonary infiltrates with eosinophilia associated with tetracycline. Chest 76:33, 1979.

105. Goodwin SD, Glenny RW: Nonsteroidal anti-inflammatory drug–associated pulmonary infiltrates with eosinophilia. Review of the literature and Food and Drug Administration adverse drug reaction reports. Arch Intern Med 152:1521, 1992.

106. Khalil H, Molinary E, Stoller JK: Diclofenax (Voltaren)-induced eosinophilic pneumonitis. Arch Intern Med 153:1649, 1993.

107. Yamakado S, Yoshida Y, Yamada T, et al: Pulmonary infiltration and eosinophilia associated with sulfasalazine therapy or ulcerative colitis: A case report and review of literature. Int Med 31:108, 1992.

108. Panayiotou BN: Pulmonary infiltrates and eosinophilia associated with sulphasalazine administration. Aust N Z J Med 21:348, 1991.

109. Oh PI, Balter MS: Cocaine induced eosinophilic lung disease. Thorax 47:478, 1992.

110. Nadeem S, Nasir N, Israel RH: Löffler's syndrome secondary to crack cocaine. Chest 105:1599, 1994.

111. Brander PE, Tukiainen P: Acute eosinophilic pneumonia in a heroin smoker. Eur Respir J 6:750, 1993.

112. Philen RM, Hill RH, Flanders WD, et al: Tryptophan contaminants associated with eosinophilia-myalgia syndrome. Am J Epidemiol 138:154, 1993.

113. Martin RW, Duffy J, Engel AG, et al: The clinical spectrum of the eosinophilia-myalgia syndrome associated with L-tryptophan ingestion. Ann Intern Med 113:124, 1990.

114. Ivey M, Eichenhorn M, Glasberg MR, et al: Hypercapnic respiratory failure due to L-tryptophan–induced eosinophilic polymyositis. Chest 99:756, 1991.

115. Strumpf IJ, Drucker RD, Anders KH, et al: Acute eosinophilic pulmonary disease associated with the ingestion of L-tryptophan–containing products. Chest 99:8, 1991.

116. Tazelaar HD, Myers JL, Drage CW, et al: Pulmonary disease associated with L-tryptophan–induced eosinophilic myalgia syndrome. Chest 97:1032, 1990.

117. Yakovlevitch M, Siegel M, Hoch DH, et al: Pulmonary hypertension in a patient with tryptophan-induced eosinophilia-myalgia syndrome. Am J Med 90:272, 1991.

118. Campagna AC, Blanc PD, Criswell LA, et al: Pulmonary manifestations of the eosinophilia-myalgia syndrome associated with tryptophan ingestion. Chest 101:1274, 1992.

119. Read CA, Clauw D, Weir C, et al: Dyspnea and pulmonary function in the L-tryptophan–associated eosinophilia-myalgia syndrome. Chest 101:1282, 1992.

120. Sarinas PS, Chitkara RK: Ascariasis and hookworm. Semin Respir Infect 12:130, 1997.

121. Marcy TW: Eosinophilia in patients presenting with pulmonary infiltrates and fever. Semin Respir Infect 3:247, 1988.

122. Rohatgi PK, Smirniotopoulos TT: Tropical eosinophil. Semin Respir Med 12:98, 1991.

122a. Ong RK, Doyle RL: Tropical pulmonary eosinophilia. Chest 113:1673, 1998.

123. Maini VK, Bhatia AS, Singh AP: Atypical radiological presentation of tropical pulmonary eosinophilia. Indian J Chest Dis Allied Sci 36:45, 1994.

124. Sandhu M, Mukhopadhyay S, Sharma SK: Tropical pulmonary eosinophilia: A comparative evaluation of plain chest radiography and computed tomography. Australas Radiol 40:32, 1996.

125. Saran R: Cytoplasmic vacuoles of eosinophils in tropical pulmonary eosinophilia. Am Rev Respir Dis 108:1283, 1973.

126. Connell JT: Morphological changes in eosinophils in allergic disease. J Allergy Clin Immunol 41:1, 1968.

127. Vijayan V, Kuppurao KV, Venkatesan P, et al: Pulmonary membrane diffusing capacity and capillary blood volume in tropical eosinophilia. Chest 97:1386, 1990.

128. Rom WN, Vijayan VK, Cornelius MJ, et al: Persistent lower respiratory tract inflammation associated with interstitial lung disease in patients with tropical pulmonary eosinophilia following conventional treatment with diethylcarbamazine. Am Rev Respir Dis 142:1088, 1990.

128a. Chitkara RK, Sarinas PS: Dirofilaria, visceral larva migrans, and tropical pulmonary eosinophilia. Semin Respir Infect 12:138, 1997.

129. deLeon EP, Pardo de Tavera M: Pulmonary schistosomiasis in the Philippines. Dis Chest 53:154, 1968.

130. Lombard CM, Tazelaar HD, Krasner DL: Pulmonary eosinophilia in coccidioidal infections. Chest 91:734, 1987.

131. Miyazaki E, Sugisaki K, Shigenaga T, et al: A case of acute eosinophilic pneumonia caused by inhalation of Trichosporon terrestre. Am J Respir Crit Care Med 151:541, 1995.

132. Cooney TP: Interrelationship of chronic eosinophilic pneumonia, bronchiolitis obliterans, and rheumatoid disease: A hypothesis. J Clin Pathol 34:129, 1981.

133. Payne CR, Connellan SJ: Chronic eosinophilic pneumonia complicating long-standing rheumatoid arthritis. Postgrad Med J 56:519, 1980.

134. Bergstrand H: Morphological equivalents in polyarthritis rheumatica, periarteritis nodosa, transient eosinophilic infiltration of the lung and other allergic syndromes. J Pathol Bacteriol 58:399, 1946.

135. Crofton JW, Livingstone JL, Oswald NC, et al: Pulmonary eosinophilia. Thorax 7:1, 1952.

136. Yousem SA, Lombard CM: The eosinophilic variant of Wegener's granulomatosis. Hum Pathol 19:682, 1988.

137. Incaprera FP: Pulmonary eosinophilia. Am Rev Respir Dis 84:730, 1981.

138. Warring FC Jr, Howlett KS Jr: Allergic reactions to para-aminosalicylic acid: Report of seven cases, including one of Löffler's syndrome. Annu Rev Tuberc 65:235, 1952.

139. Goodwin DD, Glenny RW: Nonsteroidal anti-inflammatory drug–associated pulmonary infiltrates with eosinophilia. Arch Intern Med 152:1521, 1992.

140. Rich MW, Thomas RA: A case of eosinophilic pneumonia and vasculitis induced by diflunisal. Chest 111:1767, 1997.

141. Pfitzenmeyer P, Meier M, Zuck P, et al: Piroxicam induced pulmonary infiltrates and eosinophilia. J Rheumatol 21:1573, 1994.

142. Cooper JAD Jr, White DA, Matthay RA: Drug-induced pulmonary disease. Part 2: Noncytotoxic drugs. Am Rev Respir Dis 133:488, 1986.

143. Holoye PY, Luna MA, MacKay B, et al: Bleomycin hypersensitivity pneumonitis. Ann Intern Med 88:47, 1978.

144. Yousem SA, Lifson JD, Colby TV: Chemotherapy-induced eosinophilic pneumonia: Relation to bleomycin. Chest 88:103, 1985.

145. Watanabe K, Nishimura K, Shiode M, et al: Captopril, an angiotensin-converting enzyme inhibitor, induced pulmonary infiltration with eosinophilia. Intern Med 35:142, 1996.

146. Schatz PL, Mesologites D, Hyun J, et al: Captopril-induced hypersensitivity lung disease. Chest 95:685, 1989.

147. Taylor TL, Ostrum H: The roentgen evaluation of systemic lupus erythematosus. Am J Roentgenol 82:95, 1959.

148. Burgher LW, Kass I, Schenken JR: Pulmonary allergic granulomatosis: A possible drug reaction in a patient receiving cromolyn sodium. Chest 66:84, 1974.

149. Wong PC, Yew WW, Wong CF, et al: Ethambutol-induced pulmonary infiltrates with eosinophilia and skin involvement. Eur Respir J 8:866, 1995.

150. Gould PW, McCormack PL, Palmer DG: Pulmonary damage associated with sodium aurothiomalate therapy. J Rheumatol 4:252, 1977.

151. Morley TF, Komansky HJ, Adelizzi RA, et al: Pulmonary gold toxicity. Eur J Respir Dis 65:627, 1984.

152. Beaudry C, Laplante L: Severe allergic pneumonitis from hydrochlorothiazide. Ann Intern Med 78:251, 1973.

153. Wilson IC, Gambill JM, Sandifer MG: Löffler's syndrome occurring during imipramine therapy. Am J Psychiatry 119:892, 1963.

154. Rokseth R, Storstein O: Pulmonry complications during mecamylamine therapy. Acta Med Scand 167:23, 1960.

155. White DA, Rankin JA, Stover DE, et al: Methotrexate pneumonitis. Bronchoalveolar lavage findings suggest an immunologic disorder. Am Rev Respir Dis 139:18, 1989.

156. Seebach J, Speich R, Fehr J, et al: GM-CSF–induced eosinophilic pneumonia. Br J Haematol 90:963, 1995.

157. Bentur L, Bar-Kana Y, Livni E, et al: Severe minocycline-induced eosinophilic pneumonia: Extrapulmonary manifestations and the use of *in vitro* immunoassays. Ann Pharmacother 31:733, 1997.

158. Toyoshima M, Sato A, Hayakawa H, et al: A clinical study of minocycline-induced pneumonitis. Intern Med 35:176, 1996.

159. Penn RG, Griffin JP: Adverse reactions to nitrofurantoin in the United Kingdom, Sweden, and Holland. BMJ 284:1440, 1982.

160. Wold DE, Zahn DW: Allergic (Löffler's) pneumonia occurring during antituberculous chemotherapy: Report of three cases. Annu Rev Tuberc 74:445, 1956.

161. Lazoglu AH, Boglioli LR, Dorsett B: Phenytoin-related immunodeficiency associated with Loeffler's syndrome. Ann Allergy Asthma Immunol 74:479, 1995.

162. Coyle T, Bushanow P, Winfield J, et al: Hypersensitivity reactions to procarbazine with mechlorethamine, vincristine and procarbazine chemotherapy in the treatment of glioma. Cancer 69:2532, 1992.

163. Salerno SM, Strong JS, Roth BJ, et al: Eosinophilic pneumonia and respiratory failure associated with a trazodone overdose. Am J Respir Crit Care Med 152:2170, 1995.

164. Paré JAPP: Unpublished data, 1975.

165. Phills JA, Harrold AJ, Whiteman GV, et al: Pulmonary infiltrates, asthma, and eosinophilia due to *Ascaris suum* infestation in man. N Engl J Med 286:965, 1972.

166. Bahk YW: Pulmonary paragonimiasis as a cause of Löffler's syndrome. Radiology 78:598, 1962.

167. Fanning M, Hill A, Langer HM, et al: Visceral larva migrans (toxocariasis) in Toronto. Can Med Assoc J 124:21, 1981.

168. Chitkara RK, Sarinas PS: Dirofilaria, visceral larva migrans, and tropical pulmonary eosinophilia. Semin Respir Infect 12:138, 1997.

169. Butland RJA, Coulson IH: Pulmonary eosinophilia associated with cutaneous larva migrans. Thorax 40:76, 1985.

170. McAleer R, Kroenert DB, Elder JL, et al: Allergic bronchopulmonary disease caused by *Curvularia lunata* and *Drechslera hawaiiensis*. Thorax 36:338, 1981.

171. Benatar SR, Allan B, Hewitson RP, et al: Allergic bronchopulmonary stemphyliosis. Thorax 35:515, 1980.

172. Ricker DH, Taylor SR, Gartner JC Jr, et al: Fatal pulmonary aspergillosis presenting as acute eosinophilic pneumonia in a previously healthy child. Chest 100:875, 1991.

173. Vijayan V, Reetha A, Jawahar MS, et al: Pulmonary eosinophilia in pulmonary tuberculosis. Chest 101:1708, 1992.

174. Wright JL, Paré PD, Hammond M, et al: Eosinophilic pneumonia and atypical mycobacterial infection. Am Rev Respir Dis 127:497, 1983.

175. Garofalo R, Kimpen JL, Welliver RC, et al: Eosinophil degranulation in the respiratory tract during naturally acquired respiratory syncytial virus infection. J Pediatr 120:28, 1992.

176. Bascom R, Fisher JF, Thomas RJ, et al: Eosinophilia, respiratory symptoms and pulmonary infiltrates in rubber workers. Chest 93:154, 1988.

177. Kelly KJ, Ruffing R: Acute eosinophilic pneumonia following intentional inhalation of Scotchguard. Ann Allergy 71:358, 1993.

178. Toyoshima M, Sato A, Taniguchi M, et al: A case of eosinophilic pneumonia caused by inhalation of nickel dusts. Jpn J Thorac Dis 32:480, 1994.

179. Shah PKD, Lakhotia M, Chittora M, et al: Pulmonary infiltration with blood eosinophilia after scorpion sting. Chest 95:691, 1989.

180. Marnocha KE, Maglinte DDT, Kelvin FM, et al: Eosinophilic enteritis associated with chronic eosinophilic pneumonia. Am J Gastroenterol 81:1205, 1986.

181. Camus SP, Piard F, Ashcroft T, et al: The lung in inflammatory bowel disease. Medicine (Baltimore) 72:151, 1993.

182. Gross TG, Hoge FJ, Jackson JD: Fatal eosinophilic disease following autologous bone marrow transplantation. Bone Marrow Transplant 14:333, 1994.

183. Sugiyama H, Kotajima F, Kamimura M, et al: Pulmonary involvement in immunoblastic lymphadenopathy: Case reports and review of literature published in Japan. Jpn J Thorac Dis 33:1276, 1995.

# CHAPTER 47

# Goodpasture's Syndrome and Idiopathic Pulmonary Hemorrhage

Although Goodpasture's syndrome and idiopathic pulmonary hemorrhage are separate entities,[1] the fact that their thoracic manifestations are identical justifies their simultaneous consideration in a book on chest disease. Both conditions are characterized by repeated episodes of pulmonary hemorrhage, iron-deficiency anemia, and acute or chronic pulmonary insufficiency. Goodpasture's syndrome includes renal disease in addition to the pulmonary manifestations. It is distinguished from other pulmonary-renal syndromes associated with diffuse alveolar hemorrhage and glomerulonephritis by the presence of an anti–basement membrane antibody in the circulation. (The original case reported by Goodpasture was in a young man who had repeated hemoptysis, which the author considered to be a complication of influenza.[2]) Because hemorrhage is the principal abnormality in the idiopathic variety of diffuse pulmonary hemorrhage and because hemosiderosis is only one of the pathologic consequences of the disease—sometimes a minor one—we regard the term *idiopathic pulmonary hemorrhage* (IPH) as preferable to the more traditional *idiopathic pulmonary hemosiderosis.*

The epidemiologic features of IPH and Goodpasture's syndrome show important differences. IPH occurs most commonly in children, usually younger than 10 years of age (although cases developing during adulthood or extending from childhood to adulthood are well described).[3–9] In the younger age group, the disease shows no sex predominance;[1] in adults, it occurs twice as often in men as in women. By contrast, Goodpasture's syndrome is primarily a disease of young adults older than 16 years,[11, 12] although elderly people can also be affected.[11, 13] Early reviews revealed a striking

male predominance, ranging, for example, from 3.6 to 1 to 9 to 1 in three reports;[1, 11, 14] such preponderance has not been as dramatic in later studies,[12, 13, 15] in which the proportion of men to women has been about 2 to 1. Both conditions are uncommon; for example, IPH accounts for less than 5% of all cases of pulmonary hemorrhage during infancy.[16]

## ETIOLOGY AND PATHOGENESIS

### Goodpasture's Syndrome

Goodpasture's syndrome has been reported in brothers aged 24 and 25 years[17] and in identical twins,[18] suggesting a possible hereditary factor in its pathogenesis. The finding of a strong association between the abnormality and HLA-DR2, particularly subtypes DRw15[19–22] and DR4[21, 22] (which shares a 6–amino acid sequence with DRw15), provides further support for this hypothesis. Despite these observations, most cases occur sporadically, and factors other than or in addition to heredity are likely important.

Immunologic factors are clearly implicated in the pathogenesis of Goodpasture's syndrome, which by definition is characterized by the presence of an antibody directed at collagen in glomerular and alveolar basement membrane.[13, 23–27, 35] The antibody reacts with the carboxyl-terminal region (noncollagenous region or NC1) of the alpha-3 chain of type IV collagen;[24] the amino moiety also has an important role in antibody binding *in vivo*.[10, 24] Pathogenic antibodies to other components of basement membrane are not found,[23] although antibodies may develop as a secondary response to injured basement membrane.[13] The anti–basement membrane antibody is not found in patients who have other forms of kidney disease.[23] The gene encoding the affected basement membrane protein is found on chromosome 2.[26] When T cells of patients who have Goodpasture's syndrome are exposed to the antigen *in vitro*, they demonstrate the expected proliferative response.[28]

Although type IV collagen is present throughout the body, Goodpasture's syndrome almost invariably involves only the lung and kidney. This selectivity may be the result of greater accessibility of the antigen to the antibody, to greater expression of the alpha-3 chain in alveoli and glomeruli than in other tissues, or to both factors.[13] Another unexplained feature of the immunologic reaction is the fact that some patients who have the antibody develop only alveolar hemorrhage or glomerulonephritis, instead of the more usual combination of the two. This finding may be related to structural differences between alveoli and glomeruli; for example, alveolar capillaries lack the openings (fenestrae) present in glomerular endothelium that could allow antibodies increased access to the basement membrane.[13] Increased capillary permeability may be necessary for the antibody to gain access to the alveolar basement membrane. This hypothesis is supported by data from experimental animal studies[13] and by the clinical observations that recurrent pulmonary hemorrhage may develop after infection,[29, 30] fluid overload, cigarette smoking,[31] and exposure to toxins such as high concentrations of inspired oxygen,[13] hydrocarbons,[32] industrial solvents,[13] irritant gases,[13] smoke in a house fire,[33] and hard metal dust.[34]

Although it is generally assumed that the primary target organ is the kidney, with the lung being only secondarily involved, several observations make this assertion suspect. For example, some patients have pulmonary symptoms that antedate evidence of renal disease by many months or develop recurrent pulmonary disease accompanied by relatively little evidence of renal involvement.[36, 37] Moreover, other patients who do not fulfill the strict definition of Goodpasture's syndrome have pulmonary hemorrhage associated with the presence of anti–basement membrane antibodies in the absence of renal involvement.[38–40] Finally, the illness occasionally appears to follow an upper respiratory tract viral infection.[2, 41] These observations favor the concept that the primary damage is in the lung.

The pathogenesis of the pulmonary hemorrhage in Goodpasture's syndrome is also uncertain. In the kidney, complement activation and inflammatory cell enzymes are responsible for glomerular damage. Because capillaritis has been seen in human biopsy material[42, 43] and because an early influx of neutrophils in alveolar septa has been documented in experimental animals,[44] it is possible that similar mechanisms are involved in the lung. One group of investigators found a significant correlation between the level of circulating anti–glomerular basement membrane antibody and the severity of renal abnormalities but not the severity of pulmonary hemorrhage, suggesting that factors other than antibody concentration might be important in causing pulmonary hemorrhage.[45] The results of an experimental animal model of disease suggest that expression of CD44 by endothelial cells may contribute to leukocyte recruitment and subsequent alveolar septal injury.[45a]

### Idiopathic Pulmonary Hemorrhage

The etiology and pathogenesis of IPH are even less clear than those of Goodpasture's syndrome. The disease has been reported in a mother and son[46] and in siblings,[47, 48] raising the possibility of a hereditary factor; however, as with Goodpasture's syndrome, the number of such cases is so small that the importance of such a factor is uncertain. Although some findings suggest that an autoimmune process is involved in the pathogenesis, evidence for this is not present in all cases. For example, in a study of fetal and

maternal tissues from a patient who died from IPH during pregnancy, no evidence was found of the passage of a causative antibody through the placental barrier.[49] Immunologic and ultrastructural studies of lung tissue usually fail to reveal evidence of deposition of immunoglobulin or complement components.[46, 48, 50–55] On the other hand, both circulating[56] and tissue[57] immune complexes have been identified in some patients, and the abnormality has been found in association with a number of well-recognized immune disorders,[8] including celiac disease,[9, 58–60] thyrotoxicosis,[8] and hypothyroidism.[61] In one investigation, three of the four patients with IPH and celiac disease had HLA-B8 haplotype, suggesting a genetic link.[60] Antineutrophil cytoplasmic antibodies (ANCA) were described in three of four patients with IPH in one report, none of whom developed evidence of systemic vasculitis during follow-up;[62] however, another patient did do so after suffering for 8 years with apparent IPH.[63] It is likely that such cases are in fact variants of microscopic polyangiitis or another vasculitic syndrome and represent fundamentally different abnormalities than IPH. Allergy to cow's milk protein has been described in some patients, but the association has not been a consistent one.[16]

Although structural alterations of the alveolar basement membrane have been found in some electron microscopic investigations of IPH (*see* farther on), it is not clear which, if any, of the changes represents a primary defect rather than damage secondary to an unknown agent. Structural and histochemical alterations of pulmonary elastic fibers appear to be the consequence of intra-alveolar bleeding rather than its cause.

### PATHOLOGIC CHARACTERISTICS

The histologic features of the lung in Goodpasture's syndrome[1, 12, 33, 64] and IPH[51, 53, 65–67] are virtually identical. The most prominent abnormality is hemorrhage confined largely to the alveolar air spaces and smaller airways; in fact, massive blood loss can occur into the lungs without associated hemoptysis, and the trachea and major bronchi may contain little or no blood. Other histologic changes depend on the duration and severity of the disease at the time of examination but usually include the presence of hemosiderin-laden macrophages in alveolar air spaces and interstitial tissue, mild to moderate interstitial fibrosis, and type II cell hyperplasia (Fig. 47–1). Iron may also be found apparently free within interstitial tissue, encrusted on elastic fibers in the walls of small vessels and in the basement membrane itself.[68] The quantity of sequestered iron may be large; the fact that it is not available for hemoglobin synthesis explains the chronic iron-deficiency anemia that is characteristic of these diseases.[69]

A lymphocytic interstitial infiltrate, typically mild, is seen in some cases. Focal or (less commonly) diffuse acute interstitial inflammation can also be seen.[42, 43] This is manifested as capillaritis identical to that of Wegener's granulomatosis and microscopic polyangiitis and appears as a neutrophil infiltrate intimately associated with alveolar septa with or without fibrin thrombi and necrosis. In addition to blood, a proteinaceous exudate, hyaline membranes, or both can be seen in the alveolar air spaces and transitional air-

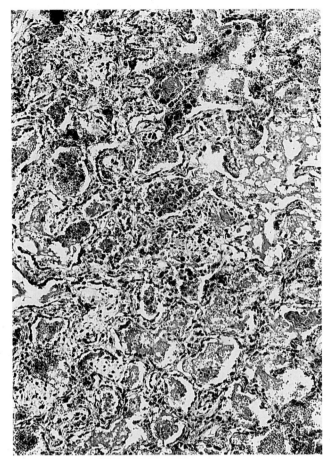

**Figure 47–1. Goodpasture's Syndrome.** The section shows diffuse, moderately severe alveolar interstitial fibrosis and extensive type II cell hyperplasia. Air spaces are filled by fresh blood and hemosiderin-laden macrophages (black cells in this illustration). The patient was a 25-year-old man who died in the early 1970s following several weeks of hemoptysis and hematuria ($\times 100$).

ways; occasionally, these findings are so extensive that they suggest a diagnosis of diffuse alveolar damage.[42]

Electron microscopic studies of alveolar walls in both Goodpasture's syndrome and IPH have shown variable results, with some investigators finding no abnormality[33, 48, 51, 53] and others finding thickening,[55, 67, 70] splitting, discontinuity,[50, 52, 54] or smudging of the basement membrane. Epithelial cell abnormalities have also been noted in cases of IPH.[55] As indicated previously, whether these findings are primary (i.e., pathogenetically related to the alveolar hemorrhage) or are simply a reflection of nonspecific alveolar wall damage has not been determined. At any rate, there is nothing specific about the electron microscopic findings in either disease. Electron-dense deposits suggestive of immune complexes have generally not been demonstrated.[33, 48, 50, 53]

Immunofluorescence studies of fresh lung tissue obtained from patients with Goodpasture's syndrome by either open or transbronchial biopsy typically show diffuse linear staining along the alveolar wall (Fig. 47–2).[33, 71–74] Immunoglobulin G (IgG) is the usual antibody detected, although IgA and IgM are occasionally present as well. Cases have also been reported in which there was isolated IgA positivity in both kidney and lung.[75, 76] The third component of complement (C3) is variably present and may be seen

in a granular, as opposed to linear, pattern.[42] In distinct contrast to the positive immunofluorescent studies in Goodpasture's syndrome, the results in IPH are almost always negative.[46, 48, 50–54]

In Goodpasture's syndrome, the kidneys show focal or diffuse necrotizing glomerulonephritis;[12] associated vasculitis is typically absent, although rare cases with this feature have been reported.[77, 78] As with the lung, immunofluorescent study reveals linear staining for immunoglobulin along the basement membrane.

## RADIOLOGIC MANIFESTATIONS

The radiologic manifestations of Goodpasture's syndrome and IPH are identical and depend in large measure on the number of hemorrhagic episodes that have occurred. In the early stages of the disease, the radiographic pattern is one of patchy areas of air-space consolidation scattered fairly evenly throughout the lungs (Fig. 47–3). An air bronchogram is usually identifiable in areas of major consolidation. At this stage, the pattern simulates pulmonary edema (*see* Fig. 47–3). Opacities are usually widespread but may be more prominent in the perihilar areas and in the middle and lower lung zones. The apices and costophrenic angles are almost invariably spared;[79] should they show evidence of consolidation, superimposed pneumonia is likely.[80] Although parenchymal involvement is usually bilateral, it is commonly asymmetric; occasionally, it is unilateral.[80] We have seen one patient with IPH in whom repeated episodes of hemorrhage in the right lung had resulted in irreversible interstitial fibrosis and increased vascular resistance (Fig. 47–4); during the period of our observation, she suffered repeated episodes of hemorrhage into both lungs, but more severely the left. Less common radiographic findings include ground-glass opacities and migratory areas of consolidation.[81, 82] The chest radiograph also may be normal; in one review of 25 patients with Goodpasture's syndrome, normal findings were documented in 7 (18%) of 39 episodes.[80] CT scanning may demonstrate parenchymal abnormalities in patients with normal or questionable radiographic findings.[82]

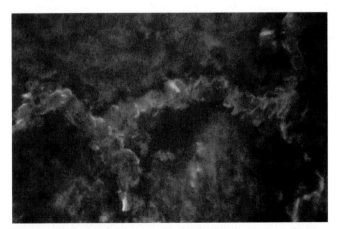

**Figure 47–2. Goodpasture's Syndrome.** This is a section of lung incubated with anti-IgG from a 43-year-old woman who presented with hemoptysis. Weak linear fluorescence is evident, corresponding to the site of the alveolar basement membrane. Adjacent air spaces contain blood.

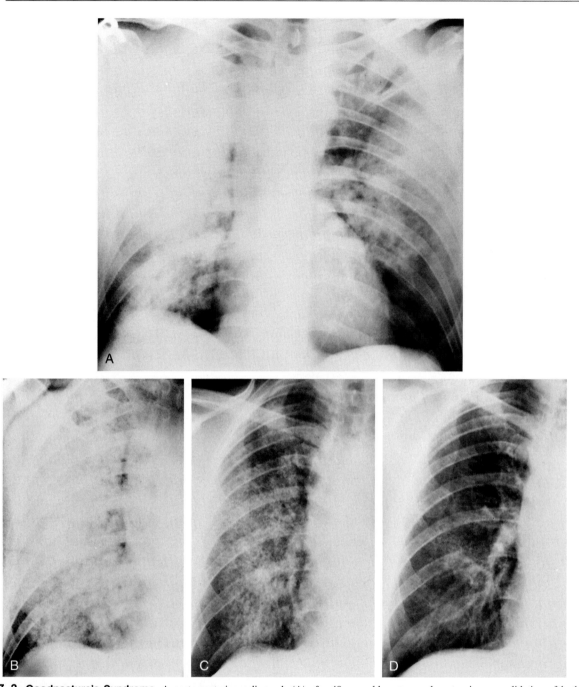

**Figure 47–3. Goodpasture's Syndrome.** A posteroanterior radiograph *(A)* of a 49-year-old man reveals extensive consolidation of both lungs. A well-defined air bronchogram is evident. Three days later *(B)*, the pattern was somewhat more granular, and 10 days after the initial episode *(C)*, it has become distinctly reticular. Six days later *(D)*, only a fine reticular pattern remains in an anatomic distribution identical to the original involvement. The sequence of changes illustrated by this patient with Goodpasture's syndrome is typical of massive pulmonary hemorrhage.

The CT manifestations of acute pulmonary hemorrhage consist of areas of ground-glass attenuation or consolidation; these may be patchy or diffuse[82, 83] but tend to involve mainly the dependent lung regions.[84] The potential diagnostic value of magnetic resonance (MR) imaging has been assessed in a 2½-year-old boy who had IPH associated with diffuse air-space consolidation.[85] The T1-weighted images showed diffusely increased signal intensity, whereas the T2-weighted images showed a markedly reduced signal intensity. The latter finding is related to the presence of paramagnetic ferric iron in the pulmonary parenchymal hemosid-

erin.[85] The MR imaging diagnosis allowed initiation of therapy and stabilization of the patient before the diagnosis was confirmed by open-lung biopsy.

Serial radiographs obtained during the several days after an acute episode of pulmonary hemorrhage usually reveal a highly predictable progressive change in the pattern (*see* Fig. 47–3): the fluffy deposits characteristic of air-space consolidation disappear within 2 to 3 days and are replaced by a reticulonodular pattern with a distribution identical to that of the air-space disease.[86, 87] In one study of six patients, HRCT performed during this resolving phase showed poorly

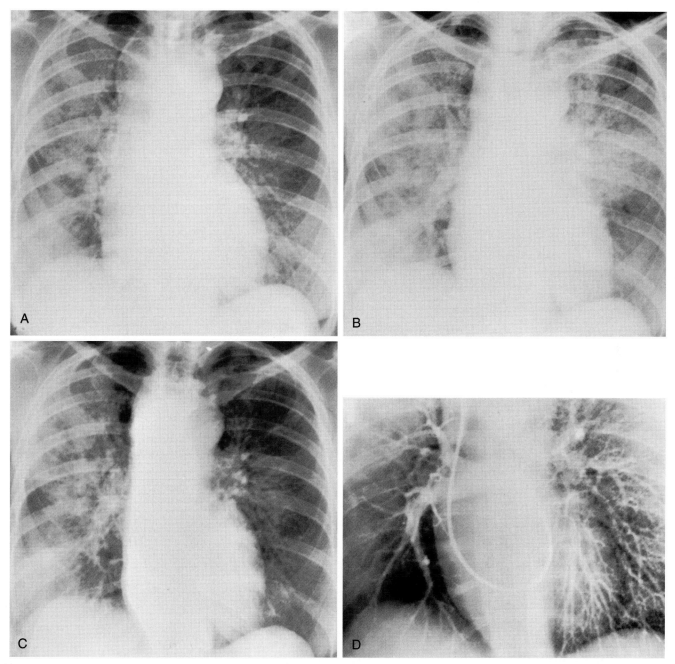

**Figure 47–4. Idiopathic Pulmonary Hemorrhage.** This 52-year-old woman had a history of increasing shortness of breath on exertion for several years. On admission, a posteroanterior radiograph *(A)* revealed a diffuse fine reticular pattern involving the right lung and associated with loss of volume; the left lung was relatively clear. (A prominent longitudinal shadow paralleling the right heart border represents severe esophageal dilation due to achalasia.) While in the hospital, the patient had a brisk hemoptysis of approximately 100 ml. Following this, a radiograph *(B)* revealed patchy air-space consolidation throughout the left lung consistent with alveolar hemorrhage; a well-defined air bronchogram is evident. Additional shadows throughout the right lung probably represent the same process. Nuclear medicine scans of both lungs following the intravenous injection of 250 ml of packed red blood cells tagged with $^{59}$Fe revealed high readings over the left lung and low readings over the right. Five days later *(C)*, most of the blood had been absorbed from the left lung, the pattern in the right remaining unchanged from the original examination. (This radiograph was exposed following ingestion of barium and reveals severe esophageal dilation.) Biopsy of the right lung at this time revealed diffuse, nonspecific interstitial fibrosis. A pulmonary angiogram *(D)* shows the bulk of pulmonary artery flow passing to the left lung, the vessels on the right being thin and attenuated; this finding is thought to indicate increase in resistance in the right lung as a result of repeated episodes of pulmonary hemorrhage and subsequent interstitial fibrosis. The predominance of the process in the right lung was unexplained.

defined 1- to 3-mm diameter centrilobular nodules in all patients, patchy areas of ground-glass attenuation in four, and interlobular septal thickening in four (Fig. 47–5).[83] This reticular pattern gradually diminishes during the next several days, and the appearance of the chest radiograph usually returns to normal about 10 to 12 days after the original episode.[80–82]

With repeated episodes, increasing amounts of hemosiderin are deposited within the interstitial tissue and are associated with progressive fibrosis (*see* Fig. 47–4). In most cases, the chest radiograph shows only partial clearing after each fresh hemorrhage, revealing persistence of a fine reticulonodular pattern indicative of the irreversible interstitial disease.[88–92] HRCT of the chest at this stage demonstrates 1- to 3-mm centrilobular nodules throughout the lung parenchyma (Fig. 47–6);[85, 85a, 85b] interlobular septal thickening also may be seen.[85c] Once these irreversible changes have developed, fresh episodes of pulmonary hemorrhage usually result in the typical pattern of air-space consolidation superimposed on the diffuse interstitial disease (*see* Fig. 47–4);[1, 93] rarely, acute episodes occur without significant variation in the radiologic pattern.[3] Uncommonly, pulmonary hypertension and chronic cor pulmonale develop as a result of diffuse pulmonary fibrosis.[1]

Pleural effusion is rare, and its presence usually indicates cardiac decompensation or superimposed pneumonia.[79] Hilar and, rarely, paratracheal lymph node enlargement has been described in IPH.[90, 94]

## CLINICAL MANIFESTATIONS

Although the morphologic and radiologic manifestations of IPH and Goodpasture's syndrome in the lungs are virtually identical, there are some important differences in their clinical manifestations. Mention has already been made of differences in age and sex incidence: IPH tends to occur in children of either sex, whereas Goodpasture's syndrome occurs more commonly in young adult men.[16]

### Idiopathic Pulmonary Hemorrhage

The onset of IPH may be insidious, with anemia, pallor, weakness, lethargy, and (sometimes) a dry cough. In other cases, the onset is acute, with fever and hemoptysis. As indicated previously, the typical changes of air-space hemorrhage may be apparent radiographically without a history of hemoptysis.[95] Some investigators have recognized two clinical forms of the disease:[10, 90, 96, 97] (1) recurrent acute episodes of intra-alveolar hemorrhage associated with mild hemoptysis, dyspnea, cough, weakness, tachycardia, cyanosis, fever, and pallor, with progression of disease associated with finger clubbing, hepatosplenomegaly, and jaundice; and (2) more prolonged illness associated with milder exacerbations, in which hemoptysis may be represented only by intermittent blood streaking, and with infrequent complete remissions.

Physical examination during the acute stage of pulmonary hemorrhage may reveal fine crackles and dullness to percussion over the affected areas of lung; the liver, spleen, and lymph nodes are palpably enlarged in 20% to 25% of patients.[1] Finger clubbing and hepatosplenomegaly usually are regarded as late manifestations of the disease,[90] although the former has been reported as a transient phenomenon associated with an acute episode of hemorrhage.[98] Myocarditis develops in a few cases.[66, 88] One case was reported of a 14-year-old boy in whom rheumatoid arthritis developed after the episodes of hemoptysis ceased.[98]

Iron-deficiency anemia develops in most patients[16] but may not be detectable when intrapulmonary hemorrhage is small and does not severely deplete the bone marrow iron stores.[99] Bilirubinemia, predominantly of the indirect fraction, and the excretion of excessive amounts of urobilinogen are often present and suggest a hemolytic process; however, iron studies characteristically reveal iron-deficiency

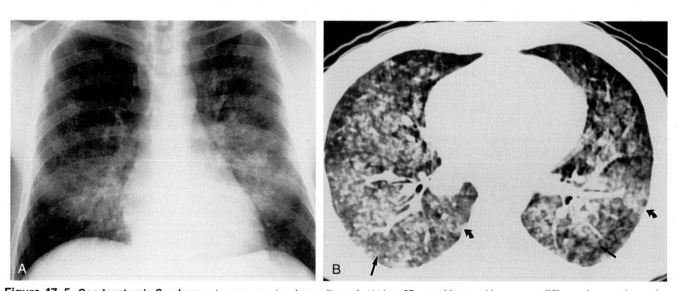

**Figure 47–5. Goodpasture's Syndrome.** A posteroanterior chest radiograph *(A)* in a 27-year-old man with recurrent diffuse pulmonary hemorrhage due to Goodpasture's syndrome reveals an extensive bilateral reticulonodular pattern with superimposed ground-glass opacities in the perihilar regions. A CT scan at the level of the inferior pulmonary veins *(B)* demonstrates numerous 1- to 3-mm diameter centrilobular nodules *(straight arrows)*. Focal areas of ground-glass attenuation are present in the lower lobes *(curved arrows)*.

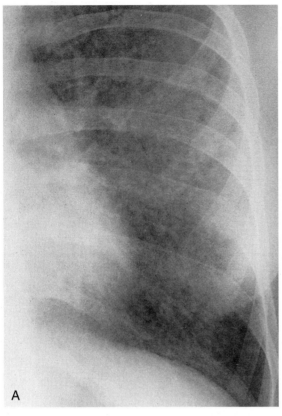

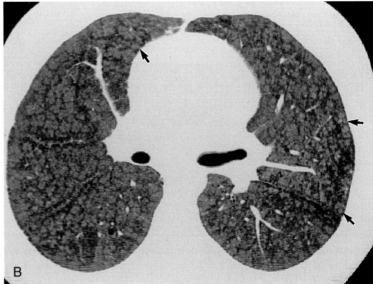

**Figure 47–6. Idiopathic Pulmonary Hemorrhage.** A view of the left lung from a posteroanterior chest radiograph in a 22-year-old woman *(A)* reveals numerous poorly defined small nodular opacities. A high-resolution CT scan *(B)* demonstrates the centrilobular distribution of the opacities *(arrows)*. The patient had a history of recurrent pulmonary hemorrhage since the age of 4 years; the opacities had remained unchanged over the previous 3 years.

anemia, and it is generally believed that hemolysis does not occur,[1, 89] except in the rare circumstance in which IPH is associated with autoimmune hemolytic anemia.[100] When associated with celiac disease, steatorrhea may be present.[59] Occasionally, a discrepancy between the degree of hemoptysis and the severity of the anemia can be explained by unrecognized malabsorption caused by celiac disease.[58] Peripheral eosinophilia was present in 12% of patients in one series, and cold agglutinins were detected in 10 of the 20 patients tested.[1]

### Goodpasture's Syndrome

Hemoptysis is the most common presenting symptom of patients who have Goodpasture's syndrome, occurring in about 80% to 95%.[13] Although it may be life-threatening, it is seldom as copious as in IPH. It may occur late in the course of the disease or be absent altogether,[1, 91, 101–103] and typically precedes the clinical manifestations of renal disease by several months.[13] The latter observation is helpful in distinguishing Goodpasture's syndrome from hemoptysis associated with chronic renal failure of other etiology.

Other presenting symptoms include dyspnea, fatigue, weakness, lassitude, pallor, cough, and (occasionally) frank hematuria.[11] Acute hemorrhage may be associated with chills, fever, and diaphoresis.[13] Chest pain, often worsened by cough, is not uncommon.[13] Flank tenderness related to renal vein thrombosis was described as the first manifestation of disease in one patient.[104]

Physical findings are similar to those of IPH; hypertension may accompany renal failure. Retinal hemorrhages and exudates have been described in about 10% of cases;[11] retinal detachment[105] and the development of subretinal neovascular membranes[106] have also been reported. Other rare manifestations include myocarditis,[107] skin rash,[108] and systemic necrotizing vasculitis.[109]

Although results of the initial urinalysis may be normal, proteinuria, hematuria, and cellular and granular casts almost invariably develop at some stage. Repeated and careful urine analyses are mandatory. Occasionally, urinary sediment findings are normal, and the presence of renal involvement is established by biopsy.[52, 110, 111] Of 51 cases in one review, anemia was present in all and leukocytosis (with a shift to the left) in half.[11]

### PULMONARY FUNCTION TESTS

There are few reports of the pulmonary function findings in patients with either IPH or Goodpasture's syndrome. Some patients, tested during remission, have had a predominantly restrictive pattern, with decreased diffusing capacity and (sometimes) a fall in resting $PaO_2$.[112–115] Such a pattern has been said to persist in both diseases after the chest radiograph has returned to normal.[52] However, in patients with previous lung hemorrhage, only the diffusing capacity result may be abnormal in the long term.[116] Air-flow limitation, air-trapping, and a low diffusing capacity have been described in cases associated with celiac disease.[60] The greater than normal uptake of carbon monoxide in patients who have active bleeding is helpful in confirming that the air-space opacities observed radiographically are in fact blood.[117, 118]

## DIAGNOSIS

The diagnosis of Goodpasture's syndrome should be suspected when a patient in the late second or third decade of life presents with hemoptysis and radiologic evidence of air-space hemorrhage, particularly when there are also manifestations of renal disease. Confirmation is obtained by the demonstration of circulating or tissue-bound anti–basement membrane antibodies by enzyme-linked immunosorbent assay or immunofluorescent examination.[119] Most other disorders characterized by hemoptysis and renal dysfunction can be recognized by associated clinical and laboratory manifestations of vasculitis[120] or by the observation of immunoglobulin and complement deposition in a granular pattern on indirect immunofluorescence examination of a kidney biopsy specimen.[120] Several authors have stressed the feasibility of making the diagnosis of Goodpasture's syndrome based on examination of a transbronchial biopsy specimen;[33, 71] however, a negative result of this examination does not exclude the diagnosis,[121] because anti–glomerular basement membrane antibody may not be identified in alveolar septa and yet still be present in glomeruli.[74, 122] Although rare, some patients with Goodpasture's syndrome have subsequently developed other forms of renal disease, such as membranous or mesangiocapillary glomerulonephritis.[123, 124]

The lack of specific morphologic or other findings in patients with IPH makes this diagnosis largely one of exclusion. This is particularly true of adults and of patients who do not manifest iron-deficiency anemia. Before ascribing the clinical and radiographic findings to IPH in these patients, thorough investigation is indicated to search for a site of localized bleeding, employing the most sophisticated clinical and imaging techniques available to exclude cardiac or vascular malformations; the condition that is most likely to mimic it is widespread aspiration of blood. Patients who appear to have IPH and whose renal function and histology are normal but who have linear deposition of immunoglobulin on alveolar and glomerular basement membranes should be designated early cases of Goodpasture's syndrome.[52, 110, 111] The criteria for the diagnosis of IPH should thus consist of clinical or laboratory evidence of repeated pulmonary hemorrhage, episodic air-space abnormalities on chest radiographs, a histologically normal renal biopsy specimen showing negative immunofluorescence, and the absence of a detectable cause of bleeding. Biopsy material should be examined by light and electron microscopy and by immunofluorescence using anti-IgG, anti-IgM, and anti-IgA antibodies.

Most authorities agree that the term *Goodpasture's syndrome* should be restricted to disease characterized by glomerulonephritis associated with a linear immunofluorescent pattern on renal biopsy, the presence of circulating anti–basement membrane antibodies, and evidence of pulmonary hemorrhage. The differential diagnosis of the pulmonary-renal syndromes—that is, the association of glomerulonephritis with diffuse alveolar hemorrhage—is broad.[125] The most common cause is probably vasculitis associated with such entities as Wegener's granulomatosis,[126, 127] rheumatoid disease,[128, 129] systemic lupus erythematosus (SLE),[130–133] and microscopic polyangiitis (systemic necrotizing vasculitis).[134] In some patients, immune complexes, cryoglobulins, or both are found in the kidneys in the absence of clinical criteria for SLE;[135–138] some of these have penicillamine-induced

toxicity[139–144] or Henoch-Schönlein purpura.[145–147] Mitomycin C[148] and products employed by hairdressers to give permanent waves[149] have also been incriminated; whether these have a pathogenesis similar to that associated with penicillamine is unclear. In still other patients, immune complexes cannot be identified by immunofluorescent examination, and yet findings such as hypocomplementemia and vasculitis clearly support the possibility of disturbed immunologic activity.[150] Rare cases of pulmonary-renal syndrome have also been described in patients who have apparent thinning of basement membrane and no evidence of glomerulonephritis.[151]

When all patients with glomerulonephritis and pulmonary hemorrhage are considered, about 20% are found to have Goodpasture's syndrome[120, 152–154] and 50% some form of systemic vasculitis;[154] most of the remainder have diffuse alveolar hemorrhage in association with other forms of glomerulonephritis.[154–158a]

Because renal involvement in Goodpasture's syndrome may not be apparent initially,[38–40] the diagnosis must still be considered in any patient who has radiologic and clinical findings consistent with diffuse alveolar hemorrhage and no evidence of kidney disease. The differential diagnosis in this situation is also large and includes the following:

1. Inhalation of toxic substances, such as epoxy resin containing the catalyst trimellitic anhydride (TMA),[159–161] isocyanates,[162] and crack cocaine;[163–165] there is evidence that the first of these is immunologically mediated[166]
2. Systemic vasculitides, including Takayasu's arteritis,[167] classic polyarteritis nodosa,[168] Churg-Strauss syndrome,[168a] and ANCA-positive vasculitis such as microscopic polyangiitis[169–171]
3. Rarely, in association with isolated pulmonary capillaritis in the absence of clinical, serologic, or histologic evidence indicating accompanying systemic disease[172]
4. A variety of autoimmune disorders, including chronic active hepatitis,[173] progressive systemic sclerosis,[174] bullous pemphigoid,[175] rheumatoid arthritis,[175a] mixed connective tissue disease,[175a] antiphospholipid antibody syndrome,[176–177a] and polymyositis[178]
5. Pulmonary neoplasms, such as epithelioid hemangioendothelioma,[179, 180] metastatic choriocarcinoma,[181] angiosarcoma,[182, 183] and (in one patient) multiple myeloma[184]
6. Aspirated blood following vascular disruption (e.g., spontaneous rupture of a bronchial artery,[185] tracheoesophageal fistula following placement of a Blakemore tube,[186] aortic dissection,[187–189] ruptured mycotic subclavian artery aneurysm in the setting of bacterial endocarditis,[190] and obstruction of a mitral prosthetic valve[191])
7. A variety of coagulation disturbances,[192–195] including as a complication of the administration of streptokinase[196–198] and other anticoagulants[198a] in the treatment of myocardial infarction (a setting in which it is often a neglected diagnosis)
8. Bone marrow transplantation (*see* page 1726)[199–203]

## PROGNOSIS AND NATURAL HISTORY

The prognosis varies considerably in patients who have IPH. For example, in one series, the average interval from onset of symptoms until death was only 2.5 years;[1] however, individual patients are known to have survived for as long as 18 to 20 years.[3, 4] The prognosis appears to be better when the disease is acquired in adulthood rather than in childhood.[204, 205] Of seven adults reported in one series (four of whom had associated celiac disease), the disease seemed remarkably benign, with five of the seven surviving for 10 to 40 years.[60]

Although spontaneous remission and long-term survival in the absence of effective therapy were occasionally noted,[206–210] the prognosis of Goodpasture's syndrome was poor before the availability of plasmapheresis and immunosuppressive therapy. For example, in one series of 25 patients reported in the early 1960s, 24 died, within an average period of 6 months.[1] Some investigators have estimated that the outcome at that time was death or renal failure in about 90% of cases.[211] Fortunately, current therapy with corticosteroids, immunosuppressive agents, and plasmapheresis has substantially improved the outlook.[211–214] Overall, more than half of patients are long-term survivors, although some are dependent on dialysis;[13, 214] preservation of renal function is favored by early diagnosis. Rarely, patients whose disease remits spontaneously or as a result of therapy manifest recurrences years later.[37, 215–218] An even more unusual and perhaps spurious association is the presence of Wegener's granulomatosis and Goodpasture's syndrome in the same patient.[219]

# REFERENCES

1. Soergel, H, Sommers SC: Idiopathic pulmonary hemosiderosis and related syndromes. Am J Med 32:499, 1962.
2. Goodpasture EW: The significance of certain pulmonary lesions in relation to the etiology of influenza. Am J Med Sci 158:863, 1919.
3. Boyd DHA: Idiopathic pulmonary hemosiderosis in adults and adolescents. Br J Dis Chest 53:41, 1959.
4. Bronson SM: Idiopathic pulmonary hemosiderosis in adults: Report of a case and review of the literature. Am J Roentgenol 83:260, 1960.
5. Ognibene AJ, Johnson DE: Idiopathic pulmonary hemosiderosis in adults: Report of case and review of literature. Arch Intern Med 111:503, 1963.
6. Cooper AS: Idiopathic pulmonary hemosiderosis: Report of a case in an adult treated with triamcinolone. N Engl J Med 263:1100, 1960.
7. Rezkalla MA, Simmons JL: Idiopathic pulmonary hemosiderosis and alveolar hemorrhage syndrome: Case report and review of the literature. S D J Med 48:79, 1995.
8. Bain SC, Bryan RL, Hawkins JB: Idiopathic pulmonary haemosiderosis and autoimmune thyrotoxicosis. Respir Med 83:447, 1989.
9. Pacheco A, Casanova C, Fogue L, et al: Long-term clinical follow-up of adult idiopathic pulmonary hemosiderosis and celiac disease. Chest 99:1525, 1991.
10. Ryan JJ, Mason PJ, Pusey CD, et al: Recombinant alpha-chains of type IV collagen demonstrate that the amino terminal of the Goodpasture autoantigen is crucial for antibody recognition. Clin Exp Immunol 113:17, 1998.
11. Proskey AJ, Weatherbee L, Easterling RE, et al: Goodpasture's syndrome: A report of five cases and review of the literature. Am J Med 48:162, 1970.
12. Teague CA, Doak PB, Simpson IJ, et al: Goodpasture's syndrome: An analysis of 29 cases. Kidney Int 13:492, 1978.
13. Kelly PT, Haponik EF: Goodpasture syndrome: Molecular and clinical advances. Medicine 73:171, 1994.
14. Benoit FL, Rulon DB, Theil GB, et al: Goodpasture's syndrome: A clinicopathologic entity. Am J Med 37:424, 1964.
15. Herody, M, Bobrie G, Gouarin C, et al: Anti-GBM disease: Predictive value of clinical histological and serological data. Clin Nephrol 40:249, 1993.
16. Dearborn DG, Infeld MD, Smith P, et al: Leads from the morbidity and mortality weekly report, Atlanta, Ga: Acute pulmonary hemorrhage/hemosiderosis among infants—Cleveland, January 1993–November 1994. JAMA 273:281, 1995.
17. Gossain VV, Gerstein AR, Janes AW: Goodpasture's syndrome: A familial occurrence. Am Rev Respir Dis 105:621, 1972.
18. D'Apice AJ, Kincaid-Smith P, Becker GH, et al: Goodpasture's syndrome in identical twins. Ann Intern Med 88:61, 1978.
19. Rees AJ, Peters DK, Compston DAS, et al: Strong association between HLA-DRW2 and antibody-mediated Goodpasture's syndrome. Lancet 1:966, 1978.
20. Rees AJ, Peters DK, Amos N, et al: The influence of HLA-linked genes on the severity of anti-GBM antibody-mediated nephritis. Kidney Int 26:445, 1984.
21. Dunckley H, Chapman JR, Burke J, et al: HLA-DR and -DQ genotyping in anti-GBM disease. Dis Markers 9:249, 1991.
22. Burns AP, Fisher M, Li P, et al: Molecular analysis of HLA class II genes in Goodpasture's disease. Q J Med 88:93, 1995.
23. Kalluri R, Wilson CB, Weber M, et al: Identification of the alpha 3 chain of type IV collagen as the common autoantigen in antibasement membrane disease and Goodpasture syndrome. J Am Soc Nephrol 6:1178, 1995.
24. Penades JR, Bernal D, Revert F, et al: Characterization and expression of multiple alternatively spliced transcripts of the Goodpasture antigen gene region: Goodpasture antibodies recognize recombinant proteins representing the autoantigen and one of its alternative forms. Eur J Biochem 229:754, 1995.
25. Hellmark T, Johansson C, Wieslander J: Characterization of anti-GBM antibodies involved in Goodpasture's syndrome. Kidney Int 46:823, 1994.
26. Kefalides NA, Ohno N, Wilson CB: Heterogeneity of antibodies in Goodpasture syndrome reacting with type IV collagen. Kidney Int 43:85, 1993.
27. Neilson EG, Kalluri R, Sun MJ, et al: Specificity of Goodpasture autoantibodies for the recombinant noncollagenous domains of human type IV collagen. J Biol Chem 268:8402, 1993.
28. Derry CJ, Ross CN, Lombardi G, et al: Analysis of T cell responses to the autoantigen in Goodpasture's disease. Clin Exp Immunol 100:262, 1995.
29. Rees AJ, Lockwood CM, Peters DK: Enhanced allergic tissue injury in Goodpasture's syndrome by intercurrent bacterial infection. BMJ 2:723, 1977.
30. Lucas Guillen E, Martinez Ruiz A, Alegria Fernandez M, et al: Goodpasture syndrome: Re-exacerbations associated with intercurrent infections. Rev Clin Esp 195:761, 1995.
31. Donaghy M, Rees AJ: Cigarette smoking and lung hemorrhage in glomerulonephritis caused by autoantibodies to glomerular basement membrane. Lancet 2:1390, 1983.
32. Bombassei GJ, Kaplan AA: The association between hydrocarbon exposure and anti-glomerular basement membrane antibody-mediated disease (Goodpasture's syndrome). Am J Ind Med 21:141, 1992.
33. Abboud RT, Chase WH, Ballon HS, et al: Goodpasture's syndrome: Diagnosis by transbronchial lung biopsy. Ann Intern Med 89:635, 1978.
34. Lechleitner P, Defregger M, Lhotta K, et al: Goodpasture's syndrome: Unusual presentation after exposure to hard metal dust. Chest 103:956, 1993.
35. Martinez-Hernandez A, Amenta PS: The basement membrane in pathology. Lab Invest 48:656, 1983.
36. Dahlberg PJ, Kurtz SB, Donadio JV Jr, et al: Recurrent Goodpasture's syndrome. Mayo Clin Proc 53:533, 1978.
37. Mehler PS, Brunvand MW, Hutt MP, et al: Chronic recurrent Goodpasture's syndrome. Am J Med 82:833, 1987.
38. Bell DD, Moffatt SL, Singer M, et al: Antibasement membrane antibody disease without clinical evidence of renal disease. Am Rev Respir Dis 142:234, 1990.
39. Tobler A, Schürch, Altermatt HJ, et al: Anti-basement membrane antibody disease with severe pulmonary haemorrhage and normal renal function. Thorax 46:68, 1991.
40. Carre PH, Lloveras JJ, Didier A, et al: Goodpasture's syndrome with normal renal function. Eur Respir J 2:911, 1989.
41. Wilson CB, Smith RC: Goodpasture's syndrome associated with influenza A2 virus infection. Ann Intern Med 76:91, 1972.
42. Lombard CM, Colby TV, Elliott CG: Surgical pathology of the lung in antibasement membrane antibody-associated Goodpasture's syndrome. Hum Pathol 20:445, 1989.
43. Travis WD, Colby TV, Lombard C, et al: A clinicopathologic study of 34 cases of diffuse pulmonary hemorrhage with lung biopsy confirmation. Am J Surg Pathol 14:1112, 1990.
44. Lan HY, Paterson DJ, Hutchinson P, et al: Leukocyte involvement in the pathogenesis of pulmonary injury in experimental Goodpasture's syndrome. Lab Invest 64:330, 1991.
45. Simpson IJ, Doak PB, Williams LC, et al: Plasma exchange in Goodpasture's syndrome. Am J Nephrol 2:301, 1982.
45a. Hill PA, Lan HY, Atkins RC, et al: Ultrastructural localization of CD44 in the rat lung in experimental Goodpasture's syndrome. Pathology 29:380, 1997.
46. Thaell JF, Greipp PR, Stubbs SE, et al: Case reports. Idiopathic pulmonary hemosiderosis: Two cases in a family. Mayo Clin Proc 53:113, 1978.
47. Breckenridge RL Jr, Ross JS: Idiopathic pulmonary hemosiderosis: A report of familial occurrence. Chest 75:636, 1979.
48. Beckerman RC, Taussig LM, Pinnas JL: Familial idiopathic pulmonary hemosiderosis. Am J Dis Child 133:609, 1979.
49. Slager UT: Idiopathic pulmonary hemosiderosis in adults: A study of fetal and maternal tissues in a case of death during pregnancy. Am Rev Respir Dis 91:915, 1965.
50. Hyatt RW, Adelstein ER, Halazun JF, et al: Ultrastructure of the lung in idiopathic pulmonary hemosiderosis. Am J Med 52:822, 1972.
51. Irwin RS, Cottrell TS, Hsu KC, et al: Idiopathic pulmonary hemosiderosis: An electron microscopic and immunofluorescent study. Chest 65:41, 1974.
52. Donald KJ, Edwarda RL, McEvoy JDS: Alveolar capillary basement membrane lesions in Goodpasture's syndrome and idiopathic pulmonary hemosiderosis. Am J Med 59:642, 1975.
53. Donlan CJ, Srodes CH, Duffy FD: Idiopathic pulmonary hemosiderosis: Electron microscopic, immunofluorescent, and iron kinetic studies. Chest 68:577, 1975.
54. Yeager H Jr, Powell D, Weinberg RM, et al: Idiopathic pulmonary hemosiderosis: Ultrastructural studies and response to azathioprine. Arch Intern Med 136:1145, 1976.
55. Corrin B, Jagusch M, Devar A, et al: Fine structural changes in idiopathic pulmonary haemosiderosis. J Pathol 153:249, 1987.
56. Louie S, Russell LA, Richeson RB, et al: Circulating immune complexes with pulmonary hemorrhage during pregnancy in idiopathic pulmonary hemosiderosis. Chest 104:1907, 1993.
57. van der Ent CK, Walenkamp MJ, Donckerwolcke RA, et al: Pulmonary hemosiderosis and immune complex glomerulonephritis. Clin Nephrol 43:339, 1995.
58. Lane DJ, Hamilton WS: Idiopathic steatorrhoea and idiopathic pulmonary haemosiderosis. BMJ 2:89, 1971.
59. Wright PH, Menzies IS, Pounder RE, et al: Adult idiopathic pulmonary haemosiderosis and coeliac disease. Q J Med 50:95, 1981.
60. Wright PH, Buxton-Thomas M, Keeling PW, et al: Adult idiopathic pulmonary haemosiderosis: A comparison of lung function changes and the distribution of pulmonary disease in patients with and without coeliac disease. Br J Dis Chest 77:282, 1983.
61. Bouros D, Panagou P, Arseniou P, et al: Idiopathic pulmonary haemosiderosis and autoimmune hypothyroidism: Bronchoalveolar lavage findings after cimetidine treatment. Respir Med 89:307, 1995.
62. Blanco A, Solis P, Gomez S, et al: Antineutrophil cytoplasmic antibodies (ANCA) in idiopathic pulmonary hemosiderosis. Pediatr Allergy Immunol 5:235, 1994.
63. Leaker B, Cambridge G, du Bois RM, et al: Idiopathic pulmonary haemosiderosis: A form of microscopic polyarteritis? Thorax 47:988, 1992.
64. Canfield CJ, Davis TE, Herman RH: Hemorrhagic pulmonary-renal syndrome: Report of three cases. N Engl J Med 268:230, 1963.
65. Soergel KH, Sommers SC: The alveolar epithelial lesion of idiopathic pulmonary hemosiderosis. Am Rev Respir Dis 85:540, 1962.
66. Murphy KJ: Pulmonary haemosiderosis (apparently idiopathic) associated with myocarditis, with bilateral penetrating corneal ulceration, and with diabetes mellitus. Thorax 20:341, 1965.
67. Gonzalez-Crussi F, Hull MT, Grosfeld JL: Idiopathic pulmonary hemosiderosis: Evidence of capillary basement membrane abnormality. Am Rev Respir Dis 114:689, 1976.
68. Brambilla CG, Brambilla EM, Stoebner P, et al: Idiopathic pulmonary hemorrhage: Ultrastructural and mineralogic study. Chest 81:120, 1982.
69. Hammond D, Crane J, with the assistance of Murphy A: Sequestration of iron in the lungs in idiopathic pulmonary hemosiderosis. J Dis Child 96:503, 1958.

70. Botting AJ, Brown AL, Divertie MB: The pulmonary lesion in a patient with Goodpasture's syndrome, as studied with the electron microscope. Am J Clin Pathol 42:387, 1964.

71. Beechler CR, Enquist RW, Hunt KK, et al: Immunofluorescence of transbronchial biopsies in Goodpasture's syndrome. Am Rev Respir Dis 121:869, 1980.

72. Hogan PG, Donald KJ, McEvoy JDS: Immunofluorescence studies of lung biopsy tissue. Am Rev Respir Dis 118:537, 1978.

73. Briggs WA, Johnson JP, Teichman S, et al: Antiglomerular basement membrane antibody-mediated glomerulonephritis and Goodpasture's syndrome. Medicine 58:348, 1979.

74. Wilson CB, Dixon FJ: Anti-glomerular basement membrane antibody-induced glomerulonephritis. Kidney Int 3:74, 1973.

75. Border WA, Baehler RW, Bhathena D, et al: IgA antibasement membrane nephritis with pulmonary hemorrhage. Ann Intern Med 91:21, 1979.

76. Espinosa-Melendez E, Forbes RDC, Hollomby DJ, et al: Goodpasture's syndrome treated with plasmapheresis: Report of a case. Arch Intern Med 140:542, 1980.

77. Wu M-J, Rajaram R, Shelp WD, et al: Vasculitis in Goodpasture's syndrome. Arch Pathol Lab Med 104:300, 1980.

78. Kondo N, Tateno M, Yamaguchi J, et al: Immunopathological studies of an autopsy case with Goodpasture's syndrome and systemic necrotizing angitis. Acta Pathol Jpn 36:595, 1986.

79. Slonim L: Goodpasture's syndrome and its radiological features. Australas Radiol 13:164, 1969.

80. Bowley NB, Steiner RE, Chin WS: The chest X-ray in antiglomerular basement membrane antibody disease (Goodpasture's syndrome). Clin Radiol 30:419, 1979.

81. Albelda SM, Gefter WB, Epstein DM, et al: Diffuse pulmonary hemorrhage: A review and classification. Radiology 154:289, 1985.

82. Müller NL, Miller RR: Diffuse pulmonary hemorrhage. Radiol Clin North Am 29:965, 1991.

83. Chea FK, Sheppard MN, Hansell DM: Computed tomography of diffuse pulmonary hemorrhage with pathologic correlation. Clin Radiol 48:89, 1993.

84. Niimi A, Amitani R, Kurasawa T, et al: Two cases of idiopathic pulmonary hemosiderosis: Analysis of chest CT findings. Nippon Kyobu Shikkan Gakkai Zasshi 30:1749, 1992.

85. Rubin GD, Edwards III DK, Reicher MA, et al: Diagnosis of pulmonary hemosiderosis by MR imaging. Am J Roentgenol 152:573, 1989.

85a. Seely JM, Effmann EL, Müller NL: High-resolution CT in pediatric lung disease: Imaging findings. Am J Roentgenol 168:1269, 1997.

85b. Engeler CE: High-resolution CT of airspace nodules in idiopathic pulmonary hemosiderosis. Eur Radiol 5:663, 1995.

85c. Lynch DA, Brasch RC, Hardy KA, et al: Pediatric pulmonary disease: Assessment with high-resolution ultrafast CT. Radiology 176:243, 1990.

86. Hodson CJ, France NE, Gordon I: Idiopathic juvenile pulmonary haemosiderosis. J Fac Radiol 5:50, 1953.

87. Theros EG, Reeder, MM, Eckert JF: An exercise in radiologic-pathologic correlation. Radiology 90:784, 1968.

88. Kennedy WPU, Shearman DJC, Delamore IW, et al: Idiopathic pulmonary haemosiderosis with myocarditis: Radioisotope studies in a patient treated with prednisone. Thorax 21:220, 1966.

89. Denson HB: Idiopathic pulmonary hemosiderosis: An adult case with acute onset, short course and sudden, fatal outcome. Ann Intern Med 53:579, 1960.

90. Bruwer AJ, Kennedy RLJ, Edwards JE: Recurrent pulmonary hemorrhage with hemosiderosis: So-called idiopathic pulmonary hemosiderosis. Am J Roentgenol 76:98, 1956.

91. Sybers RG, Sybers JL, Dickie HA, et al: Roentgenographic aspects of hemorrhagic pulmonary-renal disease (Goodpasture's syndrome). Am J Roentgenol 94:674, 1965.

92. Buerger L, Hathaway J: Idiopathic pulmonary haemosiderosis with allergic pulmonary vasculitis. Thorax 19:311, 1964.

93. Brannan HM, McCaughey WTE, Good CA: The roentgenographic appearance of pulmonary hemorrhage associated with glomerulonephritis. Am J Roentgenol 90:83, 1963.

94. Case Records of the Massachusetts General Hospital. N Engl J Med 319:227, 1988.

95. Aledort LM, Lord GP: Idiopathic pulmonary hemosiderosis: Severe anemia without hemoptysis—one year follow-up of pulmonary function. Arch Intern Med 120:220, 1967.

96. Coates JR, Bellamy JC: Idiopathic pulmonary hemosiderosis: A case report and discussion. Ann Intern Med 55:672, 1961.

97. Sprecace GA: Idiopathic pulmonary hemosiderosis: Personal experience with six adults treated within a ten-month period, and a review of the literature. Am Rev Respir Dis 88:330, 1963.

98. Smith BS: Idiopathic pulmonary haemosiderosis and rheumatoid arthritis. BMJ 1:1403, 1966.

99. Ditto WR, Ognibene AJ: Idiopathic pulmonary hemosiderosis without anemia: Report of two cases. Arch Intern Med 114:490, 1964.

100. Rafferty JR, Cook MK: Idiopathic pulmonary haemosiderosis with autoimmune haemolytic anaemia. Br J Dis Chest 78:282, 1984.

101. Silverman M, Hawkins D, Ackman CFD: Bilateral nephrectomy for massive pulmonary hemorrhage in Goodpasture's syndrome. Can Med Assoc J 108:336, 1973.

102. Elder JL, Kirk GM, Smith WG: Idiopathic pulmonary hemosiderosis and the Goodpasture syndrome. BMJ 2:1152, 1965.

103. Powell AH, Bettez PH: Goodpasture's syndrome: Pulmonary hemosiderosis with glomerulonephritis. Can Med Assoc J 90:5, 1964.

104. Gottehrer A, Reynolds SD, Libys JJ, et al: Renal vein thrombosis: Initial manifestations of Goodpasture's syndrome. Chest 99:239, 1991.

105. Hoscheit AM, Austin JK, Jones WL: Nonrhegmatogenous retinal detachment in Goodpasture's syndrome: A case report and discussion of the clinicopathologic entity. J Am Optom Assoc 64:563, 1993.

106. Rowe PA, Mansfield DC, Dutton GN: Opthalmic features of fourteen cases of goodpasture's syndrome. Nephron 68:52, 1994.

107. Mori R, Corvaglia AG, Frustaci A: An unusual chronic microvasculitis: Goodpasture's syndrome with late myocardial involvement. Recent Prog Med 83:649, 1992.

108. Ross JB, Cohen AD, Ghose T: Goodpasture's syndrome associated with skin involvement. Arch Dermatol 121:1442, 1985.

109. Kondo N, Tateno M, Yamaguchi J, et al: Immunopathological studies of an autopsy case with Goodpasture's syndrome and systemic necrotizing angiitis. Acta Pathol Jpn 36:595, 1986.

110. Wilson CB, Dixon FJ: Diagnosis of immunopathologic renal disease. Kidney Int 5:389, 1974.

111. Mathew TH, Hobbs JB, Kalowski S, et al: Goodpasture's syndrome: Normal renal diagnostic findings. Ann Intern Med 82:215, 1975.

112. Bates DV, Macklem PT, Christie RV: Respiratory Function in Disease: An Introduction to the Integrated Study of the Lung. 2nd ed. Philadelphia, WB Saunders, 1971.

113. Allue X, Wise MB, Beaudry PH: Pulmonary function studies in idiopathic hemosiderosis in children. Am Rev Respir Dis 107:410, 1973.

114. Roberts LN, Montessori G, Patterson JG: Idiopathic pulmonary hemosiderosis: Case report with pulmonary function tests and cardiac catheterization data. Am Rev Respir Dis 106:904, 1972.

115. Fuleihan FJD, Abboud RT, Hubaytar R: Idiopathic pulmonary hemosiderosis: Case report with pulmonary function tests and review of the literature. Am Rev Respir Dis 98:93, 1968.

116. Conlon PJ Jr, Walshe JJ, Daly C, et al:: Antiglomerular basement membrane disease: The long-term pulmonary outcome. Am J Kidney Dis 23:794, 1994.

117. Ewan PW, Jones HA, Rhodes CG, et al: Detection of intrapulmonary hemorrhage with carbon monoxide uptake: Application in Goodpasture's syndrome. N Engl J Med 295:1391, 1976.

118. Addleman M, Logan AS, Grossman RF: Monitoring intrapulmonary hemorrhage in Goodpasture's syndrome. Chest 87:119, 1985.

119. van Dorp R, Daha MR, Muizert Y, et al: A rapid ELISA for measurement of anti-glomerular basement membrane antibodies using microwaves. J Clin Lab Immunol 40:135, 1993.

120. Leatherman JW: Immune alveolar hemorrhage. Chest 91:891, 1987.

121. Pozo-Rodriguez F, Freire-Campo JM, Gutierrez-Millet V, et al: Idiopathic pulmonary haemosiderosis treated by plasmapheresis. Thorax 35:399, 1980.

122. Kurki P, Helve T, von Bonsdorff M, et al: Transformation of membranous glomerulonephritis into crescentic glomerulonephritis with glomerular basement membrane antibodies. Nephron 38:134, 1984.

123. Deodhar HA, Marshall RJ, Sivathondan Y, et al: Recurrence of Goodpasture's syndrome associated with mesangiocapillary glomerulonephritis. Nephrol Dial Transplant 9:72, 1994.

124. Elder G, Perl S, Yong JL, et al: Progression from Goodpasture's disease to membranous glomerulonephritis. Pathology 27:233, 1995.

125. Bonsib SM, Walker WP: Pulmonary-renal syndrome: Clinical similarity amidst etiologic diversity. Mod Pathol 2:129, 1989.

126. Travis WD, Carpenter HA, Lie JT: Diffuse pulmonary hemorrhage: An uncommon manifestation of Wegener's granulomatosis. Am J Surg Pathol 11:702, 1987.

127. Sauvaget F, Le Thi, HD, Piette JC, et al: Intra-alveolar hemorrhage in Wegener's granulomatosis. Presse Med 22:709, 1993.

128. Torralbo A, Herrero JA, Portolés J, et al: Alveolar hemorrhage associated with antineutrophil cytoplasmic antibodies in rheumatoid arthritis. Chest 105:1590, 1994.

129. Naschitz JE, Yeshurun D, Scharf Y, et al: Recurrent massive alveolar hemorrhage, crescentic glomerulonephritis, and necrotizing vasculitis in a patient with rheumatoid arthritis. Arch Intern Med 149:406, 1989.

130. Myers JL, Katzenstein AA: Microangiitis in lupus-induced pulmonary hemorrhage. Am J Clin Pathol 85:552, 1986.

131. Abud-Mendoza C, Diaz-Jouanen E, Alarcon-Segovia D: Fatal pulmonary hemorrhage in systemic lupus erythematosus: Occurrence without hemoptysis. J Rheumatol 12:558, 1985.

132. Schwab EP, Schumacher HR Jr, Freundlich B, et al: Pulmonary alveolar hemorrhage in systemic lupus erythematosus. Semin Arthritis Rheum 23:8, 1993.

133. Zamora MR, Warner ML, Tuder R, et al: Diffuse alveolar hemorrhage and systemic lupus erythematosus: Clinical presentation, histology, survival and outcome. Medicine (Baltimore) 76:192, 1997.

134. Imoto EM, Lombard CM, Sachs DPL: Pulmonary capillaritis and hemorrhage: A clue to the diagnosis of systemic necrotizing vasculitis. Chest 96:927, 1989.

135. Rossen RD, Hersh EM, Sharp JT, et al: Effect of plasma exchange on circulating immune complexes and antibody formation in patients treated with cyclophosphamide and prednisone. Am J Med 63:674, 1977.

136. Bocanegra TS, Espinoza LR, Vasey FB, et al: Pulmonary hemorrhage in systemic necrotizing vasculitis associated with hepatitis-B. Chest 80:102, 1981.

137. Yum MN, Lampton LM, Bloom PM, et al: Asymptomatic IgA nephropathy associated with pulmonary hemosiderosis. Am J Med 64:1056, 1978.

138. Buchanan GR, Moore GC: Pulmonary hemosiderosis and immune thrombocytopenia: Initial manifestations of collagen-vascular disease. JAMA 246:861, 1981.

139. Sternlieb I, Bennett B, Scheinberg IH: D-Penicillamine induced Goodpasture's syndrome in Wilson's disease. Ann Intern Med 82:673, 1975.

140. Hill HFH: Penicillamine in rheumatoid arthritis: Adverse effects. Scand J Rheumatol 28(Suppl):94, 1979.

141. Gavaghan TE, McNaught PJ, Ralston M, et al: Penicillamine-induced "Goodpasture's syndrome": Successful treatment of a fulminant case. Aust N Z J Med 11:261, 1981.

142. Gibson T, Burry HC, Ogg C: Goodpasture's syndrome and D-penicillamine. Ann Intern Med 84:100, 1976.

143. Louie S, Gamble CN, Cross CE: Penicillamine associated pulmonary hemorrhage. J Rheumatol 13:963, 1986.

144. Peces R, Riera JR, Arboleya LR, et al: Goodpasture's syndrome in a patient receiving penicillamine and carbimazole. Nephron 45:316, 1987.

145. Payton CD, Allison ME, Boulton-Jones JM: Henoch-Schönlein purpura presenting with pulmonary haemorrhage. Scott Med J 32:26, 1987.

146. Shichiri M, Tsutsumi K, Yamamoto I, et al: Diffuse intrapulmonary hemorrhage and renal failure in adult Henoch-Schönlein purpura. Am J Nephrol 7:140, 1987.

147. Markus HS, Clark JV: Pulmonary haemorrhage in Henoch-Schönlein purpura. Thorax 44:525, 1989.

148. Chang-Poon VY, Hwang WS, Wong A, et al: Pulmonary angiomatoid vascular changes in mitomycin C-associated hemolytic-uremic syndrome. Arch Pathol Lab Med 109:877, 1985.

149. Bernis P, Hamels J, Quoidbach A, et al: Remission of Goodpasture's syndrome after withdrawal of an unusual toxin. Clin Nephrol 23:312, 1985.

150. Thomashow BM, Felton CP, Navarro C, et al: Diffuse intrapulmonary hemorrhage, renal failure and a systemic vasculitis: A case report and review of the literature. Am J Med 68:299, 1980.

151. Coleman M, Stirling JW, Langford LR, et al: Glomerular basement membrane thinning in a patient with hematuria and hemoptysis mimicking Goodpasture's syndrome. Am J Nephrol 14:47, 1994.

152. Leatherman JW, Sibley RK, Davies SF: Diffuse intrapulmonary hemorrhage and glomerulonephritis unrelated to antiglomerular basement membrane antibody. Am J Med 72:401, 1982.

153. Holdsworth S, Boyce N, Thomson NM, et al: The clinical spectrum of acute glomerulonephritis and lung haemorrhage (Goodpasture's syndrome). Q J Med 55:75, 1985.

154. Boyce NW, Holdsworth SR: Pulmonary manifestations of the clinical syndrome of acute glomerulonephritis and lung hemorrhage. Am J Kidney Dis 8:31, 1986.

155. Zell SC, Duxbury G, Shankel SW: Alveolar hemorrhage associated with a membranoproliferative glomerulonephritis and smooth muscle antibody. Am J Med 82:1073, 1987.

156. Masson RG, Rennke HG, Gottlieb MN: Pulmonary hemorrhage in a patient with fibrillary glomerulonephritis. N Engl J Med 326:36, 1992.

157. Calls Ginesta J, Torras A, Ricart MJ, et al: Fibrillary glomerulonephritis and pulmonary hemorrhage in a patient with renal transplantation. Clin Nephrol 43:180, 1995.

158. Lai FM, Li EK, Suen MW, et al: Pulmonary hemorrhage: A fatal manifestation in IgA nephropathy. Arch Pathol Lab Med 118:542, 1994.

158a. Afessa B, Cowart RG, Koenig SM: Alveolar hemorrhage in IgA nephropathy treated with plasmapheresis. South Med J 90:237, 1997.

159. Ahmad D, Patterson R, Morgan WKC, et al: Pulmonary hemorrhage and haemolytic anaemia due to trimellitic anhydride. Lancet 2:328, 1979.

160. Manson MM: Epoxides: Is there a human health problem? Br J Ind Med 37:317, 1980.

161. Herbert FA, Orford R: Pulmonary hemorrhage and edema due to inhalation of resins containing tri-mellitic anhydride. Chest 76:546, 1979.

162. Patterson R, Nugent KM, Harris KE, et al: Immunologic hemorrhagic pneumonia caused by isocyanates. Am Rev Respir Dis 141:226, 1990.

163. Murray RJ, Albin RJ, Mergner W, et al: Diffuse alveolar hemorrhage temporally related to cocaine smoking. Chest 93:427, 1988.

164. Godwin JE, Harley RA, Miller KS, et al: Cocaine, pulmonary hemorrhage and hemoptysis. Ann Intern Med 110:843, 1989.

165. Forrester JM, Steele AW, Waldron JA, et al: Crack lung: An acute pulmonary syndrome with a spectrum of clinical and histopathologic findings. Am Rev Respir Dis 142:462, 1990.

166. Patterson R, Addington W, Banner AS, et al: Antihapten antibodies in workers exposed to trimellitic anhydride fumes: A potential immunopathogenetic mechanism for the trimellitic anhydride pulmonary disease—anemia syndrome. Am Rev Respir Dis 120:1259, 1979.

167. Koyabu S, Isaka N, Yada T, et al: Severe respiratory failure caused by recurrent pulmonary hemorrhage in Takayasu's arteritis. Chest 104:1905, 1993.

168. Bocanegra TS, Espinoza LR, Vasey FB, et al: Pulmonary hemorrhage in systemic necrotizing vasculitis associated with hepatitis B. Chest 80:102, 1981.

168a. Lai RS, Lin SL, Lai NS, et al: Churg-Strauss syndrome presenting with pulmonary capillaritis and diffuse alveolar hemorrhage. Scand J Rheumatol 27:230, 1998.

169. Bosch X, Font J, Mirapeix E, et al: Antimyeloperoxidase autoantibody–associated necrotizing alveolar capillaritis. Am Rev Respir Dis 146:1326, 1992.

170. Kikawada M, Ichinose Y, Minemura K, et al: Diffuse alveolar hemorrhage associated with proteinase 3-specific anti-neutrophil antibodies. Intern Med 36:430, 1997.

171. ter Maaten JC, Franssen CF, Gans RO, et al: Respiratory failure in ANCA-associated vasculitis. Chest 110:357, 1996.

172. Jennings CA, King TE, Tuder R, et al: Diffuse alveolar hemorrhage with underlying isolated, pauciimmune pulmonary capillaritis. Am J Respir Crit Care Med 155:1101, 1997.

173. Kagalwalla AF, Abu Taleb ARM, Kagalwalla YA, et al: Pulmonary hemorrhage in association with autoimmune chronic active hepatitis. Chest 103:634, 1993.

174. Griffin MT, Robb JD, Martin JR: Diffuse alveolar haemorrhage associated with progressive systemic sclerosis. Thorax 45:903, 1990.

175. Kariya ST, Stern RS, Schwartzstein RM, et al: Pulmonary hemorrhage associated with bullous pemphigoid of the lung. Am J Med 86:127, 1989.

175a. Schwarz MI, Zamora MR, Hodges TN, et al: Isolated pulmonary capillaritis and diffuse alveolar hemorrhage in rheumatoid arthritis and mixed connective tissue disease. Chest 113:1609, 1998.

176. Crausman RS, Achenbach GA, Pluss WT, et al: Pulmonary capillaritis and alveolar hemorrhage associated with the antiphospholipid antibody syndrome. J Rheumatol 22:554, 1995.

177. Gertner E, Lie JT: Pulmonary capillaritis, alveolar hemorrhage, and recurrent microvascular thrombosis in primary antiphospholipid syndrome. J Rheumatol 20:1224, 1993.

177a. Asherson RA, Cervera R, Piette JC, et al: Catastrophic antiphospholipid syndrome. Clinical and laboratory features of 50 patients. Medicine 77:195, 1998.

178. Schwarz MI, Sutarik JM, Nick JA, et al: Pulmonary capillaritis and diffuse alveolar hemorrhage: A primary manifestation of polymyositis. Am J Respir Crit Care Med 151:2037, 1995.

179. Struhar D, Sorkin P, Greif J, et al: Alveolar haemorrhage with pleural effusion as a manifestation of epithelioid hemangioendothelioma. Eur Respir J 5:592, 1992.

180. Carter EJ, Bradburne RM, Jhung JW, et al: Alveolar hemorrhage with epithelioid hemangioendothelioma. Am Rev Respir Dis 142:700, 1990.

181. Benditt JO, Farber HW, Wright J, et al: Pulmonary hemorrhage with diffuse alveolar infiltrates in men with high-volume choriocarcinoma. Ann Intern Med 109:674, 1988.

182. Segal SL, Lenchner GS, Cichelli AV, et al: Angiosarcoma presenting as diffuse alveolar hemorrhage. Chest 94:214, 1988.

183. Nara M, Sasaki T, Shimura S, et al: Diffuse alveolar hemorrhage caused by lung metastasis of ovarian angiosarcoma. Intern Med 35:653, 1996.

184. Russi E, Odermatt B, Joller-Jemelka HI, et al: Alveolar haemorrhage as a presenting feature of myeloma. Eur Respir J 6:267, 1992.

185. Sheffield EA, Moore-Gillon J, Murday AR, et al: Massive haemoptysis caused by spontaneous rupture of a bronchial artery. Thorax 43:71, 1988.

186. Akgun S, Lee DE, Weissman PS, et al: Hemoptysis and tracheoesophageal fistula in a patient with esophageal varices and Sengstaken-Blakemore tube. Am J Med 85:450, 1988.

187. Guidetti AS, Pik A, Peer A, et al: Haemoptysis as the sole presenting symptom of dissection of the aorta. Thorax 44:444, 1989.

188. Favre JP, Gournier JP, Adham M, et al: Aortobronchial fistula: Report of three cases and review of the literature. Surgery 115:264, 1994.

189. Casadevall J, Alvarez-Sala R, Prados C, et al: Dissection of ascending aorta: A new cause of alveolar hemorrhage? J Cardiovasc Surg (Torino) 35:327, 1994.

190. Cosmo LY, Risi G, Nelson S, et al: Fatal hemoptysis in acute bacterial endocarditis. Am Rev Respir Dis 137:1223, 1988.

191. Michelon G, Mullany CJ, Viggiano RW, et al: Massive pulmonary hemorrhage complicating mitral prosthetic valve obstruction. Chest 103:1903, 1993.

192. Nathan PE, Torres AV, Smith AJ, et al: Spontaneous pulmonary hemorrhage following coronary thrombolysis. Chest 101:1150, 1992.

193. Brown DL, MacIsaac AI, Topol EJ: Pulmonary hemorrhage after intracoronary stent placement. J Am Coll Cardiol 24:91, 1994.

194. Barnett VT, Bergmann F, Humphrey H, et al: Diffuse alveolar hemorrhage secondary to superwarfarin ingestion. Chest 102:1301, 1992.

195. Saka H, Ito T, Ito M, et al: Diffuse pulmonary alveolar hemorrhage in acute promyelocytic leukemia. Intern Med 31:457, 1992.

196. Swanson GA, Kaeley G, Geraci SA: Diffuse pulmonary hemorrhage after streptokinase administration for acute myocardial infarction. Pharmacotherapy 17:390, 1997.

197. Gopalakrishnan D, Tioran T, Emanuel C, et al: Diffuse pulmonary hemorrhage complicating thrombolytic therapy for acute myocardial infarction. Clin Cardiol 20:298, 1997.

198. Awadh N, Ronco JJ, Bernstein V, et al: Spontaneous pulmonary hemorrhage after thrombolytic therapy for acute myocardial infarction. Chest 106:1622, 1994.

198a. Khanlou H, Tsiodras S, Eiger G, et al: Fatal alveolar hemorrhage and Abciximab (ReoPro) therapy for acute myocardial infarction. Cathet Cardiovasc Diagn 44:313, 1998.

199. Chao NJ, Duncan Sr, Long GD, et al: Corticosteroid therapy for diffuse alveolar hemorrhage in autologous bone marrow transplant recipients. Ann Intern Med 114:145, 1991.

200. Robbins RA, Linder J, Stahl MG, et al: Diffuse alveolar hemorrhage in autologous bone marrow transplant recipients. Am J Med 87:511, 1989.

201. Mulder POM, Meinesz AF, de Vries EGE, et al: Diffuse alveolar hemorrhage in autologous bone marrow transplant recipients. Am J Med 90:278, 1991.

202. Sisson JH, Thompson AB, Anderson JR, et al: Airway inflammation predicts diffuse alveolar hemorrhage during bone marrow transplantation in patients with Hodgkin disease. Am Rev Respir Dis 146:439, 1992.

203. Agusti C, Ramirez J, Picado C, et al: Diffuse alveolar hemorrhage in allogenic bone marrow transplantation: A postmortem study. Am J Respir Crit Care Med 151:1006, 1995.

204. Morgan PGM, Turner-Warwick M: Pulmonary haemosiderosis and pulmonary haemorrhage. Br J Dis Chest 75:225, 1981.

205. Chryssanthopoulos C, Cassimos C, Panagiotidou C: Prognostic criteria in idiopathic pulmonary hemosiderosis in children. Eur J Pediatr 140:123, 1983.

206. Scheer RL, Grossman MA: Immune aspects of the glomerulonephritis associated with pulmonary hemorrhage. Ann Intern Med 60:1009, 1964.

207. Azen EA, Clatanoff DV: Prolonged survival in Goodpasture's syndrome. Arch Intern Med 114:453, 1964.
208. Walker JM, Joekes AM: Survival after haemoptysis and nephritis. Lancet 2:1199, 1963.
209. McCall CB, Harris TR, Hatch FE: Non-fatal pulmonary hemorrhage and glomerulonephritis. Am Rev Respir Dis 91:425, 1965.
210. Teichman S, Briggs WA, Kniesser MR, et al: Goodpasture's syndrome: Two cases with contrasting early course and management. Am Rev Respir Dis 113:223, 1976.
211. Rosenblatt SG, Knight W, Bannayan GA, et al: Treatment of Goodpasture's syndrome with plasmapheresis: A case report and review of the literature. Am J Med 66:689, 1979.
212. Erickson SB, Kurtz SB, Donadio JV Jr, et al: Use of combined plasmapheresis and immunosuppression in the treatment of Goodpasture's syndrome. Mayo Clin Proc 54:714, 1979.
213. Walker RG, Scheinkestel C, Becker GJ, et al: Clinical and morphological aspects of the management of crescentic anti-glomerular basement antibody (anti-GBM) nephritis/Goodpasture's syndrome. Q J Med 54:75, 1985.
214. Merkel F, Pullig O, Marx M, et al: Course and prognosis of anti-basement membrane antibody (anti-BM-Ab)–mediated disease: Report of 3 cases. Nephrol Dial Transplant 9:372, 1994.
215. Hind CRK, Bowman C, Winearis CG, et al: Recurrence of circulating anti-glomerular basement membrane antibody three years after immunosuppressive treatment and plasma exchange. Clin Nephrol 21:244, 1984.
216. Burke BR, Bear RA: Recurrent Goodpasture's syndrome. Can Med Assoc J 129:978, 1983.
217. Keller F, Nekarda H: Fatal relapse in Goodpasture's syndrome 3 years after plasma exchange. Respiration 48:62, 1985.
218. Klasa RJ, Abboud RT, Ballon HS, et al: Goodpasture's syndrome: Recurrence after a five-year remission. Am J Med 84:751, 1988.
219. Wahls TL, Bonsib SM, Schuster VL: Coexistent Wegener's granulomatosis and anti-glomerular basement membrane disease. Hum Pathol 18:202, 1987.

# PART VIII

# EMBOLIC LUNG DISEASE

# CHAPTER 48

# *Thrombosis and Thromboembolism*

## PULMONARY THROMBOSIS

Although embolization is undoubtedly the most frequent mechanism invoked to explain the presence of intrapulmonary thrombus, *in situ* thrombosis of pulmonary vessels is probably more common than is generally appreciated. However, because of the difficulty in distinguishing thromboemboli from foci of *in situ* thrombus, both radiologically and pathologically, and because the predisposing conditions for pulmonary thrombosis are frequently the same as those for systemic venous thrombosis, it can be difficult to state with certainty which of the two processes is operative in a specific case.

The pathogenesis and the effects of pulmonary vascular thrombosis are related to a large extent to its site and can be discussed conveniently under three headings: (1) arteries, (2) arterioles and capillaries, and (3) veins. As with other such classifications, it should be remembered that these categories are not mutually exclusive, and thrombosis occurs in more than one site in some cases.

### Pulmonary Arteries

The most common cause of *in situ* arterial thrombosis is probably infectious pneumonia, in which vascular damage occurs adjacent to abscesses or foci of active granulomatous inflammation. Thrombosis related to a primary or metastatic neoplasm is also frequent; it can result from invasion of the vessel by the neoplasm or vascular compression by expanding tumor. Less common causes include immune-mediated vasculitis,[1] trauma,[2] aneurysms,[3] indwelling catheters,[4] congenital heart anomalies associated with decreased pulmonary blood flow (e.g., tetralogy of Fallot),[5] and sickle cell trait or disease (*see* page 1832).[6–8] Other pulmonary and cardiac diseases, such as emphysema,[9] pneumoconiosis, mitral stenosis, and primary hypertension,[10] have also been associated with pulmonary arterial thrombosis; however, thromboemboli occur with such frequency in these conditions that it is difficult, if not impossible, to estimate with any degree of accuracy the true incidence of thrombosis. It is also likely that propagation of thrombus proximal to peripheral thromboemboli is responsible for some cases of chronic thrombosis of major pulmonary arteries.[11] Finally, it is possible that *in situ* thrombosis of small pulmonary arteries is involved in the pathogenesis of primary pulmonary hypertension (*see* page 1898).

Grossly, *in situ* arterial thrombosis should be suspected if there is adjacent parenchymal disease or if there is extensive and continuous thrombus in multiple vessels (the formation of a cast of the arterial tree being unlikely with the multiple fragments of thrombus characteristic of emboli). Histologically, *in situ* arterial thrombosis should be considered when there is associated vasculitis or when the thrombus is located eccentrically on the side of the vessel wall adjacent to a focus of parenchymal inflammation (Fig. 48–1). The genesis of isolated thrombi unassociated with pneumonia or other active inflammatory pulmonary disease cannot be determined histologically in most instances; although such *in situ* thrombi undoubtedly occur, they are usually considered thromboemboli.

Thrombosis is most often identified in small elastic or muscular arteries supplying lung that is already the site of disease; as a result, the relationship of the thrombus to radiologic or clinical manifestations is often difficult to evaluate. It is likely, however, that its effects are slight or absent in the majority of cases. Exceptions are the necrosis and cavitation that occur in some cases of pneumonia (lung "gangrene") or vasculitis, the pathogenesis of the tissue destruction being related at least partly to the thrombosis and resulting ischemia. In addition, thrombus occasionally extends proximally from a focus of active parenchymal in-

flammation, especially in tuberculosis;[10] such extension can sometimes occur as far as the pulmonary trunk and contralateral main pulmonary artery, resulting in severe obstruction of pulmonary blood flow and cor pulmonale. Thrombosis associated with sickle cell disease has also been implicated as a cause of sudden death.[12]

### Pulmonary Arterioles and Capillaries

Thrombosis of small pulmonary vessels is common in immunologically mediated capillaritis (microangiitis) (*see* page 1513); in this situation, it is usually associated with other evidence of vascular damage, particularly parenchymal hemorrhage. Fibrin thrombi can also be found in small vessels of patients who have disseminated intravascular coagulation (DIC) related to such conditions as septicemia and amniotic fluid embolism.[13, 14] Such fibrin thrombi may be obvious histologically as elongated, densely eosinophilic structures filling the vessel lumen; sometimes, however, they are relatively small and admixed with blood cells (Fig. 48–2), in which case they may be overlooked. The pulmonary parenchyma in cases of DIC may be normal or may show a variable degree of air-space hemorrhage.[15] In one autopsy study of 87 patients with the condition, microscopic fibrin thrombi were detected in 43 (approximately 50%), compared with 13 of 64 (20%) in the control patients.[16] (In this study, the frequency of macroscopic and microscopic "thromboemboli" and pulmonary infarction and hemorrhage was also greater in patients who had DIC than in the controls.)

Pulmonary microvascular thrombosis (sometimes associated with DIC) is also frequent in the early stage of the adult respiratory distress syndrome (ARDS) and, in fact, has been implicated in its pathogenesis. *In situ* thrombosis of small as well as large pulmonary vessels can also occur in sickle cell disease[6, 17] and may be responsible for some cases of the acute chest syndrome seen in patents with this condition (*see* page 1832).

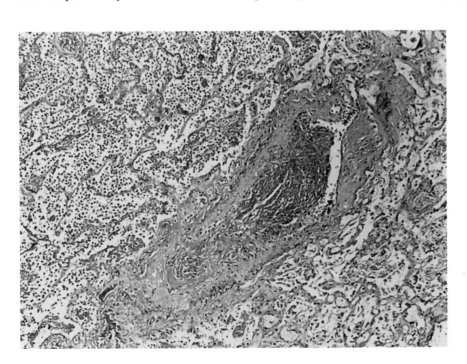

**Figure 48–1. Pulmonary Artery Thrombosis *in Situ*.** The left portion of the figure shows alveolar air spaces full of polymorphonuclear leukocytes, representing an acute bacterial pneumonia. A pulmonary artery at the junction of affected and unaffected lung reveals eccentric thrombosis in relation to the pneumonia (×80).

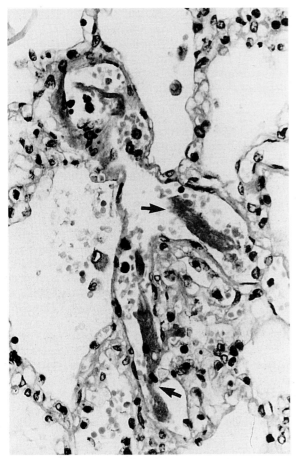

**Figure 48–2. Disseminated Intravascular Coagulation.** A magnified view of lung parenchyma shows an arteriole containing several elongated partially occlusive plugs of fibrin *(arrows)*.

Although fibrin thrombi are probably the most common histologic manifestation of pulmonary microvascular thrombosis, in some cases the only abnormality is the presence of platelet aggregates. Sometimes no clear-cut clinical association is evident, in which case it is possible that the aggregates represent no more than a premortem agonal phenomenon. However, their association with sudden postoperative death has been reported in patients undergoing liver transplantation (*see* page 1734).[18]

### Pulmonary Veins

As in the arterial circulation, pulmonary venous thrombosis commonly develops secondary to a focus of infectious pneumonia or a neoplasm. Other related conditions include those in which there is decreased blood flow (e.g., tetralogy of Fallot),[5] fibrosing mediastinitis (occasionally associated with pulmonary infarction),[19–21] and veno-occlusive disease; in fact, venous thrombosis has been considered to be intimately involved in the pathogenesis of the last-named disorder (*see* page 1734).

## PULMONARY THROMBOEMBOLISM

Emboli of fragments of thrombus to the pulmonary vasculature are common and range from minute fibrin-plate-let aggregates unassociated with clinical, radiologic, or functional consequences to massive clots that completely occlude the pulmonary trunk or a main pulmonary artery and cause sudden death. Because pulmonary thromboembolism (PTE) by definition implies the formation of thrombus elsewhere than the lungs, the two processes are frequently discussed together under the term *venous thromboembolic disease* (VTED). The term *deep venous thrombosis* (DVT) usually implies thrombosis of the deep veins of the leg, and it is used here in that sense; however, it should be noted that although clinically significant thrombosis is most common at this site, many of the factors involved in the pathogenesis of thrombosis and their consequences are similar at other sites.

### Epidemiology

It is difficult to be certain of the precise incidence of DVT and PTE and of the importance of the two with respect to morbidity and mortality. There are many reasons for this uncertainty, including the following:

1. Reported data are relatively scarce; incidence rates in population-based studies have been published in only a few countries, and the use of different diagnostic criteria makes comparison among them difficult.[22]

2. The condition is difficult to diagnose ante mortem,[22] largely as a result of the lack of specificity of signs, symptoms, radiographic manifestations, and electrocardiogram (ECG) abnormalities that may accompany it;[23, 24] in fact, many of the conditions that increase the risk for PTE, such as congestive heart failure or severe pneumonia, have symptoms that are identical to those of embolism itself.[24]

3. Signs and symptoms are absent in many patients;[25–27] in fact, some investigators have suggested that as many as 80% of patients who have PTE are asymptomatic.[28, 29] There are several reasons for this, the major one probably being that most emboli occur in subsegmental or smaller arteries; because most of these do not cause pulmonary infarction and because the vascular reserve of the lung is such that hemodynamic changes are usually minor and transient, clinical signs and symptoms are often minimal or lacking altogether. In addition, some patients who die of PTE are unable to communicate owing to sedation or coma or do so precipitously as a result of massive vascular obstruction.[30]

4. Diagnostic testing for PTE may be insufficient. Although it is recognized that 90% of emboli originate in the lower extremity,[31] many physicians fail to appreciate the poor sensitivity of the clinical examination to detect DVT at this site;[31] as a result, the diagnosis of PTE may not be considered in patients without clinical signs of DVT, whose pulmonary symptoms are consequently attributed to another condition.

**Incidence of Deep Venous Thrombosis.** As with PTE, reported figures on the incidence of DVT are variable and depend on several factors, including how the condition has been diagnosed (e.g., by phlebography, ultrasonography, scintigraphy), the specific risk factors of the population under study (e.g., postoperative state, use of the contraceptive pill, presence of cancer), whether the diagnosis is made during screening or at the onset of symptoms, and whether heparin prophylaxis has been practiced. For example, in one study of 160 patients undergoing total hip replacement, evidence of DVT was found in the legs in 81 (50%).[32] In another investigation of 72 patients followed prospectively after total hip replacement, 11 of 12 not given anticoagulation developed DVT;[33] however, 18 of the 60 patients who received anticoagulation as prophylaxis also developed DVT. These figures contrast with a much lower incidence (1.9%) in another series of 1162 patients who underwent hip replacement and in whom diagnostic testing was confined to those who were symptomatic.[34] In an investigation of 350 patients admitted to a regional trauma unit in Toronto, 63 (18%) developed proximal DVT;[35] only 3 had symptoms and signs suggesting the diagnosis.

**Incidence of Pulmonary Thromboembolism.** The incidence of PTE is very high when lung specimens from autopsies performed in hospitalized patients are examined in detail prospectively. For example, in one series of 61 such autopsies, the lungs were found to contain organized or recent thromboemboli in 39 (64%).[36] In another investigation of 263 right lungs, emboli were found in approximately 50%;[37] as the researchers indicated, the overall incidence must have been even higher, because only one lung was examined. Although the results of these autopsy studies indicate that PTE is a common finding in patients dying in hospital, it should be remembered that the majority of emboli are incidental findings that have not contributed to death.

More information is available concerning the incidence and case-fatality rates of clinically recognized PTE in hospitalized patients. Based on extrapolation of limited data concerning the fatality rate of untreated PTE and on autopsy studies that indicate that in-hospital PTE is usually not diagnosed before death, Dalen and Alpert concluded that there were approximately 630,000 cases of PTE annually in the United States;[38] of these, it was estimated that 163,000 (about 25%) had both a diagnosis and an initiation of therapy. However, it is likely that silent PTE does not have the 30% mortality of untreated PTE to which Dalen and Alpert referred. For example, in one study of 87 patients who had venographically proven DVT and no chest symptoms and who were randomized to receive treatment with anticoagulation or placebo, lung scintigraphy was performed at 10 and 60 days to assess the development of silent PTE;[39] no patient died in either group, and there was no significant difference in the rate of silent PTE (13% in the anticoagulated group and 8% in the coagulated group)!

In another study, which included data from 16 short-stay community hospitals in Massachusetts, investigators found an average annual incidence of PTE of 23 per 100,000 population and an in-hospital case-fatality rate of 12%.[40] Extrapolation of this data led to the conclusion that there are 170,000 new cases of clinically recognized DVT or PTE or both in patients treated in short-stay hospitals each year, an estimate substantially less than that proposed by Dalen and Alpert. On the other hand, it has been estimated that the incidence of PTE in the Pisa region of Italy is in the order of 100 per 100,000 population, approximately eight times the estimate from Massachusetts;[41] this high incidence was attributed to the presence of a PTE referral center in the area, with a consequent sensitization of physicians to the diagnosis. The prevalence of diagnosed acute PTE among

51,645 patients hospitalized over a 21-month period in a single institution in Detroit was about 1%.[42]

The reported incidence of PTE following surgical procedures has not been consistent. A review of data available from the untreated arms of patients in studies of the use of heparin prophylaxis in a variety of surgical patients (general, urologic, and orthopedic) revealed an incidence of PTE of approximately 2%; around one third of this 2% died.[43] However, in one series of 1,162 patients from Bristol, England, who underwent total hip replacement without the routine use of prophylactic anticoagulation, the death rate from PTE was only 0.34%.[34] A somewhat disturbing 3.2% incidence of PTE was found in a series of 1,033 consecutive patients who underwent cardiac surgery (mostly coronary bypass surgery);[44] the mortality rate in the patients who had PTE was approximately 19%, compared with 3% in those without. These findings contrast with those of much larger groups of patients undergoing a variety of open heart procedures;[45, 46] only 41 patients had a diagnosis of PTE while in hospital among more than 10,000 patients in one series,[45] and 0.56% of 5,694 patients were recognized as having PTE in a second.[46]

The incidence of PTE increases with age.[40, 47, 48, 48a] Using a random sample of claims from Medicare enrollees in the United States, the annual incidence rate for the complication was found by one group of investigators to be 1.3 per thousand between the ages of 65 and 69 years and 2.8 between 85 to 89 years;[47] 21% of affected patients died during the initial hospitalization, and an additional 18% died in the following year, reflecting the association of PTE with substantial comorbidity. Whether age is a risk factor independent of the conditions that commonly accompany aging, such as heart failure, cancer, and surgical immobilization, has not been determined. Ethnicity may also be a factor in the risk for VTED; in one study, Asians and Pacific Islanders living in California had a very low risk for DVT and a very low relative risk for PTE compared with the rates for white individuals.[48b] In another study of the records of almost 400,000 Medicare beneficiaries in the United States who had a primary or secondary diagnosis of PTE between 1984 and 1991, a decline of 10% to 15% was seen in white patients;[48c] a similar decline was not evident in African Americans.

**Pulmonary Thromboembolism as a Cause of Death.** A number of studies have been undertaken to identify the frequency with which PTE causes or contributes to death; extrapolation from the reported figures implies that the population studied is representative of the population at large, an assumption that is suspect in most series. One of the most widely quoted estimates in the United States was provided by Dalen and Alpert in the early 1970s. According to these authors, the annual number of deaths from PTE was estimated to be 200,000;[38] of these, embolism was said to be the sole cause of death in half the cases and a major contributing cause in the remainder. These figures suggest that PTE was the third most frequent cause of death in the United States at that time! The conclusions were based on extrapolation of the findings of two autopsy studies in which it was considered that 7% of deaths in hospital were due solely to PTE and that an additional 7% to 10% of autopsied persons had embolism as a major contributing cause. In the Dalen and Alpert study, it was assumed that patients in chronic care institutions would have a higher prevalence of PTE as a sole or contributing cause of death and that 5% of sudden deaths outside the hospital (not due to heart disease, stroke, or accident) were the result of PTE.

The results of subsequent investigations suggest that these 1970 estimates may have exaggerated the importance of PTE as a cause of death. For example, in one review of 21,529 autopsies performed between 1960 and 1984 in a Norwegian institution that had an autopsy rate of 75% to 80%, PTE was found in 9% of cases.[49] Overall, 3.5% of deaths were thought to be solely the result of embolism. Although the incidence of PTE did not change during the study period, the frequency with which it was considered to be the sole cause of death increased significantly with time. The diagnosis was missed clinically in approximately 85% of cases overall; it was made before death in about 20% of patients from 1960 to 1969 and in only 11% of cases in the last 5 years of the study.

Analysis of another series of 3,412 autopsies (out of a total of 6,858 deaths) in a Tennessee hospital revealed massive PTE to be the cause of death in 3.8% of patients in the last 5 years of the study;[50] this incidence was significantly lower than in the initial period of observation, possibly reflecting refined diagnostic techniques, prevention strategies, and therapy. Among 2,427 autopsies performed at the Mayo Clinic between 1985 and 1989, only 92 (approximately 4%) patients had deaths ascribed clinically and pathologically to PTE.[30] However, this figure may be an overestimation, because 54% of the 92 patients whose death was attributed to PTE had an underlying condition that might by itself have caused death. In another review of 11,044 autopsies in Singapore performed over a 5-year period, death was considered to be the result of PTE in only 116 patients (about 1%);[51] the diagnosis was unsuspected in 77% of patients. Among 404 autopsies performed at the Henry Ford Hospital in Detroit, PTE was observed in 59 (15%);[42] 20 patients (5%) were felt to "have died from pulmonary embolism." Most patients had "advanced associated disease," with death occurring within hours of the onset of symptoms; embolization was unsuspected in 14 patients. Of 260 autopsies showing PTE over a 1-year period in a Swedish hospital, only 21 fatal or "contributory" events were found in postoperative patients,[52] a group in whom one might suspect that the burden of significant comorbidity was relatively light.

Undoubtedly, the classification of PTE at autopsy as the cause of death, as a contributory factor, or as an incidental finding is somewhat arbitrary. Nevertheless, the results of the studies cited previously suggest that the estimate of Dalen and Alpert that 7% of deaths in acute care hospitals are the result of PTE alone is too high; instead, an incidence of 2% or less is likely to be more accurate.

It might be expected that the incidence of PTE as a cause of sudden death would be substantially less in nonhospitalized than in hospitalized patients. Some investigators have confirmed this hypothesis; for example, in one autopsy series of 9,785 sudden "natural deaths" in Florida, only 1.5% of cases were considered to be the result of PTE.[53] However, others have found substantially higher figures (e.g., 9.5% of 507 patients brought to the emergency department of an Italian hospital following sudden death outside the hospital).[54]

In conclusion, the true incidence of PTE and DVT is not known. Most emboli never come to medical attention, and the performance of community-based prospective trials with objective endpoints would be logistically difficult.[43] Estimates based on autopsy material, hospital discharge diagnosis, or death certificate diagnosis are inconsistent and limited by patient selection, inaccuracy, and frequent lack of objective corroboration of clinical impressions.[43] Despite this, there can be little doubt that with even the most conservative of estimates, PTE is an important illness.

## Etiology and Pathogenesis

The pathogenesis of PTE can be conveniently considered under two headings: (1) factors determining the development of thrombus and (2) effects on the lungs of the thromboemboli that follow.

### Development of Thrombus

Because of the effects of gravity and immobility, the legs are the most vulnerable site for an alteration in venous blood flow, and the frequency of PTE directly parallels thrombosis in this site; in fact, more than 90% of thromboemboli originate in the lower extremity.[31] The specific site in the leg in which thrombi are located is important: those confined to the calf generally do not embolize to the lung, whereas those that extend to or arise from the popliteal veins or higher are at risk to do so.[55–58] A popliteal artery aneurysm is an uncommon but well-described abnormality associated with PTE, presumably because of associated venous obstruction.[59] Most thrombi appear to begin as fibrin-platelet–red blood cell (RBC) aggregates, often in the region of a valve pocket, where velocity is relatively slow.[60–64]

Although the leg is by far the most common source of thromboemboli, other sites are seen occasionally. The most frequent of these are the pelvic veins (including the periprostatic veins in men), the inferior vena cava, and the right atrium; the right ventricle[65, 66] (rarely in association with a right ventricular myxoma),[67, 68] right-sided heart valves, superior vena cava,[69, 70] and veins of the neck and arms[71] are relatively infrequent sources. The incidence of thrombosis in the arms has been estimated to be less than 2% of all cases of DVT;[72] however, complicating PTE is not uncommon, being reported in 3 of 25 patients in one series[73] and in 4 of 19 with catheter-related thrombosis in another.[74]

When carefully assessed at autopsy, foci of peripheral thrombosis are sometimes multiple, making determination of the precise source of an embolus difficult; for example, in one study of 78 patients known to have had PTE, peripheral thrombi were found in 62, with multiple sites in more than a third;[75] the leg veins were involved in 46%, the right atrium in 23%, the inferior vena cava in 19%, and the pelvic veins in 16%. It should be emphasized that the source of thrombus is not found during life in up to 50% of cases of ultimately fatal embolism[76, 77] and may not be identifiable even at autopsy.[76]

The eponymous "Virchow's" triad of venous stasis, intimal injury, and alteration in coagulation remains the basis of our understanding of the mechanisms of venous thrombosis. Most instances of venous thrombosis and PTE, particularly those that are acute and massive, are associated with medical, surgical, or obstetric conditions that have well-defined risk factors for one or more of these three abnormalities.[78, 79] For example, in a chart review of 1,000 patients hospitalized in 1 of 16 Massachusetts acute care institutions, one or more risk factors were identified in 78%.[79] Of 1,231 patients who had PTE in another study, 96% had one or more recognized risk factors.[78] The risk of developing DVT also increases proportionately to the number of risk factors present in hospitalized patients.[80] In addition, a history of VTED combined with one of the risk factors is associated with a greatly increased chance of a new thrombotic event.[43, 81]

### Altered Blood Flow

The velocity of blood flow through the systemic veins to the heart depends on the cardiac output, the resistance to venous flow, the milking action of the local musculature, and, in those veins in which they are present, intraluminal valves. An alteration in any of these can lead to a decrease in blood flow that may predispose to thrombus formation.

Many of the clinical conditions associated with venous thrombosis, particularly in the legs, are associated with an abnormality of one or more of these factors. Such conditions include left-sided heart failure and shock (decreased cardiac output, immobilization),[81] obesity, pregnancy,[82, 83] intra-abdominal tumors, right-sided heart failure, external pressure from leg casts or bandages (increased resistance to flow),[81] strokes,[43] the postsurgical or paraplegic state (immobility with loss or decrease of muscle activity), and varicose veins.[43, 81, 84] Although unsupported by appropriate controlled studies, it seems likely that prolonged travel also constitutes a risk for PTE.[85, 86] Slowing of blood flow that is caused by intrinsic abnormality of the blood itself, such as in multiple myeloma[87, 88] or sickle cell anemia,[89] also predisposes to thrombosis.

An alteration in blood flow resulting in localized areas of turbulence may also be partly related to the formation of thrombus associated with foreign objects such as indwelling Swan-Ganz arterial catheters,[90, 91] central vein catheters,[74, 92] pacing catheters,[93] Hickman catheters,[94, 95] and cerebrospinal fluid shunt[96] or inferior vena cava filter devices.[97]

### Endothelial Injury

The role of endothelial injury in the pathogenesis of DVT appears to be of little importance in most situations.[60, 63, 98] In a study of 50 small thrombi in the pockets of femoral vein valves, no evidence of antecedent intimal damage was identified; however, microscopic foci of fibrin thrombi were found within apparently normal valves, which the investigator speculated were the precursors of future macroscopic thrombi.[61] In addition, although experimental venous trauma is associated with platelet adherence to exposed subendothelial tissue, it has been found to be a weak promoter of fibrin thrombus formation.[63] Thus, venous thrombosis secondary to injury or inflammation of the vessel wall (thrombophlebitis) is probably uncommon compared with the typical bland thrombosis unassociated with these events. Despite these observations, endothelial injury can be a significant factor in some situations in which there is localized venous trauma, such as total hip replacement.[32] It is also likely to be im-

portant in the thrombosis associated with bacterial endocarditis, immunologically mediated vasculitis, and trauma associated with intravenous devices.

Despite the typical absence of evidence of overt endothelial injury in association with venous thrombosis, it is likely that endothelial cells have a role in pathogenesis. For example, studies of endothelial cells lining fresh thrombi excised from patients who have chronic thromboembolic pulmonary hypertension have shown a very high level of expression of type I plasminogen activator inhibitor compared with that in endothelial cells not associated with thrombi.[99] It is possible that this inhibitor plays a role in the stabilization of thrombus, because these patients have a diminished fibrinolytic response to venous thrombosis compared with that in normal individuals.[100] In addition, an alteration in thrombomodulin, a membrane-bound protein cofactor on endothelial cells that is involved in the thrombin-mediated activation of protein C, has been found to be associated with the development of thrombosis in some individuals.[101]

Paradoxically, the contrast medium used to detect venous thrombosis can itself initiate thrombosis, presumably as a result of endothelial damage;[102, 103] it has been estimated that this complication occurs in 3% to 5% of patients undergoing the procedure.[103] In a follow-up study of a group of patients 5 to 10 years after proven venous thrombosis in a lower limb, a surprising incidence of filling defects was identified in previously normal veins, presumably representing organized thrombi;[104] the investigators suggested that the initial diagnostic venography might have been responsible.

### Coagulation Abnormalities

Occasionally, an alteration in the normal coagulation cascade renders a patient hypercoagulable and increases the risk of VTED, either in association with other risk factors[105, 106] or in their absence. Such abnormalities have been identified in less than 10% of patients who have VTED studied prospectively,[107] and they may be inherited or acquired.[107a] Although investigation of a possible coagulation disorder may be appropriate in a patient who develops PTE at a young age[108] or in whom there is a family history of VTED,[109] these clinical features have been found to have a poor predictive value for discovering such disorders in unselected populations of patients who have DVT alone.[107]

**Inherited Coagulation Abnormalities.** Activated protein C resistance constitutes the most common inherited cause of an underlying predisposition to VTED.[110, 111] In most cases, it is related to the presence of factor V Leiden (FV:Q$^{506}$),[112, 113] a substance that is resistant to degradation by activated protein C. The abnormal protein results from a single point mutation in the factor V gene. The mutation itself is present heterozygously in about 2% to 6% of normal individuals.[112, 114, 115] It was identified in approximately 12% of men who developed VTED in the Physicians' Health Study,[114] in 24 of 165 (15%) French patients admitted to hospital for DVT (compared with 4% of control patients),[116] and in 41 of 251 (16%) unselected patients studied in Padua, Italy, who had a first symptomatic episode of DVT.[117] In the last group, the risk of recurrent PTE in those carrying the gene was double that of those who did not. In contrast to these studies was a review of unselected patients who underwent investigation for possible PTE in Geneva, in which the prevalence of the trait was 5.5% in those in whom the diagnosis was confirmed and 4.0% in those in whom it was excluded;[115] the calculated odds ratio of 1.36 for presence of the trait was not statistically significant.

Factor V Leiden seems to confer increased risk for thrombosis in patients with other (albeit not all[119a]) risk factors for VTED.[43, 105, 106, 118] For example, in one study of 50 women who developed VTED during pregnancy or oral contraceptive use, 6 of 10 with the mutation developed first-trimester PTE compared with 3 of 40 without it.[110] The increase in risk for thrombotic events conferred by factor V Leiden is also associated with increasing age,[119] an observation that supports the hypothesis that the pathogenesis of PTE in this setting involves acquired as well as genetic factors.

Protein S is a vitamin K–dependent protein that serves as a cofactor for activated protein C.[43] Its absence is also an important risk factor for VTED. For example, in one study of 71 individuals who had a heterozygous deficiency (derived from 136 members of 12 families with protein S deficiency), 55 (77%) had manifestations of VTED;[105] the mean age of onset was 28 years. In another investigation of 141 young, unrelated patients evaluated at a thrombosis referral clinic in Germany, a heterozygous deficiency was identified in seven (5%).[120] An acquired deficiency of protein S also may be related to the increased frequency of DVT in some patients who have idiopathic inflammatory bowel disease.[121] The impact of inherited proteins deficiency seems to be particularly marked in patients who have a concomitant reduction in fibrinolytic capacity as a result of an increase in plasminogen activator inhibitor-1 (PAI-1). In one study of 46 such individuals, 12 (26%) had a history of PTE compared with only 7 of 97 patients (7%) who were protein S deficient and heterozygous for the PAI allele.[121a]

Antithrombin III is an $\alpha_2$-globulin that inactivates thrombin[43] as well as other procoagulants, such as factors XIIa, IXa, and Xa.[109] Previous estimates of thrombosis risk in individuals who have a deficiency of this substance may have been exaggerated as a result of the lack of objective diagnostic tests,[106] and it is now believed that deficiency of antithrombin III is less prevalent than proteins C or S among patients who are referred to specialized centers for evaluation of VTED.[43] In one review of 31 heterozygous family members of individuals who had VTED, only 6 had had thrombotic complications;[106] in 5 cases, there was an additional risk factor. However, more extended follow-up of these individuals would likely have led to the appreciation of an increased risk for the development of these complications.[118]

The role of the antiphospholipid antibodies in VTED is discussed in detail in Chapter 39 (see page 1430). When affected patients who do not have systemic lupus erythematosus (SLE) experience thrombotic events, they are said to have the primary antiphospholipid syndrome.[122] Histories of venous thrombosis, PTE, arterial thrombosis, thrombocytopenia, livedo reticularis, and pulmonary hypertension are similar to those of patients with SLE who have these antibodies.[123, 123a] In unselected patients in whom the diagnosis of SLE has been excluded and who have a first episode of VTED, only the lupus anticoagulant seems to be pathogenetically important among the antiphospholipid antibodies.[124] This antibody was found in a surprising 9 of 65 such patients in one series.[124] Recurrent thrombotic events are common in affected individuals.[125]

Hyperhomocystinemia has been reported to increase the risk of DVT.[126, 126a] In one group of 269 patients studied during their first such episode, the odds ratio of finding a plasma homocysteine level above the 95th percentile was 2.5 compared with that in a group of normal controls;[126] none of the patients had another coagulation disturbance. Children who have concurrent homocystinuria and factor V Leiden seem to be at very high risk for the development of venous or arterial thrombosis.[127] Other rare coagulation disorders associated with familial VTED include dysfibrinogenemia[43, 128] and altered thrombomodulin expression.[101]

**Acquired Coagulation Abnormalities.** A variety of noninherited factors that affect coagulation also predispose to thrombus formation. Two of the most common are neoplasms and oral contraceptives. The widely used eponym "Trousseau's syndrome" describes the paraneoplastic phenomenon of recurrent arterial and venous thrombosis; the condition may lead to death in the absence of heparin anticoagulation.[129] Neoplasms of the lung,[130, 131] gastrointestinal tract, pancreas,[132] and genitourinary tract are particularly associated with the complication; affected patients have an approximately fourfold increased incidence of PTE.

Although prospective studies controlling for other risk factors for VTED, such as immobilization, have not been performed,[133] a number of coagulation abnormalities have been found in patients with malignancy. In addition, cancer is found at the initial evaluation in patients who have "idiopathic" PE[134] or DVT[135] more frequently than in patients who have other risk factors for these disorders. For example, in one study of 21 patients who had PTE and no recognized risk factors, 6 (29%) were found to have cancer;[134] by contrast, only 3 of 51 patients (6%) who had other risk factors were discovered to have malignancy. In another study of 136 patients hospitalized for the treatment of DVT, 16 (12%) were discovered to harbor a malignancy.[136] In some of these patients, thrombus has been shown to be intimately associated with intravascular mucus secreted by the tumor, suggesting that this substance might be the initiator of thrombosis;[137] in others, an alteration in platelet aggregation or in the normal level of coagulation factors or inhibition, such as fibrinogen, antithrombin, and thromboplastin, has been identified.[138] These abnormalities are probably more common than generally appreciated; for example, in one investigation of 42 patients who had pulmonary carcinoma, "thrombosis-inducing activity (TIA)" was detected in the blood of 13 (31%), a prevalence far in excess of that in control patients;[130] injection of plasma into mice caused their death from multiple thromboses. Similar "TIA" was identified in 41 of 73 patients (56%) who had non–small cell carcinoma in another investigation;[139] among patients who died, the incidence of DIC and ARDS was much higher in those with TIA than in those without. Whether these data justify a search for underlying malignancy in the absence of clinical evidence of cancer is open to question.[139a, b] Based on an analysis of data from the Danish Cancer Registry for the years 1977 and 1992, an elevated risk for cancer was identified in the first 6 months following a diagnosis of VTED (standardized incidence ratio, 1.3); 40% of affected patients had widespread metastases at the time of diagnosis, leading the authors to conclude that an aggressive search for a hidden cancer is not warranted. Nevertheless, we feel that a limited search for a primary malignancy, including mammography and pelvic ultrasonography in women and a test for prostate-specific antigen in men, is justified.[139b, c]

Although most studies have been flawed by methodologic errors—particularly the failure to confirm the diagnosis objectively[43]—there have been consistent reports since the 1960s of an increased risk of VTED in women taking oral contraceptives.[140–145, 145a] The results of older studies suggested that the risk of death from venous or cerebral thromboembolism in young women taking oral contraceptives was seven- to eightfold that of women not taking these agents.[141] A more recent World Health Organization review of 1,143 patients who had nonfatal VTED confirmed the conclusions of previous studies,[146] although the increased risk (odds ratio 3 to 4) was lower than that found 3 decades ago.[142] Similarly, among women enrolled in the prospective investigation of pulmonary embolism diagnosis (PIOPED) study, those using oral contraceptives had an increased risk of developing postoperative pulmonary embolism (PE).[147] The risk is dose-related[143] and has been considered to be especially elevated in patients who have congenital left-to-right intracardiac shunts.[148] The culpable ingredient in the hormone pill is thought to be estrogen,[149] which both augments clotting and impairs fibrinolysis.[150]

Patients who have myeloproliferative disorders associated with thrombocytosis (e.g., polycythemia vera and essential thrombocythemia) are prone to develop both thrombotic and hemorrhagic complications,[151] whereas those with reactive thrombocytosis are less at risk.[152] In addition to *in situ* pulmonary thrombosis, patients who have DIC have an increased incidence of VTED.[16] Chemotherapy for a variety of malignancies has also been associated with increased risk for the development of VTED as a result of a drug-related increase in coagulability.[43, 153, 154]

### Miscellaneous Factors

A number of other conditions have also been associated with VTED; their pathogenesis is varied and generally less well understood than that of the risk factors previously discussed. Blood group O has been shown to be the least likely to be associated with venous thrombosis, particularly in postoperative and pregnant or puerperal women.[155, 156] Similarly, the excess risk of VTED for women taking oral contraceptives does not seem to apply to those who have blood group O, being seen instead particularly in women who have blood group A.[43] Although the reason for this is not certain, it may be related to the lower levels of antithrombin III and higher levels of factor VIII found in the latter individuals.

It is possible that defecation may trigger PTE; in one retrospective review of all patients who had a discharge diagnosis of PTE over a 3-year period, approximately 7% had symptoms of PTE that developed in close association with defecation.[157]

Certain diseases seem to be associated with a *decreased* risk of VTED. For example, PTE appears to be an infrequent cause of mortality in patients who have chronic renal failure, likely as a result of abnormalities of platelet function. In one series of 2,255 autopsies, the overall incidence of PTE was 32% (18% microscopic, 4% macroscopic, and 10% both);[158]

by contrast, in the 95 patients who had chronic renal failure (serum creatinine level over 5.0 mg/dl), the incidence was only 9% (all microscopic). In a similar vein, no diagnoses of DVT or PTE were recorded among 228 patients hospitalized with multiple sclerosis at one hospital over a 3.5-year period.[159]

### Consequences of Pulmonary Thromboembolism

A fragment of embolized thrombus lodged within a pulmonary artery has two immediate consequences—an increase in pressure proximal to the thrombus and a decrease or cessation of flow distal to it. Although the effects of thromboemboli are largely a result of these two consequences, the final clinical, radiologic, and pathologic manifestations are modified by a number of factors, including the size of the embolus, the presence of bacteria within the thrombus (septic embolism, *see* page 1829), the presence and extent of underlying lung abnormality (including previous thromboemboli), and the presence of extrapulmonary disease, particularly of the cardiovascular system. These manifestations can be discussed under five headings: (1) hemorrhage and infarction, (2) bronchoconstriction and atelectasis, (3) acute hypertension, (4) chronic hypertension, and (5) edema. The contribution of these abnormalities to the gas exchange derangements that follow PTE is discussed at the end of this section.

#### Hemorrhage and Infarction

Parenchymal consolidation secondary to sudden occlusion of a pulmonary artery is the result of one or more of three processes: (1) hemorrhage alone, (2) hemorrhage with necrosis of lung parenchyma (infarction),* or (3) pneumonia. The last-named occurs in association with septic thromboemboli or with infection superimposed on infarcted lung. The first two are a direct consequence of a deficiency of pulmonary arterial blood flow and represent different manifestations of the severity of the vascular occlusion.

Although the precise pathogenesis of pulmonary hemorrhage following PTE has not been established clearly, ischemic damage to endothelial and alveolar epithelial cells, permitting the passage of RBCs and fluid into the air spaces, is clearly involved. The blood has been considered to be derived from the bronchial arteries via bronchopulmonary

---

*Because clinical and radiographic findings seldom permit reliable differentiation between hemorrhage and infarction, at least in their early stages, the two are usually referred to in living patients by the single term *infarction*. In the past, pulmonary hemorrhage has also been referred to as "incipient" or "incomplete" infarction;[160] although it is likely that some such lesions do represent true tissue necrosis as well as hemorrhage at a stage before pathologic or radiologic identification is possible, it is clear that others are the result of reversible ischemic damage to the lung parenchyma. Despite this fundamental pathogenetic distinction, we feel it is appropriate to use the word *infarct* radiologically in all situations in which a pulmonary opacity develops within one or more bronchopulmonary segments or subsegments distal to an occluded pulmonary artery. Should follow-up examinations show rapid clearing, it would be reasonable to consider the lesion to be the result of hemorrhage alone. Should the opacity clear more slowly (i.e., over several weeks), it is reasonable to infer that the vascular insult resulted in tissue death. On the other hand, from a pathologic point of view, a precise distinction between hemorrhage and infarction is usually possible, and in the following pathologic descriptions these terms are used according to their specific connotation.

anastomoses,[161] but it can also come from the pulmonary artery itself (when the vessel is only partly occluded by the thrombus or after clot retraction or fibrinolysis has partly reopened the vessel) or from the pulmonary vein via retrograde flow. In fact, there is evidence that retrograde flow from pulmonary veins may be important in preventing infarction.[162]

Although it is not known precisely what proportion of PTEs result in infarction, autopsy reviews have provided evidence that the incidence is as low as 10% to 15%.[36, 163] Clinical and experimental findings suggest that pulmonary vascular occlusion, particularly of one of the main pulmonary arteries, usually results in no permanent tissue damage unless other factors coexist.[164] The most common underlying condition predisposing to infarction is congestive heart failure,[160] an association believed to be explained by increased pulmonary venous pressure and resulting decreased bronchial artery blood flow. The results of some animal studies have supported this hypothesis.[164, 165]

Other conditions or findings associated with an increased incidence of infarction include shock (possibly by decreasing blood flow through the bronchial arteries),[166] malignancy (especially of the lung in one series),[167] multiple thromboemboli, more than one lobe containing thromboemboli, peripheral as opposed to central thromboemboli,[161, 166] and chest wall compression and pleural effusion.[164] In one study in which the factors associated with pulmonary infarction were examined, the major determinants were the functional status of the patient, the number of lobes containing emboli, the presence of left ventricular failure, and the coexistence of pulmonary carcinoma.[167] Using discriminant analysis on a group of 21 patients, the combination of these four variables predicted the presence of infarction with 70% accuracy; the size of the infarct was correlated most strongly with the use of vasodilators and the embolic burden.

### Bronchoconstriction and Atelectasis

The pathophysiologic consequences of sudden occlusion of a pulmonary artery include a local decrease in compliance and ventilation, caused at least partly by bronchoconstriction resulting from decreased partial pressure of carbon dioxide ($Pco_2$) within the bronchus supplying the occluded segment.[168–170] In an experimental study of PTE in dogs, airway resistance was found to increase, whereas bronchography showed no change in caliber of the large bronchi,[171] suggesting that the obstruction occurs in small conducting airways.[172] In another investigation, again in dogs, radiographic opacification with powdered tantalum of airways as small as 0.5 mm in diameter showed that all outlined intrapulmonary airways constricted equally after either ipsilateral or contralateral vascular occlusion by thromboembolus.[173] Subsequently, it was shown that autologous thrombi injected into the pulmonary artery of the left diaphragmatic lobe of dogs resulted in narrowing of right-sided airways of 0.4 to 15 mm in inner diameter, indicating reflex bronchoconstriction;[174] section of the left cervical vagus nerve reduced contralateral bronchoconstriction significantly.

Using a similar technique plus bronchial pressure measurements, another group of investigators used aged, fresh, and "inert" (agarose) clots as emboli to assess the mechanical and humoral factors in the pathogenesis of bronchocon-

striction.[175] The latter occurred in airways 0.3 to 3.0 mm in diameter in all three groups; because humoral effects derived from the thrombus could be discounted or minimized in the inert agarose and aged clots, it was concluded that mechanical factors were the common denominator. Bronchoconstriction was usually transient, the airways returning to normal dimensions within 5 minutes; the time of bronchoconstriction correlated with a drop in pulmonary compliance and an increase in airway resistance. This transient bronchoconstriction has also been demonstrated by radionuclide imaging, unilateral pulmonary artery occlusion resulting in immediate diminution in ventilation of the ischemic lung and return to normal in 4 to 6 hours.[176]

Despite the results of the previous study, it is likely that humoral reactions related to thrombi themselves are also involved in the pathogenesis of bronchoconstriction. Animal experiments have provided evidence that thrombi passing through the bloodstream to the lungs collect platelets; when exposed to fresh thrombin, these can release serotonin and histamine, giving rise to bronchoconstriction.[177] Clinical and physiologic studies in humans have also indicated that pulmonary emboli are associated with the release of vasoactive and bronchoconstrictive substances such as serotonin, prostaglandins, and histamine; in addition to causing bronchoconstriction and vasoconstriction, they may result in altered pulmonary microcirculatory permeability.[178] In both animals[177] and humans,[179] these responses can be prevented with heparin.

Despite the frequency of bronchoconstriction associated with PTE, clinical signs of airway compromise are uncommon. For example, in one study of 72 patients who had PTE, physiologic evidence of bronchoconstriction was found in 61, whereas only a few had a wheeze.[180] In another investigation of 250 patients who had acute PTE confirmed by angiography, only 12 had sufficient wheezing to suggest a diagnosis of asthma; in 6 of the 12, asthma had been diagnosed several years before embolism occurred.[181] Therefore, although physiologic evidence of bronchoconstriction is common in patients who have PTE, wheezing is uncommon and is more likely to be evident in patients who have asthma.

Loss of lung volume is a common radiographic finding of PTE and is usually more striking when accompanied by infarction.[182] An alteration in surfactant almost certainly plays a role in this process,[183] because ligation of either the right or left pulmonary artery results in a reduction in lung volume and an increase in surface tension of the alveolar lavage fluid on the affected side.[184] Presumably, surfactant depletion results from the failure of delivery of the necessary substrates to alveolar type II cells.[31]

### Acute Hypertension

Information regarding the precise hemodynamic changes in humans following PTE is of necessity imprecise. Measurements that have been obtained are from a survivor population, and premorbid data regarding baseline hemodynamics in affected patients are not available for comparison with postembolic findings.[185] Nevertheless, certain observations concerning hemodynamic changes can be made.

In patients who do not have underlying cardiopulmonary disease, PTE increases pulmonary arterial pressure, the pressure rise depending on both mechanical blockage and increase in venous return as a result of hypoxemia-induced increase in sympathetic tone.[186] Initially, the cardiac index rises in previously healthy individuals,[185] aided by Starling's mechanisms as the right atrial pressure rises and by an increase in the heart rate. In fact, the presence of a depressed cardiac index without elevation of the right atrial pressure implies the presence of comorbid cardiac pathology.[185]

The observation that the pressure rise associated with obstruction of 25% to 30% of the vascular bed by thrombus is greater than that produced by experimental obstruction of 50% of the vascular bed by other means in normal individuals suggests that neural or humoral factors, or both, are also important.[187] The precise nature of these factors has not been determined; however, patients who have acute PTE have been found to have high blood levels of the potent vasoconstrictor endothelin, presumably as a result of increased synthesis or defective pulmonary handling of this peptide, or both.[188] In previously healthy individuals, the severity of pulmonary hypertension correlates with the severity of vascular occlusion; however, mean pulmonary artery pressures greater than 40 mm Hg are rarely seen.[189] In fact, the finding of pressures above this level implies the presence of pre-embolic cardiopulmonary disease or a history of unrecognized recurrent PTE.

Although patients with small PTEs may have no symptoms or signs, occlusion of a major portion of the pulmonary arterial system almost invariably results in acute pulmonary hypertension and right-sided heart failure. (A small atrial or ventricular septal defect may be sufficient to relieve the right-sided hypertension and is the rare exception to this general rule.) Even in the presence of multiple emboli, pulmonary hypertension is not sustained in patients without prior cardiopulmonary disease until at least 50% (probably closer to 70%) of the pulmonary vascular tree is occluded.[190–195]

As right ventricular afterload increases, right ventricular work rises with the increase in pulmonary artery pressure. If the right ventricle cannot tolerate this work, its end-diastolic pressure will rise.[31] This is associated with an increase in the oxygen requirement of the right ventricle, such that its dependence on coronary perfusion becomes critical.[31] A fall in systemic blood pressure may result in decreased right ventricular coronary perfusion, establishing a vicious cycle leading to right ventricular infarction or death. As cardiac output decreases, the pulmonary artery pressure may fall deceptively toward a more normal value. Although systemic blood pressure falls as the blood delivered to the left ventricle falls, the results of some animal experiments indicate that left ventricular preload may also be impaired by leftward shift of the interventricular septum and by pericardial constraint caused by right ventricular dilation.[196]

The sequence of events described previously may not hold for patients who have underlying cardiopulmonary disease. A fall in cardiac index is the general rule in such patients and appears to occur independently of the degree of vascular obstruction.[189] Right ventricular failure is more common in patients who have coronary artery disease and PTE, even in the absence of a previous history of left ventricular failure, than in patients who had no previous history of cardiopulmonary disease.[197] In practice, it may be difficult to determine to what extent pulmonary hypertension

is the result of thromboemboli and to what extent it can be attributed to prior disease. The presence of pulmonary hypertension in patients who have chronic obstructive pulmonary disease (COPD) is an indication of advanced disease; a simple measurement of the forced expiratory volume in 1 second ($FEV_1$) as an indicator of the severity of disease may be useful in distinguishing underlying disease from embolic disease as the cause of the rise in pulmonary artery pressure.[198]

### Chronic Hypertension

Chronic thromboembolic pulmonary hypertension is rare, being found in less than 0.5% of routine autopsies in several studies (*see* page 1904).[199] However, increased awareness of the abnormality and aggressive diagnostic intervention have led to more frequent diagnoses than previously; in fact, it has been estimated that about 1% of patients with PTE will develop chronic hypertension as a consequence.[200]

Although classically the development of pulmonary hypertension has been attributed to recurrent emboli,[201] clinical and pathologic observations and findings at surgery suggest that it is more often the result of retrograde propagation of clot *in situ* and of secondary structural changes in the pulmonary vasculature not directly affected by thrombus.[200–202] Vasoconstriction may also be important, because in some patients the hypertension is partially reversible following the administration of vasodilating agents.[204] Although thrombin-induced changes in the vascular endothelium might promote the development of a local procoagulant environment,[203] systemic procoagulant states are identified in less than 10% of cases.[205, 206] In one retrospective review of 216 patients who had chronic thromboembolic pulmonary hypertension and who were being considered for surgical intervention, approximately 10% were found to have lupus anticoagulant;[206] more than half of these developed heparin-associated thrombocytopenia, an association that remains unexplained.

### Edema

Diffuse pulmonary edema is sometimes seen in patients who have PTE.[207] In many, this is the result of heart failure at the time of the embolic episode.[208, 209] However, embolization of only one lung in animal experiments has been shown to result in bilateral pulmonary edema in some cases, suggesting the possibility of neurogenic or humoral mechanisms.[210, 211] Embolization of microthrombi in animals induces pulmonary vascular injury, which leads to an increase in vascular permeability.[212–214] These effects involve neutrophil sequestration and oxygen radical generation[212, 214–217] and are blunted by prostaglandin inhibition.[212, 213, 218] Although these experimental observations are more closely related to ARDS, it is possible that similar mechanisms are involved in the pathogenesis of the edema associated with PTE.

Generally speaking, mechanical factors do not seem to play a role in edema formation, because pulmonary artery pressure is poorly transmitted to the capillaries.[219] However, under exceptional circumstances such as congenital absence of the right or left pulmonary artery,[220] this mechanism might be important. Pulmonary edema localized to the left upper lobe has been well documented in a patient with massive embolism affecting the left lower lobe and right lung.[221] Sparing of the nonperfused areas of lung in both acute and chronic pulmonary embolization has also been reported in patients who develop noncardiogenic pulmonary edema.[222, 223]

## Gas Exchange Abnormalities

Hypoxemia and hypocapnia are common in patients who have PTE.[31, 185, 224] Obstruction of the vascular bed leads to an increase in dead space ventilation.[31, 224] Although this impairs the efficient elimination of carbon dioxide, compensatory hyperventilation in unaffected units more than compensates for this.[224] The magnitude of elevation of dead space ventilation does not correlate with the degree of vascular obstruction,[225] a finding that is likely explained by regional reflex bronchoconstriction in affected areas;[226] however, a normal ratio of dead space to tidal volume ($V_D/V_T$) is very uncommon in this setting.[227]

Areas of low ventilation-perfusion ($\dot{V}/\dot{Q}$) account for most of the hypoxemia seen in patients who have PTE. Although mechanical diversion of blood to unobstructed vessels explains part of this phenomenon,[225, 226, 228] reflex and humorally mediated bronchoconstriction, as previously discussed, is likely more significant. Shunt may become important as a cause of hypoxemia when perfusion of atelectatic areas occurs or when pulmonary hypertension is associated with the opening of the foramen ovale.[224] When the cardiac index falls, a low mixed venous oxygen tension can augment the hypoxemia caused by areas of shunt and $\dot{V}/\dot{Q}$ mismatch.[229, 230] Diffusion impairment seems to have little role.[228]

## Pathologic Characteristics

### Lung Parenchyma

In the majority of instances, lung parenchyma distal to a pulmonary thromboembolus is either normal or shows only mild atelectasis and minimal intra-alveolar hemorrhage or edema. When changes are more marked, they consist of either hemorrhage alone or a combination of hemorrhage and necrosis.

Parenchymal hemorrhage is grossly similar to infarction in its early stage and consists of a more or less wedge-shaped area of red, consolidated lung. In the absence of tissue death, the blood usually disappears fairly rapidly, and its residue may not be grossly detectable if the lung is examined a week or more after the embolic episode. Occasionally, deposition of hemoglobin-derived pigment in parenchymal and vascular interstitial tissue imparts a distinct yellow appearance to the previously affected lung that may remain for weeks after the initial event. In the early stages, histologic examination shows only intra-alveolar hemorrhage and edema, with intact alveolar walls. Later on, hemosiderin-laden macrophages or interstitial pigment usually is the only evidence of prior damage.

Within 1 or 2 days of thromboembolism, an infarct becomes easily recognizable as a firm, more or less wedge-shaped area of hemorrhagic consolidation typically abutting the pleura (Fig. 48–3). Although it is usually well demarcated, patchy areas of parenchymal hemorrhage may be present adjacent to it (a feature that accounts for the poor definition of infarcts radiographically). Overlying fibrinous pleuritis is often present (see Fig. 48–3). Multiple foci of infarction are not infrequent (Fig. 48–4). With time, the necrotic parenchyma becomes clearly demarcated from adjacent lung by a zone of organization tissue that may be red in appearance (reflecting its pronounced vascularity) or distinctly white (as a result of the influx of a large number of polymorphonuclear leukocytes (see Fig. 48–3). Eventually, the infarcted parenchyma is completely replaced by fibrous tissue, resulting in a contracted, somewhat elongated scar frequently associated with pleural puckering (see Fig. 48–3).

Cavitation within the infarct usually (but not invariably[231, 232]) indicates the presence of superimposed infection (although it may be difficult to distinguish this from primary pneumonia with secondary vascular thrombosis. Whatever the etiology, cavitation is typically associated with a prominent leukocytic infiltrate, the enzymes from these cells presumably causing liquefaction of necrotic tissue as a precursor to drainage and cavity formation. As a result, cavities are sometimes seen at the periphery of an infarct where they are adjacent to granulation tissue (Fig. 48–5). Occasionally, the hemorrhagic appearance of a partly organized infarct is lacking, the affected parenchyma appearing white and resembling a pulmonary carcinoma.

Histologically, infarcted lung is manifested by coagulative necrosis, which, in its early stage, may be somewhat obscured by alveolar hemorrhage and edema. Organization by granulation tissue is identifiable at the periphery after several days (Fig. 48–6). Reactive epithelial changes, particularly of type 2 pneumocytes, are often present at the margin of the infarct; when expectorated, these cells occasionally give rise to a false-positive cytologic diagnosis of malignancy.[233] Long-standing infarcts show dense parenchymal fibrosis in which the underlying lung architecture often can still be recognized. Airways within the fibrotic region may remain patent and viable, reflecting the preservation of the bronchial circulation; evidence of recanalized thrombus may be seen in pulmonary arteries (Fig. 48–7). The pleura in the vicinity of the infarct typically shows a prominent increase in vascularity as well as fibrosis and retraction into the lung (see Fig. 48–7).

Experimental investigations in dogs and observations on humans who have protracted pulmonary artery occlusion reveal a gradual increase in the bronchial circulation, which anastomoses freely with the pulmonary vasculature.[234, 235] Such systemic pulmonary arterial anastomoses are usually inapparent on postmortem aortography 3 to 7 days after embolization but are well formed by 3 to 4 weeks.[75]

### Thromboemboli and Pulmonary Vessels

The fate of pulmonary thromboemboli depends on multiple factors, including the status of the patient's fibrinolytic system, the degree of organization of the thrombus before its embolization, and the amount of new thrombus added in situ. Although emboli occasionally change little in size, thereby causing chronic vascular obstruction,[236] the vast majority are largely degraded by one or more of three

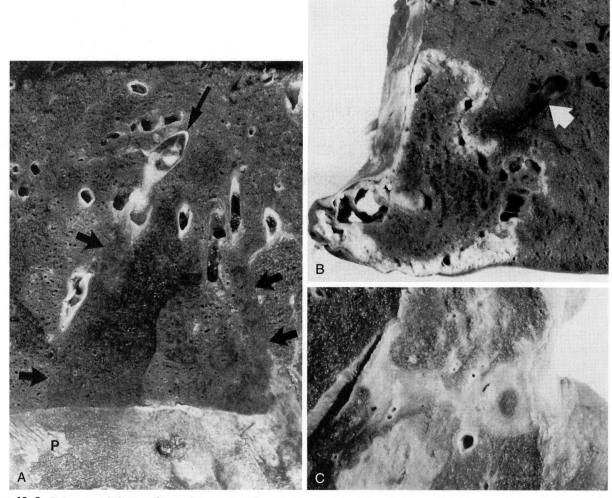

**Figure 48–3. Pulmonary Infarcts: Gross Appearance.** Recent *(A)*, organizing *(B)*, and remote *(C)* infarcts are illustrated. In *A*, a relatively ill-defined but roughly triangular focus of hemorrhagic and necrotic lung parenchyma can be seen adjacent to the pleura *(small arrows)*. Note the thrombus in the feeding pulmonary artery *(large arrow)* and the fibrinous pleuritis (P). The basal aspect of a lower lobe *(B)* shows a distinct zone of white tissue at the junction of necrotic and viable parenchyma, representing an acute inflammatory reaction to the presence of necrotic tissue; focal cavitation is also evident. Note again the pulmonary artery thrombus *(arrow)* and the residual pleuritis. An appearance such as this suggests an interval of several weeks since the original thromboembolic episode. In *C*, an organized infarct in a superior segment of a lower lobe is manifested by a roughly linear band of fibrous tissue associated with pleural puckering. (*C* from Fraser RS: Pathologic characteristics of venous thromboembolism. *In* Leclerc JR [ed]: Venous Thromboembolic Disorders. Philadelphia, Lea & Febiger, 1991. Reproduced with permission.)

mechanisms—lysis, fragmentation and peripheral embolization, and organization and recanalization.

**Lysis.** Both radiographic[237] and perfusion scanning[238] studies have shown that in many cases the flow through obstructed arteries returns relatively rapidly in the first few days after embolization. These clinical observations have been substantiated experimentally by several workers. For example, in one investigation in which serial radiographs were obtained of dogs following administration of thromboemboli labeled with powdered tantalum, a gradual decrease in the breadth of the radiopaque labels in the individual clots was found, particularly during the first 2 to 4 days after embolization.[239] In another study of fresh clot emboli in dogs, the volume of the embolized clot was seen to diminish by 50% in 3 hours.[240] Such rapid and extensive dissolution suggests the effect of fibrinolysis.

**Fragmentation and Peripheral Embolization.** In the study utilizing powdered tantalum that was cited previously, clots

were observed to fragment into small pieces that embolized farther toward the periphery of the lung;[239] this process was observed somewhat later than lysis and was most prominent after the first week following embolization. The pathogenesis of this fragmentation may be related to splitting of the thrombus into smaller and smaller pieces as a result of ingrowth of endothelial cells and macrophages from the vessel wall.[241]

**Organization and Recanalization.** Ingrowth of myofibroblasts, macrophages, and endothelial cells from the vessel wall into the peripheral portion of a thrombus can result in its organization and eventual incorporation into the wall as a fibrous plaque, typically in an eccentric location (Fig. 48–8). Alternatively, some thrombi undergo lysis and organization in their central portion at the same time as they undergo peripheral organization, resulting in the formation of multiple small vascular channels within the original lumen (recanalization) (Fig. 48–9). Although the lumens of such

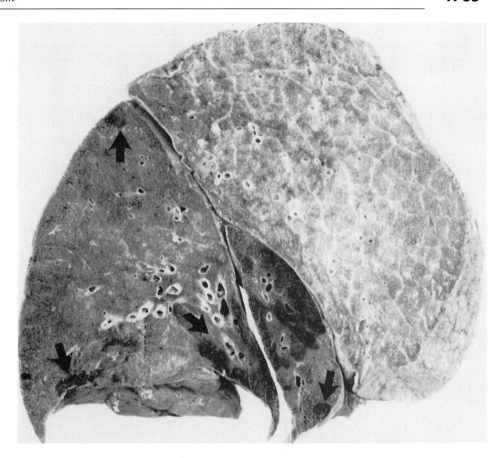

**Figure 48–4. Thromboembolism with Multiple Pulmonary Infarcts.** A sagittal slice of right lung shows multiple recent pleural-based infarcts in the middle and lower lobes *(arrows)*. (The prominent interlobular septa in the upper lobe are the result of lymphangitic carcinomatosis related to metastatic breast carcinoma.)

embolized vessels are inevitably diminished in cross-sectional area, these processes undoubtedly result in a much greater flow than would have been possible without organization.

In addition to changes attributable to organization of

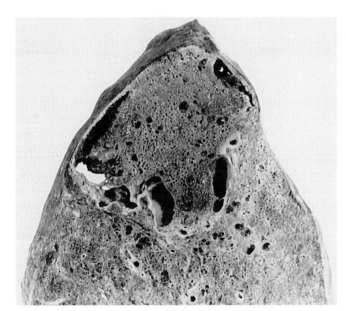

**Figure 48–5. Pulmonary Infarct: Peripheral Cavitation.** A magnified view of the superior segment of a lower lobe shows a well-delineated infarct that has separated from the adjacent viable lung in several places. A thin layer of white tissue (representing a pyogenic exudate) is evident adjacent to most of the separated tissue.

the thromboembolus, the pulmonary artery wall itself can undergo several alterations in the acute stage of embolization. Occasionally, necrosis and inflammation are seen[242, 243] (Fig. 48–10), possibly as a result of local ischemia induced by the impacted thrombus. Splits in the intimal and medial elastic laminae, focal areas of medial fibrosis, and both true and false saccular aneurysms have also been attributed to thromboemboli.[242, 244] It has been speculated that at least some of these changes might be caused by mechanical stretching at the time of embolic impaction.[244]

Despite the angiographic evidence of rapid dissolution in many cases, some recent thromboemboli remain intact and can be recognized grossly at autopsy by one or more of three characteristics: (1) the presence of distinct laminations (Fig. 48–11*A* and *B*), corresponding to alternating bands of RBCs and platelet-fibrin aggregates developed during the initial stage of venous thrombosis; (2) adherence to the vessel wall, sometimes associated with a white appearance indicative of organization and fibrosis (*see* Fig. 48–11*C*); and (3) in larger vessels, the presence of a coiled appearance as a result of imperfect fit and folding of the thrombus as it lodges in the artery (*see* Fig. 48–11*D*). If these features are lacking, it may be difficult to distinguish with certainty a recent thromboembolus from a postmortem clot. Organizing or organized thromboemboli can also be recognized in many cases as foci of intraluminal fibrous tissue containing small hemorrhagic spaces (representing areas of recanalization) or as fibrous bands or webs traversing the lumen (Fig. 48–12).[245, 246, 249]

Histologic examination of thrombi shows various degrees of organization, depending both on the extent of pul-

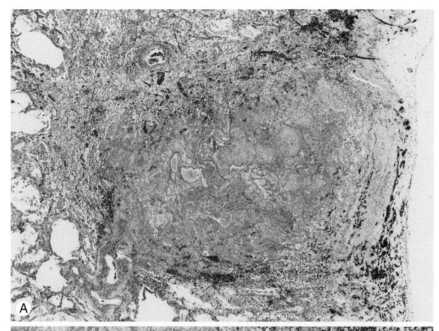

**Figure 48–6. Organizing Pulmonary Infarct.**
A histologic section at low power *(A)* reveals a fairly well demarcated focus of necrotic lung parenchyma surrounded by granulation tissue. Note the prominent vascularity in the adjacent pleura. A magnified view *(B)* shows coagulative necrosis of lung tissue on the left and granulation tissue on the right. (*A,* ×25; *B,* ×100.)

monary arterial reaction and on the degree of organization that occurred at the initial venous site of thrombosis. Medium- to large-sized muscular arteries are most commonly affected; in one autopsy study of 54 patients who had PTE, the muscular arteries were involved in all cases, elastic arteries in only 20, and the arterioles in 22.[75] Determining the precise time at which a particular thromboembolic episode occurred is difficult in most cases; however, evidence of organization in the vessel and contiguous thrombus indicates a duration of at least several days and is sufficient to exclude an embolus as the immediate cause of death. The absence of this reaction, however, does not necessarily imply a more recent event, because organization may not proceed at the same rate in all parts of the thrombus. Partially organized thrombi, particularly those in large elastic arteries, may show more than one histologic pattern (Fig. 48–13); in such cases,

the different areas are usually clearly separated, with the most recent appearing thrombus being present near the residual lumen, suggesting one or more episodes of *in situ* thrombosis adjacent to the original thromboembolus. Completely organized thromboemboli should be suspected by the presence of eccentric areas of intimal fibrosis or fibrous bands traversing the lumen[248, 249] (*see* Figs. 48–9 and 48–12). Intimal thickening originating from pulmonary emboli may also undergo transformation to an atherosclerotic plaque.[250]

## Radiographic Manifestations

Consideration of the manifestations of pulmonary thromboembolic disease should be prefaced by a further reminder that most episodes are asymptomatic and produce

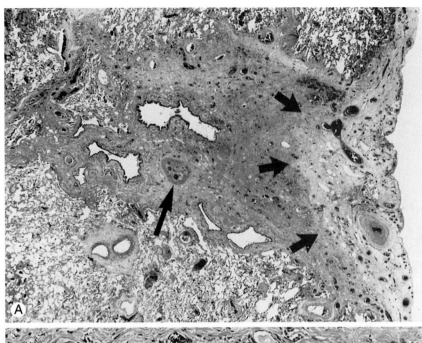

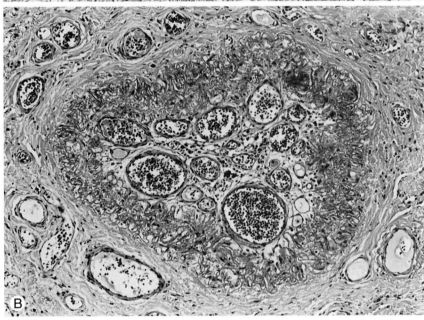

**Figure 48–7. Remote Pulmonary Infarct.** A histologic section *(A)* reveals a well-demarcated area of parenchymal fibrosis that abuts the pleura; the latter is fibrotic and retracted into the lung *(short arrows* denote the pleura-lung interface). Note the histologically viable bronchi within the infarct and the partly occluded pulmonary artery *(large arrow* and magnified in *B)* containing recanalized thrombus. *(A,* ×10; *B,* ×120.)

no detectable changes on the chest radiograph. Even if the diagnosis is suspected clinically and confirmed angiographically, no abnormalities are seen on plain films in approximately 10% to 15% of cases. For example, in one review of the chest radiographs of 383 patients who had angiographically proven PTE and 680 patients who had negative angiogram results, the chest radiograph was interpreted as normal in 12% of patients with PE;[251] the negative predictive value of a normal radiograph was 74%. In another study, a review of the findings in 123 patients who had acute PTE demonstrated that patients with normal radiographic results had a higher partial pressure of oxygen in arterial blood ($PaO_2$) and a lower mean pulmonary arterial pressure than patients who had abnormal radiographic results (16 ± 5 mm Hg compared with 21 ± 9 mm Hg).[252]

### Thromboembolism without Infarction or Hemorrhage

Changes related to thromboembolism without infarction include oligemia, change in vessel size, loss of lung volume, and alteration in size and configuration of the heart.

#### Oligemia

Peripheral oligemia (Westermark's sign) may be local, in which case it is caused by occlusion of a fairly large lobar or segmental pulmonary artery (Fig. 48–14), or general, as a result of widespread small vessel involvement.[182, 253] In a study of 25 patients who had massive PTE in whom plain film and angiographic abnormalities were correlated, local oligemia was observed in all—in fact, 79% of such zones

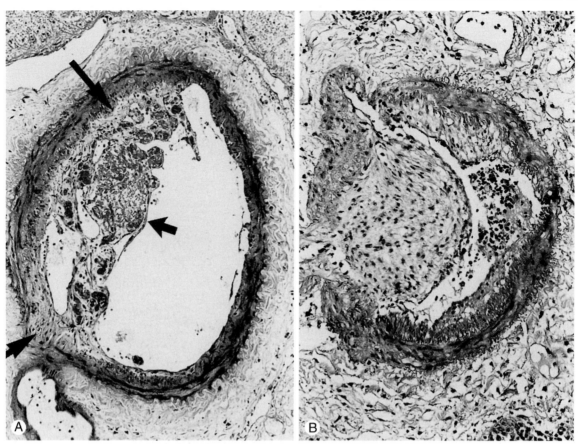

**Figure 48–8. Pulmonary Thromboemboli: Organization.** A histologic section of a muscular artery of medium size *(A)* shows a small amount of thrombus *(short arrow)* covered by endothelial cells; the thrombus has been partly replaced by fibrous tissue *(long arrows),* which is continuous with the intima. A section of another vessel *(B)* shows a more advanced stage of organization, the thrombus being completely replaced by an eccentric plaque of fibrous tissue.

apparent on the arteriogram were recognizable on the plain radiograph in retrospect.[182] The abnormality is most often detected when a whole lung or a major part of it is deprived of its arterial circulation, the unilateral oligemia contrasting markedly with the pleonemia of the other lung.[254]

General pulmonary oligemia in thromboembolic disease is usually the result of widespread occlusion of small arteries. It is nearly always accompanied by signs of pulmonary artery hypertension—enlargement of the central pulmonary arteries, cor pulmonale, cardiac decompensation, and dilation of the superior vena cava and azygos vein[255] (Fig. 48–15). Absence of pulmonary overinflation distinguises the condition from diffuse emphysema.

Although oligemia is a reliable sign in massive PE, it is not sensitive in the detection of smaller thromboemboli. For example, in one review of the radiographic findings in 123 patients who had acute PTE, oligemia was present in only 7 (5%) cases.[252] In another study of 1,063 patients suspected of having acute PTE who underwent pulmonary angiography, oligemia had a sensitivity of 14% and a specificity of 92% in the diagnosis.[251]

### Changes in the Pulmonary Arteries

Enlargement of a major pulmonary artery (Fleischner's sign) is a helpful sign in the diagnosis of PTE (Fig. 48–16), particularly when serial radiographs reveal progressive en-

largement of the affected vessel[254] *(see* Fig. 48–14). In a study of 25 patients who had massive PTE (defined arteriographically as involvement of at least half the major pulmonary arterial branches), enlarged hilar pulmonary arteries were seen in 14, 13 of which were on the right.[182] The investigators experienced difficulty (as have we) in appreciating dilation of the left interlobar artery on a posteroanterior chest radiograph, probably because of overlap by the heart; however, this vessel is often clearly seen posterior to the left upper lobe bronchus on a lateral radiograph, and a diameter greater than 18 mm can be regarded as reasonable evidence of dilation.

In the right hilum, the presence of a thrombus can be assessed by measuring the diameter of the descending branch of the pulmonary artery where it relates to the bronchus intermedius. The normal maximal diameter of this artery at total lung capacity is 16 mm in adult men and 15 mm in adult women; when values are exceeded, it may be reasonably concluded that the vessel is enlarged.[256] Perhaps more reliable than this absolute measurement is an increase in the size of the affected vessel in serial examinations, a finding that is strong evidence of thromboembolism, especially if peripheral oligemia is present *(see* Fig. 48–14). As a result of lysis and fragmentation of the thrombus, arterial widening usually diminishes rapidly and the artery reverts to normal size within a few days.[257]

In one study in which conventional chest radiographs

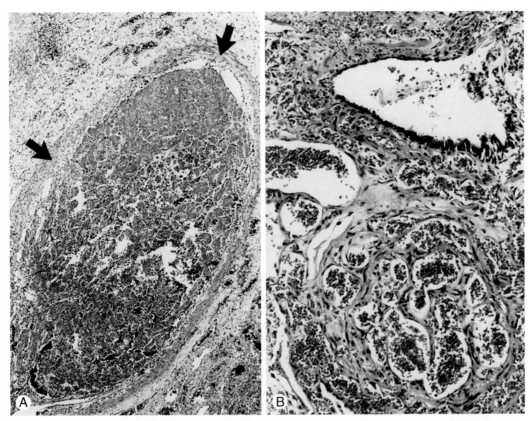

**Figure 48–9. Pulmonary Thromboemboli: Recanalization.** The photomicrograph on the left *(A)* shows a large muscular pulmonary artery that is almost completely occluded by thrombus. Adherence of the thrombus to the vessel wall as a result of fibroblastic ingrowth is evident at several places *(arrows)*. The central portion of the thrombus is partly subdivided into numerous small fragments secondary to lysis and organization; the end result of such processes is often multiple small intraluminal channels (as illustrated in a small muscular artery in *B*). (*A*, ×40; *B*, ×150.)

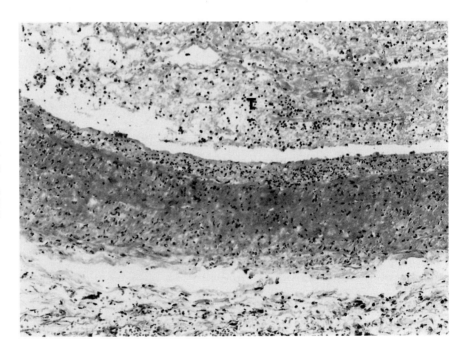

**Figure 48–10. Thromboembolism with Arterial Wall Necrosis.** A section of an elastic pulmonary artery shows fibrinoid necrosis of the media associated with an acute inflammatory infiltrate. The lumen is mostly occluded by thrombus (T), the gross appearance of which was that of a typical thromboembolus. This was a focal lesion in an otherwise normal artery (×120).

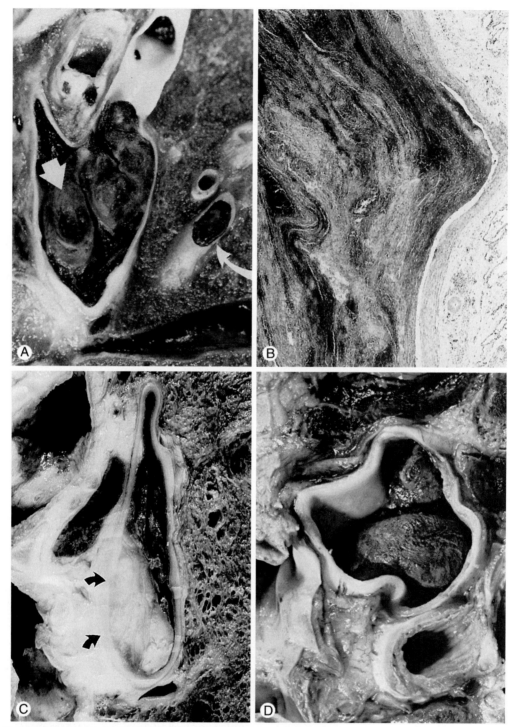

**Figure 48–11. Thromboemboli: Variable Appearance.** The illustration shows three gross features characteristic of thromboemboli. In *A,* a recent embolus has a laminated appearance *(arrow)* corresponding to alternating layers of red blood cells and fibrin platelet aggregates (also seen in a corresponding histologic section in *B*). Occlusion of a small segmental artery is also apparent *(curved arrow).* In *C,* a remote thromboembolus is largely organized, as evidenced by its fibrous (white) appearance and the indistinct junction between the thrombus and adjacent vessel wall *(arrows).* In *D,* the right interlobar artery is completely occluded by a smooth surfaced, curled thrombus. (*B,* ×25). (*D* from Fraser RS: Pathologic characteristics of venous thromboembolism. *In* Leclerc JR [ed]: Venous Thromboembolic Disorders. Philadelphia, Lea & Febiger, 1991.)

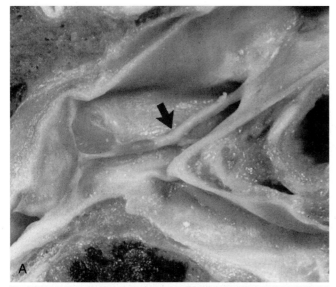

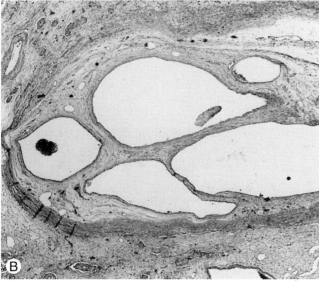

**Figure 48–12. Remote Thromboembolus: Intraluminal Fibrous Bands.** A gross specimen of a lobar pulmonary artery and its proximal branches *(A)* shows a cordlike fibrous band traversing the vessel lumen *(arrow)*. This appearance is diagnostic of organized thrombus, most often caused by embolism. A histologic section through a medium-sized elastic artery *(B)* reveals several broad fibrous bands separating the lumen into several compartments. There is no evidence of residual thrombus (×25).

of 73 patients who had PTE (confirmed by perfusion lung scanning) were compared with those of 85 age-matched patients in whom an original suspicion of embolism was not confirmed, significant dilation of the proximal portion of the right interlobar artery was found in the former group.[258] The transverse diameter of the vessel was measured at the junction of the right superior pulmonary vein with the interlobar artery and at three 1-cm intervals distally; only at the proximal two points did increased diameters reach statistical significance. In the patients who had emboli, the mean diameter of the vessel at the venoarterial junction was 17.8 mm (SD 3.94 mm) compared with a mean diameter in the patients who did not have emboli of 15.7 mm (SD 3.14 mm). At a point 1 cm distal to the venoarterial junction, comparable

figures for the patients who had emboli were 16.3 mm (SD 4.10) and 14.0 mm (SD 3.05) for those who did not.

It is almost certain that the increase in size of the interlobar artery is the result of distention of the vessel by the thrombus itself, rather than increased vascular pressure because any increase in resistance due to local embolization causes immediate redistribution of blood flow to areas of normal vascular resistance; in fact, this redistribution of blood flow may be reflected on plain radiographs by an increase in the size of vessels other than those containing the thromboembolus. In one study of 25 patients who had massive embolism, such local "hyperemia" was observed in at least one zone in 10 patients.[182] Only when there is widespread involvement in both lungs (70% of the cross-sectional area of the vascular bed) does the increased resistance increase the size of the hilar artery; in this situation, the enlargement is bilateral and symmetric (*see* Fig. 48–15).

Of equal diagnostic importance as increased size of an interlobar artery is the abrupt tapering of the occluded vessel distally, creating the so-called knuckle sign[170, 259] (Figs. 48–16 and 48–17). In the study of 73 patients who had perfusion scan–confirmed PTE cited previously, approximately 25% demonstrated this sign.[258] In addition to abrupt termination, occluded vessels may be more sharply deline-

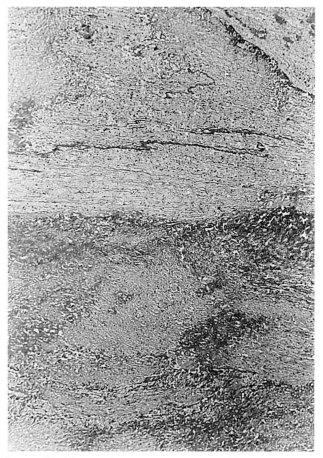

**Figure 48–13. Pulmonary Artery Thrombus: Biphasic Appearance.** A section of a thrombus within the pulmonary artery to the left lower lobe shows two quite distinct patterns—the one on the top suggests recently formed thrombus, whereas that on the bottom suggests one that is partially organized.

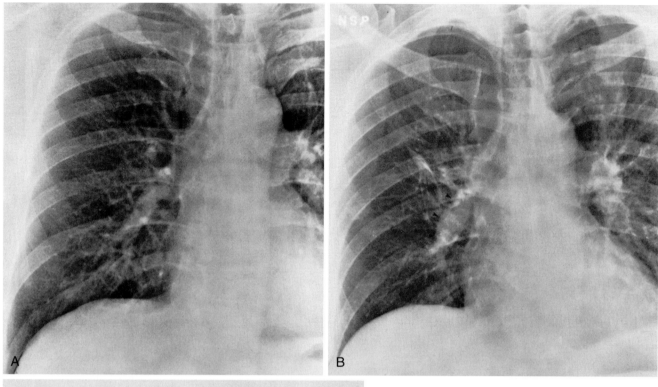

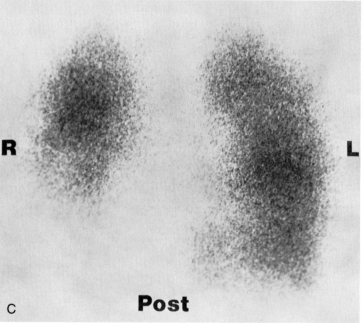

**Figure 48–14. Pulmonary Thromboembolism without Infarction: Westermark's Sign.** On admission of a 52-year-old man to the hospital, a posteroanterior radiograph *(A)* revealed no significant abnormalities. Several days following abdominal surgery, he experienced abrupt onset of right chest pain and dyspnea. A radiograph at this time *(B)* showed an obvious increase in diameter and a change in configuration of the right interlobar artery *(arrowheads)*; also, the distal end of this artery appeared "knuckled" and the vessels peripheral to it diminutive. The right lower zone showed increased radiolucency, indicating diminished perfusion (Westermark's sign). A lung scan *(C)* revealed absence of perfusion of the lower half of the right lung.

ated than normal, a sign probably relating to diminished pulsation.

As with oligemia, enlargement of a hilar pulmonary artery is usually seen only in patients who have massive PTE, and therefore this sign has a relatively low sensitivity in diagnosis. In one investigation of 123 patients who had angiographically proven acute embolism, a prominent central pulmonary artery was seen in only 20 (16%); the mean pulmonary artery pressure in these patients was 30 ± 14 mm Hg, compared with a mean pressure of 16 ± 5 mm Hg in those who had normal results on chest radiographs.[252] In another review of the chest radiographic findings in 1,063 patients suspected of having acute PE who underwent pulmonary angiography, a prominent central pulmonary artery was found to have a diagnostic specificity of 80% but a sensitivity of only 20%.[251]

### Volume Loss

Loss of volume of a lower lobe in PTE may be manifested radiographically by elevation of the hemidiaphragm, downward displacement of the major fissure, or both. The

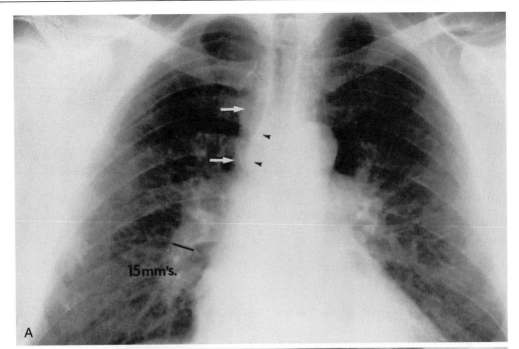

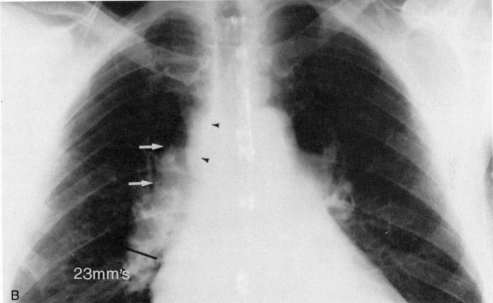

**Figure 48–15. "Acute Cor Pulmonale" and Systemic Venous Hypertension Caused by Massive Pulmonary Thromboembolism.** A posteroanterior radiograph *(A)* shows no abnormality; note the appearance of the superior vena cava *(arrows),* azygos vein *(arrowheads),* and right interlobar artery (measuring 15 mm in transverse diameter). Two months later, this elderly man suffered the sudden onset of retrosternal pain and dyspnea 10 days after prostatic surgery; a repeat chest radiograph *(B)* discloses marked enlargement of the vena cava *(arrows)* and the azygos vein *(arrowheads);* the hilar arterial vasculature is distinctly dilated, the right interlobar artery now measuring 23 mm. The combined features are highly suggestive of "cor pulmonale" associated with massive thromboembolism. A perfusion lung scan (not shown) disclosed an absence of perfusion in the right lung and large deficits in the left mid and lower lung zones.

former was observed in 25% of 123 patients with angiographically proven PTE in one study.[252] In a review of the radiographic findings in 1,063 patients, elevation of the diaphragm had diagnostic sensitivity and specificity of 20 and 85%, respectively.[251] Loss of volume is a more frequent finding when infarction is present *(see* farther on); for example, in one study of eight patients with massive PTE who showed loss of volume, seven had infarction.[182]

Another relatively common finding is the presence of line shadows representing linear atelectasis, described in 22% of patients in one study.[260] These shadows are roughly horizontal, usually occur in the lower lung zones, are 1 to 3 mm thick and several cm long, and abut the pleural surface. In a study of 10 patients who had linear atelectasis present

on their last antemortem radiograph, 6 had acute pulmonary emboli at autopsy.[261]

Cardiac Changes

Radiographic findings suggestive of acute pulmonary arterial hypertension are not a common accompaniment of PTE, being observed in only 10% of 126 patients in one study[262] and 12% of 123 in another.[252] They occur most often with widespread peripheral emboli *(see* Fig. 48–15) and sometimes—when a large enough area of the arterial system is occluded—with massive central embolization. The signs are those of cardiac enlargement due to dilation of the right ventricle, increase in size of the main pulmonary artery, and,

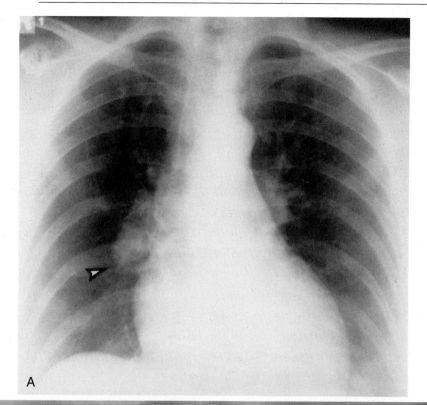

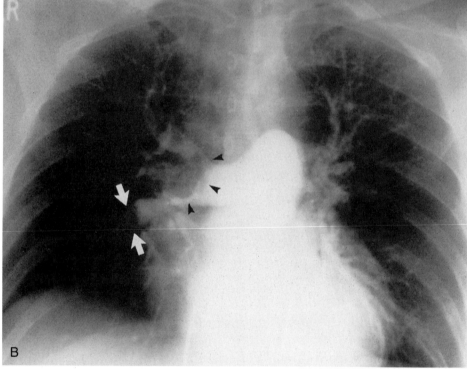

**Figure 48–16. Pulmonary Thromboembolism: Dilation and Amputation of the Right Interlobar Artery.** A conventional posteroanterior chest radiograph *(A)* reveals an enlarged cardiac shadow. The lungs are normal except for a suggestion of oligemia in the right upper and lower lung zones. The hilar arteries are dilated, and the right interlobar artery tapers rapidly and appears to terminate abruptly *(arrowhead)*. This constitutes a positive knuckle sign. A pulmonary angiogram in anteroposterior projection *(B)* discloses a large saddle embolus *(arrowheads)* partly obstructing the bifurcation of the ascending and descending branches of the right pulmonary artery. The right interlobar artery is completely occluded *(arrows)*, accounting for the features illustrated in *A*. Several segmental arterial branches in the left upper lobe and lingula are also obstructed. The patient was a middle-aged woman with a history of progressive dyspnea.

usually, increase in size and rapidity of tapering of the hilar pulmonary vessels.[254, 259] Dilation of the azygos vein and superior vena cava may also be apparent, reflecting systemic venous hypertension *(see* Fig. 48–15). It may be very difficult to recognize any of these signs, particularly cardiac enlargement, in a patient with restricted ventilation whose chest radiograph was exposed at the bedside in the supine position.[257]

## Thromboembolism with Infarction or Hemorrhage

### Parenchymal Consolidation and Volume Loss

The radiographic changes in PTE with infarction or hemorrhage consist of segmental areas of consolidation associated with volume loss (Fig. 48–18). Their relative frequency is influenced by the time interval between the onset of symptoms and the performance of radiography. In a study

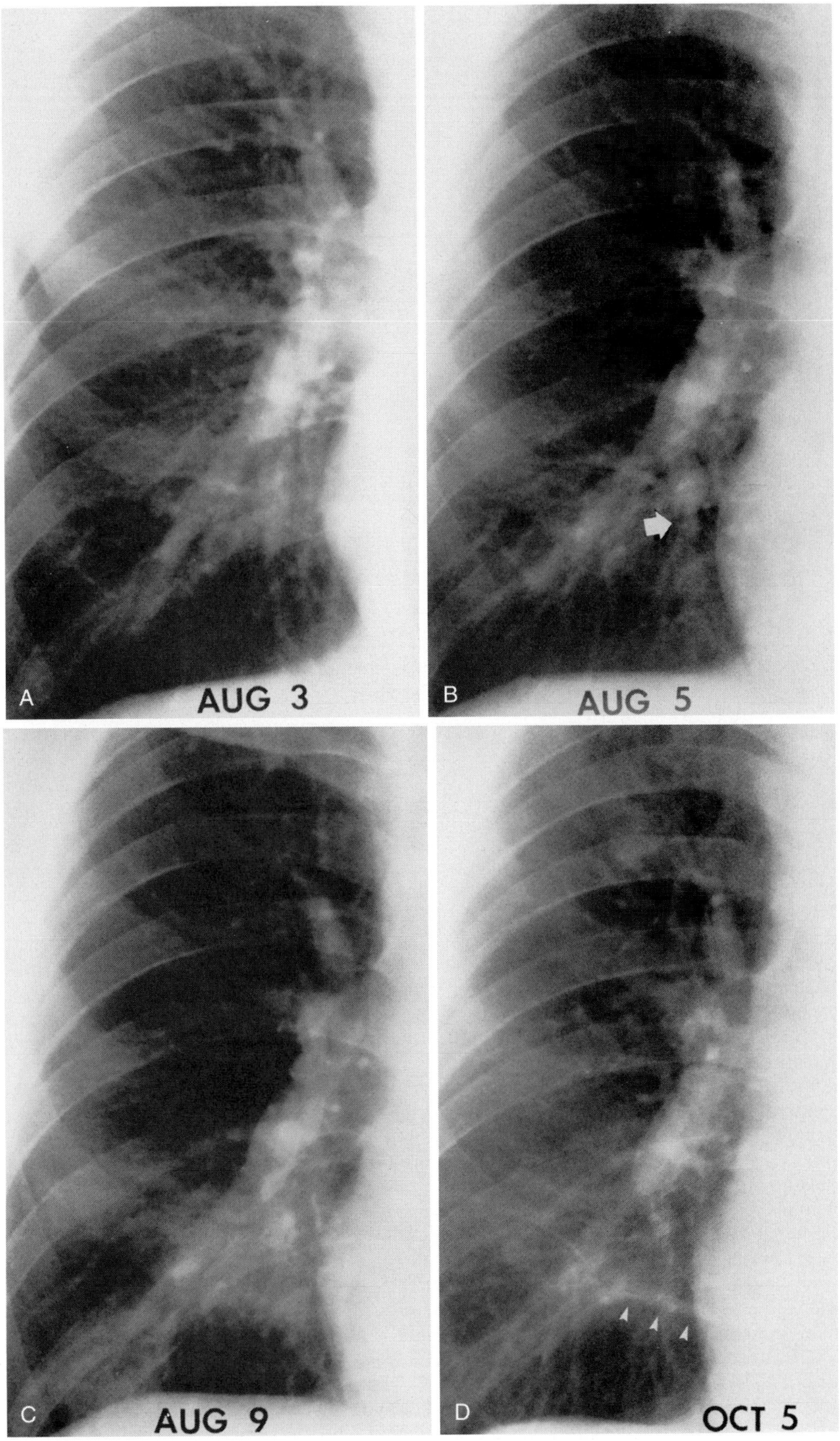

**Figure 48–17. Thromboembolism, Infarction, and Healing.** A view of the right lung from a postero-anterior chest radiograph *(A)* reveals no abnormality. Two days later *(B)*, a segmental branch in the lower lobe is focally enlarged and abruptly tapered *(arrow)*. This feature is highly suggestive of an impacted thromboembolism in a segmental artery. Four days later *(C)*, an ill-defined parenchymal opacity had appeared in the posterior basal segment of the lower lobe, representing an infarct. Approximately 2 months later *(D)*, the only residuum is a linear opacity *(arrowheads)* at the site of the previous area of consolidation, consistent with a scar. The patient was a 35-year-old renal transplant recipient who complained of the acute onset of mild dyspnea the day before the radiograph in *B*.

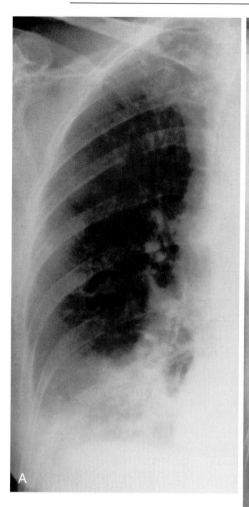 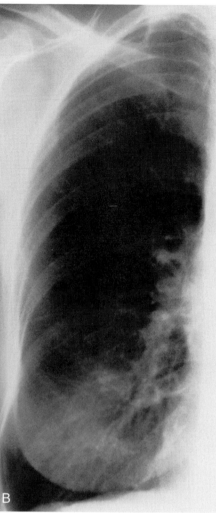

**Figure 48–18. Pulmonary "Infarction" with Rapid Resolution.** A view of the right lung from a conventional posteroanterior chest radiograph *(A)* reveals a homogeneous opacity occupying the lower half of the right lower lobe. The right hemidiaphragm is moderately elevated, and the right interlobar artery is enlarged. Eight days later *(B)*, the lower lobe consolidation has resolved and the hemidiaphragm has descended to its normal position. The patient was an elderly woman who had an acute onset of dyspnea and hemoptysis. The rapidity of resolution is compatible with pulmonary hemorrhage secondary to thromboembolism.

of 50 patients who had angiographically documented acute PTE, loss of lung volume as evidenced by elevation of a hemidiaphragm was observed in 50% within 24 hours of onset of symptoms and in only 15% when symptoms had been present longer.[263] By contrast, pulmonary opacities were found in 37% of patients within 24 hours and 57% thereafter.

The reported frequency of an elevated hemidiaphragm in association with an acute PTE is variable. Of 25 patients who had massive PTE in one study, eight (including seven with pulmonary infarction) had elevation of the ipsilateral hemidiaphragm.[182] In a retrospective study of 66 autopsy-proven cases of PTE with infarction, elevation of the hemidiaphragm was present in 26 (39%).[264] Elevation of the hemidiaphragm occurs with roughly equal frequency following emboli that result in lung necrosis and those associated with simple hemorrhage and edema.[194, 265] Because tissue necrosis is most common in patients who have cardiorespiratory disease, concomitant radiographic signs of cor pulmonale, pulmonary venous hypertension, and edema increase the likelihood that an opacity represents tissue necrosis rather than simple hemorrhage.

In the early stages of pulmonary infarction, parenchymal opacities are ill defined. They are commonest in the base of the right lower lobe, often nestled in the costophrenic sulcus (Fig. 48–19). The majority of cases involve one or perhaps two segments, thus affecting a relatively small volume of lung parenchyma; however, the process occasionally involves the whole or a major portion of a lobe.[264, 266] The interval between the embolic episode and the development of an opacity ranges from 10 to 12 hours[267, 268] to several days after vascular occlusion;[267] in one series, the opacity developed in equal numbers of cases within 24 hours and later.[260]

The configuration of a pulmonary infarct usually resembles a truncated cone, an appearance that has come to bear the euphonious eponym of Hampton's hump.[160, 251] This configuration consists of homogeneous wedge-shaped consolidation in the lung periphery, with its base contiguous to a visceral pleural surface and its rounded, convex apex toward the hilum[267, 269] (Figs. 48–20 and 48–21). The size of the consolidated area varies from patient to patient and, in the case of multiple infarctions, from one area to another (Fig. 48–22). They are usually 3 to 5 cm in diameter but may be as large as 10 cm.[267] An air bronchogram is rarely seen;[270] this absence, combined with the presence of peripheral homogeneous consolidation, should strongly suggest infarction rather than acute air-space pneumonia. However, an air bronchogram does not rule out infarction completely. Cavitation is rare[271] and usually indicates septic emboli (*see* page 1829).[231, 232]

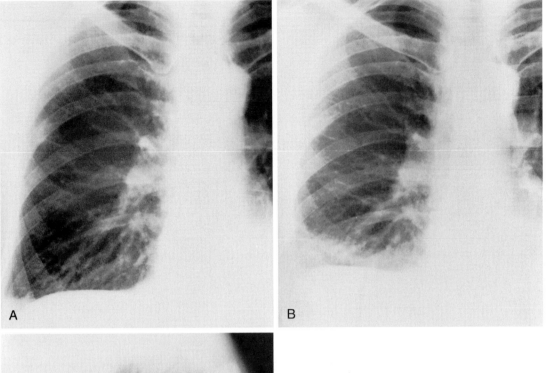

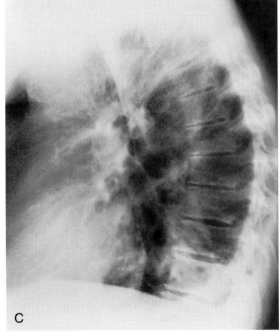

**Figure 48–19. Pulmonary Infarct, Right Lower Lobe.** Three days after laparotomy, this 57-year-old man suffered the abrupt onset of right-sided chest pain. A view of the right hemithorax from a posteroanterior radiograph exposed 24 hours later *(A)* reveals a rather poorly defined shadow of homogeneous density nestled in the costophrenic sulcus; there is a small pleural effusion. Three days later, posteroanterior *(B)* and lateral *(C)* radiographs demonstrate considerable increase in the extent of parenchymal consolidation. The right hemidiaphragm has risen since the previous examination. Although the shadow is poorly visualized in lateral projection, the presence of disease is indicated by obliteration of the posterior portion of the hemidiaphragm. Radiographic resolution was incomplete 3 weeks later, indicating that the process was one of necrosis rather than hemorrhage alone.

The time course of resolution of infarction varies widely and is a reliable indicator of the nature of the consolidative process. If embolism results only in parenchymal hemorrhage and edema, clearing may occur within 4 to 7 days, often without residua;[272] when it leads to necrosis, resolution, when it occurs, averages 20 days[257] and may take as long as 5 weeks.[273] The pattern of resolution can also be a valuable sign in differentiating pulmonary infarction from acute pneumonia.[274] In the latter, the shadow appears to break up, rendering an originally homogeneous opacity inhomogeneous as scattered areas of radiolucency appear within it; with infarction, the shadow gradually diminishes while maintaining its homogeneity and (roughly) its original shape. This pattern of resolution of pulmonary infarcts has been

likened to a melting ice cube ("the melting sign")[274] (Fig. 48–23). However, this sign is applicable only in the resolving stages of either lesion and, therefore, of no value at a time when the institution of appropriate therapy is vital.

The short- and long-term appearance of healed infarcts varies considerably. In a follow-up study of 32 patients who had 58 angiographically proven pulmonary infarcts, complete radiographic resolution occurred in 29 (50%) of the 58 infarcts; of the remainder, residual findings included linear scars (14), pleurodiaphragmatic adhesions (9), and localized pleural thickening (6).[275] In all cases, the residual features were diminutive when compared with the original abnormality. Follow-up perfusion lung images performed at time intervals similar to those of the chest radiographs were

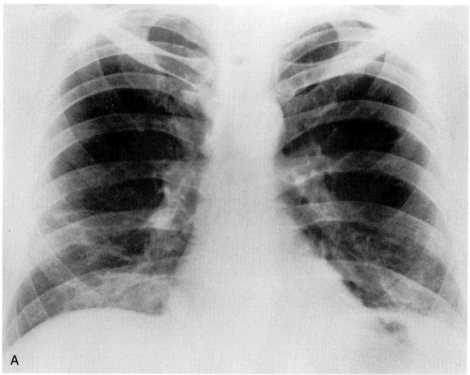

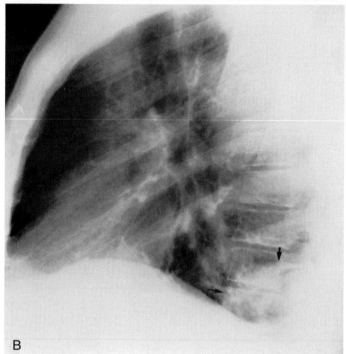

**Figure 48–20. Pulmonary Infarct, Right Lower Lobe.** Posteroanterior *(A)* and lateral *(B)* radiographs of a 40-year-old man reveal a fairly well-circumscribed shadow of homogeneous opacity occupying the posterior basal segment of the right lower lobe. In lateral projection, the shadow has the shape of a truncated cone with its apex directed toward the hilum (Hampton's hump) *(arrows)*. A small effusion can be identified in lateral projection. This combination of changes is highly suggestive of pulmonary infarction.

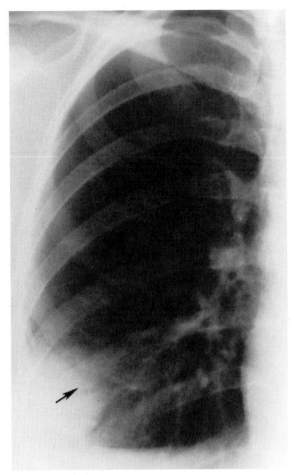

**Figure 48–21. Pulmonary Infarction: Hampton's Hump.** A view of the right lung from a posteroanterior chest radiograph reveals a homogeneous opacity in the right costophrenic angle possessing a convex contour *(arrow)* toward the hilum. This constitutes the typical features of Hampton's hump and is highly suggestive of a pulmonary infarct. The patient was a young man who had a history of acute chest pain and thrombophlebitis of the right leg.

available for 44 infarcts; 7 of these showed complete resolution, and the remaining 37 showed a residual but much smaller perfusion defect.

### Pleural Effusion

Pleural effusion is seen in 35% to 55% of patients who have acute PTE.[251, 252] It is noted most commonly in patients who have infarction or hemorrhage but may be present in those who do not have parenchymal consolidation.[194, 251, 259] (With respect to the latter, it is important to remember that the parenchymal shadow may be diminutive or hidden by the fluid.[265, 276]) The amount of pleural fluid is usually small, but it may be abundant. It is more often unilateral.[254, 267] When predominantly infrapulmonary, it may be mistaken for hemidiaphragmatic elevation.[267] The effusion usually develops and absorbs synchronously with the consolidation; occasionally, it appears later and clears sooner.[257]

### Pneumothorax

Pneumothorax is a rare complication of PTE with infarction.[265] It is thought to develop most often during posi-

tive-pressure ventilation or when an infarct has become infected.[277, 278]

### *Validity of Radiographic Findings*

Two groups of investigators have assessed the accuracy of the various radiographic findings in the diagnosis of acute PTE.[251, 279] In one study, the authors reviewed the chest radiographs of 152 patients who were suspected at one time of having acute PTE but in whom only 108 proved to have embolism on the basis of a positive pulmonary angiogram.[279] The radiographs were randomized and presented for interpretation to nine readers (seven of whom were radiologists specializing in pulmonary disease). The question "Does this patient have pulmonary embolism?" required a "yes," "no," or "don't know" answer. The average true-positive ratio (sensitivity) was 0.33 (range 0.08 to 0.52), and the average true-negative ratio (specificity) was 0.59 (range 0.31 to 0.80). A predictive index, reflecting the overall accuracy of diagnosis, was little better than chance (0.40, range 0.17 to 0.57) for the entire group.[279]

In a second study, chest radiographs of 1,063 patients who had suspected acute PTE were interpreted independently by two chest radiologists.[251] The study was based on the data obtained from the PIOPED study and included 383 patients who had angiographically proven PTE and 680 patients who had normal pulmonary angiogram results.[251] The most common parenchymal abnormalities in patients who had PE were atelectasis and focal areas of increased opacity. However, the prevalence of these findings was not significantly different from that in patients who did not have embolism; atelectasis, with elevation of the hemidiaphragm, had a sensitivity of 20% and a specificity of 85%, and pleural-based areas of increased opacity (Hampton's hump) had a sensitivity of 22% and a specificity of 82%. Similarly, oligemia (Westermark's sign), prominent central pulmonary artery (Fleischner's sign), vascular redistribution, and pleural effusion were poor predictors of PTE. The chest radiograph was interpreted as normal in 12% of patients who had PTE and in 18% of those in whom it was absent.

As these studies show, chest radiography is of limited value in the diagnosis of PTE. Its major importance lies in excluding other disease processes such as pneumonia and pneumothorax that can mimic thromboembolism and in providing correlation with V̇/Q̇ lung scans.[251, 269, 279]

### Special Diagnostic Techniques

Despite the hundreds of studies that have been performed over the past three decades, the optimal approach to the diagnosis of PTE remains controversial. As discussed previously, the chest radiograph is associated with poor sensitivity and specificity. As will become evident later, clinical symptoms and signs and the results of laboratory investigation are also of limited diagnostic value. Although it is well recognized that pulmonary angiography is the definitive method of establishing the diagnosis and of demonstrating the extent of embolism, the procedure is expensive and time-consuming and may lead to significant morbidity. For more than 2 decades, ventilation-perfusion scintigraphy was the technique of choice as the initial screening proce-

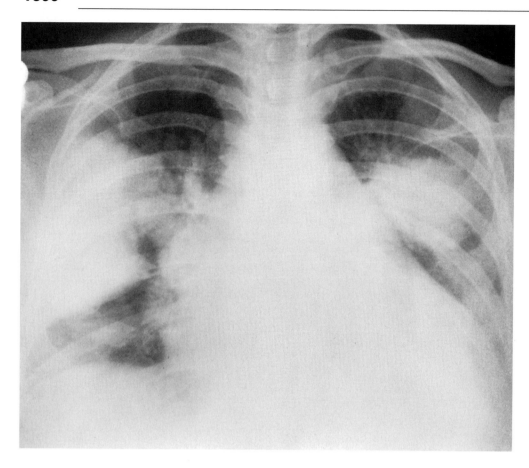

**Figure 48–22. Multiple Pulmonary Infarcts.** An anteroposterior radiograph demonstrates several homogeneous opacities in both lungs. Those on the right possess a configuration suggesting a truncated cone (Hampton's hump) with their apices directed toward the hilum. The main shadow in the left lung is roughly circular in shape, suggesting that its base may be contiguous to the anterior or posterior chest wall. At autopsy, multiple infarcts were present in both lungs, the major lesion on the left being in the superior segment of the lower lobe.

dure. More recently, contrast-enhanced computed tomography (CT) using spiral or electron-beam technique has become the method of choice in several centers. Other imaging techniques that may play a role include magnetic resonance (MR) imaging (for the diagnosis of both PTE and DVT) and a variety of other techniques used for the diagnosis of DVT, such as venography, ultrasonography, and CT.

### Scintigraphy

The V̇/Q̇ lung scan has been shown to be a safe, noninvasive technique for the evaluation of regional pulmonary perfusion and ventilation, and it has been used widely in the evaluation of patients who are believed to have PTE.

Technique

Currently, the radiopharmaceuticals of choice for perfusion lung scanning are either technetium-99m–labeled human albumin microsphere (Tc-99m HAM) particles or macroaggregated albumin (Tc-99m MAA) particles.[269, 280, 281] Tc-99m MAA particles vary in size from 10 to 150 μm, with more than 90% of particles measuring between 10 and 90 μm. Tc-99m HAM particles are more uniform in size and range from 35 to 60 μm. The biologic half-life of Tc-99m MAA within the lung is between 2 and 6 hours.

The intravenous administration of either Tc-99m HAM or Tc-99m MAA should be performed over 5 to 10 respiratory cycles with the patient in the supine position, which limits the effect of gravity on regional pulmonary arterial blood flow. Following injection, particles pass through the right atrium and ventricle and lodge within precapillary arterioles in the lungs. The distribution of particles is proportional to regional pulmonary blood flow at the time of injection. The usual administered activity is between 74 to 148 MBq (2 to 4 mCi) and contains 200,000 to 500,000 particles. It has been estimated that the particles cause transient blockage of approximately 0.1% of precapillary pulmonary arterioles,[282] providing a static image of regional flow.

When performing scintigraphy to assess pulmonary perfusion, at least six views of the lungs should be obtained, including anterior, posterior, right and left lateral, and right and left posterior oblique. Additional right and left anterior oblique views may be helpful in selected cases and are used routinely by many physicians.[269, 280, 281] In animal studies, it has been demonstrated that perfusion imaging can detect more than 90% of the emboli that completely occlude pulmonary arterial vessels greater than 2 mm in diameter.[283]

Perfusion scintigraphy is a sensitive but nonspecific technique for diagnosing pulmonary disease: virtually all parenchymal lung diseases and airway diseases such as COPD and asthma can cause decreased pulmonary arterial blood flow within the affected lung zone. Because thromboemboli characteristically cause abnormal perfusion with preserved ventilation (mismatched defects) (Fig 48–24), whereas parenchymal lung disease most often causes both ventilation and perfusion abnormalities in the same lung region (matched defects), combined ventilation and perfusion scintigraphy is performed routinely in most centers to improve diagnostic specificity. Most experience with ventilation imaging has been with xenon 133.[269] Alternative techniques using agents such as xenon 127, krypton 81m, techne-

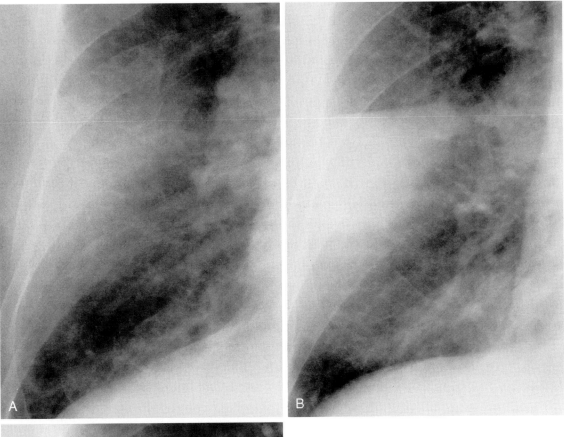

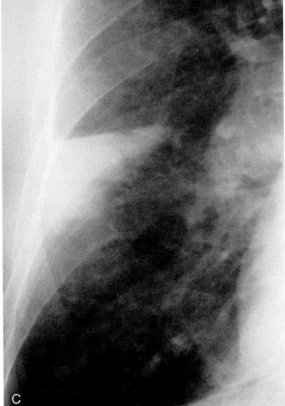

**Figure 48–23. "Melting Ice Cube" Sign.** A view of the right lung from an anteroposterior chest radiograph *(A)* in a 79-year-old man shows a pleural-based segmental area of consolidation with poorly defined margins. A radiograph 1 week later *(B)* demonstrates decrease in size but increase in radiopacity of the area of consolidation, which now also has more sharply defined borders. A radiograph 3 weeks later *(C)* shows further reduction in size of the opacity. The diagnosis of pulmonary thromboembolism was proven by angiography.

Right Posterior                                   Right Posterior

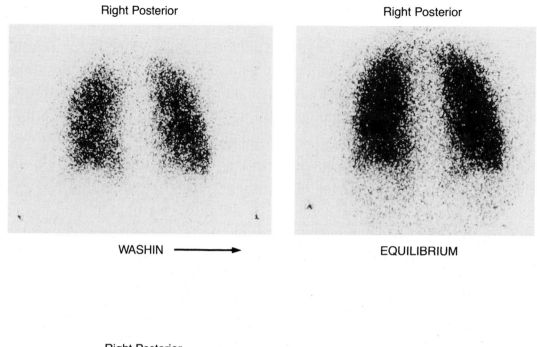

WASHIN ⟶                                        EQUILIBRIUM

Right Posterior

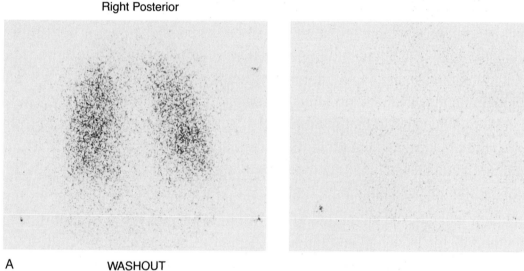

A                    WASHOUT

**Figure 48–24. The Value of Ventilation-Perfusion Lung Scans in the Diagnosis of Thromboembolism.** A xenon-133 posterior inhalation lung scan *(A)* discloses normal ventilation parameters during the washin, equilibrium, and washout phases.

tium-99m aerosols, technegas, or pertechnegas have not been as extensively evaluated;[269, 284] however, the available data suggest that there is no major diagnostic difference among them.

With xenon 133, ventilation imaging is generally performed before perfusion imaging.[269] An initial posterior washin or first breath image is acquired for 100,000 counts or 10 to 15 seconds following the inhalation of 550 to 770 MBq of xenon 133. Equilibrium images are then obtained while the patient rebreathes the gas within a closed system for at least 4 minutes. The washin or breath-hold images demonstrate regional lung ventilation. Regions of the lungs that appear defective on the washin images may appear normal on the equilibrium image as a result of collateral ventilation. Finally, serial washout images are acquired while

the patient breathes ambient air, allowing for regional air trapping to be detected as focal areas of retained activity. Serial washout images should be performed initially in the posterior projection rather than in the left and right posterior oblique positions to maximize the number of lung segments that can be visualized. To optimize the diagnostic performance of the test, images should be taken of patients in the erect position; however, if necessary, images can be made of patients who are supine or on ventilatory assistance.

### Diagnostic Criteria

The diagnosis of PTE on scintigraphy is based on the presence of $\dot{V}/\dot{Q}$ mismatch, that is, the presence of ventila-

Anterior

Posterior

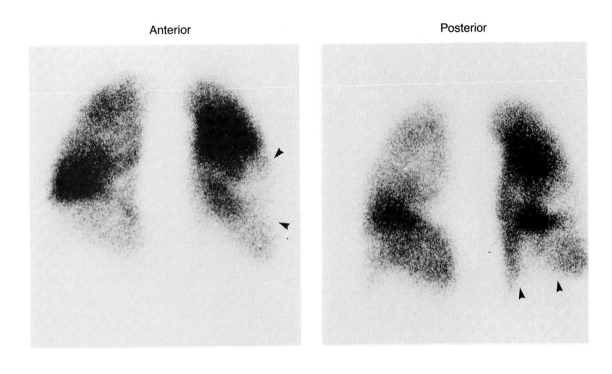

Right Posterior Oblique

Left Posterior Oblique

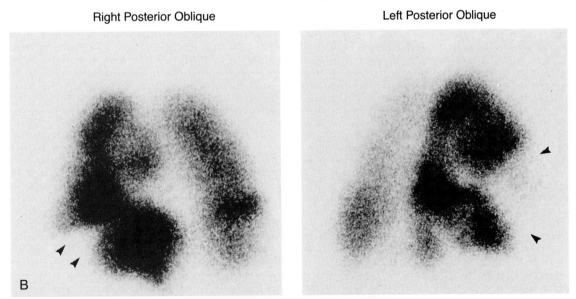

B

**Figure 48–24** *Continued.* Corresponding technetium Tc-99m MAA perfusion lung scans (B) in anterior, posterior, and right and left posterior oblique projections identify multiple segmental filling defects throughout both lungs *(arrowheads)*. These findings, in concert with the ventilation study, are virtually diagnostic (high probability) of pulmonary thromboembolism. The patient was a 65-year-old man who presented with acute dyspnea.

tion in the absence of perfusion distal to obstructing emboli (Fig. 48–25). The findings are classified in terms of probability of embolism, the most commonly used reporting terms being normal, near normal, low, intermediate, and high.

Several diagnostic criteria have been suggested for the interpretation of V̇/Q̇ lung scans.[285–288] In an investigation comparing these algorithms, the original PIOPED criteria had the highest likelihood ratio for predicting the presence of emboli on pulmonary angiography.[289] However, the PIOPED criteria also had the highest proportion of V̇/Q̇ scans interpreted as intermediate probability. Several amendments of the original PIOPED criteria have been made[288, 290] (Table 48–1). By utilizing the revised criteria, it is possible to

decrease the number of intermediate interpretations and classify them correctly as low probability. The use of these revised PIOPED criteria in clinical practice, instead of the original criteria, has been shown to provide a more accurate assessment of angiographically proven PTE.[290, 291]

### Diagnostic Accuracy

The first large-scale study that utilized perfusion lung scanning as a screening test for the diagnosis of PTE was the urokinase pulmonary embolism trial (UPET).[292] In more than 90% of the patients enrolled in this trial, perfusion lung scanning was performed following the intravenous adminis-

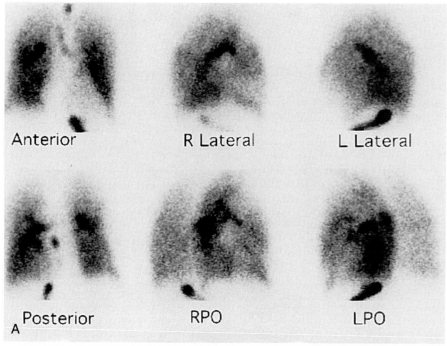

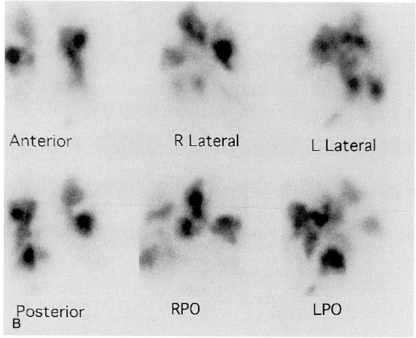

**Figure 48–25. Acute Pulmonary Thromboembolism.** Technetium-99m DTPA aerosol ventilation *(A)* and technetium Tc-99m MAA perfusion *(B)* images demonstrate multiple segmental perfusion defects that are ventilated normally (ventilation-perfusion mismatches) within both lungs. (Courtesy of Dr. Daniel Worsley, Vancouver Hospital and Health Sciences Centre, Vancouver, British Columbia.)

### Table 48–1. REVISED PIOPED CRITERIA FOR INTERPRETATION OF V̇/Q̇ IMAGES

| PROBABILITY OF PULMONARY EMBOLISM | DIAGNOSTIC CRITERIA |
|---|---|
| High probability (≥80%) | Two or more large mismatched segmental perfusion defects or the arithmetic equivalent in moderate or large and moderate defects, i.e., one large plus two or more moderate defects or four or more moderate mismatches. |
| Intermediate probability (20%–79%) | One moderate plus one large mismatched segmental perfusion defect or the arithmetic equivalent in moderate defects. |
| | One matched ventilation-perfusion defect and a normal chest radiograph result. |
| | Difficult to categorize as low or high, or not described as low or high. |
| Low probability (≤19%) | Nonsegmental perfusion defects (e.g., cardiomegaly, enlarged aorta, enlarged hila, elevated diaphragm). Any perfusion defect with a substantially larger abnormality at chest radiography. |
| | Perfusion defects matched by ventilation abnormality provided that there are (a) normal chest radiograph results and (b) some areas of normal perfusion in the lungs. |
| | Any number of small perfusion defects and a normal chest radiograph result. |
| Normal | No perfusion defects or perfusion defects that outline exactly the shape of the lungs seen on the chest radiograph (hilar and aortic impressions may be seen, and the chest radiograph and/or ventilation scan result may be abnormal). |

Modified from Gottschalk A, Sostman HD, Juni JE, et al: Ventilation-perfusion scintigraphy in the PIOPED study. II. Evaluation of criteria and interpretations. J Nucl Med 34:1119, 1993; and Sostman HD, Coleman RE, DeLong DM, et al: Evaluation of revised criteria for ventilation-perfusion scintigraphy in patients with suspected pulmonary embolism. Radiology 193:103, 1994.

tration of radioiodinated MAA ([131]IMAA). Because scanning was accomplished with a rectilinear scanner, no ventilation imaging was performed. Despite utilizing suboptimal radiopharmaceuticals and instrumentation, as judged by current standards, the UPET study established perfusion lung scanning as an effective technique to diagnose PTE and to assess restoration of pulmonary blood flow following an embolic event.[292] In this study, approximately 75% to 80% of perfusion defects resolved by 3 months; those that did not resolve by this time remained largely persistent when followed for 1 year. (The amount of clot resolution observed in this study is likely an underestimate, because ventilation scanning was not performed and many of the unresolved perfusion defects might have been related to pre-existing chronic obstructive lung disease.)

More recently, data from three large investigations using modern imaging agents and instrumentation have been reported.[293–295] In one prospective study of 874 patients suspected of having PTE, V̇/Q̇ scan interpretations were grouped into three diagnostic categories: normal, non-high probability, and high probability (mismatch defect involving at least 75% of a segment).[293] Anticoagulants were withheld in 371 patients who had a non–high probability scan result, adequate cardiorespiratory reserve, and absent proximal vein thrombosis as determined by negative serial impedance plethysmography; only 10 (2.7%) of these patients had evidence of PTE during a 3-month follow-up period, suggesting to the authors of the study that this select group of patients can be managed safely without anticoagulation. Their results also confirmed findings from previous studies that suggested that the incidence of recurrent PTE is very low in the absence of proximal lower extremity venous thrombus. However, when the clinical suspicion for PTE is high, and the V̇/Q̇ scan result is low or intermediate probability, we prefer to perform spiral CT.

Another group of investigators prospectively examined 1564 consecutive patients who had suspected PTE and who underwent both V̇/Q̇ scanning and impedance plethysmography of the lower extremities.[294] In 627 patients (40%), scans were interpreted as nondiagnostic and serial impedance plethysmography study results were negative; all had an adequate cardiorespiratory reserve and were managed without anticoagulation; only 12 (2%) had evidence of either DVT or PTE on follow-up. As indicated previously, we still favor proceeding with further testing when the clinical suspicion for PTE is high.

In a random sample of 931 patients who underwent scintigraphy in the PIOPED study, 13% had high-probability scan results, 39% had intermediate-probability scan results, 34% had low-probability scan results, and 14% had normal or near-normal scan results.[295] There was good interobserver agreement for classifying ventilation-perfusion scans as high probability (95%) or as normal (94%); however, there was a 25% to 30% disagreement in interpreting intermediate- and low-probability scans.[295] Seven hundred and fifty-five of the 931 patients underwent pulmonary angiography. Of the patients who had high-probability scan results and definitive diagnosis at angiography, 88% had PE, compared with 33% of patients with intermediate-probability scan results, 16% of patients with low-probability scan results, and 9% of patients with near-normal or normal scan results. The sensitivity, specificity, and positive predictive values of V̇/Q̇ scanning for detecting acute PTE in this study are presented in Table 48–2. The diagnostic value was not significantly different between men and women and among patients of different ages.[296, 297] The diagnostic utility was also similar among patients who had pre-existing cardiac or pulmonary disease compared with those who had no such disease. In a subset of patients who had COPD, the sensitivity of a high-probability scan interpretation was significantly lower than that in patients who had no pre-existing cardiopulmonary disease.[298] However, the positive predictive value of a high-probability scan interpretation was 100%, and the negative predictive value of a low- or very low probability scan interpretation was 94% in this group.

Although the clinical assessment of patients with suspected PTE is not diagnostic in most instances, the results from the PIOPED study emphasize the importance of incorporating the pretest clinical likelihood of PE in the overall

### Table 48–2. SENSITIVITY, SPECIFICITY AND POSITIVE PREDICTIVE VALUE (PPV) OF V̇/Q̇ LUNG SCANNING FOR DETECTING ACUTE PULMONARY EMBOLISM USING ORIGINAL PIOPED INTERPRETATION CRITERIA

| V̇/Q̇ SCAN INTERPRETATION | SENSITIVITY | SPECIFICITY | PPV |
|---|---|---|---|
| High | 40% | 98% | 87% |
| High, intermediate | 82% | 64% | 49% |
| High, intermediate, low | 98% | 12% | 32% |

The results are based on the study by Worsley DF, Palevsky HI, Alavi A: Clinical characteristic of patients with pulmonary embolism and low or very low probability lung scan interpretations. Arch Intern Med 154:2737, 1994. Copyright 1994, American Medical Association.

diagnostic evaluation (Table 48–3). In patients who had low- or very low probability V̇/Q̇ scan interpretations and no history of immobilization, recent surgery, trauma to the lower extremities, or central venous instrumentation, the prevalence of PE was only 4.5%.[299] In patients who had low- or very low probability scan interpretations and one risk factor, the prevalence of PE was 12%, whereas in patients who had two or more risk factors the prevalence was 21%. However, in the PIOPED study the majority of patients had intermediate- or low-probability V̇/Q̇ scan results and an intermediate clinical likelihood of PE; for these patients, the combination of clinical assessment and V̇/Q̇ scan interpretation does not provide adequate information to direct patient management accurately and further investigation using peripheral venous studies, spiral CT, or pulmonary angiography is warranted.

As the results of these studies suggest, the finding of a ventilation-perfusion match does not rule out PTE,[300, 301] nor is the observation of a mismatch definitive evidence for its presence. A relatively common cause of V̇/Q̇ mismatch in patients who do not have acute PTE is chronic or unresolved PE. Other causes include extrinsic vascular compression (mass lesions, adenopathy, mediastinal fibrosis), vessel wall abnormalities (pulmonary artery sarcoma, vasculitis), intraluminal obstruction by tumor or foreign body emboli, and congenital vascular abnormalities (pulmonary artery agenesis or hypoplasia).

Because of the limitations of the ventilation-perfusion

### Table 48–3. EFFECT OF SELECTED RISK FACTORS ON THE PREVALENCE OF PULMONARY EMBOLISM

| V̇/Q̇ SCAN INTERPRETATION | 0 RISK FACTORS* | 1 RISK FACTOR* | ≥2 RISK FACTORS* |
|---|---|---|---|
| High | 63/77 (82%) | 41/49 (84%) | 56/58 (97%) |
| Intermediate | 52/207 (25%) | 40/107 (37%) | 77/173 (45%) |
| Low/very low | 14/315 (4%) | 19/155 (12%) | 37/179 (21%) |

*Risk factors include immobilization, trauma to the lower extremities, surgery, or central venous instrumentation within 3 months of enrollment.

The results are based on the study by Worsley DF, Palevsky HI, Alavi A: Clinical characteristic of patients with pulmonary embolism and low or very low probability lung scan interpretations. Arch Intern Med 154:2737, 1994. Copyright 1994, American Medical Association.

scan, it has been suggested that the combination of perfusion scanning without ventilation imaging and assessment of the clinical probability of PTE may be superior to ventilation-perfusion scans in minimizing the number of pulmonary angiograms.[281] In one study, 890 consecutive patients who had suspected PTE were prospectively evaluated using perfusion scanning alone.[281] Before lung scanning, each patient was assigned a clinical probability of embolism: very likely, possibly, and unlikely, corresponding to a clinical probability of approximately 90%, 50%, and 10%, respectively. The clinical probability was based on evaluation of clinical history, physical examination, chest radiography, ECG, and arterial blood gas data.[281, 302] Perfusion scan results were classified independently as normal, near-normal, abnormal compatible with PE (PE+: single or multiple wedge-shaped perfusion defects), or abnormal not compatible with PE (PE−: perfusion defects other than wedge shaped). The study design required pulmonary angiography and clinical and scintigraphic follow-up in all patients with abnormal scan results. Of 890 scans, 220 were classified as normal or near-normal and 670 as abnormal. A definitive diagnosis was established in 563 (84%) patients who had abnormal scan results.

The overall prevalence of PTE in this study was 39%. Most patients who had angiographically proven emboli had PE+ scan results (sensitivity: 92%); conversely, most patients who did not have emboli on angiography had PE− scan results (specificity: 87%). A PE+ scan result associated with a very likely or possible clinical presentation of PTE had positive predictive values of 99% and 92%, respectively. A PE− scan result paired with an unlikely clinical presentation had a negative predictive value of 97%. The investigators concluded that clinical assessment combined with the perfusion scan evaluation established or excluded PTE in the majority of patients who had abnormal scan results. It should be noted, however, that by study design, angiography was not performed in patients who had normal or near-normal perfusion scan interpretations; in the PIOPED study, PTE was diagnosed in 5 (9%) of 57 patients who had normal or near-normal scan results and who had pulmonary angiography.[295] It is therefore likely that several cases of PTE were missed and that the sensitivity of scintigraphy was overestimated.

The value of ventilation-perfusion scans in patients who have COPD is controversial. In one combined ventilation-perfusion-angiographic study of 83 patients who had COPD and suspected PTE, the overall sensitivity and specificity of V̇/Q̇ imaging were 0.83 and 0.92, respectively.[303] False-negative interpretations occurred in 3 of the 16 patients who showed ventilation abnormalities in more than 50% of their lungs, whereas in the 67 patients who had ventilation abnormalities affecting 50% or less of their lungs, the sensitivity (0.95) and specificity (0.94) for detecting PTE were high. The researchers concluded that V̇/Q̇ imaging is a reliable method for detecting PTE in patients who have regions of V̇/Q̇ match as long as ventilation abnormalities are limited in extent.

In a later study aimed at assessing the accuracy of chest radiographs in predicting the extent of airway disease in patients with suspected PTE, investigators found that V̇/Q̇ scan results were indeterminate in all 21 patients who had radiographic evidence of widespread COPD, in 35% of those who had focal obstructive disease, and in only 18% of those whose chest radiographs revealed no evidence of COPD.[304] The investigators concluded that ventilation imaging is probably not warranted in patients who have radiographic evidence of widespread COPD. When an attempt is made to distinguish $\dot{V}/\dot{Q}$ matching that is compatible with PTE from that caused by COPD, a computation of the actual $\dot{V}/\dot{Q}$ ratio may be useful: in one study in which a $\dot{V}/\dot{Q}$ ratio of 1.25 or higher was used to define an area of mismatch, the percentage of patients classified correctly as having either PTE or COPD increased from 56% to 88% based simply on a consideration of the matched or mismatched character of perfusion.[305]

In another study of 108 patients who had COPD and who were suspected of having PTE (21 of whom had the diagnosis confirmed by angiography), it was impossible to distinguish between patients who had and who did not have thromboemboli by clinical assessment alone.[306] Among the 108 patients, high-, intermediate-, low-, and normal-probability scan results were present in 5%, 60%, 30%, and 5%, respectively. The frequency of PTE in these categories was 100%, 22%, 2%, and 0%, respectively. Therefore, although high-probability and low-probability ventilation-perfusion scan results have good predictive values, the majority of patients who have COPD have intermediate-probability scan results and require further investigation, which may include spiral CT and angiography.

Serial scanning may provide information not available from a single scan.[307] Changing patterns of perfusion defects indicate multiple emboli, some areas regaining normal activity and other previously normal zones becoming unperfused.[308, 309] In one study, new perfusion defects, developed in 22 of 63 patients under treatment for PTE;[238] most appeared within 2 weeks after the initial episode. This frequency suggests that anticoagulants are not very effective in preventing thromboembolism, although the incidence of new defects was even higher in untreated patients. However, it should be noted that diagnostic errors can be made by assuming that all new areas of hypoperfusion represent new emboli in patients who have pulmonary hypertension.[310] A region of lung whose feeding artery is partly occluded by an embolus may be well perfused on an initial scan at a time when neighboring branches are completely occluded; however, fragmentation and peripheral embolization of the thrombus in the completely occluded vessels may render a previously "normal" segment relatively underperfused and engender an erroneous interpretation of recurrent embolism.

Serial scans are also useful in following patients who have known PTE to assess resolution. In one investigation of 74 patients who had a clinical diagnosis of PTE, one third showed almost complete recovery, one third improved 25% or more, and the other third remained the same or worsened.[238] Perfusion was restored most rapidly in the first few days and more slowly during the next 2 to 3 weeks. The degree of recovery in individual patients varied greatly but tended to be most rapid initially and slower later; it was almost nil after 3 to 4 months. Patients who had large perfusion defects (greater than 30% of one lung) showed considerable improvement but, on average, recovered less completely than those with small defects.

In another study of 70 patients, the scan result became normal in one third of 34 patients who had small emboli (on average, 10 days after onset of symptoms), in 3 of 14 who

had medium-sized defects (average, 18 days), and in only 4 of 22 patients who had large defects (average, 23 days).[311] Correlation of recovery with age showed a return to normal perfusion in 57% of patients younger than 40 years but in none older than 60 years; in fact, less than half of the latter group had significant scan improvement. A similar follow-up of 40 patients who had PTE showed that, within 4 months, blood flow had returned to normal in 27 (67%) and had improved in 3 others;[308] of the 31 patients with an embolism of "intermediate" severity, 13 had normal scan results later and 16 showed improvement; of the 9 patients with "severe" embolism, only 2 had normal scan results later and 6 improved.

It should be borne in mind that in other diseases (e.g., pneumonia, congestive heart failure, and atelectasis) sequential scanning can also show rapid improvement in regional perfusion. Asthma in particular is easily confused with PTE without infarction because of its characteristic fleeting areas of reduced ventilation and perfusion, even in patients who have few symptoms and normal chest radiograph results.[312]

In summary, approximately 15% of patients who have PTE have high-probability ventilation-perfusion scan results, 40% have intermediate-probability scan results, 30% have low-probability scan results, and 15% have normal or near-normal scan results.[295] Approximately 90% of patients who have high-probability scan results have PTE compared with 30% of those who have intermediate-probability scan results, 15% of those who have low-probability scan results, and 9% of those who have normal or near-normal scan results.[295, 313]

The diagnostic accuracy can be improved by combining the results of ventilation-perfusion scanning with the clinical impression. In the PIOPED study, a clinical probability of PTE was estimated before lung scanning.[295] Three probabilities were considered: low (0% to 19%), intermediate (20% to 79%), and high (80% to 100%). A low-probability scan result paired with a low clinical index of suspicion had a negative predictive value of 96%. Conversely, a concordant high-probability ventilation-perfusion scan result and a high clinical index of suspicion had a positive predictive value of 96%. However, only 25% of patients fit into these clinico-scintigraphic categories, 75% of patients having an unresolved diagnosis.[295] Therefore, even under optimal circumstances of excellent clinical assessment and expert interpretation of lung scan results, further investigation is often required to evaluate the presence or absence of emboli.

### Computed Tomography

Initial studies assessing the potential role of CT in the diagnosis of PTE used conventional CT scanners that required a 1- to 2-second breath-hold for each transverse slice and a 6- to 8-second delay between slices. The slow imaging per section resulted in considerable cardiac and respiratory motion artifacts, and the long time required to image the entire chest (several minutes) did not allow optimal contrast enhancement of the pulmonary arteries throughout the duration of the scan. As a consequence, only relatively large emboli that affected the main or interlobar pulmonary arteries could be visualized.[314–317]

The introduction of spiral CT and ultrafast electron beam CT technology has made it possible to image the entire chest in a short period of time, often during a single breath-hold. This allows imaging of pulmonary arteries during peak enhancement with intravenous contrast and direct visualization of PTE. Several groups of investigators have shown a greater than 90% sensitivity and specificity of the two techniques in the detection of emboli in the main, lobar, and segmental pulmonary arteries, results that approximate those of angiography in the PIOPED study.[318–321a]

## Technique

Optimal assessment of pulmonary vessels on spiral and electron beam CT requires careful attention to technique. For adequate assessment of the pulmonary arteries, images should be obtained from the level of the aortic arch to 1 cm above the level of the lowest hemidiaphragm.[322] Depending on the severity of the patient's dyspnea, scans may be obtained during a breath-hold at end-inspiration or during shallow breathing. The collimation (section thickness) in various studies has ranged from 3 to 6 mm.[318–320] A section thickness greater than 3 mm leads to suboptimal visualization of segmental and subsegmental arteries as a result of partial volume averaging;[322, 323] because of this, we routinely use 3-mm collimation scans and reconstruct the images at 1.5-mm intervals. However, the technique is rapidly evolving, and preliminary results suggest that visualization of subsegmental emboli may be improved with the use of 2-mm collimation scans.[322, 324] To speed the examination, the rate of table feed may be increased to 5 mm per second, which, with 3-mm collimation, corresponds to a pitch of 1.7.

Optimal contrast enhancement of the pulmonary arteries requires selection of the most appropriate contrast agent, optimal concentration of the agent, and optimal timing and speed of contrast injection. Injection of highly concentrated contrast material (35% to 40% iodine) may result in streak artifacts originating at the level of the superior vena cava, which may radiate to the adjacent right pulmonary artery and preclude detection of intraluminal filling defects. Injection of low concentrations (12% to 15% iodine), on the other hand, requires rapid intravenous injection (up to 7 ml per second).[318] We recommend using 30% iodinated contrast (300 mg iodine/ml) at 3 to 4 ml per second for a total of 120 to 150 ml. A 12- to 15-second delay between the start of contrast injection and the start of the scan is recommended.[318, 321, 323] This time delay allows adequate contrast enhancement in the vast majority of cases. However, in patients who have decreased cardiac output, the time delay may have to be increased to 15 seconds or more.[322]

An alternate technique, which we favor, consists of using a test injection to determine the circulation time. The main pulmonary artery is located with preliminary noncontrast images. A total of 20 ml of contrast is injected at 4 ml per second, and images are obtained at the level of the main pulmonary artery at 3- to 5-second intervals for up to 20 seconds. A time-density curve is plotted by placing a region of interest (i.e., region in which the computer plots the attenuation values) over the main pulmonary artery to determine the time required for peak contrast enhancement. Current scanners automatically assess the time for enhancement, which can be used to optimize the delay between the start of intravenous contrast injection and the start of the diagnostic CT scan.

Images are viewed at lung parenchymal (window width

1500; level −700 HU) and soft tissue (window width 250 to 350 HU; level 35 to 50 HU) window settings. Assessment of both window settings is essential for accurate identification of the vessels, particularly the segmental and subsegmental pulmonary arteries, which can only be identified reliably by their location adjacent to the accompanying bronchi.

## Vascular Findings

**Acute Thromboembolism.** The diagnosis of acute PTE on contrast-enhanced CT is based on the presence of partial or complete filling defects.[314, 318–320] The former is defined as an intravascular central or marginal area of low attenuation surrounded by a variable amount of contrast material (Fig. 48–26); the latter is defined as an intraluminal area of low attenuation that occupies the entire arterial section, that is, by the abrupt absence of contrast material in a visible vessel[314, 318, 320] (Fig. 48–27). The most reliable sign of an acute embolism is a filling defect that forms an acute angle with the vessel wall and is outlined by contrast material. Although filling defects that form a smooth, obtuse angle with the vessel wall or complete cut-offs of contrast opacification of a vessel may be caused by acute thromboemboli, they may also be seen with chronic thromboemboli.

The first blinded prospective study comparing the results of spiral CT with pulmonary angiography for the detection of acute PTE included 24 patients without embolism and 18 who had angiographically proven disease.[318] Spiral CT results were correctly interpreted as positive in all 18 patients who had angiographically proven embolism (sensitivity 100%) and as negative in 23 of 24 patients who did not have embolism (specificity 96%). In this study, 112 central emboli—8 involving the main pulmonary arteries, 28 the lobar, and 76 the segmental—identified on spiral CT corresponded exactly to the angiographic findings; however, 9 intersegmental lymph nodes were erroneously interpreted as filling defects. It should be noted that the researchers excluded from the analysis arterial branches that were not identified adequately in the plane of section because of partial volume averaging. In a subsequent study of 75 patients in whom all pulmonary arteries were assessed to the level of the segmental branches, the sensitivity of spiral CT was found to be 91%, the specificity 78%, the positive predictive value 100%, and the negative predictive value 89% (compared with pulmonary angiography).[323] In both studies the analysis did not include emboli limited to subsegmental pulmonary arteries.

The accuracy of spiral CT has been assessed for both central and subsegmental pulmonary arteries in a number of other studies.[320, 321] In one series, 149 patients whose clinical assessment suggested PE were investigated by spiral CT and ventilation-perfusion scintigraphy; angiography was performed when the results of the ventilation-perfusion scan were indeterminate.[321] The spiral CT scans were assessed by two independent observers. Imaging results were compared and validated against normal perfusion scan results in 40 patients, high-probability scan results in 53 patients, and pulmonary angiography results in 56 patients. The sensitivity of spiral CT for the detection of PTE was 94% for observer 1 and 82% for observer 2; the specificity was 96% and 93%, respectively. There was good interobserver agreement on

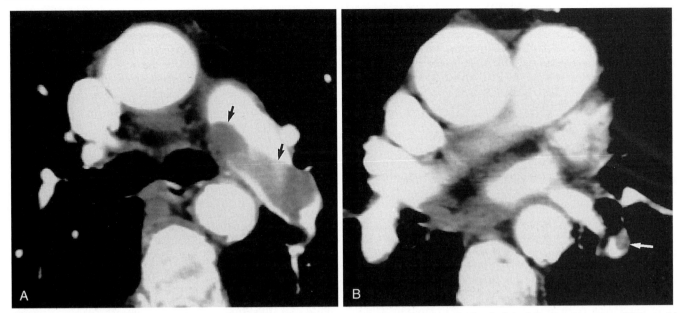

**Figure 48–26. Acute Pulmonary Thromboembolism.** A contrast-enhanced spiral CT scan at the level of the left pulmonary artery *(A)* in an 84-year-old woman demonstrates a large intraluminal filling defect *(arrows).* Contrast is present around and distal to the embolus, indicating partial occlusion of the artery. A CT image at a more caudad level *(B)* demonstrates an embolus *(arrow)* within the left lower lobe artery.

interpretation of the spiral CT results. Isolated subsegmental pulmonary emboli accounted for three false-negative spiral CT interpretations by both observers. Similar results have been reported with the use of ultrafast electron beam CT.[319, 325]

The low sensitivity of CT in the detection of emboli limited to subsegmental vessels may explain its lower diagnostic accuracy in patients who have low-probability V̇/Q̇ scan results.[326] In one study, the diagnostic accuracy of contrast-enhanced spiral CT was assessed in 20 patients who

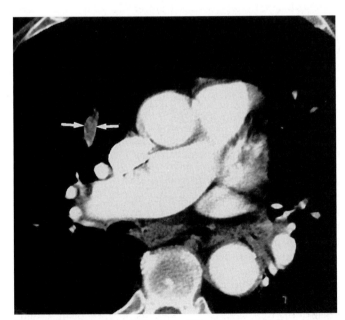

**Figure 48–27. Acute Pulmonary Thromboembolism.** A contrast-enhanced spiral CT scan in an 83-year-old man demonstrates an absence of contrast material within the medial segmental artery of the right middle lobe *(arrows),* consistent with complete occlusion of the artery by an embolus. Also note the increased diameter of the occluded vessel.

had uncertain clinical and scintigraphic diagnosis of acute PTE.[320] Patients who had normal or low-probability ventilation-perfusion scan results and a low clinical index of suspicion for PTE, and patients who had high-probability scan results were excluded from the study. Eleven of the 20 patients had angiographically proven pulmonary emboli, 4 of whom had involvement of only subsegmental vessels. When only segmental or larger vessels were analyzed, the sensitivity based on the CT findings was 86% and the specificity 92%, compared with pulmonary angiography; however, when subsegmental vessels were included, the CT results were 63% and 89%, respectively. CT allowed diagnosis of only one of four cases limited to the subsegmental vessels.

In another prospective comparison of spiral CT and ventilation-perfusion scintigraphy in 142 patients, the results of both procedures were independently assessed by two experienced observers.[327] The combination of a high-probability ventilation-perfusion scan result plus a spiral CT finding of PTE was considered diagnostic, and no further imaging studies were performed. The combination of a normal, very low, or low-probability ventilation-perfusion scan result and a negative result on spiral CT in a patient who had a low clinical index of suspicion for PTE was considered sufficient to exclude the disease. All other patients underwent pulmonary angiography. Twelve patients had discordant spiral CT and ventilation-perfusion scan results; using angiographic results as the gold standard, the spiral CT interpretation was correct in 11 and the ventilation-perfusion scan in 1. Overall, spiral CT had a sensitivity of 87% and a specificity of 98% in the diagnosis of acute PTE, compared with a sensitivity of 65% and a specificity of 94% for a high-probability ventilation-perfusion scan result. Also, there was better interobserver agreement in the interpretation of the results of the spiral CT scans than the results of the ventilation-perfusion scans. In another investigation, spiral CT and angiography were performed in 24 patients who had indeterminate V̇/Q̇ scans or discordant clinical and scintigraphic results;[324a] 6 patients (25%) had PTE. The sensitivity and specificity of spiral CT in detecting segmental and subsegmental emboli were 67% and 100%, respectively; the positive predictive value was 100%, and the negative predictive value 90%.

It can be concluded from these studies that contrast-enhanced CT has a high sensitivity and specificity for the detection of PTE. The procedure allows not only direct visualization of the intraluminal thrombi but also assessment of the mediastinum and pulmonary parenchyma and therefore evaluation of vascular changes related to nonembolic causes such as neoplasm and emphysema. In a prospective randomized trial of 78 patients who had suspected PTE, either spiral CT or V̇/Q̇ scans were performed as part of the initial investigation.[321a] A confident diagnosis of PTE was made in 35 of 39 patients (90%) who underwent spiral CT, compared with 21 of 39 patients (54%) who underwent scintigraphy first. The main reason for this difference was the ability of CT to demonstrate lesions other than PTE that were considered to be responsible for the symptoms of 13 of 39 (33%) patients.

Potential pitfalls in the diagnosis of PTE on CT include confusion with hilar lymph nodes, poor opacification of the pulmonary arteries, increased image noise in large patients, and obscuring of vessels by surrounding parenchymal opacification.[318, 322, 327, 328] The technique allows excellent assessment of the presence of emboli down to the level of the segmental arteries (Fig. 48–28). Although emboli limited to subsegmental arteries are often missed, these are relatively uncommon;[320, 327] for example, solitary emboli located distal to the segmental level were identified in only 14 of 251 patients (5.6%) in the PIOPED study.[295] Furthermore, even on pulmonary angiography, there is relatively poor agreement among experienced observers in the interpretation of subsegmental pulmonary emboli. For example, data derived from the PIOPED study showed interobserver agreement on pulmonary angiography of 98% for lobar em-

boli, 90% for segmental emboli, and only 66% for subsegmental emboli.[329]

Analysis of a cost-effectiveness decision model, based on the available data in the literature, has shown that the use of spiral CT is likely to improve cost effectiveness in the workup of PTE and to decrease mortality.[330] Investigators assessed various diagnostic algorithms consisting of combinations of ventilation-perfusion scintigraphy, ultrasound, D-dimer assay, spiral CT, and conventional angiography; for all realistic values of the pretest probability of PTE and coexisting DVT and of the diagnostic accuracy of spiral CT, all of the best diagnostic strategies included spiral CT.[330]

Although there is little doubt that contrast-enhanced CT can be helpful in the assessment of patients with suspected PTE, there is considerable controversy about the specific indications for its use.[326, 331–334] Most investigators recommend that contrast-enhanced spiral CT should be performed in patients who have indeterminate ventilation-perfusion scan results or low-probability scan results and a high clinical index of suspicion for PTE.[318, 321, 327] Various researchers have also suggested that spiral CT should replace scintigraphy in the assessment of patients whose symptoms are suggestive of acute PTE and who have no symptoms or signs of DVT (lower extremity ultrasonography being recognized as the primary imaging modality in the assessment of patients who have suspected DVT),[324a, 331, 334a] in the assessment of all patients whose symptoms are suggestive of acute PTE,[332] or in the evaluation of patients who have underlying cardiopulmonary disease and abnormal chest radiograph.[321a, 334, 335] Multicenter prospective studies are required to determine the optimal diagnostic strategy in these situations.

Currently, we perform contrast-enhanced spiral CT in patients who have symptoms that are suggestive of acute PTE and intermediate-probability ventilation-perfusion scan results and in patients who have low-probability or normal scan results and a high clinical index of suspicion. We also believe that contrast-enhanced spiral CT is the initial imaging modality of choice and should replace ventilation-perfusion scintigraphy in patients who have severe COPD or who show extensive parenchymal abnormalities on the chest radiograph. It should be noted, however, that the diagnostic accuracy of spiral CT scans in the latter group of patients has not been assessed.

Instances of clinically unsuspected PTE are occasionally found incidentally on CT scans performed in the assessment of patients who have trauma, thoracic tumors, aortic disease, or pulmonary abnormalities.[336, 337] In one study, a computer search of reports of 1,879 consecutive contrast material–enhanced spiral CT scans identified 18 such patients.[337] (In 11 of the 18 patients, the diagnosis was confirmed by angiography, ventilation-perfusion scintigraphy, or demonstration of DVT; in 6, the diagnosis was considered unequivocal on CT, and in 1 in whom the diagnosis considered probable on CT no further evaluation was performed.) The prevalence was 0.4% (6 of 1,320) among outpatients and 2% (12 of 559) among inpatients. All 18 patients had at least one risk factor for PTE, including carcinoma, atrial fibrillation, hypercoagulable state, or use of birth control pills. In another prospective investigation of 785 patients, the prevalence of PTE was evaluated on routine contrast medium–enhanced thoracic CT scans.[337a] Twelve (1.5%) patients had unsuspected PTE, with an inpatient prevalence of

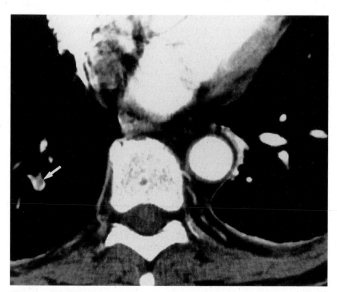

**Figure 48–28. Acute Pulmonary Thromboembolism.** A contrast-enhanced spiral CT scan in a 65-year-old man demonstrates an embolus (*arrow*) in the posterobasal segmental artery of the right lower lobe. The segmental arteries of the left lower lobe are also well seen and are normal.

5% (8 of 160) and an outpatient prevalence of 0.6% (4 of 625). Of the 12 patients who had unsuspected PTE, 10 (83%) had cancer; of the 81 inpatients with cancer, 7 (9%) had unsuspected PTE.

**Chronic Thromboembolism.** Although the majority of patients treated for acute PTE improve, some show only partial improvement and others develop chronic or recurrent embolism. In one study of 62 patients, spiral CT scans were performed 1 to 53 months (median, 8 months) after initial diagnosis.[338] All patients had been admitted to a cardiology intensive care unit and treated with anticoagulants for massive PTE; 31 had received fibrinolytic therapy initially. On the follow-up spiral CT scan, emboli were considered acute if they partially or completely occluded the arterial lumen and the arterial diameter was not reduced. They were considered chronic if at least two of the following features were present: (1) an eccentric location contiguous to the vessel wall, (2) evidence of recanalization within the intraluminal filling defect, (3) arterial stenosis or webs, (4) reduction of more than 50% of the arterial diameter, and (5) complete occlusion at the level of the stenosed arteries.[338] In 30 of 62 patients (48%), there was complete resolution of the initial embolus on the follow-up CT, and in 24 (39%) there was partial resolution; 8 (13%) developed CT features of chronic PE. The clinical presentations, risk factors at diagnosis, and treatment did not differ between the patients who had complete resolution and the other patients; however, the group of patients who showed residual abnormalities or developed chronic emboli had more extensive embolization at initial diagnosis.

As it does with acute PTE, contrast-enhanced spiral CT allows confident diagnosis of chronic thromboembolism in the majority of patients.[339–341] In one study of 75 patients who had this abnormality, the CT findings were compared with those at pulmonary angiography.[341] Chronic PE was diagnosed on CT by visualization of thrombi within the pulmonary arteries or by indirect signs such as irregular or nodular arterial walls, abrupt narrowing of the arterial diameter, or abrupt cut-off of distal lobar or segmental artery branches[341] (Fig. 48–29). CT demonstrated thrombi in the pulmonary trunk, right and left main pulmonary arteries, or lobar pulmonary arteries in 53 patients; thromboendarterectomy performed in 48 of these confirmed the CT findings of surgically resectable central chronic embolism. In 22 of the 75 patients, CT failed to demonstrate central emboli; however, organized thrombi were excised at surgery in 14 of these. Therefore, CT had a 78% sensitivity and a 100% specificity in the diagnosis of surgically resectable chronic PTE.[340]

## Parenchymal Findings

**Acute Thromboembolism.** Parenchymal manifestations of acute PTE on CT are similar to those on chest radiography and include oligemia, loss of lung volume, and wedge-shaped pleural-based opacities.[342–345] Localized areas of decreased attenuation secondary to oligemia are uncommon, except in patients who have massive thromboemboli (Fig. 48–30). Moreover, this finding is an unreliable sign of embolization; in a study of 88 patients who had suspected PTE, areas of decreased attenuation were seen in 3 of 26 (11%) patients who had acute PTE but also in 6 of 62 (10%)

patients who did not have emboli.[344] In the same study, findings that were most commonly seen in patients who had PTE included wedge-shaped pleural-based opacities (present in 62% of those who had emboli but in only 27% of those who did not) and linear opacities (in 46% and 21%, respectively).

As a manifestation of PTE, a wedge-shaped pulmonary opacity abutting the pleural surface is seen more commonly on a CT scan than on a chest radiograph.[342] The opacities may have the configuration of a full triangle or a truncated cone with concave or convex apex (Fig. 48–31). It has been postulated that the latter appearance may be related to sparing of the apex of the cone from infarction as a result of collateral circulation from bronchial arteries.[342] On CT, most infarcts can be seen to be partially or completely reabsorbed after 1 month, sometimes leaving a scar.[342]

Although characteristic of infarction, it should be remembered that a wedge-shaped pleural-based opacity on CT may be the result of a variety of other abnormalities, including hemorrhage, pneumonia, neoplasm, or edema.[346] In one study in which high-resolution CT (HRCT) findings were correlated with histologic abnormalities in 83 postmortem lung specimens, a thickened vessel leading to the apex of the pleural-based, wedge-shaped opacity was seen more commonly in patients who had infarction (10 of 12) than in those who had pneumonia (3 of 20), neoplasm (3 of 18), or hemorrhage (2 of 13) (Fig. 48–32).[346] Rarely, pulmonary infarcts cavitate (Fig. 48–33).[346a]

**Chronic Thromboembolism.** Although parenchymal abnormalities on CT are of limited value in the diagnosis of acute PTE, they are relatively common in patients who have chronic thromboembolism and are often sufficiently characteristic to suggest the diagnosis.[341, 347–350] The most common finding consists of localized areas of decreased attenuation and vascularity that are sharply marginated from adjacent areas with increased or normal attenuation and vessel size, a pattern known as *mosaic perfusion*.[351] Although this pattern can also be seen with airway diseases, particularly obliterative bronchiolitis and asthma, when associated with enlarged central pulmonary arteries or asymmetry in the size of the central or segmental pulmonary arteries, it is suggestive of pulmonary hypertension secondary to chronic thromboembolism (Fig. 48–34).[346a, 350, 351]

In a review of the CT findings in 75 patients who had angiographically proven chronic PTE, a mosaic perfusion pattern was found in 58 (77%).[341] The mean attenuation of the relatively dark areas was −868 HU and that of the relatively light areas −727 HU. After intravenous administration of contrast, the areas with decreased attenuation showed less enhancement (mean 30 HU increase after intravenous contrast) than the areas with increased attenuation (mean 45 HU). In the same study, 54 of 75 patients (72%) had nodular or wedge-shaped, pleural-based areas of increased attenuation on unenhanced scans that remained unchanged after the administration of contrast. These 54 patients had a total of 76 pleural-based areas of increased attenuation, 10 of which involved the upper lobes, 14 the middle lobe or lingula, and 48 the lower lobes. In another investigation of 33 patients who had chronic PTE, 18 (55%) had areas of mosaic perfusion and 22 (67%) had linear areas of increased attenuation.[349]

Chronic PTE may also be associated with airway abnor-

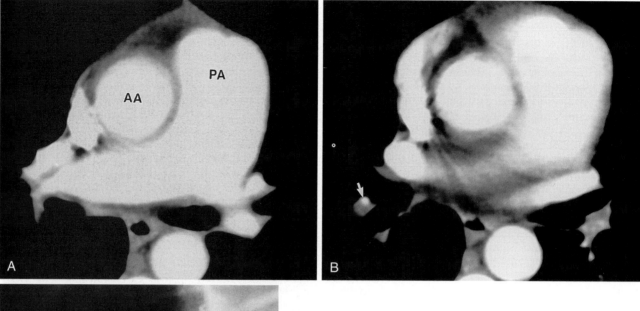

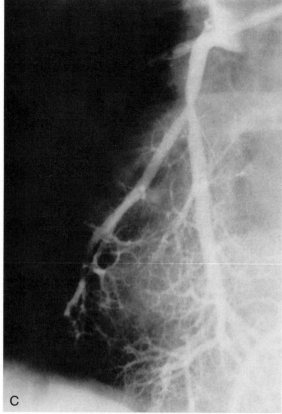

**Figure 48–29. Chronic Pulmonary Thromboembolism.** A contrast-enhanced spiral CT scan *(A)* demonstrates increased diameter of the main pulmonary artery (PA) (3.2 cm), a size larger than that of the ascending aorta (AA). Rapid tapering of the interlobar pulmonary arteries is also evident. A CT scan at a more caudad level *(B)* demonstrates a decreased diameter of the right and left interlobar pulmonary arteries. A small area of arterial enhancement *(arrow)* is present in the right interlobar artery and the left is completely occluded. A selective pulmonary angiogram *(C)* confirms the decreased size of the right pulmonary artery and demonstrates lack of perfusion in multiple areas of the right arterial bed. (From Remy-Jardin M, Remy J, Deschildre F, et al: Diagnosis of pulmonary embolism with spiral CT: Comparison with pulmonary angiography and scintigraphy. Radiology 200:699, 1996.)

malities.[349] In one study, CT findings in 33 patients who had chronic PTE were compared with those in a control group of 19 patients who had acute thromboembolism.[349] Cylindrical bronchiectasis was seen on HRCT in 21 of 33 patients (64%) with chronic embolism but in only 2 of 19 (11%) with acute disease. In the patients who had chronic PTE, the abnormal bronchi were located next to the completely obstructed and retracted pulmonary arteries. Although the pathogenesis of bronchiectasis in these cases is unclear, it has been postulated that it may be similar to that of traction bronchiectasis seen in interstitial pulmonary fibrosis, with the scarring of

the severely narrowed pulmonary arteries causing dilation of the adjacent bronchi.[349]

The diagnostic accuracy of HRCT in identifying chronic PTE based on the parenchymal findings was assessed in a study of 67 patients.[350] Seventeen had pulmonary arterial hypertension secondary to chronic PTE, 11 had pulmonary arterial hypertension due to other causes, and 39 had various interstitial, air-space, or airway abnormalities. Two independent observers had a sensitivity of 94% and 100%, respectively, and a specificity of 96% and 98%, respectively, in distinguishing patients who had chronic PTE from patients

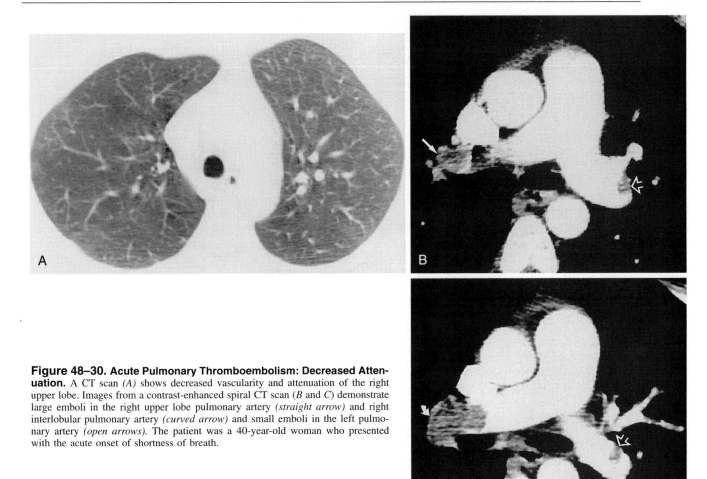

**Figure 48–30. Acute Pulmonary Thromboembolism: Decreased Attenuation.** A CT scan *(A)* shows decreased vascularity and attenuation of the right upper lobe. Images from a contrast-enhanced spiral CT scan *(B* and *C)* demonstrate large emboli in the right upper lobe pulmonary artery *(straight arrow)* and right interlobular pulmonary artery *(curved arrow)* and small emboli in the left pulmonary artery *(open arrows)*. The patient was a 40-year-old woman who presented with the acute onset of shortness of breath.

who had other abnormalities, including those with nonthromboembolic hypertension. Mosaic perfusion was identified in all patients who had chronic PTE, compared with 22% (Observer 1) and 14% (Observer 2) in patients who did not. Another finding that was helpful in differential diagnosis was the ratio of the diameter of corresponding right and left segmental pulmonary arteries, the average ratios of segmental vessel size being 2.2 ± 1 for patients who had chronic PTE and 1.1 ± 0.5 for those who did not.

### Magnetic Resonance Imaging

As with CT, MR imaging allows direct visualization of PTE. It has the additional advantage of not requiring radiation or the use of iodinated intravenous contrast; however, it is more expensive and less readily available. Initial studies using a spin-echo technique showed that large central pulmonary emboli could be visualized;[352–354] on conventional spin-echo MR images, vessels containing flowing blood at velocities greater than 15 to 20 cm per second are usually devoid of signal,[355] whereas emboli result in increased signal intensity within the vessel lumen. Despite these observations, the results of these initial studies were poor because artifacts related to respiratory motion did not allow adequate assess-

ment of segmental vessels and because slow blood flow, as may be seen with pulmonary arterial hypertension, also results in increased signal intensity on spin-echo MR images.[328, 356]

In the early 1990s, several techniques were developed to decrease artifacts due to respiratory motion and to improve the contrast between PTE and flowing blood. Important advances include the use of phase-array surface coils that allow single breath-hold MR imaging,[357–359] specialized gradient-recalled echo (GRE) sequences,[360–362] two- and three-dimensional time-of-flight imaging,[362a, b] and intravenous gadolinium for contrast enhancement.[328, 362] These techniques have allowed excellent visualization of vessels down to the level of segmental and subsegmental pulmonary arteries.[328, 362, 362b, 363]

Several groups of investigators have assessed the potential role of MR angiography in the diagnosis of PTE.[364–368] In one study of 18 patients, MR angiography had a sensitivity of 85% in the detection of PTE;[364] however, as with the other MR techniques, only emboli 1 cm or larger in anteroposterior (AP) diameter were diagnosed confidently by three independent readers. In another investigation, customized spin-echo MR images were obtained in 86 patients who had suspected PTE;[366] in 25 patients, additional custo-

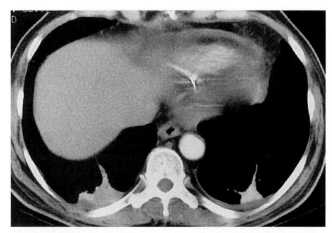

**Figure 48–31. Pulmonary Infarcts on Computed Tomography.**
A contrast-enhanced spiral CT scan in a 57-year-old patient demonstrates pleural-based wedge-shaped opacities in both lower lobes. The triangular opacity in the right lower lobe did not enhance with intravenous contrast. A small left pleural effusion is evident.

mized GRE sequences were also obtained. Only 35 of the 86 patients underwent pulmonary angiography, 21 of whom were shown to have PTE; the sensitivity of MR imaging in this subset of patients was 90% and the specificity 77%. In 29 patients, positive diagnoses were based on the results of high-probability ventilation-perfusion scans and negative ones on the results of low-probability scans with low clinical index of suspicion; in the remaining 12 patients, no definitive diagnosis was established. Of note was the fact that MR imaging had a diagnostic sensitivity of 100% (12 of 12 patients who had PTE) and a specificity of 78% (7 of 9 patients who did not) in 21 patients who had intermediate-probability ventilation-perfusion scan results and who underwent pulmonary angiography.

The use of intravenous contrast enhancement with gadolinium has great potential in MR diagnosis[367–369] (Fig. 48–35). In one study of 30 consecutive patients who had suspected PTE, MR angiography was performed during the pulmonary arterial phase of an intravenous bolus of gadolinium.[368] The procedure was carried out using a coronal three-dimensional gradient-echo pulse sequence with a slice thickness of 3 to 4 mm and an imaging time of 27 seconds. The MR images were reviewed by three independent observers and the results compared with those of standard pulmonary angiography. All 5 lobar emboli and 16 of 17 segmental emboli identified on conventional pulmonary angiography were also identified on MR angiography. Two of the three observers reported one false-positive MR angiogram each. Using conventional angiography as the gold standard, the three observers had diagnostic sensitivities of 100%, 87%, and 75% and specificities of 95%, 100%, and 95%, respectively, on MR angiography.

Preliminary studies suggest that MR may also have a role in the assessment of parenchymal abnormalities in both acute and chronic PTE.[370, 371] In one investigation, seven patients who had a clinical suspicion of PTE underwent cardiac-gated spin-echo MR imaging;[370] in three patients with angiographically confirmed emboli, opacities seen on the plain chest radiograph (presumably representing infarcts) were shown to have increased signal intensity on T1-weighted images. By contrast, in the three patients who had normal pulmonary angiography results, opacities on the radiograph did not show high signal intensity on T1-weighted images (in these patients the final diagnosis was "infectious pneumopathy"). One patient had no parenchymal abnormalities on the radiograph or MR imaging. Because of its high cost and limited availability, MR imaging currently plays a restricted role in the diagnosis of PTE.

### Pulmonary Angiography

Technique

Pulmonary angiography is the most definitive technique for diagnosing PTE.[295, 372–374] Best results are obtained if contrast medium is injected through a catheter whose tip is

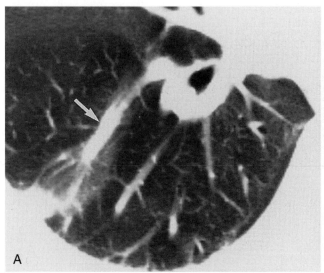

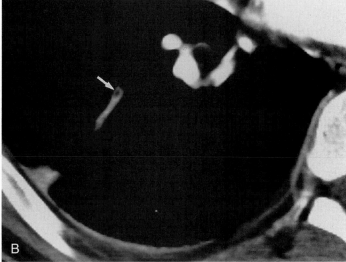

**Figure 48–32. Pulmonary Infarct on Computed Tomography.** A view of the right lower lobe *(A)* from a spiral CT scan in a 65-year-old patient shows a pleural-based opacity. Note the increased diameter of the subsegmental vessel *(arrow)* leading to it. Soft tissue windows *(B)* demonstrate a poorly enhancing subsegmental artery with a filling defect *(arrow),* consistent with recent thromboembolism.

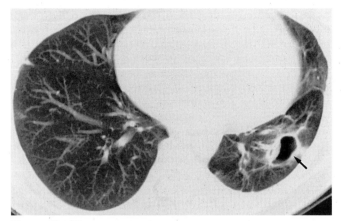

**Figure 48–33. Cavitated Infarct.** A CT scan in a 43-year-old woman demonstrates a cavitated lesion *(arrow)* in the left lower lobe. The diagnosis of sterile cavitated pulmonary infarct was made at thoracotomy.

in the right or left pulmonary artery (Fig. 48–36), a procedure that permits not only a clear view of the ipsilateral arterial tree but also the measurement of pulmonary artery pressure. The study may reveal partial or complete occlusion of lobar or segmental vessels but is seldom useful when the obstructed vessels are subsegmental or smaller.[194, 375, 376] These vessels are inadequately seen for several reasons, including dilution of contrast medium during cardiac systole, obscuring of vessel detail by overlap of many opacified vessels, and diversion of blood flow away from embolized vessels. In these situations, it may be necessary to perform segmental arteriography, first in AP projection and then in other projections if the AP study is inconclusive.[377] In one review of 57 positive pulmonary arteriogram results, it was found that additional views—the right posterior oblique projection for the right lung and the left posterior oblique or lateral projection for the left—were necessary in 26 (51%) cases.[378]

In a study of the reliability of selective pulmonary angiography in the diagnosis of PTE, three angiographers reviewed the arteriograms of a series of 60 patients retrospectively, independently, and without benefit of additional data;[379] although the interobserver agreement was 100% for emboli involving the main, lobar, and segmental vessels, it was only 13% for subsegmental emboli. Among 1,111 patients who underwent catheterization for pulmonary angiography in the PIOPED study, 61% had negative angiogram results, 35% had positive angiogram results, and 3% had nondiagnostic (poor quality) angiogram findings; in 1%, the angiogram was not completed, usually owing to complications. The overall agreement on the interpretation of angiogram results as positive, negative, or nondiagnostic among independent readers was 81%. Again, however, the interobserver agreement was related to the size of the affected vessel, being 98% for lobar vessels, 90% for segmental vessels, and 66% for subsegmental vessels.[329]

Pulmonary angiography may be performed using conventional film technique or digital subtraction (digital subtraction angiography [DSA]) (Fig. 48–37). The main advantage of DSA is the elimination of overlapping projection of other structures, thus allowing better visualization of pulmonary vessels. Use of DSA also allows an approximately 25% reduction in the volume of contrast material that is necessary to obtain optimal images,[380] a feature associated with a reduced risk of right-sided heart failure in patients who have severe pulmonary hypertension.[381]

Initial studies in which DSA was used after intravenous injection of contrast material showed it to be inferior to conventional pulmonary angiography.[382, 383] For example, in a prospective investigation of 33 patients who had suspected PTE, intravenous DSA was performed as the initial examination followed immediately by conventional pulmonary arteriography with selective right or left main pulmonary artery injections.[382] Intravenous studies of diagnostic quality were obtained in 31 patients, in whom PTE was correctly diagnosed using DSA in 12 and excluded in 18; emboli were detected in major and second-order branches and occasionally in third-order branches. There was one false-positive DSA examination. The overall accuracy was 91% (consider-

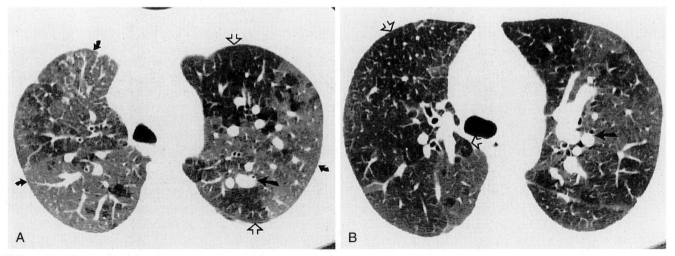

**Figure 48–34. Chronic Pulmonary Thromboembolism: Mosaic Perfusion.** High-resolution CT scans *(A and B)* demonstrate localized areas of decreased attenuation *(open arrows)* and vascularity and areas with increased attenuation and vascularity *(curved arrows)*, a pattern known as mosaic perfusion. Note the markedly increased pulmonary artery-to-bronchus diameter ratios *(straight arrows)*, particularly in the left upper lobe. The patient was a 43-year-old woman who had pulmonary arterial hypertension as a result of chronic pulmonary thromboembolism.

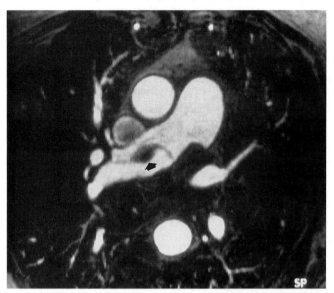

**Figure 48–35. Acute Pulmonary Thromboembolism: MR Imaging.** An MR image demonstrates an embolus *(arrow)* in the right pulmonary artery. The image was obtained using a breath-hold gradient-echo pulse sequence (TR 7.0, TE 2.2, flip angle 40 degrees) and gadolinium enhancement. (Courtesy of Dr. Pamela Woodard, Mallinckrodt Institute of Radiology, St. Louis, Missouri.)

ing all studies) and 97% (excluding the two inadequate intravenous examinations). In another study of 54 patients suspected of having PTE and studied by DSA, 13 (24%) had technically unsatisfactory examinations; of the interpretable angiograms, 27% had false-positive results.[383]

In the studies described previously, DSA was performed after intravenous injection of contrast material, dilution of which resulted in poor opacification of small pulmonary artery branches. Much better opacification is obtained with the use of selective intra-arterial injection.[384] In addition, developments in digital technique have improved the quality of DSA images markedly, with spatial resolution approaching that of conventional film angiography and image acquisition up to 30 frames per second.[385] These developments provide image quality that is comparable to that of conventional film angiography when using pulmonary arterial injection at a considerably lower cost and with the use of less contrast material. In one study in which both intra-arterial DSA and conventional pulmonary angiography were performed in 10 patients, no difference was detected in the degree of visualization of pulmonary artery branches.[386] In another investigation of 397 consecutive patients who had nondiagnostic ventilation-perfusion scans, the interobserver agreement in the interpretation of DSA images and conventional angiograms was assessed.[384] All angiograms were read immediately by the attending radiologist, by two radiologists after 6 months, and later by means of consensus of the two radiologists. The percentage agreement on conventional angiography was 80% between immediate and consensus reading, 80% between Observer 1 and consensus reading, 84% between Observer 2 and consensus reading, and 64% between Observer 1 and 2.[384] By comparison, the percentage agreements on DSA images were 88%, 96%, 95%, and 92%, respectively. Initial diagnoses were changed after the images were reviewed by consensus in 12% of patients with DSA

images compared with 20% of patients with conventional angiograms. The investigators concluded that interobserver agreement was better with intra-arterial DSA than with conventional pulmonary angiography.

In a more recent investigation, conventional film angiography and DSA were performed in identical posteroanterior and oblique projections in one lung of 80 patients undergoing pulmonary angiography.[386a] Diagnoses based on the results of blinded review of each study by three independent observers were compared with the diagnoses made by the physician who performed the procedure and with the consensus diagnoses obtained by group review of both studies. The investigation included 13 patients who had PTE. The sensitivity of DSA (i.e., correct identification of emboli by all three observers) was 92% and that of conventional film angiography, 69%; the specificities of the two modalities were not statistically significantly different. In another investigation of 39 patients, receiver operating characteristic (ROC) analysis showed similar performance for DSA and conventional film angiography.[386b] A limitation of these studies is the weak standard of reference, the final diagnosis being based on review of the angiogram by a group of experts. To overcome this, one group compared DSA and conventional angiography with the results of histopathologic examination in a porcine model;[386c] no significant difference was found between the two modalities. In summary, although it has lower spatial resolution, DSA performed using selective intra-arterial injection is comparable or slightly superior to conventional film angiography in the diagnosis of PTE. The main advantages of DSA are lower cost, the need for a lesser amount of contrast material, greater speed, and the ability to electronically magnify and view images in both subtracted and nonsubtracted modes.[386d]

### Complications

Although pulmonary angiography is considered to be the gold standard for the diagnosis of PTE, the procedure is requested for only a small percentage of patients who have clinically suspected emboli. For example, in one review of 316 consecutive cases of suspected PTE in a large university medical center in the United States, only 17% of 141 patients who had indeterminate ventilation-perfusion scan results underwent angiography.[387] In another survey of 360 acute care hospitals in the United Kingdom, it was found that approximately 47,000 ventilation-perfusion lung scans had been obtained compared with only 490 pulmonary angiograms.[388]

The reluctance to request pulmonary angiograms stems to some extent from the concern over the perceived risks from the procedure.[387, 389] This reluctance is still present in spite of a considerable decrease in the number of complications over the years.[389–391] In 1980, the complications seen in 1,350 patients who underwent pulmonary angiography at Duke University were reported.[390] There were three deaths (0.2%) directly attributable to the procedure, all in patients who had pulmonary arterial hypertension. The most common nonlethal serious complications were cardiac perforation and endocardial and myocardial injury, seen in 20 patients (1.5%). In a second study from the same institution based on 1,434 patients published in 1987, 2 deaths directly attributable to the procedure were identified.[391] Additional complications included reversible cardiac arrest in 5 patients and

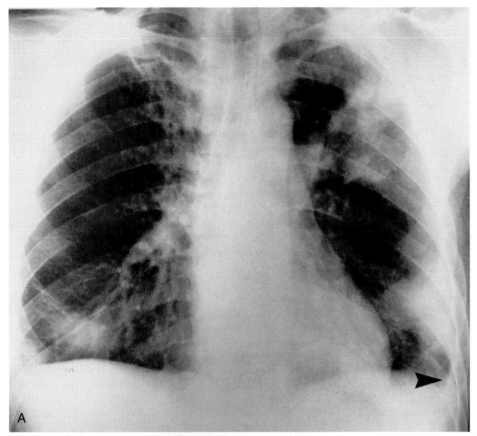

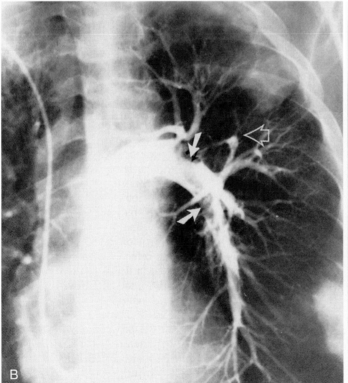

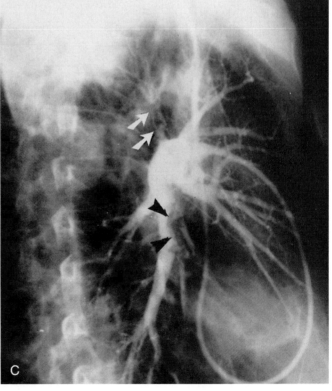

**Figure 48–36. Value of Oblique Arteriography in the Demonstration of Pulmonary Thromboembolism.** A conventional posteroanterior chest radiograph *(A)* shows multiple well- and poorly defined homogeneous opacities in both lungs, involving predominantly the lower lobes. The lesions are closely related to visceral pleura and on the left are associated with a small pleural effusion *(arrowhead)*. Cardiac size and configuration are normal. A selective left pulmonary arteriogram in left *(B)* and right *(C)* anterior oblique projections reveal multiple intraluminal filling defects, both central *(arrows)* and eccentric *(arrowheads)*. A segmental artery *(open arrow)* in the upper lobe in *B* is amputated. These features are diagnostic of pulmonary thromboemboli.

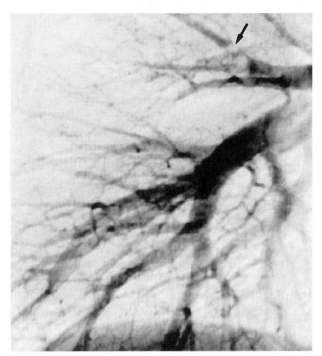

**Figure 48–37. Digital Subtraction Angiograph.** A view from a selective right pulmonary angiogram using digital subtraction technique demonstrates a localized filling defect *(arrow)* in a subsegmental artery in the right middle lobe.

cardiac arrhythmias in 15. Other researchers have also reported an increased risk of complications in patients who have pulmonary arterial hypertension. For example, in the study of 1,350 patients undergoing pulmonary angiography, the 3 deaths directly attributable to the procedure occurred in patients with pulmonary arterial hypertension (systolic pressures of 75, 70, and 160 mm).[390]

Since 1987, two major technical developments have occurred: the replacement of stiff end-hole catheters by mul-tiple side-hole pigtail[389] or flow-directed catheters[380] and the use of low-osmolar nonionic intravenous contrast medium.[389] Stiff end-hole catheters should be avoided because of the risk of cardiac perforation[392] (Fig. 48–38). In a 1996 review of 1,434 patients who underwent pulmonary angiography with nonionic contrast medium injected through multiple side-hole pigtail catheters (also at Duke university), major complications were found in only four patients (0.3%);[389] no deaths were attributed to the procedure. The major complications included respiratory arrest requiring ventilatory support (in two patients) and recurrent ventricular arrhythmias (in two more). Minor complications were seen in 11 patients (0.8%) and included arrhythmias responsive to lidocaine, catheter-induced vasovagal syncope, chest pain, and contrast-induced urticaria. In another study of 211 patients assessed by selective pulmonary DSA performed with an 8 French Swan-Ganz–type flow-directed catheter and non-ionic contrast material, no mortality or morbidity as a direct result of pulmonary angiography was observed.[380] In a third investigation of 728 patients who underwent selective angiography with a 7 French pigtail catheter and low-osmoler contrast media, there were no deaths and only one major complication (bleeding in the groin, necessitating surgery).[392a]

### Angiographic Abnormalities

The angiographic criteria for the diagnosis of PTE include primary and secondary signs[393] (Table 48–4). It should be noted that the latter reflect nothing more than diminished pulmonary arterial perfusion, a common manifestation of several pulmonary and cardiac diseases from which PTE must be differentiated.[394] However, the secondary signs listed in Table 48–4 may be useful by directing attention to areas in which manifestations of embolism may be subtle; in such cases, segmental arteriography, especially with magnification, may reveal intraluminal defects in smaller vessels. Care must be taken not to misinterpret an opacified artery seen

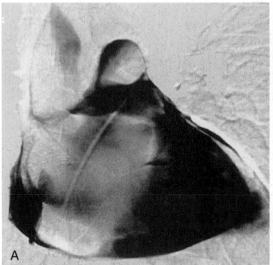
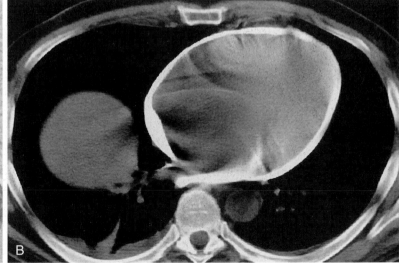

**Figure 48–38. Cardiac Perforation during Pulmonary Angiography.** A 58-year-old patient experienced sudden chest pain following injection of 40 ml of contrast during pulmonary angiography. Images from digital subtraction angiogram *(A)* and a CT scan performed immediately afterward *(B)* demonstrate contrast outlining the pericardial sac. The complication presumably was the result of perforation of the right ventricular outflow tract by the stiff-end catheter. The patient had no complications and was discharged from the hospital 2 days later.

## Table 48–4. ANGIOGRAPHIC CRITERIA REPORTED FOR THE DIAGNOSIS OF PULMONARY EMBOLISM

### PRIMARY SIGN

A. Filling defect
1. Persistent intraluminal radiolucency, central or marginal, without complete obstruction of blood flow
2. Trailing edge of an intraluminal radiolucency when there is complete obstruction of distal blood flow

### SECONDARY SIGNS

A. Abrupt occlusion ("cutoff") of a pulmonary artery without visualization of an intraluminal filling defect
B. Perfusion defect (asymmetric filling)
1. Areas of oligemia or avascularity
2. Focal areas in which the arterial phase is prolonged (especially when localized to the lower lung zones); this is usually accompanied by slow filling and emptying of the pulmonary veins
3. Tortuous, abruptly tapering peripheral vessels, with a paucity of branching vessels ("pruning")

Reprinted from Sagel SS, Greenspan RH: Nonuniform pulmonary arterial perfusion: Pulmonary embolism? Radiology 99:541, 1971, with permission of the authors and editor.

end-on as a blunt obstruction due to acute thromboembolism. A number of diseases may affect the pulmonary vasculature and result in nonuniform pulmonary arterial perfusion[393] (Table 48–5, Fig. 48–39).

The angiographic findings of chronic thromboembolic disease were assessed in a study of 250 patients and correlated with findings at pulmonary thromboendarterectomy.[395] The abnormalities consisted of abrupt vascular narrowing, complete vascular obstruction, webs or bands, intimal irregularities, and "pouching" defects (Fig. 48–40). The last was defined as the presence of obstructing or partially occlusive chronic thromboemboli that organized in a concave configuration toward the lumen of the artery. Such pouches opacify early in the angiographic sequence and may be associated with partial or complete vascular obstruction; occasionally, the appearance mimics that of unilateral pulmonary artery agenesis.[395, 396] Tapering of vessels usually connotes circumferential organization and recanalization and, therefore, an old thromboembolic episode.[397] Abrupt narrowing of a major pulmonary vessel is also a characteristic finding of chronic thromboembolism, the normal gentle tapering of the vessel being replaced by an abrupt decrease in the diameter of the opacified lumen.[395, 398] Pulmonary artery webs or bands are lines of low opacity that traverse the width of the contrast material within the pulmonary vessel and are often associated with narrowing of the vessels and poststenotic dilation (*see* Fig. 48–39).[395, 399] They have been shown in followup angiographic studies to be present at the precise sites of intra-arterial filling defects previously shown angiographically.[399] Another common finding of chronic thromboembolism is the presence of intimal irregularity, giving a scalloped appearance to the pulmonary arterial wall; at surgery this abnormality has been shown to be the result of irregularly organized thrombus lining the vessel wall.[395]

### Measurement of Pulmonary Artery Pressure

Measurement of the right ventricular and pulmonary arterial pressures is often very helpful in the evaluation of patients who have PTE,[400] and these pressures should always

be recorded carefully before pulmonary angiography is performed. Even if the angiogram reveals no evidence of major vessel occlusion, the pulmonary arterial pressure may be raised, suggesting the presence of small emboli throughout the lungs or comorbid cardiac or pulmonary disease. The pulmonary arterial pressure probably is raised in most patients who have positive angiographic findings.[401] When the main pulmonary arterial pressure is raised and the differential diagnosis is between acute thromboembolism and myocardial infarction with shock, capillary wedge pressure can be obtained with much less risk than an angiogram and usually distinguishes between the two conditions, being normal in embolism and raised in myocardial infarction.[402]

### Methods of Diagnosis of Deep Vein Thrombosis

#### Conventional Venography

Conventional contrast venography is used to outline the deep veins extending from the calf to the inferior vena cava and has been considered the gold standard imaging modality in the diagnosis of DVT.[403–406] In one prospective study, 70% of patients with PTE proven by angiography showed evidence of thrombosis of the deep veins of the legs;[407] it must be assumed either that the remaining 30% had other sources for embolism (e.g., the deep pelvic veins, inferior vena cava, or right atrium) or that all or most of the thrombus in the legs had embolized.[407, 408] Usually, the veins are opacified by injecting contrast medium into a foot vein; the iliac veins can be visualized by femoral vein injection.[409]

In one prospective study, patients clinically suspected of having PTE whose perfusion lung scan result was abnormal underwent pulmonary angiography and venography;[407] some of the patients with normal angiogram results had proximal vein thrombosis, suggesting that such thrombosis could have been associated with pulmonary emboli that were undetected by selective angiography, either for technical reasons or because of lysis of the thrombi.

Venography has several disadvantages: (1) it can be painful; (2) it actually induces thrombosis in 3% to 4% of patients when ionic contrast medium is used; (3) inadequate examinations as a result of incomplete venous filling and other technical problems occur in up to 5% of cases; and (4) there is an approximately 10% interobserver disagreement in the assessment of the presence of thrombus.[410–413] The incidence of complications is decreased with the use of nonionic contrast medium.[410, 411] In one study of 463 consecutive patients who underwent venography with a nonionic contrast agent, serious side effects (bronchospasm) were seen in only 2 (0.4%) and minor side effects (such as local pain and discomfort, nausea and vomiting, and superficial phlebitis) in 83 (18%);[411] postvenographic thrombosis confirmed by repeat venography occurred in 1 of 41 patients (2%) who had a previous normal venogram finding.

Because of the potential complications and limitations of conventional venography, it has largely been replaced by other imaging techniques, particularly ultrasound, in the investigation of patients with suspected DVT.

#### Ultrasonography

Studies of the use of ultrasound in the diagnosis of DVT in the 1980s were based on the observation that the

**Table 48–5. CONDITIONS ASSOCIATED WITH NONUNIFORM PULMONARY ARTERIAL PERFUSION**

I. *Emphysema (focal or diffuse)*
II. *Inflammatory diseases*
   Pneumonia (including tuberculosis)
   Lung abscess
   Bronchiectasis
   Pulmonary fibrosis:
      Interstitial fibrosis
      Fibrothorax
III. *Congenital*
   Absence or hypoplasia of a pulmonary artery
   Peripheral pulmonary stenosis
   Bronchopulmonary sequestration
IV. *Extrinsic obstruction of a pulmonary artery or vein by compression or actual invasion*
   Neoplasms:
      Benign
      Malignant
   Inflammatory:
      Fibrosing mediastinitis
   Aortic aneurysms
V. *Intrinsic obstruction of a pulmonary artery*
   Thromboembolic disease:
      Blood clot
      Tumor
      Fat
   The Eisenmenger reaction: superimposed obliterative arteriolitis
      develops in large left-to-right intracardiac and extracardiac shunts
   Arteritis
VI. *Postcapillary pulmonary (venous) hypertension*
   Left ventricular failure
   Mitral valvular disease
   Pulmonary veno-occlusive disease
VII. *Focal hypoventilation (frequently associated with atelectasis or air trapping)*
   Bronchial obstruction:
      Inflammatory processes
      Neoplasm
      Reflex bronchoconstriction
         Asthma
         Pulmonary embolism
   Splinting from pleural irritation:
      Inflammation ("pleuritis")
      Rib fractures

Reprinted from Sagel SS, Greenspan RH: Nonuniform pulmonary arterial perfusion: Pulmonary embolism? Radiology, 99:541, 1971, with permission of the authors and editor.

normal vein lumen is obliterated following compression by the ultrasound probe whereas a vein containing thrombus remains distended, the thrombus often being seen as an echogenic area within the normal nonechoic vein lumen.[406] Such studies showed a sensitivity of approximately 90% and a specificity of 97% to 100% in the diagnosis of popliteal and femoral vein thrombosis.[414–416]

Assessment of DVT by ultrasound improved with the advent of color flow technology in the late 1980s.[406] In the normal vein, color-coded flow completely fills the lumen. Thrombosis results in the absence of flow or the presence of isoechoic or echogenic thrombus within the lumen, with absence or persistent underfilling of color-coded flow.[406] Color Doppler ultrasound has a sensitivity of greater than 95% and a specificity of greater than 98% in the diagnosis of popliteal and femoral vein thrombosis.[417–420]

The clinical value of the assessment of calf vein thrombosis is controversial.[406] Most investigators believe that isolated calf vein thrombosis is not associated with a significant risk of PTE;[421] however, proximal propagation of calf vein thrombus has been shown to occur in up to 20% of cases.[422] It has been shown that color Doppler ultrasound allows a similar sensitivity and specificity in the diagnosis of calf vein thrombosis as those of above-knee lesions.[423, 424] In one prospective, double-blind study of 287 legs in 206 patients, investigators used contrast venography as the gold standard.[424] The study included 110 asymptomatic patients who were at increased risk for DVT following orthopedic hip or knee surgery and 26 patients who had signs or symptoms of DVT. In the postoperative patients, Doppler ultrasound had a sensitivity of 92%, a specificity of 100%, a negative predictive value of 98%, and a positive predictive value of 100% in detecting DVT in the calf with or without extension to the veins above the calf; in the symptomatic group, sensitivity was 86%, specificity 96%, negative predictive value 94%, and positive predictive value 90%. The researchers concluded that sonography is a highly accurate test in the detection of DVT in calf veins in both postoperative and symptomatic patients and that technically adequate assessment can be achieved in the majority of cases if the examination is performed with the patient sitting.

Because of its ready accessibility, low cost, and high diagnostic accuracy, ultrasonography has become the imaging modality of choice in the diagnosis of DVT in the majority of centers. In fact, in hospitalized patients with symptoms of both acute PTE and DVT, a lower extremity ultrasound has been recommended as the initial imaging modality of choice.[332, 333] A positive ultrasound result in this clinical setting allows confident diagnosis of PE with no need for further investigation.[332, 333] In patients without symptoms or signs of DVT, lower extremity Doppler ultrasound plays a limited role: several studies have shown poor sensitivity in the detection of asymptomatic nonocclusive thrombi in a variety of patients, including those who are postoperative.[406, 415, 425, 426]

## Computed Tomography

Spiral CT venography is performed by placing a 22-gauge intravenous cannula in the dorsal vein of each foot and a tourniquet around each ankle. Diluted intravenous contrast is injected simultaneously into both legs. After a 35-second delay, spiral CT is performed from the ankle to the inferior vena cava using a collimation of 10-mm and a table increment of 20-mm (pitch of 2). The images are reconstructed at 5-mm intervals.[427] The diagnosis of DVT is based on visualization of a filling defect in an opacified vein or a nonopacified venous segment interposed between a proximally and distally opacified vein.[427]

Preliminary reports suggest that the procedure is both sensitive and specific in the diagnosis of DVT.[427–429] In one study, 52 consecutive patients who had clinically suspected DVT were assessed using both spiral CT and conventional venography;[427] in cases in which the latter was nondiagnostic, color-coded duplex ultrasound was performed to establish a definitive diagnosis. CT had a sensitivity of 100%, a specificity of 96%, a positive predictive value of 91%, and a negative predictive value of 100% in the diagnosis of DVT. It was superior to conventional venography in demonstrating

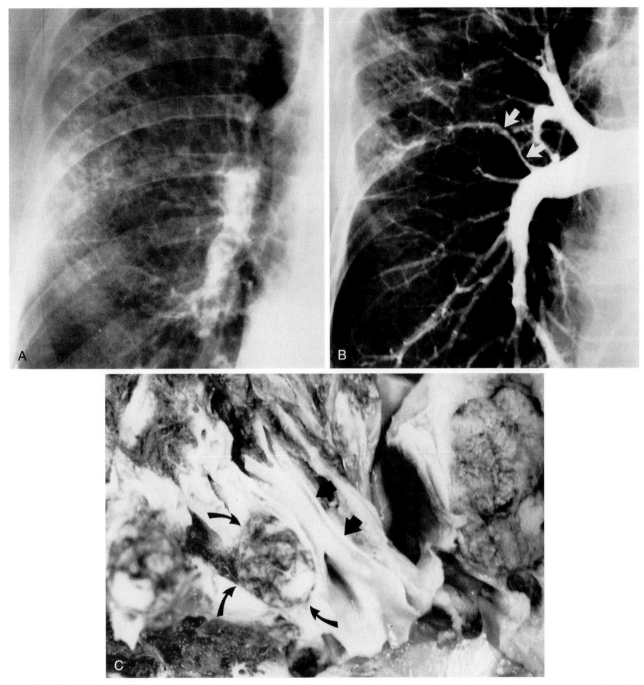

**Figure 48–39. Metastatic Pulmonary Carcinoma Mimicking Thromboembolism.** A view of the right lung from a posteroanterior radiograph *(A)* reveals a number of poorly defined opacities in the axillary portion of the right upper lobe. This 60-year-old man presented with a history of abrupt onset of right-sided chest pain, and a provisional diagnosis of acute pulmonary thromboembolism was made. A selective right pulmonary arteriogram *(B)* revealed no evidence of embolism but showed diffuse concentric narrowing of a branch of the right interlobar artery *(arrows)* extending toward the axillary opacity. At autopsy a few days later, the arterial narrowing was shown to be caused by compression by enlarged lymph nodes containing small cell carcinoma. A magnified view of the medial portion of the right lung *(C)* shows the narrowed artery *(arrows)* and the contiguous enlarged nodes *(curved arrows)*. The peripheral opacities were caused by the carcinoma.

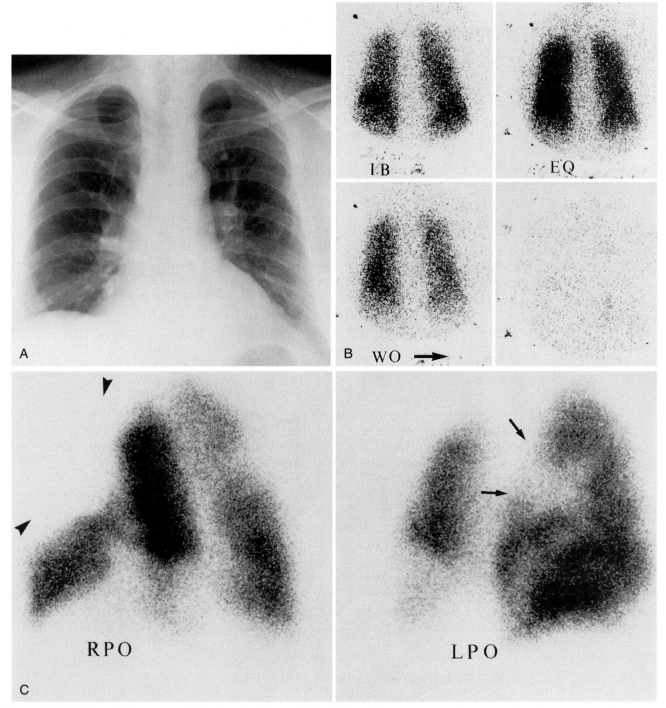

**Figure 48–40. Chronic Pulmonary Thromboembolism and Cor Pulmonale.** A posteroanterior chest radiograph *(A)* shows enlargement and increased rapidity of tapering of the hilar pulmonary arteries, indicating precapillary pulmonary hypertension. The lungs are otherwise normal. The heart is slightly enlarged. A ventilation scintigram result *(B)* is normal; however, perfusion scans in left posterior oblique (LPO) and right posterior oblique (RPO) positions *(C)* reveal a total lack of activity in the right upper lobe *(arrowheads)* and segmental defects in the right lower and left upper lobes *(arrows)*. IB, inspiratory breath hold; EQ, equilibrium; WO, washout.

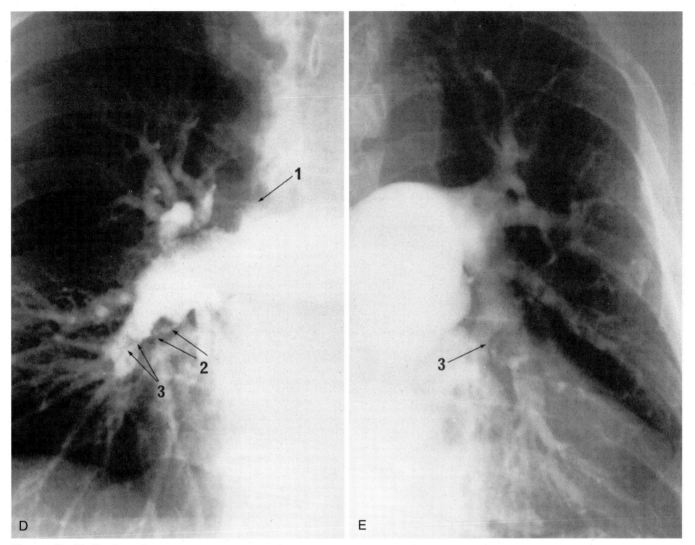

**Figure 48–40** *Continued.* Detail views of the right *(D)* and left *(E)* lungs from a pulmonary arteriogram reveal occlusion of the ascending branch of the right pulmonary artery (1), plaquelike defects in the right interlobar artery (2), and intraluminal curvilinear defects (3) consistent with organized thrombi (webs). These features are indicative of chronic thromboemboli.

extension of thrombus into the pelvic veins and inferior vena cava.

Advantages of spiral CT venography over conventional venography include simultaneous visualization of all veins in both extremities and better visualization of pelvic, peroneal, and posterior tibial veins and the inferior vena cava.[429a] It has also been suggested that adequate visualization of lower extremity veins can be obtained following intravenous injection of contrast material into an arm vein.[429b] In one study of five patients, spiral CT of the pelvis and lower extremities was obtained after spiral CT of the chest;[429b] the protocol thus allowed assessment of the presence of both PTE and DVT without the need for injection of additional intravenous contrast. This technique may be particularly useful in patients who are suspected clinically of having PTE and who have a negative spiral CT of the chest.

### Magnetic Resonance Imaging

Several studies have shown that MR imaging is comparable or superior to conventional venography or ultrasound in the diagnosis of DVT.[430–433] In a prospective study of 16 patients, GRE MR imaging was compared with conventional venography;[430] using this MR technique, thrombosed vessels showed decreased to absent signal intensity, whereas patent vessels were characterized by high signal intensity. In 16 of 17 extremities, MR imaging allowed accurate detection and localization of the thrombi that had been identified by venography.[430] In another prospective study, GRE MR imaging was compared with venography in 61 patients who had clinically suspected DVT.[432] The diagnosis on MR imaging was based on the presence of an intravascular filling defect with low signal intensity surrounded by high signal intensity due to flowing blood or on the presence of occlusion of an enlarged vein with a clot that had decreased or absent signal intensity. Compared with venography, MR imaging had a sensitivity and specificity of 87% and 97%, respectively, for the calf veins, 100% and 100% for the thigh veins, and 100% and 95% for the pelvic veins. In another series of 79 patients, GRE MR imaging had a sensitivity of 97% and a specificity of 95% compared with conventional venography.[433]

Because of its high diagnostic accuracy, MR imaging is recommended in patients with suspected DVT following a nondiagnostic ultrasound result, in patients with suspected pelvic vein thrombosis, and in the differential diagnosis of DVT from nonvascular disease such as ruptured Baker's cyst.

### Scintigraphy

Several radionuclide techniques have been assessed for the detection of DVT, including radioactive iodine ($^{125}$I)–labeled fibrinogen,[434] radioactive indium ($^{111}$In)–labeled autologous platelets,[435, 436] technetium Tc-99m MAA[437, 438] and technetium Tc 99m–modified recombinant tissue plasminogen activator.[439] The techniques have a number of limitations, including difficulty in interpretation, and have been used rarely in clinical practice.

### Impedance Plethysmography

This technique is based on variations in blood volume measured by a change in electrical resistance between electrodes fastened to the calf.[440, 441] Because blood is an excellent conductor of electricity, the change in limb venous blood volume when a thigh cuff is inflated normally results in decreased resistance; when the cuff pressure is released, a prompt increase in resistance follows. Constant dilation of the deep venous system caused by thrombotic occlusion results in little or no change in resistance with this maneuver.

In symptomatic patients, impedance plethysmography allows detection of approximately 95% of acute venous thrombi (less than 5 days old) that affect the popliteal or more central veins, including the common iliac vein.[402, 442, 443] However, the technique is of limited value, in the diagnosis of chronic venous thrombosis and acute or chronic calf vein thrombosis.[404, 444] The false-negative results in chronic thrombosis are related to the formation of collateral vessels that relieve the venous obstruction. As a result of these limitations, impedance plethysmography is seldom used for the diagnosis of DVT in clinical practice.

### Summary

Given the data in the literature and our own experience, we believe that the following recommendations are reasonable for the evaluation of patients suspected of having acute PTE:

1. All patients should have a chest radiograph, its role being mainly to exclude abnormalities such as acute pneumonia or pneumothorax that may mimic PTE clinically.

2. Patients who have symptoms or signs of DVT should undergo Doppler ultrasound of the legs; if the result of this examination is positive, the patient can be considered to have PTE and no further investigation is required.

3. Patients who have no symptoms or signs of DVT and symptomatic patients who have a negative Doppler ultrasound examination result and who do not have extensive underlying parenchymal lung disease or COPD should undergo ventilation-perfusion scintigraphy. A high-probability or a normal $\dot{V}/\dot{Q}$ scan result can be considered definitive. A low-probability finding together with a low clinical index of

suspicion can also be considered adequate to exclude PTE. All other patients should undergo further evaluation with contrast-enhanced spiral CT.

4. Patients who have extensive pulmonary parenchymal disease or COPD and patients who have nondiagnostic ventilation-perfusion scan results should undergo contrast-enhanced spiral CT.

5. Patients whose CT scan results are suboptimal and patients whose CT scan results are negative but who demonstrate a high clinical index of suspicion for PTE should undergo pulmonary angiography.

### Clinical Manifestations

As with pathologic and radiologic features, the clinical manifestations of VTED depend on several factors that, individually or in combination, influence the effect of vascular occlusion on the lung parenchyma: (1) the presence or absence of associated cardiopulmonary disease; (2) the size, number, and location of emboli; (3) whether vessel occlusion is complete or partial; (4) the presence of multiple embolic episodes and the time interval between them;[191] and (5) the rate of thrombus organization or lysis, whether spontaneously or with therapy.[445]

Most pulmonary thromboemboli produce no symptoms or cause such minimal distress that they are recognized only in retrospect, regardless of whether the occlusion has occurred in the smaller vessels, the segmental arteries, or even the lobar arteries. Among symptomatic patients, the severity of symptoms varies: at one extreme, an ostensibly healthy individual may die suddenly,[446, 447] but at the other extreme, even a large embolus obstructing a major vessel may give rise to only minor disturbances in circulatory dynamics and minimal clinical and radiographic findings.[448] The latter outcome is more likely in younger patients;[25] in older individuals, particularly those who have cardiovascular disease, a similar episode is more likely to lead to complications such as infarction, cardiac arrhythmia, and systemic hypotension, or to death.

The most common symptoms are dyspnea, tachypnea, and pleuritic chest pain. Among patients who have angiographically confirmed PTE, at least one of the three is present in 97%;[449] thus, the absence of all of these features in otherwise symptomatic individuals mitigates against the diagnosis. (This observation does not contradict the observation that most patients who have PTE are asymptomatic, a finding based on unexpected findings of thromboembolic disease at autopsy and on the findings of investigation in asymptomatic individuals at high risk of PTE, such as those who have DVT.[450, 451]) Physical findings of thromboembolism are usually nonspecific and include tachypnea, crackles, tachycardia (with or without arrhythmia), and manifestations of pulmonary arterial hypertension.[452] Fever is fairly common and should not be regarded as a useful sign in distinguishing infarction from pneumonia.

The vast majority of symptomatic patients have one of three clinical presentations:[453] (1) sudden onset of chest pain and dyspnea with or without hemoptysis (a picture associated with pulmonary infarction), (2) dyspnea in the absence of other symptoms, or (3) sudden circulatory collapse.[449, 454] Findings of acute pulmonary hypertension may accompany massive thromboembolism, whereas chronic pulmonary hypertension may be the result of recurrent thromboemboli or the failure to resolve emboli following a single significant episode.

Although the radiologic and other techniques available for the diagnosis of VTED yield important diagnostic information, it is important to remember that clinical evaluation of patients with suspected PTE has an important role in their evaluation; for example, the accuracy of V̇/Q̇ scanning is enhanced when physicians combine clinical assessment with the results of scan interpretation (*see* page 1807).[455]

**Dyspnea.** Dyspnea is the most common symptom of angiographically proven PTE, occurring in more than 80% of patients; cough is seen in more than 50%, apprehension in approximately 60%, and pleural pain in about 70%.[40, 445, 449, 452, 456, 457] In the absence of pulmonary infarction or circulatory collapse, dyspnea was the presenting syndrome in 26 of 117 patients (22%) in the PIOPED study.[449]

The onset of dyspnea is usually abrupt, an observation that aids in differentiating PTE from pneumonia, in which the onset is usually more gradual and is accompanied by cough productive of purulent material. Rarely, dyspnea is sporadic and is associated with wheezing, thus simulating asthma.[179, 181, 458, 459] In about 50% of patients, close questioning will elicit a history of one or more transitory episodes of dyspnea in the past, harbingers of later, more distressing embolism.[460–462] In fact, from information available in the preanticoagulant era, it has been estimated that a patient who has had a pulmonary thromboembolus has a 30% chance of a further embolic episode.[463, 464]

**Pulmonary Infarction.** This is seen most commonly following occlusion of segmental or subsegmental arteries.[166] In this situation, the patient complains of dyspnea of acute onset, pain on breathing, and (sometimes) hemoptysis. In the PIOPED study, this was the most common presenting clinical syndrome, occurring in 76 of 117 (65%) patients. However, among the 119 PIOPED patients who had a clinical picture of infarction, chest pain was unaccompanied by dyspnea and tachypnea in 14.[453] Hemoptysis is relatively uncommon (less than 30% of cases).[40, 449, 452, 457] When chest pain is pleuritic in type, it is usually the result of infarction; occasionally, retrosternal pain similar to that of angina pectoris results from large thromboemboli.[164, 193] Rarely, acute PE may be associated with the development of acute pericarditis;[465] the pathogenesis is a matter of speculation.

Tachycardia and fever often accompany the pain. The latter is usually low grade (37.2 to 37.7° C) but may be as high as 39.5° C; however, high fever persisting longer than 6 days should suggest a diagnosis other than PTE.[466] Fever has been described in approximately 20%[194] to 60% of patients.[466] Physical findings in patients who have pulmonary infarction include locally decreased breath sounds, crackles, rhonchi, friction rub, and signs of pleural effusion.[452, 457, 467]

The differential diagnosis includes pneumonia, atelectasis, and pleural effusion of other etiology. A cavitated infarct may be mistaken for an acute lung abscess.[278, 468] Pneumonia usually causes higher fever and purulent expectoration and has a more insidious onset; embolism may be difficult to differentiate from atelectasis, because both complications are common postoperatively. The pleural effusion of pulmonary infarction is usually grossly bloody unless it is diluted with the transudate of heart failure.

**Massive Pulmonary Thromboembolism.** This results when a thrombus lodges in the main pulmonary artery at its bifurcation or its right or left branch, with obstruction of at least 50% of the pulmonary vascular bed. It is an uncommon event, being observed in only 9 of 117 (8%) patients in the PIOPED study.[449] As a result of right ventricular failure, central venous pressure rises and cardiac output falls. Although peripheral venous vasoconstriction may initially prevent systemic hypotension, the decreased blood flow through the pulmonary circulation results in decreased left heart filling pressure and ultimately in systemic hypotension; the clinical presentation is thus that of circulatory collapse or shock.[402]

Characteristically, patients complain of severe dyspnea and retrosternal pain; tachycardia, tachypnea, and, at times, cyanosis are evident on examination. Occasionnally, circulatory collapse is unaccompanied by dyspnea, tachypnea, or chest pain.[469] Auscultation may reveal bronchial breathing; rarely crackles or a friction rub can be appreciated. The jugular veins are distended, a gallop rhythm may be audible, and there may be a diffuse systolic lift at the left sternal edge, with accentuation of the pulmonic component of the second heart sound. If the right ventricle fails acutely—a finding often associated with severe systemic hypotension—signs of pulmonary hypertension may be absent.[402, 409, 470–472] On occasion, some of the signs of right-sided heart failure are the result of right ventricular infarction secondary to increased myocardial oxygen requirements and decreased coronary blood flow.[473] Rare physical findings include pulsus alternans, pulsus paradoxus, and intensification of cyanosis caused by development of a right-to-left shunt through a patent foramen ovale.

Massive PE must be distinguished from myocardial infarction[474] and, when neurologic manifestations predominate,[475] from a cerebrovascular accident. Paradoxical embolism is another cause of neurologic abnormalities in patients with VTED, and DVT should be considered in patients who have embolic neurologic disease, even in the absence of other findings suggestive of PTE.[476, 477] In one investigation of 264 patients who were believed to have had embolic events (mostly neurologic), 49 were found to have a patent foramen ovale by transesophageal echocardiography;[476] the majority of these had clinically silent DVT.

**Chronic Pulmonary Hypertension.** As indicated previously, repeated episodes of PTE may result in increasing obstruction of the vascular bed; when this reaches about 50%, hypertension is almost inevitable. Affected patients may complain of episodic transient dyspnea, presumably a result of intermittent microembolism; others have a history of progressive breathlessness with or without clear-cut evidence of prior acute thromboembolic events.[200, 478] Recurrent attacks of cardiac arrhythmia, particularly atrial flutter, may occur,[479] and substernal chest pain is common.[480] Unusual clinical findings include a continuous murmur (believed to be caused by partial obstruction of major pulmonary arteries)[200, 481] and paralysis of the left vocal cord (Ortner's syndrome, caused by compression of the recurrent laryngeal nerve between the aorta and the enlarged pulmonary artery).[482] The latter condition has been reported more often in association with primary pulmonary hypertension,[483, 484] a disease that may be difficult to differentiate from chronic thromboembolic pulmonary hypertension (*see* page 1805).

Chronic thromboembolic pulmonary hypertension is sometimes imitated by agenesis of a pulmonary artery[485] or by pulmonary artery sarcoma.[486–488]

**Deep Venous Thrombosis.** The presence of signs and symptoms of DVT, particularly in the legs, is supportive evidence for the diagnosis of PTE and must be assessed carefully in all patients in whom this diagnosis is considered. Localized pain or tenderness in the calf, popliteal fossa, or thigh, especially if associated with a discrepancy in the diameter of the legs, suggests venous thrombosis. In some cases, pain may be elicited by dorsiflexion of the foot (Homans' sign). Although these findings are helpful when present, their absence does not in any way exclude a diagnosis of PTE: approximately 50% of patients who suffer a fatal embolism show no clinical evidence of DVT,[489, 490] and it is not unusual for persons who recover from PTE to have had no symptoms or signs of peripheral thrombosis.

**Extrathoracic Manifestations.** Although the clinical manifestations of PTE and infarction are chiefly respiratory, cardiac, or both,[491, 492] they can also mimic acute abdominal or cerebral disease.[254, 276, 460, 475, 491] Diaphragmatic pleuritis, paralytic ileus, and a rise in serum bilirubin may suggest a diagnosis of acute cholecystitis. Neurologic signs include restlessness, anxiety, syncope, convulsions, irrational behavior, hemiparesis or monoparesis, confusion, and coma.[164, 475, 491, 493, 494] They appear mainly in elderly, bedridden, or cardiac patients and almost certainly are caused by a combination of previous cerebrovascular disease, hypoxemia, and diminished cerebral oxygen delivery as a result of decreased cardiac output or cerebral vasospasm due to hypocarbia. A case report describes a single patient who had exercise-induced hypotension as a major manifestation of occult thromboembolic disease.[495] A patient who had ectopic adrenocorticotropic hormone syndrome associated with recurrent pulmonary infarction has also been described.[496]

## Laboratory Findings

Laboratory testing in the setting of suspected PTE is potentially useful in two situations: (1) the provision of additional information when the results of ventilation-perfusion studies are indeterminate or discordant with the clinical impression[497] and (2) the provision of prognostic information in patients who have established thromboembolism. Unfortunately, few tests are able to accomplish these tasks.

One of the first "tests" to be examined was the combination of an increased level of lactate dehydrogenase, a normal level of serum glutamic-oxaloacetic transaminase, and a slightly increased level of serum bilirubin (Wacker's triad).[498, 499] Unfortunately, the sensitivity of the "test" for PTE is poor, because it is positive in only about 10% of cases;[263] more important, it is unable to distinguish embolism from myocardial infarction or pneumonia.[263, 501]

Total creatine kinase (CK) may be elevated in patients who have PTE.[502] However, the hope that elevation of the MB fraction would enable reliable exclusion of a diagnosis of PTE has not been sustained,[503] because an elevation of CK-MB can occur in patients who have PTE with associated right ventricular infarction.[502]

Assays of several markers of coagulation and fibrinolysis have also been evaluated. The most promising of these are plasma D-dimers, which are circulating cross-linked fibrin degradation products that are specific markers for plasmin activity.[504] Because of the lack of specificity of the finding of elevated levels of D-dimer for the diagnosis of PTE,[505–508] its value, if any, lies in its high sensitivity.[505–510] In theory, it might be used in patients who have an intermediate probability for PTE based on clinical assessment and V̇/Q̇ scans to help select those who do not need pulmonary angiography.[510–512] However, the results of reported studies are not consistent, and is not yet clear whether the test will be useful in this respect.

In a review of studies in the English literature addressing these issues, considerable variability was found in assay sensitivity, heterogeneity of subjects tested, and inconsistency of diagnostic criteria;[513] the authors concluded that the clinical usefulness of the test remained uncertain. For example, a latex agglutination test for D-dimer, which could provide rapid results, has not provided the consistently high sensitivity required in patients who have symptoms suggestive of PTE.[506, 507, 514] In a prospective study of 179 patients in which four different techniques for the measurement of D-dimer were assessed, VTED could be excluded in only 8% to 18% of patients, using values for D-dimer that had a 100% sensitivity;[511] the investigators calculated that for every 2% decrease in sensitivity of the test, 1 per 1,000 evaluated patients would die as a result of inadequately treated PTE. Cost savings were modest, even assuming the levels of D-dimer used were confirmed as appropriate in subsequent studies.

On the other hand, using enzyme-linked immunosorbent assay (ELISA), another group of investigators found that values of plasma D-dimer below 500 μg per liter virtually exclude the diagnosis of PTE (i.e., a high negative predictive value for the test);[505, 515] a similar favorable evaluation has been documented by other workers using ELISA[497, 516, 517] or other immunoassays.[517a] One group concluded that the measurement of D-dimer was useful to exclude the diagnosis of PTE in patients who have otherwise nondiagnostic noninvasive study results; of 199 such patients, only 2 had a thromboembolic event (one a DVT, and the other PTE) in the 6 months following their initial evaluation.[512] The result was confirmed in a subsequent study involving a larger group of patients by the same group of investigators.[508] Given the numerous unfavorable study findings reported in the literature, results such as these require confirmation in other prospective studies before the test should be applied widely.

In patients who have DVT, the platelet count often falls with the onset of PTE;[518] however, a decrease may also occur with pneumonia or as a side effect of antibiotic therapy.[24] The leukocyte count seldom exceeds 15,000/mm³; in one study, 44 of 47 patients who had angiographically proven PTE had counts below this, and in almost half the count was less than 10,000/mm³.[519] However, pulmonary infarction may cause fever and neutrophilia greater than 15,000/mm³; therefore, these findings are not helpful in excluding a diagnosis of PTE.

Pleural fluid is grossly bloody in approximately two thirds of patients who have PTE and effusion.[520] This finding strongly suggests pulmonary infarction, particularly if malignancy has been excluded. In other cases, the effusion is a serous exudate or transudate; the latter is likely due to associated heart failure.[521]

## Pulmonary Function Tests

The interpretation of the results of pulmonary function studies in thromboembolic disease requires consideration of many factors. Many patients are extremely ill and cannot cooperate. A predisposing condition, such as heart failure, obesity, recent major surgery, or pregnancy, may influence lung function. Pleural pain may prevent full expansion of the thoracic cage, creating a degree of functional impairment that does not truly reflect the state of the lung parenchyma. The very nature of thromboembolic disease as a dynamic process renders comparison difficult between the results in two series or even between two patients. Pulmonary function studies may reveal restrictive disease: resting lung volume is decreased, airway resistance is increased, and lung compliance and diffusing capacity are reduced. However, in one study carried out 7 to 30 days after onset of an embolic episode, the most striking pulmonary function abnormality was its minimal disturbance, even in elderly, apparently very ill patients who had had recurrent emboli.[522]

Patients who have chronic thromboembolic pulmonary hypertension may have restriction due to parenchymal scarring, which may be apparent only with HRCT scanning.[523] In one study, 20 patients with PTE and no other apparent cardiopulmonary pathology were found to have a diffusing capacity below 75% predicted.[524] In the setting of chronic thromboembolic pulmonary hypertension, a reduced diffusing capacity is common. This is principally the result of reduced pulmonary membrane diffusing capacity (Dm);[525] a reduction in pulmonary capillary blood volume (Vc) also contributes. These changes might be related to changes in the pulmonary microcirculation caused by the hypertension; they are not reversible by surgical removal of thrombus.[525]

Arterial hypoxemia is common in acute PTE. In fact, the finding of an arterial $Po_2$ of 80 mm Hg or lower in 36 patients with angiographically proven disease raised the expectation that blood gas measurement would be a sensitive diagnostic test, with a high negative predictive value.[526] However, it is clear that arterial $Po_2$ values may be greater than 80 mm Hg, even in patients who have massive emboli.[470, 527] A normal $Pao_2$ is more likely to occur in patients who have a syndrome of pulmonary infarction than in those who present with isolated dyspnea; among the patients in the PIOPED study, a $Pao_2$ of greater than 80 mm Hg was found in 27 of 99 of the former and only 2 of 19 of the latter.[453] The lack of specificity of this test is self-evident. An attempt to increase the value of arterial blood gas analysis has been made by measuring the alveolar-arterial (A-a) gradient for oxygen. Some investigators have reported that a normal A-a gradient, while the patient breathes room air, virtually excludes a diagnosis of PTE.[528, 529] However, analysis of data from the PIOPED study showed this conclusion to be false:[530, 531] among patients with PE and no previous cardiopulmonary disease, 16 of 42 (38%) had normal gas exchange; by contrast, 4 of 28 patients (14%) with previous cardiopulmonary disease had similar normal values. Some investigators have found monitoring of pulse oximetry in critically ill trauma patients to be useful in diagnosis;[532] of

48 patients who had sudden drops in arterial oxygen saturation of 10% or more with simultaneous stability of lung compliance, 21 (44%) had angiographically confirmed emboli; in all 21, the chest radiograph results were normal or unchanged from the previous examination.

Most patients who have established PTE hyperventilate.[170, 533] Several investigators have advocated determining the difference between end-tidal and arterial $Pco_2$ as a measure of large areas of ventilated but unperfused lung.[533–537] However, because it is estimated that at least 20% to 30% of lung parenchyma must be nonperfused before the $Pco_2$ difference exceeds 6 mm Hg and because compensatory measures that restrict ventilation of the unperfused lung develop rapidly after embolism, this test is almost valueless in the diagnosis of PTE.[519]

## Electrocardiographic Abnormalities

ECG changes are common in patients who have PTE. In the PIOPED study 62 of 89 patients (70%) with PTE and no history of previous cardiopulmonary disease had an abnormal ECG result;[449] of these, 44 (49%) had nonspecific ST segment or T-wave changes. Ten patients had supraventricular arrhythmias; less than 6% had electrocardiographic evidence of p pulmonale, right ventricular hypertrophy, right axis deviation, or right bundle branch block. Left axis deviation occurred as often as right axis deviation, and this finding should in no way exclude the diagnosis of PTE. Among patients in the PIOPED study, a normal ECG result was more likely to be seen in those who had a clinical presentation of pulmonary infarction (45 of 97 [46%]) than in those who presented with dyspnea alone (2 of 21 [10%]).[453]

In another study of 49 patients who had acute symptoms subsequently shown to be caused by PTE, the ECG at the time of hospital admission (read in a blinded fashion) revealed evidence of right ventricular overload in 37 (76%).[538] This was defined as the presence of three or more of the following findings: (1) complete or incomplete right bundle branch block (n = 33) associated with ST segment elevation (n = 17) and a positive T wave in lead $V_1$ (n = 3); (2) S waves in lead I and aVL of more than 1.5 mm (n = 36 patients); (3) a shift in the transition zone in the precordial leads to $V_5$ (n = 25 patients); (4) Q waves in lead III and aVF but not in lead II (n = 24 patients); (5) right axis deviation, with a frontal QRS axis of more than 90 degrees (n = 16 patients) or an indeterminate axis (n = 15 patients); (6) a low-voltage QRS complex of less than 5 mm in the limb leads (n = 10 patients); and (7) T-wave inversion in leads 3 and aVF (n = 16 patients) or leads $V_1$ to $V_4$ (n = 13 patients), which occurred more often in patients with symptoms for more than 7 days. Of the 12 patients who initially had normal ECG results, 3 developed features suggesting embolism in follow-up studies.[538] Echocardiography revealed tricuspid valve regurgitation and increased right ventricular end-diastolic volume in all cases, and it seems likely that this group of patients had an important degree of pulmonary vascular obstruction.

In the appropriate clinical setting, ECG changes lend strong support to the diagnosis of PE. ST-T changes suggesting early myocardial infarction[24] or electrical alternans[539] can also be seen in patients with extensive PTE. In one study of 80 consecutive patients hospitalized for PTE, anterior T-wave inversion was associated with severe thromboembolic events and pulmonary hypertension;[540] early reversibility of the ECG abnormality was associated with good response to therapy and a favorable prognosis.

### Prognosis and Natural History

As discussed previously, most thromboembolic episodes are unrecognized clinically:[492, 541, 542] careful search of the pulmonary vascular tree at autopsy has revealed organized thrombi in more than 50% of unselected patients, most of whom had neither a clinical history suggestive of PTE nor pathologic evidence that the emboli had caused morbidity or mortality.[36, 37, 247] In most of these cases, the emboli were small and lodged in subsegmental or segmental vessels. One can only conclude from this that the prognosis in the majority of clinically unrecognized thromboembolic events is good.

The short-term outcome of patients who have clinically evident PTE depends to a large extent on the size of the embolus and on the presence or absence of underlying disease, particularly of the heart and lungs. For example, younger patients generally have a much better prognosis than older ones, largely because of the absence of comorbidity. In one series, 2.5% of treated patients younger than 40 died, whereas 18% of patients older than 40 expired.[25] In another series of 399 patients who had PTE and who were followed prospectively, only 2.5% died directly from PE in the year following diagnosis;[543] however, almost 25% died during this time as a result of disease that had rendered them susceptible to VTED in the first place. Whether PTE worsens the prognosis of the underlying comorbid process is not clear. Data from the PIOPED study suggest that this might be true for patients who have COPD;[544] however, information concerning baseline disease severity in the affected patients compared with patients who had COPD without PE is not available.[545] As discussed previously, many fatal pulmonary emboli are massive and occur without warning; in such cases, death typically occurs within minutes to several hours.[193, 546]

Patients who have massive embolism and shock and who survive long enough for confirmation of the diagnosis also have a poor prognosis. In a review of 144 patients with angiographically proven PTE, 45 had massive disease (defined as obstruction of 50% or more of the vascular bed);[547] of these, death occurred in 6 of 19 patients (32%) who were in shock but in only 2 of 26 (8%) who had a normal systemic arterial pressure. Similar results have been noted by other investigators.[548, 549] In patients who do not have shock, there is a correlation between the finding of right ventricular hypokinesis as assessed echocardiographically and degree of vascular obstruction as assessed by lung scan.[543] The finding of right ventricular dysfunction has also been associated with an increased risk of recurrent thromboemboli[550] and, not surprizingly, a significant increase in early and late mortality.[126a]

Although it is likely that therapy also affects the long-term outcome of patients who have PTE, the only randomized, controlled study that included a nontreatment control arm dates from 1960.[551] In this, 5 of 19 untreated patients

(26%) died as a result of PTE, and 5 had recurrent emboli; by contrast, none of the 16 patients who received anticoagulants died or had recurrence of disease. However, in the absence of prolonged anticoagulation, it is important to recognize that patients whose risk for VTED is transient are at substantially less risk of having recurrent events than those who have a persisting risk.[552]

In one investigation, the presence of a patent foramen ovale as detected by echocardiography was found to confer a very high risk of death (odds ratio 11.4) and of arterial thromboembolic complications in patients who had had a major PTE.[552a]

In nearly all patients who survive the acute event, clinical and hemodynamic resolution is complete within 4 to 6 weeks;[553–556] however, radiologic resolution may take somewhat longer. For example, in one study of 69 patients serial perfusion scans revealed that most had complete or nearly complete return of pulmonary blood flow by 4 months.[308] In another investigation of 33 patients at 30 months after PTE, residual angiographic abnormalities were evident in only 4 and chronic cor pulmonale in none.[557] Most patients show improvement in the perfusion lung scan within 2 weeks of initiation of therapy.[307, 308, 450, 549, 557] Despite these observations, patients who have larger emboli or associated cardiopulmonary disease may never show complete recovery.[549, 558, 559]

The prognosis of patients who have chronic thromboembolic pulmonary hypertension, whether treated or untreated, is poor.[200, 203] The majority of patients among those meeting selection criteria for surgery improve significantly; however, the mortality rate of attempted surgical embolectomy has varied from 6% to 40%, and not all survivors have hemodynamic improvement.[200, 203, 205, 560] Furthermore, only a small percentage of patients who have chronic thromboembolic pulmonary hypertension meet selection criteria for surgery.

## MICROTHROMBOEMBOLISM

Microscopic emboli of fibrin-platelet thrombus occur in association with all recognized sites of extrapulmonary thrombosis, including the deep veins, prosthetic heart valves, and arteriovenous cannulas.[561] The process is essentially identical to that of emboli of larger fragments of thrombus, but because of their small size, the clinical and radiologic manifestations are generally absent or minimal.[562] Rarely, the number of aggregates may be sufficient to cause significant effects, typically in situations in which blood has been present outside the vascular system for some period of time, such as in hemodialysis,[563] plasmapheresis,[564] and massive transfusions of stored blood.[563, 565–567] Identical emboli can be seen in the systemic vessels in patients in whom extracorporeal circulation is employed during cardiac surgery;[567] filters can dramatically decrease the number of such emboli.[566]

Histologic examination of the lungs in such cases shows platelet-fibrin aggregates within capillaries and precapillary arterioles, apparently occluding their lumens.[564, 567] Because many patients with these findings are critically ill from their primary disease, the role of the microemboli in morbidity and mortality is seldom clear. Occasional cases of rapid death have occurred, associated with dyspnea, bronchospasm, and hypotension. In addition to a mechanical occlusive effect, it has been speculated that platelet-derived chemical mediators may play a role in the pathogenesis of such disease.[564]

## SEPTIC EMBOLISM

Septic embolism occurs when fragments of thrombus contain organisms, usually bacteria and occasionally fungi or parasites. The pulmonary manifestations of such emboli may be the only indication of serious underlying infection; because the radiologic changes are often distinctive, their recognition early in the disease should permit diagnosis and prompt institution of therapy.[568] Although most cases of pulmonary infection associated with thromboembolism are the result of the presence of organisms within the thrombus itself (true septic emboli), it should be appreciated that secondary bacterial infection of initially sterile infarcts occasionally results in a similar pathologic and radiographic appearance (Fig. 48–41).

Septic PE occurs most often in young adults; in one study of 17 patients, the majority were younger than 40 years of age.[569] The organism most often grown on blood cultures was coagulase-positive *Staphylococcus aureus*, *Streptococcus* being the next most common; in four patients, blood culture results were negative. A predisposing factor is nearly always present, most often drug addiction, alcoholism, generalized infection in patients with immunologic deficiencies (particularly lymphoma), congenital heart disease, and skin infection.[570]

Most emboli originate from the heart (in association with endocarditis of the tricuspid valve or a ventricular septal defect[571, 572]) or the peripheral veins (septic thrombophlebitis). Because tricuspid endocarditis may not give rise to signs implicating this valve,[573] septic pulmonary emboli may be the first clue to this diagnosis. Occasionally, emboli originate in the pharynx and the infection extends to the parapharyngeal space and internal jugular venous system, resulting in a clinical presentation referred to as Lemierre's syndrome or postanginal sepsis.[574–577] A similar syndrome has been seen with mastoiditis.[578] The oral anaerobes, particularly *Bacteroides* and *Fusobacterium* species, are the most common pathogens associated with this syndrome. Staphylo-

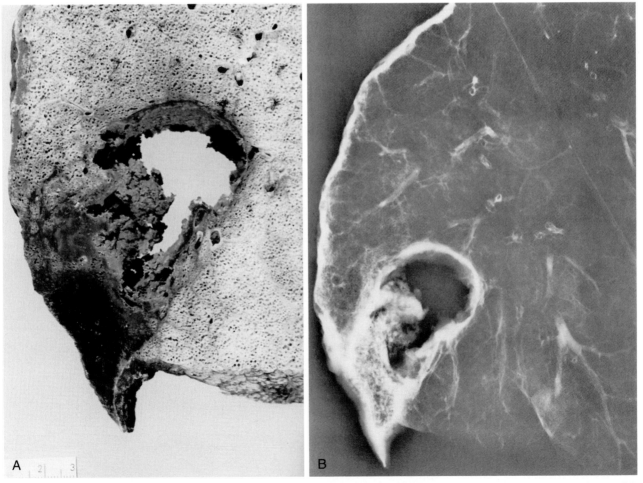

**Figure 48–41. Pulmonary Infarct with Cavitation Secondary to Bacterial Superinfection.** A magnified view of a slice of left lower lobe *(A)* shows a well-defined recent infarct with proximal cavitation. Note the focus of shaggy necrotic lung projecting into the cavity. A radiograph of the specimen *(B)* shows an appearance that simulates an intracavitary fungus ball. The patient had multiple foci of bronchopneumonia and bland infarction but no evidence of extrathoracic infection; thus, the cavitation was considered to represent secondary infection of a previously sterile infarct rather than septic embolization.

coccal osteomyelitis may also be the primary site of origin, 10 such cases having been reported in one review.[579] In this report, it was emphasized that in many cases the osteomyelitis is overlooked and that primary therapy directed toward the pulmonary complications may be unsuccessful until the osteomyelitis is recognized and treated directly.

Additional uncommon sites of septic thrombophlebitis include the arm veins in patients who have a history of intravenous drug abuse, pelvic veins in association with pelvic infection,[568] the portal vein,[580] and veins near infected indwelling catheters and arteriovenous shunts such as those used for hemodialysis.[581–584] There have also been reports of septic emboli in association with a transvenous pacemaker,[585] pyogenic liver abscess,[586, 587] and periodontal disease.[588] A single case has been described of candidiasis and septic emboli in a patient who swallowed a toothpick that traversed the duodenum, penetrated the inferior vena cava, and became impacted in the right ventricle.[589] Septic embolism has been described in a patient with toxic shock syndrome and disseminated intravascular coagulation due to β-hemolytic *Streptococcus.*[590]

Radiographically, pulmonary disease secondary to septic emboli is usually manifested by multiple, rather ill-defined, round or wedge-shaped opacities in the periphery of the lungs (Fig. 48–42). They may be uniform or may vary widely in size, reflecting recurrent showers of emboli. The opacities may be migratory in nature, appearing first in one area and then in another as older lesions resolve and new ones appear.[569] Cavitation is frequent and may occur rapidly; the cavities are usually thin-walled, and many have no fluid level. The opacities are usually bilateral, although they may be asymmetric and occasionally unilateral[591] (Fig. 48–43). Sometimes, a central loose body develops within one or more cavities (the "target sign");[592, 593] these represent pieces of necrotic lung that have been sequestered within the cavity and radiographically simulate the intracavitary

bodies that develop in some patients who have invasive aspergillosis (*see* page 940). It is important to realize that such intracavitary loose bodies can be associated with secondary bacterial infection of a "bland" infarct and, rarely, with "bland" infarcts themselves (Fig. 48–44). Acute septic embolism may be associated with hilar and mediastinal lymph node enlargement that may be massive;[594] empyema is an infrequent complication.

Radiographs sometimes show multiple, small, poorly defined opacities that simulate diffuse bronchopneumonia, and alertness is necessary to make the diagnosis, particularly if the emboli are derived from a focus of bacterial endocarditis. In questionable cases, the diagnosis can be confirmed by CT[591, 595] (Fig. 48–45). In one study, the radiographic and CT findings were compared in 15 patients who had clinically documented septic pulmonary emboli.[591] On the radiograph, diffuse bilateral nodules in various stages of cavitation were identified in 47% of cases, usually in association with focal areas of consolidation in the lower lobes; the remaining cases had only unilateral or bilateral areas of consolidation that were not identified either as being subpleural or as suggestive of pulmonary infarcts. On CT, discrete nodules in various stages of cavitation were identified in 67% of cases. In each of the patients in whom nodules were present, at least some of the nodules were located at the end of a pulmonary vessel (feeding vessel sign). In 73% of cases, the areas of consolidation were shown to be subpleural and wedge-shaped on CT. Central areas of heterogeneous lucency or frank cavitation were identified in 91% of the areas of consolidation on CT compared with only 7% of cases on the radiograph. After administration of intravenous contrast material, a rimlike pattern of peripheral enhancement could be identified along the borders of all the wedgelike areas of consolidation. Sixty-seven per cent of patients had pleural effusions, and 27% had hilar or mediastinal lymphadenopathy identified on CT.

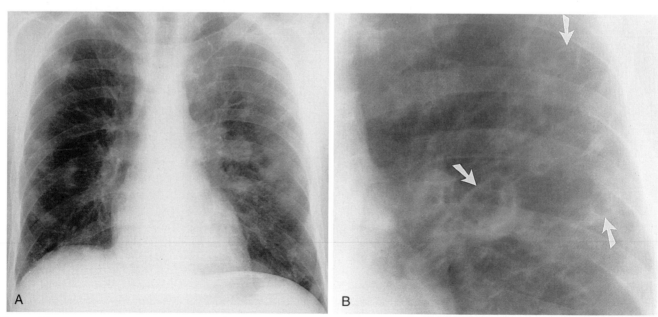

**Figure 48–42. Septic Embolism.** A view of a posteroanterior chest radiograph *(A)* in a 28-year-old man presenting with fever shows poorly defined bilateral nodular opacities. Blood cultures grew *Staphylococcus aureus.* Over the following days the nodules cavitated. A view of the left lung *(B)* from a chest radiograph performed 1 week later demonstrates multiple thin-walled cavities *(arrows).*

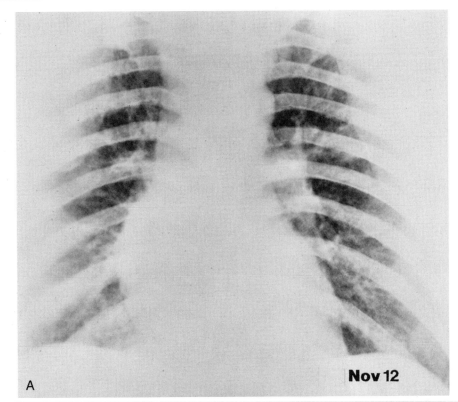

**Figure 48–43. Massive Septic Embolism.** Shortly before the radiograph illustrated in *A*, a 31-year-old man suffered a massive embolism related to severe thrombophlebitis of one leg. This film reveals relatively clear lungs, a normal left hilum, and an almost absent right hilum. A lung scan performed shortly thereafter *(B)* reveals a total lack of perfusion of the right lung and a segmental defect in the midportion of the left lung.

*Illustration continued on
following page*

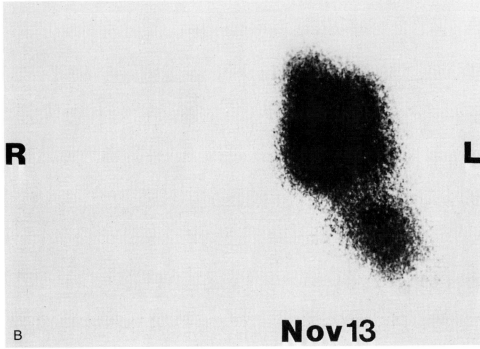

In another study of 18 patients who had documented septic PTE, multiple peripheral nodules ranging in size from 0.5 to 3.5 cm in diameter and wedged-shaped peripheral areas of consolidation abutting the pleura were identified on CT in 83% and 50% of patients, respectively;[595] 80% of patients with peripheral nodules had a feeding vessel sign. In 30% of cases the diagnosis of septic embolism was first suggested based on the CT findings.

Affected patients are often young, and many have a history of drug addiction. Those with Lemierre's syndrome may present with a sore throat, although the initial pharyngitis may have cleared by the time the infection reaches the retropharyngeal space.[574] Fever, cough (with or without expectoration of purulent material), and hemoptysis are the most common symptoms. Hemoptysis may be massive—in one report of three addicts with this complication, two died from asphyxia.[596] The presence of fever in drug addicts should always raise the suspicion of infective endocarditis;

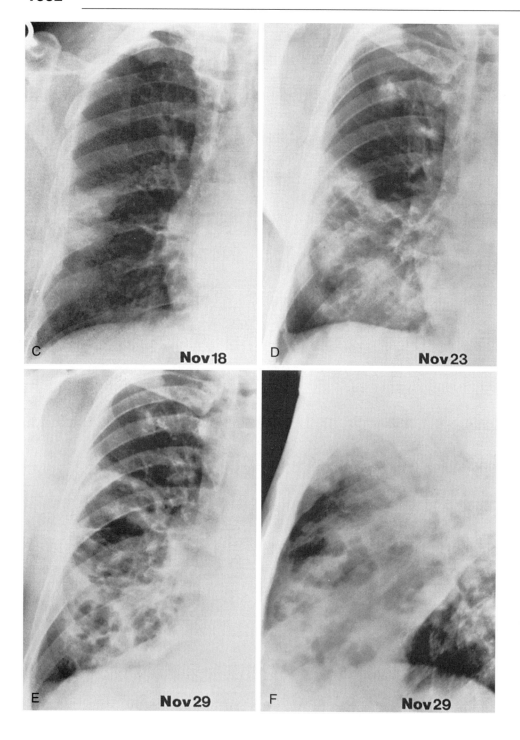

**Figure 48–43** *Continued.* Five days after the acute episode *(C)*, a poorly defined opacity has appeared in the axillary portion of the right lung in a configuration compatible with a pulmonary infarct; there is a small right pleural effusion. Five days later *(D)*, much of the lower half of the right lung has become consolidated, several areas of radiolucency scattered throughout the consolidated lobe suggesting cavitation. After another 6 days *(E* and *F)*, numerous shaggy cavities have appeared in the consolidation, representing multiple abscesses as a result of septic infarction. The disease is situated predominantly in the right middle and upper lobes.

in one series of 87 consecutive admissions of drug abusers with a temperature of 38.1° C or higher, 13% proved to have endocarditis.[597] Although infection originating in a right-sided heart valve may give rise to a murmur, in many cases it is soft and atypically located.[570]

## PULMONARY COMPLICATIONS OF SICKLE CELL DISEASE

Sickle cell lung disease occurs in all of the more common sickle hemoglobinopathies, including homozygous he-

moglobin SS and the compound heterozygous states of hemoglobin S/C, and hemoglobin S/β–thalassemia.[598] Approximately 85% of affected individuals survive into the second decade of life and therefore come to the attention of chest physicians and internists treating adults.[598] The sickle cell gene is carried by 8% of African Americans, so that the disease is relatively common in the United States.[599]

Several pulmonary complications occur in affected individuals. The most common, termed *acute chest syndrome*, is characterized by fever, pleuritic chest pain, dyspnea, leukocytosis, and new lung opacities on radiographs. The abnormality occurs in up to 50% of patients who have sickle cell

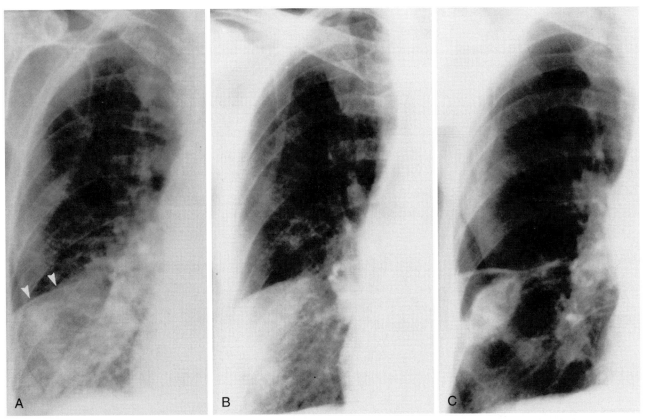

**Figure 48–44. Pulmonary Thromboembolism, Infarction, and Cavitation.** A view of the right lung from a posteroanterior chest radiograph *(A)* reveals extensive consolidation in the lateral segment of the middle lobe. Note the absence of an air bronchogram. The minor fissure *(arrowheads)* is slightly thickened and depressed. Four days later *(B)*, the consolidation has partly resolved at its hilar aspect, suggesting that it represents hemorrhagic edema. However, 18 days later *(C)*, a cavity appeared that contained an eccentrically situated fragment of necrotic lung or a hematoma. At autopsy several days later, these features were shown to be caused by a bland infarct associated with tissue necrosis and cavitation. The intracavitary mass consisted of sloughed noninfected lung parenchyma. The patient was a 72-year-old bedridden man who initially complained of cough, chest pain, and hemoptysis.

disease and is often recurrent.[598, 599] It is second only to pain as a cause for hospitalization and is responsible for 25% of all deaths in sickle cell disease.[598]

The pathogenesis of acute chest syndrome is probably multifactorial. Although there is little doubt that patients who have sickle cell disease are more susceptible to infection by a variety of organisms, including *Streptococcus pneumoniae*, *Haemophilus influenzae*, and *Mycoplasma pneumoniae*, most workers have found them to be a relatively uncommon cause of the acute chest syndrome,[600–602] except in young children.[603] One group of investigators has documented a possible association with *Parvovirus* B19 infection.[604] A more common cause of the syndrome is likely fat embolism derived from bone infarcts. In one study of 27 patients who had the syndrome, 12 were diagnosed as having fat embolism according to the results of quantitative evaluation of alveolar macrophage fat content;[605] of these, all had bone pain, 11 had chest pain, and 6 had neurologic symptoms (only 6 of 15 patients without a diagnosis of fat embolism had bone or chest pain, and none had neurologic symptoms). Another group of investigators found the level of secretory phospholipase A$_2$ (an enzyme that liberates free fatty acids) to correlate with the clinical severity of the acute chest syndrome.[606]

As indicated previously, a third potential cause of the syndrome is pulmonary infarction secondary to *in situ* thrombosis.[598] The pathogenesis of the vascular occlusion in these cases is likely complicated and may be related to increased blood viscosity as a result of RBC sickling, changes in blood coagulability, abnormal RBC-endothelial cell interactions, or a combination of these.[17] The vascular endothelium is activated in patients who have sickle cell disease;[607] it seems likely that adhesion molecules on these cells interact in an important way with plasma factors and RBC adhesion molecules. Activation of endothelial cells may also favor the development of a procoagulant state.[608] Evidence of vascular occlusion on HRCT in some patients during an episode of acute chest syndrome supports the hypothesis that this is a causative mechanism.[609] In one study of two patients, blood levels of the potent vasoconstrictor endothelin-1 were high during the syndrome, fell with resolution, and remained slightly elevated during routine clinic visits.[610] The levels were highest in one patient 4 days before the onset of acute chest syndrome, suggesting that this peptide might have a role in precipitating early microvascular occlusion. The observations that narcotics adversely affect the course of the syndrome in some patients and that incentive spirometry prevents progressive pulmonary complications in those presenting with chest pain due to early acute chest syndrome or rib infarcts[611] are in keeping with an important role for regional hypoxia precipitating sickling in the pulmonary vasculature. Despite these observations, infarcts and *in situ* thrombosis have been uncommonly documented pathologi-

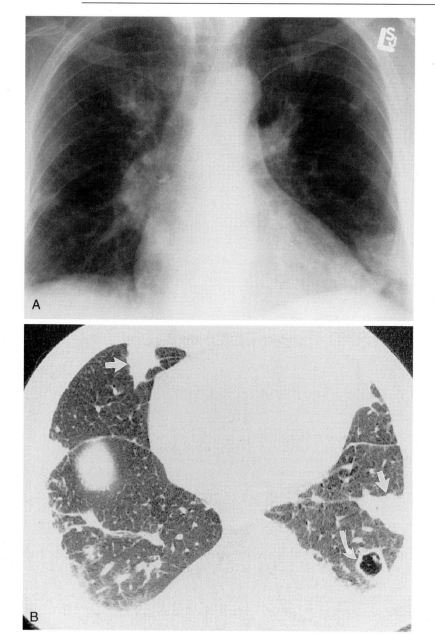

**Figure 48–45. Septic Embolism.** A posteroanterior chest radiograph *(A)* in a 64-year-old man demonstrates poorly defined bilateral opacities and small bilateral pleural effusions. A CT scan at the level of the dome of the right hemidiaphragm *(B)* demonstrates bilateral pleural-based wedge-shaped opacities *(straight arrows)* and a cavitated nodule *(curved arrow)* in the left lower lobe. Bilateral pleural effusions are also evident. Blood cultures grew *Streptococcus viridans.*

cally.[17, 382] Other potential causes of the syndrome are cigarette smoking[612] and rib infarcts.[613]

Some patients who have recurrent episodes of acute chest syndrome develop chronic parenchymal lung disease, in its most severe form with pulmonary hypertension.[599] Restrictive lung function changes, a low diffusing capacity, and hypoxemia[599, 614] precede the development of frank respiratory failure.[614] Children who have sickle cell anemia may also demonstrate an excess ventilatory response to exercise, in part as a result of an increase in physiologic dead space ventilation.[615] The cardiac response to exercise is characterized by an excessive increase in stroke volume and mixed venous oxygen desaturation, both of which are related to the severity of anemia.[616]

The radiographic findings in acute chest syndrome consist of bilateral patchy areas of consolidation, which have been attributed to edema and infarction. Rib infarcts are seen

rarely.[613] In addition to consolidation, HRCT demonstrates areas of vascular attenuation attributed to hypoperfusion.[609] Patients who have repeated pulmonary infections and episodes of acute chest syndrome may develop focal or, rarely, diffuse interstitial fibrosis.[617–619] HRCT findings of chronic sickle cell lung disease were assessed in a prospective study of 29 patients.[619] Patients were solicited from collaborating sickle cell centers and selected for the study based on a history of at least one previous episode of acute chest syndrome or pneumonia. They ranged from 5 to 54 years of age (mean 22 years) and included 27 patients with homozygous sickle cell disease and 2 with hemoglobin SC disease. Twelve of the 29 (41%) patients had multifocal interstitial changes consisting of interlobular septal thickening, parenchymal bands of attenuation, and pleural tags with associated architectural distortion; none had honeycombing or diffuse interstitial fibrosis.

# REFERENCES

1. Slavin RE, de Groot WJ: Pathology of the lung in Behcet's disease. Am J Surg Pathol 5:779, 1981.
2. Dimond EG, Jones TR: Pulmonary artery thrombosis simulating pulmonic valve stenosis with patent foramen ovale. Am Heart J 47:105, 1954.
3. Chiu B, Magil A: Idiopathic pulmonary arterial trunk aneurysm presenting as cor pulmonale: Report of a case. Hum Pathol 16:947, 1985.
4. Connors AF, Castele RJ, Farhat NZ, et al: Complications of right heart catheterization. Chest 88:567, 1985.
5. Ferencz C: The pulmonary vascular bed in tetralogy of Fallot. I. Changes associated with pulmonic stenosis. Bull Johns Hopkins Hosp 106:81, 1960.
6. Haupt HM, Moore GW, Bauer TW, et al: The lung in sickle cell disease. Chest 81:332, 1982.
7. Israel RH, Salipante JS: Pulmonary infarction in sickle cell trait. Am J Med 66:867, 1979.
8. Nussbaum RL, Rice L: Morbidity of sickle cell trait at high altitude. South Med J 77:1049, 1984.
9. Ryan SF: Pulmonary embolism and thrombosis in chronic obstructive emphysema. Am J Pathol 43:767, 1963.
10. Savacool JW, Charr R: Thrombosis of the pulmonary artery. Am Rev Tuberc 44:42, 1941.
11. Presti B, Berthrong M, Sherwin RM: Chronic thrombosis of major pulmonary arteries. Hum Pathol 21:601, 1990.
12. Heath D, Thompson IM: Bronchopulmonary anastomoses in sickle-cell anaemia. Thorax 24:232, 1969.
13. Robboy SJ, Colman RW, Minna JD: Pathology of disseminated intravascular coagulation. Hum Pathol 3:327, 1972.
14. Cramer SF, Tomkiewicz ZM: Septic pulmonary thrombosis in streptococcal toxic shock syndrome. Hum Pathol 26:1157, 1995.
15. Saka H, Ito T, Ito M, et al: Diffuse pulmonary alveolar hemorrhage in acute promyelocytic leukemia. Intern Med 31:457, 1992.
16. Katsumura Y, Ohtsubo K: Incidence of pulmonary thromboembolism, infarction and haemorrhage in disseminated intravascular coagulation: A necroscopic analysis. Thorax 50:160, 1995.
17. Weil JV, Castro O, Malik AB, et al: Pathogenesis of lung disease in sickle hemoglobinopathies. Am Rev Respir Dis 148:249, 1993.
18. Sankey EA, Crow J, Mallett SV, et al: Pulmonary platelet aggregates: Possible cause of sudden perioperative death in adults undergoing liver transplantation. J Clin Pathol 46:222, 1993.
19. Nasser WK, Feigenbaum H, Fisch C: Clinical and hemodynamic diagnosis of pulmonary venous obstruction due to sclerosing mediastinitis. Am J Cardiol 20:725, 1967.
20. Katzenstein A-LA, Mazur MT: Pulmonary infarct: An unusual manifestation of fibrosing mediastinitis. Chest 77:521, 1980.
21. Berry DF, Buccigrossi D, Peabody J, et al: Pulmonary vascular occlusion and fibrosing mediastinitis. Chest 89:296, 1986.
22. Goldhaber SZ, Morpurgo M: Diagnosis, treatment, and prevention of pulmonary embolism. JAMA 268:1727, 1992.
23. Dalen JE: Clinical diagnosis of acute pulmonary embolism—when should a VQ scan be ordered? Chest 100:1185, 1991.
24. Hampson NB: Pulmonary embolism: Difficulties in the clinical diagnosis. Semin Respir Med 10:123, 1995.
25. Green RM, Meyer TJ, Dunn M, et al: Pulmonary embolism in younger adults. Chest 101:1507, 1992.
26. Huisman MV, Büller HR, ten Cate JW, et al: Unexpected high prevalence of silent pulmonary embolism in patients with deep venous thrombosis. Chest 95:498, 1989.
27. Monreal M, Ruiz J, Olazabal A, et al: Deep venous thrombosis and the risk of pulmonary embolism—a systematic study. Chest 102:677, 1992.
28. Coon WW, Coller FA: Clinicopathologic correlation in thromboembolism. Surg Gynecol Obstet 109:259, 1959.
29. Spittell JA Jr: Pulmonary thromboembolism—some editorial comments. Dis Chest 54:401, 1968.
30. Morgenthaler TI, Ryu JH: Clinical characteristics of fatal pulmonary embolism in a referral hospital. Mayo Clin Proc 70:417, 1995.
31. Moser KM: Venous thromboembolism. Am Rev Respir Dis 141:235, 1990.
32. Stamatakis D, Kakkar VV, Sagar S, et al: Femoral vein thrombosis and total hip replacement. BMJ 2:223, 1977.
33. Kalodiki E, Domjan JM, Nicolaides AN: V/Q defects and deep venous thrombosis following total hip replacement. Clin Radiol 50:400, 1995.
34. Warwick D, Williams MH, Bannister GC: Death and thromboembolic disease after total hip replacement. A series of 1162 cases with no routine chemical prophylaxis. J Bone Joint Surg Br 77:6, 1995.
35. Geerts WH, Code KI, Jay RM, et al: A prospective study of venous thromboembolism after major trauma. N Engl J Med 331:1601, 1994.
36. Lindblad B, Sternby NH, Bergqvist D: Incidence of venous thromboembolism verified by necropsy over 30 years. BMJ 302:709, 1991.
37. Morrell MT, Dunnill MS: The post-mortem incidence of pulmonary embolism in a hospital population. Br J Surg 55:347, 1968.
38. Dalen JE, Alpert JS: Natural history of pulmonary embolism. In Sasahara AA, Sonnenblick EH, Lesch M (eds): Pulmonary Emboli. A Progress in Cardiovascular Diseases reprint (Vol. XVII, Nos. 3, 4, and 5). New York, Grune & Stratton, 1975, p 77.
39. Nielsen HK, Husted SE, Krusell LR, et al: Silent pulmonary embolism in patients with deep venous thrombosis. Incidence and fate in a randomized controlled trial of anticoagulation versus no anticoagulation. J Intern Med 235:457, 1994.
40. Anderson FA Jr, Wheeler HB, Goldberg RJ, et al: A population-based perspective of the hospital incidence and case-fatality rates of deep vein thrombosis and pulmonary embolism. Arch Intern Med 151:933, 1991.
41. Giuntini C, Di Ricco G, Melillo E, et al: Epidemiology. Chest 107:3, 1995.
42. Stein PD, Henry JW: Prevalence of acute pulmonary embolism among patients in a general hospital and at autopsy. Chest 108:978, 1995.
43. Paltiel O: Epidemiology of venous thromboembolism. In Leclerc JR (ed): Venous Thromboembolic Disorders. Philadelphia, Lea & Febiger, 1991, p 141.
44. Josa M, Siouffi SY, Silverman AB, et al: Pulmonary embolism after cardiac surgery. J Am Coll Cardiol 21:990, 1993.
45. DeLaria G, Hunter JA: Deep venous thrombosis. Implications after open heart surgery. Chest 99:284, 1991.
46. Gillinov AM, Davis EA, Alberg AJ, et al: Pulmonary embolism in the cardiac surgical patient. Ann Thorac Surg 53:988, 1992.
47. Kniffin WD Jr, Baron JA, Barrett J, et al: The epidemiology of diagnosed pulmonary embolism and deep venous thrombosis in the elderly. Arch Intern Med 154:861, 1994.
48. Gillum RF: Pulmonary embolism and thrombophlebitis in the United States, 1970–1985. Am Heart J 114:1262, 1987.
48a. Silverstein MD, Heit JA, Mohr DN, et al: Trends in the incidence of deep vein thrombosis and pulmonary embolism: A 25-year population-based study. Arch Intern Med 158:585, 1998.
48b. White RH, Zhou H, Romano PS: Incidence of idiopathic deep venous thrombosis and secondary thromboembolism among ethnic groups in California. Ann Intern Med 128:737, 1998.
48c. Siddique RM, Siddique MI, Rimm AA: Trends in pulmonary embolism mortality in the US elderly population: 1984 through 1991. Am J Public Health 88:478, 1998.
49. Karwinski B, Svendsen E: Comparison of clinical and postmortem diagnosis of pulmonary embolism. J Clin Pathol 42:135, 1989.
50. Dismuke SE, Wagner EH: Pulmonary embolism as a cause of death. The changing mortality in hospitalized patients. JAMA 255:2039, 1986.
51. Lau G: Pulmonary thromboembolism is not uncommon—results and implications of a five year study of 116 necropsies. Ann Acad Med Singapore 24:356, 1995.
52. Lindblad B, Sternby NH, Bergqvist D: Incidence of venous thromboembolism verified by necropsy over 30 years. BMJ 302:709, 1991.
53. Copeland AR: Sudden natural death due to pulmonary thromboembolism in the medical examiner's jurisdiction. Med Sci Law 27:288, 1987.
54. Gallerani M, Manfredini R, Ricci L, et al: Sudden death from pulmonary thromboembolism. Eur Heart J 13:661, 1992.
55. Beckering RE Jr, Titus JL: Femoral-popliteal venous thrombosis and pulmonary embolism. Am J Clin Pathol 52:530, 1969.
56. Le Quesne LP: Relation between deep vein thrombosis and pulmonary embolism in surgical patients. N Engl J Med 291:1292, 1974.
57. Mavor GE, Galloway JMD: The iliofemoral venous segment as a source of pulmonary emboli. Lancet 1:871, 1967.
58. Kakkar VV, Howe CT, Flanc C, et al: Natural history of postoperative deep-vein thrombosis. Lancet 2:230, 1969.
59. Aldridge SC, Comerota AJ, Katz ML, et al: Popliteal venous aneurysm: Report of two cases and review of the world literature. J Vasc Surg 18:708, 1993.
60. Stamatakis D, Kakkar VV, Sagar S, et al: Femoral vein thrombosis and total hip replacement. BMJ 2:223, 1977.
61. Sevitt S: The structure and growth of valve-pocket thrombi in femoral veins. J Clin Pathol 27:517, 1974.
62. Browse NL, Thomas ML: Source of non-lethal pulmonary emboli. Lancet 1:258, 1974.
63. Thomas DP: Venous thrombogenesis. Ann Rev Med 36:39, 1985.
64. Mammen EF: Pathogenesis of a venous thrombosis. Chest 102:640, 1992.
65. Waller BF, Dean PJ, Mann O, et al: Right ventricular outflow obstruction from thrombus with small peripheral pulmonary emboli. Chest 79:224, 1981.
66. Crowell RH, Adams GS, Koilpillai CJ, et al: In vivo right heart thrombus—precursor of life-threatening pulmonary embolism. Chest 94:1236, 1988.
67. Gonzalez A, Altieri PI, Marquez E, et al: Massive pulmonary embolism associated with a right ventricular myxoma. Am J Med 69:795, 1980.
68. Bortolotti U, Mazzucco A, Valfre C, et al: Right ventricular myxoma: Review of the literature and report of 2 patients. Ann Thorac Surg 33:277, 1982.
69. Goldstein MF, Nestico P, Olshan AR, et al: Superior vena cava thrombosis and pulmonary embolus: Association with right atrial mural thrombus. Arch Intern Med 142:1726, 1982.
70. Adelstein DJ, Hines JD, Carter SG, et al: Thromboembolic events in patients with malignant superior vena cava syndrome and the role of anticoagulation. Cancer 62:2258, 1988.
71. Sundqvist S-B, Hedner U, Kullenberg HKE, et al: Deep venous thrombosis of the arm: A study of coagulation and fibrinolysis. BMJ 283:265, 1981.
72. Coon WW, Willis PW III: Thrombosis of axillary and subclavian veins. Arch Surg 94:657, 1967.
73. Adams JT, McEvoy RK, deWeese JA: Primary deep venous thrombosis of upper extremity. Arch Surg 91:29, 1965.

74. Monreal M, Lafoz E, Ruiz J, et al: Upper-extremity deep venous thrombosis and pulmonary embolism. Chest 99:280, 1991.

75. Smith GT, Dexter L, Dammin GJ: Postmortem quantitative studies in pulmonary embolism. *In* Sasahara AA, Stein M (eds): Pulmonary Embolic Disease. New York, Grune & Stratton, 1965, pp 120–130.

76. Greenberg H: Refractory dyspnea and orthopnea. Evidence of recurrent pulmonary embolism and infarction. Am Rev Respir Dis 92:215, 1965.

77. Sevitt S: Venous thrombosis and pulmonary embolism. Their prevention by oral anticoagulation. Am J Med 33:703, 1962.

78. Anderson FA Jr, Wheeler HB: Physician practices in the management of venous thromboembolism: A community-wide survey. J Vasc Surg 16:707, 1992.

79. Anderson FA, Wheeler B, Goldberg RJ, et al: The prevalence of risk factors for venous thromboembolism among hospital patients. Arch Intern Med 152:1660, 1992.

80. Wheeler HB, Anderson FA Jr, Cardullo PA, et al: Suspected deep vein thrombosis. Management by impedance plethysmography. Arch Surg 117:1206, 1982.

81. Anderson Jr FA, Wheeler HB: Venous thromboembolism—risk factors and prophylaxis. Clin Chest Med 16:235, 1995.

82. Demers C, Ginsberg JS: Deep venous thrombosis and pulmonary embolism in pregnancy. Clin Chest Med 13:645, 1992.

83. Toglia MR, Weg JG: Venous thromboembolism during pregnancy. N Engl J Med 335:108, 1996.

84. Pangrazzi J, Donati MB, Romero M, et al: Is there still an avoidable fraction of post-operative thromboembolic complications with heparin prophylaxis? The results of a case-control surveillance. Collaborative Group on Heparin Prophylaxis in Surgery (S.E.P.E.C.). J Clin Epidemiol 46:371, 1993.

85. Milne R: Venous thromboembolism and travel: Is there an association? J R Coll Physicians Lond 26:47, 1992.

86. Cruickshank JM, Gorlin R, Jennett B: Air travel and thrombotic episodes: The economy class syndrome. Lancet 2:497, 1988.

87. Catovsky D, Ikoku NB, Pitney WR, et al: Thromboembolic complications in myelomatosis. BMJ 3:438, 1970.

88. Monta LE, Ramanan SV: Recurrent pulmonary embolism. A sign of multiple myeloma. JAMA 233:1192, 1975.

89. Barrett-Connor E: Pneumonia and pulmonary infarction in sickle cell anemia. JAMA 224:997, 1973.

90. Yorra FH, Oblath R, Jaffe H, et al: Massive thrombosis associated with use of the Swan-Ganz catheter. Chest 65:682, 1974.

91. Goodman DJ, Rider AK, Billingham ME, et al: Thromboembolic complications with the indwelling balloon-tipped pulmonary arterial catheter. N Engl J Med 291:777, 1974.

92. Monreal M, Raventos A, Lerma R, et al: Pulmonary embolism in patients with upper extremity DVT associated to venous central lines—a prospective study. Thromb Haemost 72:548, 1994.

93. Prozan GB, Shipley RE, Madding GF, et al: Pulmonary thromboembolism in the presence of an endocardiac pacing catheter. JAMA 206:1564, 1968.

94. Leiby JM, Purcell H, DeMaria JJ, et al: Pulmonary embolism as a result of Hickman catheter-related thrombosis. Am J Med 86:228, 1989.

95. Anderson AS, Krasnow SH, Boyer MW, et al: Thrombosis: The major Hickman catheter complication in patients with solid tumour. Chest 95:71, 1989.

96. Gibney RTN, Donovan F, Fitzgerald MX: Recurrent symptomatic pulmonary embolism caused by an infected Pudenz cerebrospinal fluid shunt device. Thorax 33:662, 1978.

97. Braun TI, Goldberg SK: An unusual thromboembolic complication of a Greenfield vena caval filter. Chest 87:127, 1985.

98. Sevitt S: Pathology and pathogenesis of deep vein thrombosis. *In* Poller L (ed): Recent Advances in Thrombosis. London, Churchill Livingstone, 1973, p 17.

99. Lang IM, Marsh JJ, Olman MA, et al: Expression of type 1 plasminogen activator inhibitor in chronic pulmonary thromboemboli. Circulation 89:2715, 1994.

100. Huber KM, Beckmann R, Frank H, et al: Fibrinogen, t-PA, and PAI-1 plasma levels in patients with pulmonary hypertension. Am J Respir Crit Care Med 150:929, 1994.

101. Ohlin AK, Marlar RA: The first mutation identified in the thrombomodulin gene in a 45-year-old man presenting with thromboembolic disease. Blood 85:330, 1995.

102. Winter JH, Fenech A, Bennett B, et al: Thrombosis after venography in familial antithrombin III deficiency. BMJ 283:1436, 1981.

103. Hull R, Hirsh J, Sackett DL, et al: Cost effectiveness of clinical diagnosis, venography, and noninvasive testing in patients with symptomatic deep-vein thrombosis. N Engl J Med 304:1561, 1981.

104. Browse NL, Clemenson G, Thomas ML: Is the postphlebitic leg always postphlebitic? Relation between phlebographic appearances of deep-vein thrombosis and late sequelae. BMJ 281:1167, 1980.

105. Engesser L, Broekmans AW, Briet E, et al: Hereditary protein S deficiency: Clinical manifestations. Ann Intern Med 106:677, 1987.

106. Demers C, Ginsberg JS, Hirsh J, et al: Thrombosis in antithrombin-III–deficient persons. Ann Intern Med 116:754, 1992.

107. Heijboer H, Brandjes DPM, Büller HR, et al: Deficiencies of coagulation-inhibiting and fibrinolytic proteins in outpatients with deep-vein thrombosis. N Engl J Med 323:1512, 1990.

107a. Appleby RD, Olds RJ: The inherited basis of venous thrombosis. Pathology 29:341, 1997.

108. Nuss R, Hays T, Manc-Johnson M: Childhood thrombosis. Pediatrics 96:291, 1995.

109. Otoya J, Nemcek AI Jr, Green D: Venous thromboembolism. Chest 96:1169, 1989.

110. Hirsh DR, Mikkola KM, Marks PW, et al: Pulmonary embolism and deep venous thrombosis during pregnancy or oral contraceptive use: Prevalence of factor V Leiden. Am Heart J 131:1145, 1996.

111. Svensson PJ, Dahlbäck B: Resistance to activated protein C as a basis for venous thrombosis. N Engl J Med 330:517, 1994.

112. De Stefano V, Leone G: Resistance to activated protein C due to mutated factor V as a novel cause of inherited thrombophilia. Haematologica 80:344, 1995.

113. Otterson GA, Monahan BP, Harold N, et al: Clinical significance of the FV:Q mutation in unselected oncology patients. Am J Med 101:406, 1996.

114. Ridker PM, Hennekens CH, Lindpaintner K, et al: Mutation in the gene coding for coagulation factor V and the risk of myocardial infarction, stroke, and venous thrombosis in apparently healthy men. N Engl J Med 332:912, 1995.

115. Desmarais S, de Moerloose P, Reber G, et al: Resistance to activated protein C in an unselected population of patients with pulmonary embolism. Lancet 347:1374, 1996.

116. Leroyer C, Mercier B, Escoffre M, et al: Factor V Leiden prevalence in venous thromboembolism patients. Chest 111:1603, 1997.

117. Simioni P, Prandoni P, Lensing AW, et al: The risk of recurrent venous thromboembolism in patients with an Arg$^{506}$-Gln mutation in the gene for factor V (factor V Leiden). N Engl J Med 336:399, 1997.

118. Pabinger I, Schneider B: Thrombotic risk in hereditary antithrombin III, protein C, or protein S deficiency. A cooperative, retrospective study. Arterioscler Thromb Vasc Biol 16:742, 1996.

119. Ridker PM, Glynn RJ, Miletich JP, et al: Age-specific incidence rates of venous thromboembolism among heterozygous carriers of factor V Leiden mutation. Ann Intern Med 126:528, 1997.

119a. Ryan DH, Crowther MA, Ginsberg JS, et al: Relation of factor V Leiden genotype to risk for acute deep venous thrombosis after joint replacement surgery. Ann Intern Med 128:270, 1998.

120. Gladson CL, Scharrer I, Hach V, et al: The frequency of type I heterozygous protein S and protein C deficiency in 141 unrelated young patients with venous thrombosis. Thromb Haemost 59:18, 1988.

121. Wyshock E, Caldwell M, Crowley JP: Deep venous thrombosis, inflammatory bowel disease, and protein S deficiency. Am J Clin Pathol 90:633, 1988.

121a. Zoller B, Garcia de Frutos P, Dahlback B: A common 4G allele in the promoter of the plasminogen activator inhibitor-1 (PAI-1) gene as a risk factor for pulmonary embolism and arterial thrombosis in hereditary protein S deficiency. Thromb Haemost 79:802, 1998.

122. Sasahara AA: The clinical and hemodynamic features of acute pulmonary embolism. *In* Simmons DH (ed): Current Pulmonology. Chicago, Year Book, 1988.

123. Vianna JL, Khamashta MA, Ordi-Ros J, et al: Comparison of the primary and secondary antiphospholipid syndrome. Am J Med 96:3, 1994.

123a. Brucato A, Baudo F, Barberis M, et al: Pulmonary hypertension secondary to thrombosis of the pulmonary vessels in a patient with the primary antiphospholipid syndrome. J Rheumatol 21:942, 1994.

124. Ginsberg JS, Wells PS, Brill-Edwards P, et al: Antiphospholipid antibodies and venous thromboembolism. Blood 86:3685, 1995.

125. Rosove MH, Brewer PMC. Antiphospholipid thrombosis: Clinical course after the first thrombotic event in 70 patients. Ann Intern Med 117:303, 1992.

126. Heijer MD, Koster T, Blom HJ, et al: Hyperhomocysteinemia as a risk factor for deep vein thrombosis. N Engl J Med 334:759, 1996.

126a. Goldhaber SZ: Pulmonary embolism. New Engl J Med 339:93, 1998.

127. Mandel H, Brenner B, Berant M, et al: Coexistence of hereditary homocystinuria and factor V Leiden—effect on thrombosis. N Engl J Med 334:763, 1996.

128. Wada Y, Lord ST: A correlation between thrombotic disease and a specific fibrinogen abnormality (A alpha 554 Arg–>Cys) in two unrelated kindred, Dusart and Chapel Hill III. Blood 84:3709, 1994.

129. Bell WR, Starksen NF, Tong S, et al: Trousseau's syndrome: Devastating coagulopathy in the absence of heparin. Am J Med 79:423, 1985.

130. Maruyama M, Yagawa K, Hayashi S, et al: Presence of thrombosis-inducing activity in plasma from patients with lung cancer. Am Rev Respir Dis 140:778, 1989.

131. Ogino H, Hayashi S, Kawasaki M, et al: Association of thrombosis-inducing activity (TIA) with fatal hypercoagulable complications in patients with lung cancer. Chest 105:1683, 1994.

132. Andrén-Sandberg A, Lecander I, Martinsson G, et al: Peaks in plasma plasminogen activator inhibitor-1 concentration may explain thrombotic events in cases of pancreatic carcinoma. Cancer 69:2884, 1992.

133. Rahr HB, Sorensen JV: Venous thromboembolism and cancer. Blood Coagul Fibrinolysis 3:451, 1992.

134. Monreal M, Casals A, Boix J, et al: Occult cancer in patients with acute pulmonary embolism. Chest 103:816, 1993.

135. Prandoni P, Lensing AWA, Büller HR, et al: Deep-vein thrombosis and the incidence of subsequent symptomatic cancer. N Engl J Med 327:1128, 1992.

136. Cornuz J, Pearson SD, Creager MA, et al: Importance of findings on the initial evaluation for cancer in patients with symptomatic idiopathic deep venous thrombosis. Ann Intern Med 125:785, 1996.

137. Min K-W, Gyorkey F, Sato C: Mucin-producing adenocarcinomas and nonbacterial thrombotic endocarditis. Pathogenice role of tumor mucin. Cancer 45:2374, 1980.

138. Patterson WP, Ringenberg QS: The pathophysiology of thrombosis in cancer. Semin Oncol 17:140, 1990.

139. Ogino H, Hayashi S, Kawasaki M, et al: Association of thrombosis-inducing

activity (TIA) with fatal hypercoagulable complications in patients with lung cancer. Chest 105:1639, 1994.

139a. Sørenson HT, Mellemkjaer L, Steffensen FH, et al: The risk of a diagnosis of cancer after primary deep venous thrombosis or pulmonary embolism. New Engl J Med 338:1169, 1998.

139b. Büller H, ten Cate JW: Primary venous thromboembolism and cancer screening. New Engl J Med 338:1221, 1998.

139c. Oefelein MG, Brant M, Crotty K: Idiopathic thromboembolism as the presenting sign of occult prostate cancer. Urology 51:775, 1998.

140. Royal College of General Practitioners Report by Records Unit and Research Advisory Service of RCGP: Oral contraception and thrombo-embolic disease. J Coll Gen Pract 13:267, 1967.

141. Inman WHW, Vessey MP: Investigation of deaths from pulmonary, coronary, and cerebral thrombosis and embolism in women of child-bearing age. BMJ 2:193, 1968.

142. Vessey MP, Doll R: Investigation of relation between use of oral contraceptives and thromboembolic disease. BMJ 2:199, 1968.

143. Inman WHW, Vessey MP, Westerholm B, et al: Thromboembolic disease and the steroidal content of oral contraceptives. A report to the committee on safety of drugs. BMJ 2:203, 1970.

144. Report from the Boston Collaborative Drug Surveillance Programme: Oral contraceptives and venous thromboembolic disease, surgically confirmed gallbladder disease, and breast tumours. Lancet 1:1399, 1973.

145. Vessey MP, Doll R: Investigation of relation between use of oral contraceptives and thromboembolic disease. A further report. BMJ 2:651, 1969.

145a. Grady D, Sawaya G: Postmenopausal hormone therapy increases risk of deep vein thrombosis and pulmonary embolism. Am J Med 105:41, 1998.

146. Venous thromboembolic disease and combined oral contraceptives: Results of international multicentre case-control study. World Health Organization collaborative study of cardiovascular disease and steroid hormone contraception. Lancet 346:1575, 1995.

147. Quinn DA, Thompson BT, Terrin ML, et al: A prospective investigation of pulmonary embolism in women and men. JAMA 268:1689, 1992.

148. Oakley C, Somerville J: Oral contraceptives and progressive pulmonary vascular disease. Lancet 1:890, 1968.

149. Oral contraceptives and thromboembolism. BMJ 2:187, 1968.

150. Blood clotting and the pill. BMJ 4:378, 1972.

151. Bucalossi A, Marotta G, Bigazzi C, et al: Reduction of antithrombin III, protein C, and protein S levels and activated protein C resistance in polycythemia vera and essential thrombocythemia patients with thrombosis. Am J Hematol 52:14, 1996.

152. Wu KK: Platelet hyperaggregability and thrombosis in patients with thrombocythemia. Ann Intern Med 88:7, 1978.

153. Glenn LD, Armitage JO, Goldsmith JC, et al: Pulmonary emboli in patients receiving chemotherapy for non-Hodgkin's lymphoma. Chest 94:589, 1988.

154. Hayashi S, Ogino H, Ogata K, et al: Hypercoagulopathy induced by chemotherapy in a patient with lung cancer. Chest 101:277, 1992.

155. Jick H, Westerholm B, Vessey MP, et al: Venous thromboembolic disease and ABO blood type: A cooperative study. Lancet 1:539, 1969.

156. Talbot S, Wakley EJ, Ryrie D, et al: ABO blood-groups and venous thromboembolic disease. Lancet 1:1257, 1970.

157. Kollef MH, Schachter DT: Acute pulmonary embolism triggered by the act of defecation. Chest 99:373, 1991.

158. Mossey RT, Kasabian AA, Wilkes BM, et al: Pulmonary embolism: Low incidence in chronic renal failure. Arch Intern Med 142:1646, 1982.

159. Kaufman J, Khatri BO, Riendl P: Are patients with multiple sclerosis protected from thrombophlebitis and pulmonary embolism? Chest 94:998, 1988.

160. Hampton AO, Castleman B: Correlation of postmortem chest teleroentgenograms with autopsy findings. With special reference to pulmonary embolism and infarction. Am J Roentgenol 43:305, 1940.

161. Dalen JE, Haffajee CI, Alpert JS, et al: Pulmonary embolism, pulmonary hemorrhage and pulmonary infarction. N Engl J Med 296:1431, 1977.

162. Butler J, Obermiller T, Willoughby S, et al: Reflux pulmonary vein flow prevents pulmonary infarction after pulmonary artery obstruction. Cor Vasa 32:183, 1990.

163. Smith GT, Dammin GJ, Dexter L: Postmortem arteriographic studies of the human lung in pulmonary embolization. JAMA 188:143, 1964.

164. Parker BM, Smith JR: Pulmonary embolism and infarction. A review of the physiologic consequences of pulmonary arterial obstruction. Am J Med 24:402, 1958.

165. Agostoni PG, Deffebach ME, Kirk W, et al: Upstream pressure for systemic to pulmonary flow from bronchial circulation in dogs. J Appl Physiol 63:485, 1987.

166. Tsao M, Schraufnagel D, Wang N: Pathogenesis of pulmonary infarction. Am J Med 72:599, 1982.

167. Schraufnagel DE, Tsao M, Yao YT, et al: Factors associated with pulmonary infarction. Am J Clin Pathol 84:15, 1985.

168. Comroe JH Jr: Pulmonary arterial blood flow: Effects of brief and permanent arrest. Am Rev Respir Dis 85:179, 1962.

169. Newhouse MT, Becklake MR, Macklem PT, et al: Effect of alterations in end-tidal $CO_2$ tension on flow resistance. J Appl Physiol 19:745, 1964.

170. Llamas R, Swenson EW: Diagnostic clues in pulmonary thromboembolism evaluated by angiographic and ventilation-blood flow studies. Thorax 20:327, 1965.

171. Jaffe RB, Figley MM: Roentgenographic evaluation of bronchial size following pulmonary embolization. Radiology 88:425, 1967.

172. Nadel JA, Colebatch HJH, Olsen CR: Location and mechanism of airway constriction after barium sulfate microembolism. J Appl Physiol 19:387, 1964.

173. Austin JHM, Sagel SS: Alterations of airway caliber after pulmonary embolization in the dog. Invest Radiol 7:135, 1972.

174. Austin JHM: Intrapulmonary airway narrowing after pulmonary thromboembolism in dogs: Partial control by the parasympathetic nervous system. Invest Radiol 8:315, 1973.

175. Robinson AE, Puckett CL, Green JD, et al: In vivo demonstration of small-airway bronchoconstriction following pulmonary embolism. Radiology 109:283, 1973.

176. Isawa T, Taplin GV, Beazell J, Criley JM: Experimental unilateral pulmonary artery occlusion: Acute and chronic effects on relative inhalation and perfusion. Radiology 102:101, 1972.

177. Thomas DP, Tanabe G, Khan M, et al: Humoral factors mediated by platelets in experimental pulmonary embolism. In Sasahara AA, Stein M (eds): Pulmonary Embolic Disease. New York, Grune & Stratton, 1965, pp 59–64.

178. Meth RF, Tashkin DP, Hansen KS, et al: Pulmonary edema and wheezing after pulmonary embolism. Am Rev Respir Dis 111:693, 1975.

179. Gurewich V, Sasahara AA, Stein M: Pulmonary embolism, bronchoconstriction and response to heparin. In Sasahara AA, Stein M (eds): Pulmonary Embolic Disease. New York, Grune & Stratton, 1965, pp 162–169.

180. Sasahara AA, Cannilla JE, Morse RL, et al: Clinical and physiologic studies in pulmonary thromboembolism. Am J Cardiol 20:10, 1967.

181. Windebank WJ, Boyd G, Moran F: Pulmonary thromboembolism presenting as asthma. BMJ 1:90, 1973.

182. Kerr IH, Simon G, Sutton GC: The value of the plain radiograph in acute massive pulmonary embolism. Br J Radiol 44:751, 1971.

183. Clements JA: Surfactant in pulmonary disease. N Engl J Med 272:1336, 1965.

184. Smith FB: Role of the pulmonary surfactant system in lung diseases of adults. N Y State J Med 83:851, 1983.

185. Colman NC: Pathophysiology of pulmonary embolism. In Leclerc JR (ed): Venous Thromboembolic Disorders. Philadelphia, Lea & Febiger, 1991, p 65.

186. Soloff LA, Rodman T: Acute pulmonary embolism: I. Review. Am Heart J 74:710, 1967.

187. McIntyre KM, Sasahara AA: The hemodynamic response to pulmonary embolism in patients without prior cardiopulmonary disease. Am J Cardiol 28:288, 1971.

188. Sofia M, Faraone S, Alifano M, et al: Endothelin abnormalities in patients with pulmonary embolism. Chest 111:544, 1997.

189. Sasahara AA: The clinical and hemodynamic features of acute pulmonary embolism. In Simmons DH (ed): Current Pulmonology. Chicago, Year Book, 1988.

190. Dexter L, Smith GT: Quantitative studies of pulmonary embolism. Am J Med Sci 247:641, 1964.

191. Davison P: Functional aspects of the cor pulmonale syndrome. Br J Dis Chest 54:186, 1960.

192. Baker RR, Wagner HN Jr: Pulmonary embolectomy in the treatment of massive pulmonary embolism. Surg Gynecol Obstet 122:513, 1966.

193. Gorham LW: A study of pulmonary embolism: Part II. The mechanism of death; based on a clinicopathological investigation of 100 cases of massive and 285 cases of minor embolism of the pulmonary artery. Arch Intern Med 108:189, 1961.

194. Wiener SN, Edelstein J, Charms BL: Observations on pulmonary embolism and the pulmonary angiogram. Am J Roentgenol 98:859, 1966.

195. Wood P: Pulmonary hypertension with special reference to the vasoconstrictive factor. Br Heart J 20:557, 1958.

196. Belenkie I, Dani R, Smith ER, et al: Ventricular interaction during experimental acute pulmonary embolism. Circulation 78:761, 1988.

197. McIntyre KM, Sasahara AA: The ratio of pulmonary arterial pressure to pulmonary vascular obstruction: Index of preembolic cardiopulmonary status. Chest 71:692, 1977.

198. Fanta CH, Wright TC, McFadden ER: Differentiation of recurrent pulmonary emboli from chronic obstructive lung disease as a cause of cor pulmonale. Chest 79:92, 1981.

199. Widimsky J: Acute pulmonary embolism and chronic thromboembolic pulmonary hypertension: Is there a relationship? Eur Respir J 4:137, 1991.

200. Moser KM, Auger WR, Fedullo PF, et al: Chronic thromboembolic pulmonary hypertension: Clinical picture and surgical treatment. Eur Respir J 5:334, 1992.

201. Benotti JR, Dalen JE: The natural history of pulmonary embolism. Clin Chest Med 5:403, 1985.

202. Moser KM, Bloor CM: Pulmonary vascular lesions occurring in patients with chronic major vessel thromboembolic pulmonary hypertension. Chest 103:685, 1993.

203. Rich S, Levitsky S, Brundage BH: Pulmonary hypertension from chronic pulmonary thromboembolism. Ann Intern Med 108:425, 1988.

204. Dantzker DR, Bower JS: Partial reversibility of chronic pulmonary hypertension caused by pulmonary thromboembolic disease. Am Rev Respir Dis 124:129, 1981.

205. Fedullo PF, Auger WR, Channick RN, et al: Chronic thromboembolic pulmonary hypertension. Clin Chest Med 16:353, 1995.

206. Auger WR, Permpikul P, Moser KM: Lupus anticoagulant, heparin use, and thrombocytopenia in patients with chronic thromboembolic pulmonary hypertension: A preliminary report. Am J Med 99:392, 1995.

207. Dombert MC, Rouby JJ, Smiejan JM, et al: Pulmonary oedema during pulmonary embolism. Br J Dis Chest 81:407, 1987.

208. Short DS: A survey of pulmonary embolism in a general hospital. BMJ 1:790, 1952.

209. Yuceoglu YZ, Rubler S, Eshwar KP, et al: Pulmonary edema associated with pulmonary embolism: A clinicopathological study. Angiology 22:501, 1971.

210. Swenson EW, Llamas R, Ring GC: Hypoxemia and edema of the lungs in experimental pulmonary thromboembolism. *In* Sasahara AA, Stein M (eds): Pulmonary Embolic Disease. New York, Grune & Stratton, 1965, pp 170–180.

211. Singer D, Hesser C, Pick R, et al: Diffuse bilateral pulmonary edema associated with unilobar miliary pulmonary embolization in the dog. Circ Res 6:4, 1958.

212. Perlman MB, Johnson A, Malik AB: Ibuprofen prevents thrombin-induced lung vascular injury: Mechanism of effect. Am J Physiol 252:605, 1987.

213. Garcia-Szabo R, Johnson A, Malik AB: Thromboxane increases pulmonary vascular resistance and transvascular fluid and protein exchange after pulmonary microembolism. Prostaglandins 35:707, 1988.

214. Perlman MB, Johsnon A, Jubiz W, et al: Lipoxygenase products induce neutrophil activation and increase endothelial permeability thrombin-induced pulmonary microembolism. Circ Res 64:62, 1989.

215. Garcia JG, Perlman MB, Ferro TJ, et al: Inflammatory events after fibrin microembolization. Alterations in alveolar macrophage and neutrophil function. Am Rev Respir Dis 137:630, 1988.

216. Johnson A, Perlman MB, Blumenstock FA, et al: Superoxide dismutase prevents the thrombin-induced increase in lung vascular permeability: Role of superoxide in mediating the alterations in lung fluid balance. Circ Res 59:405, 1986.

217. Malik A, Horan MJ: Mechanisms of thrombin-induced lung vascular injury and edema. Am Rev Respir Dis 136:467, 1987.

218. Johnson A, Malik AB: Pulmonary transvascular fluid and protein exchange after thrombin-induced microembolism. Differential effects of cyclooxygenase inhibitors. Am Rev Respir Dis 132:70, 1985.

219. Ehrhart IC, Granger WM, Hofman WF: Effects of arterial pressure on lung capillary pressure and edema after microembolism. J Appl Physiol 60:133, 1986.

220. Hackett PH, Creagh CE, Grover RF, et al: High-altitude pulmonary edema in persons without the right pulmonary artery. N Engl J Med 302:1070, 1980.

221. Hyers TM, Fowler AA, Wicks AB: Focal pulmonary edema after massive pulmonary embolism. Am Rev Respir Dis 123:232, 1981.

222. Jackson J, Thompson N, Miller YE: Chronic pulmonary emboli: Sparing of affected regions of lung from noncardiogenic pulmonary edema. Chest 89:463, 1986.

223. Bedard CK, Bone RC: Westermark's sign in the diagnosis of pulmonary emboli in patients with the adult respiratory distress syndrome. Crit Care Med 5:137, 1977.

224. Elliot CG: Pulmonary physiology during pulmonary embolism. Chest 101:163, 1992.

225. D'Alonzo GE, Dantzker DR: Gas exchange alterations following pulmonary thromboembolism. Clin Chest Med 5:411, 1984.

226. Santolicandro A, Prediletto R, Fornai E, et al: Mechanisms of hypoxemia and hypocapnia in pulmonary embolism. Am J Respir Crit Care Med 152:336, 1995.

227. Burki NK: The dead space to tidal volume ratio in the diagnosis of pulmonary embolism. Am Rev Respir Dis 133:679, 1986.

228. Huet Y, Lemaire F, Brun-Buisson C, et al: Hypoxemia in acute pulmonary embolism. Chest 88:829, 1985.

229. Manier G, Castaing Y: Influence of cardiac output on oxygen exchange in acute pulmonary embolism. Am Rev Respir Dis 145:130, 1992.

230. Kapitan KS, Buchbinder M, Wagner PD, et al: Mechanisms of hypoxemia in chronic thromboembolic pulmonary hypertension. Am Rev Respir Dis 139:1149, 1989.

231. Redline S, Tomashefski JF Jr, Altose MD: Cavitating lung infarction after bland pulmonary thromboembolism in patients with the adult respiratory distress syndrome. Thorax 40:915, 1985.

232. Libby LS, King TE, LaForce FM, et al: Pulmonary cavitation following pulmonary infarction. Medicine 64:342, 1985.

233. Bewtra C, Dewan N, O'Donahue WJ Jr: Exfoliative sputum cytology in pulmonary embolism. Acta Cytol 27:489, 1983.

234. Gahagan T, Manzor A, Isaac B, et al: Reestablishment of pulmonary-artery flow after prolonged complete occlusion: Studies in dogs. JAMA 198:639, 1966.

235. Liebow AA, Hales MR, Bloomer W, et al: Studies on the lung after ligation of the pulmonary artery: II. Anatomical changes. Am J Pathol 26:177, 1950.

236. Moser KM, Spragg RG, Utley J, et al: Chronic thrombotic obstruction of major pulmonary arteries: Results of thromboendarterectomy in 15 patients. Ann Intern Med 99:299, 1983.

237. Dalen JE, Banas JS Jr, Brooks HL, et al: Resolution rate of acute pulmonary embolism in man. N Engl J Med 280:1194, 1969.

238. Secker-Walker RH, Jackson JA, Goodwin J: Resolution of pulmonary embolism. BMJ 4:135, 1970.

239. Austin JHM, Wilner GD, Dominguez C: Natural history of pulmonary thromboemboli in dogs: Serial radiographic observation of clots labeled with powdered tantalum. Radiology 116:519, 1975.

240. Moser KM, Guisan M, Bartimmo EE, et al: *In vivo* and post mortem dissolution rates of pulmonary emboli and venous thrombi in the dog. Circulation 48:170, 1973.

241. Sevitt S: Organic fragmentation in pulmonary thrombo-emboli. J Pathol 122:95, 1977.

242. Salyer WR, Salyer DC, Hutchins GM: Local arterial wall injury caused by thromboemboli. Am J Pathol 75:285, 1974.

243. Meyer JS: Thromboembolic pulmonary arterial necrosis and arteritis in man. Arch Pathol 70:63, 1960.

244. Sevitt S: Arterial wall lesions after pulmonary embolism, especially ruptures and aneurysms. J Clin Pathol 29:665, 1976.

245. Freiman DG: Pathologic observations on experimental and human thromboembolism. *In* Sasahara AA, Stein M (eds): Pulmonary Embolic Disease. New York, Grune & Stratton, 1965, pp 81–85.

246. Korn D, Gore I, Blenke A, et al: Pulmonary arterial bands and webs: An unrecognized manifestation of organized pulmonary emboli. Am J Pathol 40:129, 1962.

247. Morrell MT, Dunnill MS: The post-mortem incidence of pulmonary embolism in a hospital population. Br J Surg 55:347, 1968.

248. Brucato A, Baudo F, Barberis M, et al: Pulmonary hypertension secondary to thrombosis of the pulmonary vessels in a patient with the primary antiphospholipid syndrome. J Rheumatol 21:942, 1994.

249. Vanek J: Fibrous bands and networks of postembolic origin in the pulmonary arteries. J Pathol Bacteriol 81:537, 1961.

250. Sevitt S, Walton KW: Atherosclerotic lesions from the reduction of pulmonary emboli. Atherosclerosis 59:173, 1986.

251. Worsley DF, Alavi A, Aronchick JM, et al. Chest radiographic findings in patients with acute pulmonary embolism: Observations from the PIOPED study. Radiology 189:133, 1993.

252. Stein PD, Athanasoulis C, Greenspan RH, et al: Relation of plain chest radiographic findings to pulmonary arterial pressure and arterial blood oxygen levels in patients with acute pulmonary embolism. Am J Cardiol 69:394, 1992.

253. Westermark N: On the roentgen diagnosis of lung embolism. Acta Radiol 19:357, 1938.

254. Fleischner FG: Pulmonary embolism. Clin Radiol 13:169, 1962.

255. Fleischner FG: Recurrent pulmonary embolism and cor pulmonale. N Engl J Med 276:1213, 1967.

256. Chang CH, Davis WC: A roentgen sign of pulmonary infarction. Clin Radiol 16:141, 1965.

257. Figley MM, Gerdes AJ, Ricketts HJ: Radiographic aspects of pulmonary embolism. Semin Roentgenol 2:389, 1967.

258. Palla A, Donnamaria V, Petruzzelli S, et al: Enlargement of the right descending pulmonary artery in pulmonary embolism. Am J Roentgenol 141:513, 1983.

259. Williams JR, Wilcox WC: Pulmonary embolism: Roentgenographic and angiographic considerations. Am J Roentgenol 89:333, 1963.

260. Stein GN, Chen JT, Goldstein F, et al: The importance of chest roentgenography in the diagnosis of pulmonary embolism. Am J Roentgenol 81:255, 1959.

261. Westcott JL, Cole S: Plate atelectasis. Radiology 155:1, 1985.

262. Laur A: Roentgen diagnosis of pulmonary embolism and its differentiation from myocardial infarction. Am J Roentgenol 90:632, 1963.

263. Szucs MM Jr, Brooks HL, Grossman W, et al: Diagnostic sensitivity of laboratory findings in acute pulmonary embolism. Ann Intern Med 74:161, 1971.

264. Talbot S, Worthington BS, Roebuck EJ: Radiographic signs of pulmonary embolism and pulmonary infarction. Thorax 28:198, 1973.

265. Torrance DJ Jr: Roentgenographic signs of pulmonary artery occlusion. Am J Med Sci 237:651, 1959.

266. Jacoby CG, Mindell HJ: Lobar consolidation in pulmonary embolism. Radiology 118:287, 1976.

267. Fleischner FG: Roentgenology of the pulmonary infarct. Semin Roentgenol 2:61, 1967.

268. Beilin DS, Fink JP, Leslie LW: Correlation of postmortem pathological observations with chest roentgenograms. Radiology 57:361, 1951.

269. Alderson PO, Martin EC: Pulmonary embolism: Diagnosis with multiple imaging modalities. Radiology 164:297, 1987.

270. Bachynski JE: Absence of the air bronchogram sign: A reliable finding in pulmonary embolism with infarction or hemorrhage. Radiology 100:547, 1971.

271. Coke LR, Dundee JC: Cavitation in bland infarcts of the lung. Can Med Assoc J 72:907, 1955.

272. Castleman B: Pathologic observations on pulmonary infarction in man. *In* Sasahara AA, Stein M (eds): Pulmonary Embolic Disease. New York, Grune & Stratton, 1965, pp 86–92.

273. Fleischner FG: Observations on the radiologic changes in pulmonary embolism. In Sasahara AA, Stein M (eds): Pulmonary Embolic Disease. New York, Grune & Stratton, 1965, pp 206–213.

274. Woesner ME, Sanders I, White GW: The melting sign in resolving transient pulmonary infarction. Am J Roentgenol 111:782, 1971.

275. McGoldrick PJ, Rudd TG, Figley MM, et al: What becomes of pulmonary infarcts? Am J Roentgenol 133:1039, 1979.

276. Fleischner FG: Pulmonary embolism. Can Med Assoc J 78:653, 1958.

277. Blundell JE: Pneumothorax complicating pulmonary infarction. Br J Radiol 40:226, 1967.

278. McFadden ER Jr, Luparello F: Bronchopleural fistula complicating massive pulmonary infarction. Thorax 24:500, 1969.

279. Greenspan RH, Ravin CE, Polansky SM, et al: Accuracy of the chest radiography in diagnosis of pulmonary embolism. Invest Radiol 17:539, 1982.

280. Sostman HD, Coleman RE, DeLong DM, et al: Evaluation of revised criteria for ventilation-perfusion scintigraphy in patients with suspected pulmonary embolism. Radiology 193:103, 1994.

281. Miniati M, Pistolesi M, Marini C, et al: Value of perfusion lung scan in the diagnosis of pulmonary embolism: Results of the prospective investigative study of acute pulmonary embolism diagnosis (PISA-PED). Am J Respir Crit Care Med 154:1187, 1996.

282. Heck LL, Duley JW: Statistical considerations in lung scanning with Tc-99m albumin particles. Radiology 113:675, 1975.

283. Alderson PO, Doppman JL, Diamond SS, et al: Ventilation-perfusion lung imaging and selective pulmonary angiography in dogs with experimental pulmonary emboli. J Nucl Med 19:164, 1978.

284. James JM, Herman KJ, Lloyd JJ, et al: Evaluation of 99Tcm Technegas ventilation scintigraphy in the diagnosis of pulmonary embolism. Br J Radiol 64:711, 1991.

285. Biello DR, Mattar AG, McKnight RC, et al: Ventilation-perfusion studies in suspected pulmonary embolism. Am J Roentgenol 133:1033, 1979.

286. Carter WD, Brady TM, Keyes JW Jr, et al: Relative accuracy of two diagnostic schemes for detection of pulmonary embolism by ventilation-perfusion scintigraphy. Radiology 145:447, 1982.

287. Sostman HD, Rapoport S, Gottschalk A, et al: Imaging of pulmonary embolism. Invest Radiol 21:443, 1986.

288. Gottschalk A, Sostman HD, Juni JE, et al: Ventilation-perfusion scintigraphy in the PIOPED study. II. Evaluation of criteria and interpretations. J Nucl Med 34:1119, 1993.

289. Webber MM, Gomes AS, Roe D, et al: Comparison of Biello, McNeil, and PIOPED criteria for the diagnosis of pulmonary emboli on lung scans. Am J Roentgenol 154:975, 1990.

290. Sostman HD, Coleman RE, DeLong DM, et al: Evaluation of revised criteria for ventilation-perfusion scintigraphy in patients with suspected pulmonary embolism. Radiology 193:103, 1994.

291. Freitas FE, Sarosi MG, Nagle CC, et al: The use of modified PIOPED criteria in clinical practice. J Nucl Med 36:1573, 1995.

292. UPET Investigators: The urokinase pulmonary embolism trial. A national cooperative. Circulation 47(Suppl 2):46, 1973.

293. Hull RD, Raskob GE, Coates G, et al: A new noninvasive management strategy for patients with suspected pulmonary embolism. Arch Intern Med 149:2549, 1989.

294. Hull RD, Raskob GE, Ginsberg JS, et al: A noninvasive strategy for the treatment of patients with suspected pulmonary embolism. Arch Intern Med 154:289, 1994.

295. The PIOPED Investigators: Value of the ventilation/perfusion scan in acute pulmonary embolism: Result of the Prospective Investigation of Pulmonary Embolism Diagnosis (PIOPED). JAMA 263:2753, 1990.

296. Quinn DA, Thompson BT, Terrin ML, et al: A prospective investigation of pulmonary embolism in women and men. JAMA 268:1689, 1992.

297. Worsley DF, Alavi A, Palevsky HI: Comparison of the diagnostic performance of ventilation/perfusion lung scanning in different patient populations. Radiology 199:481, 1996.

298. Lesser BA, Leeper KV Jr, Stein PD, et al: The diagnosis of acute pulmonary embolism in patients with chronic obstructive pulmonary disease. Chest 102:17, 1992.

299. Worsley DF, Palevsky HI, Alavi A: Clinical characteristic of patients with pulmonary embolism and low or very low probability lung scan interpretations. Arch Intern Med 154:2737, 1994.

300. Hull RD, Raskob GE: Low-probability lung scan findings: A need for change. Ann Intern Med 114:142, 1991.

301. Bone RC: The low-probability scan: A potentially lethal reading. Arch Intern Med 153:2621, 1993.

302. Celi AA, Palla S, Petruzzelli L, et al: Prospective study of a standardized questionnaire to improve clinical estimate of pulmonary embolism. Chest 95:332, 1989.

303. Alderson PO, Biello DR, Sachariah KG, et al: Scintigraphic detection of pulmonary embolism in patients with obstructive pulmonary disease. Radiology 138:661, 1981.

304. Smith R, Ellis K, Alderson PO: Role of chest radiography in predicting the extent of airway disease in patients with suspected pulmonary embolism. Radiology 159:391, 1986.

305. Meignan M, Simonneau G, Oliveira L, et al: Computation of ventilation-perfusion ratio with Kr-81m in pulmonary embolism. J Nucl Med 25:149, 1984.

306. Lesser BA, Leeper KV, Stein PD, et al: The diagnosis of acute pulmonary embolism in patients with chronic obstructive pulmonary disease. Chest 102:17, 1992.

307. Alderson PO, Dzebolo NN, Biello DR, et al: Serial lung scintigraphy: Utility in diagnosis of pulmonary embolism. Radiology 149:797, 1983.

308. Tow DE, Wagner HN Jr: Recovery of pulmonary arterial blood flow in patients with pulmonary embolism. N Engl J Med 276:1053, 1967.

309. Moser KM, Miale A Jr: Interpretive pitfalls in lung photoscanning. Am J Med 44:366, 1968.

310. Moser KM, Longo AM, Ashburn WL, et al: Spurious scintiphotographic recurrence of pulmonary emboli. Am J Med 55:434, 1973.

311. Winebright JW, Gerdes AJ, Nelp WB: Restoration of blood flow after pulmonary embolism. Arch Intern Med 125:241, 1970.

312. Vernon P, Burton GH, Seed WA: Lung scan abnormalities in asthma and their correlation with lung function. Eur J Nucl Med 12:16, 1986.

313. Ralph DD: Pulmonary embolism: The implications of prospective investigation of pulmonary embolism diagnosis. Radiol Clin North Am 32:679, 1994.

314. Sinner WN: Computed tomography of pulmonary thromboembolism. Eur J Radiol 2:8, 1982.

315. Godwin JD, Webb WR, Gamsu G, et al: Computed tomography of pulmonary embolism. Am J Roentgenol 135:691, 1980.

316. Breatnach E, Stanley RJ: CT diagnosis of segmental pulmonary artery embolus. J Comput Assist Tomogr 8:762, 1984.

317. Kölebo P, Wallin J: Computed tomography in massive pulmonary embolism. Acta Radiol 30:105, 1989.

318. Remy-Jardin M, Remy J, Wattinne L, et al: Central pulmonary thromboembolism: Diagnosis with spiral volumetric CT with the single-breath-hold technique: Comparison with pulmonary angiography. Radiology 185:381, 1992.

319. Teigen CL, Maus TP, Sheedy PF II, et al: Pulmonary embolism: Diagnosis with electron-beam CT. Radiology 188:839, 1993.

320. Goodman LR, Curtin JJ, Mewissen MW, et al: Detection of pulmonary embolism in patients with unresolved clinical and scintigraphic diagnosis: Helical CT versus angiography. Am J Roentgenol 164:1369, 1995.

321. van Rossum AB, Pattynama PMT, Ton ERTA, et al: Pulmonary embolism: Validation of spiral CT angiography in 149 patients. Radiology 201:467, 1996.

321a. Cross JJL, Kemp PM, Walsh CG, et al: A randomized trial of spiral CT and ventilation perfusion scintigraphy for the diagnosis of pulmonary embolism. Clin Radiol 53:177, 1998.

322. Remy-Jardin M, Remy J, Artaud D, et al: Spiral CT of pulmonary embolism: Technical considerations and interpretive pitfalls. J Thorac Imaging 12:103, 1997.

323. Remy-Jardin M, Remy J, Deschildre F, et al: Diagnosis of pulmonary embolism with spiral CT: Comparison with pulmonary angiography and scintigraphy. Radiology 200:699, 1996.

324. Remy-Jardin M, Remy J, Artaud D, et al: Peripheral pulmonary arteries: Optimization of the spiral CT acquisition protocol. Radiology 204:157, 1997.

324a. Garg K, Welsh CH, Feyerabend AJ, et al: Pulmonary embolism: Diagnosis with spiral CT and ventilation-perfusion scanning—correlation with pulmonary angiographic results or clinical outcome. Radiology 208:201, 1998.

325. Teigen CL, Maus TP, Sheedy PF II, et al: Pulmonary embolism: Diagnosis with contrast-enhanced electron-beam CT and comparison with pulmonary angiography. Radiology 194:313, 1995.

326. Stein PD: Opinion response to acute pulmonary embolism: The role of computed tomographic imaging. J Thorac Imaging 12:86, 1997.

327. Mayo JR, Remy-Jardin M, Müller NL, et al: Prospective comparison of spiral CT and ventilation-perfusion scintigraphy in the diagnosis of pulmonary embolism. Radiology 205:447, 1997.

327a. Gosselin MV, Rubin GD, Leung AN, et al: Unsuspected pulmonary embolism: Prospective detection on routine helical CT scans. Radiology 208:209, 1998.

328. Gefter WB, Hatabu H, Holland GA, et al: Pulmonary thromboembolism: Recent developments in diagnosis with CT and MR imaging. Radiology 197:561, 1995.

329. Stein PD, Athanasoulis C, Alavi A, et al: Complications and validity of pulmonary angiography in acute pulmonary embolism. Circulation 85:462, 1992.

330. van Erkel AR, van Rossum AB, Bloem JL, et al: Spiral CT angiography for suspected pulmonary embolism: A cost-effectiveness analysis. Radiology 201:29, 1996.

331. Goodman LR, Lipchik RJ: Diagnosis of acute pulmonary embolism: Time for a new approach. Radiology 199:25, 1996.

332. Goodman LR, Lipchik RJ, Kuzo RS: Acute pulmonary embolism: The role of computed tomographic imaging. J Thorac Imaging 12:83, 1997.

333. Sostman HD: Opinion response to acute pulmonary embolism: The role of computed tomographic imaging. J Thorac Imaging 12:89, 1997.

334. Gefter WB, Palevsky HI: Opinion response to acute pulmonary embolism: The role of computed tomographic imaging. J Thorac Imaging 12:97, 1997.

334a. van Rossum AB, Pattynama PMT, Mallens WMC, et al: Can helical CT replace scintigraphy in the diagnostic process in suspected pulmonary embolism? A retrospective-prospective cohort study focusing on total diagnostic yield. Eur Radiol 8:90, 1998.

335. Goodman LR, Lipchik RJ, Kuzo RS: Reply to opinions. J Thorac Imaging 12:100, 1997.

336. Romano WM, Cascade PN, Korobkin MT, et al: Implications of unsuspected pulmonary embolism detected by computed tomography. Can Assoc Radiol J 46:363, 1995.

337. Winston CB, Wechsler RJ, Salazar AM, et al: Incidental pulmonary emboli detected at helical CT: Effect on patient care. Radiology 201:23, 1996.

337a. Gosselin MV, Rubin GD, Leung AN, et al: Unsuspected pulmonary embolism: Prospective detection on routine helical CT scans. Radiology 208:209, 1998.

338. Remy-Jardin M, Louvegny S, Remy J, et al: Acute central thromboembolic disease: Posttherapeutic follow-up with spiral CT angiography. Radiology 203:173, 1997.

339. Kereiakes DJ, Herfkens RJ, Brundage BH, et al: Computerized tomography in chronic thromboembolic pulmonary hypertension. Am Heart J 106:1432, 1983.

340. Tardivon AA, Musset D, Maitre S, et al: Role of CT in chronic pulmonary embolism: Comparison with pulmonary angiography. J Comput Assist Tomogr 17:345, 1993.

341. Schwickert HC, Schweden F, Schild HH, et al: Pulmonary arteries and lung parenchyma in chronic pulmonary embolism: Preoperative and postoperative CT findings. Radiology 191:351, 1994.

342. Sinner WN: Computed tomographic patterns of pulmonary thromboembolism and infarction. J Comput Assist Tomogr 2:395, 1978.

343. Greaves SM, Hart EM, Brown K, et al: Pulmonary thromboembolism: Spectrum of findings on CT. Am J Roentgenol 165:1359, 1995.

344. Coche E, Müller NL, Kim KI, et al: Acute pulmonary embolism: Ancillary findings on spiral CT. Radiology 207:753, 1998.

345. Frazer CK, Cameron DC: Computed tomography demonstration of mosaic oligaemia in pulmonary embolism. Australas Radiol 39:14, 1995.

346. Ren H, Kuhlman JE, Hruban RH, et al: CT of inflation-fixed lungs: Wedge-shaped density and vascular sign in the diagnosis of infarction. J Comput Assist Tomogr 14:82, 1990.

346a. King MA, Ysrael M, Bergin CJ: Chronic thromboembolic pulmonary hypertension: CT findings. Am J Roentgenol 170:955, 1998.

347. Martin KW, Sagel SS, Siegel BA: Mosaic oligemia simulating pulmonary infiltrates on CT. Am J Roentgenol 147:670, 1986.

348. King MA, Bergin CJ, Yeung DWC, et al: Chronic pulmonary thromboembolism: Detection of regional hypoperfusion with CT. Radiology 191:359, 1994.

349. Remy-Jardin M, Remy J, Louvegny S, et al: Airway changes in chronic pulmonary embolism: CT findings in 33 patients. Radiology 203:355, 1997.

350. Bergin CJ, Rios G, King MA, et al: Accuracy of high-resolution CT in identifying chronic pulmonary thromboembolic disease. Am J Roentgenol 166:1371, 1996.

351. Austin JHM, Müller NL, Friedman PJ, et al: Glossary of terms for CT of the lungs: Recommendations of the Nomenclature Committee of the Fleischner Society. Radiology 200:327, 1996.

352. Moore EH, Gamsu G, Webb WR, et al: Pulmonary embolus: Detection and follow-up using magnetic resonance. Radiology 153:471, 1984.

353. Fisher MR, Higgins CB: Central thrombi in pulmonary arterial hypertension detected by MR imaging. Radiology 158:223, 1986.

354. Szucs RA, Rehr RB, Tatum JL: Pulmonary artery thrombus detection by magnetic resonance imaging. Chest 95:232, 1989.

355. Webb WR, Gamsu G, Golden JA, et al: Nuclear magnetic resonance of pulmonary arteriovenous fistula: Effects of flow. J Comput Assist Tomogr 8:155, 1984.

356. Woodard PK, Sostman HD, MacFall JR, et al: Detection of pulmonary embolism: Comparison of contrast-enhanced spiral CT and time-of-flight MR techniques. J Thorac Imaging 10:59, 1995.

357. Foo TKF, MacFall JR, Hayes CE, et al: Pulmonary vasculature: Single breath-hold MR imaging with phased-array coils. Radiology 183:473, 1992.

358. Hatabu H, Gefter WB, Listerud J, et al: Pulmonary MR angiography utilizing phased-array surface coils. J Comput Assist Tomogr 16:410, 1992.

359. MacFall JR, Sostman HD, Foo TK: Thick section, single breath-hold magnetic resonance pulmonary angiography. Invest Radiol 27:318, 1992.

360. Posteraro RH, Sostman HD, Spritzer CE, et al: Cine-gradient-refocused MR imaging of central pulmonary emboli. Am J Roentgenol 152:465, 1989.

361. Gefter WB, Hatabu H, Dinsmore BJ, et al: Pulmonary vascular cine MR imaging: A noninvasive approach to dynamic imaging of the pulmonary circulation. Radiology 176:761, 1990.

362. Rubin GD, Herfkens RJ, Pelc NJ, et al: Single breath-hold pulmonary magnetic resonance angiography: Optimization and comparison of three imaging strategies. Invest Radiol 29:766, 1994.

362a. Isoda H, Masui T, Hasegawa S, et al: Pulmonary MR angiography: A comparison of 2D and 3D time-of-flight. J Comput Assist Tomogr 18:403, 1994.

362b. Scialpi M, Scapati C, Carriero A, et al: Segmental pulmonary arteries: Two-dimensional and three-dimensional time-of-flight magnetic resonance angiography. J Thorac Imaging 13:123, 1998.

363. Wielopolski PA, Haacke EM, Adler LP: Three dimensional MR pulmonary vascular imaging: Preliminary experience. Radiology 183:465, 1992.

364. Schiebler ML, Holland GA, Hatabu H, et al: Suspected pulmonary embolism: Prospective evaluation with pulmonary MR angiography. Radiology 189:125, 1993.

365. Grist TM, Sostman HD, MacFall JR, et al: Pulmonary angiography with MR imaging: Preliminary clinical experience. Radiology 189:523, 1993.

366. Erdman WA, Peshock RM, Redman HL, et al: Pulmonary embolism: Comparison of MR images with radionuclide and angiographic studies. Radiology 190:499, 1994.

367. Loubeyre P, Revel D, Douek P, et al: Dynamic contrast-enhanced MR angiography of pulmonary embolism: Comparison with pulmonary angiography. Am J Roentgenol 162:1035, 1994.

368. Meaney JFM, Weg JG, Chenevert TL, et al: Diagnosis of pulmonary embolism with magnetic resonance angiography. N Engl J Med 336:1422, 1997.

369. Amundsen T, Kvaerness J, Jones RA, et al: Pulmonary embolism: Detection with MR perfusion imaging of lung: A feasibility study. Radiology 203:181, 1997.

370. Kessler R, Fraisse P, Krause D, et al: Magnetic resonance imaging in the diagnosis of pulmonary infarction. Chest 99:298, 1991.

371. Bergin CJ, Hauschildt J, Rios G, et al: Accuracy of MR angiography compared with radionuclide scanning in identifying the cause of pulmonary arterial hypertension. Am J Roentgenol 168:1549, 1997.

372. Kelley MA, Carson JL, Palevsky HI, et al: Diagnosing pulmonary embolism: New facts and strategies. Ann Intern Med 114:300, 1991.

373. Stein PD, Hull RD, Saltzman HA, et al: Strategy for diagnosis of patients with suspected acute pulmonary embolism. Chest 103:1553, 1993.

374. Oudkerk M, van Beek EJR, van Putten WLJ, et al: Cost-effectiveness analysis of various strategies in the diagnostic management of pulmonary embolism. Arch Intern Med 153:947, 1993.

375. Weidner W, Swanson L, Wilson G: Roentgen techniques in the diagnosis of pulmonary thromboembolism. Am J Roentgenol 100:397, 1967.

376. Ormond RS, Gale HH, Drake EH, et al: Pulmonary angiography and pulmonary embolism. Radiology 86:658, 1966.

377. Bookstein JJ: Segmental arteriography in pulmonary embolism. Radiology 93:1007, 1969.

378. Gomes AS, Grollman JH, Mink J: Pulmonary angiography for pulmonary emboli: Rational selection of oblique views. Am J Roentgenol 129:1019, 1977.

379. Quinn MF, Lundell CJ, Klotz TA, et al: Reliability of selective pulmonary arteriography in the diagnosis of pulmonary embolism. Am J Roentgenol 149:469, 1987.

380. van Rooij WJ, den Heeten GJ, Sluzewski M: Pulmonary embolism: Diagnosis in 211 patients with use of selective pulmonary digital subtraction angiography with a flow-directed catheter. Radiology 195:793, 1995.

381. Nicod P, Peterson K, Levine M, et al: Pulmonary angiography in severe chronic pulmonary hypertension. Ann Intern Med 107:565, 1987.

382. Pond GD, Ovitt TW, Capp MP: Comparison of conventional pulmonary angiography with intravenous digital subtraction angiography for pulmonary embolic disease. Radiology 147:345, 1983.

383. Musset D, Rosso J, Petitpretz P, et al: Acute pulmonary embolism: Diagnostic value of digital subtraction angiography. Radiology 166:455, 1988.

384. van Beek EJR, Bakker AJ, Reekers JA: Pulmonary embolism: Interobserver agreement in the interpretation of conventional angiographic and DSA images in patients with nondiagnostic lung scan results. Radiology 198:721, 1996.

385. Matsumoto AH, Tegtmeyer CJ: Contemporary diagnostic approaches to acute pulmonary emboli. Radiol Clin North Am 33:167, 1995.

386. van Rooij WJ, den Heeten GJ: Intra-arterial digital subtraction angiography of the pulmonary arteries using a flow-directed balloon catheter in the diagnosis of pulmonary embolism. Rofo Fortschr Geb Rontgenstr Neuen Bildgeb Verfahr 156:333, 1992.

386a. Johnson MS, Stine SB, Shah H, et al: Possible pulmonary embolus: Evaluation with digital subtraction versus cut-film angiography—prospective study in 80 patients. Radiology 207:131, 1998.

386b. Hagspiel KD, Polak JF, Grassi CJ, et al: Pulmonary embolism: Comparison of cut-film and digital pulmonary angiography. Radiology 207:139, 1998.

386c. Schlueter FJ, Zuckerman DA, Horesh L, et al: Digital subtraction versus film-screen angiography for detecting acute pulmonary emboli: Evaluation in a porcine model. J Vasc Intern Radiol 8:1015, 1997.

386d. Darcy MD: Pulmonary digital subtraction angiography: Ready for prime time. Radiology 207:11, 1998.

387. Schluger N, Henschke C, King T, et al: Diagnosis of pulmonary embolism at a large teaching hospital. J Thorac Imaging 9:180, 1994.

388. Cooper TJ, Hayward MWJ, Hartog M: Survey on the use of pulmonary scintigraphy and angiography for suspected pulmonary thromboembolism in the UK. Clin Radiol 43:243, 1991.

389. Hudson ER, Smith TP, McDermott VG, et al: Pulmonary angiography performed with Iopamidol: Complications in 1,434 patients. Radiology 198:61, 1996.

390. Mills SR, Jackson DC, Older RA, et al: The incidence, etiologies, and avoidance of complications of pulmonary angiography in a large series. Radiology 136:295, 1980.

391. Perlmutt LM, Braun SD, Newman GE, et al: Pulmonary arteriography in the high-risk patient. Radiology 162:187, 1987.

392. Dalen JE, Brooks HL, Johnson LW, et al: Pulmonary angiography in acute pulmonary embolism: Indications, techniques, and results in 367 patients. Am Heart J 81:175, 1971.

392a. Nilsson T, Carlsson A, Måre K: Pulmonary angiography: A safe procedure with modern contrast media and technique. Eur Radiol 8:86, 1998.

393. Sagel SS, Greenspan RH: Nonuniform pulmonary arterial perfusion: Pulmonary embolism? Radiology 99:541, 1971.

394. Goldhaber SZ, Hennekens CH, Evans DA, et al: Factors associated with correct antemortem diagnosis of major pulmonary embolism. Am J Med 73:822, 1982.

395. Auger WR, Fedullo PF, Moser KM, et al: Chronic major-vessel thromboembolic pulmonary artery obstruction: Appearance at angiography. Radiology 182:393, 1992.

396. Moser KM, Olson KL, Schlusselberg M, et al: Chronic thromboembolic occlusion in the adult can mimic pulmonary artery agenesis. Chest 95:503, 1989.

397. Williams JR, Wilcox WC: Pulmonary embolism: Roentgenographic and angiographic considerations. Am J Roentgenol 89:333, 1963.

398. Moser KM, Bloor CM: Pulmonary vascular lesions occurring in patients with chronic major vessel thromboembolic pulmonary hypertension. Chest 103:685, 1993.

399. Peterson KL, Fred HL, Alexander JK: Pulmonary arterial webs. A new angiographic sign of previous thromboembolism. N Engl J Med 277:33, 1967.

400. MacLean LD, Shibata HR, McLean APH, et al: Pulmonary embolism: The value of bedside scanning, angiography and pulmonary embolectomy. Can Med Assoc J 97:991, 1967.

401. Del Guercio LRM, Cohn JD, Feins NR, et al: Pulmonary embolism shock: Physiologic basis of a bedside screening test. JAMA 196:751, 1966.

402. Oakley CM: Diagnosis of pulmonary embolism. BMJ 2:773, 1970.

403. Hull R, Hirsh J, Sackett DL, et al: Clinical validity of a negative venogram in patients with clinically suspected venous thrombosis. Circulation 64:622, 1981.

404. Moser KM: State of the art: Venous thromboembolism. Am Rev Respir Dis 141:235, 1990.

405. Weinmann EE, Salzman EW: Deep-vein thrombosis. N Engl J Med 331:1630, 1994.

406. Baxter GM: The role of ultrasound in deep venous thrombosis. Clin Radiol 52:1, 1997.

407. Hull RD, Hirsh J, Carter CJ, et al: Pulmonary angiography, ventilation lung scanning, and venography for clinically suspected pulmonary embolism with abnormal perfusion lung scan. Ann Intern Med 98:891, 1983.

408. Bell WR: Pulmonary embolism: Progress and problems. Am J Med 72:181, 1982.

409. Managment of pulmonary embolism. BMJ 4:133, 1968.

410. Bettmann MA, Robbins A, Braun SD, et al: Contrast venography of the leg: Diagnostic efficacy, tolerance, and complication rates with ionic and nonionic contrast media. Radiology 165:113, 1987.

411. Lensing AWA, Prandoni P, Büller HR, et al: Lower extremity venography with Iohexol: Results and complications. Radiology 177:503, 1990.

412. Wheeler HB, Anderson FA: Diagnosis approaches for deep vein thrombosis. Chest 89:407, 1986.

413. McLachlan MSF, Thomas JG, Taylor DW, et al: Observer variation in the interpretation of lower limb venograms. Am J Roentgenol 132:227, 1979.

414. Aitken AGF, Godden DJ: Real time ultrasound diagnosis of deep vein thrombosis: A comparison with venography. Clin Radiol 38:309, 1987.

415. Cronan JJ, Dorfman GS, Scola FH, et al: Deep venous thrombosis: US assessment using vein compression. Radiology 162:191, 1987.

416. Lensing AWA, Prandoni P, Brandjes D, et al: Detection of deep vein thrombosis by real time B-mode ultrasonography. N Engl J Med 320:342, 1989.

417. Baxter GM, MacKechnie S, Duffy P: Colour Doppler ultrasound in deep venous thrombosis: A comparison with venography. Clin Radiol 42:32, 1990.
418. Foley WD, Middleton WD, Lawson TL, et al: Colour Doppler ultrasound imaging of lower extremity venous disease. Am J Roentgenol 152:371, 1989.
419. Rose SC, Zwiebel WJ, Nelson BD, et al: Symptomatic lower extremity deep venous thrombosis: Accuracy, limitations, and role of color Duplex flow imaging in diagnosis. Radiology 175:639, 1990.
420. Lewis BD, Meredith JE, Welch TJ, et al: Diagnosis of acute deep venous thrombosis of the lower extremities: Prospective evaluation of color Doppler flow imaging versus venography. Radiology 192:651, 1994.
421. Moser KM, LeMoine JR: Is embolic risk conditioned by location of deep venous thrombosis? Ann Intern Med 94:439, 1981.
422. Lagerstedt CI, Fagher BO, Olsson CG, et al: Need for long term anticoagulant treatment in symptomatic calf vein thrombosis. Lancet 2:515, 1985.
423. Baxter GM, Duffy P, Partridge E: Color flow imaging of calf vein thrombosis. Clin Radiol 46:198, 1992.
424. Atri M, Herba MJ, Reinhold C, et al: Accuracy of sonography in the evaluation of calf deep vein thrombosis in both postoperative surveillance and symptomatic patients. Am J Roentgenol 166:1361, 1996.
425. Borris LC, Christiansen HM, Lassen MR, et al: Comparison of real-time B-mode ultrasonography and bilateral ascending phlebography for detection of postoperative deep vein thrombosis following elective hip surgery. Thromb Haemost 61:363, 1989.
426. Ginsberg JS, Caco CC, Brill-Edwards PA, et al: Venous thrombosis in patients who have undergone major hip or knee surgery: Detection with compression US and impedance plethysmography. Radiology 181:651, 1991.
427. Baldt MM, Zontsich T, Stümpflen A, et al: Deep venous thrombosis of the lower extremity: Efficacy of spiral CT venography compared with conventional venography in diagnosis. Radiology 200:423, 1996.
428. Stehling MK, Rosen MP, Weintraub J, et al: Spiral CT venography of the lower extremity. Am J Roentgenol 163:451, 1994.
429. Lomas DJ, Britton PD: CT demonstration of acute and chronic iliofemoral thrombosis. J Comput Assist Tomogr 15:861, 1991.
429a. Baldt MM, Zontsich T, Kainberger F, et al: Spiral CT evaluation of deep venous thrombosis. Semin Ultrasound CT MR 18:369, 1997.
429b. Loud PA, Grossman ZD, Klippenstein DL, Ray CE: Combined CT venography and pulmonary angiography: A new diagnostic technique for suspected thromboembolic disease. Am J Roentgenol 170:951, 1998.
430. Spritzer CE, Sussman SK, Blinder RA, et al: Deep venous thrombosis evaluation with limited-flip-angle, gradient-refocused MR imaging: Preliminary experience. Radiology 166:371, 1988.
431. Erdman WA, Jayson HT, Redman HC, et al: Deep venous thrombosis of extremities: Role of MR imaging in the diagnosis. Radiology 174:425, 1990.
432. Evans AJ, Sostman HD, Knelson MH, et al: Detection of deep venous thrombosis: Prospective comparison of MR imaging with contrast venography. Am J Roentgenol 161:131, 1993.
433. Spritzer CE, Norconk JJ Jr, Sostman HD, et al: Detection of deep venous thrombosis by magnetic resonance imaging. Chest 104:54, 1993.
434. Browse NL: Prophylaxis of pulmonary embolism. BMJ 2:780, 1970.
435. Davis HH, Heaton WA, Siegel BA, et al: Scintigraphic detection of atherosclerotic lesions and venous thrombi in man by indium-111 labelled autologous platelets. Lancet 1:1185, 1978.
436. Sostman HD, Neumann RD, Loke J, et al: Detection of pulmonary embolism in man with 111 In-labeled autologous platelets. Am J Roentgenol 138:945, 1982.
437. Gomes AS, Webber MM, Buffkin D: Contrast venography vs. radionuclide venography: A study of discrepancies and their possible significance. Radiology 142:719, 1982.
438. Ryo UY, Qazi M, Srikantaswamy S, et al: Radionuclide venography: Correlation with contrast venography. J Nucl Med 18:11, 1977.
439. Butler SP, Boyd SJ, Parker SZ: Technetium-99m–modified recombinant tissue plasminogen activator to detect deep venous thrombosis. J Nucl Med 37:744, 1996.
440. Mullick SC, Wheeler HB, Songster GF: Diagnosis of deep venous thrombosis by measurement of electrical impedance. Am J Surg 119:417, 1970.
441. Wheeler HB, Mullick SC, Anderson JN, et al: Diagnosis of occult deep vein thrombosis by a noninvasive bedside technique. Surgery 70:20, 1971.
442. Hull R, Hirsh J, Sackett DL, et al: Replacement of venography in suspected venous thrombosis by impedance plethysmography and ¹²⁵I-fibrogen leg scanning: A less invasive approach. Ann Intern Med 94:12, 1981.
443. Hull R, Taylor DW, Hirsh J, et al: Impedance plethysmography: The relationship between venous filling and sensitivity and specificity for proximal vein thrombosis. Circulation 58:896, 1978.
444. Huisman MV, Buller HR, ten Cate JW: Utility of impedance plethysmography in the diagnosis of recurrent deep vein thrombosis. Arch Intern Med 148:681, 1988.
445. Benatar SR, Immelman EJ, Jeffery P: Pulmonary embolism. Br J Dis Chest 80:313, 1986.
446. Breckenridge RT, Ratnoff OD: Pulmonary embolism and unexpected death in supposedly normal persons. N Engl J Med 270:298, 1964.
447. Cohen H, Daly JJ: Unheralded pulmonary embolism. BMJ 2:1209, 1957.
448. Cooley RN: Pulmonary thromboembolism—the case for the pulmonary angiogram. Am J Roentgenol 92:693, 1964.
449. Stein PD, Terrin ML, Hales CA, et al: Clinical, laboratory, roentgenographic and electrocardiographic findings in patients with acute pulmonary embolism and no pre-existing cardiac or pulmonary disease. Chest 100:598, 1991.
450. Huisman MV, Buller KR, ten Cate JW, et al: Unexpected high prevalence of silent pulmonary embolism in patients with deep venous thrombosis. Chest 95:498, 1989.
451. Doyle DJ, Turpie AG, Hirsh J, et al: Adjusted subcutaneous heparin or continuous intravenous heparin in patients with acute deep vein thrombosis. A randomized trial. Ann Intern Med 107:441, 1987.
452. Stein PD, Willis PW III, DeMets DL: History and physical examination in acute pulmonary embolism in patents without preexisting cardiac or pulmonary disease. Am J Cardiol 47:218, 1981.
453. Stein PD, Henry JW: Clinical characteristics of patients with acute pulmonary embolism stratified according to their presenting syndromes. Chest 112:974, 1997.
454. Stein PD, Gottschalk A, Saltzman HA, et al: Diagnosis of acute pulmonary embolism in the elderly. J Am Coll Cardiol 18:1452, 1991.
455. Patil S, Henry JW, Rubenfire M, et al: Neural network in the clinical diagnosis of acute pulmonary embolism. Chest 104:1685, 1993.
456. Hirsh J, Hull RD, Raskob GE: Diagnosis of pulmonary embolism. J Am Coll Cardiol 8:128, 1986.
457. Bell WR, Simon TL, DeMets DL: The clinical features of submassive and massive pulmonary emboli. Am J Med 62:355, 1977.
458. Webster JR Jr, Saadeh GB, Eggum PR, et al: Wheezing due to pulmonary embolism: Treatment with heparin. N Engl J Med 274:931, 1966.
459. Olazábal F Jr, Román-Irizarry LA, Oms JD, et al: Pulmonary emboli masquerading as asthma. N Engl J Med 278:999, 1968.
460. Goodwin JF: The clinical diagnosis of pulmonary thromboembolism. In Sasahara AA, Stein M (eds): Pulmonary Embolic Disease. New York, Grune & Stratton, 1965, pp 239–255.
461. Prevention of pulmonary embolism. BMJ 2:1, 1973.
462. Nielsen TT, Lund O, Hedegaard M, et al: Clinical picture of acute pulmonary embolism. Relations to the degree of vascular obstruction. Ugeskr Laeger 154:2019, 1992.
463. Barker NW, Nygaard KK, Walters W, et al: A statistical study of post-operative venous thrombosis and pulmonary embolism. II. Predisposing factors. Mayo Clin Proc 16:1, 1941.
464. Barker NW, Nygaard KK, Walters W, et al: A statistical study of post-operative venous thrombosis and pulmonary embolism. III. Time of occurrence during the postoperative period. Mayo Clin Proc 16:17, 1941.
465. McAlister FA, Al-Jahlan M, Fisher B: Postpulmonary embolism pericarditis: A case report and review of the literature. Can Respir J 3:13, 1996.
466. Murray HW, Ellis GC, Blumenthal DS, et al: Fever and pulmonary thromboembolism. Am J Med 67:232, 1979.
467. Manganelli D, Palla A, Donnamaria V, et al: Clinical features of pulmonary embolism—doubts and certainties. Chest 107:25, 1995.
468. Grieco MH, Ryan SF: Aseptic cavitary pulmonary infarction. Am J Med 45:811, 1968.
469. Stein PD, Henry JW: Clinical characteristics of patients with acute pulmonary embolism stratified according to their presenting syndromes. Chest 112:974, 1997.
470. Wenger NK, Stein PD, Willis PW III: Massive acute pulmonary embolism: The deceivingly nonspecific manifestations. JAMA 220:843, 1972.
471. Sutton GC, Honey M, Gibson RV: Clinical diagnosis of acute massive pulmonary embolism. Lancet 1:271, 1969.
472. Dalen JE, Dexter L: Pulmonary embolism. JAMA 207:1505, 1969.
473. Coma-Canella I, Gamallo C, Martinez Onsurbe P, et al: Acute right ventricular infarction secondary to massive pulmonary embolism. Eur Heart J 9:534, 1988.
474. Shaw RA, Schonfeld SA, Whitcomb ME: Pulmonary embolism presenting as coronary insufficiency. Arch Intern Med 141:651, 1981.
475. Fred HL, Willerson JT, Alexander JK: Neurological manifestations of pulmonary thromboembolism. Arch Intern Med 120:33, 1967.
476. Stöllberger C, Slany J, Schuster I, et al: The prevalence of deep venous thrombosis in patients with suspected paradoxical embolism. Ann Intern Med 119:461, 1993.
477. Ward R, Jones D, Haponik EF: Paradoxical embolism—an underrecognized problem. Chest 108:549, 1995.
478. Benotti JR, Ockene IS, Alpert JS, et al: The clinical profile of unresolved pulmonary embolism. Chest 84:669, 1983.
479. Johnson JC, Flowers NC, Horan LG: Unexplained atrial flutter: A frequent herald of pulmonary embolism. Chest 60:29, 1971.
480. Palla A, Formichi B, Santolicandro A, et al: From not detected pulmonary embolism to diagnosis of chronic thromboembolic pulmonary hypertension: A retrospective study. Respiration 60:9, 1993.
481. Fraser RS, Lynne-Davies P: Continuous chest murmur acquired following pulmonary thromboembolism. Chest 65:562, 1974.
482. Albertini RE: Vocal cord paralysis associated with pulmonary emboli. Chest 62:508, 1972.
483. Brinton WD: Primary pulmonary hypertension. Br Heart J 12:305, 1950.
484. Soothill JF: A case of primary pulmonary hypertension with paralyzed left vocal cord. Guys Hosp Rep 100:232, 1951.
485. Moser KM, Olson LK, Schlusselberg M, et al: Chronic thromboembolic occlusion in the adult can mimic pulmonary artery agenesis. Chest 95:503, 1989.
486. Delany SG, Doyle TCA, Bunton RW, et al: Pulmonary artery sarcoma mimicking pulmonary embolism. Chest 103:1631, 1993.
487. Promisloff RA, Segal SL, Lenchner GS, et al: Sarcoma of the pulmonary artery. Chest 92:207, 1988.
488. Sleyster TJ, Heystraten FM: Malignant fibrous histiocytoma mimicking pulmonary embolism. Thorax 43:580, 1988.

489. Stein PD, Henry JW, Gopalakrishnan D, et al: Asymmetry of the calves in the assessment of patients with suspected acute pulmonary embolism. Chest 107:936, 1995.

490. Kearon C, Hirsh J: The diagnosis of pulmonary embolism. Haemostasis 25:72, 1995.

491. Israel HL, Goldstein F: The varied clinical manifestations of pulmonary embolism. Ann Intern Med 47:202, 1957.

492. Hildner FJ, Ormond RS: Accuracy of the clinical diagnosis of pulmonary embolism. JAMA 202:567, 1967.

493. Wolfe TR, Allen TL: Syncope as an emergency department presentation of pulmonary embolism. J Emerg Med 16:27, 1998.

494. Marine JE, Goldhaber SZ: Pulmonary embolism presenting as seizures. Chest 112:840, 1997.

495. Sigal SL, Kolansky DM, Hughes S, et al: Pulmonary embolism presenting as exercise-induced hypotension. Chest 99:500, 1991.

496. Sparagana M: Episodic ectopic ACTH syndrome associated with pulmonary infarctions. Chest 93:1110, 1988.

497. Harrison KA, Haire WD, Pappas AA, et al: Plasma D-dimer: A useful tool for evaluating suspected pulmonary embolus. J Nucl Med 34:896, 1993.

498. Wacker WEC, Snodgrass PJ: Serum LDH activity in pulmonary embolism diagnosis. JAMA 174:2142, 1960.

499. Wacker WEC, Rosenthal M, Snodgrass PJ, et al: A triad for the diagnosis of pulmonary embolism and infarction. JAMA 178:8, 1961.

500. Ruckley CV, Das PC, Leitch AG, et al: Serum fibrin/fibrinogen degradation products associated with postoperative pulmonary embolus and venous thrombosis. BMJ 4:395, 1970.

501. Snodgrass PJ, Amador E, Wacker WEC: Serum enzymes in the diagnosis of pulmonary embolism. In Sasahara AA, Stein M (eds): Pulmonary Embolic Disease. New York, Grune & Stratton, 1965, pp 93–100.

502. Adams JE III, Siegel BA, Goldstein JA, et al: Elevations of CK-MB following pulmonary embolism—a manifestation of occult right ventricular infarction. Chest 101:1203, 1992.

503. Coodley EL: Enzyme profiles in the evaluation of pulmonary infarction. JAMA 207:1307, 1969.

504. Leitha T, Speiser W, Dudczak T: Pulmonary embolism—efficacy of D-dimer and thrombin-antithrombin III complex determinations as screening tests before lung scanning. Chest 100:1536, 1991.

505. Perrier A, Bounameaux H: Contribution of laboratory tests and venous investigations in the diagnosis of pulmonary embolism. Arch Mal Coeur Vaiss 88:1699, 1995.

506. Gavaud C, Ninet J, Ville D, et al: Diagnosis of venous thrombosis and/or pulmonary embolism by determination of D-dimer using ELISA. Review based on a study of 80 consecutive patients hospitalized in an emergency unit. J Mal Vasc 21:22, 1996.

507. Flores J, Lancha C, Perez Rodriguez E, et al: Efficacy of D-dimer and total fibrin degradation products evaluation in suspected pulmonary embolism. Respiration 62:258, 1995.

508. Perrier A, Desmarais S, Goehring C, et al: D-dimer testing for suspected pulmonary embolism in outpatients. Am J Respir Crit Care Med 156:492, 1997.

509. Rochemaure JM, Laaban JP, Achkar A et al: Value of the determination of D-dimers in the diagnostic approach of venous thrombo-embolic disorders. Bull Acad Natl Med 179: 299, 1995.

510. Perrier A, Bounameaux H, Morabia A, et al: Contribution of D-dimer plasma measurement and lower-limb venous ultrasound to the diagnosis of pulmonary embolism: A decision analysis model. Am Heart J 127:624, 1994.

511. van Beek EJ, Schenk BE, Michel BC, et al: The role of plasma D-dimer concentration in the exclusion of pulmonary embolism. Br J Haematol 92:725, 1996.

512. Perrier A, Bounameaux H, Morabia A, et al: Diagnosis of pulmonary embolism by a decision analysis-based strategy including clinical probability, D-dimer levels, and ultrasonography: A management study. Arch Intern Med 156:531, 1996.

513. Becker DM, Philbrick JT, Bachhuber TL, et al: D-dimer testing and acute venous thromboembolism. A shortcut to accurate diagnosis? Arch Intern Med 156:939, 1996.

514. Bouman CS, Ypma ST, Sybesma JP: Comparison of the efficacy of D-dimer, fibrin degradation products and prothrombin fragment 1+2 in clinically suspected deep venous thrombosis. Thromb Res 77:225, 1995.

515. Perrier A: Diagnosis of acute pulmonary embolism. Rev Prat 46:1218, 1996.

516. Ginsberg JS, Brill-Edwards PA, Demers C, et al: D-dimer in patients with clinically suspected pulmonary embolism. Chest 104:1679, 1993.

517. Goldhaber SZ, Simons GR, Elliot CG, et al: Quantitative plasma D-dimer levels among patients undergoing pulmonary angiography for suspected pulmonary embolism. JAMA 270:2819, 1993.

517a. Oger E, Leroyer C, Bressollette L, et al: Evaluation of a new, rapid, and quantitative D-dimer test in patients with suspected pulmonary embolism. Am J Respir Crit Care Med 158:65, 1998.

518. Monreal M, Lafoz E, Casals A, et al: Platelet count and venous thromboembolism—a useful test for suspected pulmonary embolism. Chest 100:1493, 1991.

519. Sasahara AA: Clinical studies in pulmonary thromboembolism. In Sasahara AA, Stein M (eds): Pulmonary Embolic Disease. New York, Grune & Stratton, 1965, pp 256–264.

520. Bynum LJ, Wilson JE III: Characteristics of pleural effusions associated with pulmonary embolism. Arch Intern Med 136:159, 1976.

521. Griner PF: Bloody pleural fluid in pulmonary infarction. JAMA 202:947, 1967.

522. Colp CR, Williams MH Jr: Pulmonary function following pulmonary embolization. Am Rev Respir Dis 85:799, 1962.

523. Morris TA, Auger WR, Ysrael MZ, et al: Parenchymal scarring is associated with restrictive spirometric defects in patients with chronic thromboembolic pulmonary hypertension. Chest 110:399, 1996.

524. Wimalaratna HSK, Farrell J, Lee HY: Measurement of diffusing capacity in pulmonary embolism. Respir Med 83:481, 1989.

525. Bernstein RJ, Ford RL, Clausen JL, et al: Membrane diffusion and capillary blood volume in chronic thromboembolic pulmonary hypertension. Chest 110:1430, 1996.

526. Szucs MM Jr, Brooks HL, Grossman W, et al: Diagnostic sensitivity of laboratory findings in acute pulmonary embolism. Ann Intern Med 74:161, 1971.

527. Urokinase pulmonary embolism trial: Phase I results. A cooperative study. JAMA 214:2163, 1970.

528. Cvitanic O, Marino PL: Improved use of arterial blood gas analysis in suspected pulmonary embolism. Chest 95:48, 1989.

529. McFarlane MJ, Imperiale TF: Use of the alveolar-arterial oxygen gradient in the diagnosis of pulmonary embolism. Am J Med 96:57, 1994.

530. Stein PD, Goldhaber SZ, Henry JW, et al: Arterial blood has analysis in the assessment of suspected acute pulmonary embolism. Chest 109:78, 1996.

531. Stein PD, Goldhaber SZ, Henry JW: Alveolar-arterial oxygen gradient in the assessment of acute pulmonary embolism. Chest 107:139, 1995.

532. Brathwaite CE, O'Malley KF, Ross SE, et al: Continuous pulse oximetry and the diagnosis of pulmonary embolism in critically ill trauma patients. J Trauma 33:528, 1992.

533. Sasahara AA, Stein M, Simon M, et al: Pulmonary angiography in the diagnosis of thromboembolic disease. N Engl J Med 270:1164, 1964.

534. Robin ED, Julian DG, Travis DM, et al: A physiologic approach to the diagnosis of acute pulmonary embolism. N Engl J Med 260:586, 1959.

535. Robin ED, Forkner CE Jr, Bromberg PA, et al: Alveolar gas exchange in clinical pulmonary embolism. N Engl J Med 262:283, 1960.

536. MacKeen AD, Landrigan PL, Dickson RC: Early diagnosis of acute pulmonary embolism. Can Med Assoc J 85:233, 1961.

537. Eriksson L, Wollmer P, Olsson CG, et al: Diagnosis of pulmonary embolism based upon alveolar dead space analysis. Chest 96:357, 1989.

538. Sreeram N, Cheriex EC, Smeets JL, et al: Value of the 12-lead electrocardiogram at hospital admission in the diagnosis of pulmonary embolism. Am J Cardiol 73:298, 1994.

539. Tighe DA, Chung EK, Park CH: Electric alternans associated with acute pulmonary embolism. Am Heart J 128:188, 1994.

540. Ferrari E, Imbert A, Chevalier T, et al: The ECG in pulmonary embolism—predictive value of negative T waves in precordial leads—80 case reports. Chest 111:537, 1997.

541. Modan B, Sharon E, Jelin N: Factors contributing to the incorrect diagnosis of pulmonary embolic disease. Chest 62:388, 1972.

542. Paraskos JA, Adelstein SJ, Smith RE, et al: Late prognosis of acute pulmonary embolism. N Engl J Med 289:55, 1973.

543. Carson JL, Kelley MA, Duff A, et al: The clinical course of pulmonary embolism. N Engl J Med 326:1240, 1992.

544. Carson JL, Terrin ML, Duff A, et al: Pulmonary embolism and mortality in patients with COPD. Chest 110:1212, 1996.

545. Stein PD: COPD, pulmonary embolism, and death. Chest 110:1135, 1996.

546. Donaldson GA, Williams C, Scannell JG, et al: A reappraisal of the application of the Trendelenburg operation to massive fatal embolism. Report of a successful pulmonary-artery thrombectomy using a cardiopulmonary bypass. N Engl J Med 268:171, 1963.

547. Alpert JS, Smith RE, Ockene IS, et al: Treatment of massive pulmonary embolism: The role of pulmonary embolectomy. Am Heart J 89:413, 1975.

548. Miller GA, Hall RJ, Paneth M: Pulmonary embolectomy, heparin, and streptokinase: Their place in the treatment of acute massive pulmonary embolism. Am Heart J 93:568, 1977.

549. Urokinase pulmonary embolism trial: Phase I results. A cooperative study. JAMA 214:2163, 1970.

550. Wolfe MW, Lee RT, Feldstein ML, et al: Prognostic significance of right ventricular hypokinesis and perfusion lung scan defects in pulmonary embolism. Am Heart J 127:1371, 1994.

551. Barritt DW, Jordan SC: Anticoagulant drugs in the treatment of pulmonary embolism: A controlled trial. Lancet 1:1309, 1960.

552. Egermayer P: Follow-up for death or recurrence is not a reliable way of assessing the accuracy of diagnostic tests for thromboembolic disease. Chest 111:1410, 1997.

552a. Konstantinides S, Geibel A, Kasper W, et al: Patent foramen ovale is an important predictor of adverse outcome in patients with major pulmonary embolism. Circulation 97:1946, 1998.

553. Benotti JR, Ockene IS, Alpert JS, et al: The clinical profile of unresolved pulmonary embolism. Chest 84:669, 1983.

554. Riedel M, Stanek V, Widimsky J, et al: Longterm follow-up of patients with pulmonary thromboembolism: Late prognosis and evolution of hemodynamic and respiratory data. Chest 81:151, 1982.

555. Wilson JE III: Pulmonary embolism: Diagnosis and treatment. Clin Notes Respir Dis 20:3, 1981.

556. Donnamaria V, Palla A, Petruzzelli S, et al: Early and late follow-up of pulmonary embolism. Respiration 60:15, 1993.

557. Paraskos JA, Adelstein SJ, Smith RE, et al: Late prognosis of acute pulmonary embolism. N Engl J Med 289:55, 1973.

558. Yoo HS, Intenzo CM, Park CH: Unresolved major pulmonary embolism: Importance of follow-up lung scan in diagnosis. Eur J Nucl Med 12:252, 1986.

559. Menendez R, Nauffal D, Cremades MJ: Prognostic factors in restoration of pulmonary flow after submassive pulmonary embolism: A multiple regression analysis. Eur Respir J 11:560, 1998.

560. Daily PO, Dembitsky WP, Peterson KL, et al: Modifications of techniques and early results of pulmonary thromboendarterectomy for chronic pulmonary embolism. J Thorac Cardiovasc Surg 93:221, 1987.

561. Pulmonary microembolism (editorial). Lancet 1:429, 1967.

562. Harker LA, Slichter SJ: Studies of platelet and fibrinogen kinetics in patients with prosthetic heart valves. N Engl J Med 283:1302, 1970.

563. Bischel MD, Scoles BG, Mohler JG: Evidence for pulmonary microembolization during hemodialysis. Chest 67:335, 1975.

564. Rubenstein MD, Wall RT, Wood GS, et al: Complications of therapeutic apheresis, including a fatal case with pulmonary vascular occlusion. Am J Med 75:171, 1983.

565. Reul GJ Jr, Beall AC Jr, Greenberg SD: Protection of the pulmonary microvasculature by fine screen blood filtration. Chest 66:4, 1974.

566. Patterson RH Jr, Twichell JB: Disposable filter for microemboli: Use in cardiopulmonary bypass and massive transfusion. JAMA 215:76, 1971.

567. Jenevein EP, Weiss DL: Platelet microemboli associated with massive blood transfusion. Am J Pathol 45:313, 1964.

568. Fred HL, Harle TS: Septic pulmonary embolism. Dis Chest 55:483, 1969.

569. Jaffe RB, Koschmann EB: Septic pulmonary emboli. Radiology 96:527, 1970.

570. Roberts WC, Buchbinder NA: Right-sided valvular infective endocarditis. A clinicopathologic study of twelve necropsy patients. Am J Med 53:7, 1972.

571. Iwama T, Shigemaatsu S, Asami K, et al: Tricuspid valve endocarditis with large vegetations in a non-drug addict without underlying cardiac disease. Intern Med 35:203, 1996.

572. Clifford CP, Eykyn SJ, Oakley CM: Staphylococcal tricuspid valve endocarditis in patients with structurally normal hearts and no evidence of narcotic abuse. QJM 87:755, 1994.

573. Bain RC, Edwards JE, Scheifley CH, et al: Right-sided bacterial endocarditis and endarteritis. A clinical and pathologic study. Am J Med 24:98, 1958.

574. Hadlock FP, Wallace RJ Jr, Rivera M: Pulmonary septic emboli secondary to parapharyngeal abscess: Postanginal sepsis. Radiology 130:29, 1979.

575. Celikel TH, Muthuswamy PP: Septic pulmonary emboli secondary to internal jugular vein phlebitis (postanginal sepsis) caused by *Eikenella corrodens*. Am Rev Respir Dis 130:510, 1984.

576. Weesner CL, Cisek JE: Lemierre syndrome: The forgotten disease. Ann Emerg Med 22:256, 1993.

577. Ahkee S, Srinath L, Huang A, et al: Lemierre's syndrome: Postanginal sepsis due to anaerobic oropharyngeal infection. Ann Otol Rhinol Laryngol 103:208, 1994.

578. Hughes CE, Spear RK, Shinabarger CE, et al: Septic pulmonary emboli complicating mastoiditis: Lemierre's syndrome. Clin Infec Dis 18:633, 1994.

579. Felman AH, Shulman ST: Staphylococcal osteomyelitis, sepsis, and pulmonary disease: Observations of 10 patients with combined osseous and pulmonary infections. Radiology 117:649, 1975.

580. Plemmons RM, Dooley DP, Longfield RN: Septic thrombophlebitis of the portal vein (pylephlebitis): Diagnosis and management in the modern era. Clin Infect Dis 21:1114, 1995.

581. Goodwin NJ, Castronuovo JJ, Friedman EA: Recurrent septic pulmonary embolization complicating maintenance hemodialysis. Ann Intern Med 71:29, 1969.

582. Levi J, Robson M, Rosenfeld JB: Septicaemia and pulmonary embolism complicating use of arteriovenous fistula in maintenance haemodialysis. Lancet 2:288, 1970.

583. Shparago NI, Bruno PP, Bennett J: Systemic *Malassezia furfur* infection in an adult receiving total parenteral nutrition. J Am Osteopath Assoc 95:375, 1995.

584. Kelly RF, Yellin AE, Weaver FA: *Candida* thrombosis of the innominate vein with septic pulmonary emboli. Ann Vasc Surg 7:343, 1993.

585. Waisser E, Kuo C-S, Kabins SA: Septic pulmonary emboli arising from a permanent transvenous cardiac pacemaker. Chest 61:503, 1972.

586. Zenda T, Araki I, Hiraiwa Y, et al: Septic pulmonary emboli secondary to pyogenic liver abscess in a diabetic patient. Intern Med 34:42, 1995.

587. Chowdhury P, Stein DS: Pyogenic hepatic abscess and septic pulmonary emboli associated with *Klebsiella ozaenae* bacteremia. South Med J 85:638, 1992.

588. Christensen PJ, Kutty K, Adlam RT, et al: Septic pulmonary embolism due to periodontal disease. Chest 104:1927, 1993.

589. Noble J Jr, Cohen RB: *Candida* septicemia and pulmonary lesions. N Engl J Med 286:1309, 1972.

590. Cramer SF, Tomkiewicz ZM: Septic pulmonary thrombosis in streptococcal toxic shock syndrome. Hum Pathol 26:1157, 1995.

591. Huang RM, Naidich DP, Lubat E, et al: Septic pulmonary emboli: CT-radiographic correlation. Am J Roentgenol 153:41, 1989.

592. Zelefsky MN, Lutzker LG: The target sign: A new radiologic sign of septic pulmonary emboli. Am J Roentgenol 129:453, 1977.

593. Silingardi V, Canossi GC, Torelli G, et al: The radiology "target sign" of septic pulmonary embolism in a case of acute myelogenous leukemia. Respiration 42:61, 1981.

594. Gumbs RV, McCauley DI: Hilar and mediastinal adenopathy in septic pulmonary embolic disease. Radiology 142:313, 1982.

595. Kuhlman JE, Fishman EK, Teigen C: Pulmonary septic emboli: Diagnosis with CT. Radiology 174:211, 1990.

596. Webb DW, Thadepalli H: Hemoptysis in patients with septic pulmonary infarcts from tricuspid endocarditis. Chest 76:99, 1979.

597. Marantz PR, Linzer M, Feiner CJ, et al: Inability to predict diagnosis in febrile intravenous drug abusers. Ann Intern Med 106:823, 1987.

598. Dreyer ZE: Chest infections and syndromes in sickle cell disease of childhood. Semin Respir Infect 11:163, 1996.

599. Verdegem TD, Yee SJ: Lung disease in sickle cell anemia: A tropical disease with a twist. Sem Respir Med 12:107, 1991.

600. Charache S, Scott JC, Charache P: "Acute chest syndrome" in adults with sickle cell anemia. Microbiology, treatment, and prevention. Arch Intern Med 139:67, 1979.

601. Poncz M, Kane E, Gill FM: Acute chest syndrome in sickle cell disease: Etiology and clinical correlates. J Pediatr 107:861, 1985.

602. Powers D, Weidman JA, Odom-Maryon T, et al: Sickle cell chronic lung disease: Prior morbidity and the risk of pulmonary infection. Medicine 67:66, 1988.

603. Haynes J Jr, Kirkpatrick MB: The acute chest syndrome of sickle cell disease. Am J Med Sci 305:326, 1993.

604. Lowenthal EA, Wells A, Emanuel PD, et al: Sickle cell acute chest syndrome associated with parvovirus B19 infection: Case series and review. Am J Hematol 51:207, 1996.

605. Vichinsky E, Williams R, Das M, et al: Pulmonary fat embolism: A distinct cause of severe acute chest syndrome in sickle cell anemia. Blood 83:3107, 1994.

606. Styles LA, Schalkwijk CG, Aarsman AJ, et al: Phospholipase A2 levels in acute chest syndrome of sickle cell disease. Blood 85:2573, 1996.

607. Solovey A, Lin Y, Browne P, et al: Circulating activated endothelial cells in sickle cell anemia. N Engl J Med 337:1584, 1997.

608. Lubin BH: Sickle cell disease and the endothelium. N Engl J Med 337:1623, 1997.

609. Bhalla M, Abboud MR, McLoud TC, et al: Acute chest syndrome in sickle cell disease: CT evidence of microvascular occlusion. Radiology 187:45, 1993.

610. Hammerman SI, Kourembanas S, Conca T, et al: Endothelin-1 production during acute chest syndrome in sickle cell disease. Am J Respir Crit Care Med 156:280, 1997.

611. Bellet PS, Kalinyak KA, Shukla R, et al: Incentive spirometry to prevent acute pulmonary complications in sickle cell diseases. N Engl J Med 333:699, 1995.

612. Young RC Jr, Rachal RE, Hackney RL Jr, et al: Smoking is a factor in causing acute chest syndrome in sickle cell anemia. J Natl Med Assoc 84:267, 1992.

613. Cockshott WP: Rib infarcts in sickling disease. Eur J Radiol 14:63, 1992.

614. Johnson CS, Verdegem TD: Pulmonary complications of sickle cell disease. Semin Respir Med 9:287, 1988.

615. Pianosi P, D'Souza SJA, Esseltine DW, et al: Ventilation and gas exchange during exercise in sickle cell anemia. Am Rev Respir Dis 143:226, 1991.

616. Pianosi P, D'Souza SJA, Charge TD, et al: Cardiac output and oxygen delivery during exercise in sickle cell anemia. Am Rev Respir Dis 143:231, 1991.

617. Haupt H, Moore GW, Bauer TW, et al: The lung in sickle cell disease. Chest 81:332, 1982.

618. Powars D, Weidman J, Odom-Maryon T, et al: Sickle cell chronic lung disease: Prior morbidity and the risk of pulmonary failure. Medicine 67:66, 1988.

619. Aquino SL, Gamsu G, Fahy JV, et al: Chronic pulmonary disorders in sickle cell disease: Findings at thin-section CT. Radiology 193:807, 1994.

# CHAPTER 49

# Emboli of Extravascular Tissue and Foreign Material

Theoretically, fragments of virtually any organ, tissue, or body secretion can gain access to the systemic circulation and be transported to the lungs (Table 49–1). Some, such as megakaryocytes and trophoblast cells, do this with such frequency that the process can be considered a normal phenomenon (*see* page 132). Others are found only in pathologic conditions, in which circumstance tissue disruption with vascular laceration is a necessary precondition; thus, the underlying pathogenesis is usually trauma, most often associated with labor, accidental or battlefield injuries, or medical procedures such as venipuncture or surgery. Occasionally, a necrotizing inflammatory process can release small tissue fragments into the bloodstream and produce similar results. With the exception of amniotic fluid and fat, the clinicopathologic effects of such emboli are almost invariably nil; however, they are rarely implicated in the pathogenesis of clinically evident disease.[1–3]

In addition to normal body tissues, abnormal tissue can also embolize to the pulmonary circulation. Perhaps the most common such substance is neoplastic cells, which, because of their inherent invasive properties, can gain access to the circulation without the aid of trauma; although such emboli are usually microscopic and of no direct vascular consequence, large fragments or numerous small ones occasionally cause significant pulmonary arterial obstruction. Similar obstruction can occur with embolized parasites, either as eggs to the microvasculature (as in schistosomiasis) or as whole or fragmented adult worms to large arteries (as in ascariasis).

Foreign particulate material can also enter the venous side of the systemic circulation and embolize to the lungs. In some situations, this material is introduced by the patient directly into the vasculature (as in intravenous talcosis); in most cases, however, material gains access to the circulation as the result of a medical procedure. The vast majority of these emboli are discovered incidentally at autopsy and are of little or no clinical or radiologic importance; rarely, they are sufficient in number or size to result in pathophysiologic consequences identical to those of tissue or thromboemboli.

## FAT EMBOLISM

Although intact fragments of adipose tissue (usually with admixed hematopoietic cells) are often found in the pulmonary arteries following severe trauma, the term *fat embolism* traditionally refers to the presence of globules of free fat within the vasculature.[4–8] Exogenous fatty material, such as ethiodized oil used as radiographic contrast media and vegetable oil, is also usually excluded from the definition and is discussed separately (*see* page 1861).

The presence of numerous fat globules in the small pulmonary vessels results in dyspnea and hypoxemia. From the pulmonary circulation, the globules pass into the systemic circulation and embolize to many organs, notably the brain and skin, where they result in a variety of neurologic

**Table 49–1. PULMONARY EMBOLI OF TISSUE AND TISSUE SECRETIONS**

| EMBOLIZED TISSUE/ SECRETION | PREDISPOSING CONDITION | SELECTED REFERENCE(S) |
|---|---|---|
| Skin | Venipuncture | 320 |
| Liver | Massive hepatic necrosis or trauma | 321 |
| Bone | Bone marrow transplantation; fracture | 322 |
| Bone marrow | Accidental fracture or external cardiac massage | *See* page 1850 |
| Fat | Trauma; uncommonly fatty liver, drugs, hyperalimentation | *See* page 1845 |
| Cartilage | Fracture | 323 |
| Myocardium | Cardiac surgery | 324 |
| Transitional epithelium | Urethritis | 325 |
| Neural tissue | Head trauma or surgery | 1, 326 |
| Gastrointestinal contents | Budd-Chiari syndrome and ileal diverticulitis | 327 |
| Bile | Hepatic trauma in patients with biliary tract obstruction (often iatrogenic) | 328 |
| Retroperitoneal soft tissue | Pancreatic transplantation | 2 |
| Amniotic fluid | Older multiparous women with fetal distress and (sometimes) tumultuous labor | *See* page 1850 |

manifestations and cutaneous petechiae. The combination of respiratory, neurologic, and cutaneous disease constitutes the fat embolism syndrome.

### Epidemiology

The precise incidence of pulmonary fat embolism is difficult to ascertain, partly because diagnostic criteria are variable and partly because the majority of cases result in no clinical manifestations. It is likely, however, that asymptomatic emboli are very common; autopsy studies of patients who have experienced severe trauma reveal them in the vast majority of cases,[9] and measurement of fat globules in the venous circulation shows that they occur almost invariably during orthopedic prosthesis insertion.[5] (Despite this, there is experimental evidence that the severity of fat embolization is the same whether fractures are stabilized by intramedullary nailing or external plate fixation.[10]) The incidence of clinically significant disease in patients who have simple tibial or femoral fractures is generally believed to be about 1% to 3%[4, 11] (although some investigators have found a much higher value[12]). In individuals who have more severe trauma, the incidence of clinically evident embolism is probably in the range of 10% to 20%.[4, 5]

Severe accidental or battlefield trauma is the most common antecedent of pulmonary fat embolism; autopsy series of patients who have died after such injury show an incidence as high as 90%,[9, 11, 13] and the majority of cases of clinically significant disease occur in this setting. Despite this, it is important to remember that the syndrome can occur in patients with a history of relatively minor injury, such as tibial fracture[12] or even simple falling and bruising;[14] development of clinical symptoms in the latter situation may be more frequent in patients in whom the pulmonary vasculature is already compromised by disease, such as emphysema or kyphoscoliosis.[14] Pulmonary fat embolism has also been reported in patients and in experimental animals that have suffered crush injury,[15] suggesting an origin from nonosseous fat; however, such emboli are unlikely to be important unless extensive areas of the body are involved,

in which circumstance it is difficult to exclude concomitant bone trauma.

In addition to these forms of trauma, a wide variety of surgical procedures and medical conditions that disrupt the marrow can cause fat emboli (Table 49–2). One of the more important of these is sickle cell disease, in which fat emboli have been hypothesized to be a cause of some cases of the acute chest syndrome seen in this condition[16, 17] (*see* page 1832). The same complication has been reported rarely in patients who have thalassemia.[18] Diseases that involve adipose tissue outside the marrow are also rarely complicated by fat emboli.

### Pathogenesis

There are two theories concerning the origin of fat in the fat embolism syndrome. As is evident from the foregoing discussion, epidemiologic features suggest that the commonest source is the bone marrow, embolism developing after entry of disrupted fat into lacerated medullary veins. Although intuitively one might expect an increase in intramedullary pressure to accompany the entry of fat into the torn veins, experimental evidence suggests that this may not be necessary.[19] Observations in favor of the bone marrow as the origin of emboli include the following:[15] (1) the detection of free fat in the vicinity of recent fractures; (2) the development of pulmonary fat emboli in experimental animals after fracture or marrow disruption; (3) the presence of fat globules in the blood of humans after fractures and a variety of orthopedic procedures; (4) the frequency with which embolized bone marrow fragments are present in association with fat emboli (*see* page 1850); (5) the presence of a positive correlation between the extent of pulmonary fat embolism and the severity of bone injury; (6) the prevention of fat embolism in experimental fractures by prior venous ligation or application of a tourniquet on the affected limb; and (7) experiments in which marrow fat stained with a dye has been traced to the lung.

It has also been postulated that embolized fat can be derived from altered blood lipoproteins or chylomicrons or

**Table 49–2. PULMONARY FAT EMBOLISM**

| ETIOLOGY | COMMENT | SELECTED REFERENCE(S) |
|---|---|---|
| *External Trauma* | | |
| Major accident/battlefield trauma | The most common cause of clinically significant emboli | 9, 37, 44 |
| Isolated long bone fracture | | 12 |
| External cardiac massage | | 329–331 |
| *Surgery or Medical Procedures* | | |
| Orthopedic procedures | Intramedullary prosthesis insertion and reaming, arthroplasty | 332–334 |
| Intraosseous venography | | 53 |
| Liposuction | | 335, 336 |
| Bone marrow transplantation and harvesting | | 337, 338 |
| Venous hyperalimentation | | 339 |
| Lung transplantation | Following trauma-related embolism in the donor lung | 341 |
| Drug therapy | Cyclosporine, cisplatin | 340, 342 |
| *Underlying Disease* | | |
| Pancreatitis | | 343 |
| Diabetes mellitus | | 344 |
| Acute osteomyelitis | | 345 |
| Osteoporosis | Compression fracture | 346 |
| Sickle cell disease | | 64 |
| Thalassemia | | 347 |
| Hepatic steatosis | Secondary to drugs (e.g., steroids), poisons (e.g., carbon tetrachloride), and alcohol | 15, 348–350 |
| Epilepsy | | 351, 352 |
| Burns | | 353 |
| Decompression sickness | | 354 |
| Teratoma (ovarian dermoid tumor) | | 355 |
| Immobilization | Experimental animal study | 356 |

from stress-induced lipemia.[11, 15, 20] According to this hypothesis, a substance in the blood—the most likely being C-reactive protein—causes agglutination of plasma lipid into particles sufficient in size to obstruct pulmonary capillaries. Although it seems unlikely that this mechanism is involved in most cases of fat embolism, the possibility that it occurs in some cannot be excluded.

The pathogenetic mechanisms involved in the production of the pulmonary component of the fat embolism syndrome are probably twofold. The first is mechanical obstruction of pulmonary vessels, predominantly by fat globules themselves and possibly enhanced in some cases by platelet or red blood cell aggregates.[21] Evidence suggesting the importance of this effect includes the histologic identification of fat in the small pulmonary vessels and the observation that pulmonary arterial pressure rises transiently in experimental animals soon after embolization.[10, 22–24]

A second, biochemically mediated, process likely ensues after this initial obstructive effect has subsided (presumably due in part to passage of fat through the pulmonary capillaries into the pulmonary veins and, ultimately, systemic vasculature). Fat appears to be transported to the lungs as neutral triglycerides,[25] and it has been proposed that these triglycerides are converted by endothelial lipases into free fatty acids that then exert a direct toxic effect on the alveolar wall.[26] The resulting damage could in turn lead to the activation of complement or the release of toxins from leukocytes, further exaggerating the injury.[27] Supporting this argument are experimental investigations in which severe pulmonary edema and hemorrhage have resulted from the injection of free fatty acids into the pulmonary arteries.[28–30] However, in other experimental studies in which neutral fat has been injected into the systemic veins evidence for conversion to free fatty acids has not been found.[29, 31–33] It is also possible that intravascular coagulation, possibly instituted by thromboplastin released from the fat itself, may be important in the pathogenesis of the syndrome.[34, 35] The results of one experimental investigation suggested that endothelin and atrial natriuretic peptide have little, if any, pathogenetic role.[36]

Typically, the full clinical syndrome of fat embolism develops 1 to 2 days after trauma. Although the reasons for this delay are unclear, it has been suggested that they may be explained by (1) continuing embolization from the initial site of injury, (2) a time delay in the conversion of neutral triglycerides to unsaturated fatty acids, and (3) an imbalance between coagulation and fibrinolysis, leading to increasing deposition of fibrin in pulmonary vessels.[15]

Although the experimental observations cited previously and the presence of radiographic changes and clinical signs and symptoms shortly after trauma have understandably led to the belief that intravascular fat is responsible for the pulmonary disease that develops in patients who have fat embolism, there is evidence that this conclusion may not be entirely correct. For example, in some autopsy[37, 38] and clinical investigations[39] little correlation has been found between the presence of intravascular fat and clinical manifestations. In addition, although there is some indication that early surgical stabilization of extensive long bone fractures can decrease the incidence and severity of post-traumatic pulmonary insufficiency,[40, 41] when pelvic or long bone fractures are unaccompanied by sepsis or by severe injuries to the brain, chest, or abdomen, the severity of pulmonary disease appears to be relatively mild and recovery is common.[42] As a result of these observations, the significance of pulmonary fat emboli in previously healthy individuals has been questioned, and it has been hypothesized that the clinical findings associated with the emboli may in fact be the result of a concomitant disease process.[15, 39]

### Pathologic Characteristics

Pathologically, the lungs of patients who have died with fat emboli are frequently heavy—ranging from 870 to 1400 gm in one series of approximately 100 cases[37]—and show patchy areas of hemorrhage and edema.[15] On hematoxylin and eosin–stained sections, the presence of fat within arterioles and capillaries can be suspected when there are round-to-oval spaces, 20 to 40 μm in diameter, apparently compressing red blood cells to one side (Fig. 49–1). Fat can also be seen within macrophages in alveolar air spaces. Definitive diagnosis requires the use of fat-soluble dyes on unfixed (frozen) tissue or osmium tetroxide on formalin-fixed tissue handled by an "en bloc" technique.[43]

Fat can appear within pulmonary capillaries very rapidly after trauma;[15, 44] histologic evidence of its presence is rare if the interval between injury and death is more than 4 weeks.[45]

### Radiologic Manifestations

As indicated previously, pulmonary fat embolism is unrecognized in many cases if it is not severe, partly because symptoms are mild or absent but also because the chest radiograph result is often normal—as, for example, in 87% of patients in one series in whom the diagnosis was based on the presence of lipiduria.[46] When present, the radiographic findings are those of adult respiratory distress syndrome (ARDS) of any cause, consisting of widespread air-space consolidation (Fig. 49–2). The distribution is predominantly

peripheral rather than central[47, 48] and usually affects the basal regions to a greater degree than does pulmonary edema of cardiac origin. Further differentiation from cardiogenic edema is provided by the absence of cardiac enlargement and signs of pulmonary venous hypertension; however, in one study of 30 patients, diffuse linear opacities resembling interstitial edema were just as common as air-space opacities.[49] Pleural effusions are typically absent.

The time lapse between trauma and radiographic signs is usually 1 to 2 days.[47, 50] This delay differentiates fat embolism from traumatic lung contusion, in which the radiographic opacity invariably appears immediately after injury. In addition, whereas the latter opacity usually clears rapidly (in about 24 hours), the resolution of fat embolism usually takes 7 to 10 days and occasionally up to 4 weeks.[51] Further differentiation lies in the extent of lung involvement: contusion seldom affects both lungs diffusely and symmetrically; when both lungs are involved, the radiographic findings are usually more severe in the lung deep to the site of maximal trauma.

In one case, multiple small nodular opacities developed following fat embolism and ARDS that were shown to be calcified on computed tomography (CT) scans;[52] the majority of calcifications were interpreted on CT as being located in branches of the pulmonary arteries. A technetium-99m diphosphonate bone scan demonstrated diffuse uptake over the lungs. The patient had no symptoms except for mild dyspnea on exertion.

### Clinical Manifestations

Although symptoms may appear almost immediately after the event causing embolization,[53, 54] in most cases there is a delay of 12 to 24 hours; sometimes, the delay is as long as 3 days.[55] The most common pulmonary symptom is dyspnea; cough, hemoptysis, and pleural pain occur occasionally. Signs include pyrexia, tachypnea, tachycardia, fine

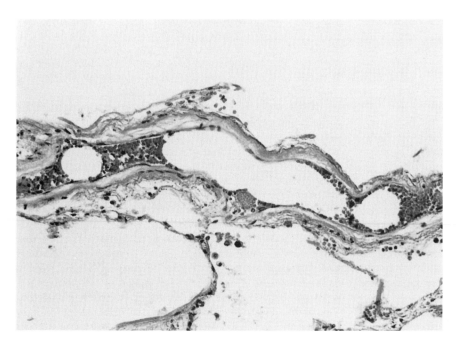

**Figure 49–1. Fat Emboli.** The lumen of this pulmonary arteriole shows one elongated and two circular spaces that are devoid of blood cells. Such an appearance is suggestive of fat and was confirmed by lipid stains. This histologic section is from a young man who died several hours after a motor vehicle accident; there was no clinical or pathologic evidence of acute lung damage. (×190.)

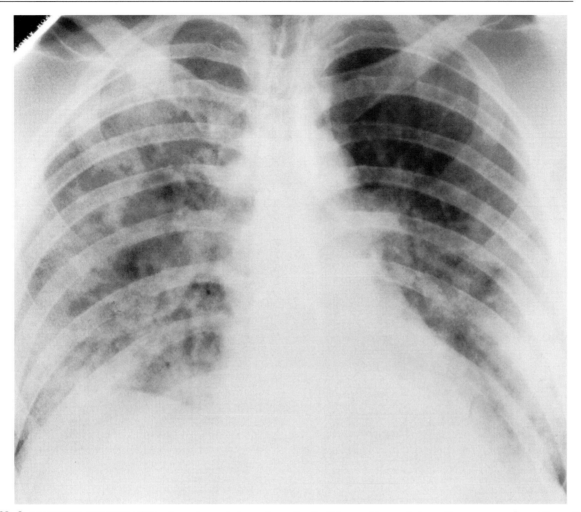

**Figure 49–2. Traumatic Fat Embolism.** An anteroposterior radiograph of a 21-year-old man 3 days after a severe automobile accident reveals extensive involvement of both lungs by patchy shadows of unit density. In many areas the shadows are confluent, but in some they are relatively discrete. For some unknown reason, the left upper lung is less severely involved. Complete radiographic resolution occurred 7 days later.

inspiratory crackles, and (occasionally) rhonchi and friction rub.[11, 55] Acute cor pulmonale with cardiac failure, cyanosis, and circulatory shock may occur.[55]

Symptoms of systemic fat embolism are seen in up to 85% of patients who have pulmonary disease.[4] They are chiefly related to the central nervous system and include confusion, restlessness, stupor, delirium, seizures, and coma. Skin involvement is also frequent (20% to 50% of cases[4]) and typically manifests as a petechial rash appearing 2 to 3 days after embolization.[55] The petechiae are particularly prominent along the anterior axillary folds[56] and in the conjunctiva and retina, a distribution that has been attributed to fat floating in the bloodstream and thus affecting vessels that are uppermost.[57] Although these systemic manifestations are usually the result of fat traversing the pulmonary circulation, rarely they follow paradoxical embolization directly through a patent foramen ovale.[58]

### Laboratory Findings and Diagnosis

Hypocalcemia may develop because of the affinity of calcium ions for free fatty acids released by the hydrolysis of embolized fat.[55] Thrombocytopenia is common[56] and may be associated with disseminated intravascular coagulation.[49] Hemolytic anemia occurs in some cases.[55, 59] Lipiduria is not uncommon,[55] and hematuria and proteinuria are seen occasionally.[4] Fat droplets are found rarely in cerebrospinal fluid.[60]

Pulmonary function tests reveal decreased compliance and an increased A-a $O_2$ gradient as a result of $\dot{V}/\dot{Q}$ inequality.[55, 61] Severe hypoxemia may persist despite inhalation of 100% oxygen.[61] Decreased diffusing capacity[62] and $Pa_{O_2}$[63] have been observed in patients with fractures of the long bones who have no chest symptoms, possibly reflecting subclinical fat embolism.

The antemortem diagnosis of pulmonary fat embolism can be difficult, partly because of the relative nonspecificity of signs and symptoms and partly because clinical abnormalities may be related more directly to the cause of the emboli (e.g., trauma-associated shock). Several techniques for identifying fat in the lungs or vasculature have been employed in an attempt to improve the accuracy of diagnosis. Some investigators have advocated the use of bronchoalveolar lavage (BAL) and analysis of harvested macrophages for the presence of fat.[64–66] However, patients who do not have fat embolism syndrome may also have lipid-laden macrophages in their BAL fluid (including some who have not experienced trauma),[66-69] and it has been suggested that the diagnosis is supported only when the percentage of abnormal macrophages is greater than a defined threshold; unfortunately, the definitive level of such a threshold is unclear, some investigators proposing a value as low as 5%[65] and others one as high as 30%.[66]

Analysis of blood aspirated from a wedged pulmonary artery catheter has also been used to identify the presence of fat in both experimental animals[70] and patients.[71] However, serum fat globules are probably present in the majority of patients with skeletal trauma whether or not they have fat embolism syndrome,[5] and controlled studies investigating the specificity of the test have not been performed. Transesophageal echocardiography has been used by some investigators to detect emboli during bone marrow reaming.[35, 72]

Several diagnostic schema based on a combination of clinical and laboratory findings have been proposed;[67, 73, 74] however, their practical usefulness has not been established clearly.

### Prognosis

It has been estimated that approximately 10% of patients who have pulmonary symptoms of fat embolism syndrome progress to respiratory failure.[75] As might be expected, those who develop features of ARDS are the most likely to succumb.[55] Rarely, patients die rapidly following trauma as a result of cardiovascular collapse.[54] Follow-up generally shows a return to normal pulmonary function.[11]

### BONE MARROW EMBOLISM

Not uncommonly, fragments of bone marrow are present in the pulmonary arteries of individuals who have sustained fractures or experienced external cardiac massage. In one investigation of 51 patients who had undergone the latter procedure, eight (15%) showed such emboli.[76] In another review of 203 consecutive autopsies of patients who had sustained multiple fractures, bone marrow emboli were identified in 13 (6%).[77] We expect that if a larger number of tissue sections were examined, the number of affected individuals would be even greater. The incidence is also likely influenced by the severity of the trauma; for example, in a study of lungs from 205 victims of an airplane crash (in which injury was undoubtedly severe), emboli were found in 60 (29%).[44]

Although most common following accidental fractures and external cardiac massage, a number of other conditions in which bone disruption may occur have been associated with bone marrow emboli, including convulsions (caused by electroconvulsive therapy, epilepsy, eclampsia, or tetanus[77]), bone biopsy,[78] and even vertebral compression fractures related to osteoporosis.[79] It is likely that emboli are also frequent but unrecognized in individuals who sustain solitary and nonlethal fractures or who undergo certain orthopedic procedures such as total hip replacement. Fragments of infarcted marrow, in the absence of known trauma, can also be found in patients who have sickle cell disease.[80]

As in fat embolism, the pathogenesis of bone marrow embolism is related to traumatic fragmentation of marrow and its entry under pressure into disrupted sinusoids or veins. Free fat emboli are probably also present in the majority of cases; in fact, in the study of plane crash victims cited previously, a positive correlation was found between the extent of fat and bone marrow embolization.[44]

The embolized fragments usually are identified histologically as incidental findings within small muscular arteries or arterioles. Tissue may fill the lumen completely or partly; in the latter case, thrombus may develop at its periphery. Experimental studies have documented periarterial interstitial edema in vessels distal to the emboli;[81] the adjacent pulmonary parenchyma shows no consistent abnormality. When emboli are recent, the histologic appearance is that of normal marrow; occasionally, spicules of bone can be identified[77, 82] (Fig. 49–3). With time, the hematopoietic cells degenerate and disappear and the residual fat and necrotic cells become incorporated into the vessel wall as a fibrous plaque.[82, 83] Infarction of lung parenchyma has not been documented.

The vast majority of bone marrow emboli are of no clinical or radiographic significance, being discovered incidentally at autopsy or in surgically excised lungs. Although they have been implicated as a major or contributory cause of death by some investigators[79] and experimental studies in rabbits have suggested that they may lead to chronic pulmonary hypertension,[83] we feel that physiologic and clinical effects are more likely related to associated free fat embolism or to concomitant systemic disease than to marrow fragments themselves.

### AMNIOTIC FLUID EMBOLISM

Amniotic fluid embolism is a highly lethal complication of pregnancy in which amniotic fluid enters the bloodstream through tears in the uterine veins and results in rapid cardiopulmonary collapse.[4, 5, 84, 85] The precise incidence of the condition is difficult to establish. In one review of cases from 1984 to 1993 in Brisbane, the incidence of fatal disease was 3.37 per 100,000 pregnancies;[86] this figure can be compared with an incidence of 1.03 per 100,000 in Australia as a whole over a 27-year period. However, because of the difficulty in unequivocally confirming the diagnosis, both during life and at autopsy, and because of the presence of nonlethal but unsubstantiated disease in an unspecified number of women,[87, 88] the true incidence is almost certainly greater than these figures suggest. It has been estimated that about 10% of peripartum maternal deaths in the United States are caused by the disease.[89] The abnormality has been documented in association with saline amnioinfusion[90] and in the presence of an intrauterine contraceptive device.[85]

### Pathogenesis

Amniotic fluid is composed of fetal urine, secretions from the amniotic membrane, and a variety of particulate material, including squames and lanugo hairs from the fetal skin, fat from the vernix caseosa, and mucin and bile from the meconium. At term, the normal volume is approximately

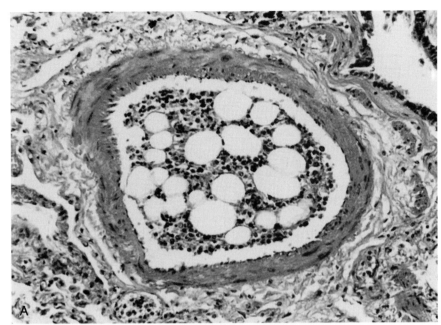

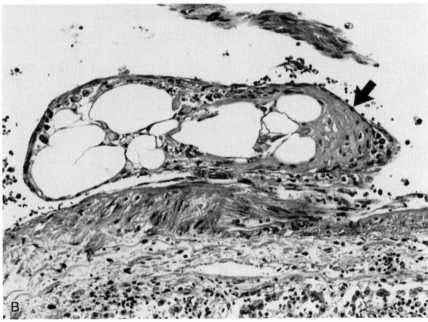

**Figure 49–3. Bone Marrow Emboli.** A section of a muscular pulmonary artery (A) contains a recent bone marrow embolus from a patient with myocardial infarction who underwent unsuccessful resuscitation. In a section from another patient who had successful resuscitation but died approximately 4 weeks later (B), the embolus is partly organized; note the loss of marrow cells, focal fibrosis (arrow), and adherence of the embolus to the vessel wall. (A and B, ×180.)

1 liter. There is reasonable evidence suggesting that little, if any, amniotic fluid enters the maternal circulation during normal pregnancy, labor, or delivery. For example, histologic studies of the lungs of mothers dying in the peripartum period without clinical evidence of amniotic fluid embolism have found microscopic evidence of embolism in only about 1% of cases.[91, 92] In addition, in one investigation of normal women in whom isotopically labeled red blood cells were injected into the amniotic sac before childbirth, no radioactivity was found in maternal blood in the peri- or postpartum periods.[93]

The results of these studies indicate that significant amniotic fluid embolism probably occurs only when there is disruption of the uterine wall in association with rupture of the placental membranes. Such disruption can occur at several sites, the most common probably being the endocervix or lower uterine segment. Traumatic tears in the small veins in these regions can occur during normal labor but are of no significance if covered by fetal membranes; however, if these have separated, uterine contractions against a head impacted in the birth canal can repeatedly "pump" amniotic fluid into the maternal venous circulation. Amniotic fluid can also enter the maternal circulation at the placental site—usually in cases of uterine rupture, placenta previa, or cesarean section when the incision involves the placental implantation site—and rarely elsewhere in the uterine wall in association with myometrial trauma.

The pathophysiologic consequences of intravascular amniotic fluid are complex and related to several potential mechanisms.

**Pulmonary Vascular Obstruction.** Once amniotic fluid enters the maternal circulation, particulate matter is quickly filtered out in the pulmonary vascular bed. It has been speculated that vascular obstruction by such particulates—particularly meconium[87, 94]—leads to an acute rise in pulmonary artery pressure and right heart failure. In support of this hypothesis are animal experiments documenting a transient increase in pulmonary artery pressure after embolization, as well as studies in which the injection of filtered amniotic fluid into the peripheral and pulmonary circulation has resulted in no significant harmful effect.[94, 95] However, the methodology of these animal studies has been questioned.[4] Moreover, hemodynamic investigations in humans have found little evidence of a significant change in pulmonary artery pressure,[4, 84] and autopsy studies have shown little correlation between the amount of intravascular particulate matter and clinical findings.[96] Thus, although it is not possible to exclude vascular obstruction as a pathogenetic factor in amniotic fluid embolism, its contribution is uncertain. It is also possible that when pulmonary hypertension does develop, it is the result of a direct effect on the pulmonary vasculature of mediators such as endothelin.[97]

**Left Ventricular Dysfunction.** Hemodynamic studies of some patients who have amniotic fluid embolism have shown decreased cardiac index and elevated pulmonary capillary wedge pressure consistent with acute left ventricular failure.[98, 99] Echocardiographic evidence of cardiomyopathy has also been documented in some of these patients.[100] Although the mechanism of such myocardial dysfunction is unclear, it has been speculated that it may be important in the development of pulmonary edema.[98]

**Adult Respiratory Distress Syndrome.** The pathogenesis of pulmonary edema in amniotic fluid embolism is probably multifactorial. In some patients, it may be related to left ventricular dysfunction as described previously or to the effects of increased extracellular fluid and decreased plasma oncotic pressure normally found at term, or to both. However, studies of some patients with pulmonary edema have revealed a normal left ventricular function[101] and an edema fluid-to-plasma protein ratio greater than 0.9,[102] both of which are consistent with ARDS. As a result, it has been speculated that some constituent of amniotic fluid may directly damage the vascular endothelium and produce capillary leakage. The nature of this agent is uncertain; however, in addition to the various particulate materials, several potent chemical substances are present in normal amniotic fluid, including prostaglandins $E_2$ and $F_{2a}$[103] and leukotriene $B_4$,[104] which theoretically may be involved.

**Anaphylaxis.** The findings in early experiments of amniotic fluid embolism were thought to simulate anaphylactic shock.[94] Although it has been speculated that substances such as meconium or blood group antigens might act as agents triggering such an immunologic reaction,[4, 87] definite evidence that such a mechanism truly exists is lacking. However, a review of cases of the National Amniotic Fluid Embolism Registry in the United States led investigators to conclude that the clinical and hemodynamic features of the disease are similar to those of both anaphylaxis and septic shock, suggesting common pathogenetic mechanisms.[105]

**Infection and Septic Shock.** Some cases of amniotic fluid embolism are associated with the prolonged rupture of membranes and the presence of infected amniotic fluid,[87] in which circumstance systemic hypotension might be related in part to endotoxemia. In the appropriate clinical setting, the presence of positive blood cultures and histologic evidence of chorioamnionitis should suggest this possibility.

**Coagulation Disturbances.** Amniotic fluid is a powerful coagulant; 1 ml of a thrombokinase-like constituent (possibly tissue factor[106]) within it is capable of coagulating 10 liters of blood.[107] Because of this property, introduction of even small amounts of fluid into the systemic circulation can cause profound disturbances in coagulation. Such disturbances occur in up to 40% of patients who survive the first hour after embolization[108] and are manifested by severe fibrin depletion and the clinical and pathologic picture of disseminated intravascular coagulation.[109, 110]

## Pathologic Characteristics

Grossly, the lungs may be edematous and show focal areas of hemorrhage, but frequently the findings are unremarkable;[87, 111] in one series of 40 cases, the average combined lung weight was only 750 gm.[112] The most striking histologic abnormality is the presence of foreign material within capillaries, arterioles, and (occasionally) medium- to small-sized pulmonary arteries. This material consists of squames, fragments of hair (which are refractile and can be demonstrated by polarization microscopy), and somewhat amorphous basophilic material (sometimes containing greenish-yellow pigment) that is considered to represent mucin and bile derived from meconium. Identical material can be seen in the systemic circulation, particularly in the brain and kidney; however, in these sites it is generally considered to be without clinical or pathologic importance.[87, 112, 113] In experimental animals, squames can be identified up to 3 weeks and lanugo hairs and mucin up to 7 months after the intravenous injection of human amniotic fluid;[114] in most instances, little histologic reaction is present. In one patient, a lung biopsy performed 1 month after the embolic episode confirmed the suspected diagnosis.[115]

Although much intravascular foreign material can be recognized with hematoxylin and eosin stain, its presence is more easily demonstrated using special techniques, which should always be performed before excluding a diagnosis of amniotic fluid embolism pathologically. Several techniques can be employed, including histochemical staining for acid mucopolysaccharides or fat[116] and immunohistochemical reactions for keratin (to identify squames),[117] fetal isoantigen (in cases in which it differs from that of the mother),[118] or sialyl Tn (an antigen related to a glycoprotein found in amniotic fluid).[119]

Pathologic evidence of uterine trauma is present in many cases, either as cervical lacerations[111] or as amniotic fluid within vessels in the myometrium, cervix, or broad ligament.[112] Occasionally, the identification of such fluid in these vessels has been the definitive diagnostic procedure.[120]

## Radiologic Manifestations

Radiographic changes in the lungs are poorly documented; in most cases, the condition is fatal so rapidly that radiographs are not obtained, and few of the rare nonfatal cases are diagnosed. In line with the pathologic characteristics, the principal radiographic finding is air-space edema indistinguishable from acute pulmonary edema of other cause.[115, 121–124] Whether cardiac enlargement accompanies the edema depends on the severity of pulmonary arterial hypertension and consequent cor pulmonale with or without left ventricular failure. The consolidation may progress to ARDS or resolve within a few days.[124] Because the predominant radiographic manifestation is widespread air-space consolidation, the chief differential diagnoses are massive pulmonary hemorrhage and aspiration of liquid gastric contents.

### Clinical Manifestations

The vast majority of patients are in the 35th to 42nd week of pregnancy at the time of embolization. The clinical manifestations are typically abrupt in onset and rapid in progression.[112, 125] Although symptoms begin during spontaneous labor in most patients, they occur after delivery in about 30% (10% spontaneous and 20% postcesarean section).[105] In one series of 40 cases, disease was heralded by dyspnea and cyanosis in 20 patients, sudden profound shock disproportionate to blood loss in 12, and signs of central nervous system irritability (convulsions, hyperreflexia, and other signs) in 8.[112] Nonspecific symptoms such as shivering, anxiety, cough, vomiting, and sensation of a bad taste may also be elicited.[4] Clinical evidence of consumptive coagulopathy is present in as many as 40% of patients and is the presenting feature in 10% to 15%.[4]

Predisposing factors that have been identified include tumultuous labor, meconium in the amniotic fluid, intrauterine fetal distress and death, older age of the mother, premature placental separation, and multiparity.[112] The first is theoretically important because of the attendant increase in uterine pressure; however, it is important to recognize that tumultuous labor is not a prerequisite for amniotic fluid embolism, being described in less than 30% of patients in one series[112] and in only 28% of reported cases in a review of the literature.[85] In addition, in the analysis of the National Registry cases, no association with prolonged labor was evident.[105] Interestingly, investigators in the last-named review found a significant association with male fetal sex. Prolonged gestation, large infants, and type of delivery do not appear to be important risk factors.

### Laboratory Findings and Diagnosis

Fibrinogen levels are low in many patients, even in the absence of clinical features of disseminated intravascular coagulation. A decreased platelet count as well as increased prothrombin and partial thromboplastin times may be evident. Arterial blood gas analysis generally shows hypoxemia and a mixed metabolic and respiratory acidosis.

Because of the frequently rapid and lethal course, the initial diagnosis should be considered seriously on the basis of the appropriate clinical findings alone. Confirmation may follow by cytologic examination of blood aspirated from a Swan-Ganz catheter (pulmonary microvascular cytology),[88, 126] the diagnosis being supported by identifying squames (particularly when associated with neutrophils), mucin, or hair fragments. The validity of this technique has been questioned by investigators who have documented the presence of squames in aspirated blood of patients who

clearly do not have amniotic fluid embolism (the squames believed to be contaminants from the patient's or operator's skin).[127] However, the methodology of these studies has in turn been questioned,[84] and it seems reasonable to consider the presence of large numbers of squames in blood samples aspirated from the pulmonary microvasculature to be at least supportive of the diagnosis.

Other relatively recent techniques for diagnosis of amniotic fluid embolism involve measurement of substances in maternal blood. One group of investigators has advocated quantification of serum sialyl Tn antigen using the monoclonal antibody TKH-2;[128] according to their findings, such determination is both easy to perform and sensitive. Another group has made similar claims concerning the fluorometric measurement of zinc coproporphyrin I (also a characteristic component of amniotic fluid) in maternal plasma.[129]

### Prognosis

Amniotic fluid embolism is a serious and frequently fulminant disease: the mortality rate of clinically recognized cases varies from 60% to 85%,[105, 130] 25% to 50% of patients dying within the first hour of the disease and most of the rest within 12 hours.[4, 125] Cardiopulmonary collapse is the most common cause of death; disseminated intravascular coagulation is an important additional factor in some patients. There are few follow-up studies of survivors; those that have been done have found little, if any, functional pulmonary disability.[131, 132] However, serious neurologic sequelae are common.[105] Subsequent uneventful pregnancies have been documented.[132]

## EMBOLIC MANIFESTATIONS OF PARASITIC INFESTATION

Immature forms of many human metazoan parasites travel through the systemic circulation to the lungs, where they lodge within pulmonary arterioles and capillaries. In most such cases, the clinical and pathologic effects are not related to vascular obstruction or damage; instead, pulmonary disease typically occurs in the adjacent lung parenchyma and represents a host reaction to the migrating organism during part of its life cycle. Examples of parasites that cause this form of disease include *Ascaris lumbricoides*, *Strongyloides stercoralis*, *Ancylostoma duodenale*, *Necator americanus*, *Toxocara canis* and *Toxocara cati*, *Paragonimus* species, *Wuchereria bancrofti*, and *Brugia malayi*.

Occasionally, embolized parasites cause disease that is related directly to pulmonary vascular obstruction. Undoubtedly, the most important such disease is schistosomiasis, in which eggs released into the systemic or portal venous circulation lodge within pulmonary arteries and arterioles and cause endarteritis obliterans and pulmonary arterial hypertension. Embolized *Ascaris suum* eggs rarely have the same effect.[133] Fragmented or whole mature parasites also can be transported to the lung and become lodged within larger pulmonary vessels. The commonest of these is *Dirofilaria immitis*, which is typically associated with parenchymal necrosis manifested radiographically as a solitary pulmonary nodule. Rarely, other adult worms such as *Schistosoma* species behave similarly.[134] An unusual complication of hepatic hydatid disease occurs when a cyst ruptures into the hepatic veins and its contents are embolized to the lungs.[135] A thorough discussion of these parasites and the diseases they cause is given in Chapter 30 (*see* page 1033).

## EMBOLISM OF NEOPLASTIC TISSUE

Because all cases of hematogenous pulmonary metastases must be derived from tumor fragments lodged within pulmonary vessels, it is evident that these are one of the most common forms of emboli. Because of the small size of most tumor fragments, however, effects related to vascular obstruction are seldom apparent. However, when tumor emboli are of sufficient size or number, the clinical, pathologic, and radiographic manifestations are identical to those of thromboemboli and include pulmonary infarction, acute cor pulmonale and sudden death, and a slowly progressive syndrome of dyspnea and pulmonary hypertension.[136] Although the diagnosis is rarely made on conventional radiography,[137] it may be suspected on CT by the presence of multifocal nodular opacities in the distribution of peripheral pulmonary arteries, leading to a beaded appearance of these vessels.[138, 139] The subject is considered in greater detail in Chapter 38 (*see* page 1397).

## AIR EMBOLISM

As with thrombi and other solid material, embolism of air* within the circulation can have important consequences,

---

*Although air itself is frequently the substance that enters the vasculature, in some cases the causative agent is gas, either altered air from the lungs or pure gas such as carbon dioxide, oxygen, or helium.[142-144] Although strictly speaking the appropriate term for the abnormality is thus *gas embolism*, because of conventional use we retain the designation *air embolism* in this text.

including stroke, cardiovascular collapse, and death. Although such emboli are uncommonly recognized clinically, it is likely that subclinical emboli occur much more frequently than is generally appreciated.[140, 141]

### Pathogenesis

Air emboli may have their origin in either the greater or the lesser circulation, the predisposing situations and pathophysiologic effects differing significantly between the two sites. In *systemic (arterial)* air embolism, air typically enters the pulmonary venous circulation and passes to the left side of the heart and then to the systemic arteries; the effects are therefore manifested chiefly in the heart, the spinal cord, and the brain. By contrast, in *pulmonary (venous)* air embolism, air usually enters the systemic venous circulation and passes to the right side of the heart and then to the lungs; clinical and functional manifestations are thus related to obstruction of the pulmonary circulation and are felt predominantly by the lungs.[145]

### *Systemic Air Embolism*

Air can gain access to the pulmonary veins only when there is an opening in a vessel exposed to air and the pressure of the air exceeds that in the vessel lumen. These two criteria are met in a variety of circumstances (Table 49–3). The easiest to comprehend and possibly the most common is penetrating thoracic trauma, either accidental or iatrogenic (e.g., the insertion of a needle into the thoracic cavity for thoracentesis or needle biopsy[146, 147] or bronchoscopic laser surgery[148]). Less commonly, nonpenetrating thoracic trauma leads to the same complication.[149]

Systemic air embolism is also a feared complication of

## Table 49–3. SYSTEMIC (ARTERIAL) AIR EMBOLISM

| ETIOLOGY | COMMENT | SELECTED REFERENCE(S) |
|---|---|---|
| *Cardiac Surgery* | | |
| Open heart | Most common; residual air in pulmonary veins released into circulation after cross-clamping terminated | 140 |
| Coronary artery bypass | | |
| Iatrogenic fistula | Between lung and left atrium | 357 |
| *Penetrating Thoracic Trauma* | | |
| Transthoracic needle aspiration | | 147, 201 |
| Thoracentesis | | |
| YAG laser bronchial surgery | Laser-related bronchovascular fistula | 359, 360 |
| Accidents | | |
| *Intrinsic Lung Disease* | | |
| Asthma | | 155 |
| Neonatal respiratory distress syndrome | | 156, 157 |
| Pulmonary abscess | Fistula between pulmonary vessel and bronchus | 193 |
| *Barotrauma* | | |
| Positive pressure ventilation | | 161 |
| Compressed air diving | | 150 |
| Air travel | | 154a |
| *Miscellaneous* | | |
| Hydrogen peroxide ingestion | | 361 |
| Prosthetic aortic valves | | 358 |

scuba diving that can occur if a diver fails to expel pressurized gas from the lung during ascent.[150, 151] Most commonly, the resulting pulmonary overpressurization syndrome is related to the presence of mediastinal or subcutaneous air and is characterized by chest pain, hoarseness, and/or neck fullness; more serious consequences develop if there is also dissemination of air through the systemic circulation. Gas trapped in a bulla or behind completely or partially obstructed airways also may undergo expansion during ascent and rupture into the pulmonary vasculature, allowing access of gas to the pulmonary veins and ultimately the systemic vasculature. Asthmatic patients may be especially susceptible to this complication: two cases of cerebral air emboli have been reported in such individuals practicing scuba diving in a swimming pool.[152] The volume of gas in a space distal to a partly or completely occluded bronchus doubles every 33 feet of a diver's ascent and can produce sufficient distention to "explode" the air space.[153] In fact, the diving depth need not be nearly as much as 33 feet to produce this complication; for example, a case has been described of a 21-year-old man who died during an attempt to swim across a 25-yard pool at a depth of 6 feet.[154] The barotrauma of ascent can also occur in airplane passengers, typically in association with a large underlying cyst or bulla.[154a]

In addition to systemic air embolism secondary to barotrauma, systemic "emboli" can occur following decompression as a result of nitrogen coming out of solution in systemic veins and body tissues and bypassing the pulmonary circulation through atrial septal defects or a patent foramen ovale (*see* farther on).[150] Systemic air embolism also occurs in a variety of situations in which there is underlying lung disease, such as severe asthma[155] and neonatal respiratory distress syndrome,[156, 157] and during assisted positive pressure breathing, particularly in neonates[158] but also in adults.[159] In all these situations, the sequence of events probably consists of alveolar rupture, interstitial emphysema, and pneumomediastinum and/or pneumothorax; as air dissects through the perivenous interstitial tissue, it also extends into the vein wall and lumen.

Although systemic air embolization originates most commonly in the pulmonary veins, occasionally air is introduced in the systemic circulation. In this case, it gains access to the systemic arteries via a patent foramen ovale (paradoxical embolism)[160–162] or an intrapulmonary shunt.[162] It is also possible that an abundance of air in the pulmonary arterioles and capillaries can "spill over" into the pulmonary venous and, ultimately, systemic circulation.[163, 164]

### Pulmonary Air Embolism

Pulmonary air embolism occurs most commonly as a result of air entering the systemic venous circulation and passing to the right side of the heart and the lungs;[145] rarely, it is caused by air entering the pulmonary arteries directly.[165] The abnormality occurs in a wide variety of circumstances (Table 49–4). Iatrogenic causes are by far the most common and include surgery (particularly of the head and neck in which the wound is above the level of the heart, i.e., with the patient in the sitting position), insertion and maintenance of intravenous apparatus, and diagnostic and therapeutic air insufflation procedures. In the case of infusion catheters, the usual mode of entry is by direct injection through the cathe-

ter; however, air has also been reported to pass along the catheter wire and through the fibrous tract formed around the catheter after the latter has been withdrawn.[166–168] A number of cases have been associated with breakage or disconnection of the catheter hub[4] and following cardiopulmonary bypass surgery.[169] Rare cases have also been associated with the use of hydrogen peroxide in wound irrigation, the presumed mechanism being the introduction of oxygen generated by the chemical into the surgically disrupted vasculature.[143] Venous air embolism has been reported to occur in more than half of all cesarean sections.[170]

As with systemic embolism, pulmonary air embolism requires both vascular disruption and a pressure gradient between the source of extravascular gas and the vascular lumen. This gradient can occur by two mechanisms: (1) positive pressure forcing gas into the veins, as seen in such situations as inadvertent force on an infusion bag,[171] pressurized infusion of CT contrast material,[172] or $CO_2$ insufflation of the peritoneal cavity before laparoscopy;[142] and (2) movement of gas into the veins as a result of a pressure gradient between the site of entry and the pulmonary vessels, a situation best exemplified by head and neck surgery in the sitting position in which the incidence of emboli may be as high as 40%.[173] (However, it is important to remember that embolization can also occur in patients who assume a prone position.[174])

In experimental animals, the physiologic effects of embolized air depend on its quantity and rate of entry into the vasculature and on the position of the animal.[175] Approximately 6 to 8 ml/kg are necessary to produce death in animals.[4] (As might be expected, a much smaller amount can produce significant disease or death in systemic embolism.) The pathogenesis of pulmonary disease is multifactorial.[4] Rapid injection of a large amount of air may result in formation of an air block in the outflow tract of the right ventricle, preventing pulmonary arterial blood flow. Smaller amounts infused slowly appear to exert an effect at the level of the distal pulmonary arteries and arterioles.[4] Some of this effect is probably related to vascular obstruction by air bubbles themselves; however, reflex vasoconstriction[176] and the formation of fibrin emboli as blood and air are whipped together in the right heart chambers[177, 178] appear to be at least as important. The overall effect of these processes is to produce a transient increase in pulmonary vascular resistance and arterial pressure.[179]

Both clinical[180–182] and experimental observations[183] indicate that pulmonary edema complicates some cases of pulmonary air embolism. Measurements of protein clearance suggest that the abnormality is related to increased microvascular permeability.[183] Although the underlying mechanism is not known, there is evidence for the involvement of neutrophils;[184] possible mediators of damage that have been investigated include superoxide anion[185] and hydrogen peroxide.[186] Whatever the mechanism, the edema results in decreased lung compliance and the development of ventilation-perfusion mismatching with a corresponding decrease in $\dot{V}/\dot{Q}$ ratio and alterations in blood gases.[187]

Another cause of pulmonary air embolism is related to the air that reaches the pulmonary vasculature as part of the decompression syndrome. When a diver spends a prolonged period breathing gas at greater than ambient air pressure, excess air dissolves in the blood and tissue fluids. With a

## Table 49–4. PULMONARY (VENOUS) AIR EMBOLISM

| ETIOLOGY | COMMENT | SELECTED REFERENCE(S) |
|---|---|---|
| *Surgery* | | |
| Central nervous system | Particularly in sitting (Fowler's) position in which the incidence is as high as 40% | 173, 213 |
| Uterus | Curettage, hysterectomy, cesarean section, laser ablation | 141, 362, 363 |
| Lung | Following bronchus/azygous vein fistula | 364 |
| Bone and joint | Dental implantation, intramedullary nailing, arthroscopic knee surgery, laminectomy | 182, 365–368 |
| Prostate | Transurethral resection, radical prostatectomy | 369, 370 |
| Kidney | Percutaneous nephrostomy | 371 |
| *Diagnostic/Therapeutic Air Injection* | | |
| Laparoscopic intra-abdominal surgery | Related to pneumoperitoneum; particularly cholecystectomy | 142, 372 |
| Arthrography | | 373 |
| Pneumoperitoneum | Historical therapy for tuberculosis | 374 |
| Pulsatile saline wound irrigation | | 375 |
| *Intravenous Devices* | | |
| Cardiac pacemaker | | 376 |
| Central venous catheters for hyperalimentation/chemotherapy | | 377, 378 |
| Pressurized infusion of intravenous fluids | Foe example, CT contrast material, blood | 172, 379 |
| Hemodialysis catheters | | 380 |
| Vena cava filters | | 381 |
| *Miscellaneous* | | |
| Vaginal inflation | Most common in pregnant women after orogenital sex; rarely manual sex or vaginal cocaine insufflation | 382–384 |
| Penis/scrotal inflation | | 385, 386 |
| Hydrogen peroxide ingestion/irrigation | Following accidental ingestion of $H_2O_2$ (with gastric catabolism producing excessive oxygen) or wound irrigation | 143, 387 |
| Positive pressure ventilation | | 388 |
| Head trauma | | 389 |
| Air-turbine dental drilling | | 390 |
| Recovery and readministration of blood products | | 391 |
| Decompression syndrome | Rapid ascent after diving or loss of cockpit pressure at high altitude | 151, 189 |

too-rapid ascent and a return of partial pressures to lower values, air comes out of solution and forms small bubbles that can be carried in the systemic veins to the right heart and pulmonary vasculature. Oxygen coming out of solution can be disposed of easily by metabolic consumption, but the inert nitrogen is much slower to be cleared. The bubbles cause lung microvascular damage and noncardiac pulmonary edema in the same manner as discussed earlier. This form of pulmonary decompression sickness, which has been called the "chokes," is a relatively uncommon form of decompression illness that is sometimes fatal.[151] Rarely, the abnormality develops during so-called Type 2 decompression sickness, which occurs when airline or air force personal undergo sudden decompression due to loss of cockpit pressure at high altitudes.[188, 189]

### Pathologic Characteristics

The gross morphologic changes caused by pulmonary air embolism have been documented in both humans[190] and experimental animals.[177] Bloody froth formed by the whipping action of the right atrium and ventricle partly fills these chambers and extends into the proximal branches of the pulmonary artery and (sometimes) the superior and inferior venae cavae. The pulmonary veins are virtually empty of blood as are the left atrium and left ventricle, which are typically contracted. Repeated sublethal intravenous injections of air in rabbits has been shown to produce pulmonary arterial intimal fibrosis.[191, 192]

### Radiologic Manifestations

The radiographic manifestations of air embolism in living patients have been documented in a small number of reports.[158, 166, 193–195] As expected, the principal sign is the presence of gas in cardiac chambers or pulmonary or systemic vessels. In pulmonary air embolism, the gas is present in the right heart chambers, central pulmonary arteries, and (sometimes) hepatic veins;[156] in systemic air embolism, it can be identified in the left heart chambers, aorta, or more peripheral branches of the systemic arterial tree such as the neck, shoulder girdles, or upper abdomen. Other manifestations of pulmonary air embolism include pulmonary edema, focal oligemia, enlarged central pulmonary arteries, and atelectasis.[195] The diagnosis has been confirmed by postmortem radiography, albeit with difficulty.[196] Systemic air embolism can also be identified on plain radiographs.[197]

The radiographic findings associated with air embolism

in scuba divers were documented in a review of 31 patients;[199] 13 (42%) had abnormalities evident on chest radiographs, including pneumomediastinum in 8, subcutaneous emphysema in 3, pneumocardium in 2, pneumothorax in 1, and pneumoperitoneum in 1. We observed an unusual case of noncardiogenic pulmonary edema developing in a scuba diver after a rapid ascent from 75 feet.[200] Immediately after surfacing, the patient became dyspneic. A chest radiograph a few hours later demonstrated bilateral consolidation. The clinical and radiographic abnormalities showed rapid improvement with hyperbaric therapy. The edema was presumably due to accumulation of air bubbles within the pulmonary vasculature, leading to release of vasoactive substances that resulted in increased vascular permeability.[200] The radiographic findings of fatal air embolism have been reported in two scuba divers;[201] in both cases, gas could be seen in the cardiac chambers, pulmonary vessels, and portal system.

Pulmonary air embolism is seen particularly well on CT. In one study of 100 patients who received intravenous contrast material that was injected by hand and followed by a drip infusion, asymptomatic venous air embolism was documented in 23.[202] The most common site (12 cases) was the main pulmonary artery. In 20 patients, the amount of air was considered to be minimal, the findings consisting of small bubbles within blood. In three patients in whom a moderate amount of air was present, air-fluid levels were identified within the vessels. In another series of 677 patients who underwent contrast-enhanced CT, air emboli were detected in 79 (12%);[203] they were located in the main pulmonary artery in 54 patients (8%), the superior vena cava in 12 (1.8%), the right ventricle in 10 (1.5%), the subclavian or brachiocephalic vein in 6 (0.9%), and the right atrium in 5 (0.7%). (Seven patients [1%] had emboli at more than one site.) CT has also revealed the presence of subpleural emphysema ("blebs") not visible on radiographs in some patients who have experienced arterial embolism during compressed air diving.[204]

### Clinical Manifestations

The vast majority of patients with pulmonary air embolism are asymptomatic. However, when the amount of air entering the lung is considerable, particularly if the entry is rapid, clinical manifestations may ensue. Symptoms are nonspecific and include faintness, lightheadedness, and dyspnea; chest pain occurs occasionally. One group of investigators has described a "gasp" reflex consisting of a cough followed by a short expiration and several seconds of inspiration.[205]

Physical findings include tachycardia, tachypnea, and systemic hypotension. A precordial murmur resembling the sound of a "mill wheel" has been described in some patients.[206] Signs of pulmonary edema also may be evident. Occasionally, the intrusion of air into the pulmonary circulation is followed by its migration to systemic vessels supplying vital organs, particularly the heart and brain; this in turn may result in convulsions, coma, and chest pain. Bubbles can be visualized in the retinal vessels in some cases.[5] Similar findings are evident in "primary" systemic air embolism.

### Laboratory Findings and Diagnosis

Laboratory findings are nonspecific. Elevated levels of lactate dehydrogenase and transaminases have been found in some patients who have had arterial air embolism following underwater diving.[207] If coronary vessels are obstructed, electrocardiographic changes may indicate myocardial ischemia or ventricular dysrhythmia.[208] Arterial blood gas analysis may show hypoxemia and hypercarbia.

The most commonly used techniques for confirming the diagnosis during life are precordial Doppler ultrasonography[209] and transesophageal echocardiography.[140] The former is probably the more sensitive, being able to detect air bubbles as small as 0.1 ml because of the high echogenic interface between air and blood.[4] However, the technique has been criticized as being too sensitive, because it detects emboli of inconsequential size[4] and may misinterpret venous turbulence as emboli.[141] Other techniques that have been utilized to detect air emboli include transcutaneous monitoring of $O_2$ and $CO_2$[210] and measurement of end-tidal $P_{CO_2}$ (as a reflection of changes in $\dot{V}/\dot{Q}$ ratio and physiologic dead space).[211] Continuous monitoring of expired nitrogen has also been employed in studies of both experimental animals[212] and humans[141] (the rationale being that the presence of air in pulmonary capillaries results in a sudden increase in expiratory nitrogen).

### Prognosis

As indicated, pulmonary air embolism is usually a benign event unrecognized by the patient or physician. For example, in one review of approximately 250 patients undergoing neurosurgery in the sitting position, air embolism was detected in 30%;[213] none of the affected patients showed clinical sequelae. Nevertheless, it is clear that if sufficient air is introduced into either pulmonary or systemic circulations over a short enough period of time that serious clinical consequences, including death, can occur. The precise incidence of this last outcome is uncertain because of difficulty in diagnosis, both during life and after death.

## EMBOLISM OF TALC, STARCH, AND CELLULOSE

Emboli of talc, starch, and cellulose are seen almost invariably in individuals who have engaged in intravenous drug abuse over a long period.[214, 215] In most instances, the complication occurs with medications intended solely for oral use; pills are crushed in a spoon or bottle top, water is added, and the mixture is drawn into a syringe and injected. The habit is usually a result of a shortage of available heroin, although some addicts use the drugs in this manner to counteract the sedative effect of the narcotic drugs themselves. Oral medications misused in this way include amphetamines[216] and closely related drugs such as methylphenidate hydrochloride (Ritalin) and tripelennamine,[217–219] methadone hydrochloride,[214, 220–222] hydromorphone hydrochloride (Dilaudid),[223] phenyltoloxamine,[224] propoxyphene (Darvon), secobarbital, pentazocine (Talwin),[225–227] meperidine,[228, 229] and propylhexedrine.[230]

All these medications have in common the addition of

an insoluble filler to bind the medicinal particles together and to act as a lubricant to prevent the tablets from sticking to punches and dyes during manufacture.[231] The most widely used filler is talc. Cornstarch is used in secobarbital and pentazocine and is also occasionally mixed with heroin and other illicit drugs. Microcrystalline cellulose is a prominent component of pentazocine.[232] The most hazardous fillers are talc and cellulose; although cornstarch alone can cause a histiocytic and foreign body giant cell reaction, it appears to be relatively innocuous.[233, 234] Illegally acquired "street" heroin may also contain diluents such as maltose, lactose, and quinine; however, most of these are water soluble and induce no pulmonary damage.[235]

Because of the association of intravenous drug abuse with acquired immunodeficiency syndrome, clinical, radiographic, and pathologic findings characteristic of this disorder may be seen in addition to those of talc emboli.[236, 237]

### Pathogenesis

When injected intravenously, the fillers become trapped within pulmonary arterioles and capillaries and cause vascular occlusion, sometimes associated with thrombosis. Presumably related to this, transient pulmonary hypertension has been reported following the intravenous injection of pentazocine;[238] rare cases of sudden death have also been attributed to acute occlusion of the pulmonary vasculature after the intravenous injection of talc.[224, 239] A more common sequela is the development of chronic pulmonary hypertension. Although this may be related in part to vascular alterations directly caused by the talc emboli, it is possible that parenchymal fibrosis and emphysema are also involved (*see* farther on). In time, the foreign particles migrate through the vessel wall and come to lie in the adjacent perivascular and parenchymal interstitial tissue, where they engender a foreign body giant cell reaction and fibrosis. As might be predicted, the severity of radiographic and pulmonary function abnormalities is related to the quantity of drug injected.[214]

### Pathologic Characteristics

In the early stages of disease, the lungs show variable numbers of more or less discrete parenchymal nodules measuring up to 1 mm in diameter[215, 226, 240] (Fig. 49–4). In long-standing disease, there is a tendency for the nodules to become confluent, especially in the upper lobes, producing large foci of consolidation resembling the progressive massive fibrosis seen in the pneumoconioses[214, 215, 241, 242] (Fig. 49–5). Panacinar emphysema, sometimes with bulla formation, is often evident.[215, 243]

Histologically, the small nodules consist of loosely formed granulomas composed largely of multinucleated giant cells and surrounded by a small amount of fibrous tissue (*see* Fig. 49–4). Although some granulomas affect the lumens and walls of smaller muscular arteries and arterioles, in most instances they are present in the perivascular or parenchymal interstitium. Evidence of recent, organizing, or organized thrombus can be seen[233] but is uncommon.

Occasionally, focal vascular dilation ("angiomatoid" lesions) and medial muscular hypertrophy have been observed.[233, 239] Sections of the large foci of upper lobe consolidation seen in long-standing disease show sheets of multinucleated giant cells separated by a variable amount of fibrous tissue (*see* Fig. 49–5).

Foreign material is readily identifiable within the giant cells and is particularly well seen by polarization microscopy. Talc can be identified as irregular, birefringent aggregates of platelike crystals ranging from 5 to 15 μm in length. Cellulose crystals tend to be larger (10 to 40 μm) and to show characteristic reactions with Congo red and methenamine silver stains.[225, 233] Starch crystals are characteristically round and contain a central Maltese cross.[233, 234]

Because of the tremendous number of injected particles characteristic of this condition, some foreign material commonly passes through the pulmonary circulation and is deposited in organs and tissues throughout the body, including the liver, bone marrow, lymph nodes, skin, and eyes.[244]

### Radiologic Manifestations

In our experience based on a 10-year follow-up of a group of affected patients, the intravenous abuse of drugs containing talc or cellulose and intended for oral use may result in a sequence of changes that are likely dose related and that can progress following cessation of the intravenous abuse.[214, 215] The earliest finding is a widespread micronodulation, the diameter of individual nodules ranging from barely visible to about 1 mm (Fig. 49–6). The pattern does not have a reticular component, the opacities being distinct and "pinpoint" in character, simulating alveolar microlithiasis. Although some authors have described a midzonal predominance of these micronodules,[220, 245] the distribution we have observed has been diffuse and uniform throughout the lungs. In our experience, the profusion of nodules does not vary from patient to patient, severity of involvement being evident from size alone: Radiographs revealing the earliest discernible changes and those of advanced disease seem to show the same number of nodules, the only difference being that the older ones are larger and therefore more clearly visible. In some patients, the widespread nodularity is associated with loss of volume, sometimes severe.

In the later stages of the disease, the opacities in the upper lobes may coalesce to form an almost homogeneous opacity that closely resembles the progressive massive fibrosis of silicosis or coal workers' pneumoconiosis except for the frequent presence of an air bronchogram.[215, 241, 246, 247] Pulmonary arterial hypertension and cor pulmonale may develop[245, 248, 249] (Fig. 49–7). In the very late stages of the disease, increasing disability and deteriorating function are associated with radiographic evidence of emphysema and bullae;[215] the chest radiograph may be diagnostic at this stage, revealing a combination of micronodular opacities, coalescent upper lobe lesions resembling progressive massive fibrosis, and lower lobe emphysema or bullae (Fig. 49–8). Pneumothorax, sometimes recurrent, has been described,[214] and mediastinal lymph node enlargement occurs occasionally.[214, 220] Gallium 67 scan results may be positive.[250, 251]

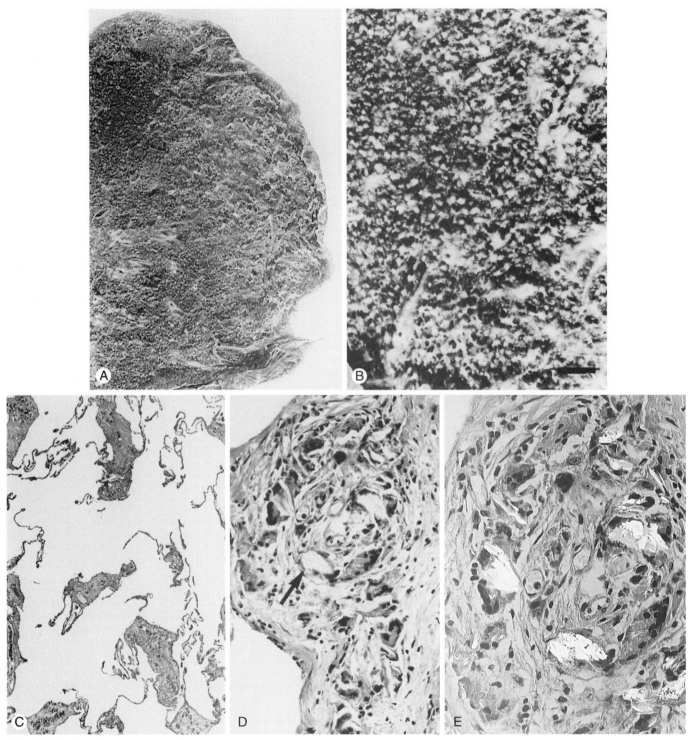

**Figure 49–4. Intravenous Talcosis.** A slice of an upper lobe *(A)* shows severe panacinar emphysema in its anterior portion and a fine nodularity in the remaining parenchyma (seen better in the magnified view *[B]*). A section from the anterior portion *(C)* shows panacinar emphysema and scattered, largely perivascular foci of fibrosis. A magnified view of one of the latter areas *(D)* shows aggregates of multinucleated giant cells containing talc crystals *(arrow)*. A photomicrograph taken with polarized light *(E)* shows the refractile talc to better advantage. *(B,* Bar = 1 cm; *C,* ×40; *D,* ×250; *E,* ×400.)

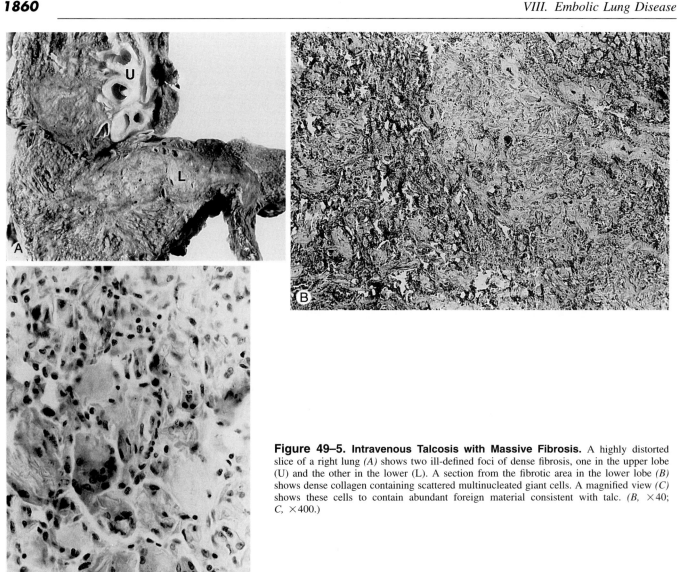

**Figure 49–5. Intravenous Talcosis with Massive Fibrosis.** A highly distorted slice of a right lung *(A)* shows two ill-defined foci of dense fibrosis, one in the upper lobe (U) and the other in the lower (L). A section from the fibrotic area in the lower lobe *(B)* shows dense collagen containing scattered multinucleated giant cells. A magnified view *(C)* shows these cells to contain abundant foreign material consistent with talc. *(B,* ×40; *C,* ×400.)

The high-resolution CT findings consist of diffuse ground-glass attenuation (Fig. 49–9), small, well-defined nodules, and perihilar upper lobe conglomerate areas of fibrosis.[252] Localized areas of high attenuation consistent with talc deposition can be seen within the conglomerate masses[252] (Fig. 49–10).

The radiographic and CT findings of intravenous abuse of methylphenidate (crushed Ritalin tablets) differ somewhat from those of other types of intravenous drug abuse.[253] The main abnormality consists of emphysema, characteristically bilateral and symmetric, that affects mainly the lower lung zones. There is no associated bullae formation. In one investigation, follow-up chest radiographs showed progression of emphysema over several years.[253]

### Clinical Manifestations

Most addicts who inject oral medications or heroin doctored with insoluble fillers are asymptomatic, granulomas being found incidentally at necropsy in those who die from other causes.[216, 231, 235] Typically, symptoms develop only in very heavy users (not infrequently with a history of injection of thousands of pills) and consist of slowly progressive dyspnea and (occasionally) persistent cough.[214, 220] Although rhonchi are heard in some patients, they are most likely related to the cigarette smoking that is almost invariably present. Cor pulmonale may be evident as a result of extensive disease. As in silicosis, the reaction to intravenously injected talc may progress and disability may increase after cessation of exposure.[214]

Organized thrombi and scars are visible on the forearms of nearly all addicts who inject drugs intravenously. Glistening particles can be seen in the fundi, principally at the posterior pole surrounding the foveal area; these may be the earliest clue to illicit use of such drugs, because they may be detected in addicts whose chest radiograph and pulmonary function test results are normal.[214, 254] Although tissue analysis is usually not required to confirm the diagnosis, foreign

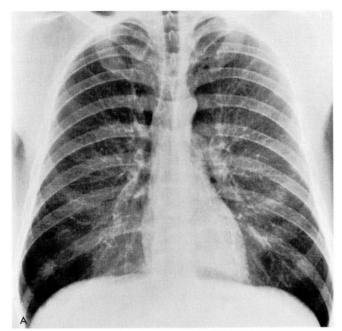

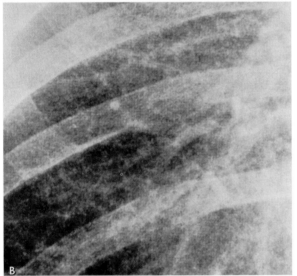

**Figure 49–6. Pulmonary Talcosis in Intravenous Drug Abuse.** This asymptomatic 22-year-old man had been "shooting" heroin and methadone for 4 years at the time these radiographs were obtained. There is widespread involvement of both lungs by tiny micronodular opacities (A), seen to better advantage on a magnified image (2:1) of the right lower zone (B). There is no anatomic predominance. The pattern is similar to the discrete opacities of alveolar microlithiasis.

material can be identified in samples obtained by fine needle aspiration[255] or BAL[250] if necessary.

Although a number of studies have assessed pulmonary function in intravenous drug users, many of them have not indicated clearly whether persons who have (or have not) abused oral medications are included.[223, 256] In one investigation of more than 500 intravenous drug abusers (96% of whom were cigarette smokers), pulmonary function test results were normal in approximately 50%;[257] in 190 patients (38%), the diffusing capacity was less than 75% of normal, and in the remainder there was obstructive or restrictive impairment with or without some reduction in diffusion. Studies of addicts who admit intravenous abuse of oral

medications have found significant impairment of gas transfer,[227] accompanied by a combination of obstructive and restrictive defects but little or no hyperinflation or air trapping, at least in the early stages.[214] In more advanced disease, severe reduction of flow rates and diffusion accompanied by hyperinflation and air trapping may become evident.[215]

## IODIZED OIL EMBOLISM

Pulmonary oil embolism is usually a complication of lymphangiography with ethiodized poppy seed oil (Ethiodol); occasionally, it has been seen after procedures such as hysterosalpingography, urethrography, and myelography.[258–260] In one case, it followed iophendylate (Pantopaque) ventriculography in a young patient with a ventriculoatrial shunt.[261] The complication has also been described in six patients undergoing transcatheter oily chemoembolization via the hepatic artery using an infusion of iodized oil and doxorubicin hydrochloride (Adriamycin).[262]

Postlymphangiographic oil emboli are undoubtedly common; both postmortem studies shortly after the procedure[263, 264] and photoscans of sputum after lymphangiography with [131]I-labeled oil[265] have shown that a considerable quantity of oil may be present in the lungs, even without radiographically demonstrable signs.

Pathologic findings have been described infrequently. In one study, lung biopsy performed 12 hours after the lymphatic oil injection showed lipid droplets widely distributed throughout the pulmonary capillary bed, corresponding to fine granular stippling observed throughout both lungs radiologically.[266] Some investigators have found reactive changes in pulmonary endothelial cells and an interstitial histiocytic and giant cell reaction, indicating passage of lipid outside the vascular space.[263] A staining technique has been described for distinguishing neutral fat from lipiodol.[267]

In one investigation of 80 patients, radiographic evidence of oil embolism was found in 44 (56%), most of whom had pelvic or abdominal lymphatic obstruction.[268] It has been postulated that such obstruction permits uptake of the contrast medium by systemic veins, so that the oil arrives in the lungs earlier and in greater concentration than it would otherwise. The findings usually consist of a fine reticular pattern,[268] which may persist for up to 11 days[260] (Fig. 49–11). In addition, small peripheral vessels may be so filled with contrast material that they present an arborizing pattern similar to that seen on pulmonary arteriography.[264] In one study of pulmonary oil embolism after transcatheter chemoembolization of hepatocellular carcinoma, radiographic abnormalities were diffuse and bilateral and ranged from a fine reticulonodular pattern to dense parenchymal consolidation.[262] The findings were most severe 2 to 10 days after chemoembolization and slowly disappeared thereafter, except in one patient who died of respiratory failure.

In another investigation of five patients undergoing lymphangiography with [131]I-labeled ethiodized oil, deposition in the lungs was maximal in the first 24 hours;[269] in three patients, more than 40% of the total dose was found in the lungs. Mean biologic half-life in the lung was 8 days (range, 5.2 to 12.6 days). Clearance was slower from the upper zones, seemingly correlating with blood flow. Interestingly, clearance was most rapid in the two active ambulant

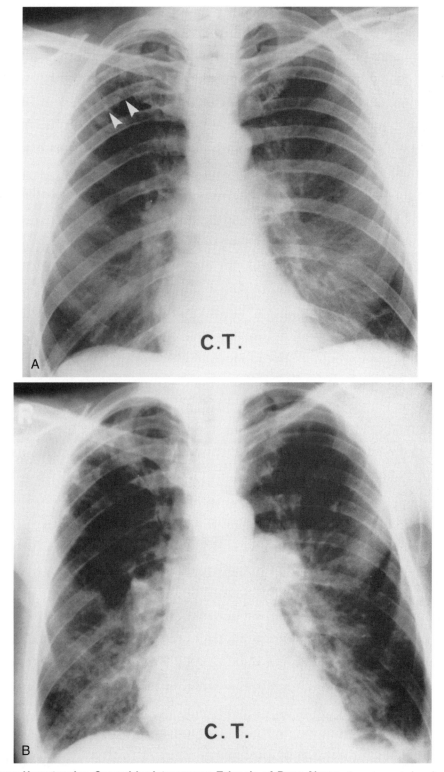

**Figure 49–7. Pulmonary Hypertension Caused by Intravenous Talcosis of Drug Abuse.** A posteroanterior chest radiograph *(A)* discloses minimal enlargement of the hilar pulmonary arteries consistent with precapillary hypertension. Cardiac size is normal. The lungs show no convincing evidence of emphysema. A few small nodular opacities are visible in the right apex *(arrowheads)*, subsequently proven to be of tuberculous origin. A multitude of micronodular opacities could be identified by visual inspection of the original radiograph but could not be reproduced. Approximately 14 months later, a chest radiograph *(B)* shows a considerable increase in the size of the hilar arteries. Cardiac size has increased, and its configuration suggests right atrial and ventricular predominance. The features are those of worsening cor pulmonale. Several months later, autopsy revealed a moderate degree of centrilobular emphysema in the upper lobes; however, the dominant histopathologic feature was extensive interstitial talc-induced granulomatosis and talc- and starch-related small vessel thrombosis.

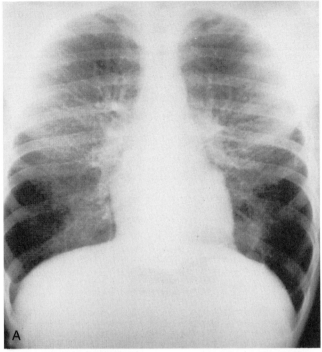

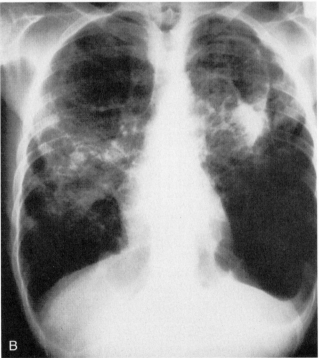

**Figure 49–8. Progressive Massive Fibrosis as a Long-Term Effect of Intravenous Talcosis of Drug Abuse.** A conventional chest radiograph *(A)* reveals a diffuse micronodular pattern throughout both lungs with considerable upper and midzonal predominance. The patient was a chronic intravenous drug abuser, and the pattern is characteristic of intravenous talcosis. Three years later *(B)*, large irregular opacities had appeared in both midlung zones, simulating the progressive massive fibrosis seen in silicosis. A pneumothorax is present on the left.

outpatients, who remained in a relatively upright semi-Fowler's position for 48 hours after lymphangiography.

Few patients have symptoms. Mild fever may develop within 48 hours after lymphangiography; rarely, cough,

chills, dyspnea, cyanosis, hemoptysis, or hypotension develop.[262, 268] Few deaths have been reported as a result of lymphangiography, the majority in patients who were known to have had pulmonary insufficiency previously.[270] In some patients, there is prolonged expectoration of oil.[271]

Several investigators have documented decreased diffusing capacity after lymphangiography, the abnormality being most marked at 24 to 48 hours.[266, 269, 270, 272, 273] This effect has been attributed to reduced pulmonary capillary blood flow in the early stage followed by interference with the membrane component of diffusion when the oil moves into the interstitial tissue.[270, 273] The reduction in diffusing capacity may persist even after most of the oil has cleared,[269, 273] possibly as the result of an inflammatory reaction in the alveolar wall as the oil is metabolized to cytotoxic fatty acid. In one study of nine patients, serial measurements of diffusing capacity showed a return to normal levels in 1 month or less.[273] Additional abnormalities include a reduction in lung compliance[272] and in arterial $Po_2$, particularly after a high dose of a contrast agent.[266, 274] As might be expected, ventilatory ability is not altered despite impairment of gas exchange and decreased pulmonary compliance.[266, 273]

## METALLIC MERCURY EMBOLISM

Pulmonary embolization of mercury may occur accidentally after injury from a broken thermometer or (formerly) during venous blood sampling with a mercury-sealed syringe, and intentionally after injection by drug abusers or individuals who attempt suicide or try to increase muscular strength.[275–277] Although the substance is moderately viscous, it flows readily through a 22-gauge needle into the veins and thence to the right heart and small pulmonary vessels. The incidence of such emboli is low but not insignificant—in one series of 1,063 patients who had cardiac catheterization or blood gas determination, it developed in 9 (0.9%).[278]

Pathologically, the inflammatory reaction in the lungs is relatively mild.[279] The mercury may remain within the pulmonary arteries, eventually becoming encased in thrombus, or may emigrate into the adjacent interstitium and alveolar air spaces, where it causes a foreign body giant cell reaction.

The radiographic appearance is distinctive because of the very high density of mercury[275, 278–281] (Fig. 49–12). The appearance may be that of spherules or of short tubular structures representing mercury-filled arterial segments. The distribution is usually bilateral and fairly symmetric. Because it is denser than plasma, mercury flows to dependent portions of the lung, so that the predominant distribution depends on the body position at the moment of injection. A local collection of mercury may be apparent in the heart, usually near the apex of the right ventricle, distinguishing it from aspirated mercury in the bronchi (see Fig. 49–12). Radiographs of the abdomen may reveal scattered mercury deposits in the liver, spleen, or kidney as a result of passage through the pulmonary capillaries into the systemic circulation. In patients in whom the mercury has been self-administered, radiographs of the forearms may reveal mercury droplets within the soft tissues at the site of injection.[280] Pulmonary, cardiac, and systemic localization of mercury droplets has also been described on CT.[282]

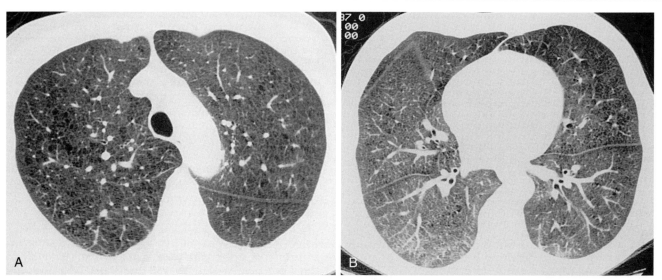

**Figure 49–9. Talcosis: Ground-Glass Attenuation on CT.** High-resolution CT scans (*A* and *B*) demonstrate a diffuse ground-glass pattern throughout all lung zones. No discrete nodules were seen at any levels. The diagnosis of talcosis was proved by open lung biopsy. The patient was a 49-year-old man with a 25-year history of intravenous drug abuse who presented with increasing shortness of breath. Over the years he had used intravenous heroin, Ritalin, and pentazocine (Talwin) on a daily basis. He also had a 70 pack-year smoking history.

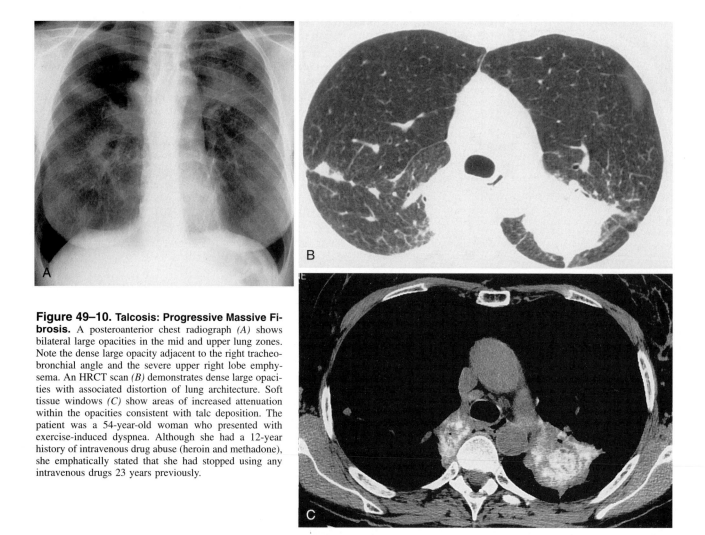

**Figure 49–10. Talcosis: Progressive Massive Fibrosis.** A posteroanterior chest radiograph *(A)* shows bilateral large opacities in the mid and upper lung zones. Note the dense large opacity adjacent to the right tracheobronchial angle and the severe upper right lobe emphysema. An HRCT scan *(B)* demonstrates dense large opacities with associated distortion of lung architecture. Soft tissue windows *(C)* show areas of increased attenuation within the opacities consistent with talc deposition. The patient was a 54-year-old woman who presented with exercise-induced dyspnea. Although she had a 12-year history of intravenous drug abuse (heroin and methadone), she emphatically stated that she had stopped using any intravenous drugs 23 years previously.

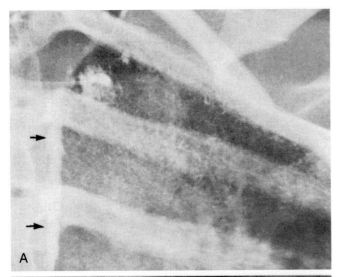

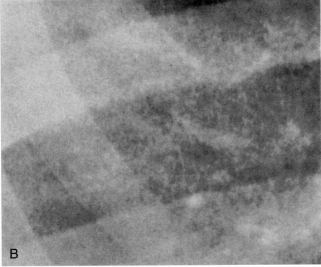

**Figure 49–11. Lipiodol Emboli.** A magnified view *(A)* of the apex of the left upper lobe approximately 1½ hours following the injection of 7 ml of Lipiodol into the lymphatics of each leg reveals a fine network of shadows of high density. This network is caused by the presence of contrast medium in the microvascular circulation of the lung. The thoracic duct can be identified on the left *(arrows)*. Twenty-four hours later *(B)* a fine stippled pattern is present.

Clinically, the body's reaction to mercury emboli is manifested by a metallic taste, excessive salivation, gingivitis, stomatitis, diarrhea, nephrosis, tremor (Hatter's shakes), and erethism.[279] These manifestations are believed to occur when sufficient metallic mercury is oxidized to the soluble mercuric ion $Hg^{2+}$, which has a selective affinity for sulfhydryl groups and acts by inhibiting enzymes containing them.[279] Pulmonary symptoms and function abnormalities are very mild or absent.[283, 284] The mercury may persist in the pulmonary vasculature for many years without apparent serious effects.[283, 284]

## MISCELLANEOUS FOREIGN BODY EMBOLISM

**Liquid Acrylate.** Liquid acrylate glues—most commonly isobutyl-2-cyanoacrylate and *n*-butyl-2-cyanoacrylate—are frequently used in embolization therapy of vascular malformations.[198, 285] Asymptomatic pulmonary embolism associated with the procedure is probably more common than is clinically and radiographically appreciated.[285, 286] Symptomatic embolization is relatively uncommon; for example, in one review of the clinical records of 182 patients treated for brain arteriovenous malformations, only 3 were noted to develop pulmonary symptoms within 48 hours of glue injection.[285] In this study, the radiographic findings consisted of subsegmental areas of consolidation (seen in all three cases) and a small left pleural effusion (seen in one).[285] CT scans demonstrated subsegmental, predominantly pleural-based wedge-shaped areas of consolidation consistent with pulmonary embolism and infarction.

Because the acrylate glue is radiolucent, it is mixed with radiopaque substances, either tantalum or Pantopaque, at the time of injection to allow accurate localization during embolization therapy. CT in all three cases discussed previously allowed identification of the punctate radiodensities representing IBCA-tantalum emboli within the pulmonary arteries.[285] In patients with asymptomatic pulmonary migration of embolic material, multiple small radiopacities can be seen throughout both lungs[286] (Fig. 49–13).

A small percentage of patients develop respiratory symptoms, usually pleuritic chest pain with or without associated cough and bloody sputum;[285] death from respiratory failure has been reported rarely.[287] Two patients developed a significant drop in $PaO_2$.[285]

**Cotton Fibers.** It is probable that in the majority of cases, fragments of cotton fibers are introduced into the pulmonary circulation by contamination of needles or intravenous catheters from clothing, bedding, or gauze used to wipe the needle. Rare examples secondary to cardiac catheterization[288] and angiography[289] have also been described, and it has been suggested that the material can occasionally be derived from intravenous fluid itself.[290] In one autopsy study of 74 children who had received intravenous fluid strained through a cotton filter, intrapulmonary fibers were demonstrated in 61;[291] there was a direct correlation between the amount of fluid administered and the number of cotton fibers per unit area of lung. These emboli result in no clinical or radiographic findings and are invariably discovered incidentally at autopsy or in a lung biopsy specimen.

Histologically, the fibers can be recognized as elongated, refractile foreign material associated with a variable inflammatory reaction. In the early stages,[289, 292] this consists simply of platelet thrombus within an acute inflammatory cellular exudate; later, the inflammation becomes granulomatous and is associated with large, multinucleated foreign body–type giant cells (Fig. 49–14). Although initially the granulomatous focus containing the cotton is located within the lumen and wall of small arteries and arterioles, it can eventually emigrate outside the vessel wall into the perivascular or alveolar interstitium;[288, 292] in these sites, it can be confused with inhaled foreign material.

**Barium.** Rarely, barium embolization to the lungs has been observed as a complication of routine barium enema[293, 294] and of barium "enema" performed inadvertently via the vagina.[295] Mucosal lacerations can usually be identified,[295] allowing entry of injected barium into the venous system. Pathologically, the barium can be seen within pulmonary arterioles and capillaries as refractile, angulated, crys-

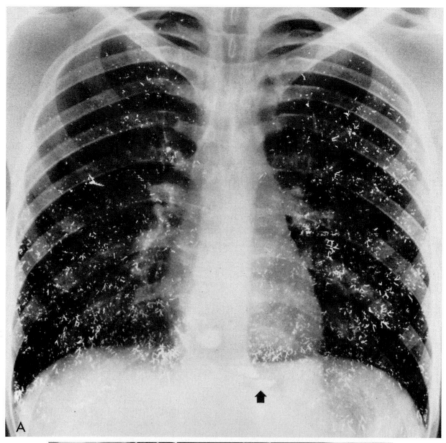

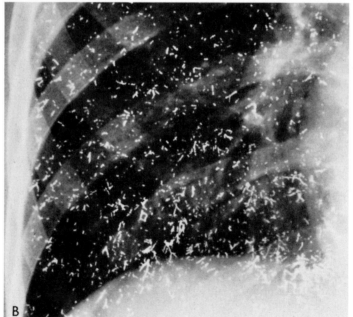

**Figure 49–12. Metallic Mercury Embolization.** A posteroanterior chest radiograph *(A)* reveals a multitude of short linear and branching opacities of metallic density distributed widely throughout both lungs, seen to better advantage in a magnified view of the lower portion of the right lung *(B)*. It would be difficult to be certain whether the material was within the vessels or the airways if it were not for the presence of a pool of mercury lying in the inferior aspect of the right ventricular chamber *(arrow in A)*. This young male drug addict injected metallic mercury into an antecubital vein for a special "kick." (Courtesy of Dr. William Beamish, University Hospital, Edmonton, Alberta.)

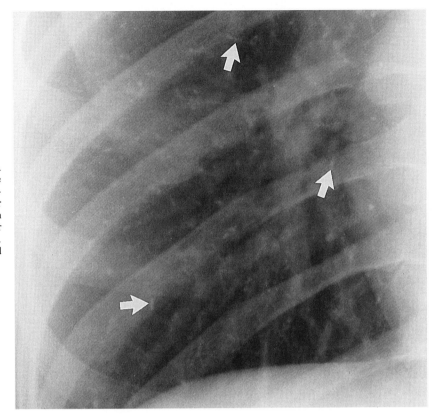

**Figure 49–13. Acrylate Pulmonary Emboli.** A 29-year-old woman had embolization therapy of a large intracerebral vascular malformation with *n*-butyl-2-cyanoacrylate (NBCA). A magnified view of the right lower lung zone performed immediately after the embolization demonstrates numerous bilateral small nodular and linear opacities of greater than soft tissue density *(arrows)*, representing emboli of tantalum and pantopaque-coated cyanoacrylate. The patient remained asymptomatic.

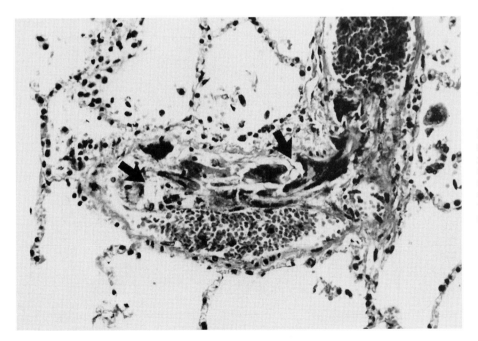

**Figure 49–14. Cotton Fiber Embolism.** A section of a small pulmonary artery shows several multinucleated foreign body giant cells adjacent to one wall. In their midst are multiple irregularly shaped spaces *(arrows)* that showed the presence of refractile material on polarization microscopy. The appearance is most suggestive of cotton fiber embolism. (×250.)

talline material. In one case, it was present within pulmonary endothelial cells that were enlarged and showed a finely vacuolated appearance.[295] The condition is serious, the majority of reported patients dying within 24 hours of the event.

**Bullets and Shrapnel.** Uncommonly, these agents enter the extrathoracic systemic veins or the right side of the heart and are carried to the lungs to lodge within pulmonary arteries[296-298] (Fig. 49–15). Both clinical observations and experimental studies have shown that such foreign bodies can remain within the pulmonary vasculature for prolonged periods without untoward effects;[299] rarely, there is complicating infarction.[296]

**Radiopaque Foreign Bodies.** A variety of devices such as wire loops and balloons filled with contrast medium have been used therapeutically in both the pulmonary and systemic circulations to obliterate arteriovenous malformations or to control intractable hemorrhage. Escape of such material into the systemic veins can result in opacities of metallic density within the lungs.[300, 301]

**Plastic Intravenous Catheters.** These devices, either whole or in fragments, usually embolize to the lungs when cut by the sharp bevel of the needle housing them[302, 303] (Fig. 49–16); occasionally, they are detached from their connector or fracture spontaneously.[304] There is evidence that such fragments should be removed;[305, 306] in one literature review,

17 of 28 patients who received no treatment died of directly related cardiopulmonary complications, whereas all 34 patients from whom catheters were removed survived and were asymptomatic.[302]

**Microscopic Particulates.** A variety of minute particulate materials, including glass, rubber, plastic, and cellulose, have been found in fluid destined for intravenous injection.[290, 307, 308] In one study, between 100 and 1,500 particles larger than 5 μm in diameter per liter of fluid were identified from four different manufacturers.[308] Although some of these particles are undoubtedly retained within the lungs after infusion, they appear to result in no clinical or radiologic manifestations. However, as with cotton, the granulomatous reaction that may develop in relation to some of the material may theoretically be a source of confusion in the interpretation of biopsy specimens.

**Silicone and Teflon.** Foreign material resembling a silicone antifoaming agent was detected within the pulmonary vasculature in 7 of 11 patients who had undergone extracorporeal circulation;[309] although there was no histologic reaction, the longest postoperative survival was only 90 hours. Pulmonary granulomas and isolated interstitial giant cells containing foreign material have been detected in patients on long-term hemodialysis[310, 311] (Fig. 49–17); although the nature of the foreign material has not been identified in all

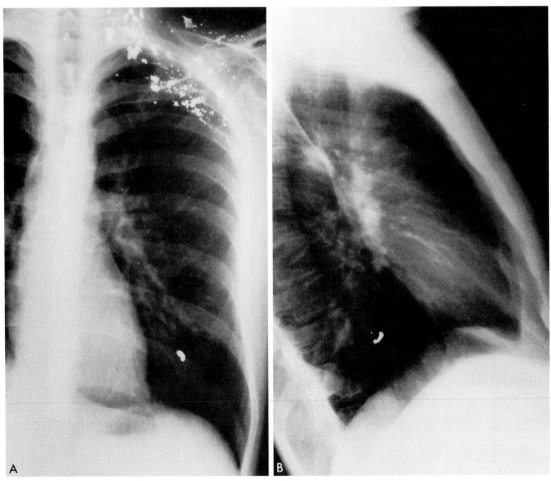

**Figure 49–15. Bullet Fragment Embolus to the Lung.** Posteroanterior *(A)* and lateral *(B)* radiographs reveal multiple metallic foreign bodies in the soft tissues of the left shoulder. In addition, a solitary metallic fragment is situated in the midportion of the left lower lobe. It is assumed that this fragment gained entry to a vein in the shoulder and embolized to the lung by way of the right heart.

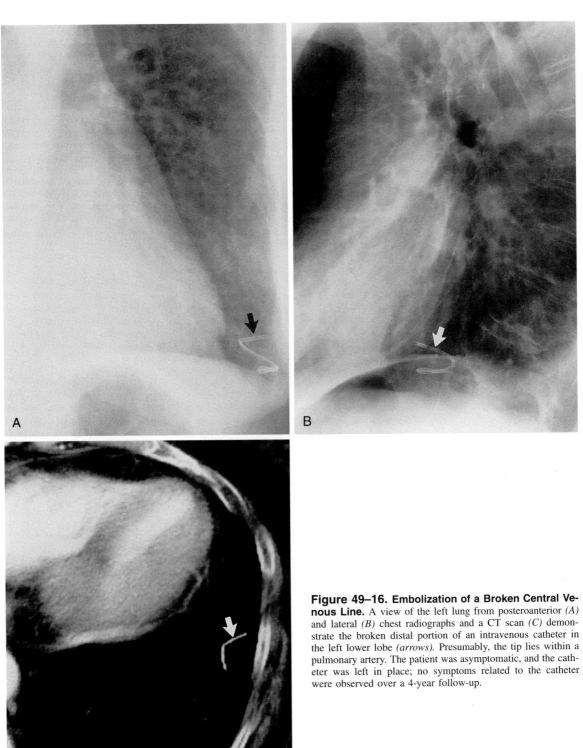

**Figure 49–16. Embolization of a Broken Central Venous Line.** A view of the left lung from posteroanterior *(A)* and lateral *(B)* chest radiographs and a CT scan *(C)* demonstrate the broken distal portion of an intravenous catheter in the left lower lobe *(arrows)*. Presumably, the tip lies within a pulmonary artery. The patient was asymptomatic, and the catheter was left in place; no symptoms related to the catheter were observed over a 4-year follow-up.

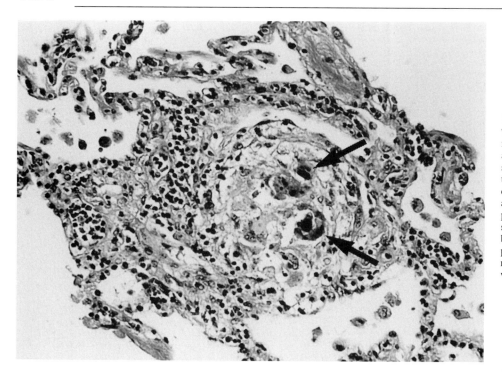

**Figure 49–17. Chronic Hemodialysis with Granulomatous Pneumonitis.** A magnified view of lung parenchyma shows an interstitial lymphocytic infiltrate and a single well-circumscribed granuloma containing several ill-defined, nonrefractile foreign particles *(arrows)*. Similar granulomas and patchy interstitial pneumonitis were present throughout both lungs and were considered to represent a reaction to microemboli related to long-term hemodialysis. The patient was a 65-year-old woman with no respiratory symptoms; the chest radiograph was normal. (×250.)

cases, in some it has been shown to be silicone, apparently derived from the dialysis tubing. In one patient, minute fragments of embolized polytef (Teflon) from a tricuspid Beall prosthesis have resulted in a similar pulmonary granulomatous reaction.[312] Clinical and radiographic manifestations have been absent in most patients.

Silicone fluid (polydimethylsiloxane) embolism has also been reported in some patients in whom the substance has been injected subcutaneously for breast augmentation.[313, 314]

Radiographs have shown a combination of interstitial and air-space disease, which, in severe cases, progresses to a pattern of ARDS. In one case, CT showed peripheral areas of ground-glass attenuation and consolidation.[314a] Patients present with progressive dyspnea, cough, and chest tightness. The disease can lead to death and to residual fibrosis in survivors.[313] The diagnosis has been made by identifying silicone-laden macrophages in specimens obtained by BAL.[314]

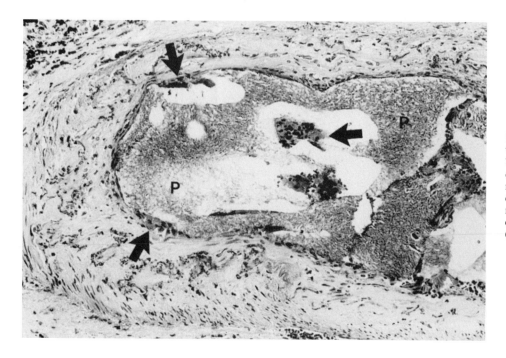

**Figure 49–18. Bronchial Artery Polyvinyl Alcohol Embolus.** A portion of a bronchial artery shows complete luminal occlusion by clumps of polyvinyl alcohol (P) rimmed by occasional multinucleated foreign body giant cells *(arrows)*. The specimen was from an autopsy 6 weeks after embolization for massive hemoptysis. (×160.)

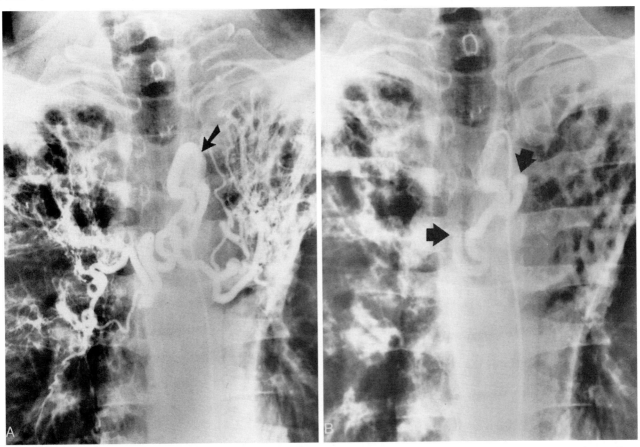

**Figure 49–19. Bronchial Artery Embolization for Life-Threatening Pulmonary Hemorrhage.** A bronchial artery angiogram *(A)* reveals marked dilation of the vessel within the mediastinum and a remarkable increase in flow to a partly atelectatic left upper lobe; note the origin of the bronchial artery from the top of the aortic arch *(arrow)*. The left upper lobe is the site of severe bronchiectasis and scarring. This 40-year-old man had cystic fibrosis and presented with hemoptysis amounting to 600 ml during the previous 24 hours. Bronchoscopy revealed a great deal of blood in the left upper lobe bronchus. Following the injection of polyvinyl alcohol foam (Ivalon) particles, a repeat injection of contrast medium *(B)* reveals total obstruction of both left and right branches of the bronchial artery *(arrows)* and an absence of flow to the left upper lobe. The embolization resulted in cessation of the hemoptysis.

**Oil.** We are aware of one report of pulmonary embolism of vegetable oil injected for augmentation mammaplasty.[315]

## BRONCHIAL ARTERY EMBOLISM

The vast majority of bronchial artery emboli consist of foreign material introduced therapeutically in an attempt to control recurrent or massive hemoptysis.[316] The embolic material is varied and includes absorbable gelatinous sponge (Gelfoam), polyvinyl alcohol (Ivalon), isobutyl-2-cyanoacrylate (bucrylate), and Gianturco coils.[317]

Pathologic examination of bronchial arteries recently embolized with such substances usually shows thrombus related to the material; in one experimental study on the effects of polyvinyl alcohol, vasculitis was also observed.[318]

Chronically, there may be fibrosis and mild inflammation, including a foreign body giant cell reaction[317] (Fig. 49–18). Spicules of polyvinyl alcohol have also been identified in the perivascular connective tissue, presumably the result of transmural migration by a process similar to that seen with embolized talc and cotton.[317] Experimentally, bronchial wall necrosis has been produced after bronchial artery occlusion by glass microspheres.[319] Despite this, the long-term effects of therapeutic emboli on the bronchial wall itself appear to be minimal.

Radiographically, the appearances are as might be anticipated: initial opacification of the bronchial artery and its peripheral arborization usually reveals a markedly dilated, hypertrophied vascular tree (Fig. 49–19); following embolization, the artery can be seen to be completely blocked at a variable distance from its origin, peripheral flow being nonexistent.

# REFERENCES

1. Collins KA, Davis GJ: A retrospective and prospective study of cerebral tissue pulmonary embolism in severe head trauma. J Forensic Sci 39:624, 1994.
2. Ho K-J: Diffuse fatal pulmonary microembolism of retroperitoneal extravascular origin. Arch Pathol Lab Med 113:1401, 1989.
3. Pyun KS, Katzenstein RE: Widespread bone marrow embolism with myocardial involvement. Arch Pathol 89:378, 1970.
4. Dudney TM, Elliott CG: Pulmonary embolism from amniotic fluid, fat and air. Prog Cardiovasc Dis 36:447, 1994.
5. King MB, Harmon KR: Unusual forms of pulmonary embolism. Clin Chest Med 15:561, 1994.
6. Muller C, Rahn BA, Pfister U, et al: The incidence, pathogenesis, diagnosis, and treatment of fat embolism. Orthop Rev 23:107, 1994.
7. Richards RR: Fat embolism syndrome. Can J Surg 40:334, 1997.
8. Johnson MJ, Lucas GL: Fat embolism syndrome. Orthopedics 19:41, 1996.
9. Palmovic V, McCarrol JR: Fat embolism in trauma. Arch Pathol 80:630, 1965.
10. Schemitsch EH, Jain R, Turchin DC, et al: Pulmonary effects of fixation of a fracture with a plate compared with intramedullary nailing. A canine model of fat embolism and fracture fixation. J Bone Joint Surg Am 79:984, 1997.
11. Benatar SR, Ferguson AD, Goldschmidt RB: Fat embolism—some clinical observations and a review of controversial aspects. Q J Med 41:85, 1972.
12. Ganong RB: Fat emboli syndrome in isolated fractures of the tibia and femur. Clin Orthop 291:208, 1993.
13. Sevitt S: The significance and classification of fat-embolism. Lancet 2:825, 1960.
14. Lessells AM: Fatal fat embolism after minor trauma. BMJ 282:1586, 1981.
15. Sevitt S: Fat Embolism. London, Butterworths, 1962.
16. Vichinsky E, Williams R, Das M, et al: Pulmonary fat embolism: A distinct cause of severe acute chest syndrome in sickle cell anemia. Blood 83:3107, 1994.
17. Castro O: Systemic fat embolism and pulmonary hypertension in sickle cell disease. Hematol Oncol Clin North Am 10:1289, 1996.
18. Kolquist KA, Vnencak-Jones CL, Swift L, et al: Fatal fat embolism syndrome in a child with undiagnosed hemoglobin S/beta+ thalassemia: A complication of acute parvovirus B19 infection. Pediatr Pathol Lab Med 16:71, 1996.
19. Wozasek GE, Simon P, Redl H, et al: Intramedullary pressure changes and fat intravasation during intramedullary nailing: An experimental study in sheep. J Trauma 36:202, 1994.
20. Hulman G: The pathogenesis of fat embolism. J Pathol 176:3, 1995.
21. Thompson PL, Williams KE, Walters MN-I: Fat embolism in the microcirculation: An in-vivo study. J Pathol 97:23, 1969.
22. Jacobovitz-Derks D, Derks CM: Pulmonary neutral fat embolism in dogs. Am J Pathol 95:29, 1979.
23. Pape HC, Dwenger A, Grotz M, et al: Does the reamer type influence the degree of lung dysfunction after femoral nailing following severe trauma? J Orthop Trauma 8:300, 1994.
24. Rautanen M, Gullichsen E, Gronroos J, et al: Catalytic activity of phospholipase A2 in serum in experimental fat embolism in pigs. Eur J Surg 163:449, 1997.
25. Hallgren B, Kerstall J, Rudenstam C-M, et al: A method for the isolation and chemical analysis of pulmonary fat embolism. Acta Chir Scand 132:613, 1966.
26. Peltier LF: Fat embolism. III. The toxic properties of neutral fat and free fatty acids. Surgery 40:665, 1956.
27. Kapur MM, Jain P, Gidh M: The effect of trauma on serum C3 activation and its correlation with injury severity score in man. J Trauma 26:464, 1986.
28. Derks CM, Jacobovitz-Derks D: Embolic pneumopathy induced by oleic acid. Am J Pathol 87:143, 1977.
29. Jones JG, Minty BD, Beeley JM, et al: Pulmonary epithelial permeability is immediately increased after embolisation with oleic acid but not with neutral fat. Thorax 37:169, 1982.
30. Syrbu S, Thrall RS, Smilowitz HM: Sequential appearance of inflammatory mediators in rat bronchoalveolar lavage fluid after oleic acid–induced lung injury. Exp Lung Res 22:33, 1996.
31. Jacobovitz-Derks D, Derks CM: Pulmonary neutral fat embolism in dogs. Am J Pathol 95:29, 1979.
32. Reidbord HE: Pulmonary fat embolism. Arch Pathol 98:122, 1974.
33. Thompson PL, Williams KE, Walters MN-I: Fat embolism in the microcirculation: An in-vivo study. J Pathol 97:23, 1969.
34. Saldeen T: Fat embolism and signs of intravascular coagulation in posttraumatic autopsy material. J Trauma 10:273, 1970.
35. Christie J, Robinson CM, Pell AC, et al: Transcardiac echocardiography during invasive intramedullary procedures. J Bone Joint Surg 77:450, 1995.
36. Rautanen M, Gullichsen E, Kuttila K, et al: Plasma levels of atrial natriuretic peptide and endothelin-1 in experimental fat embolism. Eur Surg Res 29:124, 1997.
37. Scully RE: Fat embolism in Korean battle casualties: Its incidence, clinical significance, and pathologic aspects. Am J Pathol 32:379, 1956.
38. Dines DE, Burgher LW, Okazaki H: The clinical and pathologic correlation of fat embolism syndrome. Mayo Clin Proc 50:407, 1975.
39. Gitin TA, Seidel T, Cera PJ, et al: Pulmonary microvascular fat: The significance? Crit Care Med 21:673, 1993.
40. Gustilo RB, Corpuz V, Sherman RE: Epidemiology, mortality and morbidity in multiple trauma patients. Orthopedics 8:1523, 1985.
41. Johnson KD, Cadambi A, Seibert GB: Incidence of adult respiratory distress syndrome in patients with multiple musculoskeletal injuries: Effect of early operative stabilization of fractures. J Trauma 25:375, 1985.
42. Modig J, Hedstrand U, Wegenius G: Determinants of early adult respiratory distress syndrome. A retrospective study of 220 patients with major fractures. Acta Chir Scand 151:413, 1985.
43. Abramowsky CR, Pickett JP, Goodfellow BC, et al: Comparative demonstration of pulmonary fat emboli by "en bloc" osmium tetroxide and oil red O methods. Hum Pathol 12:753, 1981.
44. Bierre AR, Koelmeyer TD: Pulmonary fat and bone marrow embolism in aircraft accident victims. Pathology 15:131, 1983.
45. Sevitt S: Fat embolism in patients with fractured hips. BMJ 2:257, 1972.
46. Glas WW, Grekin TD, Musselman MM: Fat embolism. Am J Surg 85:363, 1953.
47. Berrigan TJ Jr, Carsky EW, Heitzman ER: Fat embolism. Roentgenographic pathologic correlation in 3 cases. Am J Roentgenol 96:967, 1966.
48. Heitzman ER: The Lung: Radiologic-Pathologic Correlations. St. Louis, CV Mosby, 1973, pp 127, 137.
49. Curtis A McB, Knowles GD, Putnam CE, et al: The three syndromes of fat embolism: Pulmonary manifestations. Yale J Biol Med 52:149, 1979.
50. Maruyama Y, Little JB: Roentgen manifestations of traumatic pulmonary fat embolism. Radiology 79:945, 1962.
51. Williams JR, Bonte FJ: Pulmonary damage in nonpenetrating chest injuries. Radiol Clin North Am 1:439, 1963.
52. Hamrick-Turner J, Abbitt PL, Harrison RB, et al: Diffuse lung calcifications following fat emboli and adult respiratory distress syndromes: CT findings. J Thorac Imaging 9:47, 1994.
53. Thomas ML, Tighe JR: Death from fat embolism as a complication of intraosseous phlebography. Lancet 2:1415, 1973.
54. Peter RE, Schopfer A, Le Coultre B, et al: Fat embolism and death during prophylactic osteosynthesis of a metastatic femur using an unreamed femoral nail. J Orthop Trauma 11:233, 1997.
55. Burgher LW, Dines DE, Linscheid RL: Fat embolism and the adult respiratory distress syndrome. Mayo Clin Proc 49:107, 1974.
56. Hoare EM: Platelet response in fat embolism and its relationship to petechiae. BMJ 2:689, 1971.
57. Tachakra SS: Distribution of skin petechiae in fat embolism rash. Lancet 1:284, 1976.
58. Pell AC, Hughes D, Keating J, et al: Brief report: Fulminating fat embolism syndrome caused by paradoxical embolism through a patent foramen ovale. N Engl J Med 329:926, 1993.
59. Evarts CM: Diagnosis and treatment of fat embolism. JAMA 194:899, 1965.
60. Cross HE: Examination of CSF in fat embolism. Report of a case. Arch Intern Med 115:470, 1965.
61. Wiener L, Forsyth D: Pulmonary pathophysiology of fat embolism. Am Rev Respir Dis 92:113, 1965.
62. Davidson FF, Murray JF: Use of pulmonary diffusing capacity measurements to detect unsuspected fat embolism. Am Rev Respir Dis 106:715, 1972.
63. Hutchins PM, Macnicol MF: Pulmonary insufficiency after long bone fractures: Absence of circulating fat or significant immunodepression. J Bone Joint Surg 67:835, 1985.
64. Vichinsky E, Williams R, Das M, et al: Pulmonary fat embolism: A distinct cause of severe acute chest syndrome in sickle cell anemia. Blood 83:3107, 1994.
65. Chastre J, Fagon JY, Soler P, et al: Bronchoalveolar lavage for rapid diagnosis of the fat embolism syndrome in trauma patients. Ann Intern Med 113:583, 1990.
66. Mimoz O, Edouard A, Beydon L, et al: Contribution of bronchoalveolar lavage to the diagnosis of posttraumatic pulmonary fat embolism. Intensive Care Med 21:973, 1995.
67. Schonfeld SA, Ploysongsang Y, DiLisio R, et al: Fat embolism prophylaxis with corticosteroids: A prospective study in high risk patients. Ann Intern Med 99:438, 1983.
68. Stanley JD, Hanson RR, Hicklin GA, et al: Specificity of bronchoalveolar lavage for the diagnosis of fat embolism syndrome. Am Surg 60:537, 1994.
69. Roger N, Xaubet A, Agusti C, et al: Role of bronchoalveolar lavage in the diagnosis of fat embolism syndrome. Eur Respir J 8:1275, 1995.
70. Teng QS, Li G, Zhang BX, et al: Experimental study of early diagnosis and treatment of fat embolism syndrome. J Orthop Trauma 9:183, 1995.
71. Castella X, Valles J, Cabezuelo MA, et al: Fat embolism syndrome and pulmonary microvascular cytology. Chest 101:1710, 1992.
72. Pell AC, Christie J, Keating JF, et al: The detection of fat embolism by transoesophageal echocardiography during reamed intramedullary nailing. A study of 24 patients with femoral and tibial fractures. J Bone Joint Surg Br 75:921, 1993.
73. Gurd AR, Wilson RI: The fat embolism syndrome. J Bone Joint Surg Br 56:408, 1974.
74. Vedrienne JM, Guillaume C, Gagnieu MC: Bronchoalveolar lavage in trauma patients for diagnosis of fat embolism syndrome. Chest 102:1323, 1992.
75. Guenter CA, Braun TE: Fat embolism syndrome: Changing prognosis. Chest 79:143, 1981.
76. Carstens PHB: Pulmonary bone marrow embolism following external cardiac massage. Acta Pathol Microbiol Scand 76:510, 1969.
77. Rappaport H, Raum M, Horrell JB: Bone marrow embolism. Am J Pathol 27:407, 1951.
78. Yoell JH: Bone marrow embolism to lung following sternal puncture. AMA Arch Pathol 67:373, 1959.
79. Pyun KS, Katzenstein RE: Widespread bone marrow embolism with myocardial involvement. Arch Pathol 89:378, 1970.

80. Haupt HM, Moore GW, Bauer TW, et al: The lung in sickle cell disease. Chest 81:332, 1982.
81. Yamamoto M: Pathology of experimental pulmonary bone marrow embolism. I. Initial lesions of the rabbit lung after intravenous infusion of allogeneic bone marrow with special reference to its pathogenesis. Acta Pathol Jpn 35:45, 1985.
82. Schinella RA: Bone marrow emboli: Their fate in the vasculature of the human lung. Arch Pathol 95:386, 1973.
83. Yamamoto M: Pathology of experimental pulmonary bone marrow embolism. II. Post-embolic pulmonary arteriosclerosis and pulmonary hypertension in rabbits receiving an intravenous infusion of allogeneic bone marrow. Acta Pathol Jpn 37:705, 1987.
84. Masson RG: Amniotic fluid embolism. Clin Chest Med 13:657, 1992.
85. Morgan M: Amniotic fluid embolism. Anaesthesia 34:20, 1979.
86. Burrows A, Khoo SK: The amniotic fluid embolism syndrome: 10 years' experience at a major teaching hospital. Aust N Z J Obstet Gynecol 35:245, 1995.
87. Attwood HD: Amniotic fluid embolism. Pathol Ann 7:145, 1972.
88. Karetzky M, Ramirez M: Acute respiratory failure in pregnancy. An analysis of 19 cases. Medicine 77:41, 1998.
89. Philip RS: Amniotic fluid embolism. N Y State J Med 67:2085, 1967.
90. Maher JE, Wenstrom KD, Hauth JC, et al: Amniotic fluid embolism after saline amnioinfusion: Two cases and review of the literature. Obstet Gynecol 83:851, 1994.
91. Roche WD Jr, Norris HJ: Detection and significance of maternal pulmonary amniotic fluid embolism. Obstet Gynecol 43:729, 1974.
92. Attwood HD, Park WW: Embolism to the lungs by trophoblast. J Obstet Gynecol Br Commonw 68:611, 1961.
93. Sparr RA, Pritchard JA: Studies to detect the escape of amniotic fluid into the maternal circulation during parturition. Surg Gynecol Obstet 107:560, 1958.
94. Steiner PE, Lushbaugh CC: Maternal pulmonary embolism by amniotic fluid as a cause of obstetric shock and unexpected deaths in obstetrics. JAMA 117:1245, 1941.
95. Attwood HD, Downing SE: Experimental amniotic fluid and meconium embolism. Surg Gynecol Obstet 120:255, 1965.
96. Liban E, Raz S: A clinicopathologic study of fourteen cases of amniotic fluid embolism. Am J Clin Pathol 51:477, 1969.
97. Maradny E, Kanayama N, Halim A, et al: Endothelin has a role in early pathogenesis of amniotic fluid embolism. Gynecol Obstet Invest 40:14, 1995.
98. Clark SL: New concepts of amniotic fluid embolism: A review. Obstet Gynecol Surv 45:360, 1990.
99. Dib N, Bajwa T: Amniotic fluid embolism causing severe left ventricular dysfunction and death: Case report and review of the literature. Cathet Cardiovasc Diagn 39:177, 1996.
100. Girard P, Mal H, Laine J-F, et al: Left heart failure in amniotic fluid embolism. Anesthesiology 64:262, 1986.
101. Koegler A, Sauder P, Marolf A, et al: Amniotic fluid embolism: A case with non-cardiogenic pulmonary edema. Intensive Care Med 20:45, 1994.
102. Masson RG, Ruggieri J, Siddiqui M: Amniotic fluid embolism: Definitive diagnosis in a survivor. Am Rev Respir Dis 120:187, 1979.
103. Dray F, Frydman R: Primary prostaglandin in amniotic fluid in pregnancy and spontaneous labor. Am J Obstet Gynecol 126:13, 1976.
104. Romero R, Emamian M, Wan M, et al: Increased concentrations of arachidonic acid lipoxygenase metabolites in amniotic fluid during parturition. Obstet Gynecol 70:849, 1987.
105. Clark SL, Hankins GD, Dudley DA, et al: Amniotic fluid embolism: Analysis of the national registry. Am J Obstet Gynecol 172:1158, 1995.
106. Lockwood CJ, Bach R, Guha A, et al: Amniotic fluid contains tissue factor, a potent initiator of coagulation. Am J Obstet Gynecol 165:1335, 1991.
107. Weiner AE, Reid DE, Roby CC: The hemostatic activity of amniotic fluid. Science 110:190, 1949.
108. Aguillon A, Andjus T, Grayson A, et al: Amniotic fluid embolism: A review. Obstet Gynecol Surv 17:619, 1962.
109. Woodfield DG, Galloway RK, Smart GE: Coagulation defect associated with presumed amniotic fluid embolism in the mid-trimester of pregnancy. J Obstet Gynecol Br Commonw 78:423, 1971.
110. Laforga JB: Amniotic fluid embolism. Report of two cases with coagulation disorder. Acta Obstet Gynecol Scand 76:805, 1997.
111. Lau G, Chui PP: Amniotic fluid embolism: A review of 10 fatal cases. Singapore Med J 35:180, 1994.
112. Peterson EP, Taylor HB: Amniotic fluid embolism: An analysis of 40 cases. Obstet Gynecol 35:787, 1970.
113. Liban E, Raz S: A clinicopathologic study of fourteen cases of amniotic fluid embolism. Am J Clin Pathol 31:477, 1969.
114. Attwood HD: A histological study of experimental amniotic-fluid and meconium embolism in dogs. J Pathol Bacteriol 88:285, 1964.
115. Wasser WG, Tessler S, Kamath CP, et al: Nonfatal amniotic fluid embolism: A case report of postpartum respiratory distress with histopathologic studies. Mount Sinai J Med 46:388, 1979.
116. Roche WD Jr, Norris HJ: Detection and significance of maternal pulmonary amniotic fluid embolism. Obstet Gynecol 43:729, 1974.
117. Garland IWC, Thompson WD: Diagnosis of amniotic fluid embolism using an antiserum to human keratin. J Clin Pathol 36:625, 1983.
118. Ishiyama I, Mukaida M, Komuro E, et al: Analysis of a case of generalized amniotic fluid embolism by demonstrating the fetal isoantigen (A blood type) in maternal tissues of B blood type, using immunoperoxidase staining. Am J Clin Pathol 85:239, 1986.
119. Kobayashi H, Ooi H, Hayakawa H, et al: Histological diagnosis of amniotic fluid embolism by monoclonal antibody TKH-2 that recognizes NeuAc alpha 2-6Ga1NAc epitope. Hum Pathol 28:428, 1997.
120. Cheung AN, Luk SC: The importance of extensive sampling and examination of cervix in suspected cases of amniotic fluid embolism. Arch Gynecol Obstet 255:101, 1994.
121. Rodgers GP, Heymach GJ III: Cryoprecipitate therapy in amniotic fluid embolization. Am J Med 76:916, 1984.
122. Cornell SH: Amniotic pulmonary embolism. Am J Roentgenol 89:1084, 1963.
123. Lumley J, Owen R, Morgan M: Amniotic fluid embolism: A report of three cases. Anaesthesia 34:33, 1979.
124. Fidler JL, Patz EF Jr, Ravin CE: Cardiopulmonary complications of pregnancy: Radiographic findings. Am J Roentgenol 161:937, 1993.
125. Anderson DG: Amniotic fluid embolism: A re-evaluation. Am J Obstet Gynecol 98:336, 1967.
126. Lee KR, Catalano PM, Ortiz-Giroux S: Cytologic diagnosis of amniotic fluid embolism. Report of a case with a unique cytologic feature and emphasis on the difficulty of eliminating squamous contamination. Acta Cytol 30:177, 1986.
127. Giampaolo C, Schneider V, Kowalski BH, et al: The cytologic diagnosis of amniotic fluid embolism: A critical reappraisal. Diagn Cytopathol 3:126, 1987.
128. Kobayashi H, Ohi H, Tarao T: A simple, noninvasive, sensitive method for diagnosis of amniotic fluid embolism by monoclonal antibody TKH-2 that recognizes NeuAc alpha 2-6Ga1NAc. Am J Obstet Gynecol 168:848, 1993.
129. Kanayama N, Yamazaki T, Naruse H, et al: Determining zinc coproporphyrin in maternal plasma—a new method for diagnosing amniotic fluid embolism. Clin Chem 38:526, 1992.
130. Morgan M: Amniotic fluid embolism. Anaesthesia 34:20, 1979.
131. Masson RG, Ruggieri J, Siddiqui M: Amniotic fluid embolism: Definitive diagnosis in a survivor. Am Rev Respir Dis 120:187, 1979.
132. Clark SL: Successful pregnancy outcomes after amniotic fluid embolism. Am J Obstet Gynecol 167:511, 1992.
133. Piggott J, Hansbarger EA Jr, Neafie RC: Human ascariasis. Am J Clin Pathol 53:223, 1970.
134. Shaw AFB, Ghareeb AA: The pathogenesis of pulmonary schistosomiasis in Egypt with special reference to Ayerza's disease. J Pathol Bacteriol 146:401, 1938.
135. Richmond DR, Bernstein L: Hydatid pulmonary embolism. Case report. Aust Ann Med 17:270, 1968.
136. Schriner RW, Ryu JH, Edwards WD: Microscopic pulmonary tumor embolism causing subacute cor pulmonale: A difficult antemortem diagnosis. Mayo Clin Proc 66:143, 1991.
137. Chan CK, Hutcheon MA, Hyland RH, et al: Pulmonary tumor embolism: A critical review of clinical, imaging and hemodynamic features. J Thorac Imaging 2:4, 1987.
138. Case records of the Massachusetts General Hospital: Weekly clinicopathological exercises—case 27-1987. N Engl J Med 317:35, 1987.
139. Shepard JO, Moore EH, Templeton PA, et al: Pulmonary intravascular tumor emboli: Dilated and beaded peripheral pulmonary arteries at CT. Radiology 187:797, 1993.
140. Tingleff J, Joyce FS, Pettersson G: Intraoperative echocardiographic study of air embolism during cardiac operations. Ann Thorac Surg 60:673, 1995.
141. Lew TW, Tay DH, Thomas E: Venous air embolism during cesarean section: More common than previously thought. Anesth Analg 77:448, 1993.
142. Lantz PE, Smith JD: Fatal carbon dioxide embolism complicating attempted laparoscopic cholecystectomy—case report and literature review. J Forensic Sci 39:1468, 1994.
143. Despond O, Fiset P: Oxygen venous embolism after the use of hydrogen peroxide during lumbar discectomy. Can J Anaesth 44:410, 1997.
144. Pao BS, Hayden SR: Cerebral gas embolism resulting from inhalation of pressurized helium. Ann Emerg Med 28:363, 1996.
145. Palmon SC, Moore LE, Lundberg J, et al: Venous air embolism: A review. J Clin Anesth 9:251, 1997.
146. Tolly TL, Feldmeier JE, Czarnecki D: Air embolism complicating percutaneous lung biopsy. Am J Roentgenol 150:555, 1988.
147. Wong RS, Ketai L, Temes RT, et al: Air embolus complicating transthoracic percutaneous needle biopsy. Ann Thorac Surg 59:1010, 1995.
148. Tellides G, Ugurlu BS, Kim RW, et al: Pathogenesis of systemic air embolism during bronchoscopic Nd:YAG laser operations. Ann Thorac Surg 65:930, 1998.
149. Saada M, Goarin JP, Riou B, et al: Systemic gas embolism complicating pulmonary contusion. Diagnosis and management using transesophageal echocardiography. Am J Respir Crit Care Med 152:812, 1995.
150. Moon RE, Vann RD, Bennett PB: The physiology of decompression illness. Sci Am 273:70, 1995.
151. Kizer KW: Diving medicine. Emerg Med Clin North Am 2:513, 1984.
152. Weiss LD, Van Meter KW: Cerebral air embolism in asthmatic scuba divers in a swimming pool. Chest 107:1653, 1995.
153. Smith FR: Air embolism as a cause of death in scuba diving in the Pacific Northwest. Dis Chest 22:15, 1967.
154. Bayne CG, Wurzbacher T: Can pulmonary barotrauma cause cerebral air embolism in a non-diver? Chest 81:648, 1982.
154a. Zaugg M, Kaplan V, Widmer URS, et al: Fatal air embolism in an airplane passenger with a giant intrapulmonary bronchogenic cyst. Am J Respir Crit Care Med 157:1686, 1998.
155. Segal AJ, Wasserman M: Arterial air embolism: A cause of sudden death in status asthmaticus. Radiology 99:271, 1971.

156. Vinstein AL, Gresham EL, Lim MO, et al: Pulmonary venous air embolism in hyaline membrane disease. Radiology 105:627, 1972.

157. Siegle RL, Eyal FG, Rabinowitz JG: Air embolus following pulmonary interstitial emphysema in hyaline membrane disease. Clin Radiol 27:77, 1976.

158. Kogutt MS: Systemic air embolism secondary to respiratory therapy in the neonate: Six cases including one survivor. Am J Roentgenol 131:425, 1978.

159. Weaver LK, Morris A: Venous and arterial gas embolism associated with positive pressure ventilation. Chest 113:1132, 1998.

160. Gronert GA, Messick JM, Cucchiara RF, et al: Paradoxical air embolism from a patent foramen ovale. Anesthesiology 50:548, 1979.

161. Michel L, Pokanzer DC, Mckusick KA, et al: Fatal paradoxical air embolism to the brain: Complication of central venous catheterization. J Parenter Enterol Nutr 6:68, 1982.

162. Black M, Calvin J, Chan KL, et al: Paradoxic air embolism in the absence of an intracardiac defect. Chest 99:754, 1991.

163. Marquez J, Sladen A, Gendell H, et al: Paradoxical cerebral air embolism without an intracardiac septal defect. J Neurosurg 55:997, 1981.

164. Tommasino C, Rizzardi R, Beretta L, et al: Cerebral ischemia after venous air embolism in the absence of intracardiac defects. J Neurosurg Anesthesiol 8:30, 1996.

165. Baugh SL: Venous air embolism: Clinical and experimental considerations. Crit Care Med 20:1169, 1992.

166. Tuddenham WJ, Paskin DL: Radiographic demonstration of air embolism. Med Radiogr Photogr 50:16, 1974.

167. Paterack KA, Aggarwal A: Central venous air embolism without a catheter. Can J Anaesth 38:338, 1991.

168. Marcus RH, Weinert L, Neumann A, et al: Venous air embolism: Diagnosis by spontaneous right-sided contrast echocardiography. Chest 99:784, 1991.

169. Tuxen DV, Scheinkestel CD, Salamonson R: Air embolism—a neglected cause of stroke complicating cardiopulmonary bypass (CPB) surgery. Aust N Z J Med 24:732, 1994.

170. Lowenwirt IP, Chi DS, Handwerker SM: Nonfatal venous air embolism during cesarean section: A case report and review of the literature. Obstet Gynecol Surv 49:72, 1994.

171. Rothenberg F, Schumacher JR, Rosenthal RL: Near-fatal pulmonary air embolus from presumed inadvertent pressure placed on a partially empty plastic intravenous infusion bag. Am J Cardiol 73:1035, 1994.

172. Woodring JH, Fried AM: Nonfatal venous air embolism after contrast-enhanced CT. Radiology 167:405, 1988.

173. Matjasko J, Petrozza P, Cohen M, et al: Anesthesia and surgery in the seated position: Analysis of 554 cases. Neurosurgery 17:695, 1985.

174. Sutherland RW, Winter RJ: Two cases of fatal air embolism in children undergoing scoliosis surgery. Acta Anaesthesiol Scand 41:1073, 1997.

175. Durant TM, Long J, Oppenheimer MJ: Pulmonary (venous) air embolism. Am Heart J 33:269, 1947.

176. O'Quin RJ, Lakshminarayan S: Venous air embolism. Arch Intern Med 142:2173, 1982.

177. Hartveit F, Lystad H, Minken A: The pathology of venous air embolism. Br J Exp Pathol 49:81, 1968.

178. Warren BA, Philp RB, Inwood MJ: The ultrastructural morphology of air embolism: Platelet adhesion to the interface and endothelial damage. Br J Exp Pathol 54:163, 1973.

179. Butler BD, Hills BA: Transpulmonary passage of venous air emboli. J Appl Physiol 59:543, 1985.

180. Clark MC, Flick MR: Permeability pulmonary edema caused by venous air embolism. Am Rev Respir Dis 129:633, 1984.

181. Smelt WL, Baerts WD, de Langhe JJ, et al: Pulmonary edema following air embolism. Acta Anaesthesiol Belg 38:201, 1987.

182. Burrowes P, Wallace C, Davies JM, et al: Pulmonary edema as a radiologic manifestation of venous air embolism secondary to dental implant surgery. Chest 101:561, 1992.

183. Pou NA, Roselli RJ, Parker RE, et al: Effects of air embolism on sheep lung fluid volumes. J Appl Physiol 75:986, 1993.

184. Wang D, Li MH, Hsu K, et al: Air embolism-induced lung injury in isolated rat lungs. J Appl Physiol 72:1235, 1992.

185. Flick MR, Hoeffel JM, Staub NC: Superoxide dismutase with heparin prevents increased lung vascular permeability during air emboli in sheep. J Appl Physiol 55:1284, 1983.

186. Flick MR, Milligan SA, Hoeffel JM, et al: Catalase prevents increased lung vascular permeability during air emboli in unanesthetized sheep. J Appl Physiol 64:929, 1988.

187. Hlastala MP, Robertson HT, Ross BK: Gas exchange abnormalities produced by venous gas embolism. Respir Physiol 36:1, 1979.

188. Wirjosemito SA, Touhey JE, Workman WT: Type II altitude decompression sickness (DCS): US Air Force experience with 133 cases. Aviat Space Environ Med 60:256, 1989.

189. Bason R, Yacavone D, Bellenkes AH: Decompression sickness: USN operational experience 1969–1989. Aviat Space Environ Med 62:994, 1991.

190. Gottleib JD, Ericsson JA, Sweet RB: Venous air embolism: A review. Anesth Analg 44:773, 1965.

191. Boerema B: Appearance and regression of pulmonary arterial lesions after repeated intravenous injection of gas. J Pathol Bacteriol 89:741, 1965.

192. Balk AG, Mooi WJ, Dingemans KP, et al: Development and regression of pulmonary arterial lesions after experimental air embolism. A light and electron-microscopic study. Virchows Arch 406:203, 1985.

193. Cholankeril JV, Joshi RR, Cenizal JS, et al: Massive air embolism from the pulmonary artery. Case report. Radiology 142:33, 1982.

194. Faer JM, Messerschmidt GL: Nonfatal pulmonary air embolism: Radiographic demonstration. Am J Roentgenol 131:705, 1978.

195. Kizer KW, Goodman PC: Radiographic manifestations of venous air embolism. Radiology 144:35, 1982.

196. Taylor JD: Post-mortem diagnosis of air embolism by radiography. BMJ 1:890, 1952.

197. Roobottom CA, Hunter JD, Bryson PJ: The diagnosis of fatal gas embolism: Detection by plain film radiography. Clin Radiol 49:805, 1994.

198. Berenstein AB, Krall R, Choi IS: Embolization with n-butyl cyano-acrylate in management of CNS lesions (a). AJNR Am J Neuroradiol 10:883, 1989.

199. Harker CP, Neuman TS, Olson LK, et al: The roentgenographic findings associated with air embolism in sport scuba divers. J Emerg Med 11:443, 1993.

200. Zwirewich CV, Müller NL, Abboud RT, et al: Noncardiogenic pulmonary edema caused by decompression sickness: Rapid resolution following hyperbaric therapy. Radiology 163:81, 1987.

201. Aberle DR, Gamsu G, Golden J: Fatal systemic air embolism following lung needle aspiration. Radiology 165:351, 1987.

202. Woodring JH, Fried AM: Nonfatal venous air embolism after contrast-enhanced CT. Radiology 167:405, 1988.

203. Groell R, Schaffler GJ, Rienmueller R, et al: Vascular air embolism: Location, frequency, and cause on electron-beam CT studies of the chest. Radiology 202:459, 1997.

204. Tetzlaff K, Reuter M, Leplow B, et al: Risk factors for pulmonary barotrauma in divers. Chest 112:576, 1997.

205. Adornato DC, Gildenberg PL, Ferrario CM, et al: Pathophysiology of intravenous air embolism in dogs. Anesthesiology 49:120, 1978.

206. Ericsson JA, Gottlieb JD, Sweet RB: Closed-chest cardiac massage in the treatment of venous air embolism. N Engl J Med 270:1353, 1964.

207. Smith RM, Neuman TS: Abnormal serum biochemistries in association with arterial gas embolism. J Emerg Med 15:285, 1997.

208. Campkin TV, Perks JS: Venous air embolism. Lancet 1:235, 1973.

209. Chang JL, Albin MS, Bunegin L, et al: Analysis and comparison of venous air embolism detection methods. Neurosurgery 7:135, 1980.

210. Glenski JA, Cucchiara RF: Transcutaneous $O_2$ and $CO_2$ monitoring of neurosurgical patients: Detection of air embolism. Anesthesiology 64:546, 1986.

211. Hurter D, Sevel P: Detection of venous air embolism: A clinical report using end tidal carbon dioxide monitoring during neurosurgery. Anesthesiology 34:578, 1979.

212. Matjasko J, Petrozza P, Mackenzie CF: Sensitivity of end-tidal nitrogen in venous air embolism detection in dogs. Anesthesiology 63:418, 1985.

213. Young ML, Smith DS, Murtaugh F, et al: Comparison of surgical and anesthetic complications in neurosurgical patients experiencing venous air embolism in the sitting position. Neurosurgery 18:157, 1986.

214. Paré JA, Fraser RG, Hogg JC, et al: Pulmonary "mainline" granulomatosis: Talcosis of intravenous methadone abuse. Medicine 58:229, 1979.

215. Paré JP, Cote G, Fraser RS: Long-term follow-up of drug abusers with intravenous talcosis. Am Rev Respir Dis 139:233, 1989.

216. Kalant H, Kalant OJ: Death in amphetamine users: Causes and rates. Can Med Assoc J 112:299, 1975.

217. Hopkins GP, Taylor DG: Pulmonary talc granulomatosis. A complication of drug abuse. Am Rev Respir Dis 101:101, 1970.

218. Lewman LV: Fatal pulmonary hypertension from intravenous injection of methylphenidate (Ritalin) tablets. Hum Pathol 3:67, 1972.

219. Willey RF: Abuse of methylphenidate (Ritalin). N Engl J Med 285:464, 1971.

220. Douglas FG, Kafilmout KJ, Patt NL: Foreign particle embolism in drug addicts: Respiratory pathophysiology. Ann Intern Med 75:865, 1971.

221. Soin JS, Wagner HN, Thomashaw D, et al: Increased sensitivity of regional measurements in early detection of narcotic lung disease. Chest 67:325, 1975.

222. Zientara M, Moore S: Fatal talc embolism in a drug addict. Hum Pathol 1:324, 1970.

223. Camargo G, Colp C: Pulmonary function studies in ex-heroin users. Chest 67:331, 1975.

224. Gross EM: Talc embolism: Sudden death following intravenous injection of phenyltoloxamine. Forensic Sci 2:475, 1973.

225. Tomashefski JF Jr, Hirsch CS, Jolly PN: Microcrystalline cellulose pulmonary embolism and granulomatosis. Arch Pathol Lab Med 105:89, 1981.

226. Zeltner TB, Nussbaumer U, Rudin O, et al: Unusual pulmonary vascular lesions after intravenous injections of microcrystalline cellulose. Virchows Arch 395:207, 1982.

227. Itkonen J, Schnoll S, Daghestani A, et al: Accelerated development of pulmonary complications due to illicit intravenous use of pentazocine and tripelennamine. Am J Med 76:617, 1984.

228. Smith RH, Graf MS, Silverman JF: Successful management of drug-induced talc granulomatosis with corticosteroids. Chest 73:552, 1978.

229. Schwartz IS, Bosken C: Pulmonary vascular talc granulomatosis. JAMA 256:2584, 1986.

230. Sturner WO, Spruill FG, Garriott JC: The propylhederine-associated fatalities: Benzedrine revisited. J Forensic Sci 19:372, 1974.

231. Hopkins GB: Pulmonary angiothrombotic granulomatosis in drug offenders. JAMA 221:909, 1972.

232. Houck RJ, Bailey GL, Daroca PJ Jr, et al: Pentazocine abuse: Report of a case with pulmonary arterial cellulose granulomas and pulmonary hypertension. Chest 77:227, 1980.

233. Tomashefski JF Jr, Hirsch CS: The pulmonary vascular lesions of intravenous drug abuse. Human Pathol 11:133, 1980.

234. Johnston WH, Waisman J: Pulmonary corn starch granulomas in a drug user. Arch Pathol 92:196, 1971.

235. Siegel H, Bloustein P: Continuing studies in the diagnosis and pathology of death from intravenous narcotism. J Forensic Sci 15:179, 1970.

236. Lewis JH, Sundeen JT, Simon GL, et al: Disseminated talc granulomatosis. An unusual finding in a patient with acquired immunodeficiency syndrome and fatal cytomegalovirus infection. Arch Pathol Lab Med 109:147, 1985.

237. Ben-Haim SA, Ben-Ami H, Edoute Y, et al: Talcosis presenting as pulmonary infiltrates in an HIV-positive heroin addict. Chest 94:656, 1988.

238. Farber HW, Falls R, Glauser FL: Transient pulmonary hypertension from the intravenous injection of crushed, suspended pentazocine tablets. Chest 80:178, 1981.

239. Waller BF, Brownlee WJ, Roberts WC: Self-induced pulmonary granulomatosis: A consequence of intravenous injection of drugs intended for oral use. Chest 78:90, 1980.

240. Groth DH, Mackay GR, Crable JV, et al: Intravenous injection of talc in a narcotics addict. Arch Pathol 94:171, 1972.

241. Feigin DS: Talc: Understanding its manifestations in the chest. Am J Roentgenol 146:295, 1986.

242. Crouch E, Churg A: Progressive massive fibrosis of the lung secondary to intravenous injection of talc: A pathologic and mineralogic analysis. Am J Clin Pathol 80:520, 1983.

243. Schmidt RA, Glenny RW, Godwin JD, et al: Panlobular emphysema in young intravenous Ritalin abusers. Am Rev Respir Dis 143:649, 1991.

244. Allaire GS, Goodman ZD, Ishak KG, et al: Talc in liver tissue of intravenous drug abusers with chronic hepatitis. A comparative study. Am J Clin Pathol 92:583, 1989.

245. Genereux GP, Emson HE: Talc granulomatosis and angiothrombotic pulmonary hypertension in drug addicts. J Can Assoc Radiol 25:87, 1974.

246. Stern WZ, Subbarao K: Pulmonary complications of drug addiction. Semin Roentgenol 18:183, 1983.

247. Sieniewicz DJ, Nidecker AC: Conglomerate pulmonary disease: A form of talcosis in intravenous methadone abusers. Am J Roentgenol 135:697, 1980.

248. Robertson CH Jr, Reynolds RC, Wilson JE: Pulmonary hypertension and foreign-body granulomas in intravenous drug abusers: Documentation by cardiac catheterization and lung biopsy. Am J Med 61:657, 1976.

249. Arnett EN, Battle WE, Russo JV, et al: Intravenous injection of talc-containing drugs intended for oral use: A cause of pulmonary granulomatosis and pulmonary hypertension. Am J Med 60:711, 1976.

250. Farber HW, Fairman RP, Glauser FL: Talc granulomatosis: Laboratory findings similar to sarcoidosis. Am Rev Respir Dis 125:258, 1982.

251. Brown DG, Aguirre A, Weaver A: Gallium-67 scanning in talc-induced pulmonary granulomatosis. Chest 77:561, 1980.

252. Padley SPG, Adler BD, Staples CA, et al: Pulmonary talcosis: CT findings in three cases. Radiology 186:125, 1993.

253. Stern EJ, Frank MS, Schmutz JF, et al: Panlobular pulmonary emphysema caused by IV injection of methylphenidate (Ritalin): Findings on chest radiographs and CT scans. Am J Roentgenol 162:555, 1994.

254. Murphy SB, Jackson WB, Paré JAP: Talc retinopathy. Can J Opthalmol 13:152, 1978.

255. Tao L, Morgan RC, Donat EE: Cytologic diagnosis of intravenous talc granulomatosis by fine needle aspiration biopsy. Acta Cytol 28:737, 1984.

256. Thomashow D, Summer WR, Soin J, et al: Lung disease in reformed drug addicts: Diagnostic and physiologic correlations. Johns Hopkins Med J 141:1, 1977.

257. Overland ES, Nolan AJ, Hopewell PC: Alteration of pulmonary function in intravenous drug abusers: Prevalence, severity, and characterization of gas exchange abnormalities. Am J Med 68:231, 1980.

258. Ulm AH, Wagshul EC: Pulmonary embolization following urethrography with an oily medium. N Engl J Med 263:137, 1960.

259. Clouse ME, Hallgrimsson J, Wenlund DE: Complications following lymphography with particular reference to pulmonary oil embolism. Am J Roentgenol 96:972, 1966.

260. Gough JH, Gough MH, Thomas ML: Pulmonary complications following lymphography with a note on technique. Br J Radiol 37:416, 1964.

261. Allen WE, D'Angelo CM: Pulmonary oil embolism following pantopaque ventriculography in a patient with a ventriculovenous shunt. Case report. J Neurosurg 35:623, 1971.

262. Chung JW, Park JH, Im JG, et al: Pulmonary oil embolism after transcatheter oily chemoembolization of hepatocellular carcinoma. Radiology 187:689, 1993.

263. Hallgrimsson J, Clouse ME: Pulmonary oil emboli after lymphography. Arch Pathol 80:426, 1965.

264. Takahashi M, Abrams HL: Arborizing pulmonary embolization following lymphangiography: Report of three cases and an experimental study. Radiology 89:633, 1967.

265. Richardson P, Crosby EH, Bean HA, et al: Pulmonary oil deposition in patients subjected to lymphography: Detection by thoracic photoscan and sputum examination. Can Med Assoc J 94:1086, 1966.

266. Fraimow W, Wallace S, Lewis P, et al: Changes in pulmonary function due to lymphangiography. Radiology 85:231, 1965.

267. Felton WL II: A method for the identification of lipiodol in tissue sections. Lab Invest 1:364, 1952.

268. Bron KM, Baum S, Abrams HL: Oil embolism in lymphangiography: Incidence, manifestations, and mechanism. Radiology 80:194, 1963.

269. Fallat RJ, Powell MR, Youker JE, et al: Pulmonary deposition and clearance of [131]I-labeled oil after lymphography in man: Correlation with lung function. Radiology 97:511, 1970.

270. Weg JG, Harkleroad LE: Aberrations in pulmonary function due to lymphangiography. Dis Chest 53:534, 1968.

271. Belin RP, Shea MA, Stone NH, et al: Iodolipisputosis following lymphangiography. Report of a case. Dis Chest 48:543, 1965.

272. Gold WM, Youker J, Anderson S, et al: Pulmonary-function abnormalities after lymphangiography. N Engl J Med 273:519, 1965.

273. White RJ, Webb JAW, Tucker AK, et al: Pulmonary function after lymphography. BMJ 4:775, 1973.

274. LaMonte CS, Lacher MJ: Lymphangiography in patients with pulmonary dysfunction. Arch Intern Med 132:365, 1973.

275. Zillmer EA, Lucci K-A, Barth JT, et al: Neurobehavioral sequelae of subcutaneous injection with metallic mercury. Clin Toxicol 24:91, 1986.

276. Johnson HRM, Koumides O: Unusual case of mercury poisoning. BMJ 1:340, 1967.

277. Hill DM: Self-administration of mercury by subcutaneous injection. BMJ 1:342, 1967.

278. Buxton JT Jr, Hewitt JC, Gadsden RH, et al: Metallic mercury embolism. Report of cases. JAMA 193:573, 1965.

279. Naidich TP, Bartelt D, Wheeler PS, et al: Metallic mercury emboli. Am J Roentgenol 117:886, 1973.

280. Vas W, Tuttle RJ, Zylak CJ: Intravenous self-administration of metallic mercury. Radiology 137:313, 1980.

281. Cowan NC, Kane P, Karani J: Case report: Metallic mercury embolism: Deliberate self-injection. Clin Radiol 46:357, 1992.

282. Maniatis V, Zois G, Stringaris K: IV mercury self-injection: CT imaging. Am J Roentgenol 169:1197, 1997.

283. Hohage H, Otte B, Westermann G, et al: Elemental mercurial poisoning. South Med J 90:1033, 1997.

284. Torres-Alanis O, Garza-Ocanas L, Pineyro-Lopez A: Intravenous self-administration of metallic mercury: Report of a case with a 5-year follow-up. J Toxicol Clin Toxicol 35:83, 1997.

285. Pelz DM, Lownie SP, Fox AJ, et al: Symptomatic pulmonary complications from liquid acrylate embolization of brain arteriovenous malformations. AJNR Am J Neuroradiol 16:19, 1995.

286. Takasugi JE, Shaw C: Inadvertent bucrylate pulmonary embolization: A case report. J Thorac Imaging 4:71, 1989.

287. Goldman ML, Philip PK, Sarrafizadeh MS, et al: Transcatheter embolization with bucrylate (in 100 patients). Radiographics 2:340, 1982.

288. Johnston B, Smith P, Heath D: Experimental cotton-fibre pulmonary embolism in the rat. Thorax 36:910, 1981.

289. Adams DF, Olin TB, Kosek J: Cotton fiber embolization during angiography. Radiology 84:678, 1965.

290. Garvan JM, Gunner BW: The harmful effects of particles in intravenous fluids. Med J Aust 2:1, 1964.

291. Jaques WE, Mariscal GG: A study of the incidence of cotton emboli. Bull Int Assoc Med Museums 32:63, 1951.

292. von Glahn WC, Hall JW: The reaction produced in the pulmonary arteries by emboli of cotton fibers. Am J Pathol 25:575, 1949.

293. Truemner KM, White S, Vanlandingham H: Fatal embolization of pulmonary capillaries. JAMA 173:119, 1960.

294. Roman PW, Wagner JH, Steinbach SH: Massive fatal embolism during barium enema study. Radiology 59:190, 1952.

295. David R, Berezesky IK, Bohlman M, et al: Fatal barium embolization due to incorrect vaginal rather than colonic insertion. Arch Pathol Lab Med 107:548, 1983.

296. Collins DH: Bullet embolism: A case of pulmonary embolism following the entry of a bullet into the right ventricle of the heart. J Pathol Bacteriol 60:205, 1948.

297. Straus R: Pulmonary embolism caused by a lead bullet following a gunshot wound of the abdomen. Arch Pathol 33:63, 1942.

298. Hafez A, Dartevelle P, Lafont D, et al: Pulmonary arterial embolus by an unusual wandering bullet. Thorac Cardiovasc Surg 31:392, 1983.

299. Brewer LA III, Bai AF, King EL, et al: The pathologic effects of metallic foreign bodies in the pulmonary circulation. J Thorac Cardiovasc Surg 38:670, 1959.

300. Terry PB, Barth KH, Kaufman SL, et al: Balloon embolization for treatment of pulmonary arteriovenous fistulas. N Engl J Med 302:1189, 1980.

301. Leitman BS, McCauley DI, Firooznia H: Multiple metallic pulmonary densities after therapeutic embolization. JAMA 248:2155, 1982.

302. Bernhardt LC, Wegner GP, Mendenhall JT: Intravenous catheter embolization to the pulmonary artery. Chest 57:329, 1970.

303. Ross AM: Polyethylene emboli: How many more? Chest 57:307, 1970.

304. Prager D, Hertzberg RW: Spontaneous intravenous catheter fracture and embolization from an implanted venous access port and analysis by scanning electron microscopy. Cancer 60:270, 1987.

305. Edelstein J: Atraumatic removal of a polyethylene catheter from the superior vena cava. Chest 57:381, 1970.

306. Soni J, Osatinsky M, Smith T, et al: Nonsurgical removal of polyethylene catheter from the right cardiac cavities. Chest 57:398, 1970.

307. Editorial: Glass embolism. Lancet 2:1300, 1972.

308. Turco SJ, Davis NM: Detrimental effects of particulate matter on the pulmonary circulation. JAMA 217:81, 1971.

309. Thomassen RW, Houbert JP, Winn DF Jr, et al: The occurrence and characterization of emboli associated with the use of a silicone antifoaming agent. J Cardiovasc Thorac Surg 41:611, 1961.

310. Leong AS-Y, Disney APS, Gove DW: Spallation and migration of silicone from blood-pump tubing in patients on hemodialysis. N Engl J Med 306:135, 1982.

311. Krempien B, Bommer J, Ritz E: Foreign body giant cell reaction in lungs, liver and spleen. Virchows Arch 392:73, 1981.

312. Robinson MJ, Nestor M, Rywlin AM: Pulmonary granulomas secondary to embolic prosthetic valve material. Hum Pathol 12:759, 1981.

313. Chen Y-M, Lu C-C, Perng R-P: Silicone fluid-induced pulmonary embolism. Am Rev Respir Dis 147:1299, 1993.

314. Lai YF, Chao TY, Wong SL: Acute pneumonitis after subcutaneous injections of silicone for augmentation mammaplasty. Chest 106:1152, 1994.

314a. Duong T, Schonfeld AJ, Yungbluth M, et al: Acute pneumopathy in a nonsurgical transsexual. Chest 113:1127, 1998.

315. Kiyokawa H, Utsumi K, Minemura K, et al: Fat embolism syndrome caused by vegetable oil injection. Intern Med 34:380, 1995.

316. Uflacker R, Kaemmerer A, Picon PD, et al: Bronchial artery embolization in the management of hemoptysis: Technical aspects and long-term results. Radiology 157:637, 1985.

317. Tomashefski JF Jr, Cohen AM, Doershuk CF: Longterm histopathologic follow-up of bronchial arteries after therapeutic embolization with polyvinyl alcohol (Ivalon) in patients with cystic fibrosis. Hum Pathol 19:555, 1988.

318. Castaneda-Zuniga WR, Sanchez R, Amplatz K: Experimental observations on short- and long-term effects of arterial occlusion with Ivalon. Radiology 126:783, 1978.

319. Boushy SF, Helgason AH, North LB: Occlusion of the bronchial arteries by glass microspheres. Am Rev Respir Dis 103:249, 1971.

320. Nosanchuk JS, Littler ER: Skin embolus to lung. Arch Pathol 87:542, 1969.

321. Straus R: Pulmonary embolism caused by liver tissue. Arch Pathol 33:69, 1942.

322. Abrahams C, Catchatourian R: Bone fragment emboli in the lungs of patients undergoing bone marrow transplantation. Am J Clin Pathol 79:360, 1983.

323. Veinot JP, Edwards WD: Trauma-related embolization of cartilage to the lungs. Case report of a 41-year-old man. Am J Forensic Med Pathol 15:138, 1994.

324. Lie JT: Myocardium as emboli in the systemic and pulmonary circulation. Arch Pathol Lab Med 111:261, 1987.

325. Becker SSN, Seo IS, Cornog J: Atypical transitional epithelial cells in a pulmonary embolus. Chest 61:198, 1972.

326. Bohm N, Keller KM, Kloke WD: Pulmonary and systemic cerebellar tissue embolism due to birth injury. Virchows Arch 398:229, 1982.

327. Smith RRL, Hutchins GM: Pulmonary fecal embolization complicating the Budd-Chiari syndrome. N Engl J Med 298:1069, 1978.

328. Balogh K: Pulmonary bile emboli: Sequelae of iatrogenic trauma. Arch Pathol Lab Med 108:814, 1984.

329. Walley VM, Guindi MM, Stinson WA: Regurgitation of fat and marrow emboli into coronary veins during resuscitation. Arch Pathol Lab Med 115:65, 1991.

330. Jackson CT, Greendyke RM: Pulmonary and cerebral fat embolism after closed-chest cardiac massage. Surg Gynecol Obstet 120:25, 1965.

331. Fiallos M, Kissoon N, Abdelmoneim T, et al: Fat embolism with the use of intraosseous infusion during cardiopulmonary resuscitation. Am J Med Sci 314:73, 1997.

332. Herndon JH, Bechtol CO, Crickenberger DP, et al: Fat embolism during total hip replacement. J Bone Joint Surg (Am) 56:1350, 1974.

333. Caillouette J, Anzel S: Fat embolism syndrome following the intramedullary alignment guide in total knee arthroplasty. Clin Orthop 251:198, 1990.

334. Hagley SR, Lee FC, Blumbergs PC: Fat embolism syndrome with total hip replacement. Med J Aust 145:541, 1986.

335. Laub DR Jr, Laub DR: Fat embolism syndrome after liposuction: A case report and review of the literature. Ann Plast Surg 25:48, 1990.

336. Ross RM, Johnson GW: Fat embolism after liposuction. Chest 93:1294, 1988.

337. Lipton JH, Russell JA, Burgess KR, et al: Fat embolization and pulmonary infiltrates after bone marrow transplantation. Med Pediatr Oncol 15:24, 1987.

338. Baselga J, Reich L, Doherty M, et al: Fat embolism syndrome following bone marrow harvesting. Bone Marrow Transplant 7:485, 1991.

339. Kitchell CC, Balogh K: Pulmonary lipid emboli in association with long-term hyperalimentation. Hum Pathol 17:83, 1986.

340. Menendez LR, Bacon W, Kempf RA, et al: Fat embolism syndrome complicating intraarterial chemotherapy with cis-platinum. Clin Orthop Rel Res 254:294, 1990.

341. Waller DA, Bennett MK, Corris PA, et al: Donor-acquired fat embolism causing primary organ failure after lung transplantation. Ann Thorac Surg 59:1565, 1995.

342. Krupp P, Busch M, Cockburn I, et al: Encephalopathy associated with fat embolism induced by solvent for cyclosporin. Lancet 1:168, 1989.

343. Guardia SN, Bilbao JM, Murray D, et al: Fat embolism in acute pancreatitis. Arch Pathol Lab Med 113:503, 1989.

344. Cuppage FE: Fat embolism in diabetes mellitus. Am J Clin Pathol 40:270, 1963.

345. Broder G, Ruzumna L: Systemic fat embolism following acute primary osteomyelitis. JAMA 199:1004, 1967.

346. Day JD, Walden SM, Stuart SR, et al: Fatal fat embolism syndrome after numerous vertebral body compression fractures in a lung transplant recipient. J Heart Lung Transplant 13:785, 1994.

347. Desselle BC, O'Brien T, Bugnitz M, et al: Fatal fat embolism in a patient with sickle-beta+ thalassemia. Pediatr Hematol Oncol 12:159, 1995.

348. Hill RB Jr: Fatal fat embolism from steroid-induced fatty liver. N Engl J Med 265:318, 1961.

349. Durlacher SH, Meier JR, Fisher RS, et al: Sudden death due to pulmonary fat embolism in persons with alcoholic fatty liver. Am J Pathol 30:633, 1954.

350. Lynch MJG, Raphael SS, Dixon TP: Fat embolism in chronic alcoholism. Arch Pathol 67:68, 1959.

351. Kaufman HD, Finn R, Bourdillon RE: Fat embolism following an epileptic seizure. BMJ 1:1089, 1966.

352. Todd N: Fatal fat embolism during ritual initiation. Can Med Assoc J 113:133, 1975.

353. Rosen JM, Braman SS, Hasan FM, et al: Nontraumatic fat embolization: A rare cause of new pulmonary infiltrates in an immunocompromised patient. Am Rev Respir Dis 134:805, 1986.

354. Jones JP Jr, Ramirez S, Doty SB: The pathophysiologic role of fat in dysbaric osteonecrosis. Clin Orthop 296:256, 1993.

355. DeMonte F, al-Mefty O: Ruptured dermoid tumor of the cavernous sinus associated with the syndrome of fat embolism. Case report. J Neurosurg 77:312, 1992.

356. Xue H, Zhang YF: Pulmonary fat embolism in rabbits induced by forced immobilization. J Trauma 32:415, 1992.

357. Kole SD, Saksena DS, Oswal DH: Fat cerebral air embolism during open heart surgery caused by lung parenchyma to left atrial communication. J Heart Valve Dis 3:583, 1994.

358. Kaps M, Hansen J, Weiher M, et al: Clinically silent microemboli in patients with artificial prosthetic aortic valves are predominantly gaseous and not solid. Stroke 28:322, 1997.

359. Lang NP, Wait GM, Read RR: Cardio-cerebrovascular complications from Nd-YAG laser treatment of lung cancer. Am J Surg 162:629, 1991.

360. Golish JA, Pena CM, Mehta AC: Massive air embolism complicating Nd-YAG laser endobronchial photoresection. Lasers Surg Med 12:338, 1992.

361. Ijichi T, Itoh T, Sakai R, et al: Multiple brain gas embolism after ingestion of concentrated hydrogen peroxide. Neurology 48:277, 1997.

362. Lowenwirt IP, Chi DS, Handwerker SM: Nonfatal venous air embolism during cesarean section: A case report and review of the literature. Obstet Gynecol Surv 49:72, 1994.

363. Kelly M, Mathews HM, Weir P: Carbon dioxide embolism during laser endometrial ablation. Anaesthesia 52:65, 1997.

364. Cleveland JC: Fatal air embolism to the right side of the heart during pneumonectomy for carcinoma: Result of broncho-azygous vein communication and positive-pressure ventilation. Chest 71:556, 1977.

365. Girdler NM: Fatal sequel to dental implant surgery. J Oral Rehabil 21:721, 1994.

366. Karachalios T, Geeurickx A, Newman JH: Fatal air embolism after prophylactic intramedullary nailing. A case report. J Bone Joint Surg 74:1101, 1992.

367. Kieser C: A review of the complications of arthroscopic knee surgery. Arthroscopy 8:79, 1992.

368. Albin MS, Ritter RR, Pruett CE, et al: Venous air embolism during lumbar laminectomy in the prone position: Report of three cases. Anesth Analg 73:346, 1991.

369. Razvi HA, Chin JL, Bhandari R: Fatal air embolism during radical retropubic prostatectomy. J Urol 151:433, 1994.

370. Vacanti CA, Lodhia KL: Fatal massive air embolism during transurethral resection of the prostate. Anesthesiology 74:186, 1991.

371. Cadeddu JA, Arrindell D, Moore RG: Near fatal air embolism during percutaneous nephrostomy placement. J Urol 158:1519, 1997.

372. Fatal gas embolism caused by overpressurization during laparoscopic use of argon enhanced coagulation. Health Devices 23:257, 1994.

373. Kobayashi S, Takei T: Venous air embolism during knee arthrography. A case report. Arch Orthop Trauma Surg 110:311, 1991.

374. Dasher WA, Black JPM, Weiss W, et al: Air embolism complicating pneumoperitoneum: A review. Am Rev Tuberc 69:396, 1954.

375. Buxbaum JL, Muravchick S, Chen L: Intraoperative air embolism with pulse irrigation device. J Clin Anesth 8:519, 1996.

376. Cooper JP, Swanton RH: Complications of transvenous temporary pacemaker insertion. Br J Hosp Med 53:155, 1995.

377. McCarthy PM, Wanga N, Birchfield F, et al: Air embolism in single-lung transplant patients after central venous catheter removal. Chest 107:1178, 1995.

378. Mennim P, Coyle CF, Taylor JD: Venous air embolism associated with removal of central venous catheter. BMJ 305:171, 1992.

379. Ruesch M, Miyatalse S, Ballinger C: Continuing hazard of air embolism during pressure transfusion. JAMA 172:1476, 1960.

380. Dunbar EM, Fox R, Watson B, et al: Successful late treatment of venous air embolism with hyperbaric oxygen. Postgrad Med J 66:469, 1990.

381. Eagle CJ, Davies JM: Lethal air embolism during placement of a Kimray-Greenfield filter. J Cardiothorac Anesth 4:616, 1990.

382. Collins KA, David GJ, Lantz PE: An unusual case of maternal-fetal death due to vaginal insufflation of cocaine. Am J Forensic Med Pathol 15:335, 1994.

383. Hill BF, Jones JS: Venous air embolism following orogenital sex during pregnancy. Am J Emerg Med 11:155, 1993.

384. Eckert WG, Katchis S, Dotson P: The unusual accidental death of a pregnant woman by sexual foreplay. Am J Forensic Med Pathol 12:247, 1991.

385. Cooke RT: Self-induced air embolism in a man. BMJ 2:2297, 1961.

386. Adelson L: Fatal air embolism following intrascrotal injection in a transvestite. J Forensic Sci 2:291, 1957.

387. Cina SJ, Downs JC, Conradi SE: Hydrogen peroxide: A source of lethal oxygen embolism. Case report and review of the literature. Am J Forensic Med Pathol 15:44, 1994.

388. Morris WP, Butler BD, Tonnesen AS, et al: Continuous venous air embolism in patients receiving positive end-expiratory pressure. Am Rev Respir Dis 147:1034, 1993.

389. Rabl W, Auer M: Unusual death of a farmer. Am J Forensic Med Pathol 13:238, 1992.

390. Kost M: Thoracic complications associated with utilization of the air turbine dental drill. AANA J 64:288, 1996.

391. Linden JV, Kaplan HS, Murphy MT: Fatal air embolism due to perioperative blood recovery. Anesth Analg 84:422, 1997.

# PART IX

# PULMONARY HYPERTENSION AND EDEMA

# CHAPTER 50

# Pulmonary Hypertension

## GENERAL FEATURES OF PULMONARY HYPERTENSION

### Anatomic and Physiologic Considerations

The anatomy of the pulmonary circulation and the principles that govern blood flow through the pulmonary vascular tree are discussed in detail in Chapter 2 (*see* page 71). Only a brief overview is given here.

The pulmonary vasculature consists of a highly branched system of arteries, arterioles, capillaries, venules, and veins that can accommodate the entire cardiac output at low driving pressures. There are approximately 17 generations of arterial vessels between the main pulmonary artery (PA) and arterioles, measuring 10 to 15 $\mu$m in diameter.[1, 2] In the tracheobronchial tree most of the resistance to air flow is in the large airways, but in the PA tree the majority of the resistance is in the smaller blood vessels (muscular arteries and arterioles).

The relationship between the total cross-sectional areas of the tracheobronchial tree and the pulmonary arterial tree and the distance from the alveolar surface can be seen in Figure 50–1.[3] It is apparent that the two "trees" begin with similar-sized "trunks" but that the total cross-sectional area of the airways greatly exceeds that of the blood vessels in the periphery of the lung. Vessels in this location contain the majority of vascular smooth muscle, and it is the change in the caliber of these vessels that regulates arterial blood flow to cause the best match of ventilation and perfusion. Pulmonary capillaries arise from the arterioles and form an extensive, almost sheetlike layer of blood that is situated in the alveolar septa in intimate contact with alveolar gas. The pulmonary venules begin at the distal end of the capillary bed and course in the intralobular septa back to the hilum. Anastomoses between the bronchial and pulmonary vascular systems occur primarily at the capillary and postcapillary levels.

The pulmonary vascular circuit is a low-pressure system, the mean arterial pressure being only about one sixth

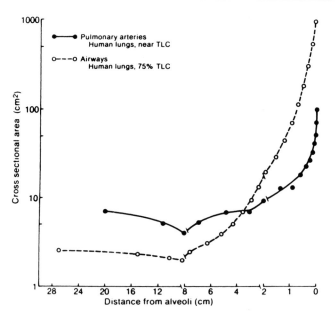

**Figure 50–1. Pulmonary Arterial and Airway Cross-Sectional Area.** The total cross-sectional area of the tracheobronchial tree and the pulmonary vascular tree increases greatly as they branch toward the gas-exchanging portion of the lung. These data show that the total area occupied by small airways exceeds that occupied by small pulmonary vessels. (From Culver BH, Butler J: Mechanical influences on the pulmonary microcirculation. Reproduced with permission, from the Annual Review of Physiology, Vol. 40, p. 187. © 1980 by Annual Reviews, Inc.)

of the systemic arterial pressure; the circuit has a remarkable capacity to compensate for a large physiologic increase in blood flow (e.g., during exercise) with little corresponding increase in pressure. This reduction in vascular resistance is achieved mainly by "recruiting" pulmonary vessels that are not perfused at rest. The ability to recruit vessels with minor increases in pressure results in a pulmonary vascular pressure-flow curve that does not have a zero flow intercept (i.e., there is no flow while there is still a positive arterial pressure) (*see* Fig. 2–27, page 105). For practical purposes, this means that any intervention that changes cardiac output will change the calculated pulmonary vascular resistance, regardless of whether there has been an actual change in pulmonary vascular smooth muscle tone. Because many pulmonary vascular smooth muscle relaxant agents may have an effect on cardiac output, these physiologic considerations are important in interpreting the results of interventions designed to increase pulmonary vascular caliber. To prove the presence of pulmonary "vasodilation," it is necessary to show a decrease in pressure at a fixed flow or a shift in the position or slope of the pressure-flow curve.

Pulmonary vascular resistance is calculated by dividing the driving flow by the cardiac output:

$$PVR = P_{Pa} - P_{La} / \dot{Q}$$

where PVR = pulmonary vascular resistance, $P_{Pa}$ = pulmonary artery pressure, $P_{La}$ = left atrial pressure, and $\dot{Q}$ = cardiac output. The driving pressure is the difference between mean pulmonary arterial pressure and mean left atrial pressure. In practice, the pulmonary wedge pressure provides a reliable estimate of left atrial pressure in the absence of large vein obstruction. The pulmonary arterial wedge pres-

sure is the pressure that is measured when pulmonary arterial flow is obstructed by wedging a catheter in a PA; the measured value approximates the pressure in the left atrium in the absence of venous obstruction. Pulmonary vascular resistance calculated in this way represents the summed resistances of the arteries, capillaries, and veins in series. An increase in pulmonary arterial pressure can occur because of an increase in blood flow; an increase in resistance to flow through arteries, capillaries, or veins; or an increase in left atrial pressure.

Pulmonary arterial hypertension may be defined as an increase above normally accepted values for pressure in the main PA at rest or during exercise. Generally accepted normal upper limits for these pressures are 30 mm Hg systolic and 18 mm Hg mean.[4] Pulmonary venous hypertension is present when the pressure in the pulmonary veins measured indirectly by a catheter wedged in a PA exceeds 12 mm Hg. Slight increases in pulmonary arterial pressure generally cause no clinical, radiographic, or electrocardiographic signs, even with mean pulmonary arterial pressures as high as 24 mm Hg.[5] However, as the pulmonary arterial pressure rises, the increased impedance to right ventricular ejection produces clinical and electrocardiographic signs and, eventually, radiographic changes indicative of hypertrophy of the right ventricle. With a further increase in pressure, catheterization studies may show elevation not only of pulmonary arterial and right ventricular systolic pressures but also of right ventricular diastolic pressure, indicating the onset of right ventricular failure.

### Pathogenesis

The pressure drop across any vascular bed is directly related to the blood flow through and the blood viscosity in that particular bed; an increase in flow or viscosity will cause an increase in pressure for any given vascular geometry. The pressure across the vascular bed is also indirectly related to the radius of its vessels; the total cross-sectional area of the vascular tree can decrease because of a loss of pulmonary vessels, intraluminal occlusion of a proportion of the vessels, vascular smooth muscle contraction and shortening, or vascular wall thickening and remodeling. Finally, pulmonary arterial pressure can be increased as a result of an increase in the downstream or venous pressure. The pathophysiologic mechanisms that can result in pulmonary hypertension are listed in Table 50–1.

The mechanism of production of pulmonary hypertension varies from patient to patient, and multiple factors are responsible in many. In some instances, such as in the early stages of primary pulmonary hypertension (PPH), there is reason to believe that the rise in pulmonary arterial pressure is caused by vasoconstriction and therefore is reversible.[6, 7] In other situations, obstruction of the pulmonary vascular tree is largely or completely caused by structural changes and is therefore irreversible.

Vasoconstriction may be produced by hypoxemia or acidosis, either metabolic or respiratory in origin;[8–11] there is evidence that this type of vasoconstriction may be reversed, at least partly, by the administration of oxygen or acetylcholine or by raising the pH of the blood.[8, 9, 12] In healthy people dwelling at very high altitudes, pulmonary hypertension can develop that disappears when the person is acclimatized at

## Table 50–1. MECHANISMS AND CAUSES OF PULMONARY HYPERTENSION

### PRECAPILLARY HYPERTENSION
#### *Primary Vascular Disease*

Increased flow (unrestricted left to right shunts)
Decreased flow (tetralogy of Fallot)
Primary pulmonary hypertension
Multiple pulmonary artery stenoses or coarctation
Compression of the main pulmonary artery or its branches
Pulmonary thrombotic and embolic disease
   Thromboembolism
   *In situ* thrombosis
   Metastatic neoplasm
   Parasites
   Miscellaneous (e.g., fat, talc, amnionic fluid)
Human immunodeficiency virus infection
Pulmonary capillary hemangiomatosis
Immunologic abnormalities (e.g., systemic lupus erythematosus,
   progressive systemic sclerosis)
High altitude
Persistent pulmonary hypertension of the newborn

#### *Pleuropulmonary Disease*

Emphysema
Bronchiectasis, bronchiolitis, and cystic fibrosis
Postpulmonary resection
Diffuse interstitial or air-space disease
   Fibrosis (e.g., granulomatous disease, pneumoconiosis,
    idiopathic pulmonary fibrosis)
   Adult respiratory distress syndrome
   Neoplasm
   Miscellaneous (e.g., alveolar microlithiasis, idiopathic
    hemosiderosis, alveolar proteinosis)
Pleural disease (fibrothorax)
Chest wall deformities
   Thoracoplasty
   Kyphoscoliosis

#### *Alveolar Hypoventilation*

Neuromuscular disease
Obesity
Obstructive sleep apnea
Chronic upper airway obstruction in children
Idiopathic (Ondine's curse)

### POSTCAPILLARY HYPERTENSION
#### *Cardiac Disease*

Left ventricular failure
Mitral valve disease
Myxoma (or thrombus) of the left atrium
Cor triatriatum

#### *Pulmonary Venous Disease*

Congenital stenosis of the pulmonary veins
Chronic sclerosing mediastinitis
Idiopathic veno-occlusive disease
Anomalous pulmonary venous return
Neoplasms
Thrombosis

---

sea level.[13] Pulmonary arterial constriction can also be caused by a variety of mediators of inflammation, including serotonin, histamine, angiotensin, catecholamines, prostaglandins, and leukotrienes.[14] The release of such mediators partly explains the acute pulmonary hypertension that develops in pulmonary thromboembolic disease. The increase in pressure in the PAs resulting from postcapillary hypertension (*see* farther on) also is initially vasospastic in origin, probably mediated through a vasovagal reflex originating from a rise in left atrial and pulmonary venous pressure. The rapid fall to normal pulmonary arterial pressure following mitral valve replacement in some cases of severe pulmonary hypertension caused by mitral stenosis can be explained only on the basis of pulmonary arterial vasoconstriction.[15]

Increasingly, the pulmonary vascular endothelium is being recognized as having an important role in the control of the pulmonary circulation. Far from being a passive bystander, it is a metabolically active tissue that responds to generalized and local changes in oxygen partial pressure, blood flow, and transmural pressure.[16] Different forms of pulmonary hypertension may exhibit particular patterns of endothelial cell dysfunction, possibly related to distinct initiating "injuries."[17] The endothelium can produce a variety of substances that affect the tone in the underlying vascular smooth muscle cells and can secrete cytokines and mitogens that play a role in the vascular wall remodeling that occurs in chronic hypertensive states.[18] The substances that have been most studied include prostanoid, prostacyclin, endothelin (ET), and nitric oxide (NO).

Prostacyclin ($PGI_2$) is produced from arachidonic acid by the action of the enzyme cyclooxygenase I. It is secreted by endothelial cells in response to increased blood flow and following stimulation by a number of specific agonists. It is both a powerful vasodilator and an inhibitor of platelet aggregation. Platelet-derived thromboxane $A_2$ and prostaglandin $F_{2\alpha}$ are also products of arachidonic acid but have the opposite effects on smooth muscle and platelets. In one study of 14 patients who had PPH and 9 patients who had secondary pulmonary hypertension as a result of severe chronic obstructive pulmonary disease (COPD), the urinary metabolites of thromboxane $A_2$ and prostacyclin were increased and decreased respectively, suggesting that an imbalance in their secretion may be a cause or a result of pulmonary hypertension.[19] Platelets also contain serotonin (5-hydroxytryptamine), which may be an important PA vasoconstrictor, especially in PPH.

ET actually represents a family of at least three different peptides—ET-1, ET-2, and ET-3—the first of which is produced by endothelial cells. It is a 21–amino acid peptide that is the most powerful vasoconstrictor known; it also has important mitogenic activity that could contribute to vascular remodeling. Levels of ET-1 are increased in the blood of patients who have PPH;[20] in addition, increased ET-1 immunoreactivity and messenger RNA have been found in the pulmonary endothelial cells of patients who have pulmonary hypertension.[21] Plasma ET levels are also increased acutely when normal subjects ascend to high altitudes, the increase correlating with the increase in PA pressure assessed by Doppler echocardiography.[22]

There has been considerable interest in the role of NO in the control of pulmonary vascular tone in health and disease.[23] This molecule has been identified as the *endothelial-derived or -dependent relaxant factor*. It is generated from the amino acid L-arginine via one of several isoforms of the enzyme NO synthase. A constitutive form of this enzyme (cNOS) is present in vascular endothelial cells and NO is released in response to the shear stress caused by flowing blood, as well as via receptor-operated mechanisms activated by acetylcholine, bradykinin, substance P, histamine, adenosine diphosphate, and platelet-derived products. NO acts via guanylate cyclase to increase the concentration of cyclic guanosine monophosphate in smooth muscle cells;

the latter in turn mediates vascular smooth muscle relaxation. NO is also released into the vascular lumen, where it can act to decrease platelet aggregation; thus, it may protect against vascular thrombosis as well as vasoconstriction. A second type of NO synthase (iNOS) is induced in inflammatory cells, smooth muscle cells, and endothelial cells in response to endotoxin and certain inflammatory cytokines. iNOS is capable of generating very high concentrations of NO, which, in inflammatory conditions, may act not only as a vasodilator but also as a mediator of cell toxicity.[24]

NO may be important in maintaining the normally low PA pressure;[25] it is also clear that it can oppose the vasoconstriction induced by various stimuli, including hypoxia.[26] Most important for the present discussion, a variety of observations suggest that impairment of NO production may contribute to the development of pulmonary hypertension. Chronic hypoxia leads to decreased NO release; PAs recovered at the time of lung transplantation from patients who have COPD and chronic hypoxemia show impaired NO generation in response to agonists such as acetylcholine.[27, 28] Although strong immunostaining for cNOS is normally detectable in pulmonary vascular endothelium, patients who have pulmonary hypertension and vascular remodeling have little or no detectable immunoreactivity.[29] Vasodilation occurs when arginine, the substrate for NO synthase, is infused intravenously into patients who have pulmonary hypertension. The magnitude of vasodilation is less in individuals who have primary, rather than secondary, pulmonary hypertension, which has led to speculation that a defect in endothelial NO production could be a basic mechanism in the idiopathic form of the disease.[16] Inhalation of NO and infusion of prostacyclin have also become important therapeutic interventions in the treatment of various forms of pulmonary hypertension,[30, 31] and the vasodilatory response to these substances has been used to assess the reversibility of increased vascular resistance in the primary form of disease.[32, 33]

Persistent pulmonary hypertension of the newborn is a syndrome in which the high PA pressure and extensive pulmonary arterial muscularization of the fetal lung do not regress in the early postnatal period. In most instances, the syndrome is due to a structural defect in the lung or heart, but in some patients the mechanism is unknown.[34] In the latter situation, it is likely that this failure is related to a disturbance in the normal regulation of one or a combination of ET, prostaglandins, and NO.[35, 36]

Endothelial dysfunction and release of vasoactive mediators are also the likely causes of the pulmonary hypertension that is frequently associated with adult respiratory distress syndrome (ARDS). The presence of pulmonary hypertension appears to be associated with a worse prognosis in this setting.[37] In fact, patients who have sepsis can have pulmonary hypertension before the onset of ARDS.[38] In experimental animals, infusion of endotoxin causes an acute increase in pulmonary arterial pressure, an effect that is blocked by cyclooxygenase inhibitors, which inhibit the formation of thromboxane $A_2$.[39] In humans with ARDS, the pulmonary hypertension is not completely reversed with cyclooxygenase inhibitors, and additional mediators, including the leukotrienes, serotonin, angiotensin II, and bradykinin, have been implicated.[40, 41] Other factors contributing to acute pulmonary hypertension in this clinical setting include

microvascular thrombi and emboli, interstitial pulmonary edema, and hypoxemia. If prolonged pulmonary dysfunction follows ARDS, vascular remodeling contributes to the persistence of pulmonary hypertension.

It is useful conceptually to divide the causes of pulmonary hypertension into three general groups, each of which shows somewhat different clinical, physiologic, and radiographic characteristics (*see* Table 50–1): those in which the major mechanisms of production are precapillary in location, those in which the significant physiologic disturbance arises from disease in the postcapillary vessels, and those in which the hypertension reflects a disturbance in vessels on both sides of the capillary bed—combined precapillary and postcapillary hypertension. In each of these groups, the capillaries may be involved to some extent and may contribute considerably to the increase in vascular resistance. For example, a major contribution to increased pulmonary vascular resistance in emphysema is the destruction of the capillary bed; also, chronic pericapillary edema can be associated with fibrosis, thereby limiting distensibility of the capillary bed in postcapillary venous hypertension.

### Pathologic Characteristics

The pathologic abnormalities seen in the pulmonary vasculature differ somewhat depending on the etiology of the hypertension. However, partly because of the limited response that can occur in the pulmonary vessels and partly because some of the abnormalities are secondary to the hypertension,[42] some findings are common to all causes. This is particularly true for changes in the large muscular and elastic arteries in patients who have hypertension of many etiologies and in the smaller arteries in patients who have primary (idiopathic) pulmonary hypertension or hypertension related to congenital cardiovascular disease, hepatic disease, acquired immunodeficiency syndrome (AIDS), connective tissue disease, and some anorexigenic drugs—conditions that are characterized by a group of vascular changes collectively known as *plexogenic pulmonary arteriopathy*. General pathologic features that occur in these and other forms of pulmonary arterial hypertension are described at this point; additional information about features specific to individual etiologies is discussed in the appropriate sections. Further details of morphologic features can be found in comprehensive texts and review articles.[43–48]

In pulmonary arterial hypertension of significant degree, the large elastic arteries, especially the main PA, are often dilated and are sometimes larger in diameter than the aorta; the dilation may be so severe that localized aneurysm formation is the result. If the hypertension is related to congenital cardiovascular disease and thus is present at birth, the fetal configuration of elastic laminae (consisting of fairly uniform concentric bands) tends to be preserved;[49] by contrast, if the hypertension is acquired, elastic laminae tend to possess an irregular, fragmented appearance similar to that of the normal adult vessel. An increase in acidic ground substance and a focal loss of elastic tissue in the media (so-called cystic medial necrosis) are sometimes present; as in the aorta, they may be associated with dissecting aneurysm.[50]

Pulmonary arterial atherosclerosis, usually mild and affecting predominantly the large elastic vessels, is a relatively common finding in older individuals; however, in the presence of pulmonary hypertension, atherosclerotic foci tend to be larger and to involve more distal branches.[51, 52] Grossly, they appear as yellow streaks or slightly elevated plaques similar to those seen in the systemic arteries. Histologically, they consist of intimal fibrous tissue containing aggregates of lipid-laden macrophages (Fig. 50–2); complicating features such as necrosis, calcification, and ulceration are uncommon. Intimal fibrosis of elastic and large muscular arteries is also frequent in pulmonary hypertension of any cause and may be so severe that it virtually obliterates the vascular lumen; in such cases, larger vessels may be identified grossly as thick-walled, rigid, pipelike structures projecting above the surface of the lung (Fig. 50–3). Paradoxically, the media in such cases may be atrophic, apparently as a consequence of the intimal fibrosis (*see* Fig. 50–3).

Histologic abnormalities can be seen in any part of the arterial or arteriolar wall. Adventitial thickening, predominantly as a result of an increase in fibrous tissue, has been documented in infants who have congenital diaphragmatic hernia and in adults who have PPH.[53, 54] It has been hypothesized that this may represent a reaction to the increased luminal pressure.[54]

Thickening of the media of small muscular arteries is a characteristic feature of many forms of pulmonary hypertension (Fig. 50–4). It is most often caused by a combination of muscle hypertrophy and hyperplasia; an increase in connective tissue between muscle cells is also seen in many cases.[55, 56] Additional smooth muscle cells are usually arranged in the same fashion as the normal circular muscle coat; however, new bundles of longitudinal muscle are also fairly common, often situated in an intimal location (*see* Fig. 50–4). Although there is obviously variation, the degree of medial thickening roughly corresponds to the severity of hypertension.[57–59] Muscle hypertrophy also occurs in pulmonary arterioles. In some cases, it is caused by an increase in the size and number of muscle fibers already present in the

arteriolar wall; in others, it represents extension of muscle into vessels that formerly contained none ("arterialization" of pulmonary arterioles).[60, 61] These new muscle cells appear to be derived from pericytes and "intermediate cells" normally present in the arteriolar wall[62] and can be associated with a substantial increase in wall thickness. As with arteries, such muscle may have a longitudinal orientation, a feature that may be related to alveolar hypoxia.[61]

In addition to muscle hypertrophy-hyperplasia, several abnormalities are often present in small- to medium-sized muscular arteries that together characterize plexogenic pulmonary arteriopathy.[45] These include cellular intimal proliferation and fibrosis, plexiform and dilation lesions, fibrinoid "necrosis," and vasculitis. Intimal thickening of muscular arteries in the early stages of plexogenic arteriopathy is characterized by the presence of loose connective tissue containing cells that are often elongated and arranged in more or less concentric layers encompassing the entire vascular lumen, resulting in a distinctive "onion skin" appearance (Fig. 50–5). The development of these lesions is a complex process that appears to involve a combination of migration of smooth muscle cells from the media, proliferation of endothelial cells, recruitment of inflammatory cells, and deposition of extracellular matrix proteins.[63–65] With time, the connective tissue component—particularly collagen and sometimes elastin—becomes prominent. This intimal thickening tends to occur more frequently in conventional than in supernumerary branches,[66] is often out of proportion to the degree of medial hypertrophy, and can result in almost complete luminal obliteration (*see* Fig. 50–5). Its recognition is important because there is evidence that its presence, at least when extensive, is associated with progressive pulmonary vascular disease despite repair of cardiovascular anomalies or treatment with vasodilator agents.[67, 68] Intimal fibrosis can also be eccentric rather than concentric, in which case the pathogenesis is likely to be related to organized throm-

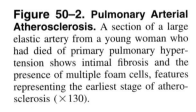

**Figure 50–2. Pulmonary Arterial Atherosclerosis.** A section of a large elastic artery from a young woman who had died of primary pulmonary hypertension shows intimal fibrosis and the presence of multiple foam cells, features representing the earliest stage of atherosclerosis (×130).

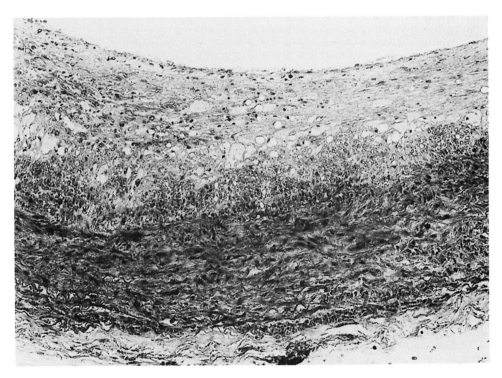

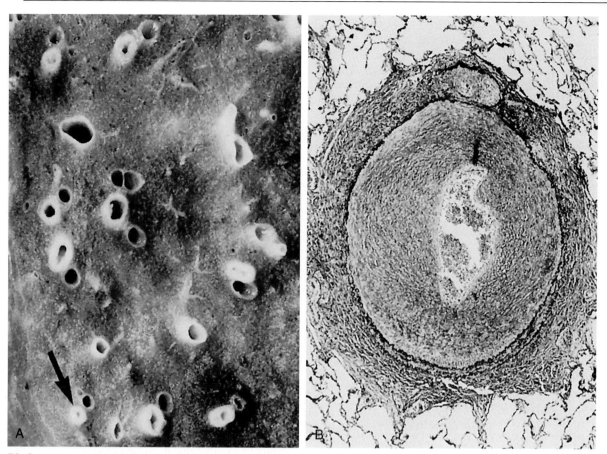

**Figure 50–3. Pulmonary Hypertension: Intimal Fibrosis.** Autopsy specimen of a 25-year-old woman who had systemic lupus erythematosus. A magnified view of peripheral lung parenchyma *(A)* shows marked thickening of the walls of many muscular arteries; in some *(arrow)*, the lumen is almost obliterated. A corresponding histologic section demonstrates the thickening to be caused predominantly by intimal fibrosis; marked medial atrophy is also evident. (*B*, Verhoeff–van Gieson, ×52.)

bus; although this pattern of fibrosis can be seen in association with plexogenic arteriopathy, it is more characteristic of pulmonary hypertension related to thrombosis ("thromboembolic" hypertension).[48, 68]

Plexiform lesions consist of distinctive abnormalities of small muscular arteries (usually 100 to 200 μm in diameter) that most often develop in a supernumerary artery a short distance beyond its origin from its parent vessel.[66] There is evidence that the distribution of lesions within the lung may vary with the underlying cause of hypertension; in one morphometric investigation of five cases of primary hypertension and six in which hypertension was associated with congenital cardiovascular disease, a preacinar location of plexiform lesions was twice as common (67% versus 34%) in the latter than in the former.[70] The lesion itself consists of a localized focus of vascular dilation associated with an intraluminal plexus of numerous slitlike vascular channels (Fig. 50–6); the latter are separated by a small amount of connective tissue and a variable number of plump fibroblast-like cells. The plexus itself often continues distally into a thin-walled, somewhat tortuous and dilated vascular channel.

The pathogenesis of plexiform lesions has been debated. Some investigators have theorized that it results from organization of intraluminal thrombus, possibly secondary to "fibrinoid necrosis," or inflammation of the adjacent vessel wall, or both.[45] The presence of intraluminal thrombus in relation to some plexiform lesions (*see* Fig. 50–6) is consis-

tent with this hypothesis. It has also been speculated that individual factors, perhaps genetic, related to reactivity of the pulmonary vasculature may be important in pathogenesis.[46] An increase in bronchiolar neuroendocrine cells, particularly those immunoreactive to bombesin, have been identified in patients who have pulmonary hypertension;[71] although this increase has been seen with various etiologies, it appears to be especially prominent in plexogenic arteriopathy, and it has been speculated that it may be involved in the pathogenesis of the lesions.

Dilation lesions may consist of separate, dilated, and often thin-walled veinlike vessels arising from a thick-walled artery or of a relatively compact cluster of tortuous, thin-walled vascular channels resembling an angioma (the latter appearance sometimes being designated *angiomatoid lesion*,[45] Fig. 50–7). These abnormalities are very uncommon and may result from a combination of elevated pressure and damage to medial cells.[45]

The term *fibrinoid necrosis* is used to describe the presence of homogeneous eosinophilic material in the wall of small PAs and arterioles (Fig. 50–8). As with plexiform lesions, the abnormality is most often seen in a small vessel close to its origin in a parent artery. Although there may be luminal thrombosis adjacent to the site of "necrosis," there is usually no inflammation of the vessel wall and the lesion most likely represents the accumulation of fibrin and other proteins within the media as a result of endothelial damage.

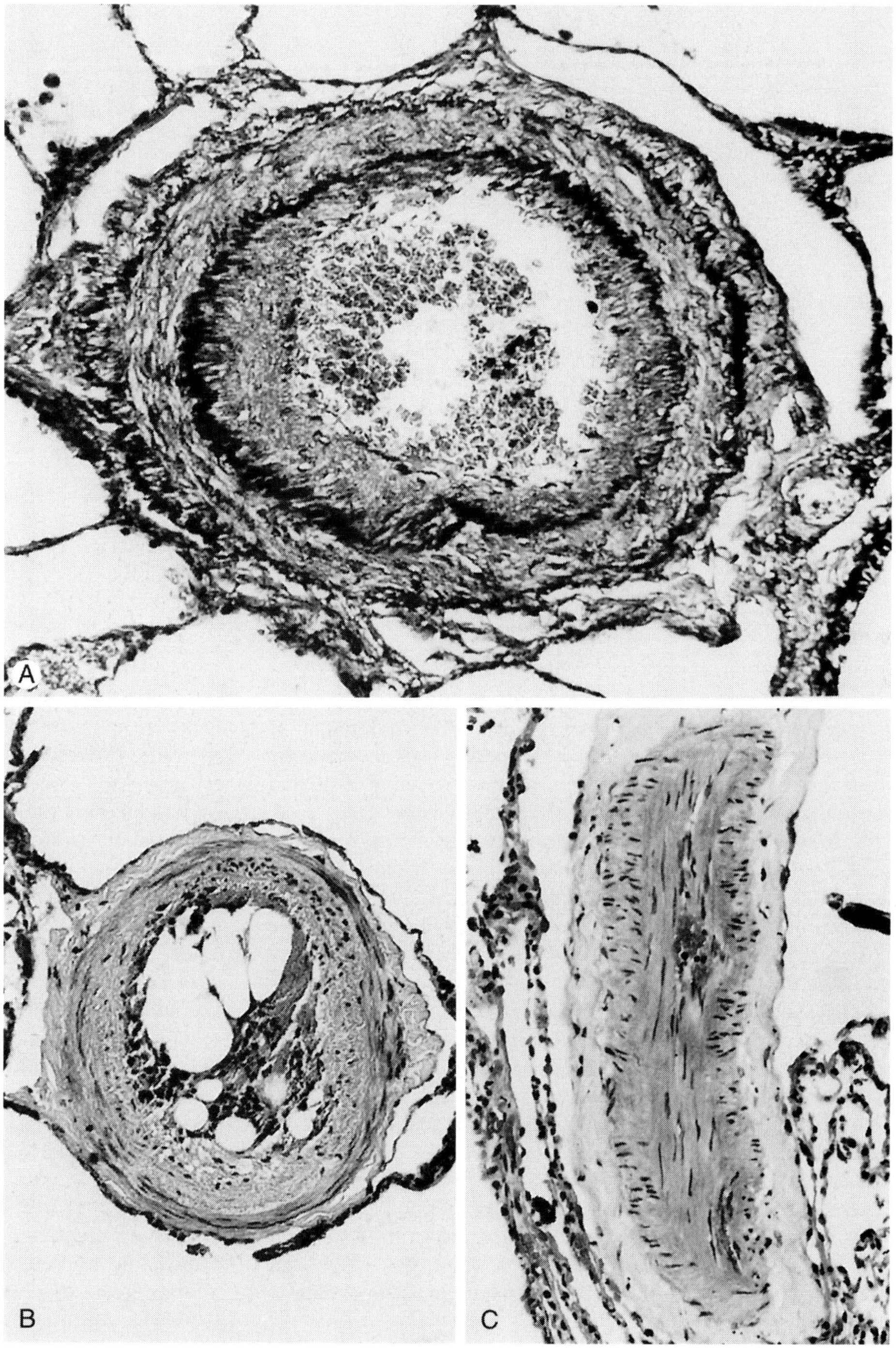

**Figure 50–4. Pulmonary Hypertension: Muscular Hyperplasia.** A section *(A)* of a medium-sized muscular artery from a 27-year-old woman who had primary pulmonary hypertension shows a moderate degree of medial thickening and mild intimal fibrosis. Cross- *(B)* and longitudinal *(C)* sections through two small arteries from a 63-year-old woman who had severe chronic obstructive pulmonary disease and cor pulmonale demonstrate clearly defined outer circular and inner longitudinal muscle. (A fragment of embolized bone marrow is present in *B.*) *(A,* Verhoeff–van Gieson, ×200; *B* and *C,* H&E, ×160.)

Whatever its nature, fibrinoid "necrosis" is relatively common in plexogenic arteriopathy in the presence of high pulmonary arterial pressures. Rarely, a vessel wall contains an acute inflammatory infiltrate, either with or without fibrinoid necrosis, indicating true vasculitis (Fig. 50–9).

Interestingly, pulmonary veins are also affected in some cases of plexogenic arteriopathy. For example, some degree of adventitial and intimal thickening was identified in veins less than 250 μm in about 50% of cases in one investigation of 19 patients.[54] Another rare and unusual finding is the presence of small nodules histologically resembling arachnoid villi adjacent to pulmonary venules;[72] these lesions have been reported in patients who have mitral stenosis and pulmonary thromboembolic disease as well as plexogenic arteriopathy, and it has been hypothesized that they may absorb excess water from the alveolar interstitium.

Two grading schemes have been suggested for quantifying the pulmonary vascular changes associated with the vascular obstruction in congenital heart disease. The Heath and Edwards system consists of six grades:[73] (1) medial hypertrophy, (2) cellular intimal proliferation, (3) progressive occlusion involving fibrosis of the intima, (4) dilation lesions associated with atrophy of the media, (5) adventitial angiomas, and (6) fibrinoid necrosis. A more recently proposed

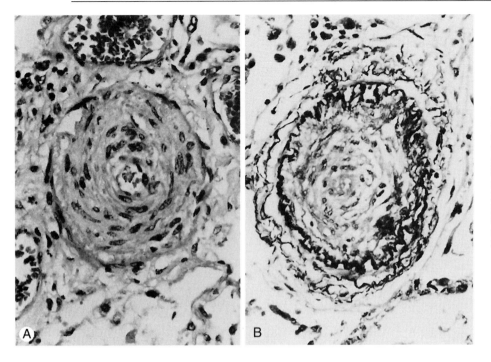

**Figure 50–5. Pulmonary Hypertension: Cellular Intimal Fibrosis.** A section of a pulmonary artery *(A)* from a young man with an atrial septal defect shows almost complete obliteration of its lumen by cellular fibrous tissue. The cell nuclei are somewhat elongated and arranged roughly in concentric layers, resulting in a somewhat whorled appearance. A section of the same vessel stained for elastic tissue *(B)* shows the cellular proliferation to be entirely within the intima. (*A,* H&E, ×160; *B,* Verhoeff–van Gieson, ×160.)

schema incorporates only three grades:[59] (A) extension of muscle into normally nonmuscular peripheral vessels, (B) medial hypertrophy of the more proximal muscular PAs, and (C) reduction in the concentration of distal vessels.

Both schemes have been used to predict the response of the pulmonary vascular hemodynamics to correction of associated congenital abnormalities; for example, with mild degrees of Grade B change there is little or no postoperative pulmonary hypertension, and regression of the vasculopathy is the rule.[44] The Heath-Edwards pathologic grading of pulmonary vascular changes has been compared with findings obtained at autopsy from *in vitro* intravascular ultrasound imaging in PAs of patients who had pulmonary hypertension.[74] In patients who had Grade 1 and 2 lesions, intravascular ultrasound demonstrated increased thickness of the echolucent zone due to increased medial thickness; patients who had Grade 3 or higher lesions also showed a bright inner layer due to intimal thickening. There was a good correlation ($r = 0.89$) of percent wall thickness derived from ultrasound and histologic examination. This technique has also been used to describe PA atherosclerotic changes in one patient *in vivo*.[75]

Scanning and transmission electron microscopic studies have revealed striking changes in the presence of pulmonary hypertension, the endothelium of small and large vessels having a "corduroy-like" and "cabled" configurations, respectively;[76] such a disfigured endothelial surface offers an increased opportunity for interaction of the endothelium with circulating platelets and inflammatory cells.

### Radiologic Considerations

The characteristic radiologic features of pulmonary arterial hypertension consist of enlargement of the central PAs and rapid tapering of the vessels as they extend to the periphery of the lungs (Fig. 50–10). This discordance in caliber between central and peripheral pulmonary vessels

is a distinctive feature of pulmonary arterial hypertension regardless of etiology.[77–79] The heart may be normal in size or enlarged. An unusual manifestation of severe chronic hypertension is the presence of PA calcification (Fig. 50–11). This usually is located in the main PA and its hilar branches; occasionally, it affects the lobar vessels.[80] Although such calcification is usually regarded as evidence of high pulmonary vascular resistance and irreversible vascular disease (most often in association with Eisenmenger syndrome), a case has been reported in which a large left-to-right shunt secondary to a ventricular septal defect was associated with extensive calcification but with near-normal pulmonary vascular resistance and reversible hypertension.[81]

Enlargement of the hilar PAs can be assessed by measuring the diameter of the interlobar arteries. The upper limit of the transverse diameter of the right interlobar artery from its lateral aspect to the air column of the intermediate bronchus is 16 mm in men and 15 mm in women.[82] Because the transverse diameter of the left interlobar artery is often impossible to measure on the posteroanterior view, a useful alternative is to measure the vessel on a lateral radiograph from the circular lucency created by the left upper lobe bronchus viewed end-on to the posterior margin of the vessel as it loops over the bronchus; the accepted upper limit of normal for this measurement is 18 mm.

Although it is clear that the presence of pulmonary hypertension can be recognized radiographically, the sensitivity and degree of accuracy with which its severity can be estimated is controversial.[77, 83–91] Measurements of the interlobar PAs are affected by the variable magnification related to patient size, distance between the x-ray tube and the film, and distance between the PA and the film. Measurement also may be difficult or impossible in the presence of extensive parenchymal lung disease. Furthermore, assessment of vascular pruning is subjective, and the degree of pruning does not correlate well with the level of pulmonary hypertension.[92] In fact, rapid tapering is usually a late mani-

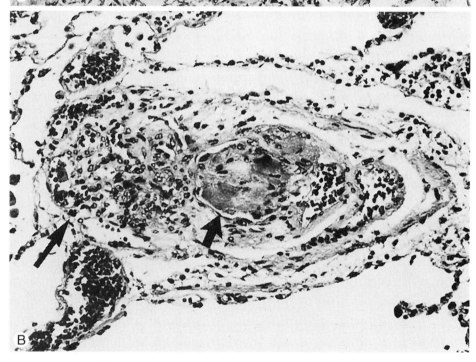

**Figure 50–6. Pulmonary Hypertension: Plexiform Lesion.** A section of a medium-sized pulmonary artery *(A)* from a young patient who had cirrhosis and portal hypertension reveals moderate intimal fibrosis *(short arrow)* continuous with a plexus of small, irregularly shaped vascular channels. These are separated by fibrous tissue containing many plump cells resembling fibroblasts *(long arrow)*. The plexus itself is continuous with a dilated, relatively thin-walled vascular channel *(curved arrows)*. Another lesion from a patient who had progressive systemic sclerosis *(B)* shows a similar vascular plexus *(long arrow)* associated with thrombus in the proximal artery *(short arrow)*. (A, ×130; B, ×140.)

festation, being seen less commonly than enlargement of the central PAs.[89, 91]

Because the main PA is intrapericardial, it cannot be measured on conventional radiography; however, it can be identified readily on computed tomography (CT) and magnetic resonance (MR) imaging. In a study of 32 patients who had cardiopulmonary disease and 26 age- and sex-matched control subjects believed but not proved to have normal PA pressure, the upper limit diameter of the main PA in normal subjects was 28.6 mm; in a patient group in which diameters were correlated with data from cardiac catheterization, a diameter of the main PA greater than 29 mm predicted the presence of pulmonary arterial hypertension.[93] Using multiple regression analysis, the investigators found that the best correlation with mean pulmonary arterial pressure was the combination of main PA and right interlobar PA cross-sectional area normalized for body surface area. However, in a subsequent study based on 24 patients who had undergone both chest CT and right-sided heart catheterization, only a trend toward correlation of main PA diameter with mean PA pressure was found.[94]

In another investigation, the findings on chest CT were compared with those at right heart catheterization in 55 patients being assessed for lung and heart-lung transplanta-

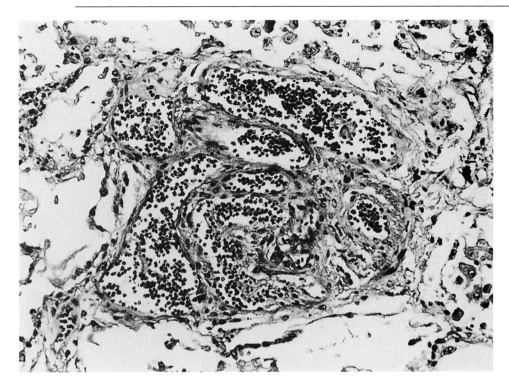

**Figure 50–7. Pulmonary Hypertension: Angiomatoid Lesion.** A plexus of interconnecting thin-walled dilated vascular channels resembles a small "angioma." From a patient with primary pulmonary hypertension (×180).

tion.[95] The study included 45 patients who had chronic lung disease, including emphysema, idiopathic pulmonary fibrosis, sarcoidosis, scleroderma, cystic fibrosis, and lymphangioleiomyomatosis, and 10 who had pulmonary vascular disease (PPH, Eisenmenger's syndrome, and chronic thromboembolism). In this study, the cutoff diameter of the main PA at or below which there was a 95% certainty of normal mean pressure was 28 mm. However, because the diameter of the main PA in patients who had normal mean arterial pressure ranged from 22 to 36 mm, the researchers con-

cluded that the cutoff diameter of 28 mm had questionable clinical utility. Multiple regression analysis revealed that the combination of main PA and left PA cross-sectional area normalized for body surface area showed the best correlation with mean PA pressure ($r = 0.81$). The multiple regression equations helped predict mean PA pressure within 5 mm Hg in 50% of patients who had chronic lung disease but in only 8% of patients who had pulmonary vascular disease. Right interlobar artery diameter did not correlate well with pulmonary arterial pressure; it was postulated that this might be

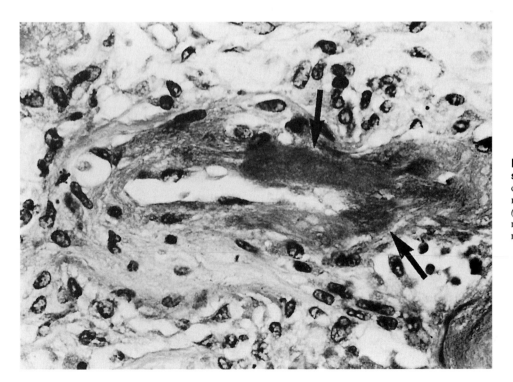

**Figure 50–8. Pulmonary Hypertension: Fibrinoid "Necrosis."** The wall of a small pulmonary artery contains homogeneous finely granular material (*arrows*) consisting of fibrin and other serum proteins. There is no inflammatory reaction or intraluminal thrombus (×520).

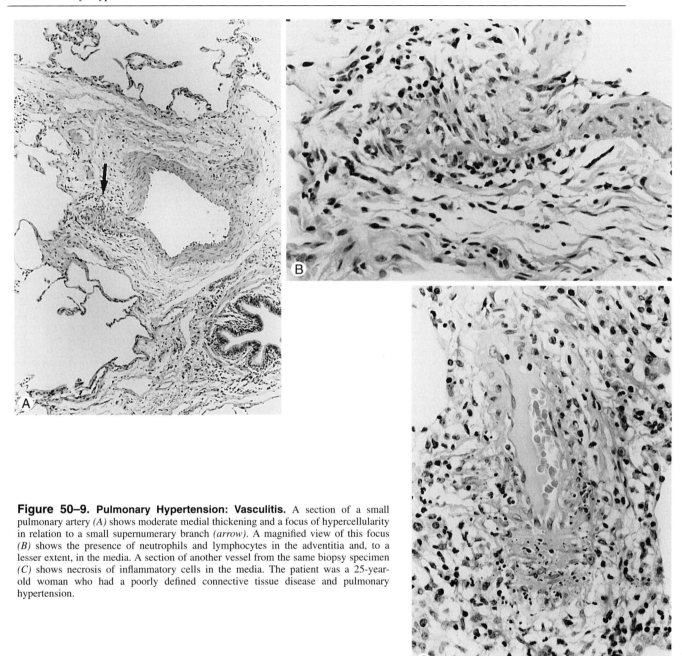

**Figure 50–9. Pulmonary Hypertension: Vasculitis.** A section of a small pulmonary artery *(A)* shows moderate medial thickening and a focus of hypercellularity in relation to a small supernumerary branch *(arrow)*. A magnified view of this focus *(B)* shows the presence of neutrophils and lymphocytes in the adventitia and, to a lesser extent, in the media. A section of another vessel from the same biopsy specimen *(C)* shows necrosis of inflammatory cells in the media. The patient was a 25-year-old woman who had a poorly defined connective tissue disease and pulmonary hypertension.

the result of difficulty in accurately measuring the diameter of the artery because of associated parenchymal lung disease or lymphadenopathy.

In another study of 36 patients who had pulmonary arterial hypertension, main PA diameter measurements on CT were correlated with right heart hemodynamic data.[95a] (Twenty patients had hypertension secondary to interstitial lung disease, 4 to COPD, 7 to chronic thromboembolism, and 3 to portal hypertension; 2 patients had primary pulmonary hypertension. Nine patients who had normal PA pressure were used as controls.) A main PA diameter on CT equal to or greater than 29 mm had a sensitivity of 87%, a specificity of 89%, and a positive predictive value of 97% for pulmonary arterial hypertension. There was no linear correlation between the degree of hypertension and main PA

diameter. Based on the results of these various studies, it is reasonable to conclude that a main PA diameter greater than 29 mm is suggestive of but not diagnostic for the presence of hypertension or increased pulmonary blood flow as a result of a left-to-right shunt. It has also been suggested that a segmental artery-to-bronchus diameter ratio greater than 1 in three or more lobes is helpful in predicting the presence of hypertension.[95a]

The most accurate noninvasive method of assessing the presence of pulmonary arterial hypertension is echocardiography. A number of variables derived from continuous wave or pulsed Doppler echocardiography can be employed to determine right ventricular peak systolic pressure, which is used as an estimate of PA pressure. These include calculation of the transtricuspid or transpulmonary valve pressure gradi-

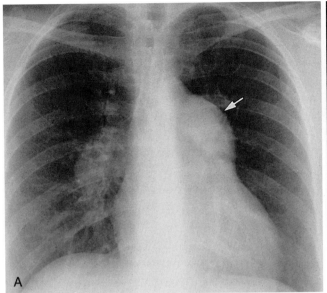

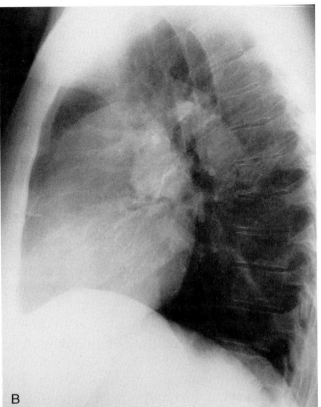

**Figure 50–10. Pulmonary Arterial Hypertension.** Posteroanterior (PA) *(A)* and lateral *(B)* chest radiographs demonstrate enlargement of the central pulmonary arteries with rapid tapering of the vessels. On the PA view, marked enlargement of the main pulmonary artery results in a focal convexity *(arrow)* immediately below the level of the aortic arch. On the lateral view, right ventricular enlargement and dilation of the pulmonary outflow tract result in filling of the lower retrosternal air space. The patient was a 36-year-old woman who had primary pulmonary arterial hypertension.

ent based on the velocity of the tricuspid or pulmonary regurgitant jets, the evaluation of right ventricular outflow tract velocity profiles, and the measurement of right ventricular isovolumic relaxation time.[96–98] The use of the tricuspid regurgitant jet is probably the most accurate.

In one study of 100 patients who had pulmonary hypertension secondary to COPD, echographic assessment was useful for estimation of PA pressure in 30;[96] in these patients, the correlation with mean PA pressure was 0.73. In the same study, the correlation coefficients for the relationships of PA

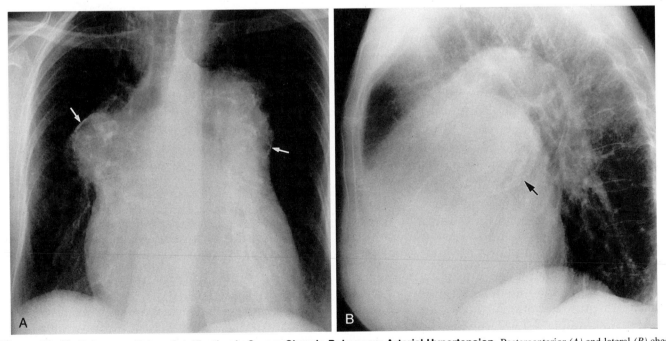

**Figure 50–11. Pulmonary Artery Calcification in Severe Chronic Pulmonary Arterial Hypertension.** Posteroanterior *(A)* and lateral *(B)* chest radiographs show cardiomegaly, marked dilation of the central pulmonary arteries, and peripheral oligemia. Note the presence of calcification *(arrows)* in the wall of the central pulmonary arteries. The patient was a 57-year-old woman who had an atrial septal defect and long-standing Eisenmenger syndrome.

pressure versus right ventricular acceleration time and right ventricular isovolumic relaxation were 0.65 and 0.61, respectively. The number of patients in whom the technique can be employed successfully is increased by injecting a small bolus of agitated saline into a peripheral vein during the test. The saline bolus contains microbubbles, which act as a echocardiographic contrast agent to enhance the detection of small tricuspid regurgitant jets.[99] Using data derived from measurements of pulmonary valve regurgitation, one group reported a correlation of PA diastolic pressure and Doppler-derived end-diastolic pressure gradient of 0.91.[100] Using a different approach, another group of investigators found that a combination of right ventricular dimensions, reflecting the presence of chronic pulmonary hypertension, was significantly correlated ($r = 0.97$) with mean PA pressure in a group of patients who had COPD.[101, 101a] The ratio of acceleration time to ejection time has been shown to be predictive of mean PA pressure in children who have pulmonary hypertension related to congenital heart disease ($r$ values of 0.92 and 0.94 in two separate groups).[101]

An advantage of echocardiographic assessment of pulmonary hemodynamics is that the dynamic response of the pulmonary circulation and right heart can be assessed by performing the measurements during increased cardiac work in response to exercise or to an inotropic agent (stress echocardiography).[102] Although the echocardiographic technique may underestimate true peak PA pressure in patients who have severe pulmonary hypertension, it is accurate enough to categorize patients as having mild, moderate, or severe disease.[103] Transesophageal echocardiography is more sensitive than transthoracic echocardiography in detecting the site of intracardiac shunts in patients who present with pulmonary hypertension of unknown cause[104] and often provides additional hemodynamic data in patients who have severe pulmonary hypertension who are being considered for lung transplantation.[105]

MR imaging can be used to define the direction and velocity of blood flow within the cardiac chambers and great vessels in addition to providing images of cardiovascular structure[106] (Fig. 50–12). Reviews of MR imaging in pulmonary hypertension and right ventricular dysfunction and in congenital heart disease have been published.[107, 108] The procedure has been shown to predict accurately right heart hemodynamics in patients who have PPH.[109] Velocity-encoded cine gradient-echo magnetic resonance imaging can also provide two-dimensional velocity maps of the cross-sectional area of a vessel. Peak systolic PA blood velocity estimated by this method correlates well with that measured using Doppler echocardiography;[110] it also shows substantial differences in velocity across the vascular lumen in patients who have pulmonary hypertension. Using MR imaging estimates of pulmonary blood flow ejection velocity, pulmonary arterial pressure has been estimated noninvasively ($r = 0.82$) in a small group of 12 patients who had different pulmonary vascular abnormalities.[111] In another group of 12 subjects who had PPH, the ratio of mean PA to aortic caliber was found to correlate significantly with the degree of hypertension ($r = 0.7$).[112] MR imaging has also been employed to make measurements of end-systolic and end-diastolic right ventricular volume and to calculate ejection volume and fraction;[113, 114] potentially it may be useful as a noninvasive supplemental method for evaluating patent ductus arteriosus and pulmonary arterial dissection.[115]

The role of ventilation-perfusion scintigraphy is mainly in distinguishing PPH from hypertension associated with chronic thromboembolism, a normal or low probability scan virtually excluding the latter process. For example, in one study of 75 patients, 24 of 25 (96%) who had chronic thromboembolic disease had high probability scans and one had an intermediate probability scan;[116] by contrast, of 35 patients who had PPH, 33 (94%) had low probability scans, one had an intermediate probability scan, and one had a high probability scan. Ten of 15 (67%) patients who had nonthromboembolic secondary pulmonary arterial hypertension had low probability scans, three (20%) had intermediate probability scans, and two (13%) had high probability scans. In patients who have intermediate or high probability scans, the diagnosis of chronic pulmonary thromboembolic disease can usually be confirmed using contrast-enhanced spiral CT[117–120] (Fig. 50–13). Preliminary results also suggest a role for MR imaging in the assessment of these patients[120] (see Fig. 50–13). In a small number of patients, pulmonary angiography may be required for definitive diagnosis.

Although fatalities have been reported following lung scanning in patients who have PPH,[121, 122] none of the 163 patients who had perfusion scans in the National Institutes of Health (NIH) study reported adverse effects.[123] Similarly, although it has been said that patients who have severe pulmonary hypertension are subject to sudden death during or following cardiac catheterization,[124] only one of the 50 patients who had pulmonary angiography in the NIH study had an adverse effect (transient hypotension). Complications are reduced by performing selective left and right main PA injections.[125] In one study in which this procedure was performed in 67 consecutive patients who had pulmonary hypertension, either primary or secondary to chronic thromboembolism, no major disturbances in cardiac rhythm, no episodes of significant systemic hypotension, and no fatalities were found; this approach has now become the standard.

## PRECAPILLARY PULMONARY HYPERTENSION

### Primary Vascular Disease

#### Increased Flow

Included in this category are the congenital heart defects with left-to-right shunt (atrial septal defect [ASD], ventricular septal defect [VSD], patent ductus arteriosus [PDA], aorticopulmonary window, transposition of the great vessels, and partial anomalous pulmonary venous drainage) and conditions associated with an increase in total blood volume or cardiac output, or both, such as thyrotoxicosis and chronic renal failure. A relative increase in pulmonary blood flow caused by extensive lung resection can also result in hypertension, presumably by similar mechanisms.[126] Rare causes include communication between the left ventricle and the right atrium[127] and communication between the aorta or its branches and the PA, right heart chambers, or superior vena cava;[128] the latter frequently involves the right coronary artery, the diagnosis being made in infancy by angiography following discovery of a continuous murmur on auscultation.

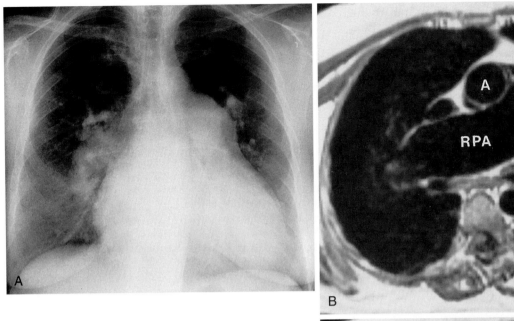

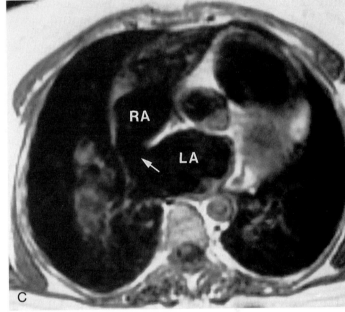

**Figure 50–12. Pulmonary Arterial Hypertension Caused by an Atrial Septal Defect.** A posteroanterior chest radiograph *(A)* shows cardiomegaly and marked enlargement of the central pulmonary arteries. Although there is rapid tapering, increased vascularity is still present in the lung periphery, particularly evident on the right side. A cardiac-gated spin-echo MR image *(B)* shows enlargement of the main (MPA) and right (RPA) pulmonary arteries. The diameter of the main pulmonary artery is considerably larger than that of the aorta (A). An MR image at the level of the right (RA) and left (LA) atrium *(C)* demonstrates an atrial septal defect *(arrow)*. The patient was a 61-year-old woman.

Pulmonary arterial flow may be increased greatly for a long time before increased resistance results in hypertension. It is assumed that the elevated resistance is caused initially by an increase in vasomotor tone and is subsequently related to more irreversible morphologic changes in the vasculature. Increased production of thromboxane and serotonin has been implicated as a potential contributing mechanism to the vasospastic phase in children with left-to-right shunts.[129, 130]

Ultimately left-to-right shunting can lead to the development of severe irreversible pulmonary arterial hypertension with dilation of the central PAs and reversal of the left-to-right shunt at the atrial, ventricular, or aortopulmonary level (Eisenmenger's syndrome).[131] This complication develops only in patients who have large, nonrestrictive defects (i.e., defects in which there is no pressure difference between the left and right atrium, left and right ventricle, or aorta and PA for ASD, VSD, and PDA, respectively). In one

autopsy investigation of 53 cases, the minimal defect sizes associated with Eisenmenger syndrome were found to be 3 cm, 1.5 cm, and 0.7 cm at the atrial, ventricular, and aortopulmonary levels.[132] In addition to the size of the defect, a critical determinant of the clinical consequences of a shunt is whether it occurs before (ASD) or after (VSD and PDA) the tricuspid valve. Eisenmenger's syndrome occurs mostly in patients who have large post-tricuspid defects beginning in infancy and is uncommon in patients who have pretricuspid defects; when it occurs in the latter group, it usually does so in adult life.[131] These different outcomes are explained by the hemodynamic changes that occur in the neonatal period: with post-tricuspid defects, PA pressure does not decrease in the postnatal period and the muscular hypertrophy normally present in the fetal pulmonary circulation never regresses; by contrast, with pretricuspid lesions, the pulmonary circulation is protected from excessive flow in the immediate post-

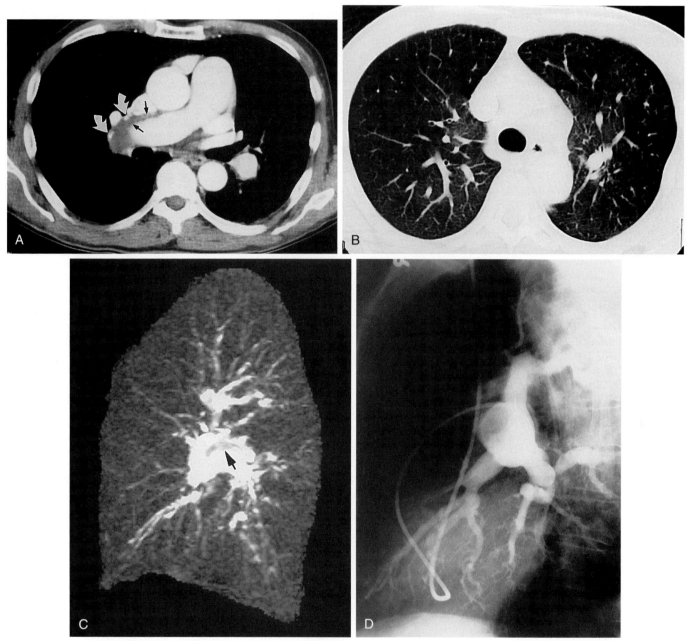

**Figure 50–13. Thromboembolic Pulmonary Arterial Hypertension.** A contrast-enhanced spiral CT *(A)* in a 65-year-old man with pulmonary arterial hypertension demonstrates a thrombus within the right pulmonary artery *(straight arrows)*. The thrombus is contiguous with the arterial wall, a finding that is characteristic of an organized embolus. Focal calcification of the intima is also evident *(curved arrows)*. Lung windows *(B)* demonstrate localized areas with decreased attenuation and vascularity and areas with increased attenuation and vascularity (a pattern known as mosaic perfusion). This pattern is seen in the majority of patients who have pulmonary arterial hypertension due to chronic thromboembolism. A sagittal gradient-recalled-echo (GRE) MR image *(C)* demonstrates thrombus lining the upper aspect of the right pulmonary artery *(arrow)*. Abnormal segmental vessels are evident in the right upper and lower lobes). A sagittal view of a selective right pulmonary angiogram *(D)* demonstrates corresponding abnormal segmental vessels. (Courtesy of Dr. Colleen Bergin, University of California, San Diego, Medical Center.)

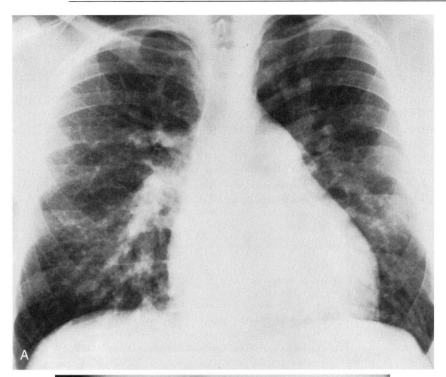

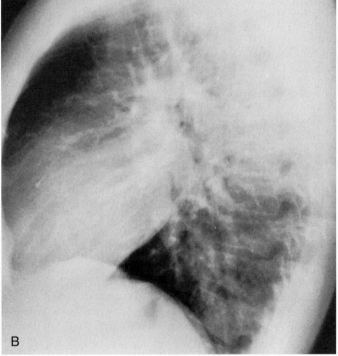

**Figure 50–14. Pulmonary Pleonemia: Atrial Septal Defect.** Posteroanterior *(A)* and lateral *(B)* radiographs of an asymptomatic 19-year-old man reveal an increase in the caliber of the pulmonary arteries and veins throughout both lungs; the vessels taper normally. The heart is moderately enlarged, possessing a contour consistent with enlargement of the right atrium and right ventricle. An atrial septal defect was corrected surgically.

natal period as a result of the low compliance of the right ventricle, allowing normal postnatal vascular muscular regression.[133]

### Pathologic Characteristics

The pathologic features of pulmonary hypertension associated with increased flow are those of plexogenic arteriopathy. As indicated previously, the fetal configuration of elastic laminae in proximal arteries (consisting of fairly uniform concentric bands) tends to be preserved.[134] Despite

this, there may fragmentation of the internal elastic lamina,[135] an effect possibly related to increased expression of a specific serine protease responsible for extracellular matrix remodeling in response to the increased pressure, flow, or both.[136]

### Radiologic Manifestations

The main radiographic sign in all these conditions is an increase in caliber of all of the PAs throughout the lungs (Fig. 50–14). Because the hemodynamic change is one of increased flow, the degree of enlargement of the main and hilar PAs usually is proportional to the degree of distention of the intrapulmonary vessels. Thus, when peripheral resistance is normal, the arteries taper gradually and proportionately distally. Vascular markings that normally are invisible in the peripheral 2 cm of the lungs may become visible. Clinical observations,[137] as well as the results of some experimental animal studies,[138] suggest that the pulmonary veins increase in size to the same extent as the PAs in conditions that cause increased flow. Very uncommonly, large left-to-right shunts are not associated radiographically with enlargement of the pulmonary vascular bed or cardiomegaly. For example, in one study of 596 patients who had ASDs proven by either cardiac catheterization or surgery, 14 (2.3%) had a normal heart size and a normal pulmonary vascular pattern;[139] all 14 had secundum ASDs of large size, the smallest shunt amounting to 50%.

It may be extremely difficult radiographically to recognize the presence of pulmonary arterial hypertension in cases of left-to-right shunt. Although increased rapidity of tapering or a disparity between proximal and peripheral pulmonary vessel size or both (Fig. 50–15) are valuable signs when present,[140, 141] peripheral oligemia is a late manifestation usually indicating reversal of the left-to-right shunt due to increased vascular resistance.[142] The difficulty is compounded by the fact that other signs of pulmonary arterial hypertension, such as enlargement of the main and hilar PAs, are unreliable because these structures may be greatly enlarged when resistance is normal.

The diagnosis of a left-to-right shunt can be made readily using echocardiography or MR imaging[143–145] (*see* Fig. 50–12). Both modalities can demonstrate the presence of shunt and the underlying anatomic features of both simple and complex cardiovascular anomalies. However, cardiac catheterization, with or without angiocardiography, is often required, particularly in the presence of suspected pulmonary arterial hypertension. When the appearance of hilar and peripheral arteries is within normal limits, arteriography may be essential to evaluate changes in the pulmonary vasculature (Fig. 50–16). In an experimental study on dogs in which the aorta was anastomosed to a single segmental PA, severe pulmonary hypertension developed in the segment;[146] direct magnification angiography revealed vascular tortuosity and the development of sclerotic vessels that were characterized angiographically by diminished fine branching and a poor capillary phase as well as by slow flow. Pathologic studies showed typical proliferative lesions of severe pulmonary hypertension with abundant bronchial arterial-pulmonary arterial anastomoses in the later stages.

### Clinical Manifestations

Clinically, many patients who have left-to-right shunts are asymptomatic. If the shunt is large, some physical underdevelopment and a tendency to respiratory infections may occur. The patient may complain of fatigue, palpitations, and dyspnea on exertion and may exhibit signs of cardiac failure. Examination of the heart and systemic vessels may provide valuable clues regarding the nature of the shunt. Uncomplicated ASD is characterized by an ejection murmur, an early systolic click, and a wide splitting of the second cardiac sound (0.05 seconds or more) that does not vary with respiration; cardiac enlargement and bulging of the precordial chest cage may develop. A VSD may be associated with a pansystolic murmur maximal at the third or fourth left interspace close to the sternum; the second sound is normally split or

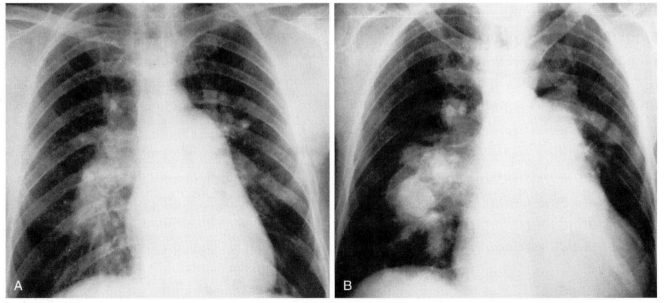

**Figure 50–15. Eisenmenger Syndrome Caused by Atrial Septal Defect.** This man presented for the first time at the age of 32 with a history of increasing shortness of breath on exertion. A radiograph *(A)* revealed marked enlargement of the hilar pulmonary arteries, which tapered rapidly as they proceeded distally. The peripheral vasculature was diminished, and the size and configuration of the heart were consistent with cor pulmonale. Cardiac catheterization revealed a secundum-type atrial septal defect. Pressures in the main pulmonary artery were 113/42 mm Hg and those in the ascending aorta 99/56 mm Hg. Eleven years later *(B)* the main pulmonary arteries and the heart had undergone remarkable enlargement; the peripheral oligemia was much more evident. The patient showed severe cyanosis and polycythemia. Despite supportive therapy, he died shortly after this examination. At autopsy the lumen of the main pulmonary artery was considerably larger than that of the ascending aorta. Mural thrombi were present in the major pulmonary arteries.

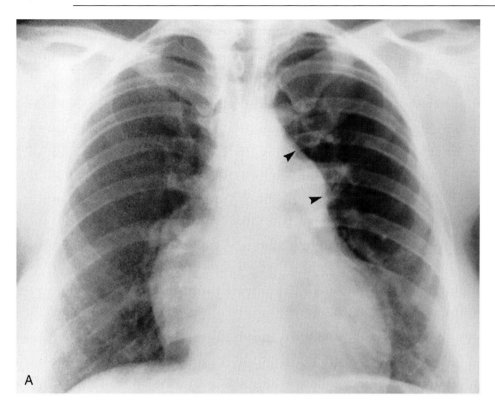

**Figure 50–16. Precapillary Hypertension Secondary to a Left-to-Right Intracardiac Shunt (Atrial Septal Defect).** A posteroanterior chest radiograph *(A)* reveals moderate cardiomegaly consistent with enlargement of right heart chambers; there is no evidence of enlargement of the left atrium. The main pulmonary artery *(arrowheads)* is very prominent, although the hilar arteries appear normal. The upper lobe vessels are roughly equal in size to those in the lower lobes, indicating the presence of increased flow to the upper lobes.

widened but, unlike its behavior in ASD, varies with respiration. The murmur of PDA before the development of pulmonary hypertension usually is long and rumbling and occupies most of systole and diastole. It is loudest in the second left interspace near the sternum and sometimes is associated with crescendo accentuation in late systole; the second pulmonic sound is increased in amplitude but is normally split and changes with respiration. A widely patent left-to-right shunt caused by PDA produces systemic peripheral vascular signs of a high pulse pressure.

The development of pulmonary hypertension in cases of left-to-right shunt gives rise to changes in the physical findings. In ASD, atrial fibrillation is a frequent occurrence and may be followed by tricuspid regurgitation and heart failure; the fixed splitting of the second heart sound becomes much narrower, and the systolic murmur may become fainter. In VSD, the systolic murmur decreases in length, and an ejection systolic murmur and click may appear. In PDA, as the pressure in the pulmonary circulation rises and the shunt and shunt gradient decrease, the murmur is reduced in intensity and, in many cases, the diastolic component disappears.

A number of additional symptoms and signs are related to cor pulmonale and right heart failure, including retrosternal pain identical to angina pectoris, parasternal thrust, a murmur of tricuspid insufficiency, and liver and neck pulsations. Pulmonary hypertension also causes accentuation of the second pulmonic sound and early diastolic murmur along the left sternal border as a result of pulmonary valvular insufficiency. A variety of additional manifestations, such as cyanosis, clubbing, and cachexia, may also be seen.

### Prognosis and Natural History

The hemodynamic consequences and clinical outcome in patients who have severe pulmonary hypertension due to

Eisenmenger's syndrome appear to be better than those in patients who have PPH of similar magnitude: in 37 patients who had Eisenmenger's syndrome and 57 who had PPH and who had similar levels of pulmonary hypertension (mean PA pressure 107 ± 20 and 97 ± 21, respectively), the patients who had Eisenmenger's syndrome had lower right atrial pressure (5 ± 2 versus 12 ± 5 mm Hg), higher cardiac index (2.7 ± 0.6 versus 2.2 ± 0.8 liters per minute/m²), and prolonged survival.[147]

### Primary Pulmonary Hypertension

PPH was first described in 1951 in a report of three young women who had severe exertional dyspnea and radiographic and clinical evidence of pulmonary hypertension and right ventricular hypertrophy.[148] Since then it has been the subject of many additional investigations and reviews.[149–152] The abnormality is very uncommon,[123] having an incidence of only about 1 per 1 million population. This low incidence has prevented individual centers from gathering sufficiently large groups of patients to permit an adequate description of epidemiologic and clinical features. However, in 1981 the Division of Lung Disease of the National Heart, Lung, and Blood Institute of NIH initiated a patient registry for the characterization of pulmonary hypertension.[123] During the next 5 years, 187 patients who had presumed PPH were entered into this registry. The mean age of the patients was 36 ± 15 years with a female-to-male predominance of 1.7 to 1.

#### Etiology and Pathogenesis

By definition, the etiology of PPH is unknown; however, the observation that similar disease occurs in association with some drugs and with cirrhosis (*see* farther on)

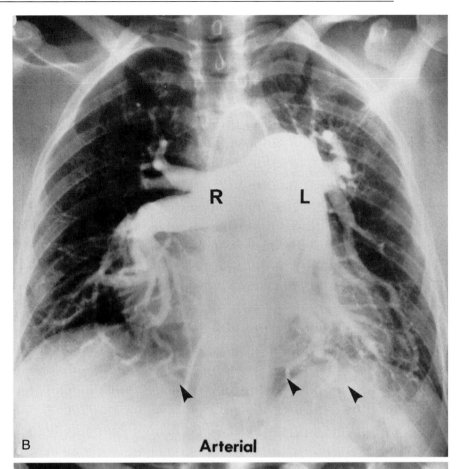

**Figure 50–16** *Continued.* A right ventricular pulmonary angiogram during the arterial *(B)* and venous *(C)* phases shows the characteristic features of precapillary hypertension: the right (R) and left (L) interlobar arteries are dilated, intrapulmonary arterial branches are tortuous and sinuous *(arrowheads),* and the veins *(open arrows)* are of normal caliber. The patient was a 32-year-old woman.

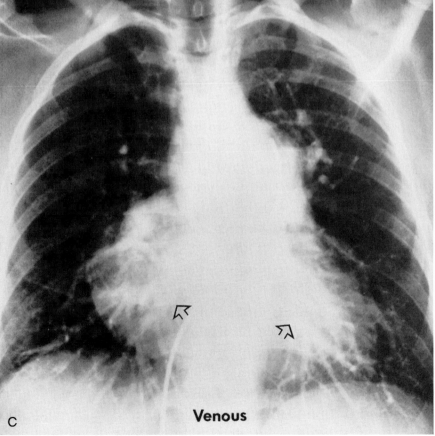

suggests that as yet unidentified toxic exogenous or endogenous substances may also be involved in the idiopathic form of disease. The possibility of an immunologic component in the pathogenesis is also theoretically possible, although there is little direct supportive evidence. A hereditary influence is well established in a small number of cases; however, the precise mechanism by which it affects the development of the disease is uncertain.

**Genetic Factors.** Although the majority of cases appear to be sporadic, there is a definite subset in which PPH is clearly familial.[153–156] The disease has been reported in 52 patients from 14 North American families,[150] in twins,[157] and in members of three-generation families.[158] Six per cent of the patients in the National Heart, Lung, and Blood Institute's Primary Pulmonary Hypertension Registry were judged to have a family history.[123] In fact, it has been suggested that many cases considered to be sporadic could be proved to be familial if the medical records of family members who died prematurely were examined; this suggestion is supported by the occasional instance of a shared ancestry in "sporadic cases."[159] Although these cases could be the result of recessive gene transmission,[160] the inheritance most closely conforms to an autosomal dominant pattern;[161, 162] in fact, some investigators have identified a locus on the long arm of chromosome 2 that is strongly linked to pulmonary hypertension and acts as a dominant gene.[163, 164] There is no evidence for a sex-linked transmission.[165] An association of familial PPH with certain HLA-DR and DQ major histocompatibility loci has been reported by one group.[166]

A number of families have been described in which the inheritance of a low-oxygen affinity–beta-chain hemoglobin variant has been associated with the development of pulmonary hypertension;[167, 168] one group has also described an association with β-thalassemia.[169] Although these associations may be coincidental, it is possible that the gene for the familial PPH could be close to and coinherited with the beta-chain gene in these families. One case of PPH has also been reported in a man who had a familial platelet storage disease associated with high plasma levels of serotonin, a substance that has been implicated in the pathogenesis of PPH.[170] In one kindred, familial pulmonary hypertension was associated with elevated levels of antiplasmin,[171] and in another pulmonary hypertension occurred in an individual with familial deficiency in plasminogen.[172] These isolated reports have led to the suggestion that PPH might be related to an inability to lyse pulmonary microthrombi or microemboli.

In one study of 24 families with 429 members in whom 124 were known to carry the gene for PPH, the age of death was significantly less ($36 \pm 13$ versus $46 \pm 15$ years) in the younger generation than in the parental generation.[165] This phenomenon (i.e., younger age at onset and more rapid progression in successive generations) is termed *genetic anticipation* and is seen in some diseases with excessively long mutant DNA repeat sequences; however, such a sequence has not yet been identified in PPH. In familial cases of PPH, there is an approximate 2-to-1 female-to-male predominance, a finding that may reflect loss of male fetuses.[165]

**Immunologic Factors.** As mentioned previously, another possible pathogenetic mechanism for the development of PPH is an immunologically mediated angiopathic process.[173] In support of this hypothesis is the observation that pulmonary hypertension is well documented as a complication of several connective tissue diseases, particularly systemic lupus erythematosus[174] and progressive systemic sclerosis[175] (*see* farther on). In addition, the incidence of Raynaud's phenomenon in patients who have PPH is higher than would be expected. The pathogenesis of the hypertension in these cases is unclear and may be related to one or more of a number of factors, such as antibody-mediated endothelial damage, vasculitis, or thrombosis.

**Vascular Factors.** It is believed that the early stages of PPH are characterized by constriction of pulmonary vascular smooth muscle; with prolonged vasoconstriction, vascular remodeling and the changes of plexogenic pulmonary arteriopathy eventually ensue. A role for vasoconstriction as a predisposing factor to the development of the full-blown picture is supported by the observation that PPH is more common at higher altitudes than at sea level.[176] In pulmonary hypertension induced by aminorex, withdrawal of the drug has resulted in symptomatic and hemodynamic improvement in some patients; similarly, spontaneous reversal has been reported,[177] suggesting that the early stage of pulmonary hypertension is related to vasospasm unassociated with irreparable anatomic alteration in the pulmonary vasculature. Theoretically, such a mechanism might also be important in PPH.

There is evidence that *in situ* thrombosis contributes to progression of disease in patients who have both primary and drug-related pulmonary hypertension.[178] This evidence is derived from pathologic studies and from the observation that anticoagulant therapy is known to improve the survival rate in patients who have PPH. For example, in one retrospective investigation of 172 patients who had pulmonary hypertension, 104 of whom had taken the appetite suppressant aminorex, anticoagulant therapy had a positive influence on long-term survival and quality of life, particularly in patients who had a history of anorectic drug intake.[179] The best mean survival time of 8.3 years was found in anticoagulated aminorex-treated patients, compared with 6.1 years in nonanticoagulated aminorex-treated patients. Moreover, aminorex-treated patients who received anticoagulant therapy soon after the onset of symptoms showed significantly better prognosis (10.9 years) than those who commenced treatment 2 years thereafter (5.9 years).

### Pathologic Characteristics

Pathologic findings in PPH are those of plexogenic arteriopathy (*see* page 1884). Not all histologic manifestations of this complex of abnormalities are identified in every case; for example, in one investigation of 19 patients (in whom lungs were obtained at autopsy in 17 and at transplantation in 2), concentric intimal thickening and plexiform lesions were found in 18 and 6, respectively;[54] arterial adventitial thickening was also found in all patients and venous intimal and adventitial thickening in about 50%. The identification of plexiform lesions is related to the number of sections examined; in a pathologic study of the lungs of 25 patients in the Primary Pulmonary Hypertension Registry of the National Heart, Lung, and Blood Institute, plexiform lesions were identified in only 3% to 4% of vessels examined.[48] It it is important to remember that evidence of previous arterial thrombosis is not uncommon in plexogenic arteriopathy and does not necessarily imply thromboembolic disease.[48, 68]

## Radiologic Manifestations

The radiographic findings consist of enlargement of the central PAs, rapid tapering, and peripheral oligemia (Fig. 50–17).[123, 180] Overinflation does not occur, permitting ready differentiation from the diffuse pulmonary oligemia associated with emphysema. In the NIH study mentioned previously, the chest radiographs of 187 patients were graded subjectively:[123] prominence of the main PA was found in 90%, enlarged hilar vessels in 80%, right ventricular hypertrophy in 74%, and decreased peripheral vascularity in 51%; the radiographic appearance was felt to be normal in 6%.

Echocardiography typically shows right ventricular and right atrial enlargement, with a normal or small left ventricle.[181] It also allows assessment of the systolic pulmonary arterial pressure[182] and exclusion of left-to-right shunts and of valvular heart disease. In the NIH study, the procedure showed right ventricular enlargement in 75% of patients and paradoxical septal wall motion in 59%.[123]

The results of ventilation-perfusion scans may be normal, or they may show patchy nonsegmental perfusion defects. In the NIH study, perfusion scan results were abnormal in 58% of cases; the majority of the abnormalities consisted of diffuse, patchy defects that were estimated to have a low probability of representing pulmonary thromboembolism[123] (Fig. 50–18). In another study based on a retrospective assessment of 35 patients who had PPH, 33 (94%) had low probability ventilation-perfusion scan results;[116] one each had intermediate and high probability scan results. Contrast-en-

hanced spiral CT or pulmonary angiography is required to rule out chronic thromboembolism in such patients.

## Clinical Manifestations

The main symptom in patients who have PPH is dyspnea on exertion, which is often insidious in onset.[183] In one series of 23 patients in whom the diagnosis was established at autopsy and in whom the clinical history did not suggest the presence of pulmonary thromboembolic disease, there was a female predominance of 5 to 1 and the median age at the time of death was 34 years; symptoms consisted of dyspnea (in 22 patients), Raynaud's phenomenon (in 7), and syncope (in 6).[180] In another report of 38 patients, the most frequent presenting symptoms were dyspnea (60%), fatigue (19%), and syncope or near syncope (13%).[184] Raynaud's phenomenon was observed in 10% of patients, virtually all of whom were female. The mean interval from the onset of symptoms to diagnosis was 2 years. Other symptoms noted during the course of disease included easy fatigability, chest pain, and cough. A positive antinuclear antibody test result was found in 29%, 69% of whom were female.

Signs of cor pulmonale and cardiac failure may be present, including giant jugular A waves, right atrial gallop, a loud pulmonary ejection click, an accentuated pulmonic sound, a palpable lift along the left sternal border, and, in some cases, murmurs caused by pulmonic and tricuspid insufficiency.[180] In the 187 patients from the multicenter NIH study, an increase in the pulmonary component of the second heart sound was found in 93%, a right-sided third or fourth heart sound in 61%, tricuspid regurgitation in 40%, pulmonic

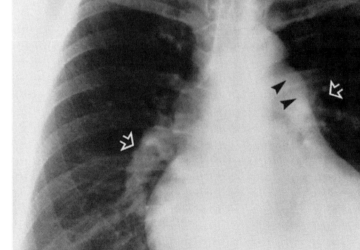

**Figure 50–17. Primary Pulmonary Hypertension.** A posteroanterior chest radiograph (*A*) shows enlargement of the right ventricle, dilation of the main *(arrowheads)* and hilar *(open arrows)* pulmonary arteries, and increased rapidity of tapering of pulmonary arteries as they proceed distally.

*Illustration continued on following page*

A

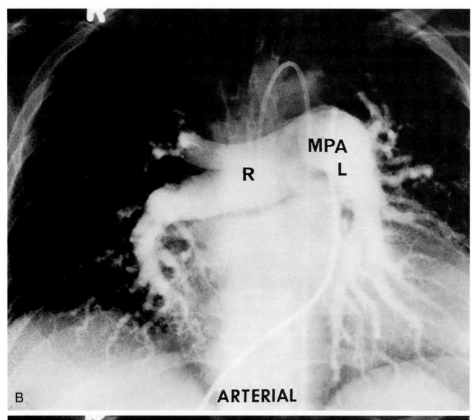

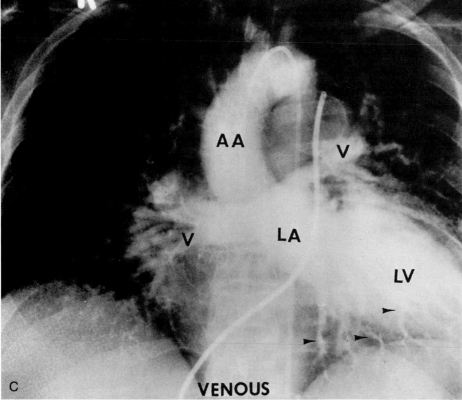

**Figure 50–17** *Continued.* These findings are confirmed on a pulmonary angiogram during the arterial *(B)* and venous *(C)* phases (main pulmonary artery [MPA], right [R] and left [L] pulmonary arteries); the middle and distal pulmonary arteries taper rapidly, displaying a sinuous ("corkscrew") appearance. Pulmonary veins (V) are normal. Some of the lower lobe arteries are persistently opacified *(arrowheads)* during the venous phase, indicating an increased resistance to blood flow in the lower lobes. The left atrium (LA), left ventricle (LV), and ascending aorta (AA) are opacified. The patient was a young woman.

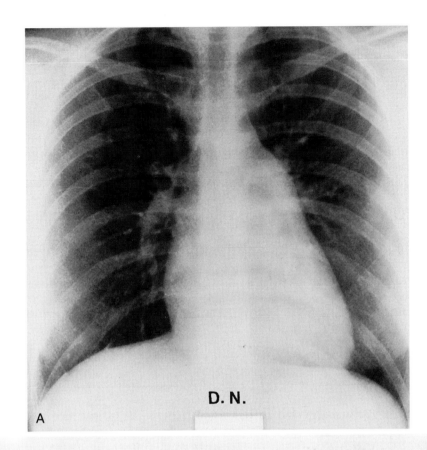

**Figure 50–18. Primary Pulmonary Hypertension: Scintigraphic Findings.** A posteroanterior chest radiograph *(A)* shows right ventricular and main pulmonary artery enlargement; the hila, pulmonary vessels, and parenchyma are normal. Cardiac catheterization in this young woman disclosed severe precapillary hypertension; there was no evidence of a gradient across either the aortic or pulmonic valves. A four-view pulmonary scintigraphic study *(B)* in anterior (A), posterior (P), left lateral (LL), and right lateral (RL) projections demonstrates shallow subpleural perfusion deficits *(arrowheads)* interpreted as low probability for thromboembolic disease.

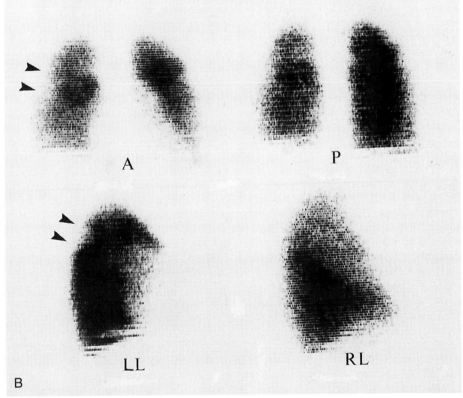

insufficiency in 13%, cyanosis in 20%, and peripheral edema in 32%.[123]

### Hemodynamic and Pulmonary Function Tests

In addition to pulmonary arterial hypertension, catheterization of the right side of the heart reveals a normal pulmonary wedge pressure, high pulmonary vascular resistance, and, in patients who have right ventricular failure, a low cardiac output.[180, 185] In the patients from the NIH study, the mean pulmonary arterial pressure was $60 \pm 18$ mm Hg, the pulmonary wedge pressure averaged approximately 9 mm Hg, and the cardiac index was mildly reduced at $2.27 \pm 0.9$ liters per minute/m².[123]

Although pulmonary function may be completely normal, arterial oxygen saturation[186] and diffusing capacity are often decreased.[187] A relatively high incidence of a restrictive ventilatory defect has been observed in some studies.[188, 189] In one retrospective study of 19 patients who had precapillary pulmonary hypertension and who were examined in the pulmonary function laboratory, the most common pattern of abnormality was a mild reduction in diffusing capacity;[190] a restrictive pattern was seen in only 20%. A severe drop in arterial oxygen saturation during exercise was the most discriminating diagnostic test.

In the NIH study, total lung capacity and vital capacity were mildly decreased, and there was a moderate decrease in pulmonary diffusing capacity (68% predicted), arterial $P_{O_2}$ ($Pa_{O_2} = 70$ mm Hg), and arterial $P_{CO_2}$ ($Pa_{CO_2} = 30$ mm Hg).[123] Using the multiple inert gas technique, it has been shown that the gas exchange abnormalities are predominantly the result of $\dot{V}/\dot{Q}$ mismatching;[191, 192] significant hypoxemia occurs only when mixed venous $P_{O_2}$ is decreased secondary to a drop in cardiac output. The fall in arterial $P_{O_2}$ that occurs during exercise is caused by a failure of cardiac output to increase sufficiently, resulting in a decrease in the mixed venous oxygen saturation;[192] the desaturated mixed venous blood passes through shunts and low $\dot{V}/\dot{Q}$ regions, worsening the arterial $P_{O_2}$.

### Prognosis and Natural History

The majority of patients who have PPH experience progressive dyspnea, cor pulmonale, and death within a few years.[150] Exceptions occur occasionally; for example, repeated catheterization may reveal no change in hemodynamics[186] or even improvement,[185] and patients have been reported to survive as long as 18 years after the onset of symptoms.[158] On the basis of data acquired in the U.S. NIH study on PPH, a prognostic equation was developed and tested retrospectively on a large cohort of patients followed at the Mexican National Institute of Cardiology between 1977 and 1992.[193] A multivariate Cox proportional-hazards regression analysis was used to assess the adjusted hazard ratios. Survival as computed by the equation correlated with real survival, with positive predictive values of 87%, 91%, and 89% at 1, 2, and 3 years, respectively.

A number of clinical, functional, and pathologic features have been associated with the natural history of the disease. In one investigation of lung specimens from 19 patients, the presence of an intimal area greater than 18% of the vascular cross-sectional area was found to have an 85%

predictive value in identifying patients who had a poor prognosis.[68] In the NIH study, a reduced forced vital capacity and cardiac index and increased right atrial pressure were significant risk factors for decreased survival after diagnosis.[193] A reduced cardiac index and symptoms such as syncope that reflect decreased cardiac output have also been found to be indicators of a poor prognosis.[194] In one retrospective cohort study of 61 patients who had PPH diagnosed by strict clinical and hemodynamic criteria, 2-, 5-, and 10-year survivals were 48%, 32%, and 12%, respectively.[195] Median survival duration from the time of diagnosis was 22 months. The survivors had significantly higher age of onset and cardiac index and significantly lower right atrial mean pressure, right ventricular end-diastolic pressure, cardiothoracic ratio from chest radiographs, and calculated pulmonary vascular resistance compared with nonsurvivors. Although PA systolic pressure was not significantly different, PA diastolic and PA mean pressures were significantly lower in survivors than in nonsurvivors.

The short-term vasodilator response to $PGI_2$ in patients who have PPH is also predictive of long-term survival on a therapeutic regimen of oral vasodilators and anticoagulants. In one study of 91 consecutive patients who underwent a short-term vasodilator trial using $PGI_2$ (5 to 10 ng/kg$^{-1}$/min$^{-1}$), the subgroup of 9 patients who showed more than 50% decrease in total pulmonary resistance index had an improved 2-year survival (62%) compared with those whose total pulmonary resistance index decreased between 20% and 50% and less than 20% (survivals of 38% and 47%, respectively).[196]

### Toxin and Drug-Related Pulmonary Hypertension

A variety of toxins and drugs have been implicated in the pathogenesis of pulmonary hypertension. In the exposure to contaminated rapeseed oil that occurred in Spain in 1981, hypertension was the principal pulmonary manifestation during the later stages of disease (*see* page 2587).[197] Eosinophilia-myalgia syndrome, a condition similar to Spanish oil toxicity, is also accompanied by pulmonary hypertension and has been reported following the ingestion of medicinal preparations containing large amounts of the amino acid L-tryptophan.[198, 199]

Pyrrolizidine alkaloids—chemicals found in the plants *Senecio jacobea* and *Crotalaria* (*C. spectabilis, C. fulva, C. laburnifolia*)—have been shown to cause pulmonary hypertension in rats.[200–203] Although these substances are readily available for human consumption,[200, 203] there is no convincing evidence that implicates them in the development of pulmonary hypertension in humans. However, *C. fulva* is ingested in the West Indies as a component of bush tea and causes veno-occlusive disease of the liver.[200] The administration of the alkaloid fulvine to rats results in vasoconstriction, medial hypertrophy, and necrotizing arteritis of PAs and thickening of the walls and proliferation of muscle fibers of pulmonary veins and venules.[202]

The possibility that some cases formerly considered to be examples of PPH might be drug induced was suggested by the finding of a 20-fold increase in the incidence of pulmonary hypertension in certain European countries in the 1960s;[204, 205] in most affected patients, symptoms of rapidly progressive exertional dyspnea and syncope developed 6 to

12 months after the institution of treatment of obesity with an anorectic drug, aminorex fumarate. Although it is presumed that the drug acted directly on the pulmonary vasculature, a few patients showed evidence of pulmonary and peripheral thromboembolic disease.[205] Whatever the pathogenesis, withdrawal of the drug from the market resulted in a decline in the incidence of pulmonary hypertension in the regions where it had been used.[205, 206]

In the 1970s, another class of appetite suppressors, the fenfluramine derivatives, was introduced and was again followed by sporadic reports and small series of cases of pulmonary hypertension.[207–210] A recent multicenter case control study in which 95 sequentially selected patients who had "PPH" were matched with 355 controls for sex and age, the use of anorectic drugs (mainly fenfluramine and dexfenfluramine) was clearly associated with an increased risk of pulmonary hypertension (odds ratio of 6.5);[211] when the drugs were used for 12 months or more, the odds ratio increased to 23.

The mechanism by which these anorectic drugs cause pulmonary hypertension is unknown. However, patients who have PPH have high plasma levels and low platelet levels of the potent pulmonary vasoconstrictor serotonin, an abnormality that persists after heart and lung transplantation. This observation has led to the suggestion that a failure of platelets to retain their serotonin content contributes to the development of PPH.[212] Because anorexigenic agents are believed to cause early satiety by blocking reuptake of serotonin in the central nervous system, they may theoretically exert an effect on the pulmonary vasculature via the action of serotonin. It is also possible that the drugs may have a direct action on the pulmonary vasculature.

In rats aminorex, fenfluramine, and dexfenfluramine have also been shown to inhibit potassium current and cause reversible membrane depolarization in smooth muscle cells taken from small PAs.[213] These actions are similar to those of hypoxia, which initiates pulmonary vasoconstriction by inhibiting a potassium current in pulmonary vascular smooth muscle.[213] In late 1997, the report of an association between valvular heart disease and use of fenfluramine in combination with another appetite suppressant "phentermine" caused these agents to be withdrawn from the market in the United States and Canada.[214] The report describes 24 young women who were found to have thickening and/or insufficiency of the mitral, aortic, or tricuspid valve at surgery or on echocardiography after taking the medication for 1 to 2 years. The pathologic findings in the five patients who underwent valvular heart surgery were similar to those reported in carcinoid syndrome, again implicating a possible role for excessive serotonin in the pathogenesis.[215]

Pulmonary hypertension has also followed the ingestion or inhalation of cocaine,[216] amphetamines,[217] and phenformin.[218] The pathogenesis of the disease with the last agent may be related to the lactic acidosis it sometimes causes.[219]

Pathologic features of toxin or drug-related pulmonary hypertension are those of plexogenic arteriopathy. Radiologic and clinical manifestations are identical to those of primary disease.

### Pulmonary Hypertension Associated with Hepatic Disease

In 1979, 9 patients were described who had combined portal and pulmonary hypertension and an additional 14 patients who had this combination of abnormalities were gleaned from the medical literature.[220] Of these 23 patients, 15 had had a surgical portacaval shunt established because of esophageal varices. Since this initial publication, there have been numerous reports of an association of liver disease and pulmonary hypertension particularly, but not invariably,[221, 222] when accompanied by portal hypertension.[221–226] In fact, the complication can occur a variable time after portosystemic shunting in patients who have noncirrhotic portal hypertension secondary to portal fibrosis[227] or multifocal nodular hyperplasia.[228]

As might be expected, the overall prevalence of pulmonary hypertension in patients who have cirrhosis is low; in one large autopsy study it was 0.73%, and in a clinical series of 2,459 patients who had biopsy-proven cirrhosis it was 0.61%.[229] In patients whose liver disease is severe enough that they are considered for liver transplantation, the prevalence may be much higher.[230] For example, in one study of 226 transplant recipients from Barcelona, eight (3.5%) were considered to have hemodynamically significant pulmonary hypertension.[231] In another study of 362 transplant candidates from the Mayo Clinic, all patients had a right heart catheterization after induction of anesthesia;[232] 72 (20%) had a mean PA pressure greater than 25 mm Hg (although only 15 [4%] had pulmonary hypertension defined as a PA pressure greater than 25 mm Hg and a pulmonary vascular resistance in excess of 120 dynes/second/cm$^5$). In neither of these studies was pulmonary hypertension shown to be an independent risk factor for a worse prognosis after transplantation; in fact, slow but steady improvement in pulmonary hemodynamics has been reported after successful liver transplantation.[233]

The pathogenesis of pulmonary hypertension in liver disease is likely to be related to several mechanisms. It has been hypothesized that vasoactive or vasotoxic substances produced in the gut and normally metabolized by the liver can reach the pulmonary circulation in patients who have cirrhosis, portal hypertension, and a portosystemic shunt;[234] however, the nature of such substances is unclear. It is also possible that a component of the pulmonary hypertension is secondary to hemodynamic alterations. In one investigation of 16 patients undergoing transjugular intrahepatic portosystemic shunting for recurrent ascites or variceal bleeding, cardiac index, PA pressure, and pulmonary vascular resistance increased from 4.5 ± 1.2 to 5.0 ± 1.1 liters per minute/m$^2$, 12 ± 3 to 20 ± 5 mm Hg, and 60 ± 30 to 82 ± 35 dynes × seconds/cm$^5$, respectively.[235] One month after placement of the transjugular intrahepatic portosystemic shunting, the PA pressure remained elevated and the cardiac index increased further. In support of a mechanical cause for the pulmonary hypertension is the observation that inhalation of NO in concentrations between 0 and 80 parts per million had no effect on PA pressure in a group of liver transplant recipients who had moderate pulmonary hypertension (mean PA pressure = 37 mm Hg).[236] Pulmonary thromboemboli originating in a congested portal circulation can reach the lung via varices and are a rare cause of pulmonary hypertension in patients who have advanced liver disease.[237]

The radiologic manifestations range from normal to the characteristic findings of pulmonary arterial hypertension[91] (Fig. 50–19). The symptoms and signs of pulmonary hypertension in patients who have liver disease are similar to

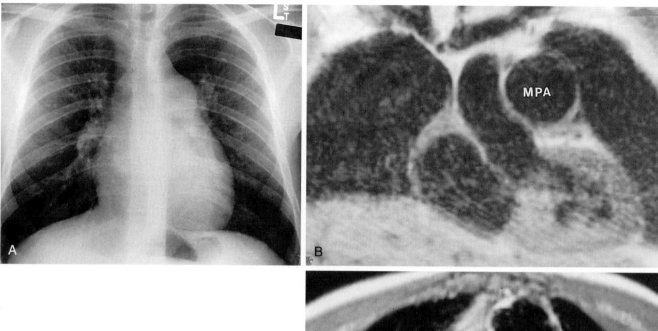

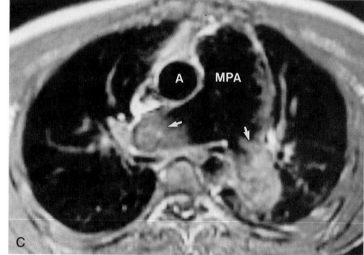

**Figure 50–19. Pulmonary Arterial Hypertension Related to Cirrhosis.** A posteroanterior chest radiograph *(A)* of a 17-year-old man demonstrates cardiomegaly and enlargement of the central pulmonary arteries. A coronal spin-echo MR image *(B)* shows marked enlargement of the main pulmonary artery (MPA). A transverse MR image *(C)* shows enlargement of the main pulmonary artery (MPA), which has a greater diameter than that of the aorta (A). Increased signal is evident within the right and left pulmonary arteries *(arrows)*, reflecting the presence of slow blood flow due to hypertension.

those in persons who have pulmonary hypertension from other causes, although they may be masked by the inactivity caused by the underlying liver disease. One interesting report describes the development of severe hypoxemia, unresponsive to oxygen, in two cirrhotic patients who were being treated with long-term beta-blocker therapy.[238] Although such hypoxemia is usually related to intrapulmonary microvascular shunts, the shunt in these patients was found to be through a patent foramen ovale due to pulmonary hypertension; the pulmonary hypertension and the right-to-left shunt eventually resolved after discontinuation of the beta-blocker therapy. The coexistence of pulmonary hypertension and noncirrhotic portal hypertension has been reported in systemic lupus erythematosus.[222]

### Pulmonary Hypertension Associated with Pulmonary Artery Thrombosis and Thromboembolism

It is inevitable that hypertension will develop if a sufficient portion of the pulmonary arterial system is occluded by thrombus. Such a situation can occur by at least three mechanisms: (1) multiple recurrent embolic episodes involving small thrombi and occurring over a number of months or years; (2) one or a few embolic episodes involving a large

thrombus that either occludes a significant proportion of the proximal pulmonary vasculature directly or does so by propagation of clot *in situ*;[239–241] such thrombi may or may not be associated with evidence of thromboembolism in small vessels; and (3) *in situ* thrombosis of small or large PAs unassociated with emboli. Although the first of these mechanisms has been thought to be the most common etiology of pulmonary hypertension of thrombotic origin,[242] a number of clinical and pathologic observations suggest that it may be an infrequent cause[68, 243] and that most cases are instead the result of the other two.

As discussed previously (*see* page 1783), the most common natural history of a pulmonary thromboembolic episode is resolution with restoration of normal pulmonary hemodynamics, gas exchange, and exercise tolerance;[244] occasionally, however, thrombi lodged in proximal arteries fail to undergo significant recanalization or dissolution, resulting in chronic pulmonary hypertension (Fig. 50–20).[245–248] This condition, which has been called *chronic thromboembolic pulmonary hypertension* (CTEPH), is important to distinguish from hypertension associated with predominantly peripheral pulmonary vascular disease because, in specialized centers, surgical removal of the central thrombi is possible with a reasonably low surgical mortality.[247] It is unclear why

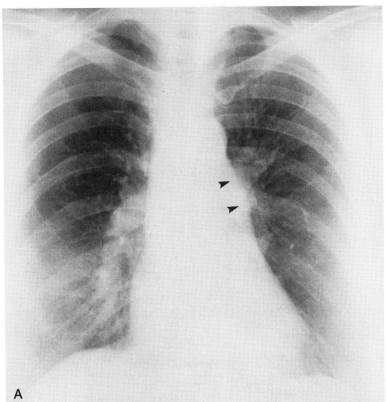

**Figure 50–20. Precapillary Pulmonary Hypertension Caused by Massive Pulmonary Thromboembolism.** A posteroanterior chest radiograph *(A)* shows moderate enlargement of the main pulmonary artery *(arrowheads)*, dilation of hilar pulmonary arteries, and slight enlargement of the heart. There is a suggestion of oligemia in the right upper lobe. The patient, a middle-aged woman, had experienced only vague chest discomfort several days before this examination. Approximately 6 weeks later, following the sudden onset of severe chest pain and circulatory collapse, a chest radiograph *(B)* disclosed an increase in the size of the heart, diffuse oligemia of the right lung, and elevation of the right hemidiaphragm. These features are consistent with acute cor pulmonale caused by thromboembolism.

*Illustration continued on following page*

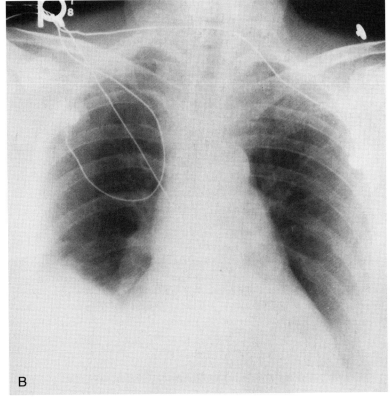

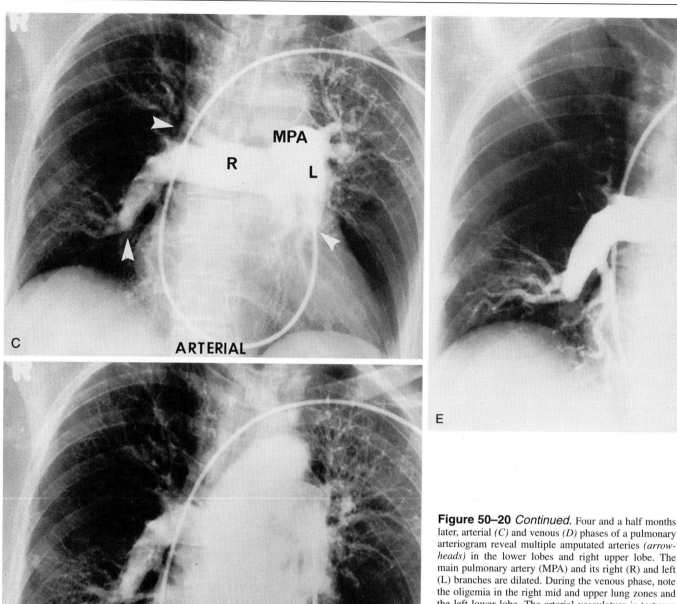

**Figure 50–20** *Continued.* Four and a half months later, arterial *(C)* and venous *(D)* phases of a pulmonary arteriogram reveal multiple amputated arteries *(arrowheads)* in the lower lobes and right upper lobe. The main pulmonary artery (MPA) and its right (R) and left (L) branches are dilated. During the venous phase, note the oligemia in the right mid and upper lung zones and the left lower lobe. The arterial vasculature is tortuous and sinuous, characteristic of chronic precapillary hypertension, a feature better shown on a detail view from a selective right pulmonary arteriogram *(E).*

some patients go on to develop CTEPH rather than recanalize or lyse their thrombi; the only definite risk factor appears to be the presence of lupus anticoagulant.[248] The abnormality is uncommon; it has been estimated that only 0.1% to 0.5% of patients who suffer an acute thromboembolic episode go on to develop CTEPH.[247]

Primary thrombosis in the pulmonary arterial circulation can occur in association with a number of conditions, including polycythemia, hemoglobin SC and hemoglobin SS disease, eclampsia,[249, 250] and disseminated fibromuscular dysplasia[251] *(see* page 1773). In addition to these abnormalities, histologic examination of the lungs of some patients

who have pulmonary hypertension and no discernible underlying disease shows fresh, organizing, and organized thrombi in small vessels more or less diffusely throughout the lungs. This finding may be present in association with the lesions of plexogenic arteriopathy (in which case the patient is considered to have PPH);[68, 252] however, in many cases no such lesions are apparent. Although traditionally these latter cases have been considered to be the result of thromboemboli, it has been hypothesized that they are instead manifestations of *in situ* thrombosis.[48, 68] Whatever the pathogenesis, it is important to distinguish pulmonary hypertension associated with these small vessel thrombi from that related to thromboemboli in the proximal arteries because of the differences in therapy and prognosis.

Because thrombotic lesions in small pulmonary vessels can be seen in plexogenic arteriopathy, it has also been speculated that they may be simply another manifestation of this disease process.[252] However, a number of observations suggest that patients who have thrombotic lesions in the pulmonary microvasculature in the absence of the usual features of plexogenic arteriopathy may be suffering from a different entity. For example, in one investigation, patients who had only thrombotic lesions had a better prognosis than those who had plexogenic arteriopathy (mean survival of 1,070 days compared with 297 days).[68] Differences in the onset of disease and sex ratio have also been documented (29 years versus 37 years and male-to-female ratio of 1:3 versus 1:1 in plexiform and thrombotic groups, respectively).[68]

In addition to vascular obstruction as a result of thrombus or its residue (i.e., fibrous tissue following organization), it is likely that vascular remodeling plays a role in the pathogenesis of the hypertension in these cases.

### Pathologic Characteristics

Cases hypothesized to represent *in situ* thrombosis of small pulmonary vessels are characterized by foci of eccentric intimal fibrosis and transluminal fibrous bands (colander or cribriform pattern)[68, 253] (Fig. 50–21). Thrombus itself is relatively sparse but often can be identified focally. When interpreting the presence of such fresh or organized thrombi, it is important to remember that they can also be found in pulmonary hypertension of other etiology, especially in older individuals, in which situation they may represent a consequence of endothelial injury or incidental thromboembolism.[254]

Examination of tissue removed from large PAs by endarterectomy shows thrombi in various stages of organization;[255] histologic evidence of recurrent (*in situ*) thrombosis adjacent to partially organized emboli may be seen. It is important to note that the small pulmonary vessels may also be abnormal in patients who have CTEPH,[255, 256] the most common features being medial hypertrophy and intimal fibrosis (which may be eccentric, concentric, or in a colander pattern consistent with recanalized thrombus). The presence of such abnormalities on lung biopsy specimens is not itself a contraindication to endarterectomy; in one study of 31 patients, the extent and nature of the changes did not relate to age, symptom duration, or hemodynamic parameters and did not preclude a good clinical and hemodynamic result following surgical resection of the central thrombi.[256]

### Radiologic Manifestations

The characteristic radiographic findings of thromboembolic pulmonary arterial hypertension include right ventricular enlargement, prominence of the central PAs, rapid taper-

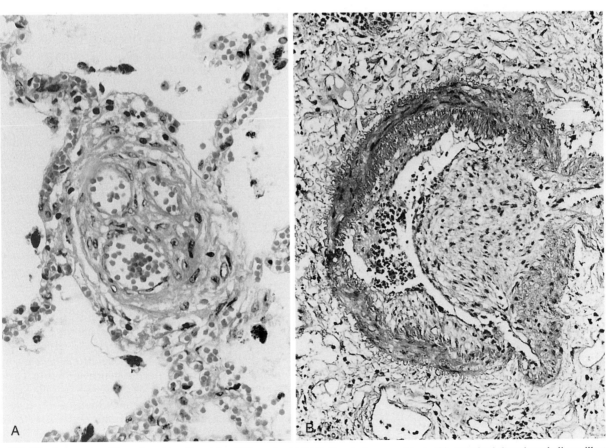

**Figure 50–21. Pulmonary Hypertension: Organized Thromboemboli.** Two lesions consistent with organized thromboemboli are illustrated. In *A*, a small artery is subdivided by fibrous bands into three small channels (colander lesion). In *B*, a somewhat nodular focus of loose fibroblastic tissue is present on one side of the vessel wall (eccentric fibrosis).

ing, and areas with decreased vascularity (mosaic oligemia)[89, 257] (*see* Fig. 50–13). In one review of 22 patients, cardiomegaly was identified in 19 (86%), right descending PA enlargement in 12 (54%), and localized areas of diminished vascularity in 15 (68%).[89] The areas of decreased vascularity on plain radiographs were confirmed by pulmonary angiography to be associated with chronic emboli. When either thrombosis or embolism occurs in the major hilar PAs, the combination of bulging hilar PAs, severe peripheral oligemia, and cor pulmonale constitutes a virtually pathognomonic triad[258] (Fig. 50–22). However, large emboli within the main PAs are occasionally associated with small hilar vessels.[89]

As indicated previously, ventilation-perfusion scintigraphy is a safe and highly sensitive test to use in evaluating patients suspected of having thromboembolic pulmonary arterial hypertension (Fig. 50–23);[116, 258a–c] despite this, it should be remembered that the extent of abnormalities on a perfusion lung scan can underestimate the severity of angiographic and hemodynamic compromise significantly.[259] In one investigation of 75 patients, including 25 who had chronic thromboembolic pulmonary arterial hypertension, 35 who had primary hypertension, and 15 who had secondary nonthromboembolic pulmonary arterial hypertension, a high probability $\dot{V}/\dot{Q}$ scan interpretation had a sensitivity of 96% and a specificity of 94% for detecting thromboembolic hypertension.[116] A combination of high and intermediate probability scan interpretations had a sensitivity of 100% and a specificity of 86%. In another study, the usefulness of the conventional chest radiograph and perfusion scintigraphy

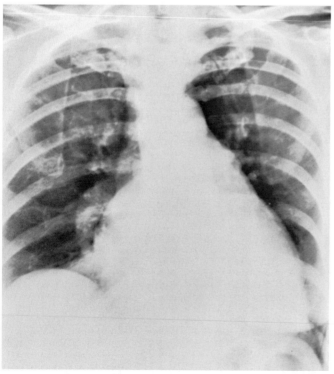

**Figure 50–22. Pulmonary Hypertension: Massive Pulmonary Artery Thromboembolism without Infarction.** Marked oligemia of both lungs is associated with moderate enlargement of both hila and rapid tapering of the pulmonary arteries as they proceed distally. The cardiac contour is typical of cor pulmonale.

using technetium-99m–labeled albumin macroaggregates was assessed in 19 patients who had biopsy-proven plexogenic pulmonary hypertension, thromboembolic pulmonary hypertension, or veno-occlusive disease.[260] Chest radiograph results were normal in patients who had plexogenic and thromboembolic hypertension; perfusion lung scan results were abnormal in seven of the eight patients who had thromboembolic disease and in none of the nine patients who had plexogenic hypertension. In the two patients who had veno-occlusive disease, the chest radiographs revealed evidence of pulmonary venous hypertension. The investigators suggested that a combination of chest radiographs and perfusion scintigraphy could be useful in distinguishing these three conditions.

The diagnosis of chronic thromboembolism can also be suggested on the basis of alterations in pulmonary vascularity and attenuation on high-resolution computed tomography (HRCT).[261–263] Such alterations consist of patchy areas of decreased vascularity and attenuation associated with blood flow redistribution to uninvolved areas, a pattern known as *mosaic attenuation* or *mosaic perfusion* (Fig. 50–24). In one study of five patients who had chronic pulmonary thromboembolism in which HRCT scan results were compared with axial single photon emission CT perfusion scan results obtained at similar levels, 176 localized areas of hypoperfusion were identified on single photon emission CT;[262] 133 were abnormal on HRCT (sensitivity 76% and specificity 50%). In another investigation of 67 patients (17 having chronic thromboembolic hypertension, 6 PPH, 5 secondary nonthromboembolic hypertension, and 39 a variety of airway, interstitial, or air-space parenchymal abnormalities), HRCT had a sensitivity and specificity of approximately 97% in separating pulmonary hypertension caused by chronic thromboembolic disease from other pulmonary abnormalities, including other causes of pulmonary hypertension.[263] The two features that allowed the accurate differentiation were disparity in the size of segmental arteries at corresponding levels in the right and left lungs and mosaic pattern of attenuation. The average ratios of segmental vessel size were 2.2 for patients who had chronic thromboembolic hypertension and 1.1 for the remaining patients.

Another group of investigators has shown a somewhat lower diagnostic accuracy of HRCT in distinguishing the various causes of pulmonary arterial hypertension.[264] In their study, which included 64 patients who had pulmonary arterial hypertension (15 chronic thromboembolism, 4 idiopathic pulmonary arterial hypertension, 21 underlying lung disease, 17 cardiac disease, and the remaining miscellaneous causes), a mosaic pattern of lung attenuation was present in 12 of 15 (80%) patients who had thromboembolic pulmonary arterial hypertension, 2 of 4 (50%) who had PPH, 2 of 2 (100%) who had pulmonary veno-occlusive disease, 1 of 21 (5%) who had underlying lung disease, and 2 of 17 (12%) who had underlying cardiac disease. The difficulty in distinguishing mosaic attenuation due to chronic thromboembolism from mosaic attenuation due to parenchymal lung disease or airway disease has been confirmed by another group.[265]

Contrast-enhanced spiral CT is currently the imaging modality of choice for the evaluation of patients who have pulmonary arterial hypertension and suspected chronic thromboembolism based on a combination of radiographic and scintigraphic findings or HRCT. Chronic emboli are

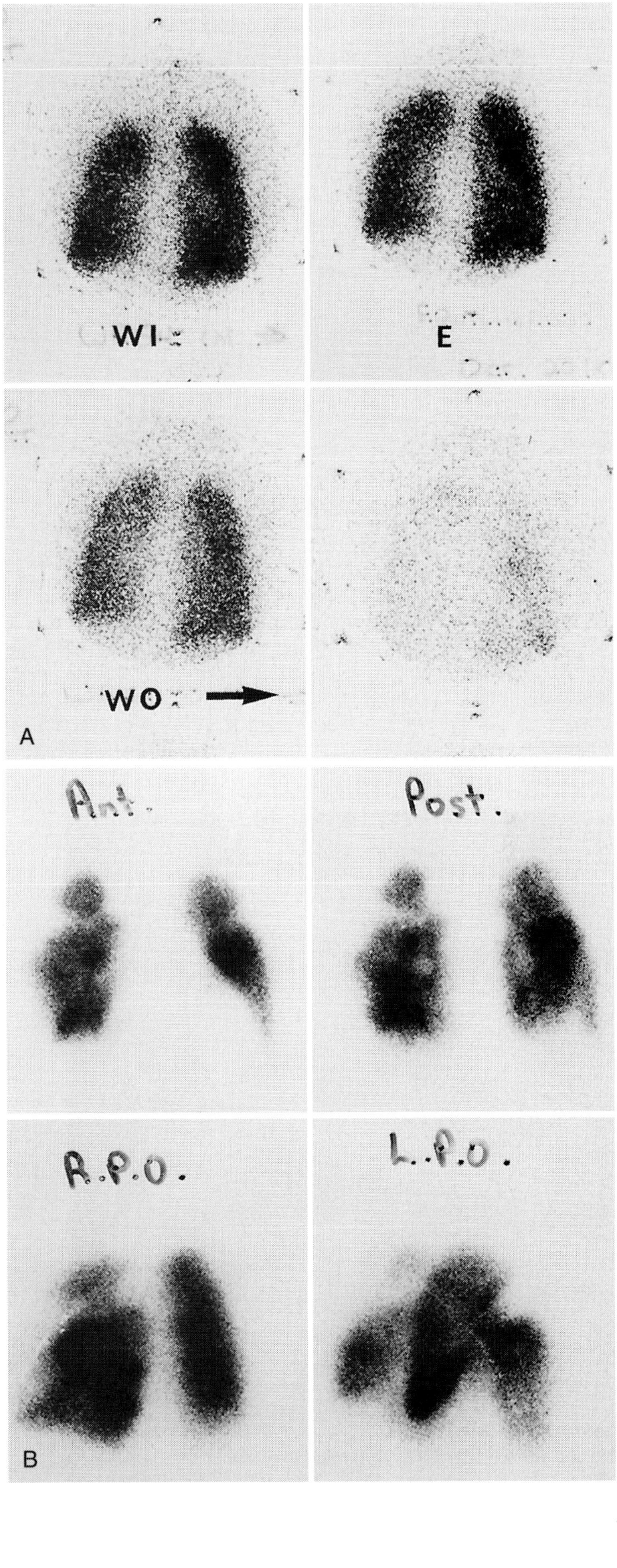

**Figure 50–23. Pulmonary Hypertension: Perfusion Pattern on Scintigraphy in Chronic Thromboembolism without Infarction.** Ventilation *(A)* and perfusion *(B)* lung scintigrams reveal features that are considered "high probability" for thromboembolism. WI, E, and WO represent the washin, equilibrium, and washout phases, respectively, of the perfusion scintigraphic study. The patient was a 64-year-old man.

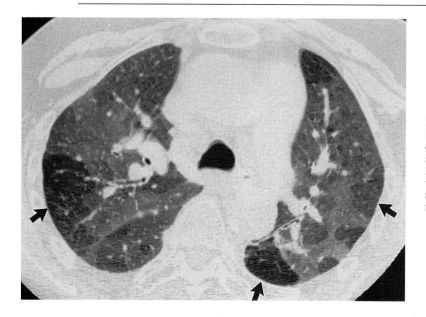

**Figure 50–24. Mosaic Perfusion in Thromboembolic Pulmonary Arterial Hypertension.** HRCT in a 73-year-old woman demonstrates localized areas that have decreased attenuation and vascularity *(arrows)* and areas with increased lung attenuation and increase in size and number of pulmonary vessels (mosaic perfusion). Note the large size of the pulmonary arteries compared with that of the adjacent bronchi, a finding consistent with pulmonary hypertension.

considered to be present on CT when at least two of the following features are identified: (1) an eccentric location contiguous to the vessel wall (Fig. 50–25), (2) evidence of recanalization within the intraluminal filling defect, (3) arterial stenosis or web, (4) abrupt narrowing of the artery with reduction of more than 50% of the arterial diameter (Fig. 50–26), and (5) complete occlusion at the level of the stenosed arteries.[266] The most common finding is an eccentric location of the thrombus, resulting in a crescentic, often irregularly margined, filling defect adjacent to the vessel

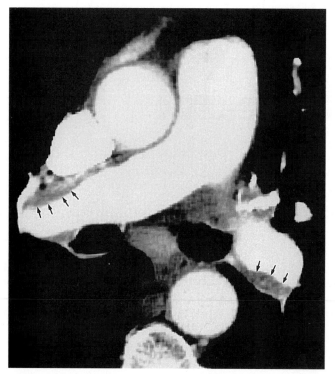

**Figure 50–25. Chronic Thromboembolism.** A contrast-enhanced spiral CT scan in a 56-year-old woman demonstrates filling defects adjacent to the wall of the right and left interlobar pulmonary arteries *(arrows)*. This eccentric location is characteristic of chronic thromboembolism.

wall.[267, 268] Calcification within the thrombus has been reported in up to 10% of cases.[268, 269]

In one study, investigators compared CT results with those of pulmonary angiography in 21 consecutive patients who had chronic pulmonary thromboembolism.[119] Contrast-enhanced CT was found to be superior to angiography in demonstrating the presence and extent of proximal clots as confirmed by surgery. It also demonstrated more peripheral thrombi than were apparent on angiography. Angiography was superior to CT in demonstrating vascular distortion and stenosis. In another study of 63 patients who underwent thromboendarterectomy, CT had a sensitivity of 77% and a specificity of 100% in confirming the diagnosis of chronic thromboembolism and ensuring operability.[118] In a third study, contrast-enhanced spiral CT was compared with MR imaging and pulmonary angiography in 55 patients who had chronic thromboembolic pulmonary hypertension[120] *(see* Fig. 50–13). MR imaging was performed using both gadolinium-enhanced spin-echo and gradient-recalled echo techniques; surgical correlation for the presence of central vessel disease was available in 40 of the 55 patients. Out of a total of 56 abnormal central arterial portions, abnormalities were identified on spiral CT in approximately 80%, compared with 70% on angiography and 35% on MR imaging. Central abnormalities were seen more clearly on the gradient-recalled echo MR images than on images using the spin-echo technique. Spiral CT has also been used to identify enlarged bronchial arteries in some patients who had chronic thromboembolic hypertension; in one study, the visualization of prominent bronchial arteries was a predictor of a favorable outcome after thromboendarterectomy.[270]

Pulmonary angiography is recommended when there is a discrepancy between the CT and the clinical findings and in the assessment of selected patients undergoing thromboendarterectomy.[120] It is safe when performed with nonionic contrast medium and selective bolus injection directly into pulmonary arterial branches.[271] In one study of 250 patients in whom pulmonary angiography was performed for assessment of chronic major vessel thromboembolic PA obstruction, the findings most suggestive of chronic thromboem-

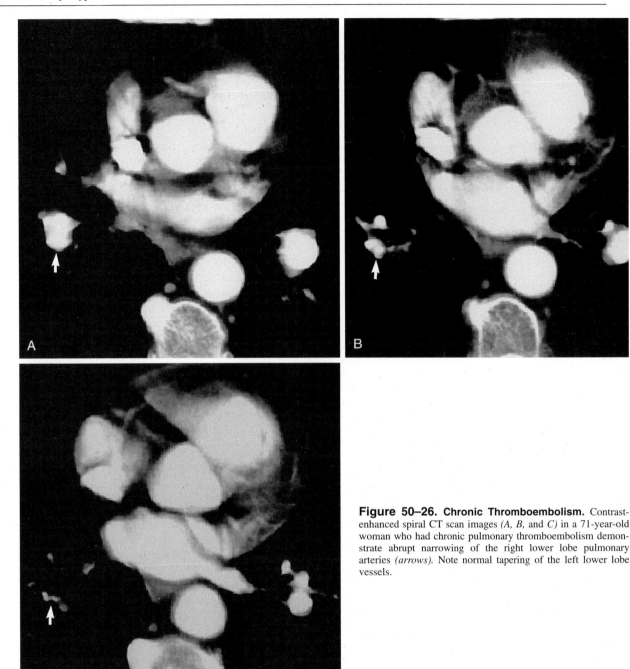

**Figure 50–26. Chronic Thromboembolism.** Contrast-enhanced spiral CT scan images *(A, B,* and *C)* in a 71-year-old woman who had chronic pulmonary thromboembolism demonstrate abrupt narrowing of the right lower lobe pulmonary arteries *(arrows).* Note normal tapering of the left lower lobe vessels.

bolic disease were "pouch defects," webs or bands, intimal irregularities, abrupt vascular narrowing, and complete vascular obstruction[272] (Fig. 50–27). A pouch defect refers to a partially or completely occlusive chronic thrombus that organizes in a concave configuration toward the lumen. Pulmonary arterial webs or bands are seen as lines of decreased opacity that traverse the width of the PA, usually at the lobar or segmental level;[273] they are often associated with vessel narrowing or poststenotic dilation.

Pulsed Doppler echocardiography permits assessment of right ventricular size and systolic function in patients who have recent or chronic pulmonary emboli. Thromboemboli within the heart or PA or both may also be detected; if

a tricuspid regurgitant jet develops as a consequence of embolization, ultrasonographic assessment of PA pressure can also be made.[274] In a study of 60 patients who had pulmonary hypertension, 35 of whom had central pulmonary emboli, transesophageal echocardiography was 97% sensitive and 88% specific in detecting this cause of hypertension.[275]

Clinical Manifestations

The symptoms and signs of pulmonary thromboemboli are described in Chapter 48 *(see* page 1824). Pulmonary function changes include an increase in the physiologic dead

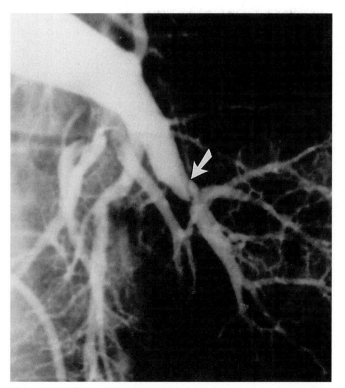

**Figure 50–27. Thromboembolic Pulmonary Arterial Hypertension.** A view from a left pulmonary angiogram demonstrates areas with decreased perfusion, irregularity of the segmental vessels, and a focal linear filling defect (arterial web) *(arrow)*, findings that are characteristic of pulmonary arterial hypertension secondary to chronic thromboembolism.

space and the arterial-alveolar gradient.[276] Exercise can increase these abnormalities and in some cases results in a worsening of pulmonary hypertension. Lung function studies in patients who have CTEPH frequently show evidence of lung restriction, especially in those who show evidence of parenchymal scarring on HRCT;[277] a reduction in the diffusing capacity for carbon monoxide attributable to a decrease in both the membrane diffusing capacity and pulmonary capillary blood volume is also seen.[258]

### Prognosis and Natural History

In specialized centers, surgical removal of thrombi from large PAs has been associated with a surgical mortality of about 10%, a value that has been decreasing.[247] However in centers whose personnel have less experience with surgical therapy for this condition, the operative mortality may be considerably higher (23%), especially in patients who have higher PA pressures (more than 50 mm Hg) and pulmonary vascular resistance (more than 1,100 dynes·s·cm$^{-5}$).[278] The causes of in-hospital mortality in these patients are unrelieved pulmonary hypertension (50%), intraoperative cardiac arrest (17%), and reperfusion pulmonary edema or stroke (8% each).[247]

As indicated previously, the prognosis of patients who have histologic features of small vessel thrombosis or thromboembolism in the absence of proximal vessel disease appears to be better than that of those who have plexogenic arteriopathy; in one study of 49 patients, those who had plexogenic lesions survived a mean 297 days, whereas those

who had only thrombotic lesions lived an average of 1,070 days.[68]

### Pulmonary Hypertension Associated with Systemic Immunologic Disorders

Pulmonary arterial hypertension, unaccompanied by parenchymal lung disease and manifested pathologically by plexogenic arteriopathy, occurs occasionally in immunologically mediated connective tissue disorders, particularly progressive systemic sclerosis (PSS), mixed connective tissue disease, and systemic lupus erythematosus (SLE) (Fig. 50–28). Raynaud's phenomenon is often present, suggesting that the pulmonary disease represents part of a generalized vasculopathy. Pulmonary hypertension also occurs in some individuals with immunologically mediated interstitial lung disease such as rheumatoid disease and PSS; in these cases, radiographic and pathologic features are identical to those associated with chronic interstitial lung disease of other etiologies. Rarely, hypertension is a complication of pulmonary vasculitis, most often Takayasu's arteritis or Behçet's disease; in these cases, the pathogenesis of the hypertension is probably related to *in situ* arterial thrombosis. This subject is considered in greater detail in relation to the specific disease entities in their respective chapters.

### Pulmonary Hypertension Associated with Antiphospholipid Syndrome

Pulmonary hypertension is being reported with increasing frequency in patients who have circulating antiphospholipid antibodies.[279, 280] The presence of antiphospholipids may be primary or secondary. The former (primary antiphospholipid syndrome) is a rare condition that is associated with widespread thrombotic and embolic phenomena.[281] In addition to pulmonary hypertension, the syndrome may be associated with pulmonary hemorrhage and ARDS.[282] Secondary antiphospholipid syndrome occurs in association with connective tissue diseases, particularly SLE. The concurrence of portal hypertension and portal venous thrombosis in association with pulmonary hypertension and thrombosis has also been reported in patients who have SLE and the antiphospholipid syndrome.[280, 283]

The importance of these antibodies in the pathogenesis of pulmonary hypertension may be greater than generally appreciated. In one study of 38 consecutive patients who had pulmonary hypertension (primary and secondary, pre- and postcapillary), 11 were found to have antibodies directed against one or more phospholipids (including 4 of 9 [44%] of those who were thought to have had primary hypertension and 7 of 29 (24%) of those who had secondary disease);[284] antibodies were detected only in those who had precapillary hypertension. The antibodies are directed against phospholipids in the endothelial cell plasma membrane, including cardiolipins, phosphatidylserine, inositol, and ethanolamine. A disturbance of the thromboxane-prostacyclin balance may be the underlying pathogenetic mechanism: both of these prostanoids can be secreted by endothelial cells, prostacyclin decreasing and thromboxane increasing platelet adhesiveness to the endothelium.[284a]

The pathologic appearance is identical to that of pulmonary hypertension associated with multiple thromboemboli,

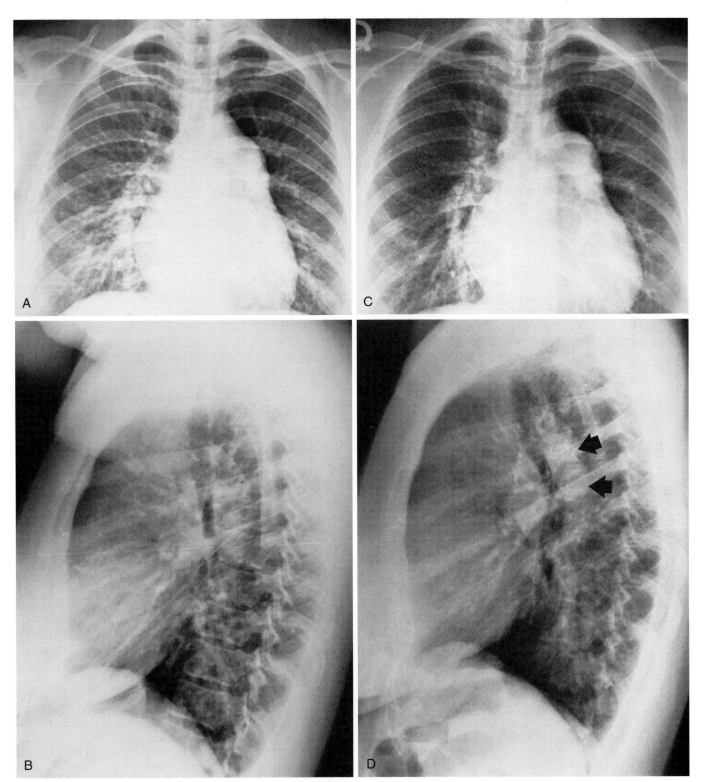

**Figure 50–28. Pulmonary Arterial Hypertension Secondary to Systemic Lupus Erythematosus (SLE).** The first chest radiographs in posteroanterior *(A)* and lateral *(B)* projection on this 32-year-old woman with SLE reveals exceptional prominence of the main pulmonary artery and mild to moderate cardiomegaly consistent with right ventricular enlargement. The pulmonary vasculature looks plethoric, but the lungs are otherwise unremarkable. Eight months later, repeat chest radiographs *(C* and *D)* showed an increase in the size of the heart and greater prominence of the main and hilar pulmonary arteries; note the markedly dilated left interlobar artery in *D (arrows).* However, a more remarkable change has occurred in the pulmonary vasculature, which now displays diffuse oligemia. These changes are characteristic of severe pulmonary arterial hypertension and cor pulmonale, attributable in this patient to vasculopathy associated with SLE. (Courtesy of Dr. M. O'Donovan, Montreal General Hospital.)

consisting of recent, organizing, and organized thrombi in the small and medium-sized pulmonary vessels.[279] Thrombosis of major PAs accessible to thromboendarterectomy has also been reported.[285, 286] Radiologic manifestations are also those of thromboembolic hypertension. The onset of respiratory symptoms may be insidious, without any features suggestive of thromboembolic episodes.[287] Although the outcome of pulmonary hypertension in association with antiphospholipid syndrome is usually fatal, long survival has been reported.[288]

### Pulmonary Hypertension Associated with Human Immunodeficiency Virus Infection

There have been an increasing number of reports of an association between pulmonary hypertension and human immunodeficiency virus (HIV) infection.[289, 290, 291] Although it was first believed that this association was related to opportunistic infection, only about 33% of affected patients have a prior AIDS-defining illness and most have no evidence of an accompanying pulmonary infection.[292] There is also no evidence of a direct effect on the pulmonary vasculature by the virus, leading to the speculation that the disease is a result of an immunologic response.[290] There is evidence that patients who have specific HLA class II antigens (HLA-DR6) may be at particular risk for the complication.[293] In most cases, the pathologic appearance is that of plexogenic pulmonary hypertension;[294, 295] however, cases of thrombus-associated hypertension[296] and of veno-occlusive disease have also been reported.[295, 297]

The clinical manifestations are identical to those of PPH, except that the age of onset is younger ($32 \pm 5$ years versus $42 \pm 13$ years in one study)[289] and the degree of hypertension tends to be less at the time of diagnosis, perhaps because these patients are under close medical supervision.[289] In most cases, the hypertension develops in the absence of other manifestations of HIV infection; however, associations with lymphocytic interstitial pneumonia,[298] membranous glomerulonephritis,[299] cirrhosis, and cryoglobulinemia have been documented.[300] The CD4 count is usually greater than $200/\mu L$. The natural history of the pulmonary hypertension is one of rapid deterioration.[289, 301] In one review of the literature published in 1998, the 1-year survival rate was approximately 50%;[291] hypertension was considered to be the direct cause of death in 29 (76%) of the 38 fatal cases.

### Pulmonary Capillary Hemangiomatosis

Pulmonary capillary hemangiomatosis is an unusual and rare form of pulmonary hypertension.[302–304] In a literature review published in 1994, only 16 cases were identified;[305] the authors added a 17th case, only the fourth in which the diagnosis had been established antemortem. The fundamental nature of the condition is uncertain; however, the infiltrative nature of the vessels on histologic examination has suggested to some that it may represent a low-grade, locally aggressive neoplasm of the pulmonary endothelial cell.[305] A familial association has been documented in some cases.[306]

Pathologically, the most striking feature is a patchy interstitial proliferation of thin-walled blood vessels the size of capillaries.[302] The vessels appear to invade the walls of pulmonary veins and to a lesser extent PAs; perineural infiltration has also been reported.[307] The venular infiltration is often accompanied by intimal fibrosis, which may lead to significant stenosis; as a result, interstitial edema and recent or remote air-space hemorrhage (manifested by hemosiderin-laden macrophages) are common. The major differential diagnosis is thus veno-occlusive disease; the use of a reticulin stain can be particularly useful in distinguishing between the two.[303]

Chest radiographs may demonstrate a predominantly reticulonodular or micronodular pattern, or the appearance may be normal except for the evidence of pulmonary hypertension.[308–310] HRCT demonstrates peribronchial cuffing, thickening of the interlobular septa and centrilobular nodular opacities,[310] or a mosaic pattern of attenuation similar to that seen with chronic pulmonary thromboembolism[311] (Fig. 50–29). Perfusion lung scans may show bilateral, nonhomo-

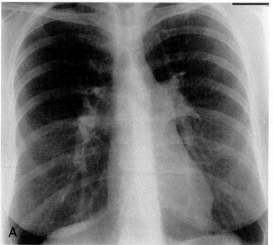
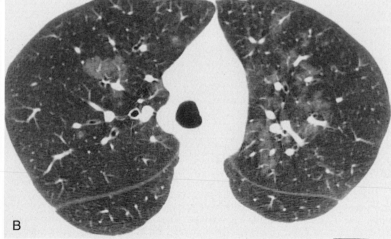

**Figure 50–29. Pulmonary Capillary Hemangiomatosis.** A posteroanterior chest radiograph *(A)* in a 52-year-old woman who had chronic pulmonary arterial hypertension demonstrates enlargement of the central pulmonary arteries. An HRCT scan *(B)* shows mosaic perfusion with localized areas of increased attenuation and vessel size. The diagnosis of pulmonary capillary hemangiomatosis was proven at lung transplantation.

geneous, subsegmental perfusion defects or segmental defects suggestive of thromboembolism.[308, 309]

Patients are generally young adults and present with a clinical picture of pulmonary hypertension; the course is one of slow progression. In one case, pulmonary function tests showed moderate restrictive impairment with decreased lung compliance and a pressure-volume curve suggestive of increased venous pressure.[308] The condition can be confused with PPH and veno-occlusive disease, in that both are associated with hemoptysis and progressive dyspnea.[304]

### Multiple Pulmonary Artery Stenosis or Coarctation

This rare abnormality of PAs may occur as a developmental anomaly (*see* page 642) or can result from intrauterine rubella infection (*see* page 993). It may be associated with diminished vascularity in the lungs and sometimes with pulmonary arterial hypertension[312–317] (Fig. 50–30).

### Compression of the Main Pulmonary Artery or Its Branches

Occasionally, an acquired disease results in diffuse pulmonary oligemia of "central" origin. For example, a mediastinal mass lying contiguous to the main PA may compress this vessel to a degree sufficient to compromise pulmonary arterial flow.[318] In one of our patients, an aneurysm of the ascending arch of the aorta compressed the pulmonary outflow tract so severely that cor pulmonale ensued; there was clear-cut radiographic evidence of pulmonary oligemia. Dissecting aneurysms of the PA[319, 320] or of the aorta[321, 322] can also compress the PA. Other reported causes include primary chondrosarcoma of the sternum[318] and fibrosing mediastinitis.[323]

### Primary Pleuropulmonary Disease

A wide variety of primary diseases of the lungs, pleura, chest wall, and respiratory control center may cause a rise in pulmonary arterial pressure without significant change in pulmonary venous pressure (*see* Table 50–1, page 1881). However, pulmonary arterial pressures seldom reach the levels attained in cases of primary vascular disease, and the arterial and arteriolar narrowing due to intimal thickening and medial hypertrophy is less; histologic features of plexogenic arteriopathy are absent. In fact, the hypertension may be transient, reflecting episodes of pulmonary infection and its associated hypoxia.

It is probable that the main cause of pulmonary arterial hypertension in this group of conditions is hypoxemia, with or without respiratory acidosis. The reduction in arterial oxygen saturation may be secondary to ventilation-perfusion inequality, shunt or generalized alveolar hypoventilation. In the majority of cases, the PA pressure decreases significantly when arterial oxygen saturation is increased as a result of treatment of pulmonary infections or administration of supplemental oxygen. Other probable contributory factors include hypervolemia, polycythemia, pulmonary capillary destruction (especially in cases of severe COPD), and increased flow through the anastomoses between the bronchial and pulmonary arterial circulations (in which case the trans-

mission of higher systemic pressure to the pulmonary circulation may raise PA pressure). Many patients who have pulmonary disease of sufficient severity to cause pulmonary hypertension are at risk for the development of pulmonary thromboemboli, and in some cases these also contribute to worsening of the hypertension.[324]

### Chronic Obstructive Pulmonary Disease

Pulmonary hypertension in patients who have COPD appears to be caused predominantly by a combination of hypoxemia and destruction of the microvasculature.[325] Acute and reversible worsening of pulmonary hypertension can occur during exacerbations of respiratory insufficiency.[326] The degree that hypertension contributes to exercise impairment is independent of the degree of ventilatory impairment.[327] Physiologic studies have shown a close correlation among pulmonary vascular resistance, oxygen saturation, and diffusing capacity during exercise.[328] In one pathologic investigation of lungs that were derived from patients enrolled in the NIH nocturnal oxygen therapy trial, significant intimal and medial thickening was identified in the medium and large muscular arteries;[329] however, these abnormalities did not correlate with premortem measurements of either the severity of pulmonary hypertension or the response of the vasculature to oxygen.

The radiographic manifestations of pulmonary hypertension in emphysema are identical to those of primary vascular disease; however, the invariable presence of overinflation permits ready differentiation (Fig. 50–31). In one study of 61 men with COPD and 42 normal control subjects, a strong positive correlation was found between the diameters of the right and left interlobar arteries and the presence and severity of pulmonary arterial hypertension.[330] The measurements were made on the right interlobar artery at its widest diameter on a posteroanterior radiograph and the left interlobar artery on the left lateral radiograph at its widest diameter posterior to the circular shadow of the left upper lobe bronchus. Right-sided heart catheterization was performed on all 61 men with COPD, and in 46 the mean PA pressure was elevated: of these 46, the right interlobar artery was dilated (> 16 mm) in 43 and the left interlobar artery (> 18 mm) in a similar number. When both arteries were dilated, the presence of PA hypertension was predicted correctly in 45 of the 46 patients, including the 26 in whom elevation of mean PA pressure was mild (21 to 30 mm Hg).

Even in the presence of cor pulmonale, the electrocardiogram (ECG) usually does not show the characteristic pattern of right ventricular hypertrophy that is associated with primary pulmonary vascular disease. Tall R waves in V1 are seldom seen, and the pattern of extreme right axis deviation, with tall, peaked P waves, may be the result of rotation of the heart rather than right ventricular hypertrophy.

### Diffuse Interstitial or Air-Space Disease

In most conditions associated with diffuse interstitial or air-space disease, elevation of PA pressure probably is related to hypoxemia and the limited distensibility of the pulmonary vascular tree; as a result, hypertension becomes particularly manifest during exercise-induced increases in cardiac output. The radiologic changes are dominated almost

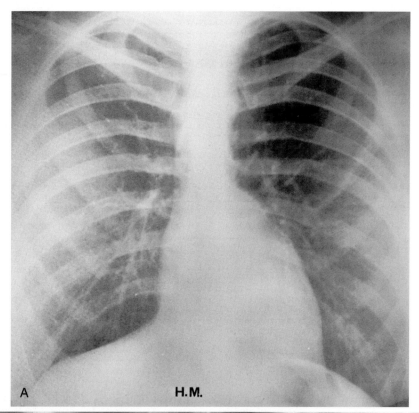

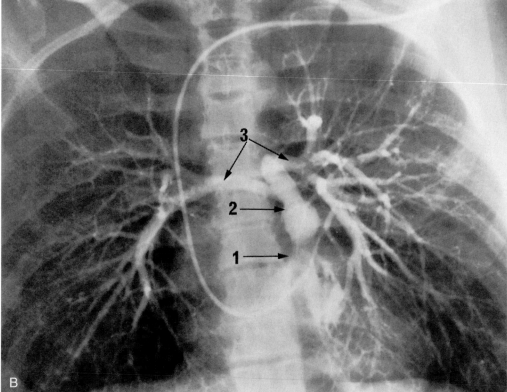

**Figure 50–30. Precapillary Pulmonary Hypertension Caused by Diffuse Pulmonary Artery Stenosis.** A posteroanterior chest radiograph *(A)* reveals cardiomegaly with a configuration consistent with right ventricular enlargement. The hila are diminutive, and the main pulmonary artery segment is barely discernible. The lungs are diffusely oligemic but otherwise unremarkable. A right ventricular angiogram *(B)* shows multilevel pulmonary artery stenosis affecting infundibular (1), valvular (2), and supravalvular (3) components. The distal (intraparenchymal) arteries are small but otherwise show no abnormality. The patient was a young woman with exertional dyspnea.

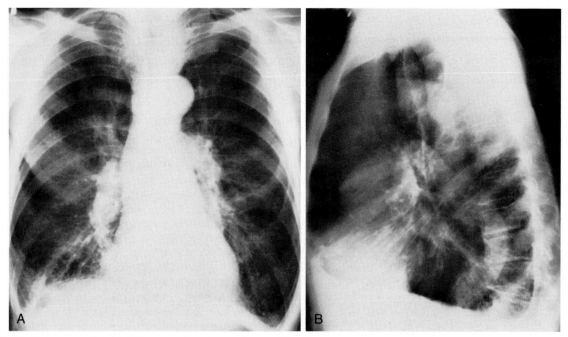

**Figure 50–31. Pulmonary Arterial Hypertension Secondary to Emphysema.** Posteroanterior *(A)* and lateral *(B)* radiographs reveal marked overinflation of both lungs, with a low flat position of the diaphragm and an increase in the depth of the retrosternal air space. The lungs are diffusely oligemic, the peripheral vessels being narrow and attenuated. A discrepancy in the size of the central and peripheral pulmonary vessels is caused not only by a decrease in caliber peripherally but by an increase in size centrally; the latter constitutes convincing evidence of pulmonary arterial hypertension. At autopsy, the parenchymal changes were predominantly those of panacinar emphysema.

invariably by the underlying pulmonary disease, and, in many cases, the peripheral vascular markings are obscured.

In one study of the radiologic findings in 29 patients who had diffuse interstitial disease (PSS in 20, sarcoidosis in 6, and miscellaneous causes in 3) and in whom cardiac catheterization had revealed pulmonary arterial hypertension and normal pulmonary wedge pressures, PA pressure was significantly related to the size of the central PAs, and pulmonary hemodynamic abnormalities were roughly proportional to the radiologic severity of parenchymal disease.[331] Perhaps because of the difficulty in objectively measuring the diameter of the right interlobar artery (mainly because of imprecise identification of the margins of the vessels as a result of contiguous disease), the transhilar-thoracic ratio proved to be a moderately accurate predictor of pulmonary arterial pressure (the transhilar distance was defined as the sum of distances from the midsagittal line to the most lateral point of junction between each interlobar artery and upper lobe vessels). Subjective evaluation of the size of the main PA proved to be of only moderate value as a predictor of pulmonary arterial pressure. In their estimation of pulmonary blood volume in the same patients, the researchers found three vascular signs to be most useful—the transhilar-thoracic ratio, the size of the right interlobar artery, and the diversion of blood flow to upper lung zones. Of these three signs, only the transhilar-thoracic ratio proved to be of value in assessing both pulmonary arterial pressure and pulmonary blood volume. Of considerable interest was the observation that diversion of blood flow to upper zones was significantly related to restriction of the pulmonary vascular bed but was not necessarily a sign of increased pulmonary arterial pressure.

In another retrospective review of 41 patients who had

PSS, the degree of pulmonary arterial hypertension was found to be out of proportion to the severity of interstitial pulmonary fibrosis, suggesting the possibility of a concomitant primary vasculopathy.[332] In this series, pulmonary arterial hypertension was evident radiographically or clinically in 15 patients (37%). Hilar PA enlargement is seldom as marked in pulmonary arterial hypertension secondary to parenchymal lung disease as it is in primary vascular disease; however, evidence of progressive enlargement on serial radiographs should suggest the diagnosis of pulmonary hypertension.

Usually, symptoms are attributable to the underlying disease, and the presence of pulmonary hypertension may not be clinically detectable until cor pulmonale and cardiac failure develop.

### Pneumonectomy

Although pneumonectomy does not appear to cause a rise in pressure in a remaining normal lung in the immediate postoperative period, pathologic and physiologic evidence of hypertension can be found in patients living for several years after surgery; the complication may result from small vessel sclerosis secondary to increased blood flow.[333]

### Fibrothorax

Chronic pleural thickening rarely is associated with pulmonary arterial hypertension and cor pulmonale. However, we have seen patients who had bilateral fibrothorax who also had hypoxemia, hypercapnia, secondary polycythemia, and cor pulmonale and no apparent parenchymal lung disease.

### Chest Deformity

Severe degrees of kyphoscoliosis and thoracoplasty may lead to pulmonary arterial hypertension and cor pulmonale, again on the basis of ventilation-perfusion imbalance and hypoventilation. A similar mechanism, along with failure of lung development, contributes to the severe pulmonary hypertension that occurs in neonates with congenital diaphragmatic hernia.[334]

### Alveolar Hypoventilation Syndromes

Underventilation of normal lungs, with consequent decreased arterial blood $Po_2$ and increased $Pco_2$, may result in pulmonary hypertension. This syndrome may be primary in origin (Ondine's curse—Fig. 50–32) or related to obesity-hypoventilation syndrome, obstructive sleep apnea,[335–339] loss of altitude acclimatization,[13] or continuous depression of the respiratory center by drugs.[340] In obstructive sleep apnea, hemodynamically significant pulmonary hypertension is more often seen in patients who have more severe daytime hypoxemia,[341] a higher body mass index, and worse lung function.[100]

## POSTCAPILLARY PULMONARY HYPERTENSION

Postcapillary pulmonary hypertension results from any condition that increases pulmonary venous pressure above a critical level. Undoubtedly, the most common of these are diseases of the left side of the heart, usually those that cause left ventricular failure, such as systemic hypertension and coronary artery disease. Less common causes include mitral stenosis, congenital cardiac anomalies such as cor triatriatum, capillary hemangiomatosis, chronic sclerosing mediastinitis, atrial myxoma, total anomalous venous drainage, and primary veno-occlusive disease.[342–344]

The mechanism by which an increase in pulmonary venous pressure causes an increase in PA pressure is not as simple as might be imagined. If the increase in pulmonary arterial pressure was simply a passive response to the increase in venous pressure, pulmonary vascular resistance would be expected to remain normal or to decrease (owing to vascular distention). In fact, there is usually an increase in pulmonary vascular resistance. In the early stages of left heart failure, this increased resistance is related to pulmonary arterial vasoconstriction (which may be related to the in-

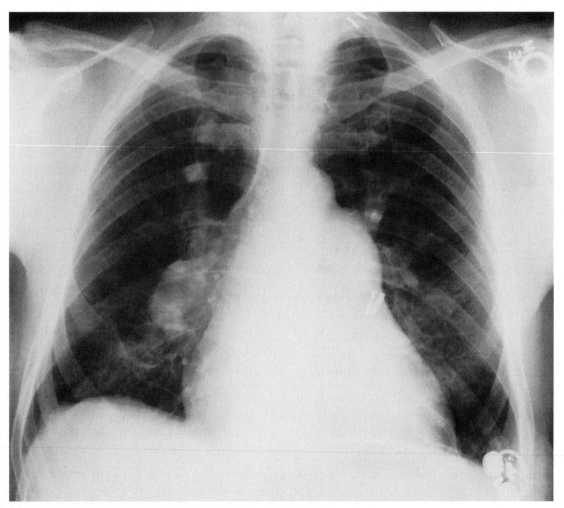

**Figure 50–32. Severe Pulmonary Arterial Hypertension in Primary Alveolar Hypoventilation (Ondine's Curse).** A posteroanterior radiograph of a 55-year-old man reveals marked dilation of the main pulmonary artery and its hilar branches, with rapid diminution in caliber of pulmonary arteries as they proceed distally. The heart is moderately enlarged in a configuration compatible with cor pulmonale. The lungs are not overinflated and show no evidence of primary disease. The pacemaker projected over the base of the left lung was pacing the left phrenic nerve to achieve repeated diaphragmatic contraction. (Courtesy of Dr. Richard Greenspan, Yale University, New Haven.)

creased plasma levels of ET-1 found in congestive heart failure).[345] When postcapillary hypertension is severe and long-standing, it induces structural changes within the pulmonary arterial circulation that perpetuate the increased resistance. These changes are radiographically indistinguishable from those of other forms of precapillary hypertension (apart from the changes in cardiac contour, which almost always permit differentiation). This has led to the suggestion that this condition be referred to as *combined precapillary and postcapillary hypertension.*[346]

### Pathologic Characteristics

Morphologic abnormalities in chronic postcapillary hypertension can be seen in the arteries, veins, and lung parenchyma. Muscular arteries usually show medial hypertrophy, and muscularization of arterioles is not uncommon;[347] concomitant intimal fibrosis is usual. Although some of the medial hypertrophy may be caused by an increase in smooth muscle, there is evidence that an increase in connective tissue itself may be more important.[55] Fibrinoid necrosis and vasculitis of small vessels have been reported but are rare;[347, 348] dilation and plexiform lesions do not occur.

Because the primary site of the hypertension is postcapillary, changes in veins and venules are almost always apparent, although they are often not as pronounced as those on the arterial side of the circulation. Medial hypertrophy and intimal fibrosis are common;[347, 349] in addition, the elastic laminae, which are normally irregular in distribution, may become concentrated into internal and external laminae, similar to the appearance of PAs (so-called arterialization of pulmonary veins) (Fig. 50–33). Dilation of the veins, especially the larger veins and those on the right side, can result in varicosities.

The pulmonary parenchyma itself is also usually abnormal. Foci of air-space hemorrhage, either recent or old, are invariably present in individuals who have died of the disease. Remote hemorrhage appears grossly as patchy foci of red-brown discoloration 1 to 3 mm in diameter corresponding to intra-alveolar accumulation of hemosiderin-laden macrophages.[349] In severe cases, hemosiderin may also be identified lying free in the interstitial tissue. In some cases, the hemorrhage occurs as a result of leakage of red blood cells from distended pulmonary capillaries; in others, it is related to rupture of bronchial vein varicosities (formed by anastomoses between pulmonary and bronchial veins).[350]

Parenchymal interstitial fibrosis and Type 2 cell hyperplasia are common in postcapillary hypertension (Fig. 50–34). The pathogenesis of the fibrosis is unclear; it has been suggested that it may be caused by organization of intra-alveolar exudate,[351] but it is perhaps more likely related to chronic leakage of fluid into the parenchymal interstitium. The combination of fibrosis and hemosiderin accumulation is responsible for use of the term *brown induration* to describe the gross appearance of these lungs. Organization of intra-alveolar fibrinous edema may be responsible for the presence of mature bone within alveolar air spaces or the lumen of alveolar ducts (*see* Fig. 50–34), a finding that is particularly common in mitral stenosis; although usually too small to be visible with the naked eye, the bone fragments are occasionally large enough to be demonstrable radiographically. The same pathogenetic mechanism is probably responsible for the peribronchial fibrosis that is seen in some patients;[352] this pathologic change may be the basis for the obstructive ventilatory pattern that is often present in these patients.[353, 354]

### Radiologic Manifestations

In 1958, Simon made the initial empiric observation that pulmonary venous hypertension from any cause produces a distinctive alteration in the pulmonary vascular pat-

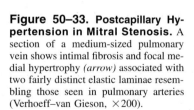

**Figure 50–33. Postcapillary Hypertension in Mitral Stenosis.** A section of a medium-sized pulmonary vein shows intimal fibrosis and focal medial hypertrophy *(arrow)* associated with two fairly distinct elastic laminae resembling those seen in pulmonary arteries (Verhoeff–van Gieson, ×200).

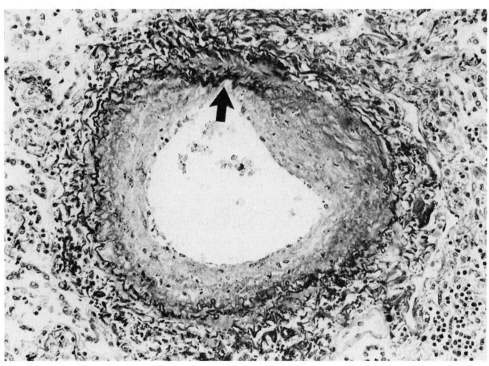

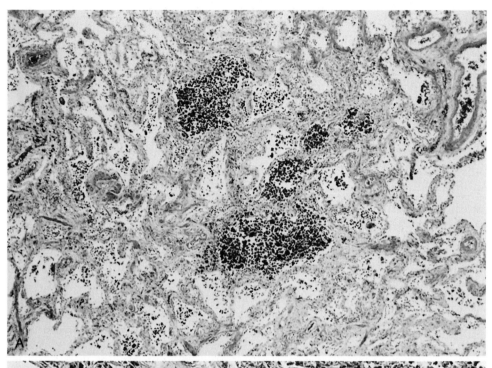

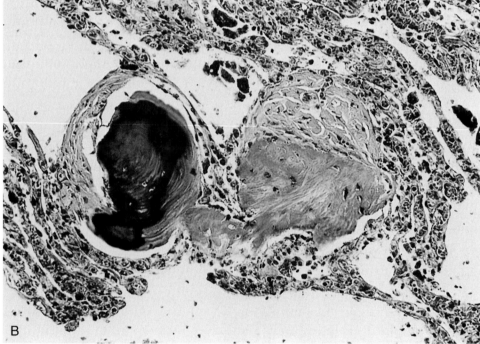

**Figure 50–34. Postcapillary Hypertension in Mitral Stenosis.** A section of lung parenchyma from a 68-year-old woman with long-standing mitral stenosis *(A)* shows several intra-alveolar aggregates of hemosiderin-laden macrophages (black cells) and a moderate degree of interstitial fibrosis. A section from another region *(B)* shows a lobulated fragment of mature bone within alveolar air spaces. (*A,* ×40; *B,* ×160.)

tern.[355] He observed that in mitral stenosis or left ventricular failure the lower lobe pulmonary vessels are narrowed and the upper lobe ones are distended, and postulated that increase in pulmonary venous pressure above a critical level results in venous vasoconstriction. In erect humans, pulmonary venous pressure is higher in the lower lobes than in the upper lobes because of a difference in hydrostatic pressure (averaging approximately 12 to 15 mm Hg in adult subjects). Therefore, the critical level is reached first in lower lung zones and the resultant vasoconstriction diverts blood flow to upper lung regions, producing the radiographic picture of upper lobe pleonemia and lower lobe oligemia (Figs. 50–35

and 50–36). This is in striking contrast to the normal situation, in which pulmonary perfusion and pulmonary vascular caliber increase from apex to base. With continued increase in venous pressure, the reduction in venous caliber progresses upward from the lung bases and eventually affects the upper lobes, constricting the engorged upper lobe veins and producing a diffuse alteration in the pulmonary vasculature. The inevitable result is generalized elevation of pulmonary arterial resistance and pulmonary arterial hypertension[356] (Fig. 50–37).

Simon's hypothesis that reflex vasoconstriction constitutes the mechanism by which vascular resistance rises in

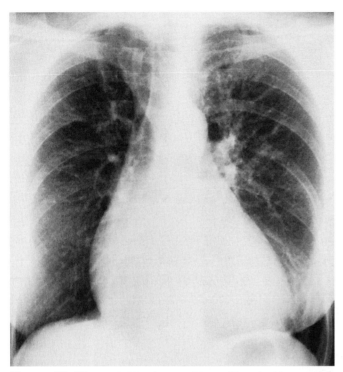

**Figure 50–35. Redistribution of Blood Flow to Upper Lung Zones Caused by Pulmonary Venous Hypertension.** A postero-anterior radiograph reveals unusually prominent vascular markings in the upper zones and rather sparse markings in the lower zones. The patient, a 42-year-old woman, had recurrent episodes of left ventricular decompensation as a result of a congestive cardiomyopathy.

the lower lobes, although never proven convincingly, was an invaluable spur to further research, and several alternative theories have been advanced to explain the observations. For example, it has been proposed that an accumulation of edema fluid around the small arteries and veins causes increased resistance by interfering with the tethering effect of the lung parenchyma that normally holds these vessels open.[357] However, this theory has been put into question by the results of studies that showed that distribution of blood flow may remain normal when the perivascular interstitial tissues are markedly distended with fluid.[358]

Another group found that reduction of blood flow to the base of the lungs occurred only when alveolar edema was produced and caused a reduction in local lung volume; the more marked the alveolar edema, the greater the reduction in flow.[359, 360] They explained the phenomenon by an increase in interstitial pressure as a result of the local reduction in expansion of lung parenchyma in the lower zones. Although this explanation has been supported by the results of additional animal experiments,[361] it must be emphasized that the findings in these studies relate only to acute left ventricular decompensation and that they should not be extrapolated to other conditions. Blood flow redistribution with an increase in the number and size of upper lobe vessels is most striking in the setting of chronic venous hypertension rather than secondary to an acute hemodynamic change.[78] Clinical experience with chronically elevated left atrial pressure, as in mitral stenosis, suggests that redistribution of flow in this circumstance does occur in the absence of alveolar edema. In such cases, the mechanism for flow

redistribution may be either the interstitial fibrosis that develops in the lower lung zones or the narrowing of vessels by hypertensive vascular lesions rather than reflex vasoconstriction, perivascular interstitial edema, or lung deflation secondary to local alveolar edema.[361]

Regardless of the mechanism, there is no doubt that a disparity between the caliber of upper and lower lobe vessels represents one of the most useful radiographic signs of pulmonary venous hypertension (Fig. 50–38). Although it is common to hear the term *upper lobe venous engorgement* used to describe redistribution of blood flow from lower to upper zones, in fact both arteries and veins show distention, since such distention is caused by increased resistance to blood flow through the lower zones. Thus, it is conceptually preferable to employ the phrase *upper zone vascular distention* to indicate redistribution of blood flow. In fact, because distention of upper zone vessels occurs in five situations other than pulmonary venous hypertension (a supine position, predominantly lower zonal parenchymal disease, left-to-right shunt, hypervolemia, and pulmonary arterial hypertension), it is advisable as a first approximation to refer to the abnormality as *recruitment of upper zone vessels*; after other aspects of the radiographic appearance have been evaluated, it will be possible to ascribe the recruitment to a specific etiology.

It is customary for radiologists to assess the caliber of upper zone vessels by comparing them with lower zone vessels. Although it is clear that a disparity must exist for redistribution of flow to be present, we feel that it is often exceedingly difficult to be convinced of an increase in upper zonal vessel caliber by such a comparison. Instead, it has been our experience that subjective assessment of the caliber of vessels in the upper zones, based on our experience of what constitutes the normal, is more dependable. Such an assessment is obviously facilitated by comparison with previous radiographs, but with few exceptions (chiefly patients who have left-to-right shunts or whose radiographs have been obtained in the recumbent position), subjective assessment is reasonably reliable even without comparison.

Although the presence of upper lobe vascular distention usually is evident from simple subjective assessment (or from comparison with lower lobe vascular caliber in patients in whom the severity or chronicity of venous hypertension has led to arterial hypertension), some investigators have proposed criteria to assess it objectively.[362] In a study of 100 pulmonary angiograms, 50 of which were performed in the recumbent and 50 in the sitting position, the mean pulmonary vein diameter at the level of the main PA was 7 mm in the supine position and 4 mm in the erect position. (More than one third of opacified pulmonary veins were too small to be measured in the erect position.) From a review of the range of normal variation in the caliber of this vessel, the investigators suggested that a pulmonary vein whose diameter is greater than 8 mm at the level of the main PA is abnormal (Fig. 50–39). They also showed that upper lobe pulmonary veins are usually too small to identify on plain chest radiographs of normal subjects exposed in the erect position. Further, they found a considerable variation in the diameters of opacified upper lobe pulmonary veins, ranging from too small to measure to 15 mm. It is thus apparent that very occasionally a moderately distended upper lobe pulmonary vein may be identified on the chest radiograph

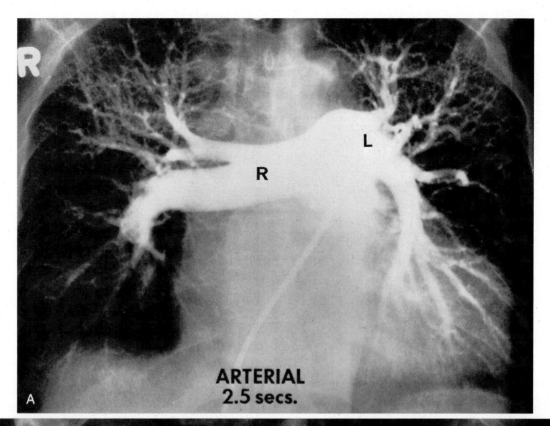

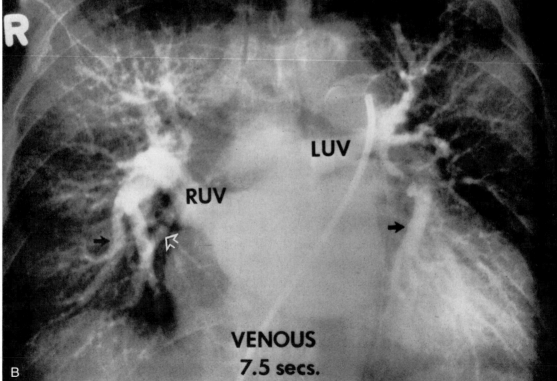

**Figure 50–36. Precapillary and Postcapillary Pulmonary Hypertension: Angiographic Features.** A main pulmonary artery angiogram during the arterial phase *(A)* reveals enlarged right (R) and left (L) pulmonary arteries. The middle and upper zone arteries are slightly tortuous, whereas lower lobe arteries are less well opacified and straightened, displaying few side branches. During the venous phase *(B)*, the right (RUV) and left (LUV) superior veins are well opacified, whereas there is only slight filling of lower lobe veins *(open arrow)*. Note the persistent opacification of the lower lobe arteries *(arrows)* during the late venous phase. The findings indicate increased resistance to blood flow through the lower lobe vasculature, resulting in preferential blood flow redistribution to upper lobe vessels.

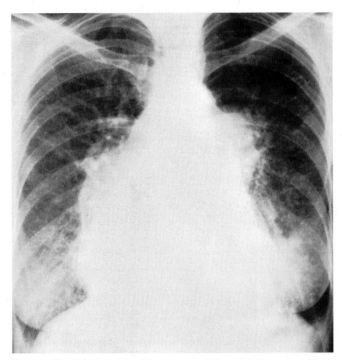

**Figure 50–37. Combined Venous and Arterial Hypertension in Mitral Stenosis.** A posteroanterior radiograph of a 40-year-old woman with a 20-year history of rheumatic heart disease reveals severe pulmonary arterial hypertension as evidenced by a moderate increase in the size of the hilar pulmonary arteries and by the rapid tapering of these vessels as they proceed distally. A slight discrepancy in the size of the upper lobe and lower lobe pulmonary vessels and well-defined Kerley B lines indicate associated pulmonary venous hypertension. When these signs are considered in the light of the character of the cardiac enlargement, the diagnosis of chronic mitral valvular disease with pulmonary venous and arterial hypertension may be made with confidence. Following commissurotomy, several of the Kerley B lines persisted, indicating that the septal thickening was the result of fibrosis as well as edema.

of an individual who does not have pulmonary venous hypertension or redistribution of blood flow related to disease.

In a review of the chest radiographs of 111 patients who had critical mitral stenosis (valve openings of 1.5 × 1.0 cm or less), dilated upper zone vessels were found in all but six persons.[363] The PA and left atrial pressures and the degree of valve narrowing were no different in these six persons from those of the group as a whole. It is apparent, therefore, that critical mitral stenosis can be present without dilation of the upper lobe vessels, although such an occurrence is very uncommon. Some researchers have suggested that a change in contour of the right hilum may supply useful confirmatory evidence of vascular redistribution.[364, 365] Because the superior pulmonary vein forms the upper rim of the right hilar concavity, distention of this vein flattens the concavity and may render it convex when ballooning is severe; however, we have seldom found this sign to be of value.

The alteration in pulmonary vascular pattern that is seen in mitral stenosis may also be observed transiently in mild left ventricular failure; for example, in a study of the chest radiographs of 50 consecutive patients admitted to a coronary care unit, redistribution of blood flow to the upper zones was found to be the commonest abnormality (76% of

patients).[366] Radiographic signs of left ventricular failure may be apparent without clinical evidence of decompensation. In another study of 94 patients who had chest radiographs obtained on admission to a coronary care unit, 31 (33%) were found to have radiographic evidence of pulmonary venous hypertension (manifested most commonly by distention of upper zone vessels) without associated clinical signs;[367] in 23 of these, however, clinically evident failure developed subsequently. In a study of 30 patients who had recent myocardial infarction, the severity of radiographic abnormality generally correlated well with levels of pulmonary capillary wedge pressure.[368] It was found that redistribution of blood flow was the earliest manifestation of elevated wedge pressure, followed sequentially by loss of the normal sharp margins of the pulmonary vessels, development of perihilar haze, and, finally, overt air-space edema.

It has been suggested that the pattern of blood flow redistribution may be different in mitral insufficiency from that in other forms of pulmonary venous hypertension.[369] Instead of symmetric dilation of vessels in both upper zones, there occurs a more prominent dilation of the right upper zone vessels, presumably as a result of reflux from the insufficient valve whose orientation posteriorly, superiorly, and to the right results in dominant flow to the right upper lobe. In fact, of 50 cases of mitral insufficiency proved surgically or angiographically in one study, 7 showed such localized dilation of right pulmonary vessels.

In addition to the typical alteration in vascular pattern observed in pulmonary venous hypertension, particularly in mitral stenosis, other pulmonary changes occur that are worthy of note. Frequently, signs of interstitial pulmonary edema are visible, including septal edema (Kerley A and B lines) and perivascular edema (manifested by loss of definition of pulmonary vascular markings; Fig. 50–40). Hemosiderosis, although often visible pathologically, is not readily identifiable radiographically unless it is severe; it is manifested by tiny punctate shadows situated mainly in the midlung and lower lung zones (Fig. 50–41). Pulmonary fibrosis may be apparent as a rather coarse, poorly defined reticulation, again predominantly in the middle and lower lung zones (Fig. 50–41).

Foci of bone formation in the lung parenchyma occur in about 5% to 15% of patients who have mitral stenosis;[370, 371] however, such foci are seldom visible on the chest radiograph. Although they are virtually pathognomonic of mitral stenosis,[372] they have also been described in pulmonary veno-occlusive disease.[373] Radiographically, foci of parenchymal ossification appear as densely calcified nodules, 2 to 5 mm in diameter, mainly in the midlung zones and sometimes containing demonstrable trabeculae (Fig. 50–42). They occur more commonly in men[371, 374] and are more numerous in the right lung.[375] Although pulmonary venous hypertension is invariably present, there is no apparent relationship between the development of ossific nodules and the degree of hypertension or associated hemosiderosis.[371]

Although it might be anticipated that radiographic evidence of redistribution of blood flow to upper lung zones in patients who have severe mitral stenosis might disappear relatively rapidly following adequate surgical correction by closed commissurotomy or valve replacement, this is not the case. In a study that was designed to determine the radiographic criteria most helpful in the evaluation of the postop-

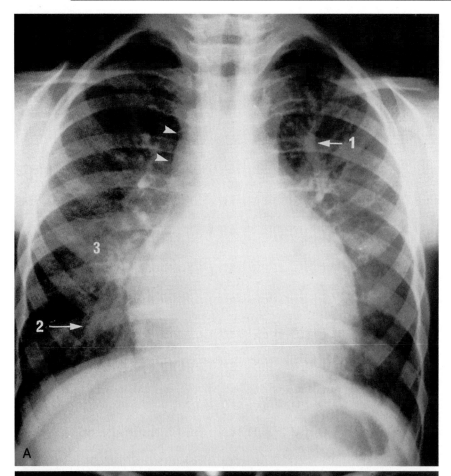

**Figure 50–38. Severe Postcapillary Pulmonary Hypertension and Edema Caused by Mitral Valve Prolapse.** A posteroanterior chest radiograph *(A)* demonstrates features typical of postcapillary pulmonary hypertension—dilated upper lobe vessels (1), ill-defined lower lobe vessels (2), and diffuse interstitial edema (3). The cardiac size is increased in a nonspecific fashion. The vascular pedicle is increased in width as a result of distention of the superior vena cava *(arrowheads),* indicating systemic venous hypertension. Anteroposterior views of the thorax from a selective main pulmonary angiogram during the arterial *(B)* and venous *(C)* phases reveal increased blood flow to the upper lobes (compare the degree of contrast-filling of the upper lobe arteries to the relatively branchless lower lobe arterial vasculature). The mid and upper zones show a "background blush"; the lower lobes do not. Note the persistence of the lower lobe arterial pattern, the well-distended upper lobe veins (V1), and the poorly filled lower lobe veins (V2) during the venous phase.

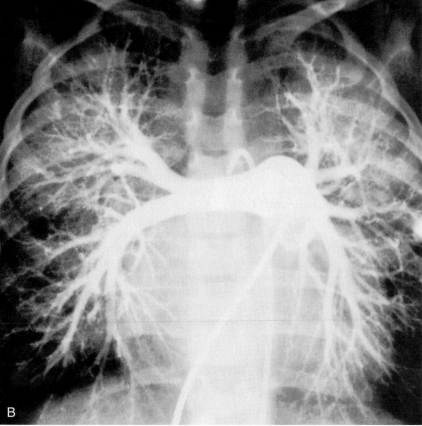

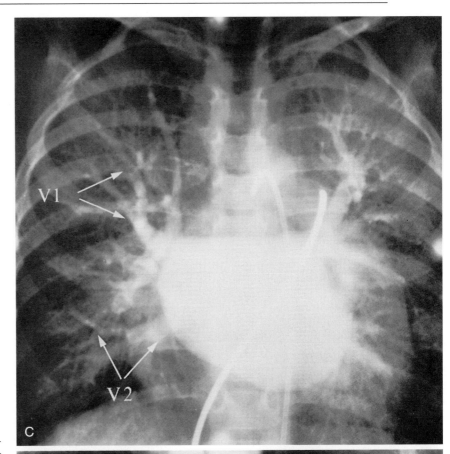

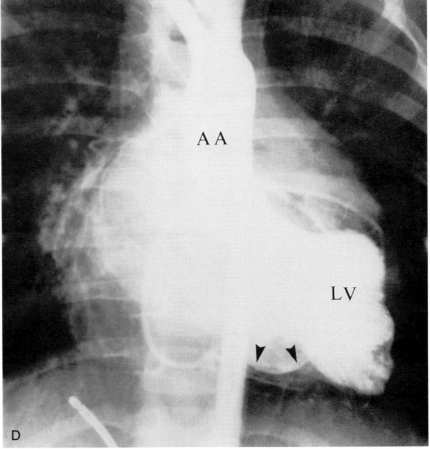

**Figure 50–38** *Continued.* A left ventricular angiogram *(D)* shows a prolapsed mitral valve *(arrowheads)* as the cause of the above-described features. LV and AA represent the left ventricle and ascending aorta, respectively. The patient was a young woman.

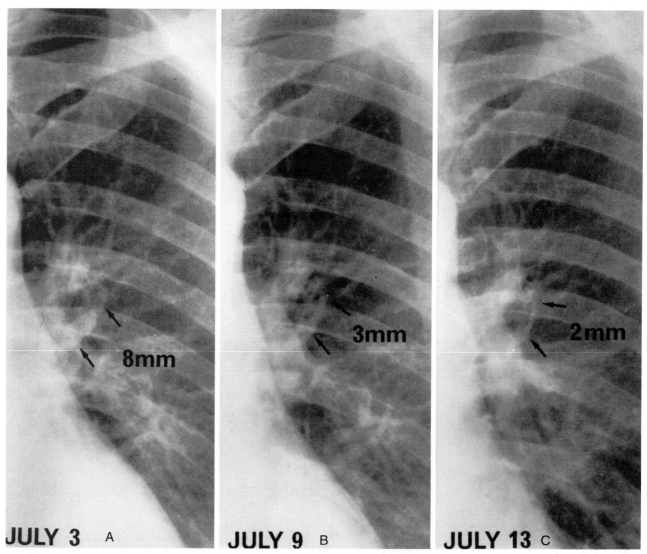

**Figure 50–39. Distention of the Left Superior Pulmonary Vein as a Sign of Pulmonary Venous Hypertension.** A detail view of the left hemithorax *(A)* from a posteroanterior chest radiograph reveals a slightly dilated superior pulmonary vein *(arrows)* that measures 8 mm in transverse diameter. Six days later, following diuretic therapy *(B)*, the vein *(arrows)* has diminished in size to 3 mm; subsequently, 4 days later *(C)*, it has diminished to 2 mm. Note the decreasing prominence of the left heart border in the illustrative sequence. The patient was an elderly man who was admitted to the hospital for a transurethral prostatectomy.

erative hemodynamic and clinical status, five radiographic signs were used in an analysis of preoperative and postoperative radiographs of 25 patients who had pure mitral stenosis:[376] (1) septal (Kerley B) lines, (2) abnormal pulmonary vascular pattern (redistribution of blood flow), (3) left atrial enlargement, (4) the ratio of the diameter of the main PA to the diameter of the left hemithorax, and (5) the diameter of the right interlobar artery. The most useful postoperative changes were found to be the left atrial size, the ratio of the width of the main PA from the midline divided by the diameter of the left hemithorax at the diaphragm, and the diameter of the right interlobar artery distal to the right middle lobe artery. The use of these signs resulted in prediction of significant hemodynamic and clinical improvement in 100% and 86% of cases, respectively.

A change from the abnormal vascular pattern observed preoperatively—that is, a disappearance of signs of redistri-

bution of blood flow—was found to be less reliable, a finding for which the investigators gave two reasons: (1) hemodynamic improvement secondary to decreased pulmonary vasoconstriction may not be accompanied by a decrease in tissue of the vessel wall; and (2) considerable time is required for relatively fixed anatomic changes in vessels to regress.[377] This observation is of considerable importance, in that the radiographic demonstration of persisting upper zonal vascular distention several months following corrective surgery does not necessarily indicate elevated levels of left atrial and pulmonary venous pressure. As pointed out in the chapter on pulmonary edema, persistence of septal or Kerley B lines may also be a poor indicator of hemodynamic or clinical improvement, because such lines may be caused by fibrosis secondary to chronic or recurrent edema and thus will not regress or disappear despite a return to normal pulmonary hemodynamics.

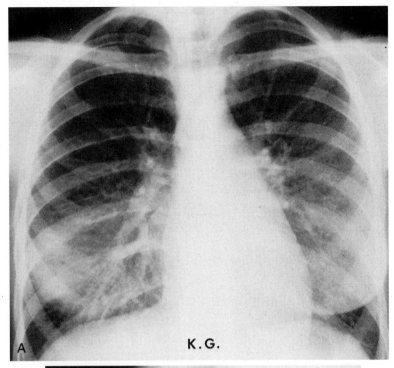

K.G.

**Figure 50–40. Postcapillary Hypertension Caused by a Left Atrial Myxoma.** Posteroanterior *(A)* and lateral *(B)* chest radiographs show perihilar and lower-lobe parenchymal haze, ill-defined lower-lobe bronchovascular bundles, and thickening of interlobar fissures as a result of pleural edema *(arrowheads)*. On the posteroanterior projection, the heart does not appear enlarged; however, on the lateral view, there is a suggestion of left atrial *(open arrows)* and right ventricular enlargement. The findings are consistent with obstruction at or proximal to the mitral valve.

*Illustration continued on following page*

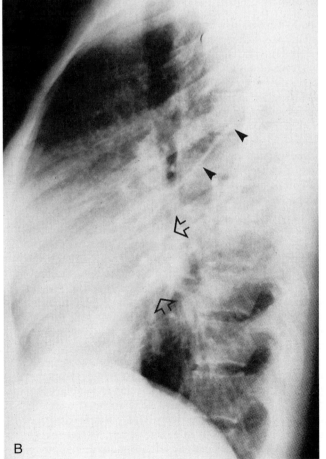

B

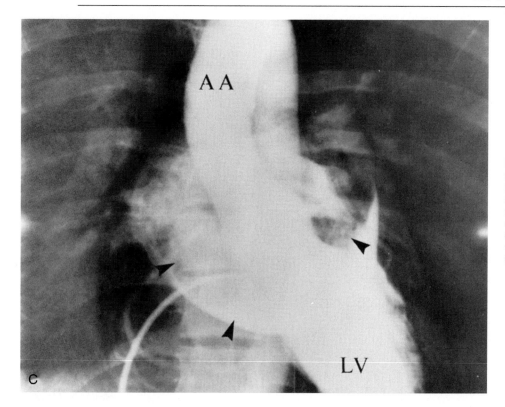

**Figure 50–40** *Continued.* A transseptal left atrial angiogram *(C)* discloses a large intra-atrial filling defect *(arrowheads)* consistent with a myxoma (subsequently confirmed). The left ventricle (LV) and ascending aorta (AA) are opacified with contrast medium. The patient was a young woman with intermittent episodes of exertional dyspnea.

### Clinical Manifestations

The symptoms associated with postcapillary hypertension usually are differentiated readily from those of precapillary origin. In left ventricular failure, which is the most common cause of pulmonary venous hypertension, symptoms and signs are predominantly those arising from acute or subacute pulmonary edema, including dyspnea, orthopnea, and paroxysmal nocturnal dyspnea. Expectoration of pink frothy fluid may be present; occasionally (particularly in mitral stenosis), bright red blood may be coughed up. When pulmonary venous hypertension develops as a result of a myxoma or thrombus blocking the mitral valve orifice, the clinical course usually is punctuated by episodes of pulmonary edema or syncope that can be relieved by a change in position. In some instances, myxomas give rise to systemic emboli or are associated with constitutional findings, such as fever, weight loss, raised sedimentation rate, anemia, or elevation of gamma globulin levels.[378, 379]

Some patients who have chronic congestive heart failure[380] or pulmonary veno-occlusive disease[381] do not present with these typical symptoms, and their radiographic findings and hemodynamic measurements may be equivocal; in such circumstances, an erroneous diagnosis of primary pulmonary arterial or interstitial disease may be made. The same situation can be seen with a severe degree of mitral stenosis, which can be differentiated from PPH only by the symptoms and signs of pulmonary edema, by the loud opening snap, and by the rumbling diastolic murmur associated with this valvular abnormality. Patients who have postcapillary pulmonary hypertension due to an increased resistance between the pulmonary capillaries and the left atrium have symptoms identical to those of mitral stenosis but without the characteristic accentuation of the first heart sound, the opening snap, or the rumbling diastolic murmur.

The degree of pulmonary arterial hypertension that develops in patients who have pulmonary venous hypertension due to left ventricular dysfunction is highly variable and is an important predictor of outcome.[382] In one study of 102 consecutive patients who had primary left ventricular dysfunction (ejection fraction < 50%), the best predictors of pulmonary hypertension (as assessed by Doppler echocardiography using tricuspid regurgitant velocity) were the degree of mitral regurgitation and a measure of left ventricular diastolic stiffness.[382]

### Electrocardiographic and Pulmonary Function Tests

The ECG findings in postcapillary hypertension reflect the cause of the hypertension and the rapidity of increase in pressure. In pure mitral stenosis, the changes may be identical to those of primary arterial hypertension with right ventricular hypertrophy. In mitral insufficiency, the ECG usually shows left ventricular hypertrophy, with or without evidence of right ventricular hypertrophy; rarely, only the latter is evident.

In the early stages of mitral stenosis, the diffusing capacity for carbon monoxide may be increased, presumably as a result of an increase in pulmonary capillary blood volume; however, in patients who have moderate or severe disease it is reduced significantly.[383] Pulmonary function studies in patients who have mitral valve disease show a progressive decrease in vital capacity and diffusing capacity and, with advancing disease, in expiratory flow rates.[384] Mitral valve repair by surgical or balloon valvotomy does not result in an improvement in diffusing capacity;[385, 386] however, a considerable reduction in minute ventilation during exercise and a more nearly normal oxygen uptake may be observed.[387] The degree of normalization of pulmonary

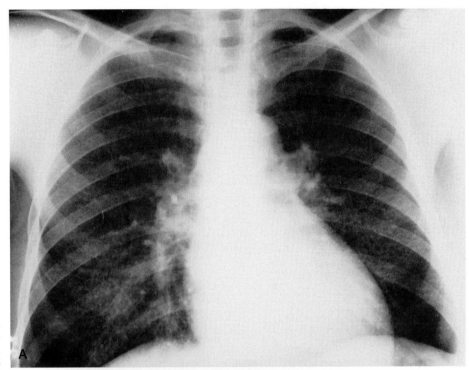

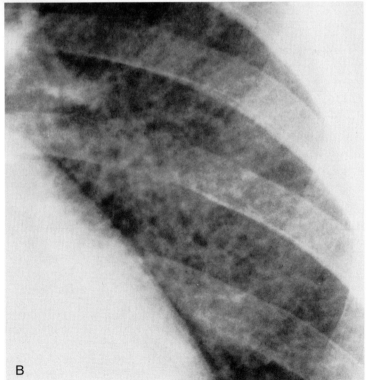

**Figure 50–41. Pulmonary Hemosiderosis and Fibrosis Secondary to Recurrent Episodes of Pulmonary Edema.** A posteroanterior radiograph *(A)* and a magnified view of the midportion of the left lung *(B)* reveal a medium reticular pattern throughout both lungs, most evident in the mid and lower zones. This pattern did not change on sequential examinations. The patient was a 29-year-old man who had severe aortic stenosis and repeated episodes of pulmonary edema.

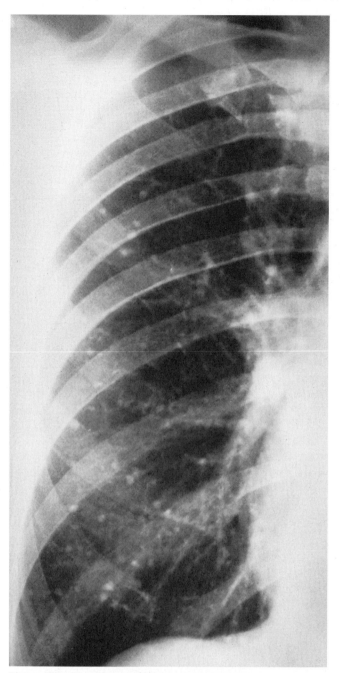

**Figure 50–42. Ossific Nodules in Mitral Stenosis.** A view of the right lung from a posteroanterior chest radiograph demonstrates multiple, sharply defined 1- to 3-mm calcific (ossific) nodules most numerous in the mid and lower thirds of the lung. The patient was a middle-aged man with long-standing mitral stenosis.

hemodynamics after mitral balloon valvotomy is dependent on the degree of preoperative pulmonary hypertension; in one study of 100 patients, pulmonary vascular resistance remained abnormally high in 91% of the 23 patients whose preoperative mean systolic pressure was greater than 50 mm Hg.[379] These data and the lack of improvement in diffusing capacity suggest that significant structural remodeling of the pulmonary vasculature must occur after prolonged increases in pulmonary venous pressure.

## PULMONARY VENO-OCCLUSIVE DISEASE

Pulmonary veno-occlusive disease (PVOD) is a rare abnormality characterized pathologically by evidence of repeated pulmonary venous thrombosis and clinically by pulmonary arterial hypertension, pulmonary edema, or both. In most of the cases described in the literature before 1990, the diagnosis was made at autopsy;[388, 389] however, as a result of the more widespread recognition of the variable presentations of the disease and the availability of HRCT, it is now being made more frequently ante mortem. The condition can occur at any age but is most common during childhood and adolescence. In adolescent patients, the sex incidence is approximately equal; however, in older individuals, there appears to be a slight male predominance.[390]

### Etiology and Pathogenesis

The etiology and pathogenesis are unknown and may be related to more than one source or mechanism. Electron-dense deposits have been found in the alveolar capillary walls by some investigators, suggesting the possibility of immune complex deposition;[391, 392] however, it is possible that these deposits represent simply degenerated red blood cells.[391] The disorder has been reported in association with a variety of diseases known to have an autoimmune basis, including chronic active hepatitis, celiac disease,[393] Raynaud's disease,[394] and SLE,[395] and it is thus possible that some abnormality of immune function may be involved in PVOD.

Although a possible association with viral infection has been documented by some investigators,[396] apart from occasional cases of HIV infection,[397] no specific organism has been implicated. Familial clusters of the disease suggest a genetic predisposition;[398, 399] however, such clusters are unusual, and a common environmental agent has not been excluded definitively.

A variety of ingested substances have been implicated in the causation of PVOD. The most important of these are medications, including bleomycin and mitomycin.[400, 401] Herbal "bush" teas containing *Senecio*, *Crotalaria*, and *Heliotropium* species may cause hepatic veno-occlusive disease, and in some persons who have this disease pulmonary venous involvement has also been described.[402, 403] PVOD has also been reported following the use of oral contraceptives,[406] an association that has been reported with hepatic veno-occlusive disease as well.[407] The basis of this relationship may be related to pulmonary vascular prostaglandin balance, especially of prostacyclin. The latter acts as both a vasodilator and an inhibitor of coagulation and is normally produced by the pulmonary vascular endothelium (as evidenced by the higher left ventricular, as opposed to pulmonary arterial, levels of 6-oxo-PGF$_1$-$\alpha$, a stable metabolite of prostacyclin). This pulmonary arterial-systemic gradient of prostacyclin may be a mechanism by which thrombosis of pulmonary veins is prevented. The use of oral contraceptives causes a reduction in pulmonary endothelial prostacyclin production, leading to speculation that alteration of prostaglandin metabolism may be partly responsible for an increased risk of venous thrombosis.[408] The same mechanism might be responsible for the pulmonary venous obstruction and occlusion observed in patients who have either hepatic or pulmonary veno-occlusive disease.

PVOD has also been reported after bone marrow transplantation[404] and after radiation therapy to the thorax.[405]

### Pathologic Characteristics

Pathologically, the most prominent feature is stenosis or complete obliteration of the lumens of small pulmonary veins and venules by intimal fibrous tissue[390, 393] (Fig. 50–43). Larger pulmonary veins are usually spared. The fibrous tissue may have a loose (active) or mature appearance; not uncommonly, it is present as trabeculae that subdivide the lumen into several channels, suggesting recanalized thrombus. Occasionally, an inflammatory infiltrate can be identified in the adjacent wall;[396, 409] however, recent or organizing thrombus is uncommon.

Histologic evidence of pulmonary arterial hypertension is usually present in the form of medial hypertrophy of small PAs, with or without intimal proliferation, fibrosis, and thrombi.[390] Although the plexiform lesions characteristic of PPH are absent,[410] capillary proliferation in the alveolar walls has been reported, suggesting that angiogenesis of the pulmonary circulation can occur in this setting.[411] The lung parenchyma may show evidence of remote hemorrhage (interstitial and air-space hemosiderin-laden macrophages); some degree of interstitial fibrosis and chronic inflammation are also often evident.[412]

### Radiologic Manifestations

Radiographically, signs of pulmonary arterial hypertension are no different from those associated with primary or thromboembolic disease but with the important addition of signs of postcapillary hypertension, chiefly pulmonary edema[413, 414] (Fig. 50–44). In a review of the radiographic findings in 26 patients, evidence of pulmonary edema was present in 20 (77%). The left atrium is not enlarged, and there is no evidence of redistribution of blood flow to upper lung zones, both important signs in distinguishing PVOD from mitral stenosis. Similar to the radiograph, HRCT demonstrates smooth thickening of the interlobular septa and interlobar fissures and areas of ground-glass attenuation consistent with interstitial pulmonary edema[415, 416] (Fig. 50–45). Small pleural effusions are present in the majority of patients.[416] Ventilation-perfusion scans can show segmental areas of V̇/Q̇ mismatch.[417]

### Clinical Manifestations

Patients typically have slowly progressive dyspnea and orthopnea punctuated by attacks of acute pulmonary edema; hemoptysis may occur. Crackles may be heard over the lung bases, and the second pulmonic sound is accentuated in most cases. As the condition progresses, a right ventricular heave develops, together with murmurs indicative of pulmonic and tricuspid insufficiency. The presence of additional conditions, such as HIV infection, connective tissue disease, malignancy and bone marrow transplantation,[418] may complicate the differential diagnosis. Most patients die within 2 years of the onset of symptoms.[389]

### Pulmonary Function Tests

Pulmonary function tests reveal arterial oxygen desaturation and a reduction in diffusing capacity and lung compli-

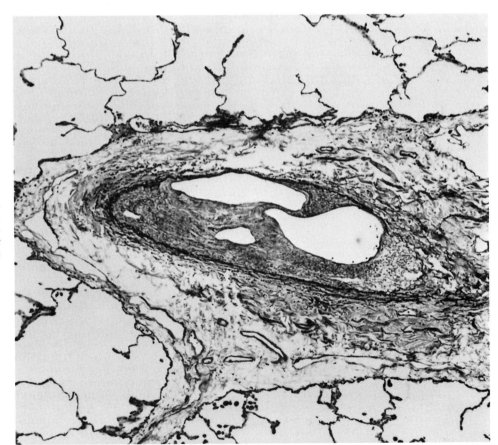

**Figure 50–43. Veno-occlusive Disease.** A section of a medium-sized pulmonary vein shows intraluminal fibrosis and multiple variable-sized vascular spaces suggesting recanalized thrombus (×40).

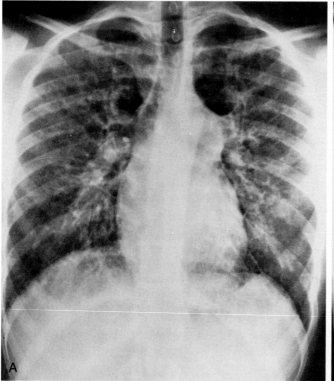

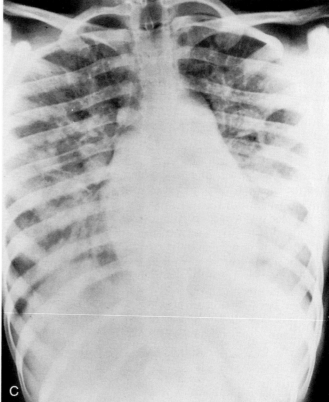

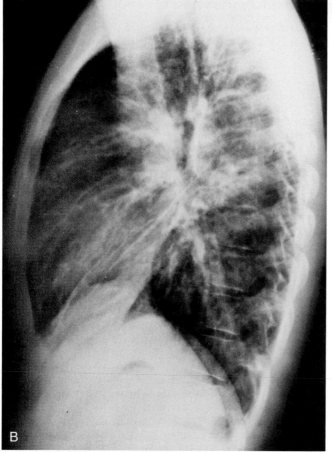

**Figure 50–44. Primary Veno-occlusive Disease.** Posteroanterior *(A)* and lateral *(B)* chest radiographs of this 16-year-old man reveal dilated main and hilar pulmonary arteries and diffuse interstitial edema (septal lines were visible on the original radiographs but have not reproduced). Echocardiography showed a dilated right ventricular chamber consistent with cor pulmonale but no other structural abnormality; specifically, the mitral valve and left atrium were normal in appearance. This combination of findings is virtually diagnostic of veno-occlusive disease, in a patient of this age almost certainly of the primary variety. Two weeks later, a chest radiograph *(C)* revealed massive air-space edema, and the patient died shortly thereafter. At autopsy, there were characteristic features of veno-occlusive disease.

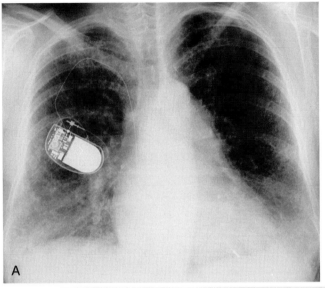

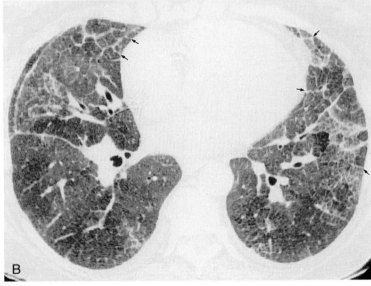

**Figure 50–45. Primary Veno-occlusive Disease.** A posteroanterior chest radiograph *(A)* in a 51-year-old woman demonstrates enlargement of the central pulmonary arteries and extensive interstitial pulmonary edema. A permanent pacemaker with a right ventricular lead in place is evident. An HRCT scan *(B)* essentially confirms the radiographic findings, demonstrating interlobular septal thickening *(arrows)* and areas of ground-glass attenuation consistent with interstitial pulmonary edema.

ance.[343] In one patient, the pressure-volume curve showed a decrease in elastic recoil at low lung volumes and an increase at high lung volumes. This pattern has also been observed in patients who have pulmonary venous hypertension secondary to mitral stenosis[419] and may be the result of pulmonary vascular congestion. The pulmonary arterial wedge pressure is usually normal or low,[420] a finding best explained by the fact that the wedged PA catheter measures the pressure not in the small pulmonary veins (which are narrowed by the obliterative process) but in the large pulmonary veins (which are usually distal to the site of obstruction); the wedge pressure therefore reflects the pressure in the large pulmonary veins and left atrium, which is normal, and not the pressure in the pulmonary capillaries, which is elevated.[410, 421] Although the triad of normal wedge pressure, pulmonary arterial hypertension, and pulmonary edema is virtually diagnostic of PVOD, left atrial myxoma can cause

similar findings *(see* Fig. 50–40): the patient can present with intermittent pulmonary edema during times of mitral valve obstruction but can have a normal PA wedge pressure when obstruction is not present.

## MISCELLANEOUS CAUSES OF PULMONARY HYPERTENSION

Numerous additional causes of pulmonary hypertension or associations of pulmonary hypertension with specific clinical entities have been described (Table 50–2). In addition to the conditions listed in Table 50–2, pulmonary hypertension has been reported in a patient who had Loeffler's endocarditis and endomyocardial fibrosis;[422] multiple pulmonary emboli originating in the right ventricle appeared to be the cause of the hypertension. A combination of pulmonary

## Table 50–2. MISCELLANEOUS CAUSES OF PULMONARY HYPERTENSION

|  | REFERENCE |
| --- | --- |
| Pierre Robin syndrome | 490 |
| Crow-Fukase syndrome | 491, 492 |
| Williams syndrome | 493 |
| POEMS syndrome* | 494 |
| Alveolar capillary dysplasia | 495 |
| Polycythemia rubra vera | 496 |
| Endocardial fibroelastosis in pregnancy | 497 |
| Idiopathic pulmonary hilar fibrosis | 498 |
| Prolonged exposure to domestic wood smoke | 499 |
| Schistosomiasis | 500 |
| Sarcoidosis | 501 |
| Amyloidosis | 502 |
| Sickle cell disease | 503 |

*POEMS, polyneuropathy, organomegaly, endocrinopathy, M protein, skin changes.

vasculitis, hypereosinophilia, and episodic pulmonary hypertension was described in three siblings in one report.[423] Finally, an unusual form of pulmonary hypertension has been described that is associated histologically with smooth muscle proliferation in the walls of bronchioles, alveoli, small PAs, and pulmonary veins.[424]

## CHRONIC COR PULMONALE

Although the presence of pulmonary hypertension does not necessarily imply cor pulmonale, it does indicate that there is a strain on the right ventricle that, if prolonged, will lead inevitably to right ventricular hypertrophy. Strictly speaking, the term *cor pulmonale* should be restricted to instances in which abnormality of lung structure or function results in right ventricular hypertrophy. Although disease of the left side of the heart and congenital cardiac disease may closely mimic true cor pulmonale, they are not generally accepted under this definition.[425] Approximately 80% of cases of chronic cor pulmonale result from COPD and emphysema.[426]

Radiographically, cardiac enlargement is not always apparent, even when right ventricular hypertrophy is evident at post mortem.[425] This failure to appreciate cardiac enlargement is particularly notable in the presence of pulmonary emphysema, when only serial radiography may reveal the increase. Advances in radionuclide and echocardiographic techniques have greatly expanded our understanding of right ventricular function in health and disease.[427–430]

Clinically, right ventricular thrust, usually felt along the left sternal border, may also be obscured by pulmonary overinflation in emphysema. A systolic heave or thrill may be felt over the pulmonary area. A loud $P_2$ sound with a pulmonary systolic ejection click and, in some cases, harsh systolic and diastolic murmurs may be heard over the same area. As right-sided heart failure develops, a systolic murmur, which may be louder during inspiration (Carvallo's sign), becomes audible along the left sternal border. It may be associated with a palpable pulse in the (enlarged) liver, a systolic venous pulse in the neck, and, in many cases, peripheral edema and ascites. Although this systolic murmur has

been attributed to tricuspid regurgitation, catheterization studies in patients who have cor pulmonale suggest that it more likely denotes sudden reversal of flow from the right atrium to major veins as a result of the large pressure variation originating in a congested right atrium.[431] The right ventricular enlargement associated with chronic cor pulmonale has a secondary effect on left ventricular function by causing leftward deviation of the interventricular septum and impairment of diastolic filling.[433]

The ECG results may be normal, even in patients who have severe disease; for example, in one study of 40 patients who had pathologically proven cor pulmonale, only two thirds had ECG tracings typical of right ventricular hypertrophy.[432] The Expert Committee Report for the World Health Organization suggested the following criteria for right ventricular hypertrophy, indicating that at least two of these signs should be present: R/S less than one in $V_5$ and $V_6$; predominant S wave in lead I or incomplete right bundle branch block; P waves taller than 2 mm in lead II; right axis deviation greater than 110 degrees; and inversion of T waves in $V_1$ to $V_4$ or $V_2$ and $V_3$.[434] This last finding is of less diagnostic value.[425]

Because these criteria have low sensitivity, another formula for detection of right ventricular hypertrophy has been developed and tested for sensitivity and specificity in a group of 50 patients who had right ventricular hypertrophy secondary to mitral stenosis.[435] Three criteria were identified: (1) an increase in the anterior (A) and rightward (R) forces and a decrease in the posterolateral forces (criterion A + R − PL ≥ 0.7 mV); (2) an R wave less than or equal to 0.2 mV in lead I; and (3) a P wave less than 0.25 mV in leads II, III, aVF, $V_1$, or $V_2$. These were associated with a specificity of 94% and a sensitivity of 64% for the diagnosis of right ventricular hypertrophy. When the criteria were applied to a group of patients who had cor pulmonale secondary to COPD, the sensitivity was 89%.[436] It has also been suggested that recording right chest leads $V_1$ to $V_6R$ increases the sensitivity of detecting cor pulmonale in patients who have COPD and a hyperinflated thorax.[437]

As mentioned earlier, the term *cor pulmonale*, strictly speaking, is reserved for the presence of right ventricular hypertrophy secondary to pulmonary disease; however, it is increasingly being used to describe right heart failure secondary to pulmonary hypertension caused by pulmonary vascular obstruction. In fact the term *acute cor pulmonale* has been used to describe the syndrome of acute right ventricular pressure overload and failure, which occurs in a variety of clinical settings, including massive pulmonary embolism, severe asthma, episodes of primary lactic acidosis or (infrequently) during the course of ARDS.[438] The sequence of hemodynamic events that characterizes acute cor pulmonale is best appreciated using continuous wave and pulsed Doppler echocardiography. The echocardiogram shows evidence of acute right ventricular enlargement, which flattens and causes paradoxical motion of the interventricular septum and inhibits diastolic filling of the left ventricle. Because acute right ventricular dilation usually causes tricuspid regurgitation and because the peak velocity of the regurgitant jet is proportional to the pressure gradient between the right ventricle and the atrium, the acute rise in PA pressure can be estimated.[438]

# PULMONARY ARTERY ANEURYSMS

Aneurysms of the main and lobar branches of the PA are rare.[439-441] For example, in a review published in 1947, only 8 examples were found in 109,571 autopsies, an incidence of 1 in 13,696;[442] only 147 pathologically proven cases had been reported in the literature to that date. If tuberculosis-related aneurysms and microscopic mycotic aneurysms associated with septic emboli or pneumonia are excluded, aneurysms of the intrapulmonary branches of the PA are even less common. Additional exceptionally rare aneurysms are those that involve a pulmonary vein[443] or a feeding vessel to sequestered lung.[444]

## Etiology and Pathogenesis

The etiology and pathogenetic mechanisms are diverse (Table 50–3) and are discussed only briefly here; more detailed information can be found elsewhere in the book where specific diseases are discussed. In some cases, more than one pathogenetic factor is involved.

**Congenital Factors.** Congenital anomalies of the heart and great vessels are not infrequently associated with PA aneurysms, in which circumstance the pathogenesis can be difficult to establish precisely. In most cases, the aneurysm is related to stenosis of the pulmonary valve, right ventricular infundibulum, or a portion of the PA itself and represents poststenotic dilation caused by disturbed hemodynamics.[445, 446] However, the degree of stenosis in some cases appears to be insufficient to account for the aneurysm,[447] raising the possibility of a concomitant structural weakness of the vessel wall. In other cases—for example, in association with a patent ductus arteriosus—increased pulmonary blood flow and eventual arterial hypertension likely play an important role by causing distention in areas of focal vascular weakness. Although, a congenital structural abnormality of the arterial wall may be an important underlying cause of such weakness, histologic evidence of this has been reported rarely.[448]

**Genetic Factors.** Rarely, aneurysmal dilation occurs in association with a hereditary disease such as Marfan's syndrome[449] or hereditary hemorrhagic telangiectasia.[450] An abnormality of mural connective tissue leading to focal areas of structural weakness is likely the pathogenetic mechanism in such cases.

**Trauma.** Trauma to the chest wall or directly to a vessel (e.g., via an intravascular catheter or a surgical procedure) can result in pulmonary arterial damage and, occasionally, residual aneurysm formation;[451, 452] however, the walls of many of these lesions are probably formed by blood clot and they are in fact better described as pseudoaneurysms. Small aneurysms about 0.5 to 1.0 mm in diameter have been seen adjacent to thromboemboli, and it has been suggested that they might be caused by physical damage resulting from impact;[453] it is perhaps more likely that local ischemia of the arterial wall adjacent to a thromboembolus causes necrosis and subsequent aneurysmal dilation (*see* page 1785).[454, 455]

**Infection.** Infection is an important pathogenetic factor in many PA aneurysms. A variety of microorganisms can be responsible. In "developed" countries, syphilis[442] and tuberculosis (Rasmussen's aneurysm)[456] were relatively common causes until the middle of the 20th century;[439] with control of these diseases, pyogenic organisms such as *Staphylococcus aureus* and *Streptococcus* have become increasingly important.[457-459] Rarely, fungi such as *Aspergillus* or *Candida* are the cause.[460, 461]

Organisms can gain access to the arterial wall by three routes:

1. By direct continuity from a focus of pulmonary parenchymal infection. Aneurysms that develop this way occur most often in chronic fibrocaseous tuberculosis; rupture with hemorrhage is a relatively common cause of death in affected patients.[456]

2. Via the vasa vasorum derived from the bronchial arteries, a pathway that is probably the mechanism of aneurysm formation in syphilis.

3. By direct extension into a vessel wall from an intraluminal septic thromboembolus or the blood itself (i.e., in bacteremia). This is probably the most common mechanism of mycotic aneurysm formation in industrialized countries today. The source of thromboemboli is usually endocarditis, particularly of the tricuspid valve in drug abusers,[459] and of valvular, cardiac, or vascular endothelium in patients who have a variety of congenital anomalies.[457] Infectious thrombophlebitis and infected thrombi associated with intravenous catheters are occasional sources.

## Table 50–3. ETIOLOGY AND PATHOGENESIS OF PULMONARY ARTERY ANEURYSMS

| TYPE | CAUSES | SELECTED REFERENCES |
|---|---|---|
| Congenital | Deficiency of vessel wall | 458 |
| | Postvalvular or arterial stenosis | 445 |
| Degenerative/metabolic | Marfan's syndrome | 449 |
| | "Cystic medial necrosis" (dissecting aneurysm) | 50 |
| Traumatic | | 451, 453 |
| Infectious (mycotic) | Syphilis | 442 |
| | Tuberculosis | 456 |
| | Pyogenic bacterial | 457, 458, 475 |
| | Others (e.g., fungi) | 460 |
| Immunologic | Behçet's disease (?Hughes-Stovin syndrome) | 462 |
| | Polyarteritis nodosa (bronchial arteries) | |
| Secondary to pulmonary disease | Hypertension (including dissecting aneurysms) | 467, 468 |
| | Bronchiectasis | |
| Idiopathic | Hughes-Stovin syndrome | 469, 471 |

**Immunologic Factors.** Immunologically mediated vasculitis is uncommonly associated with PA aneurysm formation, most often in Behçet's disease.[462, 463] It has been suggested that many cases of Hughes-Stovin syndrome (see farther on) in fact represent Behçet's disease.[462] Isolated cases of aneurysm formation have also been reported in giant cell arteritis,[464] unclassified vasculitis,[465] and, occasionally, in the bronchial arteries in classic polyarteritis nodosa.

**Pulmonary Hypertension.** Pulmonary arterial hypertension secondary to cardiovascular or pulmonary disease is undoubtedly an important factor in the formation of many aneurysms.[441] The most common underlying condition is a left-to-right cardiovascular shunt, usually a patent ductus arteriosus or a ventricular septal defect; occasionally, pulmonary hypertension is primary. Rare cases have been associated with plexogenic arteriopathy.[466] Although dissecting aneurysms are a rare complication of pulmonary hypertension, they usually have this as an underlying cause.[467, 468]

**Idiopathic.** Hughes-Stovin syndrome is a rare disorder characterized by aneurysms of the large and small PAs and thrombosis of peripheral veins and dural sinuses.[469] It is possible that the syndrome has several pathogenetic mechanisms, some cases being associated with congenital cardiovascular defects and others representing a manifestation of Behçet's disease. An infectious basis for the aneurysms has not been substantiated by the discovery of organisms at autopsy.[470] Most affected patients are young men.[471] Pulmonary thromboembolism is a common complication.

### Pathologic Characteristics

Aneurysms may be solitary or multiple and usually range in size from several millimeters to 5 cm in diameter; enlargement to a huge size (16 × 9 × 8 cm) has been reported rarely.[472] Atherosclerosis, thrombosis, and "cystic medial necrosis" are evident in many of the larger lesions.[473, 474] Attenuation and fragmentation of elastic laminae are also not uncommon.[475] Inflammation of the vessel wall is seen uncommonly and should suggest the possibility of Behçet's disease or infectious (mycotic) aneurysm.

### Radiologic Manifestations

Radiographic findings include pulmonary nodules ranging from 2 to 8 cm in diameter or dense focal parenchymal consolidation[475–479] (Fig. 50–46). The nodules may have well- or poorly defined margins as a result of associated hemorrhage. Areas of consolidation may persist or may evolve into a nodule or mass.[478] The diagnosis may be confirmed using contrast-enhanced CT,[479–482] MR imaging,[482, 483] or angiography[478, 479, 482] (Fig. 50–47). CT may demonstrate a halo of ground-glass attenuation surrounding the aneurysm, again due to pulmonary hemorrhage.[484] In addition to being helpful in diagnosis, angiography is integral to treatment with embolotherapy using wire coils or detachable balloons.[485–488]

### Clinical Manifestations

In many patients, pulmonary signs and symptoms are absent or are overshadowed by underlying cardiac or pulmonary disease; in some, cough, dyspnea, and hemoptysis are present.[475] Rarely, the aneurysm projects into the bronchial lumen as an endobronchial mass.[488a] A more common manifestation of such extension is rupture with massive hemorrhage;[463, 475] in fact, it has been estimated that as many as 3% to 6% of patients who have massive hemoptysis have an underlying PA aneurysm.[439] It has been stressed that hemoptysis is an indicator of aneurysm "instability" and the need for prompt intervention.[439]

Physical examination may reveal a thrill or murmur over the aneurysm. Propagation of thrombus from an aneurysm in the main PA may lead to cor pulmonale.[489] Dis-

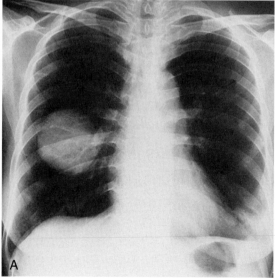
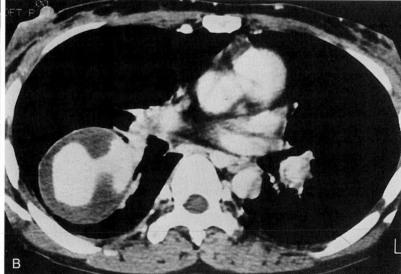

**Figure 50–46. Pulmonary Artery Aneurysm: Behçet's Disease.** A posteroanterior chest radiograph *(A)* in a 37-year-old woman who had Behçet's disease shows a round, well-defined mass in the right lower lobe and a localized area of consolidation in the left lower lobe. A contrast-enhanced CT scan *(B)* demonstrates a large aneurysm of the right pulmonary artery with enhancement of the patent lumen and a circumferential thrombus. The resected right lower lobe demonstrated aneurysmal dilation of the right pulmonary artery with perianeurysmal fibrosis and mural blood clots. (Courtesy of Dr. Jung Gi-Im, Seoul National University Hospital, Seoul, South Korea. From Ahn JM, Im JG, Ryoo JW, et al: Thoracic manifestations of Behçet syndrome: Radiographic and CT findings in nine patients. Radiology 194:199, 1995.)

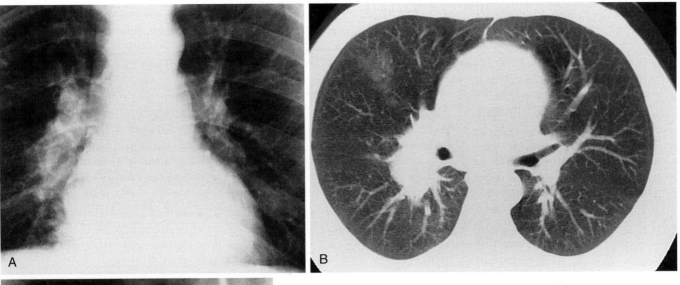

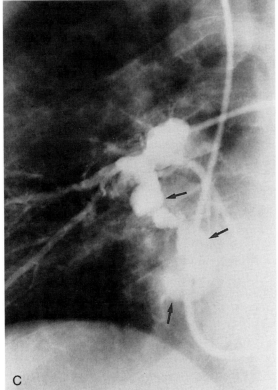

**Figure 50–47. Pulmonary Artery Aneurysm: Behçet's Disease.** A 28-year-old patient who had Behçet's disease presented with massive hemoptysis. A view from a posteroanterior chest radiograph *(A)* shows prominence of the inferior aspect of the right hilum. A CT scan *(B)* demonstrates focal enlargement of the right hilum and localized areas of ground-glass attenuation due to pulmonary hemorrhage in the right middle lobe. A selective right pulmonary angiogram *(C)* demonstrates irregular aneurysm formation involving the right interlobar, right lower lobe, and right posterior basal segmental pulmonary arteries *(arrows)*. The hemoptysis resolved following occlusion of the right interlobar pulmonary artery with coils. (Courtesy of Professor Martine Remy-Jardin, Universitaire de Lille, Lille, France.)

secting aneurysms may be manifested by precordial pain; proximal extension with intrapericardial hemorrhage and tamponade is a frequent cause of death.[467, 468, 473] In Hughes-Stovin syndrome, recurrent episodes of fever, lack of re- sponse to antibiotics, hemoptysis, and respiratory symptoms resulting from recurrent PA occlusions have been prominent clinical features;[470] a common terminal event is massive hemoptysis.

# REFERENCES

1. Cumming G: The structure of the pulmonary circulation. *In* Scadding G, Cumming G, Thurlbeck WM (eds): Scientific Foundations of Respiratory Medicine. London, Heinemann, 1981, p 71.
2. Horsfield K: Morphometry of the small pulmonary arteries in man. Circ Res 42:593, 1978.
3. Culver BH, Butler J: Mechanical influences on the pulmonary microcirculation. Annu Rev Physiol 42:187, 1980.
4. Fowler NO, Westcott RN, Scott RC: Normal pressure in the right heart and pulmonary artery. Am Heart J 46:264, 1953.
5. Sasamoto H, Hosono K, Katayama K, et al: Electrocardiographic findings in patients with chronic cor pulmonale. Respir Circ 9:55, 1961.
6. Shepherd JT, Wood EH: The role of vessel tone in pulmonary hypertension. Circulation 19:641, 1959.
7. Lupi-Herrera E, Bialostozky D, Sobrino A: The role of isoproterenol in pulmonary artery hypertension of unknown etiology (primary). Short- and long-term evaluation. Chest 79:293, 1981.
8. Richards DW: The J Burns Amberson Lecture: The right heart and lung: With some observations on teleology. Am Rev Respir Dis 94:691, 1966.
9. Harvey RM, Enson Y, Ferrer MI: A reconsideration of the origins of pulmonary hypertension. Chest 59:82, 1971.
10. Youssef HH, Edeen HE, Elgammal MY: Hypercapnic pulmonary hypertension. (A preliminary report.) Dis Chest 53:328, 1968.
11. Vogel JHK, Blount SG Jr: The role of hydrogen ion concentration in the regulation of pulmonary artery pressure. Observations in a patient with hypoventilation and obesity. Circulation 32:788, 1965.
12. Fritts HW Jr, Harris P, Clauss HH, et al: The effect of acetylcholine on the human pulmonary circulation under normal and hypoxic conditions. J Clin Invest 37:99, 1958.
13. Penazola D, Sime F: Chronic cor pulmonale due to loss of altitude acclimatization (chronic mountain sickness). Am J Med 50:728, 1971.
14. Rounds S, Hill NS: Pulmonary hypertensive diseases. Chest 85:397, 1984.
15. Harris P, Heath D: The Human Pulmonary Circulation: Its Form and Function in Health and Disease. Baltimore, Williams & Wilkins, 1962.
16. Stewart DJ: Endothelial dysfunction in pulmonary vascular disorders. Arzneimittelforschung 44:451, 1994.
17. Higenbottam T: Pathophysiology of pulmonary hypertension: A role for endothelial cell dysfunction. Chest. 105:7S, 1994.
18. Emery CJ: Vascular remodelling in the lung. Eur Respir J 7:217, 1994.
19. Christmas BW, McPherson CD, Newman JH, et al: An imbalance between the excretion of thromboxane and prostacyclin metabolites in pulmonary hypertension. N Engl J Med 327:70, 1992.
20. Stewart DJ, Levy RD, Cernacek P, et al: Increased plasma endothelin-1 in pulmonary hypertension: Marker or mediator of disease? Ann Intern Med 114:464, 1991.
21. Giaid A, Yanagisawa M, Langleben D, et al: Expression of endothelin-1 in the lungs of patients with pulmonary hypertension. N Engl J Med 328:1732, 1993.
22. Goerre S, Wenk M, Bartsch P, et al: Endothelin-1 in pulmonary hypertension associated with high-altitude exposure. Circulation 91:359, 1995.
23. Adnot S, Raffestin B, Eddahibi S: NO in the lung. Respir Physiol 101:109, 1995.
24. Moncada S, Palmer R, Higgs E: Nitric oxide: Physiology, pathophysiology and pharmacology. Pharmacol Rev 43:109, 1991.
25. Dinh-Xuan AT: Endothelial modulation of pulmonary vascular tone. Eur Respir J 5:757, 1992.
26. Brashers VL, Peach MJ, Rose CE: Augmentation of hypoxic pulmonary vasoconstriction in isolated perfused rat lung by in vitro antagonists of endothelium-dependent relaxation. J Clin Invest 82:1495, 1988.
27. Dinh-Xuan AT, Higenbottam TW, Clelland CA, et al: Impairment of endothelium-dependent pulmonary-artery relaxation in chronic obstructive lung disease. N Engl J Med 324:1539, 1991.
28. Higenbottam, CG: Acute and chronic hypoxic pulmonary hypertension. Eur Respir J 6:1207, 1993.
29. Giaid A, Saleh D: Reduced expression of endothelial nitric oxide synthase in the lungs of patients with pulmonary hypertension. N Engl J Med 333:214, 1995.
30. Zapol W, Rimer S, Gillis N, et al: Nitric oxide and the lung. Am J Respir Crit Care Med 149:1375, 1994.
31. Barst RJ, Rubin LJ, Long WA, et al: A comparison of continuous intravenous epoprostenol (prostacyclin) with conventional therapy for primary pulmonary hypertension. The primary pulmonary hypertension study group. N Engl J Med 334:296, 1996.
32. Pepke-Zaba J, Higenbottam TW, Dinh-Xuan AT, et al: Inhaled nitric oxide as a cause of selective vasodilatation in pulmonary hypertension. Lancet 338:1173, 1991.
33. Sitbon O, Brenot F, Denjean A, et al: Inhaled nitric oxide as a screening vasodilator agent in primary pulmonary hypertension. A dose-response study and comparison with prostacyclin. Am J Respir Crit Care Med 151:384, 1995.
34. Soifer SJ: Pulmonary hypertension: Physiologic or pathologic disorder? Crit Care Med 21:S370, 1993.
35. Ziegler JW, Ivy DD, Kinsella JP, et al: The role of nitric oxide, endothelin, and prostaglandins in the transition of the pulmonary circulation. Clin Perinatol 22:387, 1995.
36. Kumar P, Kazzi NJ, Shankaran S: Plasma immunoreactive enothelin-1 concentra-
37. Romand JA, Donald FA, Suter PM: Cardiopulmonary interactions in acute lung injury: Clinical and prognostid importance of pulmonary hypertension. New Horiz 2:457, 1994.
38. Sibbald WJ, Paterson NAM, Holliday RL, et al: Pulmonary hypertension in sepsis. Measurement by pulmonary arterial diastolic-pulmonary wedge pressure gradient and the influence of passive and active factors. Chest 73:583, 1978.
39. Begley CJ, Ogletree ML, Meyrick BO, et al: Modification of pulmonary responses to endtoxemia in awake sheep by steroidal and nonsteroidal anti-inflammatory agents. Am Rev Respir Dis 130:1140, 1984.
40. Spapen H, Vincken W: Pulmonary arterial hypertension in sepsis and the adult respiratory distress syndrome. Acta Clin Belg 47:30, 1992.
41. Fox GA, McCormack DG: A new look at the pulmonary circulation in acute lung injury. Thorax 47:743, 1992.
42. Meyrick B: Structure function correlates in the pulmonary vasculature during acute lung injury and chronic pulmonary hypertension. Toxicol Pathol 19:447, 1991.
43. Wagenvoort CA, Wagenvoort N: Pathology of Pulmonary Hypertension. New York, John Wiley & Sons, 1977.
44. Collins-Nakai RL, Rabinovitch M: Pulmonary vascular obstructive disease. Cardiol Clin 11:675, 1993.
45. Wagenvoort CA: Plexogenic arteriopathy. Thorax 49:S39, 1994.
46. Pietra GG: The pathology of primary pulmonary hypertension. *In* Rubin LJ, Rich S (eds): Primary Pulmonary Hypertension. Vol. 99 of Lenfant C (executive ed): Lung Biology in Health and Disease. New York, Marcel Dekker, 1997.
47. Burke AP, Farb A, Virmani R: The pathology of primary pulmonary hypertension. Mod Pathol 4:269, 1991.
48. Pietra GG, Edwards WD, Kay JM, et al: Histopathology of primary pulmonary hypertension. A qualitative and quantitative study of pulmonary blood vessels from 58 patients in the National Heart, Lung, and Blood Institute, Primary Pulmonary Hypertension Registry. Circulation 80:1198, 1989.
49. Heath D, DuShane JW, Wood EH, et al: The structure of the pulmonary trunk at different ages and in cases of pulmonary hypertension and pulmonary stenosis. J Pathol Bacteriol 77:443, 1959.
50. Shilkin KB, Low LP, Chen BTM: Dissecting aneurysm of the pulmonary artery. J Pathol 98:25, 1969.
51. Moore GW, Smith RRL, Hutchins GM: Pulmonary artery atherosclerosis. Correlation with systemic atherosclerosis and hypertensive pulmonary vascular disease. Arch Pathol Lab Med 106:378, 1982.
52. Botney MD, Kaiser LR, Cooper JD, et al: Extracellular matrix protein gene expression in atherosclerotic hypertensive pulmonary arteries. Am J Pathol 140:357, 1992.
53. Yamataka T, Puri P: Pulmonary artery structural changes in pulmonary hypertension complicating congenital diaphragmatic hernia. J Pediatr Surg 32:387, 1997.
54. Chazova I, Loyd JE, Zhdanov VS, et al: Pulmonary artery adventitial changes and venous involvement in primary pulmonary hypertension. Am J Pathol 146:389, 1995.
55. Wagenvoort CA, Wagenvoort M: Smooth muscle content of pulmonary arterial media in pulmonary venous hypertension compared with other forms of pulmonary hypertension. Chest 81:581, 1982.
56. Hall SM, Haworth SG: Onset and evolution of pulmonary vascular disease in young children: Abnormal postnatal remodeling studied in lung biopsies. J Pathol 166:183, 1992.
57. Yamaki S, Wagenvoort CA: Plexogenic pulmonary arteriopathy: Significance of medial thickness with respect to advanced pulmonary vascular lesions. Am J Pathol 105:70, 1981.
58. Wagenvoort CA, Nauta J, Van der Schaar PJ, et al: Effect of flow and pressure on pulmonary vessels. A semiquantitative study based on lung biopsies. Circulation 35:1028, 1967.
59. Rabinovitch M, Haworth S, Nadas A, et al. Lung biopsy in congenital heart disease: A morhpometric approach to pulmonary vascular disease. Circulation 58:1107, 1978.
60. Rabinovitch M, Haworth SG, Vance Z, et al: Early pulmonary vascular changes in congenital heart disease studied in biopsy tissue. Hum Pathol 11(Suppl):449, 1980.
61. Heath D, Williams D, Rios-Dalenz J, et al: Small pulmonary arterial vessels of Aymara Indians from the Bolivian Andes. Histopathology 16:565, 1990.
62. Meyrick B, Reid L: Ultrastructural findings in lung biopsy material from children with congenital heart defects. Am J Pathol 101:527, 1980.
63. Heath D, Smith P, Gosney J: Ultrastructure of early plexogenic pulmonary arteriopathy. Histopathology 12:41, 1988.
64. Smith P, Heath D, Yacoub M, et al: The ultrastructure of plexogenic pulmonary arteriopathy. J Pathol 160:111, 1990.
65. Jones PL, Cowan KN, Rabinovitch M: Tenascin-C, proliferation and subendothelial fibronectin in progressive pulmonary vascular disease. Am J Pathol 150:1349, 1997.
66. Yaginuma G, Mohri H, Takahashi T: Distribution of arterial lesions and collateral pathways in the pulmonary hypertension of congenital heart disease: A computer aided reconstruction study. Thorax 45:586, 1990.
67. Wagenvoort CA: Open lung biopsies in congenital heart disease for evaluation

of pulmonary vascular disease. Predictive value with regard to corrective operability. Histopathology 9:417, 1985.

68. Palevsky HI, Schloo BL, Pietra GG, et al: Primary pulmonary hypertension. Vascular structure, morphometry, and responsiveness to vasodilator agents. Circulation 80:1207, 1989.

69. Yaginuma G, Mohri H, Takahashi T: Distribution of arterial lesions and collateral pathways in the pulmonary hypertension of congenital heart disease: A computer aided reconstruction study. Thorax 45:586, 1990.

70. Jamison BM, Michel RP: Different distribution of plexiform lesions in primary and secondary pulmonary hypertension. Hum Pathol 26:987, 1995.

71. Heath D, Yacoub M, Gosney JR, et al: Pulmonary endocrine cells in hypertensive pulmonary vascular disease. Histopathology 16:21, 1990.

72. Heath D, Smith P: Nodules resembling arachnoid villi in pulmonary venules in plexogenic pulmonary arteriopathy. Cardioscience 3:161, 1992.

73. Health D, Edwards JE: The pathology of hypertensive pulmonary vascular disease: A description of six grades of structural changes in the pulmonary artery with special reference to congenital cardiac septal defect. Circulation 18:533, 1958.

74. Ishii M, Kato H, Kawano T, et al: Evaluation of pulmonary artery histopathologic findings in congenital heart disease: An in vitro study using intravascular ultrasound imaging. J Am Coll Cardiol 26:272, 1995.

75. Kravitz KD, Scharf GR, Chandrasekaran K: In vivo diagnosis of pulmonary atherosclerosis. Role of intravascular ultrasound. Chest 106:632, 1994.

76. Rabinovitch M, Bothwell T, Hayakawa BN, et al: Pulmonary artery endothelial abnormalities in patients with congenital heart defects and pulmonary hypertension: A correlation of light with scanning electron microscopy and transmission electron microscopy. Lab Invest 55:632, 1986.

77. Chen JTT, Capp MP, Johnsrude IS, et al: Roentgen appearance of pulmonary vascularity in the diagnosis of heart disease. Am J Roentgenol 112:559, 1971.

78. Ravin CE: Pulmonary vascularity: Radiographic considerations. J Thorac Imaging 3:1, 1988.

79. Randall PA, Heitzman ER, Bull MJ, et al: Pulmonary hypertension: A contemporary review. Radiographics 9:905, 1989.

80. Mallamo JT, Baum RS, Simon AL: Diffuse pulmonary artery calcifications in a case of Eisenmenger's syndrome. Radiology 99:549, 1971.

81. Gutierrez FR, Moran CJ, Ludbrook PA, et al: Pulmonary arterial calcification with reversible pulmonary hypertension. Am J Roentgenol 135:177, 1980.

82. Chang CH: The normal roentgenographic measurement of the right descending pulmonary artery in 1,085 cases. Am J Roentgenol 87:929, 1962.

83. Jacobson G, Turner AF, Balchum OJ, et al: Vascular changes in pulmonary emphysema: The radiologic evaluation by selective and peripheral pulmonary wedge angiography. Am J Roentgenol 100:374, 1967.

84. Viamonte M Jr, Parks RE, Barrera F: Roentgenographic prediction of pulmonary hypertension in mitral stenosis. Am J Roentgenol 87:936, 1962.

85. Milne ENC: Physiological interpretation of the plain radiograph in mitral stenosis, including a review of criteria for the radiological estimation of pulmonary arterial and venous pressures. Br J Radiol 36:902, 1963.

86. Turner AF, Lau FYK, Jacobson G: A method for the estimation of pulmonary venous and arterial pressures from the routine chest roentgenogram. Am J Roentgenol 116:97, 1972.

87. Anderson G, Reid L, Simon G: The radiographic appearances in primary and in thromboembolic pulmonary hypertension. Clin Radiol 24:113, 1973.

88. Matthay RA, Schwarz MI, Ellis JH Jr, et al: Pulmonary artery hypertension in chronic obstructive pulmonary disease: Determination by chest radiography. Invest Radiol 16:95, 1981.

89. Woodruff WW III, Hoeck BE, Chitwood WR Jr, et al: Radiographic findings in pulmonary hypertension from unresolved embolism. Am J Roentgenol 144:681, 1985.

90. Rich S, Dantzker DR, Ayres SM, et al: Primary pulmonary hypertension: A national prospective study. Ann Intern Med 107:216, 1987.

91. Chan T, Palevsky HI, Miller WT: Pulmonary hypertension complicating portal hypertension: Findings on chest radiographs. Am J Roentgenol 151:909, 1988.

92. Ormond RS, Drake EH, Hildner FJ: Pulmonary hypertension: An angiographic study. Radiology 88:680, 1967.

93. Kuriyama K, Gamsu G, Stern RG, et al: CT-determined pulmonary artery diameters in predicting pulmonary hypertension. Invest Radiol 19:16, 1984.

94. Moore NR, Scott JP, Flower CDR, et al: The relationship between pulmonary artery pressure and pulmonary artery diameter in pulmonary hypertension. Clin Radiol 39:486, 1988.

95. Haimovici JBA, Trotman-Dickenson B, Halpern EF, et al: Relationship between pulmonary artery diameter at computed tomography and pulmonary artery pressures at right-sided heart catheterization. Acad Radiol 4:327, 1997.

95a. Tan RT, Kuzo R, Goodman LR, et al: Utility of CT scan evaluation for predicting pulmonary hypertension in patients with parenchymal lung disease. Chest 113:1250, 1998.

96. Tramarin R, Torbicki A, Marchandise B, et al: Doppler echocardiographic evaluation of pulmonary artery pressure in chronic obstructive pulmonary disease. A European multicentre study. Working Group on Noninvasive Evaluation of Pulmonary Artery Pressure. Eur Heart J 12:103, 1991.

97. Burghuber OC, Brunner CH, Schenk P, et al: Pulsed Doppler echocardiography to assess pulmonary artery hypertension in chronic obstructive pulmonary disease. Monaldi Arch Chest Dis 48:121, 1993.

98. Brecker SJ, Xiao HB, Stojnic BB, et al: Assessment of the peak tricuspid regurgitant velocity from the dynamics of retrograde flow. Int J Cardiol 34:267, 1992.

99. Torres F, Tye T, Gibbons R, et al: Echocardiographic contrast increases the yield for right ventricular pressure measurement by Doppler echocardiography. J Am Soc Echocardiogr 2:419, 1989.

100. Lei MH, Chen JJ, Ko YL, et al: Reappraisal of quantitative evaluations of pulmonary regurgitation and estimation of pulmonary artery pressure by continuous wave Doppler echocardiography. Cardiology 86:249, 1995.

101. Chotivittayatarakorn P, Pathmanand C, Thisyakorn C, et al: Doppler echocardiographic predictions of pulmonary artery pressure in children with congenital heart disease. J Med Assoc Thailand 75:79, 1992.

101a. Trivedi HS, Joshi MN, Gamade AR: Echocardiography and pulmonary artery pressure: correlation in chronic obstructive pulmonary disease. J Postgrad Med 38:24, 1992.

102. Bach DS: Stress echocardiography for evaluation of hemodynamics: Valvular heart disease, prosthetic valve function, and pulmonary hypertension. Prog Cardiovasc Dis 39:543, 1997.

103. Brecker SJ, Gibbs JS, Fox KM, et al: Comparison of Doppler derived haemodynamic variables and simultaneous high fidelity pressure measurements in severe pulmonary hypertension. Br Heart J 71:384, 1994.

104. Chen WJ, Chen JJ, Lin SC, et al: Detection of cardiovascular shunts by transesophogeal echocardiography in patients with pulmonary hypertension of unexplained cause. Chest 107:8, 1995.

105. Gorcsan J, Edwards TD, Ziady GM, et al: Transesophageal echocardiography to evaluate patients with severe pulmonary hypertension for lung transplantation. Ann Thoracic Surg 59:717, 1995.

106. Frank H, Globits S, Glogar D, et al: Detection and quantification of pulmonary artery hypertension with MR imaging: Results in 23 patients. Am J Roentgenol 161:27, 1993.

107. Boxt LM: MR imaging of pulmonary hypertension and right ventricular dysfunction. MRI Clin North Am 4:307, 1996.

108. Rebergen SA, Niezen RA, Helbing WA, et al: Cine gradient-echo MR imaging and MR velocity mapping in the evaluation of congenital heart disease. Radiographics 16:467, 1996.

109. Tardivon AA, Mousseaux E, Brenot F, et al: Quantification of hemodynamics in primary pulmonary hypertension with magnetic resonance imaging. Am J Respir Crit Care Med 150:1075, 1994.

110. Kondo C, Caputo GR, Masui T, et al: Pulmonary hypertension: Pulmonary flow quantification and flow profile analysis with velocity-encoded cine MR imaging. Radiology 183:751, 1992.

111. Wacker CM, Schad LR, Gehling U, et al: The pulmonary artery acceleration time determined with the MR-RACE-technique: Comparison to pulmonary artery mean pressure in 12 patients. Magn Reson Imaging 12:25, 1994.

112. Murray TI, Boxt LM, Katz J, et al: Estimation of pulmonary artery pressure in patients with primary pulmonary hypertension by quantitative analysis of magnetic resonance images. J Thorac Imaging 9:198, 1994.

113. Boxt LM, Katz J, Kolb T, et al: Direct quantitation of right and left ventricular volumes with nuclear magnetic resonance imaging in patients with primary pulmonary hypertension. J Am Coll Cardiol 19:1508, 1992.

114. Boxt LM, Katz J: Magnetic resonance imaging for quantitation of right ventricular volume in patients with pulmonary hypertension. J Thorac Imaging 8:92, 1993.

115. Stern EJ, Graham C, Gamsu G, et al: Pulmonary artery dissection: MR findings. J Comput Assist Tomogr 16:481, 1992.

116. Worsley DF, Palevsky HI, Alavi A: Ventilation-perfusion lung scanning in the evaluation of pulmonary hypertension. J Nucl Med 35:793, 1994.

117. Falaschi F, Palla A, Formichi B, et al: CT evaluation of chronic thromboembolic pulmonary hypertension. J Comput Assist Tomogr 16:897, 1992.

118. Schwickert HC, Schweden F, Schild HH, et al: Pulmonary arteries and lung parenchyma in chronic pulmonary embolism: Preoperative and postoperative CT findings. Radiology 191:351, 1994.

119. Tardivon AA, Musset D, Maitre S, et al: Role of CT in chronic pulmonary embolism: Comparison with pulmonary angiography. J Comput Assist Tomogr 17:345, 1993.

120. Bergin CJ, Sirlin CB, Hauschildt JP, et al: Chronic thromboembolism: Diagnosis with helical CT and MR imaging with angiographic and surgical correlation. Radiology 204:695, 1997.

121. Williams JO: Death following injection of lung scanning agent in a case of pulmonary hypertension. Br J Radiol 47:61, 1974.

122. Child JS, Wolfe JD, Tashkin D, et al: Fatal lung scan in a case of pulmonary hypertension due to obliterative pulmonary vascular disease. Chest 67:308, 1975.

123. Rich S, Dantzker DR, Ayres SM, et al: Primary pulmonary hypertension: A national prospective study. Ann Intern Med 107:216, 1987.

124. Caldini P, Gensini GG, Hoffman MS: Primary pulmonary hypertension with death during right heart catheterization: A case report and a survey of reported fatalities. Am J Cardiol 4:519, 1959.

125. Nicod P, Peterson K, Levine M, et al: Pulmonary angiography in severe chronic pulmonary hypertension. Ann Intern Med 107:565, 1987.

126. Cachecho R, Isik FF, Hirsch EF: Pathologic consequences of bilateral pulmonary lower lobectomies: Case report. J Trauma 32:268, 1992.

127. Komai H, Naito Y, Fujiwara K, et al: An unusual variation of left ventricular-right atrial communication. Surg Today 26:825, 1996.

128. Wheatley D, Coleman EN, Reid JM: Coronary artery fistula: Report of three cases. Thorax 30:535, 1975.

129. Breuer J, Georgaraki A, Sieverding L, et al: Increased turnover of serotonin in children with pulmonary hypertension seconday to congenital heart disease. Pediatr Cardiol 17:214, 1996.

130. Fuse S, Kamiya T: Plasma thromboxane $B_2$ concentration in pulmonary hypertension associated with congenital heart disease. Circulation 90:2952, 1994.

131. Hopkins WE: Severe pulmonary hypertension in congential heart disease: A review of Eisenmenger syndrome. Curr Opin Cardiol 10:517, 1995.

132. Wood P: The Eisenmenger syndrome or pulmonary hypertension with reversed central shunt. BMJ 2:701, 755, 1958.

133. Perloff JK: The Clinical Recognition of Congenital Heart Disease. 4th ed. Philadelphia, WB Saunders, 1994.

134. Heath D, DuShane JW, Wood EH, et al: The structure of the pulmonary trunk at different ages and in cases of pulmonary hypertension and pulmonary stenosis. J Pathol Bacteriol 77:443, 1959.

135. Rabinovitch M, Bothwell BT, Hayakawa BN, et al: Pulmonary arterial endothelial abnormalities in patients with congenital heart defects and pulmonary hypertension: A correlation of light with scanning electron microscopy and transmssion electron microscopy. Lab Invest 55:632, 1986.

136. Collins-Nakai RI, Rabinovitch M: Pulmonary vascular obstructive disease. Cardiol Clin 11:675, 1993.

137. Ormond RS, Poznanski AK, Templeton AW: Pulmonary veins in congenital heart disease in the adult. Radiology 76:885, 1961.

138. Milne ENC: Some new concepts of pulmonary blood flow and volume. Radiol Clin North Am 16:515, 1978.

139. Baltaxe HA, Amplatz K: The normal chest roentgenogram in the presence of large atrial septal defects. Am J Roentgenol 107:322, 1969.

140. Rees RSO, Jefferson KE: The Eisenmenger syndrome. Clin Radiol 18:366, 1967.

141. Rees S: The chest radiograph in pulmonary hypertension with central shunt. Br J Radiol 41:172, 1968.

142. Doyle AE, Goodwin JF, Harrison CV, et al: Pulmonary vascular patterns in pulmonary hypertension. Br Heart J 19:353, 1957.

143. Brenner LD, Caputo GR, Mostbeck GH, et al: Quantification of left-to-right atrial shunts with velocity-encoded cine nuclear magnetic resonance imaging. J Am Coll Cardiol 20:1246, 1992.

144. Wexler L, Higgins CB, Herfkens RJ: Magnetic resonance imaging in adult congenital heart disease. J Thorac Imaging 9:219, 1994.

145. Rebergen SA, Niezen RA, Helbing WA, et al: Cine gradient-echo MR imaging and MR velocity mapping in the evaluation of congenital heart disease. Radiographics 16:467, 1996.

146. Friedman PJ: Direct magnification angiography and correlative pathophysiology in experimental pulmonary hypertension. Invest Radiol 7:474, 1972.

147. Hopkins WE, Ochoa LL, Richardson GW, et al: Comparison of the hemodynamics and survival of adults with severe primary pulmonary hypertension or Eisenmenger syndrome. J Heart Lung Transplant 15:100, 1996.

148. Dresdale DT, Schultz M, Michtom RJ: Primary pulmonary hypertension I. Clinical and haemodynamic study. Am J Med 11:686, 1951.

149. Fishman AP, Pietra GG: Primary pulmonary hypertension. Annu Rev Med 31:421, 1980.

150. Hughes JD, Rubin LJ: Primary pulmonary hypertension: An analysis of 28 cases and a review of the literature. Medicine 65:56, 1986.

151. D'Alonzo GE, Dantzker DR: Diagnosing primary pulmonary hypertension. *In* Rubin LJ, Rich S (eds): Primary Pulmonary Hypertension. Vol. 99 of Lenfant C (executive ed): Lung Biology in Health and Disease. New York, Marcel Dekker, 1997.

152. Rubin LJ, Rich S (eds): Primary Pulmonary Hypertension. Vol. 99 of Lenfant C (executive ed): Lung Biology in Health and Disease. New York, Marcel Dekker, 1997.

153. Langleben D: Familial primary pulmonary hypertension. Chest 105(Suppl):13S, 1995.

154. Kodama K, Hamada M, Shigematsu Y, et al: Familial primary pulmonary hypertension. Jpn J Med 30:273, 1991.

155. Morse JH, Barst RJ, Fotino M: Familial pulmonary hypertension: Immunogenetic findings in four Caucasian kindreds. Am Rev Respir Dis 145:787, 1992.

156. Loyd JE, Newman JH: Familial primary pulmonary hypertension. *In* Rubin LJ, Rich S (eds): Primary Pulmonary Hypertension. Vol. 99 of Lenfant C (executive ed): Lung Biology in Health and Disease. New York, Marcel Dekker, 1997.

157. Porter CM, Creech BJ, Billings FT Jr: Primary pulmonary hypertension occurring in twins. Arch Intern Med 120:224, 1967.

158. Melmon KL, Braunwald E: Familial pulmonary hypertension. N Engl J Med 269:770, 1963.

159. Elliott G, Alexander G, Leppert M, et al: Coancestry in apparently sporadic primary pulmonary hypertension. Chest 108:973, 1995.

160. Squarcia U, Carano N, Agnetti A, et al: Primary pulmonary hypertension in childhood: Familial aspects. Pediatr Med Chir 3:467, 1981.

161. Loyd JE, Primm RK, Newman JH: Familial primary pulmonary hypertension—clinical patterns. Am Rev Respir Dis 129:194, 1984.

162. Thompson P, McRae C: Familial pulmonary hypertension: Evidence of autosomal dominant inheritance. Br Heart J 32:758, 1970.

163. Nichols WC, Koller DL, Slovis B, et al: Localization of the gene for familial primary pulmonary hypertension to chromosome 2Q 31–31. Nat Genet 15:277, 1997.

164. Morse JH, Jones AC, Barst RJ, et al: Mapping of familial primary pulmonary hypertension locus (PPH1) to chromosome 2q31–q32. Circulation 95:2603, 1997.

165. Loyd JE, Butler MG, Foroud TM, et al: Genetic anticipation and abnormal gender ratio at birth in familial primary pulmonary hypertension. Am J Respir Crit Care Med 152:93, 1995.

166. Morse JH, Barst RJ, Fotino M: Familial pulmonary hypertension: Immunogenetic findings in four Caucasian kindreds. Am Rev Respir Dis 145:787, 1992.

167. Rich S, Hart K: Familial pulmonary hypertension in association with an abnormal hemoglobin. Insights into the pathogenesis of primary pulmonary hypertension. Chest 99:1208, 1991.

168. Wille RT, Krishnan K, Cooney KA, et al: Familial association of primary pulmonary hypertension and a new low-affinity beta-chain hemoglobinopathy, Hb Washtenaw. Chest 109:848, 1996.

169. Aessopos A, Stamatelos G, Skoumas V, et al: Pulmonary hypertension and right heart failure in patients with beta-thalassemia intermedia. Chest 107:50, 1995.

170. Ribeiro PA, Muthusamy R, Duran CM: Right-sided endomyocardial fibrosis with recurrent pulmonary emboli leading to irreversible pulmonary hypertension. Br Heart J 68:326, 1992.

171. Inglesby TV, Singer JW, Gordon DS: Abnormal fibrinolysis in familial pulmonary hypertension. Am J Med 55:5, 1973.

172. Okamura T, Tsuda Y, Murakawa M, et al: A patient with congenital plasminogen deficiency manifesting primary pulmonary hypertension. Intern Med 32:332, 1993.

173. Berliner S, Schoenfeld Y, Dean H, et al: Primary pulmonary hypertension: A facet of a diffuse angiopathic process? Respiration 43:76, 1982.

174. Perez HD, Kramer N: Pulmonary hypertension in systemic lupus erythematosus: Report of four cases and review of the literature. Semin Arthritis Rheum 11:117, 1981.

175. Salerni R, Rodman GP, Leon DF, et al: Pulmonary hypertension in the CREST syndrome variant of progressive systemic sclerosis. Ann Intern Med 86:394, 1977.

176. Blount SG Jr, Vogel JHK: Pulmonary hypertension. Mod Concepts Cardiovasc Dis 36:61, 1987.

177. Gurtner HP: Pulmonary hypertension "plexigenic pulmonary arteriopathy," antiappetite depressant drug Aminorex: Post or propter. Bull Eur Physiopathol Respir 15:897, 1979.

178. Chaouat A, Weitzenblum E, Higenbottam T: The role of thrombosis in severe pulmonary hypertension. Eur Respir J 9:356, 1996.

179. Frank H, Mlczoch J, Huber K, et al: The effect of anticoagulant therapy in primary and anorectic drug-induced pulmonary hypertension. Chest 112:714, 1997.

180. Walcott G, Burchell HB, Brown AL Jr: Primary pulmonary hypertension. Am J Med 49:70, 1970.

181. Goodman J, Harrison DC, Popp RL: Echocardiographic features of primary pulmonary hypertension. Am J Cardiol 33:438, 1974.

182. Martin-Duran R, Larman M, Trugeda A, et al: Comparison of Doppler-determined elevated pulmonary arterial pressure with pressure measured at cardiac catheterization. Am J Cardiol 57:859, 1986.

183. Selby CL: Living with primary pulmonary hypetension. *In* Rubin LJ, Rich S (eds): Primary Pulmonary Hypertension. Vol. 99 in Lenfant C (executive ed): Lung Biology in Health and Disease. New York, Marcel Dekker, 1997, pp 319–325.

184. Gupta BD, Moodie DS, Hodgman JR: Primary pulmonary hypertension in adults. Cleve Clin Q 47:275, 1980.

185. Yu N: Primary pulmonary hypertension: Report of six cases and review of literature. Ann Intern Med 49:1138, 1958.

186. Sleeper JC, Orgain ES, McIntosh HD: Primary pulmonary hypertension. Review of clinical features and pathologic physiology with a report of pulmonary hemodynamics derived from repeated catheterization. Circulation 26:1358, 1962.

187. Williams MH Jr, Adler JJ, Colp C: Pulmonary function studies as an aid in the differential diagnosis of pulmonary hypertension. Am J Med 47:378, 1969.

188. Scharf SM, Feldman NT, Graboys TB, et al: Restrictive ventilatory defect in a patient with primary pulmonary hypertension. Am Rev Respir Dis 118:409, 1978.

189. Horn M, Ries A, Neview C, et al: Restrictive ventilatory pattern in precapillary pulmonary hypertension. Am Rev Respir Dis 128:163, 1983.

190. Romano AM, Tomaselli S, Gualtieri G, et al: Respiratory function in precapillary pulmonary hypertension. Monaldi Arch Chest Dis 48:201, 1993.

191. Dantzker DR, Bower JS: Mechanisms of gas exchange abnormality in patients with chronic obliterative pulmonary vascular disease. J Clin Invest 64:1050, 1979.

192. Dantzker DR, D'Alonzo GE, Bower JS, et al: Pulmonary gas exchange during exercise in patients with chronic obliterative pulmonary hypertension. Am Rev Respir Dis 130:412, 1984.

193. Sandoval J, Bauerle O, Palomar A, et al: Survival in primary pulmonary hypertension. Validation of a prognostic equation. Circulation 89:1733, 1994.

194. Rich S, Levy PS: Characteristics of surviving and non-surviving patients with primary pulmonary hypertension. Am J Med 76:573, 1984.

195. Rajasekhar D, Balakrishnan KG, Venkitachalam CG, et al: Primary pulmonary hypertension: Natural history and prognostic factors. Indian Heart J 46:165, 1994.

196. Raffy O, Azarian R, Brenot F, et al: Clinical significance of the pulmonary vasodilator response during short-term infusion of prostacyclin in primary pulmonary hypertension. Circulation 93:484, 1996.

197. Kilbourne EM, Posada de la Paz M, Borda IA, et al: Toxic oil syndrome: A current clinical and epidemiologic summary, including comparisons with eosinophilia-myalgia syndrome. J Am Coll Cardiol 18:711, 1991.

198. Yakovlevitch M, Siegel M, Hoch DH, et al: Pulmonary hypertension in a patient with tryptophan-induced eosionphilia-myalgia syndrome. Am J Med 90:272, 1991.

199. Kay JM: Dietary pulmonary hypertension. Thorax 49(Suppl):S33, 1994.

200. Kay JM, Heath D, Smith P, et al: Fulvine and the pulmonary circulation. Thorax 26:249, 1971.

201. Kay JM, Smith P, Heath D: Electron microscopy of *Crotalaria* pulmonary hypertension. Thorax 24:511, 1969.

202. Wagenvoort CA, Wagenvoort N, Dijk HJ: Effect of fulvine on pulmonary arteries and veins of the rat. Thorax 29:522, 1974.
203. Heath D, Shaba J, Williams A, et al: A pulmonary hypertension-producing plant from Tanzania. Thorax 30:399, 1975.
204. Gurtner HP, Gertsch M, Salzmann C, et al: Häufen sich die primär vaskulären formen des chronischen cor pulmonale? Schweiz Med Wochenschr 98:1579, 1968.
205. Follath F, Burkart F, Schweizer W: Drug-induced pulmonary hypertension? BMJ 1:265, 1971.
206. Kay JM, Smith P, Heath D: Aminorex and the pulmonary circulation. Thorax 26:262, 1971.
207. Douglas JG, Munro JF, Kitchin AH, et al: Pulmonary hypertension and fenfluramine. BMJ 283:881, 1981.
208. McMurray J, Bloomfield P, Miller HC: Irreversible pulmonary hypertension after treatment with fenfluramine. BMJ 293:51, 1986.
209. Brenot F, Herve P, Petitpretz P, et al: Primary pulmonary hypertension and fenfluramine use. Br Heart J 70:537, 1993.
210. Thomas SH, Butt AY, Corris PA, et al: Appetite suppressants and primary pulmonary hypertension in the United Kingdom. Br Heart J 74:660, 1995.
211. Abenhaim L, Moride Y, Brenot F, et al: Appetite-suppressant drugs and the risk of primary pulmonary hypertension. N Engl J Med 335:609, 1996.
212. Herve P, Launay JM, Scrobohaci ML, et al: Increased plasma serotonin in primary pulmonary hypertension. Am J Med 99:249, 1995.
213. Weir EK, Reeve HL, Huang JM, et al: Anorexic agents aminorex, fenfluramine, and dexfenfluramine inhibit potassium current in rat pulmonary vascular smooth muscle and cause pulmonary vasoconstriction. Circulation 94:2216, 1996.
214. Connolly HM, Crary JL, McGoon MD, et al: Valvular heart disease associated with fenflurmamine-phentermine. N Engl J Med 337:581, 1997.
215. Pellikka PA, Tajik AJ, Khandheria BK, et al: Carcinoid heart disease: Clinical and echocardiographic spectrum in 74 patients. Circulation 87:1188, 1993.
216. Albertson TE, Walby WF, Derlet RW: Stimulant-induced pulmonary toxicity. Chest 108:1140, 1995.
217. Schaiberger PH, Dennedy TC, Miller FC, et al: Pulmonary hypertension associated with long-term inhalation of "crank" methamphetamine. Chest 104:614, 1993.
218. Fahlen M, Bergman H, Helder G, et al: Phenformin and pulmonary hypertension. Br Heart J 35:824, 1973.
219. Latif M, Weil M: Circulatory defects during phenformin lactic acidosis. Intensive Care Med 5:135, 1979.
220. Lebrec D, Capron JP, Dhumeaux D, et al: Pulmonary hypertension complicating portal hypertension. Am Rev Respir Dis 120:849, 1979.
221. Yoshida EM, Erb SR, Ostrow DN, et al: Pulmonary hypertension associated with primary biliary cirrhosis in the absence of portal hypertension: A case report. Gut 35:280, 1994.
222. Woolf D, Voigt MD, Jaskiewicz K, et al: Pulmonary hypertension associated with non-cirrhotic portal hypertension in systemic lupus erythematosus. Postgrad Med J 70:41, 1994.
223. van der Heijde RM, Lameris JS, van den Berg B, et al: Pulmonary hypertension after transjugular intrahepatic portosystemic shunt (TIPS). Eur Respir J 9:1562, 1996.
224. Shah HA, Piris J, Finlayson ND: Primary pulmonary hypertension developing 11 years after a splenorenal shunt for portal hypertension in hepatic cirrhosis. Eur J Gastroenterol Hepatol 7:283, 1995.
225. Schraufnagel DE, Kay JM: Structural and pathologic changes in the lung vasculature in chronic liver disease. Clin Chest Med 17:1, 1996.
226. Mandell MS, Groves BM: Pulmonary hypertension in chronic liver disease. Clin Chest Med 17:17, 1996.
227. Rossi SO, Gilbert-Barness E, Saari T, et al: Pulmonary hypertension with coexisting portal hypertension. Pediatr Pathol 12:433, 1992.
228. Portmann B, Stewart S, Higenbottam TW, et al: Nodular transformation of the liver associated with portal and pulmonary arterial hypertension. Gastroenterology 104:616, 1993.
229. McDonnell PJ, Toye PA, Hutchins GM: Primary pulmonary hypertension and cirrhosis: Are they related? Am Rev Respir Dis 127:437, 1983.
230. Kup P: Pulmonary hypertension: Considerations in the liver transplant candidate. Transpl Int 9:141, 1996.
231. Taura P, Garcia-Valdecasas JC, Beltran J, et al: Moderate primary pulmonary hypertension in patients undergoing liver transplantation. Anesth Analg 83:675, 1996.
232. Castro M, Krowka MJ, Schroeder DR, et al: Frequency and clinical implications of increased pulmonary artery pressures in liver transplant patients. Mayo Clin Proc 71:543, 1996.
233. Levy MT, Torzillo P, Bookallil M, et al: Case report: Delayed resolution of severe pulmonary hypertension after isolated liver transplantation in a patient with cirrhosis. J Gastroenterol Hepatol 11:734, 1996.
234. Kibria G, Smith P, Heath D: Observations on the rare association between portal and pulmonary hypertension. Thorax 35:945, 1980.
235. Van der Linden P, Le Moine O, et al: Pulmonary hypertension after transjugular intrahepatic portosystemic shunt: Effects on right ventricular function. Hepatology 23:982, 1996.
236. Ramsay MA, Schmidt A, Hein HA, et al: Nitric oxide does not reverse pulmonary hypertension associated with end-stage liver disease: A preliminary report. Hepatology 25:524, 1997.
237. King PD, Rumbaut R, Sanchez C: Pulmonary manifestations of chronic liver disease. Dig Dis 14:73, 1996.
238. Raffy O, Sleiman C, Vachiery F, et al: Refractory hypoxemia during liver cirrhosis. Hepatopulmonary syndrome or "primary" pulmonary hypertension? Am J Respir Crit Care Med 153:1169, 1996.
239. Moser KM, Auger WR, Fedullo PF, et al: Chronic thromboembolic pulmonary hypertension: Clinical picture and surgical treatment. Eur Respir J 5:334, 1992.
240. Moser KM, Bloor CM: Pulmonary vascular lesions occurring in patients with chronic major vessel thromboembolic pulmonary hypertension. Chest 103:685, 1993.
241. Rich S, Levitsky S, Brundage BH: Pulmonary hypertension from chronic pulmonary thromboembolism. Ann Intern Med 108:425, 1988.
242. Benotti JR, Dalen JE: The natural history of pulmonary embolism. Clin Chest Med 5:403, 1985.
243. Rich S, Levitsky S, Brundage BH: Pulmonary hypertension from chronic pulmonary thromboembolism. Ann Intern Med 108:425, 1988.
244. Benotti JR, Dalen JE: The natural history of pulmonary embolism. Clin Chest Med 5:403, 1984.
245. de Soyza NDB, Murphy ML: Persistent post-embolic pulmonary hypertension. Chest 62:665, 1972.
246. Moser KM, Spragg RG, Utley J, et al: Chronic thrombotic obstruction of major pulmonary arteries. Results of thromboendarterectomy in 15 patients. Ann Intern Med 99:299, 1983.
247. Fedullo PF, Auger WR, Channick RN, et al: Chronic thromboembolic pulmonary hypertension. Clin Chest Med 16:353, 1995.
248. Auger WR, Moser KM, Fedullo PF, et al: The association of heparin-induced thrombocytopenia and the lupus anticoagulant in patients with chronic thromboembolic pulmonary hypertension. Am Rev Respir Dis 143:A-403, 1991.
249. Starkie CM, Harding LK, Fletcher DJ, et al (The Birmingham eclampsia study group): Intravascular coagulation and abnormal lung-scans in pre-eclampsia and eclampsia. Lancet 2:889, 1971.
250. Littler WA, Redman CWG, Bonnar J, et al: Reduced pulmonary arterial compliance in hypertensive pregnancy. Lancet 1:1274, 1973.
251. Fukuhara H, Kitayama H, Yokoyama T, et al: Thromboembolic pulmonary hypertension due to disseminated fibromuscular dysplasia. Pediatr Cardiol 17:340, 1996.
252. Loyd JE, Atkinson JB, Pietra GG, et al: Heterogeneity of pathologic lesions in familial primary pulmonary hypertension. Am Rev Respir Dis 138:952, 1988.
253. Pietra GG, Ruttner JR: Specificity of pulmonary vascular lesions in primary pulmonary hypertension. A reappraisal. Respiration 52:81, 1987.
254. Wagenvoort CA, Mulder PG: Thrombotic lesions in primary plexogenic arteriography. Similar pathogenesis or complication? Chest 103:844, 1993.
255. Presti B, Berthrong M, Sherwin RM: Chronic thrombosis of major pulmonary arteries. Hum Pathol 21:601, 1990.
256. Moser KM, Bloor CM: Pulmonary vascular lesions occurring in patients with chronic major vessel thromboembolic pulmonary hypertension. Chest 103:685, 1993.
257. Chitwood WR Jr, Sabiston DC Jr, Wechsler AS: Surgical treatment of chronic unresolved pulmonary embolism. Clin Chest Med 5:507, 1984.
258. Bernstein RJ, Ford RL, Clausen JL, et al: Membrane diffusion and capillary blood volume in chronic thromboembolic pulmonary hypertension. Chest 110:1430, 1996.
258a. Woodruff WW III, Hoeck BE, Chitwood WR Jr, et al: Radiographic findings in pulmonary hypertension from unresolved embolism. AJR 144:681, 1985.
258b. Lisbona R, Kreisman H, Novales-Diaz J, et al: Perfusion lung scanning: differentiation of primary from thromboembolic pulmonary hypertension. AJR 144:27, 1985.
258c. Powe JE, Palevsky HI, McCarthy KE, et al: Pulmonary arterial hypertension: value of perfusion scintigraphy. Radiology 164:727, 1987.
259. Ryan KI, Fedullo PF, Davis GB, et al: Perfusion scan findings understate the severity of angiographic and hemodynamic compromise in chronic thromboembolic pulmonary hypertension. Chest 93:1180, 1988.
260. Rich S, Pietra GG: Primary pulmonary hypertension: Radiographic and scintigraphic patterns of histologic subtypes. Ann Intern Med 105:499, 1986.
261. Martin KW, Sagel SS, Siegel BA: Mosaic oligemia simulating pulmonary infiltrates on CT. Am J Roentgenol 147:670, 1986.
262. King MA, Bergin CJ, Yeung DWC, et al: Chronic pulmonary thromboembolism: Detection of regional hypoperfusion with CT. Radiology 191:359, 1994.
263. Bergin CJ, Rios G, King MA, et al: Accuracy of high-resolution CT in identifying chronic pulmonary thromboembolic disease. Am J Roentgenol 166:1371, 1996.
264. Sherrick AD, Swensen SJ, Hartman TE: Mosaic pattern of lung attenuation on CT scans: Frequency among patients with pulmonary artery hypertension of different causes. Am J Roentgenol 169:79, 1997.
265. Worthy SA, Müller NL, Hartman TE, et al: Mosaic attenuation pattern on thin-section CT scans of the lung: Differentiation among infiltrative lung, airway, and vascular diseases as a cause. Radiology 205:465, 1997.
266. Remy-Jardin M, Louvegny S, Remy J, et al: Acute central thromboembolic disease: Post-therapeutic follow-up with spiral CT angiography. Radiology 203:173, 1997.
267. Teigen CL, Maus TP, Sheedy PE, et al: Pulmonary embolism: Diagnosis with electron-beam CT. Radiology 188:839, 1993.
268. Roberts HC, Kauczor HU, Schweden F, et al: Spiral CT of pulmonary hypertension and chronic thromboembolism. J Thorac Imaging 12:118, 1997.
269. Schwickert H, Schweden F, Schild H, et al: Demonstration of chronic recurrent pulmonary emboli with spiral CT. Fortschr Roentgenstr 158:308, 1993.
270. Kauczor H-U, Schwickert HC, Mayer E, et al: Spiral CT of bronchial arteries in chronic thromboembolism. J Comput Assist Tomogr 18:855, 1994.

271. Pitton MB, Duber C, Mayer E, et al: Hemodynamic effects of nonionic contrast bolus injection and oxygen inhalation during pulmonary angiography in patients with chronic major-vessel thromboembolic pulmonary hypertension. Circulation 94:2485, 1996.

272. Auger WR, Fedullo PF, Moser KM, et al: Chronic major-vessel thromboembolic pulmonary artery obstruction: Appearance at angiography. Radiology 182:393, 1992.

273. Peterson KL, Fred HL, Alexander JK: Pulmonry arterial webs: A new angiographic sign of previous thromboembolism. N Engl J Med 277:33, 1967.

274. Come PC: Echocardiographic evaluation of pulmonary embolism and its response to therapeutic interventions. Chest 101(4 Suppl):151S, 1992.

275. Wittlich N, Erbel R, Eichler A, et al: Detection of central pulmonary artery thromboemboli by transesophageal echocardiography in patients with severe pulmonary embolism. J Am Soc Echocardiogr 5:515, 1992.

276. Nadel JA, Gold WM, Burgess JH: Early diagnosis of chronic pulmonary vascular obstruction. Value of pulmonary function tests. Am J Med 44:16, 1968.

277. Morris TA, Auger WR, Ysrael MZ, et al: Parenchymal scarring is associated with restrictive spirometric defects in patients with chronic thromboemboic pulmonary hypertension. Chest 110:399, 1996.

278. Hartz RS, Byrne JG, Levitsky S, et al: Predictors of mortality in pulmonary thrombendarterectomy. Ann Thorac Surg 62:1255, 1996.

279. Brucato A, Baudo F, Barberis M, et al: Pulmonary hypertension secondary to thrombosis of the pulmonary vessels in a patient with the primary antiphospholipid syndrome. J Rheumatol 21:942, 1994.

280. De Clerck LS, Michielsen PP, Ramael MR, et al: Portal and pulmonary vessel thrombosis associated with systemic lupus erythematosus and anticardiolipin antibodies. J Rheumatol 18:1919, 1991.

281. Asherson RA, Khamashta MA, Ordi-Ros J, et al: The "primary" antiphospholipid syndrome: Major clinical and serological features. Medicine (Baltimore) 68:366, 1989.

282. Gertner E, Lie JT: Pulmonary capillaritis, alveolar haemorrhage, and recurrent microvacular thrombosis in primary antiphospholipid syndrome. J Rheumatol 20:1224, 1993.

283. Mackworth-Young CG, Gharavi AE, Boey ML, et al: Portal and pulmonary hypertension in a case of systemic lupus erythematosus: Possible relationship with clotting abnormality. Eur J Rhematol Inflamm 7:71, 1984.

284. Karmochkine M, Cacoub P, Dorent R, et al: High prevalence of antiphospholipid antibodies in precapillary pulmonary hypertension. J Rheumatol 23:286, 1996.

284a. Asherson RA, Cervera R: Review: Antiphospholipid antibodies and the lung. J Rheumatol 22:62, 1995.

285. Sandoval J, Amigo MC, Barragan R, et al: Primary antiphospholipid syndrome presenting as chronic thromboembolic pulmonary hypertension. Treatment with thromboendarterectomy. J Rheumatol 23:772, 1996.

286. Luchi ME, Asherson RA, Lahita RG: Primary idiopathic pulmonary hypertension complicated by pulmonary arterial thrombosis. Association with antiphospholipid antibodies. Arthritis Rheum 35:700, 1992.

287. Miyashita Y, Koike H, Misawa A, et al: Asymptomatic pulmonary hypertension complicated with antiphospholipid syndrome. Intern Med 35:912, 1996.

288. Nagai H, Yasuma K, Katsuki T, et al: Primary antiphospholipid syndrome and pulmonary hypertension with prolonged survival. A case report. Angiology 48:183, 1997.

289. Petitpretz P, Brenot F, Azarian R, et al: Pulmonary hypertension in patients with human immunodeficiency virus infection. Comparison with primary pulmonary hypertension. Circulation 89:2722, 1994.

290. Mette SA, Palevsky HI, Pietra GG, et al: Primary pulmonary hypertension in association with human immunodeficiency virus infection. A possible viral etiology for some forms of hypertensive pulmonary arteriopathy. Am Rev Respir Dis 145:1196, 1992.

291. Mesa RA, Edell ES, Dunn WF, et al: Human immunodeficiency virus infection and pulmonary hypertension: Two new cases and a review of 86 reported cases. Mayo Clin Proc 73:37, 1998.

292. Weiss JR, Pietra GG, Schraf SM: Primary pulmonary hypertension and the human immunodeficiency virus: Report of two cases and a review of the literature. Arch Intern Med 155:2350, 1995.

293. Morse JH, Barst RJ, Itescu S, et al: Primary pulmonary hypertension in HIV infection: An outcome determined by particular HLA class II alleles. Am J Respir Crit Care Med 153:1299, 1996.

294. Cool CD, Kennedy D, Voelkel NF, et al: Pathogenesis and evolution of plexiform lesions in pulmonary hypertension associated with scleroderma and human immunodeficiency virus infection. Hum Pathol 28:434, 1997.

295. Jacques C, Richmond G, Tierney L, et al: Primary pulmonary hypertension and human immunodeficiency virus infection in a non-hemophiliac man. Hum Pathol 23:191, 1992.

296. Heron E, Laaban JP, Capron F, et al: Thrombotic primary pulmonary hypertension in an HIV+ patient. Eur Heart J 15:394, 1994.

297. Escamilla R, Hermant C, Berjaud J, et al: Pulmonary veno-occlusive disease in a HIV-infected intravenous drug abuser. Eur Respir J 8:1982, 1995.

298. Polos PG, Wolfe D, Harley RA, et al: Pulmonary hypertension and human immunodeficiency virus infection. Two reports and a review of the literature. Chest 101:474, 1992.

299. de Chadarevian JP, Lischner HW, Karmazin N, et al: Pulmonary hypertension and HIV infection: New observations and review of the syndrome. Mod Pathol 7:685, 1994.

300. Mani S, Smith GJ: HIV and pulmonary hypertension: A review. South Med J 87:357, 1994.

301. Duchesne N, Gagnon JA, Fouquette B, et al: Primary pulmonary hypertension associated with HIV infection. Can Assoc Radiol J 44:39, 1993.

302. Wagenvoort CA, Beetstra A, Spijker J: Capillary hemangiomatosis of the lung. Histopathology 2:401, 1978.

303. Tron V, Magee F, Wright JL, et al: Pulmonary capillary hemangiomatosis. Hum Pathol 17:1144, 1986.

304. Masur Y, Remberger K: Pulmonary capillary hemangiomatosis as a rare cause of pumonary hypertension. Pathol Res Pract 192:290, 1996.

305. Eltorky MA, Headley AS, Winer-Muram H, et al: Pulmonary capillary hemangiomatosis: A clinicopathologic review. Ann Thorac Surg 57:772, 1994.

306. Langleben D, Heneghan JM, Batten AP, et al: Familial pulmonary capillary hemangiomatosis resulting in primary pulmonary hypertension. Ann Intern Med 109:106, 1988.

307. Faber CN, Yousem SA, Dauber JH, et al: Pulmonary capillary hemangiomatosis: A report of three cases and a review of the literature. Am Rev Respir Dis 140:808, 1989.

308. Magee F, Wright JL, Kay JM, et al: Pulmonary capillary hemangiomatosis. Am Rev Respir Dis 132:922, 1985.

309. Langleben D, Heneghan JM, Batten AP, et al: Familial pulmonary capillary hemangiomatosis resulting in primary pulmonary hypertension. Ann Intern Med 109:106, 1988.

310. Eltorky MA, Headley AS, Winer-Muram H, et al: Pulmonary capillary hemangiomatosis: A clinicopathologic review. Ann Thorac Surg 57:772, 1994.

311. Primack SL, Müller NL, Mayo JR, et al: Pulmonary parenchymal abnormalities of vascular origin: High-resolution CT findings. Radiographics 14:739, 1994.

312. Arvidsson H, Karnell J, Möller T: Multiple stenosis of the pulmonary arteries associated with pulmonary hypertension, diagnosed by selective angiocardiography. Acta Radiol 44:209, 1955.

313. Dighiero J, Fiandra O, Barcia A, et al: Multiple pulmonary stenoses with pulmonary hypertension: Report of a case. Acta Radiol 48:439, 1957.

314. Gyllenswärd A, Lodin H, Lundberg A, et al: Congenital, multiple peripheral stenoses of the pulmonary artery. Pediatrics 19:399, 1957.

315. Orell SR, Karnell J, Wahlgren F: Malformation and multiple stenoses of the pulmonary arteries with pulmonary hypertension. Acta Radiol 54:449, 1960.

316. Gay BB Jr, Franch RH, Shuford WH, et al: The roentgenologic features of single and multiple coarctations of the pulmonary artery and branches. Am J Roentgenol 90:599, 1963.

317. Winfield ME, McDonnel GM, Steckel RJ: Multiple coarctations of the pulmonary arteries with associated infundibular pulmonic stenosis. Case report with serial right-heart catheterization studies obtained at a three-year interval. Radiology 83:854, 1964.

318. del Castillo JJ, Gianfrancesco H, Mannix EP Jr: Pulmonic stenosis due to compression by sternal chondrosarcoma. J Thorac Cardiovasc Surg 52:255, 1966.

319. Tikoff G, Bloom S: Complete interruption of the aortic arch in an adult associated with a dissection aneurysm of the pulmonary artery. Am J Med 48:782, 1970.

320. Best J: Dissecting aneurysm of the pulmonary artery with multiple cardiovascular abnormalities and pulmonary hypertension. Med J Austral 2:1129, 1967.

321. Nasraliah A, Goussous Y, El-Said G, et al: Pulmonary artery compression due to acute dissecting aortic aneurysm: Clinical and angiographic diagnosis. Chest 67:228, 1975.

322. Buja LM, Ali N, Fletcher RD, et al: Stenosis of the right pulmonary artery: A complication of acute dissecting aneurysm of the ascending aorta. Am Heart J 83:89, 1972.

323. Cheris DN, Dadey JL: Fibrosing mediastinitis. An unusual cause for cor pulmonale. Am J Roentgenol 100:328, 1967.

324. Baum GL, Fisher FD: The relationship of fatal pulmonary insufficiency with cor pulmonale, rightsided mural thrombi and pulmonary emboli: A preliminary report. Am J Med Sci 240:609, 1960.

325. MacNee W: Pathophysiology of cor pulmonale in chronic obstructive pulmonary disease. Am J Respir Crit Care Med 150:833, 1994.

326. Weitzenblum E: The pulmonary circulation and the heart in chronic lung disease. Mondali Arch Chest Dis 49:231, 1994.

327. Fujii T, Kurihara N, Fujimoto S, et al: Role of pulmonary vascular disorder in determining exercise capacity in patients with severe chronic obstructive lung disease. Clin Physiol 16:521, 1996.

328. Emirgil C, Sobol BJ, Herbert WH, et al: Routine pulmonary function studies as a key to the status of the lesser circulation in chronic obstructive pulmonary disease. Am J Med 50:191, 1971.

329. Wright JL, Petty T, Thurlbeck WM: Analysis of the structure of the muscular pulmonary arteries in patients with pulmonary hypertension and COPD: National Institutes of Health nocturnal oxygen therapy trial. Lung 170:109, 1992.

330. Matthay RA, Schwarz MI, Ellis JH Jr, et al: Pulmonary artery hypertension in chronic obstructive pulmonary disease: Determination by chest radiography. Invest Radiol 16:95, 1981.

331. Austin JHM, Young BG Jr, Thomas HM, et al: Radiologic assessment of pulmonary arterial pressure and blood volume in chronic, diffuse, interstitial pulmonary diseases. Invest Radiol 14:9, 1979.

332. Steckel RJ, Bein ME, Kelly PM: Pulmonary arterial hypertension in progressive systemic sclerosis. Am J Roentgenol 124:461, 1975.

333. Fry WA, Archer FA, Adams WE: Long-term clinical-pathologic study of the pneumonectomy patient. Dis Chest 52:720, 1967.

334. O'Toole SJ, Irish MS, Holm BA, et al: Pulmonary vascular abnormalilties in congenital diaphragmatic hernia. Clin Perinatol 23:781, 1996.

335. Massumi RA, Sarin RK, Pooya N, et al: Tonsillar hypertrophy, airway obstruction, alveolar hypoventilation, and cor pulmonale in twin brothers. Dis Chest 55:110, 1969.

336. Obstruction by tonsils and adenoids. BMJ 4:5, 1968.
337. Levin DL, Muster AJ, Pachman LM, et al: Cor pulmonale secondary to upper airway obstruction. Cardiac catheterization, immunologic, and psychometric evaluation in nine patients. Chest 68(Suppl):166, 1975.
338. Gerald B, Dungan WT: Cor pulmonale and pulmonary edema in children secondary to chronic upper airway obstruction. Radiology 90:679, 1968.
339. Levy AM, Tabakin BS, Hanson JS, et al: Hypertrophied adenoids causing pulmonary hypertension and severe congestive heart failure. N Engl J Med 277:506, 1967.
340. Marks CE Jr, Goldring RM: Chronic hypercapnia during methadone maintenance. Am Rev Respir Dis 108:1088, 1973.
341. Sajkov D, Cowie RJ, Thorton AT, et al: Pulmonary hypertension and hypoxemia in obstructive sleep apnea syndrome. Am J Respir Crit Care Med 149:416, 1994.
341a. Chaouat A, Weitzenblum E, Krieger J, et al: Pulmonary hemodynamics in the obstructive sleep apnea syndrome. Results in 220 consecutive patients. Chest 109:380, 1996.
342. Bindelglass IL, Trubowitz S: Pulmonary vein obstruction: An uncommon sequel to chronic fibrous mediastinitis. Ann Intern Med 48:876, 1958.
343. Stovin PGI, Mitchinson MJ: Pulmonary hypertension due to obstruction of intrapulmonary veins. Thorax 20:106, 1965.
344. Singshinsuk SS, Hartmann AF Jr, Elliott LP: Stenosis of the individual pulmonary veins: A rare cause of pulmonary hypertension? Radiology 87:514, 1966.
345. Cody RJ: The potential role of endothelin as a vasoconstrictor substance in congestive heart failure. Eur Heart J. 13:1573, 1992.
346. Simon M: The pulmonary vessels: Their hemodynamic evaluation using routine radiographs. Radiol Clin North Am 1:363, 1963.
347. Wagenvoort CA: Pathology of congestive pulmonary hypertension. Prog Respir Res 9:195, 1975.
348. Symmers WSC: Necrotizing pulmonary arteriopathy associated with pulmonary hypertension. J Clin Pathol 5:36, 1952.
349. Wagenvoort CA: Morphologic changes in intrapulmonary veins. Hum Pathol 1:205, 1970.
350. Heath D, Edwards JE: Histological changes in the lung in diseases associated with pulmonary venous hypertension. Br J Dis Chest 53:8, 1959.
351. Heard BE, Path FC, Steiner RE, et al: Oedema and fibrosis of the lungs in left ventricular failure. Br J Radiol 41:161, 1968.
352. Spencer H: Pathology of the Lung. Vol 2. 4th ed. Oxford, Pergamon Press, 1985, p 667.
353. Wood TE, McLeod P, Anthonisen NR, et al: Mechanics of breathing in mitral stenosis. Am Rev Respir Dis 104:52, 1971.
354. Collins JR, Clark TJH, Brown DJ: Airway function in healthy subjects and patients with left heart disease. Clin Sci (Colch) 49:217, 1975.
355. Simon M: The pulmonary veins in mitral stenosis. J Fac Radiol 9:25, 1958.
356. Milne ENC: Pulmonary blood flow distribution. Invest Radiol 12:479, 1977.
357. West JB, Dollery CT, Heard BE: Increased pulmonary vascular resistance in the dependent zone of the isolated dog lung caused by perivascular edema. Circ Res 17:191, 1965.
358. Ritchie BC, Schauberger G, Staub NC: Inadequacy of perivascular edema hypothesis to account for distribution of pulmonary blood flow in lung edema. Circ Res 24:807, 1969.
359. Muir AL, Hall DL, Despas P, et al: Distribution of blood flow in the lungs in acute pulmonary edema in dogs. J Appl Physiol 33:763, 1972.
360. Hughes JMB, Glazier JB, Maloney JE, et al: Effect of interstitial pressure on pulmonary blood-flow. Lancet 1:192, 1967.
361. Surette GD, Muir AL, Hogg JC, et al: Roentgenographic study of blood flow redistribution in acute pulmonary edema in dogs. Invest Radiol 10:109, 1975.
362. Burko H, Carwell G, Newman E: Size, location, and gravitational changes of normal upper lobe pulmonary veins. Am J Roentgenol 111:687, 1971.
363. Simon G: The value of radiology in critical mitral stenosis—an amendment. Clin Radiol 23:145, 1972.
364. Lavender JP, Doppman J, Shawdon H, et al: Pulmonary veins in left ventricular failure and mitral stenosis. Br J Radiol 35:293, 1962.
365. Doppman JL, Lavender JP: The hilum and the large left ventricle. Radiology 80:931, 1963.
366. Tattersfield AE, McNicol MW, Shawdon H, et al: Chest x-ray film in acute myocardial infarction. BMJ 3:332, 1969.
367. Chait A, Cohen HE, Meltzer LE, et al: The bedside chest radiograph in the evaluation of incipient heart failure. Radiology 105:563, 1972.
368. McHugh TJ, Forrester JS, Adler L, et al: Pulmonary vascular congestion in acute myocardial infarction: Hemodynamic and radiologic correlations. Ann Intern Med 76:29, 1972.
369. Bryk D: Dilated right pulmonary veins in mitral insufficiency. Chest 58:24, 1970.
370. Kerley P: Lung changes in acquired heart disease. Am J Roentgenol 80:256, 1958.
371. Galloway RW, Epstein EJ, Coulshed N: Pulmonary ossific nodules in mitral valve disease. Br Heart J 23:297, 1961.
372. Legge DA, Miller WE, Ludwig J: Pulmonary findings associated with mitral stenosis. Chest 58:403, 1970.
373. Heath D, Scott O, Lynch J: Pulmonary veno-occlusive disease. Thorax 26:663, 1971.
374. Wilson WR, Sasaki R, Johnson CA: Disseminated nodular pulmonary ossification in patients with mitral stenosis. Circulation 19:323, 1959.
375. Whitehouse G: Tracheopathia osteoplastica: Case report. Br J Radiol 41:701, 1968.
376. Seningen RP, Chen JTT, Peter RH, et al: Roentgen interpretation of postoperative changes (clinical and hemodynamic) in pure mitral stenosis. Am J Roentgenol 113:693, 1971.
377. Ramirez A, Grimes ET, Abelmann WH: Regression of pulmonary vascular changes following mitral valvuloplasty. An anatomic and physiologic case study. Am J Med 45:975, 1968.
378. Symbas PN, Abbott OA, Logan WD, et al: Atrial myxomas: Special emphasis on unusual manifestations. Chest 59:504, 1971.
379. Ribeiro PA, al Zaibag M, Abdullah M: Pulmonary artery pressure and pulmonary vascular resistance before and after mitral balloon valvotomy in 100 patients with severe mitral valve stenosis. Am Heart J 125:1110, 1993.
380. Rosenow EC III, Harrison CE Jr: Congestive heart failure masquerading as primary pulmonary disease. Chest 58:28, 1970.
381. Thadani U, Burrow C, Whittaker W, et al: Pulmonary veno-occlusive disease. Q J Med 44:133, 1975.
382. Enriquez-Sarano, Rossi M, Seward JB, et al: Determinants of pulmonary hypertension in left ventricular dysfunction. J Am Coll Cardiol 29:152, 1997.
383. Rhodes KM, Evemy K, Nariman S, et al: Effects of mitral valve surgery on static lung function and exercise performace. Thorax 40:107, 1985.
384. Palmer WH, Gee JBL, Mills FC, et al: Disturbances of pulmonary function in mitral valve disease. Can Med Assoc J 89:744, 1963.
385. Singh T, Dinda P, Chatterjee SS, et al: Pulmonary function studies before and after closed mitral valvotomy. Am Rev Respir Dis 101:62, 1970.
386. Ray S, Dodds P, Wilson G, et al: Effects of balloon commissurotomy on the diffusing capacity of the alveolar capillary membrane and pulmonary capillary blood volume in patients with mitral stenosis. Am J Cardiol 74:1068, 1994.
387. Donald KW, Bishop JM, Wade OL, et al: Cardiorespiratory functions two years after mitral valvotomy. Clin Sci 16:325, 1957.
388. Carrington CD, Liebow AA: Pulmonary veno-occlusive disease. Hum Pathol 1:322, 1970.
389. Shackelford GD, Sacks EJ, Mullins JD, et al: Pulmonary veno-occlusive disease. Case report and review of the literature. Am J Roentgenol 128:643, 1977.
390. Wagenvoort CA, Wagenvoort N, Takahashi T: Pulmonary veno-occlusive disease. Involvement of pulmonary arteries and review of the literature. Hum Pathol 16:1033, 1985.
391. Kay JM, deSa DJ, Mancer JFK: Ultrastructure of lung in pulmonary veno-occlusive disease. Hum Pathol 14:451, 1983.
392. Corrin B, Spencer H, Turner-Warwick M, et al: Pulmonary veno-occlusion—an immune complex disease? Virchows Arch 364:81, 1974.
393. Hasleton PS, Ironside JW, Whittaker JS, et al: Pulmonary veno-occlusive disease. A report of four cases. Histopathology 10:933, 1986.
394. Leinonen H, Pohjola-Sintonen S, Krogerus L: Pulmonary veno-occlusive disease. Acta Med Scand 221:307, 1987.
395. Kishida Y, Kanai Y, Kuramochi S, et al: Pulmonary veno-occlusive disease in a patient with systemic lupus erythematosus. J Rheumatol 20:2161, 1993.
396. McDonnell PJ, Summer WR, Hutchins GM: Pulmonary veno-occlusive disease. Morphological changes suggesting a viral cause. JAMA 246:667, 1981.
397. Ruchelli ED, Nojadera G, Rutstein RM, et al: Pulmonary veno-occlusive disease: Another vascular disorder associated with human immunodeficiency virus infection? Arch Pathol Lab Med 118:664, 1994.
398. Voordes CG, Kuipers JRG, Elema JD: Familial pulmonary veno-occlusive disease: A case report. Thorax 32:763, 1977.
399. Davies P, Reid L: Pulmonary veno-occlusive disease in siblings: Case reports and morphometric study. Hum Pathol 13:911, 1982.
400. Lombard C, Churg A, Winokur S: Pulmonary veno-occlusive disease following therapy for malignant neoplasms. Chest 92:871, 1987.
401. Waldhorn R, Tsou E, Smith F, et al: Pulmonary veno-occlusive disease associated with microangiopathic hemolytic anemia and chemotherapy of gastric adenocarcinoma. Med Pediatr Oncol 12:394, 1984.
402. Stuart KL, Bras G: Veno-occlusive disease of the liver. Q J Med 26:219, 1957.
403. Mehta MJ, Karmody AM, McKneally MF: Mediastinal veno-occlusive disease associated with herbal tea ingestion. N Y State J Med 86:604, 1986.
404. Williams LM, Fussell S, Veith RW, et al: Pulmonary veno-occlusive disease in an adult following bone marrow transplantation. Case report and review of the literature. Chest 109:1388, 1996.
405. Kramer MR, Estenne M, Berkman N, et al: Radiation-induced pulmonary veno-occlusive disease. Chest 104:1282, 1993.
406. Townend JN, Roberts DH, Jones EL, et al: Fatal pulmonary veno-occlusive disease after use of oral contraceptives. Am Heart J 124:1643, 1992.
407. Alpert LI: Veno-occlusive disease of the liver associated with oral contraceptives: Case reports and review of literature. Hum Pathol 7:709, 1976.
408. Hensby CN, Dollery CT, Barnes PJ, et al: Production of 6-oxo-PGF$_1$ alpha by human lung *in vivo*. Lancet 2:1162, 1979.
409. Crissman JD, Koss M, Carson RP: Pulmonary veno-occlusive disease secondary to granulomatous venulitis. Am J Surg Pathol 4:93, 1980.
410. Case records of the Massachusetts General Hospital. Case 14–1983. N Engl J Med 308:825, 1983.
411. Schraufnagel DE, Sekosan M, McGee T, et al: Human alveolar capillaries undergo angiogenesis in pulmonary veno-occlusive disease. Eur Respir J 9:346, 1996.
412. Wagenvoort CA, Wagenvoort N: The pathology of pulmonary veno-occlusive disease. Virchows Arch 364:69, 1974.
413. Shackleford GD, Sacks EJ, Mullins JD, et al: Pulmonary veno-occlusive disease: Case report and review of the literature. Am J Roentgenol 128:643, 1977.
414. Rambihar VS, Fallen EL, Cairns JA: Pulmonary veno-occlusive disease: Antemortem diagnosis from roentgenographic and hemodynamic findings. Can Med Assoc J 120:1519, 1979.

415. Cassart M, Gevenois PA, Kramer M, et al: Pulmonary venoocclusive disease: CT findings before and after single-lung transplantation. Am J Roentgenol 160:759, 1993.

416. Swensen SJ, Tashjian JH, Myers JL, et al: Pulmonary venoocclusive disease: CT findings in eight patients. Am J Roentgenol 167:937, 1996.

417. Weisser K, Wyler F, Gloor F: Pulmonary veno-occlusive disease. Arch Dis Child 42:322, 1967.

418. Salzman D, Adkins DR, Craig F, et al: Malignancy-associated pulmonary veno-occlusive disease: Report of a case following autologous bone marrow transplantation and review. Bone Marrow Transplant 18:755, 1996.

419. Bates DV, Macklem PT, Christie RV: Respiratory Function in Disease: An Introduction to the Integrated Study of the Lung. 2nd ed. Philadelphia, WB Saunders, 1971.

420. Rambihar VS, Fallen EL, Cairns JA: Pulmonary veno-occlusive disease: Antemortem diagnosis from roentgenographic and hemodynamic findings. Can Med Assoc J 120:1519, 1979.

421. Wiedmann HP: Wedge pressure in pulmonary veno-occlusive disease (letter). N Engl J Med 315:1233, 1986.

422. Ribeiro PA, Muthusamy R, Duran CM: Right-sided endomyocardial fibrosis with recurrent pulmonary emboli leading to irreversible pulmonary hypertension. Br Heart J 68:326, 1992.

423. Kawashima A, Kimura A, Katsuda S, et al: Pulmonary vasculitis with hypereosinophilia and episodic pulmonary hypertension: Report of three siblings. Pathol Int 45:66, 1995.

424. Kay JM, Kahana LM, Rihal C: Diffuse smooth muscle proliferation of the lungs with servere pulmonary hypertension. Hum Pathol 27:969, 1996.

425. Chronic cor pulmonale. Report of an expert committee (reprinted from World Health Organization Technical Report Series No. 213). Circulation 27:594, 1963.

426. Stevens PM, Terplan M, Knowles JH: Prognosis of cor pulmonale. N Engl J Med 269:1289, 1963.

427. Schulman DS, Matthay RA: The right ventricle in pulmonary disease. Cardiol Clin 10:111, 1992.

428. Setaro JF, Cleman MW, Remetz MS: The right ventricle in disorders causing pulmonary venous hypertension. Cardiol Clin 10:165, 1992.

429. Lee FA: Hemodynamics of the right ventricle in normal and disease states. Cardiol Clin 10:59, 1992.

430. Jain D, Zaret BL: Assesment of right ventricular function: Role of nuclear imaging techniques. Cardiol Clin 10:23, 1992.

431. Sherman WT, Ferrer MI, Harvey RM: Competence of the tricuspid valve in pulmonary heart disease (cor pulmonale). Circulation 31:517, 1965.

432. Sepúveda G, Riös E, León J, et al: Clinico-pathologic correlation in chronic cor pulmonale. Dis Chest 52:205, 1967.

433. Schena M, Clini E, Errera D, et al: Echo-Doppler evaluation of left ventricular impairment in chronic cor pulmonale. Chest 109:1446, 1996.

434. World Health Organization, Report of an Expert Committee: Definition and diagnosis of pulmonary diseases with special reference to chronic bronchitis and emphysema. *In* Chronic Cor Pulmonale, WHO Technical Report Series No. 213, 1961, pp 14–19.

435. Butler PM, Leggett SI, Howe CM, et al: Identification of electrocardiographic criteria for diagnosis of right ventricular hypertrophy due to mitral stenosis. Am J Cardiol 57:639, 1986.

436. Behar JV, Howe CM, Wagner NB, et al: Performance of new criteria for right ventricular hypertrophy and myocardial infarction in patients with pulmonary hypertension due to cor pulmonale and mitral stenosis. J Electrocardiol 24:231, 1991.

437. Bhan AK, Mittal SR, Lalgadiya M: Importance of recording lead V1 in the seventh right intercostal space in diagnosing cor pulmonale. Int J Cardiol 43:99, 1994.

438. Jardin F, Dubourg O, Bourdarias J-P: Echocardiographic pattern in acute cor pulmonale. Chest 111:209, 1997.

439. Bartter T, Irwin RS, Nash G: Aneurysms of the pulmonary arteries. Chest 94:1065, 1988.

440. Lopez-Candales A, Kleiger RE, Aleman-Gomez J, et al: Pulmonary artery aneurysm: Review and case report. Clin Cardiol 18:738, 1995.

441. Charlton RW, Du Plessis LA: Multiple pulmonary artery aneurysms. Thorax 16:364, 1961.

442. Deterling RA Jr, Clagett OT: Aneurysm of the pulmonary artery: Review of the literature and report of a case. Am Heart J 34:471, 1947.

443. DeBoer DA, Margolis ML, Livornese D, et al: Pulmonary venous aneurysm presenting as a middle mediastinal mass. Ann Thorac Surg 61:1261, 1996.

444. Janssen DP, Schilte PP, De Graaff CS, et al: Bronchopulmonary sequestration associated with an aneurysm of the aberrant artery. Ann Thorac Surg 60:193, 1995.

445. Baum D, Khoury GH, Ongley PA, et al: Congenital stenosis of the pulmonary artery branches. Circulation 29:680, 1964.

446. Tami LF, McElderry MW: Pulmonary artery aneurysm due to severe congenital pulmonic stenosis. Case report and literature review. Angiology 45:383, 1994.

447. Shindo T, Kuroda T, Watanabe S, et al: Aneurysmal dilatation of the pulmonary trunk with mild pulmonic stenosis. Intern Med 34:199, 1995.

448. Plokker HWM, Wagenaar S, Bruschke AVG, et al: Aneurysm of a pulmonary artery branch: An uncommon cause of a coin lesion. Chest 68:258, 1975.

449. Tung H, Liebow AA: Marfan's syndrome. Lab Invest 1:382, 1952.

450. Koh KK, Kim SS, Park CS, et al: Pulmonary artery aneurysm associated with hereditary hemorrhagic telangiectasia. Int J Cardiol 45:227, 1994.

451. Symbas PN, Scott HW Jr: Traumatic aneurysm of the pulmonary artery. J Thorac Cardiovasc Surg 45:645, 1963.

452. Kumar RV, Roughneen PT, de Leval MR: Mycotic pulmonary artery aneurysm following pulmonary artery banding. Eur J Cardiothorac Surg 8:665, 1994.

453. Sevitt S: Arterial wall lesions after pulmonary embolism, especially ruptures and aneurysms. J Clin Pathol 29:665, 1976.

454. Salyer WR, Salyer DC, Hutchins GM: Local arterial wall injury caused by thromboemboli. Am J Pathol 75:285, 1974.

455. Meyer JS: Thromboembolic pulmonary arterial necrosis and arteritis in man. Arch Pathol 70:63, 1960.

456. Auerbach O: Pathology and pathogenesis of pulmonary arterial aneurysm in tuberculous cavities. Am Rev Tuberc 39:99, 1939.

457. Kauffman SL, Lynfield J, Hennigar GR: Mycotic aneurysms of the intrapulmonary arteries. Circulation 35:90, 1967.

458. Jaffe RB, Condon VR: Mycotic aneurysms of the pulmonary artery and aorta. Radiology 116:291, 1975.

459. Navarro C, Dickinson PCT, Kondlapoodi P, et al: Mycotic aneurysms of the pulmonary arteries in intravenous drug addicts. Am J Med 76:1124, 1984.

460. Choyke PL, Edmonds PR, Markowitz RI, et al: Mycotic pulmonary artery aneurysm: Complication of aspergillus endocarditis. Am J Roentgenol 138:1172, 1982.

461. Rousch K, Scala-Barnett DM, Donabedian H, et al: Rupture of a pulmonary artery associated with candidal endocarditis. Am J Med 84:142, 1988.

462. Slavin RE, de Groot WJ: Pathology of the lung in Behcet's disease. Am J Surg Pathol 5:779, 1981.

463. de Montpreville VT, Macchiarini P, Dartevelle PG, et al: Large bilateral pulmonary artery aneurysms in Behcet's disease: Rupture of the contralateral lesion after aneurysmorrhaphy. Respiration 63:49, 1996.

464. Dennison AR, Watkins RM, Gunning AJ: Simultaneous aortic and pulmonary artery aneurysms due to giant cell arteritis. Thorax 40:156, 1985.

465. Hartley JPR, Dinnen JS, Seaton A: Pulmonary and systemic aneurysms in a case of widespread arteritis. Thorax 33:493, 1978.

466. Nienaber CA, Spielman RP, Monyz R, et al: Development of pulmonary aneurysm in primary pulmonary hypertension: A case report. Angiology 37:319, 1986.

467. Luchtrath H: Dissecting aneurysm of the pulmonary artery. Virchows Arch 391:241, 1981.

468. Shilkin KB, Low LP, Chen BTM: Dissecting aneurysm of the pulmonary artery. J Pathol 98:25, 1968.

469. Hughes JP, Stovin PGI: Segmental pulmonary artery aneurysms with peripheral venous thrombosis. Br J Dis Chest 53:19, 1959.

470. Kopp WL, Green RA: Pulmonary artery aneurysms with recurrent thrombophlebitis. The "Hughes-Stovin syndrome." Ann Intern Med 56:105, 1962.

471. Teplick JG, Haskin ME, Nedwich A: The Hughes-Stovin syndrome: Case report. Radiology 113:607, 1974.

472. Chen YF, Chiu CC, Lee CS: Giant aneurysm of main pulmonary artery. Ann Thorac Surg 62:272, 1996.

473. Shanks JH, Coup A, Howat AJ: Dissecting aneurysm of the pulmonary artery associated with a large facial cavernous haemangioma. Histopathology 30:390, 1997.

474. Butto F, Lucas RV JR, Edwards JE: Pulmonary artery aneurysm: A pathologic study of five cases. Chest 91:237, 1987.

475. Ungaro R, Saab S, Almond CH, et al: Solitary peripheral pulmonary artery aneurysms. J Thorac Cardiovasc Surg 71:566, 1976.

476. Chung CW, Doherty JU, Kotler R, et al: Pulmonary artery aneurysm presenting as a lung mass. Chest 108:1164, 1995.

477. Gavant ML, Winer-Muram HT: Traumatic pulmonary artery pseudoaneurysm. J Can Assoc Radiol 37:108, 1986.

478. Dieden JD, Friloux LA III, Renner JW: Pulmonary artery false aneurysms secondary to Swan-Ganz pulmonary artery catheters. Am J Roentgenol 149:901, 1987.

479. Loevner LA, Andrews JC, Francis IR: Multiple mycotic pulmonary artery aneurysms: A complication of invasive mucormycosis. Am J Roentgenol 158:761, 1992.

480. Crivello MS, Hayes C, Thurer RL, et al: Traumatic pulmonary artery aneurysm: CT evaluation. J Comput Assist Tomogr 10:503, 1986.

481. Ahn JM, Im JG, Ryoo JW, et al: Thoracic manifestations of Behcet syndrome: Radiographic and CT findings in nine patients. Radiology 194:199, 1995.

482. Numan F, Islak C, Berkmen T, et al: Behcet disease: Pulmonary arterial involvement in 15 cases. Radiology 192:465, 1994.

483. Jeang MK, Adyanthaya AV, Schwepe I, et al: Multiple pulmonary artery aneurysms: New use for magnetic resonance imaging. Am J Med 81:1001, 1986.

484. Guttentag AR, Shepard JAO, McLoud TC: Catheter-induced pulmonary artery pseudoaneurysm: The halo sign on CT. Am J Roentgenol 158:637, 1992.

485. Remy J, Smith M, Lamaitre L, et al: Treatment of massive hemoptysis by occlusion of a Rasmussen aneurysm. Am J Roentgenol 135:605, 1980.

486. Davidoff AB, Udoff EJ, Schonfeld SA: Intraaneurysmal embolization of a pulmonary artery aneurysm for control of hemoptysis. Am J Roentgenol 142:1019, 1984.

487. Bartter T, Irwin RS, Phillips DA, et al: Pulmonary artery aneurysm: A potentially fatal but treatable cause of pulmonry artery catheterization. Arch Intern Med 148:471, 1988.

488. Bartter T, Irwin RS, Nash G: Aneurysms of the pulmonary arteries. Chest 94:1065, 1988.

488a. Gibbs PM, Hami A: Pulmonary arterial aneurysm presenting as an endobronchial mass. Thorax 50:1013, 1995.

489. Chiu B, Magil A: Idiopathic pulmonary arterial trunk aneurysm presenting as cor pulmonale: Report of a case. Hum Pathol 16:947, 1985.

490. Himmelmann AW, Speich R, Real F, et al: Unusual course of pulmonary hypertension of vascular origin. Respiration 60:292, 1993.
491. Iwasaki H, Ogawa K, Toshida H, et al: Crow-Fukase syndrome associated with pulmonary hypertension. Intern Med 32:556, 1993.
492. Okura H, Gohma I, Hatta K, et al: Thiamine deficiency and pulmonary hypertension in Crow-Fukase syndrome. Intern Med 34:674, 1995.
493. Land SD, Shah MD, Berman WF: Pulmonary hypertension associated with portal hypertension in a child with Williams syndrome—a case report. Pediatr Pathol 14:61, 1994.
494. Ribadeau-Dumas S, Tillie-Leblond I, Rose C, et al: Pulmonary hypertension associated with POEMS syndrome. Eur Respir J 9:1760, 1996.
495. Sirkin W, O'Hare BP, Cox PN: Alveolar capillary dysplasia: lung biopsy diagnosis, nitric oxide responsiveness, and bronchial generation count. Pediatr Pathol Lab Med 17:125, 1997.
496. Nand S, Orfei E: Pulmonary hypertension in polycythemia vera. Am J Hematol 47:242, 1994.
497. Mandel RI, Bruner JP: Endocardial fibroelastosis: An unusual cause of pulmonary hypertension in pregnancy. Am J Perinatol 12:319, 1995.
498. Espinosa RE, Edwards WD, Rosenow EC, et al: Idiopathic pulmonary hilar fibrosis: An unusual cause of pulmonary hypertension. Mayo Clin Proc 68:778, 1993.
499. Sandoval J, Salas J, Martinez-Guerra ML, et al: Pulmonary arterial hypertension and cor pulmonale associated with chronic domestic wood smoke inhalation. Chest 103:12, 1993.
500. Barbosa MM, Lamounier JA, Oliveria EC, et al: Pulmonary hypertension in schistosomiasis mansoni. Trans R Soc Trop Med Hyg 90:663, 1996.
501. Salazar A, Mana J, Sala J, et al: Combined portal and pulmonary hypertension in sarcoidosis. Respiration 61:117, 1994.
502. Shive ST, McNally DP: Pulmonary hypertension from prominent vascular involvement in diffuse amyloidosis. Arch Intern Med 148:687, 1988.
503. Castro O: Systemic fat embolism and pulmonary hypertension in sickle cell disease. Hematol Oncol Clin North Am 10:1289, 1996.

# *Pulmonary Edema*

The anatomic and physiologic features of the lungs are such that a constant interstitial water content is normally maintained, resulting in dry or, perhaps more correctly, ideally moist alveoli. Despite the relative constancy of fluid content within the interstitium and alveolar air spaces, there is considerable transport of water between different tissue compartments within the lung. Normally, an ultrafiltrate of plasma moves from the pulmonary microvessels into the interstitial tissue, from which it enters lymphatic channels and is eventually returned to the systemic circulation through the right lymphatic and thoracic ducts. The volume of water and protein movement depends on the balance of pressures across the pulmonary microvasculature and the permeability of the microvascular membrane. A disturbance of sufficient magnitude in one or both of these factors will result in an increase in the transudation and/or exudation of fluid from the microvessels into the interstitium. Accumulation of fluid in this compartment constitutes interstitial edema; when the storage capacity of the interstitial space is exceeded, alveolar flooding and air-space edema develop. In normal circumstances, the balance of hydrostatic and osmotic forces across microvascular walls is so precise that the escape of water and protein into the interstitial tissue is exactly balanced by the removal of fluid by pulmonary lymphatics that absorb the fluid and return it to the systemic circulation. Additional routes for removal of lung fluid include evaporative water loss from the alveolar and bronchial surfaces, reabsorption into pulmonary and bronchial microvessels, and transport into the pleural space.

The most common cause of pulmonary edema is elevation of pulmonary microvascular pressure secondary to elevated pulmonary venous pressure caused by left ventricular decompensation. This form of edema is called cardiogenic, hemodynamic, hydrostatic, or elevated microvascular pressure pulmonary edema. A less common, but nevertheless significant, mechanism for the formation of pulmonary edema is an increase in the permeability of the microvascular endothelial barrier as a result of toxic injury. In its pure form, this mechanism results in the accumulation of excess water and protein in the lungs in the absence of elevated microvascular pressure and is thus termed *permeability, normal microvascular pressure,* or *noncardiogenic edema.* Many causes can lead to this form of pulmonary edema, and the clinical syndrome that results has been termed the *adult respiratory distress syndrome* (ARDS).[1, 2]

Before a discussion of these types of pulmonary edema and the diseases with which they are associated, it is desirable to review certain anatomic and physiologic considerations relating to lung fluid and solute exchange. Much of the following material has been gleaned from the many reviews on the subject.[3–20]

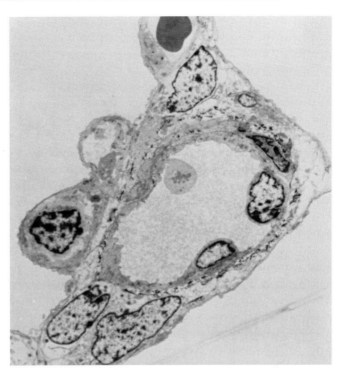

**Figure 51–1. A Corner Vessel: Ultrastructure.** Corner vessels are pulmonary capillaries that behave like extra-alveolar vessels. Because they are situated at the junction of three alveolar walls, lung inflation causes them to dilate while compressing alveolar wall vessels. (Courtesy of Dr. David Walker, Department of Pathology, University of British Columbia, Vancouver.)

## GENERAL PATHOGENETIC FEATURES

### Anatomic Considerations

#### The Pulmonary Circulation and Microvascular Endothelium

Because gas exchange takes place solely by diffusion, the lungs have an enormous surface area for transport of oxygen and carbon dioxide. In fact, the surface area available for gas exchange is approximately 70 square meters in the average adult,[21, 22] an area that is also potentially available for fluid exchange. The microcirculation is composed primarily of the pulmonary capillaries. Although it is believed that most of the fluid exchange in the lungs takes place across the alveolocapillary endothelium, there is abundant evidence that precapillary and postcapillary vessels also take part; as a result, the most appropriate term for this process is *microvascular fluid exchange.*[23–25]

Conceptually, the pulmonary vasculature can be divided into two compartments based on the vascular response to an increase in alveolar pressure: (1) *alveolar vessels,* which are affected directly by an increase in alveolar pressure that compresses them and narrows their lumen; and (2) *extra-alveolar vessels,* which are affected indirectly by alveolar pressure, in that they expand during pulmonary distention as a result of the development of a more negative interstitial pressure. Although most pulmonary capillaries function as alveolar vessels, some (termed *corner vessels*) behave like extra-alveolar vessels and remain patent despite an increase in alveolar pressure to values that exceed pulmonary microvascular pressure (Fig. 51–1). These corner vessels, as well as small arterioles and venules, contribute to fluid exchange.[26] In fact, under Zone I conditions (*see* page 108),

the rate of fluid filtration into the lung can be as much as half that in Zone III, suggesting that a considerable proportion of the pulmonary microvessels that exchange fluid remain patent under these conditions and therefore function as extra-alveolar vessels.[9]

The alveolar septum has two distinct anatomic and functional zones: a thin side for gas exchange and a thick side that serves for both structural support and fluid exchange. On the thin side, the alveolocapillary membrane measures no more than 0.3 to 0.5 μm in thickness and consists of three layers—the alveolar epithelium, the capillary endothelium, and the fused basement membranes in between (Fig. 51–2). This arrangement provides the lung with an enormous area for gas exchange without the encumbrance of excessive mass. By contrast, between the basement membranes on the thick side is a relatively thick interstitial tissue compartment that contains collagen and elastic fibers, proteoglycans, contractile interstitial cells (myofibroblasts), and inflammatory cells (principally macrophages). This compartment not only provides support for the capillary network but also constitutes an essential component of the water-exchanging apparatus of the lung, operating to expedite the removal of water and proteins from the interstitial space toward the lymphatic capillaries.[3] When excess water and protein accumulate in the alveolar septa, as in interstitial pulmonary edema, they do so exclusively or predominantly on the thick side (Fig. 51–3).[27]

Electron microscopic and freeze-fracture studies have shown that the pulmonary capillaries are virtually indistinguishable from those found in muscle.[28] Unlike endothelial

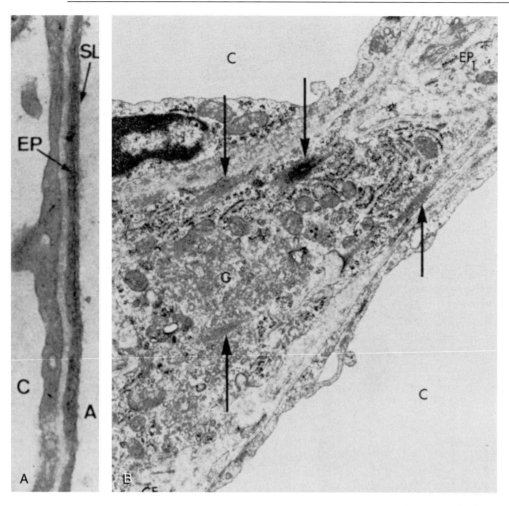

**Figure 51–2. The Air-Blood Barrier.** *A*, Thin portion. A capillary (C) is present on the left and the alveolar space (A) on the right. A type I alveolar epithelial cell (EP) is covered by a clearly extracellular osmiophilic layer (SL). (TEM, ×48,420.) (From Gil J, Weibel ER: Resp Physiol 8:13, 1969.) *B*, Thick portion. Capillaries (C) and epithelial cells (EP₁) are separated by collagen fibers (CF) and a prominent interstitial cell (myofibroblast) containing a Golgi apparatus (G) and numerous fibrillar bundles *(arrows)*. (Rat lung; TEM, ×24,000.) (From Kapanci Y, Assimacopoulos A, Irle C, et al: J Cell Biol 60:375, 1974. Copyright, The Rockefeller University Press.)

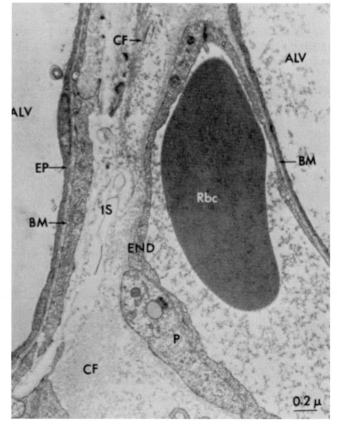

**Figure 51–3. Interstitial Pulmonary Edema.** The interstitial space (IS) of the thick portion of the alveolar septum has been considerably widened by edema fluid during hydrostatic pulmonary edema, whereas the opposite thin part, containing the fused basement membranes (BM), remains unchanged in thickness. ALV, alveolar space; EP, alveolar epithelium; IS, interstitial space; CF, collagen fibers; END, capillary endothelium; Rbc, red blood cell. Transmission electron microscope (TEM) section stained with uranil acetate and lead citrate (×12,000). (Reprinted from Fishman A: Circulation 46:389, 1972. With permission of the author and The American Heart Association Inc.)

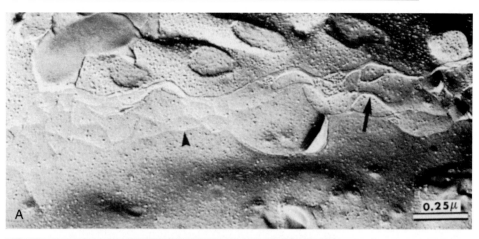

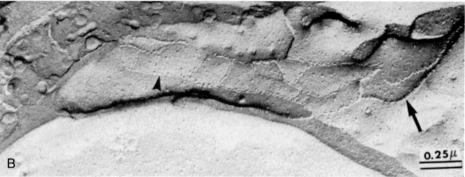

**Figure 51–4. Epithelial and Endothelial Cell Junctions.** A tight junction between a type I and a type II pneumocyte is shown in *A*. On the ectoplasmic fracture face, the tight junction is a reticulum of furrows *(arrowhead)*. On the protoplasmic fracture face, it is a reticulum of continuous fibers *(arrow)*. An endothelial tight junction between two alveolar capillary endothelial cells is shown in *B*. On ectoplasmic fracture faces, the tight junction is a reticulum of furrows containing particles *(arrowhead)*. On the protoplasmic fracture face, the junctional complex consists of discontinuous particles *(arrow)*. The differences in the complexity of the tight junction structure between endothelial and epithelial cells are believed to relate to the different permeability of these tissues. (Courtesy of Dr. David Walker, University of British Columbia, Vancouver.)

cells in visceral capillaries, those in the pulmonary capillaries do not have large fenestrations and are held together by tight junctions that extend around the cells in a zipper-like fashion, thereby keeping them in close approximation (Fig. 51–4). Strands are evident on freeze fracture through the junctional complex of endothelial cell contacts, representing protein particles within the cell membrane of opposing cells; it is these structural proteins that provide endothelial integrity. Discontinuities in these strands form the paracellular pathway or "pores" through which the bulk of water transport and all of the solute transport occurs across the endothelium. The junctional complexes of the capillary endothelium are much less well developed than those of the alveolar epithelial cells; because there is a correlation between the number of junctional strands and the permeability of a cellular membrane, this explains the known differences in pulmonary capillary and epithelial permeability.[29] The results of some studies suggest that large discontinuities in the tight junctions can exist at the junction between three adjacent capillary endothelial cells, such "pores" being visible on electron microscopy.[30] There are relatively fewer junctional strands (and by inference, more permeable endothelium) on the venous than on the arterial end of the capillary membrane.[28]

To cross the endothelium, water-soluble substances must be transported by pinocytosis or must pass through the paracellular pathway just described. The selective sieving of protein molecules according to their molecular size suggests that the primary pathway for protein movement across the endothelium is by means of the paracellular pathway. Small molecules traverse the pulmonary capillary endothelium with ease, whereas larger molecules are excluded in direct propor-

tion to their molecular size; very large molecules do not reach the pulmonary interstitium at all. There have been a number of attempts to model and calculate the size of the "pores" between pulmonary endothelial cells by measuring transendothelial flux of different-sized tracer molecules and water, as a function of varying microvascular pressures. No simple pore model can adequately explain the transport characteristics, and it is probable that "pores" in the capillary endothelium possess a wide variety of sizes. The results of calculations suggest that there are a large number of small "pores" that only allow transport of water and many fewer large "pores" that permit transport of protein.[31–34] For example, the data in one model were best explained by a large population of pores 12 to 14 nm in diameter and a small number of pores measuring 40 to 44 nm;[35] the ratio of small to large pores was estimated to be 200:1.

It has been hypothesized that a rise in pulmonary microvascular pressure can increase the size of the gaps between endothelial cells, thus increasing protein permeability (the "stretched pore theory"). Although this theory remains controversial, it is probable that within a range of moderately elevated microvascular pressures, pulmonary endothelial permeability is not directly affected by pressure.[36] However, when pulmonary capillary pressure exceeds a critical value (about 30 cm $H_2O$), stress failure of the capillary endothelial membrane can result, leading to the development of increased permeability edema and intra-alveolar hemorrhage.[37, 38] It should be appreciated that the "pores" through which fluid movement normally occurs in the pulmonary microvasculature represent a minute fraction of the total capillary surface area; in fact, the surface area occupied by "pores" may be as little as one millionth of the total endothelial surface area.[39] As a result, a doubling or tripling of the surface area occupied by "pores" might not be detected by conventional microscopic techniques, whereas it would markedly enhance fluid and solute transport.

### The Bronchial Circulation and Endothelium

The bronchial circulation and the structures it supplies are described in detail in Chapter 2 (*see* page 119). Briefly, the bronchial arteries supply the airway walls, the peribronchial and perivascular connective tissue, the visceral pleura over the mediastinal and diaphragmatic surfaces of the lungs, mediastinal and hilar lymph nodes, and the vasa vasorum of the large arteries and veins within the thorax. Within the airway walls, the bronchial vessels form two extensive plexuses, one inside the smooth muscle (the submucosal plexus) and the other outside it (the peribronchial plexus). At the level of the respiratory bronchioles, the bronchial capillary network meshes with the pulmonary capillary and venous system. The majority of the bronchial blood drains to the left side of the heart by means of capillary and venous anastomoses with the pulmonary circulation;[40] the portion that supplies the large airways returns through bronchial veins to the azygos and hemiazygos veins and ultimately reaches the right atrium.

Although the total blood flow through the bronchial circulation is small relative to that through the pulmonary circulation, the bronchial microcirculation may still play an important role in fluid exchange within the lung. In some animal species, the surface area of the bronchial microvessels has been calculated to be as much as one half of the corresponding airway epithelial surface area.[41] If a similar anatomic arrangement were to exist in humans, these vessels would provide a large surface area for fluid exchange.[42] Unfortunately, there are few data concerning either this variable or the permeability of the bronchial microvascular endothelium in humans.

The microscopic anatomy of the bronchial microvessels is quite different from that of the pulmonary capillaries. The bronchial capillary endothelium is similar to that in microvessels in the liver, gut, and kidney with respect to the presence of fenestrae between the cells, an anatomic feature that suggests increased permeability compared with the pulmonary endothelium. In addition, bronchial microvessels respond to pharmacologic agents differently from those of the pulmonary circulation.[43] The endothelial lining cells of the bronchial capillaries and venules contain a rich network of contractile fibers. Administration of histamine, bradykinin, or the mast cell degranulating substance 48–80 causes contraction of these intracellular fibers, resulting in enlargement of paracellular pathways and increased permeability of the microvessels to large-molecular-weight substances and tracers such as colloidal carbon.[42] Flow through the bronchial circulation is strongly controlled by the endothelial secretion of nitric oxide, a potent vasodilator; if nitric oxide synthesis is inhibited, marked vasoconstriction occurs, whereas if it is stimulated (as occurs during inflammation), a marked increase in bronchial blood flow is the result.[44]

Although these anatomic and functional features make the bronchial circulation a potentially important contributor to pulmonary fluid exchange, there is little direct evidence to implicate the bronchial circulation in the production of pulmonary edema. In one study in sheep, there was a modest increase in lung lymph flow and microvascular permeability when histamine was infused directly into the bronchial artery;[45] however, the investigators attributed this to the effects of the drug on the pulmonary circulation, which it could have reached through anastomotic channels.

### The Pulmonary Interstitium

The interstitial connective tissue of the lung can be considered as a branching system that supports alveoli and airways on the one hand and the large and small vessels on the other. The interstitial space can be divided into two functionally distinct compartments—an alveolar wall (parenchymal) compartment and a peribronchovascular (axial) compartment. The latter is in continuity with the interstitial tissue surrounding the pulmonary veins and in the interlobular septa and pleura. As discussed previously, the alveolar wall compartment consists of the thick side of the alveolocapillary membrane. Despite the fact that there are no qualitative differences in the connective tissue in the two "compartments," their compliance and ability to store fluid are quite different; the parenchymal compartment is very noncompliant, so that interstitial edema tends to accumulate to a lesser extent in alveolar walls than in the peribronchovascular compartment. Staub and coworkers have shown that not only does an interstitial phase of edema exist for a variable period before alveolar flooding occurs but edema also develops in the connective tissue around the airways and vessels before it accumulates in the alveolar septa (Fig. 51–5).[46]

Pulmonary interstitial tissue is a gel that contains both connective tissue fibers and cells. The gel itself is composed of a matrix of highly polymerized glycosaminoglycans that, in combination with proteins, form glycoproteins that are called proteoglycans. The principal glycosaminoglycans are chondroitin sulfate and hyaluronic acid. The glycoprotein complexes are extremely hydrophilic and can bind large amounts of water with weak hydrogen bonds; the combination of the loosely bound water molecules and the large complex macromolecules forms the gel. A significant portion of the water within the interstitial space is inaccessible to large-molecular-weight solutes such as serum proteins. This portion of the interstitial water volume is called the *excluded volume*. The latter can be likened to water contained within "capsules" that have semipermeable membranes (i.e., permeable to water and small-molecular-weight solutes but not to proteins). As a result of the excluded volume, the protein concentration (and therefore the osmotic pressure) of the interstitial fluid is greater than would be calculated from the known quantities of protein and water. It has been suggested that during swelling of the interstitial space, some of the "excluded" water is released from the proteoglycans;[47] by diluting interstitial protein, it lowers the interstitial osmotic pressure, thereby providing a safety factor that retards the further development of pulmonary edema. It has also been suggested that proteoglycans may be fragmented during the development of edema, resulting in an increased compliance of the interstitial space.[47a] However, it has been argued that water bound to the proteoglycans cannot be made "available" during swelling of the gel and that only a washout of interstitial proteoglycan can decrease the excluded volume.[48]

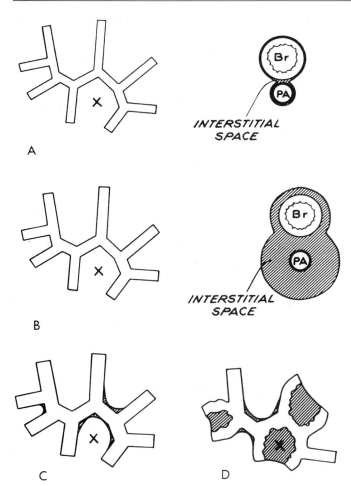

**Figure 51–5. Schematic Representation of the Sequence of Fluid Accumulation in Acute Pulmonary Edema.** *A*, Normal lung (alveolar wall and alveoli on the left, bronchovascular bundle on the right); *B*, interstitial edema in which fluid has accumulated preferentially in the interstitial space around the conducting blood vessels and airways without affecting the alveolar walls; *C*, early alveolar edema showing interstitial spaces filled and fluid present in alveoli, preferentially at the corners at which the curvature is greatest; *D*, alveolar flooding in which individual alveoli have reached a critical configuration at which existing inflation pressure can no longer maintain stability and the alveolar gas volume rapidly passes to a new configuration with much reduced curvature. (Slightly modified from Staub NE, Nagano H, Pearce ML: J Appl Physiol 22:227, 1967, with permission.)

It has been estimated that 40% of the extravascular water of the lung is in the extracellular interstitial compartment. During the development of interstitial pulmonary edema, this volume can more than double before alveolar flooding occurs. In fact, the fluid storage capacity of the interstitial space increases as lung volume is increased. One group found that the interstitium contained less than 1 ml of water per gm of dry lung at a transpulmonary pressure of 5 cm $H_2O$ as compared with 6 ml of water per gm of dry lung at a transpulmonary pressure of 15 cm $H_2O$.[49] Pulmonary inflation in an already edematous lung can also redistribute the edema fluid, shifting it from alveolar air spaces to the peribronchovascular interstitial compartment. This phenomenon has been demonstrated in animal models of both hydrostatic[50] and permeability[51] pulmonary edema and may be a practical explanation for the beneficial effect of positive end-expiratory pressure (PEEP).

## The Alveolocapillary Membrane

The alveolar side of the alveolocapillary membrane consists of a continuous epithelium composed predominantly of thin cytoplasmic extensions of type 1 alveolar epithelial cells. A continuous, well-defined basement membrane is shared with the basement membrane of the capillary endothelium on the thin side of the alveolar wall. The intercellular junctions of the alveolar epithelium are much more developed than those of the capillary endothelium, a morphologic complexity that is reflected in impermeability to all lipid-insoluble substances other than water.[29, 52] The permeability of the alveolar membrane can be tested by measuring the appearance of intravenously administered tracer molecules in the alveolar fluid or by measuring the appearance of tracers placed into the alveolar air spaces in the blood. Only small molecules, such as urea and sucrose, and ions, such as sodium and calcium, are able to diffuse across the alveolar epithelium; however, like the capillary endothelium, there appears to be a sieving that is based on molecular size.[11, 53] This size selectivity allows the calculation of an equivalent "pore" radius, which in lambs has been found to range from 0.7 to 1.4 nm; however, the permeability of the membrane increases during lung inflation as a result of an increase in calculated "pore" radius to 3 to 4 nm.[53] This estimated range of alveolar epithelial pore size contrasts to the calculated range of "pore" size in the capillary endothelium, in which a proportion of "pores" as large as 100 nm is required to explain the difference in lymph and plasma protein concentration.[33, 34]

The alveolar air spaces are lined by a layer of fluid 0.2 to 0.3 μm thick, the total volume having been estimated to be approximately 20 ml.[11] In air-filled lungs, the liquid smoothes out any irregularities in the alveolar wall and transforms the air-fluid interface into a smooth regular membrane with a constant radius of curvature.[54] This smoothing effect is caused by the surface tension generated at the air-liquid interface.

## The Lymphatic System

Pulmonary lymphatic capillaries are similar to those in other organs with a discontinuous or absent basement membrane and attenuated, irregular endothelial lining cells that have poorly developed intercellular junctions.[55] The lymphatic endothelium is thought to offer no significant impedance to the flow of water or protein from the lung interstitium,[12] and it is generally believed that the concentration of solute in the "nonexcluded" portion of the interstitial liquid is the same as that in lymph;[7] however, it is possible that the protein concentration of lymph may be altered during its passage through regional lymph nodes.[56]

The lymphatics begin as blind-ended vessels in the region of the alveolar ducts and respiratory bronchioles,[57] close to alveolar walls.[58] Tissue fluid enters the terminal lymphatics through the gaps between endothelial cells. The lymphatic walls are tethered to the surrounding connective tissue by a mesh of fine filaments so that when the tissue swells there is increased traction on the lymphatics that keeps them patent and facilitates drainage.[59] Once the tissue fluid has entered the peripheral ends of the lymphatic vessels, it is pumped centrally, any bidirectional movement being prevented by valves. The pumping is partly passive, being related to the respiratory motion of the lungs; however, it is also active, the larger pulmonary lymphatics being surrounded by a layer of smooth muscle that contracts rhythmically, propelling lymph centripetally.[11] Pulmonary lymphatics can generate considerable pressure when obstructed (up to 60 cm $H_2O$), and lymph continues to empty into the systemic circulation despite an elevation in systemic venous pressure.[11] However, it has been suggested that high venous pressure can impair lymphatic function to some extent; in one experimental study in dogs, hydrostatic pulmonary edema increased in severity when superior vena caval pressure was increased to 30 cm $H_2O$.[60]

## Physiologic Considerations

### The Starling Equation

The factors that govern the formation and removal of extravascular water within the lungs are described by the fluid transport equation, originally proposed by Starling (Fig. 51–6).[61] This equation describes the net flux of fluid across a membrane under steady state conditions, transport being almost entirely by bulk flow:

$$\dot{Q}f = Kf\,[(Pmv - Ppmv) - \sigma(\pi mv - \pi pmv)]$$

where $\dot{Q}f$ = the net transvascular fluid flow, a value that should be equivalent to the net lymphatic flow from the lung in the absence of edema formation; $Kf$ = the filtration coefficient, a measure of fluid conductance; $Pmv$ = the

hydrostatic pressure in the lumen of the fluid-exchanging microvessels; $Ppmv$ = the hydrostatic pressure in the interstitial tissue surrounding the fluid-exchanging microvessels; $\sigma$ = the osmotic reflection coefficient (i.e., a number between 0 and 1 that describes the effectiveness of the membrane in preventing the flow of protein compared with the flow of water); $\pi mv$ = the protein osmotic pressure in the microvascular lumen; and $\pi pmv$ = the protein osmotic pressure in the interstitial fluid surrounding the microvessels.

The factors governing the net flux of a given solute across the membrane are described in the solute transport equation:

$$\dot{Q}s = PS(\pi mv - \pi pmv) + (1 - \sigma)\,\overline{C}s\dot{Q}f$$

where $\dot{Q}s$ = the net transport of a specific protein; $PS$ = the net permeability surface area product, a measure of the permeability of the membrane to protein; $\pi mv$ and $\pi pmv$ = the microvascular and perimicrovascular concentrations of the specific protein; $\sigma$ = the reflection coefficient for the specific protein; and $\overline{C}s$ = the average protein concentration in the membrane. Because the endothelium is freely permeable to small molecules, such as electrolytes, which flow across the membrane with water and exert no net osmotic effect, this equation applies only to the transport of plasma proteins.[6]

Because the endothelial permeability and the reflection coefficient are different for protein molecules of different sizes, their net flux will be inversely related to molecular weight; the steady-state interstitial concentrations of proteins relative to their plasma concentration will also vary as a

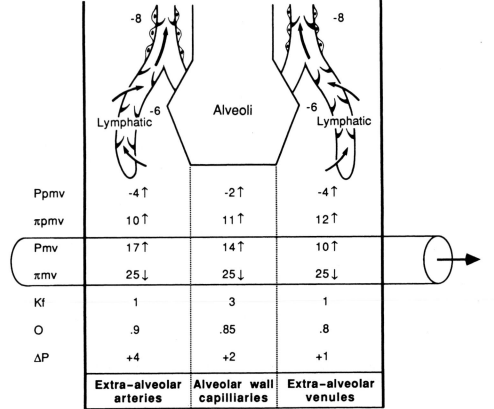

**Figure 51–6. A Three-Compartment Model of Starling's Forces.** The values for microvascular and perimicrovascular hydrostatic and osmotic pressures represent rough estimates and have been chosen to illustrate the longitudinal variation of the net driving pressure ($\Delta P$) within the exchanging vessels. The arbitrary values for $Kf$ illustrate the relative importance of the different compartments to overall lung fluid exchange, and the values for the reflection coefficient ($\sigma$) reflect the morphometric complexity of endothelial intercellular junctions on the arterial and venous side of the microcirculation. A value of 1.0 for $\sigma$ would represent a membrane that was freely permeable to water but completely impermeable to protein. The driving pressure is greatest in the precapillary vessels and least in the postcapillary venules. There is a gradient in interstitial pressure that drives fluid from the pericapillary interstitial space toward the hilum. (Modified from Staub NC: Pathophysiology of pulmonary edema. *In* Staub NC, Taylor AE [eds]: Edema. New York, Raven Press, 1984, p 719.)

|  | Extra-alveolar arteries | Alveolar wall capilliaries | Extra-alveolar venules |
|---|---|---|---|
| Ppmv | -4 ↑ | -2 ↑ | -4 ↑ |
| πpmv | 10 ↑ | 11 ↑ | 12 ↑ |
| Pmv | 17 ↑ | 14 ↑ | 10 ↑ |
| πmv | 25 ↓ | 25 ↓ | 25 ↓ |
| Kf | 1 | 3 | 1 |
| σ | .9 | .85 | .8 |
| ΔP | +4 | +2 | +1 |

function of molecular size. When pulmonary microvascular permeability and pressures are normal, the ratios of lymphatic (representing interstitial) to plasma protein concentrations for albumin, globulin, and fibrinogen are approximately 0.8, 0.5, and 0.2, respectively.[9] As microvascular pressure is increased, the ratios for proteins of all sizes decrease as the transport of fluid outstrips protein transport. The net result is a dilution of interstitial proteins and a decrease in the perimicrovascular interstitial osmotic pressure; this phenomenon represents one of the safety factors that limit edema formation.

Under normal steady-state conditions, there is a continual net outward flow of fluid and protein from the pulmonary microvasculature to the interstitium; these substances are then returned to the bloodstream by the lymphatics. When this balance is disrupted, edema results, initially in the interstitial space but eventually in air spaces when the imbalance of forces becomes more severe or more prolonged. Although an increase in capillary hydrostatic pressure (Pmv) or an increase in endothelial permeability (Kf) are the most common causes of edema, it is useful to discuss each of the factors in the Starling equation individually because all are important determinants of transvascular fluid flux.

### Microvascular Hydrostatic Pressure (Pmv)

A gradient in intraluminal hydrostatic pressure exists in the pulmonary vasculature from the main pulmonary arteries to the large pulmonary veins and left atrium. The hydrostatic pressure in the fluid-exchanging vessels must be somewhere between the mean pulmonary arterial pressure (about 20 cm $H_2O$) and the mean left atrial pressure (about 5 cm $H_2O$). The actual value is predominantly dependent on the relative resistances of the vessels upstream and downstream from the fluid-exchanging vessels. If arterial resistance is high relative to venous resistance, a large arterial frictional pressure loss will occur and microvascular pressure will be close to venous pressure. Conversely, if venous resistance is large relative to arterial resistance and the majority of the pressure drop occurs across the venous system, pulmonary microvascular pressure will approach arterial pressure. In Zone III conditions,

$$Pmv = PLa + RV(PPa - PLa)/RA + RV$$

where Pmv = microvascular pressure; PLa = left atrial pressure; RV and RA = venous and arterial resistances, respectively; and PPa = pulmonary arterial pressure.[7] The results of most studies show that venous resistance is slightly less than arterial resistance, and it has been suggested that the value of 0.4 can be used for the normal fractional contribution of venous resistance in the calculation of Pmv.[7] Although it is true that most pathologic conditions increase microvascular pressure by increasing outflow pressure (PLa) and/or outflow resistance (RV), microvascular pressure can also be increased by an increase in pulmonary arterial pressure or pulmonary blood flow.[15] An increase in hydrostatic pressure may be important in the pathogenesis of neurogenic pulmonary edema and the edema that is occasionally seen after pulmonary thromboembolism,[61a] catecholamine administration,[61b] or increased cardiac output in the presence of pulmonary hypertension.[62]

If mean pulmonary arterial pressure is 20 cm $H_2O$ and mean left atrial pressure is 4 cm $H_2O$:

$$Pmv = 4 + 0.4 \times (20 - 4) = 10.4 \ cm \ H_2O$$

In Zone I and II conditions, the relative contributions of arterial and venous resistance will change.

Indirect measurements of the arterial and venous resistances have been made using techniques that employ a fluid bolus of low viscosity or that use rapid inflow and outflow occlusion.[63, 64] Direct measurements of microvascular pressure have also been made in subpleural vessels using micropuncture techniques, allowing calculation of the serial distribution of vascular resistance within the lung.[65] According to these measurements, approximately 40% of the total pressure drop between the pulmonary artery and left atrium occurs within the alveolar wall capillaries themselves; in addition, there is very little resistance in arterial vessels larger than 50 $\mu m$ in diameter or in veins larger than 20 $\mu m$. These results mean that there must be substantial variation in microvascular pressure along the relatively short length of the pulmonary capillaries and that fluid filtration may occur at the arterial end of the capillary while reabsorption from the interstitial space to the capillary lumen could occur at the venous end. As indicated previously, fluid transport across the pulmonary vascular endothelium occurs in pulmonary arterioles and venules as well as capillaries. A three-compartment model of lung fluid exchange in which the balance of forces and microvascular permeability vary from arterial microvessels to venous microvessels has been suggested.[9]

Although it is customary to talk of a single microvascular pressure within the pulmonary vasculature, it is obvious that there must be a large regional variation caused by the effects of gravity. Measurements of vascular pressures are normally referenced to the level of the left atrium; in the erect position, there is approximately 15 cm of lung above and 10 cm below this level. Pulmonary arterial and venous pressures decrease or increase by 1 cm $H_2O$ pressure for each centimeter that the vessel in question is above or below the left atrium. If the pulmonary microvessels were noncompressible, the capillary pressure would also vary directly as a function of lung height. However, because they can be compressed or distended, the hydrostatic gradient affects the ratio of arterial to venous resistance that also influences capillary pressure. Nevertheless, it has been demonstrated that most of the lung is within 5 cm above and below the level of the left atrium in the erect as well as in the prone or supine positions.[9] Because there is as much lung above as below this level, the integrated microvascular pressure over the height of the lung is not much different from that which would be calculated from the average PPa and PLa at the level of the left atrium.

### Perimicrovascular Interstitial Hydrostatic Pressure (Ppmv)

Just as there is no unique value for microvascular pressure, there is also no unique value that describes pulmonary interstitial pressure. Direct measurements of pressure in the connective tissue near the hilum have shown it to be subatmospheric (about −5 cm $H_2O$ at functional residual capacity [FRC]), being more negative than pleural or alveolar pressure; it becomes progressively more negative during lung inflation (about $-12$ cm $H_2O$ at total lung capacity).[66-68]

Direct measurements of interstitial pressure have been made using a micropuncture technique in the subpleural parenchyma in close proximity to alveolar vessels; the pressures in this location were less than in the perihilar region, although still subatmospheric (about $-3$ cm $H_2O$).[65] Presumably, the pericapillary pressure is even less negative, because there must be a gradient in pressure that drives fluid from the pericapillary to the perihilar (axial) interstitial compartment (*see* Fig. 51-6).[9] Theoretically, alveolar wall pressure should be equal to alveolar pressure minus the pressure generated by alveolar wall and surface tension. Using known values for alveolar surface tension and the radius of curvature of the alveoli, an estimate of 1 cm $H_2O$ negative relative to alveolar pressure has been calculated.[69]

There is probably a vertical gradient in interstitial pressure from the top to the bottom of the lung. In a study of dogs in which an indirect method was used to measure interstitial pressure, the vertical gradient in interstitial pressure was 0.6 cm $H_2O$/cm.[70] Interestingly, there is no gradient in interstitial pressure in excised lungs, in which there is a uniform transpulmonary pressure; this suggests that the gradient in interstitial pressure *in situ* is a reflection of the vertical gradient in transpulmonary pressure.[19] The fact that microvascular pressure changes by 1.0 cm $H_2O$ for each centimeter and interstitial pressure by only 0.6 cm $H_2O$/cm probably explains the tendency for pulmonary edema to occur preferentially in dependent lung. In addition, as edema fluid forms, the resistance to fluid flow through the interstitial space decreases, so that gravity-dependent downward flow in this space may exceed lymphatic clearance, causing an accumulation of fluid at the lung bases.[71, 72]

### Plasma Protein Osmotic Pressure ($\pi$mv)

The osmotic pressure exerted by plasma proteins is dependent on their concentration and on the permeability of the endothelial membrane to protein. The maximal potential osmotic pressure can be calculated using standard equations[73, 74] or measured with an osmometer.[75] This value represents the osmotic pressure that would be produced by that concentration of protein acting across a membrane that was completely impermeable to protein (i.e., reflection coefficient of 1.0). To calculate osmotic pressure accurately, the albumin and globulin fractions of the serum protein should be known. Osmotic pressure increases alinearly with protein concentration and linearly with the albumin fraction.[74]

### Interstitial Protein Osmotic Pressure ($\pi$pmv)

Although plasma protein concentration (and therefore osmotic pressure) is constant throughout the microvasculature, substantial regional variations in protein concentration and osmotic pressure probably exist within the interstitium. It is assumed that the protein concentration of lung lymph represents the average protein concentration within the interstitium; however, this assumption may be invalid if there is significant inhomogeneity of protein concentration within the interstitial space.[48] Interstitial protein concentration decreases as fluid filtration increases, so that it is probable that the concentration is lowest at the base of the lung where

gravity promotes the largest fluid filtration rate.[31] As discussed previously, the longitudinal variation in net filtration pressure and microvascular permeability from the arterial to the venous sides of the microvasculature favors the development of differences in protein concentration between the two sides. Like the osmotic pressure of the plasma, the interstitial osmotic pressure is related to protein concentration; however, because of the alinear relationship between osmotic pressure and solute concentration, a halving in protein concentration results in more than a 50% decrease in osmotic pressure.

### The Filtration Coefficient (Kf)

The filtration coefficient is a measure of endothelial permeability to water. It is analogous to the pulmonary airway conductance for air flow or diffusing capacity of the alveolocapillary membrane for a gas. The units for the filtration coefficient are ml per minute per cm $H_2O$ per unit lung weight; the more permeable the endothelium, the larger is the value for Kf (i.e., the greater the fluid flux for a given net driving pressure). For the lung as a whole, Kf is influenced by both the permeability of the endothelium and the surface area available for fluid transport. If closed microvessels are opened (recruited) as a result of an increase in microvascular pressure, Kf will increase without an actual increase in "permeability"; for this reason, the whole-organ filtration coefficient is often spoken of as the permeability–surface area product.

It is impossible to measure Kf *in vivo*. In fact, even in excised lung preparations the reported values simply represent the best estimates, because to calculate Kf precisely, it is necessary to know the four pertinent pressures (Pmv, Ppmv, $\pi$mv, and $\pi$pmv) as well as the permeability of the endothelium to protein ($\sigma$) and the net fluid flux.[9, 12]

### The Osmotic Reflection Coefficient ($\sigma$)

A solute will exert a net osmotic pressure across a membrane only if the membrane is less permeable to the solute than it is to the solvent and if there is a difference in the concentration of solute on the two sides of the membrane. If the pulmonary capillary endothelium were impermeable to ions such as $Na^+$ and $Cl^-$, these solutes would exert an enormous osmotic pressure across the microvascular endothelium (about 5,000 cm $H_2O$ at normal plasma ion concentrations).[11] Because these ions freely traverse the endothelium, there is no difference in ion concentration between plasma and interstitial fluid and thus no osmotic pressure gradient. The reflection coefficient is a numerical estimate of the permeability of the membrane to a solute and therefore is also an estimate of the effectiveness with which a given concentration of solute can exert osmotic pressure. A reflection coefficient of 1 means that the membrane is completely impermeable to the solute and that the osmotic pressure exerted by that solute will be equal to that measured in an osmometer. When the reflection coefficient is zero, the membrane is completely permeable to the solute and the solute exerts no osmotic pressure. A coefficient of 0.5 means that one half of the potentially available osmotic pressure is exerted by the solute.[11]

Although it is often assumed that the reflection coefficient for plasma proteins is 1, experimental data suggest that more appropriate values are approximately 0.85, 0.9, and 0.98 for albumin, globulin, and fibrinogen, respectively.[9] The values for osmotic reflection coefficient vary according to the method that is used to measure it. Values between 0.3 and 0.98 have been reported for albumin in different experimental preparations.[15] In the presence of noncardiogenic pulmonary edema, the capillary endothelial permeability for water (Kf) and protein ($\sigma$) is altered; when the endothelium is severely damaged, the reflection coefficient approaches zero so that plasma proteins exert no effective pressure across the endothelium and the most powerful force preventing the formation of edema is lost.

### Fluid Transport across the Alveolar Epithelium

The morphologic appearance of the alveolar epithelial tight junctions suggests that the alveolar epithelium is much less permeable than the endothelium to water and solute, an hypothesis confirmed by physiologic studies.[29] Although the principles that govern fluid and solute transport across the endothelium are the same as those that operate across the epithelium, the fluid conductivity is at least one order of magnitude lower; since the membrane is so restrictive, solutes that do not exert osmotic pressure across the endothelium (electrolytes) can have important effects on fluid balance across the epithelium. Although the protein content of the fluid lining the alveoli is unknown, the electrolyte content is probably quite different from that in the plasma and interstitium as a result of active transport of chloride across epithelial cells into the alveolar liquid.[76, 77]

The transport of fluid and solute across the alveolar epithelium can be measured accurately only when the air spaces are full of liquid, a state that occurs normally only in the fetus. In the normal adult lung, the surface tension present at the interface between alveolar liquid and air exerts a pressure that tends to suck fluid from the interstitium into the air spaces. Because of the ability of surfactant to lower surface tension, this pressure is small (about 15 cm $H_2O$); however, when surfactant is deficient or inactivated, the increase in surface tension can play an important role in the formation of alveolar edema fluid.[78]

### Fluid Transport across the Bronchial Endothelium

The components of the Starling equation that are necessary to calculate fluid transport across the bronchial vascular endothelium are largely unknown. However, there are a number of features that, taken together, suggest that the bronchial microvasculature may be an important site of fluid exchange, including (1) the morphologic evidence of large intercellular gaps; (2) the likelihood that capillary hydrostatic pressure in these systemic microvessels is considerably higher than in the pulmonary microvasculature;[11] and (3) the probability that a more negative interstitial fluid pressure surrounds these vessels as they pass through the peribronchovascular connective tissue.

### The Safety Factors

Normally, the alveolar air spaces remain ideally moist despite substantial changes in microvascular and interstitial pressure related to posture, gravity, variations in hydration, and changes in lung volume. The homeostasis is provided by a number of safety factors that tend to minimize accumulation of fluid in the lung.[9]

### The Lymphatic System

Lung lymph flow is the first and most important safety factor. In the presence of an acute increase in microvascular pressure or permeability, lymph flow from the lung can increase 10-fold or more before there is significant accumulation of edema fluid.[7] The rate of lung lymph flow during pulmonary edema is unknown in humans. However, in one study in which *Pseudomonas aeruginosa* bacteremia was used to induce endothelial permeability in sheep, steady-state lymph flows were found to increase 10 times from baseline and absolute flows were as high as 70 ml per hour.[79] Scaling these results up to those of adult humans suggests that steady-state lung lymph flows of up to 200 ml per hour may be achieved.

It is curious that excess water should ever accumulate in the lungs in the face of such an elaborate drainage system.[3] Whether or not a "ceiling" exists for lymphatic drainage is disputable. In the experiments on sheep described earlier, the investigators were unable to demonstrate a maximal lymph flow.[79] However, others have suggested that a ceiling for lymphatic drainage exists and is set by the relatively small caliber of the thoracic and right lymphatic ducts.[80] In chronic left ventricular failure, the lymphatic vessels proliferate and increase in caliber.[81] These effects have been shown in a series of studies in dogs in which acute pulmonary edema was produced by partial obstruction of the left atrium by a balloon and chronic heart failure by creation of an aortocaval anastomosis.[82–84] During acute pulmonary edema there was only a small increase in lymph flow in the right lymphatic duct; however, during chronic heart failure there was a major increase in pulmonary lymph flow ranging from 300% to 2,800% more than the normal flow of 4 ml/hour. Thus, in these experiments, at least, the lymphatics were relatively ineffectual in removing acute accumulations of lung water; however, they showed important functional expansion over a period of time and acted as a compensatory mechanism for the prevention of overt alveolar edema. These experiments are analogous to the clinical states of acute pulmonary edema (e.g., after acute myocardial infarction) on the one hand and chronic left atrial hypertension (e.g., from chronic mitral stenosis) on the other.

When lymphatic drainage is impaired because of obstruction in the lymphatic channels or the draining lymph nodes, fluid accumulates within the lungs. However, this is seldom, if ever, the sole cause of pulmonary edema. For example, partial ligation of pulmonary lymphatics causes pulmonary edema in animals only after a simultaneous increase in left atrial pressure has been produced by production of a mitral valve lesion.[85, 86] One might anticipate that the systemic venous hypertension that occurs in isolated right ventricular failure might impede lymph flow from the lung to a degree that would result in pulmonary edema; however, this is seldom, if ever, the case.[87, 88] The combination of tachypneic ventilatory movements and muscular contraction of the walls of the large lymphatics presumably suffices to keep the lungs free of edema under these circumstances.[3]

The ability of the lymphatic system to remove fluid and protein from the lung is enhanced in the presence of damage to the pulmonary endothelium; it has been estimated that the maximal lymph flow can be four times higher in the presence of capillary endothelial damage than can be achieved during comparable edematous states induced by increasing microvascular pressure.[89] The mechanism for this stimulation of lymphatic clearance is not known; however, it has been speculated that mediators may be released by the damaged endothelial cells, which cause the lymphatic system to become more efficient in removing fluid.[15]

### Protein Sieving

A second safety factor that operates in hydrostatic but not in permeability edema is dilution of the interstitial protein, resulting in a decrease in interstitial osmotic pressure during increased fluid transport. This effect is dependent on the relative impermeability of the microvascular endothelium to protein. As transvascular fluid movement increases as a result of elevated microvascular hydrostatic pressure, water transport outstrips protein transport; the resulting dilution of interstitial protein decreases the osmotic pressure and attenuates the driving pressure.[90] A corollary to the dilution of interstitial proteins is the concentration of plasma proteins that must result if the exit of water exceeds that of protein.

### Interstitial Compliance

The third safety factor that tends to minimize the accumulation of edema within the lungs is the increase in tissue pressure that accompanies the swelling of the interstitium. Although the precise pressure-volume relationship of the interstitial space is unknown, there is some agreement regarding its overall nature.[11] As fluid accumulates in the interstitial space, the structure of the tightly compacted gel resists deformation and pressure increases sharply after only a slight increase in volume. Once a certain amount of fluid has accumulated, the compliance of the gel appears to increase, so that further swelling occurs despite only a slight increase in pressure. In most tissues, an additional final phase of the pressure-volume relationship exists in which the interstitial compartment again becomes stiff; in the lung, the development of alveolar flooding at this stage opens up an enormous reserve for fluid accumulation and edema can accumulate rapidly accompanied by little increase in pressure. The results of morphologic studies suggest that the pressure-volume characteristics of the peribronchovascular interstitium are such that this space may be more compliant than that of the alveolar walls, because it is in this connective tissue that fluid first accumulates.[46]

It has been suggested that the integrity of the alveolar epithelium is an important component of this safety factor; the evidence for this concept comes from experimental studies on dogs in which it was found that there was more alveolar flooding and less accumulation of interstitial lung water in pulmonary edema induced by oleic acid than in hydrostatic pulmonary edema.[91] To the extent that the epithelium resists alveolar flooding, interstitial pressure will increase as fluid accumulates in this space. If the epithelium is damaged, as occurs in ARDS, alveolar flooding can occur at a much lower interstitial pressure.

Increased interstitial pressure may also serve as a protection against impaired gas exchange in the setting of edema. If interstitial pressure is high in edematous lung regions, vessels in that region will be compressed and blood flow will be redistributed to less edematous regions, minimizing the mismatching of ventilation and perfusion. This increase in interstitial pressure associated with fluid accumulation may be an explanation for the redistribution of pulmonary blood "flow" evident on erect chest radiographs in patients who have pulmonary venous hypertension; presumably, the interstitial edema is predominant in lower lung zones. When interstitial pressure fails to increase because of generalized damage to the alveolar epithelium, blood flow to the edematous regions will not decrease; as a consequence, arterial desaturation caused by pulmonary shunt will be more severe than that associated with equivalent degrees of hydrostatic edema.

### Active Transport of Water and NaCl

Another mechanism that serves to keep the alveolar air spaces free of excessive fluid is active transport of solute and water from the alveolar surface into the interstitium and, ultimately, the pulmonary capillary blood. Distal airway epithelial cells and alveolar type II cells express amiloride-sensitive $Na^+$ channels on their apical (luminal) surface and oubain-sensitive $Na^+,K^+$-ATPase pumps on their basal (abluminal) surfaces. Both of these ion channels can be stimulated to remove $Na^+$ from the alveoli and airways; water follows passively through specialized channels called aquaporins, which are made up of channel-forming integral membrane proteins.[16, 92] The process of active sodium and water transport appears to be enhanced in the early stages of alveolar capillary damage, as shown in experimental studies in which the degree of edema produced after an ischemia-reperfusion injury was markedly enhanced after administration of amiloride and oubain.[93] The increase in clearance during injury appears to be mediated by a beta-adrenergic mechanism; in an animal model of sepsis-induced lung injury the increased alveolar clearance of fluid was blocked by propranolol.[94]

### The Development and Clearance of Pulmonary Edema

The sequence of events that occurs during the development of pulmonary edema has been described in experimental animal models[46] and is similar for both hydrostatic and permeability edema.

The earliest manifestation of pulmonary edema observed by light microscopy is expansion of the connective tissue space around conducting airways, their accompanying vessels, and the interlobular septa (Fig. 51–7). Excess fluid also distends the lymphatics within the peribronchovascular interstitium. The appearance of fluid within these tissues occurs before there is alveolar flooding and when measurements of alveolar wall thickness are virtually normal. Fluid accumulation can markedly increase airway and vascular wall thickness; in experimental animals, the maximal fluid volume has been estimated to be 5% to 10% of air-space volume.[95, 96]

As the volume of edema fluid increases, there is a

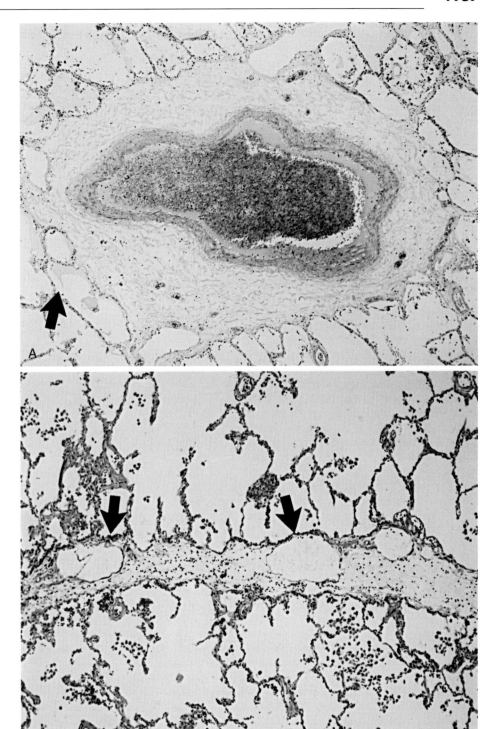

**Figure 51–7. Interstitial Pulmonary Edema.** A section of a medium-sized pulmonary artery *(A)* reveals widening of the perivascular interstitial tissue as a result of the presence of abundant fluid separating the connective tissue fibers. Mild air-space edema is also evident *(arrow)*. In the periphery of the lung, a section of an interlobular septum *(B)* shows similar widening as well as dilated lymphatic channels *(arrows)*. (*A*, ×40; *B*, ×60.)

progressive increase in alveolar wall thickness as fluid accumulates in the thick side of the alveolocapillary membrane. A transition has been observed between this phase and overt alveolar edema, characterized by the accumulation of small amounts of fluid within the air spaces confined to the alveolar "corners."[46]

Alveolar flooding begins after the extravascular water content of the lung has increased by approximately 50%.[71] The results of morphologic studies indicate that such flooding is an all-or-nothing phenomenon, alveoli being either liquid filled or air filled.[46, 97, 98] The lack of intermediate grades of filling suggests that flooding of individual alveoli occurs rapidly. In addition, alveolar flooding is patchy in nature; some alveoli fill with fluid whereas immediately adjacent alveoli remain dry. The walls of fluid-filled alveoli lose their circular shape and are folded, indicating loss of volume resulting from disruption of the normal surfactant layer by the edema fluid.

In both hydrostatic and permeability edema, the protein content of the fluid in the alveolar air spaces is the same as that in the interstitium,[99, 100] implying that the epithelium loses all ability to sieve during alveolar flooding and thus permits the outpouring of pure tissue fluid. It is easy to see how this could occur in permeability edema, in which the epithelium of the alveolar wall is damaged; however, exactly how the epithelial barrier gives way in hydrostatic edema is unresolved. It has been suggested that the fluid may enter the peripheral air spaces by airway epithelial junctions rather than the alveoli;[101] according to this theory, if interstitial pressure becomes sufficiently positive during edema formation, fluid may breach the epithelium of the small airways and flow peripherally to the alveoli ("the overflowing bathtub theory").[101] However, the results of anatomic studies in which fluorescent probes were used as tracers suggest that the site of leakage is the alveolar wall.[102]

Once the increase in microvascular pressure or microvascular permeability resolves, it is necessary to remove the accumulated edema fluid from the lung to restore normal function. Lymphatic clearance alone cannot account for the rate of clearance of pulmonary edema. Alternate pathways include reuptake into pulmonary microvessels, clearance up the tracheobronchial tree, flow into the mediastinum, and transport across the pleural surface into the pleural space.[18] Once edema fluid reaches the pleural space it is returned to the systemic circulation through the pleural lymphatics. This pathway was shown to account for between 23% and 29% of fluid clearance in a model of hydrostatic edema[103] and 21% clearance in oleic acid induced edema.[104] It is also necessary to remove protein from the alveoli. Most evidence suggests that this occurs by passive diffusion, although the results of some studies suggest that alveolar epithelial cells express specific albumin- and immunoglobulin-binding molecules that might aid in the transcellular clearance of these proteins.[17] Alveolar macrophages may also play a role by ingesting and degrading proteins.[105]

## CLASSIFICATION OF PULMONARY EDEMA

As indicated previously, it is convenient to classify the causes of pulmonary edema into two major categories on the basis of underlying pathogenetic abnormality (Table 51–1). In the first category are those conditions in which the edema results from an increase in the pulmonary microvascular pressure or a decrease in plasma oncotic pressure (hydrostatic edema). Left ventricular failure is by far the most common cause of high-pressure pulmonary edema (hemodynamic edema, cardiogenic edema). A decrease in the serum osmotic pressure or in interstitial fluid pressure can contribute to the development of hydrostatic edema, although these disorders do not cause edema by themselves. The basic abnormality in hydrostatic edema is an exaggeration of the normal transvascular fluid flux and an overwhelming of the safety factors that normally control the volume of pulmonary extravascular water.

The second category includes conditions in which the edema results from an increase in microvascular permeability (normal-pressure pulmonary edema, low-pressure pulmonary edema, capillary-leakage pulmonary edema, noncardiogenic pulmonary edema). We prefer to call this form of

## Table 51–1. CLASSIFICATION OF PULMONARY EDEMA

**HYDROSTATIC PULMONARY EDEMA**

*Cardiogenic*

   Left ventricular failure
   Mitral valve disease
   Left atrial myxoma or thrombus
   Cor triatriatum

*Disease of the Pulmonary Veins*

   Primary (idiopathic) veno-occlusive disease
   Chronic fibrosing mediastinitis

*Neurogenic (Combined Hydrostatic and Permeability Pulmonary Edema)*

   Head trauma
   Increased intracranial pressure
   Postictal

*Decreased Capillary Osmotic Pressure*

   Renal disease
   Fluid overload
   Cirrhosis

**INCREASED PERMEABILITY PULMONARY EDEMA (ARDS)**

   Systemic sepsis
   Pulmonary infection
   Trauma
   Inhalation of noxious fumes and gases
   Aspiration of noxious fluids
   Ingestion or injection of drugs or poisons

pulmonary edema increased permeability edema or permeability edema. Although many specific insults can cause sufficiently widespread endothelial or epithelial damage (or both) to result in generalized pulmonary edema, the resulting clinical, radiologic, and pathologic manifestations are remarkably similar.[1, 2]

It is not always possible to assign individual patients who have pulmonary edema to one of these two categories; in fact, a combination of permeability and cardiogenic edema is common. Such coexistence is particularly serious, because many of the safety factors that impede the accumulation of excess extravascular water are lost when the endothelium loses its selectivity for solutes.

## PULMONARY EDEMA ASSOCIATED WITH ELEVATED MICROVASCULAR PRESSURE (HYDROSTATIC PULMONARY EDEMA)

### Cardiogenic Pulmonary Edema

Undoubtedly, the most common cause of interstitial and air-space pulmonary edema is a rise in pulmonary venous pressure secondary to disease of the left side of the heart. Increased pressure within the left atrium can be transmitted to the pulmonary veins as a result of back pressure from the left ventricle (secondary to long-standing systemic hypertension, aortic valvular disease, cardiomyopathy, and coronary artery disease with or without myocardial infarction) or can be caused by obstruction to the left atrial outflow (as a result of mitral valve stenosis, left atrial myxoma, or cor triatriatum). Rarely, pulmonary venous hypertension develops as a result of stenosis of the pulmonary veins themselves, such as occurs in congenital or acquired veno-occlusive disease or fibrosing mediastinitis.

### Radiologic Manifestations

Hydrostatic pulmonary edema results in two principal radiologic patterns related to whether the fluid remains localized in the interstitial space or whether it also occupies the air spaces of the lung.

#### Predominantly Interstitial Edema

Transudation of fluid into the interstitial spaces of the lung inevitably constitutes the first stage of pulmonary edema, because the capillaries are situated in this compartment. However, it is often not the first radiographic sign of cardiac decompensation or pulmonary venous hypertension. As discussed previously (*see* page 1919), pulmonary venous hypertension is usually manifested by a redistribution of blood "flow" from the lower to the upper lung zones, so that an increase in caliber of upper zone vessels typically precedes evidence of overt edema (Fig. 51–8).[106–108] However, it is important to remember that such upper-lobe vessel "recruitment" also occurs in a number of other situations (e.g., intracardiac left-to-right shunts) (Fig. 51–9) and is

seen more commonly in patients who have chronic venous hypertension than in those who have acute left ventricular failure.[108, 108a] Furthermore, redistribution of blood flow can only be assessed reliably on radiographs performed at maximal inspiration in the erect position.[107, 108] Usually, this is done subjectively by comparing the number and size of upper zone vessels to lower zone vessels at an equal distance from the hila.[107, 108] The earliest stage at which redistribution can be recognized is when the number and caliber of upper zone vessels is similar to that of those in the lower zone.[107, 109] As the redistribution becomes more pronounced, the upper zone vessels become larger.

A more objective assessment of arterial enlargement is based on the measurement of the diameter of bronchi and adjacent pulmonary arteries seen end-on. Normally, the diameter of pulmonary arteries in the upper lung zones is the same or less than the external diameter of the companion bronchus.[107, 110] When there is blood flow redistribution, the artery becomes larger than the accompanying bronchus (Fig. 51–10). In one investigation in which the pulmonary artery-to-bronchus diameter ratios were measured on the upright chest radiographs, the mean ratio in 30 normal subjects was 0.85 (standard deviation [SD] 0.15), compared with 1.62 (SD 0.31) in 30 patients who had fluid overload and 1.50 (SD 0.25) in 30 patients who had left ventricular failure.[110] The mean ratio in normal subjects in the supine position

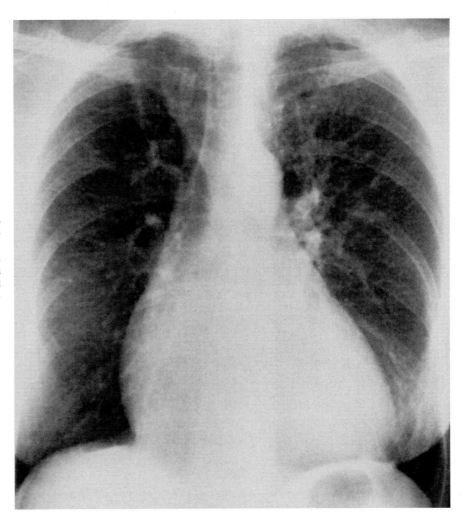

**Figure 51–8. Redistribution of Blood Flow to Upper Lung Zones Caused by Pulmonary Venous Hypertension.** A posteroanterior radiograph reveals unusually prominent vascular markings in the upper zones and rather sparse markings in the lower zones. The patient was a 42-year-old woman who had recurrent episodes of left ventricular decompensation as a result of cardiomyopathy.

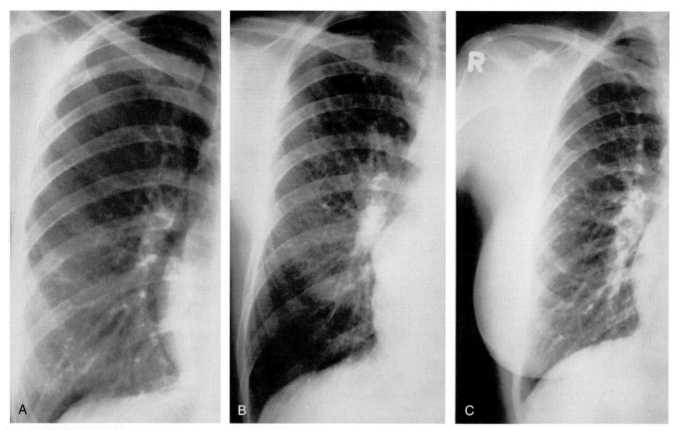

**Figure 51–9. Recruitment of Upper Lobe Vessels in Postcapillary Hypertension and Left-to-Right Shunt: Radiographic Distinction.**
A view of the right lung from a posteroanterior chest radiograph *(A)* is normal. Note that in the erect position, the upper-lobe arteries and veins are much smaller than those in the lower lobe, a reflection of the influence of gravity on blood flow. The vasculature is well defined throughout. Contrast this appearance to that in two patients with increased blood flow to the upper lobes, in *B* caused by mitral stenosis and in *C* by an atrial septal defect (ASD). Upper-lobe vessels are dilated *(B)*; lower-lobe vessels are narrowed and ill defined as a result of interstitial edema. These features are typical of postcapillary hypertension. Upper-lobe *and* lower-lobe vessels are larger than normal and are sharply defined *(C)*, findings indicative of a left-to-right shunt. Note that the cause of the upper-zone vessel recruitment in *B* and *C* cannot be distinguished by the appearance of the upper-lobe vessels alone.

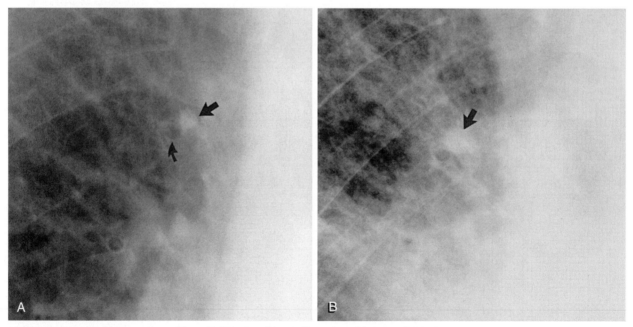

**Figure 51–10. Increased Upper Lung Zone Pulmonary Artery–Bronchus Diameter Ratio in Hydrostatic Pulmonary Edema.** A view of the right upper lung zone from an anteroposterior chest radiograph *(A)* in a healthy 87-year-old man shows a normal pulmonary artery–bronchus diameter ratio. The external diameter of the pulmonary artery *(straight arrow)* is similar to that of the external diameter of its accompanying bronchus *(curved arrow)*. Three years later the patient developed acute pulmonary edema after myocardial infarction. An erect anteroposterior chest radiograph *(B)* shows an increased diameter of the pulmonary artery *(arrow)*. A perihilar haze is also evident.

was 1.01 (SD, 0.13) compared with 1.49 (SD, 0.31) for patients who had left ventricular failure.

As discussed previously, when pulmonary venous hypertension is moderate in degree, fluid accumulates within the perivascular interstitial tissue and interlobular septa.[111] As a result of this localization, edema fluid produces the typical radiographic pattern of loss of the normal sharp definition of pulmonary vascular markings and thickening of the interlobular septa (A and B lines of Kerley, Fig. 51–11). The radiologic characteristics of septal lines (Kerley A and B lines) are discussed in detail in Chapter 18 (see page 480). Several groups of investigators have shown that they tend to develop when pulmonary venous pressure (wedge pressure) is 17 to 20 mm Hg or higher.[107, 112–116] Although the presence of septal lines can be of value in confirming the diagnosis when other signs are equivocal, in our experience the fre-

quency with which they can be identified is low compared with loss of definition of vessel markings; thus, their absence should not be construed as evidence against the diagnosis.

In circumstances in which edema fluid accumulates in the parenchymal interstitial tissues (the alveolar wall phase[46]) before the development of overt air-space edema, the accumulation usually is invisible or only faintly discernible radiographically as a "haze," which tends to be predominantly lower zonal or perihilar in distribution. The sequence of redistribution of blood flow, loss of the sharp marginal contour of pulmonary vessels, and, finally, perihilar haze and air-space consolidation was observed in one study of 30 patients who had recent myocardial infarction;[116] generally, the severity of radiographic abnormalities correlated well with pulmonary wedge pressure. Despite these findings, there is often a phase lag between elevation of pulmonary

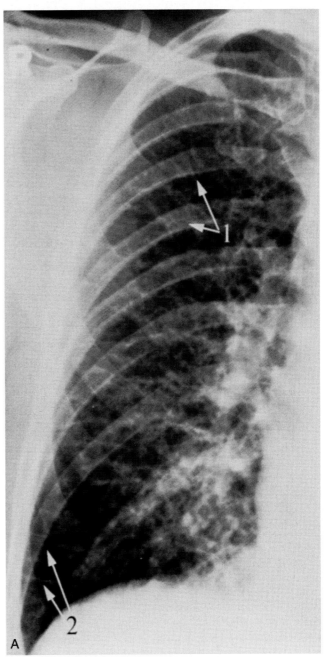

**Figure 51–11. Acute Interstitial Pulmonary Edema.** A view of the right lung from a posteroanterior chest radiograph (A) reveals the classic features of acute interstitial edema—septal A (1) and B (2) lines and thickened and ill-defined bronchovascular bundles. Evidence for recruitment of upper-zone vessels is not at all convincing, a common finding in our experience in patients with acute interstitial edema of any cause. The patient was an elderly man seen 4 hours after the onset of anterior chest pain caused by myocardial infarction.

*Illustration continued on following page*

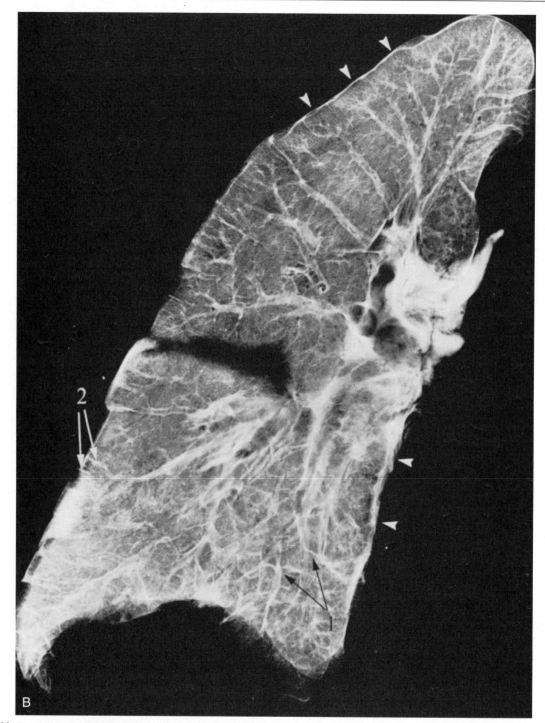

**Figure 51–11** *Continued.* A radiograph of a coronal slice through the right lung after an autopsy of a different patient *(B)* reveals similar features—septal A lines (1) and B lines (2) and thickened peribronchovascular interstitium. Note the thickened pleura *(arrowheads)*, indicating the presence of pleural edema.

wedge pressure and radiographic signs of pulmonary edema, possibly because of the time required for transudation of fluid into the extravascular space.[117] The heart usually is enlarged, but it may not be when the exciting cause of the edema is recent myocardial infarction, coronary insufficiency,[118] restrictive cardiomyopathy, left atrial myxoma, cor triatriatum, tachyarrhythmias, acute systemic hypertension such as that occasioned by an adrenal pheochromocytoma, or, occasionally, mitral stenosis or aortic stenosis.

Evidence for interstitial pulmonary edema is also pro-

vided by an increase in the thickness of the walls of bronchi seen end-on in the perihilar zones. In the absence of chronic airway disease, such as bronchitis or asthma, these structures measure less than 1 mm in thickness. When fluid accumulates in the interstitial tissue surrounding them, their shadow thickens and loses its sharp definition (Fig. 51–12). Similar thickening can occur in large central airways such as the intermediate bronchus. This sign has been employed to advantage in some cases in which other signs of interstitial edema have not been convincing;[119] however, it is important

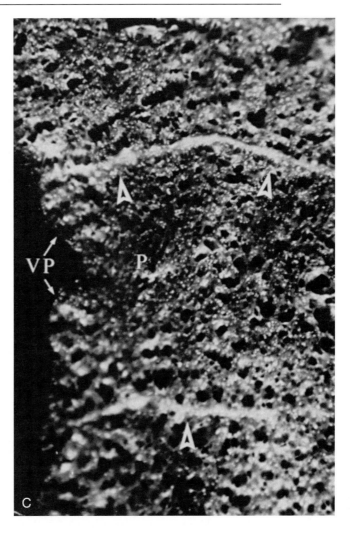

**Figure 51–11** *Continued.* A magnified view *(C)* of a portion of the parenchyma *(P)* from the gross specimen in *B* reveals two edematous interlobular septa *(arrowheads)* that extend perpendicular to the visceral pleura (VP). (*A* and *B* from Genereux GP: Pattern recognition in diffuse lung disease. A review of theory and practice. Med Radiogr Photogr 61:2, 1985. Reprinted courtesy Eastman Kodak Company.)

to exclude airway disease such as chronic bronchitis or asthma as the cause of the bronchial wall thickening. Another sign of interstitial edema is thickening of the interlobar fissures (Fig. 51–13).[108, 120, 121] Because the pleural connective tissue is in continuity with that of the interlobular septa, when fluid accumulates in the latter sites (creating Kerley B lines), it often collects in the pleural interstitium as well. In such circumstances, the excess fluid causes not only a thickening of the interlobar fissures but also a widening of the pleural layer over the convexity of the lungs, particularly in the costophrenic recesses, an abnormality that is sometimes confused with pleural effusion. Small pleural effusions may be present in addition, of course.

In a hemodynamic, electrocardiographic, and radiographic assessment of 36 acutely ill patients who had myocardial infarction or serious angina there was a very good correlation between pulmonary arterial wedge pressure and evidence of pulmonary venous hypertension as assessed from bedside chest radiographs.[122] The investigators found a normal chest radiograph to be an exceptional feature of the early stages of infarction, because evidence for pulmonary venous hypertension presented itself immediately after mean left ventricular filling pressure rose above 10 mm Hg. Similarly, in a study of 26 patients admitted to a coronary care unit suffering from recent myocardial infarction in whom abnormalities in bedside chest radiographs were correlated

with pulmonary arterial diastolic pressure (assumed to reflect left ventricular end-diastolic pressure), a normal chest radiograph was almost always associated with a pulmonary arterial diastolic pressure less than 14 mm Hg.[123] Radiographic evidence of pulmonary venous hypertension usually indicated a pulmonary diastolic pressure greater than 14 mm Hg but was seen on several occasions when pressures were below this level.

When there is adequate treatment of the edema, the radiologic signs may disappear within a matter of hours. However, a delay in resolution occurs in some patients.[116] For example, in both of the studies cited earlier, investigators observed a time lag between the fall of pressure and radiologic improvement, in some cases as long as 12 to 22 hours after left ventricular filling pressure had returned to normal as the result of treatment.[122, 123] Persistence of septal lines after adequate therapy (such as mitral commissurotomy for mitral stenosis) usually indicates irreversible fibrosis. The radiographic features that help to distinguish hydrostatic from permeability edema are the normal heart size and infrequent interstitial edema or pleural effusion in edema associated with increased microvascular permeability.[125]

Although the diagnosis of hydrostatic pulmonary edema is usually based on clinical information and conventional chest radiography, it is important to recognize the appearance of hydrostatic pulmonary edema on CT and HRCT, because

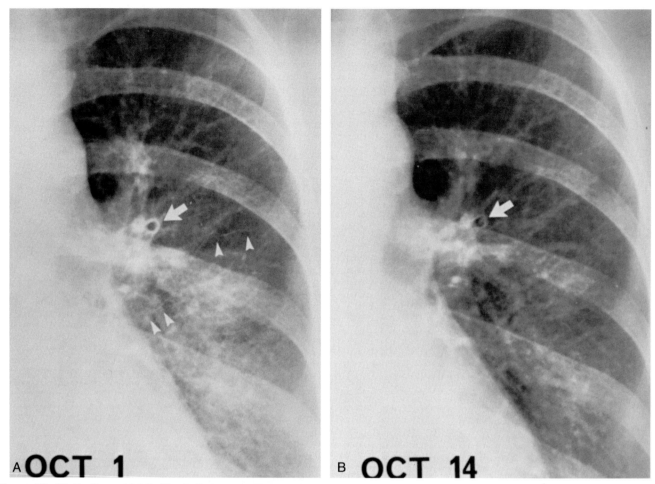

**Figure 51–12. Peribronchial Cuffing in Pulmonary Edema.** A detail view of the upper half of the left lung from a posteroanterior chest radiograph *(A)* reveals distended upper-lobe vessels, perihilar haze, septal A lines *(arrowheads)*, and a thickened bronchial wall viewed end-on *(arrow)*. A few days later, after diuretic therapy *(B)*, signs of pulmonary edema had resolved. Note the decreased thickness of the bronchial wall *(arrow)*. The patient was a middle-aged woman with renal failure.

it can mimic other diseases and sometimes occurs as an unsuspected finding in patients who are having CT for a different reason.[126–128] As on radiographs, there is disproportionate enlargement of nondependent pulmonary arteries and veins, smooth thickening of the interlobular septa, subpleural connective tissue, and peribronchovascular connective tissue (Fig. 51–14).[126–130] Areas of ground-glass attenuation can result from interstitial or air-space edema, whereas consolidation reflects the presence of air-space edema. Pleural and pericardial effusions are more easily detected than on standard radiographs.[131] Other findings that can be seen on CT include enlarged mediastinal lymph nodes and inhomogeneous attenuation of mediastinal fat.[131a]

In an experimental study in animals who had undergone fluid overload, HRCT showed an increase in arterial diameter of 20% and an increase in venous diameter of 33%;[132] a gravity-dependent increase in parenchymal attenuation was also evident. The sensitivity of HRCT in detecting heart failure was shown by one group who performed scans at rest and after treadmill exercise in 10 normal subjects and in 10 patients who had mild heart failure (New York Heart Association Class [NYHA] 1) and 10 who had moderate failure (NYHA 2 and 3).[133] After exercise, they found that

the patients who had moderate heart failure developed signs of interstitial pulmonary edema, including the presence of a pulmonary artery-to-bronchial diameter ratio greater than 1 in the upper lobes, a peripheral increase in vascular markings, interlobular septal thickening, and peribronchial cuffing. In another study, pulmonary diffusing capacity and CT were performed in a group of elite athletes after a triathlon; the diffusing capacity decreased, and the CT showed evidence of increased interstitial attenuation consistent with edema.[134]

The advent of newer imaging modalities has made it possible to derive estimates of the quantity of pulmonary edema fluid or pulmonary extravascular fluid volume (PEV). In addition to CT,[135, 136] these techniques include Compton-scatter densitometry,[137] electrical impedance tomography,[138] positron emission tomography (PET),[139, 140] magnetic resonance (MR) imaging, and thallium-201 scintigraphy.[141] PET using radiolabeled water and carbon monoxide can provide an estimate of regional pulmonary blood flow in addition to PEV but is only useful as a research tool.[142] In experimental animal studies, MR imaging has been shown to yield accurate estimates of PEV; however, as yet, this form of imaging has no advantages in the clinical assessment of patients who

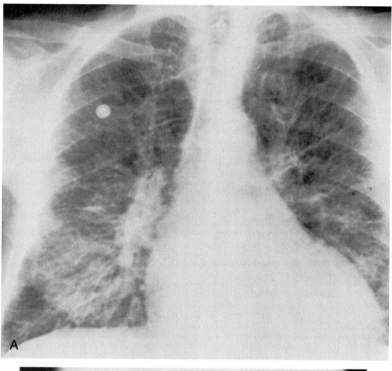

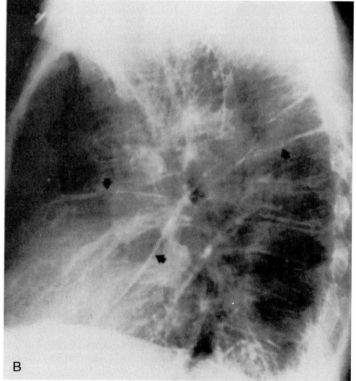

**Figure 51–13. Interstitial Pulmonary Edema.** Posteroanterior *(A)* and lateral *(B)* radiographs reveal multiple linear opacities throughout both lungs. These lines consist of a combination of long septal lines (Kerley A) and shorter peripheral septal lines (Kerley B). In the lateral projection *(B)*, the interlobar fissures are very prominent *(arrows)*, representing pleural edema.

have, or are suspected of having, pulmonary edema.[124, 143–147] PEV can also be measured using an isotope dilution technique in which two radiolabeled substances are injected intravenously; one of these remains in the intravascular compartment while the other diffuses into the interstitial compartment. In one study of 45 patients who had valvular heart disease and 9 normal subjects in which this procedure was employed, radiologic evidence of interstitial pulmonary edema was found in only 7 of the 18 patients in whom the PEV was above the normal range;[148] the increase in PEV correlated with changes in pulmonary arterial and left atrial pressures.

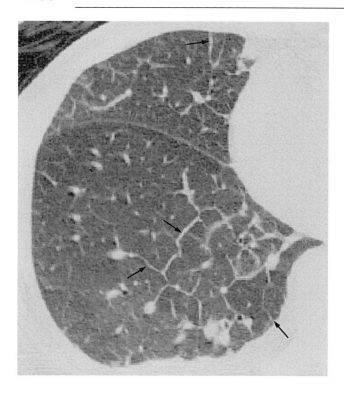

**Figure 51–14. Interstitial Pulmonary Edema.** A view of the right lung from an HRCT scan demonstrates increased diameter of the pulmonary vessels, smooth thickening of interlobular septa *(arrows)* and localized areas of ground-glass attenuation in the dependent lung regions. A small pleural effusion is also present. The patient was a 49-year-old woman who developed interstitial pulmonary edema as a result of fluid overload.

## Air-Space Edema

Interstitial edema invariably precedes air-space edema (Fig. 51–15), and in some patients the chest radiograph shows evidence of both simultaneously.[149–151] The characteristic radiographic abnormality is the presence of patchy or confluent bilateral areas of consolidation that tend to be symmetric and to involve mainly the perihilar regions and the lower lung zones. Air bronchograms can be seen in 20% to 30% of patients.[150, 151] In the majority of cases, the shadows are confluent, creating irregular, rather poorly defined, patchy opacities of unit density scattered randomly throughout the lungs; in the medial third of the lungs particularly, coalescence of areas of consolidation is common. The distribution varies from patient to patient but may be surprisingly similar during different episodes in the same individual. Patchy air-space consolidation sometimes extends to the subpleural zone or "cortex" of the lung (Fig. 51–16); however, the cortex may be completely spared, thus creating the "bat's wing" or "butterfly" pattern of edema (*see* later).

Although the effects of gravity on the distribution of blood flow and ventilation in the normal lung have been well established, its effects on the distribution of pulmonary edema are not as clear. Gravity predisposes to dependent edema both by generating higher hydrostatic pressures toward the bases and by draining interstitial fluid toward the bases through the interstitial space.[152] However, opposing these forces are the augmented ventilatory movements that promote the removal of fluid through the lymphatics and that are considerably more vigorous in lower than in upper lung zones. The net effect of these opposing forces is difficult to predict; however, from a practical point of view, they result in maximal fluid accumulation in the lower and central lung zones.

Although edema caused by cardiac disease usually is bilateral and fairly symmetric, it may be predominantly unilateral.[153, 154] The mechanisms underlying the development of unilateral hydrostatic or increased-permeability pulmonary edema were described in a study of 15 patients[155] and the literature has been reviewed.[156, 157] The causes of such edema have been divided into ipsilateral and contralateral groups.[156] The former refers to those conditions in which the pathogenetic mechanism leading to the asymmetry is on the same side as the edema. Conditions in this category include systemic-to-pulmonary shunts in congenital heart disease,[158, 159] bronchial obstruction (the "drowned" lung), unilateral veno-occlusive disease, prolonged lateral decubitus position, unilateral aspiration, pulmonary contusion, and rapid thoracentesis of either air or fluid (re-expansion pulmonary edema, *see* page 1968) (Fig. 51–17). Uncommon causes of unilateral pulmonary edema include raised intracranial pressure,[160] administration of a hypotonic saline solution through a central venous catheter inadvertently placed in a pulmonary artery,[161] ventricular septal rupture,[162] and unilateral thoracic sympathectomy.[163] Two cases have also been described in which unilateral edema developed in the remaining lobe after lobectomy, in both cases caused by thrombosis of ipsilateral veins.[164] Edema localized to the right upper lobe is sometimes seen in patients in whom mitral regurgitation is the cause of the edema (Fig. 51–18);[157, 165, 166] for example, in one study of 131 patients who had severe regurgitation, 12 (9%) demonstrated this pattern.[166] The mechanism underlying this distribution has been shown to be a predominant orientation of the regurgitant jet toward the right superior pulmonary vein.[157] A case has also been reported of predominant left upper lobe edema secondary to paravalvular leak around a prosthetic mitral valve.[166a]

Contralateral edema refers to the accumulation of excess water in a "normal" lung opposite to the abnormality. Conditions that have been reported to cause this pattern include proximal interruption of a pulmonary artery, obstruc-

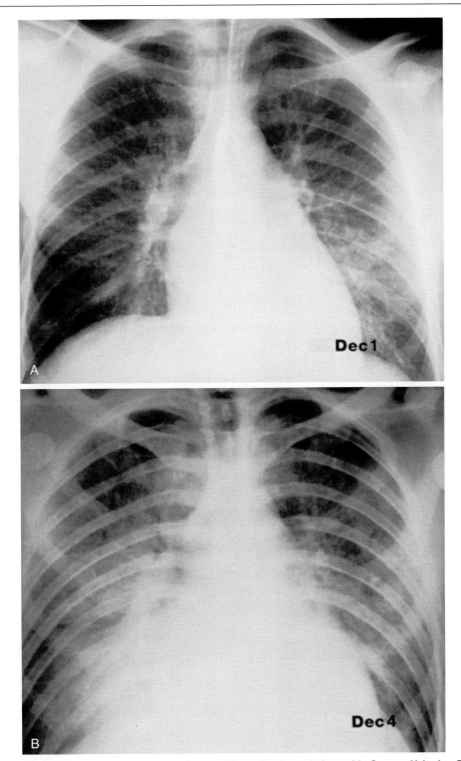

**Figure 51–15. Interstitial Edema Progressing to Air-Space Edema in Association with Severe Valvular Disease and Bacterial Endocarditis.** The initial posteroanterior radiograph of this 22-year-old man *(A)* reveals diffuse interstitial edema manifested by loss of definition of vascular markings throughout both lungs and by septal lines in both costophrenic recesses. Three days later *(B)*, the lungs had become massively consolidated by air-space edema. The heart size had increased considerably in this interval. The patient had clinical evidence of both aortic and mitral insufficiency.

tion of a pulmonary artery by an aortic aneurysm,[167, 168] Swyer-James syndrome, acute pulmonary thromboembolism, local emphysema (Fig. 51–19), lobectomy, rapid re-expansion of pneumothorax in a patient who had left-sided heart failure, systemic-to-pulmonary artery shunt, pleural disease, and unilateral sympathectomy.[156] Sparing of accessory lobes

during generalized pulmonary edema has also been reported.[169]

In patients who have cardiac decompensation, unilateral edema is probably seen most often when the affected lung is dependent for a prolonged period. In one review of 357 chest radiographs from 25 patients who had pulmonary

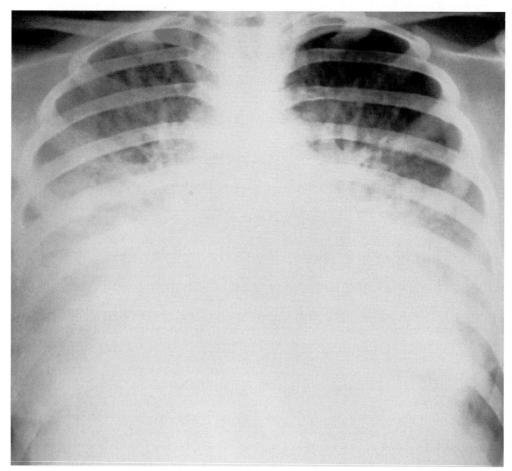

**Figure 51–16. Acute Pulmonary Edema Secondary to Left Ventricular Failure.** A posteroanterior radiograph reveals extensive consolidation of both lungs extending to the visceral pleural surfaces. The heart is moderately enlarged. Six hours before this radiograph was taken, the patient had abrupt onset of severe dyspnea, pleuritic pain, and cough productive of copious frothy sputum. Both the clinical and radiographic pictures are typical of acute pulmonary edema secondary to left ventricular failure.

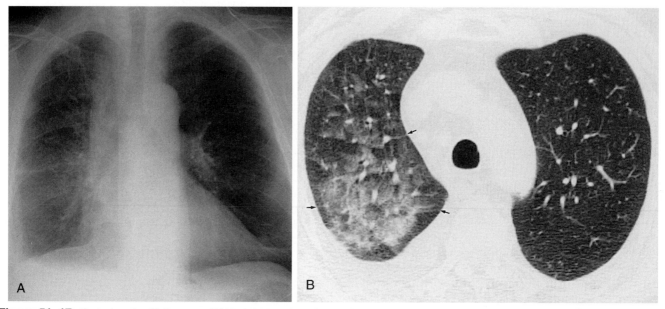

**Figure 51–17. Re-expansion Pulmonary Edema.** A posteroanterior chest radiograph *(A)* shows ground-glass opacification of the right lung and a small right pleural effusion. An HRCT scan *(B)* demonstrates areas of ground-glass attenuation, minimal thickening of interlobular septa *(arrows)*, and a small right pleural effusion. The patient was a 79-year-old man who developed edema after thoracentesis and rapid drainage of a large right pleural effusion.

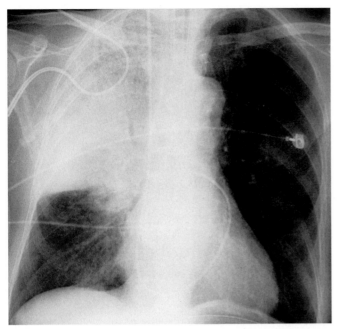

**Figure 51–18. Right Upper Lobe Pulmonary Edema Secondary to Acute Mitral Regurgitation.** An anteroposterior chest radiograph of a 66-year-old woman shows diffuse right upper-lobe consolidation. Although the appearance is most suggestive of pneumonia, it was proven to be air-space pulmonary edema secondary to acute mitral regurgitation after myocardial infarction. This is an extreme example of localized right upper-lobe edema related to mitral regurgitation.

edema, were receiving assisted ventilation, and were often positioned on their side to promote drainage of tracheobronchial secretions, 68% showed gravity-dependent asymmetric edema;[170] only 18% showed edema predominantly in the "up" lung. Sometimes the edema shifted to the contralateral lung after the patient's position was changed to the opposite side. We have seen one patient (Fig. 51–20) in whom pulmonary edema was uniquely right sided on repeated episodes of acute cardiac decompensation. When questioned, he replied that he always lay on his right side because lying on his back or left side produced marked discomfort and anxiety. Some of the apparent shift in "edema" may be related to the development of dependent atelectasis, as suggested by the results of a recent CT study in which the shifts in density have been shown to occur in a matter of minutes when patients who have ARDS are repositioned.[171]

When edema is predominantly unilateral or in other ways unusually distributed, the radiographic differentiation from pneumonia may be difficult.[172] In this situation, visualization of changes typical of interstitial edema is helpful. One group has also employed a "gravitational shift test" in differential diagnosis:[173] by comparing bedside chest radiographs of patients examined in the supine position and after prolonged lateral decubitus positioning, they were able to distinguish pneumonia and edema by observing a shift of fluid from one lung to the other while no change occurred in the anatomic location of pneumonia. Although interesting, we doubt that this form of examination is worth the trouble; in patients in whom doubt exists, a trial of diuretic therapy would appear to be more efficacious and less time consuming.

Like hydrostatic interstitial pulmonary edema, air-space edema usually clears fairly rapidly in response to adequate

treatment of the underlying condition, and resolution appears complete radiographically in not more than 3 days in most cases. It is likely that the efficiency of the lymphatic system plays a major role in clearance time. Studies of lymph flow before and after experimental induction of acute heart failure have shown lymph drainage to increase by 300% to 2,800%.[152] Pulmonary edema may clear more slowly when lymphatic drainage is hindered by factors such as systemic venous hypertension.

### The "Bat's Wing" or "Butterfly" Pattern of Edema

These terms describe an anatomic distribution of edema in which the hilum and "medulla" of the lungs are fairly uniformly consolidated and the peripheral 2 to 3 cm of lung parenchyma—the "cortex"—is relatively uninvolved (Fig. 51–21). Definition of the margin of consolidated parenchyma often is rather indistinct but may be remarkably sharp. Localization of the edema to the central lung regions may be apparent in both posteroanterior and lateral radiographic projections[174] and can be seen in the interstitium as well as the air spaces, particularly on CT. The uninvolved "cortex" usually extends along the interlobar lung fissures as well as around the convexity of the thorax, thereby creating a waistlike indentation visible in posteroanterior projection in the region of the minor fissure. Similarly, the upper and lower paramediastinal zones may be relatively free of involvement. Resolution of the edema generally begins in the periphery and spreads medially.[175] The pattern is uncommon; in one series of 110 cases of moderate to severe edema of varying etiology, it was identified in only 5%.[154]

Many theories have been propounded to explain the mechanism of the "bat's wing" distribution of pulmonary edema.[176] One is based on a division of the lung into three anatomic units: (1) the hilar root area, which contains chiefly conducting airways and vessels and little or no parenchyma; (2) the medullary area, which includes the second, third, and fourth orders of bronchial and vascular divisions, and intervening parenchymal tissue; and (3) the cortex, which measures 3 to 4 cm in thickness at the periphery of the lung and consists almost entirely of parenchyma.[175, 177] It has been suggested that the arterioles of the cortex may be particularly adapted for vasoconstriction or vasodilation, much the same as in the kidney.[177] Vasoconstriction would result in the shunting of blood to the medullary zones of the lung, thus protecting the cortex from edema. In addition, the precapillary network of the medulla is disproportionately short compared with the major branches from which it arises. Because of this, high pressure within the pulmonary arteries might be more readily transmitted to precapillaries and thence to the proximal capillaries.[178] These anatomic differences in the pulmonary vasculature of the two zones could make the medulla more susceptible to transudation of fluid.

It has also been proposed that the accumulation of fluid is dependent on the efficiency with which the lymphatics can remove an excess.[179] According to this hypothesis, the peripheral portion of the lungs undergoes greater volume change than does the medulla during respiration, an increased movement that operates in much the same way as muscular exercise in the extremities to stimulate increased lymphatic flow. Although this theory is plausible, in the only experiment designed to test it little difference was found in the degree of lengthening and shortening of segments of the

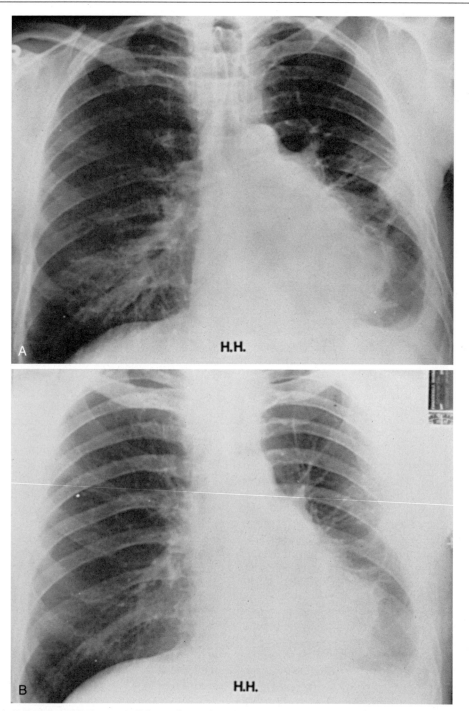

**Figure 51–19. Atypical Pattern of Pulmonary Edema Caused by Unilateral Fibrothorax.** A posteroanterior chest radiograph *(A)* shows the typical features of left heart failure in the right lung as evidenced by upper lobe redistribution of blood flow and loss of definition of bronchovascular bundles as a result of interstitial edema. However, note the absence of such findings in the left lung. The pleura is irregularly thickened over the lower half of this lung, suggesting that unilateral fibrothorax may be inhibiting ventilation with resulting hypoperfusion. Several days later, following diuretic therapy *(B)*, signs of cardiac decompensation had resolved.

bronchial tree in the cortex as compared with those in the medulla between full inspiration and expiration.[180]

### Clinical Manifestations

The clinical manifestations of cardiogenic pulmonary edema depend on whether the onset of edema is acute or insidious. When severe, the acute form is dramatic, with dyspnea developing over a short period (minutes to hours). The patient characteristically sits bolt upright in obvious respiratory distress and uses the accessory muscles of respiration. Peripheral and central cyanosis, tachycardia, pallor, cool sweaty skin, anxiety, and an elevated blood pressure are often present as a result of sympathetic stimulation. In severe cases, the patient may expectorate frothy, blood-tinged fluid; occasionally, there is frank hemoptysis. "Air

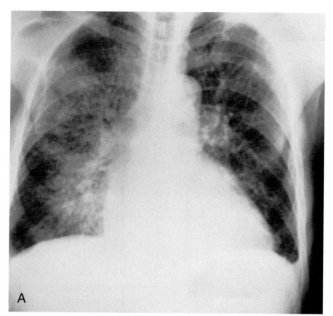

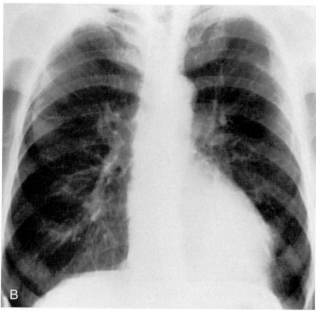

**Figure 51–20. Predominantly Unilateral Pulmonary Edema.** A posteroanterior radiograph *(A)* of a 70-year-old man admitted with an acute myocardial infarct reveals patchy air-space consolidation occupying the medial two thirds of the right lung characteristic of acute pulmonary edema. The left lung is unaffected, although there is a small left pleural effusion. The heart is moderately enlarged. A visit to the patient's bedside revealed the fact that he lay on his right side most of the time, since other positions seemed to intensify his shortness of breath. A radiograph after resolution of the edema *(B)* shows a marked increase in volume of both lungs characteristic of diffuse pulmonary emphysema. The unilaterality of the edema was clearly related to the influence of gravity. It cannot be explained on the basis of emphysema, because this disease is bilateral and symmetric.

hunger" may be sufficient to interfere with normal speech. There is a diurnal variation in the onset of pulmonary edema, the presentation being most often in the evening or early morning hours.[181]

Occasionally, the clinical manifestations of "butterfly" edema are almost as unimpressive as the radiographic appearance is dramatic. Even when there is radiographic evidence of massive consolidation of the medial two thirds of the lungs the clinical presentation may be unremarkable; even those patients who complain of dyspnea and orthopnea may have minimal or nonexistent physical signs, much the same as in diffuse interstitial edema. This dissociation of clinical and radiologic findings is attributed to the relatively mild involvement of the "cortical" parenchyma.

Physical examination may reveal an elevated jugular venous pressure; however, in severe edema the jugular veins may be difficult to evaluate, owing to the patient's use of the cervical accessory muscles of respiration and to the considerable swings in pleural pressure that are transmitted to the cervical veins. Other signs of congestive failure, such as hepatosplenomegaly and peripheral edema, may be present. Auscultation of the thorax reveals widespread crackles and expiratory wheezes. In the terminal stages, there is a decrease in the patient's level of consciousness and circulatory collapse. In patients who have mitral stenosis or left ventricular failure secondary to systemic hypertension or aortic valvular disease, the episode of acute pulmonary edema may develop only after exertion or may be caused by the increase in pulmonary blood volume associated with the assumption of the supine from the erect position. Acute cardiogenic pulmonary edema is not a static condition, and there is usually improvement or worsening during a relatively short time course. Potentially confusing differential diagnoses include fulminant pneumonia, an acute exacerbation of chronic obstructive pulmonary disease (COPD) or asthma, acute pulmonary hemorrhage, and upper airway obstruction. Findings of sympathetic hyper-reactivity suggest a diagnosis of edema.

In patients in whom pulmonary edema develops less precipitously, the onset of symptoms may be insidious and there may be few physical findings. Dyspnea in such patients may only occur during exertion; a history of orthopnea and paroxysmal nocturnal dyspnea is a helpful diagnostic feature in such patients, although these symptoms, accompanied by cough, are also common in patients who have asthma or COPD. When the edema is confined to the interstitial space, there may be no auscultatory findings, although expiratory wheezing is present in some patients at this stage. The quieter chest allows more careful auscultation of the heart, which may reveal a gallop rhythm or a murmur caused by valvular dysfunction. Although an S3 gallop rhythm is thought to be one of the more reliable signs of left ventricular failure, it may be missed by even highly trained clinicians.[182] An estimate of the right-sided heart filling pressure can be obtained by examining the jugular veins, and the increase in jugular venous pressure caused by compression of the abdomen (hepatojugular [abdominojugular] reflux) can be assessed using a standardized maneuver.[183]

Occasionally, it is necessary to use a pulmonary artery catheter and measure the pulmonary arterial wedge pressure to establish that the cause of pulmonary edema is an increase in pulmonary venous pressure. However, echocardiographic techniques such as transesophageal echo and pulsed Doppler are increasingly being used to provide estimates of ventricular function; pulsed Doppler evaluation has been shown to provide a fairly accurate estimate of pulmonary capillary wedge pressure.[184] Blood levels of atrial and brain natriuretic peptide are increased in dyspneic patients who are in mild

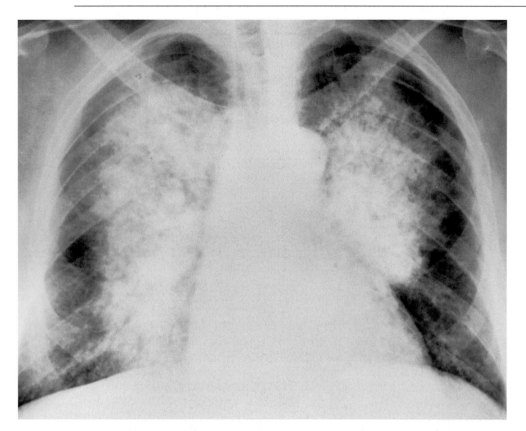

**Figure 51–21. The "Bat's Wing" Pattern of Pulmonary Edema.** A posteroanterior radiograph demonstrates consolidation of the parahilar and "medullary" portions of both lungs, creating a bat's wing or "butterfly" appearance; the "cortex" of both lungs is relatively unaffected. The margins of the edematous lung are rather sharply defined. The consolidation is fairly homogeneous and is associated with well-defined air bronchograms on both sides. This 59-year-old man had suffered a massive myocardial infarct 48 hours previously; he had a cough productive of pinkish sputum and was able to lie flat in bed.

heart failure but not in similarly dyspneic patients whose symptoms are secondary to primary lung diseases.[185]

### Pulmonary Function Tests

The abnormalities of lung function that occur in pulmonary edema are caused by the effects of pulmonary vascular engorgement, interstitial fluid accumulation, and alveolar flooding.

#### Pulmonary Compliance and Lung Volumes

Pulmonary vascular congestion by itself stiffens the lung,[186, 187] probably as a result of an erectile effect of vascular distention; the reduced compliance is rapidly reversed when microvascular pressure is decreased. During the stage of interstitial edema, compliance undergoes little further decrease; however, coincident with the development of overt alveolar flooding, compliance, vital capacity, and total lung capacity are all diminished further as a result of replacement of alveolar gas by fluid and disruption of the surfactant-air interface.[188] Despite the foregoing, the relationship between changes in lung compliance and volumes and the severity of pulmonary edema is inconsistent.[189]

#### Airway Resistance and Closing Volume

Clinical findings suggestive of airway narrowing are frequent in patients who have pulmonary edema. Although the pathogenesis of this is not certain, there is evidence that it is related to the continuity of the interstitial tissue that surrounds pulmonary arteries and airways. Because fluid that accumulates in this compartment relates to both structures, "competition" for space may lead to preferential narrowing of the relatively more compressible airway. Airway resistance is increased in both acute and chronic pulmonary edema.[190, 191] In an experimental study in dogs in which pulmonary edema was induced by elevating microvascular pressure, the investigators measured resistance of central and peripheral (<2 mm internal diameter) airways and showed that there was a small, reversible increase in small airway resistance when pulmonary venous pressure was increased acutely;[191] this presumably represented airway narrowing caused by vascular engorgement. However, when the venous pressure elevation was prolonged, a progressive and dramatic increase in the peripheral but not central airway resistance was observed that was thought to be secondary to peribronchovascular edema. These small airways are those that close at low lung volumes; if interstitial edema caused them to narrow significantly, one would predict that the closing volume test would be able to detect the change. In fact, closing volume is acutely increased in normal subjects subjected to volume overload[192] and is also increased in patients who have recent myocardial infarction, possibly due to the development of mild interstitial pulmonary edema.[193] Closing volume is also increased in patients on renal hemodialysis and decreases after removal of excess extracellular fluid.[194]

Another manifestation of the airway effects of chronic pulmonary edema is the bronchial hyper-responsiveness, which has been reported in both children[195] and adults.[196, 197] It is believed that the hyper-responsiveness is secondary to congestion and fluid accumulation in the airway walls that exaggerates the effects of pharmacologically induced airway smooth muscle contraction.

### Ventilation-Perfusion Mismatching and Gas Exchange

In excised dog lungs, there is normally an apex-to-base gradient in regional blood flow such that flow at the base of the lung is greater. When pulmonary venous pressure is raised sufficiently to produce pulmonary edema, this pattern is altered to a point where flow to upper lung zones almost equals that to lower zones.[198] The exact mechanism of this reversal of the normal distribution of flow is unclear. It has been suggested that perivascular edema forms first at the lung base and that edema in this location increases the regional pulmonary vascular resistance.[199] However, one group of investigators, who studied blood flow distribution during the development of pulmonary edema in dogs, found a reversal in the apex-to-base flow pattern only when overt alveolar edema developed.[98] Another mechanism that has been hypothesized to explain the phenomenon is reflex vasoconstriction of lower lung vessels.[200]

The distribution of ventilation is also affected in the presence of pulmonary edema.[201] However, because the effects of edema on perfusion and ventilation distribution are inhomogeneous, $\dot{V}/\dot{Q}$ mismatching develops and arterial hypoxemia results. When edema is confined to the interstitium, arterial hypoxemia is usually mild; when air spaces are involved, true shunting of pulmonary blood combines with the $\dot{V}/\dot{Q}$ mismatching to cause more severe hypoxemia. The $\dot{V}/\dot{Q}$ mismatching and shunt can be improved by having patients in a prone position.[202] The improvement is seen in both hydrostatic and permeability edema and appears to occur because the gradient in pleural, and therefore transpulmonary pressure, is less in the prone than in the supine position, so that more uniform alveolar inflation occurs.[203]

In patients who have interstitial and mild-to-moderate air-space edema, the arterial $PCO_2$ is normal or low, reflecting an overall increase in alveolar ventilation. The increase in ventilation during these stages of edema is out of proportion to the degree of hypoxemia, and it is thought that the hyperventilation may be mediated by stimulation of the "J receptors."[204] Although most patients who have acute pulmonary edema are hypocapnic or eucapnic, the majority are acidemic as a result of hypoperfusion of peripheral tissues and the development of lactic acidosis.[205, 206] Approximately 10% of patients in whom arterial blood gas analysis has been performed are hypercapnic; almost invariably, this respiratory acidosis is accompanied by metabolic acidosis. In the majority of patients, the hypercapnia cannot be attributed to pre-existing obstructive pulmonary disease, as has been demonstrated by subsequent assessment of pulmonary function. Although many such patients are extremely ill and the mortality rate is high,[207, 208] particularly in the older age group,[209] edema often appears to be no more severe than that in patients who have normal or low arterial $PCO_2$, and they may respond readily to appropriate therapy.[205]

### Pulmonary Edema Associated with Renal Disease, Hypervolemia, or Hypoproteinemia

Both acute and chronic renal disease—with or without uremia—can be associated with acute pulmonary edema.[110, 210, 211] It is likely that the major contributing cause to the development of edema in these cases is left ventricular failure, although it is probable that decreased protein osmotic

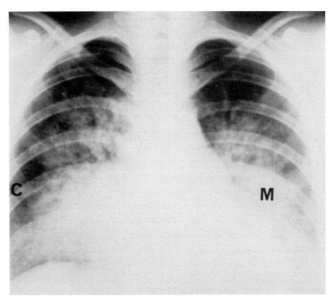

**Figure 51–22. Acute Air-Space Pulmonary Edema: The "Bat's Wing" Pattern.** A posteroanterior chest radiograph reveals a classic bat's wing pattern of air-space consolidation, consisting of a dense central core (medulla, M) surrounded by a radiolucent peripheral zone of normal lung (cortex, C). The heart is moderately enlarged.

pressure, hypervolemia, and increased capillary permeability also have a role (Fig. 51–22). In fact, in some patients who have uremia, normal pulmonary capillary pressures have been recorded in the presence of pulmonary edema.[212]

The contributing factors to hydrostatic pulmonary edema in uremic patients include a constant high cardiac output secondary to anemia and arteriovenous fistula (in patients on chronic hemodialysis), coronary artery disease, fluid overload, and left ventricular hypertrophy.[213] The last-named is itself related to several factors, including the increased output state, systemic hypertension, and poorly understood neurohumoral alterations.[214] Left ventricular hypertrophy is a significant risk factor for death in patients who are on chronic hemodialysis; the hypertrophy may present as a dilated cardiomyopathy or as a concentric or asymmetric septal hypertrophy.[213] The acute onset of pulmonary edema appears to be a particularly frequent manifestation in patients whose renal disease, hypertension, or both are the result of bilateral renal artery stenosis.[215, 216] Patients on dialysis often have subclinical interstitial pulmonary edema that can be detected using indicator dilution methods;[217] the abnormality is normalized during dialysis.

Pulmonary function studies in patients who have severe renal failure have shown a significant reduction in diffusing capacity;[218, 219] in one study, this was presumed to be caused by increased permeability pulmonary edema, because affected patients showed no evidence of left ventricular failure.[218] In another investigation, hemodialysis resulted in an improvement in midexpiratory flow rates and a reduction in gas trapping;[219] the authors concluded that these changes could be attributed to the resolution of peribronchial edema at the lung bases. A quantitative estimate of the volume of pulmonary edema removed at the time of dialysis can be made by plotting the distribution of density in lung pixels before and after the procedure; in 10 patients in whom the ultrafiltrate volumes were between 1 and 4.5 liters, this estimate correlated with increases in total lung capacity and functional residual capacity after dialysis.[220]

The administration of large volumes of intravenous fluids has been shown to cause pulmonary edema in patients who do not have underlying heart disease,[221–223] particularly during the postoperative period and in the elderly. In many of these patients, the edema develops in the absence of known pulmonary injury and has usually been attributed to volume overload of the left ventricle, resulting in temporary high-output left ventricular failure. However, it has also been shown that, in some patients, fluid infusion results in pulmonary edema without functional impairment of the left ventricle and without an increase in left ventricular filling pressures or pulmonary arterial wedge pressure;[222] in these cases, the edema has been attributed at least in part to a decrease in colloid osmotic pressure. In one study, large volumes of normal saline were administered in six dogs until obvious pulmonary edema was observed radiographically.[224] After the volume overload, a statistically significant increase occurred in the size of the heart, left atrium, pulmonary arteries and veins, and systemic veins, unaccompanied by an elevation in left ventricular end-diastolic pressure or by a decrease in cardiac output or stroke volume. The authors concluded that in the absence of left ventricular failure, acute volume overload can simulate the radiographic changes produced by congestive heart failure; they suggested that the pulmonary edema may have occurred at least partly as a result of a marked decrease in serum colloid osmotic pressure.

Although radiographic changes simulating congestive heart failure have also been observed in normal male volunteers whose blood volume was expanded by administration of large amounts of sodium chloride solution,[225] the changes were largely those of systemic venous engorgement and pulmonary congestion in the absence of overt edema. There is little doubt that the effects on the lungs of volume overload are amplified in patients who are on the verge of cardiac or renal failure. The intravenous route is not the only avenue by which excessive fluid can be administered. For example, pulmonary edema has been reported as a consequence of absorption of the hypotonic fluid used during hysteroscopy;[226] a case of pulmonary edema has also been described in a patient who received 7,900 ml of fluid subcutaneously during the course of cosmetic tumescent liposuction![227]

Pulmonary edema occurs with increased frequency in patients who have hepatic disease[11] and who have undergone liver transplantation.[228] Tests of regional lung function suggest that pulmonary extravascular water is increased in patients who have chronic hepatic failure and cirrhosis.[229] Pulmonary edema also frequently accompanies the development of acute hepatic failure.[230] It is unclear whether increased capillary pressure, increased endothelial permeability, or decreased plasma osmotic pressure is the major contributor to the development of edema in these patients; however, it is likely that a combination of factors is responsible. In chronic end-stage hepatic failure, the development of noncardiogenic edema is often associated with sepsis and carries a poor prognosis, death usually occurring before liver transplantation.[231]

### Pulmonary Edema Secondary to Abnormalities of the Pulmonary Veins

Obstructive disease of the pulmonary veins is a relatively rare cause of pulmonary venous hypertension and edema that has a number of causes, including (1) congenital heart disease of both high and low flow types; (2) congenital stenosis or atresia of the pulmonary veins at their junction with the left atrium (*see* page 642); (3) idiopathic veno-occlusive disease involving the small- and medium-sized veins (*see* page 1930); (4) fibrosing mediastinitis, in which the pulmonary veins are involved in a cicatricial process (*see* page 2856); (5) anomalous pulmonary venous drainage, above or below the diaphragm, in which venous compression, stenosis, or increased resistance of the hepatic sinusoids leads to a rise in pulmonary venous pressure (*see* page 647);[232] (6) invasion or compression of pulmonary veins (e.g., by a malignant neoplasm such as left atrial leiomyosarcoma,[233] by enlarged lymph nodes,[234] or by a bronchogenic cyst [Fig. 51–23]); and (7) pulmonary vein thrombosis (as in the cases of postlobectomy edema.)[164]

The clinical, physiologic, and radiographic manifestations of pulmonary edema are usually indistinguishable from those of pulmonary venous hypertension from cardiac causes except that in most cases the heart is of normal size and, in cases in which only one or two veins are affected, the edema may be localized to a specific portion of lung (e.g., a single lobe or lung). The edema is predominantly interstitial in location, although associated periodically with air-space filling. The chronic elevation of venous pressure may result in pulmonary arterial hypertension indistinguishable from that associated with chronic mitral stenosis.

### Neurogenic and Postictal Pulmonary Edema

Acute pulmonary edema in association with raised intracranial pressure, head trauma, and seizures is a well-described but infrequent phenomenon. Although its mechanism is poorly understood, clinical and experimental studies indicate that both increased microvascular pressure and increased permeability are involved. In experiments on rats and rabbits in which increased intracranial pressure was produced acutely by injection of fibrin into the cisterna magna, it was concluded that left atrial and pulmonary venous hypertension caused the edema;[235] increased left-sided heart pressures were thought to be the result of peripheral systemic vasoconstriction, bradycardia, and reduced cardiac output. The role of the vagus nerve in neurogenic pulmonary edema is not clear. In one experimental model, edema did not develop when the vagus nerves were sectioned before the increase in intracranial pressure;[236] however, previous cervical vagotomy failed to prevent the development of edema in dogs and monkeys subjected to increased intracranial pressure in another investigation.[237]

In an experimental animal model of neurogenic pulmonary edema, measurements of left ventricular pressure were taken before and after transection of the spinal cord at T4, bilateral stellectomy, or vagotomy (or a combination of these).[238] The investigators concluded that (1) systemic vasoconstriction resulted in increased venous return, which overloaded the heart and caused severe pulmonary congestion, and (2) levels of left ventricular diastolic pressure were raised chiefly because of neural adrenergic stimuli but also because of circulating catecholamines and the increased venous return resulting from systemic vasoconstriction. In an experimental study of status epilepticus in sheep, a massive increase in plasma epinephrine and norepinephrine concen-

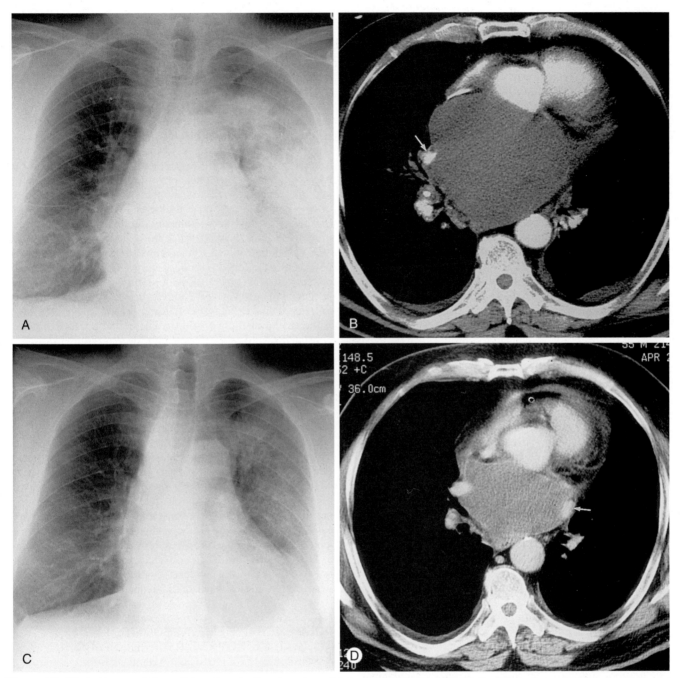

**Figure 51–23. Pulmonary Edema Secondary to Compression of Pulmonary Vein by a Mediastinal Bronchogenic Cyst.** A posteroanterior chest radiograph *(A)* in a 55-year-old man demonstrates extensive consolidation of the left upper lobe and a small left pleural effusion. A CT scan *(B)* demonstrates a large cystic mass with homogeneous water density in the subcarinal region, consistent with a mediastinal bronchogenic cyst. Note that the right superior pulmonary vein is seen *(straight arrow)* but that the left superior pulmonary vein is not visualized as a result of compression by the mass. Small bilateral pleural effusions are also evident. A chest radiograph performed 3 days later *(C)* shows marked improvement in the left upper-lobe consolidation. In the interval, the patient has developed increased opacity in the right paratracheal region associated with displacement of the trachea as a result of accumulation of fluid from spontaneous rupture of the cyst. A contrast-enhanced CT scan *(D)* demonstrates a marked decrease in size of the subcarinal cyst. Note that the left superior pulmonary vein now shows contrast enhancement *(arrow)*. The consolidation in the left upper lobe presumably represented pulmonary edema related to compression of the left superior pulmonary vein; it resolved within 3 days after spontaneous rupture of the cyst. (Courtesy of Dr. Carole Dennie, Department of Radiological Sciences, Ottawa Civic Hospital, Ottawa, Canada.)

trations (150 times baseline levels) was found and was associated with increased right- and left-sided vascular pressure;[239] when the increase in pressure was prevented using a reservoir system, the twofold increase in lung lymph flow caused by seizures was completely abolished, suggesting that, in this model at least, the increased transcapillary fluid flux is purely hydrostatic.[240] These experimental studies suggest that neurogenic pulmonary edema may be caused by transient, massive sympathetic discharge from the central nervous system, which results in generalized vasoconstriction, a shift of blood volume into the pulmonary vascular compartment, and consequent elevation of pulmonary microvascular pressure.

Clinical studies have suggested that there is also an alteration in microvascular permeability. A number of investigators have reported normal microvascular pressures and protein-rich edema fluid in patients who have neurogenic pulmonary edema.[241–243] The combination of increased pressure and increased permeability have led to the following hypothesis for the production of neurogenic pulmonary edema:[244] an acute increase in intracranial pressure causes a generalized sympathetic discharge that results in a massive increase in pulmonary vascular pressures, barotrauma to the endothelium, and consequent increased permeability; by the time microvascular pressures have been measured, they may have returned to control levels, leaving barotrauma-induced changes in permeability as the major culprit. This hypothesis has been supported by individual case reports in which patients who had neurogenic pulmonary edema have been observed to develop episodic systemic and pulmonary vascular hypertensive crises during which pulmonary arterial wedge pressure increased to 50 mm Hg.[245] In one investigation, plasma and edema fluid protein concentrations were measured, and the pattern was characterized as being suggestive of either hydrostatic- or permeability-type based on the ratio of alveolar fluid to plasma protein concentration (hydrostatic = a ratio < 0.65 and increased permeability = a ratio > 0.70);[246] seven patients had a ratio suggestive of hydrostatic edema, and five had a ratio suggestive of permeability edema. Those who had increased permeability edema had worse gas exchange and the edema took longer to resolve.

There is also experimental evidence to support the barotrauma hypothesis. For example, two groups of investigators have examined the effect of increased intracranial pressure in sheep on pulmonary lymphatic flow and lymphatic protein clearance.[247, 248] Although both groups found a moderate and transient increase in pulmonary vascular pressures, there was also a prolonged and substantial increase in lung lymph flow and an increase in the ratio of lymph-to-plasma protein concentration, suggesting an increase in microvascular permeability. The vasoconstriction and increase in permeability were blocked by prior administration of the alpha-adrenergic blocking agent phentolamine, suggesting that both effects were mediated through the sympathetic nervous system.

There is increasing evidence that a direct negative inotropic effect on the heart also contributes to the pathogenesis of neurogenic pulmonary edema.[249] Both the cardiac index and left ventricular stroke work index were markedly depressed in 12 of 20 patients admitted to one intensive care unit;[250] the hemodynamic abnormalities were improved by administration of dobutamine. Echocardiographic evidence of cardiac dysfunction develops in 10% to 30% of patients

who have subarachnoid hemorrhage.[251, 252] The dysfunction occurs in young women who are at no risk of coronary artery disease, is unassociated with an elevation of cardiac enzymes, and appears to be completely reversible.[253, 254] Although the mechanism of the cardiac injury is incompletely understood, it is related to the massive overactivity of the autonomic nervous system because it can be prevented by adrenergic blockade.[249]

Of the various causes of neurogenic edema, head trauma is one of the most frequent; although it is often severe, it may be relatively mild and nonfatal.[160] In nontraumatized patients in whom edema develops as a consequence of raised intracranial pressure, the rise in pressure may or may not be abrupt. In three cases, edema developed from a relatively insidious elevation of intracranial pressure caused by cerebellar astrocytoma, postmeningitic hydrocephalus, and leukemic infiltration of the meninges.[160] The mechanism of development of postictal pulmonary edema is undoubtedly the same as that after trauma and increased intracranial pressure. It can develop immediately after an epileptic seizure or can be delayed for several hours. This type of edema occurs most often in young patients who have idiopathic epilepsy and in those in whom seizures relate to expanding intracranial lesions.[255–258] Neuroanatomic studies of affected individuals have suggested that the critical area of the brain is the caudal medulla where the nuclei that regulate systemic arterial pressure and afferent and efferent pathways to and from the lungs are located.[259]

The radiographic distribution of neurogenic pulmonary edema is usually generalized;[243] however, an atypical pattern (e.g., predominantly upper zonal or unilateral) is seen in some cases.[160] The atypical distribution could be related to positional factors and gravity effects. Characteristically, the edema disappears within several days after surgical relief of increased intracranial pressure. Most patients are comatose and experience frequent periods of apnea when pulmonary edema develops. Thus, they are likely to aspirate gastric secretions and suffer prolonged hypoxemia. (In fact, it is possible that aspiration is the cause of the edema in some cases.) Patients who are unconscious after head trauma and who do not develop overt pulmonary edema have been found to have abnormalities in gas exchange characterized by $\dot{V}/\dot{Q}$ mismatching and an increase in shunt;[260] it is possible that these abnormalities represent subclinical pulmonary edema.

## PULMONARY EDEMA ASSOCIATED WITH NORMAL MICROVASCULAR PRESSURE (PERMEABILITY PULMONARY EDEMA)

Following a variety of direct or indirect pulmonary insults, a number of patients develop progressive respiratory distress characterized by tachypnea, dyspnea, cough, and the physical findings of air-space consolidation. The chest radiograph reveals diffuse air-space disease, blood gas analysis demonstrates severe arterial desaturation that is resistant to high concentrations of inhaled oxygen, the lungs become stiff and difficult to ventilate, pulmonary vascular pressures and resistance increase, and it becomes necessary to institute prolonged ventilatory support. Pathologic changes are similar despite the varying inciting events, consisting of interstitial and alveolar edema, hyaline membrane formation, and destruction of type I epithelial cells in the early stage and interstitial and air-space fibrosis later on.

Although a number of terms have been used to describe this group of clinicopathologic abnormalities,[261, 262] the term *adult respiratory distress syndrome*, originally coined by Petty and Ashbaugh in 1971,[263] is now in general usage. A second relatively common designation is *permeability edema;* although *increased permeability edema* is more appropriate, the abbreviated nomenclature serves to distinguish this form of edema from that resulting primarily from increased microvascular pressure. Because of their familiarity and brevity, "permeability edema" and "ARDS" are employed throughout this text.

### Epidemiology

Although estimates in the early 1970s implied that there were as many as 150,000 new cases of ARDS each year in the United States (75 per 100,000 population),[264] more recent evidence suggests that the incidence of the disorder, as presently defined, is about 1.5 cases per 100,000 people per year.[265] Major risk factors include sepsis, aspiration of liquid gastric contents, severe trauma (including long-bone and pelvic fractures and pulmonary contusion), multiple blood transfusions, near-drowning, pancreatitis, prolonged hypotension, overwhelming pneumonia, and disseminated intravascular coagulation (DIC) (often associated with sepsis).[266, 267] Less common risk factors are drug overdose, major burns,[268] and coronary artery bypass surgery.[267]

In one study, 993 patients who had at least one of eight risk factors known to predispose to the development of permeability pulmonary edema were followed prospectively;[269] 57 of the 993 patients (about 6%) had more than one risk factor. (ARDS was defined as acute respiratory failure requiring mechanical ventilation, accompanied by the acute onset of widespread air-space opacities on the chest radiograph; physiologic criteria included a pulmonary wedge pressure less than 12 mm Hg, a respiratory system compliance less than 50 ml cm $H_2O$, and an arterial-to-alveolar partial pressure ratio of 0.2 or less.) Of the 993 patients, 67 (7%) developed ARDS, the incidence increasing to 24% in the 57 patients who had two or more risk factors. Over the period of study, the syndrome developed in 20 additional patients from causes other than those identified for prospective evaluation, including drug overdose, pancreatitis, thoracic trauma, and presumed sepsis. The risk factor with the highest incidence of ARDS was aspiration, 16 of 45 patients (36%) being so affected.

### Pathogenesis

ARDS is often regarded as a manifestation of increased microvascular permeability localized to the lungs; however, there is abundant evidence that it is really a specific feature of a generalized inflammatory disorder termed the *systemic inflammatory response syndrome* [SIRS].*[270–273] Although an increase in microvascular permeability and the development of interstitial and air-space edema are initially the major clinical consequences of this acute inflammatory process, the injury also involves severe damage to endothelial cells in multiple organs, especially in the setting of sepsis and trauma. Initially, the generalized endothelial injury is often clinically silent; however, if the patient survives the consequences of pulmonary edema, manifestations of renal, cardiac, gastrointestinal, and/or cerebral dysfunction soon appear. In fact, patients who die of ARDS after 72 hours almost invariably have evidence of a syndrome termed *multiple system organ failure* (MSOF; multiple organ dysfunction syndrome [MODS]).*[273, 274] The pathogenesis of this syndrome involves a complex series of inflammatory events, including the participation of cytokines and chemokines, preformed plasma-derived inflammatory mediators, and newly generated arachidonic acid mediators from both the cyclooxygenase and lipoxygenase pathways.[275] Activation of the complement and blood clotting systems can also be involved. These biochemical substances, as well as integrins and selectins on endothelial cells and epithelial cells, mediate the recruitment of a variety of inflammatory cell types.

There is as yet no unifying theory to tie together the intricate inflammatory cascades and cytokine networks involved in the pathogenesis of SIRS, ARDS, and MODS, and we present only a survey of the various pathways and mechanisms that are thought to be important. Despite this complexity and the wide variety of precipitating events (Table 51–2), the similarity of the pathologic characteristics in all cases of ARDS suggest that there is a common final pathway of injury.[278]

### Pulmonary Microvascular Endothelial Cells, Alveolar Epithelial Cells, and Macrophages

The major targets for the agents that precipitate ARDS are the endothelial and epithelial cells that line the alveolar walls. The same cells also have an important role in orchestrating the inflammatory response by secreting a number of cytokines and expressing a variety of surface glycoproteins (selectins and integrins). Human pulmonary endothelial cells in culture are sensitive to the effects of bacterial endo-

---

*There is a confusing array of diagnostic labels that have been applied to patients who have evidence of a systemic inflammatory response, with or without evidence for a systemic infection. *Sepsis syndrome* is a commonly used term that has been defined as the presence of systemic bacterial infection accompanied by evidence of a deleterious systemic effect of the infection.[276] Criteria for the diagnosis of infection include significant hyperthermia or hypothermia, appreciable leukopenia or leukocytosis, and a positive blood culture of an accepted pathogen (or the identification of a suspected source of systemic infection from which a known pathogen was cultured); evidence for deleterious systemic effects includes hypotension or a decrease in systemic vascular resistance (or both) and unexplained metabolic acidosis.

In 1991, the American College of Chest Physicians and the Society of Critical Care Medicine recommended a series of labels and diagnostic criteria to describe gradations of illness in the clinical settings that lead to the development of ARDS.[273] According to these recommendations, SIRS can be defined as a clinical condition that includes, but is not limited to, hyperthermia (>38° C) or hypothermia (<36° C), tachycardia (>90 beats per minute), tachypnea (>20 breaths per minute), hyperventilation (Paco₂ <32 mm Hg), and increased or decreased white blood cell count (>12,000/cu mm or < 4,000/cu mm). When the syndrome can be shown to be associated with an infectious process the term *sepsis* is appropriate; when associated with evidence of organ dysfunction as a result of hypoperfusion the term *severe sepsis* is used. The term *septic shock* is reserved for patients who have severe sepsis and who develop systemic hypotension resistant to fluid resuscitation. As patients progress from SIRS to septic shock, an increasing proportion develop ARDS.[277] MODS refers to a process in which multiple organs develop an absolute or relative inability to maintain normal homeostasis; it can be a primary consequence of the initial insult (e.g., multiple trauma) or may be secondary to an exuberant inflammatory reaction.[273]

### Table 51–2. CAUSES OF INCREASED PERMEABILITY PULMONARY EDEMA (ARDS)

**DIRECT PULMONARY INSULTS**

*Inhalation or Aspiration*

Smoke
Toxic chemicals
Nitrogen dioxide (silo-filler's disease)
Sulfur dioxide
Carbon monoxide
Ozone
Ammonia
Chlorine
Phosgene inhalation[679]
Cocaine inhalation[680]
Lacrimator exposure (pepper spray, tear gas, or mace)[681]
Gastric acid
Polymer fumes (polytetrafluoroethylene)[682, 683]
Nitric acid inhalation[684]
$NO_2$ (from a zamboni in an enclosed skating area)[685]
Oxygen toxicity
Water (near-drowning)
Numerous community or industrial chemical gas exposures[686]

*Drugs and Chemicals*

Paraquat
Heroin and morphine[687]
Salicylates[688, 689]
Bleomycin[690]
Amiodarone[691]
Ethylene glycol[692]
Lithium[693]
Ethchlorvynol
Polyethylene glycol[694]
Methadone
Ketamine abuse (possibly a hydrostatic component)[695]
Propoxyphene
Ibuprofen (in acquired immunodeficiency syndrome)[696]
Paclitaxel therapy for breast cancer (possibly a hydrostatic component)[697]
Low-molecular-weight dextran[698]
Carbamate and organophosphate poisoning[699]
Hydrogen peroxide (used to irrigate a wound)[700]
Cocaine and amphetamines[701]
Gemcitabine antineoplastic therapy[702]
Ethanolamine oleate (used to sclerose esophageal varices)[703]
Verapamil overdose[704]
Hydrochlorothiazide[705]
Tocolytic therapy (e.g., terbutaline infused to prevent the onset of labor)[706, 707]
Ergometrine therapy for vaginal bleeding (possibly a hydrostatic component)[708]
Tricyclic antidepressants (possibly a hydrostatic component)[709]

Triazolam[710]
Interleukin-2 therapy for metastatic carcinoma (combined hydrostatic and permeability edema)[711]
Sublingual buprenorphine[712]
Scorpion envenomation[713, 714]
Stonefish envenomation[715]
Kombucha tea (mushroom-based tea)[716]
Numerous drugs and poisons[717]

*Infection*

Viral (e.g., Hantavirus[717a])
Rickettsial[719]
Bacterial (e.g., typhoid fever[720])
Babesiosis[718]
Fungal
Tuberculosis[721]
Protozoal (*Pneumocystis,* malaria)[722, 723]

*Miscellaneous*

Fat emboli
Amniotic fluid emboli[724]
Air emboli[725, 726]
Decompression sickness[727]
Pulmonary contusion
Radiologic contrast media[672]
Thoracic radiation[728]
Chronic eosinophilic pneumonia[729]

**INDIRECT PULMONARY INSULTS**

Sepsis
Anaphylaxis[730]
Multisystem trauma
Multiple transfusions
Antilymphocyte globulin therapy[731]
Disseminated intravascular coagulation
Pancreatitis
Pheochromocytoma[666–668]
Diabetic ketoacidosis[669, 670]
Cardiopulmonary bypass
High altitude
Rapid lung re-expansion
Neurogenic
Sickle-cell crisis[732]
Hyperthermia[733]
Hypothermia[734]
Hyponatremic encephalopathy[735]
Eclampsia[736]
Bone marrow transplantation[737]
Extreme physical exertion[738]
Tumor lysis syndrome[739]

---

toxin,[279] as well as many of the constituents of the cytokine "soup" that is generated by inflammatory and tissue cells during acute lung injury.[280] In such models, endothelial injury is first manifested by cell retraction, which causes a reduction in barrier function, a release of intracellular enzymes, and, ultimately, cell death. Endothelial cells exposed to endotoxin can produce a variety of cytokines, including interleukin (IL)-1, IL-6, and IL-8 as well as factors such as granulocyte-macrophage colony-stimulating factor (GM-CSF), which can influence the bone marrow to increase the production of inflammatory cells.[281] The stimulated endothelial cells also express surface molecules that cause circulating inflammatory cells to adhere to them and migrate through their intercellular junctions; these molecules include the intercellular adhesion molecules-1 and -2 (ICAM-1, and

ICAM-2), vascular cell adhesion molecule-1 (VCAM-1), and members of the selectin family (E-selectin and P-selectin).[282]

Although alveolar epithelial cells are more resistant to injury than endothelial cells, they are invariably damaged in the course of ARDS and may also have an active role in mediating the inflammatory response. Epithelial cells are capable of expressing a variety of cytokines and surface active molecules.[283] Such expression is associated with attraction of leukocytes as well as adherence to and migration across the epithelium.

Alveolar macrophages also have an important role in modulating the inflammatory reaction in ARDS. After exposure to endotoxin, they release tumor necrosis factor (TNF) and IL-1, both of which are powerful proinflammatory mediators that can initiate and perpetuate the inflammatory cascade directly and by secondary induction of additional cytokines.[280]

### Shock

Episodes of hypotension, either brief or prolonged and caused by hypovolemia, impaired cardiac output, a decrease in systemic vascular smooth muscle tone, or a combination of these, are frequent in patients who subsequently develop ARDS. Although this suggests a pathogenetic role, it is difficult to cause lung damage by shock alone,[284] and it is probable that other factors must be involved to produce the complete syndrome in most instances.

In an ultrastructural study of the lungs of dogs subjected to hemorrhagic shock, the initial change was platelet adhesiveness and aggregation.[285] These aggregates, to which leukocytes were soon added, caused extensive occlusion of the pulmonary microcirculation, followed shortly afterward by swelling and fragmentation of vascular endothelium and disintegration and disappearance of the platelets; subsequently, the leukocytes also disintegrated, freeing their lysosomes into the microcirculation, particularly the capillaries and venules. Discontinuities appeared in type I alveolar lining cells, and edema fluid and red blood cells began to accumulate in the interstitium and alveoli. The development of these pathologic abnormalities was time dependent: rapid bleeding of the dog followed by death within 20 minutes elicited platelet aggregation but no changes in the alveolar septa, whereas more prolonged hypotension or hypovolemia (up to 1 hour) permitted leukocytes to become incorporated into the aggregates, with subsequent disintegration and release of lysosomal granules. The investigators further observed that reinfusion of the withdrawn blood after the hypotensive episode increased the severity of the pulmonary lesions unless the blood was passed through a filter that removed platelet-leukocyte microemboli. By contrast, the results in a study in sheep showed that hemorrhage and reinfusion of the shed blood produced no evidence of pulmonary microvascular injury.[286]

In another study of dogs who had hemorrhagic shock, lung lymph flow remained constant or increased and the protein concentration in lymph remained high despite a decrease in the calculated microvascular pressure, indicating an increase in microvascular permeability.[39] Using horseradish peroxidase as a marker, the investigators calculated that the findings could be explained best by a sevenfold increase in pore number and no change in average pore size. As the authors pointed out, these figures might be associated with a very subtle injury that could easily be missed on ultrastructural examination.

### Polymorphonuclear Leukocytes

There is considerable evidence derived from both experimental and clinical studies that leukocytes are important in the pathogenesis of pulmonary injury in many cases of ARDS.* A large pool of marginated neutrophils reside

---

*Although the polymorphonuclear leukocyte is the most important white blood cell implicated in the pathogenesis of ARDS, eosinophil cationic protein has been demonstrated in the bronchoalveolar lavage (BAL) fluid of patients who have ARDS, suggesting that eosinophils may also participate.[291, 292]

within the normal lung. Under normal circumstances, their presence in the pulmonary circulation may simply reflect the fact that they are larger and less deformable than red blood cells, mechanical constraints that slow their transit through the pulmonary microvasculature. The size of the marginated pool of leukocytes appears to be dependent on pulmonary blood flow, at least in some species.[287–289] As a result, there is a vertical gradient in leukocyte retention in the lung; that is, more white blood cells are delayed in the lung microvasculature in a single pass through the nondependent lung (where blood flow per unit lung volume is low) than at the lung base (where blood flow per unit lung volume is high). Similarly, if pulmonary blood flow is transiently decreased, white blood cells accumulate within the lung but are released again when cardiac output is increased. This phenomenon appears to explain the leukocytosis that occurs in humans after exercise and catecholamine infusion, increased blood flow in both situations transiently "flushing" leukocytes from the marginated pool.[290] Thus, it is possible that blood flow can play an important role in the development of leukocyte-induced lung injury.

Although the initial leukocyte–endothelial cell contact is caused by mechanical factors, prolonged sequestration and adherence requires an interaction of the cellular adhesion molecules, which are expressed by both the neutrophil and the endothelial cell. Leukocyte–endothelial cell adherence is mediated by three distinct families of surface molecules; on the neutrophils, L-selectin mediates loose adherence (rolling) whereas the $\beta_2$-integrins (CD11/CD18 heterodimers) are responsible for firm adherence and are necessary for diapedesis into the pulmonary interstitium and air spaces.[293, 294] CD11/CD18 expression is increased on the surface of circulating neutrophils in patients who have ARDS.[295] These leukocyte-specific molecules interact with ICAM-1 and ICAM-2, VCAM-1, and P- and E-selectin on the endothelial and epithelial cell surfaces.

Circulating or marginated neutrophils respond to a chemotactic gradient that causes them to migrate toward a site of injury. This chemoattraction is mediated by a variety of chemotaxins and chemokines. The former include factors such as the bacterial lipopolysaccharide endotoxins, the complement anaphylatoxin C5a, leukotrienes, prostaglandins, immunoglobulin fragments, fibrinogen fragments, macrophage products such as macrophage inflammatory protein-2 (MIP-2), and platelet-activating factor. The chemokines (RANTES, IL-8, MIP-1α, and MIP-1β) are a family of low-molecular-weight peptides that are produced by a variety of cells and act on chemokine receptors expressed on a variety of leukocytes.[296] These substances and chemical compounds such as N-formylated peptides (f-MLP) and phorbol esters (e.g., phorbol myristate acetate [PMA]) cause both migration and activation of neutrophils. The latter is manifested by increased generation of oxygen free radicals, lysosomal enzymes, and arachidonate metabolites.[297] It is associated with a respiratory burst that appears to be related to the stimulation of a membrane-bound nicotinamide adenine dinucleotide phosphate (reduced form) (NADPH) oxidase and is characterized by increased oxygen consumption, increased hexose-monophosphate shunt activity, and the production of several species of oxygen radicals, including superoxide ($O_2^{*-}$), hydrogen peroxide ($H_2O_2$), and the hydroxyl radical (OH*). Oxygen radical generation by activated neutrophils is necessary for its bactericidal action on ingested microorganisms.

In addition to oxygen radicals, neutrophils can also release products of arachidonate metabolism (including prostaglandins, thromboxanes, and leukotrienes) and enzymes that are designed for bacterial digestion. Neutrophil granules contain a variety of enzymes, including elastase, collagenase, cathepsins, cationic proteins, lysozyme, lactoferrin, and myeloperoxidase, many of which can attack and degrade normal proteins and cells; regurgitation of these toxic enzymes during bacterial phagocytosis, either successful or attempted, may be an important mechanism of tissue injury. Neutrophil elastase in particular is capable of degrading every component of the extracellular matrix; it is likely that this capability is related to the evidence of active elastolysis in ARDS.[298]

There is abundant clinical and experimental evidence in support of a role for neutrophils in the pathogenesis of ARDS, including (1) the presence of animal models of acute lung injury that are dependent on the presence of neutrophils; (2) the presence of animal models in which chemotactic agents such as C5a have been shown to attract leukocytes to the pulmonary microvasculature with resulting pulmonary microvascular injury; (3) the demonstration that severe, acute leukopenia frequently predates the onset of ARDS in patients;[299, 300] (4) the presence of neutrophils in lung biopsy specimens and postmortem lung specimens from patients who have established ARDS;[301, 302] (5) the presence of increased numbers of neutrophils and of neutrophil-derived products such as neutrophil elastase in BAL fluid of similarly affected patients; (6) the recognition that many of the risk factors for ARDS are associated with complement activation and leukopenia secondary to sequestration of leukocytes within the lungs; and (7) the observation that the production of leukopenia protects against certain lung injuries.

Infusion of gram-negative bacteria[303] or microemboli[304] can cause an increase in microvascular permeability in sheep in which lung lymph flow and protein concentration are used to assess microvascular permeability. Neutrophils are necessary for the development of these permeability changes, because prior administration of chemotherapeutic agents in doses sufficient to cause neutropenia protects against the development of lung injury.[304–306] Neutrophils are also necessary for the development of pulmonary edema resulting from the injection of PMA, a substance that causes increased neutrophil adhesiveness, aggregation, degranulation, and the production of oxygen radicals. In the presence of leukocytes, PMA causes pulmonary edema in rabbit lungs, an effect that can be attenuated when dimethylthiourea (an oxygen free radical scavenger) is administered in conjunction with the PMA.[307, 308]

In experimental animals, endotoxin causes preferential neutrophil sequestration in the pulmonary vascular bed. Low doses apparently exert a direct effect on the leukocytes rather than on the pulmonary microvascular endothelium itself. A combination of minute doses of endotoxin and chemotactic factors, such as complement fragments, results in prolonged sequestration of neutrophils within the pulmonary microvascular compartment and increased microvascular permeability.[309] Endotoxin infusion in sheep has been shown to cause a combination of leukopenia, pulmonary arterial hypertension, and increased pulmonary vascular permeability;[310] a blocker of the cyclooxygenase pathway of arachidonic acid

metabolism prevents the pulmonary hypertensive effect but not the leukopenia or increased permeability.

In patients who have established ARDS, BAL fluid not only shows a considerable increase in the differential count of neutrophils but also contains chemotactic factors for human neutrophils.[311] Peripheral circulating leukocytes show signs of activation, characterized by an increased chemotactic index, increased metabolic activity, and increased superoxide anion generation.[312, 313] In one study, BAL fluid was obtained from 9 intubated control subjects who did not have ARDS, 12 patients who had risk factors for the development of ARDS (aspiration or sepsis), and 11 patients who had established ARDS caused chiefly by aspiration or sepsis;[314] the percentage of neutrophils was approximately 1 in the control group, 50 in those at risk, and 70 in patients who had established ARDS. In addition, there was a 10- to 40-fold increase in the protein content of the lavage fluid in the latter two groups, indicating a considerable increase in alveolar epithelial permeability.

In another study in which BAL was performed on 4 mechanically ventilated control subjects, 12 normal volunteers, and 11 patients who had ARDS, the percentage of neutrophils in the lavage fluid was 4%, 0.8%, and 68%, respectively;[315] moreover, the percentage correlated with the severity of the gas exchange impairment in the patients who had ARDS. In another investigation, the peripheral blood leukocyte count was monitored every 6 hours in 40 patients at high risk for the development of ARDS;[316] ARDS developed in 10 patients, in 8 of whom the clinical diagnosis was preceded by the development of transient leukopenia (defined as a total leukocyte count less than 4,200 cells/mm³). Only 4 of the 30 patients in whom ARDS did not develop showed a similar leukopenia. It has also been shown that patients who have fully developed ARDS—or even those who have factors such as sepsis that predispose to ARDS—sequester increased numbers of polymorphonuclear leukocytes in their lungs.[317]

Despite the impressive list of observations implicating neutrophils in the pathogenesis of ARDS, there is also convincing evidence that the syndrome can occur in the absence of circulating or tissue neutrophils.[318, 319] For example, in one retrospective study, 11 patients were identified in whom ARDS was accompanied by an absence of circulating neutrophils;[320] in 5 of these, lung biopsy specimens showed changes typical of ARDS unassociated with a neutrophilic infiltrate. In another investigation of 6 leukopenic patients, ARDS developed in the absence of circulating neutrophils;[321] however, it worsened appreciably when the white blood cell count eventually increased as a result of bone marrow recovery from chemotherapeutic suppression. Finally, certain specific causes of ARDS, such as Hantavirus infection, appear to be unassociated with neutrophilic activation.[322]

### Surfactant

Both qualitative and quantitative abnormalities of surfactant have been demonstrated in alveolar fluid obtained from patients who have ARDS.[323–325] These abnormalities may have several causes, including dilution of the normal amount of surface active phospholipid by the exudate within the alveoli, deficiency in phospholipid production as a result of epithelial injury, and surfactant inactivation by oxygen radicals or other substances.[326] Studies of animals subjected to acute lung injury by subcutaneous injection of N-nitroso-N-methylurethane have shown a progressive decrease in lung compliance coincident with a reduction in levels of desaturated phosphatidylcholine in alveolar lavage fluid during the early phase of the injury.[327] In addition to a reduction in the amount of surface active phospholipid that can be recovered by lavage, a decrease in intracellular desaturated phosphatidylcholine also occurs, suggesting that impaired synthesis rather than increased degradation is the major cause of the deficiency.[328] Oxygen radicals generated by activated neutrophils can also directly inactivate surfactant activity by lipid peroxidation.[329, 330]

A number of the cytokines and mediators implicated in the pathogenesis of ARDS have an effect on surfactant function or synthesis. For example, TNF-α decreases the synthesis of surfactant by isolated type II pneumocytes.[331, 332] Proteolytic enzymes such as neutrophil elastase are capable of degrading the surfactant proteins SP-A, SP-B, and SP-C, which are important for proper function of surfactant.[333] As the coagulation cascade is initiated in the air spaces during the exudative phase of ARDS, surfactant is bound within the fibrin strands and loses its surface active properties.[280, 334] Because surfactant can inhibit IL-1, IL-6, and TNF release from alveolar macrophages,[332, 335, 336] its degradation also has a proinflammatory action.

In the respiratory distress syndrome of newborns, a deficiency of surfactant production associated with a loss of the ability of alveolar lining fluid to lower surface tension is believed to be the primary cause of pulmonary injury. By contrast, the abnormalities of surfactant function and synthesis that occur in adults who have ARDS are the result rather than the cause of the injury. This has been well illustrated by the lack of a distinct benefit of exogenous surfactant replacement in large randomized trials[337, 338] and in smaller clinical[339, 340] and experimental studies.[341] This is not to say that the disruption of the surfactant layer and the resultant increase in surface tension are not important mechanisms contributing to the development and perpetuation of alveolar edema in ARDS; disruption of surfactant by itself can increase lung water, presumably by increasing the surface tension at the alveolar fluid-air interface, resulting in the suction of water from the interstitial space.[78]

### Complement

Although activation of complement is designed primarily to initiate inflammation as part of the protective response against invading microorganisms, it is clear that in some circumstances it results in host damage. For example, complement may have a direct toxic effect on certain cells; neutrophil activation can then cause a release of enzymes and oxygen radicals that can secondarily damage host cells and tissues.[342] Trauma and infection are two important causes of activation of the complement system; it may also occur after extracorporeal circulation during hemodialysis,[343] after cardiopulmonary bypass for coronary artery grafting,[344] and after plasmapheresis.[345] In fact, when patients who have established ARDS are supported by extracorporeal membrane oxygenation, further activation of complement and a decrease in the circulating leukocyte count occur.[346]

One of the components of complement activation by either the classic or alternate pathway is the "anaphylatoxin" C5a. Biologically, this substance is a highly active peptide that, in addition to having a direct effect on pulmonary capillary permeability, can release histamine from mast cells, cause contraction of smooth muscle, and act as a chemotactic agent for white blood cells.[347] Several observations suggest that this peptide may be important in the pathogenesis of ARDS. For example, administration of C5a in experimental animals induces lung injury associated with an intense acute inflammatory reaction.[348] In addition, both the blood and BAL fluid of patients who have ARDS have been shown to contain increased levels of the C5a.[349–351]

Despite these observations, the importance of complement activation in the pathogenesis of ARDS has been questioned.[352] For example, it has been shown that a large percentage of patients who have sepsis and other risk factors for the development of ARDS manifest complement activation in vivo unaccompanied by the subsequent development of pulmonary dysfunction.[353, 354] In two studies, complement fragments, and the cytokines IL-6 and IL-8, were elevated in severely injured patients at first assessment, regardless of whether they went on to experience ARDS or MSOF.[355, 356]

### The Clotting System

Abnormalities of the clotting system are common in ARDS and have been reviewed by several groups.[280, 357, 358] Clotting can be initiated by either the intrinsic or the extrinsic system. Exposure of collagen after pulmonary microvascular injury could activate the intrinsic system, whereas tissue thromboplastin generated from damaged lung could activate the extrinsic system. Activation results in the production of thrombin and fibrin, both of which have been shown experimentally to result in endothelial cell damage and increased pulmonary vascular permeability. In addition, fibrin monomers can stimulate pulmonary vasoconstriction through the arachidonic acid metabolism pathway. Once fibrin is generated, the plasminogen system is activated and fibrin is degraded by plasmin into fibrin split products, which themselves can damage the pulmonary microvascular endothelium.[359]

There is evidence of activation of the clotting cascade and inhibition of fibrinolysis in about 25% of patients who have ARDS.[360] In a study in which thrombin was infused intravenously in sheep and dogs, a transient increase in pulmonary arterial pressure and a sustained increase in pulmonary microvascular permeability, indicated by increased lung lymph flow and lung lymph protein concentration, were both documented.[361, 362] The increase in microvascular permeability was associated with a decrease in peripheral blood fibrinogen level, an increase in blood fibrin split products, and a decrease in the number of circulating leukocytes and platelets. Morphologic examination of the lungs of these animals showed neutrophils and platelets trapped within an intravascular meshwork of fibrin; in addition, there was evidence of interstitial and alveolar edema. The microvascular injury associated with thrombin infusion is dependent on activation of the coagulation cascade, because defibrinogenation before fibrin infusion attenuates both the vascular and permeability effects.[363] The permeability response can also be attenuated or abolished if polymorphonuclear leukocytes[364] or complement[365] are depleted before thrombin challenge or if there is interference with activation of the fibrinolytic pathway.[363] However, some investigators have shown that pulmonary damage is increased when fibrinolysis is blocked.[366]

The results of these experiments have suggested the following sequence of events in the pathogenesis of the vascular injury after thrombin infusion:[361]

- fibrin is generated from fibrinogen and activates the fibrinolytic system, resulting in the formation of plasmin from plasminogen;
- plasmin breaks down fibrin and causes cleavage of complement proteins and the formation of the chemotactic peptides C3a and C5a;
- the complement fragments cause sequestration of neutrophils within the lung; and
- neutrophil activation results in vascular injury and pulmonary edema.

There is also ample evidence that ARDS is associated with DIC.[284, 367, 368] For example, in a study of 30 consecutive patients who had ARDS, definite evidence of DIC was detected in 7 (23%).[359] However, it is unclear whether the association of DIC with ARDS is causative (i.e., the activation of the coagulation cascade results in pulmonary microvascular injury) or is secondary. DIC appears to be particularly related to the development of ARDS in patients who are affected by heat stroke. One group of investigators studied 52 consecutive patients who had this abnormality during the 1985 pilgrimage to Mecca.[369] Of these, 12 (23%) developed ARDS and 9 died; all of the 12 patients who had ARDS demonstrated biochemical evidence of DIC, whereas only 1 of the 40 patients who did not develop ARDS showed evidence of activation of the coagulation system.

Patients who have ARDS frequently have elevated blood levels of fibrin degradation products[370] and factor VIII,[371] accompanied by decreased levels of factor XII, prekallikrein,[372] antithrombin III,[373] and platelets.[374] Activation of the coagulation system is particularly evident when ARDS follows major trauma. In one study, 18 severely injured patients were evaluated prospectively for the development of ARDS and for biochemical evidence of coagulation and fibrinolysis;[375] the 8 patients who fulfilled the criteria for ARDS were found to have levels of antithrombin III, fibrinogen, and plasminogen that were significantly lower than those in whom the pulmonary complications of trauma did not develop. In another investigation of 29 patients who had major trauma, 5 of whom fulfilled the clinical criteria for the diagnosis of ARDS, 5 patients had a low platelet count and decreased levels of antithrombin III, fibrinogen, and plasminogen;[376] the authors suggested that after acute trauma, a decrease in platelet count may be a sensitive predictor of the development of ARDS. In a third study of 30 patients, fibrin degradation products were measured on days 1, 2, 3, and 7 after a major trauma;[377] fibrin degradation product levels were increased in all patients at the time of first measurement, but the levels were significantly lower in the individuals who went on the develop ARDS. Radiolabeled fibrinogen accumulates rapidly in the lungs of patients suffering from ARDS, but not in the lungs of patients who are equally ill but do not have ARDS.[378]

Examination of BAL fluid from patients who have ARDS reveals increased levels of a procoagulant that is capable of activation of factor X;[379] this augmented activity of the extrinsic coagulation pathway within the air spaces may partly explain the presence of extravascular fibrin deposition and hyaline membrane formation in ARDS. Additional evidence that the coagulation process may participate in the pathogenesis of ARDS comes from the morphologic observation of considerable intra-alveolar fibrin deposition and capillary obliteration by fibrin clots during the acute phase.[380]

Thrombocytopenia occurs in at least 50% of patients who have ARDS, almost certainly as a result of platelet consumption rather than decreased production. In a study in which radiolabeled platelets were injected into patients who had ARDS, platelet life span was lower than normal and the platelets were sequestered in the pulmonary vasculature.[381]

Because endothelial cells are the source of factor VIII, damage to pulmonary endothelial cells may be reflected in an alteration in the normal level of this substance. In a study of 100 patients who had ARDS, increased levels of immunoreactive factor VIII were detected (although overall coagulant ability was within the normal range);[382] the investigators suggested that endothelial damage may result in the release of a defective factor VIII molecule.

### Oxygen Radicals

Short-lived unstable species of oxygen molecules are generated by neutrophils, by certain specific enzymes normally present within the body, and by a variety of toxic substances. These oxygen free radicals include the superoxide radical ($O_2^{*-}$), hydrogen peroxide ($H_2O_2$), hydroxyl radical ($OH^*$), singlet oxygen ($O_2^*$), and peroxide radicals generated by peroxidation of lipids. These highly toxic species are generated by enzymes, such as xanthine oxidase, and by the normal mitochondrial energy transfer reactions. Under normal conditions, the body is equipped with a battery of antioxidant defense mechanisms that include specific enzymes, such as superoxide dismutase (which catalyzes the conversion of $O_2^{*-}$ to hydrogen peroxide), catalase (which catalyzes the conversion of hydrogen peroxide to oxygen and water), and glutathione peroxidase (which converts peroxide radicals to nontoxic lipids). In addition to these specific enzymes that can inactivate oxygen free radicals, nonspecific "free radical scavengers," such as ascorbic acid, β-carotene, and glutathione, can also neutralize these radicals.

Pulmonary toxicity associated with agents that produce oxygen free radicals is enhanced by hyperoxic conditions and lessened by hypoxic conditions. In many animal models, the specific enzymes that metabolize oxygen free radicals and the drugs that are known to scavenge them can protect against lung injury; the protection is effective in models in which the injurious agent appears to damage the endothelium directly by generating radicals and in those in which neutrophil sequestration and activation within the lung appear to be a prerequisite for the development of injury. Experimental studies suggest that oxygen free radical damage may be the final common pathway in a variety of acute lung injuries, whether they are related to direct toxicity or to neutrophil-mediated toxicity.[383] However, it is difficult to gather direct evidence that incriminates oxygen free radical formation in the pathogenesis of ARDS in humans. Oxygen free radicals are extremely short-lived, and no direct methods are available either to identify them or to quantify them. Indirect evidence for their presence in the lung derives from studies that have shown an increased amount of oxidized substances, such as $\alpha_1$-proteinase inhibitor, in the BAL fluid of patients who have ARDS.[384] Hydrogen peroxide also can be detected in increased amounts in the urine of patients who have ARDS with and without sepsis, and higher levels are associated with a worse prognosis.[385]

The pulmonary sources of oxygen radicals include activated neutrophils, macrophages, and even endothelial cells themselves. Many of the proinflammatory stimuli that have already been mentioned, including endotoxin, TNF, IL-1, IL-6, IL-8, platelet-activating factor, and complement fragments, can facilitate or directly stimulate neutrophils and macrophages to produce oxygen radicals.[386] Endothelial cells convert xanthines to uric acid using a xanthine dehydrogenase/oxidase system; oxygen radicals are a byproduct of the oxidase portion of the enzyme complex, and its activity can be increased in acute lung injury.[387] Neutrophils recovered from central venous blood have a greater capacity to generate free radicals than those simultaneously collected from arterial blood, suggesting that the activated neutrophils are preferentially retained within the pulmonary circulation.[388]

### Enzymes and Mediators

There is no doubt that both the mediators of inflammation and a variety of enzymes play important roles in initiating or modifying lung injury in ARDS. The initiators of the inflammatory response appear to be the cytokines.[389] These are a diverse group of biologically active proteins and peptides that act as soluble signals between cells.[296] As mentioned previously, TNF and IL-1 generated by alveolar and tissue macrophages are the first mediators to be detected. They have the ability to alter hemodynamics and lung oxygenation, induce fever, and activate neutrophils and the coagulation cascade. They also induce the up-regulation of endothelial and epithelial adhesion molecules and cause secretion of the powerful neutrophil chemoattractant IL-8.[390] Levels of this mediator are particularly increased in patients whose ARDS is attributed to sepsis.[391] TNF and IL-1 also stimulate the liver to synthesize and secrete IL-6 and acute-phase proteins and decrease the synthesis of albumin.[392, 393] All of these cytokines are increased in the circulating blood of patients who have ARDS relative to normal subjects and to patients who have cardiogenic pulmonary edema.[280]

Cytokines also cause the generation and secretion of arachidonic acid metabolites,[394] which in turn can either cause or protect against lung injury. Arachidonic acid is a membrane-derived, free fatty acid that can be metabolized by means of the cyclooxygenase pathway to the prostaglandins and thromboxanes or by means of the lipoxygenase pathway to the leukotrienes. Thromboxane causes platelet aggregation and pulmonary vascular constriction, whereas prostacyclin is a potent pulmonary arterial dilator and is capable of causing disaggregation of platelets. The leukotrienes are a varied group of mediators that can cause edema either directly by increasing vascular permeability or indirectly by inducing vascular smooth muscle contraction and chemotaxis of leukocytes to the site of mediator release. Leukotriene B$_4$ is a potent neutrophil chemoattractant that is produced in the lung by activated macrophages and seques-

tered neutrophils, resulting in the potential for a powerful positive feedback loop to perpetuate the inflammatory response.[395, 396] Most cells have the enzymatic capacity to produce prostaglandins and leukotrienes, although different cell types preferentially generate particular products. There may be complex interactions between various arachidonic acid-derived mediators; for example, the lipoxygenase-derived product leukotriene D$_4$ causes pulmonary arterial hypertension that can be blocked by the cyclooxygenase blocker indomethacin, suggesting that it exerts its vascular effect by stimulating prostaglandin production.[397]

Although plasma levels of prostaglandins are not increased in patients who have ARDS,[398] increased levels of leukotrienes (including leukotriene D$_4$) have been identified in the pulmonary edema fluid of such patients but not in those who have hydrostatic edema of similar severity.[399] There is also evidence for decreased pulmonary removal of certain prostaglandins, such as prostaglandin E$_1$, probably secondary to the diffuse endothelial injury that constitutes the basic feature of ARDS.[400, 401] A number of attempts have been made to alter the natural course of ARDS by modulating the synthesis of arachidonic acid products. However, several randomized studies have shown no beneficial effect of any "anti-inflammatory" medications (both steroids and nonsteroidal anti-inflammatory agents).[402, 403]

A number of additional mediators and enzymes have also been implicated in the pathogenesis of ARDS. Endothelin-1 is the most powerful pulmonary arterial vasoconstrictor known, and circulating levels have been reported to average seven times the normal level during the acute exudative stage of ARDS.[404] In fact, the increased levels of endothelin-1 may be one of the explanations for the persistently elevated pulmonary artery pressure with which ARDS is associated. Prekallikrein is the inactive precursor of plasma kallikrein, which is both a component of the coagulation and fibrinolytic systems and an activator of the kinin system. There is some evidence for prekallikrein activation in the blood and BAL fluid of patients who have ARDS;[405, 406] in addition, in animal models of acute lung injury, bradykinin generation has been demonstrated and has been accompanied by increased pulmonary vascular permeability.[407] Greatly increased concentrations of elastase[406, 408–410] and other neutrophil-derived enzymes[411] can be detected in the blood and BAL fluid of patients who have ARDS. It is likely that these increased enzyme levels represent a marker of leukocyte activation, although it is possible that the enzymes themselves cause tissue injury. Increased levels of the enzyme phospholipase A$_2$ have been demonstrated in the blood of patients who have gram-negative sepsis, the levels being particularly high in those who develop ARDS.[412] If the phospholipase gained access to the alveolar air space, it could cause degradation of surfactant and thus contribute to the decreased lung compliance characteristic of ARDS. Additional cytokines and mediators that have been reported in ARDS include the platelet-derived neutrophil activating peptide-2 (NAP-2),[413] the polyamines,[414] and transforming growth factor-$\alpha$ (TGF-$\alpha$);[415] the last-named may be particularly important during the proliferative phase of the injury.

### Pathologic Characteristics

The pathologic changes in the lungs of patients who have ARDS are virtually the same regardless of etiology and are usually described by the term *diffuse alveolar damage.* Although a continuum of histologic abnormalities exists, for purposes of discussion the changes can conveniently be described in three phases: exudative, proliferative, and fibrotic.[416-418]

**The Exudative Phase.** In the early exudative phase, which in most cases occurs within hours after the initial pulmonary insult, the lungs are heavy and airless and often deep red-purple. Histologically, there is interstitial edema (affecting perivascular and interlobular interstitium as well as the alveolar wall), capillary congestion, and air-space filling by a proteinaceous exudate and a variable number of red blood cells; despite the evidence implicating neutrophils in the pathogenesis of disease, inflammatory cells are usually scarce at the time biopsy specimens are viewed. Fibrin thrombi may be present in capillaries and small arterioles and venules.[416, 419]

Somewhat later in the course of the exudative phase (2 to 7 days), the intra-alveolar edema appears more compact and eosinophilic and may contain macrophages; similar material in alveolar ducts and distal respiratory bronchioles tends to become flattened against the airway wall, producing hyaline membranes (Fig. 51–24). Ultrastructurally, these membranes are composed of necrotic cellular debris and fibrin;[420, 421] immunohistochemically, they contain immunoglobulin (predominantly IgG), fibrinogen, surfactant apoprotein, and, in the later stages, fibronectin.[420] During this period, type II alveolar epithelial cells undergo proliferation, resulting in a relining of alveolar surfaces. Such hyperplastic cells are often large and can show markedly atypical nuclear features.

**The Proliferative Phase.** Although it is not possible to put a precise time on the end of the exudative phase, changes of the proliferative phase are usually seen from 7 to 28 days after the initial pulmonary insult. This process is characterized by fibroblast (myofibroblast) proliferation, predominantly within alveolar air spaces but also in the parenchymal interstitium.[420] The cellular proliferation is accompanied by synthesis and deposition of proteoglycans such as versican in the interstitium.[422] In time, collagen is laid down within this provisional matrix. Proximal transitional airways are often spared, creating a highly characteristic gross appearance of multiple, evenly distributed spaces (representing the lumens of transitional airways) separated by more or less solid white-gray tissue (representing consolidated lung parenchyma) (Fig. 51–25). Mononuclear inflammatory cells, predominantly lymphocytes, may be apparent within the interstitium. In the lungs of patients who die of respiratory failure, focal areas of bronchopneumonia caused by bacterial superinfection are fairly common.

**The Fibrotic Phase.** In some patients, sufficient collagen is deposited to result in a significant degree of interstitial fibrosis. In those who have less severe disease, much of the fibroblastic proliferation resolves without functionally or histologically significant residual fibrosis. Pulmonary vascular abnormalities are also common and are sometimes extensive.[423, 424] They probably result from several causes, including microvascular thrombosis initiated by the initial pulmonary insult and thromboembolism.[423] In some cases, they are associated with vascular remodeling characterized by tortuous arteries and veins, a decreased number of pulmonary capillaries, intimal fibrosis, increased muscle in arterial

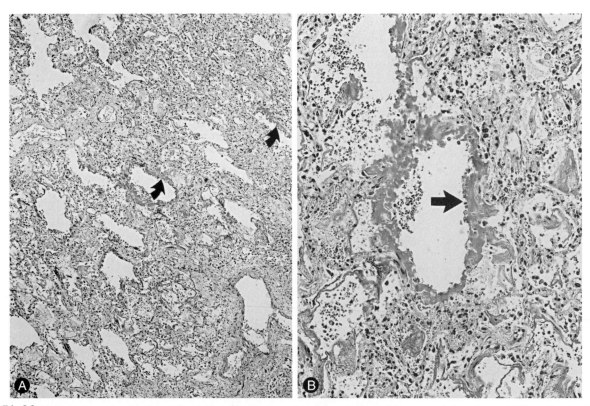

**Figure 51–24. Diffuse Alveolar Damage: Exudative Phase.** A section of lung in the full-blown exudative phase of diffuse alveolar damage *(A)* shows filling of almost all alveolar air spaces by a proteinaceous exudate containing scattered red blood cells (seen to better advantage in a section at higher magnification *[B]*). Inflammatory cells are few, and there is a mild to moderate degree of interstitial edema. Well-developed hyaline membranes *(arrows)* are present in several transitional airways. (*A,* ×40; *B,* ×120.)

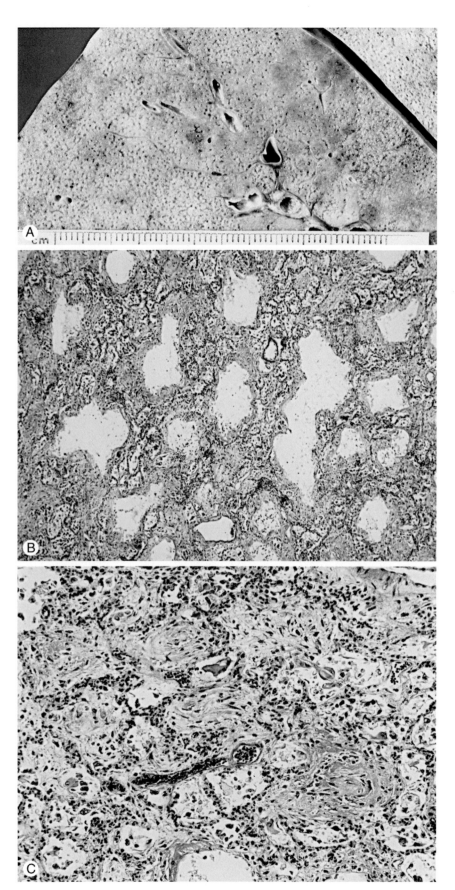

**Figure 51–25. Diffuse Alveolar Damage: Organizing Phase.** A magnified view of the superior segment of a lower lobe *(A)* shows diffuse, fairly uniform parenchymal consolidation associated with numerous minute "holes." A section *(B)* reveals that the "holes" consist of patent transitional airways. At higher magnification *(C)*, the intervening lung parenchyma is seen to be almost completely consolidated by loose connective tissue containing fibroblasts and macrophages. Alveolar walls are clearly recognizable and are only slightly thickened, indicating that the fibroblastic reaction is occurring predominantly within alveolar air spaces. *(B, ×40; C, ×120.)*

media, and extension of muscle into arterioles (neomuscularization).

### Radiologic Manifestations

Radiography

Remarkably good correlation has been reported between the radiographic patterns observed during life and the pathologic changes observed at autopsy.[416, 425–427]

**The Exudative Phase.** All observers report a characteristic delay of up to 12 hours from the clinical onset of respiratory failure to the appearance of abnormalities on the chest radiograph. The earliest findings consist of patchy, ill-defined opacities throughout both lungs. In one study, evidence of interstitial edema was remarkably infrequent (only 5 of 75 patients);[425] however, in two other series, it was more common (Fig. 51–26).[416, 426] The appearance is similar to air-space edema of cardiac origin, except that the heart size is usually normal and the edema tends to show a more peripheral distribution (Fig. 51–27).

The patchy zones of consolidation rapidly coalesce to

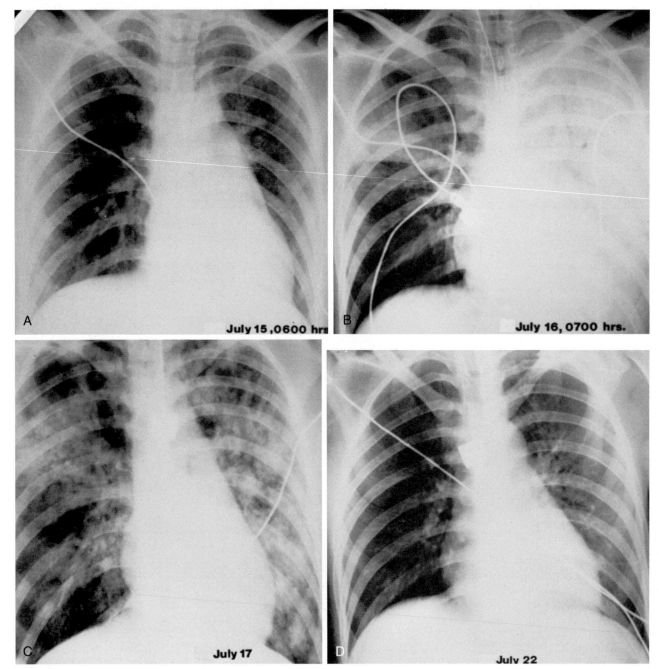

**Figure 51–26. Adult Respiratory Distress Syndrome Associated with Gram-Negative Septicemia.** Several hours before the radiograph illustrated in *A*, a 31-year-old woman had noted the onset of respiratory distress, which had increased in severity in this interval. This radiograph reveals diffuse interstitial edema but no evidence of air-space edema or of major pulmonary consolidation. Twenty-four hours later *(B)*, the right upper lobe and the whole of the left lung were extensively consolidated by acute air-space edema. Forty-eight hours later *(C)*, the lungs were uniformly involved, although in a more patchy distribution. With the institution of vigorous supportive therapy and positive end-expiratory pressure ventilation (PEEP), the patient's condition improved slowly to a point where 5 days later *(D)* the lungs were almost clear. Gram-negative septicemia occurred after laparotomy.

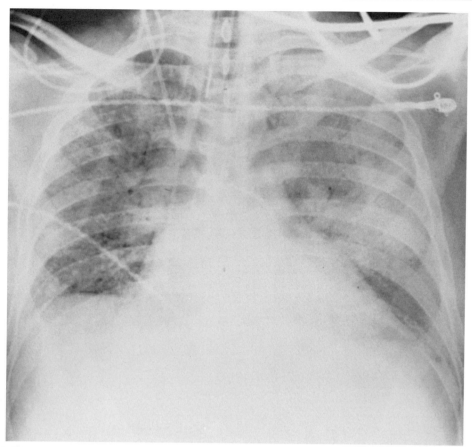

**Figure 51–27. Adult Respiratory Distress Syndrome Caused by Traumatic Shock.** A radiograph of the chest in anteroposterior projection, supine position, reveals diffuse air-space consolidation that is evenly distributed throughout both lungs; a prominent air bronchogram is visible. Heart size is within normal limits. A normal pulmonary arterial wedge pressure was recorded through a Swan-Ganz catheter. The patient died several days later, and at autopsy the lungs showed the exudative phase of diffuse alveolar damage. The patient was a young woman who was admitted to hospital in shock approximately 12 hours after a motor vehicle accident.

a point of massive air-space consolidation (Fig. 51–28). Characteristically, involvement is diffuse, affecting all lung zones from apex to base and to the extreme periphery of each lung; in our experience, this widespread distribution can be of considerable value in distinguishing ARDS from cardiogenic pulmonary edema, whose distribution is seldom as extensive. Similarly, in contrast to cardiogenic edema, an air bronchogram is frequently visible. Pleural effusion is characteristically inapparent on supine radiographs; its presence should strongly suggest concomitant hydrostatic pulmonary edema or complicating acute pneumonia or pulmonary infarction.

It is important to be aware of the potential effects of mechanical ventilation and PEEP on radiographic appearances.[427a] The institution of PEEP can result in dramatic variations in the parenchymal opacities in technically identical radiographs exposed over a 10- to 15-minute period; in fact, patients who demonstrate radiographic evidence of diffuse pulmonary edema in the absence of mechanical ventilation can show an almost complete disappearance of radiographic abnormality within minutes of the institution of PEEP (*see* Fig. 51–28). It is obvious that knowledge of ventilator settings is essential to the correct interpretation of the severity of pulmonary abnormalities in patients who have ARDS. Continuous positive-pressure ventilation can also lead to diffuse interstitial emphysema that may be readily

visible against the background of parenchymal consolidation. It is important to recognize this complication, because of the risk of ensuing pneumomediastinum or pneumothorax, or both.

In some centers, partial liquid ventilation with a perfluorocarbon chemical (perflubron) is being investigated as a method to improve gas exchange and outcome in patients who have ARDS.[428–430] Perflubron is an inert, radiopaque liquid in which oxygen readily dissolves at concentrations 20 times greater than in water.[431] Chest radiographs during ventilation with this substance show a gravity-dependent distribution of perflubron (Fig. 51–29).[430] After discontinuation of liquid ventilation, it is gradually cleared, although small amounts can remain in the lungs for several months.[430] On CT, perflubron can show a gravity-dependent, patchy, or, less commonly, diffuse distribution within the lungs (Fig. 51–30).[432] Perflubron can often be seen on CT in intrathoracic lymph nodes and, less often, in supraclavicular and axillary lymph nodes or in the mediastinal or retroperitoneal soft tissues.[432]

**The Proliferative and Fibrotic Phases.** After approximately 1 week, the lungs remain diffusely abnormal, but the pattern tends to become reticular or "bubbly."[416, 426] It is likely that this pattern represents diffuse interstitial and air-space fibrosis characteristic of the end-stage picture observed pathologically (Fig. 51–31). In the vast majority of patients who

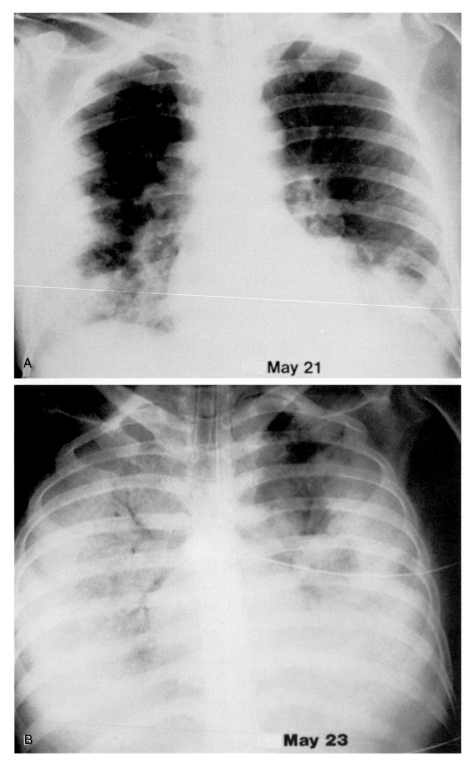

**Figure 51–28. Adult Respiratory Distress Syndrome (ARDS).** This 18-year-old girl was admitted to the intensive care unit in severe shock after a motor vehicle accident. A radiograph the day after admission *(A)* revealed homogeneous consolidation of the left lower lobe and the axillary portion of the right lung. Two days later *(B)*, both lungs were massively consolidated; note the prominent air bronchogram.

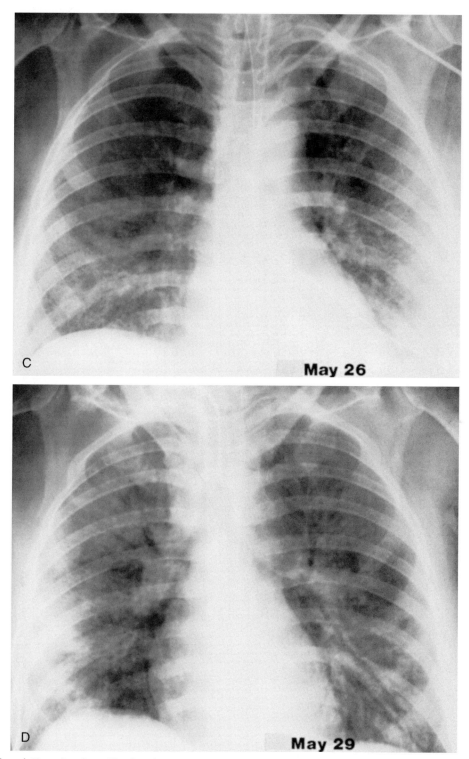

**Figure 51–28** *Continued.* Three days later *(C)*, after vigorous supportive therapy and positive end-expiration pressure (PEEP) ventilation, the patient's condition improved slightly and a radiograph revealed considerable clearing of the air-space edema. Three days later *(D)*, the radiographic appearance of the lungs had once again deteriorated and there was evidence of patchy air-space consolidation.

*Illustration continued on following page*

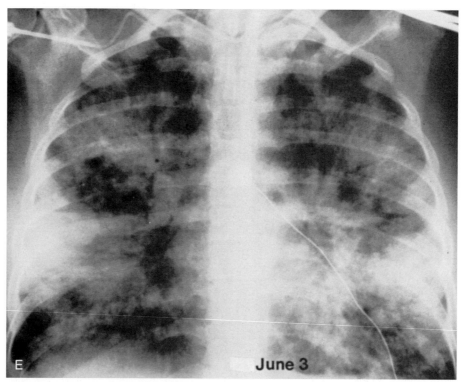

**Figure 51–28** *Continued.* Five days later *(E)*, both lungs had become massively consolidated. The patient died shortly thereafter. At autopsy, the lungs showed the organizing phase of diffuse alveolar damage.

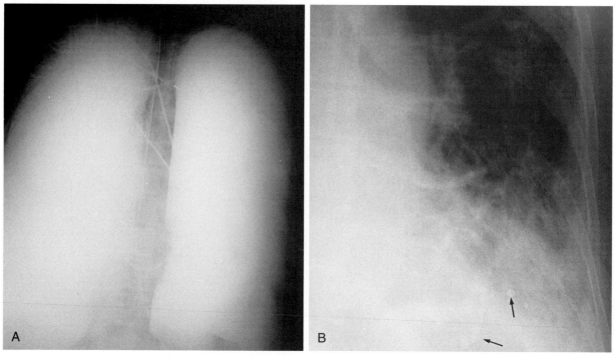

**Figure 51–29. Partial Liquid Ventilation with Perflubron.** A view from an anteroposterior chest radiograph in a 61-year-old woman undergoing liquid ventilation *(A)* demonstrates symmetric opacification of both lungs. A view of the left lung *(B)* from a chest radiograph performed 30 days after the last perflubron dose demonstrates a reticular pattern and small amounts of residual perflubron *(arrows).* (Courtesy of Dr. Ella Kazerooni, University of Michigan Medical Center, Ann Arbor, MI.)

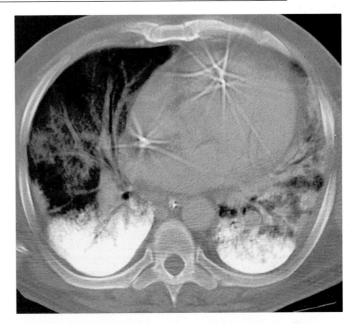

**Figure 51–30. Partial Liquid Ventilation with Perflubron.** A CT scan obtained 3 hours after administration of the last dose of perflubron demonstrates gravity-dependent distribution of the agent. The patient was a 73-year-old woman who developed respiratory failure secondary to sepsis. (Courtesy of Dr. Ella Kazerooni, University of Michigan Medical Center, Ann Arbor, MI.)

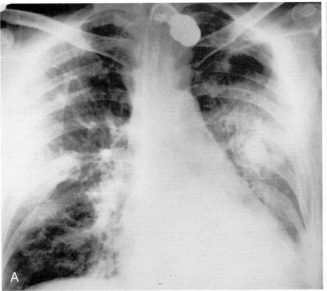

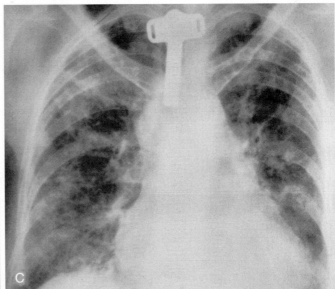

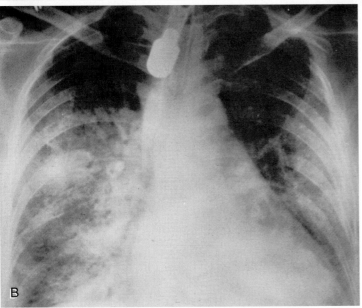

**Figure 51–31. Adult Respiratory Distress Syndrome (ARDS) with a Prolonged Course and Partial Resolution.** Twenty-four hours after admission of a young woman with multiple bone fractures sustained in a motor vehicle accident, a radiograph of the chest in anteroposterior projection, supine position *(A)* shows a mixture of reticular and air-space opacities asymmetrically distributed throughout the lungs. Endotracheal intubation is evident. Four days later, a repeat radiograph *(B)* demonstrates worsening of the air-space consolidation, a progression that is common in ARDS. Approximately 2 months later, a predischarge radiograph *(C)* shows that most of the air-space component has resolved; however, the lungs are the site of persistent coarse reticulation that almost certainly represents residual parenchymal fibrosis. Follow-up films over the ensuing months demonstrated only modest further improvement.

survive, the radiograph shows improvement within the first 10 to 14 days. Failure to improve may indicate the development of a superimposed process (e.g., pneumonia) and carries a poor prognosis.[433] Of 46 patients who were followed in one study, 8 who had a relatively long survival and continuous assisted ventilation developed a coarse reticular pattern.[416]

## Computed Tomography

The findings on CT and HRCT are also dependent on the stage of ARDS at which the examination is performed. In a study of oleic acid–induced edema in pigs, CT scans performed within the first few hours after injury showed predominantly peripheral consolidation.[443] One group of investigators recorded the CT findings in 74 patients at various stages of the disease.[434] Although the pulmonary opacities were bilateral (92%) and gravity dependent (86%) in the majority, only 25% showed a homogeneous increase in attenuation, and most showed patchy consolidation or mixed air-space and ground-glass opacification (Fig. 51–32). Air bronchograms were almost invariable (89%), and small pleural effusions were common; 22% and 28% had unilateral or bilateral pleural effusions, respectively. Early in the exudative phase of ARDS, CT commonly shows diffuse, but not uniform, ground-glass opacification or consolidation, which often does not conform to a gravity-dependent distribution (Fig. 51–33). The interspersed areas of relative sparing are not easily appreciated on chest radiographs.[108a] Later in the

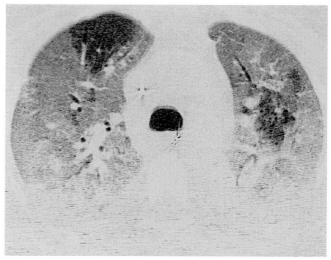

**Figure 51–33. Adult Respiratory Distress Syndrome.** An HRCT scan demonstrates extensive bilateral areas of ground-glass attenuation, air bronchograms, areas of consolidation in the dependent lung regions, and focal areas of relatively normal lung. The patient was a 45-year-old woman who developed ARDS secondary to a cytotoxic drug reaction. The diagnosis was proven at autopsy.

exudative phase, the consolidation becomes more homogeneous and gravity dependent. During the organizing phase, there is often a decrease in overall lung density and the appearance of interstitial reticulation.[131] Examination at this

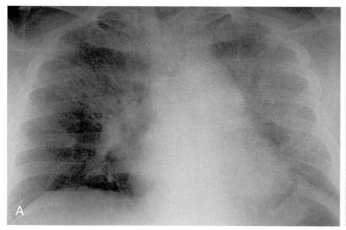

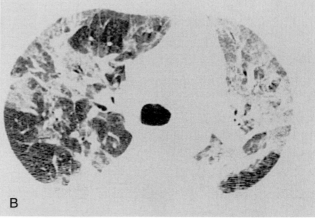

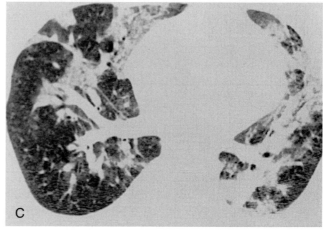

**Figure 51–32. Adult Respiratory Distress Syndrome.** An anteroposterior chest radiograph *(A)* demonstrates extensive bilateral areas of consolidation with relative sparing of the right lower lobe. HRCT scans *(B and C)* show bilateral areas of ground-glass attenuation and consolidation. Note the patchy areas of uninvolved right and left lung. The patient was a 36-year-old man who developed ARDS secondary to a cytotoxic drug reaction. The diagnosis was proven at open-lung biopsy.

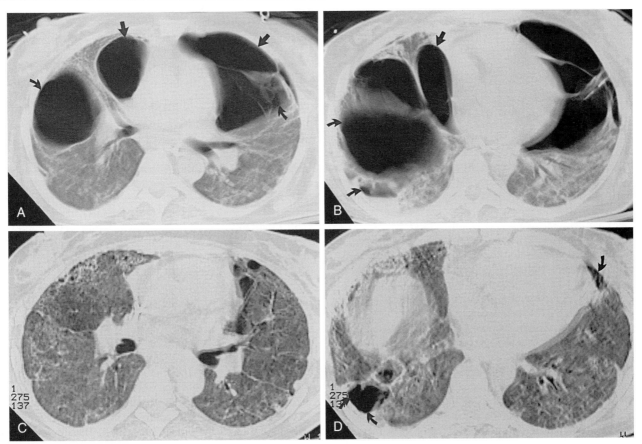

**Figure 51–34. Cystic Changes in ARDS.** A 30-year-old woman developed sepsis and ARDS after cesarean section. HRCT scans 1 week later *(A and B)* demonstrate bilateral loculated pneumothoraces *(straight arrows)* and cystic changes *(curved arrrows)* in both lungs. HRCT scans 1 month later *(C and D)* demonstrate bilateral areas of ground-glass attenuation, irregular linear opacities, and residual cystic changes *(curved arrows)*. (Courtesy of Dr. Maura Brown, Surrey Memorial Hospital, Surrey, British Columbia.)

stage often shows evidence of complications of ARDS and its treatment, such as interstitial emphysema, pneumomediastinum, pneumothorax, and subpleural bullae or cysts (Fig. 51–34).[108a, 435]

CT has the capacity to provide a quantitative estimate of the amount of pulmonary edema; because air has an attenuation of −1,000 Hounsfield Units (HU) and water has a value of 0 HU, CT densitometry and area measurement can be used to calculate lung water, lung weight, and lung density. However, in one investigation in which these calculations were compared with an assessment of the severity of edema based on the subjective examination of a portable chest radiograph, a highly significant correlation was found, indicating the robustness of the plain radiograph.[436] CT can also be used to calculate the vertical gradient in lung inflation in patients who have ARDS. In one study of 17 patients, a significant decrease in the calculated milliliters of gas per gram of tissue was found at all levels;[437] however, as in normal individuals, a vertical gradient persisted.

As with the radiograph, the CT features of ARDS are altered when the patient's lungs are inflated by the application of PEEP. Because the involvement of the lung is often patchy, PEEP tends to inflate the uninvolved, normally compliant regions but does not alter the volume of the densely consolidated regions. Less consolidated (ground-glass) or atelectatic areas of lung may show an increase in aeration if the applied PEEP exceeds a critical opening pressure.[438, 439]

This patchy inflation is the reason that application of high levels of PEEP and/or high tidal volumes frequently result in barotrauma in these patients.

The major conditions to be considered in radiologic differential diagnosis are severe cardiogenic pulmonary edema and widespread bacterial pneumonia. The latter may be impossible to differentiate from ARDS except on clinical grounds. Although involvement of the lungs is seldom as widespread and uniform in cardiogenic edema as in ARDS, differentiation between the two in the most severe cases can be made only by measuring the pulmonary arterial wedge pressure with a Swan-Ganz catheter, bearing in mind that left ventricular failure and consequent elevation of the wedge pressure can also occur as a complication of ARDS itself.

### Radiographic Differentiation of Cardiogenic and Permeability Edema

The diagnosis of pulmonary edema can usually be readily made on the chest radiograph. There is considerable controversy, however, on the ability to distinguish high-pressure (cardiogenic) from low-pressure (permeability) pulmonary edema on the basis of radiographic abnormalities.[108, 151, 440–442] Investigators have found a high degree of variability in diagnostic accuracy and in the features that are considered to constitute the most helpful signs in making the distinction. Some of this variability is related to different patient populations, differences in data analysis, and the use of posteroanterior as compared with anteroposterior chest radiographs and of upright versus supine chest radiographs.[108, 150, 440, 443] In general, the distinction is more reliably made in patients who have mild to moderate edema, on radiographs performed in posteroanterior projection, in erect or seated patients, and by analysis of changes seen in sequential radiographs.[108, 151, 440, 442]

Based on the results of the various studies in the literature, we believe that the most helpful radiographic findings in differential diagnosis are the number and caliber of pulmonary vessels (distribution of pulmonary blood flow), the distribution of pulmonary edema, vascular pedicle width, and the presence or absence of cardiomegaly, septal lines, air bronchograms, and pleural effusion.

**Pulmonary Vascular Caliber.** This may be categorized as normal, balanced (equal size of upper and lower lung zone vessels), or inverted (upper zone vessels larger than lower zone vessels).[151] In one study in which the majority of radiographs were performed in the posteroanterior projection with the patient upright or seated, approximately 50% of 61 patients who had cardiogenic pulmonary edema had an inverted blood flow pattern, compared with none of 30 patients who had fluid overload and 10% of 28 patients who had permeability pulmonary edema.[151] A balanced blood flow pattern was not found to be helpful in differential diagnosis. Distribution of blood flow has also been found inadequate in distinguishing the various forms of pulmonary edema in supine patients.[440, 442]

**Distribution of Pulmonary Edema.** In one study, the distribution of edema was even (homogeneous from chest wall to heart) in 90% of patients who had cardiac failure, 30% of patients who had renal failure, and 35% of patients who had high permeability edema.[151] A perihilar distribution was seen in 10% of patients who had cardiac failure, 70% who had renal failure, and none who had permeability edema; a peripheral predominance was seen in 45% of patients who had permeability edema. In a second investigation, a peripheral predominance was seen in 12 of 25 (48%) patients who had increased permeability edema compared with 2 of 15 (13%) who had hydrostatic pulmonary edema.[442]

**Width of the Vascular Pedicle.** A large portion of the superior mediastinal opacity on the posteroanterior chest radiograph is caused by the large systemic vessels and has therefore been called the vascular pedicle.[151] The width of this "structure" is measured from the point at which the superior vena cava crosses the right main bronchus to the point at which the left subclavian artery arises from the aortic arch. In one investigation in which the majority of radiographs were performed on posteroanterior projection in erect or seated patients, the width of the vascular pedicle was increased (greater than 53 mm on erect posteroanterior radiographs) in 60% of patients who had cardiac failure, 85% of patients who had fluid overload, and 20% of patients who had increased permeability pulmonary edema.[151] However, in two other studies in which the radiographs were performed with the patients supine, differences in the width of the vascular pedicle were not considered helpful in diagnosis.[440, 442]

**Septal Lines.** The presence of septal lines is one of the most useful findings in differential diagnosis. For example, in one investigation, they were observed in approximately 30% of patients who had either cardiac or renal overhydration edema but were identified in none of the patients who had ARDS.[151] In a second series, septal lines were identified in 21 of 49 (43%) patients who had cardiac failure and in only 3 of 33 (9%) patients who had permeability edema.[440] Although not all workers have found similar results,[442] we consider septal lines to be highly suggestive of hydrostatic pulmonary edema or a combination of hydrostatic and permeability edema.

**Air Bronchograms.** In one investigation, this sign was identified in 70% of patients who had permeability edema and in only 20% of the cardiac and renal overhydration cases.[151] In a second study, it was seen in 23 of 33 (70%) patients who had permeability edema and in only 13 of 49 (26%) patients who had hydrostatic pulmonary edema.[440]

**Pleural Effusion.** As might be expected, pleural effusion is generally more common in association with cardiogenic edema. For example, it was identified in approximately 40% of patients who had this condition in one review, as compared with only 10% of those who had permeability edema.[151] However, when specifically looked for on decubitus or upright radiographs or on CT, small effusions are not uncommon in permeability edema; for example, in one investigation, they were identified on the radiograph in 14 of 49 (29%) patients who had hydrostatic pulmonary edema and 9 of 33 (27%) who had permeability edema.[442]

**Heart Size.** Again, one might expect this to be a useful indicator of the etiology of pulmonary edema. In one investigation, after application of a 12.5% correction factor necessitated by the supine position of patients, the anteroposterior projection, and the shortened 40-inch distance, cardiac enlargement was identified in 72% of patients who had cardiogenic edema, but in only 32% of those who had capillary permeability edema.[151] In another investigation, 9 of 15 (60%) patients who had hydrostatic edema had cardiomegaly compared with 11 of 25 (44%) patients who had permeability edema.[442]

**Summary.** As these studies demonstrate, no single radiographic criterion allows reliable distinction of hydrostatic from permeability edema. However, a *combination* of findings permits correct identification of hydrostatic pulmonary edema in 80% to 90% of patients[151, 441, 442] and correct identification of permeability edema in 60% to 90%.[151, 441, 442] In the cases in which the diagnosis is equivocal, measurement of the pulmonary arterial wedge pressure with a Swan-Ganz catheter may be required, bearing in mind that elevation of the wedge pressure secondary to left ventricular dysfunction can occur as a complication of ARDS itself.

### Clinical Manifestations

The clinical manifestations of ARDS can develop either insidiously, hours or days after the initiating event (e.g., sepsis or fat emboli), or acutely, coincident with the event (e.g., aspiration of liquid gastric contents). Typical symptoms are dyspnea, tachypnea, dry cough, retrosternal discomfort, and agitation; cyanosis may be present. The expectoration of copious blood-tinged fluid signifies the presence of the full-blown syndrome. Examination of the chest reveals coarse crackles and bronchial breath sounds. Arterial blood analysis shows severe hypoxemia and a normal or decreased arterial $Pco_2$. The hypoxemia is difficult or impossible to

**Table 51–3. DIAGNOSTIC CRITERIA FOR ADULT RESPIRATORY DISTRESS SYNDROME**

| INJURY | CRITERIA |
| --- | --- |
| Acute lung injury | Acute onset<br>$Pao_2/Fio_2 \leq 300$ mm Hg<br>Bilateral pulmonary "infiltrates" on frontal chest radiograph<br>Pulmonary artery wedge pressure $\leq$ 18 mm Hg (when measured) or no clinical evidence of left atrial hypertension |
| Adult respiratory distress syndrome | Acute onset<br>$Pao_2/Fio_2 \leq 200$ mm Hg<br>Bilateral pulmonary "infiltrates" on frontal chest radiograph<br>Pulmonary artery wedge pressure $\leq$ 18 mm Hg (when measured) or no clinical evidence of left atrial hypertension |

correct even with the use of very high concentrations of inspired oxygen. Clinical deterioration is usual, requiring endotracheal intubation to maintain adequate oxygenation ($O_2$ saturation greater than 90%).

Difficulties in comparing studies of prognosis, treatment, and outcome in ARDS have been hampered by a lack of consistent diagnostic criteria. This deficiency stimulated individuals at an American-European consensus conference to develop criteria to define groups of patients on the basis of disease severity.[444] According to these criteria, patients can be separated into two groups, one that has less severe disease (termed *acute lung injury*) and one that has the more severe features of full blown ARDS. As shown in Table 51–3, the criteria are based on clinical, radiographic, and physiologic findings.

### Diagnosis

As discussed previously, the chest radiograph in patients who have ARDS typically reveals widespread air-space consolidation, raising the question of whether the edema is cardiogenic or permeability in type. Although the radiographic features described earlier can aid differentiation, the measurement of pulmonary vascular pressures is frequently required to establish definitive diagnosis. Such measurement is most often achieved using a balloon-tipped, flow-directed (Swan-Ganz) catheter.[445] When correctly measured, the wedge pressure provides an accurate estimate of the filling pressure of the left ventricle and is therefore a reflection of left ventricular preload; in addition, it provides information concerning the hydrostatic pressure in fluid-exchanging microvessels.

The principle behind the measurement is as follows: Inflation of a balloon in a pulmonary artery to a size sufficient to occlude flow results in a static column of blood that extends from the tip of the catheter to the point where the pulmonary vein subserved by that artery joins other pulmonary veins before their entrance into the left atrium. Because the pulmonary circulation has almost no precapillary collateral perfusion, the wedge pressure provides an accurate reflection of pulmonary venous pressure at the confluence of

the pulmonary veins close to the left atrium. Because an elevated left atrial pressure is the hallmark of cardiogenic pulmonary edema, the finding of a normal wedge pressure provides convincing evidence that edema is the result of increased permeability (provided that therapy with diuretics and cardiac-stimulating agents has not been instituted). Central venous pressure measurement does not provide similar information because the right and left ventricles often differ considerably in their performance characteristics and filling pressures.[446]

Correct measurement of the arterial wedge pressure as an estimate of pulmonary venous pressure requires that a column of blood extend from the peripheral end of the wedged catheter to the pulmonary venous system. When the lung is in Zone I or II conditions and alveolar pressure exceeds pulmonary arterial or pulmonary venous pressure (or both), the pulmonary wedge pressure may not be an accurate reflection of pulmonary venous pressure.[445] This artefact can occur when there is an increase in alveolar pressure (e.g., in the presence of PEEP or auto-PEEP) or when there is a decrease in intravascular pressure (e.g., in the presence of shock). The application of PEEP can also influence the measurement of pulmonary capillary wedge pressure by increasing pleural pressure around the heart and pulmonary veins. Normally, about half of the externally applied PEEP is transmitted to the pleural space; as a result, the pulmonary wedge pressure increases by approximately half of the PEEP pressure that is added. The proportion of externally applied PEEP that is transmitted to the pleural space—and therefore to the wedge catheter measurement—is dependent on the relative compliances of the lung and chest wall. If the lung is very stiff, as in patients who have ARDS, less of the externally applied PEEP is "seen" in the pleural space. Whether or not the pulmonary artery catheter is in Zone III can be determined by obtaining a lateral radiograph of the chest with a horizontal x-ray beam. If the mean pulmonary artery pressure (referenced to midthorax) and the alveolar pressure at end-expiration are known, the vertical level at which Zone I flow conditions will begin can be calculated. In addition, if the catheter is wedged in Zone I or II, the pressure will show very little cardiogenic fluctuation but will have considerable respiratory swings.

Measurements of pulmonary wedge pressure may also be elevated in association with a normal left atrial pressure if there is a significant obstruction to blood flow between the confluence of pulmonary veins and their point of entry into the left atrium.[445] Provided there is no mitral valvular obstruction, pulmonary wedge pressure also provides an accurate reflection of left ventricular end-diastolic pressure. Another rare cause for an artefactually high pulmonary wedge pressure occurs when the catheter tip is located in an area of lung in which there is anomalous pulmonary drainage into the systemic circulation, as occurs in the scimitar syndrome.[447] After pneumonectomy, the pulmonary wedge pressure can provide a falsely low estimate of left atrial pressure.[448]

In addition to giving an accurate estimate of left atrial filling pressure, the pulmonary wedge pressure provides information concerning the pulmonary microvascular pressure. As discussed earlier, pulmonary capillary pressure is dependent on the relative resistance of the arterial and venous systems. During occlusion of the pulmonary artery, any pressure drop between the pulmonary microvessels and the major pulmonary veins disappears, so that pulmonary wedge pressure will underestimate pulmonary capillary pressure. The latter must be somewhat higher than pulmonary wedge pressure, the magnitude of this difference being related directly to the pulmonary venous resistance. Because pulmonary venous resistance is relatively low and because few conditions selectively increase it, in most cases it is reasonable to use the pulmonary wedge pressure as an estimate of pulmonary microvascular pressure. The one condition in which this assumption is invalid and can lead to diagnostic errors is pulmonary veno-occlusive disease. When small pulmonary veins are obstructed, pulmonary capillary pressure can be substantially higher than pulmonary venous pressure during conditions of flow. However, when the wedge catheter is inserted, the large pressure drop between pulmonary capillary and pulmonary vein disappears; as a consequence, the wedge pressure gives an erroneously low estimate of the functional pulmonary capillary pressure.

In addition to its use as a method of determining the fundamental cause of pulmonary edema, the measurement of wedge pressure can be a very effective management tool in testing the effectiveness of agents and therapies designed to lower intravascular pressure. In the presence of increased microvascular permeability, edema formation is critically dependent on microvascular pressure; although an increase in microvascular pressure is not the primary cause of edema in such circumstances, a transient or prolonged elevation can significantly exaggerate the formation of edema (Fig. 51–35).[20] For example, in an investigation utilizing dog lungs, a 3-mm Hg increase in microvascular pressure increased lymph flow by a factor of 8 after acid aspiration but only by a factor of 2 in normal lungs.[449] The potential usefulness of measurement of pulmonary wedge pressure has led to the widespread use of flow-directed, thermistor-tipped catheters in critically ill patients. However there is no objective evidence that their use improves the outcome of

patients who have ARDS after correction for other risk factors.[450]

A normal or low pulmonary arterial wedge pressure measurement provides strong, indirect evidence that endothelial damage and increased permeability are the cause of pulmonary edema. A number of direct tests of endothelial integrity have also been devised; although none is practical for general clinical use, they are of considerable theoretical interest. Radioactive tracers can be nebulized or instilled into the lung and their appearance in the blood monitored over time as a measure of permeability.[451–456] In some studies, an increase in permeability has been demonstrated before the manifestations of ARDS became evident clinically, suggesting that tests of permeability may be useful in predicting the probability of the development of ARDS.[457] Similar results have been obtained when radiolabeled tracers have been administered intravenously and their accumulation in the lung monitored, either with external counters[454, 458] or by measurement of BAL fluid.[459, 460] The pulmonary endothelium normally metabolizes both propranolol and serotonin during their passage through the pulmonary microvasculature; pulmonary extraction after radiolabeling of both substances has been shown to be impaired in patients who have ARDS, the degree of impairment correlating with the severity of the pulmonary damage.[461]

Sampling of edema fluid through an endotracheal tube in intubated patients permits measurement of its protein concentration. The results of a number of studies have shown that the ratio of such protein concentration to that of protein in serum is significantly higher in patients who have permeability edema compared with those who have clinically diagnosed cardiogenic edema, permitting clear separation of the two entities in patients in whom the diagnosis may not be obvious.[462–466] Patients who have hydrostatic pulmonary edema have ratios of 0.65 or less, whereas those who have permeability edema have ratios between 0.75 and 1.0. Only 10% to 15% of patients who have pulmonary edema have ratios between 0.65 and 0.75; in these individuals, a combination of increased microvascular pressure and permeability may be present.[467] Protein concentration can also be measured in BAL fluid, although the effect of dilution cannot be controlled for. In addition to the measurement of protein content, the cell population of the air spaces can be assessed by examining BAL fluid and a host of assays for a variety of mediators can be carried out.[467] As discussed farther on, elevated levels of these mediators or cells is associated with an increased risk for the development of ARDS and a poorer prognosis once it is established.

The severity of the lung injury in patients who have ARDS can be followed using a number of quantitative measurements. The amount of extravascular lung water can be more directly assessed using the double indicator dilution technique,[468, 469] in which the volume of distribution of a tracer is based on the relationship between flow, volume of distribution, and transit time according to the formula

$$Volume\ of\ distribution\ =\ Flow\ \times\ transit\ time$$

If a tracer is injected into the pulmonary artery and its arrival in the aorta is determined, the volume of its distribution between those two points can be measured if the total flow through the system (i.e., cardiac output) is known and

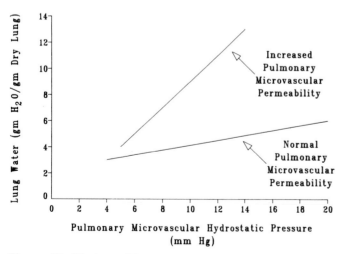

**Figure 51–35. Lung Water versus Pulmonary Microvascular Pressure.** Lung water, expressed as grams of water per gram of dry lung, is plotted against mean pulmonary microvascular pressure. When pulmonary microvascular permeability is normal, increased microvascular pressure causes a modest increase in lung water (hydrostatic edema); when microvascular permeability is increased, the same changes in pressure cause a marked accumulation of lung water.

if the transit time between the injection and sensing site can be measured. If two tracers are injected simultaneously, one of which remains confined to the intravascular space and the other diffuses throughout the interstitial space of the lung, measurement of both in the left side of the heart or aorta reveals the difference between the volumes of distribution of the diffusible and nondiffusible tracer and constitutes a measure of pulmonary extravascular water. The most practical method involves the intravenous injection of a cold green dye, with subsequent detection of the dye and measurement of blood temperature (using a thermocouple) in the arterial circulation. The dye remains confined to the intravascular space and serves as a nondiffusible indicator while the temperature dissipates readily in the entire pulmonary extravascular space. By measuring the appearance times of the dye and the cold with a specially designed catheter inserted into a systemic artery, the quantity of extravascular lung water can be estimated.[470–472] Using a similar principle, lung water can also be quantified by inhaling gases of different solubility such as acetylene and dimethyl ether.[473]

### Pulmonary Function Tests

The most important pathophysiologic effect of the edema in patients who have ARDS is on gas exchange, the profound hypoxemia rather than the ventilatory failure being the major indication for intubation and mechanical ventilation. By employing the multiple inert gas technique[474, 475] or the classic method of 100% $O_2$ ventilation,[476] it has been shown that the predominant pathogenesis of hypoxemia is pure shunt rather than other forms of $\dot{V}/\dot{Q}$ mismatching. The gas-exchange impairment is worse in patients who have ARDS than in those who have cardiogenic pulmonary edema of equal severity, an effect that is possibly the result of a failure of the mechanisms that normally tend to minimize $\dot{V}/\dot{Q}$ mismatching. As discussed previously, these mechanisms could be either a failure of interstitial pressure to increase and thus occlude vessels in the edematous lung regions or a failure of hypoxic pulmonary vasoconstriction. In one study of 14 patients who had ARDS, more abnormal gas exchange and poorer prognosis related better to an increased permeability–surface area product than to increased lung water;[477] the investigators suggested that preservation of pulmonary vascular constriction improves gas exchange and survival in patients who have ARDS. Other investigators have also shown that increased pulmonary vascular tone improves gas exchange.[478] The intrapulmonary shunt in patients who have ARDS increases when total pulmonary blood flow is increased,[479, 480] an effect that is probably related to an increase in mixed venous $Po_2$ and decreased hypoxic vasoconstriction. Interestingly, prone positioning of patients who have ARDS improves gas exchange; the results of experimental studies have shown that this effect is related to a more even distribution of blood flow[481] and to the generation of a transpulmonary pressure sufficient to exceed airway opening pressure in dorsal lung regions (i.e., in regions where atelectasis, shunt, and $\dot{V}/\dot{Q}$ heterogeneity are most severe), without adversely affecting ventral lung regions.[482] Although they are not routinely measured, lung diffusing capacity and functional residual capacity are decreased in patients who have ARDS.[483] Pulmonary resistance is also increased.[484]

There is also evidence that peripheral oxygen uptake is impaired in patients who have ARDS. In normal subjects, oxygen consumption by the body is not dependent on oxygen delivery (cardiac output $\times$ arterial $O_2$ content); if the oxygen content of arterial blood decreases, peripheral oxygen extraction increases, resulting in a larger difference in arterial-to-venous oxygen content and preservation of total oxygen consumption. In fact, oxygen consumption does not diminish in normal individuals until oxygen delivery decreases to approximately 8 ml per minute per kg.[485] By contrast, in patients who have ARDS most (albeit not all[486]) investigators have shown that $O_2$ consumption decreases linearly with $O_2$ delivery, even when it exceeds 20 ml per minute per kg.[487–490] Although the mechanism of this defect in tissue oxygen extraction is incompletely understood, it is presumably a reflection of the generalized abnormality of microvascular function seen in patients who have MSOF.

ARDS is often accompanied by pulmonary arterial hypertension, and the resultant increase in right ventricular afterload usually causes right ventricular dysfunction.[491] Abnormalities of right ventricular contractility have been demonstrated by radionuclide techniques[492, 493] and by two-dimensional echocardiography.[494] There is also evidence that right ventricular dysfunction can result in left ventricular dysfunction, most likely related to a shift in the shared interventricular septum.[493] In the late stages of ARDS, the lung becomes progressively noncompliant and although the gas exchange may improve somewhat it is harder to maintain a normal arterial $Paco_2$.[495]

### Natural History and Prognosis

ARDS is a serious disease, having a mortality rate of greater than 50% despite the availability of modern diagnostic techniques and therapies.[496, 497] In one study of 57 patients, 37 (65%) died;[269] in 90% of these, death occurred within 14 days of the onset of symptoms. Patients who die of pulmonary insufficiency usually show a progressive decrease in lung compliance and worsening gas exchange; in the terminal stages, both barotrauma and hypercapnia may develop despite an enormous minute ventilation. Pathologic examination of the lungs in these patients reveals extensive interstitial and intra-alveolar fibrosis; biochemical analysis demonstrates the presence of increased lung collagen.[498] Significant fibrosis can occur over an extremely short time course;[499] we have observed the development of ossification of pulmonary tissue over a period of 2 weeks after the onset of the syndrome.

There have been numerous studies in which prospective analyses of clinical and laboratory data have been assessed for their ability to predict progression to ARDS in patients at risk and to provide an index of prognosis in patients who have established ARDS.[267, 467] In the study of 57 patients mentioned earlier, the only clinical features and laboratory data recorded at the time of diagnosis that were significantly related to increased mortality were a decreased number of band-form polymorphonuclear leukocytes, a low arterial blood pH, and a low concentration of arterial blood bicarbonate ion;[269] direct measurements of the severity of the pulmonary injury such as arterial blood gas tensions, gas-exchange abnormalities, and pulmonary hemodynamic derangements were not predictive of survival. These results suggest that factors other than the severity of the pulmonary injury itself may be important in determining prognosis after the development of ARDS.

In a cooperative, prospective study of 713 patients who had ARDS, multiple organ failure was an important contributing factor to the 61% mortality rate:[500] only 40% of those who had pulmonary insufficiency alone died, whereas patients who had two, three, four, and five organs involved showed mortality rates of 54%, 72%, 84%, and 100%, respectively. Coincident renal failure is a particularly important complication; in one study, the mortality rate increased from 40% in patients who had pulmonary involvement alone to 89% in those who had combined renal and respiratory failure.[501] Sepsis is also a frequent, fatal complication of ARDS in addition to being the most common initiator of the syndrome; infection is most often caused by gram-negative organisms, and the most frequent sites of infection are the lung and abdominal cavity.[502]

The suggestion that mortality in ARDS is related to functional derangement of multiple organs more closely than to specific pulmonary dysfunction has been supported by a study of risk and mortality in 207 patients who were prospectively identified as being at risk for the development of ARDS.[276] The specific risk factors included the "sepsis syndrome," documented aspiration of gastric contents, near-drowning, pulmonary contusion, multiple long-bone fractures, multiple transfusions (more than 10 units of blood over 6 hours), and hypotension (systolic blood pressure less than 90 mm Hg for more than 2 hours). ARDS was defined as a $PaO_2$-to-$FIO_2$ ratio less than 150, radiographic evidence of diffuse air-space consolidation, a pulmonary artery wedge pressure less than 18 mm Hg, and no other findings to explain these abnormalities. Forty-seven (23%) of the 207 patients developed ARDS, and 32 (68%) of these died; by contrast, only 55 (34%) of the 160 patients died who had similar risk factors but did not develop ARDS. Only 5 of the 32 ARDS patients died of irreversible respiratory failure, most of the deaths that occurred during the first 3 days after entry into the study being attributed to the underlying illness or injury and most of those that occurred after 3 days being related to unremitting sepsis.

The results of this study are in contrast to those of the multicenter randomized trial of extracorporeal membrane oxygenation sponsored by the U.S. National Heart, Lung, and Blood Institute.[503] In that trial, 82 of 90 patients died; 40 were thought to have had a respiratory-related death and only 22% of these developed sepsis. The differences observed in the results of this study and the one previously cited[276] are probably related to their design: in the membrane oxygenation study, patients who had severe gas-exchange abnormalities were preferentially selected, whereas those who had significant disease involving other organs tended to be excluded.

Despite their differences, the results of these studies permit three important conclusions:[276, 503]

1. Maintenance of normal arterial blood gases throughout the period of acute lung injury does not guarantee survival, because lung repair and reversal of the injury do not necessarily occur.

2. Multiple organ failure and death from causes unrelated to, or only secondarily related to, the primary pulmonary insult are the rule rather than the exception.

3. The prognosis is dismal despite intensive medical management, and survival may depend in large measure on the institution of early prophylactic therapeutic interventions to prevent rather than treat this devastating condition.

In one prospective study of patients who had ARDS, changes in body weight and balance of fluid intake and output were important predictors of survival;[504] patients who had progressive weight gain were less likely to survive than those who lost weight, an effect that was present even after correction for serum albumin levels and renal status. There are two possible explanations for these observations: (1) patients who did not survive had a continued generalized microvascular capillary leak that resulted in progressive fluid accumulation; and (2) hemodynamic instability in those who died was sufficiently severe to require excessive fluid transfusion. Detailed formulas for calculating a patient's degree of illness or injury, such as the APACHE II score (Acute Physiology and Chronic Health Evaluation), predict the likelihood of developing ARDS with a sensitivity of 79% and a specificity of 25%.[505] Similarly, the Injury Severity Score (ISS), which is based on the severity of anatomic injury in trauma victims, is modestly predictive of the likelihood of progression to ARDS.[506]

The relatively low predictive value of clinical indices in individual patients has led to a search for cellular or molecular markers in blood or BAL fluid that will provide more precise prognostic information. Based on a knowledge of the pathogenesis of ARDS, markers of endothelial injury have been particularly investigated. Some patients at risk for ARDS show increased circulating levels of factor VIII and von Willebrand's factor, both of which are synthesized by endothelial cells.[507, 508] In one study of 45 individuals at risk for ARDS (of whom 15 developed the disease), an increase in von Willebrand's factor was found to be 87% sensitive and 77% specific for the diagnosis;[508] however, the results of other studies have not shown a similar discriminatory ability.[509] Many of the mediators and cytokines that are implicated in the pathogenesis of ARDS can be measured using sensitive assays in plasma and/or BAL. Increased plasma levels of TNF-$\alpha$,[510] IL-8,[511] and leukotriene B$_4$[512] have been shown to be predictive of ARDS with varying degrees of sensitivity and specificity in some studies; however, some investigators have found no relationship.[513] Levels of IL-1$\beta$,[514] C3a,[515] and leukotriene[516] in BAL fluid have also been associated with an increased risk for the development of ARDS. Although there are no absolute molecular predictors of the development of ARDS,[517a] a number of markers of cell activation have been found to be related to outcome.[467] Specifically, increased plasma levels of L-selectin,[518] CD11b/CD18,[519] and elastase[520] have been found to be associated with later ARDS.

The other outcome that investigators have tried to predict is the likelihood of recovery in patients who have been diagnosed as having ARDS. Increased plasma concentrations of type IV collagen,[521] von Willebrand's factor,[508] and soluble E- and P-selectin[522] and increased BAL levels of type III procollagen,[517] surfactant protein A (SP-A),[523] and IL-1$\beta$[524] have all been associated with a worse prognosis in patients who have ARDS. The initial degree of arterial desaturation is not predictive of subsequent death after correction for other clinical factors.[525]

Patients who survive ARDS manifest surprisingly little long-term impairment of lung function.[526–528] Some have a mild restrictive impairment and gas-exchange deficit;[526] occasionally, there is partly reversible airway obstruction.[529] Most of these abnormalities improve in the first year after ARDS; however, if deficits persist at 1 year, further improvement is unlikely.[530] Long-term abnormalities of function are more likely to be seen in patients who have had the most severe disturbances in lung mechanics and gas exchange during their acute illness and in those treated for prolonged periods with an $FIO_2$ greater than 0.5.[531, 532]

## Specific Forms of Permeability Edema

### High-Altitude Pulmonary Edema

Many individuals develop a symptom-complex known as high-altitude pulmonary edema (HAPE) or mountain or altitude sickness while becoming acclimatized to high altitudes.[533] Clinical features of the condition include headache, giddiness, dizziness, tiredness, weakness, body aches, anorexia, nausea, vomiting, abdominal pain, insomnia, restlessness, cough, dyspnea on exertion, and fever.[534] Physical examination of some patients reveals crackles, which may persist or increase as long as the individuals remain at high altitude. Diastolic blood pressure and pulse rate increase and peak expiratory flow rates decrease. All symptoms and signs characteristically disappear on descent to sea level. A small percentage of individuals arriving at high altitude develop severe pulmonary edema, which occasionally proves fatal.[535, 536]

The illness may become manifest on both acute[537] and prolonged[538] exposure at 3,500 to 4,000 meters (11,500 to 13,000 feet); rare cases have been documented to develop at 2,750 meters (9,000 feet).[539, 540] Usually, the move from sea level to high altitude is abrupt; for example, all but 3 of 101 patients in one report had arrived at an altitude of 3,500 meters by airplane.[536] Affected individuals are characteristically young and otherwise healthy. Although some have arrived at high altitudes for the first time, the condition appears to show a predilection for former residents who are returning after being at sea level for a few days to several weeks;[536, 541–543] in one study, 75% of affected patients were returning to high altitude where they had lived for 6 to 9 months followed by a sojourn of 30 to 60 days on the plains.[543] Edema usually develops within 2 to 3 days and almost always within the first month after arrival at high altitude. Physical exertion and cold weather are considered precipitating factors in some cases;[544–546] however, many individuals have been employed in sedentary occupations.[536]

The pathogenesis of HAPE is uncertain and somewhat controversial.[547] The results of a number of studies have clearly demonstrated that increased capillary permeability is a contributing factor.[548–551] However, the fact that the edema usually occurs in individuals who develop an inordinate degree of pulmonary arterial hypertension after exposure to normally tolerable levels of hypoxia suggests that increased intravascular pressure is also important.[3, 552] Despite this, some patients who have experienced high-altitude edema demonstrate completely normal pulmonary vascular responsiveness to hypoxemia.[551a] In one study of a group of men who were known to have had HAPE months before, susceptible persons were found to have shorter chests, smaller lung volumes, and higher pulmonary arterial pressures and pulse rates than a group of control individuals;[543] breathing of a hypoxic gas mixture lowered the oxygen saturation of the arterial blood and raised the pulmonary arterial pressures to a greater extent in the susceptible than in the normal subjects.

The pathophysiology of acute mountain sickness, HAPE, and high-altitude cerebral edema is probably interrelated and represents different manifestations of the same underlying process.[553–555] Significant changes in vital capacity can be demonstrated in individuals who manifest symptoms of acute mountain sickness in the absence of overt pulmonary edema.[556] In one study of 8 normal individuals who were exposed for 40 days to simulated altitudes of up to 8,848 meters in a hypobaric chamber, vital capacity decreased by a mean of 14%.[557] In another investigation of 32 healthy subjects, the single breath diffusing capacity was found to increase in most after ascent to altitude, presumably as a result of increased pulmonary capillary blood volume;[558] however, the increase was significantly less in subjects who developed symptoms of acute mountain sickness. The authors believed that the difference was probably related to subclinical interstitial edema. People who experience altitude sickness have lower minute ventilation and higher values of end-tidal $PCO_2$ at high altitude and also show a decreased ventilatory response to hypoxia when studied at sea level.[559] In normal individuals, the mechanical properties of the lungs do not change significantly during acclimatization to altitude;[560] there occurs a slight loss of elastic recoil and a slight increase in maximal expiratory flow rates, presumably as a result of the decreased density of air at high altitude.[561a]

A very plausible hypothesis for the pathogenesis of HAPE has been advanced.[551, 562, 563] In susceptible individuals, hypoxia secondary to the low $FIO_2$ causes intense, but inhomogeneous, vasoconstriction of a large proportion of the pulmonary arteries, forcing blood flow at high pressures through the remaining patent vessels. Thus, in regions where arterial constriction is deficient, there will be high flow and transmission of the increased pulmonary arterial pressure directly to the capillary bed. The high capillary pressure and the shear stress caused by the high flow in the unconstricted areas results in pulmonary microvascular endothelial damage and permeability edema. According to this hypothesis, the inflammatory reaction, which is recognizable by examination of BAL fluid in affected patients,[551, 564] represents a response to the injury caused by high pressure and flow. One group has suggested that the medial muscle hypertrophy seen in the pulmonary arteries of high-altitude natives involutes only partially and nonuniformly during a stay at sea level, thus accounting for the nonuniform intensity of precapillary vasoconstriction on return to high altitude.[565]

A number of experimental observations support this mechanical hypothesis. For example, obstruction of 75% of the pulmonary vascular bed in dogs has been shown to result in pulmonary edema.[566] Edema has also been demonstrated when blood flow through isolated canine lobes was increased to four to five times the normal level.[563, 567] It is also possible that venoconstriction may be involved in the pathogenesis of the edema. In one animal study, prolonged hypoxia was associated with pulmonary venous constriction as well as precapillary vasoconstriction.[568] This effect might go unnoticed in affected patients even during right-sided heart catheterization, because the wedge pressure may be normal in the face of increased pulmonary venous resistance.

The "mechanical" hypothesis for pulmonary capillary endothelial damage in HAPE has been strengthened by the development of the concept of "stress failure" in the pulmonary capillaries.[37, 38] Because the alveolocapillary membrane is extremely thin to optimize gas exchange, it is also vulnerable to excessive stress when the capillary pressure is increased above certain levels, especially when the increase is accompanied by an increase in lung volume or tidal volume. These relationships have been exemplified in a series of ultrastructural studies of rabbit lung in which disruption of the capillary endothelial and alveolar epithelial layers has been shown to be associated with an increase in capillary pressure to about 30 cm $H_2O$;[569, 570] these changes are much more pronounced at capillary pressures of 50 cm $H_2O$, and a similar degree of damage can be seen at lower capillary pressures when the lung is inflated to high volumes. The stress experienced by the capillary wall is related to the radius of the vessel, the transmural pressure, and the thickness of its wall. Although the normally low capillary pressure and small radius are associated with a low wall tension, the actual stress (tension per unit area) is quite high because of the extreme thinness of the membrane. When blood flow is increased, as occurs at altitude, capillary pressure becomes closer to arterial pressure,[571] and stress-related disruption of the vessels can occur. A similar mechanism has been postulated to explain the capillary damage seen in neurogenic pulmonary edema, exercise-induced pulmonary hemorrhage in racehorses, and the occasional instance of exercise-induced pulmonary hemorrhage in elite athletes.[37] The same process may also be responsible for the occasional cases of pulmonary edema seen in association with massive pulmonary thromboembolism,[572] balloon dilation of stenotic pulmonary arteries,[573] surgical removal of a large central thromboembolus,[574] and pneumonectomy. Additional support for the hypothesis is provided by the observations that the risk of developing HAPE is increased in patients who have congenital absence of one pulmonary artery[575, 576] or mild pulmonary hypertension[577] and that the syndrome can be precipitated by an acute thromboembolus.[578] A mild preexisting viral respiratory infection, which might be expected to enhance the inflammatory response in the lung also appears to predispose to the development of HAPE, at least in children.[579]

A number of workers have studied the normal physiologic variations that render certain individuals susceptible to the development of HAPE.[580] Patients who have previously suffered from HAPE have lower than average ventilatory response to hypoxia[581, 582] and higher resting pulmonary artery pressures at sea level; they also develop a greater increase in pulmonary artery pressure during exercise, as a result of augmented, flow-dependent pulmonary vasoconstriction and/or a reduced vascular cross-sectional area.[583] One group of investigators made careful measurements of gas exchange in seven individuals who had a previous history of HAPE and nine subjects who tolerated altitude without pulmonary symptoms.[561] At a simulated altitude of 4,150 meters, the former showed significantly lower $Pao_2$ and higher $Paco_2$ values; the hypoxemia could not be attributed solely to decreased ventilation, because the alveolar-arterial

oxygen difference was also increased. Previous victims of HAPE also show enhanced pulmonary vasoreactivity to hypoxia compared with control subjects, whereas successful high-altitude climbers have a decreased response.[584] Susceptible individuals also develop greater exercise induced $\dot{V}/\dot{Q}$ mismatch than appropriate controls.[585]

The evidence that HAPE is associated with increased microvascular permeability derives from clinical studies of vascular pressures and the characteristics of the edema fluid. Right-sided heart catheterization studies have revealed raised pulmonary arterial pressure and normal pulmonary wedge pressure.[545, 586, 587] Although there may be little evidence of increased endothelial permeability early in the course of HAPE,[588] the results of most studies support the concept of an inflammatory response and microvascular damage. The constituents of pulmonary edema fluid have been measured in a tented camp situated at 4,400 meters and equipped with bronchoscopes, ventilators, and oxygen;[548–550] when compared with the lavage fluid from healthy climbers, edema fluid from affected individuals was shown to possess a high protein content and to contain increased numbers of macrophages and neutrophils and increased amounts of arachidonic acid metabolites (including leukotriene $B_4$), complement fragments, and a variety of proteolytic enzymes. Additional mediators of inflammation, such as IL-1β, IL-6, IL-8, TNFα,[551] and endothelin-1[589] have been reported in the BAL fluid of affected individuals. Increased urinary leukotriene $E_4$ has also been detected in 38 HAPE victims compared with 10 controls.[564]

Occasional patients who die of HAPE have been found at autopsy to have diffuse pulmonary edema, with focal hemorrhage and thrombi in the smaller branches of the pulmonary artery.[542] These observations, coupled with the finding of increased circulating levels of fibrinopeptide A in severe cases, raise the possibility that activation of the clotting system also plays a role in pathogenesis. However, like the inflammation, these changes are most likely secondary to endothelial damage.[563]

The radiographic appearances are those of acute pulmonary edema of any etiology. In a retrospective study of the radiographic findings in 60 patients who had high-altitude pulmonary edema severe enough to warrant admission to the hospital, 55 (92%) had air-space consolidation (homogeneous in 40 and patchy in distribution in 15).[589a] In about 45%, the consolidation was bilaterally symmetric, in 45% it affected mainly the right lung, and in 10% it was seen mainly in the left lung. The consolidation tended to be most severe in the lower lobes and most commonly involved both central and peripheral lung regions; in some patients it was predominantly central or, less commonly, peripheral in distribution. Nearly all patients had some peribronchial and perivascular cuffing and perihilar haze, and nine (15%) had Kerley B lines. None had pleural effusion at presentation; however, four developed small effusions within 24 to 48 hours. The cardiothoracic ratio was normal or minimally increased. On CT, the edema had a patchy and predominantly peripheral distribution.[589b] Although the central pulmonary vessels may be prominent as a result of acute pulmonary hypertension, cardiac enlargement has not been noted. The edema usually resolves within 1 to 2 days,[590, 591] but may be present for as long as 10 days.[443]

Symptoms develop within 12 hours to 3 days after

arrival at high altitude[536, 542] and consist of cough, dyspnea, weakness, and hemoptysis, often associated with substernal discomfort. Cyanosis and tachycardia are common; crackles may be heard throughout the lungs. Papilledema and retinal hemorrhages have been described.[587] Fever occurs in about one third of patients, and leukocytosis is common, ranging from 13,000/mm³ to as high as 30,000/mm³.[539, 565, 592] The electrocardiogram may show nonspecific changes, such as right atrial enlargement or right-axis shift, but is usually normal.[539] Patients respond rapidly to the administration of oxygen or return to or toward sea level. The chest radiograph clears within 24 to 48 hours.[541]

In addition to the physiologic changes associated with HAPE, a variety of abnormalities have been identified in individuals at high altitude that are not clearly related to the syndrome. The ambient and arterial $PO_2$ at the summit of Mount Everest are so low that maximal exercise capacity is severely diminished because of reduced oxygen delivery.[593] Climbers who have a brisk hypoxic ventilatory response are particularly successful at extreme altitudes, presumably because the extra ventilation gives them a slightly higher $PaO_2$ and increases their $Vo_2max$.[594] Exercise at altitude is associated with a moderate retention of fluid and sodium, a factor that in addition may also contribute to the development of pulmonary edema.[595] A significant relationship exists between the symptoms of acute mountain sickness and weight gain during ascent to high altitude.[596] High-altitude climbers develop striking episodes of periodic breathing and apnea during sleep, associated as expected with severe hypoxemia.[597] Acetazolamide stimulates breathing and decreases the nocturnal hypoventilation by producing a mild metabolic acidosis.

### Postpneumonectomy Pulmonary Edema

Acute pulmonary edema is a well-recognized complication of lung resection, especially pneumonectomy.[598, 598a] In one study of 197 patients who had pneumonectomy, it was diagnosed in 2.5%;[599] in another investigation of 402 patients who had a lobectomy or pneumonectomy, it was recognized in 1% of the former and in about 5% of the latter. Risk factors include the use of fresh-frozen plasma (relative risk [RR], 4.3), high mechanical ventilation pressures (RR, 3),[599] a low preoperative diffusing capacity,[600] and right pneumonectomy.[601] In one investigation, pulmonary edema occurred in 8 of 113 patients (7%) who underwent right pneumonectomy and only 3 of 130 (2%) who had a left pneumonectomy;[602] in another study of 10 patients, 9 of the 10 had had a right pneumonectomy.[603]

Although fluid overload was formerly believed to be the major contributing factor, it is clear now that the edema is related to increased pulmonary capillary permeability.[604] It is possible that the mechanism is related to stress failure of the pulmonary capillaries, as has been suggested to occur in HAPE and neurogenic pulmonary edema. The combination of surgical reduction in the cross-sectional area of the pulmonary capillary bed to one half of normal, ventilation of one lung with high pressures, administration of fluid and inotropic agents, and pre-existing emphysema and/or pulmonary vascular disease could combine to cause transient elevations of capillary pressure to very high levels. Shear stress caused by high blood velocity through the remaining lung paren-

chyma could also contribute to the capillary damage.[605] Additional pathogenetic mechanisms that have been suggested are microemboli[606] and a reperfusion type injury;[604] however, because the affected lungs are never really ischemic, the latter explanation seems unlikely.

Postpneumonectomy pulmonary edema has been reported to have a very high mortality rate, exceeding 80% in most series.[599, 601]

### Pulmonary Edema after Lung Re-expansion

Numerous case reports have been documented of unilateral pulmonary edema developing after rapid removal of air or liquid from the pleural space in the presence of pneumothorax or hydrothorax.[607–620] The subject has been reviewed by several groups.[621, 623] It is almost certain that the complication is more common than the number of reports indicate. In one study in which arterial blood gas tensions were measured sequentially before, during, and after thoracentesis, hypoxia was observed between 20 minutes and 2 hours after thoracentesis in the majority of subjects and resolved spontaneously by 24 hours.[622] A possible explanation is subclinical pulmonary edema.

Based on a summary of 12 cases reported in 1975, three features were considered as being common to almost all cases:[612] (1) the pneumothorax or hydrothorax is moderate or large in size (amounting to at least 50% of the affected hemithorax); (2) the pulmonary edema is strictly localized to the ipsilateral lung; and (3) the pneumothorax or hydrothorax has been present for a considerable period of time, usually several days, before rapid re-expansion. In the 12 cases, the duration of pneumothorax, as judged from the onset of dyspnea, averaged 18 days, with a minimum of 3 days. Although these features are applicable to the majority of cases, it is clear that they are not seen in all. For example, cases have been documented in which edema has developed after re-expansion of pneumothoraces that have been present for only one or a few hours[607] and in which the edema has developed contralateral to the re-expanded lung.[624, 625] The edema usually develops immediately or within 1 hour of re-expansion, and all cases occur within a 24-hour period.[626]

The pathogenesis of this form of edema is unclear. Increased capillary permeability would appear to be at least one factor, as indicated by the elevated protein content of the edema fluid.[627, 628] Several mechanisms have been proposed, all of which assume a normal microvascular pressure:[621]

1. A sudden increase in negative intrapleural pressure transmitted to the interstitial space;[607] in support of this process is a report of one patient in whom the lungs were exposed inadvertently to a negative pressure of 120 mm Hg.[610]

2. A delay in venous or lymphatic return caused by stasis in the pulmonary venules and lymphatics during prolonged collapse.[176]

3. The alteration in alveolar surface tension that may accompany prolonged relaxation atelectasis could cause a more negative interstitial pressure.[608, 613]

4. Reperfusion injury to the pulmonary endothelium caused by the local production of toxic oxygen free radicals.

Although a direct anoxic effect on the pulmonary capillaries has also been considered a possible mechanism, it is now clear that hypoxia has no direct effect in producing pulmonary edema.[6]

The first of these hypotheses seems to be the most logical. Because the negative pressure within the pleural space is instantaneously transferred to the alveoli and the interstitium, it might be expected to alter the Starling forces in a manner favoring transudation of fluid from the microvasculature. However, the negative pressure will also be transmitted to the pulmonary microvessels and it is not at all clear that a net change in transvascular hydrostatic pressure would occur. In addition, the negative pressure hypothesis does not explain the finding of increased protein in the edema fluid.[628] It is certain, however, that the rapidity of re-expansion influences the development of edema. In experiments on rhesus monkeys, ipsilateral pulmonary edema developed within 2 hours in all animals in which an 80% to 100% pneumothorax had been maintained for 3 days and in which rapid re-expansion was accomplished by applying suction of $-10$ cm Hg;[629] by contrast, edema did not develop in those animals whose lungs were re-expanded after 1 hour with the application of negative pressure to the pleural space or in those in which underwater drainage of the pneumothorax was applied after 3 days of collapse.

In a rabbit model of the disease, rapid reinflation using a very negative pleural pressure was required to produce edema;[630] moreover, by using radiolabeled tracers to measure protein flux into the extravascular, extracellular space, the edema was found to be associated with increased permeability. When a lung is collapsed as a result of pneumothorax or hydrothorax, perfusion to that lung decreases because of the mechanical collapse of extra-alveolar vessels and the hypoxic vasoconstriction that accompanies the reduction in ventilation.[631] When the lung is re-expanded, there is a rapid but incomplete return of blood flow, and it is this sudden reperfusion that may cause endothelial damage. Reperfusion of the heart and kidneys has been shown to cause damage in these organs; similarly, rapid reperfusion of lung made ischemic by pulmonary artery occlusion has been shown to cause fever, leukopenia, and pulmonary edema.[632] Although the mechanism of perfusion injury of the lung is unknown, it is possibly related to the generation of oxygen free radicals by tissue enzymes, such as xanthine oxidase,[621] that were depleted of substrate and $O_2$ during ischemia and are suddenly presented with an abundance of both. Leukocytes also play a role in the reperfusion injury, because rapid re-expansion of collapsed lung can be associated with the acute development of leukopenia. In one patient, alveolar fluid sampled in the presence of re-expansion pulmonary edema contained increased numbers of polymorphonuclear leukocytes and the powerful leukocyte chemoattractants IL-8 and leukotriene $B_4$.[633]

The radiographic manifestations typically consist of unilateral air-space consolidation that develops within 2 to 4 hours after re-expansion of the lung.[634] The consolidation usually affects the entire re-expanded lung, although it occasionally involves only one lobe.[634] Rarely, both lungs are affected.[634a] CT shows a patchy distribution of the areas of consolidation (Fig. 51–36). The consolidation resolves after 5 to 7 days.

Although re-expansion pulmonary edema is unassociated with significant clinical consequences in most instances,

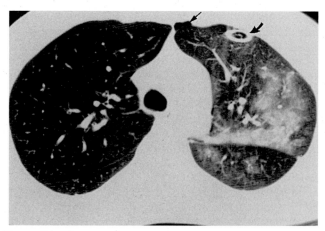

**Figure 51–36. Re-expansion Pulmonary Edema.** A high-resolution CT scan in a 23-year-old man shows patchy areas of consolidation involving the left lung. Also noted are a small residual left pneumothorax *(straight arrow)* and a left chest tube *(curved arrow)* in place. The patient developed edema after chest tube drainage of a large left pneumothorax.

severe respiratory symptoms can occur. The development of edema is often preceded by a feeling of tightness in the chest and by spasmodic coughing; when such symptoms develop, thoracentesis should be discontinued. Although the edema typically resolves spontaneously within a few days, fatalities have been reported.[608, 634–636] The complication can be prevented by slow withdrawal of gas or liquid by underwater drainage.

### Pulmonary Edema Associated with Severe Upper Airway Obstruction

This has been observed in both children and adults and occurs exclusively in lesions affecting the extrathoracic airway from the nasopharynx to the thoracic inlet (Fig. 51–37).[152, 638, 639] It is often precipitated by laryngospasm, which develops especially after surgery on or near the upper airway.[639–642] The laryngospasm characteristically develops within minutes of extubation. In the majority of cases, the edema develops a few minutes after relief of the upper airway obstruction by reintubation.[643] Upper airway obstruction may also contribute to the pulmonary edema that is often seen in victims of hanging.[644] Because the effects of airway obstruction above the thoracic inlet are manifested predominantly during inspiration, efforts to inspire are associated with an increase in negative intrathoracic pressure—in effect, a sustained Mueller maneuver. This can conceivably alter the Starling equation to cause transudation of fluid from capillaries into the interstitium and air spaces. In experiments performed on dogs in 1942, investigators showed that a large increase in negative intrathoracic pressure drew fluid from pulmonary capillaries into the parenchyma;[645] under extreme conditions, red blood cells also left the capillaries.

Although the theory that sustained negative intrathoracic pressure is attractive as an explanation for capillary leakage before the obstruction is relieved, it does not explain the development of edema after relief of obstruction. Some investigators have studied children whose chest radiographs appeared normal just before bypass of severe upper airway obstruction but who developed edema after tracheal intubation.[646, 647] The hypothesis to explain this phenomenon was

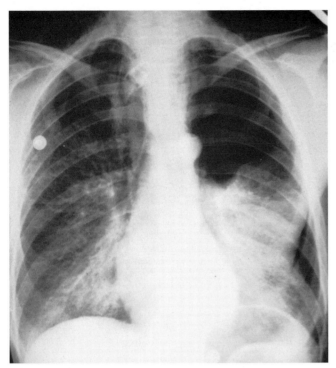

**Figure 51–37. Acute Pulmonary Edema Related to Excessive Negative Intra-alveolar Pressure.** A 52-year-old woman was brought to the emergency department in severe respiratory distress and was found to have a huge mass (subsequently proved to be a primary carcinoma) almost completely obstructing the larynx. An emergency tracheostomy was performed. A radiograph taken shortly thereafter shows diffuse interstitial and air-space pulmonary edema and a moderate-sized left pneumothorax; cardiac size and configuration are within normal limits. It is assumed that the edema resulted from prolonged, sustained negative intrathoracic pressure occasioned by the patient's futile attempts to inspire beyond the laryngeal obstruction—in essence a sustained Mueller maneuver. The edema disappeared in less than 24 hours after tracheostomy.

that the high-negative intrapulmonary pressures generated during inspiration before the obstruction is relieved are counteracted by an expiratory component akin to a modified Valsalva maneuver; when the obstruction is relieved, the counteracting force is no longer present, pulmonary blood flow rapidly increases, and pulmonary edema occurs because of the increased permeability of damaged capillaries (analogous to the proposed mechanism of re-expansion edema). Pulmonary edema developing after the relief of upper airway obstruction has also been reported in adults.[643, 648, 649]

Cardiac "dysfunction" almost certainly contributes to the development of the edema. It is not commonly recognized what a profound effect a very negative intrathoracic pressure can have on left-sided heart function: inspiratory effort against a severely narrowed, or occluded, upper airway can generate pressures of $-140$ cm $H_2O$ or greater;[642] for the left side of the heart this is analogous to adding an afterload of approximately 100 mm Hg (i.e., an increase in mean aortic pressure from 90 to 190 mm Hg!). This mechanism may contribute to the recurrent pulmonary edema that occasionally develops in patients who have obstructive sleep apnea combined with some degree of left ventricular dysfunction.[650] Regardless of the mechanism of this form of edema, its recognition is of obvious importance because vigorous treatment usually results in prompt resolution.[642, 643, 651, 652]

## Miscellaneous Causes of Permeability Edema

As indicated previously, many direct and indirect pulmonary insults have been associated with the development of ARDS (*see* Table 51–2, page 1978). The clinical features, pathophysiology, and radiographic appearance of most of these conditions are described in the sections of this text dealing directly with these causes; some of the causes that are not dealt with elsewhere are discussed briefly in the following sections.

### Transfusion

Although increased knowledge of blood type compatibility has decreased the incidence of pulmonary edema associated with blood transfusion, the risk has not been eliminated.[637, 653, 654] It is worth emphasizing that the edema is usually not a result of overloading of the circulation. Observations that support this interpretation include the relatively small amount of transfused blood that can precipitate the syndrome and a lack of clinical evidence of left ventricular failure. In fact, several groups of investigators have shown that increased capillary permeability resulting from leukoagglutinins and/or human leukocyte antigen incompatibility is the mechanism in the majority of cases.[655–658] The antibodies may be in the donor's serum directed against the recipient's leukocytes or vice versa. Rarely—when the blood product is from multiple donors, as in platelet transfusion—pulmonary injury is caused by antibodies in the plasma of one donor reacting with leukocytes from another donor.[659]

Affected patients have an abrupt onset of chills, fever, tachycardia, nonproductive cough, and dyspnea; blood eosinophilia is sometimes evident.[655] Chest radiographs show patchy opacities affecting predominantly the perihilar and lower lung zones without associated cardiac enlargement or redistribution of blood flow. Leukoagglutinins often are demonstrable in the donors, who generally are multiparous. The antibodies develop because of incompatibility with fetal leukocytes, much in the same manner as Rh antibodies develop. The differential diagnosis should include hemolytic transfusion reactions, anaphylaxis caused by IgA antibodies in the recipient reacting with IgA in the donor's blood (a reaction seen in patients who have IgA deficiency), hypervolemia, and bacterial sepsis.[659]

### Pancreatitis

ARDS develops in a small but significant proportion of patients who have acute pancreatitis unassociated with other precipitating causes such as sepsis or aspiration (Fig. 51–38). In one large autopsy study, the pulmonary complications of acute pancreatitis were the most common cause of death in the first 7 days after admission.[660] The mechanism by which pancreatitis causes pulmonary edema is unclear. However, in experiments on both sheep[661] and dogs,[662] it has been shown to result in increased transvascular fluid and protein flux related to an alteration in lung endothelial permeability. It has been proposed that the pancreatic enzymes in the blood could cause activation of the coagulation pathway, generation of kinins,[663] or activation of the complement system.[664]

It has also been suggested that patients who have ARDS

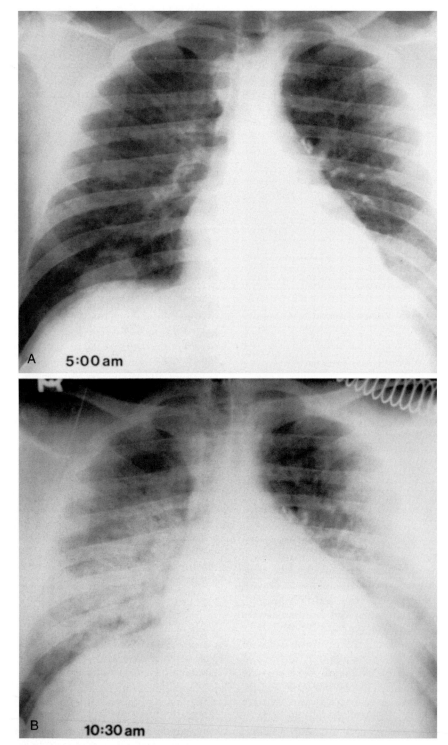

**Figure 51–38. Adult Respiratory Distress Syndrome (ARDS) Associated with Acute Pancreatitis.** This acutely ill 23-year-old man was admitted from the emergency department with a typical clinical presentation of acute pancreatitis. An anteroposterior radiograph at 5 A.M. *(A)* revealed homogeneous consolidation of the base of the left lung and a much smaller area of consolidation in the right lower lobe. Five hours later *(B)*, both lungs had become extensively consolidated in a pattern consistent with severe air-space edema. He died shortly thereafter from ventilatory failure.

of diverse causes can develop secondary pancreatic injury.[665] In a study in which patients who had ARDS were compared with those who had bronchopneumonia, cardiogenic pulmonary edema, or shock without ARDS, those who had ARDS were found to have increased blood levels of trypsin and lipase that followed rather than preceded the onset of their symptoms. These results suggest that microvascular injury may be diffuse in patients who had ARDS and that such injury may result in secondary pancreatic damage.

### Fat Embolism

ARDS frequently occurs after major trauma, particularly in the presence of multiple pelvic and long bone fractures (Fig. 51–39) (*see* page 1845). The contribution of this condition to post-traumatic ARDS is controversial; patients who have multiple trauma are frequently hypotensive, have massive transfusions, or develop sepsis, each of which by itself is a risk factor for the development of ARDS, and it is not always certain to what extent fat emboli themselves contribute to pulmonary damage.

### Pheochromocytoma

Some patients who have pheochromocytoma present with episodes of acute pulmonary edema; by the time they are examined, signs of left ventricular failure or elevated pulmonary microvascular pressure are usually absent, and the clinical syndrome has all of the features of permeability pulmonary edema. It is possible that the mechanism of edema formation in these patients is similar to that which occurs from neurogenic causes—massive adrenergic stimulation that results in a considerable (transient) increase in pulmonary microvascular pressure and subsequent pulmonary vascular leak.[666–668]

### Diabetic Ketoacidosis

Rarely, patients who have diabetic acidosis develop noncardiogenic pulmonary edema that does not appear to be related to other well-defined predisposing factors such as sepsis.[669–671] The mechanism of edema formation is unknown; however, severe leukopenia developed in one case before the onset of the edema, suggesting to the authors that complement activation associated with severe acidosis could have caused pulmonary sequestration of leukocytes and resultant lung injury.[671]

### Parenteral Contrast Media

Pulmonary edema has been described after the parenteral administration of the oil-based medium used for lymphangiography and the water-based media employed in urography, angiography, and contrast-enhanced CT. (The edema that develops occasionally after aspiration of hypertonic contrast media used for examination of the upper gastrointestinal tract is discussed in Chapter 13 [*see* page 2512].) It has been shown that the injection of an oil-based contrast medium in rabbits results in hemorrhagic pulmonary edema several days after embolization.[672] The fatty acids used in ethiodized oil are esterified; although a major proportion of the content of this material is oleic acid, esterification makes it less toxic than the free fatty acid. It is possible that the oil microemboli are acted on by esterases in the lung, causing a breakdown of the esterified compounds to free fatty acids and resultant pulmonary capillary damage.

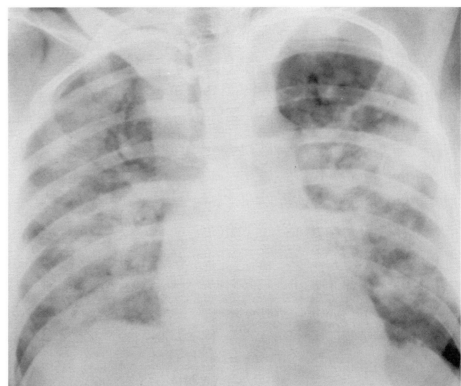

**Figure 51–39. Adult Respiratory Distress Syndrome Associated with Traumatic Fat Embolism.** A radiograph of the chest in anteroposterior projection, supine position, shows diffuse air-space consolidation with some peripheral predominance. Cardiac size is normal. The patient, a young woman with multiple leg fractures sustained in a motor vehicle accident, died shortly thereafter.

Pulmonary edema can also accompany the anaphylactic shock that occasionally occurs after intravenous administration of water-based contrast media.[673, 674, 674a] The onset of the edema is characteristically acute, occurring minutes to hours after the injection, and is associated with evidence of systemic hypotension and complement activation.[674] The complication has been reported after the administration of high osmolality,[675] ionic low osmolality,[676] and nonionic low osmolality contrast material.[677] The prognosis is generally good.[678]

# REFERENCES

1. Ashbaugh DG, Bigelow DB, Petty TL, et al: Acute respiratory distress in adults. Lancet 2:319, 1967.
2. Petty TL, Ashbaugh DG: The adult respiratory distress syndrome: Clinical features, factors influencing prognosis and principles of management. Chest 60:233, 1971.
3. Fishman AP: Pulmonary edema: The water-exchanging function of the lung. Circulation 46:390, 1972.
4. Robin ED, Carroll EC, Zelis R: Pulmonary edema (first of two parts). N Engl J Med 288:239, 1973.
5. Robin ED, Carroll EC, Zelis R: Pulmonary edema (second of two parts). N Engl J Med 288:292, 1973.
6. Staub NC: "State of the art" review: Pathogenesis of pulmonary edema. Am Rev Respir Dis 109:358, 1974.
7. Staub NC: Pulmonary edema. Physiol Rev 54:678, 1974.
8. Staub NC: Pulmonary edema due to increased microvascular permeability. Ann Rev Med 32:291, 1981.
9. Staub NC: Pathophysiology of pulmonary edema. In Staub NC, Taylor AE (eds): Edema. New York, Raven Press, 1984, p 719.
10. Staub NC: Pathways for fluid and solute fluxes in pulmonary edema. In Fishman AP, Renkin EM (eds): Pulmonary Edema. Baltimore, Williams & Wilkins, 1979, p 113.
11. Pritchard JS: Edema of the Lung. Springfield, IL, Charles C Thomas, 1982.
12. Effros RM: Pulmonary microcirculation and exchange. In Renkin EM, Michel CG (eds): Handbook of Physiology—the Cardiovascular System. Vol IV. Oxford, Oxford University Press, 1984, pp 865–915.
13. Snashall PD: Pulmonary oedema. Br J Dis Chest 74:2, 1980.
14. Staub NC (ed): Lung water and solute exchange. In Lenfant C (executive ed): Lung Biology in Health and Disease. New York, Marcel Dekker, 1978.
15. Taylor AE, Khimenko PL, Moore TM, Adkins WK: Fluid balance. In Crystal RG, West JB, et al (eds): The Lung: Scientific Foundations. 2nd ed. Philadelphia, Lippincott-Raven, 1997, pp 1549–1566.
16. Matthay MA, Folkesson HG, Verkman AS: Salt and water transport across alveolar and distal airway epithelia in the adult lung. Am J Physiol 270 (Lung Cell Mol Physiol 14):L487, 1996.
17. Folkesson HG, Matthay MA, Westrom BR, et al: Alveolar epithelial clearance of protein. J Appl Physiol 80:1431, 1996.
18. Wiener-Kronish JP, Broaddus VC: Interrelationship of pleural and pulmonary interstitial liquid. Annu Rev Physiol 55:209, 1993.
19. Lai-Fook SJ: Mechanical factors in lung liquid distribution. Annu Rev Physiol 55:155, 1993.
20. Cope DK, Grimbert F, Downey J, Taylor A: Pulmonary capillary pressure: A review. Crit Care Med 20:1043, 1992.
21. Weibel ER: Morphometry of the Human Lung. New York, Academic Press, 1963.
22. Weibel ER: Morphological basis of alveolar-capillary gas exchange. Physiol Rev 53:419, 1973.
23. Iliff LD: Extra-alveolar vessels and edema development in excised dog lungs. Circ Res 28:524, 1971.
24. Albert RK, Lakshminarayan S, Charan NB, et al: Extra-alveolar vessel contribution to hydrostatic pulmonary edema in in situ dog lungs. J Appl Physiol 54:1010, 1983.
25. Albert RK: Sites of leakage in pulmonary edema. In Said SI (ed): The Pulmonary Circulation and Acute Lung Injury. New York, Futura, 1985, p 189.
26. Bo G, Hauge A, Nicolaysen G: Alveolar pressure and lung volume as determinants of net transvascular fluid filtration. J Appl Physiol 42:476, 1977.
27. Cottrell TS, Levine OR, Senior RM, et al: Electron microscopic alterations at the alveolar level in pulmonary edema. Circ Res 21:783, 1967.
28. Schneeberger EE: Barrier function of intercellular junctions in adult and foetal lungs. In Fishman AP, Renkin EM (eds): Pulmonary Edema. Baltimore, Williams & Wilkins, 1979.
29. Claude P, Goodenough DA: Fracture faces of zonulae occludentes from "tight" and "leaky" epithelium. J Cell Biol 58:390, 1973.
30. Walker DC, MacKenzie A, Hulbert WC, et al: A reassessment of the tricellular region of epithelial cell tight junctions. Acta Anat 122:35, 1985.
31. Blake LH, Staub NC: Pulmonary vascular transport in sheep, a mathematical model. Microvasc Res 12:197, 1976.
32. Blake LH: Mathematical modelling of steady state fluid and protein exchange in lung. In Staub NC (ed): Lung Water and Solute Exchange. New York, Marcel Dekker, 1978, p 99.
33. McNamee JE, Staub NC: Pore models of sheep lung microvascular barrier using new data on protein tracers. Microvasc Res 10:229, 1979.
34. Harris TR, Roselli RJ: A theoretical model of protein, fluid, and small molecule transport in the lung. J Appl Physiol 50:1, 1981.
35. Parker JC, Parker RE, Granger DN, Taylor AE: Vascular permeability and transvascular fluid and protein transport in the dog lung. Circ Res 48:545, 1981.
36. Brigham K: Lung edema due to increased vascular permeability. In Staub NC (ed): Lung Water and Solute Exchange. New York, Marcel Dekker, 1978, p 235.
37. West JB, Mathieu-Costello O: Stress failure of pulmonary capillaries. In Crystal RG, West JB, et al (eds): The Lung. Philadelphia, Lippincott-Raven, 1997, pp 1493–1501.
38. Mathieu-Costello OA, West JB: Are pulmonary capillaries susceptible to mechanical stress? Chest 105:102S, 1994.
39. Todd TRJ, Baile E, Hogg JC: Pulmonary capillary permeability during hemorrhagic shock. J Appl Physiol 45:298, 1978.
40. Baile EM, Paré PD, Ernest D, Dodek PM: Distribution of blood flow and neutrophil kinetics in bronchial vasculature of sheep. J Appl Physiol 82:1466, 1997.
41. Renzoni A: Importanza del plesso venoso peribronchiale nel cane. Arch Ital Anat Embryol 60:111, 1955.
42. Pietra GG, Fishman AP: Bronchial edema. In Staub NC (ed): Lung Water and Solute Exchange. In Lenfant C (executive ed): Lung Biology in Health and Disease. New York, Marcel Dekker, 1978, p 407.
43. Pietra GG, Szidon JP, Leventhal MM, et al: Histamine and interstitial pulmonary edema in the dog. Circ Res 29:323, 1971.
44. Sasaki F, Paré PD, Ernest D, et al: Endogenous nitric oxide influences acetylcholine-induced bronchovascular dilation in sheep. J Appl Physiol 78:539, 1995.
45. Nakahara K, Ohkuda K, Staub NC: Effect of infusing histamine into pulmonary or bronchial artery on sheep pulmonary fluid balance. Am Rev Respir Dis 120:875, 1979.
46. Staub NC, Nagano H, Pearce ML: Pulmonary edema in dogs, especially the sequence of fluid accumulation in lungs. J Appl Physiol 22:227, 1967.
47. Parker JC, Falgout HJ, Parker RE, et al: The effect of fluid volume loading on exclusion of interstitial albumin and lymph flow in the dog lung. Circ Res 45:440, 1979.
47a. Negrini D, Passi A, de Luca G, Miserocchi G: Pulmonary interstitial pressure and proteoglycans during development of pulmonary edema. Am J Physiol 270:H2007, 1996.
48. Bert JL, Pearce RH: The interstitium and microvascular exchange. In Renkin EM, Michel CG (eds): Handbook of Physiology—the Cardiovascular System. IV. Oxford, Oxford University Press, 1984, pp 521–547.
49. Gee MH, Williams DO: Effect of lung inflation on perivascular cuff fluid volume in isolated dog lung lobes. Microvasc Res 17:192, 1979.
50. Paré PD, Warriner B, Baile EM, et al: Redistribution of pulmonary extravascular water with positive end-expiratory pressure in canine pulmonary edema. Am Rev Respir Dis 127:590, 1983.
51. Malo J, Ali J, Duke K, et al: Effects of PEEP on lung liquid distribution and pulmonary shunt in canine oleic acid pulmonary edema. Clin Res 28:703, 1980.
52. Schneeberger-Keeley EE, Karnovsky MJ: The ultrastructural basis of alveolar-capillary membrane permeability to peroxidase used as a tracer. J Cell Biol 37:781, 1968.
53. Egan EA: Effect of lung inflation on alveolar permeability to solutes. In Lung Liquids. Ciba Symposium. (New Series) 38, New York, Excerpta Medica, 1976.
54. Gil J, Weibel ER: Morphological study of pressure volume hysteresis in rat lungs fixed by vascular perfusion. Respir Physiol 15:190, 1972.
55. Lauweryns JM, Boussauw L: The ultrastructure of pulmonary lymphatic capillaries of newborn rabbits and of human infants. Lymphology 2:108, 1969.
56. Renkin EM: Lymph as a measure of the composition of interstitial fluid. In Fishman AP, Renkin EM (eds): Pulmonary Edema. Baltimore, Williams & Wilkins, 1979, p 145.
57. Lauweryns JM, Baert JH: Alveolar clearance and the role of the pulmonary lymphatics. Am Rev Respir Dis 115:625, 1977.
58. Tobin CE: Lymphatics of the pulmonary alveoli. Anat Rec 120:625, 1954.
59. Leak LV, Burke JF: Ultrastructural studies on the lymphatic anchoring filaments. J Cell Biol 36:129, 1968.
60. Paré PD, Brooks LA, Baile EM: Effect of systemic venous hypertension on pulmonary function and lung water. J Appl Physiol 51:592, 1981.
61. Starling EH: On the absorption of fluids from the connective tissue spaces. J Physiol (London) 19:312, 1896.
61a. Jobe RL, Forman MB: Focal pulmonary embolism presenting as diffuse pulmonary edema. Chest 103:644, 1993.
61b. β-Adrenergic agonists and pulmonary oedema in preterm labour. Grand Rounds—Hammersmith Hospital. J Scott, professor of medicine. BMJ 308:260, 1994.
62. Van Mieghem W, Verleden G, Demedts M: Acute pulmonary oedema in patients with primary pulmonary hypertension and normal pulmonary capillary wedge pressure. Acta Cardiol 49:483, 1994.
63. Dawson CA, Grimm DJ, Linehan JH: Effects of lung inflation on longitudinal distribution of pulmonary vascular resistance. J Appl Physiol 43:1089, 1977.
64. Hakim TS, Dawson CA, Linehan JH: Hemodynamic responses of dog lung lobe to lobar venous occlusion. J Appl Physiol 47:145, 1979.
65. Bhattacharya J, Staub MC: Direct measurement of microvascular pressures in the isolated perfused dog lung. Science 210:327, 1980.
66. Goshy M, Lai-Fook SJ, Hyatt RE: Perivascular pressure measurements by wick catheter technique in isolated dog lobes. J Appl Physiol 46:950, 1979.
67. Inoue H, Inoue C, Hildebrandt J: Vascular and airway pressures and interstitial edema affect peribronchial fluid pressure. J Appl Physiol 48:177, 1980.
68. Lai-Fook SJ: Perivascular interstitial fluid pressure measured by micro-pipettes in isolated dog lung. J Appl Physiol 52:9, 1982.
69. Schürch S, Goerke J, Clements JA: Direct determination of surface tension in the lung. Proc Natl Acad Sci U S A 73:4698, 1976.
70. Parker JC, Guyton AC, Taylor AE: Pulmonary interstitial and capillary pressures estimated from intra-alveolar fluid pressures. J Appl Physiol 44:267, 1978.
71. Lai-Fook SJ: Mechanics of lung fluid balance. Crit Rev Biomed Eng 13:171, 1986.

72. Beck KC, Lai-Fook SJ: Effect of height on alveolar liquid pressure in isolated edematous dog lung. J Appl Physiol 54:619, 1983.

73. Landis EN, Pappenheimer JR: Exchange of substances through the capillary wall. *In* Hamilton WS, Dow P (eds): Handbook of Physiology. Washington DC, American Physiological Society, 1963, p 261.

74. Nitta S, Ohnuki T, Okkuda K, et al: The corrected protein equation to estimate plasma colloid osmotic pressure and its development on a nomogram. Tohoku J Exp Med 135:43, 1981.

75. Prather JW, Gaar KA, Guyton AC: Direct continuous recording of plasma colloid osmotic pressure of whole blood. J Appl Physiol 24:602, 1968.

76. Olver RE, Strang LB: Ion fluxes across the pulmonary epithelium and the secretion of lung liquid in the foetal lamb. J Physiol 241:327, 1974.

77. Olver RE: Ion transport and water flow in the mammalian lung. *In* Lung Liquids. Ciba Symposium (New Series) 38, New York, Excerpta Medica, 1976.

78. Albert RK, Lakshminarayan S, Hildebrandt J, et al: Increased surface tension favours pulmonary edema formation in anesthetized dogs' lungs. J Clin Invest 63:115, 1979.

79. Brigham KL, Woolverton WC, Staub NV: Increased pulmonary vascular permeability after *Pseudomonas aeruginosa* bacteremia in unanesthetized sheep. Fed Proc 32:440, 1973.

80. Dumont AE, Clauss RH, Reed GE, et al: Lymph drainage in patients with congestive heart failure. N Engl J Med 269:949, 1963.

81. Sampson JJ, Leeds SE, Uhley HN, et al: Studies of lymph flow and changes in pulmonary structures as indexes of circulatory changes in experimental pulmonary edema. Isr J Med Sci 5:826, 1969.

82. Uhley HN, Leeds SE, Sampson JJ, et al: Some observations on the role of the lymphatics in experimental acute pulmonary edema. Circ Res 9:688, 1961.

83. Uhley HN, Leeds SE, Sampson JJ, et al: Role of pulmonary lymphatics in chronic pulmonary edema. Circ Res 11:966, 1962.

84. Leeds SE, Uhley HN, Sampson JJ, et al: Significance of changes in the pulmonary lymph flow in acute and chronic experimental pulmonary edema. Am J Surg 114:254, 1967.

85. Rusznyák L, Földi M, Szabó G: Lymphatics and lymph circulation: Physiology and pathology. *In* Youlten L (ed): 2nd English ed. Oxford, Pergamon Press, 1967.

86. Magno M, Szidon JP: Haemodynamic pulmonary edema in dogs with acute and chronic lymphatic edema. Am J Physiol 231:1777, 1976.

87. Turino GM, Edelman NH, Senior RM, et al: Extravascular lung water in cor pulmonale. Bull Physiopathol Respir 4:47, 1968.

88. O'Reilly G, Jefferson K: Septal lines in pure right heart failure. Br J Radiol 49:123, 1976.

89. Casley-Smith JR, Taylor AE: Increased initial lymphatic uptake in high flow, high protein oedema: An additional safety factor. Lymphology 24:2, 1991.

90. Erdmann AJ, Vaughan TR, Brigham KL, et al: Effect of increased vascular pressure on lung fluid balance in unanesthetized sheep. Circ Res 37:271, 1975.

91. Montaner JSG, Tsang J, Evans KG, et al: Alveolar epithelial damage: A critical difference between high pressure and oleic acid–induced low pressure pulmonary edema. J Clin Invest 77:1786, 1986.

92. Matthay M: Function of the alveolar epithelial barrier under pathologic conditions. Chest 105:67S, 1994.

93. Khimenko P, Barnard JW, Moore TM, et al: Vascular permeability and epithelial transport effects on lung edema formation in ischemia and reperfusion. J Appl Physiol 77:1116, 1994.

94. Pittet JF, Wiener-Kronish JP, McElroy MC, et al: Stimulation of alveolar epithelial liquid clearance by endogenous release of catecholamines in septic shock. J Clin Invest 94:663, 1994.

95. Conhaim Rl, Lai-Fook SJ, Eaton A: Sequence of perivascular liquid accumulation in liquid-inflated sheep lung lobes. J Appl Physiol 66:2659, 1989.

96. Conhaim RL, Lai-Fook SJ, Staub NC: Sequence of perivascular liquid accumulation in liquid inflated dog lung lobes. J Appl Physiol 60:513, 1986.

97. West JB, Dollery CT, Heard BE: Increased vascular resistance in the lower zone of the lung caused by perivascular oedema. Lancet 2:181, 1964.

98. Muir AL, Hall DL, Despas P, et al: Distribution of blood flow in the lungs in acute pulmonary edema in dogs. J Appl Physiol 33:763, 1972.

99. Vreim CE, Staub NC: Protein composition of lung fluid in acute alloxan edema in dogs. Am J Physiol 230:376, 1976.

100. Vreim CE, Snashall PD, Staub NC: Protein composition of lung fluid in anesthetized dogs with acute cardiogenic edema. Am J Physiol 231:1466, 1976.

101. Staub NC: Alveolar flooding and clearance. Am Rev Respir Dis 127(part 2)S:44, 1983.

102. Conhaim RL: Airway level at which edema liquid enters the air space of isolated dog lung. J Appl Physiol 67:2234, 1989.

103. Broaddus VC, Wiener-Kronish JP, Staub NC: Clearance of lung edema into the pleural space of volume-loaded, anesthetized sheep. J Appl Physiol 68:2623, 1990.

104. Julien M, Hoeffel JM, Flick MR: Oleic acid injury in sheep. J Appl Physiol 60:433, 1986.

105. Berthiaume Y, Albertine KH, Grady M, et al: Protein clearance from the air spaces and lungs of unanesthesized sheep over 144 h. J Appl Physiol 67:1887, 1989.

106. McHugh TJ, Forrester JS, Adler L, et al: Pulmonary vascular congestion in acute myocardial infarction: Hemodynamic and radiologic correlations. Ann Intern Med 76:29, 1972.

107. Ravin CE: Pulmonary vascularity: Radiographic considerations. J Thorac Imaging 3:1, 1988.

108. Morgan PW, Goodman LR: Pulmonary edema and adult respiratory distress syndrome. Radiol Clin North Am 29:943, 1991.

108a. Ketai LH, Godwin JD: A new view of pulmonary edema and acute respiratory distress syndrome. J Thorac Imaging 13:147, 1998.

109. Turner AF, Lau FYK, Jacobson G: A method for the estimation of pulmonary venous and arterial pressures from the routine chest roentgenogram. Am J Roentgenol 116:97, 1972.

110. Woodring JH: Pulmonary artery-bronchus ratios in patients with normal lungs, pulmonary vascular plethora, and congestive heart failure. Radiology 179:115, 1991.

111. Stender HS, Schermuly W: Das interstitielle Lungenödem im Röntgenbild. (Roentgen findings in interstitial pulmonary edema.) Fortschr Roentgensstr 95:461, 1961.

112. Simon M: The pulmonary vessels: Their hemodynamic evaluation using routine radiographs. Radiol Clin North Am 1:363, 1963.

113. Melheim RE, Dunbar JD, Booth RW: The "B" lines of Kerley and left atrial size in mitral valve disease: Their correlation with the mean left atrial pressure as measured by left atrial puncture. Radiology 76:65, 1961.

114. Viamonte M Jr, Parks RE, Barrera F: Roentgenographic prediction of pulmonary hypertension in mitral stenosis. Am J Roentgenol 87:936, 1962.

115. Milne ENC: Physiological interpretation of the plain radiograph in mitral stenosis, including a review of criteria for the radiological estimation of pulmonary arterial and venous pressures. Br J Radiol 36:902, 1963.

116. McHugh TJ, Forrester JS, Adler L, et al: Pulmonary vascular congestion in acute myocardial infarction: Hemodynamic and radiologic correlations. Ann Intern Med 76:29, 1972.

117. Slutsky RA, Higgins CB: Intravascular and extravascular pulmonary fluid volumes: II. Response to rapid increases in left atrial pressure and the theoretical implications for pulmonary radiographic and radionuclide imaging. Invest Radiol 18:33, 1983.

118. Dodek A, Kassebaum DG, Bristow JD: Pulmonary edema in coronary-artery disease without cardiomegaly: Paradox of the stiff heart. N Engl J Med 286:1347, 1972.

119. Heitzman ER: The Lung: Radiologic-Pathologic Correlations. St. Louis, CV Mosby, 1973, pp 127, 137.

120. Grainger RG: Interstitial pulmonary oedema and its radiological diagnosis: A sign of pulmonary venous and capillary hypertension. Br J Radiol 31:201, 1958.

121. Heitzman ER, Ziter FM: Acute interstitial pulmonary edema. Am J Roentgenol 98:291, 1966.

122. Heikkilä J, Hugenholtz PG, Tabakin BS: Prediction of left heart filling pressure and its sequential change in acute myocardial infarction from the terminal force of the P wave. Br Heart J 35:142, 1973.

123. Bennett ED, Rees S: The significance of radiological changes in the lungs in acute myocardial infarction. Br J Radiol 47:879, 1974.

124. Carroll FE Jr, Loyd JE, Nolop KB, et al: MR imaging parameters in the study of lung water: A preliminary study. Invest Radiol 20:381, 1985.

125. Milne EN, Pistolesi M, Miniati M, et al: The radiologic distinction of cardiogenic and noncardiogenic edema. Am J Roentgenol 144:879, 1985.

126. Primack SL, Müller NL, Mayo JR, et al: Pulmonary parenchymal abnormalities of vascular origin: High-resolution CT findings. Radiographics 14:739, 1994.

127. Primack SL, Remy-Jardin M, Remy J, Müller NL: High-resolution CT of the lung: Pitfalls in the diagnosis of infiltrative lung disease. Am J Roentgenol 167:413, 1996.

128. Storto ML, Kee ST, Golden JA, Webb WR: Hydrostatic pulmonary edema: High-resolution CT findings. Am J Roentgenol 165:817, 1995.

129. Forster BB, Müller NL, Mayo JR, et al: High-resolution computed tomography of experimental hydrostatic pulmonary edema. Chest 101:1434, 1992.

130. Goodman LR: Congestive heart failure and adult respiratory distress syndrome: New insights using computed tomography. Radiol Clin North Am 34:33, 1996.

131. Goodman LR: Congestive heart failure and adult respiratory distress syndrome: New insights using computed tomography. Intensive Care Med 34:33, 1996.

131a. Slanetz PJ, Truong M, Shepard JAO, et al: Mediastinal lymphadenopathy and hazy mediastinal fat: New CT findings of congestive heart failure. Am J Roentgenol 171:1307, 1998.

132. Herold CJ, Wetzel RC, Robotham JL, et al: Acute effects of increased intravascular volume and hypoxia on the pulmonary circulation: Assessment with high-resolution CT. Radiology 183:665, 1992.

133. Brasileiro FC, Vargas FS, Kavakama JI, et al: High-resolution CT scan in the evaluation of exercise-induced interstitial pulmonary edema in cardiac patients. Chest 111:1577, 1997.

134. Caillaud C, Serrecousine O, Anselme F, et al: Computerized tomography and pulmonary diffusing capacity in highly trained athletes after performing a triathlon. J Appl Physiol 79:1226, 1995.

135. Hedlund LW, Vock P, Effmann EL, et al: Hydrostatic pulmonary edema: An analysis of lung density changes by computed tomography. Invest Radiol 19:254, 1984.

136. Kato S, Nakamoto T, Lizuka M: Early diagnosis and estimation of pulmonary congestion and edema in patients with left-sided heart diseases from histogram of pulmonary CT number. Chest 109:1439, 1996.

137. Gamsu G, Kaufman L, Swann SJ, et al: Absolute lung density in experimental canine pulmonary edema. Invest Radiol 14:261, 1979.

138. Campbell JH, Harris ND, Zhang F, et al: Clinical applications of electrical impedance tomography in the monitoring of changes in intrathoracic fluid volumes. Physiol Meas Suppl 2A:A217, 1994.

139. Ahluwalia BD, Brownell GL, Hales CA: An index of pulmonary edema measured with emission computed tomography. J Comput Assist Tomogr 5:690, 1981.

140. Calandrino FS Jr, Anderson DJ, Mintun MA, et al: Pulmonary vascular permeability during the adult respiratory distress syndrome; a positron emission tomographic study. Am Rev Respir Dis 138:421, 1988.

141. Tamaki N, Itoh H, Ishii Y, et al: Hemodynamic significance of increased lung uptake of thallium-201. Am J Roentgenol 138:223, 1982.

142. Serizawa S, Suzuki T, Niino H, et al: Using $H_2(15)O$ and C15O in noninvasive pulmonary measurements. Chest 106:1145, 1994.

143. Caruthers SD, Paschal CB, Pou NA, Harris TR: Relative quantification of pulmonary edema with non–contrast-enhanced MRI. J Magn Reson Imaging 7:544, 1997.

144. Estilaei M, Mackay A, Roberts C, Mayo J: H-1 NMR measurements of wet/dry ratio and T-1, T-2 distributions in lung. J Magn Reson 124:410, 1997.

145. Skalina S, Kundel HL, Wolf G, et al: The effect of pulmonary edema on proton nuclear magnetic resonance relaxation times. Invest Radiol 19:7, 1984.

146. Wexler HR, Nicholson RL, Prato FS, et al: Quantitation of lung water by nuclear magnetic resonance imaging: A preliminary study. Invest Radiol 20:583, 1985.

147. Schmidt HC, McNamara MT, Brasch RC, et al: Assessment of severity of experimental pulmonary edema with magnetic resonance imaging: Effect of relaxation enhancement by Gd-DTPA. Invest Radiol 20:687, 1987.

148. McCredie M: Measurement of pulmonary edema in valvular heart disease. Circulation 36:381, 1967.

149. Gleason DC, Steiner RE: The lateral roentgenogram in pulmonary edema. Am J Roentgenol 98:279, 1966.

150. Milne ENC: Letter to the editor: Hydrostatic versus increased permeability pulmonary edema. Radiology 170:891, 1989.

151. Milne ENC, Pistolesi M, Miniati M, et al: The radiologic distinction of cardiogenic and noncardiogenic edema. Am J Roentgenol 144:879, 1985.

152. Uhley HN, Leeds SE, Sampson JJ, et al: Role of pulmonary lymphatics in chronic pulmonary edema. Circ Res 11:966, 1962.

153. Richman SM, Godar TJ: Unilateral pulmonary edema. N Engl J Med 264:1148, 1961.

154. Nessa CG, Rigler LG: The roentgenological manifestations of pulmonary edema. Radiology 37:35, 1941.

155. Azimi F, Wolson AH, Dalinka MK, et al: Unilateral pulmonary edema—differential diagnosis. Australas Radiol 19:20, 1975.

156. Calenoff L, Kruglik GD, Woodruff A: Unilateral pulmonary edema. Radiology 126:19, 1978.

157. Roach JM, Stajduhar KC, Torrington KG: Right upper lobe pulmonary edema caused by acute mitral regurgitation: Diagnosis by transesophageal echocardiography. Chest 103:1286, 1993.

158. Albers WH, Nadas AS: Unilateral chronic pulmonary edema and pleural effusion after systemic-pulmonary artery shunts for cyanotic congenital heart disease. Am J Cardiol 19:861, 1967.

159. Salem MR, Masud KZ, Tatooles CJ, et al: Unilateral pulmonary oedema following aorta to right pulmonary artery anastomosis (Waterston's operation). Br J Anaesth 43:701, 1971.

160. Felman AH: Neurogenic pulmonary edema: Observations in 6 patients. Am J Roentgenol 112:393, 1971.

161. Royal HD, Shields JB, Donati RM: Misplacement of central venous pressure catheters and unilateral pulmonary edema. Arch Intern Med 135:1502, 1975.

162. Akiyama K, Suetsugu F, Hidai T, et al: Left-sided unilateral pulmonary edema in postinfarction ventricular septal rupture. Chest 105:1264, 1994.

163. Flick MR, Kantzler GB, Block AJ: Unilateral pulmonary edema with contralateral thoracic sympathectomy in the adult respiratory distress syndrome. Chest 68:736, 1975.

164. Gyves-Ray KM, Spizarny DL, Gross BH: Case report: Unilateral pulmonary edema due to postlobectomy pulmonary vein thrombosis. Am J Roentgenol 148:1079, 1987.

165. Alarcon JJ, Guembe P, de Miguel E, et al: Localized right upper lobe edema. Chest 107:274, 1995.

166. Schnyder PA, Sarraj AM, Duvoisin BE, et al: Pulmonary edema associated with mitral regurgitation: Prevalence of predominant involvement of the right upper lobe. Am J Roentgenol 161:33, 1993.

166a. Rice J, Roth SL, Rossoff LJ: An unusual case of left upper lobe pulmonary edema. Chest 114:328, 1998.

167. Takahashi M, Ikeda U, Shimada K, Takeda H: Unilateral pulmonary edema related to pulmonary artery compression resulting from acute dissecting aortic aneurysm. Am Heart J 126:1225, 1993.

168. Kagele SF, Charan NB: Unilateral pulmonary edema: An unusual cause. Chest 102:1279, 1992.

169. Greatrex KV, Fisher MS: Sparing of some accessory lobes in diffuse pulmonary edema. J Thorac Imaging 12:78, 1997.

170. Leeming BWA: Gravitational edema of the lungs observed during assisted respiration. Chest 64:719, 1973.

171. Brussel T, Hachenberg T, Roos N, et al: Mechanical ventilation in the prone position for acute respiratory failure after cardiac surgery. J Cardiothorac Vasc Anesth 7:541, 1993.

172. Robin ED, Thomas ED: Some relations between pulmonary edema and pulmonary inflammation (pneumonia). Arch Intern Med 93:713, 1954.

173. Zimmerman JE, Goodman LR, St Andre AC, et al: Radiographic detection of mobilizable lung water: The gravitational shift test. Am J Roentgenol 138:59, 1982.

174. Hughes RT: The pathology of butterfly densities in uraemia. Thorax 22:97, 1967.

175. Herrnheiser G, Hinson KFW: An anatomical explanation of the formation of butterfly shadows. Thorax 9:198, 1954.

176. Rigler LG, Surprenant EL: Pulmonary edema. Semin Roentgenol 2:33, 1967.

177. Prichard MML, Daniel PM, Ardran GM: Peripheral ischaemia of the lung: Some experimental observations. Br J Radiol 27:93, 1954.

178. Reeves JT, Tweeddale D, Noonan J, et al: Correlations of microradiographic and histologic findings in the pulmonary vascular bed: Technique and application in pulmonary hypertension. Circulation 34:971, 1966.

179. Fleischner FG: The butterfly pattern of acute pulmonary edema. Am J Cardiol 20:39, 1967.

180. Wrinch J, Thurlbeck WM, Hogg J, et al: The pathogenesis of the "butterfly" shadow in pulmonary edema: A study of the effect of the lymphatic drainage. Unpublished data.

181. Fava S, Azzopardi J: Circadian variation in the onset of acute pulmonary edema and associated acute myocardial infarction in diabetic and nondiabetic patients. Am J Cardiol 80:336, 1997.

182. Ishmail AA, Wing S, Ferguson J, et al: Interobserver agreement by auscultation in the presence of a third heart sound in patients with congestive heart failure. Chest 91:870, 1987.

183. Ewy GA: The abdominojugular test: Technique and hemodynamic correlates. Ann Intern Med 109:456, 1988.

184. Berger M, Bach M, Hecht SR, et al: Estimation of pulmonary arterial wedge pressure by pulsed Doppler echocardiography and phonocardiography. Am J Cardiol 69:562, 1992.

185. Davis M, Espiner E, Richards G, et al: Plasma brain natriuretic peptide in assessment of acute dyspnoea. Lancet 343:440, 1994.

186. Frank NJ: Influence of acute pulmonary vascular congestion on the recoiling forces of excised cats' lungs. J Appl Physiol 14:905, 1959.

187. Cooke CD, Mead J, Schreiner GL, et al: Pulmonary mechanics during induced pulmonary edema in anesthetized dogs. J Appl Physiol 14:17, 1969.

188. Said SI, Longacre JW, David RK, et al: Pulmonary gas exchange during induction of pulmonary edema in anesthetized dogs. J Appl Physiol 19:403, 1964.

189. Levine OR, Mellins RB, Fishman AP: Quantitative assessment of pulmonary edema. Circ Res 17:414, 1965.

190. Sharp JG, Griffith GD, Bunnell IL, et al: Ventilatory mechanics in pulmonary edema in man. J Clin Invest 37:111, 1958.

191. Hogg JC, Agarawal JB, Gardiner AJF, et al: Distribution of airway resistance with developing pulmonary edema in dogs. J Appl Physiol 32:20, 1972.

192. Collins JV, Cochrane SN, Davis J, et al: Some aspects of pulmonary function after rapid saline infusion in healthy subjects. Clin Sci Molec Med 45:407, 1973.

193. Hales CA, Kazemi H: Small airway function in myocardial infarction. N Engl J Med 290:761, 1974.

194. Zidulka A, Despas DJ, Milic-Emili J, et al: Pulmonary function with acute loss of lung water by hemodialysis in patients with chronic uremia. Am J Med 55:134, 1973.

195. Tsubata S, Ichida F, Miyazaki A, et al: Bronchial hyper-responsiveness to inhaled histamine in children with congenital heart disease. Acta Paediatr Jpn 37:336, 1995.

196. Lockhart A, Dinh-Xuan AT, Regnard J, et al: Effect of airway blood flow on airflow. Am Rev Respir Dis 146(5 Pt 2):S19, 1992.

197. Cabanes LR, Weber SN, Matran R, et al: Bronchial hyperresponsiveness to methacholine in patients with impaired left ventricular function. N Engl J Med 320:1317, 1989.

198. West JB, Dollery CT, Heard BE: Increased pulmonary vascular resistance in the dependent zone of the isolated dog lung caused by perivascular edema. Circ Res 17:191, 1965.

199. West JB: Perivascular oedema: A factor in pulmonary vascular resistance. Am Heart J 70:570, 1965.

200. Milne EN: What is "congested" in cardiac failure? A newer approach to plain film interpretation of cardiac failure. Rays 22:94, 1997.

201. Dawson A, Kaneko K, McGregor M: Regional lung function in patients with mitral stenosis studied with 133 XE during air and oxygen breathing. J Clin Invest 44:999, 1965.

202. Langer M, Mascheroni D, Marcolin R: The prone position in ARDS patients: A clinical study. Chest 94:103, 1988.

203. Mutoh T, Guest RJ, Lamm WJ, Albert RK: Prone position alters the effect of volume overload on regional pleural pressures and improves hypoxemia in pigs *in vivo*. Am Rev Respir Dis 146:300, 1992.

204. Paintal AF: Mechanism of stimulation of type J pulmonary receptors. J Physiol 203:511, 1969.

205. Aberman A, Fulop M: The metabolic and respiratory acidosis of acute pulmonary edema. Ann Intern Med 76:173, 1972.

206. Fulop M, Horowitz M, Aberman A, et al: Lactic acidosis in pulmonary edema due to left ventricular failure. Ann Intern Med 79:180, 1973.

207. Anthonisen NR, Smith HJ: Respiratory acidosis as a consequence of pulmonary edema. Ann Intern Med 62:991, 1965.

208. Agostoni A: Acid-base disturbances in pulmonary edema. Arch Intern Med 120:307, 1967.

209. Avery WG, Samet P, Sackner MA: The acidosis of pulmonary edema. Am J Med 48:320, 1970.

210. Wilson JG: Pulmonary oedema in acute glomerulonephritis. Arch Dis Child 36:661, 1961.

211. Macpherson RI, Banerjee AK: Acute glomerulonephritis: A chest film diagnosis? J Can Assoc Radiol 25:58, 1974.

212. Gibson DG: Hemodynamic factors in the development of acute pulmonary oedema in renal failure. Lancet 2:1217, 1966.

213. Kooman JP, Leunissen KM: Cardiovascular aspects in renal disease. Curr Opin Nephrol Hypertens 2:791, 1993.

214. London GM, Guerin AP, Marchais SJ. Pathophysiology of left ventricular hypertrophy in dialysis patients. Blood Purif 12:277, 1994.

215. Lye WC, Leong SO, Lee EJ: Transplant renal artery stenosis presenting with recurrent acute pulmonary edema. Nephron 72:302, 1996.

216. Ducloux D, Jamali M, Chalopin JM: Chronic congestive heart failure associated with bilateral renal artery stenosis. Clin Nephrol 48:54, 1977.

217. Wallin CJ, Jacobson SH, Leksell LG: Subclinical pulmonary oedema and intermittent haemodialysis. Nephrol Dial Transplant 11:2269, 1996.

218. Lee HY, Stretton TB, Barnes AM: The lungs in renal failure. Thorax 30:46, 1975.

219. Zidulka A, Despas PJ, Milic-Emili J, et al: Pulmonary function with acute loss of excess lung water by hemodialysis in patients with chronic uremia. Am J Med 55:134, 1973.

220. Metry G, Wegenius G, Hedenstrom H, et al: Computed tomographic measurement of lung density—changes in lung water with hemodialysis. Nephron 75:394, 1997.

221. Cooperman LH, Price HL: Pulmonary edema in the operative and postoperative period. Ann Surg 172:883, 1970.

222. daLuz PL, Weil MH, et al: Pulmonary edema related to changes in colloid osmotic and pulmonary artery wedge pressure in patients after acute myocardial infarction. Circulation 51:350, 1975.

223. Stein L, Beraud J, Cavonilles J, et al: Pulmonary edema during fluid infusion in the absence of heart failure. JAMA 229:65, 1974.

224. Westcott JL, Rudick MG: Cardiopulmonary effects of intravenous fluid overload: Radiologic manifestations. Radiology 129:577, 1978.

225. Luft FC, Klatte EC, Weyman AE, et al: Cardiopulmonary effects of volume expansion in man: Radiographic manifestations. Am J Roentgenol 144:289, 1985.

226. Witz CA, Silverberg KM, Burns WN, et al: Complications associated with the absorption of hysteroscopic fluid media. Fertil Steril 60:745, 1993.

227. Gilliland MD, Coates N: Tumescent liposuction complicated by pulmonary edema. Plast Reconstr Surg 99:215, 1997.

228. O'Brien JD, Ettinger NA: Pulmonary complications of liver transplantation. Clin Chest Med 17:99, 1996.

229. Ruff F, Hughes JBM, Stanley M, et al: Regional lung function in patients with hepatic cirrhosis. J Clin Invest 50:2403, 1971.

230. Trewby PN, Warren R, Contini S, et al: Incidence and pathophysiology of pulmonary oedema in fulminant hepatic failure. Gastroenterology 74:859, 1978.

231. Matuschak GM, Shaw BW: Adult respiratory distress syndrome associated with acute liver allograft rejection: Resolution following hepatic retransplantation. Crit Care Med 15:878, 1987.

232. Hacking PM, Simpson W: Partially obstructed total anomalous pulmonary venous return. Clin Radiol 18:450, 1967.

233. Sande MA, Alonso DR, Smith JP, et al: Left atrial tumor presenting with hemoptysis and pulmonary infiltrates. Am Rev Respir Dis 102:258, 1970.

234. Montreal General Hospital Case Records: Dyspnea and lymphadenopathy in a patient with two PH-1 chromosomes. N Engl J Med 289:524, 1973.

235. Sarnoff SJ: Massive pulmonary edema of central nervous system origin: Hemodynamic observations and the role of sympathetic pathways. Fed Proc 10:118, 1951.

236. Cameron GR, De SN: Experimental pulmonary oedema of nervous origin. J Pathol Bacteriol 61:375, 1949.

237. Ducker TD, Simmons RL: Increased intracranial pressure and pulmonary edema: II. Hemodynamic response of dogs and monkeys to increased intracranial pressure. J Neurosurg 28:118, 1968.

238. Worthen M, Argano B, Siwadiowski W, et al: Mechanisms of intracisternal veratrine pulmonary edema. Dis Chest 55:45, 1969.

239. Benowitz NL, Simon RP, Copeland JR: Status epilepticus: Divergence of sympathetic activity and cardiovascular response. Ann Neurol 19:197, 1986.

240. Johnston SC, Darragh TM, Simon RP: Postictal pulmonary edema requires pulmonary vascular pressure increases. Epilepsia 37:428, 1996.

241. Harari A, Rapin M, Regnier B, et al: Normal pulmonary capillary pressures in the late phase of neurogenic pulmonary edema. Lancet 1:494, 1976.

242. Melon E, Bonnet F, Lepresle E, et al: Altered capillary permeability in neurogenic pulmonary oedema. Intensive Care Med 11:323, 1985.

243. Ducker TD: Increased intracranial pressure and pulmonary edema: I. Clinical study of 11 patients. J Neurosurg 28:112, 1968.

244. Theodore J, Robin E: Speculations on neurogenic pulmonary edema. Am Rev Respir Dis 113:404, 1976.

245. Wray NP, Nicotra MB: Pathogenesis of neurogenic pulmonary edema. Am Rev Respir Dis 118:783, 1978.

246. Smith WS, Matthay MA: Evidence for a hydrostatic mechanism in human neurogenic pulmonary edema. Chest 111:1326, 1997.

247. Van der Zee H, Malik AB, Lee BC, et al: Lung fluid and protein exchange during intracranial hypertension and role of sympathetic mechanisms. J Appl Physiol 48:273, 1980.

248. Bowers RE, McKeen CR, Park BE, et al: Increased pulmonary vascular permeability follows intracranial hypertension in sheep. Am Rev Respir Dis 119:637, 1979.

249. Samuels M: Neurally induced cardiac damage: Definition of the problem. Neurocardiology 11:273, 1993.

250. Deehan SC, Grant IS: Haemodynamic changes in neurogenic pulmonary oedema: Effect of dobutamine. Intensive Care Med 22:672, 1996.

251. Davie KR, Gelb AW, Manninen PH, et al: Cardiac function in aneurysmal subarachnoid haemorrhage: A study of electrocardiographic and echocardiographic abnormalities. Br J Anaesth 67:58, 1991.

252. Pollick C, Cujec B, Parker S, Tator C: Left ventricular wall motion abnormalities

253. Wells JC, Johnson D: Reversibility of severe left ventricular dysfunction in patients with subarachnoid hemorrhage. Am Heart J 129:409, 1995.

254. Mayer SA, Fink ME, Homma S, et al: Cardiac injury associated with neurogenic pulmonary edema following subarachnoid hemorrhage. Neurology 44:815, 1994.

255. Bonbrest HC: Pulmonary edema following an epileptic seizure. Am Rev Respir Dis 91:97, 1965.

256. Huff RW, Fred HL: Postictal pulmonary edema. Arch Intern Med 117:824, 1966.

257. Chang CH, Smith CA: Postictal pulmonary edema. Radiology 89:1087, 1967.

258. Teplinsky K, Hall J: Post-ictal pulmonary edema: Report of a case. Arch Intern Med 146:801, 1986.

259. Simon RP: Neurogenic pulmonary edema. Neurocardiology 11:309, 1993.

260. Schumacker PT, Rhodes GR, Newell JC, et al: Ventilation-perfusion imbalance after head trauma. Am Rev Respir Dis 119:33, 1979.

261. Addington WW, Cugell DW, Bayley ES, et al: The pulmonary edema of heroin toxicity—an example of the stiff lung syndrome. Chest 62:199, 1972.

262. Briscoe WA, Smith JP, Bergofsky E, et al: Catastrophic pulmonary failure. Am J Med 60:248, 1976.

263. Petty TL, Ashbaugh DG: The adult respiratory distress syndrome: Clinical features, factors influencing prognosis and principles of management. Chest 60:233, 1971.

264. Respiratory Diseases. Task Force Report on Problems, Research Approaches, Needs. DHEW publication No. NIH73–432. Bethesda, MD, National Heart and Lung Institute, 1972, pp 167–180.

265. Villar J, Slutsky AS: The incidence of adult respiratory distress syndrome. Am Rev Respir Dis. 140:814, 1989.

266. Petty TL: Indicators of risk, course, and prognosis in adult respiratory distress syndrome (ARDS). Am Rev Respir Dis 132:471, 1985.

267. Connelly KG, Repine JE: Markers for predicting the development of acute respiratory distress syndrome. Annu Rev Med 48:429, 1997.

268. Wittram C, Kenny JB: The admission chest radiograph after acute inhalation injury and burns. Br J Radiol 67:751, 1994.

269. Fowler AA, Hamman RF, Good JT, et al: Adult respiratory distress syndrome: Risk with common predisposition. Ann Intern Med 98:593, 1983.

270. Kreuzfelder E, Joka T, Keinecke HO, et al: Adult respiratory distress syndrome as a specific manifestation of a general permeability defect in trauma patients. Am Rev Respir Dis 137:95, 1988.

271. Hyers TM, Gee M, Andreadis NA: Cellular interactions in multiple organ injury syndrome. Am Rev Respir Dis 135:952, 1987.

272. Rinaldo JE, Christman JW: Mechanisms and mediators of the adult respiratory distress syndrome. Clin Chest Med 11:621, 1990.

273. Bone RC, Balk RA, Cerra FB, et al: ACCP/SCCM consensus conference: Definitions for sepsis and organ failure and guidelines for the use of innovative therapies in sepsis. Chest 101:1644, 1991.

274. Montgomery BR, Stager MA, Carrico CJ, Hudson LD: Causes of mortality in patients with the adult respiratory distress syndrome. Am Rev Respir Dis 132:484, 1985.

275. Bone RC: Toward a theory regarding the pathogenesis of the systemic inflammatory response syndrome: What we do and do not know about cytokine regulation. Crit Care Med 24:163, 1996.

276. Montgomery AB, Stager MA, Carrico CJ, et al: Causes of mortality in patients with the adult respiratory distress syndrome. Am Rev Respir Dis 132:485, 1985.

277. Rangel-Frausto MS, Pittet D, Costigan M, et al: The natural history of the systemic inflammatory response syndrome (SIRS): A prospective study [see comments]. JAMA 273:117, 1995.

278. Blennerhassett JB: Shock lung and diffuse alveolar damage: Pathological and pathogenetic considerations. Pathology 17:239, 1985.

279. Meyrick B, Berry LC, Christman BW: Response of cultured human pulmonary artery endothelial cells to endotoxin. Am J Physiol 12:239, 1995.

280. Canonico A, Brigham K: Biology of acute injury. *In* Crystal RG, West JB, et al (eds): The Lung. Philadelphia, Lippincott-Raven, 1997, pp 2475–2498.

281. Clinton SK, Underwood R, Hayes L, et al: Macrophage colony-stimulating factor gene expression in vascular cells and in experimental and human atherosclerosis. Am J Pathol 140:301, 1992.

282. Springer TA: Adhesion receptors of the immune system. Nature 346:425, 1990.

283. Tosi MF, Stark JM, Smith CW, et al: Induction of ICAM-1 expression on human airway epithelial cells by inflammatory cytokines: Effects on neutrophil-epithelial cell adhesion. Am J Respir Cell Mol Biol 7:214, 1992.

284. Blaisdell FW, Schlobohm RM: The respiratory distress syndrome: A review. Surgery 74:251, 1973.

285. Connell RS, Swank RL, Webb MC: The development of pulmonary ultrastructural lesions during hemorrhage shock. J Trauma 15:116, 1975.

286. Demling RH, Niehaus G, Will JA: Pulmonary microvascular response to hemorrhagic shock, resuscitation and recovery. J Appl Physiol 46:498, 1979.

287. Thommasen HB, Martin BA, Wiggs B, et al: The effect of pulmonary blood flows on white blood cell uptake and release by the dog lung. J Appl Physiol 56:966, 1984.

288. Hogg JC, Martin BA, Lee S, et al: Regional differences in red blood cell transit in normal lungs. J Appl Physiol 59:126, 1985.

289. Doerschuk CM, Allard MF, Martin BA, et al: Marginated pool of neutrophils in rabbit lungs. J Appl Physiol 63:1806, 1987.

290. Muir AL, Cruz M, Martin BA, et al: Leukocyte kinetics in the human lung: Role of exercise and catecholamines. J Appl Physiol 57:711, 1984.

291. Hallgren R, Samuelsson T, Venge P, et al: Eosinophil activation in the lung is

in subarachnoid hemorrhage: An echocardiographic study. J Am Coll Cardiol 12:600, 1988.

related to lung damage in adult respiratory distress syndrome. Am Rev Respir Dis 135:639, 1987.

292. Modig J, Hallgren R: Lethal adult respiratory distress syndrome after meningococcal septicemia biochemical markers in bronchoalveolar lavage. Resuscitation 13:159, 1986.

293. Larson RS, Springer TA: Structure and function of leukocyte integrins. Immunol Rev 114:181, 1990.

294. Springer TA: Traffic signals for lymphocyte recirculation and leukocyte emigration: The multistep paradigm. Cell 76:301, 1994.

295. Laurent T, Markert M, Von Fliedner V, et al: CD11b/CD18 expression, adherence, and chemotaxis of granulocytes in adult respiratory distress syndrome. Am J Respir Crit Care Med 149:1534, 1994.

296. Nicod LP: Cytokines: I. Overview. Thorax 48:660, 1993.

297. Cochrane CG: The enhancement of inflammatory injury. Am Rev Respir Dis 136:1, 1987.

298. Tenholder MF, Rajagopal KR, Phillips YY, et al: Urinary desmosine excretion as a marker of lung injury in adult respiratory distress syndrome. Chest 100:1385, 1991.

299. Tate RM, Repine JE: Neutrophils and the adult respiratory distress syndrome. Am Rev Respir Dis 128:552, 1983.

300. Thommasen HB: The role of the polymorphonuclear leukocyte in the pathogenesis of the adult respiratory distress syndrome. Clin Invest Med 8:185, 1985.

301. Bachofen N, Weibel ER: Alterations of the gas exchange apparatus in adult respiratory insufficiency associated with septicemia. Am Rev Respir Dis 116:589, 1977.

302. Elliott CG, Zimmerman GA, Orme JF, et al: Granulocyte aggregation in adult respiratory distress syndrome (ARDS)—serial histologic and physiologic observations. Am J Med Sci 289:70, 1985.

303. Brigham KL, Woolverton WC, Blake LH, et al: Increased sheep lung vascular permeability caused by *Pseudomonas* bacteremia. J Clin Invest 54:792, 1974.

304. Flick MR, Perel G, Staub NC: Leukocytes are required for increased lung microvascular permeability after microembolism in sheep. Circ Res 48:344, 1981.

305. Heflin AJ, Brigham KL: Prevention by granulocyte type depletion of increased vascular permeability of sheep lung following endotoxemia. J Clin Invest 68:1253, 1981.

306. Johnson A, Malik AP: Effect of granulocytopenia on extravascular lung water content after micro-embolization. Am Rev Respir Dis 122:561, 1980.

307. Shasby DM, Fox RB, Harada RN, et al: Reduction of the edema of acute hypoxic lung injury by granulocyte depletion. J Appl Physiol 52:1237, 1982.

308. Shasby DM, Van Benthuysen KM, Tate RM, et al: Granulocytes mediate acute edematous lung injury in rabbits and isolated rabbit lungs perfused with phorbol myristate acetate: Role of oxygen radicals. Am Rev Respir Dis 125:443, 1982.

309. Worthen GS, Haslett C, Rees AJ, et al: Neutrophil-mediated pulmonary vascular injury: Synergistic effect of trace amounts of lipopolysaccharide and neutrophil stimuli on vascular permeability and neutrophil sequestration in the lung. Am Rev Respir Dis 136:19, 1987.

310. Snapper JR, Bernard GR, Hinson JM, et al: Endotoxemia-induced leukopenia in sheep—correlation with lung vascular permeability and hypoxemia but not with pulmonary hypertension. Am Rev Respir Dis 127:306, 1983.

311. Parsons PE, Fowler AA, Hyers TM, et al: Chemotactic activity in bronchoalveolar lavage fluid from patients with adult respiratory distress syndrome. Am Rev Respir Dis 132:490, 1985.

312. Zimmerman GA, Renzetti AD, Hill HR: Functional and metabolic activity of granulocytes from patients with adult respiratory distress syndrome—evidence for activated neutrophils in the pulmonary circulation. Am Rev Respir Dis 127:290, 1983.

313. Miyata T, Torisu M: Plasma endotoxin levels and functions of peripheral granulocytes in surgical patients with respiratory distress syndrome. Jpn J Surg 16:412, 1986.

314. Fowler AA, Hyers TM, Fisher BJ, et al: The adult respiratory distress syndrome: Cell populations and soluble mediators in the air spaces of patients at high risk. Am Rev Respir Dis 136:1225, 1987.

315. Weiland JE, Davis WB, Holter JF, et al: Lung neutrophils in the adult respiratory distress syndrome: Clinical and pathophysiologic significance. Am Rev Respir Dis 133:218, 1986.

316. Thommasen HB, Russell JA, Boyko WJ, et al: Transient leukopenia associated with adult respiratory distress syndrome. Lancet 1:809, 1984.

317. Warshawski FJ, Sibbald WJ, Driedger AA, et al: Abnormal neutrophil-pulmonary interaction in the adult respiratory distress syndrome: Qualitative and quantitative assessment of pulmonary neutrophil kinetics in humans with *in vivo* [111]Indium neutrophil scintigraphy. Am Rev Respir Dis 133:797, 1986.

318. Maunder RJ, Hackman RC, Riff E, et al: Occurrence of the adult respiratory distress syndrome in neutropenic patients. Am Rev Respir Dis 133:313, 1986.

319. Braude S, Apperley J, Krausz T, et al: Adult respiratory distress syndrome after allogeneic bone-marrow transplantation: Evidence for a neutrophil-independent mechanism. Lancet 1:1239, 1985.

320. Ognibene RP, Martin SE, Parker MM, et al: Adult respiratory distress syndrome in patients with severe neutropenia. N Engl J Med 315:547, 1986.

321. Rinaldo JE, Borovetz H: Deterioration of oxygenation and abnormal lung microvascular permeability during resolution of leukopenia in patients with diffuse lung injury. Am Rev Respir Dis 131:579, 1985.

322. Butler JC, Peters CJ: Hantaviruses and hantavirus pulmonary syndrome. Clin Infect Dis 19:387, 1994.

323. Hallman M, Spragg R, Harrell JH, et al: Evidence of lung surfactant abnormality in respiratory failure. J Clin Invest 70:673, 1982.

324. Petty TL, Reiss OK, Paul GW, et al: Characteristics of pulmonary surfactant in adult respiratory distress syndrome associated with trauma and shock. Am Rev Respir Dis 115:531, 1977.

325. Petty TL, Silvers DW, Paul GW: Abnormalities in lung elastic properties and surfactant function in adult respiratory distress syndrome. Chest 75:571, 1979.

326. Lewis JF, Jobe AH: Surfactant and the adult respiratory distress syndrome. Am Rev Respir Dis 147:218, 1993.

327. Liau DF, Barrett CR, Bell ALL, et al: Functional abnormalities of lung surfactant in experimental acute alveolar injury in the dog. Am Rev Respir Dis 136:395, 1987.

328. Ryan SF, Liau DF, Bell ALL, et al: Correlation of lung compliance and quantities of surfactant phospholipids after acute alveolar injury from N-nitroso-N-methylurethane in the dog. Am Rev Respir Dis 123:200, 1981.

329. Seeger W, Lepper H, Wolf HRD, Neuhof H: Alteration of alveolar surfactant function after exposure to oxidative stress and oxygenated and native arachidonic acid *in vitro*. Biochim Biophys Acta 835:58, 1985.

330. Ryan SF, Ghassibi Y, Liau DF: Effects of activated polymorphonuclear leukocytes upon pulmonary surfactant in vitro. Am J Respir Cell Mol Biol 4:33, 1991.

331. Arias-Diaz J, Vara E, Garcia C, Balibrea JL: Tumor necrosis factor-alpha-induced inhibition of phosphatidylcholine synthesis by human type II pneumocytes is partially mediated by prostaglandins. J Clin Invest 94:244, 1994.

332. Arias-Diaz J, Vara E, Garcia C, et al: Tumour necrosis factor-alpha inhibits synthesis of surfactant by isolated human type II pneumocytes. Eur J Surg 159:541, 1993.

333. Pison U, Tam EK, Caughey GH, Hawgood S: Proteolytic inactivation of dog lung surfactant-associated proteins by neutrophil elastase. Biochim Biophys Acta 992:241, 1989.

334. Jacobson W, Park GR, Saich T, Holcroft J: Surfactant and adult respiratory distress syndrome. Br J Anaesth 70:522, 1993.

335. Thomassen MJ, Antal JM, Connors MJ, et al: Characterization of exosurf (surfactant)-mediated suppression of stimulated human alveolar macrophage cytokine responses. Am J Respir Cell Mol Biol 10:399, 1994.

336. Thomassen MJ, Antal JM, Divis LT, Wiedemann HP: Regulation of human alveolar macrophage inflammatory cytokines by tyloxapol: A component of the synthetic surfactant Exosurf. Clin Immunol Immunopathol 77:201, 1995.

337. Weg JG, Balk RA, Tharrat RS, et al, for the Exosurf ARDS Sepsis Study Group: Safety and potential efficacy of an aerosolized surfactant in human sepsis–induced adult respiratory distress syndrome. JAMA 272:1433, 1994.

338. Anzueto A, Baughman RP, Guntupalli KK, et al: Aerosolized surfactant in adults with sepsis-induced acute respiratory distress syndrome. Exosurf Acute Respiratory Distress Syndrome Sepsis Study Group. N Engl J Med 334:1417, 1996.

339. Spragg RG, Gilliard N, Richman P, et al: Acute effects of a single dose of porcine surfactant on patients with the adult respiratory distress syndrome. Chest 105:195, 1994.

340. Haslam PL, Hughes DA, MacNaughton PD, et al: Surfactant replacement therapy in late-stage adult respiratory distress syndrome. Lancet 343:1009, 1994.

341. Huang YC, Caminiti SP, Fawcett TA, et al: Natural surfactant and hyperoxic lung injury in primates. J Appl Physiol 76:991, 1994.

342. Till GO, Ward PA: Complement-induced lung injury. *In* Said SI (ed): The Pulmonary Circulation and Acute Lung Injury. Mount Kisco, NY, Futura, 1985, p 387.

343. Knudsen P, Nielsen AH, Pedersen JD, et al: Adult respiratory distress-like syndrome during hemodialysis: Relationship between activation of complement, leukopenia, and release of granulocyte elastase. Int J Artif Organs 8:187, 1985.

344. Lew PD, Forster A, Perrin LH, et al: Complement activation in the adult respiratory distress syndrome following cardiopulmonary bypass. Bull Eur Physiopathol Respir 21:231, 1985.

345. Boogaerts MA, Roelant C, Goossens W, et al: Complement activation and adult respiratory distress syndrome during intermittent flow apheresis procedures. Transfusion 26:82, 1986.

346. Gardinali M, Cicardi M, Frangi D, et al: Studies of complement activation in ARDS patients treated by long term extracorporeal $CO_2$ removal. Int J Artif Organs 8:135, 1985.

347. Muller-Eberhard HJ: Complement. Annu Rev Biochem 44:697, 1975.

348. Shaw JO, Henson PM, Henson J, et al: Lung inflammation induced by complement derived chemotactic fragments in the alveolus. Lab Invest 42:547, 1980.

349. Robbins RA, Russ WD, Rasmussen JK, et al: Activation of the complement system in the adult respiratory distress syndrome. Am Rev Respir Dis 135:651, 1987.

350. Weigelt JA, Chenoweth DE, Borman KA, et al: Complement and the severity of pulmonary failure. J Trauma 28:1013, 1988.

351. Langlois PF, Gawryl MS: Accentuated formation of the terminal C5b-9 complement complex in patient plasma precedes development of the adult respiratory distress syndrome. Am Rev Respir Dis 138:368, 1988.

352. Rinaldo JE, Rogers RM: Adult respiratory distress syndrome. N Engl J Med 315:578, 1986.

353. Weinberg PF, Matthay MA, Webster RO, et al: Biologically active products of complement and acute lung injury in patients with sepsis syndrome. Am Rev Respir Dis 130:791, 1984.

354. Duchateau J, Haas M, Schreyen H, et al: Complement activation in patients at risk of developing the adult respiratory distress syndrome. Am Rev Respir Dis 130:1058, 1984.

355. Donnelly TJ, Meade P, Jagels M, et al: Cytokine, complement, and endotoxin profiles associated with the development of the adult respiratory distress syndrome after severe injury. Crit Care Med 22:768, 1994.

356. Zilow G, Joka T, Obertacke U, et al: Generation of anaphylatoxin C3a in plasma and bronchoalveolar lavage fluid in trauma patients at risk for the adult respiratory distress syndrome. Crit Care Med 20:468, 1992.

357. Malik AB: Mediators of pulmonary vascular injury and edema after thrombin. *In* Said SI (ed): The Pulmonary Circulation and Acute Lung Injury. Mount Kisco, NY, Futura, 1985, p 429.

358. Saldeen T: Clotting, microembolism, and inhibition of fibrinolysis in adult respiratory distress. Surg Clin North Am 63:285, 1983.

359. Carlson RW, Schaeffer RC, Carpio M, et al: Edema fluid and coagulation changes during fulminant pulmonary edema. Chest 79:43, 1981.

360. Dorinsky PM, Gadek JE: Mechanisms of multiple nonpulmonary organ failure in ARDS. Chest 99:293, 1989.

361. Malik AB: Pulmonary microembolism. Physiol Rev 63:1114, 1983.

362. Saldeen T: The microembolism syndrome. *In* Saldeen T (ed): The Microembolism Syndrome. Stockholm, Almquist & Wiksell International, 1979, p 7.

363. Johnson A, Tahamont MB, Malik AB: Thrombin-induced lung vascular injury: Role of fibrinogen and fibrinolysis. Am Rev Respir Dis 128:38, 1983.

364. Tahamont MB, Malik AB: Granulocytes mediate the increase in pulmonary vascular permeability after thrombin embolism. J Appl Physiol 54:1489, 1983.

365. Johnson A, Blumenstock FA, Malik AB: Effect of complement depletion on lung fluid balance after thrombin. J Appl Physiol 55:1480, 1983.

366. Lo SK, Perlman MB, Niehaus GD, et al: Thrombin-induced alterations in lung fluid balance in awake sheep. J Appl Physiol 58:1421, 1985.

367. Kwaan HC: Disseminated intravascular coagulation. Med Clin North Am 56:177, 1972.

368. Bone RC, Francis PB, Pierce AK: Intravascular coagulation associated with the adult respiratory distress syndrome. Am J Med 61:585, 1976.

369. El-Kassimi FA, Al-Mashhadani DCP, Abdullah AK, et al: Adult respiratory distress syndrome and disseminated intravascular coagulation complicating heat stroke. Chest 90:571, 1986.

370. Haynes AB, Hyers TM, Giclas PC, et al: Elevated fibrin(ogen) degradation products in the adult respiratory distress syndrome. Am Rev Respir Dis 122:841, 1980.

371. Moalli R, Boyle JM, Tahhan HR, et al: Fibrinolysis in critically ill patients. Am Rev Respir Dis 140:287, 1989.

372. Carvalho ACA: Blood alterations in ARDS. *In* Zapol WM, Falke KJ (eds): Acute Respiratory Failure. New York, Marcel Dekker, 1985, pp 303–346.

373. Fourrier F, Chopin C, Goudemand J, et al: Septic shock, multiple organ failure, and disseminated intravascular coagulation. Chest 101:816, 1992.

374. Schneider RC, Zapol WM, Carvalho AC: Platelet consumption and sequestration in severe acute respiratory failure. Am Rev Respir Dis 122:445, 1980.

375. Modig J, Bagge L: Specific coagulation and fibrinolysis tests as biochemical markers in traumatic-induced adult respiratory distress syndrome. Resuscitation 13:87, 1986.

376. Alberts KA, Norén I, Rubin M, et al: Respiratory distress following major trauma: Predictive value of blood coagulation tests. Acta Orthop Scand 57:158, 1986.

377. Sorensen JV, Jensen HP, Rahr HB, et al: Fibrinogen and fibrin derivatives in traumatized patients: Relation to injury severity and posttraumatic pulmonary dysfunction. Haemostasis 23:91, 1993.

378. Quinn DA, Carvalho AC, Geller E, et al: $^{99m}$Tc-fibrinogen scanning in adult respiratory distress syndrome. Am Rev Respir Dis 135:100, 1987.

379. Idell S, Gonzalez K, Bradford H, et al: Procoagulant activity in bronchoalveolar lavage in the adult respiratory distress syndrome: Contribution of tissue factor associated with factor 7. Am Rev Respir Dis 136:1466, 1987.

380. Bachofen M, Weibel ER: Structural alterations of lung parenchyma in the adult respiratory distress syndrome. Clin Chest Med 3:35, 1982.

381. Schneider RC, Zapol WM, Carvalho AC: Platelet consumption and sequestration in severe, acute respiratory failure. Am Rev Respir Dis 122:445, 1980.

382. Carvalho ACA, Bellman SM, Saullo VJ, et al: Altered factor 8 in acute respiratory failure. N Engl J Med 307:1113, 1982.

383. Taylor AE, Martin DJ, Townsley MI: Oxygen radicals and pulmonary edema. *In* Said SI (ed): The Pulmonary Circulation and Acute Lung Injury. Mount Kisco, NY, Futura, 1985, p 307.

384. Cochrane CG, Spragg R, Revak SD: Pathogenesis of the adult respiratory distress syndrome—evidence of oxidant activity in bronchoalveolar lavage fluid. J Clin Invest 71:754, 1983.

385. Mathru M, Rooney MW, Dries DJ, et al: Urine hydrogen peroxide during adult respiratory distress syndrome in patients with and without sepsis. Chest 105:232, 1994.

386. Nakae H, Endo S, Inada K, et al: Significance of alpha-tocopherol and interleukin-8 in septic adult respiratory distress syndrome. Res Comm Chem Pathol Pharmacol 84:197, 1994.

387. Brigham KL, Meyrick B, Berry JC, Repine JE: Antioxidants protect cultured bovine lung endothelial cells from injury by endotoxin. J Appl Physiol 63:840, 1987.

388. Braun J, Pein M, Djonlagic H, Dalhoff K: Production of reactive oxygen species by central venous and arterial neutrophils in severe pneumonia and cardiac lung edema. Intensive Care Med 23:170, 1997.

389. White CW, Kumuda CD: Role of cytokines in acute lung injury. *In* Crystal RG, West JB (eds): The Lung. 2nd ed. Philadelphia, Lippincott-Raven, 1997, pp 2451–2464.

390. Sica A, Marsushima K, Van Damme J, et al: IL-1 transcriptionally activates the neutrophil chemotactic factor/IL-8 gene in endothelial cells. Immunology 69:548, 1990.

391. Miller EJ, Cohen AB, Matthay MA: Increased interleukin-8 concentrations in the pulmonary edema fluid of patients with acute respiratory distress syndrome from sepsis. Crit Care Med 24:1448, 1996.

392. Dinarello CA: Interleukin-1 and its biologically related cytokines. Adv Immunol 44:153, 1989.

393. Gauldie J, Richards C, Harnish D, et al: Interferon 2/BSF-2 shares identity with monocyte derived hepatocyte stimulating factor and regulates the major acute phase response in liver cells. Proc Natl Acad Sci U S A 84:7251, 1987.

394. Fogh K, Larsen CG, Iversen L, Kragballe K: Interleukin-8 stimulates the formation of 15-hydroxy-eicosatetraenoic acid by human neutrophils *in vitro*. Agents Actions 35:227, 1992.

395. Garcia JG, Noonan TC, Jubiz W, Malik AB: Leukotrienes and the pulmonary microcirculation. Am Rev Respir Dis 136:161, 1987.

396. Seeger W, Grimminger F, Barden M, et al: Omega-oxidized leukotriene B4 detected in the bronchoalveolar lavage fluid of patients with non-cardiogenic pulmonary edema, but not in those with cardiogenic edema. Intensive Care Med 17:1, 1991.

397. Ahmed T, Marchett B, Wanner A, et al: Direct and indirect effects of leukotriene D4 on the pulmonary and systemic circulations. Am Rev Respir Dis 131:554, 1985.

398. Slotman GJ, Burchard KW, Yellin SA, et al: Prostaglandin and complement interaction in clinical acute respiratory failure. Arch Surg 121:271, 1986.

399. Matthay MA, Eschenbacher WL, Goetzl EJ: Elevated concentrations of leukotriene D4 in pulmonary edema fluid of patients with the adult respiratory distress syndrome. J Clin Immunol 4:479, 1984.

400. Gillis CN, Pitt BR, Widemann HP, et al: Depressed prostaglandin E1 and 5-hydroxytryptamine removal in patients with adult respiratory distress syndrome. Am Rev Respir Dis 134:739, 1986.

401. Cox JW, Andreadis NA, Bone RC, et al: Pulmonary extraction and pharmacokinetics of prostaglandin E1 during continuous intravenous infusion in patients with adult respiratory distress syndrome. Am Rev Respir Dis 137:5, 1988.

402. Bernard GR, Luce JM, Sprung CL, et al: High dose corticosteroids in patients with the adult respiratory distress syndrome. New Engl J Med 317:1565, 1987.

403. Bone RC, Slotman G, Maunder R, et al: Randomized double-blind multicenter study of prostaglandin E-1 in patients with the adult respiratory distress syndrome. Chest 96:114, 1889.

404. Mitaka C, Hirata Y, Nagura T, et al: Circulating endothelin-1 concentrations in acute respiratory failure. Chest 104:476, 1993.

405. Schapira M, Gardaz JP, Py P, et al: Prekallikrein activation in the adult respiratory distress syndrome. Bull Eur Physiopathol Respir 21:237, 1985.

406. Idell S, Kucich U, Fein A, et al: Neutrophil elastase-releasing factors in bronchoalveolar lavage from patients with adult respiratory distress syndrome. Am Rev Respir Dis 132:1098, 1985.

407. O'Brodovich HM, Stalcup SA, Pang LM, et al: Bradykinin production and increased pulmonary endothelial permeability during acute respiratory failure in unanesthetized sheep. J Clin Invest 67:514, 1981.

408. McGuire WW, Spragg RG, Cohen AB, et al: Studies on the pathogenesis of the adult respiratory distress syndrome. J Clin Invest 69:543, 1982.

409. Nuytinck JK, Goris JA, Redl H, et al: Posttraumatic complications and inflammatory mediators. Arch Surg 121:886, 1986.

410. Lee CT, Fein AM, Lippmann M, et al: Elastolytic activity in pulmonary lavage fluid from patients with adult respiratory-distress syndrome. N Engl J Med 304:192, 1981.

411. Johnson AR, Coalson JJ, Ashton J, et al: Neutral endopeptidase in serum samples from patients with adult respiratory distress syndrome: Comparison with angiotensin-converting enzyme. Am Rev Respir Dis 132:1262, 1985.

412. Vadas P: Elevated plasma phospholipase A2 levels: Correlation with the hemodynamic and pulmonary changes in gram-negative septic shock. J Lab Clin Med 104:873, 1984.

413. Cohen AB, Stevens MD, Miller EJ, et al: Neutrophil-activating peptide-2 in patients with pulmonary edema from congestive heart failure or ARDS. Am J Physiol 264:L490, 1993.

414. Heffner JE, Ali R, Jeevanandam M: Urinary excretion of polyamines in the adult respiratory distress syndrome. Exp Lung Res 21:275, 1995.

415. Chesnutt AN, Kheradmand F, Folkesson HG, et al: Soluble transforming growth factor-alpha is present in the pulmonary edema fluid of patients with acute lung injury. Chest 111:652, 1997.

416. Ostendorf P, Birzle H, Vogel W, et al: Pulmonary radiographic abnormalities in shock: Roentgen-clinical pathological correlation. Radiology 115:257, 1975.

417. Hasleton PS: Adult respiratory distress syndrome—a review. Histopathology 7:307, 1983.

418. Blennerhasset JB: Shock lung and diffuse alveolar damage: Pathological and pathogenetic considerations. Pathology 17:239, 1985.

419. Putman CE, Minagi H, Blaisdell FW: The roentgen appearance of disseminated intravascular coagulation (DIC). Radiology 109:13, 1973.

420. Fukuda Y, Ishizaki M, Masuda Y, et al: The role of intraalveolar fibrosis in the process of pulmonary structural remodeling in patients with diffuse alveolar damage. Am J Pathol 126:171, 1987.

421. Nash G, Langlinais PC: Pulmonary interstitial edema and hyaline membranes in adult burn patients: Electron microscopic observations. Hum Pathol 5:149, 1974.

422. Bensadoun ES, Burke AK, Hogg JC, Roberts CR: Proteoglycan deposition in pulmonary fibrosis. Am J Respir Crit Care Med 154:1819, 1996.

423. Tomashefski JF Jr, Davies P, Boggis C, et al: The pulmonary vascular lesions of the adult respiratory distress syndrome. Am J Pathol 112:112, 1983.

424. Snow RL, Davies P, Pontoppidan H, et al: Pulmonary vascular remodeling in adult respiratory distress syndrome. Am Rev Respir Dis 126:887, 1982.

425. Joffe N: The adult respiratory distress syndrome. Am J Roentgenol 122:719, 1974.

426. Dyck DR, Zylak CJ: Acute respiratory distress in adults. Radiology 106:497, 1973.

427. Greene R: Adult respiratory distress syndrome: Acute alveolar damage. Radiology 163:57, 1987.

427a. Zimmerman JE, Goodman LR, Shahvari MBG: Effect of mechanical ventilation and positive end-expiratory pressure (PEEP) on chest radiographs. Am J Roentgenol 133:811, 1979.

428. Wolfson MR, Shaffer TH: Liquid ventilation during early development: Theory, physiologic processes and application. J Dev Physiol 13:1, 1990.

429. Leach CL, Fuhrman BP, Morin FC, et al: Perfluorocarbon-associated gas exchange (partial liquid ventilation) in respiratory distress syndrome: A prospective, randomized, controlled study. Crit Care Med 21:1270, 1993.

430. Kazerooni EA, Pranikoff T, Cascade PN, et al: Partial liquid ventilation with perflubron during extracorporeal life support in adults: Radiographic appearance. Radiology 198:137, 1996.

431. Shaffer TH, Wolfson MR, Clark LC Jr: Liquid ventilation. Pediatr Pulmonol 14:102, 1992.

432. Meaney JFM, Kazerooni EA, Garver KA, et al: Acute respiratory distress syndrome: CT findings during partial liquid ventilation. Radiology 202:570, 1997.

433. Wheeler AP, Carroll FE, Bernard GR: Radiographic issues in adult respiratory distress syndrome. New Horiz 1:471, 1993.

434. Tagliabue M, Casella TC, Zincone GE, et al: CT and chest radiography in the evaluation of adult respiratory distress syndrome. Acta Radiol 35:230, 1994.

435. Gattinoni L, Bombino M, Pelosi P, et al: Lung structure and function in different stages of severe adult respiratory distress syndrome. JAMA 271:1772, 1994.

436. Bombino M, Gattinoni L, Pesenti A, et al: The value of portable chest roentgenography in adult respiratory distress syndrome. Chest 100:762, 1991.

437. Pelosi P, D'Andrea L, Vitale G, et al: Vertical gradient of regional lung inflation in adult respiratory distress syndrome. Am J Respir Crit Care Med 149:8, 1994.

438. Zimmerman JE, Goodman LR, Shahvari MB: Effect of mechanical ventilation and positive end-expiratory pressure (PEEP) on chest radiograph. Am J Roentgenol 133:811, 1979.

439. Gattinoni L, D'Andrea L, Pelosi P, et al: Regional effects and mechanism of positive end-expiratory pressure in early adult respiratory distress syndrome. JAMA 269:2122, 1993.

440. Smith RC, Mann H, Greenspan RH, et al: Radiographic differentiation between different etiologies of pulmonary edema. Invest Radiol 22:859, 1987.

441. Miniati M, Pistolesi M, Paoletti P, et al: Objective radiographic criteria to differentiate cardiac, renal, and injury lung edema. Invest Radiol 23:433, 1988.

442. Aberle DR, Wiener-Kronish JP, Webb WR, et al: Hydrostatic versus increased permeability pulmonary edema: Diagnosis based on radiographic criteria in critically ill patients. Radiology 168:73, 1988.

443. Im JG, Yu YJ, Ahn JM, et al: Hydrostatic versus oleic acid–induced pulmonary edema: High-resolution computed tomography findings in the pig lung. Acta Radiol 1:364, 1994.

444. Bernard GR, Artigas A, Brigham KL, et al: The American-European Consensus Conference on ARDS: Definitions, mechanisms, relevant outcomes, and clinical trial coordination. Am J Respir Crit Care Med 149:818, 1994.

445. O'Quin R, Marini JJ: Pulmonary artery occlusion pressure: Clinical physiology, measurement, and interpretation. Am Rev Respir Dis 128:319, 1983.

446. Touissant GP, Burgess JH, Hanipson LG: Central venous pressure and pulmonary wedge pressure in critical surgical illness: A comparison. Arch Surg 109:265, 1974.

447. Pomerantz SM, Mirvis SE, Siegel EL, Belzberg H: False pulmonary artery catheter measurements due to the scimitar (hypogenetic lung) syndrome: Potential for iatrogenic pulmonary edema. Chest 103:1895, 1993.

448. Wittnich C, Trudel J, Zidulka A, et al: Misleading "pulmonary wedge pressure" after pneumonectomy: Its importance in postoperative fluid therapy. Ann Thorac Surg 42:192, 1986.

449. Grimbert FA, Parker JC, Taylor AE: Increased lung microvascular permeability following acid aspiration. J Appl Physiol 51:335, 1981.

450. Bender JS, Smithmeek MA, Jones CE: Routine pulmonary artery catheterization does not reduce morbidity and mortality of elective vascular surgery—results of a prospective, randomized trial. Ann Surg 226:229, 1997.

451. Jones J, Grossman RF, Berry M, et al: Alveolar-capillary membrane permeability: Correlation with functional, radiographic, and post-mortem changes after fluid aspiration. Am Rev Respir Dis 120:399, 1979.

452. Jones JG, Minty BD, Royston D: Alveolar barrier permeability and ARDS. Eur J Respir Dis 64:9, 1983.

453. Tennenberg SD, Jacobs MP, Solomkin JS, et al: Increased pulmonary alveolar-capillary permeability in patients at risk for adult respiratory distress syndrome. Crit Care Med 15:289, 1987.

454. Braude S, Nolop KB, Hughes JMB, et al: Comparison of lung vascular and epithelial permeability indices in the adult respiratory distress syndrome. Am Rev Respir Dis 133:1002, 1986.

455. Permeability of the blood-gas barrier. In Crystal RG, West JB (eds): The Lung. Philadelphia: Lippincott-Raven, 1997, pp 1567–1580.

456. Groeneveld JAB: Radionuclide assessment of pulmonary microvascular permeability. Eur J Nucl Med 24:450, 1997.

457. Groeneveld AB, Raijmakers PG, Teule GJ, Thijs LG: The 67 gallium pulmonary leak index in assessing the severity and course of the adult respiratory distress syndrome. Crit Care Med 24:1467, 1996.

458. Spicer KM, Reines DH, Frey GD: Diagnosis of adult respiratory distress syndrome with Tc-99m human serum albumin and portable probe. Crit Care Med 14:669, 1986.

459. Anderson R, Holliday L, Driedger A, et al: Documentation of pulmonary capillary permeability in the adult respiratory distress syndrome accompanying human sepsis. Am Rev Respir Dis 119:869, 1979.

460. Glauser FL, Millen JE, Falls R: Effects of acid aspiration on pulmonary alveolar epithelial membrane permeability. Chest 76:201, 1979.

461. Morel DR, Dargent F, Bachmann M, et al: Pulmonary extraction of serotonin and propranolol in patients with adult respiratory distress syndrome. Am Rev Respir Dis 132:479, 1985.

462. Sprung CL, Long WM, Marcial EH, et al: Distribution of proteins in pulmonary edema: The value of fractional concentrations. Am Rev Respir Dis 136:957, 1987.

463. Sprung CL, Rackow EC, Fein IA, et al: The spectrum of pulmonary edema: Differentiation of cardiogenic intermediate noncardiogenic forms of pulmonary edema. Am Rev Respir Dis 124:718, 1981.

464. Matthay MA, Eschenbacher WL, Goetzl EJ: Elevated concentrations of leukotrienes D4 in pulmonary edema fluid of patients with the adult respiratory distress syndrome. J Clin Immunol 4:479, 1984.

465. Miller EJ, Cohen AB, Nagao S, et al: Elevated levels of NAP-1/interleukin-8 are present in the airspaces of patients with adult respiratory distress syndrome and are associated with increased mortality. Am Rev Respir Dis 146:427, 1992.

466. Matthay MA, Wiener-Kronish JP: Intact epithelial barrier function is critical for the resolution of alveolar edema in humans. Am Rev Respir Dis 142:1250, 1990.

467. Pittet JF, Mackersie RC, Martin TR, Matthay MA: Biological markers of acute lung injury: Prognostic and pathogenetic significance. Am J Respir Crit Care Med 155:1187, 1997.

468. Rinaldo JE, Borovetz HS, Mancini MC, et al: Assessment of lung injury in the adult respiratory distress syndrome using multiple indicator dilution curves. Am Rev Respir Dis 133:1006, 1986.

469. Laggner A, Kleinberger G, Haller J, et al: Bedside estimation of extravascular lung water in critically ill patients: Comparison of the chest radiograph and the thermal dye technique. Intensive Care Med 10:309, 1984.

470. Eisenberg PR, Hansbrough JR, Anderson D, et al: A prospective study of lung water measurements during patient management in an intensive care unit. Am Rev Respir Dis 136:662, 1987.

471. Sibbald WJ, Short AK, Warshawski FJ, et al: Thermal dye measurements of extravascular lung water in critically ill patients: Intravascular Starling forces and extravascular lung water in the adult respiratory distress syndrome. Chest 87:585, 1985.

472. Feeley TW, Mihm FG, Halperin BD, et al: Failure of the colloid oncotic-pulmonary artery wedge pressure gradient to predict changes in extravascular lung water. Crit Care Med 13:1025, 1985.

473. Overland ES, Gupta RN, Huchon GJ, et al: Measurement of pulmonary tissue volume and blood flow in persons with normal and edematous lungs. J Appl Physiol 51:1375, 1981.

474. Dantzker DR, Brook CJ, Dehart P, et al: Ventilation-perfusion distributions in the adult respiratory distress syndrome. Am Rev Respir Dis 120:1039, 1979.

475. Ralph DD, Robertson HT, Weaver LJ, et al: Distribution of ventilation and perfusion during positive end-expiratory pressure in the adult respiratory distress syndrome. Am Rev Respir Dis 131:54, 1985.

476. Lemaire F, Matamis D, Lampron N, et al: Intrapulmonary shunt is not increased by 100% oxygen ventilation in acute respiratory failure. Bull Eur Physiopathol Respir 21:251, 1985.

477. Brigham KL, Kariman K, Harris TR, et al: Correlation of oxygenation with vascular permeability surface area but not with lung water in humans with acute respiratory failure and pulmonary edema. J Clin Invest 72:339, 1983.

478. Melot C, Naeije R, Mols P, et al: Pulmonary vascular tone improves pulmonary gas exchange in the adult respiratory distress syndrome. Am Rev Respir Dis 136:1232, 1987.

479. Lynch JP, Mhyre, JG, Dantzker DR: Influence of cardiac output on intrapulmonary shunt. J Appl Physiol 46:315, 1979.

480. Breen PH, Schumacker PT, Hedenstierna G, et al: How does increased cardiac output increase shunt in pulmonary edema? J Appl Physiol 53:1273, 1982.

481. Wiener CM, Kirk W, Albert RK: Prone position reverses gravitational distribution of perfusion in dog lungs with oleic acid-induced injury. J Appl Physiol 68:1386, 1990.

482. Lamm WJ, Graham MM, Albert RK: Mechanism by which the prone position improves oxygenation in acute lung injury. Am J Respir Crit Care Med 150:184, 1994.

483. Macnaughton PD, Evans TW: Measurement of lung voume and DLCO in acute respiratory failure. Am J Respir Crit Care Med 150:770, 1994.

484. Pesenti A, Pelosi P, Rossi N, et al: Respiratory mechanics and bronchodilator responsiveness in patients with the adult respiratory distress syndrome. Crit Care Med 21:78, 1993.

485. Shiabutani K, Komatsu T, Kubal K, et al: Critical level of oxygen delivery in anesthetized man. Crit Care Med 11:640, 1983.

486. Annat G, Viale JP, Percival C, et al: Oxygen delivery and uptake in the adult respiratory distress syndrome: Lack of relationship when measured independently in patients with normal blood lactate concentrations. Am Rev Respir Dis 133:999, 1986.

487. Danek SJ, Lynch JP, Weg JG, et al: The dependence of oxygen uptake on oxygen delivery in the adult respiratory distress syndrome. Am Rev Respir Dis 122:387, 1980.

488. Rashkin MC, Bosken C, Baughman RP: Oxygen delivery in critically ill patients. Relationship to blood lactate and survival. Chest 87:580, 1985.

489. Kariman K, Burns SR: Regulation of tissue oxygen extraction is disturbed in adult respiratory distress syndrome. Am Rev Respir Dis 132:109, 1985.

490. Mohsenifar Z, Goldbach P, Tashkin DP, et al: Relationship between $O_2$ delivery and $O_2$ consumption in the adult respiratory distress syndrome. Chest 84:267, 1983.

491. Zapol WM, Snider MT: Pulmonary hypertension in severe acute respiratory failure. N Engl J Med 296:476, 1977.

492. Sibbald WJ, Short AI, Driedger AA, et al: The immediate effects of isosorbide dinitrate on right ventricular function in patients with acute hypoxemic respiratory failure: A combined invasive and radionuclide study. Am Rev Respir Dis 131:862, 1985.

493. Sibbald WJ, Driedger AA, Cunningham DG, et al: Right and left ventricular performance in acute hypoxemic respiratory failure. Crit Care Med 14:852, 1986.

494. Jardin F, Gueret P, Dubourg O, et al: Right ventricular volumes by thermodilution in the adult respiratory distress syndrome: A comparative study using two-dimensional echocardiography as a reference method. Chest 88:34, 1985.

495. Gattinoni L, Bombino M, Peosi P, et al: Lung structure and function in different stages of severe adult respiratory distress syndrome. JAMA 271:1772, 1994.

496. Bernard GR, Brigham KL: The adult respiratory distress syndrome. Annu Rev Med 36:195, 1985.

497. Lee J, Turner JS, Morgan CJ, et al: Adult respiratory distress syndrome: Has there been a change in outcome predictive measures? Thorax 49:596, 1994.

498. Zapol WM, Trelstad RL, Coffey JW, et al: Pulmonary fibrosis in severe acute respiratory failure. Am Rev Respir Dis 119:547, 1979.

499. Auler JO, Calheiros DF, Brentani MM, et al: Adult respiratory distress syndrome: Evidence of early fibrogenesis and absence of glucocorticoid receptors. Eur J Respir Dis 69:261, 1986.

500. Bartlett RH, Morris AH, Fairley HB, et al: A prospective study of acute hypoxic respiratory failure. Chest 89:684, 1986.

501. Gillespie DJ, Marsh HM, Divertie MB, et al: Clinical outcome of respiratory failure in patients requiring prolonged (greater than 24 hours) mechanical ventilation. Chest 90:364, 1986.

502. Seidenfeld JJ, Pohl DF, Bell RC, et al: Incidence, site, and outcome of infections in patients with the adult respiratory distress syndrome. Am Rev Respir Dis 134:12, 1986.

503. National Heart, Lung, and Blood Institute: Extracorporeal support for respiratory insufficiency: Collaborative study. Washington, DC: National Heart, Lung, and Blood Institute, December 1979.

504. Simmons RS, Berdine GG, Seidenfeld JJ, et al: Fluid balance and the adult respiratory distress syndrome. Am Rev Respir Dis 135:924, 1987.

505. Hudson LD, Milberg JA, Anardi D, et al: Clinical risks for the development of the acute respiratory distress syndrome. Am J Respir Crit Care Med 151:298, 1995.

506. Roumen RMH, Redl H, Schlag G, et al: Scoring systems and blood lactate concentrations in relation to the development of adult respiratory distress syndrome and multiple organ failure in severely traumatized patients. J Trauma 35:349, 1993.

507. Carvalho ACA, Bellman SM, Saullo VJ, et al: Altered factor VIII in acute respiratory failure. N Engl J Med 307:1113, 1982.

508. Rubin DB, Wiener-Kronish JP, Murray JF, et al: Elevated von Willebrand factor antigen is an early plasma predictor of acute lung injury in nonpulmonary sepsis syndrome. J Clin Invest 96:474, 1990.

509. Moss M, Acherson L, Gillespie MK, et al: Von Willebrand factor antigen levels are not predictive for the adult respiratory distress syndrome. Am J Respir Crit Care Med 151:15, 1995.

510. Li XY, Donaldson K, Brown D, MacNee W: The role of tumor necrosis factor in increased airspace epithelial permeability. Am J Respir Cell Mol Biol 13:185, 1995.

511. Donnelly SC, Strieter RM, Kunkel SL, et al: Interleukin-8 development of adult respiratory distress syndrome in at-risk patients. Lancet 341:643, 1993.

512. Davis JM, Meyer JD, Barie PS, et al: Elevated production of neutrophil leukotriene B4 precedes pulmonary failure in critically ill surgical patients. Surg Gynecol Obstet 170:495, 1990.

513. Donnelly TJ, Meade P, Jagels M, et al: Cytokine, complement, and endotoxin profiles associated with the development of the adult respiratory distress syndrome after severe injury. Crit Care Med 22:768, 1994.

514. Suter PM, Sute S, Girardin E, et al: High bronchoalveolar levels of tumor necrosis factor and its inhibitors, interleukin-1, interferon, elastase, in patients with adult respiratory distress syndrome after trauma, shock or sepsis. Am Rev Respir Dis 145:1016, 1992.

515. Zilow G, Joka T, Obertake U, et al: Generation of anaphylatoxin C3a in plasma and bronchoalveolar lavage fluid in trauma patients at risk for the adult respiratory distress syndrome. Crit Care Med 20:468, 1992.

516. Stephenson AH, Lonigro AJ, Hyers TM, et al: Increased concentrations of leukotrienes in bronchoalveolar lavage fluid of patients with ARDS or at risk for ARDS. Am Rev Respir Dis 138:714, 1988.

517. Clark JG, Milberg JA, Steinberg KP, Hudson LD: Type III procollagen peptide in the adult respiratory distress syndrome: Association of increased peptide levels in bronchoalveolar lavage fluid with increased risk for death. Ann Intern Med 122:17, 1995.

517a. Connelly KG, Repine JE: Markers for predicting the development of acute respiratory distress syndrome. Annu Rev Med 48:429, 1997.

518. Donnelly SC, Haslett C, Dransfield I, et al: Role of selectins in the development of adult respiratory distress syndrome. Lancet 344:215, 1994.

519. Laurent T, Markert V, Fliedner VV, et al: CD11b/CD18 expression, adherence, chemotaxis of granulocytes in adult respiratory distress syndrome. Am J Respir Crit Care Med 149:1534, 1994.

520. Donnelly SC, McGregor I, Zamani A, et al: Plasma elastase levels and the development of the adult respiratory distress syndrome. Am J Respir Crit Care Med 151:1428, 1995.

521. Kawamura M, Yamasawa F, Ishizaka A, et al: Serum concentration of 7S collagen and prognosis in patients with the adult respiratory distress syndrome. Thorax 49:144, 1994.

522. Sakamaki F, Ishizaka A, Handa M, et al: Soluble form of P-selectin in plasma is elevated in acute lung injury. Am J Respir Crit Care Med 151:1821, 1995.

523. Pison U, Obertacke U, Seeger W, Hawgood S: Surfactant protein A is decreased in acute parenchymal lung injury associated with polytrauma. Eur J Clin Invest 22:712, 1992.

524. Goodman RB, Strieter RM, Steinberg KP, et al: Inflammatory cytokines in patients with persistence of the adult respiratory distress syndrome. Am J Respir Crit Care Med 154:602, 1996.

525. Jimenez P, Torres A, Roca J, et al: Arterial oxygenation does not predict the outcome of patients with acute respiratory failure needing mechanical ventilation. Eur Respir J 7:730, 1994.

526. Elliott CG, Morris AH, Cengiz M: Pulmonary function and exercise gas exchange in survivors of adult respiratory distress syndrome. Am Rev Respir Dis 123:492, 1981.

527. Buchser E, Leuenberger P, Chiolero R, et al: Reduced pulmonary capillary blood volume as a long-term sequel of ARDS. Chest 87:608, 1985.

528. Towne BH, Lott IT, Hicks DA, et al: Long-term follow-up of infants and children treated with extracorporeal membrane oxygenation (ECMO): A preliminary report. J Pediatr Surg 20:410, 1985.

529. Simpson DL, Goodman M, Spector SL, et al: Long-term follow-up and bronchial reactivity testing in survivors of the adult respiratory distress syndrome. Am Rev Respir Dis 117:449, 1978.

530. Hert R, Albert RK: Sequelae of the adult repiratory distress syndrome. Thorax 49:8, 1994.

531. Fanconi S, Kraemer R, Weber J, et al: Long-term sequelae in children surviving adult respiratory distress syndrome. J Pediatr 106:218, 1985.

532. Elliott CG, Rasmusson BY, Crapo RO, et al: Prediction of pulmonary function abnormalities after adult respiratory distress syndrome (ARDS). Am Rev Respir Dis 135:634, 1987.

533. Wilson R: Acute high-altitude illness in mountaineers and problems of rescue. Ann Intern Med 78:421, 1973.

534. Maggiorini M, Bärtsch P, Oelz O: Association between raised body temperature and acute mountain sickness: Cross-sectional study. BMJ 315:403, 1997.

535. Hurtado A: Some clinical aspects of life at high altitudes. Ann Intern Med 53:247, 1960.

536. Menon ND: High-altitude pulmonary edema: A clinical study. N Engl J Med 273:66, 1965.

537. Kamat SR, Banerjil BC: Study of cardiopulmonary function on exposure to high altitude: I. Acute acclimatization to an altitude of 3500 to 4000 meters in relation to altitude sickness and cardiopulmonary function. Am Rev Respir Dis 106:404, 1972.

538. Kamat SR, Rao TL, Sama BS, et al: Study of cardiopulmonary function on exposure to high altitude: II. Effects of prolonged stay at 3500 to 4000 meters and reversal on return to sea level. Am Rev Respir Dis 106:414, 1972.

539. Kleiner JP, Nelson WP: High altitude pulmonary edema: A rare disease? JAMA 234:491, 1975.

540. Leading Article: Pulmonary oedema of mountains. BMJ 3:65, 1972.

541. Hultgren HN, Spickard WB, Hellriegel K, et al: High altitude pulmonary edema. Medicine 40:289, 1961.

542. Hultgren H, Spickard W, Lopez C: Further studies of high altitude pulmonary oedema. Br Heart J 24:95, 1962.

543. Viswanathan R, Jain SK, Subramanian S, et al: Pulmonary edema of high altitude: II. Clinical, aerohemodynamic, and biochemical studies in a group with history of pulmonary edema of high altitude. Am Rev Respir Dis 100:334, 1969.

544. Houston CS: Acute pulmonary edema of high altitude. N Engl J Med 263:478, 1960.

545. Fred HL, Schmidt AM, Bates T, et al: Acute pulmonary edema of altitude: Clinical and physiologic observations. Circulation 25:929, 1962.

546. Singh I, Kapila CC, Khanna PK, et al: High-altitude pulmonary oedema. Lancet 1:229, 1965.

547. Richalet JP: High altitude pulmonary oedema: Still a place for controversy? Thorax 50:923, 1995.

548. Schoene RB: Pulmonary edema at high altitude: Review, pathophysiology, and update. Clin Chest Med 6:491, 1985.

549. Schoene RB, Hackett PH, Henderson WR, et al: High-altitude pulmonary edema: Characteristics of lung lavage fluid. JAMA 256:63, 1986.

550. Schoene RB, Roach RC, Hackett PH, et al: High altitude pulmonary edema and exercise at 4,400 meters on Mount McKinley: Effect of expiratory positive airway pressure. Chest 87:330, 1985.

551. Hultgren HN. High-altitude pulmonary edema: Current concepts. Annu Rev Med 47:267, 1996.

551a. Hohenhaus E, Paul A, McCullough RE, et al: Ventilatory and pulmonary vascular response to hypoxia and susceptibility to high altitude pulmonary oedema. Eur Respir J 8:1825, 1995.

552. Hackett PH, Roach RC, Schoene RB, et al: Abnormal control of ventilation in high-altitude pulmonary edema. J Appl Physiol 64:1268, 1988.

553. Sutton JR, Lassen N: Pathophysiology of acute mountain sickness and high altitude pulmonary oedema: An hypothesis. Bull Eur Physiopathol Respir 15:1045, 1979.

554. Hackett PH, Rennie D, Grover RF, et al: Acute mountain sickness and the edemas of high altitude: A common pathogenesis? Respir Physiol 46:383, 1982.

555. Schoene RB, Swenson ER, Pizzo CJ, et al: The lung at high altitude: Bronchoalveolar lavage in acute mountain sickness and pulmonary edema. J Appl Physiol 64:2605, 1988.

556. Anholm JD, Houston CS, Hyers TM: The relationship between acute mountain sickness and pulmonary ventilation at 2,835 meters (9,300 ft.). Chest 75:33, 1979.

557. Welsh CH, Wagner PD, Reeves JT, et al: Operation Everest: II: Spirometric and radiographic changes in acclimatized humans at simulated high altitude. Am Rev Respir Dis 147:1239, 1993.

558. Ge RL, Matsuzawa Y, Takeoka M, et al: Low pulmonary diffusing capacity in subjects with acute mountain sickness. Chest 111:58, 1997.

559. Moore LG, Harrison GL, McCullough RE, et al: Low acute hypoxic ventilatory response and hypoxic depression in acute altitude sickness. J Appl Physiol 60:1407, 1986.

560. Gautier H, Peslin R, Grassino A, et al: Mechanical properties of the lungs during acclimatization to altitude. J Appl Physiol 52:1407, 1982.

561. Hyers TM, Scoggin CH, Will DH, et al: Accentuated hypoxemia at high altitude in subjects susceptible to high-altitude pulmonary edema. J Appl Physiol 46:41, 1979.

561a. Mansell A, Powles A, Sutton J: Changes in pulmonary PV characteristics of human subjects at an altitude of 5,366 m. J Appl Physiol 49:79, 1980.

562. Hultgren HN, Flamm MD: Pulmonary edema. Mod Concepts Cardiovasc Dis 31:1, 1969.

563. Hultgren HN: High altitude pulmonary edema: Hemodynamic aspects. Int J Sports Med 18:20, 1997.

564. Kaminsky DA, Jones K, Schoene RB, Voelkel NF: Urinary leukotriene E(4) levels in high-altitude pulmonary edema—a possible role for inflammation. Chest 110:939, 1996.

565. Viswanathan R, Jain SK, Subramanian S: Pulmonary edema of high altitude: III. Pathogenesis. Am Rev Respir Dis 100:342, 1969.

566. Visscher MB: The pathophysiology of lung edema: A physical and physicochemical problem. Lancet 82:43, 1962.

567. Younes M, Bshouty Z: Effect of high blood flow, ventilation, breathing pattern, and alveolar hypoxia on lung fluid flux. In Sutton J, Coates, Remmers J (eds): Hypoxia: The Adaptations. Toronto, BC Decker, 1990, pp 155–162.

568. Welling K, Sanchez R, Rven J, et al: Effect of prolonged alveolar hypoxia on pulmonary artery pressure and segmental vascular resistance. J Appl Physiol 75:1194, 1993.

569. Costello ML, Mathieu-Costello O, West JB: Stress failure of alveolar epithelial cells studied by scanning electron microscopy. Am Rev Respir Dis 145:1446, 1992.

570. Fu Z, Costello ML, Tsukimoto D, et al: High lung volume increases stress failure in pulmonary capillaries. J Appl Physiol 73:123, 1992.

571. Younes M, Bshouty Z, Ali J: Longitudinal distribution of pulmonary vascular resistance with very high pulmonary blood flow. J Appl Physiol 62:344, 1987.

572. Combret M, Rouby J, Smiegan J, et al: Pulmonary edema during pulmonary embolism. Br J Dis Chest 81:407, 1987.

573. Arnold L, Keane J, Kan J, et al: Transient unilateral pulmonary edema after successful balloon dilatation of peripheral pulmonary artery stenosis. Am J Cardiol 62:327, 1988.

574. Levinson R, Shure D, Moser K: Reperfusion pulmonary edema after pulmonary artery thromboendarterectomy. Am Rev Respir Dis 139:1291, 1986.

575. Hackett P, Creagh C, Grover R, et al: High altitude pulmonary edema in persons without the right pulmonary artery. N Engl J Med 302:1070, 1980.

576. Sebbane M, Wuyam B, Pin I, et al: Unilateral agenesis of the pulmonary artery and high-altitude pulmonary edema (HAPE) at moderate altitude. Pediatr Pulmonol 24:111, 1997.

577. Naeije R, De Backer D, Vachiery JL, De Vuyst P: High-altitude pulmonary edema with primary pulmonary hypertension. Chest 110:286, 1996.

578. Nakagawa S, Kubo K, Koizumi T, et al: High-altitude pulmonary thromboembolism. Chest 103:948, 1993.

579. Durmowicz AG, Noordeweir E, Nicholas R, Reeves JT: Inflammatory processes may predispose children to high-altitude pulmonary edema. J Pediatr 130:838, 1997.

580. Peacock AJ: High altitude pulmonary oedema: Who gets it and why? Eur Respir J 8:1819, 1995.

581. Richalet JP, Keromes A, Dersch B, et al: The physiological characteristics of high altitude climbers. Sci Sports 3:89, 1988.

582. Hohenhaus E, Paul A, McCullough RE, et al: Ventilatory and pulmonary vascular response to hypoxia and susceptibility to high altitude pulmonary oedema. Eur Respir J 8:1825, 1995.

583. Eldridge MW, Podolsky A, Richardson RS, et al: Pulmonary hemodynamic response to exercise in subjects with prior high-altitude pulmonary edema. J Appl Physiol 81:911, 1996.

584. Vachiery JL, McDonagh T, Moraine JJ, et al: Doppler assessment of hypoxic pulmonary vasoconstriction and susceptibility to high altitude pulmonary oedema. Thorax 50:22, 1995.

585. Podolsky A, Eldridge MW, Richardson RS, et al: Exercise-induced $\dot{V}_A/\dot{Q}$ inequality in subjects with prior high-altitude pulmonary edema. J Appl Physiol 81:922, 1996.

586. Hultgren HN, Lopez CE, Lundberg E, et al: Physiologic studies of pulmonary edema at high altitude. Circulation 29:393, 1964.

587. Kobayashi T, Koyama S, Kubo K, et al: Clinical features of patients with high altitude pulmonary edema in Japan. Chest 92:814, 1987.

588. Kleger GR, Bartsch P, Vock P, et al: Evidence against an increase in capillary permeability in subjects exposed to high altitude. J Appl Physiol 81:1917, 1996.

589. Droma Y, Hayano T, Takabayashi Y, et al: Endothelin-1 and interleukin-8 in high altitude pulmonary oedema. Eur Respir J 9:1947, 1996.

589a. Vock P, Brutsche MH, Nanzer A, et al: Variable radiomorphologic data of high altitude pulmonary edema: Features from 60 patients. Chest 100:1306, 1991.

589b. Bärtsch P: High altitude pulmonary edema. Respiration 64:435, 1997.

590. Felman AH: Neurogenic pulmonary edema: Observations in 6 patients. Am J Roentgenol 112:393, 1971.

591. Colice GL, Matthay MA, Bass E, et al: Neurogenic pulmonary edema: Clinical commentary. Am Rev Respir Dis 130:941, 1984.

592. Singh I, Khanna PK, Srivastava MC, et al: Acute mountain sickness. N Engl J Med 280:175, 1969.

593. West JB, Hackett PH, Maret KH, et al: Pulmonary gas exchange on the summit of Mt. Everest. J Appl Physiol 55:678, 1983.

594. Schoene RB, Lahiri S, Hackett PH, et al: Relationship of hypoxic ventilatory response to exercise performance on Mount Everest. J Appl Physiol 56:1478, 1984.

595. Whithey WR, Milledge JS, Williams ES, et al: Fluid and electrolyte homeostasis during prolonged exercise at altitude. J Appl Physiol 55:409, 1983.

596. Hackett PH, Rennie D, Hofmeister SE, et al: Fluid retention and relative hypoventilation in acute mountain sickness. Respiration 43:321, 1982.

597. Sutton JR, Houston CS, Mansell AL, et al: Effect of acetazolamide on hypoxemia during sleep at high altitude. N Engl J Med 301:1329, 1979.

598. Shapira OM, Shahian DM: Postpneumonectomy pulmonary edema. Ann Thorac Surg 56:190, 1993.

598a. Kopec SE, Irwin RS, Umali-Torres CB, et al: The postpneumonectomy state. Chest 114:1158, 1998.

599. van der Werff YD, van der Houwen HK, Heijmans PJ, et al: Postpneumonectomy pulmonary edema: A retrospective analysis of incidence and possible risk factors. Chest 111:1278, 1997.

600. Dong S, Paré PD: Postpneumonectomy pulmonary edema and cardiac dysrhythmias are the major cause of postoperative mortality and morbidity. Am J Respir Crit Care Med 147:A740, 1993.

601. Turnage WS, Lunn JJ: Postpneumonectomy pulmonary edema: A retrospective analysis of associated variables. Chest 103:1646, 1993.

602. Verheijen-Breemhaar L, Bogaard JM, van den Berg B, Hilvering C: Postpneumonectomy pulmonary oedema. Thorax 43:323, 1988.

603. Zeldin RA, Normandin D, Landtwing D, Peters RM: Postpneumonectomy pulmonary edema. J Thorac Cardiovasc Surg 87:359, 1984.

604. Williams EA, Evans TW, Goldstraw P: Acute lung injury following lung resection: Is one lung anaesthesia to blame? Thorax 51:114, 1996.

605. Staub NC: Pulmonary edema due to increased microvascular permeability to fluid and protein. Circ Res 43:143, 1978.

606. Satur CMR, Robertson RH, DaCosta PE, et al: Multiple pulmonary microemboli complicating pneumonectomy. Ann Thorac Surg 52:122, 1991.

607. Humphreys RL, Berne AS: Rapid reexpansion of pneumothorax: A cause of unilateral pulmonary edema. Radiology 96:509, 1970.

608. Trapnell DH, Thurston JGB: Unilateral pulmonary oedema after pleural aspiration. Lancet 1:1367, 1970.

609. Carlson RI, Classen KL, Gollan F, et al: Pulmonary edema following the rapid reexpansion of a totally collapsed lung due to a pneumothorax: A clinical and experimental study. Surg Forum 9:367, 1959.

610. Ziskind MM, Weill H, George RA: Acute pulmonary edema following the treatment of spontaneous pneumothorax with excessive negative intrapleural pressure. Am Rev Respir Dis 92:632, 1965.

611. Childress ME, Moy G, Mottram M: Unilateral pulmonary edema resulting from treatment of spontaneous pneumothorax. Am Rev Respir Dis 104:119, 1971.

612. Waqaruddin M, Bernstein A: Re-expansion pulmonary oedema. Thorax 30:54, 1975.

613. Ratliff JL, Chavez CM, Jamchuk A, et al: Re-expansion pulmonary edema. Chest 64:654, 1973.

614. Saini GS: Unilateral pulmonary oedema after drainage of spontaneous pneumothorax. BMJ 1:615, 1974.

615. Grant MJA: Acute unilateral oedema following re-expansion of a spontaneous pneumothorax: Case report. NZ Med J 74:250, 1971.

616. Murphy K, Tomlanovich MC: Unilateral pulmonary edema after drainage of a spontaneous pneumothorax: Case report and review of the world literature. J Emerg Med 1:29, 1983.

617. Kassis E, Philipsen E, Clausen KH: Unilateral pulmonary edema following spontaneous pneumothorax. Eur J Respir Dis 62:102, 1981.

618. Mahajan VK, Simon M, Huber GL: Reexpansion pulmonary edema. Chest 75:192, 1979.

619. Shaw TJ, Caterine JM: Recurrent re-expansion pulmonary edema. Chest 86:784, 1984.

620. Mahfood S, Hix WR, Aaron BL, et al: Reexpansion pulmonary edema. Ann Thorac Surg 63:1206, 1997.

621. Tarver RD, Broderick LS, Conces DJ: Reexpansion pulmonary edema. J Thorac Imaging 11:198, 1996.

622. Brandstetter RD, Cohen RP: Hypoxemia after thoracentesis: A predictable and treatable condition. JAMA 242:1060, 1979.

623. Trachiotis GD, Vricella LA, Aaron BL, Hix WR: As originally published in 1988: Reexpansion pulmonary edema. Updated in 1997. Ann Thorac Surg 63:1206, 1997.

624. Steckel RJ: Unilateral pulmonary edema after pneumothorax. N Engl J Med 289:621, 1973.

625. Gascoigne A, Appleton A, Taylor R, et al: Catastrophic circulatory collapse following re-expansion pulmonary oedema. Resuscitation 31:265, 1996.

626. Mahfood S, Hix WR, Aaron BL, et al: Reexpansion pulmonary edema. Ann Thorac Surg 45:340, 1988.

627. Buczko GB, Grossman RF, Goldberg M: Re-expansion pulmonary edema: Evidence for increased capillary permeability. Can Med Assoc J 125:459, 1981.

628. Sprung CL, Loewenherz JW, Baier H, et al: Evidence for increased permeability in reexpansion pulmonary edema. Am J Med 71:497, 1981.

629. Miller WC, Toon R, Palat H, et al: Experimental pulmonary edema following re-expansion of pneumothorax. Am Rev Respir Dis 108:664, 1973.

630. Pavlin JD, Nessly ML, Cloney FW: Increased pulmonary vascular permeability as a cause of re-expansion edema in rabbits. Am Rev Respir Dis 124:422, 1981.

631. Yamazaki S, Ogawa J, Shohzu A, et al: Pulmonary blood flow to rapidly reexpanded lung in spontaneous pneumothorax. Chest 81:1, 1982.

632. Bishop MJ, Boatman ES, Ivey TD, et al: Reperfusion of ischaemic dog lung results in fever, leukopenia and lung edema. Am Rev Respir Dis 134:752, 1986.

633. Nakamura H, Ishizaka A, Sawafuji M, et al: Elevated levels of interleukin-8 and leukotriene B4 in pulmonary edema fluid of a patient with reexpansion pulmonary edema. Am J Respir Crit Care Med 149:1037, 1994.

634. Tarver RD, Broderick LS, Conces DJ: Reexpansion pulmonary edema. J Thorac Imaging 11:198, 1996.

634a. Trachiotis GD, Vricella LA, Aaron BL, et al: Reexpansion pulmonary edema: Update 1997. Ann Thorac Surg 63:1206, 1997.

635. Henderson AF, Banham SW, Moran F: Re-expansion pulmonary oedema: A potentially serious complication of delayed diagnosis of pneumothorax. BMJ 291:593, 1985.

636. Olcott EW: Fatal reexpansion pulmonary edema following pleural catheter placement. JVIR 5:176, 1994.

637. Lewis RW, Rudd N, Pittman JA: Blood transfusion complications: Leukoagglutinin reactions. Obstet Gynecol 65:785, 1985.

638. Lagler U, Russi E: Upper airway obstruction as a cause of pulmonary edema during late pregnancy. Am J Obstet Gynecol 156:643, 1987.

639. Padley SP, Downes MO: Case report: Pulmonary oedema secondary to laryngospasm following general anaesthesia. Br J Radiol 67:654, 1994.

640. Ingrams D, Burton M, Goodwin A, Graham J: Acute pulmonary oedema complicating laryngospasm. J Laryngol Otol 111:482, 1997.

641. Wilson GW, Bircher NG: Acute pulmonary edema developing after laryngospasm: Report of a case. J Oral Maxillofac Surg 53:211, 1995.

642. Goldenberg JD, Portugal LG, Wenig BL, Weingarten RT: Negative-pressure pulmonary edema in the otolaryngology patient. Otolaryngol Head Neck Surg 117:62, 1997.

643. Halow KD, Ford EG: Pulmonary edema following post-operative laryngospasm: A case report and review of the literature. Am Surg 59:443, 1993.

644. Kaki A, Crosby ET, Lui AC: Airway and respiratory management following non-lethal hanging. Can J Anaesth 44:445, 1997.

645. Warren MF, Peterson DK, Drinker CK: The effects of heightened negative pressure in the chest, together with further experiments upon anoxia in increasing the flow of lung lymph. Am J Physiol 137:641, 1942.

646. Young LW, Bowen A, Oh KS, et al: Postintubation pulmonary edema (abstract). Invest Radiol 16:428, 1981.

647. Sofer S, Bar-Ziv J, Scharf SM: Pulmonary edema following relief of upper airway obstruction. Chest 86:401, 1984.

648. Randour P, Joucken K, Collard E, et al: Pulmonary edema following acute upper airway obstruction. Acta Anaesthesiol Belg 37:225, 1986.

649. Tami TA, Chu F, Wildes TO, et al: Pulmonary edema and acute upper airway obstruction. Laryngoscope 96:506, 1986.

650. Liam CK, Liao CM, Kannan P: Recurrent acute pulmonary oedema associated with obstructive sleep apnoea. Singapore Med J 35:411, 1994.

651. Lorch DG, Sahn SA: Post-extubation pulmonary edema following anesthesia induced by upper airway obstruction. Are certain patients at increased risk? Chest 90:802, 1986.

652. McGonagle M, Kennedy TL: Laryngospasm induced pulmonary edema. Laryngoscope 94:1583, 1984.

653. Levy GJ, Shabot MM, Hart ME, et al: Transfusion-associated noncardiogenic pulmonary edema: Report of a case and a warning regarding treatment. Transfusion 26:278, 1986.

654. Popovsky MA, Moore SB: Diagnostic and pathogenetic considerations in transfusion-related acute lung injury. Transfusion 25:573, 1985.

655. Ward HN: Pulmonary infiltration associated with leukoagglutinin transfusion reactions. Ann Intern Med 73:688, 1970.

656. Thompson JS, Severson CD, Parmerly MJ, et al: Pulmonary "hypersensitivity" reactions induced by transfusion of non-HL-A leukoagglutinins. N Engl J Med 284:1120, 1971.

657. Jeter E, Spivey MA: Noninfectious complications of blood transfusion. Transfus Med 9:187, 1995.

658. Kawamata M, Miyabe M, Omote K, et al: Acute pulmonary edema associated with transfusion of packed red blood cells. Intensive Care Med 21:443, 1995.

659. Virchis AE, Patel RK, Contreras M, et al: Acute non-cardiogenic lung oedema after platelet transfusion. BMJ 314:880, 1997.

660. Renner IG, Savage WT, Pantoja JL, et al: Death due to acute pancreatitis: A retrospective analysis of 405 autopsy cases. Dig Dis Sci 30:1005, 1985.

661. Tahamont MV, Barie PS, Blumenstock FA, et al: Increased lung vascular permeability after pancreatitis and trypsin infusion. Am J Pathol 109:15, 1982.

662. Falls R, Millen JE, Galuser FL, et al: Pulmonary alveolar epithelial permeability in surgically induced hemorrhagic pancreatitis in dogs. Respiration 40:213, 1980.

663. Satake K, Rozmanith JS, Appert H, et al: Hemodynamic change and bradykinin levels in plasma and lymph during experimental acute pancreatitis in dogs. Ann Surg 178:659, 1973.

664. Minta JO, Man D, Movat HZ: Kinetic studies on the fragmentation of the third component of complement ($C_3$) by trypsin. J Immunol 118:2192, 1977.

665. Nicod L, Leuenberger P, Seydoux C, et al: Evidence for pancreas injury in adult respiratory distress syndrome. Am Rev Respir Dis 131:696, 1985.

666. deLeeuw PW, Waltman FL, Birkenhager WH: Noncardiogenic pulmonary edema as the sole manifestation of pheochromocytoma. Hypertension 8:810, 1986.

667. Blom HJ, Karsdorp V, Birnie R, et al: Phaeochromocytoma as a cause of pulmonary oedema. Anesthesia 42:646, 1987.

668. Feldman JM: Adult respiratory distress syndrome in a pregnant patient with a pheochromocytoma. J Surg Oncol 29:5, 1985.

669. Brun-Buisson CJ, Bonnet F, Bergeret S, et al: Recurrent high-permeability pulmonary edema associated with diabetic ketoacidosis. Crit Care Med 13:55, 1985.

670. Botha J, van Niekerk DJ, Rossouw DJ, et al: The adult respiratory distress syndrome in association with diabetic keto-acidosis: A case report. S Afr Med J 71:535, 1987.

671. Russell J, Follansbee S, Matthay M: Adult respiratory distress syndrome complicating diabetic ketoacidosis. West J Med 135:148, 1981.

672. Silvestri RC, Huseby JS, Rughani I, et al: Respiratory distress syndrome from lymphangiography contrast medium. Am Rev Respir Dis 122:543, 1980.

673. Solomon DR: Anaphylactoid reaction and non-cardiac pulmonary edema following intravenous contrast injection. Am J Emerg Med 4:146, 1986.

674. Boden WE: Anaphylactoid pulmonary edema ("shock lung") and hypotension after radiologic contrast media injection. Chest 81:759, 1982.

674a. Bouachour G, Varache N, Szapiro N, et al: Noncardiogenic pulmonary edema resulting from intravascular administration of contrast material. Am J Roentgenol 157:255, 1991.

675. Borish L, Matloff SM, Findlay SR: Radiographic contrast media–induced noncardiogenic pulmonary edema: Case report and review of the literature. J Allerg Clin Immunol 74:104, 1984.

676. Delacour JL, Floriot C, Wagschal G, et al: Non-cardiac pulmonary edema following intravenous contrast injection. Intensive Care Med 15:49, 1988.

677. Goldsmith SR, Steinberg P: Noncardiogenic pulmonary edema induced by nonionic low-osmolality radiographic contrast media. J Allerg Clin Immunol 96:698, 1995.

678. Ramesh S, Reisman R: Noncardiogenic pulmonary edema due to radiocontrast media. Ann Allerg Asthma Immunol 75:308, 1995.

679. Lim SC, Yang JY, Jang AS, et al: Acute lung injury after phosgene inhalation. Korean J Intern Med 11:87, 1996.

680. Batlle MA, Wilcox WD: Pulmonary edema in an infant following passive inhalation of free-base ("crack") cocaine. Clin Pediatr 32:105, 1993.

681. Vaca FE, Myers JH, Langdorf M: Delayed pulmonary edema and bronchospasm after accidental lacrimator exposure. Am J Emerg Med 14:402, 1996.

682. Silver MJ, Young DK: Acute noncardiogenic pulmonary edema due to polymer fume fever. Cleve Clin J Med 60:479, 1993.

683. Lee CH, Guo YL, Tsai PJ, et al: Fatal acute pulmonary oedema after inhalation of fumes from polytetrafluoroethylene (PTFE). Eur Respir J 10:1408, 1997.

684. Bur A, Wagner A, Roggla M, et al: Fatal pulmonary edema after nitric acid inhalation. Resuscitation 35:33, 1997.

685. Morgan WK: "Zamboni disease." Pulmonary edema in an ice hockey player. Arch Intern Med 155:2479, 1995.

686. Cordasco EM, Burns DE, Beerel F, et al: Noncardiac pulmonary edema: Newer environmental aspects. J Vasc Dis 46:759, 1995.

687. Grellner W, Madea B, Sticht G: Pulmonary histopathology and survival period in morphine-involved deaths. J Forens Sci 41:433, 1996.

688. Suarez M, Krieger BP: Bronchoalveolar lavage in recurrent aspirin-induced adult respiratory distress syndrome. Chest 90:452, 1986.

689. Yip L, Jastremski MS, Dart RC: Salicylate intoxication. J Intensive Care Med 12:66, 1997.

690. Gilson AJ, Sahn SA: Reactivation of bleomycin lung toxicity following oxygen administration: A second response to corticosteroids. Chest 88:304, 1985.

691. Wood DL, Osborn MJ, Rooke J, et al: Amiodarone pulmonary toxicity: Report of two cases associated with rapidly progressive fatal adult respiratory distress syndrome after pulmonary angiography. Mayo Clin Proc 60:601, 1985.

692. Catchings TT, Beamer WC, Lundy L, et al: Adult respiratory distress syndrome secondary to ethylene glycol ingestion. Ann Emerg Med 14:594, 1985.

693. Lawler PG, Cove-Smith JR: Acute respiratory failure following lithium intoxication: A report of two cases. Anaesthesia 41:623, 1986.

694. Paap CM, Ehrlich R: Acute pulmonary edema after polyethylene glycol intestinal lavage in a child. Ann Pharmacol 27:1044, 1993.

695. Murphy JL Jr: Hypertension and pulmonary oedema associated with ketamine administration in a patient with a history of substance abuse. Can J Anaesth 40:160, 1993.

696. Chetty KG, Ramirez MM, Mahutte CK: Drug-induced pulmonary edema in a patient infected with human immunodeficiency virus. Chest 104:967, 1993.

697. Alagaratnam TT: Sudden death 7 days after paclitaxel infusion for breast cancer. Lancet 342:1232, 1993.

698. Taylor MA, DiBlasi SL, Bender RM, et al: Adult respiratory distress syndrome

complicating intravenous infusion of low-molecular-weight dextran. Cathet Cardiovasc Diagn 32:249, 1994.

699. Saadeh AM, Farsakh NA, al-Ali MK: Cardiac manifestations of acute carbamate and organophosphate poisoning. Heart 77:461, 1997.

700. Saissy JM, Guignard B, Pats B, et al: Pulmonary edema after hydrogen peroxide irrigation of a war wound. Intens Care Med 21:287, 1995.

701. Albertson TE, Walby WF, Derlet RW: Stimulant-induced pulmonary toxicity. Chest 108:1140, 1995.

702. Pavlakis N, Bell DR, Millward MJ, et al: Fatal pulmonary toxicity resulting from treatment with gemcitabine. Cancer 80:286, 1997.

703. Lee JY, Moon SH, Lee SM, et al: A case of noncardiogenic pulmonary edema by ethanolamine oleate. Korean J Intern Med 9:125, 1994.

704. Leesar MA, Martyn R, Talley JD, et al: Noncardiogenic pulmonary edema complicating massive verapamil overdose. Chest 105:606, 1994.

705. Fine SR, Lodha A, Zoneraich S, et al: Hydrochlorothiazide-induced acute pulmonary edema. Ann Pharmacother 29:701, 1995.

706. Lampert MB, Hibbard J, Weinert L, et al: Peripartum heart failure associated with prolonged tocolytic therapy. Am J Obstet Gynecol 168:493, 1993.

707. Scott J: β-Adrenergic agonists and pulmonary oedema in preterm labour. Grand Rounds—Hammersmith Hospital. BMJ 308:260, 1994.

708. Carey M: Adverse cardiovascular sequelae of ergometrine. Br J Obstet Gynaecol 100:865, 1993.

709. Zuckerman GB, Conway EE Jr: Pulmonary complications following tricyclic antidepressant overdose in an adolescent. Ann Pharmacother 27:572, 1993.

710. Chan T, Ho S, Li PK: Noncardiogenic pulmonary edema associated with triazolam. Clin Toxicol 33:185, 1995.

711. Berthiaume Y, Boiteau P, Fick G, et al: Pulmonary edema during IL-2 therapy: Combined effect of increased permeability and hydrostatic pressure. Am J Respir Crit Care Med 152:329, 1995.

712. Thammakumpee G, Sumpatanukule P: Noncardiogenic pulmonary edema induced by sublingual buprenorphine. Chest 106:306, 1994.

713. Amaral CFS, Rezende NA: Both cardiogenic and noncardiogenic factors are involved in the pathogenesis of pulmonary oedema after scorpion envenoming. Toxicon 35:997, 1997.

714. Amaral CF, Barbosa AJ, Leite VH, et al: Scorpion sting–induced pulmonary oedema: Evidence of increased alveolocapillary membrane permeability. Toxicon 32:999, 1994.

715. Lehmann DF, Hardy JC: Stonefish envenomation. N Engl J Med 325:65, 1991.

716. Unexplained severe illness possibly associated with consumption of kombucha tea—Iowa, 1995. JAMA 275:96, 1996.

717. Parsons PE: Respiratory failure as a result of drugs, overdoses, and poisonings. Respir Emerg 15:93, 1994.

717a. Ketai LH, Kelsey CA, Jordan K, et al: Distinguishing Hantavirus pulmonary syndrome from acute respiratory distress syndrome by chest radiography: Are there different radiographic manifestations of increased alveolar permeability? J Thorac Imaging 13:172, 1998.

718. Boustani MR, Lepore TJ, Gelfand JA, et al: Acute respiratory failure in patients treated for babesiosis. Am J Respir Crit Care Med 149:1689, 1994.

719. Gotloib L, Barzilay E, Shustak A, et al: Hemofiltration in severe high microvascular permeability pulmonary edema secondary to rickettsial spotted fever. Resuscitation 13:15, 1985.

720. Buczko GB, McLean J: Typhoid fever associated with adult respiratory distress syndrome. Chest 105:1873, 1994.

721. Dyer RA, Chappel WA, Potgieter PD: Adult respiratory distress syndrome associated with miliary tuberculosis. Crit Care Med 13:12, 1985.

722. Feldman RM, Singer C: Noncardiogenic pulmonary edema and pulmonary fibrosis in falciparum malaria. Rev Infect Dis 9:134, 1987.

723. Hashimoto H, Toshima S, Hashimoto H, et al: Falciparum malaria in an overseas traveler complicated by disseminated intravascular coagulation and pulmonary edema. Intern Med 32:395, 1993.

724. Koegler A, Sauder P, Marolf A, et al: Amniotic fluid embolism: A case with non-cardiogenic pulmonary edema. Intensive Care Med 20:45, 1994.

725. Lam KK, Hutchinson RC, Gin T: Severe pulmonary oedema after venous air embolism. Can J Anaesth 40:964, 1993.

726. Frim DM, Wollman L, Evans AB, et al: Acute pulmonary edema after low-level air embolism during craniotomy. J Neurosurg 85:937, 1996.

727. Zwirewich CV, Müller NL, Abboud RT, et al: Noncardiogenic pulmonary edema caused by decompression sickness: Rapid resolution following hyperbaric therapy. Radiology 163:81, 1987.

728. Fulkerson WJ, McLendon RE, Prosnitz LR: Adult respiratory distress syndrome after limited thoracic radiotherapy. Cancer 57:1941, 1986.

729. Ivanick MJ, Donohue JF: Chronic eosinophilic pneumonia: A cause of adult respiratory distress syndrome. South Med J 79:686, 1986.

730. Lazar A: Pulmonary oedema following scorpion sting. J Assoc Physicians India 33:489, 1985.

731. Dean NC, Amend WC, Matthay MA: Adult respiratory distress syndrome related to antilymphocyte globulin therapy. Chest 91:619, 1987.

732. Haynes J, Allison RC: Pulmonary edema: Complication in the management of sickle cell pain crisis. Am J Med 80:833, 1986.

733. Stark P, Guthrie AM, Bull J: Thoracic radiographic changes after systemic hyperthermia for advanced cancer. Radiology 154:55, 1985.

734. Morales CF, Strollo PJ: Noncardiogenic pulmonary edema associated with accidental hypothermia. Chest 103:971, 1993.

735. Ayus JC, Arieff AI: Pulmonary complications of hyponatremic encephalopathy: Non-cardiogenic pulmonary edema and hypercapnic respiratory failure. Chest 107:517, 1995.

736. Mushambi MC, Halligan AW, Williamson K: Recent developments in the pathophysiology and management of pre-eclampsia. Br J Anaesth 76:133, 1996.

737. Breuer R, Lossos IS, Berkman N, et al: Pulmonary complications of bone marrow transplantation. Respir Med 87:571, 1993.

738. Young M, Sciurba F, Rinaldo J: Delirium and pulmonary edema after completing a marathon. Am Rev Respir Dis 136:737, 1987.

739. Marenco JP, Nervi A, White AC: ARDS associated with tumor lysis syndrome in a patient with non-Hodgkin's lymphoma. Chest 113:550, 1998.

PART X

# DISEASE OF THE AIRWAYS

# Upper Airway Obstruction

The upper airway can be considered as the conduit for inspired and expired gas that extends from the external nares (during nose breathing) or the lips (during mouth breathing) to the tracheal carina. It thus consists of a varied and somewhat complex system of channels arranged in series. Obstruction of this system is possible at any level; although the following discussion deals largely with anatomic abnormalities that cause such obstruction, a number of conditions can result in the same effect as a result of contraction of the muscles designed to maintain upper airway patency.[1]

## ACUTE UPPER AIRWAY OBSTRUCTION

Acute upper airway obstruction occurs most commonly in infants and young children because of the small intraluminal caliber and greater compliance of their upper airways. The cause is often apparent from the history. For example, patients who have acute upper respiratory infections generally have fever and cough (although in one series of 97 patients who had acute epiglottitis, cough was present in only one third).[2] Similarly, patients who have angioneurotic edema may give a history of allergy, with or without familial occurrence, and have usually experienced previous episodes dating back to childhood. Acute onset while eating suggests aspiration. Regardless of etiology, the cardinal symptom is a sudden onset of dyspnea, sometimes requiring emergency tracheostomy. Stridor is common; although its presence does not necessarily constitute an indication for immediate tracheostomy, it does suggest the need for immediate direct or indirect visualization of the larynx.[3]

The principal causes of acute upper airway obstruction are infection, edema, hemorrhage, foreign body aspiration, laryngeal dysfunction, and faulty placement of an endotracheal tube. However, there are many other uncommon or rare etiologies (Table 52–1).

### Infection

Infection may cause severe narrowing of the upper airways in infants and young children. Acute pharyngitis and tonsillitis, which may be complicated by retropharyngeal abscess, are caused most commonly by β-hemolytic streptococci[4] and less often by adenoviruses[5, 6] and coxsackieviruses.[7, 8] Rarely, tonsillitis or infection of the supraglottic region causes life-threatening acute upper airway obstruction in adults,[9] especially Epstein-Barr virus–related mononucleosis.[10] Acute laryngotracheitis (croup) is caused by parainfluenza or respiratory syncytial viruses and results in a characteristic narrowing of the subglottic trachea. A variant of this usual picture is seen in so-called membranous croup, in which the inflammatory narrowing of the upper trachea is associated with the presence of adherent or semiadherent mucopurulent membranes that cause marked irregularity of contour of the proximal tracheal mucosa;[11] the membranes can cause a severe degree of obstruction and sometimes require endoscopic removal.

Acute bacterial tracheitis is a rare but potentially life-threatening cause of upper airway obstruction that usually affects children[12] but has been reported in adults (*see* page 701).[13] In one study of 995 cases of measles in children, 34 showed evidence of significant upper airway obstruction;[14] in most, it appeared to be due to the virus, but in 8 it was shown to be secondary to bacterial tracheitis. *Corynebacterium pseudodiphtheriticum* has been reported to cause severe necrotizing tracheitis rarely.[15]

Acute epiglottitis usually is caused by *Haemophilus influenzae* and occasionally by *Staphylococcus aureus* or *Streptococcus pneumoniae*.[2] Although it most commonly affects infants and young children, it also occurs in adults, in whom it is often unrecognized;[16, 17] for example, in one series of 47 patients who had acute epiglottitis, 10 (21%) were adults, and of these, an initial diagnosis of epiglottitis was made in only 4.[16] Radiographic findings include swelling

### Table 52–1. RARE CAUSES OF ACUTE UPPER AIRWAY OBSTRUCTION

| CONDITION OR DISEASE PROCESS | SELECTED REFERENCES |
|---|---|
| Epiglottic prolapse after head injury and coma or head and neck surgery, rarely spontaneous | 296, 297 |
| Cervical herniation of the lung | 298 |
| Surgical emphysema | 299 |
| Complication of transesophageal echocardiography | 300 |
| Genioglossal or lingual hematoma secondary to trauma or surgery | 301–303 |
| Laryngeal hematoma | 304 |
| Acute suppurative parotitis | 305 |
| Cervical actinomycosis | 306 |
| Brown recluse spider envenomization | 307 |
| Lingual cellulitis | 308 |
| Stevens-Johnson syndrome | 309 |
| Aspiration of disinfectant (Dettol) | 310, 311 |
| "Aspiration" of a pharyngeal soft tissue tumor | 312 |
| Toxic epidermal necrolysis | 313 |

of the epiglottis, aryepiglottic folds, arytenoids, uvula, and prevertebral soft tissues; the hypopharynx and oropharynx tend to be ballooned and the valleculae obliterated. Narrowing of the subglottic trachea, simulating croup, occurs in roughly 25% of affected children.[18] In one investigation of 27 adults who had acute epiglottitis and 15 patients without symptoms, a ratio of the width of the epiglottis to the anteroposterior width of the C-4 vertebral body greater than 0.33 had a sensitivity of 96% and a specificity of 100% in the diagnosis.[19] In another investigation in which 31 patients who had epiglottitis were compared with age- and sex-matched controls, a ratio of epiglottic width to third cervical vertebral body width greater than 0.5 and a ratio of aryepiglottic fold width to third cervical body width greater than 0.35 had a 100% sensitivity and specificity for the diagnosis.[20] Although the findings are also well seen on computed tomography (CT),[21] this imaging modality is seldom indicated. The presenting symptoms are severe sore throat and difficulty in breathing. In the previously mentioned series, stridor was noted in 5 of the 10 adults and hoarseness in 4;[16] emergency tracheostomy was required in 5 of the 10 patients. All patients were much improved after 72 hours of appropriate therapy, and none died. *Bordetella pertussis* and adenovirus types I, II, III, and IV are the causative agents of whooping cough.[22, 23]

Acute retropharyngeal abscess can result in severe upper airway obstruction in both infants and adults (Fig. 52–1) and can extend into the mediastinum and cause a mediastinal abscess. In one case, a hyperextension injury was associated with the perforation of the anterior pharyngeal wall by an osteophyte, followed by retropharyngeal abscess formation and the development of upper airway obstruction.[24] A congenital laryngocele can become infected, with resulting laryngopyocele formation and acute upper airway obstruction.[25] Laryngeal stenosis due to tuberculosis infection is usually subacute rather than acute, but it may be the sole manifestation of the infection.[26] An acute severe necrotizing pseudomembranous tracheobronchitis caused by *Aspergillus* species can be seen in immunosuppressed patients,[27] including patients who have the acquired immunodeficiency syndrome.[28]

### Edema

As a cause of acute upper airway obstruction, edema of noninfective origin characteristically affects the larynx.

Underlying causes include trauma, the inhalation of irritant noxious gases, and angioneurotic edema. The last named is perhaps the most common cause of acute upper airway obstruction and has a variable etiology, including allergy (anaphylaxis) and heredity;[29, 30] some cases are idiopathic. The laryngeal edema is often associated with multiple pruritic and usually nonpainful swellings in the subcutaneous tissues of the face, hands, feet, and genitalia; urticaria is sometimes seen. Although many patients are atopic, with or without a familial history, the precise allergenic trigger for the development of angioedema is identified in less than one fifth of cases. In these, acute episodes are provoked by certain foods, inhalants, bee stings, or drugs; in this situation, antigen combines with immunoglobulin E (IgE), resulting in the release from mast cells of histamine, leukotrienes, and eosinophil-chemotactic factors, with consequent local vasodilation and exudation of edema fluid (a classical type I allergic reaction mediated by IgE). Type III reactions of a less acute nature may be caused by antiserum, certain drugs (such as penicillin), and some radiographic contrast media. Antigen-antibody complexes are formed with IgG, complement is activated, and chemical mediators are released from damaged endothelial cells. Some drugs (such as aspirin) may cause nonimmunologic mediator release, particularly in adults who have nasal polyps. Angioedema also has been reported as a complication of therapy with angiotensin-converting enzyme (ACE) inhibitors;[31, 32, 32a] it can develop after the first dose of the drug or after prolonged therapy. In one case-control study of 40 patients who presented to the emergency department with angioneurotic edema, 13 (33%) were taking ACE inhibitors;[33] the odds ratio compared with a group of age- and sex-matched controls was 5.

The hereditary form of angioneurotic edema usually begins in childhood and is characterized by recurrent attacks, often in association with abdominal cramps.[34] In one review of 69 affected members of two large families, 98% presented before the age of 30 years;[35] the attack frequency varied from less than 1 to 26 per year, and 4 subjects died of acute upper airway obstruction. Symptoms tend to worsen during pregnancy and treatment with oral contraceptives. The attacks are not precipitated by allergens but may follow local trauma, such as tonsillectomy or tooth extraction,[34] or may be associated with emotional upsets. The form of inheritance is autosomal dominant. The underlying defect is absence or abnormal function of a serum α2-globulin esterase inhibitor of the first component of complement (C1 esterase inhibitor), the increase in C1 being reflected in a decrease in C2 and C4. Numerous mutations have been found in the C1 esterase gene on chromosome 11 in affected families.[36] Normal serum levels of C4 during a symptomatic period rules out the diagnosis.[37] It is believed that the byproducts of the complement cascade are responsible for the release of vasoactive substances, which in turn produce angioedema. In 10% to 15% of patients, the $\alpha_2$-globulin inhibitor is present in normal quantity but is nonfunctional. The prognosis in the hereditary form of angioneurotic edema is grave: about one third of individuals die from acute upper airway obstruction;[29, 30] however, careful management and long-term prophylactic measures can save a considerable number of lives.[34]

Thermal injury of the upper airway is a common com-

plication of smoke inhalation and may lead to sufficient edema to cause acute upper airway obstruction; rarely, the complication is secondary to a scalding injury of the hypopharynx or epiglottis following the ingestion of hot liquid.[38, 39] Hot air and smoke inhalation account for 50% of the fire-related deaths reported annually in the United States.[40] The presence of burned or singed nasal hairs in a smoke-exposed patient indicates that mucosal damage is likely at the level of the larynx. Hoarseness is another clue that the larynx may be damaged and that fiberoptic laryngoscopy is indicated.[40] Inspiratory and expiratory flow-volume loops can be of help in assessment.[41] Although the obstruction usually occurs within 24 hours, late tracheal stenosis may also occur.[42] An unusual mechanism for the development of late upper airway obstruction consists of cutaneous burns that result in severe scar contractures of the neck; affected patients may manifest upper airway obstruc-

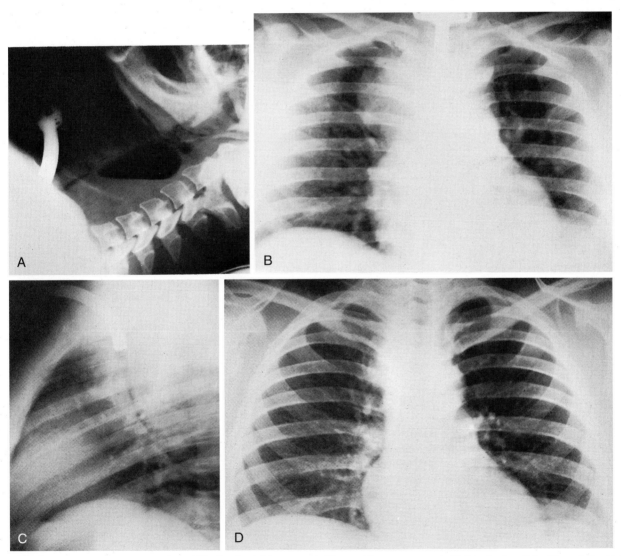

**Figure 52–1. Acute Retropharyngeal and Mediastinal Abscess.** A 29-year-old woman was admitted to the hospital with an 8-day history of increasing dyspnea, difficulty in swallowing, and loss of voice. An emergency tracheostomy was performed. A lateral radiograph of the soft tissues of the neck with a horizontal x-ray beam *(A)* revealed a large accumulation of gas and fluid in the retropharyngeal space associated with complete obliteration of the air space of the hypopharynx and anterior displacement of the cervical trachea. Anteroposterior *(B)* and lateral *(C)* radiographs showed a large mediastinal mass projecting predominantly to the right of the midline, situated mainly behind the trachea and causing anterior displacement and narrowing of this structure. The retropharyngeal and mediastinal abscesses were evacuated and drained surgically; 3 weeks later the mediastinal silhouette was almost normal *(D)*.

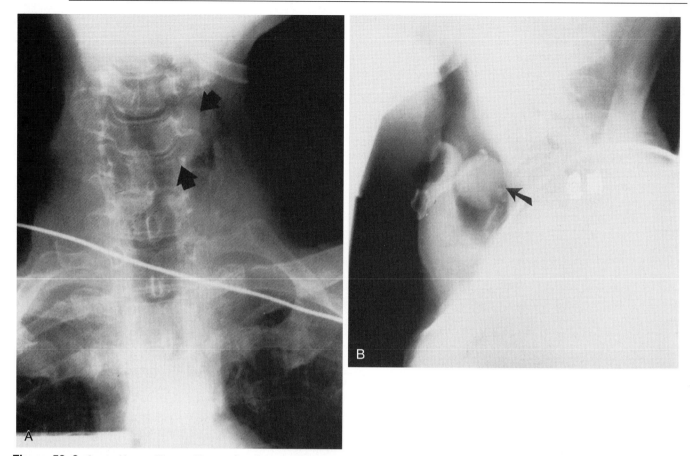

**Figure 52–2. Acute Upper Airway Obstruction Caused by a Foreign Body.** A radiograph of the neck in anteroposterior projection *(A)* reveals a grape-sized opacity *(arrows)* situated in the region of the left piriform sinus immediately above the false vocal cords. The object can be seen with greater clarity *(arrow)* on a detail lateral view of the soft tissues of the neck *(B)*. This 71-year-old woman presented in acute respiratory distress; she was cyanotic and stuporous. Direct laryngoscopy revealed a grape, the removal of which resulted in prompt improvement. (Courtesy of Dr. John Fleetham, University of British Columbia, Vancouver.)

tion when endotracheal intubation is attempted.[43] A case has been reported in which acute upper airway obstruction developed in an infant as a result of retropharyngeal edema secondary to idiopathic thrombosis of the superior vena cava and brachiocephalic veins.[44] Another rare cause is inflammatory edema of the uvula.[45]

### Retropharyngeal Hemorrhage

Acute upper airway obstruction can result from hemorrhage into the retropharyngeal space from a variety of causes, including neck surgery, external trauma, carotid angiography, transbrachial retrograde catheterization,[46] and erosion of an artery secondary to infection. Hemorrhage can also occur spontaneously in patients who have hematologic disorders, such as hemophilia, acute leukemia, or polycythemia rubra vera, or who are receiving anticoagulant therapy.[47–53] Rarely, cervical or intrathoracic hematomas resulting from rupture of an aneurysm of the great vessels cause tracheal obstruction.[54–56]

### Foreign Body Aspiration

Obstruction of the air and food passages by foreign bodies occurs most frequently in infants and young children and tends to affect the esophagus and major bronchi much more commonly than the upper airway.[57] The objects most frequently aspirated by children are peanuts, coins, plastic toys, and screws, whereas in adults, meat and bones are the most common offending agents (Fig. 52–2).[57] The aspiration of partly masticated meat and its lodgment in the larynx is the most common cause of the café-coronary syndrome (*see* page 2487). As might be anticipated, obstruction from foreign bodies occurs more often in patients who have preexisting dysfunction of pharyngeal muscles. Candies inhaled by young children can cause severe edema of the airway mucosa as a result of the hyperosmolar viscid fluid produced as they dissolve.[58] Dilation of the esophagus secondary to achalasia has been reported to compress and obstruct the intrathoracic trachea.[59] Large foreign bodies within the esophagus are also occasional causes of upper airway obstruction.[60]

### Faulty Placement of an Endotracheal Tube

Complications of endotracheal intubation are uncommon and occur more often in association with emergency resuscitation than with routine respiratory therapy.[61] The chief complication is large airway obstruction resulting from malpositioning of the tube too low in the trachea and major bronchi. In most instances, the endotracheal tube enters the right main bronchus (in 27 of 28 cases in one series),[61] and the orifice of the left main bronchus is occluded by the balloon cuff, resulting in complete obstruction and atelectasis of the left lung (Fig. 52–3). If the tube is advanced sufficiently far down the right main bronchus, the right upper lobe bronchus may be occluded, with resultant atelectasis of this lobe as well as the left lung or of the right middle lobe alone.[61] Occasionally, the tube enters the left rather than the right main bronchus, leading to obstruction of the latter. The rate at which atelectasis occurs depends on the gas content of the lung at the moment of occlusion. Total collapse requires 18 to 24 hours if the parenchyma is air containing but may occur in a matter of minutes if the lung contains 100% oxygen (as is often the case in acute respiratory emergencies). Withdrawal of the tube typically results in rapid re-expansion of the collapsed lung or lobe.

It has been suggested that the ideal location of the tip of an endotracheal tube is 3 cm distal to the vocal cords;[61] however, because the vocal cords are infrequently visualized on bedside radiographs, the carina seems a much more logical point from which to establish a reference. It has been recommended that with the head and neck in a neutral position, the ideal distance between the tip of the endotracheal tube and the carina is 5 ± 2 cm.[62] Flexion and extension of the neck can cause a 2-cm descent and ascent, respectively, of the tip of the endotracheal tube; if the position of the neck can be established from the radiograph (through visualization of the mandible), the ideal distance between the tip of the endotracheal tube and the carina should be 3 ± 2 cm with the neck flexed and 7 ± 2 cm with the neck extended. If the carina is not visualized, the endotracheal tube can be assumed to be in adequate position if its tip is aligned with the fifth, sixth, or seventh thoracic vertebra.[63]

The radiographic findings of a malpositioned endotracheal tube are typical and should present no difficulty in interpretation. Clinically, the examining physician should not be misled by hearing breath sounds transmitted from the normal or overinflated contralateral lung through the collapsed lung.

## CHRONIC UPPER AIRWAY OBSTRUCTION

### General Features

In contrast to acute upper airway obstruction, the cause of which is often apparent, chronic obstructive disease of the pharynx, larynx, and trachea frequently is misdiagnosed as asthma or chronic obstructive pulmonary disease (COPD). Dyspnea is the usual presenting complaint, often first noted on exertion and sometimes exacerbated when the patient assumes a recumbent position. In a minority of patients, obstruction results in serious impairment of alveolar ventilation, cor pulmonale, and sleep disturbance. Although the symptoms may mislead the physician into a false interpretation of acute or chronic lower airway obstruction, the application of standard and specialized radiographic procedures and the discovery of characteristic physiologic disturbances on pulmonary function testing readily permit identification of the offending lesion in most cases. The intermittent nocturnal obstruction of the hypopharynx that occurs in obstructive sleep apnea is the most common form of chronic upper airway obstruction and represents a sufficiently distinct syndrome to be considered separately (*see* page 2054).

A great variety of conditions affecting the upper airway from the nasopharynx to the tracheal carina can cause chronic upper airway obstruction (Table 52–2). The most common are hypertrophy of the tonsils and adenoids, vocal

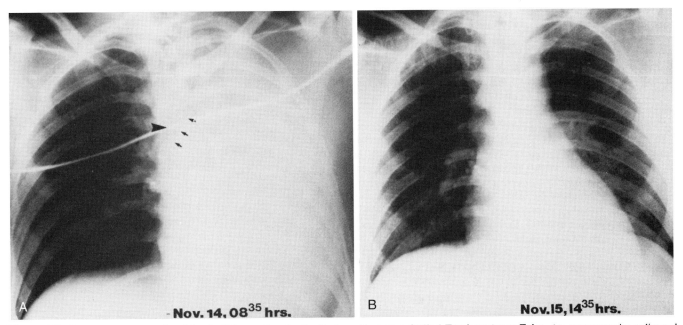

**Figure 52–3. Acute Atelectasis of the Left Lung Due to Faulty Insertion of a Cuffed Tracheostomy Tube.** An anteroposterior radiograph in the supine position *(A)* reveals complete airlessness of the left lung associated with slight displacement of the mediastinum to the left. A tracheostomy tube is in position, its tip *(arrowhead)* situated in the right main bronchus just beyond the carina (the medial wall of the right main bronchus is indicated by *arrows*). This atelectasis occurred over a very brief period of time, since a high-oxygen mixture was being administered. Following withdrawal of the tracheostomy tube *(B)*, the left lung reinflated spontaneously and rapidly.

## Table 52–2. CAUSES OF CHRONIC UPPER AIRWAY OBSTRUCTION

| CONDITION OR DISEASE PROCESS | SELECTED REFERENCES |
|---|---|
| **Infection** | |
| Chronic granulomatous infection with *Klebsiella rhinoscleromatis* | 364 |
| Laryngotracheal papillomatosis | 314, 315 |
| **Ectopic Tissue** | |
| Ectopic endotracheal thymus | 316 |
| Ectopic endotracheal thyroid | 317 |
| Lingual thyroid gland | 318 |
| **Neoplasms** | |
| **Primary neoplasms** | |
| Squamous cell carcinoma | 191, 319 |
| Tracheobronchial gland neoplasms | 319, 320 |
| Plasmacytoma | 321 |
| Lymphoma | |
| Soft tissue neoplasms (e.g., neurilemoma, granular cell tumor) | 197, 322–324 |
| Laryngeal oncocytic cystadenomas | 325 |
| Hypopharyngeal lipoma | 326 |
| Kaposi's sarcoma | 327, 328 |
| Chondroma of the thyroid cartilage | 329 |
| Metastatic carcinoma | 193 |
| **Direct extension of neoplasm** | |
| Pulmonary carcinoma | |
| Thyroid carcinoma | 330 |
| Esophageal carcinoma | 331 |
| **Cysts** | |
| Thyroglossal duct cyst | 332, 333 |
| Mediastinal bronchogenic cyst | 334 |
| Traumatic thoracic duct lymphocele | 335, 336 |
| Laryngoceles | 337 |
| **Musculoskeletal Abnormalities** | |
| Ankylosis of the cricoarytenoid joint in long-standing rheumatoid arthritis | 338 |
| Temporomandibular joint ankylosis | 339 |
| Cervical osteophytes | 340, 341 |
| Ankylosing spondylitis of the cervical spine | 342 |
| Focal muscular hypoplasia of the posterior tracheal wall | 343 |
| **Metabolic Abnormalities** | |
| Acromegaly (macroglossia and pharyngeal soft tissue hypertrophy) | 344, 345 |
| Amyloidosis | 346, 347 |
| Mucopolysaccharidosis | 348, 349 |
| **Immunologic Abnormalities** | |
| Sarcoidosis | 350 |
| Wegener's granulomatosis | 351 |
| Ulcerative colitis | 352 |
| Relapsing polychondritis | 215 |
| **Vascular Abnormalities** | |
| Right-sided aortic arch | |
| Aberrant subclavian, innominate, or common carotid artery | 353, 354 |
| Pulmonary artery sling | 355 |
| Aortic aneurysm | 356 |
| **Trauma** | |
| Intubation | |
| **Miscellaneous** | |
| Congenital macroglossia | 357 |
| Down's syndrome | 358 |
| Epidermolysis bullosa dystrophica | 359 |
| Achalasia | 360 |
| Massive phenytoin-induced gingival hypertrophy | 361 |
| Rhinoscleroma of the larynx during pregnancy | 362 |
| "Saber-sheath" trachea | 206 |
| Tracheobronchopathia osteochondroplastica | 363 |

cord paralysis, tracheal stenosis following tracheostomy or prolonged tracheal intubation, and primary and secondary neoplasms. Disturbance in the dynamic activity of the trachea as a result of increased compliance of its walls (tracheomalacia) may occur as a part of some of these conditions. Each of these possesses fairly characteristic radiologic manifestations that permit their differentiation (*see* farther on); however, certain radiologic, clinical, and physiologic manifestations are common to all, regardless of their precise nature, and these are described first.

### Physiologic Manifestations

Upper airway obstruction has historically been considered to be fixed or variable according to the effects of respiration on the severity of obstruction. *Fixed obstructions* are those in which the cross-sectional area of the airway is unable to change in response to transmural pressure differences; thus, they may be situated in either extrathoracic or intrathoracic airways without observed differences in their physiologic effects. By contrast, *variable obstructions* are those in which the airway is capable of responding to transmural pressure; because this pressure is different in the extrathoracic and intrathoracic airways, the physiologic (and to lesser extent radiographic) effects depend to a considerable extent on the anatomic location of the lesion.

In contrast to inspiratory flow, which is effort dependent at all lung volumes from residual volume (RV) to total-lung capacity (TLC), forced expiratory flow from TLC is effort dependent only over the upper 20% to 30% of vital capacity (VC) and is independent of effort over the remaining 70% to 80% down to RV. Over this effort-independent section of the forced vital capacity (FVC), flow is limited in such a way that an increase in effort with increased pleural pressure simply compresses airways downstream from the equal pressure point and does not result in increased expiratory flow. The increased resistance caused by upper airway obstruction is reflected in a reduction in expiratory flow at high lung volumes, at which flow is effort dependent, but may not be identified in measurements that measure flow at low lung volumes, at which flow is effort independent.[64–66]

An excellent method of portraying how physiologic determinants of flow can be affected by various obstructing lesions of the conducting system is the flow-volume loop, which combines maximal expiratory and inspiratory curves from TLC and RV, respectively (Fig. 52–4). In normal subjects, the maximal or peak expiratory flow rate (PEFR) occurs early in the effort-dependent portion of the curve, and a flow ratio between expiratory and inspiratory limbs at mid-VC (50%) is about 1.[66, 67] The flow-volume loop can be altered by having normal subjects breathe through fixed external resistances.[66, 68–70] Breathing through an external orifice 6 mm in diameter reduces peak flows and produces plateaus on both inspiration and expiration (*see* Fig. 52–4), a loop pattern closely resembling that of fixed airway obstruction. Asthma and COPD are predominantly diseases of the small airways; reduction in flow is apparent mainly in the effort-independent portion of the expiratory loop and the mid-VC expiratory-to-inspiratory ratio is usually less than 0.5 (*see* Fig. 52–4). By contrast, in upper airway obstruction, the reduction in flow is proportionately greater in the effort-dependent portion of the loop (both inspiratory and expiratory), with one or both limbs tending to plateau.

The dynamic effects of lesions of the upper airway depend in part on the extent to which the obstruction is fixed (i.e., the airway is unable to change cross-sectional area in response to transmural pressure differences—usually produced by circumferential benign strictures) or variable (i.e., the airway responds to transmural pressure—most often resulting from neoplasms that arise from the wall of the airway and create a crescentic lumen, thus permitting a variable cross-sectional diameter throughout the forced ventilatory cycle). Characteristic flow-volume loop patterns are produced by fixed and variable lesions (*see* Fig. 52–4). Because fixed upper airway obstructions, either intrathoracic or extrathoracic, are not influenced by transmural pressure gradients,

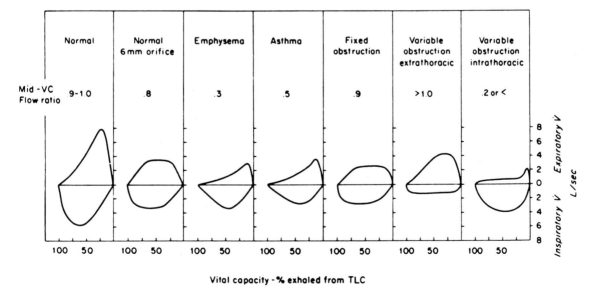

**Figure 52–4. Flow-Volume Loops of Various Obstructive Conditions Compared with Normal.** Volume is given as a percentage of vital capacity exhaled from total lung capacity. Representative mid-vital capacity flow ratios are given. (Reproduced from Miller RD, Hyatt RE, Mayo Clin Proc 44:145, 1969, with permission of the authors and editor.)

both inspiratory and expiratory flow are proportionately lowered. When a lesion causes variable obstruction, its location (intrathoracic or extrathoracic) becomes important because the airway responds to transmural pressure. When there is a variable extrathoracic tracheal obstruction, inspiratory flow is disproportionately lowered because intraluminal pressure is subatmospheric while extraluminal pressure is nearly atmospheric. However, the pressure surrounding the extrathoracic trachea may not be as close to atmospheric pressure as was once believed. Several groups of investigators have shown that pleural pressure may be transmitted to the tissue spaces in the neck; to the extent that negative pleural pressure is transmitted here, the dynamic compression of the trachea associated with upper airway obstruction is attenuated.[71, 72]

In contrast to the dynamic events that occur during inspiration in variable extrathoracic lesions, during expiration, intraluminal pressure is positive relative to extraluminal pressure, thus tending to dilate the airway and obscure the presence of the lesion. Thus, a variable extrathoracic lesion tends to cause predominant decrease in maximal inspiratory flow and relatively little effect on maximal expiratory flow.[66] This situation is reversed when a variable lesion is intrathoracic in location. During inspiration, extraluminal pressure (equivalent to pleural pressure) is negative relative to intraluminal pressure, so that transmural pressure favors airway dilation. By contrast, during expiration, extraluminal pressure is positive relative to intraluminal pressure, so that airway narrowing occurs. Thus, a variable intrathoracic lesion results in a predominant reduction in maximal expiratory flow with relative preservation of maximal inspiratory flow (*see* Fig. 52–4).[66]

The usefulness of comparing maximal flows on inspiratory and expiratory flow-volume curves has been confirmed in a study in which lesions were localized with tantalum bronchograms.[73] It was shown that expiratory-to-inspiratory flow ratios near 1 may be seen when the tracheal stenosis is near the thoracic inlet and that increased ratios may be observed with extrathoracic tracheomalacia. Periodic flow oscillations that can be identified on either volume-time or flow-volume recordings and that correspond to a fluttering of upper airway structures, either passively or as a result of periodic muscle contraction, may be an important indicator of an abnormality of control of upper airway caliber.[74–76] Such oscillations are also seen in some patients who have obstructive snoring or obstructive sleep apnea.[77] The identification of such flow oscillations should lead to the investigation of the upper airway and its surrounding musculature because these changes may be an early indicator of disorders that can eventually lead to symptomatic upper airway obstruction.

Because the clinical and radiographic diagnosis of upper airway obstruction may be exceedingly difficult, it is important to recognize the basic physiologic changes caused by lesions in this area and to know how they are reflected in pulmonary function tests. In studies of normal subjects breathing through fixed resistances (the equivalent of fixed upper airway obstruction), FVC was not reduced by an orifice as small as 4 mm, and forced expiratory volume in 1 second ($FEV_1$) did not decrease until orifice size was reduced to 6 mm in diameter.[66] These relationships between lung function tests and airway size have been confirmed in symptomatic patients who have tracheal stenosis.[66, 78]

Lesions of the larynx and trachea that produce a predominantly inspiratory obstruction may be recognized by comparing forced inspiratory (FIF) with forced expiratory (FEF) flow rates;[70, 79] these are usually measured at mid-VC and produce an FEF-to-FIF ratio of greater than 1. However, because FIF measurement is not routine in some laboratories, and because forced inspiratory flow is an effort-dependent test, it is pertinent to compare the results of tests that measure effort-dependent expiratory flow with those that reflect the effort-independent flow contribution. The diagnosis may be suggested by finding a PEFR that is reduced proportionately greater than the $FEV_1$.[64, 65, 68] An $FEV_1$-to-PEFR ratio greater than 10 ml per liter per minute is a sensitive indicator of upper airway obstruction, although the sensitivity is somewhat diminished in the presence of concomitant lower airway obstruction.[81] A reduction in the ratio of maximal voluntary ventilation to $FEV_1$ was found to be the most accurate predictor of upper airway obstruction in one study of patients who had combined lower airway obstruction; however, this test is performed rarely.[81]

Some investigators advocate measurement of other ratios of flow at small to large lung volumes, such as $FEV_1$ to $FEV_{0.5}$.[68] A comparison of $FEV_1$ and $FEF_{25-75\%}$ may be of particular benefit in detecting upper airway obstruction when flow-volume loops are not available. In the absence of airflow obstruction, the numeric values of $FEV_1$ and $FEF_{25-75\%}$ are roughly comparable; however, as lower airway obstruction develops (e.g., in asthma or COPD), the $FEF_{25-75\%}$ becomes disproportionately lowered. In upper airway obstruction, the $FEV_1$ (reflecting both effort-dependent and effort-independent flow) is decreased to the same extent as $FEF_{25-75\%}$, which reflects effort-independent flow only.[82] In one study, patients who had asthma, emphysema, or upper airway obstruction were best separated by the ratio of peak expiratory flow to flow at 50% FVC ($PEF/MEF_{50\%}$), which was lower in those who had upper airway obstruction, and the ratio of $FEV_1$ to PEF, which was higher in those who had upper airway obstruction.[83] A high index of suspicion is necessary to detect upper airway obstruction by spirometry; one group showed that it was frequently overlooked by general internists compared with respirologists.[84] In another study, 27 patients who had asthma, 20 who had emphysema, and 18 who had upper airway obstruction had measurements of $FEV_1$, PEF, and $MEF_{50\%}$, as well as airway resistance (Raw) and airway conductance (Gaw);[85] the $MEF_{50\%}$-to-Gaw ratio was the best discriminator, with mean values of 0.19, 0.44, and 0.63 in the patients who had emphysema, asthma, and upper airway obstruction, respectively.

Tests measuring the distribution (mixing) of inspired gases and the response to bronchodilators also may be useful in distinguishing upper from lower airway obstruction; despite considerable obstruction, patients who have upper airway lesions often show normal distribution of inspired gas and are unresponsive to bronchodilators. It would be anticipated that patients who have upper airway obstruction, in contrast to those who have emphysema, would have normal diffusing capacity, and a limited number of reports suggest that this is so.[78, 86] The breathing of helium-oxygen mixtures can also differentiate between upper and lower airway obstruction.[64, 87] The resistance caused by turbulent flow in the larger bronchi is reduced by the breathing of this less dense gas mixture, whereas the resistance related to laminar flow in peripheral airways remains unaffected. Although this is true in theory, patients who have asthma and COPD can show substantial increases in flow while breathing a helium-oxygen mixture, and the test is not used clinically.

Pulmonary gas exchange in patients who have upper airway obstruction is usually better preserved than that in patients who have comparable degrees of obstruction secondary to lower airway diseases. The presence of hypoxemia and hypercarbia at rest is usually indicative of an extreme degree of airway narrowing in these patients. An exercise challenge may result in a decrease in $Po_2$ and an increase in $Pco_2$ in patients who have less severe obstruction.[68]

### Radiologic Manifestations

Plain radiography plays a limited role in the assessment of patients who have pharyngeal or laryngeal abnormalities. The main exceptions are the use of lateral radiographs of the soft tissues in the neck in the evaluation of patients suspected of having acute epiglottitis, retropharyngeal abscess, or foreign body obstruction. Imaging of intrinsic abnormalities of the pharynx and larynx usually is performed using CT or magnetic resonance (MR) imaging.[88–91] Spiral CT has been shown to be superior to conventional CT in the assessment of the larynx.[92] CT has also been shown to be helpful in the assessment of extralaryngeal causes of vocal cord paralysis; for example, in one investigation of 20 patients who had left vocal cord palsy from such a cause, CT demonstrated a tumor in the aortopulmonary window (presumably involving the recurrent laryngeal nerve) in 18 (90%).[93] The chest radiograph showed an abnormality at this site in only 5 of the 18 patients. In the same study, 8 of 11 cases of right vocal cord paralysis were the result of malignant tumors involving the recurrent laryngeal nerve in the lower neck or lung apex; in all 8, CT demonstrated a mass in the expected course of the right recurrent laryngeal nerve.

The initial radiologic examination in patients suspected of having a tracheal abnormality usually consists of a frontal and lateral chest radiograph.[94, 95] Adequate visualization of the trachea, mediastinum, and lungs requires the use of high (120 to 150) kilovolts (peak). Unfortunately, the trachea is all too often a "blind spot" for the radiologist, a deficiency that can be corrected only by paying particular attention to this region. An example of this diagnostic difficulty is provided by one investigation of 44 patients who had primary tracheal carcinoma;[96] prospectively, the tumor was detected on the chest radiograph in only 8 (18%) patients, whereas it could be identified retrospectively in 29 (66%). As might be expected, CT significantly improves detection of tracheal abnormalities; for example, in one study of 35 patients who had focal or diffuse disease of the trachea or main bronchi and 5 normal controls, an abnormality was detected on the radiograph in 23 (66%) patients and on conventional CT in 33 (94%).[95]

CT allows assessment of the location and extent of tracheal abnormalities as well as the presence of mediastinal involvement.[87, 95, 97–99] Conventional CT provides excellent resolution in the transverse plane but leads to underestimation of the cephalocaudad extent of tracheal stenosis or tumor involvement.[87, 100, 101] Better assessment of the extent of disease in this plane is obtained using spiral CT with multiplanar and three-dimensional reconstructions (Fig. 52–5).[102–106] In one investigation, spiral CT with multiplanar reconstruction was compared with bronchoscopy in 25 patients who had known or suspected stenosis of the trachea or main bronchi.[103] Spiral CT demonstrated the presence, site, degree, and extent of tracheal and main bronchial stenosis with a sensitivity of 93% (14 true-positive results, one false-negative) and a specificity of 100% (3 true-negative results, 0 false-positive); in one patient, focal narrowing as a result of tracheomalacia was detected at bronchoscopy but missed on CT. Spiral CT with multiplanar reconstructions also demonstrates focal abnormalities that may not be apparent on conventional transverse sections.[102, 104, 105, 107] Optimal assessment of tracheal abnormalities on spiral CT requires the use of relatively thin sections (3-mm collimation or less) and reconstructions at 1- to 1.5-mm intervals.[103, 107] The combination of spiral technique, thin sections, and volume rendering allows depiction of endoluminal-surface views similar to those obtained with bronchography.[107a] Volume-rendered three-dimensional images have been shown to improve recognition of mild tracheal abnormalities not readily apparent on conventional cross-sectional images.[107a]

The presence and extent of tracheal abnormalities, including intrinsic stenosis, extrinsic compression, and primary and secondary neoplasms, can also be assessed using MR imaging.[94, 108] It has also been suggested that dynamic MR imaging may be helpful in the diagnosis of tracheomalacia.[108a] However, because of its inferior spatial resolution and high cost, the procedure has a limited role.

Three unusual radiographic manifestations of chronic upper airway obstruction relate to the heart and pulmonary circulation. Pulmonary edema occurs rarely but can have serious consequences. It is thought to be caused by the sustained maximal negative intrathoracic pressure created by attempted inspiration against an obstruction (Müller's maneuver); however, as pointed out in Chapter 51, there is evidence that the edema develops in some patients only after the obstruction has been relieved. The second unusual manifestation is cardiac enlargement (cor pulmonale) that results from pulmonary arterial hypertension secondary to chronic hypoxemia and acidosis;[109] in fact, some children who have certain forms of chronic upper airway obstruction, such as hypertrophied tonsils, can present in frank right ventricular failure.

The third unusual manifestation of chronic upper airway obstruction consists of a paradoxical change in heart size between inspiration and expiration. Normally, cardiac diameter is greater on expiration than inspiration; in the presence of chronic (and sometimes acute) upper airway obstruction, the heart is smaller on expiration than inspiration, a paradox that also occasionally occurs in association with chronic *lower* airway obstruction, such as in emphysema. This can be explained on the basis of Valsalva's and Müller's maneuvers. In the presence of upper airway obstruction, expiration constitutes an effective Valsalva's maneuver, raising intrathoracic pressure and reducing venous return to the thorax; the heart becomes smaller. By contrast, inspiration against the obstruction creates Müller's maneuver, with greater negativity of intrathoracic pressure and increased venous return to the thorax; in addition to increasing venous return, the very negative intrathoracic pressure functions as an afterload on the left ventricle, which must pump blood out of the thorax into the systemic circulation, which is unaffected by the negative pressure.

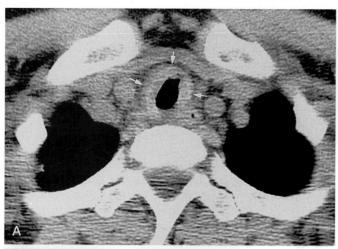

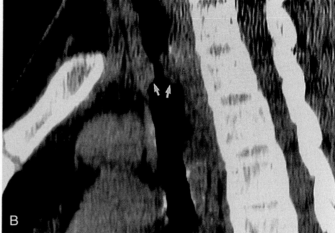

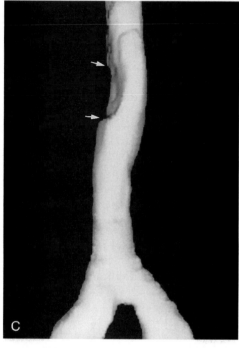

**Figure 52–5. Spiral CT with Sagittal and Three-Dimensional Reconstructions in Endotracheal Tuberculosis.** A 3-mm collimation spiral CT scan *(A)* demonstrates circumferential thickening of the trachea *(arrows)*. The sagittal reconstruction *(B)* allows better assessment of the focal nature of the thickening as well as narrowing of the lumen *(arrows)*. The focal narrowing is also well seen on the coronal 3-D reconstruction *(arrows in C)* of the trachea and main bronchi. The patient was a 27-year-old woman. (Courtesy of Dr. Kyung Soo Lee, Department of Radiology, Samsung Medical Center, Seoul, Korea.)

### Clinical Manifestations

Obviously, the symptoms and signs of chronic upper airway obstruction vary with the nature of the underlying lesion and, to some extent, with the age of the patient. As might be expected, the major complaint is dyspnea, either during exercise or at rest, depending on the severity of obstruction. Stridor also may be noted either at rest or during exercise, and its timing may be inspiratory, expiratory, or both. Nonproductive cough is common.

### Specific Causes

#### Hypertrophy of Tonsils and Adenoids

Hypertrophy of the palatine tonsils results in a characteristic radiographic appearance of a smooth, well-defined, elliptical mass of unit density extending downward from the soft palate into the hypopharynx; hypertrophy of the nasopharyngeal adenoids is commonly associated. Both ab-

normalities should be readily apparent on lateral radiographs of the soft tissues of the neck. The major effect of the chronic upper airway obstruction is alveolar hypoventilation, with resultant hypoxia, hypercapnia, and pulmonary arterial hypertension and cor pulmonale.[110–112] In one such patient, pulmonary arterial pressure was near systemic levels;[113] this pressure was halved shortly after intubation. A similar picture can be seen in obese subjects as a result of obstruction of the pharynx by the tongue when the patient is recumbent *(see* Chapter 53, page 2054).[64, 114, 115]

#### Goiter

Goiter is a relatively common cause of upper airway obstruction.[116] Although it usually causes chronic obstruction, it occasionally is associated with an acute clinical course.[117] In one study of 44 patients who had goiter and whose flow-volume loops were assessed, evidence of upper airway obstruction was present in 31%.[118] Inspection of the flow-volume loops was 78% specific and 100% sensitive in detecting upper airway obstruction, whereas an $FEV_1$-to-PEF flow ratio greater than 8 was 94% specific and 64% sensitive. Twenty-seven of 29 patients who had upper airway obstruction showed improvement after surgical removal of the goiter. In another study of 51 patients, maximal inspiratory flow increased from 3.9 to 4.9 liters per second after thyroidectomy.[119] In patients who have goiter and respiratory symptoms during recumbency, flow-volume loops performed in various body positions may reveal upper airway obstruction.[120] A large retrosternal goiter can cause upper airway obstruction in association with superior vena caval obstruction.[121]

The radiographic manifestations of goiter consist of a paratracheal mass associated with smooth eccentric or circumferential tracheal narrowing. On CT, the thyroid is often asymmetrically enlarged, shows inhomogeneous areas of attenuation, contains foci of calcification, and demonstrates marked enhancement after intravenous administration of contrast.[122–126] Tracheal narrowing may also result from thyroiditis and thyroid carcinoma. Riedel's thyroiditis is a chronic inflammatory condition associated with a marked desmoplastic reaction; it can be associated with tracheal narrowing and fibrosing mediastinitis;[126] on CT, the enlarged thyroid has poorly defined margins (Fig. 52–6). Thyroid carcinomas usually present as a focal mass, which may have homogeneous or inhomogeneous attenuation and can often

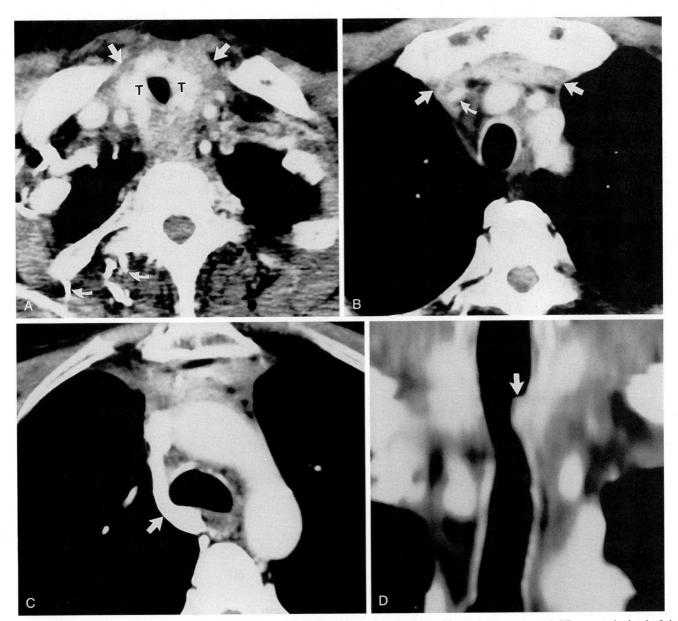

**Figure 52–6. Riedel's Thyroiditis with Tracheal Narrowing and Fibrosing Mediastinitis.** A contrast-enhanced CT scan at the level of the thoracic inlet *(A)* in a 74-year-old man demonstrates tracheal narrowing and ill-defined soft tissue density *(straight arrows)* surrounding the thyroid (T). Note venous collateral circulation *(curved arrows)* in the chest wall. An image at the level of the great vessels *(B)* shows soft tissue *(straight arrows)* in the anterior mediastinum with associated narrowing of the right brachiocephalic vein *(curved arrow)*. An image at the level of the aortic arch *(C)* shows normal diameter of the superior vena cava with collateral circulation from the azygos vein *(arrow)* bypassing the obstruction of the brachiocephalic veins. Coronal reconstruction *(D)* demonstrates localized tracheal narrowing *(arrow)*. The findings were confirmed at thoracotomy. Biopsies confirmed the diagnosis of Riedel's struma and extensive fibrosing mediastinitis. (Courtesy of Dr. Hiram Nogueira, Vitoria/ES, Brazil.)

contain foci of low attenuation as a result of cystic degeneration.[126-128] Occasionally, they cause diffuse enlargement of the thyroid (Fig. 52–7). The appearance of thyroid carcinomas can mimic that of benign conditions such as goiter or adenomas, and definitive diagnosis usually requires biopsy. Rarely, marked tracheal narrowing is secondary to an ectopic intratracheal thyroid tissue mass.[129]

### Laryngeal Dysfunction

The upper airway site with the greatest potential for deranged function is the larynx. There are 24 sets of skeletal muscles that surround the upper airway and are involved in stabilization and closure of the airway; most of these are laryngeal muscles under both voluntary and involuntary control. They are involved in speech, song, cough, defecation, and so on.[1] The major laryngeal dilator muscle (abductor) is the posterior cricoarytenoid, and the major constrictors (adductors) are the thyroarytenoid and lateral cricoarytenoid. These muscles are respiratory, in that they receive phasic neural output from brainstem respiratory neurons. During inspiration, the posterior cricoarytenoid dilates the larynx; in some instances, expiratory adductor activation narrows it. The alae nasi are also inspiratory muscles; during periods of increased ventilation, their phasic inspiratory contraction prevents collapse of the external nares.[130] Laryngeal dysfunction, either decreased activity of dilating muscle groups or increased activity of constricting muscles, can cause acute or chronic obstruction.

Paralysis of the laryngeal abductors causes fixed obstruction of the upper airway,[131-133] whereas episodic unopposed action of laryngeal adductors results in laryngospasm. Bulbar involvement in generalized neuromuscular disease causes weakness of the upper airway muscles that may be associated with inspiratory upper airway obstruction and characteristic flow oscillations on flow-volume curves.[134, 135] The importance of tonic sensory input in the maintenance of

upper airway caliber can be demonstrated by the transient increase in inspiratory (predominantly glottic) resistance that is caused by upper airway anesthesia secondary to nebulized lidocaine.[136]

In children and infants, important causes of upper airway obstruction include hypotonic larynx,[137] congenital hypoplasia of laryngeal structures, congenital cleft larynx[138] and bilateral vocal cord paralysis.[139] Chronic upper airway obstruction as a result of vocal cord paralysis also occurs in adults.[140, 141] Interruption of the superior laryngeal nerves at the time of thyroidectomy is the most common cause of bilateral vocal cord paralysis in adults. It can also occur in rheumatoid disease or poliomyelitis, following viral infections, in association with Guillain-Barré syndrome, or for no apparent reason (idiopathic). Cases of vocal cord paralysis have also been reported in intravenous drug abusers who damaged the recurrent laryngeal nerves while trying to inject into the jugular veins,[142] or after blunt trauma to the anterior neck.[143] Vocal cord paralysis predominantly affects inspiratory flow; in one investigation of 10 patients, the mean expiratory-to-inspiratory flow ratio at 50% VC was 1.65.[133] Some degree of obstruction can also be caused by unilateral vocal cord paralysis.[144]

A syndrome that mimics asthma, termed *emotional laryngeal wheezing,* occurs in emotionally disturbed patients and is caused by expiratory glottic narrowing.[145] Such narrowing, uninfluenced by general anesthesia, has also been reported in patients who are truly asthmatic.[146, 147] In one such patient, episodes of hypopharyngeal narrowing were alleviated by sedatives and psychotherapy.[148] A similar syndrome, characterized by episodic stridor (psychogenic stridor, episodic paroxysmal laryngospasm), is caused by adduction of the vocal cords during inspiration; it responds to reassurance and neurofeedback training but tends to recur.[149-153] These cases of episodic, paroxysmal inspiratory laryngeal narrowing and stridor result in a syndrome in adults that resembles croup; the abnormal laryngeal muscle

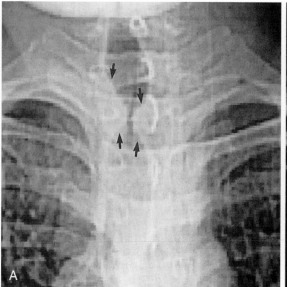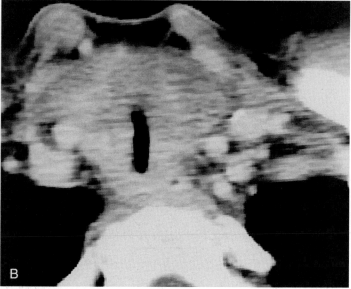

**Figure 52–7. Tracheal Narrowing Secondary to Medullary Carcinoma of the Thyroid.** A view of the thoracic inlet in a 26-year-old man *(A)* demonstrates focal circumferential narrowing of the lower cervical trachea *(arrows)*. A contrast-enhanced CT scan *(B)* demonstrates diffuse enlargement of the thyroid. The gland has poorly defined margins and lower than normal attenuation. Note the associated compression of the trachea.

activity has been documented by video recording of bronchoscopic images. In some instances, the attacks are precipitated by respiratory tract infection and histamine inhalation and abolished by continuous positive airway pressure.[154] Occasionally, episodes of apparent laryngospasm are reversed by panting; in this situation, there may be marked discrepancies between the results of flow-volume loops and airway resistance measured plethysmographically during panting. It has been suggested that this discrepancy should be a clue to the diagnosis.[155]

Laryngeal narrowing can also occur in association with lower airway obstructive diseases, such as asthma and COPD.[156] In many asthmatic patients, inspiratory resistance is paradoxically greater than expiratory resistance, and inspiratory pressure-flow curves are more curvilinear and density dependent, suggesting that the upper airway is the site of the excessive inspiratory narrowing.[157] The reasons for this are unclear. In normal subjects and asthmatic patients, histamine-induced airway obstruction is associated with expiratory glottic and oropharyngeal narrowing.[158, 159] The glottic narrowing is not caused by a direct effect on the laryngeal musculature because the larynx contains no smooth muscle, and skeletal muscles do not contract in response to histamine; it may be caused by stimulation of afferent receptors and a reflex effect. It is puzzling why the glottis should narrow in response to lower airway obstruction; one possible explanation is that such narrowing slows expiratory flow, producing a dynamic increase in functional residual capacity, thus sparing the inspiratory muscles the task of maintaining hyperinflation.[159]

Glottic inspiratory and expiratory dimensions are decreased and upper airway resistance is increased in patients who have COPD; the decreased laryngeal dimensions correlate with the severity of expiratory flow limitation.[160, 161] The expiratory narrowing may function in a manner similar to pursed-lip breathing, preventing airway closure and contributing to hyperinflation. Functional upper airway obstruction can also occur in patients who have a variety of extrapyramidal neurologic disorders.[162, 163] For example, abnormal flow-volume curves were reported in 24 of 27 patients who had extrapyramidal disorders, including essential tremor and Parkinson's disease.[162] In another study of 58 patients who had Parkinson's disease, 36 (62%) had evidence of some degree of upper airway obstruction on flow-volume loops and spirometry.[164] Although respiratory impairment in myasthenia gravis is usually attributed to respiratory muscle weakness, weakness of the bulbar and upper airway muscles can lead to upper airway obstruction; for example, in one investigation of 12 patients, 7 showed flow-volume loops characteristic of upper airway obstruction.[165] It appears that the obstruction in some of these patients was caused by rhythmic or irregular involuntary contractions of the laryngeal adductors. Endoscopy during performance of flow-volume curves showed either rhythmic or irregular changes in the glottic area as a result of alternating abduction and adduction of the vocal cords and supraglottic structures.

### Tracheal Stenosis

Even when predicted on the basis of age, height, and sex, there is considerable variation in maximal expiratory flow among normal subjects. Because central airways (trachea to segmental bronchi) are the site of flow limitation over most of the VC in normal subjects,[166, 167] part of this variation is caused by differences in the size of the central airways.[168, 169]

Tracheal cross-sectional areas can be evaluated from posteroanterior and lateral chest radiographs or from CT scans.[170–174] Assuming a normative range that encompasses three standard deviations about the mean (i.e., pertaining to 99.7% of the normal population), the upper limits of normal for coronal and sagittal diameters in men ranging in age from 20 to 79 years are 25 mm and 27 mm; in women they are 21 mm and 23 mm, respectively.[175] The lower limits of normal for both dimensions are 13 mm in men and 10 mm in women. These measurements were obtained from conventional posteroanterior and lateral chest radiographs of 808 patients who had no clinical or radiographic evidence of respiratory disease; there were 430 men and 378 women. All radiographs were exposed at TLC, and measurements were made at a point 2 cm above the projected top of the aortic arch. Deviation from these figures indicates the presence of pathologic widening or narrowing, respectively, of the caliber of the tracheal air column. Of some interest was the observation that no statistically significant correlation was found between tracheal caliber, body weight, or body height.

The diameters of the extrathoracic trachea increase during Valsalva's maneuver and decrease during Müller's maneuver.[172, 173] By contrast, the diameters of the intrathoracic trachea are not influenced by changes in pleural pressure[172] but are markedly affected by changes in lung volume.[174] In one investigation of 10 normal subjects, the mean cross-sectional area of the trachea at the level of the aortic arch as measured on CT decreased from 280 mm² at TLC (range, 221 to 382 mm²) to 178 mm² at RV (range, 115 to 236 mm²), a mean plus or minus standard deviation decrease of 35 ± 18%.[174]

One of the most common causes of chronic upper airway obstruction is tracheal stenosis occurring as a complication of intubation or tracheostomy. In one study of 342 patients who required prolonged endotracheal intubation, 5% manifested stridor after extubation, and 1.8% required reintubation or tracheostomy.[176] Although reversible laryngeal edema and inflammation were the major causes of the stridor, stricture developed as a result of fibrosis in 4 patients.

Tracheal stenosis following the prolonged use of cuffed tracheostomy or endotracheal tubes may occur at the level of the stoma, at the level of the inflatable cuff, or, rarely, where the tip of the tube impinges on the tracheal mucosa. The frequency with which stenosis occurs at these sites seems to vary from series to series; in one group of 25 clinically significant tracheal strictures, 18 occurred at the stoma and 7 at the inflatable cuff;[177] by contrast, in another group of 55 patients, the incidence of stoma (24 cases) and inflatable cuff (23 cases) stenosis was almost equal (the remaining 8 cases were at various other locations, mostly in the cervical trachea).[178]

Plastic tubes with inflatable high-compliance balloons are now the most commonly used endotracheal and tracheostomy devices. Once the tube is in position, the cuff is inflated with sufficient air to occlude the tracheal lumen to provide an airtight system at the maximal ventilatory pressure required by the patient. The cuff is usually situated 1.5 cm or more distal to the stoma.[179, 180] Because the trachea is not circular in cross-section, the circumferential cuff can attain an airtight seal only by expanding the tracheal lumen and deforming its wall (Fig. 52–8). The tracheal mucosa is easily compressed between the cuffed balloon and the underlying cartilage; because the cuff pressure may easily exceed capillary pressure, blood supply to the mucosa may be compromised, resulting in ischemic necrosis. The most susceptible portion of the trachea is where the mucosa overlies the cartilaginous rings, and it is here that necrosis occurs most often.[179] The lesion begins as a superficial tracheitis and progresses to shallow mucosal ulcerations, usually 2 days or more after inflation of the cuff. As the mucosa becomes eroded, the cartilaginous rings are exposed, become softened, split, and fragment.[179] After deflation of the cuff and removal of the tracheostomy tube, fibrosis occurs in the damaged tracheal wall, resulting in stenosis (Fig. 52–9).

Experimental studies on dogs have demonstrated both the immediate effects of intubation and the effects of prolonged use of cuffed tracheostomy tubes. In one investigation, tracheas examined by scanning electron microscopy 2 hours after intubation showed nearly complete denudation of ciliated cells along the tract of tubal insertion.[181] When cuffs were inflated, more widespread changes were observed, especially over tracheal rings. Seven days later, regeneration was nearly complete, although isolated areas of denudation could still be identified. In another study, both cuffed and uncuffed tracheostomy tubes were maintained in position for 2 weeks at low and high pressures.[182] Changes were assessed by bronchoscopy and tracheography and by histologic examination following sacrifice 8 weeks after extubation. The investigators found that the greater the size of the tracheostomy tube relative to tracheal diameter and the greater the inflating pressure, the more severe the resultant stenosis. In a third study of two low-pressure cuffs, both produced little visible damage to the tracheal wall of dogs intubated contin-

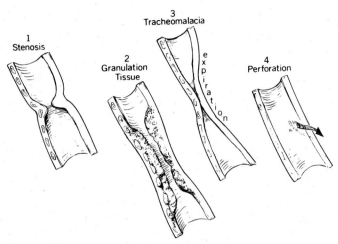

**Figure 52–9. Diagrammatic Representation of Distal Posttracheostomy Lesions That Occur in the Area of the Balloon Cuff.** (Reproduced from MacMillan AS Jr, James AE Jr, Stitik FP, Grillo HC: Thorax 26:696, 1971, with permission of the authors and editor.)

uously over a 2-week period.[183] Tracheal stenosis at the cuff level after extubation occurred far less frequently than when the stiff, unyielding, low-residual-volume cuffs were used. Although such low-pressure cuffs are less likely to cause tracheal damage and stenosis, this complication is still possi-

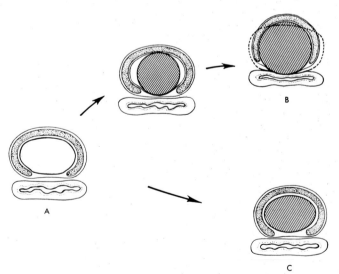

**Figure 52–8. Diagrammatic Views of the Trachea in Cross Section with Varied Inflation of a Balloon Cuff.** *A,* Without the balloon cuff; *B,* overinflation of the balloon with increased pressure on the tracheal wall; *C,* normal inflation of the balloon. (Reproduced from Cooper JD, Grillo HC: Surg Gynecol Obstet 129:1235, 1969, with permission of the authors and editor.)

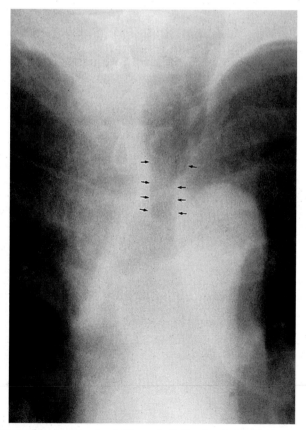

**Figure 52–10. Tracheal Stenosis Following Intubation.** A view of the trachea from a posteroanterior chest radiograph demonstrates focal circumferential tracheal narrowing *(arrows).* The patient was a 45-year-old man who developed tracheal stenosis following intubation for 24 hours.

ble after prolonged intubation, especially if the cuff pressure is not monitored.[184]

Radiographically, postintubation tracheal stenosis extends for several centimeters and typically affects the trachea above the level of the thoracic inlet (Fig. 52–10).[185] The narrowing is often concentric; multiple stenotic areas may occur.[185] Stenosis following tracheostomy typically begins 1 to 1.5 cm distal to the inferior margin of the tracheostomy stoma and involves 1.5 to 2.5 cm of tracheal wall (including two to four cartilaginous rings).[179] Three radiographic appearances have been described: (1) circumferential narrowing of the tracheal lumen over a distance of about 2 cm; (2) a thin membrane or diaphragm (caused by granulation tissue rather than mature fibrous tissue) that may project almost at right angles from the tracheal wall; and (3) a long, thickened, eccentric opacity of soft tissue density that compromises the tracheal lumen.[179] The last named results most often from impingement of the tip of the tracheostomy tube on the tracheal wall (or from an eccentric cuff), so that mucosal necrosis and subsequent fibrosis are local rather than circumferential.

The degree and extent of tracheal narrowing are often difficult to assess on the radiograph and on conventional cross-sectional CT images (Fig. 52–11).[87] With the latter procedure, a focal area of stenosis may be missed, the severity of stenosis may be overestimated, and the cephalocaudad extent is often underestimated.[87] Optimal assessment of focal trachea stenosis requires the use of spiral technique, thin sections (3- to 5-mm collimation), image reconstruction at 1- to 3-mm intervals, and multiplanar reconstructions;[102–106] such procedure allows accurate assessment of the presence, extent and severity of stenosis in most cases (Fig. 52–12).[103]

Occasionally, focal stenosis of the cervical trachea is idiopathic. In one series of 15 patients, the stenosis was 2 to 4 cm long and resulted in a tracheal lumen 3 to 5 mm in diameter at the narrowest portion.[186] The radiologic appearance was similar to that of postintubation or post-traumatic tracheal strictures: the narrowing was circumferential in 8 patients (53%) and eccentric in 7; the margins of the stenosis were smooth in 9 patients (60%) and irregular and lobulated in 6.

Sometimes, thinning of the trachea results in tracheomalacia rather than stenosis, usually as a result of excessive removal of cartilage at the time of tracheostomy or its destruction as a result of pressure and infection.[187, 188] The presence of such tracheomalacia can be missed on CT scans performed at end inspiration,[103] and the diagnosis requires the use of dynamic CT or comparison of images obtained at end inspiration and at the end of maximal expiration.[174] In one investigation of 10 individuals, the cross-sectional area of the intrathoracic trachea decreased by 11% to 61% from TLC to RV;[174] in 1 patient who had tracheomalacia, the tracheal diameter decreased from 256 to 54 mm², an 80% decrease.[174]

Clinically, most patients are symptom free for a variable period after removal of the tracheostomy tube. Eventually, they experience increasing difficulty in raising secretions and note shortness of breath on exertion; these symptoms may progress to stridor and marked dyspnea on minimal exertion.[179] Stridor may not be present at rest but may be noticed with exercise or be brought on by hyperventilation. Symptoms and signs of upper airway obstruction may not become apparent for several weeks, during which time the edema subsides and progressive fibrosis occurs; rarely, symptoms do not appear for many years.[189]

### Tracheal Neoplasms

Compared with the larynx and bronchi, the trachea is a rare site of primary cancer. At the Mayo Clinic, only 53 primary cancers of the trachea were diagnosed over a period

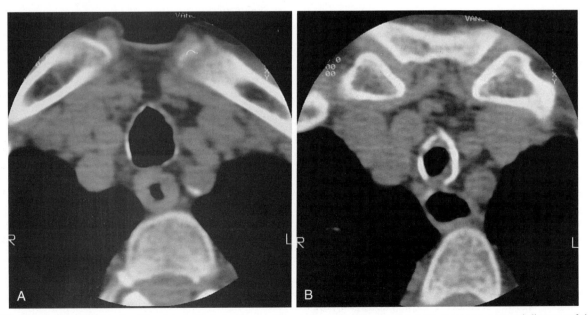

**Figure 52–11. Tracheal Stenosis After Intubation.** A CT scan through the level of the thoracic inlet *(A)* shows a normal diameter of the trachea. A scan at a more caudad level *(B)* demonstrates circumferential narrowing. The patient presented with stridor three months after extubation. (From Kwong JS, Müller NL, Miller RR: Diseases of the trachea and main-stem bronchi: Correlation of CT with pathologic findings. Radiographics 12:645, 1992, with permission.)

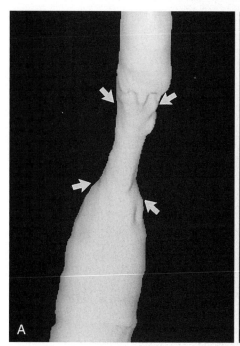
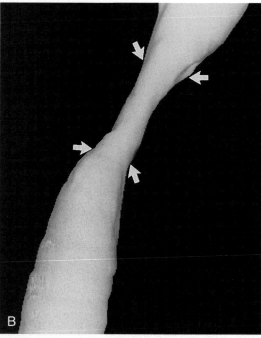

**Figure 52–12. Posttracheotomy Tracheal Stenosis.** Three-dimensional reconstructions from a spiral CT in anteroposterior *(A)* and lateral projections *(B)* demonstrate tracheal stenosis *(between arrows).* The reconstructions were performed using surface shading technique. (Courtesy of Dr. Martine Remy-Jardin, Centre Hospitalier Regional et Universitaire de Lille, Lille, France.)

of 30 years; the relative incidence compared with laryngeal cancer was 1 to 75 and with lung cancer 1 to 180.[190] The most common primary tumor is squamous cell carcinoma (Fig. 52–13), constituting 50% or more of cases in various series and being about four times as common in men as in women.[190–192] Adenoid cystic carcinoma is slightly less common and shows no sex predilection (*see* page 1253). Other neoplasms, such as lymphoma, leukemia, plasmacytoma, benign and malignant soft tissue neoplasms, and other types of primary and secondary carcinomas, are much less common.[193–200]

Radiologically, tracheal tumors manifest as intraluminal nodules that may have smooth, irregular, or lobulated margins or as eccentric or circumferential thickening of the tracheal wall associated with narrowing of the lumen.[98, 201] Benign neoplasms, such as schwannomas, neurofibromas, and leiomyomas, most commonly manifest as well-circumscribed, round soft tissue masses measuring 2 cm or less in diameter (Fig. 52–14).[98] On CT, such lesions are usually sessile or polypoid and do not extend beyond the tracheal wall.[98] Malignant tumors most commonly appear as focal or circumferential tracheal narrowing or as a relatively flat or polypoid mass; most measure between 2 and 4 cm (Fig. 52–15).[98] Associated findings include a paratracheal mass secondary to extratracheal extension, mediastinal lymph node enlargement, pulmonary nodules related to metastases, and, rarely, a tracheoesophageal fistula.[97, 98] CT is helpful in assessing the extent of tracheal neoplasms but may underestimate the cephalocaudad intramural and extratracheal tumor extent and thus not allow reliable distinction of a benign from a malignant process.[94–100] Again, spiral CT is superior to conventional CT.[102–106] Tumor extent can also be assessed using MR imaging.[94, 98] Endotracheal metastases may manifest as single or multiple polypoid lesions (Figs. 52–16 and 52–17).

Patients who have tracheal neoplasms often are treated for asthma for considerable periods of time before the correct

diagnosis is made.[190, 193, 195, 202, 203] Although dyspnea may be noted initially only on exertion, eventually its paroxysmal occurrence at night may suggest the diagnosis of asthma. Hoarseness, cough, and wheeze are common; hemoptysis may also occur. A characteristic wheeze (stridor) may be heard with or without a stethoscope placed over the trachea. The timing of stridor is characteristically inspiratory with extrathoracic lesions and expiratory with intrathoracic lesions. Rarely, granulomas or neoplasms of the trachea may result in hypoventilation, hypoxemia, hypercarbia, pulmonary hypertension, and cor pulmonale.[112, 203]

### "Saber-Sheath" Trachea

In cross-section, the resting trachea is roughly horseshoe shaped, with the open end of the cartilage rings closed by the compliant posterior sheath. Considerable variation exists in the shape of the tracheal cartilage rings, the most common being a C shape; however, U and V shapes also occur.[204, 205] On posteroanterior and lateral radiographs, the coronal and sagittal diameters of the tracheal air column are roughly equal. Occasionally, the coronal diameter is markedly reduced and the sagittal diameter correspondingly increased, a condition called *saber-sheath trachea* (Fig. 52–18). In the initial description of 13 patients who had this condition, the only criterion for selection was an internal coronal diameter of the intrathoracic trachea one half or less of the corresponding sagittal diameter;[206] measurements were made 1 cm above the level of the top of the aortic arch. All patients were men who ranged in age from 52 to 75 years. The coronal tracheal diameter ranged from 7 to 13 mm (mean, 10.5 mm) and the *tracheal index* (the ratio of coronal to sagittal diameter) from 0.5 to 0.25 (mean, 0.4). Generally, the narrow coronal diameter extended the entire length of the intrathoracic trachea; at the thoracic outlet, the coronal diameter abruptly increased and the sagittal diameter narrowed, the air column thus assuming a normal configuration.

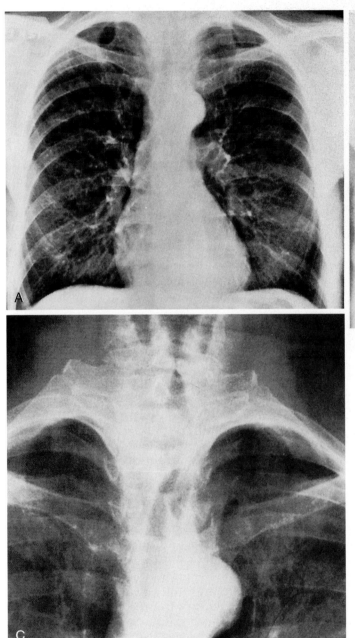

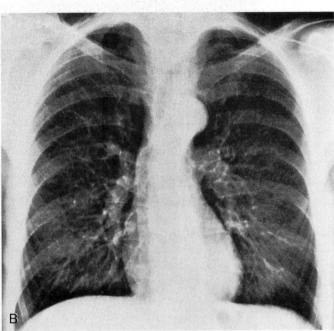

**Figure 52–13. Primary Carcinoma of the Trachea.** At the time of the normal radiograph illustrated in *A,* the patient, a 55-year-old man, had no chest symptoms. Approximately 1 year later, during which time he had noted increasing dyspnea on effort, a radiograph *(B)* revealed an increased thoracic volume, the diaphragm being approximately 2 cm lower than on the previous radiograph. In addition, the air column of the cervical trachea approximately 2 cm distal to the larynx had become markedly narrowed. A large mass can be identified arising from the right wall of the trachea and extending over a distance of at least 3 cm of its length (seen to better advantage in *C*).

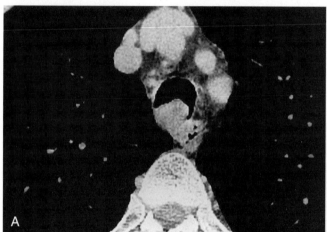

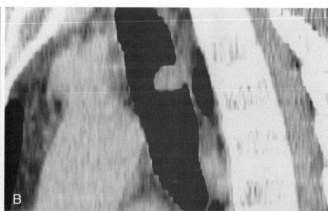

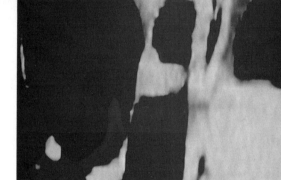

**Figure 52–14. Tracheal Neurilemoma.** A CT scan *(A)* in a 62-year-old man demonstrates a polypoid endotracheal tumor. The origin of the tumor from the posterior lateral walls of the trachea is well shown on the sagittal *(B)* and coronal *(C)* reconstructions from a spiral CT scan. (Courtesy of Dr. Kyung Soo Lee, Department of Radiology, Samsung Medical Center, Seoul, Korea.)

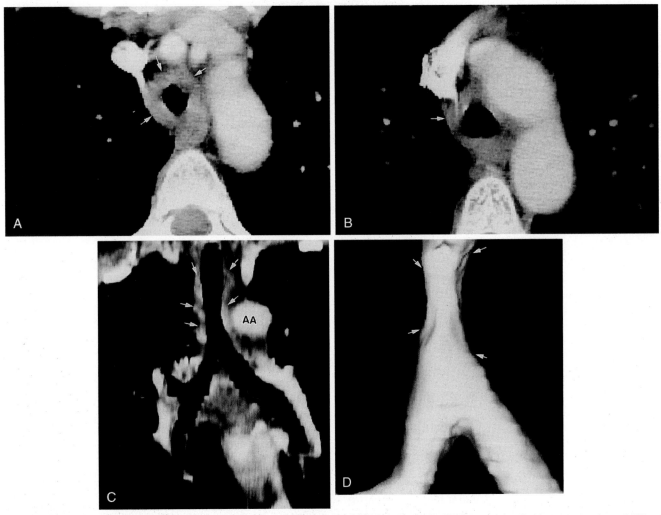

**Figure 52–15. Adenoid Cystic Carcinoma: Spiral CT with Coronal and Three-Dimensional Reconstructions.** Contrast-enhanced CT scans *(A* and *B)* in a 53-year-old woman demonstrate circumferential thickening of the tracheal wall extending for several centimeters *(arrows)* with associated narrowing of the tracheal lumen. The cephalocaudad extension of tumor can be better appreciated on the coronal reconstruction *(C),* which demonstrates tracheal wall thickening *(arrows)* extending from above the level of the aortic arch (AA) to just above the level of the tracheal carina. The patient also had subcarinal lymphadenopathy. A three-dimensional reconstruction using surface-shading technique *(D)* demonstrates the cephalocaudad extent of the tracheal narrowing *(arrows).*

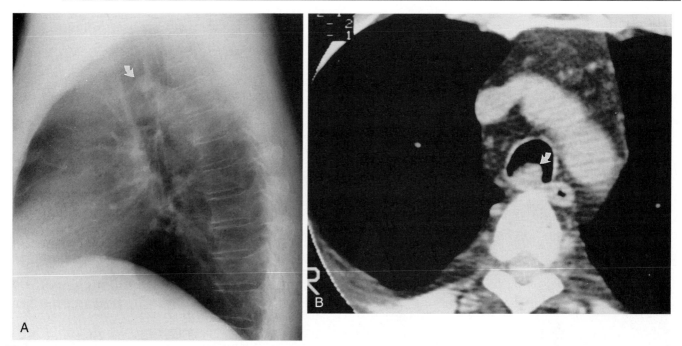

**Figure 52–16. Metastatic Melanoma.** A lateral chest radiograph *(A)* shows a well-defined nodule *(arrow)* arising from the posterior wall of the trachea. A CT scan *(B)* obtained following intravenous administration of contrast demonstrates enhancement of the nodule *(arrow)*. There is no evidence of invasion into contiguous structures. The patient was a 56-year-old man; the diagnosis of metastatic melanoma was proven by endoscopic biopsy. (From Kwong JS, Adler BD, Padley SPG, Müller NL: Diagnosis of diseases of the trachea and main bronchi: Chest radiography vs CT. Am J Roentgenol 161:519, 1993, with permission.)

This abrupt change in configuration from intrathoracic to extrathoracic trachea was a consistent finding and almost certainly reflected the influence of intrathoracic transmural pressures (Fig. 52–19). Rarely, the presence of mediastinal lipomatosis in association with a saber-sheath trachea simulates a mediastinal tumor causing tracheal compression on the chest radiograph; the correct diagnosis can be readily made on CT.[207]

In the investigation of 13 patients cited previously, obvious tracheal ring calcification was identified in 10, and the lateral tracheal walls seemed relatively thick in comparison with normal dimensions.[206] Autopsy examination of 1 patient who died from unrelated causes revealed extensive ossification of the cartilaginous rings associated with a rather rigid deformity, indicating a fixed deformity. All of the initial 13 patients were heavy smokers; 7 had a primary diagnosis of COPD and 10 an "associated diagnosis of chronic bronchitis." Despite this apparent association between chronic air-flow limitation and the saber-sheath tracheal configuration, the investigators felt insecure in establishing a definite relationship between the two conditions because of the small number of patients involved.

A subsequent case-control study was conducted in 60 male patients who had the saber-sheath tracheal configuration and 60 control subjects 50 years of age or older.[208] Of the 60 patients, 57 (95%) had clinical evidence of obstructive airway disease, compared with only 18% of the control subjects. Twenty-six (45%) of the 57 patients who had COPD lacked conventional radiographic evidence of obstructive airway disease; thus, the saber-sheath deformity provided a clue to the presence of COPD when other signs were absent. Although it was not stated whether flow-volume loops were obtained for these patients, it is probable that

they would not have been particularly informative in any event: the almost universal presence of obstructive disease of the lower airways would likely have influenced the results such that a fixed upper airway obstruction would not have been recognized. It remains unclear whether saber-sheath trachea is a result or a cause of airflow obstruction; a number of investigators have suggested that it is a consequence of hyperinflation in patients who have COPD.[209, 210] A saber-sheath trachea can also cause excessive narrowing of a endotracheal tube during surgery.[211]

### Relapsing Polychondritis

Relapsing polychondritis is an uncommon systemic disease that affects cartilage in many sites throughout the body, including the ribs, tracheobronchial tree, ear lobes, nose, and central or peripheral joints. It is now recognized as one of the autoimmune connective tissue diseases, and its characteristics are discussed in greater detail in Chapter 39.

The typical radiographic finding consists of diffuse circumferential narrowing of the trachea and main bronchi;[212–215] CT also demonstrates mild circumferential thickening of their walls (Fig. 52–20).[97, 214, 216] Similar findings are seen on MR imaging.[214] The stenosis can be fixed[97, 214, 216] or variable,[213, 217] single and localized,[218] multiple,[219] or diffuse.[216, 220] "Active" lesions have been reported to take up gallium 67.[221]

The effects on the major airways may be fixed or variable.[217] Variable obstruction is the result of increased compliance and flaccidity, so that the airway readily collapses on expiration, sometimes to such a degree that it causes death. The degree of air-flow obstruction, as judged by a reduced $FEV_1$, may be severe and does not improve

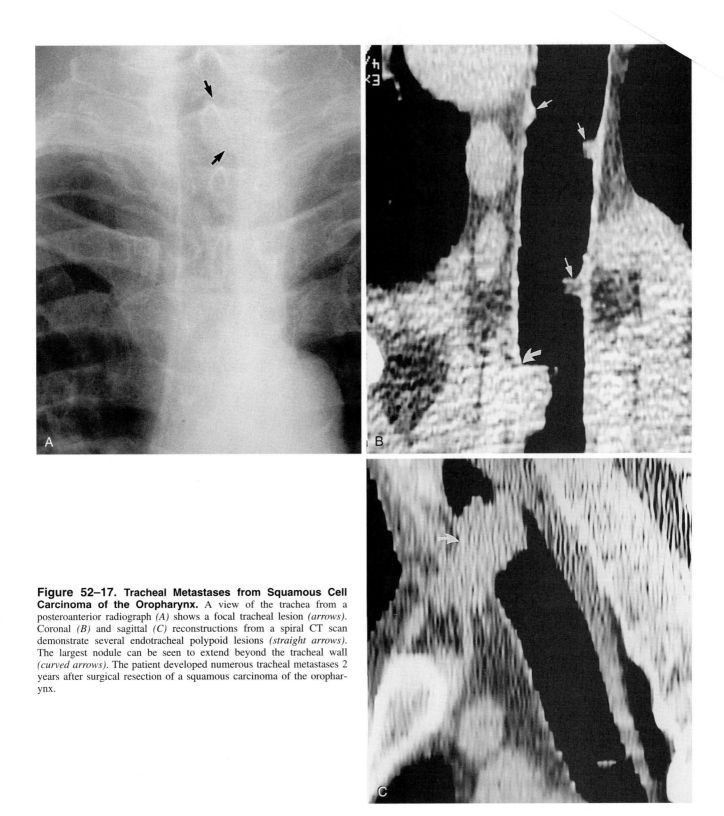

**Figure 52–17. Tracheal Metastases from Squamous Cell Carcinoma of the Oropharynx.** A view of the trachea from a posteroanterior radiograph *(A)* shows a focal tracheal lesion *(arrows).* Coronal *(B)* and sagittal *(C)* reconstructions from a spiral CT scan demonstrate several endotracheal polypoid lesions *(straight arrows).* The largest nodule can be seen to extend beyond the tracheal wall *(curved arrows).* The patient developed numerous tracheal metastases 2 years after surgical resection of a squamous carcinoma of the oropharynx.

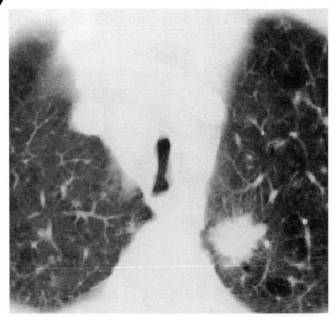

**Figure 52–18. Saber-Sheath Trachea.** A CT scan in a 73-year-old man demonstrates narrowing of the coronal diameter and increase in the sagittal diameter of the trachea. Also note evidence of emphysema and a 2-cm diameter left upper lobe nodule (subsequently shown to be pulmonary carcinoma).

after inhaled bronchodilator administration.[217] In one study of pulmonary function in five patients, flow-volume loops showed a flattening of the expiratory limb compatible with intrathoracic upper airway obstruction; however, in most subjects, there was also a decrease in inspiratory flow.[222]

Respiratory complications have accounted for the cause of 50% of the reported deaths, although they are infrequently the presenting problem.[217, 222, 223] The airway involvement can be rapidly progressive and severe; because a beneficial effect of corticosteroid therapy has been reported, prompt recognition and institution of therapy are important.[224] Rarely, an airway lesion resembling relapsing polychondritis develops without evidence of other cartilaginous involvement or systemic connective tissue disease.[225]

### Tracheobronchopathia Osteochondroplastica

Tracheobronchopathia osteochondroplastica (tracheo-osteoma, tracheitis chronica ossificans, tracheopathia osteoplastica) is a rare condition characterized by the development of nodules or spicules of cartilage and bone in the submucosa of the trachea and bronchi.[226–228] It occurs most frequently in men older than 50 years, although it has been reported in younger individuals and women.[229, 230] In most reported cases, the condition was diagnosed as an incidental finding at autopsy or during bronchoscopy;[231] for example, in a prospective bronchoscopic study of 2,180 patients over an 8-year period, the abnormality was recognized in 9.[227]

The etiology and pathogenesis are unknown. Tracheobronchial amyloidosis can cause airway narrowing (Fig. 52–21) and has been associated with tracheobronchopathia osteochondroplastica in some reports;[232–234] in view of the common occurrence of calcification and ossification in amyloidosis,[235] it has been speculated that tracheobronchopathia

osteochondroplastica may simply represent an end stage of this condition.[232, 234] However, because most cases of the classic disease,[236] as well as occasional examples of apparently early disease,[237] show no evidence of amyloid deposition, it seems unlikely that this is a valid explanation. A more likely hypothesis is that the nodules develop as enchondroses from the tracheobronchial cartilage rings.[236]

Pathologically, the nodules are usually confined to those portions of the tracheal and bronchial walls that normally contain cartilage, showing little or no tendency to develop in the posterior membranous sheath. The cartilaginous and bony masses are submucosal and produce numerous sessile and polypoid elevations that give the trachea and bronchi a beaded appearance at both autopsy and bronchoscopy. Histologically, the nodules are composed of calcified cartilage or bone.[238] Serial sections invariably demonstrate continuity with the perichondrium of the underlying cartilage rings. The rings themselves are often normal but may show focal metaplastic bone formation. The overlying mucosa usually is intact, although it may show squamous metaplasia.

The typical radiographic manifestation consists of nodular or undulating thickening of the tracheal and bronchial walls (Fig. 52–22).[201, 220, 241, 242] Foci of calcification are often not apparent on the radiograph;[220, 243] in fact, it may fail to demonstrate any abnormality.[244, 245] When apparent, the calcification is best seen on a lateral view.[220] Occasionally, the first radiologic abnormalities consist of recurrent pneumonia or atelectasis.[214, 243, 246] The characteristic CT findings consist of nodular thickening of the trachea, resulting in irregular or undulating narrowing of its lumen (Fig. 52–23). In most cases, foci of calcification are also present within the submucosal nodules;[97, 214, 242, 245] occasionally, minimal calcification is evident.[243] These CT abnormalities are typically seen in the anterior and lateral walls of the trachea and spare the posterior membranous portion; in fact, the presence of multiple calcified nodules protruding into the tracheal lumen in this distribution is considered diagnostic of the condition.[214]

Most patients do not have symptoms because the degree of osteochondromatous proliferation is insufficient to cause clinically significant airway narrowing. Occasionally, there is dyspnea, hoarseness, cough, expectoration, wheezing, and hemoptysis.[239, 240, 247] In one review of 15 patients, cough (66%), hemoptysis (60%), dyspnea on exertion (53%), and wheeze (30%) were the most common symptoms.[230] A reported association with nontuberculous mycobacterial infection is probably fortuitous.[248] Pulmonary function studies in one case revealed an increase in TLC and RV and a decrease in FEV$_1$ and maximal breathing capacity.[249]

The diagnosis can be made at bronchoscopy, the spicule-like formations of bone and cartilage producing a grating sensation as the instrument is passed. When the disease affects the more distal cartilaginous bronchi, the submucosal masses may be large enough to obstruct lumens, with resultant atelectasis or obstructive pneumonitis. Rarely, death from such bronchial obstruction has been reported.[149] The differential diagnosis includes amyloidosis, endobronchial sarcoidosis, calcific tuberculosis, papillomatosis, and Wegener's granulomatosis.[250]

### Tracheomalacia

Tracheomalacia (tracheobronchomalacia) is a descriptive term that refers to weakness of the tracheal walls and

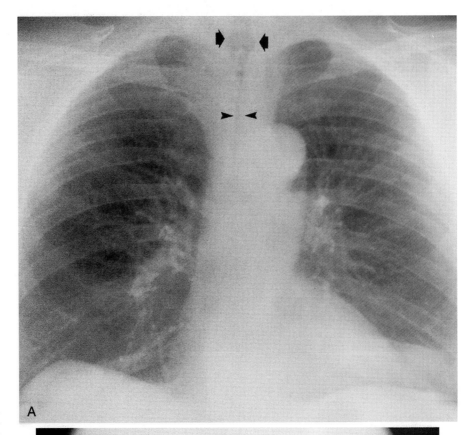

**Figure 52–19. Saber-Sheath Trachea.**
Posteroanterior *(A)* and lateral *(B)* chest radiographs reveal severe narrowing of the intrathoracic trachea in the coronal plane *(arrowheads)* and widening in the sagittal plane *(open arrows),* resulting in an abnormal "tracheal index" of 0.20 or less (see text). Note that the extrathoracic trachea *(arrows)* is normal, the narrowing beginning at the thoracic inlet.

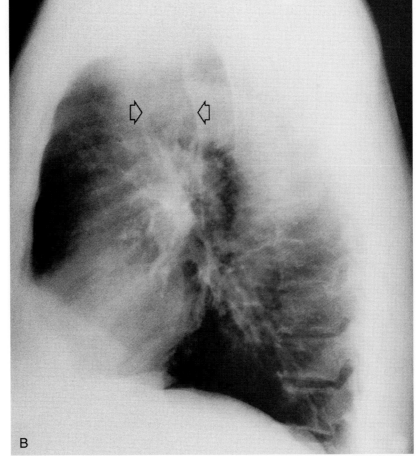

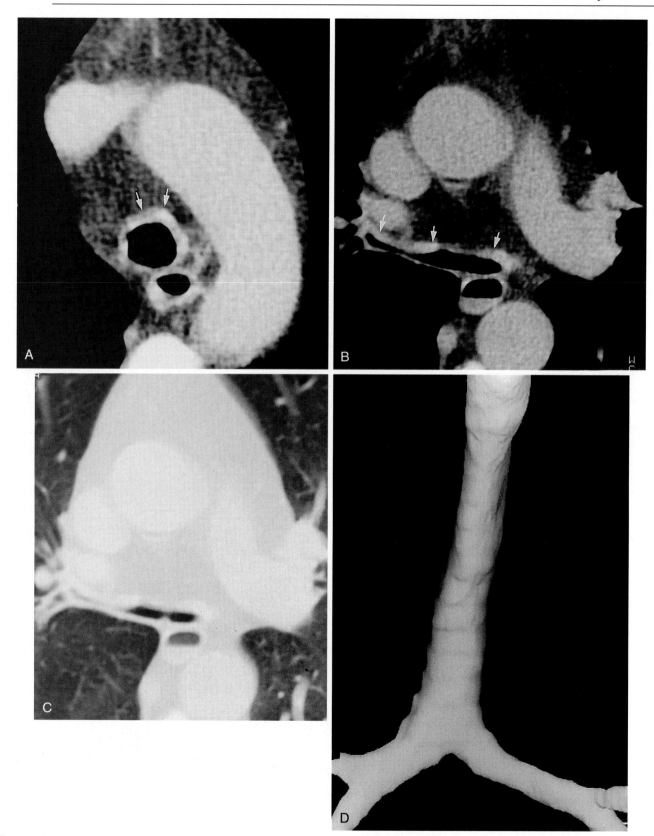

**Figure 52–20. Relapsing Polychondritis.** Spiral CT scans demonstrate mild thickening and calcification of the wall of the trachea *(arrows)* *(A)* and main and right upper lobe bronchi *(B)* *(arrows)*. Lung windows *(C)* demonstrate narrowing of the bronchial lumen. A three-dimensional reconstruction using surface shading technique *(D)* demonstrates relatively mild but extensive narrowing of the trachea and main bronchi, particularly the left. (Courtesy of Dr. Martine Remy-Jardin, Centre Hospitalier Regional et Universitaire de Lille, Lille, France.)

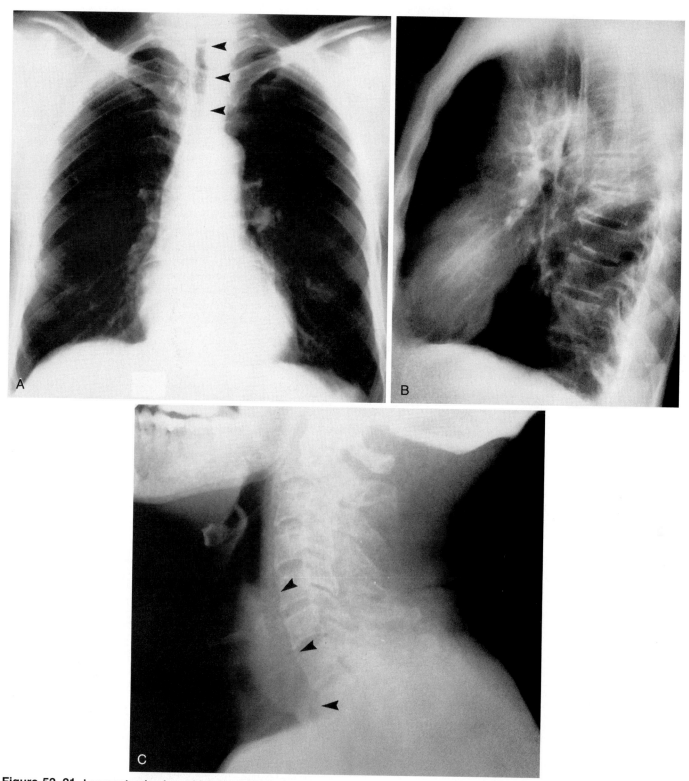

**Figure 52–21. Laryngotracheobronchial Amyloidosis.** Posteroanterior *(A)* and lateral *(B)* chest radiographs reveal diffuse narrowing and internal lobulation of the tracheal air column *(arrowheads)*. The lungs are slightly overinflated, but the pulmonary vasculature is normal. A lateral view of the neck *(C)* shows a posteriorly located laryngotracheal soft tissue mass *(arrowheads)*. Faint stippled calcification is suggested within the lesion. A biopsy of the proximal mass disclosed amyloidosis. The patient was a middle-aged man who had a forced expiratory wheeze.

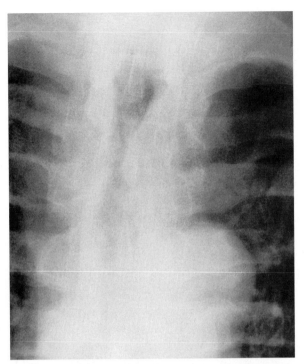

**Figure 52–22. Tracheobronchopathia Osteochondroplastica.** A view of the trachea from a posteroanterior chest radiograph in a 69-year-old man demonstrates irregular narrowing of the trachea. The wall has a nodular appearance; no definite calcification is evident.

supporting cartilage with resultant easy collapsibility. Tracheomalacia may or may not be accompanied by tracheomegaly. It is most often secondary to pressure necrosis of cartilage due to intubation, thyroid lesions,[116, 251] vascular abnormalities,[252] trauma, chronic or recurrent infection, radiation therapy,[152] or relapsing polychondritis.[253] It can also be seen as a primary condition, most often in children and usually associated with a deficiency of cartilage in the tra-

cheobronchial tree.[254–256] In this circumstance, it may be associated with other structural congenital anomalies, including vascular rings, duodenal or esophageal atresia, laryngomalacia, and cleft palate.[257–261] A similar process affecting the cartilage of the larynx, called "laryngomalacia," is the most common cause of stridor in infants.[262]

Unrecognized tracheomalacia can cause life-threatening airway obstruction after surgical repair of congenital esophageal abnormalities.[263] As with tracheobronchomegaly, abnormal flaccidity causes inefficiency of the cough mechanism, resulting in the retention of mucus, recurrent pneumonitis, and bronchiectasis. Symptoms include stridor and shortness of breath. In both tracheomalacia and tracheobronchomegaly, imaging techniques reveal dilation of the conducting airways during inspiration and their premature collapse during expiration.[255, 260, 264] During bronchoscopy of conscious normal subjects, a voluntary cough produces less than 40% narrowing of the anteroposterior tracheal diameter. In patients with acquired tracheomalacia, the narrowing is greater than 50%; in fact, in the presence of severe disease, the anterior and posterior walls can actually come in contact.[265] These changes in tracheobronchial dynamics may be particularly well illustrated cinefluorographically or during dynamic spiral CT,[266] electron-beam CT,[267] or MR imaging.[108a]

### Tracheobronchomegaly

Tracheobronchomegaly (Mounier-Kuhn syndrome) is characterized by dilation of the tracheobronchial tree that may extend all the way from the larynx to the periphery of the lung.[268–270] Although surveys of the literature do not suggest a high prevalence of this disorder,[271] some investigators have found that the condition is an often unrecognized contributor to obstructive lung disease.[264] According to these researchers, the disease occurs predominantly in men, most of whom are in their third and fourth decades of life. Few children or persons who are older than 50 years present,

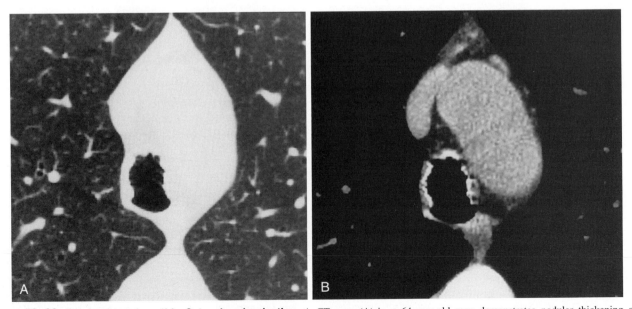

**Figure 52–23. Tracheobronchopathia Osteochondroplastica.** A CT scan *(A)* in a 64-year-old man demonstrates nodular thickening of the tracheal wall. Soft tissue windows *(B)* demonstrate extensive calcification of the submucosal nodules. Note the lack of involvement of the posterior membranous portion of the trachea, a characteristic finding of tracheobronchopathia osteochondroplastica.

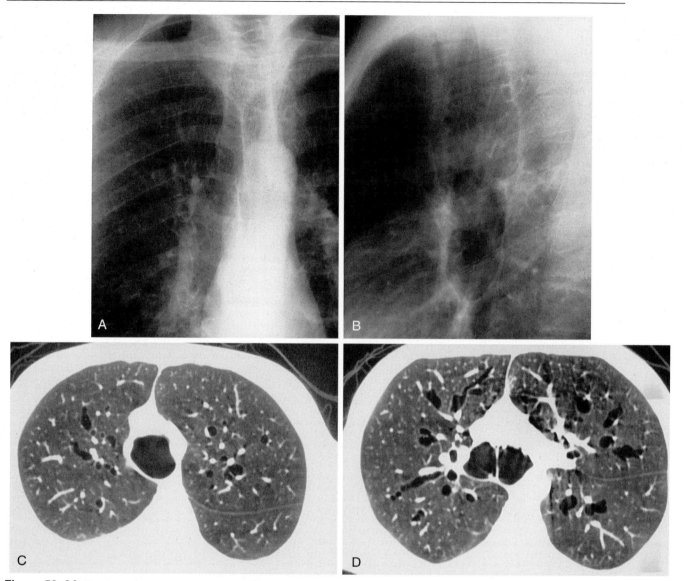

**Figure 52–24. Tracheobronchomegaly.** Views from posteroanterior *(A)* and lateral *(B)* chest radiographs demonstrate marked dilation of the trachea and main bronchi. HRCT scans through the trachea *(C)* and main bronchi *(D)* demonstrate diffuse dilation of the trachea, both main bronchi and intraparenchymal bronchi. Note that the bronchi have thin walls. The trachea measured 3.3 cm in diameter and the right and left main bronchi 3.0 and 3.4 cm, respectively. The patient was a 21-year-old man. (From Kwong JS, Müller NL, Miller RR: Diseases of the trachea and main-stem bronchi: Correlation of CT with pathologic findings. Radiographics 12:645, 1992, with permission.)

although a case has been reported in an 18-month-old child.[272]

The etiology and pathogenesis are unclear. The association of the abnormality with Ehlers-Danlos syndrome has been reported in adults,[273, 274] and it has been found in children who have congenital cutis laxa,[275] suggesting the presence of an underlying defect in elastic tissue. An adult marfanoid patient has been reported who developed hypercapnic respiratory failure secondary to the condition.[276] The abnormality has also been described in combination with congenital syndromes involving multiple skeletal abnormalities, including the Kenny-Caffey[277] and Brachmann–de Lange syndromes.[278] An acquired form of the condition has been reported as a complication of diffuse pulmonary fibrosis[279, 280] and in association with ankylosing spondylitis.[281, 282] Localized disease also has been reported in association with end-stage relapsing polychondritis.[283]

Pathologically, both the cartilaginous and membranous portions of the trachea and bronchi are affected, having thin atrophied muscular and elastic tissue.[284, 285] In one case, marked widening and flaccidity of the posterior membranous sheath of the right main bronchus and, to a lesser extent, the left main bronchus were found at autopsy. A marked decrease in airway smooth muscle and elastic tissue has also been reported in a bronchoscopic biopsy specimen in one patient.[286]

Radiographically, the diagnosis is usually apparent at a glance (Fig. 52–24). The caliber of the trachea and major bronchi generally is increased, and the air columns have an irregular corrugated appearance caused by the protrusion of mucosal and submucosal tissue between the cartilaginous rings (an appearance that has been termed *tracheal diverticulosis*). This appearance is often best visualized in lateral projection.[268, 269] In the appropriate clinical setting, tracheobronchomegaly can be diagnosed from the chest radiograph in women when the transverse and sagittal diameters of the trachea exceed 21 and 23 mm respectively and when the transverse diameters of the right and left main bronchi exceed 19.8 and 17.4 mm, respectively. In men, it can be considered to be present when the transverse and sagittal diameters of the trachea exceed 25 and 27 mm, respectively, and when the transverse diameters of the right and left main bronchi exceed 21.1 and 18.4 mm, respectively.[287]

Both CT and MR imaging can be used to identify the tracheal and bronchial dilation (*see* Fig. 52–24).[97, 288–290] Cinefluoroscopy and dynamic CT demonstrate collapse of the dilated trachea and bronchi on expiration;[290, 291] CT may also reveal dilation of the intrapulmonary bronchi.[97, 292] In patients who have bronchiectasis, the trachea tends to be larger than in normal controls. In one study in which measurement of airway dimensions were made on CT and compared with normal tracheal dimensions derived from radiographs, 7 (17%) of 42 patients who had bronchiectasis were found to fulfill criteria for tracheobronchomegaly, compared with less than 5% of control subjects.[293] In contrast to bronchiectasis, however, the dilated bronchi of patients who have tracheobronchomegaly typically have thin walls.

The increased compliance of the trachea in tracheobronchomegaly results in abnormal flaccidity and easy collapsibility during forced expiration and coughing; the abnormal behavior of the airways can be observed bronchoscopically.[264] In normal subjects, all central airways narrow during coughing, and the resultant increase in the linear velocity of expired air aids in the transport and expectoration of mucus and sputum; however, in tracheobronchomegaly, the trachea is the only portion of the tracheobronchial tree that narrows when pleural pressure increases during coughing. The inefficient cough mechanism leads to retention of mucus with resultant recurrent pneumonia, emphysema, bronchiectasis, and pulmonary parenchymal scarring.[294] It is unclear whether increased large airway compliance is a pathogenetic mechanism in patients who have COPD without an abnormally dilated trachea; at bronchoscopy, many patients who have COPD appear to have an increase in tracheal compliance manifested by large changes in the tracheal cross-sectional area during the respiratory cycle. However, it is unclear whether this is a manifestation of a more collapsible airway or simply reflects the larger pleural pressure swings in these obstructed patients.

Symptoms of tracheobronchomegaly are usually indistinguishable from those of chronic bronchitis or bronchiectasis. However, the presence of prolonged cough and a loud, harsh, rasping sound on auscultation in a patient who complains of inability to expectorate secretions should arouse suspicion of the diagnosis.[266, 285] Pulmonary function tests typically show a decrease in expiratory flow rates,[268] an enlarged dead space, and increased tidal volume.[271]

# REFERENCES

1. Proctor DF: All that wheezes. Am Rev Respir Dis 127:261, 1983.
2. Bass JW, Steele RW, Wiebe RA: Acute epiglottis: A surgical emergency. JAMA 229:671, 1974.
3. Wanner A, Cutchavaree A: Early recognition of upper airway obstruction following smoke inhalation. Am Rev Respir Dis 108:1421, 1973.
4. Evans AS: Clinical syndromes in adults caused by respiratory infections. Med Clin North Am 51:803, 1967.
5. Upper respiratory tract infections (editorial). BMJ 3:101, 1971.
6. Hobson D: Acute respiratory virus infections. BMJ 2:229, 1973.
7. Hable KA, O'Connell EJ, Herrmann EC Jr: Group B coxsackieviruses as respiratory viruses. Mayo Clin Proc 45:170, 1970.
8. Hawley HB, Morin DP, Geraghty ME, et al: Coxsackievirus B epidemic at a boys' summer camp: Isolation of a virus from swimming water. JAMA 26:33, 1973.
9. Deeb ZE. Acute supraglottitis in adults: Early indicators of airway obstruction. Am J Otolaryngol 18:112, 1997.
10. Stone CK, Thomas SH: Upper airway obstruction from tonsillar infection in adults. Eur J Emerg Med 1:37, 1994.
11. Han BK, Dunbar JS, Striker TW: Membranous laryngotracheobronchitis (membranous croup). Am J Roentgenol 133:53, 1979.
12. Seigler RS: Bacterial tracheitis: Recognition and treatment. J S C Med Assoc 89:83, 1993.
13. Valor RR, Polnitsky CA, Tanis DJ, et al: Bacterial tracheitis with upper airway obstruction in a patient with the acquired immunodeficiency syndrome. Am Rev Respir Dis 146:1598, 1992.
14. Manning SC, Ridenour B, Brown OE, et al: Measles: An epidemic of upper airway obstruction. Otolaryngol Head Neck Surg 105:415, 1991.
15. Colt HG, Morris JF, Marston BJ, et al: Necrotizing tracheitis caused by *Corynebacterium pseudodiphtheriticum:* Unique case and review. Rev Infect Dis 13:73, 1991.
16. Schabel SI, Katzberg RW, Burgener FA: Acute inflammation of epiglottis and supraglottic structures in adults. Radiology 122:601, 1977.
17. Ossoff RH, Wolff AP: Acute epiglottitis in adults. JAMA 244:2639, 1980.
18. Shackelford GD, Siegel MJ, McAlister WH: Subglottic edema in acute epiglottitis in children. Am J Roentgenol 131:603, 1978.
19. Nemzek WR, Katzberg RW, Van Slyke MA, et al: A reappraisal of the radiologic findings of acute inflammation of the epiglottis and supraglottic structures in adults. Am J Neuroradiol 16:495, 1995.
20. Rothrock SG, Pignatiello GA, Howard RM: Radiologic diagnosis of epiglottitis: Objective criteria for all ages. Ann Emerg Med 19:978, 1990.
21. Walden CA, Rogers LF: CT evaluation of adult epiglottitis. J Comput Assist Tomogr 13:883, 1989.
22. Connor JD: Evidence for an etiologic role of adenoviral infection in pertussis syndrome. N Engl J Med 283:390, 1970.
23. Connor JD: Communication in answer to a letter re pertussis syndrome. N Engl J Med 283:1174, 1970.
24. Robinson MH, Young JD, Burge PD: Retropharyngeal abscess, airway obstruction, and tetraplegia after hyperextension injury of the cervical spine: Case report. J Trauma 32:107, 1992.
25. Weissler MC, Fried MP, Kelly JH: Laryngopyocele as a cause of airway obstruction. Laryngoscope 95:1348, 1985.
26. Ramadan HH, Tarazi AE, Baroudy FM: Laryngeal tuberculosis: Presentation of 16 cases and review of the literature. J Otolaryngol 22:39, 1993.
27. Hines DW, Haber MH, Yaremko L, et al: Pseudomembranous tracheobronchitis caused by *Aspergillus.* Am Rev Respir Dis 143:1408, 1991.
28. Kemper CA, Hostetler JS, Follansbee SE, et al: Ulcerative and plaque-like tracheobronchitis due to infection with *Aspergillus* in patients with AIDS. Clin Infect Dis 17:344, 1993.
29. Sheffer AL: Urticaria and angioedema. Pediatr Clin North Am 22:193, 1975.
30. Michel RG, Hudson WR, Pope TH: Angioneurotic edema: A review of modern concepts. Arch Otolargyngol 101:544, 1975.
31. Jain M, Armstrong L, Hall J: Predisposition to and late onset of upper airway obstruction following angiotensin-converting enzyme inhibitor therapy. Chest 102:871, 1992.
32. Seidman MD, Lewandowski CA, Sarpa JR, et al: Angioedema related to angiotensin-converting enzyme inhibitors. Otolaryngol Head Neck Surg 102:727, 1990.
32a. Weng PK, Wang HW, Lin JK, Su WY: Late-onset life-threatening angioedema and upper airway obstruction caused by angiotensin-converting enzyme inhibitor: Report of a case. Ear Nose Throat J 76:404, 1997.
33. Gabb GM, Ryan P, Wing LM, et al: Epidemiological study of angioedema and ACE inhibitors. Aust N Z J Med 26:777, 1996.
34. Frank MM, Gelfand JA, Atkinson JP: Hereditary angioedema: The clinical syndrome and its management. Ann Intern Med 84:580, 1976.
35. Winnewisser J, Rossi M, Spath P, et al: Type I hereditary angio-oedema: Variability of clinical presentation and course within two large kindreds. J Intern Med 241:39, 1997.
36. Bissler JJ, Aulak KS, Donaldson VH, et al: Molecular defects in hereditary angioneurotic edema. Proc Assoc Am Physicians 109:164, 1997.
37. Sim TC, Grant JA: Hereditary angioedema: Its diagnostic and management perspectives. Am J Med 88:656, 1990.
38. Bjork L, Svensson H: Upper airway obstruction: An unusual complication following a minor scalding injury. Burns 19:85, 1993.
39. Harjacek M, Kornberg AE, Yates EW, et al: Thermal epiglottitis after swallowing hot tea. Pediatr Emerg Care 8:342, 1992.
40. Cahalane M, Demling RH: Early respiratory abnormalities from smoke inhalation. JAMA 251:771, 1984.
41. Haponik EF, Munster AM, Wise RA, et al: Upper airway function in burn patients: Correlation of flow-volume curves and nasopharyngoscopy. Am Rev Respir Dis 129:251, 1984.
42. Colice GL, Munster AM, Haponik EF: Tracheal stenosis complicating cutaneous burns: An underestimated problem. Am Rev Respir Dis 134:1315, 1986.
43. Waymack JP, Law E, Park R, et al: Acute upper airway obstruction in the postburn period. Arch Surg 120:1042, 1985.
44. Hayden CK Jr, Swischuk LE: Retropharyngeal edema, airway obstruction and caval thrombosis. Am J Roentgenol 138:757, 1982.
45. Hawke M, Kwok P: Acute inflammatory edema of the uvula (uvulitis) as a cause of respiratory distress: A case report. J Otolaryngol 16:188, 1987.
46. Eshagby B, Loeb HS, Miller SE, et al: Mediastinal and retropharyngeal hemorrhage: A complication of cardiac catheterization. JAMA 226:427, 1973.
47. Morris P, Shaw EA: Acute upper respiratory tract obstruction complicating childhood leukemia. BMJ 2:703, 1974.
48. Genovesi MG, Simmons DH: Airway obstruction due to spontaneous retropharyngeal hemorrhage. Chest 68:840, 1975.
49. Duong TC, Burtch GD, Shatney CH: Upper-airway obstruction as a complication of oral anticoagulation therapy. Crit Care Med 14:830, 1986.
50. Waldron J, Youngs RP: Respiratory arrest produced by anticoagulant-induced haemorrhage into parapharyngeal space. J Laryngol Otol 100:857, 1986.
51. Mackenzie JW, Jellicoe JA: Acute upper airway obstruction: Spontaneous retropharyngeal haematoma in a patient with polycythaemia rubra vera. Anaesthesia 41:57, 1986.
52. Tg OL, Kotecha B, Rothera MP: Upper airway obstruction secondary to anticoagulant induced haemorrhage necessitating a tracheostomy. Irish Med J 83:151,1990.
53. Joynt GM, Wickham NW, Young RJ, et al: Upper airway obstruction caused by acquired inhibitor to factor VIII. Anaesthesia 51:689, 1996.
54. Primack SL, Mayo JR, Fradet G: Perforated atherosclerotic ulcer of the aorta presenting with upper airway obstruction. Can Assoc Radiol J 46:209, 1995.
55. Nandapalan V, Dg OS, Siodlak M, et al: Acute airway obstruction due to ruptured aneurysmal arterio-venous fistula: Common carotid artery to internal jugular vein. J Laryngol Otol 109:562, 1995.
56. Meulenbroeks AA, Vos GD, van der Beek JM, et al: An unexpected cause of upper airway obstruction. J Laryngol Otol 109:252, 1995.
57. Brooks JW: Foreign bodies in the air and food passages. Ann Surg 175:720, 1972.
58. Mearns AJ, England RM: Dissolving foreign bodies in the trachea and bronchus. Thorax 30:461, 1975.
59. Given DC, Scott PH, Eigen H, et al: Achalasia and tracheal obstruction in a child. Eur J Respir Dis 66:70, 1985.
60. Handler SD, Beaugard ME, Canalis RF, et al: Unsuspected esophageal foreign bodies in adults with upper airways obstruction. Chest 80:234, 1981.
61. Twigg HL, Buckley CE: Complications of endotracheal intubation. Am J Roentgenol 109:452, 1970.
62. Conrardy PA, Goodman LR, Laing F, et al: Alteration of endotracheal tube position: Flexion and extension of the neck. Crit Care Med 4:7, 1976.
63. Goodman LR, Conrardy PA, Laing F, et al: Radiographic evaluation of endotracheal tube position. Am J Roentgenol 127:433, 1976.
64. Kryger M, Bode F, Antic R, et al: Diagnosis of obstruction of the upper and central airways. Am J Med 61:85, 1976.
65. Empey DW: Assessment of upper airways obstruction. BMJ 3:503, 1972.
66. Miller RD, Hyatt RE: Obstructing lesions of the larynx and trachea: Clinical and physiologic characteristics. Mayo Clin Proc 44:145, 1969.
67. Bass H: The flow volume loop: Normal standards and abnormalities in chronic obstructive pulmonary disease. Chest 63:171, 1973.
68. Al-bazzaz P, Grillo H, Kazemi H: Response to exercise in upper airway obstruction. Am Rev Respir Dis 111:631, 1975.
69. Gibson GJ, Pride NB, Empey DW: The role of inspiratory dynamic compression in upper airway obstruction. Am Rev Respir Dis 108:1352, 1973.
70. Shim C, Corro P, Park SS, et al: Pulmonary function studies in patients with upper airway obstruction. Am Rev Respir Dis 106:233, 1972.
71. Moreno R, Taylor R, Müller N, et al: In vivo human tracheal pressure-area curves using computerized tomographic scans. Am Rev Respir Dis 134:585, 1986.
72. Brown IG, Maclean PA, Webster PM, et al: Lung volume dependence of esophageal pressure in the neck. J Appl Physiol 59:1849, 1985.
73. Gamsu G, Borson DB, Webb WR, et al: Structure and function and tracheal stenosis. Am Rev Respir Dis 121:519, 1980.
74. Vincken W, Dollfuss RE, Cosio MG: Upper airway dysfunction detected by respiratory flow oscillations. Eur J Respir Dis 68:50, 1986.
75. Vincken W, Cosio MG: Flow oscillations on the flow-volume loop: A nonspecific indicator of upper airway dysfunction. Bull Eur Physiopathol Respir 21:559, 1985.
76. Bogaard JM, Hovestadt A, Meerwaldt J, et al: Maximal expiratory and inspira-

tory flow-volume curves in Parkinson's disease. Am Rev Respir Dis 139:610, 1989.

77. Katz I, Zamel N, Slutsky AS, et al: An evaluation of flow-volume curves as a screening test for obstructive sleep apnea. Chest 98:337, 1990.

78. Strieder DJ, Goodman ML: Cough and wheezing with radiologic abnormality involving the trachea. N Engl J Med 293:866, 1975.

79. Clark TJH: Inspiratory obstruction. BMJ 3:682, 1970.

80. Hira HS, Singh H: Assessment of upper airway obstruction by pulmonary function testing. J Assoc Physicians Ind 42:531, 1994.

81. Garcia-pachon E, Casan P, Sanchis J: Indices of upper airway obstruction in patients with simultaneous chronic airflow limitation. Respiration 61:121, 1994.

82. Paré PD, Donevan RD, Nelems JM, et al: Clues to unrecognized upper airway obstruction: A case report. Can Med Assoc J 127:39, 1982.

83. Mellisant CF, Van Noord JA, Van de Woestijne KP, et al: Comparison of dynamic lung function indices during forced and quiet breathing in upper airway obstruction, asthma, and emphysema. Chest 98:77, 1990.

84. Hnatiuk O, Moores L, Loughney T, et al: Evaluation of internists' spirometric interpretations. J Gen Intern Med 11:204, 1996.

85. Millisant CF, Van Noord JA, Van de Woestijne KP, et al: Comparison of dynamic lung function indices during forced and quiet breathing in upper airway obstruction, asthma and emphysema. Chest 98:77, 1990.

86. Sackner MA: Physiologic features of upper airway obstruction. Chest 62:414, 1972.

87. Gamsu G, Webb WR: Computed tomography of the trachea: Normal and abnormal. Am J Roentgenol 139:321, 1982.

88. Curtin HD: Imaging of the larynx: Current concepts. Radiology 173:1, 1989.

89. Phelps PD: Carcinoma of the larynx: The role of imaging in staging and pretreatment assessments. Clin Radiol 46:77, 1992.

90. Hermans R, Verschakelen JA, Baert AL: Imaging of laryngeal and tracheal stenosis. Acta Otorhinolaryngol Belg 49:323, 1995.

91. Becker M, Moulin G, Kurt A-M, et al: Non–squamous cell neoplasms of the larynx: Radiologic-pathologic correlation. Radiographics 18:1189, 1998.

92. Suojanen JN, Mukherji SK, Wippold FJ: Spiral CT of the larynx. Am J Neuroradiol 15:1579, 1994.

93. Glazer HS, Aronberg DJ, Lee JKT, et al: Extralaryngeal causes of vocal cord paralysis: CT evaluation. Am J Roentgenol 141:527, 1983.

94. Shepard JAO, McLoud TC: Imaging the airways: Computed tomography and magnetic resonance imaging. Clin Chest Med 12:151, 1991.

95. Kwong JS, Adler BD, Padley SPG, Müller NL: Diagnosis of diseases of the trachea and main bronchi: Chest radiography vs CT. Am J Roentgenol 161:519, 1993.

96. Manninen MP, Paakkala TA, Pukander JS, et al: Diagnosis of tracheal carcinoma at chest radiography. Acta Radiologica 33:546, 1992.

97. Kwong JS, Müller NL, Miller RR: Diseases of the trachea and main-stem bronchi: Correlation of CT with pathologic findings. Radiographics 12:645, 1992.

98. Mccarthy MJ, Rosado-de-Christenson ML: Tumors of the trachea. J Thorac Imaging 10:180, 1995.

99. Kittredge RD: Computed tomography of the trachea: A review. J Comput Tomogr 5:44, 1981.

100. Spizarny DL, Shepard JAO, McLoud TC, et al: CT of adenoid cystic carcinoma of the trachea. Am J Roentgenol 146:1129, 1986.

101. Morency G, Chalaoui J, Samson L, et al: Malignant neoplasms of the trachea. J Can Assoc Radiol 40:198, 1989.

102. Newmark GM, Conces DJ Jr, Kopecky KK: Spiral CT evaluation of the trachea and bronchi. J Comput Assist Tomogr 18:552, 1994.

103. Whyte RI, Quint LE, Kazerooni EA, et al: Helical computed tomography for the evaluation of tracheal stenosis. Ann Thorac Surg 60:27, 1995.

104. Lacrosse M, Trigaux JP, Van Beers BE, et al: 3D spiral CT of the tracheobronchial tree. J Comput Assist Tomogr 19:341, 1995.

105. Quint LE, Whyte RI, Kazerooni EA, et al: Stenosis of the central airways: Evaluation by using helical CT with multiplanar reconstructions. Radiology 194:871, 1995.

106. Tello R, Kruskal J, Dupuy D, et al: In vivo three-dimensional evaluation of the tracheobronchial tree. J Thorac Imaging 10:291, 1995.

107. Lee KS, Yoon JH, Kim TK, et al: Evaluation of tracheobronchial disease with helical CT with multiplanar and three-dimensional reconstruction: Correlation with bronchoscopy. Radiographics 17:555, 1997.

107a. Remy-Jardin M, Remy J, Artaud D, et al: Volume rendering of the tracheobronchial tree: Clinical evaluation of bronchographic images. Radiology 208:761, 1998.

108. Fletcher BD, Dearborn DG, Mulopulos GP: MR imaging in infants with airway obstruction: Preliminary observations. Radiology 160:245, 1986.

108a. Suto Y, Tanabe Y: Evaluation of tracheal collapsibility in patients with tracheomalacia using dynamic MR imaging during coughing. Am J Roentgenol 171:393, 1998.

109. Capitanio MA, Kirkpatrick JA: Obstructions of the upper airway in children as reflected on the chest radiograph. Radiology 107:159, 1973.

110. Massumi RA, Sarin RK, Pooya N, et al: Tonsillar hypertrophy, airway obstruction, alveolar hypoventilation, and cor pulmonale in twin brothers. Dis Chest 55:110, 1969.

111. Djalilian M, Kern EB, Brown HA, et al: Hypoventilation secondary to chronic upper airway obstruction in childhood. Mayo Clin Proc 50:11, 1975.

112. Lyons HA: Another curse of Ondine. Chest 59:590, 1971.

113. Levy AM, Tabakin BS, Hanson JS, et al: Hypertrophied adenoids causing pulmonary hypertension and severe congestive heart failure. N Engl J Med 277:506, 1967.

114. Walsh RE, Michaelson ED, Harkleroad LE, et al: Upper airway obstruction in obese patients with sleep disturbance and somnolence. Ann Intern Med 76:185, 1972.

115. Kryger M, Quesney LF, Holder D, et al: The sleep deprivation syndrome of the obese patient: A problem of periodic nocturnal upper airway obstruction. Am J Med 56:531, 1974.

116. Newman E, Shaha AR: Substernal goiter. J Surg Oncol 60:207, 1995.

117. Mettam IM, Reddy TR, Evans FE: Life-threatening acute respiratory distress in late pregnancy. Br J Anaesth 69:420, 1992.

118. Miller MR, Pincock AC, Oates GD, et al: Upper airway obstruction due to goitre: Detection, prevalence and results of surgical management. Q J Med 74:177, 1990.

119. Geraghty JG, Coveney EC, Kiernan M, et al: Flow volume loops in patients with goiters. Ann Surg 215:83, 1992.

120. Meysman M, Noppen M, Vincken W: Effect of posture on the flow-volume loop in two patients with euthyroid goiter. Chest 110:1615, 1996.

121. Promisloff RA, Pervall-Phillips GP: Superior vena cava syndrome caused by a benign retrosternal multinodular goiter. J Am Osteopath Assoc 97:409, 1997.

122. Reede DL, Bergeron RT, McCauley DA: CT of the thyroid and other thoracic inlet disorders. J Otolaryngol 11:349, 1982.

123. Reede DL, Whelan MA, Bergeron RT: CT of the soft tissue structures of the neck. Radiol Clin North Am 22:239, 1984.

124. Bashist B, Ellis K, Gold RP: Computed tomography of intrathoracic goiters. Am J Roentgenol 140:455, 1983.

125. Glazer GM, Axel L, Moss AA: CT diagnosis of mediastinal thyroid. Am J Roentgenol 138:495, 1982.

126. Yousem DM: Parathyroid and thyroid imaging. Neuroimag Clin North Am 6:435, 1996.

127. Som PM, Sacher M, Lanzieri CF, et al: Two benign CT presentations of thyroid-related papillary adenocarcinoma. J Comput Assist Tomogr 9:162, 1985.

128. Swartz JD, Yussen PS, Popky GL: Imaging of soft tissues of the neck: Nonnodal acquired disease. Crit Rev Diag Imaging 31:471, 1991.

129. Muysoms F, Boedts M, Claeys D: Intratracheal ectopic thyroid tissue mass. Chest 112:1684, 1997.

130. Brancatisano A, Engel LAV: Role of the upper airway in the control of respiratory flow and lung volume in humans. In Mathew OP, Sant 'Ambrogio G (eds): Respiratory Function of the Upper Airway. New York, Marcel Dekker, 1988.

131. Miller RD, Hyatt RE: Evaluation of obstructing lesions of the trachea and larynx by flow-volume loops. Am Rev Respir Dis 108:475, 1973.

132. Rotman HH, Lisa HP, Weg JG: Diagnosis of upper airway obstruction by pulmonary function testing. Chest 68:796, 1975.

133. Cormier Y, Kashima H, Summer W, et al: Upper airways obstruction with bilateral vocal cord paralysis. Chest 75:423, 1979.

134. Vincken W, Elleker G, Cosio MG: Detection of upper airway muscle involvement in neuromuscular disorders using the flow-volume loop. Chest 90:52, 1986.

135. Knobil K, Becker FS, Harper P, et al: Dyspnea in a patient years after severe poliomyelitis: The role of cardiopulmonary exercise testing. Chest 105:777, 1994.

136. Liistro G, Stanescu DC, Veriter C, et al: Upper airway anesthesia induces airflow limitation in awake humans. Am Rev Respir Dis 146:581, 1992.

137. Caffey J: Pediatric X-ray Diagnosis, 6th ed, Vol 1. Chicago, Year Book Medical Publishers, 1972, p 235.

138. Holinger LD, Tansek KM, Tucker GF: Cleft larynx with airway obstruction. Ann Otol Rhinol Laryngol 94:622, 1985.

139. Williams JL, Capitanio MA, Turtz MG: Vocal cord paralysis: Radiologic observations in 21 infants and young children. Am J Roentgenol 128:649, 1977.

140. Kanner RE: Bilateral vocal cord paralysis for 26 years with respiratory failure. Chest 84:304, 1983.

141. Bogaard JM, Pauw KH, Stam H, et al: Interpretation of changes in spirographic and flow-volume variables after operative treatment in bilateral vocal cord paralysis. Eur Soc Clin Respir Physiol 21:131, 1985.

142. Hillstrom RP, Cohn AM, McCarroll KA. Vocal cord paralysis resulting from neck injections in the intravenous drug use population. Laryngoscope 100:503–6,1990.

143. Levine RJ, Sanders AB, LaMear WR: Bilateral vocal cord paralysis following blunt trauma to the neck. Ann Emerg Med 25:253, 1995.

144. Cormier Y, Kashima H, Summer W, et al: Airflow in unilateral vocal cord paralysis before and after Teflon injection. Thorax 33:57, 1978.

145. Rodenstein DO, Francis D, Stanescu DC: Emotional laryngeal wheezing: A new syndrome. Am Rev Respir Dis 127:354, 1983.

146. Macklem PT, Wang KP, Summer WR: Upper airway obstruction in asthma. Johns Hopkins Med 147:233, 1980.

147. Elshami AA, Tino G: Coexistent asthma and functional upper airway obstruction: Case reports and review of the literature. Chest 110:1358, 1996.

148. Nagai A, Yamaguchi E, Sakamoto K, et al: Functional upper airway obstruction: Psychogenic pharyngeal constriction. Chest 101:1460, 1992.

149. Ophir D, Katz Y, Tavori I, et al: Functional upper airway obstruction in adolescents. Arch Otolaryngol Head Neck Surg 116:1208, 1990.

150. Heiser JM, Kahn ML, Schmidt TA: Functional airway obstruction presenting as stridor: A case report and literature review. J Emerg Med 8:285, 1990.

151. Nahmias J, Tansey M, Karetzky MS: Asthmatic extrathoracic upper airway obstruction: Laryngeal dyskinesis. N J Med 91:616, 1994.

152. Chetty KG, Kadifa F, Berry RB, Mahutte CK: Acquired laryngomalacia as a cause of obstructive sleep apnea. Chest 106:1898, 1994.

153. Gallivan GJ, Hoffman L, Gallivan KH: Episodic paroxysmal laryngospasm: Voice and pulmonary function assessment and management. J Voice 10:93, 1996.

154. Collett PW, Brancatisano T, Engel LA: Spasmodic croup in the adult. Am Rev Respir Dis 127:500, 1983.

155. Pitchenik AE: Functional laryngeal obstruction relieved by panting. Chest 100:1465, 1991.

156. Wood RP, Jafek BW, Cherniack RM: Laryngeal dysfunction and pulmonary disorder. Otolaryngol Head Neck Surg 94:374, 1986.

157. Lisboa C, Jardim J, Angus E, et al: Is extrathoracic airway obstruction important in asthma? Am Rev Respir Dis 122:115, 1980.

158. Higenbottam T: Narrowing of glottis opening in humans associated with experimentally induced bronchoconstriction. J Appl Physiol Respir Environ 49:403, 1980.

159. Collett PW, Brancatisano T, Engel LA: Changes in the glottic aperture during bronchial asthma. Am Rev Respir Dis 128:719, 1983.

160. Campbell AH, Imberger H, Jones M: Increased upper airway resistance in patients with airway narrowing. Br J Dis Chest 70:58, 1976.

161. Higenbottam T, Payne J: Glottis narrowing in lung disease. Am Rev Respir Dis 125:746, 1982.

162. Vincken WG, Gauthier SG, Dollfuss RE, et al: Involvement of upper airway muscles in extrapyramidal disorders: A cause of airflow limitation. N Engl J Med 311:438, 1984.

163. Izquierdo-alonso JL, Martinez-Martin P, Juretschke-Moragues MA, et al: Severe upper airway obstruction in essential tremor presenting as asthma. Eur Respir J 7:1182, 1994.

164. Sabate M, Gonzalez I, Ruperez F, et al: Obstructive and restrictive pulmonary dysfunctions in Parkinson's disease. J Neurol Sci 138:114, 1996.

165. Putman MT, Wise RA: Myasthenia gravis and upper airway obstruction. Chest 109:400, 1996.

166. Smaldone GC, Smith PL: Location of flow-limiting segments via airway catheters near residual volume in humans. J Appl Physiol 59:502, 1985.

167. Wilson TA, Hyatt RE, Rodarte JR, et al: The mechanisms that limit expiratory flow. Lung 158:193, 1980.

168. Osmanliev D, Bowley N, Hunter DM, et al: Relation between tracheal size and forced expiratory volume in one second in young men. Am Rev Respir Dis 126:179, 1982.

169. Montner P, Miller A, Calhoun F, et al: Tracheal diameter as a predictor of pulmonary function. Lung 162:115, 1984.

170. Gibellino F, Osmanliev DP, Watson A, et al: Increase in tracheal size with age: Implications for maximal expiratory flow. Am Rev Respir Dis 132:784, 1985.

171. Griscom N, Wohl ME: Dimensions of the growing trachea related to body height, length, anteroposterior and transverse diameters, cross-sectional area, and volume in subjects younger than 20 years of age. Am Rev Respir Dis 131:840, 1985.

172. Griscom NT, Wohl MEB: Tracheal size and shape: Effects of change in intraluminal pressure. Radiology 149:27, 1983.

173. Moreno R, Taylor R, Müller N, et al: In vivo human tracheal pressure-area curves using computerized tomography scans: correlation with maximal expiratory flow rates. Am Rev Respir Dis 134:585, 1986.

174. Stern EJ, Graham CM, Webb WR, et al: Normal trachea during forced expiration: dynamic CT measurements. Radiology 187:27, 1993.

175. Breatnach E, Abbott GC, Fraser RG: Dimensions of the normal human trachea. Am J Roentgenol 141:903, 1984.

176. Dixon TC, Sando MJW, Bolton JM, et al: A report of 342 cases of prolonged endotracheal intubation. Med J Aust 2:529, 1968.

177. Pearson FG, Goldberg M, da Silva AJ: Tracheal stenosis complicating tracheostomy with cuffed tubes: Clinical experience and observations from a prospective study. Arch Surg 97:380, 1968.

178. Hemmingsson A, Lindgren PG: Roentgenologic examination of tracheal stenosis. Acta Radiol Diagn 19:753, 1978.

179. James AE Jr, MacMillian AS Jr, Eaton SB, et al: Roentgenology of tracheal stenosis resulting from cuffed tracheostomy tubes. Am J Roentgenol 109:455, 1970.

180. Macmillan AS, James AE Jr, Stitik FP, et al: Radiological evaluation of post-tracheostomy lesions. Thorax 26:696, 1971.

181. Klainer AS, Turndorf H, Wu W-H, et al: Surface alterations due to endotracheal intubation. Am J Med 58:674, 1975.

182. Goldberg M, Pearson FG: Pathogenesis of tracheal stenosis following tracheostomy with a cuffed tube: An experimental study in dogs. Thorax 27:678, 1972.

183. Leverment JN, Pearson FG, Fae S: Tracheal size following tracheostomy with cuffed tracheostomy tubes: An experimental study. Thorax 30:271, 1975.

184. Messahel BF: Total tracheal obliteration after intubation with a low-pressure cuffed tracheal tube. Br J Anaesth 73:697, 1994.

185. Goodman LR: Post intubation tracheal stenosis. In Proto AW (ed): Chest Disease (4th series, test and syllabus). Reston VA, American College of Radiology, 1989, p 337.

186. Bhalla M, Grillo HC, McLoud TC, et al: Idiopathic laryngotracheal stenosis: Radiologic findings. Am J Roentgenol 161:515, 1993.

187. Harley HRS: Laryngotracheal obstruction complicating tracheostomy or endotracheal intubation with assisted respiration: A critical review. Thorax 26:493, 1971.

188. Silva LU, Wood GJ: Tracheomalacia from excessive cuff pressure of an endotracheal tube. King Faisal Specialist Hosp Med 4:201, 1984.

189. Mariotta S, Guidi L, Li Bianchi E, et al: Severe subglottic stenosis, well-tolerated for many years. Monaldi Arch Chest Dis 49:403, 1994.

190. Houston HW, Payne WS, Harrison EG Jr, et al: Primary cancers of the trachea. Arch Surg 99:132, 1969.

191. Hadju SI, Huvos AG, Goodner JT, et al: Carcinoma of the trachea: Clinicopathologic study of 41 cases. Cancer 25:1448, 1970.

192. Mccafferty GJ, Parker LS, Suggit SC: Primary malignant disease of the trachea. J Laryngol Otol 78:441, 1964.

193. Garces M, Tsai E, Marsan RE: Endotracheal metastasis. Chest 65:350, 1974.

194. Johnstone RE, Brooks SM: Upper airway obstruction after extubation. JAMA 218:92, 1971.

195. Hakimi M, Pai RP, Fine G, et al: Fibrous histiocytoma of the trachea. Chest 68:367, 1975.

196. Pollak ER, Naunheim KS, Little AG: Fibromyxoma of the trachea: A review of benign tracheal tumors. Arch Pathol Lab Med 109:926, 1985.

197. Slasky BS, Hardesty RL, Wilson S: Tracheal chondrosarcoma with an overview of other tumors of the trachea. J Comput Tomogr 9:225, 1985.

198. Kaplan MA, Pettit CL, Zukerberg LR, et al: Primary lymphoma of the trachea with morphologic and immunophenotypic characteristics of low-grade B-cell lymphoma of mucosa-associated lymphoid tissue. Am J Surg Pathol 16:71, 1992.

199. Prapphal N, Limudomporn S, Watana D, et al: Lymphomatoid granulomatosis with upper airway obstruction: A case report. J Med Assoc Thai 74:526, 1991.

200. Dean MG, Cunningham I, Dao LP, et al: Chronic lymphocytic leukaemia with upper airway obstruction. Leuk Lymphoma 20:505, 1996.

201. Dennie CJ, Coblentz CL: The trachea: Pathologic conditions and trauma. Can Assoc Radiol J 44:157, 1993.

202. Spivey CG Jr, Walsh RE, Perez-Guerra F, et al: Central airway obstruction: Report of seven cases. JAMA 226:1186, 1973.

203. Baydur A, Gottlieb LS: Adenoid cystic carcinoma (cylindroma) of the trachea masquerading as asthma. JAMA 234:829, 1975.

204. Mackenzie CF, McAslan TC, Shin B, et al: The shape of the human adult trachea. Anesthesiology 49:48, 1978.

205. deKock MA: Functional anatomy of the trachea and main bronchi. In deKock MA, Nadel JA, Levis CM (eds): Mechanisms of Airways Obstruction in Human Respiratory Disease. Cape Town, South African Medical Research Council, 1979.

206. Greene R, Lechner GL: "Saber-sheath" trachea: A clinical and functional study of marked coronal narrowing of the intrathoracic trachea. Radiology 115:265, 1975.

207. Hoskins MC, Evans RA, King SJ, et al: "Sabre sheath" trachea with mediastinal lipomatosis mimicking a mediastinal tumour. Clin Radiol 44:417, 1991.

208. Greene R: "Saber-sheath" trachea: Relation to chronic obstructive pulmonary disease. Am J Roentgenol 130:441, 1978.

209. Trigaux JP, Hermes G, Dubois P, et al: CT of saber-sheath trachea: Correlation with clinical, chest radiographic and functional findings. Acta Radiologica 35:247, 1994.

210. Tsao TC, Shieh WB: Intrathoracic tracheal dimensions and shape changes in chronic obstructive pulmonary disease. J Formos Med Assoc 93:30, 1994.

211. Bayes J, Slater EM, Hedberg PS, et al: Obstruction of a double-lumen endotracheal tube by a saber-sheath trachea. Anesth Analg 79:186, 1994.

212. Booth A, Dieppe PA, Goddard PL, et al: The radiological manifestations of relapsing polychondritis. Clin Radiol 40:147, 1989.

213. Goddard P, Cook P, Laszlo G, et al: Relapsing polychondritis: Report of an unusual case and a review of the literature. Br J Radiol 64:1064, 1991.

214. McLoud TC: Diffuse tracheal abnormalities. In Siegel BA (ed): Chest Disease (5th series, test and syllabus). Reston VA, American College of Radiology, 1996, p 259.

215. Dolan DL, Lemmon GB Jr, Teitelbaum SL: Relapsing polychondritis: Analytical literature review and studies on pathogenesis. Am J Med 41:285, 1966.

216. Müller NL, Miller RR, Ostrow DN, et al: Clinico-radiologic-pathologic conference: Diffuse thickening of the tracheal wall. Can Assoc Radiol J 40:213, 1989.

217. Gibson GJ, Davis P: Respiratory complications of relapsing polychondritis. Thorax 29:726, 1973.

218. Mcadam LP, O'Hanlon MA, Bluestone R, et al: Relapsing polychondritis: Prospective study of 23 patients and a review of the literature. Medicine 55:193, 1976.

219. Mohsenifar Z, Tashkin DP, Carson SA, et al: Pulmonary function in patients with relapsing polychondritis. Chest 81:711, 1982.

220. Choplin RH, Wehunt WD, Theros EG: Diffuse lesions of the trachea. Semin Roentgenol 18:38, 1983.

221. Dupont A, Bossuyt A, Sommers G, et al: Relapsing polychondritis: Gallium-67 uptake in recurrent lung lesions. J Nucl Med Allied Sci 27:57, 1983.

222. Mohsenifar Z, Tashkin DP, Carson SA, et al: Pulmonary function in patients with relapsing polychondritis. Chest 81:711, 1982.

223. Tillie-Leblond I, Wallaert B, Leblond D, et al: Respiratory involvement in relapsing polychondritis. Clinical, functional, endoscopic, and radiographic evaluations. Medicine 77:168, 1998.

224. Neilly JB, Winter JH, Stevenson RD, et al: Progressive tracheobronchial polychondritis: Need for early diagnosis. Thorax 40:78, 1985.

225. Higenbottam T, Dixon J: Chrondritis associated with fatal intramural bronchial fibrosis. Thorax 34:563, 1979.

226. Van Nierop MA, Wagenaar SS, Van den Bosch JM, et al: Tracheobronchopathia osteochondroplastica: Report of four cases. Eur J Respir Dis 64:129, 1983.

227. Baird RB, McCartney JW: Tracheopathia osteoplastica. Thorax 21:321, 1966.

228. Bowen DAL: Tracheopathia osteoplastica. J Clin Pathol 12:435, 1959.

229. Vilkman S, Keistinen T: Tracheobronchopathia osteochondroplastica: Report of a young man with severe disease and retrospective review of 18 cases. Respiration 62:151, 1995.

230. Nienhuis DM, Prakash UB, Edell ES: Tracheobronchopathia osteochondroplastica. Ann Otol Rhinol Laryngol 99:689, 1990.

231. Coetmeur D, Bovyn G, Leroux P, et al: Tracheobronchopathia osteochondroplastica presenting at the time of a difficult intubation. Respir Med 91:496, 1997.

232. Sakula A: Tracheobronchopathia osteoplastica: Its relationship to primary tracheobronchial amyloidosis. Thorax 23:105, 1968.

233. Shuttleworth JS, Self CL, Pershing HS: Tracheopathia osteoplastica. Ann Intern Med 52:234, 1960.
234. Alroy GG, Lichtig C, Kaftori JK: Tracheobronchopathia osteoplastica: End stage of primary lung amyloidosis? Chest 61:465, 1972.
235. Weiss L: Isolated multiple nodular pulmonary amyloidosis. Am J Clin Pathol 33:318, 1960.
236. Pounder DJ, Pieterse AS: Tracheopathia osteoplastica: Report of four cases. Pathology 14:429, 1982.
237. Pounder DJ, Pieterse AS: Tracheopathia osteoplastica: A study of the minimal lesion. J Pathol 138:235, 1982.
238. Akyol MU, Martin AA, Dhurandhar N, et al: Tracheobronchopathia osteochondroplastica: A case report and a review of the literature. Ear Nose Throat J 72:347, 1993.
239. Eimind K: Tracheopathia osteoplastica. Nord Med 72:1029, 1964.
240. Clee MD, Anderson JM, Johnston RN, et al: Clinical aspects of tracheobronchopathia osteochondroplastica. Br J Dis Chest 77:308, 1983.
241. Young RH, Sandstrom RE, Mark GJ: Tracheopathia osteochondroplastica: Clinical, radiologic and pathologic correlations. J Thorac Cardiovasc Surg 79:537, 1980.
242. Onitsuka H, Hirose N, Watanabe K, et al: Computed tomography of tracheopathia osteoplastica. Am J Roentgenol 140:268, 1983.
243. Williams SM, Jones ET: Tracheobronchopathia osteochondroplastica. Radiographics 17:797, 1997.
244. Lundgren R, Stjernberg NL: Tracheobronchopathia osteochondroplastica: A clinical bronchoscopic and spirometric study. Chest 80:706, 1981.
245. Mariotta S, Pallone G, Pedicelli G, et al: Spiral CT and endoscopic findings in a case of tracheobronchopathia osteochondroplastica. J Comput Assist Tomogr 21:418, 1997.
246. Hodges MK, Israel E: Tracheobronchopathia osteochondroplastica presenting as right middle lobe collapse: Diagnosis by bronchoscopy and computerized tomography. Chest 94:842, 1988.
247. Park SS, Shin DH, Lee DH, et al: Tracheopathia osteoplastica simulating asthmatic symptoms. Diagnosis by bronchoscopy and computerized tomography. Respiration 62:43, 1995.
248. Baugnee PE, Delaunois LM: *Mycobacterium avium-intracellulare* associated with tracheobronchopathia osteochondroplastica. Eur Respir J 8:180, 1995.
249. Secrest PG, Kendig TA, Beland AJ: Tracheobronchopathia osteochondroplastica. Am J Med 36:815, 1964.
250. Meyer CN, Dossing M, Broholm H: Tracheobronchopathia osteochondroplastica. Respir Med 91:499, 1997.
251. Krishnan H, May RE: An unusual cause for respiratory difficulty after thyroidectomy. Br J Clin Pract 47:47, 1993.
252. van Son JA, Julsrud PR, Hagler DJ, et al: Surgical treatment of vascular rings: The Mayo Clinic experience (see comments). Mayo Clin Proc 68:1056, 1993.
253. Feist JH, Johnson TH, Wilson RJ: Acquired tracheomalacia, etiology and differential diagnosis. Chest 68:340, 1975.
254. Cogbill TH, Moore FA, Accurso FJ, et al: Primary tracheomalacia. Am Thorac Surg 35:538, 1983.
255. Williams H, Campbell P: Generalized bronchiectasis associated with deficiency of cartilage in the bronchial tree. Arch Dis Child 35:182, 1960.
256. Santoli E, Di Biasi P, Vanelli P, et al: Tracheal obstruction due to congenital tracheomalacia in a child: Case report. Scand J Thorac Cardiovasc Surg 25:227, 1991.
257. McDonald-Mcginn DM, Driscoll DA, Bason L, et al: Autosomal dominant "Opitz" GBBB syndrome due to a 22q11.2 deletion. Am J Med Genet 59:103, 1995.
258. Rideout DT, Hayashi AH, Gillis DA, et al: The absence of clinically significant tracheomalacia in patients having esophageal atresia without tracheoesophageal fistula. J Pediatr Surg 26:1303, 1991.
259. Stratton RF, Young RS, Heiman HS, et al: Fryns syndrome. Am J Med Genet 45:562, 1993.
260. Baxter JD, Dunbar JS: Tracheomalacia. Ann Otol 72:1012, 1963.
261. Horns JW, O'Loughlin BJ: Tracheal collapse in polychondritis. Am J Roentgenol 87:844, 1962.
262. Mcclurg FL, Evans DA: Laser laryngoplasty for laryngomalacia. Laryngoscope 104:247, 1994.
263. Corbally MT, Spitz L, Kiely E, et al: Aortopexy for tracheomalacia in oesophageal anomalies. Eur J Pediatr Surg 3:264, 1993.
264. Campbell AH, Young IF: Tracheobronchial collapse, a variant of obstructive respiratory disease. Br J Dis Chest 57:174, 1963.
265. Nuutinen J: Acquired tracheobronchomalacia. Eur J Respir Dis 63:380, 1982.
266. Goh RH, Dobranowski J, Kanaha L, et al: Dynamic computed tomography evaluation of tracheobronchomegaly. Can Assoc Radiol J 46:212, 1995.
267. Kao SC, Kimura K, Smith WL, et al: Tracheomalacia before and after aortosternopexy: Dynamic and quantitative assessment by electron-beam computed tomography with clinical correlation. Pediatr Radiol 25:S187, 1995.
268. Johnston RF, Green RA: Tracheobronchiomegaly: Report of five cases and demonstration of familial occurrence. Am Rev Respir Dis 91:35, 1965.
269. Ettman IK, Keel DT Jr: Tracheal diverticulosis. Radiology 78:187, 1962.
270. Mounier-Kuhn P: Dilatation de la trachée: Constations radiographiques et bronchoscopiques. (Tracheal dilatation: Roentgenographic and bronchographic findings.) Lyon Med 150:106, 1932.
271. Bateson EM, Woo-Ming M: Tracheobronchomegaly. Clin Radiol 24:354, 1973.
272. Hunter TB, Kuhns LR, Roloff MA, et al: Tracheobronchomegaly in an 18 month old child. Am J Roentgenol 123:687, 1975.
273. Aaby GV, Blake HA: Tracheobronchomegaly. Ann Thorac Surg 2:64, 1966.
274. Ayres J, Rees J, Cochrane GM, et al: Hemoptysis and non-organic upper airways obstruction in a patient with previously undiagnosed Ehlers-Danlos syndrome. Br J Dis Chest 75:309, 1981.
275. Wonderer AA, Elliot FE, Goltz RW, et al: Tracheobronchomegaly and acquired cutis laxa in child: Physiologic and immunologic studies. Pediatrics 44:709, 1969.
276. Shivaram U, Shivaram I, Cash M: Acquired tracheobronchomegaly resulting in severe respiratory failure. Chest 98:491, 1990.
277. Sane AC, Effmann EL, Brown SD: Tracheobronchiomegaly: The Mounier-Kuhn syndrome in a patient with the Kenny-Caffey syndrome. Chest 102:618, 1992.
278. Grunebaum M, Kornreich L, Horev G, et al: Tracheomegaly in Brachmann-de Lange syndrome. Pediatr Radiol 26:184, 1996.
279. Woodring JH, Barrett PA, Rehm SR, et al: Acquired tracheomegaly in adults as a complication of diffuse pulmonary fibrosis. Am J Roentgenol 152:743, 1989.
280. Vidal C, Pena F, Rodriguez Mosquera M, et al: Tracheobronchomegaly associated with interstitial pulmonary fibrosis. Respiration 58:207, 1991.
281. Padley S, Varma N, Flower CD: Tracheobronchomegaly in association with ankylosing spondylitis. Clin Radiol 43:139, 1991.
282. Fenlon HM, Casserly I, Sant SM, et al: Plain radiographs and thoracic high-resolution CT in patients with ankylosing spondylitis. Am J Roentgenol 168:1067, 1997.
283. Choplin RH, Wehunt WD, Theros EG, et al: Diffuse lesions of the trachea. Semin Roentgenol 18:38, 1983.
284. Katz I, LeVine M, Herman P: Tracheobronchomegaly: The Mounier-Kuhn syndrome. Am J Roentgenol 88:1084, 1962.
285. Al-mallah Z, Quantock OP: Tracheobronchomegaly. Thorax 23:230, 1968.
286. Van Schoor J, Joos G, Pauwels R: Tracheobronchomegaly: The Mounier-Kuhn syndrome. Report of two cases and review of the literature. Eur Respir J 4:1303, 1991.
287. Woodring JH, Howard R II, Rehm SR: Congenital tracheobronchomegaly (Mounier-Kuhn syndrome): A report of 10 cases and review of the literature. J Thorac Imaging 6f:1, 1991.
288. Rapti A, Drossos C, Tzavelas D, et al: Mounier-Kuhn syndrome (tracheobronchomegaly). Monaldi Arch Chest Dis 50:195, 1995.
289. Dunne MG, Reiner B: CT features of tracheobronchomegaly. J Comput Assist Tomogr 12:388, 1988.
290. Doyle AJ: Demonstration on computed tomography of tracheomalacia in tracheobronchomegaly (Mounier-Kuhn syndrome). Br J Radiol 62:176, 1989.
291. Gay S, Dee P: Tracheobronchomegaly: The Mounier-Kuhn syndrome. Br J Radiol 57:640, 1984.
292. Shin MS, Jackson RM, Ho K-J: Tracheobronchomegaly (Mounier-Kuhn syndrome): CT diagnosis. Am J Roentgenol 150:777, 1988.
293. Roditi GH, Weir J: The association of tracheomegaly and bronchiectasis. Clin Radiol 49:608, 1994.
294. Smith DL, Withers N, Holloway B, Collins JV: Tracheobronchomegaly: An unusual presentation of a rare condition. Thorax 49:840, 1994.
295. Weng PK, Wang HW, Lin JK, Su WY: Late-onset life-threatening angioedema and upper airway obstruction caused by angiotensin-converting enzyme inhibitor: Report of a case. Ear Nose Throat J 76:404, 1997.
296. Woo P: Acquired laryngomalacia: Epiglottis prolapse as a cause of airway obstruction. Ann Otol Rhinol Laryngol 101:314, 1992.
297. Harries PG, Randall CJ: Adult floppy epiglottis: A simple surgical remedy. J Laryngol Otol 109:871, 1995.
298. Gonzalez del Rey J, Cunha C: Cervical lung herniation associated with upper airway obstruction. Ann Emerg Med 19:935, 1990.
299. Bellamy MC, Berridge JC, Hussain SS: Surgical emphysema and upper airway obstruction complicating recovery from anaesthesia. Br J Anaesth 71:592, 1993.
300. Saphir JR, Cooper JA, Kerbavez R, et al: Upper airway obstruction after transesophageal echocardiography. J Am Soc Echocardiogr 10:977, 1997.
301. Woodmansee VA, Rodriguez A, Mirvis S, et al: Genioglossus hemorrhage after blunt facial trauma. Ann Emerg Med 21:440, 1992.
302. Kattan B, Snyder HS: Lingual artery hematoma resulting in upper airway obstruction. J Emerg Med 9:421, 1991.
303. Williams PJ, Jani P, McGlashan J: Lingual haematoma following treatment with streptokinase and heparin: anaesthetic management. Anaesthesia 49:417, 1994.
304. Aiken TC, Collin RC: Acute airway obstruction by laryngeal haematomas in acute immune thrombocytopenic purpura. Postgrad Med J 72:233, 1996.
305. Saunders PR, Macpherson DW: Acute suppurative parotitis: A forgotten cause of upper airway obstruction. Oral Surg Oral Med Oral Pathol 72:412, 1991.
306. Balatsouras DG, Kaberos AK, Eliopoulos PN, et al: Cervicofacial actinomycosis presenting as acute upper respiratory tract obstruction. J Laryngol Otol 108:801, 1994.
307. Goto CS, Abramo TJ, Ginsburg CM: Upper airway obstruction caused by brown recluse spider envenomization of the neck. Am J Emerg Med 14:660, 1996.
308. Madden GJ, Smith OP: Lingual cellulitis causing upper airway obstruction. Br J Oral Maxillofac Surg 28:309, 1990.
309. Bhoopat T, Bhoopat L: Sudden death in Stevens-Johnson syndrome: A case report. Forensic Sci Int 67:197, 1994.
310. Chan TY, Lau MS, Critchley JA: Serious complications associated with Dettol poisoning. Q J Med 86:735, 1993.
311. Joynt GM, Ho KM, Gomersall CD: Delayed upper airway obstruction: A life-threatening complication of Dettol poisoning. Anaesthesia 52:261, 1997.
312. Penfold JB: Lipoma of the hypopharynx. BMJ (Part 1):1286, 1952.
313. Lebargy F, Wolkenstein P, Gissenbrecht M, et al: Pulmonary complications in

toxic epidermal necrolysis: A prospective clinical study. Intensive Care Med 23:1237, 1997.

314. Balazic J, Masera A, Poljak M: Sudden death caused by laryngeal papillomatosis. Acta Otolaryngol Suppl (Stockh) 527:111, 1997.

315. Kashima HK, Mounts SP, Shah K: Recurrent respiratory papillomatosis. Obstet Gynecol Clin North Am 23:699, 1996.

316. Martin KW, McAlister WH: Intratracheal thymus: A rare cause of airway obstruction. Am J Roentgenol 149:1217, 1987.

317. al-Hajjaj MS: Ectopic intratracheal thyroid presenting as bronchial asthma. Respiration 58:329, 1991.

318. Williams JD, Sclafani AP, Slupchinskij O, et al: Evaluation and management of the lingual thyroid gland. Ann Otol Rhinol Laryngol 105:312, 1996.

319. Gelder CM, Hetzel MR: Primary tracheal tumours: A national survey. Thorax 48:688, 1993.

320. Howard DJ, Haribhakti VV: Primary tumours of the trachea: Analysis of clinical features and treatment results. J Laryngol Otol 108:230, 1994.

321. Wiltshaw E: The natural history of extramedullary plasmacytoma and its relation to solitary myeloma of bone and myelomatosis. Medicine 55:217, 1976.

322. Brandwein M, LeBenger J, Strauchen J, et al: Atypical granular cell tumor of the larynx: An unusually aggressive tumor clinically and microscopically. Head Neck 12:154, 1990.

323. Stack PS, Steckler RM: Tracheal neurilemmoma: Case report and review of the literature. Head Neck 12:436, 1990.

324. Pulli RS, Coniglio JU: Subglottic nerve sheath tumor in a pediatric patient: Case report and literature review. Head Neck 19:440, 1997.

325. Brandwein M, Huvos A: Laryngeal oncocytic cystoadenomas: Eight cases and a literature review. Arch Otolaryngol Head Neck Surg 121:1302, 1995.

326. Tan KK, Abraham KA, Yeoh KH: Lipoma of hypopharynx. Singapore Med J 35:219, 1994.

327. Mouchloulis G, Irving RM, Grant HR, et al: Laryngeal Kaposi's sarcoma in patients with AIDS. J Laryngol Otol 110:1034, 1996.

328. Beitler AJ, Ptaszynski K, Karpel JP: Upper airway obstruction in a woman with AIDS-related laryngeal Kaposi's sarcoma. Chest 109:836, 1996.

329. Johnson DB, McGrath F, Ryan MJ: Laryngeal chondroma: An unusual cause of upper airway obstruction. Clin Radiol 50:412, 1995.

330. Tsumori T, Nakao K, Miyata M, et al: Clinicopathologic study of thyroid carcinoma infiltrating the trachea. Cancer 56:2843, 1985.

331. Sons HU, Borchard F: Esophageal cancer. Arch Pathol Lab Med 108:983, 1984.

332. Colohan DP, Hillborn M: An unusual case of intermittent upper airway obstruction. J Emerg Med 11:157, 1993.

333. Strachan D, Wengraf C: An unusual thyroglossal cyst causing upper airway obstruction. Br J Clin Pract 50:472, 1996.

334. Lippmann M, Solit R, Goldberg SK, et al: Mediastinal bronchogenic cyst: A cause of upper airway obstruction. Chest 102:1901, 1992.

335. Allen SJ, Koch SSM, Tonnesen AS, et al: Tracheal compression caused by traumatic thoracic duct leak. Chest 106:296, 1994.

336. Theaker NJ, Brady PW, Fisher MM: Postesophagectomy mediastinal chylothorax causing upper airway obstruction misdiagnosed as asthma: A report of two cases. Chest 111:1126, 1997.

337. Thomas DM, Madden GJ: Bilateral laryngoceles. Ear Nose Throat J 72:819, 1993.

338. Kandora TF, Gilmore IM, Sorber JA, et al: Cricoarytenoid arthritis presenting as cardiopulmonary arrest. Ann Emerg Med 14:700, 1985.

339. el-Sheikh MM, Medra AM, Warda MH: Bird face deformity secondary to bilateral temporomandibular joint ankylosis. J Craniomaxillofac Surg 24:96, 1996.

340. Solomons NB, Linton DM, Potgieter PD: Cervical osteophytes and respiratory failure: An unusual case of upper airway obstruction. S Afr Med J 71:259, 1987.

341. Demuynck K, Van Calenbergh F, Goffin J, et al: Upper airway obstruction caused by a cervical osteophyte. Chest 108:283, 1995.

342. Sidi J, Hadar T, Shvero J, et al: Respiratory distress due to diffuse cervical hyperostosis. Ann Otol Rhinol Laryngol 96:178, 1987.

343. Benisch BM, Wood WG, Kroeger GB, et al: Focal muscular hyperplasia of the trachea. Arch Otolaryngol 99:226, 1974.

344. Morewood DJ, Belchetz PE, Evans CC, et al: The extrathoracic airway in acromegaly. Clin Radiol 37:243, 1986.

345. Murrant NJ, Gatland DJ: Respiratory problems in acromegaly. J Laryngol Otol 104:52, 1990.

346. Breuer R, Simpson GT, Rubinow A, et al: Tracheobronchial amyloidosis: Treatment by carbon dioxide laser photoresection. Thorax 40:870, 1985.

347. Woo KS, Van Hasselt CA, Waldron J: Laser resection of localized subglottic amyloidosis. J Otolaryngol 19:337, 1990.

348. Belani KG, Krivit W, Carpenter BL, et al: Children with mucopolysaccharidosis: Perioperative care, morbidity, mortality, and new findings. J Pediatr Surg 28:403; discussion 408, 1993.

349. Bredenkamp JK, Smith ME, Dudley JP, et al: Otolaryngologic manifestations of the mucopolysaccharidoses. Ann Otol Rhinol Laryngol 101:472, 1992.

350. Miller A, Brown LK, Teirstein AS, et al: Stenosis of main bronchi mimicking fixed upper airway obstruction in sarcoidosis. Chest 88:244, 1985.

351. Morris CJ, Byrd RP, Roy TM: Wegener's granulomatosis presenting as subglottic stenosis. J Ky Med Assoc 88:547, 1990.

352. Rickli H, Fretz C, Hoffman M, et al: Severe inflammatory upper stenosis in ulcerative colitis. Eur Respir J 7:1899, 1994.

353. Mandell GA, McNicholas KW, Padman R, et al: Innominate artery compression of the trachea: Relationship to cervical herniation of the normal thymus. Radiology 190:131, 1994.

354. Maayan C, Mogle P, Tal A, et al: Prolonged wheezing and tracheal compression caused by an aberrant right subclavian artery. Thorax 36:793, 1981.

355. van Son JA, Julsrud PR, Hagler DJ, et al: Surgical treatment of vascular rings: The Mayo Clinic experience (see comments). Mayo Clin Proc 68:1056, 1993.

356. MacGillivray RG: Tracheal compression caused by aneurysms of the aortic arch: Implications for the anaesthetist. Anaesthesia 40:270, 1985.

357. Rimell FL, Shapiro AM, Shoemaker DL, et al: Head and neck manifestations of Beckwith-Wiedemann syndrome. Otolaryngol Head Neck Surg 113:262, 1995.

358. Jacobs IN, Gray RF, Todd NW: Upper airway obstruction in children with Down syndrome. Arch Otolaryngol Head Neck Surg 122:945, 1996.

359. Thompson JW, Ahmed AR, Dudley JP: Epidermolysis bullosa dystrophica of the larynx and trachea: Acute airway obstruction. Ann Otol 89:428, 1980.

360. Turkot S, Golzman B, Kogan J, et al: Acute upper-airway obstruction in a patient with achalasia. Ann Emerg Med 29:687, 1997.

361. Bolger WE, West CB Jr, Parsons DS, et al: Upper airway obstruction due to massive gingival hyperplasia: A case report and description of a new surgical treatment. Int J Pediatr Otorhinolaryngol 19:63, 1990.

362. Armstrong WB, Peskind SSP, Bressler KL, et al: Airway obstruction secondary to rhinoscleroma during pregnancy. Ear Nose Throat J 74:768, 1995.

363. Nienhuis DM, Prakash UB, Edell ES: Tracheobronchopathia osteochondroplastica. Ann Otol Rhinol Laryngol 99:689, 1990.

364. Amoils CP, Shindo ML: Laryngotracheal manifestations of rhinoscleroma. Ann Otol Rhinol Laryngol 105:336, 1996.

# Obstructive Sleep Apnea

A variety of respiratory disorders manifest themselves during sleep. A comprehensive review of the measurements, definitions, and severity ratings pertaining to such sleep-disordered breathing has been published;[1] the definitions that follow are derived largely from this consensus view. *Obstructive apnea* is an event characterized by complete closure of the upper airway; air flow is prevented despite continued respiratory efforts and lasts at least 10 seconds. *Central apnea* is characterized by the absence of both air flow and respiratory effort for at least 10 seconds. *Hypopnea* can be defined as a transient reduction in, but not a complete cessation of, breathing; hypopneas may be central or obstructive, the only reliable method of differentiating them being simultaneous measurement of esophageal pressure. In this chapter, we confine ourselves to the disorders that cause narrowing or obstruction of the airway during sleep and result in obstructive hypopnea or apnea. Central apnea is related to abnormalities of the respiratory control centers in the pons and medulla and is discussed in Chapter 79 (*see* page 3052).

As the name suggests, obstructive apnea is secondary to physical limitation in air flow, usually located in the upper respiratory tract. A mixed apnea is one that begins with a cessation of respiratory effort but continues during increasing respiratory efforts against a closed airway. Purely obstructive and mixed apneas characterize patients who have the obstructive sleep apnea–hypopnea syndrome. The latter is characterized by recurrent episodes of upper airway obstruction during sleep that usually result in oxygen desaturation (3% or greater decrease from baseline), recurrent arousals, and daytime symptoms.[1] Our knowledge of this abnormality has increased markedly since the 1970s, and the diagnosis and management of affected patients has achieved virtual subspecialty status among respiratory physicians. To understand its pathophysiology, it is necessary to have some knowledge of the physiologic interactions between sleep and breathing, because the former has profound effects on respiratory system mechanics, the control of breathing, metabolism, and hemodynamics.

## PHYSIOLOGIC CHARACTERISTICS OF NORMAL SLEEP

Sleep is categorized as either non–rapid eye movement (NREM) or rapid eye movement (REM) based on the electroencephalographic pattern (*see* farther on) and on the presence or absence of rapid phasic eye movements on an electro-oculogram. NREM sleep is in turn subdivided into four stages in which progressively slower electroencephalographic activity is associated with specific events termed *sleep spindles* and *K complexes*:[2] stages 1 and 2 make up light sleep, during which breathing is unsteady and irregular; stages 3 and 4 make up slow-wave sleep, during which breathing is at its most regular. During the initial 10 to 60 minutes of sleep, frequent changes occur between wakefulness and stages 1 and 2; this unsteady phase of NREM sleep is associated with periodic breathing. Major cyclic variations occur in tidal volume ($V_T$), and the breathing pattern may resemble Cheyne-Stokes or Biot's breathing.*

The periods of relative hyperpnea may be followed by brief central apneas, that is, cessation of ventilation without respiratory effort. The oscillations in breathing patterns correlate with oscillations in sleep stage and are probably related to differences in the setpoint for regulation of ventilation in the awake and asleep states.[2] During unsteady NREM sleep, the average minute ventilation ($V_E$) decreases and alveolar and arterial $P_{CO_2}$ increase slightly.

---

*\*Biot's breathing* is characterized by irregular periods of apnea alternating with periods in which four or five breaths of identical depth are taken; it is seen in patients who have increased intracranial pressure and at high altitudes.

    *Cheyne-Stokes respiration* is a breathing pattern characterized by a cyclic fluctuation in ventilation, in which periods of central apnea or hypopnea alternate with periods of hyperpnea in a gradual crescendo and decrescendo fashion.[1]

Coincident with the onset of steady NREM sleep (stages 3 and 4), breathing becomes remarkably regular, although $V_T$ and overall $V_E$ decrease further as a result of a decrease in $V_T/T_I$ (mean inspiratory flow) with little or no change in the ratio of inspiratory time to total respiratory cycle time (duty cycle). The decrease in ventilation ranges from 5% to 30% of awake $V_E$; although part of this decrease is related to a decreased metabolic rate, there is net alveolar hypoventilation as reflected in an increase in end-tidal $PaCO_2$ of 2 to 7 mm Hg.[3–5] The decrease in $V_T$ during NREM sleep is not caused by a decrease in respiratory muscle activity as measured by electromyographic activity; in fact, electromyographic activity of the intercostal muscles may actually increase during this stage.[6] Despite preserved muscle activation, a decrease in $V_E$ suggests increased impedance; during sleep, upper airway resistance increases by more than 50%, whereas lower airway resistance does not change.[7] The increased upper airway resistance is caused by decreased activation of the upper airway dilating and stabilizing muscles—the superior and inferior hyoid, the genioglossus, and the tensor palatini. In normal individuals, tensor palatini electromyographic activity decreases progressively from wakefulness to stages 3 and 4 of NREM sleep as upper airway resistance increases; the decreased neural input renders the upper airway more collapsible.[8]

Breathing becomes irregular again with the onset of REM sleep. $V_T$ decreases concomitantly with the development of episodes of REMs, and an irregular pattern of rapid shallow breathing is observed. In contrast to NREM sleep, there is a substantial decrease in intercostal electromyographic activation and in the contribution of rib cage expansion to $V_T$. Although diaphragmatic electromyographic activity may increase, there is a further overall decrease in $V_E$ with considerable fluctuation in breath-by-breath alveolar ventilation. The decreased intercostal activation is secondary to the generalized supraspinal inhibition of alpha–motor neuron drive and the depression of fusimotor function that occurs during REM sleep. The resultant muscular atonia affects most skeletal muscles, including those in the upper airways, resulting in a further increase in upper airway resistance.[2]

Ventilatory chemosensitivity decreases during all stages of sleep, both hypoxic and hypercapnic ventilatory responses being depressed. The slope describing the relationship between change in arterial oxygen saturation ($SaO_2$) and ventilation is a useful index of ventilatory chemosensitivity to hypoxia; it can decrease by one third to one half of its value during wakefulness, a drop that is particularly prominent in men.[9] Depression in the slope of the relationship between changes in $PCO_2$ and changes in ventilation that characterizes the hypercapnic response is similar in both men and women. In general, the depression in chemosensitivity is more pronounced during REM than during NREM sleep. Besides the decreased ventilatory response to $CO_2$ that accompanies the deeper stages of sleep, NREM sleep is associated with a change in the $CO_2$ apnea threshold. During wakefulness and REM sleep, the arterial $PCO_2$ can be lowered 10 to 20 mm Hg before ventilation ceases, whereas in NREM sleep, apnea occurs when the $PaCO_2$ is decreased by only 2 to 4 mm Hg.[10, 11] This increase in the apnea threshold can lead to instability of the respiratory pattern, periodic breathing, and obstructive apneas.

During wakefulness, the addition of an external resistive load results in rapid adjustment in ventilatory drive so that $V_T$ and $V_E$ are restored to their baseline values; this load detection is dependent on lung and chest wall afferent input. During sleep, the compensatory response to added external resistive loads is diminished. The effectiveness of load compensation during loaded breathing can be tested by occluding the airway and measuring the pressures generated in the first 0.1 second (P 0.1) of the occluded breath; during resistive loading, P 0.1 does not increase as much during sleep as it does during the awake state, indicating that the compensatory mechanisms that adjust for increased impedance are diminished.[9]

Thus, sleep is a time of particular vulnerability for the respiratory system—the resistance of the system is increased and at the same time both chemical and mechanical sensors are depressed. There is also a decrease in the rate of mucociliary clearance and a depression in the cough threshold. The ultimate safeguard is arousal, which results in a rapid decrease in upper airway resistance and an increase in sensitivity of the chemical and mechanical responses.[12] Alteration in arterial blood gases is relatively ineffective in causing arousal during sleep;[9, 13, 14] for example, in some individuals, arterial $PO_2$ values as low as 40 mm Hg do not induce arousal. Arousal is defined as the simultaneous presence of electromyographic activation, eye movements, and alpha encephalographic activity, that is, a short neurologic awakening; when these persist for longer than 15 seconds, they constitute a true awakening. To induce wakefulness in normal individuals, an increase in $PCO_2$ of 15 mm Hg or more may be required. Considerable individual variation exists in the threshold for arousal in response to changes in blood gases or in response to added loads, this variation in responsiveness may be an important risk factor for obstructive sleep apnea (OSA).

## EPIDEMIOLOGY

The prevalence of OSA in the general population is unclear and is very dependent on the diagnostic threshold selected.[15, 16] Epidemiologic surveys have been of three types:[17] (1) studies based solely on questionnaire data concerning habitual snoring, witnessed apneas, or both; (2) studies in which positive responses to questionnaires are followed up with full polysomnography; and (3) studies in which most or all subjects undergo a full sleep study or some form of nocturnal respiratory monitoring. The prevalence of OSA in these studies has ranged from less than 1% to higher than 10%, higher figures tending to be found using the third study design. The variability of prevalence estimates is also related to the lack of a precise definition of OSA. For example, based solely on a telephone interview and on a definition of OSA as habitual snoring, breathing pauses during sleep, and daytime drowsiness, 3.5% of men and 1.5% of women were felt to have OSA syndrome in the United Kingdom.[18] However, when the condition is defined more precisely as more than five apneas per hour of sleep (apnea being defined as the cessation of breathing for greater

**Table 53–1. SEVERITY OF OBSTRUCTIVE SLEEP APNEA**

| EVALUATION CRITERIA | MILD | MODERATE | SEVERE |
|---|---|---|---|
| Apnea-hypopnea index | 5–19 | 20–49 | > 50 |
| Min SaO$_2$ (%) | 80–90 | 70–79 | < 70 |

Min SaO$_2$ (%) = minimum oxygen saturation.

Modified from Chervin RD, Guilleminault C: Obstructive sleep apnea and related disorders. Neurol Clin 14:583, 1996.

than 10 seconds*), OSA was identified in approximately 11% of men and 6% of women in a study of 1,504 Danes.[19]

The previous definition has been modified to include the frequency of apneas and "hypopneas," which are defined as periods of nocturnal hypoventilation associated with a decrease in SaO$_2$ of 4% or greater[22] or with a significant reduction in thoracoabdominal movement.[23] The degree of OSA can be quantified as the apnea index (AI), the apnea-hypopnea index (AHI), or the respiratory disturbance index (RDI), the last being defined as the average number of apneas plus hypopneas per hour of sleep (Table 53–1). An AHI of greater than 10 is now more often used as the cut-off for definition of OSA in epidemiologic and clinical studies. Using this definition, estimates of prevalence have been 2.7% in a study of 1,510 Italian men,[24] 10% of men and 7% of women in an investigation of 400 Australian adults,[25] and 8% of men and 2.3% of women in a study of 263 American adults.[26] In the Wisconsin Sleep Cohort Study, a random sample of 602 working men and women aged 30 to 60 years was studied using overnight polysomnography; 9% of men had 15 or more episodes of apnea or hypopnea per hour of sleep. By applying a more conservative set of diagnostic criteria, the investigators concluded that 4% of men and 2% of women in the workplace suffer from OSA. In one small "population" study of 46 healthy men who snored, 13% had an AI of more than 5;[27] however, even in this "asymptomatic" group, apneic severity correlated with elevated blood pressures and with subjective evidence of sleepiness and napping frequency, suggesting that "subclinical" levels of sleep apnea may not be completely benign. The calculated prevalence decreases when the consequences of OSA are included in the definition; for example, in one Spanish study the prevalence was 2.2% among adult men and 0.8% among women when severe snoring plus excessive daytime sleepiness were added to polysomnographic indices of diagnosis.[28]

The estimated prevalence of OSA is also strongly influenced by the age, sex, and ethnicity of the study population.[17, 29, 30] For example, in one study, 80% of elderly subjects suffered more than five apneas an hour, although only a small number of these had significant clinical symptoms.[31] Using home monitoring of SaO$_2$, 16% of 40- to 64-year-old Hispanics and "other racial minorities" in the United States were found to have greater than 20 events (> 4% decrease in SaO$_2$) per hour compared with 4.9% of non-Hispanic

whites.[32] In another investigation, the odds ratio for an increased apnea index was 1.9 in African Americans even after correction for risk factors such as obesity, sex, and familial clustering; the risk was especially pronounced in younger individuals.[33] The prevalence of OSA is higher during early childhood[34] and old age.[35]

A great variety of conditions predispose to the development of OSA (Table 53–2), the most important of which is obesity. When the patient sample is made up of individuals recruited from a sleep clinic, 60% to 90% of those diagnosed as having OSA are obese (defined as a body mass index [BMI] greater than 28 kg/m$^2$).[16] Even more powerful than BMI as a predictor of OSA are measures that suggest central and visceral obesity, such as increased waist-to-hip ratio

**Table 53–2. CONDITIONS ASSOCIATED WITH OBSTRUCTIVE SLEEP APNEA**

| CONDITION | SELECTED REFERENCE |
|---|---|
| *Neurologic* | |
| Alzheimer's disease | 388 |
| Parkinson's disease | 389 |
| Syringomyelia | |
| Arnold-Chiari malformation | 390 |
| Poliomyelitis | 391 |
| Autonomic neuropathies | 392 |
| Normal pressure hydrocephalus | 393 |
| Diabetic neuropathy | 392 |
| Shy-Drager syndrome | 394 |
| Acid maltase deficiency | 395 |
| Mucopolysaccharidosis | 396 |
| Alpert's syndrome | 397, 398 |
| Myasthenia gravis | |
| Möbius' syndrome | 398a |
| Fragile X syndrome | 399 |
| Klippel-Feil sequence | 400 |
| Myotonic dystrophy | |
| Duchenne's muscular dystrophy | 401, 402 |
| Tourette's syndrome | 403 |
| Quadriplegia | 404 |
| Rubinstein-Taybi syndrome | 405 |
| *Metabolic* | |
| Obesity | |
| Hypothyroidism | 406 |
| Acromegaly | 407 |
| Diabetes | 408, 410 |
| Growth hormone therapy | 411 |
| Testosterone treatment | 412 |
| Cushing's disease | 413 |
| *Musculoskeletal* | |
| Kyphoscoliosis | 414 |
| Pectus excavatum | 415 |
| Achondroplasia | 416 |
| Fibromyalgia | 417 |
| Ollier's disease (skeletal chondromatosis) | 418 |
| *Miscellaneous* | |
| Chronic renal failure | 419, 420 |
| Hemodialysis | 421 |
| Marfan's syndrome | 188 |
| Pregnancy | 409 |
| Chronic fatigue syndrome | 422 |
| Tracheobronchomalacia and laryngomalacia | 283, 423 |
| Carcinoid syndrome | 424 |
| Obstructing upper airway tumor | 121, 425, 426 |
| Floppy eyelid syndrome | 427 |
| Sarcoidosis | 428 |
| Repaired cleft palate | 429 |

*This definition was derived from studies in which it was found that normal individuals between 18 and 60 years experienced fewer than 25 apneas a night, whereas every patient who had symptomatic OSA experienced more than 45 apneas per night.[20, 21]

and increased neck circumference.[36–39] In addition, based on measurements of skin fold thickness, patients who have OSA have a greater amount of body fat than measurements of BMI would suggest.[40]

The association of obesity with ventilatory abnormalities antedates the knowledge that nocturnal airway obstruction is the basic pathophysiologic mechanism in OSA. The association became fixed in medical teaching with the appreciation that the fat boy, Joe, in Dickens' *The Posthumous Papers of the Pickwick Club* had all the features of what we now recognize as florid OSA, including obesity, a plethoric appearance, hypersomnolence, snoring, and dropsy (right heart failure).[41] In 1956, a small series of patients was described in which a similar constellation of clinical findings was identified and described as the "pickwickian syndrome."[41] Even at that time, the pivotal role of nocturnal apnea was not appreciated; it was believed that obesity caused ventilatory depression and hypercapnia by increasing the mechanical load on the respiratory system and that it was the hypercapnia that caused the excessive daytime somnolence. It was also suggested that some primary hypothalamic defect might contribute to both the obesity and the decreased central respiratory drive.[41] Now that the pathophysiology of OSA is understood, the "retrospectoscope" has allowed identification of individuals whose personalities and behavior were shaped by OSA; for example, it has been suggested that the giant in "Jack and the Beanstalk" suffered from the disorder because he was fat and irritable and snored during sleep and fell asleep during the day;[42] undoubtedly, acromegaly also contributed to his OSA!

Although the diagnosis of OSA is now made more frequently in patients who are of normal weight or are only slightly overweight,[43] severe obesity is associated with a higher incidence and more severe form of the disorder. In fact, in individual patients the severity of OSA is logarithmically related to body weight; that is, a small decrease in body weight can result in a large decrease in the AI.[43–45] This relationship was well illustrated in a study of eight patients in which moderate dietary-induced weight loss improved oxygenation during both sleep and wakefulness, decreased the number of disordered breathing events, and decreased the collapsibility of the nasopharyngeal airway.[46]

There is an increasing prevalence of snoring and OSA with age in adults.[16, 47] Approximately 60% of men older than 40 are snorers.[48] In one report from Denmark, OSA had a prevalence of 1.5% in the fourth decade and 12% in the seventh decade;[49] a prevalence as high as 40% (AHI greater than 15) has been reported in one elderly nursing home population.[35] Although the prevalence increases as a function of age, the results of one study have suggested that the clinical severity of OSA peaks in middle age and declines thereafter.[50]

Although approximately 85% to 90% of clinically diagnosed patients are male,[51, 52] some data suggest that this striking gender imbalance may be due to diagnostic bias. The reported relative risk for OSA in women is dependent on the type of study. In investigations from sleep disorder clinics, the ratio of clinically diagnosed OSA in men and women is approximately 9 to 1.[53, 54] However, the results of epidemiologic surveys suggest that OSA is only two to three times more prevalent in men than in women.[26, 55] The reason for the discrepancy is unclear; although it likely represents

diagnostic or referral bias,[56, 57] it is also possible that women have fewer or different symptoms (more insomnia and fatigue) for the same degree of apnea and therefore are not referred to a sleep disorder clinic.[58] In women, the condition usually occurs in the postmenopausal period.

Additional risk factors for OSA include a family history of the condition (*see* farther on); lower vital capacity;[59] and the use of tobacco,[60] alcohol,[61, 62] and medications such as sedatives, antihistamines, or certain antihypertensive drugs.[16] In reports from the Wisconsin Sleep Cohort Study, current smoking was associated with an odds ratio of 4.4 for moderate or worse OSA.[63] The increased risk of OSA in alcoholics may persist after they have achieved abstinence.[64] Curiously, left-handedness is associated with an increased severity but not with an increased prevalence of OSA.[65] Cigarette smoking by the mother has been shown to increase the frequency and duration of obstructive apnea episodes in newborns.[66] Pregnancy may be associated with the development of OSA.[67] It is unclear whether there is an increased incidence of OSA in patients who have hypothyroidism;[68] if there is, it is likely to be related to the accompanying obesity or goiter rather than to a direct effect of decreased thyroid hormones.[69, 70]

In summary, the results of many studies indicate a remarkably high prevalence of OSA in the general population, a prevalence that approaches that of asthma.[71] In fact, it has been suggested that OSA represents a public health problem that consumes vast amounts of health care resources—comparable to that of cigarette smoking.[72–74] Modeling studies suggest a significant cost benefit of early diagnosis and treatment.[75] The strongest risk factors for the disease are obesity, older age, and male gender.[76] In prediction models of the presence of OSA based purely on clinical and anthropometric findings, BMI, habitual loud snoring, witnessed nocturnal choking, and (to a lessor extent) male gender and increased age are the most important variables.[16]

## ETIOLOGY AND PATHOGENESIS

It is generally accepted that OSA is caused by the normal loss of upper airway muscle tone during sleep superimposed on a degree of upper airway narrowing.[77–79] The episodes of obstruction and apnea occur during all stages of sleep but especially during stage 2 of NREM sleep and during REM sleep, when the apneas tend to be the longest and the resultant arterial desaturation most severe.[80] The precise mechanism or mechanisms that cause the obstruction are not completely understood, although its usual anatomic location at the level of the nasopharynx and oropharynx has been well established. The factors that have been implicated in pathogenesis include an anatomically narrowed airway, an abnormally collapsible airway (i.e., one that has increased compliance), decreased neural drive to upper airway dilating muscles, decreased chemoreceptor stimulation and load compensation of upper airway dilating muscles,[81] and uncoordinated activation of the upper airway muscles (Fig. 53–1).[43]

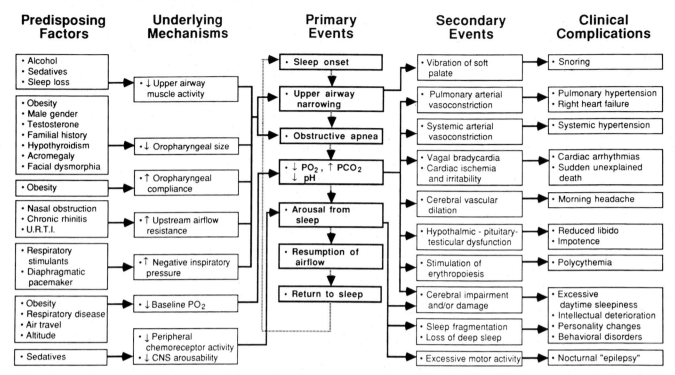

**Figure 53–1. The Pathogenesis of Obstructive Sleep Apnea.** (Modified from a table constructed by Dr. John Fleetham, Vancouver General Hospital, University of British Columbia, Vancouver.)

## Genetic Factors

There are a number of case reports of familial aggregation of OSA.[82–84] For example, in one study of three generations, the condition was described in nine nonobese individuals;[85] cephalometry showed the two subjects who had the most severe OSA to have the longest soft palates and the most inferiorly displaced hyoids. Familial aggregation of OSA has also been investigated using population studies.[86, 87] In one investigation, 105 adult offspring (66 men and 39 women) of 45 randomly selected patients who had OSA underwent overnight polysomnography;[88] 47% (36 men and 13 women) had OSA and an additional 22% were simple snorers. In a study of more than 4,000 Finnish twins, concordance for snoring among monozygotic individuals was greater than among dizygotic twins.[89]

In another study of individuals who had polysomnographically proven OSA and control subjects, loud snoring, daytime sleepiness, and witnessed apnea were reported 2 to 24 times more frequently among the first-degree relatives of the patients than among the controls;[90] these findings were independent of age, gender, weight, smoking, and alcohol consumption. In a case control study of 51 first-degree relatives of patients who had OSA and 51 age, sex, and weight-matched controls, the relatives of the patients reported snoring and daytime sleepiness more frequently and had a mean apnea plus hypopnea index of 13 per hour compared with 4 per hour for controls;[91] the relatives also had narrower upper airways, retroposed maxillae and mandibles, and longer soft palates with wider uvulas. Disproportionate craniofacial anatomy has also been found to be more common in relatives of patients who have OSA.[92]

The basis for a genetic contribution to the pathogenesis of OSA is unknown; however, there is evidence that obesity, craniofacial structure, and ventilatory control are, in part, hereditary.[93, 94] Twin studies suggest that approximately 70% of the variance in obesity is genetic,[95, 96] possibly related to variation in metabolic rate, fat storage, and eating behavior and with abnormalities in autonomic and hypothalamic function.[97, 98] Genes can also influence body fat distribution, accounting for as much as 25% of the intersubject variability in this trait.[99]

In a multivariate analysis of cephalometric data from 24 monozygotic and 21 dizygotic twins of the same gender, a high heritability was found for all 8 cephalometric parameters.[100] Many of the hereditary syndromes that are characterized by craniofacial abnormalities are accompanied by OSA, including Prader-Willi,[101] Treacher Collins, Pierre Robin, Crouzon's,[102] and Hallermann-Streiff.[103] These syndromes are associated with relatively small or deformed bones, particularly the mandible, which are important in determining upper airway size. Macroglossia, malocclusion, and tonsillar hypertrophy are also commonly found, and, singly or in combination, they may predispose to the development of OSA. Down's syndrome is the most common congenital disease associated with OSA;[104] in this abnormality, OSA is usually secondary to tonsillar hypertrophy.[105]

Family members of patients who have OSA have decreased ventilatory responses to hypoxemia and a greater increase in airway impedance in response to inspiratory loading than age- and gender-matched control subjects.[106] In addition, healthy offspring of fathers who had OSA have been found to show a greater decrease in VT when faced with an inspiratory resistive load.[107]

There has been limited investigation of genetic markers in OSA. However, one group found an increased frequency of human leukocyte antigens HLA-A2 and HLA-B39 in patients who had OSA compared with normal controls in the Japanese population.[108]

## Endocrine Factors

As indicated previously, there is a significantly increased risk of OSA in men compared with women. Although the precise basis for this is uncertain, there is abundant evidence that it is related to hormonal differences. Women who have OSA have elevated androgen levels, and administration of androgens can induce the abnormal state in previously unaffected men and women.[109–111] Androgen therapy in women can cause an increase in upper airway resistance, suggesting that these drugs can exert an effect on the structural configuration of the oropharynx.[112] Testosterone therapy has also been reported to precipitate OSA in a 13-year-old boy.[113] These observations, together with the known ventilatory stimulant effect of medroxyprogesterone, have lead to the hypothesis that the male predominance in OSA is related to a detrimental effect of the hormone testosterone and the lack of a protective effect of the hormone progesterone.[109]

The potential importance of hormones in the pathogenesis of OSA was demonstrated in one study in which seven male and seven female patients who were referred for surgery for morbid obesity participated in overnight sleep studies.[114] Six of the seven men had apneic periods and significant arterial oxygen desaturation, whereas none of the women did; the one man in whom obstruction and desaturation did not develop had hypogonadism!

## Structural Narrowing

Structural narrowing of the upper airway is a major independent risk factor in the vast majority of patients who have clinically significant OSA.[115–120] It may be caused by congenital or acquired abnormalities. Only a minority of these are grossly evident, such as enlarged adenoids and tonsils (particularly in children but also in adults who have Down's syndrome,[105] lymphomatous involvement of the tonsils,[121] or human immunodeficiency virus infection[122]), macroglossia in myxedema or acromegaly, and retrognathia or micrognathia in facial dysmorphia (e.g., in the Pierre Robin syndrome) (*see* Table 53–2).[123] Temporomandibular joint degeneration and resultant laxity can allow the jaw to fall posteriorly during sleep, contributing to airway obstruction,[124] as has been reported in patients who have rheumatoid arthritis.[125]

The airway obstruction that develops during sleep apnea usually occurs at the level of the velopharynx, nasopharynx, or oropharynx. For example, in one study of 11 patients, fluoroscopy showed that obstruction began in the oropharynx in all patients and progressed to the hypopharynx and larynx in some individuals;[126] the soft palate was seen to be sucked down into the hypopharynx, where it acted as a plug in the airway. Although nasopharyngeal obstruction does not cause apnea by itself, it can precipitate it by virtue of the more negative downstream inspiratory pressures that must be generated.[127, 128] Nasal obstruction may also necessitate

mouth breathing, which itself can precipitate obstructive apnea.[129] In normal men, mechanical nasal obstruction during sleep causes apneas and episodic arterial oxygen desaturation.[130, 131] The effect of nasal obstruction may be related in part to the bypassing of receptors for nasal air flow and temperature, because stimulation of these receptors causes reflex activation of upper airway dilating muscles; this hypothesis has been strengthened by the observations that nasal and oropharyngeal anesthesia can induce nocturnal apnea in normal subjects[132, 133] and depress the action of upper airway dilating muscles in patients who have OSA.[134] This mechanism may also be relevant to the gender difference in the prevalence of OSA; although both men and women normally breathe through the nose during sleep, a significantly greater proportion of nocturnal breathing is through the mouth in older men.[135] Breathing through the mouth may also increase risk for OSA by its effect on the tongue. The tongue forms the anterior wall of the oropharynx; both the supine posture and opening of the mouth tend to displace it posteriorly and encourage airway closure.[136]

Cephalometry has demonstrated a variety of abnormalities of craniofacial and upper airway soft tissue anatomy that may predispose patients to upper airway obstruction during sleep and affect the severity of OSA.[137] Many patients who have OSA have been shown to have a small posteriorly placed mandible, a narrow posterior airway space, an enlarged tongue and soft palate, an inferiorly placed hyoid bone, or a combination of these. For example, in one study of 155 patients who had OSA, 150 (97%) exhibited at least two significant cephalometric abnormalities,[138] the most common being retroposition of the mandible and inferior displacement of the hyoid bone. Distinctive changes in the orientation of the bony support of the upper airway are also seen when patients who have OSA assume the supine posture.[139] The length of the pharynx may also be important; in one study, it became considerably longer in patients who had OSA than in control subjects when they assumed the supine posture.[140] Differences in cephalometric parameters have been identified in some racial groups, a finding that could be relevant to the ethnic variation in the prevalence of OSA mentioned previously.[141, 142]

An important cause of upper airway narrowing is the deposition of adipose tissue in the soft tissues surrounding the pharynx. Neck circumference is a simple clinical measurement that reflects obesity in the region of the upper airway. Using an acoustic reflection technique, one group showed that the pharyngeal cross-sectional area of obese patients who have OSA is less than that of equally obese patients who do not have the disorder.[143] Patients who have OSA have been shown to have big necks when compared with both nonapneic snorers and weight-matched controls.[144, 145] Furthermore, neck circumference correlates with several soft tissue variables measured from lateral cephalometry[146] and correlates better than BMI with apnea severity.[147] These findings suggest that obesity mediates its effect in OSA through fat deposition in the neck.[148] Even nonobese patients who have OSA have a greater percentage of their body mass as fat than weight-matched non-OSA patients;[149] moreover, the distribution of the fat, as assessed by magnetic resonance (MR) imaging, shows preferential deposition in the neck, anterolateral to the upper airway. As might be expected, there is a spectrum of upper airway soft tissue and craniofacial abnormalities among patients who have OSA. There are obese patients whose upper airway soft tissue is increased in amount, nonobese patients who have abnormal craniofacial structure, and an intermediate group of patients who have abnormalities in both craniofacial structure and upper airway soft tissue structures.[125]

Deposition of adipose tissue in the submucosal connective tissue surrounding the oropharynx and the soft palate can narrow the upper airway and increase its compliance.[150] Obesity also decreases functional residual capacity (FRC) and increases airway resistance, especially in the supine posture;[151] should FRC fall to below closing capacity, nocturnal hypoxemia would result, thus contributing to more severe arterial oxygen desaturation during apneic episodes. There is also a possibility that the converse of the obesity-OSA relationship might occur, that is, sleep apnea might itself contribute to the development of obesity.[152] Successful treatment of OSA by continuous positive nasal pressure facilitates subsequent weight reduction. This has led to the hypothesis that prolonged hypoxemia, hypercapnia, and sleep fragmentation could cause changes in hypothalamic-pituitary function that favor the development of obesity. Hypoxia and sleep interruption can increase stress hormones and alter glucose metabolism and may influence the extent and pattern of deposition of adipose tissue.[153]

Besides these well-defined causes for anatomic narrowing of the upper airway, CT studies of the oropharyngeal airway sometimes show a narrowing of the airway not attributable to any specific cause. Tongue size also has a wide normal range, and individuals who have large tongues are at risk of developing OSA. Cinefluorography of the upper airways during sleep shows that the tongue and hypopharyngeal soft tissues are approximated during inspiration, obliterating the hypopharyngeal air space and causing intermittent and almost complete obstruction to air flow.[154, 155] The results of dynamic studies and MR imaging also show that there is lateral narrowing and wall thickening of the pharynx in patients who have OSA.[156, 157] In fact, there is some evidence that airway shape, independent of cross-sectional area, is a risk factor for OSA. This evidence has led to the hypothesis that an elliptic-shaped airway that has its long axis oriented in an anteroposterior direction is a risk for OSA, because the lumen area changes less in response to changes in transmural pressure.[158] The importance of upper airway geometry as a risk for OSA was demonstrated in a study of 300 consecutive patients in which a prediction model based on BMI, neck circumference, and oral cavity measurements was found to be 98% sensitive and 100% specific in detecting OSA ($\geq$ 5 apneic episodes per hour).[158a]

It is possible that some of the pharyngeal narrowing seen in patients who have OSA occurs as a result of the obstruction rather than the cause. Many patients have swollen pharyngeal walls and soft palate as well as a pendulous uvula;[43] it is possible that chronic obstruction and snoring causes edema of these structures because of the very negative intrapharyngeal pressures that are engendered. However, if swelling does occur because of these mechanisms, it could act to exacerbate the obstruction. Pathologic study of uvulas resected at the time of surgery for OSA has shown an increase in the number of inflammatory cells and thickening of the lamina propria as a result of interstitial edema (com-

pared with uvulas derived from autopsies of patients who did not have OSA).[160]

These anatomic causes of narrowing of the upper airway may be suggested by abnormalities of inspiratory and expiratory flow-volume curves.[161, 162] In one study of 60 patients referred for investigation of possible OSA, 14 of 35 who had confirmed disease had a ratio of maximal midexpiratory to midinspiratory flow greater than 1:

$$\dot{V}max_{50}E/\dot{V}max_{50}I > 1.0$$

In only 2 of the 25 patients without demonstrable obstruction was the ratio greater than 1.[163] However, given the prevalence of OSA in the population at large, the results of this study indicate the test has little diagnostic value. The measurement of maximal or tidal-breath inspiratory and expiratory flow-volume curves in the supine position increases the ability to distinguish patients who have OSA from those who do not.[164, 165] In one investigation, the presence of a "saw-toothed" curve was 92% specific in differentiating 17 patients with obstruction and 13 nonaffected individuals (Fig. 53–2).[166] "Saw-toothing" and mid–vital capacity flow ratios greater than 1 also correlate with pharyngeal airway narrowing detected during fiberoptic nasopharyngoscopy.[167] Snorers and patients who have OSA may exhibit flow-limited inspiration and expiration during sleep as a result of a flow-limiting segment in the oropharynx similar to the flow-limiting airway collapse that occurs in the intrathoracic airways during maximal expiratory flow maneuvers.[168, 169]

### Increased Compliance

Increased compliance of the upper airway is the second major factor that has been implicated in the pathogenesis of OSA.[170] The compliance of the upper airway can be measured during sleep or anesthesia by applying negative pressure at the airway opening and determining the negative pressure that will result in airway closure.[171–173] In normal individuals, negative pressures of $-25$ cm $H_2O$ or lower can be applied before closure occurs; however, in patients who have OSA, closure occurs when pressures are as small

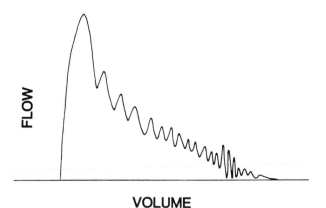

**Figure 53–2. A "Saw-Toothed" Flow-Volume Curve.** This flow-volume curve was obtained in a patient with Parkinson's disease. It shows reduced maximal expiratory flow and a rhythmic fluctuation in flow throughout expiration caused by the "tremor" in the upper airways and expiratory muscles.

as $-0.5$ cm $H_2O$. The airway is most compliant during REM sleep, during which the average closing pressure is $-2.4$ cm $H_2O$; it is most stable during slow wave sleep, when the average closing pressure is $-4.2$ cm $H_2O$. In some individuals who have OSA, a positive airway pressure is necessary to maintain airway patency when the dilator muscles are completely relaxed. In one study of 57 normal individuals and patients who had mild or moderate OSA, the velopharynx was the site of closure during anesthesia in 49 (86%,);[174] closure occurred when airway pressure was $-3.8$, $+0.9$, and $+2.8$ cm $H_2O$ in the normal, mildly obstructed, and moderately obstructed groups, respectively.

The velopharynx is the portion of the pharynx that is immediately posterior to the soft palate and is now recognized as the site of obstruction in the majority of patients who have OSA.[174] It has been shown that closing pressure is less negative in the supine than in the lateral decubitus position.[173] Opening of the mouth increases upper airway collapsibility during sleep.[175] Using the acoustic reflection technique, the pressure-area curves of the pharynx were measured in subjects who snored and who had or did not have OSA;[176] the results showed that specific compliance of the oropharynx was 2.5-fold greater in individuals who had OSA. In another study, the pharyngeal size and change in size, as a function of lung volume, were measured in 77 normal men and 98 normal women. Although men had a larger pharyngeal cross-sectional area (3.6 cm² versus 3.2 cm²), the change in area with changing lung volume was significantly greater in men (0.6 cm²) than in women (0.12 cm²).[177]

One group of investigators measured pharyngeal cross-sectional area and compliance in normal subjects and in snorers who had and did not have OSA;[178] they found that although airway size was decreased in all the snorers, those who had OSA also had unstable hypercollapsible pharyngeal airways at low lung volumes. Increased collapsibility can be demonstrated dynamically using digital fluoroscopy.[179] Once the airway closes, the pressure necessary to re-establish patency increases as a result of surface adhesive forces.[180] In human infant cadavers, the oropharynx closes when $-0.04$ cm $H_2O$ pressure is applied, whereas much more negative pressure is required to close the nasopharynx and hypopharynx;[181] pressures as low as $-60$ cm $H_2O$ are necessary to close the larynx.

Although the oropharynx has been identified as the principal site of airway narrowing in some studies,[182] there is evidence that the nasopharyngeal airway is also narrower and more compliant.[183] In studies in which endoscopic examination of the upper airway was performed during sleep, the velopharynx and nasopharynx were the principal sites of narrowing but narrowing at more than one site was common.[184, 185] The site of the major increase in resistance can differ from patient to patient, which may explain why a single surgical procedure is not universally successful therapy.[186] Oral appliances that produce protrusion of either the mandible or the tongue increase the cross-sectional area and alter the shape of the upper airway and are effective in preventing apnea in some patients.[187]

Nearly two thirds of patients who have Marfan's syndrome have OSA, an association that may relate to increased compliance of their upper airway secondary to the connective tissue abnormality.[188] It has been suggested that the presence of OSA, by increasing intrathoracic swings in pressure, contributes to the development of progressive aortic root dilation in patients who have Marfan's syndrome.[189]

## Neuromuscular Dysfunction

Dysfunction of the upper airway muscles is another factor that may contribute to the development of OSA.[190] A variety of neurologic disorders are associated with an increased prevalence of obstructive as well as central sleep apnea.[191] Twenty-three pairs of muscles encircle the pharyngeal airway, the majority of which dilate and stabilize the pharynx when they contract. These dilating muscles include the genioglossi, the geniohyoid, the hypoglossus, the tensor palatini, and the thyrohyoid. Contraction of these muscles stiffens the walls of the oropharynx, counteracting the tendency of the airway to narrow in response to the negative intraluminal pressure that develops during inspiration. The muscles display tonic and phasic respiratory electromyographic activity. Their inspiratory activation (via the 12th cranial nerve) typically precedes phrenic activity by 50 to 100 milliseconds, so that the upper airway is dilated and stiffened before the onset of the negative intraluminal pressure that develops with inspiratory air flow.[192, 193]

Periodic and parallel fluctuations in diaphragmatic and genioglossal muscle electromyographic activity occur during sleep, the nadirs of these cycles occurring simultaneously with hypopneic episodes and central or obstructive apneas.[194, 195] The onset of REM sleep is associated with maximally decreased activation (hypotonia) of upper airway muscles; because the decrease in diaphragmatic activation is less, REM sleep represents the period of maximal vulnerability for airway closure.[196, 197] Periodic breathing can be induced with hypoxic inspiratory gas mixtures and, in otherwise normal individuals, can cause both episodic increase in upper airway resistance and apneas.[198] Patients who have Cheyne-Stokes breathing also show an increased incidence of OSA, supporting the contention that periodic breathing is important in the genesis of this condition.[199]

The activity of the upper airway dilating muscles is influenced by a number of factors, including changes in lung volume, changes in chemical drive, and input from upper airway receptors.[127] The increasing lung volume that occurs during inspiration suppresses the neural drive of the upper airway muscles. The afferent information concerning these changes comes from lung mechanoreceptors that run in the vagal nerve. The neural drive to upper airway muscles also increases in response to hypercapnia and hypoxia[200–202] and to stimulation of upper airway mucosal receptors that respond to pressure, temperature, and muscle contraction.[127]

Pharyngeal patency is promoted by input from all the sources discussed previously. If the airway narrows, the more negative intraluminal pressure induced by inspiration stimulates mechanoreceptors; should the obstruction persist, a decrease in $V_T$ and changes in arterial blood gas content augment muscle activity, thus tending to restore upper airway patency. These protective mechanisms are depressed during sleep and by alcohol and sedative drugs.[203–207] It is still unclear whether a primary abnormality of these protective mechanisms is responsible for some cases of OSA. However, an abnormality in neuromuscular control of upper airway caliber could be a factor that contributes to the familial tendency for the development of OSA; in fact, a definite decrease in genioglossal activation during sleep has been reported in one family with the affliction.[208] Although the cross-sectional area of the upper airway is smaller in women,[209] they have greater electromyographic activity in the dilating muscles such as the genioglossus and demonstrate a greater increase in electromyographic activity when challenged with an inspiratory load.[210] During wakefulness the electromyographic activity of the genioglossus and tensor palatini muscles is greater in patients who have OSA than in normal individuals, presumably to compensate for a degree of structural narrowing; however, with sleep onset there is a larger decrease in electromyographic activity in patients who have OSA.[211] Patients who have OSA also demonstrate impaired enhancement of the electromyographic activity in upper airway dilating muscles when a negative pressure is applied at the mouth.[212]

The sleep deprivation and hypoxia that result from OSA can cause depression of phasic respiratory activity in the upper airway muscles and can lead to a vicious cycle of worsening obstruction and more fragmented sleep.[127, 213–215] Evidence for this observation derives from direct recordings of genioglossal electromyographic activity[214] and from clinical studies in which the prolonged use of nasal positive pressure causes improvement in sleep apnea, even when patients are studied without nasal positive pressure.[127] This improvement may be the result of the beneficial effect of adequate sleep on the respiratory control centers; however, a decrease in pharyngeal edema is also a possible explanation. It is conceivable that injury or fatigue could develop in the upper airway muscles following exposure to very negative intraluminal pressures, but there is no evidence that this occurs.[216] However, there is evidence that increased upper airway collapsibility causes compensatory metabolic and phenotypic changes in upper airway dilating muscles such as the musculus uvulae.[217, 218] Patients who have OSA have decreased central ventilatory drive and impaired load compensation in addition to decreased activation of upper airway muscles;[219] however, it is unclear whether this impairment is a result of the disorder or a predisposing factor for its development. Further support for an important role for malfunction of the upper airway dilating muscles in the pathogenesis of OSA is provided by the relatively frequent occurrence of the syndrome in patients who have generalized myopathic processes such as muscular dystrophy.[220]

The importance of coordinating the muscular dilation and stabilization of the oropharynx with the muscular contraction of the respiratory pump is illustrated by case reports of patients in whom OSA develops during diaphragmatic pacing.[221] During pacing, the diaphragmatic contraction is not associated with synchronous activation of upper airway muscles, and if the patient does not have a tracheostomy, upper airway closure can develop. A similar sequence results in the airway closure that accompanies a hiccup.

Brief periods of central hypoventilation or apnea frequently precede and initiate the obstructive episodes in patients who have OSA; the mechanism of these central depressions may be the periods of hyperventilation that terminate the previous obstructive apneic episodes. The hypocapnia that results can depress the respiratory center and initiate the next apneic episode, thus setting up a vicious

cycle.[222] Activation of upper airway dilating muscles is depressed by alcohol[223] and by hypnotic sleeping pills,[224] both of which are known to exacerbate snoring and OSA. Interestingly, narcotics that decrease ventilatory drive do not appear to increase the incidence of sleep apnea.[225]

It is not known which stimulus causes arousal during apneic episodes. Although hypoxemia seems to be the most obvious candidate, administration of oxygen does not invariably prolong the apneic episodes. Arousal frequently occurs when the amount of tension generated by the inspiratory muscles against the occluded upper airway approaches the amount of tension that causes muscle fatigue, suggesting that a message from inspiratory muscles may be an important arousal stimulus.[226] However, the results of two separate studies have shown that electromyographic evidence of diaphragmatic fatigue does not develop during an apnea episode even though very high transdiaphragmatic pressures can be achieved.[227, 228] Upper airway mechanoreceptors may be important in mediating arousals during apnea; in one study, mean apnea duration was increased from 24 to 31 seconds after local anesthesia of the upper airway mucosa.[229] Apnea duration increases progressively during the night in patients who have OSA, from 26 to 33 seconds in one study,[230] suggesting that there is a blunting of the arousal response. An experimental study in dogs suggests that sleep fragmentation is the mechanism for delayed arousal in OSA.[231]

### Summary

In summary, OSA occurs primarily because of an anatomically small or excessively collapsible upper airway coupled with the normal reduction in upper airway muscle dilator action that occurs during sleep; defective ventilatory control and arousal mechanisms may contribute in some patients.[22] The available evidence suggests that an exaggerated reduction in the activity of the upper airway dilator musculature is a primary abnormality in a minority of patients.[151] Whatever its cause, narrowing of the airway results in an increase in pharyngeal resistance that causes more negative intrapharyngeal inspiratory pressures and airway closure. Although the latter increases the neural input to the pharyngeal dilator muscles, it also increases drive to the diaphragm and intercostal inspiratory muscles, thus generating more negative intra-airway pressures that keep the oropharynx closed. The only escape from such a vicious cycle is arousal accompanied by higher center activation of the upper airway dilator muscles and consequent relief of the obstruction.[127, 232]

## RADIOLOGIC MANIFESTATIONS

Given the importance of upper airway anatomy in the pathogenesis of OSA, one might expect that upper airway imaging would play an important role in diagnosis. Although imaging techniques have greatly enhanced our understanding of the pathogenesis of OSA, there is no ideal method of examining upper airway structure, especially the changes that occur during sleep apnea;[233, 234] as a result, imaging plays a limited role in the assessment of the disorder in individual patients.[235] Despite this, cephalometry, CT, or a combination of these techniques has been used to characterize the abnormalities of soft tissue and bony structures in patients who have proven OSA, and these procedures are reported to aid in the planning of the most appropriate therapy.[236–241]

A lateral radiograph of the head and neck using soft tissue technique (sometimes referred to as lateral cephalometry) allows assessment of the upper airways, soft tissues, and bony structures (Fig. 53–3). The procedure has demonstrated a variety of abnormalities of craniofacial and upper airway soft tissue anatomy that may predispose to upper airway obstruction during sleep and that also relate to the severity of OSA.[137, 242–244] Some investigators have found that the technique allows separation of snorers who do or do not have OSA with a precision of approximately 80%;[245] however, others have not been able to distinguish reliably between patients who have sleep apnea and nonapneic, habitual snorers.[246] For example, in one investigation of 117 patients referred for evaluation of heavy snoring and possible OSA, a lateral view of the airway obtained after swallowing contrast material was used to measure pharyngeal diameters at three sites along the airway;[247] all measurements were performed with the patient standing and supine. Apneic and nonapneic snorers demonstrated a significant reduction in the retropalatal distance on assumption of the supine posture. Stepwise multiple linear regression analysis showed that the retropalatal distance and airway diameter at the tip of the palate and 1 cm distal to it were significant predictors of snoring but not apnea.

The dimensions of the upper airway can also be assessed using CT (Fig. 53–4). In one study of 25 adult men in whom three-dimensional CT reconstructions were performed, measurement of the cross-sectional area of the upper airway at different levels revealed the narrowest point to be in the oropharynx ($0.52 \pm 0.18$ cm$^2$) in the majority;[248] in some subjects, a second narrowing was seen at the level of the hypopharynx. The investigators also measured the volume of the tongue and found that subjects who had larger tongues experienced more severe OSA and had a smaller airway lumen. In another investigation of 36 patients who had OSA and 10 control subjects, measurements of the cross-sectional area of the oropharyngeal lumen were taken at the level of the narrowing;[249] 27 patients who had severe OSA (defined as a high number and prolonged episodes of OSA and 22% or greater decrease in oxygen saturation) had an oropharyngeal cross-sectional area measuring less than 50 mm$^2$. By comparison, patients who had moderate OSA had an oropharyngeal cross-sectional area of 60 to 100 mm$^2$, and the control subjects had a minimal pharyngeal cross-sectional area of 110 mm$^2$.

In another investigation of the effects of respiration on upper airway caliber using cine CT in 15 normal subjects, 14 snorer/mildly apneic subjects, and 13 patients who had OSA, all subjects were scanned in the supine position during awake nasal breathing.[250] CT images were obtained at four anatomic levels from the nasopharynx to the retroglossal region every 0.4 seconds during a respiratory cycle. The investigators found that the upper airway was significantly smaller in apneic than in normal subjects, especially at the low retropalatal and retroglossal anatomic levels; however, little airway narrowing occurred during inspiration in all three subjects groups, suggesting that the action of the upper

airway dilator muscles balanced the effects of negative intraluminal pressure. Using dynamic CT imaging, another group found the mean airway cross-sectional area to be largest at end inspiration and smallest at end expiration, consistent with relaxation of upper airway dilator muscle activity during expiration.[251] Additional findings on CT include an increase in nonfatty tissues in the pharyngeal wall, thickening of the mucosa of the naso- and oropharynx, enlargement of the lymphoid tissue, and hypertrophy of the tongue, soft tissue palate, or muscles.[235]

Upper airway dimensions can also be assessed using MR imaging (Fig. 53–5). T1-weighted spin-echo sequences show deposition of fat adjacent to the pharyngeal airway in patients who have OSA.[252, 253] Ultrafast MR imaging has great potential for providing dynamic three-dimensional images;[254, 255] the procedure is able to detect sites of airway narrowing and closure and has shown considerable differences among individuals who have OSA (*see* Fig. 53–5).[256, 257] MR imaging is also sensitive in detecting changes in upper airway water content. In one study, five patients who had moderate to severe OSA were studied with MR imaging before and 4 to 6 weeks after beginning nasal continuous positive airway pressure therapy; the results showed a significant increase in pharyngeal lumen volume (while off continuous positive airway pressure) and reductions in tongue volume and pharyngeal mucosal water content.[258]

## CLINICAL MANIFESTATIONS

The key symptoms of OSA are snoring, apneas witnessed by a bed partner, and excessive daytime sleepiness (*see* Fig. 53–1, page 2058).[17]

### Snoring and Apnea

Snoring is almost invariable and often precedes the diagnosis of OSA, sometimes by many years.[47] However, the symptom is by no means a specific indicator of the presence of the disorder. In a survey of 4,713 people, 41% of men and 28% of women were found to be occasional or habitual snorers;[259] the incidence in men and women older than 60 years of age was 60% and 40%, respectively. Despite these figures, only 1% to 3% of the population suffers from symptomatic sleep apnea. The snoring of persons who have OSA tends to be loud, irregular, and very disturbing to bed partners, roommates, or others in the household. In addition, it is typically interrupted by frequent periods of apnea, during which progressively greater inspiratory efforts are expended against a completely closed airway. The apneic periods are terminated by loud snorting and motor activity associated with arousal. With resumption of sleep, rhythmic snoring returns, punctuated by frequent apneas, explosive snorts, and arousals.

Because obtaining a history of snoring and a description of the snoring pattern is important in the investigation of patients who have suspected OSA, it is necessary to interview a spouse or bed partner. A history of loud snoring interspersed with quiet periods and ending with a loud snort and motor activity is strong evidence for the presence of the

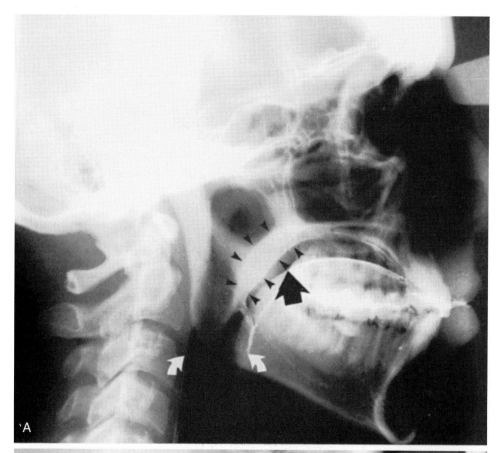

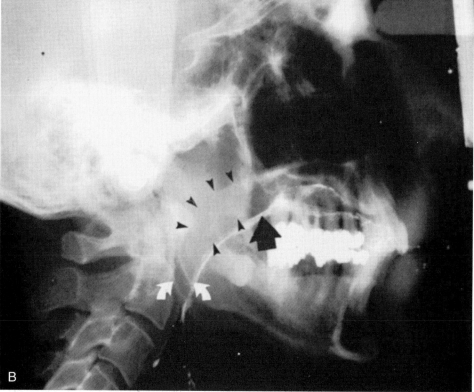

**Figure 53–3. Radiography of the Upper Airway in a Normal Subject and a Patient with Obstructive Sleep Apnea.** A lateral radiograph of the face and neck *(A)* of a normal subject after ingestion of barium paste to outline the top of the tongue *(large arrows)* reveals a widely patent oropharynx, normal uvula *(arrowheads)*, and hypopharynx *(curved arrows)*. A similar view in a patient who has obstructive sleep apnea *(B)* shows a markedly narrowed oropharynx *(large arrow)* and hypopharynx *(curved arrows)* and a very large uvula *(arrowheads)*.

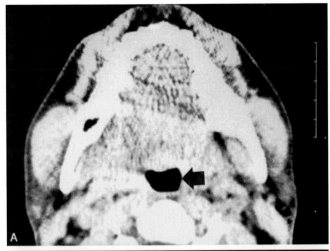

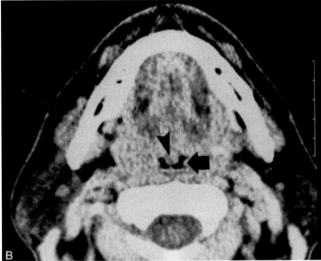

**Figure 53–4. Computed Tomography of the Upper Airway in a Normal Subject and a Patient with Obstructive Sleep Apnea.** A CT scan at the level of the oropharynx in a normal subject *(A)* reveals a widely patent oropharynx *(arrow)*. In a patient who has obstructive sleep apnea, a CT image at approximately the same level *(B)* shows a markedly reduced cross-sectional area of the airway *(arrowhead)* and a prominent uvula *(arrow)*.

condition; a more rhythmic crescendo and decrescendo pattern indicates simple heavy snoring without apnea.[43] The loud and disturbing snoring and frequent arousals associated with OSA can cause considerable disruption in the personal life of affected individuals; spouses cannot sleep in the same bed or in the same room (or occasionally in the same house!) and may actually be injured during the erratic motor activity that accompanies arousal. It is not surprising that marital problems are a frequent consequence.

### Daytime Hypersomnolence

Another characteristic symptom of OSA is excessive daytime sleepiness. Its severity correlates with the intensity of nocturnal apnea and sleep deprivation and can be estimated by taking a careful history[43] and by applying questionnaires that have been designed to test for daytime sleepiness, including the Stanford Sleepiness Scale,[260] the Rotterdam

Daytime Sleepiness Scale,[261] and the Epworth Sleepiness Scale.[262]

There are three clinical levels of increasing severity.[263] In Category 1, or mild sleepiness, the individual falls asleep only when reading, watching television, or listening to lectures; although the sleepiness is more severe when the sub-

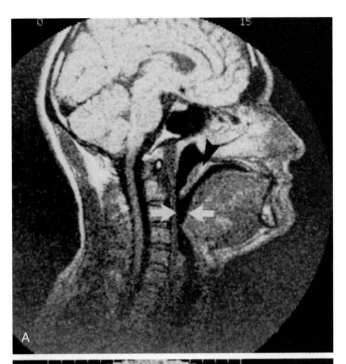

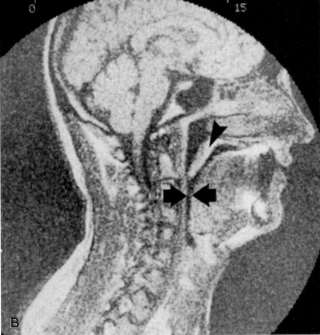

**Figure 53–5. MR Imaging of the Upper Airway in a Normal Subject and a Patient with Obstructive Sleep Apnea.** A sagittal MR image of the head and neck of a normal subject *(A)* demonstrates the uvula *(arrowhead)* and hypopharyngeal airway *(arrows)*. A similar image of a patient who has obstructive sleep apnea *(B)* reveals a slightly enlarged uvula *(arrowhead)* and a markedly narrowed hypopharyngeal airway *(arrows)*. These images were obtained at 8:00 A.M. following an overnight sleep study.

ject is overtired, it does not completely disappear despite a "good" night's sleep. The patient and family members do not view the sleepiness as a problem, and it does not interfere with the patient's work. Category 2, or moderate sleepiness, is characterized by unequivocal hypersomnolence; the patient falls asleep not only while relaxing, but also while engaged in activities such as driving. The patient and family members are aware that excessive sleepiness is a problem and is interfering with the individual's work. Category 3, or severe sleepiness, implies extreme hypersomnolence; the patient may fall asleep while talking, eating, or relating his or her medical history and is unable to work or drive a car.

The frequency and duration of nocturnal apneas and the severity of nocturnal arterial oxygen desaturation correlate well with the severity of hypersomnolence. Subjects in Category 1 typically experience 30 to 60 apneas per night, and arterial saturation rarely falls below 80%. By contrast, individuals in Category 3 have more than 400 apneic episodes a night, and arterial oxygen saturation falls below 80% during each episode; these patients spend most of the night either obstructed or awake. Hypersomnolence associated with OSA is easy to recognize in patients in Categories 2 and 3; however, it can be difficult to distinguish patients who have the mild sleepiness of Category 1 from normal individuals who are "overtired" or have postprandial lethargy.[43]

Hypersomnolence also can be estimated quantitatively by tests such as the multiple sleep latency test, which measures the rapidity with which a patient can fall asleep.[264] The patient is given the opportunity to fall asleep during several daytime nap periods of 20 minutes each and is evaluated by electroencephalography, electromyography, and electro-oculography. The "latency" to sleep is defined as the time until the beginning of any sleep stage. A significantly decreased latency is indicative of pathologic hypersomnolence.[265] Another objective test of sleepiness is the maintenance of wakefulness test, which is a measure of a subject's inability to stay awake when desired.[263]

The precise cause of the hypersomnolence of OSA is not known. Although sleep fragmentation during the night likely contributes to it, it may not be the sole explanation. In one study, four patients who had severe sleep apnea and hypersomnolence were compared with patients whose sleep apnea was equally severe but was unassociated with hypersomnolence:[266] the former patients were more obese and demonstrated significantly more severe arterial oxygen desaturation while asleep and awake. It is thus possible that the hypoxemia contributes to sleepiness.[267, 268] However, although hypersomnolence is rapidly corrected by tracheostomy or the use of continuous nasal positive pressure,[131] it is not improved by the administration of long-term nocturnal oxygen therapy.[269]

The arterial oxygen desaturation associated with apneic episodes causes pulmonary arterial hypertension and an increase in right ventricular afterload.[270] Because prolonged pulmonary hypertension can result in irreversible vascular narrowing, the pulmonary hypertension may eventually persist during the waking hours and result in cor pulmonale and, ultimately, in right ventricular failure.[271] Persistent pulmonary hypertension occurs in approximately 15% to 20% of patients who have OSA,[272] almost invariably in association with chronic obstructive lung disease.[273] Such patients

experience not only severe arterial oxygen desaturation at night but also arterial oxygen desaturation and hypercapnia during the day.[274, 275] In fact, approximately 5% of patients who have clinically recognized OSA have chronic alveolar hypoventilation characterized by the persistence of elevated arterial $P_{CO_2}$ and decreased arterial $P_{O_2}$ during wakefulness. These patients comprise a subset of OSA patients who have the pickwickian syndrome, or (as it is more often called) the obesity hypoventilation syndrome. Such patients tend to be morbidly obese and have severe and prolonged apneas, profound nocturnal oxygen desaturation, persistent pulmonary hypertension, and cor pulmonale; these complications are reversed by successful treatment of the nocturnal obstruction.[22]

Although individuals who have the obesity hypoventilation syndrome have worse lung function than those who do not develop hypercapnia,[276] the degree of abnormality is not enough to explain the alveolar hypoventilation, and it is unclear why they develop daytime ventilatory failure. It has been suggested that the chronic sleep deprivation combined with nocturnal hypoxia and hypercapnia lead to a disruption of normal central ventilatory control.[277] In some patients, daytime hypoventilation is attributable partly to concomitant obstructive pulmonary disease[278] and partly to the central ventilatory depression that may be occasioned by prolonged sleep deprivation and hypoxemia.[279, 280] The ventilatory response to $CO_2$ is not different in first-degree relatives of patients who have OSA and develop chronic hypercapnia and those who do not have hypercapnea.[281]

## Cardiovascular Manifestations

The association of OSA and cardiovascular disease is an area of intense interest and investigation.[282] Although the results of one systematic review suggest that the relevance of sleep apnea to public health has been exaggerated,[283] those of most studies support an increased prevalence of systemic hypertension,[284, 285] coronary artery disease, and stroke in patients who suffer from OSA.[286] However, many of these studies have been poorly designed and confounded by the fact that the recognized risk factors for these conditions, such as cigarette smoking, obesity, age, and male gender, are the same factors that increase the risk of OSA.[287]

Theoretically, patients who have OSA may develop systemic arterial hypertension because of smooth muscle contraction related to hypoxemia and respiratory acidosis, increased sympathetic nervous system activity,[288] or increased secretion of catecholamines.[289–294] Systemic hypertension has been reported in more than 50% of patients who have OSA;[295, 296] when multivariate analyses have been performed, this increased risk has been found to be independent of age and obesity.[297, 298] The association of hypertension and OSA persists when the prevalence of OSA is examined in hypertensive patients rather than vice versa. In one study, OSA was diagnosed in 38% of patients who were hypertensive and in only 4% of a nonhypertensive control group;[299] although part of the relationship was explained by BMI, age, and sex, there was an independent contribution of hypertension to the prediction of OSA. Thus, sleep apnea should be considered a diagnostic possibility in patients who have hypertension and should stimulate inquiry regarding snoring and daytime hypersomnolence, especially in obese male patients. However, the strength of the association does not justify mass screening for OSA among hypertensive patients.[271, 285]

OSA or snoring in the absence of apnea is also associated with an increased risk of myocardial infarction,[300] cerebrovascular accident, cardiac arrhythmia (including supraventricular tachycardia,[301] atrioventricular block, and ventricular arrhythmia[302]), and sudden death. The association of snoring and myocardial infarction persists even after correction for BMI, hypertension, and smoking, the odds ratio having been found to be 1.71.[303] Although the mechanism for this association is unknown, the results of one study showed that patients who have OSA have decreased plasma fibrinolytic activity.[304] In addition, electrocardiographic monitoring shows that episodes of apnea are frequently associated with myocardial ischemia.[305] OSA is an independent risk factor for coronary artery disease in women even after adjustment for age, BMI, hypertension, smoking, and diabetes.[306] Although during wakefulness hypoxemia and hypercapnia cause tachycardia,[307] in sleep apnea they are more often associated with bradycardia and, on rare occasions, with serious conduction defects (e.g., heart block, sinus arrest) or dysrhythmias (e.g., ventricular tachycardia).[271, 296, 308] Such serious cardiac dysrhythmias are an unusual occurrence in OSA;[309] however, they are an important indication for prompt and definitive treatment because affected patients are at risk for sudden nocturnal death.[310]

The hemodynamic and metabolic consequences of OSA may also affect cardiac muscle action. Obstructive apneas cause a transient increase in left ventricular afterload, as a result of both the catecholamine-induced systemic vasoconstriction and the progressively negative swings in intrapleural pressure associated with increasingly forceful inspiratory effort against the occluded upper airway. Because the heart is entirely within the thoracic cavity and must pump blood into the extrathoracic systemic circulation, which is surrounded by atmospheric pressure, negative intrapleural pressure acts on the left ventricle in the same way as increased systemic blood pressure.[311, 312] The cyclic increase in afterload that accompanies obstructed respiratory efforts is manifest by the development of pulsus paradoxus during apnea.[313] Patients who have OSA have a high incidence of left and right ventricular hypertrophy as assessed by echocardiography.[314]

OSA may exacerbate heart failure by virtue of the negative intrathoracic pressure that develops during periods of apnea. This negative pressure is transmitted to the chambers of the heart and acts as an increased afterload in the same way as would an increase in arterial blood pressure. In one study of eight men who had concomitant OSA and idiopathic dilated cardiomyopathy, the application of nasal continuous positive pressure during sleep successfully treated the OSA and increased the left ventricular ejection fraction from $37 \pm 4\%$ to $49 \pm 5\%$.[314a]

## Neurologic Manifestations

OSA is associated with increased risk for a variety of neurologic disorders. In one case control study, the risk for stroke in habitual snorers was increased (odds ratio = 2.1),

even after correction for the presence of hypertension or heart disease.[315] The mechanism responsible for such cerebral vascular disease may be the wide swings in cerebral blood flow and systemic arterial pressure that occur during and after apneic episodes.[316, 317] It should be remembered that patients who have had cerebral vascular accidents may also develop OSA, an occurrence that is of no value in localizing the cerebral lesion.[159] In fact, it may be unclear whether OSA precedes the development of stroke or vice versa.[318]

In addition to pronounced sleepiness, OSA may be manifested by cognitive impairment, depression, personality changes, and decreased vigilance.[319–321] Episodic hypoxemia and profound sleep fragmentation are the most likely causes of the changes in personality and behavior. Confusion with a psychiatric disorder is likely if the excessive sleepiness is attributed to depression. The consequences for the individual and for society in terms of family relations, job performance, and public safety are profound.[22, 322] For example, patients who have OSA and daytime sleepiness are at increased risk for motor vehicle accidents,[323–325] a complication that may be particularly important in long-haul truck drivers.[326] There is also a striking incidence of severe psychosocial disruption in the lives of patients who have sleep apnea.

Headache, especially on awakening, is significantly more common among snorers and patients who have OSA than among appropriate control subjects; for example, 5% of the general population in one study complained of morning headache compared with 18% of individuals who were heavy snorers and had OSA.[327] Hearing loss has also been reported and attributed to loud snoring![328]

## Miscellaneous Manifestations

Nocturia and enuresis are common in OSA, perhaps because of high nocturnal levels of atrial natriuretic factor.[329, 330] Decreased libido and impotence are additional symptoms and are probably attributable to prolonged hypoxemia and hypercapnia.[22] Although testosterone is a risk factor for the development of sleep apnea, the presence of severe OSA itself causes reduced serum testosterone levels, and successful treatment results in a return toward normal levels.[331] OSA is also associated with decreased nocturnal growth hormone levels and increased insulin levels.[332] Nocturnal hypoxemia can also stimulate erythropoietin secretion and may cause secondary polycythemia, particularly in individuals who have baseline arterial hypoxemia; in fact, nocturnal accentuation of arterial desaturation makes an important contribution to the polycythemia of obstructive pulmonary disease.[307, 333] There is a disruption of the normal circadian rhythm of secretion of the cytokine tumor necrosis factor-alpha in patients who have OSA.[334]

Although there is continued uncertainty regarding the relationship between sudden infant death syndrome and OSA, there is evidence that sudden infant death syndrome is more common in families of individuals who have OSA and that family members of infants who have died from this syndrome have anatomically narrowed upper airways.[335]

## DIAGNOSTIC TECHNIQUES

The diagnosis of OSA requires the study of breathing during sleep. The techniques of polysomnography have been reviewed;[52, 336] for physicians interested specifically in respiration, the measurements include sleep staging, respiratory effort, air flow, and changes in arterial blood gas tensions. The first of these is accomplished by recording the electroencephalogram (EEG) (usually two electrode positions), the electro-oculogram, and the electromyogram (EMG) of a skeletal muscle (usually the submental muscle). The frequency and amplitude of the brain waves are the most important signals used in sleep staging.

During wakefulness, the EEG is dominated by rapid, relatively low-amplitude waves called alpha waves (7 to 16 cycles per second). At the onset of Stage 1 sleep, periods of lower-frequency activity are interspersed with alpha waves. During Stage 2, the low-amplitude, mixed-frequency electroencephalographic activity continues but is mixed with brief episodes of high-frequency, low-amplitude rhythmic bursts (sleep spindles) and with well-defined, higher-amplitude negative deflections that are followed by sharp positive waves (K complexes). Tonic electromyographic activity is slightly decreased during Stages 1 and 2, and there are no eye movements. Approximately 50% of sleep is spent in Stage 2. Stages 3 and 4 are called slow-wave sleep and are characterized by high-amplitude, low-frequency periods of electroencephalographic activity (0.1 to 3 cycles per second). Stage 4 is distinguished from Stage 3 by a greater amount of time occupied by the low-frequency pattern, slow waves constituting more than 50%. During Stages 3 and 4, electromyographic activity decreases further and there are no eye movements. Between 8% and 20% of sleep is characterized by slow waves. The onset of REM sleep is signaled by a return to low-amplitude, rapid-frequency electroencephalographic waves and by episodic bursts of REMs detected by electro-oculography. The EMG shows a virtual absence of activity, with the exception of short bursts during REM. Approximately 20% to 25% of sleep is spent in REM sleep. Stages vary throughout sleep, and on average about 40 changes occur between stages during a sleep of 7.5 hours duration.

Sleep is staged by visually scoring the polysomnographic record and categorizing short time periods (called *epochs*) into the appropriate stage based on the EMG, electro-oculogram, and EEG. Alternatively, computer-based algorithms have been developed that automatically stage sleep stages with reasonable accuracy and a considerable saving of labor.[337, 338] In addition to the stages, it is possible to determine the total time asleep, sleep latency (the time taken to fall asleep), sleep efficiency (the time spent asleep divided by the time in bed), and number of arousals. Sleep efficiency decreases, and sleep latency and number of awakenings increase with older age.

Respiration can be assessed during sleep by measuring air flow and respiratory movement. Respiratory effort can be determined using devices that measure rib cage or abdominal movement, or both, or changes in intrathoracic pressure. Rib cage or abdominal movement can be measured by employing a circumferential strain gauge, by transthoracic impedance pneumography, or, more commonly, by respiratory inductance plethysmography (Respitrace). It is important to measure rib cage and abdominal motion separately, because the paradoxical chest wall motion that occurs during OSA can result in little change in net volume; that is, as the rib cage expands, there is an equal and opposite inward motion of the abdominal wall. Respiratory effort can also be sensitively detected by measuring changes in esophageal pressure; however, this is invasive and is not used routinely.

Respiratory air flow can be measured using a thermistor, a microphone, a pneumotachograph, or a device that measures fluctuations in expired $CO_2$. A thermistor is a thermally sensitive electrical resistor that changes its electrical resistance in response to inspiratory cooling and expiratory warming, causing a signal that is in phase with flow. The device must be positioned over the nose and mouth to detect breathing through these orifices. A microphone placed over the trachea provides a simple but effective signal of respiratory air flow.[339] A $CO_2$ sensor positioned over the nose or mouth detects expired $CO_2$ and is also a useful noninvasive means of sensing respiratory air flow. A pneumotachograph requires the use of a face mask that can interfere with sleep and may modify the breathing pattern; however, this device can also provide an estimate of VT.

Changes in arterial blood gas concentration and arterial oxygen saturation can be monitored noninvasively, the most commonly used device being a pulse-type or transmittance-type ear oximeter. A probe applied to the ear or finger provides a continuous reading of arterial oxygen saturation. There are also devices that can measure mean capillary $Po_2$ and $Pco_2$ transcutaneously. The final measurements that complete a polysomnographic record are an electrocardiogram (ECG) to record cardiac dysrhythmias and an audio signal to detect snoring. The sound power spectrum derived from the snoring of patients who have OSA is significantly different from that of those who have simple snoring.[340] Although polysomnography is the gold standard for the diagnosis of OSA, it is not infallible; for example, in one study of 11 patients who had a negative study but who were deemed to have a high probability of OSA on clinical grounds, 6 had a positive test following restudy.[341]

A complete overnight sleep study with full polysomnography is expensive and time consuming. For these reasons, as well as the long waiting lists at some centers, a number of methods have been investigated for the detection of clinically significant OSA in addition to full polysomnography. These methods include anthropometric analyses, questionnaires,[342] abbreviated sleep studies,[343] overnight home monitoring,[344, 345] video recording,[346] or a combination of these methods.[347] The results of one investigation suggest that an accurate estimate of AI, total apnea time, mean apnea time, mean oxygen saturation, sleep efficiency, and sleep staging can be achieved by examining as little as 20% of an overnight sleep record.[348] In another study, a questionnaire coupled with measurement of BMI had an area under the receiver operating curve (ROC) curve of 0.79;[349] use of BMI alone by another group was associated with an area under the curve of 0.73.[350] In 594 patients referred to a sleep clinic because of suspicion of OSA, a composite index based on age, sex, BMI, oropharyngeal examination, and questioning of the bed partner yielded a sensitivity of 60% and a specificity of 63% for an AHI greater than 10.[351] Although these various measures are not definitive, they may be useful in prioritizing patients for full sleep studies.

The British Thoracic Society has suggested that if baseline arterial saturation is greater than 90% by pulse oximetry, the presence of more than 15 episodes of 4% oxygen desaturation per hour of sleep is indicative of OSA. In one study of 69 patients, this criterion was 100% specific (albeit only 31% sensitive).[352] In another investigation, oximetry alone was 90% sensitive and 75% specific in detecting OSA among 300 patients who had suspected disease;[353] however, it was ineffective in detecting patients who had the "upper airway resistance syndrome,"* narcolepsy, and a syndrome characterized by excessive periodic limb movements. Moreover, approximately 10% of the overnight records were of insufficient quality for adequate interpretation. In a third study of 240 outpatients referred for suspected OSA, overnight oximetry was 98% sensitive (108 of 110) and 48% specific (62 of 130) for the diagnosis.[354] As with other diagnostic tests, the positive predictive value of overnight oximetry increases when the pretest probability for OSA is judged to be high on the basis of clinical history and physical examination.[355]

Studies done during a daytime nap are usually not sufficient to make a confident diagnosis and are not cost efficient because, in patients in whom there is a high clinical suspicion, negative results have to be verified with complete overnight polysomnography.[358] In addition, false-positive findings may result if daytime polysomnography is performed after a night of sleep deprivation.[359] "Split-night polysomnography" has also been employed;[360] in this technique, the diagnosis of OSA is confirmed and its severity quantified in the first half of the night and the efficacy of therapy using continuous positive pressure is assessed in the second half. Although there is a danger of missing the diagnosis if a sufficiently prolonged duration of REM sleep does not occur in the first half, the results of one study suggest that the recording of sleep stage is not essential to detect sleep-disordered breathing;[361] in this study of 200 patients referred for diagnosis of OSA, determination of sleep stage did not alter the accuracy of the test.

Sophisticated portable monitoring devices are now available that allow the in-home detection of sleep state, EOG, EMG, arterial saturation, air flow, and respiratory effort;[344, 362] for some of these, effectiveness in the diagnosis of OSA has been compared with polysomnography.[363–370] A valuable measure is wrist actigraphy; in this procedure, a simple device is used to measure movement at the wrist, giving an accurate measure of sleep duration as well as helping in the detection of periodic limb movement, one of the most important differential diagnoses in patients who have excessive daytime sleepiness. It is unclear whether the use of these devices will prove cost-effective in the diagnosis of OSA. To be cost-effective, the savings from the full polysomnographic studies that are avoided must more than offset the cost of the portable studies without a decrease in diagnostic accuracy.[371] Portable monitoring is recommended in selected patients by the American Sleep Disorders Association's Standards of Practice Committee.[372] The technique is satisfactory when the classic results of OSA are detected; however, polysomnography is required when the results are negative or equivocal. A useful two-stage approach is to conduct portable monitoring of oxygen saturation, snoring, and body position on patients selected on the basis of neck circumference, blood pressure, habitual snoring, and witnessed nocturnal choking and gasping.[347]

## PULMONARY FUNCTION TESTS

The severity of nocturnal desaturation depends not only on the length of apneic periods but also on lung function while the patient is awake and on the preobstruction arterial $PO_2$. Because of the shape of the oxygen dissociation curve, considerable hypoxemia can occur without much desaturation if arterial $PO_2$ is normal to begin with. If significant hypoxemia precedes the apneic episodes, as it may in individuals who have intrinsic pulmonary disease, a similar duration of apnea will cause more profound desaturation.[373] This may be another of the mechanisms by which obesity interacts with OSA: because obesity causes a decrease in FRC in the supine position, it tends to diminish baseline, preapneic arterial $PO_2$ and thus to exaggerate the asphyxic effects of an apnea. It is difficult to separate the effects on lung function of the sleep apnea syndrome from those due to the frequently accompanying obesity.[374] In one study, 32 moderately obese patients who had OSA were compared with 17 non-OSA patients matched for age, sex, and weight;[375] while awake, those who had OSA showed depressed ventilatory responses to $CO_2$ but not to hypoxia and had a lower $PaO_2$, a higher arterial $PCO_2$, and a significantly reduced total lung capacity. In another investigation, 52 patients who had severe OSA (AHI > 30) were compared with 56 who had moderate disease (AHI > 10 and < 30) and 62 whose AHI was < 10;[376] $FEV_1$, $FEF_{50}$ and $FEV_1$/ FVC decreased as a function of the severity of OSA, and there was a highly significant relationship between the specific conductance of the respiratory system and AHI. Interestingly, patients who have OSA may have higher than normal diffusing capacity, an effect that may be attributable to obesity rather than to nocturnal obstruction.[377]

These data suggest that patients who have OSA have smaller lungs, narrower lower and upper airways, and decreased ventilatory drive compared with similarly obese individuals who do not have OSA. In addition to the clinical manifestations described earlier, a number of other features are seen in many patients who have OSA. These are particularly evident in the cardiovascular and central nervous systems.

## PROGNOSIS

Although OSA is associated with an increased mortality, the contribution of OSA to this increase is unclear. This is in part because of variation in the experimental design of studies addressing this issue and in part because of the

---

*The upper airway resistance syndrome is characterized by episodes of partial airway collapse and hypoventilation unaccompanied by apnea or marked arterial oxygen desaturation. As with OSA, the irregular breathing is associated with frequent arousals and sleep fragmentation, and patients may have significant daytime hypersomnolence. They may also benefit from therapy for OSA. The reason for the arousals is presumably the increased ventilatory drive that stimulates respiratory muscle and upper airway mechanoreceptors.[71, 356, 357] The syndrome can be diagnosed by measuring fluctuations in esophageal pressure swings or total respiratory system resistance during sleep.[343]

confounding influences of obesity and hypertension.[16] In one multivariate analysis of 57 deaths that occurred in 1,620 adult men and women who were diagnosed as having OSA and were followed for a mean of 12 years, age, BMI, hypertension, and AI were all independent predictors of excess mortality due to cardiopulmonary disease.[378] Early studies of mortality in OSA focused on severely affected patients referred to clinics and were associated with quite alarming statistics, especially in men younger than 50 years (10% mortality over 8 years).[379, 380] In more recent studies, the confounding influences of comorbid disease have been demonstrated using multivariate analysis,[381] and the contribution of OSA to excess mortality has been shown to be lower,

especially in older individuals.[35] For example, in one study of older individuals, the presence of OSA was not a separate predictor of increased mortality after adjustment for age and cardiopulmonary disease;[382] however, this association may be biased by the possibility that OSA could have contributed to the cardiopulmonary disease.

The prospective use of cephalometry, somnofluoroscopy,[383] and CT reconstruction of the upper airway[384] has the potential to identify patients who will benefit from surgery and could aid in the planning of individual surgical procedures.[248, 385–387] However, to date the effectiveness of selection of candidates for specific surgical approaches has been disappointing.

# *REFERENCES*

1. Criteria for measurements, definitions, and severity rating of sleep-disordered breathing in adults. Report of an American Sleep Disorders Association Task Force, in conjunction with the European Respiratory Society, the Australian Sleep Association, and the American Thoracic Society. Sleep, in press.
2. Krieger J: Breathing during sleep in normal subjects. Clin Chest Med 6(4):577, 1985.
3. Bülow K, Inguar D: Respiration and state of wakefullness in normals, studied by spirography, capnography and EEG. Acta Physiol Scand 51:230, 1961.
4. Robin ED, Whaley RD, Crump CC, et al: Alveolar gas tensions, pulmonary ventilation and blood pH during physiological sleep in normal subjects. J Clin Invest 37:981, 1958.
5. Gothe B, Altose MD, Goldman MD, et al: Effect of quiet sleep on resting and $CO_2$ stimulated breathing in humans. J Appl Physiol 50:724, 1981.
6. Lopes JM, Tabachnik E, Müller NL, et al: Total airway resistance and respiratory muscle activity during sleep. J Appl Physiol 54:773, 1983.
7. Hudgel DW, Martin RJ, Johnson B, et al: Mechanics of the respiratory system and breathing pattern during sleep in normal humans. J Appl Physiol 56:133, 1984.
8. Tangel DJ, Mezzanote WA, White DP: Influence of sleep on tensor palatini EMG and upper airway resistance in normal men. J Appl Physiol 70:2574, 1991.
9. Douglas NJ: Control of ventilation during sleep. Clin Chest Med 6(4):563, 1985.
10. Remmers JE: Sleeping and breathing. Chest 3:77S, 1997.
11. Berssenbrugge A, Dempsey J, Iber C, et al: Mechanisms of hypoxia-induced periodic breathing during sleep in humans. J Physiol 343:507, 1983.
12. Phillipson EA, Sullivan CE: Arousal: The forgotten response to respiratory stimuli. Am Rev Respir Dis 118:896, 1978.
13. Berthon-Jones M, Sullivan CE: Ventilatory and arousal responses to hypoxia in sleeping humans. Am Rev Respir Dis 125:632, 1982.
14. Berthon-Jones N, Sullivan CE: Ventilation and arousal responses to hypercapnia in normal sleeping adults. J Appl Physiol 57:59, 1984.
15. Bresnitz EA, Goldberg R, Kosinski RM: Epidemiology of obstructive sleep apnea. Epidemiol Rev 16:210, 1994.
16. Strohl KP, Redline S: Recognition of obstructive sleep apnea. Am J Respir Crit Care Med 154:279, 1996.
17. McNamara SG, Grunstein RR, Sullivan CE: Obstructive sleep apnea. Thorax 48:754, 1993.
18. Ohayon MM, Guilleminault C, Priest RG, et al: Snoring and breathing pauses during sleep: Telephone interview survey of a United Kingdom population sample. BMJ 314:860, 1997.
19. Jennum P, Soul A: Epidemiology of snoring and obstructive sleep apnoea in a Danish population age 30–60. J Sleep Res 1:240, 1992.
20. Guilleminault C, Dement WC: Sleep apnea syndromes and related sleep disorders. In Williams RL, Karacon I (eds): Sleep Disorders: Diagnosis and Treatment. New York, Wiley, 1978, p 11.
21. Guilleminault C, van den Hoed J, Mitler MM: Clinical overview of the sleep apnea syndromes. In Guilleminault C, Dement WC (eds): Sleep Apnea Syndromes. New York, Alan R. Liss, 1978, p 1.
22. Wiegand L, Zwillich CW: Obstructive sleep apnea. Dis Mon 40:197, 1994.
23. Whyte KF, Allen MB, Fitzpatrick MF, et al: Accuracy and significance of scoring hypopneas. Sleep 15:257, 1992.
24. Cirignotta F, d'Alessandro R, Partinen M, et al: Prevalence of every night snoring and obstructive sleep apneas among 30–69 year old men in Bologna, Italy. Acta Neurol Scand 79:366, 1989.
25. Bearpark H, Elliott L, Cullen S, et al: Home monitoring demonstrates high prevalence of sleep disordered breathing in men in the Busselton population. Sleep Res 20A:411, 1991.
26. Young T, Zaccaro D, Leder R, et al: Prevalence and correlates of sleep disordered breathing in the Wisconsin sleep cohort study. Am Rev Respir Dis 143:A380, 1991.
27. Berry DT, Webb WB, Block AJ, et al: Sleep-disordered breathing and its concomitants in a subclinical population. Sleep 9:478, 1986.
28. Marin JM, Gascon JM, Carrizo S, et al: Prevalence of sleep apnoea syndrome in the Spanish adult population. Int J Epidemiol 26:381, 1997.
29. Berry DTR, Webb WB, Block AJ: Sleep apnea syndrome: A critical review of the apnea index as a diagnostic criterion. Chest 86:529, 1984.
30. Partinen M, Telakivi T: Epidemiology of obstructive sleep apnea syndrome. Sleep 15:S1, 1992.
31. Ancoli-Israel S, Kripke DF, Mason W, et al: Sleep apnea and periodic movements in an aging sample. J Gerontol 40:419, 1985.
32. Kripke DF, Ancoli-Israel S, Klauber MR, et al: Prevalence of sleep-disordered breathing in ages 40–64 years: A population-based survey. Sleep 20:65, 1997.
33. Redline S, Tishler PV, Hans MG, et al: Racial differences in sleep-disordered breathing in African-Americans and Caucasians. Am J Respir Crit Care Med 155:186, 1997.
34. American Thoracic Society: Standards and indications for cardiopulmonary sleep studies in children. Am J Respir Crit Care Med 153:866, 1996.
35. Ancoli-Israel S, Klauber MR, Kripke DF, et al: Sleep apnea in female patients in a nursing home. Chest 96:1054, 1989.
36. Dealberto MJ, Ferber C, Garma L, et al: Factors related to sleep apnea syndrome in sleep clinic patients. Chest 105:1753, 1994.
37. Grunstein R, Wilcox I, Yang T, et al: Snoring and sleep apnoea in men: Association with central obesity and hypertension. Int J Obes 17:533, 1993.
38. Davies RJO, Stradling J: The relationship between neck circumference, radiographic pharyngeal anatomy, and the obstructive sleep apnea syndrome. Eur Respir J 3:509, 1990.
39. Shinohara E, Kihara S, Yamashita S, et al: Visceral fat accumulation as an important risk factor for obstructive sleep apnoea syndrome in obese subjects. J Intern Med 241:11, 1997.
40. Levinson PD, McGarvey ST, Carlisle CC, et al: Adiposity and cardiovascular risk factors in men with obstructive sleep apnea. Chest 103:1336, 1993.
41. Burwell CS, Robin ED, Whaley RD, et al: Extreme obesity associated with alveolar hypoventilation—a Pickwickian syndrome. Am J Med 21:811, 1956.
42. Phillipson EA: Pickwickian, obesity-hypoventilation, or fee-fi-fo-fum syndrome? Am Rev Respir Dis 121:781, 1980.
43. Sullivan CE, Issa FG: Obstructive sleep apnea. Clin Chest Med 6(4):633, 1985.
44. Harman EM, Wynne JW, Block AJ: The effect of weight loss on sleep-disordered breathing and oxygen desaturation in morbidly obese men. Chest 82:291, 1982.
45. Smith PL, Gold AR, Meyers DA, et al: Weight loss in mildly to moderately obese patients with obstructive sleep apnea. Ann Intern Med 103:850, 1985.
46. Suratt PM, McTier RE, Findley LJ, et al: Changes in breathing and the pharynx after weight loss in obstructive sleep apnea. Chest 92:631, 1987.
47. Redline S, Young T: Epidemiology and natural history of obstructive sleep apnea. Ear Nose Throat J 72:20, 1993.
48. Lugaresi E, Cirignotta F, Montagna P, et al: Snoring: Pathogenesis, clinical and therapeutic aspects. In Kryger MH, Roth T, Dement WC, et al (eds): Principles and Practice of Sleep Medicine. 2nd ed. Philadelphia, WB Saunders, 1993, pp 621–629.
49. Jennum P, Wildschiodtz G: Epidemiology of snoring and sleep apnea. Abstracts of the Copenhagen Sleep Research Meetings 401, 1987.
50. Bixler EO, Vgontzas N, Have TT, et al: Effects of age on sleep apnea in men. 1. Prevalence and severity. Am J Respir Crit Care Med 157:144, 1998.
51. Guilleminault C, Dement WC: Sleep apnea syndromes and related disorders. In Williams RL, Katacan I (eds): Sleep Disorders: Diagnosis and Treatment. New York, Wiley, 1978.
52. Fletcher EC: History, techniques and definitions in sleep-related respiratory disorders. In Fletcher EC (ed): Abnormalities of Respiration During Sleep. Orlando, Grune & Stratton, 1986, p 1.
53. Block AJ, Boysen PG, Wynne JW, et al: Sleep apnea, hypopnea and oxygen desaturation in normal subjects. N Engl J Med 300:513, 1979.
54. Guilleminault C, Quera-Salva MA, Partinen M, et al: Women and the obstructive sleep apnea syndrome. Chest 93:104, 1988.
55. Young T, Palta M, Dempsey J, et al: The occurrence of sleep-disordered breathing among middle-aged adults. N Engl J Med 328:1230, 1993.
56. Guilleminault C, Stoohs R, Kim YD, et al: Upper airway sleep-disordered breathing in women. Ann Intern Med 122:493, 1995.
57. Sloan EP, Shapiro CM: Obstructive sleep apnea in a consecutive series of obese women. Int J Eat Disord 17:167, 1995.
58. Redline S, Kump K, Tishler PV, et al: Gender differences in sleep disordered breathing in a community-based sample. Am J Respir Crit Care Med 149:722, 1994.
59. Redline S, Hans M, Pracharktam N, et al: Differences in the age distribution and risk factors for sleep-disordered breathing in blacks and whites. Am J Respir Crit Care Med 149:577, 1994.
60. Wetter D, Young T, Bidwall T, et al: Smoking as a risk factor for sleep disordered breathing. Arch Intern Med 154:2219, 1994.
61. Stradling JR, Crosby JH: Relation between systemic hypertension and sleep hypoxemia or snoring: Analysis in 748 men drawn from general practice. BMJ 300:75, 1992.
62. Dawson A, Bigby BG, Poceta JS, et al: Effect of bedtime alcohol on inspiratory resistance and respiratory drive in snoring and nonsnoring men. Alcohol Clin Exp Res 21:183, 1997.
63. Wetter DW, Young TB, Bidwell TR, et al: Smoking as a risk factor for sleep-disordered breathing. Arch Intern Med 154:2219, 1994.
64. Le Bon O, Verbanck P, Hoffmann G, et al: Sleep in detoxified alcoholics: Impairment of most standard sleep parameters and increased risk for sleep apnea, but not for myoclonias—a controlled study. J Stud Alcohol 58:30, 1997.
65. Hoffstein V, Chan CK, Slutsky AS: Handedness and sleep apnea. Chest 103:1860, 1993.
66. Kahn A, Groswasser J, Sottiaux M, et al: Prenatal exposure to cigarettes in infants with obstructive sleep apneas. Pediatrics 93:778, 1994.
67. Lefcourt LA, Rodis JF: Obstructive sleep apnea in pregnancy. Obstet Gynecol Surv 51:503, 1996.
68. Winkelman JW, Goldman H, Piscatelli N, et al: Are thyroid function tests necessary in patients with suspected sleep apnea? Sleep 19:790, 1996.
69. Pelttari L, Rauhala E, Polo O, et al: Upper airway obstruction in hypothyroidism. J Intern Med 236:177, 1994.
70. Deegan PC, McNamara VM, Morgan WE: Goitre: A cause of obstructive sleep apnoea in euthyroid patients. Eur Respir J 10:500, 1997.
71. National Heart, Lung and Blood Institute: Fact Book: Fiscal Year 1993. Bethesda, MD, U.S. Department of Health and Human Services, U.S. Public Health Service, National Institutes of Health, 1994.
72. Philipson EA: Sleep apnea—a major public health problem. N Engl J Med 328:1271, 1993.

73. Phillips BA, Feinsilver SH, Gillin JC: Catching up on sleep. The National Sleep Disorders Research Plan (editorial). Chest 110:1132, 1996.
74. Kryger MH, Roos L, Delaive K, et al: Utilization of health care services in patients with severe obstructive sleep apnea. Sleep 19:S111, 1996.
75. Fischer J, Raschke F: Economic and medical significance of sleep-related breathing disorders. Respiration 64:39, 1997.
76. Wittels EH: Obesity and hormonal factors in sleep and sleep apnea. Med Clin North Am 69:1265, 1985.
77. White DP: Pathophysiology of obstructive sleep apnoea. Thorax 50:797, 1995.
78. Deegan PC, McNicholas WT: Pathophysiology of obstructive sleep apnoea. Eur Respir J 8:1161, 1995.
79. Douglas NJ, Polo O: Pathogenesis of obstructive sleep apnoea/hypopnoea syndrome. Lancet 344:653, 1994.
80. Findlay LJ, Wilholt SC, Suratt PM: Apnea duration and hypoxemia during REM sleep in patients with obstructive sleep apnea. Chest 87:432, 1985.
81. Parisi RA, Croce SA, Edelman NH, et al: Obstructive sleep apnea following bilateral carotid body resection. Chest 91:922, 1987.
82. Strohl KP, Saunders NA, Feldman NT, et al: Obstructive sleep apnea in family members. N Engl J Med 299:969, 1978.
83. Manon-Espaillat R, Gothe B, Adams N, et al: Familial "sleep apnea plus" syndrome: Report of a family. Neurology 38:190, 1988.
84. Wittig RM, Zorick FJ, Roehrs TA, et al: Familial childhood sleep apnea. Henry Ford Hosp Med J 36:13, 1988.
85. El Bayadi S, Millman RP, Tishler PV, et al: A family study of sleep apnea. Anatomic and physiologic interactions. Chest 98:554, 1990.
86. Williamson J, Tosteson T, Redline S, et al: Familial aggregation studies with matched proband sampling. Hum Hered 46:76, 1996.
87. Guilleminault C, Powell N, Heldt G, et al: Small upper airway in near-miss SIDS infants and their families. Lancet 8478:402, 1986.
88. Pillar G, Lavie P: Assessment of the role of inheritance in sleep apnea syndrome. Am J Respir Crit Care Med 151:688, 1995.
89. Kaprio J, Koskenvuo M, Partinen M, et al: A twin study of snoring. Sleep Res 17:365, 1988.
90. Redline S, Tosteson T, Tishler PV, et al: Studies in the genetics of obstructive sleep apnea. Am Rev Respir Dis 145:440, 1992.
91. Mathur R, Douglas NJ: Family studies in patients with the sleep apnea-hypopnea syndrome. Ann Intern Med 122:174, 1995.
92. Guilleminault C, Partinen M, Hollman K, et al: Familial aggregates in obstructive sleep apnea syndrome. Chest 107:1545, 1995.
93. Redline S, Tishler PV: Familial influences on sleep apnea. In Saunders NA, Sullivan CE (eds): Sleep and Breathing. 2nd ed. New York, Marcel Dekker, 1994, pp 363–377.
94. Osborne RH, De George FV: Genetic Variation of Morphological Variation. Cambridge, MA, Harvard University Press, 1959.
95. Bodurtha JN, Mosteller M, Hewitt JK, et al: Genetic analysis of anthropometric measures in 11 year old twins. The Medical College of Virginia Twin Study. Pediatr Res 28:1, 1990.
96. Strunkard AJ, Harris JR, Pedersen NL, et al: The body-mass index of twins who have been reared apart. N Engl J Med 322:1483, 1990.
97. Bray GA: Genetic and hypothalamic mechanisms for obesity—finding the needle in the haystack. Am J Clin Nutr 50:891, 1989.
98. Van Itallie TB: Obesity, genetics and ponderal set point. Clin Neuropharmacol 11(Suppl):S1, 1988.
99. Bouchard C: Genetic factors in obesity. Med Clin North Am 73:67, 1989.
100. Nance WE, Nakata M, Paul TD, et al: Congenital defects. In Janerich DT, Skalko RG, Porter IH (eds): New Directions in Research. New York, Academic Press, 1974, pp 23–49.
101. Clarke DJ, Waters J, Corbett JA: Adults with Prader-Willi syndrome: Abnormalities of sleep behavior. J R Soc Med 82:20, 1989.
102. Sirotnak J, Brodsky L, Pizzuto M: Airway obstruction in the Crouzon syndrome: Case report and review of the literature. Int J Pediatr Otorhinolaryngol 31:235, 1995.
103. Ryan CF, Lowe AA, Fleetham JA: Nasal continuous positive airway pressure (CPAP) therapy for obstructive sleep apnea in Hallermann-Streiff syndrome. Clin Pediatr 29:122, 1990.
104. Ferri R, Curzi-Dascalova L, Del Gracco S, et al: Respiratory patterns during sleep in Down's syndrome: Importance of central apnoeas. J Sleep Res 6:134, 1997.
105. Bower CM, Richmond D: Tonsillectomy and adenoidectomy in patients with Down syndrome. Int J Pediatr Otorhinolaryngol 33:141, 1995.
106. Redline S, Leitner J, Arnold J, et al: Ventilatory-control abnormalities in familial sleep apnea. Am J Respir Crit Care Med 156:155, 1997.
107. Pillar G, Schnall RP, Peled N, et al: Impaired respiratory response to resistive loading during sleep in healthy offspring of patients with obstructive sleep apnea. Am J Respir Crit Care Med 155:1602, 1997.
108. Yoshizawa T, Akashiba T, Kurashina K, et al: Genetics and obstructive sleep apnea syndrome: A study of human leukocyte antigen (HLA) typing. Int Med 32:94, 1993.
109. Robinson RW, Zwillich CW: The effect of drugs on breathing during sleep. Clin Chest Med 6:603, 1985.
110. Sandblom RE, Matsumoto AM, Schoene RB, et al: Obstructive sleep apnea syndrome induced by testosterone administration. N Engl J Med 108:508, 1983.
111. Matsumoto AM, Sandblom RE, Schoene RB, et al: Testosterone replacement in hypogonadal men: Effects on obstructive sleep apnoea, respiratory drives, and sleep. Clin Endocrinol (Oxf) 22:713, 1985.
112. Johnson MW, Anch AM, Remmers JE: Induction of the obstructive sleep apnea

syndrome in a woman by exogenous androgen administration. Am Rev Respir Dis 129:1023, 1984.
113. Cistulli PA, Grunstein RR, Sullivan CE: Effect of testosterone administration on upper airway collapsibility during sleep. Am J Respir Crit Care Med 149:530, 1994.
114. Harman E, Wynne JW, Block AJ, et al: Sleep-disordered breathing and oxygen desaturation in obese patients. Chest 79:256, 1981.
115. Tsuchiya M, Lowe A, Fleetham J: Obstructive sleep apnea subtypes by cluster analysis. Am J Orthod 101:533, 1992.
116. Lowe AA, Fleetham JA, Adachi S, et al: Cephalometry and computed tomography predictors of obstructive sleep apnea. Am J Orthod 107:589, 1995.
117. Lowe AA, Ono T, Ferguson KA, et al: Cephalometric comparisons of craniofacial and upper airway morphology by skeletal subtype and gender in patients with obstructive sleep apnea. Am J Orthod 110:653, 1996.
118. Bacon W, Krieger J, Turlot J-C, et al: Craniofacial characteristics in patients with obstructive sleep apnea syndrome. Cleft Palate J 25:374, 1988.
119. Jamieson A, Guilleminault, C, Partinen N, et al: Obstructive sleep apnea patients have craniomandibular abnormalities. Sleep 9(4):469, 1986.
120. Hudgel DW: The role of upper airway anatomy and physiology in obstructive sleep apnea. Clin Chest Med 13:383, 1992.
121. Abe K, Hori Y, Ohtsu SY, et al: A case of non-Hodgkin's lymphoma with macroglobulinemia. Acta Otolaryngol Suppl (Stockh) 523:259, 1996.
122. Epstein LJ, Strollo PJ Jr, Donegan RB, et al: Obstructive sleep apnea in patients with human immunodeficiency virus (HIV) disease. Sleep 18:368, 1995.
123. Spier S, Rivlin J, Rowe RD, et al: Sleep in Pierre Robin syndrome. Chest 90:711, 1986.
124. Chervin RD, Guilleminault C: Obstructive sleep apnea and related disorders. Neurol Clin 14:583, 1996.
125. Ferguson KA, Ono T, Lowe AA, et al: The relationship between obesity and craniofacial structure in obstructive sleep apnea. Chest 108:375, 1995.
126. Pepin JL, Ferretti G, Veale D, et al: Somnofluoroscopy, computed tomography, and cephalometry in the assessment of the airway in obstructive sleep apnoea. Thorax 47:150, 1992.
127. Kuna ST, Remmers JE: Pathophysiology and mechanisms of sleep apnea. In Fletcher EC (ed): Abnormalities of Respiration during Sleep. Orlando, Grune & Stratton, 1986, p 63.
128. Papsidero MJ: The role of nasal obstruction in obstructive sleep apnea syndrome. Ear Nose Throat J 72:82, 1993.
129. Young T, Finn L, Kim H: Nasal obstruction as a risk factor for sleep-disordered breathing. The University of Wisconsin Sleep and Respiratory Research Group. J Aller Clin Immunol 99:S757, 1997.
130. Zwillich CW, Picket C, Hanson FN, et al: Disturbed sleep and prolonged apnea during nasal obstruction in normal men. Am Rev Respir Dis 124:158, 1981.
131. Rajagopal KR, Bennett LL, Dillard TA, et al: Overnight nasal CPAP improves hypersomnolence in sleep apnea. Chest 90:172, 1986.
132. White DP, Cadieux RJ, Lombard RM: The effects of nasal anesthesia on breathing during sleep. Am Rev Respir Dis 132:972, 1985.
133. McNicholas WT, Coffey M, McDonnell T, et al: Upper airway obstruction during sleep in normal subjects after selective topical oropharyngeal anesthesia. Am Rev Respir Dis 135:1316, 1987.
134. Berry RB, McNellis MI, Kouchi K, et al: Upper airway anesthesia reduces phasic genioglossus activity during sleep apnea. Am J Respir Crit Care Med 156:127, 1997.
135. Gleeson K, Zwillich CW, Braier K, et al: Breathing route during sleep. Am Rev Respir Dis 134:115, 1988.
136. Masumi S, Nishigawa K, Williams AJ, et al: Effect of jaw position and posture on forced inspiratory airflow in normal subjects and patients with obstructive sleep apnea. Chest 109:1484, 1996.
137. Nelson S, Hans M: Contribution of craniofacial risk factors in increasing apneic activity among obese and nonobese habitual snorers. Chest 111:154, 1997.
138. Jamieson A, Guilleminault C, Partinen M, et al: Obstructive sleep apneic patients have craniomandibular abnormalities. Sleep 9:469, 1986.
139. Ono T, Lowe AA, Ferguson KA, Fleetham JA: Associations among upper airway structure, body position, and obesity in skeletal class I male patients with obstructive sleep apnea. Am J Orthod Dentofacial Orthop 109:625, 1996.
140. Pae EK, Lowe AA, Fleetham JA: A role of pharyngeal length in obstructive sleep apnea patients. Am J Orthod Dentofacial Orthop 111:12, 1997.
141. Will MJ, Ester MS, Ramirez SG, et al: Comparison of cephalometric analysis with ethnicity in obstructive sleep apnea patients. Sleep 18:87, 1995.
142. Lee JJ, Ramirez SG, Will MJ: Gender and racial variations in cephalometric analysis. Otolaryngol Head Neck Surg 117:326, 1997.
143. Hoffstein V, Zamel N, Phillipson EA: Lung volume dependence of pharyngeal cross-sectional area in patients with obstructive sleep apnea. Am Rev Respir Dis 130:175, 1984.
144. Katz I, Stradling J, Slutsky AS, et al: Do patients with obstructive sleep apnea have thick necks? Am Rev Respir Dis 141:1228, 1990.
145. Hoffstein V, Mateika S: Differences in abdominal and neck circumference in patients with and without obstructive sleep apnea. Eur Respir J 5:377, 1992.
146. Davies RJO, Stradling JR: The relationship between neck circumference, radiographic anatomy, and the obstructive sleep apnea syndrome. Eur Respir J 3:509, 1990.
147. Davies RJ, Ali NJ, Stradling JR: Neck circumference and other clinical features in the diagnosis of the obstructive sleep apnoea syndrome. Thorax 47:101, 1992.
148. Davies RJO, Nabeel JA, Stradling JR: Neck circumference and other clinical features in the diagnosis of the obstructive sleep apnoea syndrome. Thorax 47:101, 1992.

149. Mortimore IL, Marshall I, Wraith PK, et al: Neck and total body fat deposition in nonobese and obese patients with sleep apnea compared with that in control subjects. Am J Respir Crit Care Med 157:280, 1998.
150. Ryan CF, Love LL: Mechanical properties of the velopharynx in obese patients with obstructive sleep apnea. Am J Respir Crit Care Med 154:806, 1996.
151. Douglas NJ: The sleep apnoea/hypopnoea syndrome. Eur J Clin Invest 25:285, 1995.
152. Grunstein RR: Metabolic aspects of sleep apnea. Sleep 19:S218, 1996.
153. Strohl KP, Novak RD, Singer W, et al: Insulin levels, blood pressure and sleep apnea. Sleep 17:614, 1994.
154. Walsh RE, Michaelson ED, Harkleroad LE, et al: Upper airway obstruction in obese patients with sleep disturbance and somnolence. Ann Intern Med 76:185, 1972.
155. Felman AH, Loughlin GM, Leftridge CA Jr, et al: Upper airway obstruction during sleep in children. Am J Roentgenol 133:213, 1979.
156. Schwab RJ: Properties of tissues surrounding the upper airway. Sleep 19:S170, 1996.
157. Schwab RJ, Gupta KB, Gefter WB, et al: Upper airway and soft tissue anatomy in normal subjects and patients with sleep-disordered breathing. Significance of the lateral pharyngeal walls. Am J Respir Crit Care Med 152:1673, 1995.
158. Leiter JC: Upper airway shape. Is it important in the pathogenesis of obstructive sleep apnea? Am J Respir Crit Care Med 153:894, 1996.
158a. Kushida CA, Efron B, Guilleminault C: A predictive morphometric model for the obstructive sleep apnea syndrome. Ann Intern Med 127:581, 1997.
159. Bassetti C, Aldrich MS, Quint D: Sleep-disordered breathing in patients with acute supra- and infratentorial strokes. A prospective study of 39 patients. Stroke 28:1765, 1997.
160. Sekosan M, Zakkar M, Wenig BL, et al: Inflammation in the uvula mucosa of patients with obstructive sleep apnea. Laryngoscope 106:1018, 1996.
161. Sturani C, Barrot-Cortez E, Papiris S, et al: Respiratory flutter during carbon dioxide rebreathing in patients with obstructive sleep apnea syndrome. Eur J Respir Dis 69:75, 1986.
162. Neukirch F, Weitzenblum E, Liard R, et al: Frequency and correlates of the saw-tooth pattern of flow-volume curves in an epidemiological survey [see comments]. Chest 101:425, 1992.
163. Haponik EF, Bleecker ER, Allen RP, et al: Abnormal inspiratory flow-volume curves in patients with sleep-disordered breathing. Am Rev Respir Dis 124:571, 1981.
164. Miura C, Hida W, Miki H, et al: Effects of posture on flow-volume curves during normocapnia and hypercapnia in patients with obstructive sleep apnoea. Thorax 47:524, 1992.
165. Kayaleh RA, Dutt A, Khan A, et al: Tidal breath flow-volume curves in obstructive sleep apnea. Am Rev Respir Dis 145:1372, 1992.
166. Shore ET, Millman RP: Abnormalities in the flow-volume loop in obstructive sleep apnea sitting and supine. Thorax 39:775, 1984.
167. Tammelin BR, Wilson AF, Borowiecki BD, et al: Flow-volume curves reflect pharyngeal airway abnormalities in sleep apnea syndrome. Am Rev Respir Dis 128:712, 1983.
168. Skatrud JB, Dempsey JA: Airway resistance and respiratory muscle function in snorers during NREM sleep. J Appl Physiol 59:328, 1985.
169. Stanescu D, Kostianev S, Sanna A, et al: Expiratory flow limitation during sleep in heavy snorers and obstructive sleep apnoea patients. Eur Respir J 9:2116, 1996.
170. Isono S, Remmers JE, Tanaka A, et al: Static properties of the passive pharynx in sleep apnea. Sleep 19:S175, 1996.
171. Issa FG, Sullivan CE: Arousal and breathing responses to airway occlusion in healthy sleeping adults. J Appl Physiol 55:1113, 1983.
172. Issa FG, Sullivan CE: Upper airway closing pressures in snorers. J Appl Physiol 57:528, 1984.
173. Issa FG, Sullivan CE: Upper airway closing pressures in obstructive sleep apnea. J Appl Physiol 57:520, 1984.
174. Isono S, Remmers JE, Tanaka A, et al: Anatomy of pharynx in patients with obstructive sleep apnea and in normal subjects. J Appl Physiol 82:1319, 1997.
175. Meurice JC, Marc I, Carrier G, et al: Effects of mouth opening on upper airway collapsibility in normal sleeping subjects. Am J Respir Crit Care Med 153:55, 1996.
176. Brown I, Bradley TD, Phillipson E, et al: Pharyngeal compliance in snoring subjects with and without obstructive sleep apnea. Am Rev Respir Dis 132:211, 1985.
177. Brooks LJ, Strohl KP: Size and mechanical properties of the pharynx in healthy men and women. Am Rev Respir Dis 146:1394, 1992.
178. Bradley TD, Brown IG, Grossman RF, et al: Pharyngeal size in snorers, nonsnorers, and patients with obstructive sleep apnea. N Engl J Med 315:1327, 1986.
179. Tsushima Y, Antila J, Svedstrom E, et al: Upper airway size and collapsibility in snorers: Evaluation with digital fluoroscopy. Eur Respir J 9:1611, 1996.
180. Roberts JL, Reed WR, Mathew OP, et al: Assessment of pharyngeal airway stability in normal and micrognathic infants. J Appl Physiol 58:290, 1985.
181. Reed WR, Roberts JL, Thach BT: Factors influencing regional patency and configuration of the human infant upper airway. J Appl Physiol 58:635, 1985.
182. Katsantonis GP, Moss K, Miyazaki S, et al: Determining the site of airway collapse in obstructive sleep apnea with airway pressure monitoring. Laryngoscope 103:1126, 1993.
183. Suratt PM, McTier RF, Wilhoit SC: Collapsibility of the nasopharyngeal airway in obstructive sleep apnea. Am Rev Respir Dis 132:967, 1985.
184. Morrison DL, Launois SH, Isono S, et al: Pharyngeal narrowing and closing pressures in patients with obstructive sleep apnea. Am Rev Respir Dis 148:606, 1993.
185. Isono S, Morrison DL, Launois SH, et al: Static mechanics of the velopharynx of patients with obstructive sleep apnea. J Appl Physiol 75:148, 1993.
186. Hudgel DW: Variable site of airway narrowing among obstructive sleep apnea patients. J Appl Physiol 61:1403, 1986.
187. Ferguson KA, Love LL, Ryan CF: Effect of mandibular and tongue protrusion on upper airway size during wakefulness. Am J Respir Crit Care Med 155:1748, 1997.
188. Cistulli PA, Sullivan CE: Sleep-disordered breathing in Marfan's syndrome. Am Rev Respir Dis 147:645, 1993.
189. Cistulli PA, Wilcox I, Jeremy R, et al: Aortic root dilatation in Marfan's syndrome: A contribution from obstructive sleep apnea? Chest 111:1763, 1997.
190. Horner RL: Motor control of the pharyngeal musculature and implications for the pathogenesis of obstructive sleep apnea. Sleep 19:827, 1996.
191. Guilleminault C, Stoohs R, Quera-Salva MA: Sleep-related obstructive and nonobstructive apneas and neurologic disorders. Neurology 42:53, 1992.
192. Strohl KP, Hensley MJ, Hallett M, et al: Activation of upper airway muscles before onset of inspiration in normal humans. J Appl Physiol 49:638, 1980.
193. Suratt PM, McTier R, Wilhoit SC: Alae nasi electromyographic activity and timing in obstructive sleep apnea. J Appl Physiol 58:1252, 1985.
194. Onal E, Lopata M, O'Connor T: Pathogenesis of apneas in hypersomnia-sleep apnea syndrome. Am Rev Respir Dis 125:167, 1982.
195. Warner G, Skatrud JB, Dempsey JA: Effect of hypoxia-induced periodic breathing on upper airway obstruction during sleep. J Appl Physiol 62:2201, 1987.
196. Ingbar DH, Gee JBL: Pathophysiology and treatment of sleep apnea. Annu Rev Med 36:369, 1985.
197. Berry DT, Webb WB, Block AJ, et al: Sleep-disordered breathing and its concomitants in a subclinical population. Sleep 9:478, 1986.
198. Onal E, Burrows DL, Hart RH, et al: Induction of periodic breathing during sleep causes upper airway obstruction in humans. J Appl Physiol 61:1438, 1986.
199. Alex CG, Onal E, Lopata M: Upper airway occlusion during sleep in patients with Cheyne-Stokes respiration. Am Rev Respir Dis 133:42, 1986.
200. Parisi RA, Neubauer JA, Frank M, et al: Correlation between geniogossal and diaphragmatic responses to hypercapnia in sleeping goats. Am Rev Respir Dis 131:A295, 1985.
201. Weiner D, Mitra J, Salamone J, et al: Effect of chemical stimuli on nerves supplying upper airway muscles. J Appl Physiol 52:530, 1982.
202. Onal E, Lopata N, O'Connor T: Diaphragmatic and genioglossal electromyogram responses to isocapnic hypoxia in humans. Am Rev Respir Dis 124:215, 1981.
203. Dolly FR, Block AJ: Effect of flurazepam on sleep-disordered breathing and nocturnal oxygen desaturation in asymptomatic subjects. Am J Med 73:239, 1982.
204. Taasan VC, Block AJ, Boysen PG, et al: Alcohol increases sleep apnea and oxygen desaturation in asymptomatic men. Am J Med 71:240, 1981.
205. Bonora M, Shields GI, Knuth SL, et al: Selective depression by ethanol of upper airway respiratory motor activity in cats. Am Rev Respir Dis 130:156, 1984.
206. Remmers JE: Obstructive sleep apnea—a common disorder exacerbated by alcohol (editorial). Am Rev Respir Dis 130:153, 1984.
207. Leiter J, Knuth S, Krol R, et al: The effect of diazepam on genioglossal muscle activity in normal human subjects. Am Rev Respir Dis 132:216, 1985.
208. Strohl KP, Saunders NA, Feldman NT, et al: Obstructive sleep apnea in family members. N Engl J Med 299:969, 1978.
209. Brooks LJ, Stohl KP: Size and mechanical properties of the pharynx in healthy men and women. Am Rev Respir Dis 146:1394, 1992.
210. Popovic RM, White DP: Influence of gender on waking genioglossal electromyogram and upper airway resistance. Am J Respir Crit Care Med 152:725, 1995.
211. Mezzanotte WS, Tangel DJ, White DP: Influence of sleep onset on upper-airway muscle activity in apnea patients versus normal controls. Am J Respir Crit Care Med 153:1880, 1996.
212. Mortimore IL, Douglas NJ: Palatal muscle EMG response to negative pressure in awake sleep apneic and control subjects. Am J Respir Crit Care Med 154:867, 1997.
213. Martin RJ, Sanders MH, Gray BA, et al: Acute and long-term ventilatory effects of hyperoxia in the adult sleep apnea syndrome. Am Rev Respir Dis 125:175, 1982.
214. Leiter JC, Knuth SL, Bartlett D: The effect of sleep deprivation on activity on the genioglossus muscle in man. Am Rev Respir Dis 132:1242, 1985.
215. Bartlett D, Leiter JC, Knuth SL: Control and actions of the genioglossus muscle. Prog Clin Biol Res 345:99, 1990.
216. Petrof BJ, Hendricks JC, Pack AI: Does upper airway muscle injury trigger a vicious cycle in obstructive sleep apnea? A hypothesis. Sleep 19:465, 1996.
217. Series F, Cote C, Simoneau JA, et al: Upper airway collapsibility, and contractile and metabolic characteristics of musculus uvulae. FASEB J 10:897, 1996.
218. Series FJ, Simoneau SA, St. Pierre S, et al: Characteristics of the genioglossus and musculus uvulae in sleep apnea hypopnea syndrome and in snorers. Am J Respir Crit Care Med 153:1870, 1996.
219. Rajagopal KR, Abbrecht PH, Tellis CJ: Control of breathing in obstructive sleep apnea. Chest 85:174, 1984.
220. van Lunteren E: Muscles of the pharynx: Structural and contractile properties. Ear Nose Throat J 72:27, 1993.
221. Hyland RH, Hutcheon MA, Perl A, et al: Upper airway occlusion induced by diaphragm pacing for primary alveolar hypoventilation—implications for the pathogenesis of obstructive sleep apnea. Am Rev Respir Dis 124:180, 1981.
222. Iber C, Davies SF, Chapman RC, et al: A possible mechanism for mixed apnea in obstructive sleep apnea. Chest 89:800, 1986.

223. Bonora M, Shields G, Knuth S, et al: Selective depression by ethanol of upper airway respiratory motor activity in cats. Am Rev Respir Dis 130:156, 1984.
224. Hwang J, St. John W, Bartlett D: Respiratory-related hypoglossal nerve activity influence of anesthetics. J Appl Physiol 55:785, 1983.
225. Robinson RW, Zwillich CW, Bixler EO, et al: Effects of oral narcotics on sleep-disordered breathing in healthy adults. Chest 91:197, 1987.
226. Vincken W, Guilleminault C, Silvestri L, et al: Inspiratory muscle activity as a trigger causing the airways to open in obstructive sleep apnea. Am Rev Respir Dis 135:372, 1987.
227. Montserrat JM, Kosmas EN, Cosio MG, et al: Lack of evidence for diaphragmatic fatigue over the course of the night in obstructive sleep apnoea. Eur Respir J 10:133, 1997.
228. Cibella F, Cuttitta G, Romano S, et al: Evaluation of diaphragmatic fatigue in obstructive sleep apnoeas during non-REM sleep. Thorax 52:731, 1997.
229. Berry RB, Kouchi KG, Bower JL, et al: Effect of upper airway anesthesia on obstructive sleep apnea. Am J Respir Crit Care Med 151:1857, 1995.
230. Montserrat JM, Kosmas EN, Cosio MG, et al: Mechanism of apnea lengthening across the night in obstructive sleep apnea. Am J Respir Crit Care Med 154:988, 1996.
231. Brooks D, Horner RL, Kimoff RJ, et al: Effect of obstructive sleep apnea versus sleep fragmentation on responses to airway occlusion. Am J Respir Crit Care Med 155:1609, 1997.
232. Kuna ST, Sant'ambrogio G: Pathophysiology of upper airway closure during sleep. JAMA 266:1384, 1991.
233. Douglas NJ: Upper airway imaging. Clin Phys Physiol Meas 11:117, 1990.
234. Fleetham JA: Upper airway imaging in relation to obstructive sleep apnea. Clin Chest Med 13:399, 1992.
235. Stark P, Norbash A: Imaging of the trachea and upper airways in patients with chronic obstructive airway disease. Radiol Clin North Am 36:91, 1998.
236. Tangugsorn V, Skatvedt O, Krogstad O, et al: Obstructive sleep apnoea: A cephalometric study. Part II. Uvulo-glossopharyngeal morphology. Eur J Orthod 17:57, 1995.
237. Tangugsorn V, Skatvedt O, Krogstad O, et al: Obstructive sleep apnoea: A cephalometric study. Part I. Cervico-craniofacial skeletal morphology. Eur J Orthod 17:45, 1995.
238. Hochban W, Brandenburg U: Morphology of the viscerocranium in obstructive sleep apnoea syndrome—cephalometric evaluation of 400 patients. J Craniomaxillofac Surg 22:205, 1994.
239. Avrahami E, Englender M: Relation between CT axial cross-sectional area of the oropharynx and obstructive sleep apnea syndrome in adults. AJNR Am J Neuroradiol 16:135, 1995.
240. Lowe AA, Fleetham JA, Adachi S, et al: Cephalometric and computed tomographic predictors of obstructive sleep apnea severity (see comments). Am J Orthod Dentofacial Orthoped 107:589, 1995.
241. Battagel JM, L'Estrange PR: The cephalometric morphology of patients with obstructive sleep apnoea (OSA). Eur J Orthod 18:557, 1996.
242. Pracharktam N, Hans MG, Strohl KP, et al: Upright and supine cephalometric evaluation of obstructive sleep apnea syndrome and snoring subjects. Angle Orthod 64:63, 1994.
243. Lowe AA, Ono T, Ferguson KA, et al: Cephalometric comparisons of craniofacial and upper airway structure by skeletal subtype and gender in patients with obstructive sleep apnea. Am J Orthod Dentofacial Orthop 110:653, 1996.
244. Lowe AA, Ozbek MM, Miyamoto K, et al: Cephalometric and demographic characteristics of obstructive sleep apnea: An evaluation with partial least squares analysis. Angle Orthod 67:143, 1997.
245. Pracharktam N, Nelson S, Hans MG, et al: Cephalometric assessment in obstructive sleep apnea. Am J Orthod Dentofacial Orthoped 109:410, 1996.
246. Frohberg U, Naples RJ, Jones DL: Cephalometric comparison of characteristics in chronically snoring patients with and without sleep apnea syndrome. Oral Surg Oral Med Oral Pathol Oral Radiol Endod 80:28, 1995.
247. Hoffstein V, Weiser W, Haney R: Roentgenographic dimensions of the upper airway in snoring patients with and without obstructive sleep apnea. Chest 100:81, 1991.
248. Lowe AA, Gionhaku N, Takeuchi K, et al: Three dimensional CT reconstructions of tongue and airway in adult subjects with obstructive sleep apnea. Am J Orthod Dentofacial Orthop 90:364, 1986.
249. Avrahami E, Englender M: Relation between CT axial cross-sectional area of the oropharynx and obstructive sleep apnea syndrome in adults. Am J Neuroradiol 16:135, 1995.
250. Schwab RJ, Gefter WB, Hoffman EA, et al: Dynamic upper airway imaging during awake respiration in normal subjects and patients with sleep disordered breathing. Am Rev Respir Dis 148:1385, 1993.
251. Shepard JW Jr, Stanson AW, Sheedy PF, et al: Fast-CT evaluation of the upper airway during wakefulness in patients with obstructive sleep apnea. Prog Clin Biol Res 345:273, 1990.
252. Shelton KE, Woodson H, Gay S, et al: Pharyngeal fat in obstructive sleep apnea. Am Rev Respir Dis 148:462, 1993.
253. Shelton KE, Woodson H, Gay SB, et al: Adipose tissue deposition in sleep apnea. Sleep 16:S103, 1993.
254. Suto Y, Inoue Y: Sleep apnea syndrome. Examination of pharyngeal obstruction with high-speed MR and polysomnography. Acta Radiol 37:315, 1996.
255. Suto Y, Matsuda E, Inoue Y: MRI of the pharynx in young patients with sleep disordered breathing. Br J Radiol 69:1000, 1996.
256. Suto Y, Matsuo T, Kato T, et al: Evaluation of the pharyngeal airway in patients with sleep apnea: Value of ultrafast MR imaging. Am J Roentgenol 160:311, 1993.

257. Okada T, Fukatsu H, Ishigaki T, et al: Ultra-low-field magnetic resonance imaging in upper airways obstruction in sleep apnea syndrome. Psychiatr Clin Neurosci 50:285, 1996.
258. Ryan FC, Lowe AA, Li D, et al: Magnetic resonance imaging of the upper airway in obstructive sleep apnea before and after chronic nasal continuous positive airway pressure therapy. Am Rev Respir Dis 144:939, 1991.
259. Lugaresi E, Cirignotta F, Coccagna G, et al: Some epidemiological data on snoring and cardiocirculatory disturbances. Sleep 3:221, 1980.
260. Hoddes E, Dement W, Zarcone V: The development and use of the Stanfords Sleepiness Scale (SSS). Psychophysiology 9:150, 1972.
261. van Knippenberg FC, Passchier J, Heysteck D, et al: The Rotterdam Daytime Sleepiness Scale: A new daytime sleepiness scale. Psychol Rep 76:83, 1995.
262. Johns MW: A new method for measuring daytime sleepiness: The Epworth Sleepiness Scale. Sleep 14:540, 1991.
263. Criteria for measurements, definitions, and severity rating of sleep-disordered breathing in adults. Report of an American Sleep Disorders Association Task Force, in conjunction with the European Respiratory Society, the Australian Sleep Association, and the American Thoracic Society. Sleep, in press.
264. Pollak CP: How should the multiple sleep latency test be analyzed? Sleep 20:34, 1997.
265. Carskadon MA, Dement WC, Mither MM, et al: Guidelines for the multiple sleep latency test (MSLT): A standard measure of sleepiness. Sleep 9:519, 1986.
266. Orr WC, Martin RJ, Imes NK, et al: Hypersomnolent and nonhypersomnolent patients with upper airway obstruction during sleep. Chest 75:418, 1979.
267. Weitzman ED: Syndrome of hypersomnia and sleep-induced apnea. Chest 75:414, 1979.
268. Sink J, Bliwise DL, Dement WC: Self-reported excessive daytime somnolence and impaired respiration in sleep. Chest 90:177, 1986.
269. Gold AR, Schwartz AR, Bleecker ER, et al: The effect of chronic nocturnal oxygen administration upon sleep apnea. Am Rev Respir Dis 134:925, 1986.
270. Podszus T, Bauer W, Mayer J, et al: Sleep apnea and pulmonary hypertension. Klin Wochenschr 64:131, 1986.
271. Hudgel DW: Clinical manifestations of the sleep apnea syndrome. In Fletcher EC (ed): Abnormalities of Respiration during Sleep. Orlando, Grune & Stratton, 1986.
272. Kessler R, Chaouat A, Weitzenblum E, et al: Pulmonary hypertension in the obstructive sleep apnoea syndrome: Prevalence, causes and therapeutic consequences. Eur Respir J 9:787, 1996.
273. Chaouat A, Weitzenblum E, Krieger J, et al: Pulmonary hemodynamics in the obstructive sleep apnea syndrome. Results in 220 consecutive patients. Chest 109:380, 1996.
274. Bradley T, Rutherford R, Grossman R, et al: Role of daytime hypoxemia in the pathogenesis of right heart failure in the obstructive sleep apnea syndrome. Am Rev Respir Dis 131:835, 1985.
275. Whyte KF, Douglas NJ: Peripheral edema in the sleep apnea/hypopnea syndrome. Sleep 14:354, 1991.
276. Javaheri S, Colangelo G, Lacey W, et al: Chronic hypercapnia in obstructive sleep apnea-hypopnea syndrome. Sleep 17:416, 1994.
277. Chin K, Hirai M, Kuriyama T, et al: Changes in the arterial Pco$_2$ during a single night's sleep in patients with obstructive sleep apnea. Intern Med 36:454, 1997.
278. Bradley TD, Rutherford R, Lue F, et al: Role of diffuse airway obstruction in the hypercapnia of obstructive sleep apnea. Am Rev Respir Dis 134:920, 1986.
279. Jones J, Wilhoit S, Findley L, et al: Oxyhemoglobin saturation during sleep in subjects with and without the obesity-hypoventilation syndrome. Chest 88:9, 1985.
280. Rapoport DM, Garay SM, Epstein H, et al: Hypercapnia in the obstructive sleep apnea syndrome. A reevaluation of the "Pickwickian syndrome." Chest 89:627, 1986.
281. Javaheri S, Colangelo G, Corser B, et al: Familial respiratory chemosensitivity does not predict hypercapnia of patients with sleep apnea-hypopnea syndrome. Am Rev Respir Dis 145:837, 1992.
282. Bonsignore MR, Marrone O, Insalaco G, et al: The cardiovascular effects of obstructive sleep apnoeas: Analysis of pathogenic mechanisms. Eur Respir J 7:786, 1994.
283. Wright J, Johns R, Watt I, et al: Health effects of obstructive sleep apnoea and the effectiveness of continuous positive airway pressure: A systematic review of the research evidence. BMJ 314(7084):851, 1997.
284. Hoffstein V, Chan CK, Slutsky AS: Sleep apnea and systemic hypertension: A causal association review. Am J Med 91:190, 1991.
285. Fletcher EC: The relationship between systemic hypertension and obstructive sleep apnea: Facts and theory. Am J Med 98:118, 1995.
286. Peter JH, Koehler U, Grote L, et al: Manifestations of obstructive sleep apnoea. Eur Respir J 8:1572, 1995.
287. Wright J, Johns R, Watt I, et al: Health effects of obstructive sleep apnoea and the effectiveness of continuous positive airways pressure: A systematic review of the research evidence. BMJ 314:851, 1997.
288. Somers VK, Dyken ME, Clary MP, et al: Sympathetic neural mechanisms in obstructive sleep apnea. J Clin Invest 96:1897, 1995.
289. Fletcher EC, De Behnke RD, Lovoi MS, et al: Undiagnosed sleep apnea in patients with essential hypertension. Ann Intern Med 103:190, 1985.
290. Baruzzi A, Riva R, Cirignotta F, et al: Atrial natriuretic peptide and catecholamines in obstructive sleep apnea syndrome. Sleep 14:83, 1991.
291. Ziegler MG, Nelesen R, Mills P, et al: Sleep apnea, norepinephrine-release rate, and daytime hypertension. Sleep 20:224, 1997.
292. Tilkian AG, Guilleminault C, Schroeder RS, et al: Hemodynamics in sleep-

induced apnea. Studies during wakefulness and sleep. Ann Intern Med 85:714, 1976.

293. Fletcher EC, De Behnke RD, Lovoi MS, et al: Undiagnosed sleep apnea in patients with essential hypertension. Ann Intern Med 103:190, 1985.

294. Kales A, Bixler ED, Cadieux RJ, et al: Sleep apneas in a hypertensive population. Lancet 2:1005, 1984.

295. Stradling JR, Crosby JH: Predictors and prevalence of obstructive sleep apnoea and snoring in 1001 middle aged men. Thorax 46:85, 1991.

296. Millman RP, Redline S, Carlisle CC, et al: Daytime hypertension in obstructive sleep apnea: Prevalence and contributing risk factors. Chest 99:861, 1991.

297. Carlson JT, Hedner JA, Ejnell H, et al: High prevalence of hypertension in sleep apnea patients independent of obesity. Am J Respir Crit Care Med 150:72, 1994.

298. Young T, Peppard P, Palta M, et al: Population-based study of sleep-disordered breathing as a risk factor for hypertension. Arch Intern Med 157:1746, 1997.

299. Worsnop CJ, Naughton MT, Barter CE, et al: The prevalence of obstructive sleep apnea in hypertensives. Am J Respir Crit Care Med 157:111, 1998.

300. Hung J, Whitford EG, Parsons RW, et al: Association of sleep apnoea with myocardial infarction in men. Lancet 336:261, 1990.

301. Randazzo DN, Winters SL, Schweitzer P: Obstructive sleep apnea–induced supraventricular tachycardia. J Electrocardiol 29:65, 1996.

302. Guilleminault C, Connolly SJ, Winkle RA: Cardiac arrhythmia and conduction disturbances during sleep in 400 patients with sleep apnea syndrome. Am J Cardiol 52:490, 1985.

303. Koskenvuo M, Kaprio J, Telakivi T, et al: Snoring as a risk factor for ischemic heart disease and stroke in men. BMJ 294:16, 1987.

304. Rangemark C, Hedner JA, Carlson JT, et al: Platelet function and fibrinolytic activity in hypertensive and normotensive sleep apnea patients. Sleep 18:188, 1995.

305. Schafer H, Koehler U, Ploch T, et al: Sleep-related myocardial ischemia and sleep structure in patients with obstructive sleep apnea and coronary heart disease. Chest 111:387, 1997.

306. Mooe T, Rabben T, Wiklund U, et al: Sleep-disordered breathing in women: Occurrence and association with coronary artery disease. Am J Med 101:251, 1996.

307. Flenley DC: Sleep in chronic obstructive lung disease. *In* Kryger MH (ed): Symposium on Sleep Disorders. Philadelphia, WB Saunders, 1985.

308. Shepard JW Jr: Gas exchange and hemodynamics during sleep. Med Clin North Am 69:1243, 1985.

309. Rama PR, Sharma SC: Sleep apnea and complete heart block. Clin Cardiol 17:675, 1994.

310. Guilleminault C: Natural history, cardiac impact, and long-term follow-up of sleep apnea syndrome. *In* Guilleminault C, Lugaresi E (eds): Sleep/Wake Disorders: Natural History, Epidemiology, and Long-Term Evolution. New York, Raven Press, 1983, p 107.

311. Garpestad E, Katayama H, Parker JA, et al: Stroke volume and cardiac output decrease at termination of obstructive apneas. J Appl Physiol 73:1743, 1992.

312. Bradley TD, Floras JS: Pathophysiologic and therapeutic implications of sleep apnea in congestive heart failure. J Card Fail 2:223, 1996.

313. Shiomi T, Stoohs R, Guilleminault C: Aging, respiratory efforts during sleep, and pulsus paradoxus. Lung 171:203, 1993.

314. Noda A, Okada T, Yasuma F, et al: Cardiac hypertrophy in obstructive sleep apnea syndrome. Chest 107:1538, 1995.

314a. Malone S, Liu PP, Holloway R, et al: Obstructive sleep apnoea in patients with dilated cardiomyopathy: Effects of continuous positive airway pressure. Lancet 338(8781):1480, 1998.

315. Palomaki H: Snoring and the risk of brain infarction. Stroke 22:1021, 1991.

316. Balfors EM, Franklin KA: Impairment of cerebral perfusion during obstructive sleep apneas. Am J Respir Crit Care Med 150:1587, 1994.

317. Morgan BJ: Acute and chronic cardiovascular responses to sleep disordered breathing. Sleep 19:S206, 1996.

318. Dyken ME, Somers VK, Yamada T, et al: Investigating the relationship between stroke and obstructive sleep apnea. Stroke 27:401, 1996.

319. Naëgelé B, Thouvard V, Pépin JL, et al: Deficits of cognitive executive functions in patients with sleep apnea syndrome. Sleep 18:43, 1995.

320. Bedard MA, Montplaisir J, Richer F, et al: Nocturnal hypoxemia as a determinant of vigilance impairment in sleep apnea syndrome. Chest 100:367, 1991.

321. Naegele B, Thouvard V, Pepin JL, et al: Deficits of cognitive executive functions in patients with sleep apnea syndrome. Sleep 18:43, 1995.

322. Kales A, Caldwell AB, Cadieux RJ, et al: Severe obstructive sleep apnea—II: Associated psychopathology and psychosocial consequences. J Chronic Dis 38:427, 1985.

323. American Thoracic Society: Sleep apnea, sleepiness, and driving risk. Am J Respir Crit Care Med 150:1463, 1994.

324. George C, Nickerson P, Millar T, et al: Sleep apnea patients have more automobile accidents. Lancet 8556:447, 1987.

325. Wu H, Yan-Go F: Self-reported automobile accidents involving patients with obstructive sleep apnea. Neurology 46:1254, 1996.

326. Stoohs RA, Guilleminault C, Itoi A, et al: Traffic accidents in commercial long-haul truck drivers: The influence of sleep-disordered breathing and obesity. Sleep 17:619, 1994.

327. Ulfberg J, Carter N, Talback M, et al: Headache, snoring and sleep apnoea. J Neurol 243:621, 1996.

328. Quera-Salva MA, Guilleminault C: Health problems associated with obstructive sleep apnea. Sleep Res 16:410, 1987.

329. Lin CC, Tsan KW, Lin CY: Plasma levels of atrial natriuretic factor in moderate to severe obstructive sleep apnea syndrome. Sleep 16:37, 1993.

330. Ulfberg J, Thuman R: A non-urologic cause of nocturia and enuresis—obstructive sleep apnea syndrome (OSAS). Scand J Urol Nephrol 30:135, 1996.

331. Santamaria JC, Prior JC, Fleetham JA: Reversible reproductive dysfunction in men with obstructive sleep apnea. Clin Endocrinol 28:461, 1988.

332. Grunstein RR: Neuroendocrine function in sleep apnea: Metabolic aspects of sleep apnea. Sleep 19:S218, 1996.

333. Hoffstein V, Herridge M, Mateika S, et al: Hematocrit levels in sleep apnea. Chest 106:787, 1994.

334. Entzian P, Linnemann K, Schlaak M, et al: Obstructive sleep apnea syndrome and circadian rhythms of hormones and cytokines. Am J Respir Crit Care Med 153:1080, 1996.

335. Mathur R, Douglas NJ: Relation between sudden infant death syndrome and adult sleep apnoea/hypopnoea syndrome. Lancet 344:819, 1994.

336. West P, Kryger MH: Sleep and respiration: Terminology and methodology. Clin Chest Med 6(4):691, 1985.

337. Sangal RB, Semery JP, Belisle CL: Computerized scoring of abnormal human sleep: A validation. Clin Electroencephalogr 28:64, 1997.

338. Salmi T, Brander PE: Computer assisted detection of REM and non-REM sleep for analysis of nocturnal hypoxaemia in patients with ventilatory impairment. Int J Clin Monit Comput 11:63, 1994.

339. Commiskey J, Williams TC, Krumpe PE, et al: The detection and quantification of sleep apnea by tracheal sound recordings. Am Rev Respir Dis 126:221, 1982.

340. Fiz JA, Abad J, Jane R, et al: Acoustic analysis of snoring sound in patients with simple snoring and obstructive sleep apnea. Eur Respir J 9:2365, 1996.

341. Meyer TJ, Eveloff SE, Kline LR, et al: One negative polysomnogram does not exclude obstructive sleep apnea. Chest 103:756, 1993.

342. Flemons WW, Whitelaw WA, Brant R, et al: Likelihood ratios for a sleep apnea clinical prediction rule. Am J Respir Crit Care Med 150:1279, 1994.

343. Ruhle KH, Schlenker E, Randerath W: Upper airway resistance syndrome. Respiration 64:29, 1997.

344. Broughton R, Fleming J, Fleetham J: Home assessment of sleep disorders by portable monitoring. J Clin Neurophysiol 13:272, 1996.

345. Ferber R, Millman R, Coppola M, et al: Portable recording in the assessment of obstructive sleep apnea. ASDA standards of practice. Sleep 17:378, 1994.

346. Sivan Y, Kornecki A, Schonfeld T: Screening obstructive sleep apnoea syndrome by home videotape recording in children. Eur Respir J 9:2127, 1996.

347. Flemons WW, Remmers JE: The diagnoses of sleep apnea: Questionnaires and home studies. Sleep 19:S243, 1996.

348. Steyer BJ, Quan SF, Morgan WJ: Polysomnography scoring for sleep apnea—use of a sampling method. Am Rev Respir Dis 131:592, 1985.

349. Maislin G, Pack AI, Kribbs NB, et al: A survey screen for prediction of apnea. Sleep 18:158, 1995.

350. Pouliot Z, Peters M, Neufeld H, et al: Using self-reported questionnaire data to prioritize OSA patients for polysomnography. Sleep 20:232, 1997.

351. Hoffstein V, Szalai JP: Predictive value of clinical features in diagnosing obstructive sleep apnea. Sleep 16:118, 1993.

352. Ryan PJ, Hilton MF, Boldy DA, et al: Validation of British Thoracic Society guidelines for the diagnosis of the sleep apnoea/hypopnoea syndrome: Can polysomnography be avoided? Thorax 50:972, 1995.

353. Yamashiro Y, Kryger MH: Nocturnal oximetry: Is it a screening tool for sleep disorders? Sleep 18:167, 1995.

354. Series F, Marc I, Cormier Y, et al: Utility of nocturnal home oximetry for case finding in patients with suspected sleep apnea hypopnea syndrome. Ann Intern Med 119:449, 1993.

355. Gyulay S, Olson LG, Hensley MJ, et al: A comparison of clinical assessment and home oximetry in the diagnosis of obstructive sleep apnea. Am Rev Respir Dis 147:50, 1993.

356. Guilleminault C, Stoohs R, Clerk A, et al: A cause of excessive daytime sleepiness. The upper airway resistance syndrome. Chest 104:781, 1993.

357. Guilleminault C, Stoohs R, Duncan S: Snoring: Daytime sleepiness in regular heavy snorers. Chest 99:40, 1991.

358. American Thoracic Society: Medical Section of the American Lung Association: Indications and standards for cardiopulmonary sleep studies. Am Rev Respir Dis 139:559, 1989.

359. Persson HE, Svanborg E: Sleep deprivation worsens obstructive sleep apnea. Comparison between diurnal and nocturnal polysomnography. Chest 109:645, 1996.

360. Fanfulla F, Patruno V, Bruschi C, et al: Obstructive sleep apnoea syndrome: Is the "half-night polysomnography" an adequate method for evaluating sleep profile and respiratory events? Eur Respir J 10:1725, 1997.

361. Douglas NJ, Thomas S, Jan MA: Clinical value of polysomnography. Lancet 339:347, 1992.

362. White DP: Complex home monitoring. Sleep 19:S248, 1996.

363. Hida W, Shindoh C, Miki H, et al: Prevalence of sleep apnea among Japanese industrial workers determined by a portable sleep monitoring system. Respiration 60:332, 1993.

364. Gugger M: Comparison of ResMed AutoSet (version 3.03) with polysomnography in the diagnosis of the sleep apnoea/hypopnoea syndrome. Eur Respir J 10:587, 1997.

365. Esnaola S, Duran J, Infante-Rivard C, et al: Diagnostic accuracy of a portable recording device (MESAM IV) in suspected obstructive sleep apnea. Eur Respir J 9:2597, 1996.

366. Kiely JL, Delahunty C, Matthews S, et al: Comparison of a limited computerized diagnostic system (ResCare Autoset) with polysomnography in the diagnosis of obstructive sleep apnoea syndrome. Eur Respir J 9:2360, 1996.

367. White DP, Gibb TJ, Wall JM, et al: Assessment of accuracy and analysis time of a novel device to monitor sleep and breathing in the home. Sleep 18:115, 1995.

368. Issa FG, Morrison D, Hadjuk E, et al: Digital monitoring of sleep-disordered breathing using snoring sound and arterial oxygen saturation. Am Rev Respir Dis 148:1023, 1993.

369. Bradley PA, Mortimore IL, Douglas NJ: Comparison of polysomnography with ResCare Autoset in the diagnosis of the sleep apnoea/hypopnoea syndrome. Thorax 50:1201, 1995.

370. Tvinnereim M, Mateika S, Cole P, et al: Diagnosis of obstructive sleep apnea using a portable transducer catheter. Am J Respir Crit Care Med 152:775, 1995.

371. Parra O, Garcia-Esclasans N, Montserrat JM, et al: Should patients with sleep apnoea/hypopnoea syndrome be diagnosed and managed on the basis of home sleep studies? Eur Respir J 10:1720, 1997.

372. Practice parameters for the use of portable recording in the assessment of obstructive sleep apnea. Standards of Practice Committee of the American Sleep Disorders Association. Sleep 17:372, 1994.

373. Bradley TD, Martinez D, Rutherford R, et al: Physiological determinants of nocturnal arterial oxygenation in patients with obstructive sleep apnea. J Appl Physiol 59:1364, 1985.

374. Rubinstein I, Zamel N, DuBarry L, et al: Airflow limitation in morbidly obese, non-smoking men. Ann Intern Med 112:828, 1990.

375. Gold AR, Schwartz AR, Wise RA, et al: Pulmonary function and respiratory chemosensitivity in moderately obese patients with sleep apnea (see comments). Chest 103:1325, 1993.

376. Zerah-Lancner F, Lofaso F, Coste A, et al: Pulmonary function in obese snorers with or without sleep apnea syndrome. Am J Respir Crit Care Med 156:522, 1997.

377. Collard P, Wilputte JY, Aubert G, et al: The single-breath diffusing capacity for carbon monoxide in obstructive sleep apnea and obesity. Chest 110:1189, 1996.

378. Lavie P, Herer P, Peled R, et al: Mortality in sleep apnea patients: A multivariate analysis of risk factors. Sleep 18:149, 1995.

379. He J, Kryger M, Zorick F: Mortality and apnea index in obstructive sleep apnea. Chest 89:331, 1988.

380. Partinen M, Jamieson A, Guilleminault C: Long-term outcome for obstructive sleep apnea patients. Chest 94:1200, 1988.

381. Baltzan M, Suissa S: Mortality in sleep apnea patients: A multivariate analysis of risk factors—a response to Lavie and collaborators (letter). Sleep 20:377, 1997.

382. Ancoli-Israel S, Kripke DF, Klauber MR, et al: Morbidity, mortality and sleep-disordered breathing in community dwelling elderly. Sleep 19:277, 1996.

383. Hegstrom T, Emmons LL, Hoddes E, et al: Obstructive sleep apnea syndrome: Preoperative radiologic evaluation. Am J Roentgenol 150:67, 1988.

384. Larsson SG, Gislason T, Lindholm CE: Computed tomography of the oropharynx in obstructive sleep apnea. Acta Radiol 29:401, 1988.

385. Riley R, Guilleminault C, Powell N, et al: Palatropharyngoplasty failure, cephalometric roentgenograms, and obstructive sleep apnea. Otolaryngol Head Neck Surg 93:240, 1985.

386. Katsantonis GP, Walsh JK: Somnofluoroscopy: Its role in the selection of candidates for uvulopalatopharyngoplasty. Otolaryngol Head Neck Surg 94:56, 1986.

387. Walsh JK, Katsantonis GP, Schweitzer PK, et al: Somnofluoroscopy: Cineradiographic observation of obstructive sleep apnea. Sleep 8:294, 1985.

388. Erkinjuntti T, Partinen M, Sulkava R, et al: Sleep apnea in multi-infarct dementia and Alzheimer's disease. Sleep 10:419, 1987.

389. Apps MC, Sheaff PC, Ingram DA, et al: Respiration and sleep in Parkinson's disease. J Neurol Neurosurg Psychiatry 48:1240, 1985.

390. Arcaya J, Cacho J, Del Campo F, et al: Arnold-Chiari malformation associated with sleep apnea and central dysregulation of arterial pressure. Acta Neurol Scand 88:224, 1993.

391. Steljes DG, Kryger MH, Kirk BW, et al: Sleep in postpolio syndrome. Chest 98:133, 1990.

392. Guilleminault C, Briskin JG, Greenfield MS, et al: The impact of autonomic nervous system dysfunction on breathing during sleep. Sleep 4:263, 1981.

393. McNamara ME, Millman RP, Epstein MH, et al: The association of normal-pressure hydrocephalus with obstructive sleep apnea. J Geriatr Psychiatr Neurol 5:238, 1992.

394. McBrien F, Spraggs PD, Harcourt JP, et al: Abductor vocal fold palsy in the Shy-Drager syndrome presenting with snoring and sleep apnoea. J Laryngol Otol 110:681, 1996.

395. Margolis ML, Howlett P, Goldberg R, et al: Obstructive sleep apnea syndrome in acid maltase deficiency. Chest 105:947, 1994.

396. Shapiro J, Strome M, Crocker AC: Airway obstruction and sleep apnea in Hurler and Hunter syndromes. Ann Otol Rhinol Laryngol 94:458, 1985.

397. Schafer ME: Upper airway obstruction and sleep disorders in children with craniofacial anomalies. Clin Plast Surg 9:555, 1982.

398. Cohen MM Jr, Kreiborg S: Upper and lower airway compromise in the Alpert syndrome. Am J Med Genet 44:90, 1992.

398a. Gilmore RL, Falace P, Kanga J, Baumann R: Sleep-disordered breathing in Mobius syndrome. J Child Neurol 6:73, 1991.

399. Tirosh E, Borochowitz Z: Sleep apnea in fragile X syndrome. Am J Med Genet 43:124, 1992.

400. Rosen CL, Novotny EJ, D'Andrea LA, et al: Klippel-Feil sequence and sleep-disordered breathing in two children. Am Rev Respir Dis 147:202, 1993.

401. Khan Y, Heckmatt JZ: Obstructive apnoeas in Duchenne muscular dystrophy (see comments). Thorax 49:157, 1994.

402. Barbe F, Quera-Salva MA, McCann, et al: Sleep-related respiratory disturbances in patients with Duchenne muscular dystrophy. Eur Respir J 7:1403, 1994.

403. Sverd J, Montero G: Is Tourette syndrome a cause of sudden infant death syndrome and childhood obstructive sleep apnea? Am J Med Genet 46:494, 1993.

404. McEvoy RD, Mykytyn I, Sajkov D, et al: Sleep apnoea in patients with quadriplegia. Thorax 50:613, 1995.

405. Zucconi M, Ferini-Strambi L, Erminio C, et al: Obstructive sleep apnea in the Rubinstein-Taybi syndrome. Respiration 60:127, 1993.

406. Pelttari L, Rauhala E, Polo O, et al: Upper airway obstruction in hypothyroidism. J Intern Med 236:177, 1994.

407. Buyse B, Michiels E, Bouillon R, et al: Relief of sleep apnoea after treatment of acromegaly: Report of three cases and review of the literature. Eur Respir J 10:1401, 1997.

408. Strohl KP: Diabetes and sleep apnea. Sleep 19:S225, 1996.

409. Feinsilver S, Hertz G: Respiration during sleep in pregnancy. Clin Chest Med 13:637, 1992.

410. Katsumata K, Okada T, Miyao M, Katsumata Y: High incidence of sleep apnea syndrome in a male diabetic population. Diabetes Res Clin Pract 13:45, 1991.

411. Gerard JM, Garibaldi L, Myers SE, et al: Sleep apnea in patients receiving growth hormone. Clin Pediatr 36:321, 1997.

412. Cistulli PA, Grunstein RR, Sullivan CE: Effect of testosterone administration on upper airway collapsibility during sleep. Am J Respir Crit Care Med 149:530, 1994.

413. Shipley JE, Schteingart DE, Tandon R, et al: Sleep architecture and sleep apnea in patients with Cushing's disease. Sleep 15:514, 1992.

414. Guilleminault C, Kurland G, Winkle R, et al: Severe kyphoscoliosis, breathing and sleep: The "Quasimodo" syndrome. Chest 79:626, 1981.

415. Marcus CL, Carroll JL: Obstructive sleep apnea syndrome. *In* Loughlin GM, Eigen H (eds): Respiratory Disease in Children: Diagnosis and Management. Baltimore, Williams & Wilkins, 1993, p 475.

416. Zucconi M, Weber G, Castronovo F, et al: Sleep and upper airway obstruction in children with achondroplasia. J Pediatr 129:743, 1996.

417. May KP, West SG, Baker MR, et al: Sleep apnea in male patients with the fibromyalgia syndrome. Am J Med 94:505, 1993.

418. Clauser L, Marchetti C, Piccione M, et al: Craniofacial fibrous dysplasia and Ollier's disease: Combined transfrontal and transfacial resection using the nasal-cheek flap. J Craniofac Surg 7:140, 1996.

419. Langevin B, Fouque D, Leger P, et al: Sleep apnea syndrome and end-stage renal disease. Cure after renal transplantation. Chest 103:1330, 1993.

420. Hallett M, Burden S, Stewart D, et al: Sleep apnea in end-stage renal disease patients on hemodialysis and continuous ambulatory peritoneal dialysis. ASAIO J 41:M435, 1995.

421. Piperno JG, Francois B, Charra B: Sleep apnea incidence in maintenance hemodialysis patients: Influence of dialysate buffer. Nephron 71:138, 1995.

422. Buchwald D, Pascualy R, Bombardier C, et al: Sleep disorders in patients with chronic fatigue. Clin Infect Dis 1:S68, 1994.

423. Chetty KG, Kadifa F, Berry RB, et al: Acquired laryngomalacia as a cause of obstructive sleep apnea. Chest 106:1898, 1994.

424. Milkiewicz P, Olliff S, Johnson AP, et al: Obstructive sleep apnoea syndrome (OSAS) as a complication of carcinoid syndrome treated successfully by hepatic artery embolization. Eur J Gastroenterol Hepatol 9:217, 1997.

425. Byrd RP Jr, Roy TM, Bentz W, et al: Plasmacytoma as a cause of obstructive sleep apnea. Chest 109:1657, 1996.

426. Jakubikova J, Zitnan D, Batorova A: An unusual reason for obstructive sleep apnea in a boy with hemophilia B: Supraglottic papilloma. Int J Pediatr Otorhinolaryngol 34:165, 1996.

427. McNab AA: Floppy eyelid syndrome and obstructive sleep apnea. Ophthal Plast Reconstr Surg 13:98, 1997.

428. Turner GA, Lower EE, Corser BC, et al: Sleep apnea in sarcoidosis. Sarcoidosis Vasc Diffuse Lung Dis 14:61, 1997.

429. Schmidt-Nowara WW: Continuous positive airway pressure for long-term treatment of sleep apnea. Am J Dis Child 138:82, 1984.

# *Asthma*

One of the most concise definitions of asthma was proposed by Scadding in 1983: "a disease characterized by wide variations over short periods of time in resistance to air flow in intrapulmonary airways."[1] The changes in severity of airway narrowing can occur spontaneously or as a result of therapy. In addition to brevity, this definition has the advantage of being easily applicable to clinical practice. However, these features are also found in other conditions, such as cystic fibrosis and congestive heart failure. Because of this problem, other definitions have been proposed based on the recognition that the airways of asthmatic persons show an increased responsiveness to a variety of stimuli[2] and evidence of a chronic inflammatory reaction.[3] An example of such an extended definition is that proposed by the Global Initiative for Asthma:[4]

Asthma is a chronic inflammatory disorder of the airways in which many cells play a role, in particular mast cells, eosinophils, and T lymphocytes. In susceptible individuals this inflammation causes recurrent episodes of wheezing, breathlessness, chest tightness, and cough, particularly at night and/or in the early morning. These symptoms are usually associated with widespread but variable airflow limitation that is at least partly reversible either spontaneously or with treatment. The inflammation also causes an associated increase in airway responsiveness to a variety of stimuli.

However, because both airway inflammation and hyper-responsiveness are seen in other diseases,[5] and because information concerning morphologic abnormalities is not available in the vast majority of patients, these additional refinements are of limited value in routine clinical practice.[6] In the final analysis, it is difficult to draft a single, all-inclusive definition that is both sensitive and specific and that would satisfy epidemiologist, clinician, and basic scientist alike.

The airway narrowing that occurs in asthma is intermittent and variable; complete remission can occur between attacks, although some abnormality of function is often detectable with sensitive tests.[7, 8] There is also evidence that chronic asthma can lead to a degree of fixed air-flow obstruction in some patients.[9] During attacks, generalized narrowing of the bronchi and bronchioles results in diffuse wheezing; the wheezing is often associated with dyspnea, even at rest. Although the reversibility of airway obstruction may be suspected from the clinical history, it should always be evaluated objectively by measurement of airway function after administration of a bronchodilator or after a course of anti-inflammatory therapy.[10] Asthma should be a diagnosis of exclusion; as indicated previously, several diseases can be associated with a clinical picture that simulates asthma, including acute bronchitis and bronchiolitis, chronic bronchitis, emphysema, bronchiectasis, lymphangitic carcinomatosis, left-sided heart failure, and anatomic or functional upper airway obstruction. To apply the term "asthma" to the clinical manifestations of patients who have these disorders is incorrect and inevitably results in confusion. Although there is some overlap, asthma can be considered in two major categories: extrinsic and intrinsic.

**Extrinsic Asthma.** Extrinsic asthma (atopic asthma, allergic asthma) occurs in patients who are atopic.* As discussed in more detail further on, the inheritance of the atopic tendency is complex and usually incomplete, with a greatly increased risk of being affected if both parents are atopic. The reason for the high incidence of atopy (which appears to be harmful to the person affected) is not clear; however, it has been hypothesized that the ability to respond with IgE antibody may have survival benefit in offering protection against parasitic infestations.[11]

The prevalence of atopy increases until approximately 20 years of age, after which it gradually declines. Peak IgE levels occur at age 14; in infants and young children, atopy is twice as common in males.[11–13] Besides demonstrating increased blood levels of IgE, atopic persons have positive immediate skin test responses to a variety of antigens and a high incidence of eczema, rhinitis, and asthma. However, atopy is not synonymous with asthma: the former occurs in over 30% of the population, whereas the incidence of asthma is considerably less. Although identical twins are almost invariably concordant for the presence or absence of atopy, their individual allergic manifestations are often discordant.[14, 15]

Extrinsic asthma is associated with a number of clinical and epidemiologic findings, including[1, 15] (1) a family history of atopy, (2) onset in the first three decades of life, (3) seasonal symptoms, (4) an elevated blood level of IgE, (5) positive skin and bronchial challenge tests to specific allergens, and (6) a tendency for the disease to remit in later life. Although the airway inflammation and narrowing that occur in the extrinsic form of disease are presumably the result of inhalation of specific allergens, it is often difficult to identify the allergens that are responsible for symptoms in an individual patient.

The term *extrinsic nonatopic asthma* has been used to refer to disease in patients in whom exposure to a specific agent can be clearly shown to be the cause of reversible bronchoconstriction but in whom specific IgE does not mediate the response or in whom there is no tendency for excessive IgE production.[1] Patients who exhibit this form of disease usually have occupational asthma that occurs in response to powerful sensitizers such as plicatic acid or toluene diisocyanate.[16] On the other hand, certain antigens are powerful inducers of IgE production and can result in IgE-mediated airway responses in the absence of a genetic atopic predisposition.[16]

**Intrinsic Asthma.** Intrinsic (nonatopic, cryptogenic) asthma occurs in patients in whom atopy and specific allergic triggers of bronchoconstriction cannot be identified. The modifier *intrinsic* was initially coined because it was believed that these patients were responding to antigens released from microorganisms residing in the airways; however, this is now believed to be unlikely. In contrast to patients who have extrinsic asthma, those who have the intrinsic form of disease are characterized by (1) being older and more likely to be female, (2) having no or a less convincing family history of asthma or atopy, (3) an absence of elevated blood levels of total and specific IgE or positive skin or bronchial response to allergen challenge, (4) an increased incidence of autoantibodies to smooth muscle, (5) an increased incidence of autoimmune disease, (6) decreased responsiveness to therapy, (7) a greater risk of being aspirin-sensitive, and (8) a tendency to persistent and progressive disease resulting in fixed air-flow obstruction.[1, 17–21]

It has been suggested that intrinsic asthma represents a distinct immunopathologic entity—a conclusion based on measures of cytokine production by pulmonary and peripheral blood lymphocytes.[22] Although the T cells of atopic and nonatopic asthmatic patients both seem to be of the Th2 type, in that they secrete interleukin-5 (IL-5) and IL-2 but not interferon-γ (IFN-γ), the results of some studies suggest that only the T cells of allergic asthmatic persons secrete an increased amount of IL-4.[23, 24] However, some investigators have found no detectable differences in the T cell cytokine profiles synthesized by atopic and nonatopic asthmatics.[25] In fact, the whole concept of a separate subset of intrinsic asthmatic patients has been challenged.[5, 26] Even older, adult-onset asthmatic patients who have negative results on skin testing show elevated levels of serum IgE;[27] moreover, in one study, "intrinsic" asthmatic patients were as likely to have a positive family history as those who were allergic.[19] Despite these observations, we believe there is a small but significant number of patients who have adult-onset asthma associated with features of "intrinsic" disease, and that retention of this category is clinically useful.

**Additional Terms.** Although a number of additional "forms" of asthma have been delineated, none is in fact sufficiently distinctive to warrant separate designation. "Exercise-induced asthma" is not a separate category, because the majority of patients who have either extrinsic or intrinsic asthma develop exaggerated bronchoconstriction during exercise. Similarly, "nocturnal asthma" is no more than a manifestation of asthma that tends to occur in persons who have poorly controlled disease. The excessive bronchial la-

---

*Atopy can be defined as the genetic predisposition to respond to antigenic challenge with excessive IgE production and to exhibit the clinical expression of illnesses such as rhinitis, asthma, or eczema that involve IgE-antigen interaction. Also included in some definitions are elevations of total IgE or aeroallergen-specific IgE measured semiquantitatively using skin tests or quantitatively using enzyme-linked immunosorbent assay (ELISA) or radioallergosorbent test (RAST).

bility seen in some patients who have chronic bronchitis, chronic obstructive pulmonary disease (COPD), bronchiectasis, or cystic fibrosis should not be called asthma; although these conditions fulfill some of the features of asthma, each has a clearly defined etiologic basis.

## EPIDEMIOLOGY

Although asthma is undoubtedly a common disease, estimates of its prevalence vary considerably in different regions; for example, in children the prevalence in different countries has been estimated to range from as little as 1% or less to as much as 20%.[28–34] Part of this variation relates to the definition of asthma that has been used in epidemiologic studies. In most such studies, the identification of asthma is based on a history of compatible symptoms rather than objective determination of reversible air-flow obstruction. Different questions are associated with different estimates of prevalence;[35] for example, in one study the prevalence of "wheeze" was 25% in young adults, while the prevalence of "attacks of asthma" was only 5%.[36]

The prevalence of asthma is also related to geography, ethnicity, and age.[37–39] Although variations in allergy and asthma prevalence have been described in different ethnic groups, these are probably related more to differences in culture and lifestyle than to genetic predisposition.[40] When the diagnosis of asthma was based on the presence of wheeze in the previous 12 months, the range of positive responses varied, ranging from 2% to 5% in China and Hong Kong, to 10% to 15% in Canada, the United States, and the United Kingdom, to 20% to 27% in Fiji, Australia, and Chile;[40] it is interesting that the five countries that had the highest prevalence were in the southern hemisphere. Although some of these differences may be geographic rather than ethnic, there is also evidence for differences in ethnic groups within geographic regions. For example, the Maori people have a higher prevalence of asthma than white New Zealanders,[41] persistent wheeze is more common in African Americans than in whites,[42] and asthma is more common among the Indian and Malay populations of Singapore than among the Chinese population.[43]

Part of the ethnic variation in prevalence could be based on linguistic differences in the interpretation of words like *wheeze*; however, the results of a study that used a video questionnaire depicting the clinical signs and symptoms of asthma showed differences in prevalence among citizens of Hong Kong, England, Australia, and New Zealand comparable to those observed when verbal and written questionnaires were used.[44] A natural experiment on the effect of environment was provided by the separation of a genetically homogeneous population by the wall between West Germany and East Germany; when prevalence rates of atopy and asthma in the two countries were compared in postreunification studies, these conditions were found to be more common in West Germany, despite lower levels of industrial pollution.[45–47]

The lower incidence of asthma in some tropical countries is believed by some[31, 39, 48] but not all investigators[49] to be related to a protective effect of high serum IgE levels induced by parasitic infestation (*see* farther on). In Venezuela, the prevalence of atopy and asthma is inversely related to socioeconomic status and the likelihood of infestation with intestinal parasites; in one investigation, the treatment of worms was followed by an increase in sensitivity to aeroallergens, supporting the hypothesis of a protective effect of parasites.[50] Additional evidence that the prevalence of asthma within a population can change is illustrated by studies of Papua New Guinea Melanesians in the 1970s and 1980s, during which time the prevalence of asthma increased from 0.1% to 7.3%;[51–54] it is possible that the increase was related to the intensity of house dust mite infestation.[55] Although it is likely that the differences in prevalence of asthma and allergy between different ethnic groups represent the influence of socioeconomic, cultural, dietary, and other environmental factors rather than a difference in biologic susceptibility, it is also possible that there is a gradation of risk on a genetic basis, as is seen in other respiratory diseases such as cystic fibrosis and diffuse panbronchiolitis.

The most important risk factors for the development of asthma are atopy, cigarette smoke exposure, and childhood bronchiolitis.[56–58] In a 23-year longitudinal study of 1,836 college freshmen, positive results on allergy skin testing at baseline increased the risk of asthma at follow-up threefold.[59] In another investigation of 13-year-olds in New Zealand, the prevalence of asthma increased linearly with the size of the skin test wheal in response to house dust mite and cat allergens (about 4% with negative results on skin testing and over 60% when the combined wheal diameters exceeded 10 mm).[60] Of 198 adult asthmatics aged 18 to 50 years in the United Kingdom, 178 (90%) had a positive result on skin testing for allergy to house dust mite, grass, or cat dander.[61] In a U.S. study, the odds ratio (OR) for asthma if the result of one skin test was positive was 3.5; if results of two were positive, the relative risk increased to 4.2;[62] the risk appeared to be especially high for sensitivity to certain allergens such as house dust mite (OR = 2.9) and *Alternaria* (OR = 5.1). For example, in a sample of genetically susceptible children, the level of exposure to house dust mite in early childhood predicted the degree of sensitization and the risk of developing asthma by the age of 11 years.[63] There are also strong correlations between the serum level of IgE, the risk of asthma, and the presence of bronchial hyper-responsiveness.[26, 27, 64, 65] It has been suggested that there is a chronologic window of risk for sensitization to allergens that increases the likelihood of subsequent asthma.[66]

Passive exposure to cigarette smoke has consistently been shown to increase the risk for the development of asthma and allergic sensitization, ORs varying between 1.2 and 5.[57, 67, 68] There is also evidence that both environmental and personal exposure to cigarette smoke increases nonspecific airway responsiveness.[69]

The role of viral respiratory infections during infancy is more controversial. Although infants who develop significant respiratory syncytial virus bronchiolitis in the first two years of life have an increased risk of subsequent asthma, it is unclear whether the acute episode of bronchiolitis represents the first attack of asthma in a child destined to develop the disease or is an insult that precipitates asthma. In long-term prospective studies, it has been shown that 75% of infants who are admitted to hospital for acute bronchiolitis manifest wheezing in the first 2 years after their initial illness, and that 40% will continue to "wheeze" 5 years later.[58, 70] It is not clear whether this wheezing represents asthma or is a clinical manifestation of anatomic differences in airway caliber between children and adults.

The prevalence of asthma seems to be highest in childhood, with a decrease during adolescence and adulthood.[71] Part of this decrease is related to maturation of the respiratory system. Since airways are relatively smaller in infants and children, any process that causes edema and smooth muscle contraction in these age groups is more likely to be manifested as a wheeze; as the lung matures and the airways become larger, wheezing illnesses become less common. For example, in one study of a large cohort of infants who were studied prospectively, approximately one third had a "wheezy" illness before the age of 3 years; however, the majority of these children were asymptomatic by age 6.[72] These "transient early wheezers" showed mildly impaired lung function shortly after birth, and the attacks of wheezing appeared to be precipitated by respiratory viral infection. Children who continued to wheeze at 6 and 11 years of age were more likely to have the risk factors commonly associated with extrinsic asthma, such as positive results on skin testing with aeroallergens and a positive family history.

The prevalence of asthma before the age of 10 is higher in boys than in girls;[73] after that, it is higher in females. Females are also more likely to visit the emergency room and be admitted for acute severe asthma.[74] The first attack of asthma can occur at any age, although the onset of extrinsic asthma is almost always before the age of 30 years and that of the intrinsic variety is more commonly in middle life.[75]

Evidence is accumulating that the prevalence of asthma and other allergic diseases is increasing worldwide.[76, 77] Although the increase may be related to changes in the criteria used to diagnose the disease, this does not appear to be the most important factor:[78] in one review of 23 studies designed to determine the change in prevalence of asthma or asthma-like symptoms over time, all but one study showed an increase, the calculated annual increase ranging between 1% and 12% per year.[77] The increase was consistent whether based on the presence of symptoms, diagnosed asthma, or asthma attacks[33, 79] and was apparent across age groups.[80] The reasons for the increase are unclear; at a Ciba Foundation Symposium devoted entirely to the subject, the participants agreed that the increase had to be the result of environmental rather than genetic factors but could not agree on which factors were the most important.[81]

Environmental factors that could play a role in increased asthma prevalence include greater *in utero* and domestic exposure to tobacco smoke, alterations in diet, increased exposure to allergens (especially domestic allergens), environmental pollution, occupational sensitizing agents, and diminished frequency of bacterial and viral infections.[82, 83] Consumption of fresh fruit and vegetables has decreased over the past three decades in some "developed" countries.[84] These foodstuffs are an important source of antioxidants such as vitamin C and beta carotene, whose lack could enhance airway inflammation.[85] An increased risk of asthma and allergy is seen in populations that adopt a "western" lifestyle, and it has been suggested that a high prevalence of respiratory infection, parasitic infestations, and "poor hygiene" coupled with traditional, nonaffluent lifestyles in some way protect against the development of atopic dis-

eases.[83] Whatever the protective mechanism, it appears that migration from rural to urban areas is associated with an increase in asthma prevalence among some groups.[86]

The results of several studies suggest an inverse association between childhood respiratory infection and the development of asthma. In a study of Japanese schoolchildren, a strong inverse association was noted between skin test responses to *Mycobacterium tuberculosis* and atopy, positive tuberculin responses being associated with a lower incidence of asthma, lower serum IgE levels, and cytokine profiles biased toward Th1 type;[87] the authors suggested that exposure and response to *M. tuberculosis* may inhibit the development of atopic disorders by modification of immune profiles. A similar mechanism has been proposed for the lower prevalence of atopy in children who have had measles than in those who have not.[88, 89] There is an inverse correlation between the number of siblings and the prevalence of allergic rhinitis; one interpretation of these data is that having a lot of siblings increases exposure to viral respiratory infections and that these infections protect against the development of allergy.[90] A similar explanation has been offered for the difference in prevalence rates of allergic disease between East Germany and West Germany mentioned previously;[91] children in East Germany were routinely placed in child care at the age of 1 year, exposing them to more viral organisms.

## GENETIC CONSIDERATIONS

There is abundant evidence that heredity has an important role in the pathogenesis of asthma and allergic diseases.[92–94] The inheritance does not follow the classical mendelian pattern characteristic of single gene disorders such as cystic fibrosis; instead, the inheritance pattern is similar to that of "complex genetic disorders" such as hypertension, atherosclerosis, and diabetes. As with such disorders, the mode of inheritance of asthma cannot be simply classified as autosomal dominant, autosomal recessive, or sex-linked. Although the precise reasons for this complexity are uncertain, it is likely that a number of genes predispose to the development of the disease; according to this hypothesis, more than one abnormal gene is required in an affected person (i.e., inheritance is polygenic), and different combinations of genes produce the disease in different individuals (i.e., genetic heterogeneity). Moreover, environmental factors are also necessary for expression of the disease phenotype.

Another important feature that distinguishes complex from single gene disorders is their relatively high prevalence in the population at large. Asthma occurs in about 4% to 8% of the population, allergic rhinitis has been reported in 25% of some populations, and atopy (defined as positive results on skin testing with common aeroallergens) can be detected in approximately 40% of most populations.[95, 96] By contrast, cystic fibrosis, which is the most frequent mendelian disorder to affect the lungs, is about 100 times less frequent than asthma, occurring only once in every 2,000 live births in whites.

Any study of the genetic contribution to a disorder requires that a phenotype be defined first, so that the pattern of inheritance of the phenotype can be followed in population, family, and twin studies. Such definition is the most

## Table 54–1. ASTHMA AND ALLERGY PHENOTYPES

Atopy (defined by the presence of an allergic disorder and/or elevated total or specific IgE levels and/or positive results on skin prick tests)
Elevated specific IgE by RAST or skin prick tests
Elevated total IgE
Bronchial hyper-responsiveness
Presence of an allergic disorder: asthma, rhinitis, or eczema
Exercise-induced asthma
Nocturnal asthma
ASA-induced asthma
Occupational asthma (low- and high-molecular-weight antigens)
Asthma severity (e.g., fatal or near-fatal asthma)

ASA, acetylsalicylic acid; RAST, radio allergosorbent test.

difficult and contentious aspect of the study of the genetics of asthma and allergic disorders. The phenotype in allergic disorders can be based on symptoms (e.g., wheeze, cough, dyspnea, rhinitis, conjunctivitis, or dermatitis) or on evidence for exaggerated IgE production (e.g., positive results on allergy skin testing, increased total serum IgE, or increased serum levels of specific IgE directed against common aeroallergens). Bronchial hyper-responsiveness to nonspecific stimuli such as cold dry air, methacholine, or histamine has also been proposed as a separate phenotypic trait that can contribute to asthma. Table 54–1 shows some of the phenotypes that have been used in studies of the genetics of asthma and allergy.

The importance of genes to the expression of asthma and allergy phenotypes can be determined by studying their distribution in populations, their transmission in families, and their concordance in monozygotic and dizygotic twins. One method of determining the contribution of heredity to a disease is to calculate the relative risk of the disorder in first-degree relatives of an affected individual divided by the prevalence in the general population.[97] For asthma, the prevalence in the general population is about 5% and in first-degree relatives of asthmatics, approximately 20% (relative risk of about 5). This value can be converted to an estimate of the heritability, defined as the proportion of phenotypic variance in a population that can be attributed to genetic influence. Although the results are variable, most investigators have found the heritability of allergy and asthma to be high (between about 0.6 and 1.0).[98–101] These estimates are similar to those that have been derived by comparing the concordance rates for asthma and allergy phenotypes in twins. Concordance in monozygotic twins is between 21% and 62%, while for dizygotic twins it ranges between 13% and 44%.[102, 103]

It is also possible that the increased prevalence of a disease in the first-degree relatives of an affected individual could be the result of the shared environment. For example, certain allergies such as allergy to house dust mite or cat dander are very specific to the microenvironment of a particular household. To address this possibility, one group of investigators compared the concordance rates of allergic phenotypes in 34 monozygotic twin pairs who were raised together in the same environment with those in 53 pairs who were separated shortly after birth;[102] the twins reared apart were as concordant for allergy phenotypes (such as total IgE) as were those reared together, supporting an important

role for heredity. The results of one investigation have provided evidence that the gene for IFN-γ may be involved in the production of the atopic state.[104] The gene for this substance is a good candidate for atopy, because it acts as an antagonist to IL-4 and down-regulates the production of IgE from B cells. The authors found that low placental cord blood IFN-γ levels were predictive of atopic symptoms at 12 months of age, suggesting that reduction of IFN-γ secretion is a cause rather than a result of the atopic state.

Another feature of airway disease that may have a hereditary component is bronchial hyper-responsiveness.[101, 105] Although it is clear that nonspecific bronchial hyper-responsiveness (NSBH) can be a consequence of allergic inflammation, it is also true that atopic persons may not have airway hyper-responsiveness and that persons who have NSBH may not be atopic or may not have symptoms of asthma. This discrepancy between NSBH and symptomatic asthma has led to the hypothesis that NSBH is a separately heritable phenotype.

The results of most population studies have shown a unimodal distribution of measures of airway responsiveness, with considerable overlap between asthmatic and nonasthmatic persons.[106] However, two groups of investigators found measures of airway responsiveness to be bimodally distributed in nonasthmatic first-degree relatives of asthmatic patients;[101, 102a, 107] because this pattern is consistent with the segregation of a dominant gene, the authors suggested that this finding supports a genetic contribution to airway responsiveness that is separate from atopy. In another study of the first-degree relatives of children who had atopic asthma, a high prevalence of hyper-responsiveness was found in the relatives who had some atopic symptoms (prevalence 39%) as well as in those who were healthy (32%);[108] moreover, a direct relationship between positive results on allergy skin tests and hyper-responsiveness was not found in either group, suggesting that these were separate phenotypes. The same group of investigators also reported frequent concordance of hyper-responsiveness in monozygotic twins who were not necessarily concordant for atopy or asthma. Despite these findings, other workers have concluded that airway hyper-responsiveness is predominantly acquired.[109, 110] Taken together, the results of these studies do not prove or refute the hypothesis that bronchial hyper-responsiveness is under separate genetic control rather than a consequence of airway inflammation and remodeling; a definitive outcome awaits the results of additional, more rigorous studies.

A number of chromosomal locations have been linked to asthma and allergy phenotypes.[111, 112] The most reproducible of the linked loci have been on the long arms of chromosome 11[113–118] and chromosome 5.[119–121] Several candidate genes that could play a pathophysiologic role in asthma at both sites have been identified. The gene for the high-affinity IgE receptor (FcεRI) is located on chromosome 11q, and the linked region on 5q contains a cluster of cytokine genes (IL-4, IL-5, IL-13) as well as the beta-adrenergic receptor gene. However, specific mutations that alter the function of any of these candidate genes in a manner that would enhance the production of IgE or increase bronchial responsiveness have not been identified. Linkage has also been demonstrated between specific IgE responses and a region on chromosome 14q that contains the gene for the alpha chain of the T cell antigen receptor (TCR).[122]

Because the HLA class II molecules play a key role in antigen presentation, there have been numerous attempts to identify gene variants that control IgE responses to specific allergens.[123] Many associations between class II alleles and IgE hyper-responsiveness to specific allergens have been investigated. In general, significant associations are found with highly purified, simple allergens and not with more complex, common ones. For example, the complex allergens of house dust mite—Der p and Der f—have not been associated with a specific HLA type. However, specific epitopes of Der p have been identified at the amino acid level and have been shown to be presented by HLA-DR and -DQ gene products.[124]

Perhaps the strongest class II association is with HLA-DR2/Dw2, which is found in 95% of IgE responders to the pollen allergen Amb aV.[125] The DR2 region is known to be associated with DQw1. It has been shown that the responses of cloned T cells to Amb aV is inhibited by anti-DR antibodies and not by anti-DQ antibodies, suggesting that DR is the region involved in the presentation of Amb aV.[126] Studies involving immunogenetics and antigen-specific T cell clones have implicated the DRB1 and not the DRB5 gene of the DR2 region. Specific HLA associations have also been reported for sensitivity to house dust mite allergen in some populations.[127, 128] As discussed further on, sensitivity to certain drugs, occupational allergens, and chemicals is associated with specific MHC class II HLA alleles and haplotypes (i.e., a combination of alleles).

Associations between asthma and atopy and HLA class I antigens (designated A, B, and C) have also been investigated. HLA-B8 (which is associated with DR3) has a possible role in the pathogenesis of atopy. Although some investigators have found it to be present in patients who are atopic,[129, 130] including those who are asthmatic,[131] other workers have not.[132, 133] However, HLA-B8 is well known for its association with autoimmune diseases.[134] Since both autoimmune diseases and atopy result from hyperimmune responses, it may be that B8 is a marker for decreased immunoglobulin suppression. In fact, several groups of investigators have shown that lymphocytes from B8/DR3-positive individuals produce less INF-$\gamma$ and more IL-4 *in vitro*.[135–137]

That variations in the beta$_2$-adrenergic receptor might be implicated in the pathogenesis of asthma has been a long-standing hypothesis.[138] Four mutations have been identified in the receptor gene that cause amino acid substitutions.[139] Although none of these mutations has been found to be more prevalent in patients who have asthma than in normal controls, a number of workers have shown that one such mutation—a substitution of glycine for arginine at position 16—is associated with more severe asthma,[139, 140] increased nocturnal asthma symptoms,[141] and less bronchodilator response to beta agonists.[142] The biologic explanation for this effect appears to be an increased propensity for the GLY 16 variant to be down-regulated after stimulation with beta agonist, an effect that has been demonstrated both *in vitro*[143] and *in vivo*.[144] The results of these studies suggest that mutations in the beta$_2$-adrenergic receptor gene do not play a primary role in the pathogenesis of asthma; however, they may act to modulate the severity of symptoms in affected persons.[145] These observations could explain the decreased beta$_2$-adrenergic responsiveness observed in airway smooth muscle of patients who have died of asthma,[146] a finding that is not seen in surgically resected airway tissue derived from patients who have less severe disease.[147] Substitution of glutamic acid for glutamine at position 27 is another mutant variant that has been shown to render the receptor more resistant to agonist-induced down-regulation in the *in vitro* system;[143] this variant has been found to be associated with less marked airway hyper-responsiveness in a group of asthmatic patients.[148]

Additional associations of asthma/bronchial hyper-responsiveness and specific mutations include (1) an increased prevalence of the alpha$_1$-antiprotease ($\alpha_1$-PI) Z allele in children who have more severe disease,[149, 150] (2) an increased prevalence of PiZ heterozygotes among asthmatics compared with controls,[151, 152] (3) an increased prevalence of the M$_2$ subtype of the normal M allele of $\alpha_1$-PI in patients who have asthma,[153] (4) bronchial hyper-responsiveness and PiS heterozygosity,[154] (5) asthma and a deficiency of alpha$_1$-antichymotrypsin,[155] (6) asthma and a deletion mutation in the angiotensin-converting enzyme (ACE) gene that causes increased enzyme activity,[156] (7) asthma and a mutation in the regulatory region of the tumor necrosis factor-$\alpha$ (TNF-$\alpha$) gene that may cause an increase in secretion of this powerful proinflammatory cytokine,[157, 158] and (8) polymorphisms in the promoter regions of the IL-4 and IL-10 genes with asthma and allergy phenotypes.[159] Several groups of investigators have found evidence suggesting an increased prevalence of atopy,[160] asthma,[161] and bronchial hyper-responsiveness[162] in patients who are heterozygous for cystic fibrosis (CF); however, these findings have not always been replicated.[163, 164] One group also found evidence that heterozygosity for the most common CF allele ($\Delta F508$) *protected* against asthma.[165] They suggested that this heterozygote advantage may account for the high prevalence of the allele in the Caucasian population.

## PATHOLOGIC CHARACTERISTICS

The details of the structural changes in the lungs and airways of asthmatics come from morphometric and immuno- and histochemical analyses of the lung tissue of asthmatic persons. Tissue has been obtained at the time of autopsy after fatal attacks of asthma, from autopsy samples of the lungs of patients who had asthma but who died of other causes, and from airway wall biopsies obtained via bronchoscopy in relatively stable asthmatic patients. Unfortunately, these sources do not provide the full spectrum of pathologic material that would be necessary to describe the morphologic changes in the airway walls as a function of clinical severity, chronicity, or age. Especially lacking are specimens from patients during acute attacks of allergic bronchoconstriction and from patients who have atopy and abnormal airway responsiveness but no lower respiratory tract symptoms. In addition, the data derived from biopsies are incomplete, because only the mucosal region is normally sampled, precluding quantitative morphometry of the full thickness of the airway wall.

Because much of our knowledge of the pathologic characteristics of asthma derives from studies done at autopsy on patients who have died of asthma, the changes that have been described inevitably represent severe disease; thus, generalization to milder forms of disease could be questioned. Despite this, evidence provided by a few studies of asthmatic patients who have died of other causes and from analysis of bronchial biopsy specimens suggests that although morphologic changes can diminish between attacks,[166] considerable epithelial, muscular, inflammatory cellular, and microvascular abnormalities can persist.[167–172] Although it is impossible to follow the sequence of histologic changes that occur in the airways of asthmatic patients, animal models allow more precise chronology of morphologic features, at least following antigen challenge. In allergic rabbits, for example, the immediate reaction (30 minutes later) is characterized by edema alone;[173] at 6, 24, and 48 hours, there is a combination of edema, congestion, and cellular infiltration.

At autopsy, the lungs of patients who die of asthma are distended and typically project above the cut ends of the ribs and across the midline of the thorax when the chest is opened. Focal depressions bounded by interlobular septa are evident on the pleural surface, representing areas of subsegmental atelectasis caused by bronchiolar obstruction.[174] Cut sections of the lung characteristically show the bronchi and bronchioles to be plugged with viscid mucus, which in some cases extends into the trachea. Focal cystic bronchiectasis, often in the upper and middle lobes, has been reported in some patients[174] and should suggest the diagnosis of allergic bronchopulmonary aspergillosis.

Histologically, the mucous plugs are most frequent in bronchi and membranous bronchioles but may extend into the respiratory bronchioles.[174] They are composed of both mucoid and proteinaceous material and typically completely fill the airway lumen (Fig. 54–1). Scattered within them is a variable number of cells, most of which are eosinophils or ciliated cells derived from the airway epithelium. The latter can occur singly or in clusters of up to 100 cells; such clusters are termed Creola bodies.[175] Also present in both airway plugs and sputum[168] are Charcot-Leyden crystals and Curschmann spirals. The former are variably sized crystals ranging from 20 to 40 μm in length and from 2 to 4 μm in width (Fig. 54–2) and are believed to be composed predominantly of lysophospholipase (phospholipase B) derived from eosinophilic granules.[176] The crystals appear bright yellow-green on fluorescence microscopy.[177] Curschmann spirals are convoluted strands of mucus having a relatively compact central core surrounded by numerous delicate fibrils (Fig. 54–2); they are typically microscopic in size but may be up to 2 cm in length. Although they are generally believed to be formed by inspissation of secretions within small airways, similar structures have been seen in pleural and peritoneal fluid specimens,[178] and the precise mechanism by which they are formed is not clear. Although characteristic of asthma, neither Charcot-Leyden crystals nor Curschmann spirals are pathognomonic of the condition.[176, 179]

Histologic changes in the bronchial and bronchiolar walls are characteristic of asthma and involve the epithelium, lamina propria, muscularis mucosa, and submucosa.[169, 174] Although the epithelium may be normal, goblet cell hyperplasia is frequent and is sometimes so marked that large segments of the airway surface are composed solely of these cells (Fig. 54–3);[169] in one morphometric investigation, the presence of extensive goblet cell hyperplasia was associated with severe asthma and the presence of intraluminal mu-

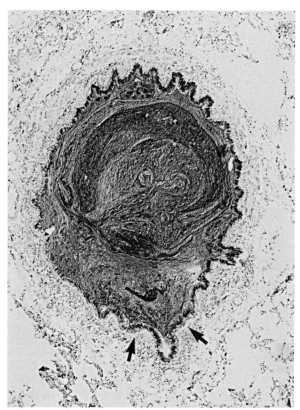

**Figure 54–1. Asthma: Mucous Plugging.** A section of a small bronchus shows it to be completely occluded by a dense plug of strongly periodic acid–Schiff (PAS)-positive mucus; variation in cellularity of the mucus causes a somewhat laminated appearance. The bronchial wall contains a moderate number of inflammatory cells; even at this magnification, thickening of the basement membrane is evident as a lightly stained subepithelial stripe *(arrows)*. Note the strong PAS positivity of the epithelium, indicating extensive goblet cell hyperplasia. The patient was a 43-year-old man who died of asthma (PAS, ×40).

cus.[180] In many cases, epithelial cells are detached, leaving only a layer of cuboidal basal cells (Fig. 54–4);[181] this feature can be seen in both autopsy[169, 174] and biopsy[182] specimens. The pathogenesis of this epithelial damage and shedding is unclear. It has been suggested that it may be caused by transudation of fluid from the subepithelial microvessels in the lamina propria into the airway lumen and epithelium and/or by damage from basic proteins and oxygen radicals released from eosinophils and other inflammatory cells.[174, 182–184] Ultrastructural evidence of such damage has been described in the ciliated cells of patients whose disease is in remission and in those who have severe persistent asthma.[169, 182] In one case of a patient who had an ovarian teratoma and who died of asthma, the tumor contained bronchial mucosa that showed all the pathologic changes typically found in pulmonary airways in asthma, including shedding of surface epithelial cells;[175] this suggests that the pathogenesis of the epithelial abnormalities is not a local phenomenon. Whatever the mechanism of epithelial damage and shedding, it is likely that the resulting loss of ciliary function is at least partly responsible for the presence of the extensive intraluminal mucus found at autopsy.

There is increasing evidence that an important contributor to the chronic nature of asthma is the structural changes that occur in the airways as a consequence of episodic and

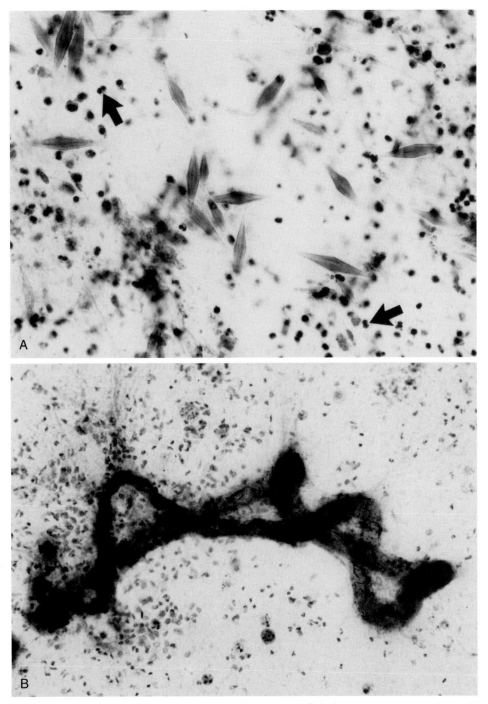

**Figure 54–2. Asthmatic Sputum: Charcot-Leyden Crystals and Curschmann Spiral.** A sputum specimen from a 20-year-old man who had an exacerbation of asthma *(A)* shows multiple uniformly shaped Charcot-Leyden crystals. Bilobed nuclei, some showing degenerative changes, indicate the presence of eosinophils *(arrows)*. Elsewhere in the same specimen *(B)*, a convoluted Curschmann spiral was evident. The dense central core and lightly stained filamentous periphery are characteristic. (Papanicolaou stain.)

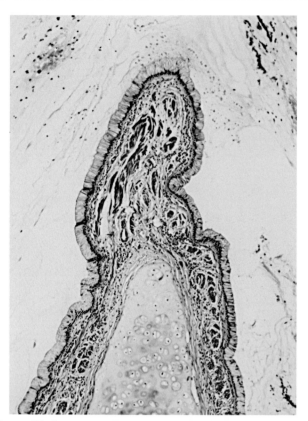

**Figure 54–3. Asthma: Goblet Cell Hyperplasia.** A section of bronchial wall at a bifurcation shows the epithelium to be composed almost entirely of goblet cells. The specimen was obtained at autopsy of the same patient as illustrated in Figure 54–1 (×60).

ongoing inflammation. These changes, which are collectively referred to as *airway wall remodeling,* include the deposition and reorganization of connective tissue components, hypertrophy and hyperplasia of various tissue cells, and hyperplasia of the bronchial vasculature. The combination of these alterations results in airway wall thickening that can have profound effects on airway function. In addition to this quantitative effect, airway mechanics may be altered as a result of changes in the biochemical composition or material properties of the various mucosal and submucosal constituents.

Figure 54–5 shows a diagrammatic representation of an airway in cross section. The wall can be divided into three compartments: (1) the inner wall, consisting of epithelium, basement membrane, and lamina propria; (2) the outer wall, consisting of the connective tissue between the cartilage and the surrounding parenchyma in bronchi and the muscle layer and parenchyma in bronchioles (the adventitia); and (3) the smooth muscle layer.[185] Although it has been recognized for some time that the airway walls of asthmatic patients are thickened,[186, 187] it was not possible to perform a systematic study of the quantitative changes in airway wall dimensions because a yardstick of airway size was not available to allow a valid comparison between normal and asthmatic persons. The demonstration that the airway basement membrane perimeter is relatively constant after smooth muscle contraction or changes in lung volume[188, 189] has allowed reliable examination of the relationship between airway wall compartment

areas and airway size.[170, 190, 191] This is done by examining the relationships between airway internal perimeter (Pi) or basement membrane perimeter (Pbm) and the areas occupied by the respective tissue components. The results of a number of studies confirm that airway wall thickness is markedly increased in patients who have had fatal asthma, with involvement of all layers of the airway wall. Less information is available for patients who have had asthma but who died for other reasons or who have had a lobectomy; however, the available data suggest that the airway wall dimensions in these patients are intermediate between those of patients who have died of asthma and normal persons.[170, 171] Thus, an increase in airway wall dimensions does not simply reflect a terminal event.

Other bronchial wall abnormalities characteristic of asthma include "basement membrane" thickening,[169, 192] edema and vascular congestion of the lamina propria and submucosa, and a more or less intense mural infiltrate of inflammatory cells, particularly eosinophilic leukocytes (*see* Fig. 54–4).[172] The first of these may be caused by repeated bouts of epithelial damage[169, 193] and in fact represents thickening of the subepithelial fibrillar collagen layer.[194] This collagenous matrix layer is typically doubled in thickness, from 5 to 8 μm to 10 to 15 μm, and contains type I, type III, and type V collagen and fibronectin but not basal lamina components (type IV collagen, laminin).[194] The matrix may be synthesized by adjacent myofibroblasts,[195, 213] because the number of the latter cells correlates with the magnitude of subepithelial thickening.[196] These structural changes have been observed in patients who have mild asthma and in those who have occupational asthma associated with exposure to a variety of chemicals.[197] Moreover, in some persons who have toluene diisocyanate (TDI)-induced asthma, cessation of exposure to TDI has been followed after 6 to 20 months by a decrease in subepithelial collagen thickness and decreased numbers of subepithelial fibroblasts, mast cells, and lymphocytes.[198] Although this suggests that these changes are reversible, the mechanism of the reversal is unknown. The collagen deposition in the subepithelial layer as well as in the adventitia probably explains the decreased airway distensibility in asthmatic patients.[9, 199] In addition to collagen, elastic fibers[195] and a variety of glycoproteins and proteoglycans, including fibronectin, tenascin, versican, and decorin,[200, 201] are increased in the airway walls of asthmatics; these substances also increase the volume of the submucosa and may also contribute to altered airway mechanics.[201]

The mechanisms underlying changes in extracellular matrix composition in asthma are incompletely understood. A number of growth factors and cytokines released by epithelial cells and inflammatory cells (including eosinophils, mast cells, and T cells) have the capacity to stimulate extracellular matrix metabolism by mesenchymal cells. Both inflammatory cells and stimulated epithelial and mesenchymal cells (including smooth muscle cells) have the capacity to release transforming growth factor-β1 (TGF-β1), a growth factor that induces matrix deposition, and to release the potent fibroblast mitogens, platelet-derived growth factor (PDGF), and insulin-like growth factor-1 (IGF-1). This combination of mitogens and growth factors is known to induce matrix synthesis and provides a potentially powerful mechanism for remodeling of airway wall architecture.[202–204] However, although TGF-β1 has been found to be abundantly

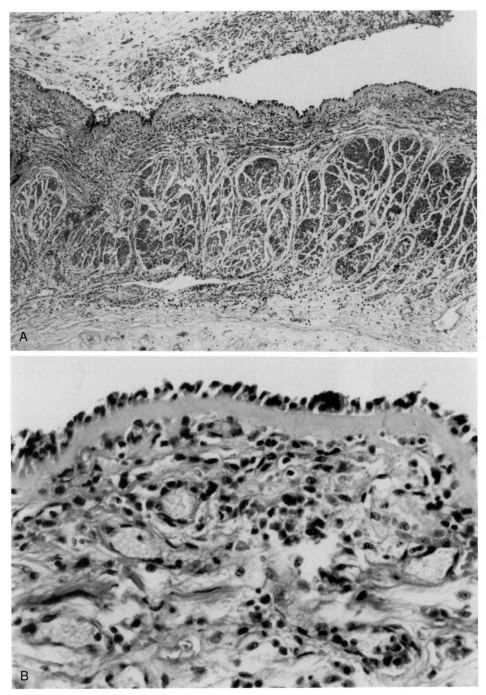

**Figure 54–4. Asthma: Bronchial Wall Abnormalities.** A section of bronchial wall *(A)* shows marked thickening of the muscularis mucosa, numerous inflammatory cells, and a uniformly thickened basement membrane. The bronchial epithelium is composed only of a row of cuboidal basal cells, the ciliated and goblet cells having been shed into the overlying mucus. A view at greater magnification *(B)* reveals to better advantage the residual epithelium, thickened basement membrane, and inflammatory cell infiltrate. The section is from the same patient as in Figure 54–1. *(A,* ×40; *B,* ×300.)

expressed in the airway walls of asthmatic patients, in one study its expression did not seem to be greater than in the airways of nonasthmatics.[203]

The airway wall remodeling that occurs in chronic asthma is also accompanied by degradation of matrix material. For example, ultrastructural evidence for elastin degradation has been reported in airway walls of some patients.[205] Degradation of such substances could alter the mechanical properties of the airways, making them more easily narrowed by the hypertrophied smooth muscle. Because the smooth muscle in the airway wall is encased in and to some extent confined by connective tissue, degradation of the latter occurring as a consequence of chronic inflammation may allow increased smooth muscle contractility.[206, 207] Rarely, local exaggeration of the submucosal inflammatory reaction results in the formation of endobronchial polyps similar to those found in the nasal passages of patients who have allergic rhinitis.[208] Some investigators believe that the bronchial mucous glands are increased in size,[169, 209] although others have not found evidence for this.[174]

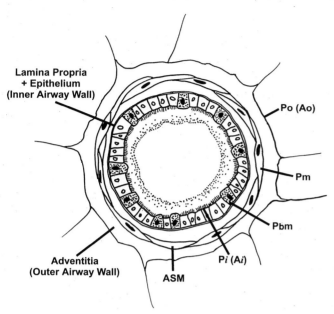

Lamina Propria
+ Epithelium
(Inner Airway Wall)

Po (Ao)

Pm

Pbm

P*i* (A*i*)

Adventitia
(Outer Airway Wall)

ASM

**Figure 54–5. Airway Wall Dimensions.** A diagrammatic representation of an airway cut in cross section is shown. Po = outer perimeter (subtending outer area Ao), Pm = smooth muscle perimeter, Pbm = basement membrane perimeter, P*i* = internal perimeter (subtending luminal area A*i*). ASM = airway smooth muscle. The airway wall can be divided into three compartments: (1) the inner wall, consisting of epithelium, basement membrane, and lamina propria; (2) the outer wall, consisting of the connective tissue between the cartilage and the surrounding parenchyma in bronchi and the smooth muscle layer and parenchyma in bronchioles (the adventitia); and (3) the smooth muscle layer. See Persson CGA: Plasma exudation. Asthma 1:917, 1997, for details.

Most, albeit not all,[171, 210] workers have reported an increase in the amount of smooth muscle in patients who have asthma.[169, 174, 209, 211, 212] In those studies in which no increase has been documented, the asthma was relatively mild and not the cause of death. On the other hand, the results of several studies show that the airway smooth muscle layer is markedly thickened in patients with severe, chronic disease.[186, 209, 214] There is evidence that the increase in smooth muscle is the result of both hypertrophy and hyperplasia of airway smooth muscle cells.[215, 216] In fact, two patterns of airway smooth muscle hypertrophy and hyperplasia were reported in one investigation.[215] In some cases, muscle was found to be increased only in central bronchi, where hyperplasia predominated; in others, the muscle was increased throughout the tracheobronchial tree as a result of both hyperplasia and hypertrophy, especially in the peripheral airways.

It has been suggested that the increase in airway smooth muscle area that has been reported in asthma could have been overestimated.[217] One group of investigators measured the airway smooth muscle area in the large central airways of five asthmatic patients and showed no significant difference compared with a matched control group. In this study, the investigators used 1.5-mm sections of plastic-embedded tissue and discriminated between smooth muscle cells and their surrounding matrix. They reasoned that the plane of section, the use of thick sections, and a failure to distinguish between smooth muscle cells and their associated extracellular matrix could explain an overestimation of smooth muscle area in other studies. However, they studied only large central air-

ways, and the predominant increase in smooth muscle area that has been reported is in peripheral airways.

Abnormalities of the bronchial vasculature are also often seen in asthma. At least three mechanisms exist by which such abnormalities could contribute to the excessive airway narrowing observed in asthma: engorgement, vascular leak, and proliferation. Both relaxation of the bronchial smooth muscle and an increase in the intravascular pressure will lead to engorgement of these vessels. The latter could result in reduction in the area of the airway lumen and/or in outward expansion of the airway wall so that it compresses the adjacent lung parenchyma. An increase in the outer diameter of the airway will "insulate" the airway smooth muscle from the load normally applied by the surrounding lung parenchyma, allowing the muscle to shorten and thereby decrease the luminal area. There is also some evidence that the size and number of bronchial vessels are increased in asthma, suggesting that angiogenesis may be a part of the airway remodeling. In one study of patients who had died of asthma, investigators showed an increase in the fraction of the submucosa and adventitia occupied by bronchial vessels and in the number of bronchial vessels within each of these compartments.[170] Another group found an increase in the number of bronchial venules in cartilaginous airways of asthmatic patients when compared with control subjects.[218]

Inflammatory cells are characteristically increased in the epithelium, lamina propria, and submucosa of patients who have asthma. Typically, they are most prominent in patients who have died of the disease, but they have also been identified in persons who have untreated disease of recent onset.[172] An increase in eosinophils is most characteristic; however, an increase in lymphocytes, macrophages, and neutrophils has also been documented.[172, 219] It should be remembered that neutrophils are occasionally more prominent than eosinophils. In one review of seven patients who died of asthma, three had this histologic finding;[220] these patients had experienced a much more rapid onset of asthma than the four who had prominent airway eosinophils. Mast cells can be found in the submucosa, airway epithelium, and airway lumen; in the latter two locations, they can be particularly important because of their potential for interacting with inhaled allergens prior to epithelial penetration.[167, 221] These cells have also been found to be increased in number in the airway epithelium of patients with newly diagnosed, untreated asthma.[172] However, in the bronchi of patients who died of asthma, a sparsity of mast cells has been reported in comparison with bronchi of nonasthmatic control subjects or asthmatic patients who died of other causes;[222] this observation may reflect a failure to recognize such cells after degranulation.

## PATHOGENESIS

The basic pathophysiologic abnormality that determines the functional and symptomatic status of an asthmatic patient is airway narrowing. This can occur by four main mechanisms: (1) airway smooth muscle contraction and shortening; (2) edema, inflammatory cell infiltration, and congestion of the airway wall; (3) mucous hypersecretion and plugging of the airway lumen; and (4) airway wall remodeling. For the most part, it is difficult if not impossible to determine in a given patient at a given time what proportion of airway obstruction is caused by each of these mechanisms. As a generalization, however, it can be reasonably concluded that when obstruction is rapidly reversible following inhalation of cholinergic antagonists or beta-adrenergic agonists, the pathogenesis is smooth muscle shortening, whereas when it responds over a period of days to steroids and other therapeutic interventions, it is caused by edema, inflammatory cell infiltration and mucous plugging.[223, 224] When given over prolonged periods, anti-inflammatory therapy may be associated with some reversal of the airway remodeling.[225]

Figure 54–6 is a schematic overview of the pathogenesis of asthma. The symptoms of asthma, including wheeze, cough, and breathlessness, are caused directly and indirectly by acute and chronic inflammation in the airways. Repeated allergic responses to inhaled aeroallergens constitute the most frequent cause of the inflammation, although there are other mechanisms that can cause a similar response and lead

to similar symptoms. The cellular and molecular mechanisms involved in the inflammatory reaction are extremely complex and are directed by an interacting group of cytokines. Many of these cytokines have been implicated in the pathogenesis of asthma and allergic disease, and reviews of the subject are available.[226–228]

In genetically susceptible individuals, the intensity, timing, and mode of exposure to aeroallergens determine the extent to which a distinct subset of antigen-specific T helper cells (Th2) cells is expanded. These cells produce a specific group of cytokines (IL-4, IL-5, and IL-10) that facilitate the production by B lymphocytes of specific IgE antibodies directed against the aeroallergens. The IgE molecules attach to mast cells and basophils; interaction with their corresponding allergen is followed by release of various stored mediators and cytokines and by the production of additional ones. The cytokines perpetuate the inflammatory response by initiating the chemotaxis and migration of circulating inflammatory cells, particularly eosinophils, and by activat-

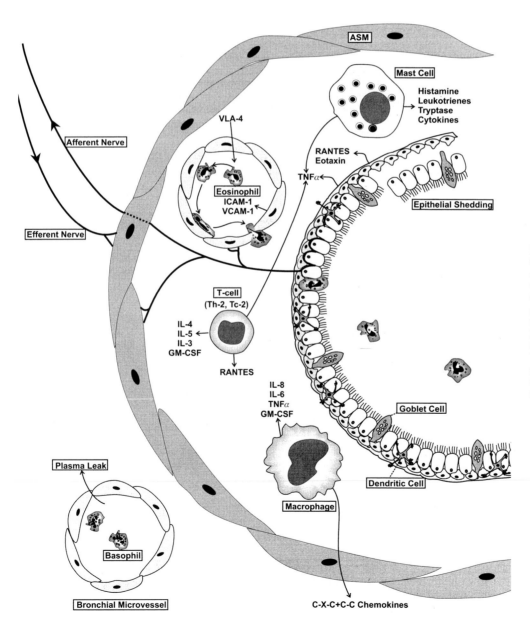

**Figure 54–6. Asthma: Mechanisms of Inflammation.** A schematic diagram of the airway wall shows some of the cells, mediators, and cytokines involved in allergic airway inflammation. TNF-α, tumor necrosis factor-α; VLA-4, very late activation antigen-4; ICAM-1, intercellular adhesion molecule-1; VCAM-1, vascular cell adhesion molecule-1; IL, interleukin; GM-CSF, granulocyte macrophage colony–stimulating factor.

ing resident cells to express and secrete molecules that enhance inflammation. The cytokines also cause an up-regulation of expression of integrins and selectins on the surface of endothelial and epithelial cells; these surface molecules interact with complementary ligands on inflammatory cells to enhance their adherence and migration.

A number of environmental agents, such as respiratory viruses and tobacco smoke, can be inhaled in addition to aeroallergens and, in genetically predisposed individuals, can aggravate the airway obstruction produced by the allergic inflammatory reaction. The acute airway inflammation caused by the release of mediators and cytokines from the resident and motile effector cells is characterized by increased vascular permeability, mucus hypersecretion, inflammatory cell chemotaxis and migration, and smooth muscle contraction. The consequences of chronic inflammation are structural and functional alterations (airway wall remodeling), which render the airways hyper-responsive to a variety of nonspecific (nonallergic) irritants. Because these structural and functional alterations are relatively irreversible, airway hyper-responsiveness and symptoms can persist despite the removal of the inciting allergens.

In this section we review the cellular and molecular mechanisms that initiate and perpetuate the inflammatory reaction in asthma, examine its consequences (bronchial hyper-responsiveness, exaggerated mucus production, and impaired mucus clearance), and discuss the various triggers of asthma.

## Cellular and Molecular Mechanisms of Inflammation

Although inflammation was recognized by Osler as an important part of asthma,[229] it is only since the 1980s that the central role of inflammation in the pathogenesis of asthma has been fully appreciated. Ample evidence confirms that airway inflammation is inevitably present in symptomatic disease; moreover, the severity of disease is generally mirrored by the intensity of inflammation.[230] The other major factor that has resulted in the increased attention placed on airway inflammation is the remarkable improvement in our understanding of the actions of the many cells, cytokines, and mediators involved in the pathogenesis of airway inflammation (see Fig. 54–6). Space does not permit a comprehensive review of these mechanisms, and the reader is referred instead to a number of review articles and texts for additional information.[231–234]

### Inflammatory, Immune, and Other Cells

#### Lymphocytes

The T lymphocyte is a key cell in the orchestration of chronic airway inflammation in asthma.[235–237] In susceptible persons, specific subsets of CD4$^+$ helper cells (Th2) and CD8$^+$ cytotoxic (Tc) cells directed against occupational agents, environmental aeroallergens or viral antigens are stimulated to proliferate, infiltrate the airway wall, and become activated. Such activated cells secrete a variety of cytokines that amplify and perpetuate the airway inflammation. The Th2 cytokines include IL-4, IL-3, IL-5, and granulocyte-macrophage colony-stimulating factor (GM-CSF).

The last three stimulate the bone marrow to produce eosinophils, attract them to the airway wall, activate them, and markedly prolong their life span.[238, 239] IL-4 stimulates B lymphocytes to differentiate into plasma cells that produce allergen-specific IgE. The Th2 lymphocytes also secrete IL-10, which suppresses the proliferation of Th1 lymphocytes, whose activation is protective against asthma. A similar cytokine profile is also apparent in patients who have nonallergic asthma, although in these patients an increase in IL-4 may not detected; in fact, it has been suggested that it is IL-5–mediated activation of eosinophils that is the common pathway linking the different forms of asthma.[237]

### Mast Cells and Basophils

The mast cell is the most important cell involved in the acute inflammatory reaction in the airways of asthmatic patients. It has a high surface density of the high-affinity IgE receptors to which IgE attaches; when allergen-specific IgE is cross-linked by interaction with allergen, the cell is activated to release pre-formed mediators and to synthesize new mediators and cytokines. Mast cells are the principal source of airway histamine and can release prostaglandins, leukotrienes, platelet-activating factor (PAF), and adenosine; these in turn cause increased vascular permeability, airway smooth muscle contraction, mucus hypersecretion, and fibroblast proliferation.[240] The release of proteolytic enzymes such as tryptase and chymase may be important in matrix degradation and airway remodeling.[241] Mast cells also secrete IL-4, which stimulates further synthesis of IgE and may influence the local T cell population via cytokine signaling.[241] Mast cell granules also contain heparin, neutral proteases, and acid hydrolases (such as N-acetyl-beta-glucosaminidase, beta-glucuronidase, and aryl sulfatase); although the role of these enzymes in the acute allergic response is unknown, they probably contribute to tissue damage and remodeling.[242]

Like mast cells, basophils have a high density of the high-affinity IgE receptor on their surface and can release their store of mediators via a signaling pathway stimulated by allergen-IgE interaction on their surface. Basophils can be detected in the lung and sputum of patients who have atopic asthma during the late phase of the allergic reaction to inhaled allergen.[244] There is evidence that basophils from asthmatic patients can release mediators more readily than those from normal persons.[245, 246] In one study, the amount of histamine released from basophils in response to anti-IgE was compared in monozygotic and dizygotic twins. The inter-twin correlation coefficient for the amount of histamine released by a similar number of basophils in the monozygotic twin pairs (r = 0.84) was significant, while that for the dizygotic pairs was not, raising the possibility that there is a genetic influence on basophil phenotype.[247]

### Eosinophils

Abundant evidence suggests that the eosinophil is a central effector cell in asthmatic airway inflammation.[248] High concentrations of eosinophils, in the absence of neutrophils, can be found in sputum, bronchoalveolar lavage (BAL) samples, and tissue biopsies from asthmatic patients.[249] Blood and tissue levels of eosinophils are increased in both intrinsic and extrinsic asthma, indicating that their presence is not necessarily related to an IgE-mediated immune response.[250]

The role of eosinophils in causing airway disease in asthma is related to their ability to release proinflammatory mediators and cytokines as well as certain unique, highly charged toxic proteins. The cells can synthesize leukotrienes, particularly leukotriene $C_4$ ($LTC_4$), which is converted to $LTD_4$.[248] When stimulated with the calcium ionophore A23187, eosinophils from patients who have either intrinsic or extrinsic asthma generate three times more $LTC_4$ than the cells of normal persons.[251] The eosinophil produces a variety of toxic cationic proteins that are important in protection against parasitic infestation but are also capable of causing profound tissue damage. These proteins include major basic protein (MBP), eosinophil cationic protein (ECP), and eosinophil protein X (EPX).[250, 252] Elevated levels of eosinophils and ECP can be detected in the sputum and BAL fluid of patients who have symptomatic asthma, levels decreasing after successful treatment.[253, 254] Although the blood eosinophil count decreases during and after antigen challenge,[254] the serum level of ECP rises—a sequence that suggests that eosinophils are sequestered in the lung and then release ECP. In some patients, there is a secondary increase in the serum level of ECP coincident with a delayed asthmatic response.[250, 255]

The selective recruitment of eosinophils to the airway as part of the inflammatory reaction in asthma is dependent on their expression of specific surface receptors as well as the expression of specific complementary molecules on the bronchial microvascular endothelium. Two of the most important of these are very late activation antigen-4 (VLA-4), which is specifically expressed on eosinophils, and vascular cell adhesion molecule-1 (VCAM-1), which is expressed on the endothelial cells and is specific for the adherence of eosinophils. Eosinophils normally have a short half-life in the circulating blood (about 12 to 24 hours), as a result of their removal by apoptosis. However, under the influence of Th2 cytokines released in the airway wall, they undergo phenotypic changes that include a dramatic increase in their life span to a period of weeks.[244, 256] Eosinophils can themselves synthesize IL-4 and IL-5 in an inflammatory milieu and could thus influence their own survival.[257] There is an association of eosinophilia and bronchial hyper-responsiveness,[258] and MBP can cause airway hyper-responsiveness in nonhuman primates.[259] A possible mechanism for this phenomenon has been suggested by the observation that eosinophil cationic proteins selectively inhibit the $M_2$ muscarinic receptors on airway cholinergic nerves;[260, 261] because it is via the $M_2$ receptor that acetylcholine mediates a down-regulation of its further release, a block of this receptor can induce increased vagally mediated bronchoconstriction.

Although the bulk of evidence suggests that eosinophils play a harmful role in asthma, they could have a beneficial effect through the production of certain enzymes and proteins. These enzymes include aryl sulfatase B, phospholipase D, and histaminase, agents that can deactivate leukotrienes, PAF, and histamine, respectively, thereby damping the allergic response.

### Macrophages and Dendritic Cells

Although T cells, mast cells, eosinophils, and basophils have received the most attention in the study of the patho-genesis of asthma, it has become increasingly evident that other cells can also play an important role. For example, both tissue and alveolar macrophages have membrane receptors that bind IgE; allergen binding, in turn, stimulates mediator release from these cells.[262–264] Alveolar macrophages can also produce a factor that releases histamine from basophils and mast cells[264] and can produce $LTB_4$, the potent leukotriene chemotaxin, which could in turn amplify the allergic reaction by attracting blood-derived inflammatory cells.[266] Both alveolar macrophages and tissue macrophages in the airway wall can also act as antigen-presenting cells (APCs) and can secrete proinflammatory cytokines such as TNF-$\alpha$ and GM-CSF.[267]

Intraepithelial dendritic cells express very high levels of the class I and II MHC antigens and are among the first cells to interact with inhaled allergen; they process the allergens and transport them to the regional lymph nodes, where they present them to T cells.[268, 269]

### Epithelial and Mesenchymal Cells

Although the bronchial vascular endothelium, airway epithelium, and airway smooth muscle are generally considered the targets for damage in airway inflammation, there is increasing evidence that they are actively involved in the process. The endothelium plays a part in controlling plasma exudation by modulating the size of the intraendothelial gaps and participates in inflammatory cell recruitment by up-regulating the expression of adhesion molecules such as VCAM-1 and intercellular adhesion molecule-1 (ICAM-1). The endothelial cell is also metabolically active, generating relaxant prostaglandins and nitric oxide (NO) as well as the potent smooth muscle constrictor endothelin-1.[270]

Airway epithelial cells synthesize arachidonic acid–derived lipid mediators including PAF, the prostaglandins, and 15-hydroxyeicosatetraenoic acid (15-HETE). They also contain a variety of catabolic enzymes such as neutral metalloendopeptidase, which is capable of inactivating small inflammatory peptides such as substance P, bradykinin, and neurokinin A. Like the endothelium, the airway epithelium is capable of synthesizing NO via a constitutively expressed NO synthase enzyme as well as an inducible enzyme (c-NOS and iNOS, respectively) and can play an active role in the movement of inflammatory cells by expressing adhesion molecules such as ICAM-1.[271]

Interstitial fibroblasts in the airway wall have also been implicated in airway inflammation. Besides their obvious ability to synthesize connective tissue proteins and proteoglycans, fibroblasts can secrete a variety of cytokines, including the chemokines IL-8 and RANTES, eosinophil stimulants such as GM-CSF, and growth factors such as PDGF and TGF-$\beta$.[272]

### Inflammatory Mediators and Cytokines

#### Histamine

In humans, histamine originates from mast cells and basophils. It produces airway smooth muscle contraction by a direct action on the muscle and indirectly by stimulation of afferent receptors that cause reflex bronchoconstriction[273] it also increases mucus production and causes bronchial vascular dilatation and leak.[274] Allergic persons challenged with allergens develop increased levels of histamine in mixed venous and arterial blood, although arterial levels are higher, indicating that histamine is metabolized in its passage through the systemic circulation.[275] Nonallergic stimuli capable of inducing histamine release include bradykinin, substance P, and complement.[276] In addition, certain cytokines and chemokines such as IL-3, IL-5, GM-CSF, and RANTES can act as histamine-releasing factors by priming mast cells and basophils to more easily release their histamine stores.[277]

The importance of local tissue concentrations has been observed in studies in which the effects of aerosol and intravenous histamine were compared:[278] histamine administered intravenously to asthmatic patients results in less bronchial response than when it is administered as an aerosol, even though the intravenous route produces systemic symptoms such as flushing and a throbbing headache. By stimulating afferent lung receptors, locally released histamine can also induce cough and changes in the breathing pattern.[279, 280]

There are three types of histamine receptors: $H_1$, $H_2$, and $H_3$. Airway smooth muscle contraction and microvascular permeability changes are mediated by the $H_1$ receptor, and mucus secretion and bronchial vascular dilation are mediated by the $H_2$ receptors.[281] $H_3$ receptors, located on mast cells, limit further histamine release by a negative feedback loop. $H_2$ receptors on suppressor T lymphocytes also may allow histamine-induced modulation of IgE production.[282] Parenteral $H_1$ receptor blockade does not significantly decrease the airway response to inhaled antigen because the blocker is ineffective in antagonizing histamine that is released locally and because other mediators are not inhibited.[283, 284]

### Leukotrienes

Since "slow-reacting substances of anaphylaxis" were chemically identified as the leukotrienes in 1979,[285, 286] an appreciation of the importance of these chemicals in the pathogenesis of asthma and other inflammatory disorders has increased tremendously. Like the prostaglandins, the leukotrienes are derived from the metabolism of arachidonic acid, which can be mobilized during the inflammatory process. The leukotrienes $LTC_4$, $LTD_4$, and $LTE_4$ are capable of inducing bronchial smooth muscle contraction, increased vascular permeability, and increased mucus production.[287, 288] Although $LTC_4$ and $LCD_4$ cause more severe bronchoconstriction in asthmatic patients than in normal persons, they are relatively more potent in normal persons than is methacholine or histamine.[289] The leukotriene $LTB_4$ has no contractile effect on muscle, but it is a powerful chemotaxin that can attract both eosinophils and neutrophils to the site of its release.[290] When administered by aerosol to human subjects, the bronchoconstricting leukotrienes cause dose-dependent airway narrowing that is maximal at 3 minutes and resolves over 1 to 3 hours—a duration of action that is longer than that produced by histamine.[291] Asthmatic patients are about 25 to 100 times more sensitive to the effects of $LTD_4$ than are normal subjects, whereas patients who have allergic rhinitis are only slightly (three to four times) more sensitive. In normal individuals and asthmatic patients, the response of the airways to $LTD_4$ correlates with the response to methacholine, although on a molar basis $LTD_4$ is 250 to 800 times more potent than methacholine.[291–293]

Leukotrienes can be synthesized by mast cells, airway epithelial cells, macrophages, and blood-derived inflammatory cells, the proportion of the various leukotrienes produced varying with the enzyme complement of the cell. They are released following antigen challenge of the respiratory tract,[294, 295] during anti-IgE challenge of purified human lung mast cells,[296] following exercise-induced asthma,[297] and during acute spontaneous attacks of asthma.[298] They appear to be especially important in the pathogenesis of aspirin (acetylsalicylic acid [ASA])-induced asthma. Even in the absence of exposure to ASA, patients who are ASA-sensitive excrete three times the normal amount of $LTE_4$ in their urine;[299] challenge with oral or inhaled ASA also causes excessive additional production of $LTE_4$ in aspirin-sensitive but not aspirin-insensitive asthmatic patients.[300, 301]

The important role of leukotrienes in the pathogenesis of asthma has been convincingly proved by the beneficial effect of leukotriene receptor blockers and synthesis inhibitors in patients who have severe asthma.[302, 303]

### Prostaglandins

Prostaglandins and thromboxane are produced by the action of the cyclooxygenase enzymes on arachidonic acid.[304, 305] Cyclooxygenase exists in two isoforms: COX-1, which produces the prostaglandins involved in normal physiologic function, and COX-2, which is induced in a restricted tissue-specific fashion by inflammatory stimuli.[306, 307] Although virtually all cells have the ability to generate prostaglandins, the amount and type produced are dependent on the enzyme content of the individual cell type.

Prostaglandins can both contract and relax airway smooth muscle. In normal persons, prostaglandins $E_1$ and $E_2$ ($PGE_1$ and $PGE_2$) usually cause bronchodilatation, although low concentrations result in bronchoconstriction.[308, 309] In asthmatic patients, administration of $PGE_2$ by aerosol produces either bronchoconstriction or dilatation.[309] Prostaglandin $F_2$ is the best known of the bronchoconstricting prostaglandins; asthmatic patients are up to 8,000 times more sensitive to $PGF_2$ than are healthy normal persons,[310–312] although some show a paradoxical bronchodilatation or tachyphylaxis with high concentrations of the inhaled drug.[313, 314] Despite these observations, the therapeutic administration of $PGF_2$ to women who have normal lung function for the purpose of inducing abortion has been shown to result in greatly reduced midexpiratory flow rates, air trapping, and hypoxemia.[315] $PGD_2$ is released in substantial amounts after IgE challenge in excised human lung and is a potent bronchoconstrictor in both normal persons and asthmatic patients.[316]

The observations that antigen challenge of lung fragments from sensitized individuals[317] and inhalation of specific allergens by asthmatic patients[318] result in the release of prostaglandins and their metabolites suggest that prostaglandin may make an important contribution to the allergic airway response. However, sodium cromoglycate is unable to inhibit bronchospasm induced by $PGF_2$,[318, 319] whereas it blocks antigen responses; moreover, in allergic nonasthmatic persons (such as those who have allergic rhinitis), pretreatment with indomethacin has been shown to increase bronchoconstriction in response to inhaled antigen, suggesting that in some persons, production of bronchodilator prostaglandins may be an important negative feedback mechanism.[320]

Prostaglandin synthesis is responsible for the refractory period after exercise or isocapnic hyperventilation–induced bronchoconstriction. Leukotrienes released during exercise appear to stimulate the production of $PGE_2$, which inhibits the bronchoconstricting effects of subsequently released leukotrienes.[321] The important role of the cyclooxygenase and lipoxygenase pathways of arachidonic acid metabolism in the production of asthma caused by administration of aspirin and other nonsteroidal anti-inflammatory agents is discussed farther on (*see* page 2112).

### Chemotactic Factors

Many mediators and cytokines, such as $LTB_4$, PAF, IL-5, IL-3, TNF-$\alpha$, and GM-CSF, that are generated by tissue and inflammatory cells in the airways of asthmatic patients exhibit chemotactic activity for eosinophils, neutrophils, monocytes, and lymphocytes. There are also a large number of low-molecular-weight substances termed *chemokines* ("chemoattractant cytokines") that act as potent inflammatory cell attractants;[322–324] among those implicated in the airway inflammation of asthma are eotaxin, RANTES, macrophage chemoattractant protein-1 (MCP-1), macrophage chemoattractant protein-3 (MCP-3), and IL-8. These chemokines act through a family of receptors between which there is ample cross-reactivity; i.e., one chemokine can bind to a variety of receptors and vice versa. Despite this cross-reactivity, certain chemokines are more or less specific for certain receptors and cell types. RANTES, synthesized by airway epithelial cells and mast cells, and eotaxin, synthesized by macrophages, are extremely potent chemoattractants for eosinophils and can be detected in the tissue and BAL fluid of asthmatics.[325, 326] Chemotactic activity for neutrophils can also be demonstrated in the BAL fluid of asthmatics; although some of this is related to complement fragments (C5a and C5a desArg) and the chemokine IL-8, there are also a number of poorly characterized agents that may contribute to neutrophil recruitment.[326]

### Platelet-Activating Factor

PAF is a phospholipid that is released from mast cells and basophils during antigen challenge. It can also be produced by macrophages, and its release stimulated by endotoxin.[327] In addition to causing platelet aggregation and degranulation, PAF is associated with a wide variety of biologic activities that may be important in the pathogenesis of asthma. For example, the substance causes airway smooth muscle contraction in the presence of platelets; by itself, it increases vascular permeability, and in aerosol form it causes prolonged inflammation and eosinophilia in animals. PAF may also release or generate mitogenic factors that could lead to airway smooth muscle hypertrophy or hyperplasia and the development of nonspecific bronchial hyperresponsiveness.[327, 328] In one study of 12 patients, the blood levels of PAF correlated with asthmatic symptoms.[329] Inhalation of an aerosol containing PAF results in a prolonged increase in nonspecific airway responsiveness in normal persons.[330]

### Neurokinins

The extensive sensory and motor neural network that innervates the tracheobronchial tree contains a variety of neuropeptide transmitters that have been implicated in airway inflammation; so-called neurogenic inflammation is particularly well documented in animal models.[331] Substance P is an 11-amino-acid peptide found primarily in afferent fibers; along with the related tachykinins, neurokinins A and B, it is a powerful airway smooth muscle contractile agonist and can increase vascular permeability and mucus secretion. These neuropeptides can be released locally following afferent nerve stimulation. The release of substance P from afferent nerve fibers is thought to be responsible for the "flare" portion of the cutaneous wheal-and-flare response, and a similar axonal reflex has been suggested as a mechanism for airway mucosal swelling in asthma.[332] The expression of substance P has been reported to be increased and that of the bronchodilating vasoactive intestinal polypeptide (VIP) to be decreased in the airways of asthmatics.[333, 334] However, in another study the quantity of immunoreactive substance P and VIP were not different in the lungs of patients who had or did not have asthma.[335] The amount of substance P that can be recovered from the airways is greater in allergic than in nonallergic persons and is increased following allergen challenge.[336] The results of these studies emphasize the uncertain role of neurokinins in the pathogenesis of asthma.

The neurokinins are normally metabolized in the airway by neutral endopeptidases (NEPs); in one study, the bronchoconstricting effects of nebulized neurokinin A was enhanced following the administration of an inhibitor of NEP.[337] Data such as these suggest that NEP depletion, perhaps following epithelial damage, might contribute to an amplification of neurogenic airway inflammation. The importance of sensory neuropeptides can be investigated using capsaicin, the pungent component of red pepper, which selectively releases and depletes tachykinins from sensory nerves. In animal models, this substance is effective in attenuating allergic inflammation;[331] however, inhalation of capsaicin causes only slight and transient bronchial narrowing in normal persons.[338]

### Nitric Oxide

There has been considerable interest in the potential role of nitric oxide (NO) in the modulation of airway inflammation in asthma.[339] NO is normally produced by the bronchial and pulmonary vascular endothelium via the action of NO synthase (NOS). In response to inflammatory stimuli, an isoform of the enzyme called inducible NOS (iNOS) also can be produced by airway epithelium, macrophages, smooth muscle cells, fibroblasts, and neutrophils.[339] NO can be detected in exhaled gas from the lungs of normal persons and is increased in asthmatic patients; this increase has been attributed to up-regulation of the expression of iNOS in the airway epithelium.[340] The potential role of NO in modulating airway inflammation is unclear; in theory, it can act as a vasodilator, enhancing airway hyperemia and edema, but if it reaches the smooth muscle, it should act as a mild bronchodilator rather than a constrictor. A more important role for NO may be as an immune modulator; the substance has been shown to inhibit the production of Th1-type cytokines, such as interferon-$\gamma$, and thus could foster an increase in Th2-type T cells and their proinflammatory cytokines.[341] It has been suggested that the measurement of NO in expired gas could be a useful noninvasive method of monitoring airway inflammation in asthma.[340, 342]

### Endothelins

In human beings, there are three separate genes that code for endothelins ET-1, ET-2, and ET-3 and two distinct receptors called ET-A and ET-B. ET-1 has a variety of effects: it stimulates airway smooth muscle contraction, principally via the ET-B receptor, causes mucus secretion from serous and mucous cells in the nasal mucosa, acts as a weak mitogen for airway smooth muscle cells, increases TNF, IL-1β, and IL-6 secretion from macrophages, and activates mast cells.[343] Increased levels of ET-1 have been detected in BAL fluid of asthmatic patients; the source, as assessed by immunohistochemistry, is probably the airway epithelium rather than the systemic vascular endothelium.[344–346]

### Miscellaneous Mediators

Bradykinin and related kinins are peptides that are formed in tissues and fluids during inflammation. They act via distinct $B_1$ and $B_2$ receptors and could influence airway function directly by stimulating smooth muscle contraction or indirectly by virtue of their proinflammatory action.[347] In asthmatic patients, nebulized bradykinin causes prolonged cough, retrosternal discomfort, and bronchoconstriction.[348] Basophils contain and may release a kallikrein-like enzyme on antigen challenge. The enzyme can react with human plasma kininogen and generate kinins that can provide an additional link among immediate anaphylaxis, the delayed allergic response, and the chronic inflammation of asthma.[349, 350]

Plasma renin levels have been reported to be increased during the acute phase of an asthmatic attack, and angiotensin levels to rise during the recovery phase.[351] Serotonin (5-hydroxytryptamine) is not present in human lung mast cells or blood-derived inflammatory cells. Although it is produced by the neuroendocrine cells of the gastrointestinal and respiratory tracts, it is not considered to have a significant role in causing anaphylaxis or asthma in human beings. However, in the carcinoid syndrome, the substance can be liberated in large quantities and can cause severe bronchospasm by its direct action on bronchial smooth muscle.

There is little evidence that complement activation or circulatory immune complexes are important in the pathogenesis of asthma.[352, 353] Oxygen radicals, specifically hydrogen peroxide ($H_2O_2$), can cause smooth muscle contraction,[354] and airway cells from asthmatic patients generate increased amounts of oxygen radicals.[355]

### Mucus and Mucociliary Clearance

There is no doubt that an important contributing factor in the pathogenesis of acute severe and prolonged asthma (status asthmaticus) is plugging of airways with mucus. Although little is known about the factors governing the type and quantity of tracheobronchial mucus in asthma, a feature of prolonged asthmatic attacks is the presence of secretions that are more viscid than those from normal persons.[355, 356] Many attempts have been made to identify a specific biochemical or rheologic abnormality in the sputum and mucus of patients who have asthma.[358, 359] Generally, studies have shown that the glycoprotein content and viscoelastic properties of mucus in patients who have asthma or other airway diseases relate more to the type of sputum—mucoid, mucopurulent, or purulent—than to the underlying disease. Patients who have asthma tend to have mucoid sputum. Sputum samples from patients who have intrinsic asthma demonstrate a variable glycoprotein content and possess viscoelastic properties similar to the sputum of patients who have chronic bronchitis; by contrast, the sputum of patients who have extrinsic asthma possesses less variability in biochemical and viscoelastic properties.[358] Many inflammatory mediators are known to increase the quantity of mucus secretion, including histamine, the prostaglandins ($PGE$, $PGF_2$, $PGD_2$, and $PGI$), alpha-adrenergic agonists, and leukotrienes.[360]

Radioaerosol techniques reveal impaired mucociliary clearance in patients who have stable asthma, the degree of impairment being related to the degree of air-flow obstruction.[361] This is true despite the fact that asthmatic patients tend to show more central deposition of inhaled radiolabeled marker, a feature that should favor faster clearance rates.[362, 363] When the Teflon disk method is used to measure mucociliary clearance, asthmatic patients in remission show tracheal mucus velocities as low as 55% of normal.[364] Mucociliary clearance can be even more markedly impaired during an acute attack; for example, in one study, 96% of an inhaled radiolabeled marker was retained in the lung after 2 hours (following recovery, the clearance of a marker distributed in an identical fashion was 71%).[365] Prolonged therapy with corticosteroids for 4 weeks has been shown to result in improved mucociliary clearance, despite more peripheral deposition of the inhaled radiolabeled marker.[366]

In atopic asthmatic patients and in sheep that have specific allergy to *Ascaris suum*, antigen challenge further decreases mucus transport. This effect cannot be attributed to bronchoconstriction alone, because challenge with histamine and acetylcholine in doses sufficient to produce bronchoconstriction comparable to that seen with allergen challenge actually increases mucociliary clearance.[359] This effect on clearance is prevented by pretreatment with either cromolyn sodium or a leukotriene antagonist.[367–371] The observation that histamine inhalation alone stimulates mucociliary clearance and that leukotriene inhibitors and cromolyn sodium block the antigen-induced decrease in mucociliary clearance suggests that the impaired clearance is caused by leukotrienes. In support of this hypothesis is experimental evidence that antigen challenge increases clearance after pretreatment with a leukotriene antagonist, suggesting that the inhibitory effect is attributable to the leukotrienes, whereas other released mediators may be stimulatory.[371] In fact, inhaled $LTD_4$ and PAF, both of which are released during allergen challenge, depress mucociliary clearance.[372]

Despite these observations, *in vitro* antigen challenge of ciliated epithelial cells of allergic sheep has been shown to result in a stimulation of ciliary activity and an increase in ciliary beat frequency.[370] The addition of leukotrienes to airway explants also results in a dose-dependent stimulation of ciliary beat frequency; this occurs despite the fact that administration of nebulized leukotrienes depresses mucociliary clearance.[367]

The results of these studies suggest that the chemical mediators of allergic asthma exert their deleterious effects on mucociliary function by altering the quantity and perhaps the rheologic properties of airway secretions. The role of antigen and the resulting mediators in modulating the secretion of the liquid in the sol phase is incompletely understood, but it is possible that these mediators interfere with epithelial water transport.[367] In fact, challenge of sheep trachea by *Ascaris suum in vitro* stimulates the production of glycoprotein secretion and transiently increases $Na^+$ and $Cl^-$ flux across the respiratory epithelium.[373]

The effect on mucociliary clearance of a single antigen challenge may be very prolonged. In allergic sheep, antigen challenge has been shown to result in an increase in pulmonary resistance, a decrease in arterial partial pressure of oxygen ($Pao_2$), and impairment of tracheal mucus velocity (measured by the radiopaque Teflon disk method);[374] although pulmonary mechanics and gas exchange return to normal by 2 to 3 hours, mucociliary clearance continues to worsen, reaching its lowest value between 5 and 7 hours and remaining depressed for up to 7 days.

Some asthmatic patients have been found to have a ciliary inhibitory compound in their sputum that possesses a low molecular weight (of 6,000 to 8,000). The inhibitory effect has been demonstrated in human bronchial explants and is more common in the sputum of asthmatic patients during clinical exacerbation; it is readily reversible on removal of the specific sol phase.[375] A variety of mediators, proteins and enzymes that have also been implicated in airway inflammation can influence ciliary beat frequency *in vitro*. Mediators that increase ciliary beat frequency include adenosine triphosphate (ATP); beta-adrenergic agents; capsaicin; acetylcholine; the endothelins ET-1, ET-2, and ET-3; leukotrienes $LTC_4$ and $LTD_4$; the prostaglandins $PGE_1$, $PGE_2$, and $PGF_{2\alpha}$; and substance P. Substances that decrease beat frequency include PAF, adenosine, the alpha-adrenergic agonists, eosinophil major basic protein (MBP), neutrophil elastase, serum proteins, and various products derived from bacteria such as *Pseudomonas aeruginosa*.[359]

### Nonspecific Bronchial Responsiveness

Airway hyper-responsiveness can be defined as an abnormality of the airways that allows them to narrow too much and too easily in response to a provoking stimulus. In practice, it is generally defined as the dose or concentration—$PD_{20}$ or $PC_{20}$, respectively—of inhaled methacholine or histamine that causes a 20% decline in forced expiratory volume in 1 second ($FEV_1$).[5]

Nonspecific bronchial hyper-responsiveness (bronchial hyper-reactivity, bronchial hyperexcitability) is the exaggerated airway narrowing that occurs in response to inhalation of a variety of nonallergic, usually pharmacologic stimuli. We use the term *nonspecific bronchial responsiveness* (NSBR) as the generic term for this phenomenon and *nonspecific bronchial hyper-responsiveness* (NSBH) for exaggerated responsiveness.[376] Although all the stimuli used to demonstrate NSBH result in some degree of airway narrowing in normal persons, it is the excessive narrowing at

very much lower doses or concentrations that characterizes NSBH. There is considerable interest in the mechanisms that cause NSBH, because many of the symptoms of asthma are related to its presence. In fact, NSBH has been considered to be a *sine qua non* of the disease.[377]

Exaggerated bronchial narrowing in response to pharmacologic agents was described many years ago, but only since the 1970s has the importance of NSBH been recognized and have techniques to demonstrate and quantify it been developed.[378, 380]

The list of substances to which asthmatic patients respond excessively is continually enlarging; the pharmacologic agents include histamine, pilocarpine, methacholine, carbachol, acetylcholine, serotonin, bradykinin, $PGF_{2\alpha}$, the leukotrienes $LTC_4$ and $LTD_4$, and adenosine.[289, 378, 381] Asthmatic patients also show excessive airway narrowing in response to inhalation of atmospheric pollutants, dust, and cold and dry air, and to certain respiratory maneuvers such as a deep inspiration or forced expiration to RV.[378] Although edema of airway walls and mucous plugging of their lumens contribute to the airway obstruction in spontaneous asthmatic episodes, the responses that result from tests of NSBR are caused predominantly by airway smooth muscle shortening because they are rapid in onset and promptly reversible with bronchodilators.[378] Moreover, in atopic persons, hyper-responsiveness may involve structures other than smooth muscle; for example, patients who have allergic rhinitis show increased nasal mucus secretion and protein exudation in response to administration of intranasal methacholine.[382, 383]

The fact that NSBH is such a characteristic feature of asthma raises the question of whether it represents a basic defect in the control of bronchial caliber that precedes and predisposes to the development of the asthmatic state or whether it is a consequence of asthma. The demonstration that bronchomotor response to pharmacologic agents in various nonasthmatic animal species as well as in human beings is highly variable raises the possibility that the exaggerated airway narrowing in asthma simply represents one end of a wide biologic spectrum determined at least in part by heredity.[384–386] A number of observations support this hypothesis. For example, certain canine species exhibit markedly increased NSBR,[387] and some strains of rats can be bred to manifest exaggerated bronchoconstriction;[388] in addition, a substantial percentage of clinically healthy, first-degree relatives of children who have asthma demonstrate NSBH.[389]

Despite these observations, the results of some studies have shown inter-twin variability of response to methacholine, supporting the role of environmental factors as determinants of nonspecific responsiveness.[390] It is also clear that NSBH is not a static phenomenon; a person's responsiveness can change considerably following exposure to infectious agents,[391] environmental pollutants,[392] and specific antigens or sensitizing agents.[393] For example, in a group of patients who had occupational asthma secondary to western red cedar exposure, NSBR decreased gradually over a period of months following cessation of exposure and increased again following re-exposure.[394] These related studies make it likely that airway hyper-responsiveness is, at least in part, a result of asthma in addition to being a genetic risk factor for it.

Patients who have allergic rhinitis without pulmonary symptoms do not invariably demonstrate NSBH.[395, 396] The NSBH manifested by some patients who have atopy and isolated nasal symptoms has been interpreted as indicating the presence of "subclinical" asthma.[395]

NSBH is so characteristic of asthma that it is questionable whether, in symptomatic patients, a diagnosis can be made in its absence.[377] Rarely, patients who have occupational asthma or nonoccupational extrinsic asthma do not show NSBH at the time of diagnosis; however, they often develop increased responsiveness with prolonged exposure.[397-400] Although the presence of NSBH is a very sensitive indicator of asthma, it is far from being specific; for example, it may be seen in patients who have sarcoidosis,[401, 402] extrinsic allergic alveolitis,[403-405] or COPD,[406-408] although in these conditions it appears to be primarily related to a baseline decrease in airway caliber.[401, 403, 407] In a comparison study of patients who had asthma or COPD, NSBH was found to be unrelated to baseline $FEV_1$ in the former but to be significantly related to pre-challenge $FEV_1$ in the latter.[407]

In one study of 876 adults in western Australia, the incidence of NSBH (defined as a histamine $PC_{20}$ of less than 3.9 μM) was approximately 11%, whereas the incidence of asthma (defined as the presence of symptoms consistent with asthma in addition to bronchial hyper-responsiveness) was only 6%.[409] Bronchial hyper-responsiveness was significantly related to respiratory symptoms, atopy, smoking, and abnormal underlying lung function. The prevalence of NSBH was even higher (19%) in another study of 1,400 Australian school children between 8 and 10 years of age;[410] not all children who had symptoms compatible with asthma (or who had asthma diagnosed by a physician) were hyper-responsive; and conversely, only about 60% of the children who had NSBH had symptoms of asthma. Similarly, in occupational surveys of airway responsiveness, the incidence of NSBH is higher than that of clinically diagnosed asthma.[411, 412]

### Measurement

The various methods that have been used to quantify nonspecific airway responsiveness are described in detail in Chapter 17 (*see* page 420). Asthmatics show exaggerated airway narrowing in whatever test is employed, but better separation between asthmatic patients and normal individuals can be achieved by using a test that includes a maximal inspiratory maneuver ($FEV_1$, peak expiratory flow rate [PEFR], or maximal expiratory flows, rather than airway or pulmonary resistance); this is so because in addition to exhibiting exaggerated narrowing, the airways of asthmatic patients show less bronchodilatation after a big breath.[413]

Asthmatics have an increase in both sensitivity and maximal airway narrowing following exposure to provoking agents. Sensitivity (or potency) is generally measured by determining the lowest dose associated with a measurable change and has been distinguished from reactivity, which is represented by the degree of change for a given arithmetic or logarithmic increase in concentration or dose of agonist.[414] Plateaus in the dose-response relationship also can be elicited *in vivo*, at least in some subjects, and this has provided another numerical value—the maximal airway narrowing (efficacy) (Fig. 54–7).[415-419] In one population study of 201 individuals, 76% of those who had no symptoms of asthma had a plateau, and 49% of those who had any symptoms had a plateau.[420] If a plateau can be demonstrated, an additional

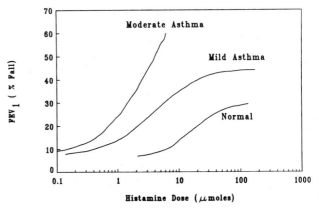

**Figure 54–7. Histamine Dose-Response Curves.** The percentage fall in the forced expiratory volume in 1 second ($FEV_1$) is plotted against the dose of inhaled histamine for a normal subject and patients with mild and moderate asthma. In the normal subject and the patient with mild asthma, a plateau is reached on the dose-response curve. In the patient with moderate asthma, there is no plateau despite a 60% decrease in $FEV_1$. Asthma is characterized by a shift of the dose-response curve to the left and an increase in the maximal response. (Modified from Woolcock AJ, Salome CM, Yan K: The shape of the dose-response curve to histamine in asthmatic and normal subjects. Am Rev Respir Dis 130:71, 1984.)

measure of sensitivity is the dose that causes a 50% maximal response ($ED_{50}$).[417] Although there is experimental evidence that the mechanisms that cause increased sensitivity and increased maximal response are different, the distinction is not used clinically at the present time.[414, 421-424]

The dose-response curve can also be analyzed by measuring the slope of a line extending from the origin to the last data point obtained. This slope has been found to enable separation of asthmatic patients from normal individuals; in one study, there was a greater than 3,000-fold difference between the least and most responsive individuals.[425] The advantage of the use of the dose-response slope is that an estimate can be obtained in all individuals, a feature that is useful in epidemiologic studies.

The most frequently used numeric estimates of NSBR are the dose or concentration of inhaled histamine or methacholine that causes a 20% decrease in $FEV_1$ ($PD_{20}$ or $PC_{20}$) or a 35% decrease in specific airway conductance; there is close concordance between the results using both agents.[426-428] These measurements do not separate sensitivity, reactivity, or maximal response; an alteration in any of these variables could cause similar changes in the estimates of responsiveness. Both agents act directly on specific receptors on airway smooth muscle—methacholine at the postganglionic muscarinic $M_3$ receptor and histamine at the $H_1$ receptor. Although histamine can potentially stimulate reflex bronchoconstriction via sensory afferents as well as smooth muscle directly, it is primarily the direct effect that is most important in clinical testing. Methacholine has been reported to cause a late or prolonged response after inhalation of very high doses, suggesting that a mechanism other than smooth muscle shortening—such as mucous plugging or edema—might be responsible.[429] Tests with both agents show very good short- and long-term reproducibility in asthmatics, provided that patients remain clinically stable between tests.[427, 430-435] Other triggers that have been used to demonstrate airway hyper-responsiveness in asthma include exercise, isocapnic hyperventilation of cold and/or dry air, and the inhalation of ultrasonically generated hypotonic or hypertonic solutions.[436–439]

A different approach to the measurement of NSBR has been to study diurnal variation in airway function and in the responsiveness to a bronchodilating rather than a bronchoconstricting stimulus. Spontaneous diurnal variation in peak expiratory flow rates, as well as exercise-induced lability and bronchodilator response to a beta-adrenergic agonist, has shown excellent correlation with responsiveness to inhaled histamine, although the histamine response is more sensitive and specific for asthma.[440, 441] The concordance between measures of the responsiveness to such a wide variety of stimuli in asthmatic patients emphasizes the nonspecific nature of the hyper-responsiveness. Any theory to explain the pathogenesis of airway hyper-responsiveness must take this nonspecificity into account.

### Pathogenesis

The various links between airway smooth muscle stimulation, airway narrowing, and an increase in airway resistance are shown diagrammatically in Figure 54–8. Abnormalities at any level of this cascade can theoretically produce an exaggeration of airway narrowing in response to a given stimulus; an increase in smooth muscle shortening or a

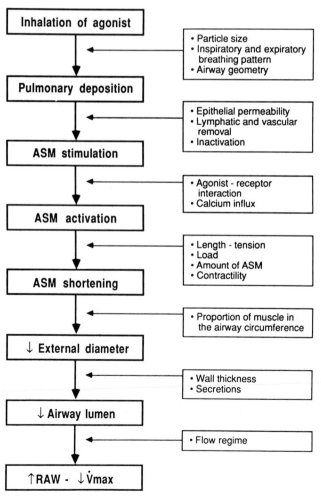

**Figure 54–8. Airway Responsiveness Cascade.** See text for description.

deficiency in one of the inhibitory relaxant systems could result in NSBH. In the following discussion, the factors that have been proposed to explain NSBH are considered individually.

### Starting Airway Caliber

Because airway resistance is alinearly related to airway radius, the effect of a given degree of narrowing is greater in previously narrowed airways; in fact, resistance is related to the fourth power of the radius during both laminar and turbulent flow regimens. In addition, turbulent flow is more likely to occur when there is prior airway narrowing and could itself result in an exaggeration of the alinear relationship between pressure and flow. These observations have led to the theory that decreased starting airway caliber may be a major contributor to NSBH, at least in persons whose airways are narrowed to begin with. It has also been suggested that normally narrower airways are the cause of the increased methacholine response observed in the very young[442] and in women.[443]

In theory, the prechallenge dimensions of the conducting airways could be decreased in asthmatic patients for a variety of reasons: (1) mural edema as a result of mucosal inflammation; (2) fixed thickening of the airway wall caused by deposition of connective tissue in the subepithelial region and submucosa, (3) alterations of bronchiolar surface tension; (4) increased vagal tone, increased muscle response to normal vagal tone, or increased smooth muscle response to inflammatory mediators; and (5) mucous plugging of the airway lumen.[444]

If starting airway caliber were an important contributor to NSBH, a relationship would be expected between the baseline resistance or expiratory flow rates and the responsiveness to challenge. Although such a relationship has been clearly shown in patients who have COPD and other nonasthmatic diseases associated with NSBH,[401, 403] studies in asthmatic patients either have failed to show such a relationship[440, 445] or have found a less striking one.[446] For a given reduction in airway caliber, as assessed using baseline $FEV_1$, asthmatic patients are much more responsive than patients who have other forms of obstructive airway disease.[447] However, these observations do not exclude an important role for initial airway caliber as a contributor to NSBH, because calculations suggest that minor and possibly unmeasurable differences in initial airway size may have a profound influence on the subsequent response.[434, 444, 448]

Airway wall thickening internal and external to the smooth muscle layer theoretically could markedly enhance the effect of a given degree of airway smooth muscle shortening.[170, 190] This amplification could occur with or without alteration in starting airway size, depending on whether the increased airway wall edema or tissue accumulates at the expense of airway luminal narrowing or airway smooth muscle lengthening (*see* Fig. 54–5).[434, 444] A similar mechanical explanation has been advanced to explain the exaggerated vascular responsiveness of essential hypertension.[450]

A number of investigators have developed computerized models of the tracheobronchial tree in an attempt to determine which structural changes are the most important contributors to exaggerated airway narrowing in asthma.[448, 450] Although all three of the major structural changes—increased mucosal thickness, increased smooth muscle thickness, and increased adventitial thickness—could contribute to increased maximal airway narrowing, the increase in muscle thickness has been shown to be the most important. The results of detailed analysis have shown that increased submucosal and adventitial thickness could increase the maximal airway narrowing by a factor of 2 to 10, whereas increased muscle thickness has the potential to increase maximal airway narrowing by two orders of magnitude. The most important, and untested, assumption on which this conclusion is based is that the increased airway smooth muscle mass that occurs in asthma is accompanied by a parallel increase in the ability of the muscle to generate force. However, as mentioned previously, there is reason to believe that the hyperplastic airway smooth muscle may be less contractile than normal.[451]

In these analyses, it was also assumed that the only load that the muscle has to overcome in order to contract is the elastic recoil of the lung. However, it is now known that the folding of the mucosa that occurs during airway smooth muscle contraction provides an additional load that impedes smooth muscle shortening; this impediment is dependent on the number of folds that develop and the thickness and stiffness of the mucosa.[452–454] Because the bending stiffness of a substance increases as the cube of its thickness, the results of the latter studies suggest that the wall thickening observed in asthma could cause sufficient stiffening to prevent excessive narrowing.

Some degree of airway smooth muscle shortening is undoubtedly present in the majority of patients who have moderate to severe asthma even prior to airway challenge, because they show a greater than normal response to inhaled bronchodilators. However, baseline smooth muscle shortening would not necessarily result in the greater maximal shortening characteristic of asthma; in fact, the results of studies designed to test this possibility suggest that increased baseline "tone" does not lead to exaggerated responsiveness.[455]

### Altered Aerosol Deposition

Airway responses are quantified *in vivo* by measuring the effect of a given nebulized dose or concentration of inhaled agonist. A more accurate relationship between dose and response could be obtained if the amount of the agonist deposited in the lung or (ideally) reaching smooth muscle could be calculated. The fraction of nebulized drug that reaches the tracheobronchial tree may in fact be small, and the amount and distribution of the inhaled agonist can vary considerably with the breathing pattern.[456, 457] Although it is convenient to think of the tracheobronchial tree as a single "resistor" and the airway narrowing in response to inhaled agonist as the response of a single tissue, in reality the airway is made up of a multitude of resistors joined in series and in parallel.[458] The response to inhaled agonists is dependent on the fractional distribution of aerosol to a given airway generation, the surface area of wall at that level of the airway, and the relative importance of that generation of airway to overall airway resistance or flow limitation.

Deposition of aerosol particles of the size used for testing airway responsiveness is dependent predominantly on impaction;[459] because impaction increases when linear velocity and turbulence are increased, altering baseline airway caliber and the air flow during aerosol inhalation will change the site of deposition of an inhaled drug. For example, rapid inspiratory or expiratory flow rates result in more central deposition of aerosol;[456, 457] this concentration of drug at a site that contributes importantly to total airway resistance and to flow limitation can shift the inhaled concentration-response curve leftward, creating an apparent hyper-responsiveness. It has been suggested that more central deposition of agonist is the mechanism responsible for the association between tracheal size (measured radiographically) and airway responsiveness in normal persons.[460] Even asymptomatic asthmatic patients can show more central deposition of inhaled aerosol; however, the importance of this in NSBH is unknown. In addition, the exaggerated responsiveness to cold and dry air in asthmatics cannot be explained by altered deposition.

### Increased Bronchial Mucosal Permeability

To have any effect, inhaled agonists must cross a layer of respiratory tract secretions and the airway epithelium to reach receptor sites on smooth muscle. Similarly, agents that cause reflex bronchoconstriction via irritant nerve endings must penetrate the bronchial epithelium through tight junctions between epithelial cells.[461] The amount or concentration of drug that reaches the smooth muscle will be dependent on the balance between penetration of these barriers and the removal of agonist by the bronchial vasculature, lymphatics, and enzymatic degradation. Since the respiratory epithelium is characteristically damaged in patients who have asthma, it seems reasonable to assume that a greater proportion of inhaled agonist might reach receptors on vagal afferents and smooth muscle.[461] In fact, one group of investigators showed a relationship between NSBR and quantitative estimates of epithelial damage in a small number of asthmatic patients;[462] similarly, patients who have sarcoidosis and extrinsic allergic alveolitis who have NSBH have epithelial damage and hyperpermeability.[463, 464]

Although the results of animal studies have shown that NSBR increases with epithelial damage induced by cigarette smoke[465] and antigen exposure,[466] studies in humans have failed to show a direct relationship between airway mucosal hyperpermeability and NSBH. In studies in which disappearance of inhaled $^{99m}$Tc-diethylenetriaminepenta-acetate (DTPA) was employed as a marker of epithelial permeability, no differences have been observed between normal persons and stable asthmatic patients, despite marked differences in airway responses to inhaled histamine.[467–469] Mucosal permeability does increase transiently during attacks of asthma, but the relationship of this change to any changes in NSBR is unclear.[470] The lack of relationship between airway epithelial permeability and NSBR has also been illustrated by the demonstration of hyperpermeability without hyper-responsiveness in cigarette smokers.[468] The inhalation of hypotonic distilled water fog produces transiently increased permeability in both normal individuals and asthmatic patients; however, airway narrowing in response to this challenge occurs only in asthmatics.[471, 472] In baboons that have been heavy cigarette smokers (two packs a day for 3 years), airway responsiveness to inhaled methacholine has been found to be decreased in comparison with that in nonsmoking control animals[473]—an effect that could be related to a protective action of tracheobronchial mucus.[474]

A difference in the rate of removal of inhaled or locally released mediators is an additional factor that has the potential to contribute to NSBH. Although very little is known about the mechanisms of mediator removal, both the pulmonary and bronchial circulations appear to contribute, at least in peripheral airways.[475]

### Abnormalities of Neurohumoral Control

Airway smooth muscle is innervated by the autonomic nervous system and is equipped with membrane receptors for a wide variety of circulating excitatory and inhibitory substances.[378] Theoretically, exaggerated excitatory or deficient inhibitory control could result in NSBH.

**Parasympathetic and Sympathetic Nerves and Neural Receptors.** Stimulation of afferent receptors in the nose, larynx, or lung causes reflex bronchoconstriction; in addition, connections between chemoreceptors and baroreceptors and the efferent vagal system have been demonstrated.[378] The lung irritant receptors are potentially the most important with respect to NSBH. The afferents begin as a network of free nerve endings located immediately below the tight junctions of the respiratory epithelium; they are mainly mechanoreceptors that respond to local irritation but are also stimulated by inhalation of dust and pollutants, by altered local osmolarity, by drugs such as histamine, and by bronchoconstriction itself. In addition to producing reflex bronchoconstriction, stimulation of these nerve endings results in a subjective sensation of irritation, cough, and—at least in animals—an altered pattern of breathing termed *rapid shallow breathing*.[378, 476, 477] The reflex bronchoconstriction can be blocked by vagal section or atropine; however, atropine does not abolish the cough or altered breathing pattern.[378] In addition to their role as the afferent limb of reflex bronchoconstriction, afferent receptors in the airway may have a more direct pathophysiologic role related to their ability to secrete inflammatory neuropeptides, including substance P, neurokinin A, neurokinin B, and calcitonin gene–related peptide, that cause increased vascular permeability and edema as well as direct smooth muscle stimulation.[478–480] Excessive afferent nerve stimulation could theoretically cause airway narrowing in the absence of a central nervous system connection via the so-called axonal reflex.[478]

The presence of a synapse between preganglionic and postganglionic cholinergic fibers within the ganglia of the airway wall allows for the possibility of presynaptic modulation of efferent cholinergic activity. In various animal species, norepinephrine-induced inhibition[481] and substance P–induced enhancement[482] of cholinergic excitation have been demonstrated. The distribution of vagal efferent fibers within the tracheobronchial tree varies among animal species and among individuals within a species.[378] The autoradiographic demonstration of cholinergic receptors suggests denser innervation of central airways and sparse or absent innervation of bronchioles,[483] consistent with the results of functional studies. Some efferent cholinergic tone can be demonstrated in normal individuals by anticholinergic-induced bronchodilatation.[484] NSBH may be magnified by exaggerated vagal tone caused by increased afferent stimulation from lung

receptors, or by increased efferent activity in response to a normal afferent input.

Early studies suggesting that much of the histamine-induced and even antigen-induced airway narrowing was vagally mediated supported the concept that exaggerated reflex bronchoconstriction could explain the entire phenomenon of NSBH.[378, 485] However, it has become clear that the major effect of histamine is directly on smooth muscle.[486, 487] In addition, asthmatic patients manifest increased bronchoconstriction in response to methacholine, a substance that has little effect on vagal afferents.[476, 477] NSBH cannot be attributed to reflex bronchoconstriction, because it fails to explain the nonspecificity of the exaggerated response; asthmatic subjects show exaggerated responsiveness to agents that do not act via efferent cholinergic pathways. Moreover, atropine does not block the accentuated NSBR that occurs after antigen exposure in allergic asthmatics.[488]

Despite these observations, it appears that there may be abnormalities of the parasympathetic system in asthmatic patients; for example, they show exaggerated reflex bradycardia in response to a deep breath or simulated dive, and this increased cholinergic reactivity correlates with NSBR.[489, 490] It is now known that there are three cholinergic receptors that have different functions. In the airways, $M_3$ receptors are localized on the airway smooth muscle and mediate bronchoconstriction, and $M_2$ receptors are localized on the efferent cholinergic nerve endings and decrease further release of acetylcholine.[491] It has been shown that allergen challenge results in a decreased effectiveness of the $M_2$ receptors in experimental animals;[492] there is also evidence suggesting that this mechanism of autonomic dysregulation could be present in the airways of asthmatic patients.[493]

**The Nonadrenergic Noncholinergic Inhibitory System.** It has been suggested that a defect in the nonadrenergic noncholinergic inhibitory system (NANCi) may be responsible for NSBH.[378] In the cat, nonadrenergic bronchodilatation has been demonstrated; *in vitro* stimulation of the vagus nerve in beta-adrenergic-blocked animals has been shown to reverse serotonin-induced bronchoconstriction.[494, 495] However, in airway tissue from a small number of patients who had COPD and a variable degree of NSBR, the magnitude of nonadrenergic smooth muscle relaxation was small in comparison to beta-adrenergic relaxation and showed no correlation with *in vivo* responsiveness to methacholine.[496] In another investigation, maximal NANCi stimulation produced only 10% to 20% of maximal theophylline-induced relaxation in human tissue, whereas it accounted for 70% of maximal relaxation in the guinea pig airway.[497] In a third study, NANCi-induced relaxation of airway smooth muscle was not less than normal in airways from patients who died of asthma.[146]

The NANCi system was first demonstrated *in vivo* in human beings by a group of investigators who also quantified its importance in bronchodilatation and compared its effectiveness in normal and asthmatic individuals.[498, 499] They stimulated the larynx mechanically during histamine-induced bronchoconstriction and showed an abrupt but transient fall in pulmonary resistance that was not mediated through the beta-adrenergic system. Although these results clearly demonstrate the presence of nonadrenergic bronchodilatation, there was incomplete relaxation of the airway smooth muscle and no significant difference between normal and asthmatic patients in the effectiveness of bronchodilatation.[499] NANCi bronchodilatation can also be demonstrated during leukotriene-induced bronchoconstriction by stimulating afferent nerves using aerosolized capsaicin;[500] however, the bronchodilatation is weak and transient.

Vasoactive intestinal polypeptide (VIP) was long thought to be the most likely neurotransmitter involved in NANCi bronchodilatation;[501–503] however, it has now been clearly demonstrated that NO is the principal and, perhaps, sole transmitter in human beings.[504, 505]

**Beta-Adrenergic Receptors.** The major inhibitory or bronchodilating influence on airway smooth muscle is stimulation of beta-adrenergic receptors. The beta-adrenergic receptors on human airway smooth muscle are not related to adrenergic innervation: adrenergic postganglionic fibers originating in the stellate ganglion enter the lung at the hila but in human beings appear to supply only pulmonary and bronchial vascular smooth muscle. As noted previously, adrenergic fibers can also innervate airway ganglia and modulate cholinergic activity, but direct airway smooth muscle innervation has not been demonstrated.[506] Human lung beta receptors have been identified autoradiographically;[507] these can be demonstrated and subtyped on alveolar and bronchial epithelium and glands as well as on airway and vascular smooth muscle. Consistent with their function, the receptors on airway smooth muscle are largely of the beta$_2$ subtype, and their density is greater in peripheral than in central airways.[508]

One possible mechanism contributing to NSBH is partial beta-adrenergic blockade.[509] This hypothesis has received support from the results of numerous studies in asthmatic patients in whom defective beta-adrenergic responsiveness[510] and decreased beta receptor number and function in isolated blood leukocytes were demonstrated.[511–514] In some studies of the ability of beta-adrenergic agonists to relax contracted normal and asthmatic airway smooth muscle *in vitro,* deficient relaxation was found in the specimens obtained from the asthmatic patients, although theophylline was equally potent in the two groups.[515–517] Beta-adrenergic responsiveness was impaired in the airway smooth muscle of patients who died of asthma.[146]

Part of this decreased beta responsiveness is believed to be the result of exogenous beta-adrenergic administration, with resulting down-regulation of beta receptor number and/or function in blood cells[518–520] and airway smooth muscle.[521–524] The hypothesis is that beta receptor number and, therefore, responsiveness are not static but vary over time in response to various stimuli: Stable asthmatics not receiving beta-adrenergic therapy show normal numbers of beta receptors on leukocytes (and presumably on airway smooth muscle); however, prolonged beta-agonist therapy[519] or acute antigen exposure[525, 526] decreases the receptor number. Despite the attractiveness of this theory, the results of one study showed that there was a threefold increase in beta-adrenergic receptor number on asthmatic airway smooth muscle detected by an autoradiographic ligand-binding technique.[527] These results mean that the down-regulation of beta-adrenergic function in asthma must be related to an abnormality of signal transduction downstream from the receptor. The potential influence of beta-adrenergic receptor down-regulation as a modifier of asthma severity has engendered increased interest because of the discovery of two common polymorphisms in the gene for the beta-adrenergic receptor

that alter its function.[139] One of the mutations increases the tendency for the receptor to be down-regulated by agonist, and the other appears to protect against this effect.

If beta-adrenergic dysfunction were an important contributor to airway hyper-responsiveness, pharmacologic beta blockade could be expected to produce NSBH in normal persons—which is in fact not the case. Exaggerated bronchoconstriction does not develop in normal persons in response to nonspecific stimuli, even when profound beta-adrenergic blockade is produced by systemic or inhaled beta-blocking agents.[386, 528–531] However, asthmatic patients can show profound bronchoconstriction following administration of beta-blocking drugs.[532–534] Clearly, despite the fact that many asthmatics have decreased beta-adrenergic function, airway patency is partly dependent on tonic beta receptor stimulation, which counteracts a tendency to ongoing bronchoconstriction. The fact that cholinergic blockade alleviates the beta blocker effect suggests that vagal tone contributes to the ongoing constrictor activity.[532, 533] Some degree of airway obstruction can even develop with the use of beta-blocking eye drops for prevention of glaucoma in elderly persons not previously suspected of having asthma.[535]

One hypothesis for the effect of beta blockade is the loss of beta-adrenergic inhibition of neural transmission at the level of the airway nerve ganglia. Such an effect, coupled with the possibility of a defective M$_2$ muscarinic response and heightened airway smooth muscle responsiveness to acetylcholine, could explain the exaggerated response.[493, 536] An additional potential mechanism for bronchial narrowing following beta blockade is inhibition of endogenous beta agonist–induced depression of mast cell mediator release. However, plasma histamine levels do not increase following propranolol infusion in asthmatic patients.[537] It is of interest that the use of the cholinesterase inhibitor pyridostigmine during military maneuvers to protect against possible exposure to nerve gas was associated with exacerbations of asthma, presumably as a result of the excessive action of acetylcholine.[538]

Evidence also suggests that endogenous release of catecholamines may be abnormal in asthmatic patients. Although stable patients show normal levels of circulating catecholamines at rest, data from some studies suggest that the exercise-induced increase in blood levels is impaired and that the response to the acute stress of an asthmatic attack is blunted.[537, 539, 540] However, no detectable increase in levels of circulating plasma epinephrine or norepinephrine occurs in response to inhaled methacholine in normal or asthmatic persons, making it unlikely that differences in catecholamine release are important in NSBH.[541]

**Alpha-Adrenergic Receptors.** Discussions concerning the role of alpha-adrenergic receptors in the control of normal and asthmatic airway caliber are confusing and controversial.[378, 542] The agonist norepinephrine does not contract normal human airway smooth muscle *in vitro,* unless the tissue is pretreated with histamine or potassium chloride; by contrast, postmortem specimens of airway smooth muscle from patients who had a variety of lung diseases respond with contraction to alpha-adrenergic stimulation without pretreatment.[543] These data suggest that human airway smooth muscle is equipped with alpha receptors, but that to be effective the receptors must be modified or unmasked in some way.

The results of *in vivo* studies also have been conflicting. For example, in one investigation, phenylephrine did not produce bronchial obstruction in asthmatic patients even after beta blockade was induced to negate any possible beta agonist effect of this largely alpha agonist agent;[544] however, inhalation of methoxamine, an alpha-adrenergic agent, consistently produces airway narrowing in some persons.[545-547] It is possible that alpha agonist–induced airway narrowing is secondary to stimulation of alpha receptors at sites other than smooth muscle. Alpha-adrenergic stimulation of mast cells may increase mediator release, whereas activation of bronchial vascular smooth muscle may produce vasoconstriction, thus decreasing the removal of mediators. It is also possible that alpha agonists may exert their effect at the level of the airway ganglia.[547] Data from studies showing exaggerated alpha-adrenergic cutaneous vascular constriction and pupillary dilatation in asthmatic and atopic patients suggest that a systemic derangement in alpha receptor function may be important.[548, 549] Alpha-adrenergic blocking agents do not appear to have a bronchodilating effect when given alone,[550] although they tend to attenuate the airway response to histamine,[551] exercise,[552] and isocapnic hyperventilation of dry air.[553] Clearly, the ultimate importance of the alpha-adrenergic component of the sympathetic nervous system in the control of airway patency requires further study; however, it is safe to say that unopposed alpha receptor stimulation is not a major mechanism of NSBH.

**Histamine Receptors.** Histamine produces bronchoconstriction in human airways by stimulating $H_1$ receptors. The demonstration in animals that $H_1$-contracting and $H_2$-relaxing histamine receptors could be present in the same airway tissue raised the possibility that an imbalance in receptor number or affinity could result in the increased histamine response seen with asthma.[554] However, despite extensive study, the presence and importance of $H_2$ receptors in human airways have not been clearly determined.[554] Although data from *in vitro* studies suggest the presence of smooth muscle–relaxing $H_2$ receptors, at least in large airways,[555] the expected increase in histamine-induced bronchoconstriction *in vivo* in the presence of specific $H_2$ blockers has not been a consistent finding.[556-560] Whatever the role of $H_1$ and $H_2$ receptors, their imbalance cannot be an important contributor to NSBH, because it can account for exaggerated responses only to this specific agonist.[554]

Another and theoretically more important role for $H_2$ receptors is histamine-induced feedback inhibition of mediator release from mast cells.[561, 562] If this were an important mechanism that modulated mediator release, $H_2$ blocker administration would be expected to worsen asthma symptoms and signs and increase the response to inhaled antigen; however, neither effect has been reported following therapeutic doses of $H_2$ blockers.[559, 563]

### Abnormalities of Smooth Muscle

In pharmacologic parlance, hyper-reactivity or supersensitivity can be prejunctional or postjunctional, the junction referring to the neural (receptor) muscle cell interface. Prejunctional supersensitivity occurs when receptor number is increased or when a greater proportion of an administered or released drug is available to interact with receptors (increased input). Postjunctional supersensitivity occurs when

there is augmentation of excitation-contraction coupling, i.e., a greater response or output for a given prejunctional input. Postjunctional supersensitivity is characteristically nonspecific;[564, 565] the nonspecificity of asthmatic airway hyper-responsiveness suggests that augmentation of excitation-contraction coupling may be important. Alternatively, a given degree of contraction may result in greater smooth muscle shortening and airway narrowing if an alteration in the smooth muscle length–tension relationship and/or a decrease in smooth muscle load occurs.[444]

To understand how changes in excitation-contraction coupling or smooth muscle length–tension relationships could result in NSBH, a brief review of the biochemistry and mechanics of airway smooth muscle contraction is desirable. The generation of tension and shortening in smooth muscle is believed to be related to actin and myosin filament interaction, similar to that producing skeletal and cardiac muscle contraction. The initiating event is influx of free intracellular calcium from a sequestered source; calcium interacts with calmodulin, activating specific enzymes that mediate actin and myosin cross-bridge formation, which is responsible for tension development and shortening. Calcium is normally sequestered extracellularly in a concentration 1,000 times greater than intracellular levels; this active exclusion is accomplished by an energy-requiring ion pump. Calcium is also stored in an inactive form within intracellular membrane–bound organelles, such as mitochondria and the sarcoplasmic reticulum. It can be released from these sources into the intracellular space to initiate contraction through transmembrane channels that respond to cell depolarization (voltage-dependent channels) or through separate channels that open in response to specific receptor activation (receptor-activated channels).[566] Calcium channel blockers inhibit smooth muscle contraction by blocking the voltage-dependent channels but have little effect on receptor-operated channels or intracellular organelle sources of $Ca^{2+}$. Once calcium is released into the cytoplasm and contraction is initiated, the free calcium is resequestered to terminate the contractile process. Cyclic adenosine monophosphate (cAMP) within the cell accelerates the removal of $Ca^{2+}$, and bronchodilating drugs may exert their effect by increasing levels of this substance.[566]

Airway hyper-responsiveness may occur as a result of either increased calcium availability from one of its sources or decreased calcium removal from an intracellular location. Increased contraction of the actin-myosin chain in response to $Ca^{2+}$ release is another possible cause of postjunctional supersensitivity.[564] An alteration in calcium handling could play a pivotal role in the pathogenesis of airway obstruction at sites other than smooth muscle. The same process of calcium sequestration and release initiates both mucus secretion and mast cell mediator release, each of which is known to be abnormal in asthma. Although the hypothesis that an abnormality of calcium handling is involved in the pathogenesis of asthma is intriguing, no convincing data are available to corroborate it.

Smooth muscle can considered to be of two types. (1) So-called single-unit smooth muscle shows spontaneous oscillations in membrane potential and the development of action potentials that spread from cell to cell via electrical interconnectors between cells called gap junctions. This form of muscle is sparsely innervated but exhibits myogenic control, responding to external forces such as stretch or distention. (2) Multi-unit smooth muscle is densely innervated and possesses little cell-to-cell communication. This type is believed to be entirely under nervous control, its mechanical activation being dependent on the magnitude and distribution of nerve firing.[567]

Although normal human tracheobronchial smooth muscle possesses some gap junctions, it behaves as the multi-unit type, being dependent on excitatory innervation to induce contraction. However, the type of smooth muscle is not static, and it is possible that inflammatory mediators alter muscle function and structure toward those of single-unit muscle; because activation of a single unit can enhance the response by spreading the effect of activation over many muscle units, hyper-responsiveness would be expected.[567] Single-unit behavior is also a possible explanation for the bronchoconstriction that characteristically occurs in asthmatics following a deep inspiration.[568] An inspiratory capacity maneuver dilates airways and stretches the smooth muscle; if the stretch results in contraction as it does in single-unit muscle, airway narrowing would ensue. Such a myogenic response to stretch has been demonstrated in isolated smooth muscle from dogs that have been sensitized to ovalbumin and demonstrate *in vivo* hyper-responsiveness.[569]

The increase in the amount of smooth muscle in patients who have asthma could also be an important factor in airway hyperresponsiveness. The increased muscle mass could have a simple geometric effect with respect to airway narrowing, much like the effect of thickening of the submucosal region. However, if the increased mass was associated with a concomitant increase in its force-generating ability, it might also be able to shorten excessively against the elastic loads provided by lung parenchymal distortion and mucosal folding.[450] In theory, an increase in the contractility of the muscle without an increase in mass could also result in exaggerated airway narrowing. Unfortunately, there have been few studies in which the functional properties of airway smooth muscle from asthmatic subjects have been measured and corrected for the amount of muscle in the preparation. However, in two studies of airway preparations from asthmatic patients obtained at the time of lung resection, increased maximal isometric force generation and isotonic shortening were demonstrated despite a normal amount of smooth muscle.[570, 571] Increased force generation and decreased relaxation of airway smooth muscle have also been shown in tissue obtained from patients who had fatal asthma.[572]

It is possible that chronic stimulation by cytokines and growth factors in the inflamed airway wall results in proliferation and "de-differentiation" of smooth muscle, making it less contractile.[573, 574] The conjecture that the basic defect underlying NSBH may reside postjunctionally at the level of the smooth muscle contractile apparatus has prompted a number of investigators to compare *in vivo* airway responses with *in vitro* smooth muscle function. These studies have generally been conducted in smokers who have COPD of variable severity and who have undergone resection of lung tissue for pulmonary carcinoma. Although these patients showed a wide range of responsiveness to inhaled bronchoconstrictors preoperatively, resected large airway tissue showed much less variability in response, with no *in vivo/in vitro* correlation.[496, 516, 575–578] In the few studies in which human asthmatic airway tissue has been studied, the results

of correlations between *in vivo* and *in vitro* behavior have also been disappointing.[579]

It is of interest that prohibition of deep inspiration during the measurement of a methacholine dose-response curve in normal persons causes excessive airway narrowing and an ineffectual reversal of bronchoconstriction when deep inspirations are ultimately allowed.[580, 581] (Normally, a deep inspiration substantially reverses pharmacologic airway narrowing by providing a stretch to the contracted smooth muscle.) Since these results mimic the altered airway function in asthmatic patients,[582–584] several investigators have suggested that the primary defect explaining airway hyperresponsiveness could be an impairment of the bronchodilator response to deep inspiration, rather than enhanced end-organ responsiveness.[580, 582, 585–587]

The response of smooth muscle to stretch could be impaired for a number of reasons. First, it has been shown that the mechanics and biochemistry of normal smooth muscle contraction change during the course of stimulation. Early in such stimulation, there is rapid cycling of cross-bridges and rapid velocity of shortening, although the muscle is relatively compliant. Later in contraction, there is less rapid cycling of cross-bridges, but the muscle is stiffer, presumably as a result of a greater percentage of attached cross-bridges. Without periodic deep inspiration, such stiffer cross-bridges could develop; a facilitation of this process, which has been termed the "latch bridge state," could be the mechanism by which excessive airway narrowing and deficient response to deep inspiration develop in asthma.[588] An alternate explanation for the enhanced response could be an accumulation of fluid in the peribronchial space. During prolonged smooth muscle contraction, a decrease in peribronchial interstitial pressure will increase the transudation of fluid into the airway wall. Such increased fluid could affect airway function by increasing airway wall thickness and thereby reduce the effectiveness of the stretch provided by deep inspiration.[589, 590] Because microvascular permeability is increased in the inflamed airways of asthmatic patients, this mechanism could be exaggerated.

Although the difference between normal individuals and asthmatic patients in the effect of a deep inspiration can partly explain NSBH, it is unlikely to be the sole explanation, because measurements such as pulmonary resistance obtained prior to a deep inspiration can be altered to a much greater extent in asthmatic patients at much lower concentrations of an inhaled drug.[591]

### Decreased Smooth Muscle Load

Once activated, smooth muscle narrows the airway by shortening. The degree to which it shortens in response to a stimulus depends on several factors, including receptor number and occupancy, the effectiveness of excitation-contraction coupling, and the load against which the muscle must shorten.

Isometric contraction occurs when smooth muscle contracts against an immovable load and the energy of contraction results in tension without shortening; by contrast, a purely isotonic contraction occurs when smooth muscle is completely unloaded, so that the total energy is transferred into shortening. As smooth muscle is progressively loaded, both the speed and magnitude of shortening progressively decrease, the ultimate load resulting in a purely isometric contraction. The magnitude of shortening of stimulated smooth muscle is also dependent on its initial length. All muscle—smooth, striated, and cardiac—displays a characteristic length-tension relationship, there being a unique length at which stimulation will result in the greatest shortening or tension generation. This optimal length, Lmax, is determined by the optimal geometric relationship for interaction between actin and myosin filaments within the muscle; at lengths longer or shorter than Lmax, the same stimulus will result in less shortening or tension.[592, 593]

The loads and operating lengths of smooth muscle *in vivo* are unknown. Airway smooth muscle at optimal length will shorten 70% when allowed to contract isotonically *in vitro*.[594] If the muscle completely surrounds an airway, is at optimal length, and contracts isotonically, it can be calculated that muscle shortening of approximately 45% will result in luminal occlusion. Because maximal pharmacologic stimulation in normal subjects results in only a 4- to 10-fold increase in resistance (approximately 25% smooth muscle shortening), it is unlikely that isotonic contraction from Lmax can occur *in vivo*.[444, 594a]

The vast potential for airway narrowing that these mechanical considerations imply has led to the speculation that the key to understanding the hyper-responsiveness of asthma is to understand the apparent hyporesponsiveness of normal persons.[595] The mechanism by which airway smooth muscle shortening is limited in normal persons is not certain; however, the most likely explanation is that contraction is not isotonic, because the muscle is contracting against loads that impede shortening and, consequently, airway narrowing. In large airways, the muscle is loaded by the outward recoil of mural cartilage,[596] whereas in smaller airways, this load is provided by the elastic recoil of the lung and the folding of the airway mucosa. As the airway narrows, local lung parenchyma becomes distorted, increasing transmural pressure and converting more of the smooth muscle activation to tension generation rather than to shortening.[444]

The load dependency of smooth muscle shortening is most graphically illustrated by the effect of lung volume on maximal airway narrowing: although airway resistance varies only slightly with lung volume in the absence of smooth muscle stimulation, marked changes in resistance occur with changes in lung volume when the muscle is contracted.[597] These mechanical details of airway smooth muscle contraction suggest additional potential explanations for NSBH; if airway smooth muscle length was moved toward Lmax *in vivo* or if the loads impeding shortening were decreased, a similar activation would produce greater narrowing.

It is possible that changes in smooth muscle afterload could be important in the airway hyper-responsiveness of patients who have COPD, in whom the loss of lung elastic recoil and decrease in cartilage would be expected to increase the potential for shortening;[598] however, it is more difficult to envisage how the resting length or afterload could be deranged in the airways of patients who have asthma. Besides lung recoil and airway cartilage, another load on smooth muscle is provided by the connective tissue components of the airway wall, which run parallel to the muscle fibers and need to be deformed during shortening. As noted previously, the folding of the mucosa uses up some of the force generated by the muscle and therefore can limit its

shortening. It has been suggested that proteolytic digestion of mucosal connective tissue by enzymes released from inflammatory cells could decrease this component of the load on airway smooth muscle and contribute to hyper-responsiveness.[599] In fact, incubation of human airway smooth muscle preparations from normal individuals with collagenase causes an increase in shortening in response to maximal stimuli.[600]

The degree of shortening of smooth muscle in response to a stimulus depends on muscle strength, starting length, and load. If muscle shortening is limited by elastic loads, hyperplasia produced by adding fibers could increase the shortening for a given stimulus while not necessarily altering the maximally obtainable shortening of unloaded muscle.[601] The effect of the increased smooth muscle strength that accompanies hyperplasia and hypertrophy is separate from the effect of increasing wall thickness discussed previously but is possibly additive.[444, 449]

### Inflammation

Bronchial hyper-responsiveness develops in normal persons following viral respiratory tract infections[602] or exposure to ozone or other atmospheric pollutants.[392] NSBH also increases during infection and pollutant exposure in asthmatic patients and is enhanced following specific antigen challenge[603–605] and inhalation of ultrasonically nebulized distilled water.[606, 607] The increased responsiveness associated with antigen exposure occurs in the laboratory as well as naturally. It appears to be dependent on the development of a late response to antigen; patients who have an isolated immediate response do not show a change, although NSBH may be increased in the interval between the immediate and delayed response.[608–611] NSBH increases during the pollen season in asthmatic patients who are sensitive to ragweed and grass[611a] and correlates with domestic levels of house dust mite Der p 1 protein antigen in persons who have an isolated sensitivity to this allergen.[612]

Perhaps the clearest demonstration of acquired airway hyper-responsiveness occurs in occupational asthma.[613] The NSBH that occurs with the development of sensitivity to plicatic acid in western red cedar sawdust can be profound. Similarly, exposure to toluene diisocyanate (TDI) in the plastic and paint industries induces increased airway responsiveness in sensitive persons.[614] In the majority of affected persons, the hyper-responsiveness decreases slowly after cessation of exposure.[378, 394] The ability of these substances to enhance or produce hyper-responsiveness has led to the suggestion of a more precise terminology for bronchoactive agents.[615] According to this terminology, *inciters* are considered to be the agents that cause a primary response, the most common being histamine, methacholine, exercise, and isocapnic dry air hyperventilation; an inciter produces bronchoconstriction without altering subsequent responses to bronchoactive agents. *Inducers* are substances or processes that augment the nonspecific response to inciters, usually after producing their own bronchoconstrictive effect; included among the inducers are allergen exposure (when accompanied by a late asthmatic response), substances that cause occupational asthma, endotoxin, and viruses.

A number of mechanisms have been postulated to explain the relationship between NSBH and inflammation. The increased permeability of endothelium and epithelium may result in greater exposure of airway smooth muscle and irritant receptors to inhaled or injected agonist. However, failure to demonstrate hyperpermeability in stable but hyper-responsive asthmatic patients makes this unlikely to be the sole explanation.[467, 603] Alternatively, the increased vascular permeability and secondary airway wall edema may unload the smooth muscle and/or enhance the airway narrowing effect of a given degree of smooth muscle shortening. Finally, the release of secondary mediators from inflammatory cells could directly alter smooth muscle responsiveness.[392, 616]

The relationship between inflammation and increased smooth muscle response has been described in animals exposed to ozone and antigen. The evidence suggests that ozone causes acute airway epithelial damage and that the damaged epithelium responds by producing chemotactic substances such as the leukotriene $LTB_4$ and chemokines. The neutrophils that migrate to the airway release additional leukotrienes and prostaglandins that act on the smooth muscle and airway nerves to enhance its responsiveness to subsequently administered challenges. Allergen exposure of sensitized animals also causes airway inflammation and increased airway responsiveness.[617] Following antigen challenge, the inflammatory cell infiltrate is composed predominantly of eosinophils attracted by cytokines, such as IL-5, and chemokines, such as RANTES and macrophage inflammatory protein-1α (MIP-1α), which are released from mast cells, T cells, and epithelial cells. The release of IL-4 also seems to be important, because its inhibition decreases the hyper-responsiveness.[618] In addition to the effects of leukotrienes and prostaglandins, the enzymes released from mast cells and the toxic cationic proteins derived from eosinophils may directly or indirectly affect airway smooth muscle function.[617] Incubation of normal human airway smooth muscle with serum containing high concentrations of IgE has been shown to enhance its *in vitro* contractile response to a variety of agonists;[619–621] however, it is unclear how this comes about and whether the enhanced contractility relates in any way to the airway hyper-responsiveness associated with airway inflammation.

Although inflammation-induced modification of airway responsiveness is an attractive theory, some observations suggest that it is only part of the explanation.[622] Correlations between quantitative markers of inflammation and measures of hyper-responsiveness are weak.[623, 624] In addition, the increase in NSBR caused by manipulations that produce airway inflammation is small compared with the large increases in sensitivity and maximal response apparent in asthmatic patients. Finally, the small changes in sensitivity and response that can be produced are transient, whereas the NSBH of asthmatic patients is prolonged.

### Consequences and Clinical Usefulness of Measurements of Nonspecific Bronchial Hyper-responsiveness

Although the pathogenesis of NSBH is not completely understood, its physiologic and clinical manifestations have been clearly established. NSBH renders asthmatic persons susceptible to excessive airway narrowing in response to a wide variety of otherwise trivial exposures. Its importance in this respect is most clearly defined for allergic reactions.

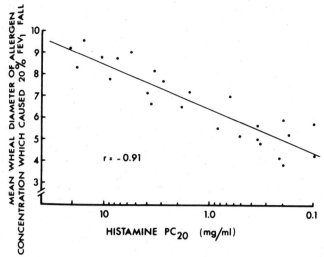

**Figure 54–9. Relationship of Allergic and Nonallergic Airway Responsiveness.** The magnitude of the airway allergic response is determined by an individual's degree of sensitization to the inhaled antigen and by nonspecific bronchial hyper-responsiveness. This plot shows the mean wheal diameter raised in a skin test using the concentration of allergen that caused a 20% fall in $FEV_1$ during inhalation challenge in individual asthmatic subjects versus the nonspecific bronchial hyper-responsiveness as determined by the histamine concentration that provoked a 20% decrease in $FEV_1$. Individuals with increased nonspecific bronchial responsiveness (low values for $PC_{20}$) require only low concentrations of inhaled antigen, whereas those without increased nonspecific bronchial responsiveness (higher values for $PC_{20}$) require a larger concentration of antigen. (From Cockcroft DW, Ruffin, RE, Frith PA, et al: Determinants of allergen-induced asthma: Dose of allergen, circulating IgE antibody concentration, and bronchial responsiveness to inhaled histamine. Am Rev Respir Dis 120:1053, 1979.)

The magnitude of the airway response to an inhaled specific allergen is related to the severity of allergy as assessed by the size of the skin response to a given dose of allergen, and to the degree of NSBH as measured by a histamine dose-response curve.[625, 626] The severity of antigen-induced bronchoconstriction can be appreciated better when a combination of the two measures is used rather than either alone (Fig. 54–9).[627–629] This observation emphasizes the vicious circle of specific and nonspecific airway responses that tend to perpetuate and potentiate the asthmatic state: on the one hand, allergen exposure induces increased nonspecific airway response; on the other, the degree of response to allergen is related to the NSBH. In fact, it is probable that most symptoms experienced by asthmatic patients are the result of excessive airway narrowing in response to otherwise trivial inhalational exposures. These nonspecific episodes occur on a background of episodic exposure to inducing inflammatory agents, such as allergens and viruses.[630–632]

Patients who have NSBH also tend to experience greater diurnal variation in lung function, greater increases in flow rates after inhaling a bronchodilator, and symptoms that are more difficult to control.[633] In addition to its use in epidemiologic studies and in the investigation of the basic mechanisms of asthma, the measurement of NSBR is employed clinically to establish a diagnosis of asthma and to follow its severity in relation to treatment or exposure to occupational sensitizing substances.

Although the diagnosis of asthma is usually made from a knowledge of the history, spirometry, and the response to bronchodilating drugs, some patients have normal spirometric values at the time of examination, thus precluding assessment of bronchodilator response. In these persons, demonstration of NSBH (defined, for example, by a $PC_{20}$ of less than 8 mg/ml) is a useful adjunct to diagnosis.[634] Tests of NSBR are particularly useful in patients who have the isolated symptom of chronic cough; this can be the sole presenting symptom in some patients. The demonstration of increased nonspecific airway responsiveness is useful in predicting whether the patient will respond symptomatically to antiasthmatic therapy.[634, 635] However, as discussed previously, the lack of NSBH, even in symptomatic patients, does not exclude the diagnosis; some patients, especially those with seasonal symptoms or occupational asthma, may develop detectable hyper-responsiveness only following exposure to sufficient inducing agents.[634] Similarly, the demonstration of NSBH alone does not make the diagnosis, particularly if baseline airway function is abnormal.[401, 403] Population studies consistently show that a significant subset of the population (2% to 14%) have airway hyper-responsiveness in the absence of symptoms.[633, 634] It is unclear if asymptomatic airway hyper-responsiveness has any prognostic implications for future disease manifestations.[635]

Although tests of NSBR may be useful in diagnosing asthma in patients who have normal or near-normal baseline lung function, they are of less help and potentially dangerous in patients whose airways are already severely obstructed; in such patients, the history and response to bronchodilators are usually diagnostic.[636] Because NSBH can be altered by treatment, it is theoretically possible to use the degree of hyper-responsiveness as an indicator of the effectiveness of therapy and the need for more or less intensive therapy.[637] However, some investigators have found that a single measure of airway responsiveness is not a good indicator of asthma severity.[638] In an occupational setting, serial measurement of NSBH may be of particular value; i.e., the development or worsening of NSBH during occupational exposure and its gradual improvement following withdrawal of exposure constitute strong evidence that the symptoms are work-related.[639]

### Summary

NSBH is the exaggerated airway narrowing demonstrated by asthmatic patients in response to inhalation of pharmacologic bronchoconstricting agents and a variety of irritant substances. It can be quantified by measuring the dose or concentration of inhaled histamine or methacholine that causes a 20% decrease in $FEV_1$. Rather than being a congenital defect that increases the risk of developing asthma, NSBH is probably an acquired abnormality; however, its pathogenesis remains unknown despite considerable research. The majority of evidence suggests that it is a consequence of inflammation in the airway mucosa, with attendant epithelial damage and increased airway permeability, wall edema and thickening, and alteration of the amount and contractility of airway smooth muscle. NSBH is almost invariable in patients who have asthma, and measurement of the degree of hyper-responsiveness is a useful diagnostic test. However, although its presence is virtually diagnostic of asthma in patients who have compatible symptoms and a normal baseline $FEV_1$, increased bronchial responsiveness also occurs in other airway diseases associated with baseline airway narrowing, such as COPD, cystic fibrosis, and bron-

chiectasis. In addition to its diagnostic usefulness, NSBH is important because it is probably responsible for the majority of asthmatic symptoms.

### Provoking Factors

Asthmatic individuals are prone to episodic airway obstruction that can be precipitated in a variety of ways. The most thoroughly studied of these provoking factors is the inhalation of antigenic material, resulting in an extrinsic allergen-induced asthmatic attack that may have both early (10 to 60 minutes in duration) and late components (3 to 8 hours or longer). Bronchospasm can also occur in association with anaphylaxis, which consists of a generalized allergic reaction precipitated by ingestion, inhalation, or parenteral administration of a specific allergen. Additional provoking factors include infection, exercise, certain analgesic drugs (notably acetylsalicylic acid [ASA]), nonspecific irritants in the atmosphere, ingested antigens (such as food additives), altered climatic conditions, and a variety of substances encountered in occupational settings. Psychologic factors also are probably responsible for initiating or modifying the course of some attacks.

### Allergens

Specific antigens provoke asthmatic attacks in sensitized persons. The same people also frequently suffer from other allergic manifestations, such as hay fever and eczema, and usually manifest positive results on prick or intradermal skin testing with a variety of allergens. Despite these indicators of a state of hypersensitivity, antigen exposure is not often identified as being responsible for a specific attack of spontaneous asthma. In a minority of patients, the timing of attacks with exposure to certain antigens and the amelioration experienced with their avoidance[640] leave little doubt as to the cause of the attacks; such antigens are often pollens, animal dander, or food. More frequently, incrimination of a suspected allergen requires confirmation by more reliable means such as radioallergosorbent test (RAST)[613, 641] or inhalation challenge.[613] RAST is an *in vitro* radioimmunoassay in which anti-IgE prepared in animals is used to detect IgE antibodies to specific allergens in human serum.[613]

When a sensitized person inhales antigen in the laboratory, there is an immediate or early response characterized by bronchoconstriction, which reaches a maximum in 15 to 30 minutes and is followed by a return toward normal lung function even without treatment.[642] In some patients, this early response is followed by a late or delayed response that develops 3 to 8 hours after the initial challenge and may persist for 48 hours (Fig. 54–10). In other patients, a single-antigen inhalation challenge is followed by recurrent nocturnal episodes of asthma.[643] Occasional individuals develop only a delayed response to inhaled antigen.

Besides being more prolonged, the late asthmatic response differs from the immediate response with respect to the effect of pharmacologic interventions. Beta-adrenergic agonists in sufficient concentration block the immediate response but are much less effective against the delayed response; on the other hand, corticosteroids do not influence the immediate response but attenuate the late response. Diso-

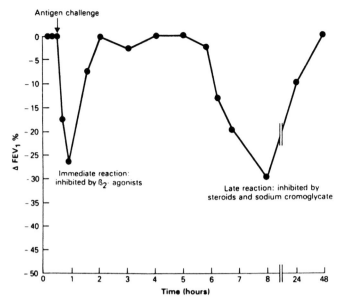

**Figure 54–10. Immediate and Late Allergic Airway Response.**
This graph reveals the response when asthmatic patients are challenged with a specific antigen to which they are allergic: they can develop an immediate bronchoconstriction that generally wanes by 1 hour, followed by a late reaction that begins 4 to 6 hours after challenge and can last as long as 24 hours. Beta-adrenergic agonists effectively inhibit the immediate allergic reaction but have less effect on alleviating the late response. Both the immediate and late responses can be inhibited by sodium cromoglycate, whereas steroid therapy attenuates the late response but has no influence on the immediate response.

dium cromoglycate inhibits both reactions.[644] Increased blood levels of histamine and chemotactic factors can be found during both the immediate and delayed responses.[645] The physiologic changes associated with the two responses are also similar; however, there is evidence of more peripheral airway participation during the delayed response, in which the pulmonary function changes closely resemble those found in spontaneous exacerbations of asthma.[646] The delayed response in human skin and in the airways of animals is characterized histologically by edema and a perivascular eosinophil infiltrate.[173, 647] Examination of BAL fluid during this phase of the allergic response shows an increase in the amount of albumin and in the number of eosinophils and neutrophils; an increased number of desquamated epithelial cells is also evident.[648] It has been suggested that such inflammation may result in irreversible structural and functional changes in the airway after repeated late responses to naturally occurring antigen. A similar common final pathway of airway inflammation may explain the similarity of airway function and pathology in patients in whom asthma is triggered by occupational exposure to low-molecular-weight compounds.[649]

The cellular and molecular mechanisms of the immediate and delayed allergic responses are well worked out. Both reactions are mediated through an interaction of an allergen and specific IgE bound to mast cells and circulating basophils via a high-affinity IgE receptor. The antibody also binds to eosinophils, macrophages, neutrophils, and platelets; however, the relevance of this finding to the pathogenesis of allergen responsiveness is less clear than is mast cell and basophil binding.[650–652] Inhaled antigen first comes in contact

with mast cells in the respiratory epithelium. Its interaction with the IgE on the mast cell surface is followed by linking of receptors, which in turn triggers the release and synthesis of cytokines and mediators. These can alter epithelial permeability, allowing penetration of antigen through the mucosal barrier, where it can interact with IgE on tissue mast cells and circulating basophils.

The detection of specific antigens responsible for asthma involves the measurement of tissue-bound IgE by skin prick tests and specific serum IgE. Although many asthmatic patients have raised levels of total IgE,[652, 653] there is considerable overlap with values obtained in normal persons.[654] In fact, serum levels of IgE do not distinguish asthmatics from control populations nearly as well as do skin tests and RAST.[655] The serum concentration of IgE also gives little indication of the severity of the disease; in fact, very high levels of IgE (such as are found in patients with parasitic infestation) are thought to block the binding sites on the mast cells from aeroallergen specific IgE molecules and thus to protect against asthma.[48, 656] In population studies, peak IgE levels occur between 6 and 14 years of age and decline progressively thereafter. Males have higher levels than females, and persons who have positive skin responses to antigens have levels four to five times higher than those who are non–skin test–sensitive.[657] Although there is general agreement that antigen activation of an IgE-sensitized target cell releases mediators by a noncytotoxic secretory process with the initiation of immediate anaphylaxis, some workers have also demonstrated immediate reactions to skin prick and inhalation challenge with the house mite *Dermatophagoides pteronyssinus,* mediated by a short-term–sensitizing IgG.[658, 659]

The environment contains innumerable potential antigens, exposure to which is often governed by geographic and seasonal variation. As discussed previously, the prevalence of allergic sensitization to environmental and occupational allergens is increasing worldwide. Population surveys from different countries using immediate skin test reactivity to a variety of antigens show a wide variability (e.g., between 8% and 69% in one review[78]). In most large surveys, the prevalence is between 20% and 45% with definite increases over the last two decades in Europe, the United States, New Zealand, and Australasia.[79, 660–662] Many of these sensitized persons are asymptomatic; in those who have symptoms, the most common manifestation is seasonal or perennial rhinitis. Positive skin test reactions show a definite age relationship, the peak incidence being in the third decade of life and decreasing rapidly after the age of 50 years.[660]

As might be expected, surveys of atmospheric pollens and fungal spores (and skin test reactions to them) reveal geographic variation. Grass and tree pollens are universal and are the most common causes of hay fever.[660, 663–665] However, although they cause positive skin reactions and inhalation challenge in many atopic asthmatics,[666, 667] they are not thought to be common causes of asthmatic attacks. Moreover, when it does occur, seasonal asthma caused by pollens usually is not severe. Ragweed pollen grains, one of the most common causes of hay fever, are approximately 20 μm in diameter; thus, only fragmented pollen grains can gain access to the lower respiratory tract.[668] The association of outbreaks of asthma with thunderstorms has been hypothesized to be the result of the osmotic release of "submicronic," allergen-containing starch granules from grass pollen.[669] In one such outbreak, visits to hospital emergency rooms increased 10-fold over baseline, and persons who were pollen-sensitive were preferentially affected.[669] In addition to pollens, fungal spores are a major source of airborne allergens, outnumbering the former by up to 1,000:1. The most commonly recognized agents are imperfect fungi, including *Alternaria, Aspergillus, Cladosporium, Mucor* species, and *Penicillium*; however, additional entire families have been relatively ignored and may be important.[670]

Increasing evidence indicates that indoor allergens are the most important cause of chronic allergic asthma.[671] Animal dander from a variety of household pets, especially cats but also dogs, gerbils, guinea pigs, rats, and (rarely) birds, can cause ocular and nasal symptoms as well as asthma.[670, 672, 673] The principal cat allergen is a protein called Fel d I. The most important of the insect allergens are those derived from house dust mites. Many asthmatics show positive skin test reactions to house dust; although such dust contains many substances, including potentially allergenic molds and disintegrating fibers, studies have shown that various house mites, notably *D. pteronyssinus,* are present in especially large numbers, particularly in dust from mattresses.[674-678] This organism measures approximately 300 μm in length and thrives in homes that are usually damp. It is found worldwide, except in very dry climates and at high altitudes.[679, 680] It yields several antigens, the most important of which is Der p 1. Numerous investigators have shown that sensitivity to house dust mite is a very significant risk factor for asthma.[671] Several workers have shown that persons sensitive to house dust tend to manifest increased sensitivity to extracts of dust mites;[674, 681, 682] most of the 30% of patients who do not have such mite extract sensitivity respond to animal danders present in the dust.[683]

Another indoor insect that appears to be important in chronic asthma is the cockroach.[684] In one study of 476 asthmatic children from eight inner-city areas in the United States, skin tests for sensitivity to cockroach, house dust mite, and cat allergens yielded a positive result in 37%, 35%, and 23%, respectively;[685] it was hypothesized that cockroach allergy and exposure to high levels of this allergen may help explain the high frequency of asthma-related health problems in inner-city children. Certain insects such as the caddis fly (mayfly) and the mushroom fly have also been held responsible for epidemic asthma in certain areas during the spring and autumn.[686, 687]

A variety of foods, especially eggs, fish, shellfish, nuts, spices, and chocolate, tend to cause immediate wheal and flare reactions to intracutaneous skin testing, particularly in children. Evidence of hypersensitivity to the specific food may be corroborated by the occurrence of an asthmatic attack following ingestion of the food in question and, in some cases, by the absence of attacks when the specific allergens are avoided. However, some persons who manifest positive skin test reactions to specific food allergens can consume these foods repeatedly with apparent impunity. Although asthmatic patients associate symptoms with the ingestion of specific foods in about 20% of attacks, objective evidence incriminating them is obtained only rarely.[688, 689] From a clinical point of view, it is relatively rare that wheeze is the sole manifestation of food allergy; the majority of

affected persons also have atopic eczema, gastrointestinal food intolerance, and/or angioedema or urticaria.[690]

Approximately 10% of patients undergoing chronic hemodialysis develop IgE antibody in response to human serum albumin–ethylene oxide conjugates. (The latter is used in sterilization of the dialysis equipment.) Some of these patients develop chronic asthma, and others experience, anaphylactoid reactions during dialysis.[692, 693] Although latex allergy is primarily an occupational risk (*see* farther on), there is an increasing prevalence of such allergy in nonoccupational settings; affected persons often have cross-reacting hypersensitivity to avocado, banana, kiwi fruit, and chestnuts.[693a]

### Anaphylaxis

Anaphylaxis is a particularly virulent form of allergic reaction that, in addition to bronchoconstriction, has a variety of systemic manifestations. The reaction typically develops rapidly, reaching a maximum within 5 to 30 minutes. Early symptoms include nausea and vomiting, pruritus, and substernal tightness; these are followed quickly by generalized urticaria, angioedema, shortness of breath, weakness, hypotension, choking, and loss of consciousness. Death is not uncommon, usually as a result of asphyxia related to laryngeal edema or bronchoconstriction; sometimes, the clinical presentation is one of circulatory collapse and hypovolemia.[694, 695]

As with asthma, many agents are known to be responsible for initiating an anaphylactic attack. A particularly serious and sometimes fatal manifestation of anaphylaxis can occur following administration of drugs.[696] The reaction usually occurs when the drug is administered intravenously or intramuscularly, although oral, percutaneous, or even respiratory exposure may produce a response in highly sensitive persons. The most commonly implicated agent is penicillin. For example, in a study of 809 cases of anaphylactic shock resulting from parenteral administration of antibiotics, all but 16 were judged to be related to penicillin;[698] 74 (9%) of the patients died. Sensitive persons also may develop asthmatic attacks from inhaled medications, including acetylcysteine, pancreatic dornase,[700] lidocaine,[701] and even disodium cromoglycate[702, 703] and beclomethasone dipropionate administered for the treatment of the asthma![703a]

Another well-known cause of potentially fatal anaphylaxis is a sting from one of the insects of the Hymenoptera order, including bees, wasps, hornets, and yellow jackets.[697] In the United States, stings from these insects are said to cause as many deaths as snake bites.[697] Usually, the victim has an atopic background;[705] for example, in one study of 249 affected patients, 53% had a history of rhinitis, asthma, or cutaneous allergy.[697]

Other substances that occasionally cause systemic anaphylactic reactions in human beings include heterologous proteins in the form of antiserum, hormones, enzymes, extracts, foods, and diagnostic agents such as iodinated contrast media.[705] A rare cause is passive sensitization by blood transfusion from an atopic donor.[706, 707]

### *Exercise*

Exercise-induced asthma (EIA) can be defined as excessive airway narrowing and reduction in maximal expiratory flow rates in the setting of moderate or vigorous exercise.[708–711] Although EIA occurs in the majority of asthmatic patients, the term "exercise-induced asthma" is unfortunate because it implies that exercise induces the asthmatic state; in fact, exercise is no more than one of many provoking stimuli in patients who have asthma. However, the label is so well established in the literature that any attempt to introduce a more reasonable nomenclature such as "exercise asthmatic response" would be futile.[376, 712,713]

A decrease of 10% or more in PEFR or $FEV_1$ or a greater than 35% decrease in specific airway conductance (SGaw), mean forced expiratory flow at mid–forced vital capacity ($FEF_{25-75}$), or instantaneous forced expiratory flow at 50% of vital capacity ($Vmax_{50}$) following exercise is considered diagnostic of EIA.[714] Although some airway narrowing can occur during exercise,[715] the maximal impairment in lung function characteristically occurs 5 to 10 minutes after exercise or hyperventilation.[716] In one study, $FEV_1$ was measured during and after 4, 8, and 16 minutes of isocapnic hyperventilation;[717] the mean declines in $FEV_1$ were 13 ± 10%, 22 ± 7%, and 29 ± 12% at 4, 8, and 16 minutes, but no significant bronchoconstriction occurred until the hyperventilation was stopped, regardless of its duration. These results suggest either that hyperventilation itself inhibits bronchoconstriction or that the mechanisms that induce bronchoconstriction operate after, rather than during, hyperventilation.

The bronchoconstriction of EIA spontaneously remits within 30 to 60 minutes, although rarely the attack can be prolonged. The majority of patients are refractory to the induction of a second episode of EIA for approximately 2 hours. Late bronchoconstriction in response to exercise has been reported, particularly in children, although it is less frequent and severe than the late response following antigen challenge.[712, 713, 718] The response to allergen challenge may be increased 24 hours after an exercise challenge in some patients.[719]

The degree of obstruction produced by exercise or hyperventilation can be calculated as the *percentage fall index* (PFI):

$$PFI = \frac{pre\text{-}exercise\ value\ -\ lowest\ postexercise\ value}{pre\text{-}exercise\ value} \times 100$$

Defined in this way, EIA occurs in 70% to 80% of patients who have asthma and exercise at 80% to 90% of their maximal work load for 6 to 8 minutes.[712, 720] In both normal and asthmatic persons, bronchodilation occurs during the first few minutes of exercise, and the magnitude of bronchodilation is calculated as the *percentage rise index* (PRI):[712, 721, 722]

$$PRI = \frac{highest\ intraexercise\ value\ -\ pre\text{-}exercise\ value}{pre\text{-}exercise\ value} \times 100$$

The physiologic abnormalities of lung function and gas exchange that accompany EIA do not differ from those that occur in response to other inciters of asthmatic episodes.[712] A number of investigators have attempted to localize the site of the airway narrowing using density dependence of maximal expiratory flow and have found that both large and small airways participate;[723, 724] the degree of peripheral airway narrowing appears to be greater in patients who have more severe EIA.[725] However, the uncertainty regarding the usefulness of density dependence measurements in determining the site of obstruction and the poor reproducibility of the response in some asthmatic patients at different times makes these conclusions questionable.[726]

Although it was formerly believed that EIA was equally common in athletes and unfit persons,[727, 728] the results of some studies suggest that trained athletes are more likely to develop exercise-induced bronchoconstriction than the population at large.[709] In one investigation of 124 figure skaters, 43 (35%) had a greater than 10% decrease in $FEV_1$ following their usual routine.[729] Sixty-seven of the 596 (11%) members of the 1984 United States Summer Olympics team had asthma based on history or challenge testing;[730] 41 of these won medals. In another study of 42 elite cross-country skiers, 33 (79%) had symptoms of asthma or were taking asthma medications.[731] Even highly trained swimmers appear to have an increased prevalence of EIA; however, in such persons this may be related, at least in part, to exposure to chlorine in swimming pools.[732]

Patients who have asthma can show excessive bronchodilation during exercise in addition to the exaggerated postexercise bronchoconstriction. An increase in PEFR or $FEV_1$ greater than 22% is considered abnormal. In general, the lower the starting flow rate, the greater the degree of exercise-induced bronchodilation; however, the degree of bronchoconstriction cannot be predicted from baseline studies. The mechanism of exercise-induced bronchodilation is not completely understood, but the phenomenon is partly related to decreased vagal tone and increased circulating catecholamines.[712, 722, 733]

An index of overall bronchial lability in response to exercise can be obtained by combining the percentage fall index and the percentage rise index to give the *exercise lability index* (ELI):

$$ELI = \frac{highest\ flow\ rate\ during\ exercise\ -\ lowest\ postexercise\ value}{initial\ value} \times 100$$

The ELI tends to be higher than normal both in patients who have allergic rhinitis and in asymptomatic relatives of asthmatic patients.[734] In the latter group, the ELI is abnormal chiefly as a result of excessive exercise-induced bronchodilation; in asthmatic patients, the main contributor is exaggerated bronchoconstriction.[735]

The degree of bronchoconstriction in response to either exercise or isocapnic hyperventilation (ISH) depends on the level of NSBR.[736–740] In fact, the responses correlate with NSBH so closely that exercise has been suggested as a test for NSBH, although it does not appear as sensitive as histamine and methacholine in separating normal persons from those with asthma.[741]

Exercise and ISH of cold and/or dry air cause cough as well as bronchoconstriction. The time course of the cough is very similar to that of bronchoconstriction, peaking 5 minutes after exercise or ISH and lasting for approximately 30 minutes. It correlates better with respiratory water loss than with heat loss and occurs in both normal persons and asthmatic patients. Cough also occurs in response to inhaled hypertonic aerosols, suggesting that the stimulus is the change in airway fluid osmolarity attendant on evaporative water loss. Pretreatment with beta agonist blocks bronchoconstriction but not cough, suggesting that cough is not secondary to the bronchoconstriction induced by stimulation of irritant receptors.[742, 743]

### Pathogenesis

Our understanding of the mechanism responsible for EIA is based on the observation that airway narrowing can be completely abolished if the inspired air during exercise is warmed to body temperature and saturated with water vapor (37° C and a water content of about 46 mg/liter).[744–747] In addition, the degree of airway obstruction following identical exercise challenges can be modified by altering the inspired air conditions: the colder and drier the air breathed during exercise, the greater the subsequent response.[747, 748] In fact, the airway response can be elicited by ISH of cold and/or dry air in the absence of exercise.[749–751] The severity of EIA can also be diminished by the use of masks that recover exhaled heat and water during frigid air breathing.[752] Body cooling without alteration in inspired air conditions also may produce bronchoconstriction;[753, 754] in fact, even consumption of cold drinks has been shown to enhance nonspecific responsiveness to histamine, although direct effects on the airway have not been demonstrated.[755] It is not known whether the airway narrowing that occurs with somatic cooling is related to EIA.

When the inspired air conditions are constant, there is a dose-response relationship between ventilation and the severity of bronchoconstriction in patients who have asthma, whether the increased ventilation is associated with exercise or with ISH. Even normal persons develop some airway narrowing in response to cold dry air hyperventilation, although much greater ventilation is required to produce much smaller changes in expiratory flow rates.[756–758] When the water content and temperature of inspired air are held constant, the mode of exercise is not important as a determinant of obstruction in asthmatic patients; at matched levels of minute ventilation, the bronchoconstriction that occurs during treadmill walking, bicycling, or swimming is similar.

The fact that EIA is related to the breathing of cold and/or dry air has rekindled interest in inspired air conditioning. Because inspired air temperature is almost always below body temperature and less than 100% saturated with water vapor, and because alveolar gas is 100% saturated at body temperature, the airways must give up heat and water to the inspired air. During resting ventilation and nasal breathing, the conditioning process is almost completed by the time inspired gas reaches the lower airways;[759] however, during the increased ventilation and mouth breathing that occur during exercise, incompletely conditioned air can penetrate deeply into the lung, especially if cold dry air is breathed.[760] The consequences are cooling and drying of the airway wall. The degree of cooling is determined by the combination of convective heat loss from the airway wall as the inspired air is warmed and evaporative heat loss that results from its humidification. The total heat lost can be calculated as follows:

$$RHL = VE \cdot HC\,(TI - TE) + VE \cdot HV\,(WCE - WCI)$$

where RHL = total respiratory heat loss in kilocalories (kcal)/min; VE = minute ventilation in liters/min; HC = heat capacity of air ($0.304 \times 10^{-3}$ kcal/1° C); TI and TE = inspired and expired air temperature, respectively; HV = the latent heat of vaporization of water ($0.58 \times 10^{-3}$ kcal/mg), and WCI and WCE = inspired and expired water content, respectively, of air (mg/liter).[747]

Obviously, the total heat loss will be greater when inspired air is cooler or drier. The temperature and water content of expired gas differ from those of alveolar gas because a countercurrent exchange mechanism serves to recover a portion of the heat and water added to inspired air. The upper airway mucosa cools during inspiration as a result of convective and evaporative heat loss; the cooled mucosa, in turn, recovers heat and water during expiration by cooling expired gas and condensing expired water vapor. The effectiveness of the countercurrent exchange is dependent on the surface area of the upper airway mucosa and its blood flow: an increase in mucosal blood flow by warming the surface of the airway would decrease the penetration of cool air into the lung but would result in a larger expired heat and water loss; on the other hand, a decrease in mucosal blood flow would serve to cool the upper airway surface further, facilitating the recovery of heat and water from expired air but also resulting in greater penetration of unconditioned air into the lung.[761]

An increase in tracheobronchial blood flow has been reported in the dog following inspiration of cold and/or dry air during ISH.[761] Based on observations of blanching of the tracheobronchial mucosa during cold air breathing in human beings, it has been postulated that the bronchial vasculature constricts, although no direct measurements of airway blood flow have been made.[762] It is clear, however, that cooling of the airway occurs for a variable distance into the lung; although evidence for this was initially obtained indirectly by measuring retrotracheal esophageal temperature,[763] subsequent mapping of airway thermal profiles in human beings has shown that during cold air hyperventilation, temperature does not equilibrate with body temperature until the air reaches airways 2 mm in diameter.[764] Of some interest is the observation that airway cooling is identical for a given level of ventilation whether it is achieved during exercise or ISH, suggesting that variations in overall cardiac output do not affect inspired air conditioning.[748]

In individual asthmatic patients, the degree of bronchoconstriction produced by exercise or ISH correlates with the calculated respiratory heat loss and with changes in retrotracheal esophageal temperature, although the slope of the relationship differs among subjects.[763, 765, 766] The bronchoconstriction that occurs in asthmatics in response to the ventilation of unconditioned air appears to result not from a defect in inspired air conditioning but rather from an abnormal response to a normal stimulus. Healthy persons do not seem to have more efficient air conditioning, because they develop equivalent airway cooling at matched levels of ventilation and inspired air conditions.[763] When the levels of ventilation and inspired air conditions are identical, nasal breathing results in much less airway cooling and bronchoconstriction than that noted during oral breathing.[767, 768]

The observations that airways cool during exercise and ISH and that there is a dose-response relationship between cooling and bronchoconstriction suggest that in some way cooling of the airway is responsible for the bronchoconstriction.[759, 765] However, because it is difficult to produce cooling without drying, it is also possible that airway drying is the inciting stimulus.[769–771] In fact, hyperventilation of dry air at different temperatures results in approximately equivalent degrees of bronchoconstriction.[748] Moreover, when the temperature and water content of inspired air are varied so as to produce a range of total respiratory heat and water loss, the magnitude of bronchoconstriction correlates more closely with calculated water loss than with heat loss.[769, 770, 772, 773]

To the extent that water loss from the airway mucosa exceeds water replacement, the fluid lining the airway will become hyperosmolar relative to plasma. This has led some investigators to postulate that it is the osmolarity of the periciliary fluid that in some way mediates the bronchoconstriction of EIA and ISH.[756] This hypothesis has been strengthened by studies showing that inhalation of hyperosmolar aerosols elicit bronchoconstriction in patients with EIA.[774, 775] A significant relationship between the severity of EIA and the responsiveness to inhaled hypertonic aerosols has also been demonstrated.[776] Despite these observations the results of some studies have cast doubt on this hypothesis; no increase in histamine, tryptase, prostaglandin, or mast cells was found in BAL fluid when hypertonic saline was nebulized or directly delivered to the airways of a small group of asthmatic patients.[777] In addition, in one *in vitro* study of human airway tissue, hyperosmolar and hypo-osmolar conditions did not produce smooth muscle contraction or alter the responsiveness to added agonists.[778]

How airway cooling or drying results in airway narrowing is also incompletely understood. The most widely discussed potential mechanisms have been (1) release of mediators from mast cells or other sources, (2) stimulation of afferent receptors with resultant reflex bronchoconstriction, and (3) bronchial vascular dilatation and mucosal edema.

**Release of Mediators.** Although there is some variation among studies, most investigators have been able to detect inflammatory mediators in the peripheral blood of asthmatic patients who have bronchoconstriction following exercise or ISH.[779–781] The mediators that have been detected include histamine and the high-molecular-weight chemotactic substance neutrophil chemotactic factor of anaphylaxis (NCFA), both of which are thought to be derived from pulmonary mast cells.[712, 780, 782] Their release appears to be causally related to the bronchoconstriction, because a similar magnitude of methacholine-induced bronchial obstruction does not result in detectable levels of these mediators and because the breathing of warm humid air during exercise blocks both the bronchoconstriction and the mediator release.[783, 784] Exercise and ISH result in similar plasma histamine levels at matched levels of ventilation, but the rise in NCFA is less or absent with ISH—one of the few differences between the two challenges.[785] Although normal persons develop equivalent degrees of airway cooling (and presumably drying), they do not show increased plasma levels of histamine or NCFA during exercise; this suggests that the mast cells of asthmatic patients may release mediators more readily.[786] There is also evidence that leukotrienes are generated and released during exercise- and ISH-induced bronchoconstriction, and treatment with blockers of leukotriene production or action have a therapeutic benefit.[787] The same is not true for blockers of thromboxane.[788] Patients who have EIA also show evidence of inflammatory cell and platelet activation after exercise.[784, 789]

Mediator release from mast cells in the airway may be triggered by the change in osmolarity accompanying evaporative water loss. Basophils and mast cells release preformed mediators *in vitro* in response to both hyperosmolar and hypo-osmolar challenges.[790–792] This is not associated with cell disruption or death; in fact, very high levels of osmolarity inhibit mediator release. Because cells from normal and asthmatic patients appear to respond equally to alterations in osmolarity *in vitro,* the link with the abnormal increase in plasma mediators *in vivo* remains speculative. Of some interest is the fact that the osmolar mediator release is dependent on temperature, the maximal effect occurring at 32° C—a temperature that can easily develop in the airway wall during exercise or ISH.[790]

In some persons, exercise appears to produce generalized release of mast cell mediators that results in anaphylaxis; this rare entity is associated with "generalized body warmth, pruritus, erythema and urticaria, laryngeal edema, hoarseness, gastrointestinal colic, and vascular collapse."[793] In these people, increased blood levels of histamine and degranulation of skin mast cells have been demonstrated.[793, 794] Exercise-induced anaphylaxis occurs more frequently after ingestion of a foodstuff to which the affected person is allergic.[795–797] The eating of celery before exercising appears to be a particular risk factor for the syndrome.[798] Bronchoconstriction can also accompany a less severe form of systemic mast cell mediator release known as cholinergic urticaria, characterized by generalized punctate wheals and itchiness that follow hot showers or accompany pyrexia.[799]

The release of vasoactive and chemotactic substances from the lung during exercise suggests the development of an inflammatory response. However, although mucosal inflammation and epithelial damage have been shown to develop in animals breathing dry air through a tracheostomy,[800] evidence of similar effects in response to exercise in human asthma is conflicting. In some studies, no increase in chemical or cellular markers has been detected in BAL fluid;[801, 802] however, one group of investigators found an increased number of eosinophils in such fluid as well as a greater percentage of degranulated mast cells in bronchial biopsy specimens from asthmatics at 3 hours following an exercise challenge.[803]

Additional evidence that the release of inflammatory mediators may be important in the pathogenesis of exercise- and ISH-induced airway obstruction derives from studies in which anti-inflammatory drugs have proved effective in preventing bronchoconstriction. Mediator release from mast cells can be attenuated by administration of heparin,[804] disodium cromoglycate, beta agonists, and calcium channel blockers, each of which has provided effective prophylaxis against exercise- and ISH-induced asthma.[804, 805] Although beta agonists and calcium channel blockers may also have a relaxant effect on smooth muscle, it has not been established whether this action or inhibition of mediator release is the more important. It is also possible that these agents may have a dilating effect on the bronchial vasculature, resulting in a decreased airway cooling for a given ventilation; however, this does not appear to be the case for disodium cromoglycate, at least.[807] In addition to the evidence for a contribution from mast cell mediators, the observation that leukotriene receptor antagonists attenuate exercise-induced bronchoconstriction in some persons supports a role for the generation of new mediators during challenge.[808]

**Stimulation of Afferent Receptors.** A second mechanism by which airway cooling or drying might produce bronchoconstriction is by cold or hyperosmolar stimulation of afferent nerve endings in the airway. The evidence for such a mechanism comes largely from *in vivo* studies of pharmacologic blockade of the afferent or efferent vagal pathway; however, reports of the data relating to both limbs of the reflex are conflicting and controversial. For example, interruption of the afferent limb by inhalation of local anesthetic agents appears to decrease the subsequent airway response to exercise, at least as reported by some investigators.[809, 810] However, despite objective evidence of afferent interruption (decreased gag reflex and decreased citric acid–induced cough), other workers have shown no decrease in response at matched levels of ventilation.[811, 812] It is possible that airway anesthesia decreases ventilation at any level of exercise, thus decreasing the stimulus for EIA rather than the response to it.[809] Another pharmacologic approach to the determination of the importance of sensory neuropeptides in the pathogenesis of EIA was used in a study in which thiorphan, an inhibitor of neutral endopeptidase (NEP), was administered prior to exercise in asthmatic patients;[813] the response to exercise was actually attenuated following the treatment, suggesting that the release of bronchodilating neuropeptides such as atrial natriuretic peptide and vasoactive intestinal polypeptide (VIP) normally modulates the response.

Interruption of the efferent limb of the reflex pathway has been produced by aerosol and parenteral administration of atropine or ipratropium bromide. Although cholinergic blockade has been found to attenuate the response to exercise or ISH in most studies, the effect is small, and it is difficult to separate an "apparent" protection (secondary to increased baseline airway size) from a direct effect.[814–816] In one study in which hypertonic saline was used as the stimulant, the provocative concentration of aerosol required to cause a 20% decrease in $FEV_1$ was increased 2.5-, 2.0-, and 2.6-fold after administration of intramuscular atropine, inhaled ipratropium bromide, and inhaled lidocaine, respectively.[817] However, in other studies, parenteral administration of atropine has been shown to be more effective in attenuating airway responses despite baseline bronchodilation equivalent to that achieved following inhalation, suggesting that complete cholinergic blockade is not achieved with the inhaled drug.[818, 819]

It is possible that a cholinergic reflex is the major cause of obstruction in some persons, whereas mediator release is more important in others. In one study, asthmatic patients who were refractory to repeated ISH challenges derived no protective effect from inhaled ipratropium bromide, whereas those who did not show a refractory period were helped by the inhaled anticholinergic agent.[820] Because the refractory period is thought to be caused by mediator release and depletion, such release may be the major mechanism only in patients who show a refractory period and lack of anticholinergic protection.

**Bronchial Vascular Dilatation.** Although it is generally believed that airway smooth muscle contraction is the major cause of airway narrowing in EIA, at least some of the effect could be secondary to bronchial vascular dilatation and mucosal edema.[821, 822] This hypothesis is lent some credence by the observation that rapid changes in caliber can occur in the nose; because the latter has no encircling layer of smooth muscle, these changes are entirely attributable to vasomotion. Like the nose, the lower airway mucosa possesses a complex and extensive mucosal plexus of blood vessels, and it is quite possible that cold-induced vascular constriction followed by vasodilation and mucosal edema may play a role in the airway obstruction of EIA.

A number of clinical and experimental observations support the hypothesis. As mentioned previously, blanching of the airway mucosa has been observed bronchoscopically in human beings during cold dry air hyperventilation,[762] and bronchial vascular dilatation occurs after isocapnic hyperventilation in dogs.[761] Following cessation of exercise or hyperventilation, asthmatic patients show a more rapid rewarming of expired air, which may indicate a more brisk and/or exaggerated rebound bronchial vascular dilatation.[823] In addition, when bronchial vascular dilatation is inhibited by administration of inhaled norepinephrine, the degree of airway narrowing following ISH is attenuated.[824] On the other hand, experiments in dogs have suggested that bronchial vascular dilatation could play a *protective* role in dry air–induced bronchoconstriction, perhaps by more rapidly removing locally released mediators.[825]

### Refractory Period

About 50% to 80% of asthmatic patients who develop EIA show a refractory period following challenge, during which similar levels of exercise produce no response or an attenuated response.[718, 826] Similar degrees of refractoriness are produced by matched levels of ISH.[827, 828] The degree of attenuation of the second response is dependent on the intensity of the initial exercise and on time; although such a response is considerably less 30 minutes after an initial episode, by 4 hours the protective effect has completely disappeared.[826] A more prolonged protective effect can be achieved by using short bursts of cold air hyperventilation over a 12-week training period; however, in some patients, this protocol caused a reduction of prechallenge expiratory flows and a worsening of symptoms.[829]

There are a number of possible explanations for the refractory period, including[712] (1) mediator depletion of the cells that respond to airway cooling and/or drying, (2) decreased responsiveness of airway smooth muscle to released mediator, (3) decreased respiratory heat and water loss despite similar exercise, (4) decreased response resulting from exercise-induced sympathoadrenal activation, and (5) release of secondary bronchodilating mediators such as prostaglandins. Some of these possibilities have been tested experimentally. Exercise produces refractoriness to subsequent antigen challenge in some patients who have asthma[830] but does not affect methacholine and histamine responses.[831, 832] This finding suggests that mediator depletion may be important and excludes a direct effect on smooth muscle responsiveness. However, although such depletion is an attractive hypothesis, decreased blood levels have not been demonstrated by direct measurement of NCFA during initial and subsequent challenges.[833]

The calculated heat and water losses are the same

during the initial and second exercise periods, making an adaptation of air-conditioning mechanisms unlikely.[834] Because ISH results in a refractory period without causing the increase in circulating catecholamines associated with exercise, a protective effect of beta-adrenergic stimulation is also unlikely to be the only explanation.[835] The fact that indomethacin abolishes the refractory period supports the hypothesis that exercise-induced release of bronchodilating prostaglandins, such as PGE[2], may be the cause.[836, 837]

Refractoriness following challenge is also seen with repeated exposure to inhaled sodium metabisulfite and the leukotriene LTD[4].[838] In one study, exercise attenuated the subsequent response to metabisulfite and *vice versa*, indicating that the mechanisms of refractoriness are partially shared.[839] Cross-refractoriness also exists for exercise and LTD[4], supporting the contention that exercise causes an increase in LTD[4], which secondarily releases prostaglandins, which in turn attenuate subsequent bronchoconstriction.[838]

There is controversy about whether the refractory period depends on the development of bronchoconstriction during the initial exercise period. Some investigators have found that a refractory period persists even if bronchoconstriction is prevented during the initial exercise by breathing warm humid air,[840, 841] whereas others have shown the absence of a refractory period with a similar sequence of challenges.[842] Although it has been suggested that hypoxia accentuates and hyperoxia attenuates EIA, in one study eucapnic hypoxia did not enhance the bronchoconstriction that occurred following dry air hyperventilation.[843] The hyperoxic attenuation of EIA may be caused by decreased ventilation and resultant heat and water loss at similar exercise levels.[844, 845]

### Delayed Exercise Responses

Although a late or delayed bronchoconstrictive response has been reported following EIA (but not ISH), it does not appear as frequently (occurring in 30% to 50% of patients) as the late response to antigen inhalation and does not result in as severe airway narrowing as in the late allergen response.[846–849] In some studies, no late response was detected in children,[850] whereas in other studies, a late response—occurring from 4 to 12 hours after the initial reaction—was reported, especially in persons who had a severe initial response.[851] Another difference noted between the late exercise-induced and antigen-induced responses was the lack of change in subsequent nonspecific airway responsiveness following the former.[852–854]

### Summary

EIA is the bronchial narrowing that occurs in association with vigorous exercise in asthmatic patients. It is common to virtually all asthmatics and thus is not a specific form of the disease. In susceptible persons, it can be mimicked by the hyperventilation of air that is not completely humidified or warmed to body temperature. There is abundant evidence that the stimulus for EIA is not exercise itself but the cooling or drying of the airway mucosa that occurs on inhalation of incompletely conditioned air; however, it is uncertain whether the pertinent stimulus is the cooling of the airway or the drying of the mucosa and subsequent development of hyperosmolarity in the surface-lining liquid. In addition, the mechanism by which cooling or drying causes bronchoconstriction is unclear; although it may be related to stimulation of irritant receptors within the airway wall, release of bronchoconstricting mediators may also be important. Following one episode of EIA, the majority of patients remain refractory in a second challenge for a period of up to 4 hours. From a clinical point of view, it is important to remember that exercise-induced bronchospasm or cough may be the only manifestation of the disease in some patients who have asthma.

### Infection

Viral respiratory tract infection can cause abnormal airway function in normal people, increased nonspecific bronchial responsiveness (NSBR) in normal and asthmatic patients, and exacerbation of symptoms in patients who have asthma. Although most normal persons develop only cough without wheezing or dyspnea, abnormalities of airway function can be detected in the majority.[855] Children are particularly susceptible to the development of airway narrowing, as a result of their relatively smaller peripheral airways.[855] In otherwise healthy adults, small but measurable transient changes in airway function and NSBR have been shown after infection by respiratory syncytial virus (RSV) and influenza A virus and after vaccination with live attenuated virus;[856–860] killed virus vaccination is not associated with any change in lung function.[861] In asthmatic patients, heat-killed and live attenuated influenza vaccination as well as naturally occurring infection with RSV, rhinovirus, and influenza A virus has been reported to cause increased NSBR.[391, 862–865] This phenomenon could be related to several factors, including epithelial damage and enhanced mucosal permeability and/or edema and inflammatory cell infiltration.[866]

Viral and mycoplasmal but not bacterial respiratory tract infection can also precipitate symptomatic exacerbation in asthmatic patients, although the importance of such infection varies in different series.[867–869] In one study of 16 children aged 3 to 11 years who had a history of wheezing associated with apparent symptomatic respiratory infection, 42 (70%) of 61 episodes of asthma were coincident with viral infections, mostly caused by rhinoviruses and influenza A virus.[870] By contrast, in an adult population, careful sputum culture for bacterial and viral agents and assessment of viral antibody titers showed that infection was a triggering stimulus in only 11% of 111 exacerbations of asthma.[871] In another investigation, increased levels of specific antibodies to *Mycoplasma pneumoniae* were detected in 21% of 95 adult patients who had acute exacerbations.[872] When experimental rhinovirus infection was induced in 19 patients who had asthma, typical upper respiratory tract coryzal symptoms developed in 17;[391] however, a greater than 10% decrease in FEV[1] developed in only 4. Allergic persons develop more severe "cold" symptoms in response to an experimental rhinoviral infection than do nonallergic controls, suggesting that there is synergy between viral and allergen-induced inflammation.[873]

The development of the polymerase chain reaction (PCR) for detection of viral genome has facilitated studies designed to test the importance of viral infection as a precipitant of acute asthma attacks, particularly infection due to viruses such as human rhinovirus, which has over 100 serotypes. In one prospective longitudinal study, a respiratory virus was detected by PCR of nasal secretions in 73% of children during asthmatic exacerbations, compared with a prevalence of 13% in a control population.[874] Using similar methodology, RSV and parainfluenza viruses have also been shown to cause exacerbations of asthma.[867] The duration of symptoms following these infectious exacerbations is longer than that related to noninfectious exacerbations.[875]

Not only does bacterial infection fail to precipitate exacerbations of asthma, but it also does not appear to have an increased incidence in asthmatic patients. In a comparative study of normal persons and patients who had either bronchitis or asthma, bacterial precipitins were identified in 50% of those who had bronchitis but in only 6% of the asthmatic patients—an incidence identical to that found in the normal population.[876]

How viral or mycoplasmal respiratory tract infection precipitates an attack of asthma is not clear;[877] however, several mechanisms are theoretically possible, including interaction with cholinergic or sensory nerves, epithelial damage, and stimulation of cytokine synthesis.[878–880] Little evidence exists to support an immunologic mechanism. It is conceivable that airway wall edema and increased secretions within bronchial lumens induced by the response to virus further diminish the caliber of already narrowed airways. Another possibility is that the mucosal inflammation associated with viral infection results in airway smooth muscle contraction secondary to mediator release from inflammatory cells in the same way that is postulated for the airway response to ozone.[392]

Although the subject is complicated and controversial,[881, 882] there is evidence that a number of cases of asthma that develop in adolescents and young adults are related to a history of infections bronchiolitis in infancy or childhood.[883] Theoretically, the immaturity of the infant lung leaves it particularly vulnerable to long-term harmful effects of such infection. In fact, the results of some studies suggest that as many as 50% of children who have an episode of RSV bronchiolitis during infancy develop recurrent wheezing and asthma;[884, 885] moreover, the more severe the initial episode of bronchiolitis, the higher the subsequent risk.[886] In another 10-year follow-up study of 27 children who had had type 7 adenoviral pneumonia, 16 had persistently abnormal lung function.[887] However, as discussed previously, it is not always clear whether the bronchiolitis in these cases precipitates the onset of asthma or whether what is diagnosed as bronchiolitis is in fact the first attack of asthma in a genetically susceptible child.[888–890]

In one study in which 61 patients who developed bronchiolitis were matched with 47 controls and compared 5½ years after the initial infection, the index cases were more likely to have cough (43% versus 17%), wheeze (34% versus 13%), and a history of bronchodilator use (33% versus 3%);[891] the incidence of atopy was not increased (as assessed by skin tests and family history), supporting the notion that it was viral bronchiolitis that initiated the subsequent airway dysfunction. On the other hand, support for a familial tendency was provided by another study, in which investigators found a significant bronchodilator response to salbutamol in 24% of the parents of children who had bronchiolitis com-

pared with a response rate of zero in a control group.[892] In another study conducted 3 years after infantile RSV infection, bronchiolitis was found to be a significant risk factor for physician-diagnosed asthma (11/47 [23%] versus 1/93 [1%] in controls) and for increased serum IgE titers to common allergens (14/44 [32%] versus 8/92 [9%] in controls).[893] The development of a high titer of RSV-specific IgE at the time of the acute bronchiolitis may be a marker for subsequent atopic airway disease.[894]

The mechanisms by which viral respiratory infection might predispose to subsequent asthma are unclear. It is possible that the bronchiolitis alters the subsequent immune response to aeroallergens in genetically susceptible persons. Alternatively, it has been shown in animal models of adenoviral and RSV bronchiolitis that the viral genome can persist or become latent within the airways, establishing a potentially persistent inflammatory stimulus.[866, 895, 896]

### Analgesics

Acetylsalicylic acid (ASA) and several other unrelated analgesics and anti-inflammatory agents are capable of provoking attacks in an appreciable proportion of patients who have asthma. The incidence of ASA sensitivity in the nonasthmatic population is less than 1%, whereas in the general asthmatic population it has been reported to range from about 5% to 28%.[897–900] The typical ASA-sensitive asthmatic patient is a nonatopic woman over the age of 20 years who has a long history of rhinitis and nasal polyps.[901] The incidence of migraine headaches is high (almost 50% in some studies).[902] Long-standing asthma and rhinitis usually precede the development of ASA sensitivity, and the intolerance increases with age, being six times more common after age 50 than before age 20.[899] The asthma in these patients is often severe, requiring systemic steroids to control symptoms.[903] Peripheral eosinophilia is observed in over 50% of patients, although serum IgE levels are usually normal[898, 900] and specific IgE directed toward ASA is not detectable.[904]

Symptoms and signs develop anywhere from 20 minutes to 3 hours after ingestion of the drug. Two forms of response have been described: a primarily respiratory pattern and an urticarial-angioedema form; only rarely do both occur in the same person.[900] The respiratory response is dominated by bronchoconstriction but is often associated with rhinitis, conjunctivitis, and a scarlet flushing of the head and neck.[903] In a study of patients with a history of ASA intolerance who were subjected to oral challenge, 72% developed bronchial narrowing;[905] 92% of this group showed concomitant nasal symptoms, and 12% showed rhinitis alone. Sixteen per cent of all patients had no response, indicating that tolerance can develop spontaneously. ASA or another nonsteroidal anti-inflammatory drug can precipitate life-threatening asthma;[906] in one study, 25% of 145 asthmatic patients who required mechanical ventilation for acute attacks were shown to be sensitive to ASA.[907]

Although ASA can act as an antigen and stimulate antibody production, there is abundant evidence that the airway narrowing it induces is nonallergic in nature.[898, 904, 908] Indirect evidence has been obtained that mast cell mediator release may play a role; for example, neutrophil chemotactic factor derived from these cells can be detected in the blood 60 to 120 minutes after the ingestion of ASA, coincident with or following maximal bronchoconstriction.[909, 910] However, the fact that its appearance does not precede the airway narrowing raises the possibility that it is released secondary to the bronchoconstriction.[910] Disodium cromoglycate, which is believed to exert a beneficial effect by decreasing mast cell mediator release following antigen challenge, is also partly effective in decreasing ASA-induced and indomethacin-induced airway responses when administered prior to challenge.[911, 912]

The accepted mechanism by which ASA and other nonsteroidal anti-inflammatory agents cause bronchoconstriction is related to their ability to block metabolism of arachidonic acid via the cyclooxygenase pathway. A number of clinical and experimental observations support this hypothesis. Several drugs are also able to induce bronchoconstriction in ASA-sensitive persons, including indomethacin, aminopyrine, mefenamic acid, ibuprofen, naproxen, sulfinpyrazone, phenylbutazone, ketorolac,[913] and (rarely) tartrazine; all inhibit prostaglandin synthesis.[903] On the other hand, acetaminophen, sodium salicylate, and trisalicylates have little anti-cyclooxygenase activity and can be safely used in most ASA-sensitive patients.[914–916]

Of the two cyclooxygenase enzymes, the constitutively expressed COX-1 and the inducible COX-2, inhibition of the former is evidently required for ASA sensitivity.[917] The degree of bronchoconstriction these drugs induce *in vivo* has been shown to be proportional to their ability to retard prostaglandin synthesis *in vitro*.[908, 918, 919] It has been postulated that patients who have ASA-sensitive asthma produce large amounts of the bronchodilator $PGE_2$ in compensation for continued bronchoconstriction; when ASA or another anti-inflammatory agent is administered, an acute drop in $PGE_2$ synthesis precipitates an acute asthmatic attack.[908] Alternatively, it has been suggested that blockade of the cyclooxygenase series of enzymes diverts more arachidonic acid toward the lipoxygenase metabolic pathway, resulting in excessive production of bronchoconstricting leukotrienes. In fact, aspirin challenge causes a temporary increase in the urinary excretion of the leukotriene $LTE_4$,[920] and inhalation of lysine-aspirin causes increased release of leukotrienes into BAL fluid of sensitive persons.[921] Urinary leukotriene excretion has also been found to decrease during an ASA-desensitization protocol.[301] The importance of increased leukotriene production in the induction of ASA-sensitive asthma has been confirmed by the finding that pretreatment with either a lipoxygenase inhibitor or a leukotriene receptor antagonist markedly attenuates the response to ASA.[300, 922, 923]

Studies of HLA phenotype and aspirin-induced asthma have yielded conflicting results. One group showed that the HLA-DQw2 phenotype is a marker for aspirin-sensitive asthma;[924] however, this was not confirmed by two other groups of investigators[925, 926] (although an increased prevalence of the *DPB1*0101* allele was found in one of the studies[926]). In another study of 59 ASA-sensitive asthmatic patients, *HLA-DPB1*0301* was associated with a 4.4-fold increased risk, and *DPB1*0401,* with a 50% reduction in risk for ASA sensitivity compared with that in normal persons and in non–ASA-sensitive asthmatics.[927] The diagnosis of ASA-sensitive asthma can be made by challenging the patient via the oral, nasal, or inhaled route; lysine-aspirin is used for the inhaled challenges and can cause early and late asthmatic responses.[902]

From 10% to 30% of patients who have ASA-induced bronchoconstriction also show a paradoxical bronchial narrowing following intravenous administration of the corticosteroid hydrocortisone.[928, 929] Although it was initially believed that this reaction might be caused by preservative additives, bronchial narrowing clearly occurs with pure drug and may be secondary to an effect on prostaglandin metabolism. The effect is rarely marked and should not interfere with the therapeutic administration of systemic corticosteroids if they are otherwise indicated.[929, 930] In a very small number of patients who have asthma, treatment with aspirin or another nonsteroidal anti-inflammatory drug leads to improvement; in one such patient, the administration of a lipoxygenase inhibitor caused an acute asthmatic attack![931]

### Gastroesophageal Reflux

The association of asthma and gastroesophageal reflux (GER) is common, various investigators having estimated the concordance to be from 30% to over 80%.[932–934] There is evidence that GER can induce asthma, and that asthma can cause a worsening of GER. It is possible that GER triggers airway narrowing in susceptible persons by reflex bronchoconstriction secondary to stimulation of afferent nerves in the esophagus or pharynx and/or by direct aspiration of a small amount of esophageal contents.[934–937] In an animal model of GER, minute quantities of acid instilled into the tracheobronchial tree caused considerably greater bronchoconstriction than did acid in the esophagus, suggesting that such aspiration could be a powerful stimulus.[936] It is difficult to prove that reflux results in direct aspiration into the lung; however, in one study of four asthmatic patients who complained of GER, simultaneous decreases in esophageal and tracheal pH and profound decreases in PEFR were seen in 14% of 37 episodes of reflux.[938]

GER without aspiration is common in both normal and asthmatic persons[935, 939] and may or may not[940] precipitate airway narrowing. When acid is instilled into the esophagus of asthmatic patients, it is primarily those who develop symptoms of esophagitis who experience bronchoconstriction;[941–944] however, this can be seen even in those who have no symptoms of reflux.[945, 946] It has been suggested that because reflux is exacerbated during sleep as a result of recumbency and decreased tone in the lower esophageal sphincter, this could contribute to nocturnal asthma;[935, 947] however, a direct test of this hypothesis yielded negative results in one study.[948] GER reflux can transiently increase NSBR as well as causing bronchoconstriction in its own right.[949] Antacids and $H_1$ blockers reduce the esophageal and respiratory symptoms caused by GER,[941, 950] and some data indicate long-term improvement in respiratory function following antireflux therapy.[951] For example, in one study of 13 asthmatic patients who underwent surgical therapy for chronic GER, improvement in asthmatic symptoms and medication usage was seen in 11.[951a]

Asthma could exacerbate GER by causing dysfunction of the lower esophageal sphincter; the more negative intrathoracic pressure associated with hyperinflation decreases the effectiveness of the sphincter, and in severe cases of airway obstruction, there may actually be herniation of the sphincter into the thoracic cavity.[952] Methacholine-induced bronchoconstriction can cause a worsening of reflux.[953] Both beta-adrenergic agonists and theophylline can cause relaxation of the sphincter, thereby contributing to GER in asthma.[932] There is also a strong association of cough and GER in patients who have and those who do not have asthma (*see* Chapter 16, page 381).[932]

### Emotion

Emotional distress can trigger an attack in a patient who has asthma. In fact, mild bronchoconstriction and bronchodilation can be produced by suggestion, presumably as a result of changes in cholinergic vagal activity.[954–956] In some of the studies designed to test the effect of suggestion,[957] it is possible that airway cooling or drying caused by hyperventilation may have acted as a true physiologic stimulus for bronchoconstriction. Hyperventilation provoked by anxiety is common in asthmatics and can lead to a vicious circle, the hyperventilation causing bronchoconstriction as a result of hypocapnia and airway drying, which is then followed by an increase in anxiety.[958] Despite these observations, the emotional instability or dependence exhibited by some asthmatic patients is almost always a result of their disease rather than a factor predisposing to its development. Although emotional distress can trigger an attack in a patient who has asthma, there is no evidence that it plays a role in the basic pathophysiologic process that causes the asthmatic state. This was illustrated in one study in which patients who had urticaria had a similar degree of "psychologic distress" as in those who had asthma.[22] Besides the direct connection of the brain and the lung via the vagus nerve, there is abundant evidence for neural effects on the immune response, resistance to infection, and endocrine function, all of which could also have an influence on the development of asthma.[959]

### Environmental Factors

The importance of air pollution as a trigger of asthmatic attacks is not known precisely; however, a number of observations suggest that it has a significant effect in some patients. Although general atmospheric pollution is by far the most important in this regard, symptoms of asthma can also be related to "domestic air pollution." In fact, in one study of 164 asthmatics, the use of wood stoves, fireplaces, and gas stoves was associated with increased morbidity.[960]

It is clear that low levels of atmospheric chemical pollutants can cause functional abnormalities in patients who have hyper-reactive airways. A number of investigators have shown that emergency department visits and hospital admission rates for asthma are related to atmospheric levels of pollution, especially with sulfate aerosol and ozone ($O_3$).[961, 961a] In nonasthmatic individuals, cough and phlegm are more common in communities in which there are high ambient sulfur dioxide ($SO_2$) levels.[962a] In the ambient Los Angeles air, which contains, among other things, 0.14 part per million (ppm) of $O_3$, exercise has been found to cause a significant decrease in maximal expiratory flow when compared with a similar level of exercise in purified air.[963, 964] In another investigation of the relationship between air pollution and asthma in the Los Angeles area, investigators found the peak period of attacks to be during the early morning, despite the fact that maximal oxidant levels were recorded between 10

A.M. and 4 P.M.[965] However, a significantly greater number of persons had attacks on days when oxidant levels were high enough to cause eye irritation and damage to plants. Studies in the New Orleans area showed a sharp increase in the incidence of asthmatic attacks during June–July and October–November, periods during which atmospheric pollution also increased.[966–968]

A notable example of the relationship between air pollution and a syndrome characterized by acute respiratory distress resembling asthma was observed in U.S. armed forces in the Tokyo and Yokohama regions of Japan in the 1970s.[969, 970] The syndrome, which was called "Tokyo-Yokohama asthma," ceased when the patients were removed from the area. Since that time a number of striking examples of periodicity in asthma attack rates have been reported; however, they cannot all be explained by fluctuating levels of pollution.[971] For example, a peak in asthma emergency department visits was noted in Vancouver, Canada, starting in the last week of September and continuing for 3 weeks over 3 consecutive years;[972] in these periods, the number of patients seen weekly for asthma reached 130, compared with between 30 and 90 during the rest of the year. The peak affected children and adults between the ages of 15 and 60 years of age. The increased rate could not be explained by variations in atmospheric $SO_2$, nitrogen dioxide ($NO_2$), or $O_3$ measured at 11 monitoring stations in the city, suggesting that there are additional environmental causes of asthma periodicity. The spring and early summer increase in asthma attacks that occurs in Melbourne, Australia, also cannot be explained by atmospheric pollution; it occurs in temporal association with high grass pollen levels.[973] Large hatches of certain allergenic insects can also be responsible for outbreaks of asthma.[686, 687]

Environmental pollution has been considered as a potential culprit to explain the increase in the prevalence of asthma over the past three decades. However, there is little evidence to support the hypothesis of a direct effect of pollution.[974, 975] Nevertheless, it is possible that certain pollutants may alter the immunologic response to inhaled allergen, thus fostering an increase in allergic airway disease;[976, 977] in one study, low $O_3$ concentrations similar to those commonly occurring in urban areas increased the bronchial response to allergen in atopic asthmatic persons.[978]

The major respirable atmospheric chemicals that affect lung function are $O_3$ and the oxides of sulfur and nitrogen. As with viral infections, these agents can cause mild airway obstruction and increased NSBR in normal persons and can precipitate symptomatic exacerbations in asthmatic patients. In normal persons, exposure to $SO_2$ in concentrations of 0.5 to 1.0 ppm causes mild, transient, asymptomatic bronchoconstriction during exercise (when the dose of $SO_2$ reaching the airways is increased).[979–981] The effect is partly blocked by atropine and disodium cromoglycate, so that both reflex and mediator-related mechanisms may be operative.[982]

As might be expected, patients who have asthma are more sensitive than normal persons to the bronchoconstricting effects of $SO_2$; a concentration as low as 0.25 ppm can cause detectable obstruction during mild exercise,[983–986] and 5 minutes of heavy exercise in 0.4 or 0.5 ppm of $SO_2$ can cause transient symptomatic exacerbation (followed by recovery within 24 hours).[987] There may be some tachyphylaxis with repeated bouts of exercise at the same $SO_2$

concentration;[986, 988] for the same level of ventilation and $SO_2$ exposure, nasal breathing is protective, presumably because the very soluble $SO_2$ dissolves in the fluid lining the nasal mucosa and fails to reach the lower respiratory tract.[989, 990] The degree of bronchoconstriction caused by inhalation of $SO_2$ in asthmatic patients cannot be predicted by their response to histamine suggesting that the pollutant acts by different mechanisms.[991] The bronchoconstriction caused by $SO_2$ as well as that caused by breathing cold dry air is synergistic: when cold dry air is inspired, a concentration of $SO_2$ as low as 0.1 ppm will produce detectable airway obstruction.[992–994] On the basis of these observations, it can be concluded that $SO_2$ can cause airway narrowing and symptoms in asthmatic patients at concentrations well below accepted "standards"; such concentrations are frequently reached in urban industrial areas, and the effects are accentuated by exercise, mouth breathing, and cold dry air.

Ozone causes a dose-dependent decrease in expiratory flow rates and volumes as well as in total lung capacity (TLC) in both normal persons and asthmatic patients at a concentration as low as 0.12 ppm (0.000012%), making it the most potent irritant gas.[995–1005] As with $SO_2$, the effects are enhanced by exercise,[995, 1003–1005] and tolerance can develop with repeated exposure.[999] Of more interest than direct $O_3$-induced airway narrowing is the ability of brief $O_3$ exposure to increase subsequent NSBR in normal persons: 2 hours of exposure to 0.6 ppm of $O_3$ increases the subsequent response to inhaled histamine and methacholine for at least 24 hours without significantly increasing baseline values of airway resistance.[1006, 1007] Atropine blocks the effect of $O_3$ on NSBR, suggesting that the effect could be related to increased reactivity of cholinergic postganglionic pathways; however, atropine also substantially reduces the baseline airway resistance (prehistamine or premethacholine), creating difficulty in comparing these results with those for the nonatropine experiments.[1006]

A more likely explanation for the $O_3$-induced increase in airway responsiveness is the airway inflammatory response that follows exposure. As discussed previously, animal models and human studies of the $O_3$ effect suggest that the enhanced NSBR is mediated by airway inflammation.[1008–1011] In one study, analysis of nasal fluid of normal persons and asthmatic patients revealed increased levels of $LTB_4$, PAF, and IL-8 after exposure to ozone;[1012] the increase was greater in the asthmatics than in the controls. The degree of shift in histamine and methacholine response is small, and these exposures certainly do not alter the airway responsiveness of normal persons to the same extent as in patients who have spontaneous asthma; however, it is possible that the mechanism of the altered response is similar to that which occurs in asthma. In one study of 1,215 school children selected from a polluted industrial town and from a rural area, the prevalence of airway hyper-responsiveness was related to the level of pollution.[1013]

The oxides of nitrogen are another component of smog and industrial pollution that in low concentrations can precipitate symptomatic episodes in hyper-responsive persons. A transient increase in nitrogen dioxide ($NO_2$) levels to greater than 500 parts per billion (ppb) was blamed for an acute outbreak of asthma in Barcelona, Spain, in which 44 patients required hospital admission over a 2- to 3-hour period.[962] Inhalation of $NO_2$ at a concentration of 0.3 ppm

increases the severity of exercise-induced bronchoconstriction in asthmatic patients.[1014] In most studies, low-level $NO_2$ exposure (0.1 ppm for 1 hour or 910 μg/m³ for 20 minutes) has been found to enhance nonspecific airway responsiveness in asthmatic but not in normal individuals.[963, 964, 1015]

### Deep Inspiration

The effect of a deep inspiration on airway caliber in normal and asthmatic persons varies between individuals and is dependent on whether there is spontaneous or pharmacologically induced airway narrowing before the deep breath. Without previous administration of bronchoconstrictors, normal persons show a transient decrease in airway resistance and an increase in anatomic dead space after a deep inspiration, suggesting that large central airways dilate.[1016] Maximal expiratory flows also increase slightly, as judged by a comparison of flow rates on partial and complete flow-volume curves (Fig. 54–11). These effects decrease as a function of age.[1017] The situation is reversed in many patients who have asthma: when airway resistance is used as the test of airway caliber, there is a paradoxical narrowing and a decrease in dead space after a deep inspiration.[568, 1018] Maximal expiratory flows are not increased following deep inspiration, even when the overall flow is abnormally low; in fact, in some patients, the maximal flows can be less on a complete than on a partial flow-volume curve.[591, 1019, 1020] The bronchoconstrictor effect of a deep inspiration correlates with the severity of airway inflammation in asthmatic patients[1021] and with the severity of symptoms and the intensity of therapy in individual patients.[1022]

In normal persons, a deep breath also has a profound bronchodilating effect during pharmacologically induced airway narrowing, regardless of whether airway resistance

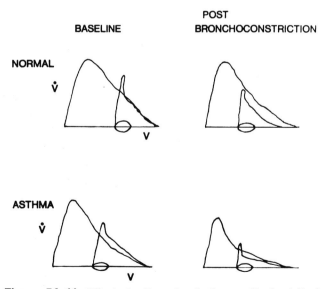

**Figure 54–11. Effect of a Deep Inspiration on Maximal Expiratory Flow.** Partial and complete flow-volume (V-V) curves before and after pharmacologically induced bronchoconstriction are shown for a normal subject and an asthmatic patient. At baseline, a deep inspiration does not increase maximal flow in the normal subject but causes a decrease in maximal flow in the asthmatic. Following bronchoconstriction, the normal subject shows marked reversibility following a deep inspiration, a feature shown by the asthmatic patient as well but to a lesser extent.

(Raw) or flows on a maximal flow-volume curve are used to estimate airway caliber (*see* Fig. 54–11). By contrast, the bronchodilating effect of a deep inspiration during induced bronchoconstriction is less than in normal persons and may not occur at all in asthmatic patients;[413, 1023, 1024] any effect is enhanced by a rapid deep inspiration and is attenuated by an end-inspiratory breath-hold.[1025, 1026]

The mechanisms responsible for changes in airway size associated with deep inspiration are incompletely understood and may be related to several factors. Normally, a deep breath can stimulate airway irritant and stretch receptors, the former mediating reflex bronchoconstriction and the latter dilatation. It has been suggested that excessive stimulation of irritant receptors in asthmatic patients is responsible for the paradoxical response to a deep breath in the nonchallenged condition; a study in which inhaled local anesthetic was shown to decrease the degree of bronchoconstriction supports this hypothesis.[1026] On the other hand, cholinergic blockade in normal persons has not been found to decrease the bronchodilating effect of a deep inspiration, suggesting that withdrawal of vagal efferent activity is not responsible for the dilatation.[1027]

During a deep breath, lung recoil is increased, thereby stretching airway smooth muscle. This effect would be expected to dilate the airways and reverse pharmacologically induced muscle shortening; however, because of lung pressure-volume hysteresis, the lung recoil at FRC is transiently decreased following a deep inspiration, thus tending to unload airway smooth muscle and allow increased shortening. It has been proposed that the variable response to a deep breath in asthmatic patients is related to a variation in the effects of smooth muscle and parenchymal stretch.[1028] In persons in whom a deep breath has little effect on smooth muscle tone but produces a decrease in lung recoil (and therefore smooth muscle load), narrowing of the airways would be expected. Bronchodilation would occur in those persons in whom a deep inspiration stretches smooth muscle considerably but reduces lung recoil only slightly.

A third possibility to explain the differences in the effect of a deep breath between normal and asthmatic patients is a change in the intrinsic smooth muscle response to stretch. Certain kinds of smooth muscle (such as the urinary bladder) show a "myogenic" response, consisting of a contraction following stretch. Although trachealis muscle in normal dogs relaxes when stretched, that from allergic dogs shows myogenic behavior. When smooth muscle from human airways is passively sensitized by incubating it overnight in a medium containing high levels of IgE to house dust mite, there is an enhancement of the myogenic response to a quick stretch.[1029] These data suggest that smooth muscle response to stretch could be altered in patients who have asthma.

As discussed previously (*see* page 2096), it has been proposed that the absent or deficient bronchodilating effect of a deep breath may be a major contributor to the nonspecific bronchial hyper-responsiveness (NSBH) of asthma.[413, 580, 1018] When histamine or methacholine dose-response curves from asthmatic and nonasthmatic persons are compared, there is much more overlap between the groups in decreases in expiratory flow and specific airway conductance measured before a deep inspiration than for isovolume flow and $FEV_1$ measured after a deep inspiration.[580, 584] These observations have led to the suggestion that NSBH in asthma may be related more to an impaired capacity to bronchodilate with increased lung volume than to enhanced end-organ responsiveness.[413]

### Miscellaneous Factors

**Food Additives.** Certain food additives can precipitate acute bronchoconstriction in asthmatic patients.[1030] The most commonly implicated is metabisulfite, to which approximately 4% of asthmatic patients demonstrate sensitivity.[1031] As a result of their antioxidant activity, salts of this substance prevent discoloration and thus are used as preservatives in a wide variety of foods and beverages, including wine, beer, fruit juices, fresh fruits and vegetables, and seafood.[1032] They cause bronchoconstriction by producing $SO_2$, which is inhaled during swallowing. The response to wine depends on its $SO_2$ content; the higher the level, the greater the response.[1033] Sensitivity can be documented by careful oral challenges using capsules containing increasing amounts of metabisulfite.[1032] Paradoxical dose-dependent bronchoconstriction has also been reported in response to a beta-adrenergic agonist containing sodium bisulfite.[1034] Monosodium glutamate and the food coloring additive tartrazine can also cause attacks.[1030, 1035] ASA-sensitive asthmatic subjects frequently are also sensitive to tartrazine, suggesting that the mechanism of action of the two substances may be similar.

**Alcohol.** Alcohol-containing beverages have been reported to precipitate attacks of bronchoconstriction in some asthmatic patients: in a questionnaire study of 168 patients, 32% reported that alcohol, usually in the form of beer, wine, or whiskey, worsened their symptoms, whereas 23% suggested that they received some benefit, usually from whiskey or brandy.[1036] Although in some cases the bronchoconstriction is caused by the metabisulfite, adverse responses to pure ethanol administered orally have also been documented. Because acetaldehyde leads to degranulation of mast cells and/or basophils, alcohol may have its effect by elevating blood acetaldehyde levels;[1037] clearly, this effect would be especially likely in individuals who have a genetic defect in the metabolism of acetaldehyde. Asians, who have a very high incidence of acetaldehyde dehydrogenase deficiency, often manifest vasomotor responsiveness to ethanol and may be particularly sensitive to its bronchoconstricting effects.[1038] Affected persons develop rapid onset of flushing, nasal congestion, and wheeze; the response is attenuated by histamine $H_1$ and cyclooxygenase blockers but not by atropine.[1038, 1039] Red wine is a not infrequent precipitant; although its effect could also be related to metabisulfite, one group of investigators attributed it to the histamine content of the wine coupled with diminished histamine degradation.[1040]

**Drugs.** Beta-adrenergic blocking agents are widely used for the treatment of hypertension, anxiety, tremor, glaucoma, and arrhythmias and cause acute attacks of asthma in as many as 50% of asthmatic patients, even when used topically in the eye.[914] Although angiotensin-converting enzyme (ACE) inhibitors can cause cough and angioedema, presumably as a result of the inhibition of metabolism of substance P and bradykinin, they do not seem to cause these complications more often in asthmatic patients than in nonasthmatic patients.[1041] Despite this, the results of one investigation suggest that asthmatic patients are in danger of worsening disease within the first few weeks of therapy using an ACE inhibitor.[1042] Additional studies on the relationships between ACE therapy, cough, and bronchospasm are reviewed in Chapter 63, page 2570.

Asthmatic patients are at increased risk of a serious adverse response to radiographic contrast agents.[1043] Severe asthma has been reported following ingestion of ergometrine for the control of postpartum hemorrhage;[1044] because ergometrine in low concentration causes contraction of canine tracheal smooth muscle, its effect on human airway smooth muscle could be direct.[1044]

**Perfumes.** A large number of asthmatics report a worsening of symptoms in the presence of certain odors, of which perfume and cologne are the most frequently mentioned offenders; in fact, exposure to these aromas has been associated with objective evidence of worsening air-flow obstruction.[1045, 1046] Even perfume-scented strips in magazines can cause exacerbations of symptoms and airway obstruction; severe and atopic asthma increases the risk of such reactions.[1047]

**Cigarette Smoke.** Patients who have asthma frequently complain of an exacerbation of symptoms following passive exposure to cigarette smoke. In one study of 10 subjects, side-stream smoke sufficient to increase carboxyhemoglobin by only 0.4% resulted in an average 21% decline in $FEV_1$.[1048] In addition, asthmatic children of smoking women have been shown to have more symptoms and lower expiratory flow rates than do children of women who do not smoke.[1049] Despite these observations, in one investigation of approximately 50 smokers who also had asthma, little change in flow rates was recorded after one cigarette.[1050]

**Menstruation.** Up to 30% of women who have asthma experience increased symptoms in the premenstrual period; these are associated with a decrease in maximal expiratory flow and are not attributable to the use of ASA.[1051–1053] Some asthmatic women have been unaware that their asthma was worsening during the premenstrual period until there was formal documentation;[1054] estradiol therapy was associated with a significant reduction in asthma symptoms and improvement in dyspnea index scores. In another study, intramuscular progesterone therapy eliminated severe premenstrual declines in peak flow in three women and allowed a reduction in corticosteroid therapy.[1055]

**Environmental Temperature and Pressure.** Outbreaks of asthma have been reported following thunderstorms and sudden changes in barometric pressure, temperature, and humidity.[1056] Although these outbreaks could be the result of the climatic changes, they could also be secondary to enhanced exposure to specific allergens; heavy rain can cause a massive release of fungal spores[1057] and of allergen particles from grass pollen.[669]

## Occupational Asthma

The observation that asthma can be caused by exposure to inhaled substances in the workplace has been appreciated for a long time, and more than 250 chemicals have now been implicated (Table 54–2).[1058–1061] The condition is important: it has been estimated that as many as 15% to 20% of all cases of asthma can be attributed to occupational exposure,[1058] although to the average chest physician, even one with a high index of suspicion for occupational asthma, these estimates will seem excessive. At least 7.8 million U.S. workers have potential contact with one or more causative agents.[1062] In addition, occupational asthma is now the most common form of occupational lung disease, accounting for as many as 50% of all cases.[1063–1065] The discovery of new occupations or compounds associated with asthma requires a high index of suspicion and careful history taking; it should not be forgotten that the offending exposure is not necessarily associated with the patient's primary occupation but may instead be related to a hobby. It is important to recognize that asthma related solely to occupational exposure can sometimes be "cured" by avoiding exposure to the specific causative agent, making its early recognition especially important; recognition also allows for the protection of other workers.

Various mechanisms contribute singly or in combination to the production of asthmatic symptoms and airway narrowing during occupational exposure. In one comprehensive review, the authors defined categories based on four mechanisms:[16] reflex, acute inflammatory, pharmacologic, and immunologic. The last-named was in turn subdivided into two groups: (1) exposures associated with proven allergic pathophysiology, in which a high-molecular-weight substance or a low-molecular-weight hapten, combined with a protein, can be implicated; and (2) exposures in which an immunologic mechanism was likely but unproved and in which low-molecular-weight substances are the offending agents. We prefer to limit the designation "occupational asthma" to those cases that predominantly fit in the immunologic category (both high- and low-molecular-weight groups), in which the patient's asthma is caused by exposure to a specific sensitizing agent in the workplace; we do not include in this designation cases in which pre-existing asthma is worsened by nonspecific bronchoconstriction in response to irritants in the workplace (reflex), or those in which a single exposure to a toxic substance causes an "acute inflammatory" reaction leading to persistent reactive airways disease (reactive airways dysfunction syndrome [RADS]). Finally, there are a variety of occupational lung diseases that affect airway function (e.g., byssinosis) but that we do not believe fulfill the diagnostic criteria for asthma. These are discussed separately.

The proven and possible allergic forms of occupational asthma are the most important in terms of the numbers of affected persons; although only a small subset of exposed workers develop sensitization (i.e., the response is idiosyncratic), the prevalence of affected workers in any specific work environment is related to the level of exposure to the offending agent.[1066, 1067]

### *Proven Allergic Bronchoconstriction*

Table 54–1 contains a list of agents and occupations in which a specific IgE-induced allergic mechanism has been proved. For the most part, the antigens are high-molecular-weight proteins, polysaccharides, or glycoproteins derived from plants or animals. However, the IgE may also be directed against a complex of a host protein and a low-molecular-weight agent that acts as a hapten; examples of this mechanism include sensitivity to platinum salts and acid anhydrides. Sensitivity develops predominantly in workers who are atopic and have a positive immediate skin test or

## Table 54–2. CAUSES AND MECHANISMS OF OCCUPATIONAL ASTHMA

| AGENT | OCCUPATION |
|---|---|

### PROVEN ALLERGIC

*Animals and Animal Products*

| | |
|---|---|
| Laboratory animals (rats, mice, rabbits, guinea pigs, and monkeys), hair, and urine | Laboratory workers, veterinarians, animal handlers[1576] |
| Birds (pigeons, chickens, budgerigars) | Bird breeders and poultry workers |
| Mink | Mink breeder[1577] |
| Alpha-lactalbumin | Chocolate manufacture[1578] |
| Cow dander | Agricultural worker[1579] |
| Pig | Butcher[1580] |
| Frog | Frog catcher[1581] |
| Chicken | Poultry worker[1582] |
| Casein (cow's milk) | Tanner[1583] |

*Insects*

| | |
|---|---|
| Poultry mites | Poultry workers[1584] |
| Grain mites, flour weevils | Grain and mill workers[1079] |
| Storage mites | Farmers[1586] |
| Locusts | Research laboratory |
| River fly | Power plants along rivers |
| Screw worm fly | Flight crews and entomologists |
| Cockroaches | Laboratory workers[1587] |
| Crickets | Field contact |
| Bee moth | Fish bait breeder |
| Moths, butterflies, and blow flies | Entomologists[1588, 1589] |
| Sewer flies | Sewer workers[1590] |
| Silkworm larvae | Sericulture[1588] |
| Honeybees and honeybee pollen | Apiary workers[1591, 1592] |
| *Dactylopius coccus* | Dye manufacture[1593] |
| Red spider mite (*Tetranychus urticae*) | Flower industry[1594] |
| *Chrysoperla carnea, Leptinotarsa decemlineata, Ostrinia nubilalis, Ephestia kuehniella* | "Bio-factories" for production of beneficial arthropods for use in pest control[1595] |
| Sheep blow fly | Technicians[1596] |
| *Daphnia* | Fish food store[1597] |
| Acarian | Apple growers[1598] |
| Fruit fly | Laboratory worker[1599] |
| Mexican bean weevil | [1600] |

*Marine Animals*

| | |
|---|---|
| Snow crabs and prawns | Crab and prawn processing[1070, 1601] |
| Hoya (sea squirt) | Oyster farming |

*Plants and Plant Products*

| | |
|---|---|
| Grain dust | Grain elevator and storage workers, dock workers |
| Wheat, rye, and buckwheat flour | Bakers and millers[1602] |
| Green coffee beans | Coffee bean handlers[1603, 1604] |
| Castor bean, soybean | Oil industry, felt industry,[1605] and seamen[1606] |
| Tea | Tea workers |
| Tulips and narcissi | Gardeners[1079] |
| Tobacco leaf | Tobacco handling and cigarette manufacture |
| Baby's breath (*Gypsophila paniculata*) | Florists[1607] |
| Hops | Beer brewers |
| Garlic | Spice manufacture[1608, 1609] |
| Curry, coriander, and mace | Spice industry[1610] |
| Buckwheat | Bakers, cooks[1611] |
| Cacao | Chocolate manufacture[1612] |
| Guar gum | Carpet manufacture |
| Pectin | Manufacture of jam[1613] |
| Green tea (epigallocatechin gallate) | Tea factory[1614] |
| Soybean lecithin | Bakers[1615] |
| *Pfaffia paniculata* root powder | Manufacture of ginseng capsules[1616] |

*Biologic Products and Enzymes*

| | |
|---|---|
| *Bacillus subtilis* | Detergent industry |
| Trypsin, pancreatin, papain, pepsin, flaviastase, bromelin, fungal amylase | Plastics, pharmaceutical, and laboratory personnel[1114, 1617] |
| Lactase | Plastics, pharmaceutical, and laboratory personnel[1114, 1617, 1618] |
| Subtilisin | Plastics, pharmaceutical, and laboratory personnel[1114, 1617, 1619] |
| Bovine serum albumin | Plastics, pharmaceutical, and laboratory personnel[1114, 1617, 1620] |
| Senna | Plastics, pharmaceutical, and laboratory personnel[1114, 1617, 1621] |
| Psyllium (*Ispaghula* husks) | Plastics, pharmaceutical, and laboratory personnel[1114, 1617, 1621] |
| Erythropoietin (EPO60) | Plastics, pharmaceutical, and laboratory personnel[1114, 1617, 1622] |
| Human corticotropin-releasing factor | Plastics, pharmaceutical, and laboratory personnel[1114, 1617, 1623] |

*Vegetables*

| | |
|---|---|
| Gum acacia | Printers |
| Gum tragacanth | Gum manufacturing[1624] |
| Cellulase | |

**Table 54–2. CAUSES AND MECHANISMS OF OCCUPATIONAL ASTHMA** *Continued*

| AGENT | OCCUPATION |
|---|---|
| *Metals and Other Haptens* | |
| Ninhydrin | Forensic laboratory worker[1625] |
| Platinum | Platinum refinery workers |
| Anhydrides (phthalic, trimellitic, pyromellitic tetrachlorophthalic, hexahydrophthalic) | Epoxy resin and plastics manufacture and use[1626–1628] |

**NOT PROVEN ALLERGIC**

| AGENT | OCCUPATION |
|---|---|
| *Diisocyanates* | |
| Toluene, 1,5-naphthylene, diphenylmethane, and hexamethylene diisocyanate | Polyurethane industry, plastics manufacture, foundry, paint, rubber, and varnish workers[1629–1634] |
| *Wood Dusts* | |
| Western red cedar, eastern white cedar, California redwood, cedar of Lebanon, Cocabolla, Iroko oak, Mahogany, abiruana, African maple, Tanganyika aningie, Central American walnut, kejaat, and African zebra wood | Carpenters, cabinet makers, construction and sawmill workers[1117, 1635] |
| *Metals* | |
| Nickel | Metal plating; dental workers[1636] |
| Chromium | Tanning |
| Aluminum salts | Aluminum manufacture[1170, 1171, 1637] |
| Cobalt, vanadium, and tungsten carbide | Hard metal workers, diamond polishers[1638] |
| *Fluxes* | |
| Aminoethyl ethanolamine | Aluminum soldering |
| Colophony | Electronics industry |
| *Drugs* | |
| Penicillin, cephalosporins, phenylglycine acid chloride, piperazine hydrochloride, methyldopa, spiramycin, amprolium hydrochloride, tetracycline, sulfone chloramides | Pharmaceutical industry, chemists, nurses, brewers, poultry feed mixture |
| Morphine | Pharmaceutical industry, chemists, nurses, brewers, poultry feed mixture[1639] |
| Hydralazine | Pharmaceutical industry, chemists, nurses, brewers, poultry feed mixture[1640] |
| Ipecacuanha | Pharmaceutical industry, chemists, nurses, brewers, poultry feed mixture[1641] |
| Salbutamol | Pharmaceutical industry, chemists, nurses, brewers, poultry feed mixture[1642] |
| Ceftazidime | Pharmaceutical industry, chemists, nurses, brewers, poultry feed mixture[1643] |
| Piperacillin | Pharmaceutical industry, chemists, nurses, brewers, poultry feed mixture[1644] |
| Methacholine | Pharmaceutical industry, chemists, nurses, brewers, poultry feed mixture[1645] |
| *Other Chemicals* | |
| Dimethyl ethanolamine | Spray painters, cleaners[1646] |
| Persulfate salts and henna | Hairdressers[1647, 1648] |
| Ethylene diamine | Photographers, chemical workers[1649] |
| Azobisformamide | Plastics industry[1650] |
| Azodicarbonamide | Plastic and rubber industry[1650] |
| Diazonium salt | Photocopying and dyeing[1651] |
| Glutaraldehyde, hexachlorophene and formalin | Hospital staff[1652] |
| Urea formaldehyde | Insulation and resin workers |
| Freon | Refrigeration |
| Paraphenylene diamine | Fur dyeing |
| Furfuryl alcohol | Foundry mold making[1653] |
| Polyvinylchloride | Plastics manufacture and meat wrappers[1183, 1654] |
| Oil mists | Machinists[1655] |
| Hydroquinones and methionine | Chemical workers[1656] |
| Acid vapors | Mineral analysis laboratory workers[1657] |
| Isothiazolinone | Chemical plant operator[1658] |
| Triglycidyl isocyanurate | Spray painter[1659] |
| Benzisothiazolin | Detergent plant[1660] |
| Lauryl dimethyl benzyl ammonium chloride | Cleaning agent[1661] |
| Sodium iso-nonanoyl oxybenzene sulfonate (SINOS) | Bleach manufacture[1662] |
| Styrene | Chemical plant[1663] |
| Remazol dyes | Textile dyeing[1664] |
| Lanasol yellow 4G dye | Cotton dyeing[1665] |
| Blue dye number 2 (indigotin) | Food processing[1666] |
| Quaternary amines (benzalkonium chloride) | Janitorial work[1667] |
| Aliphatic polyamines | Chemical factory workers[1668] |
| Aliphatic and cycloaliphatic diamines | Resin hardening[1669] |
| Tetrachloroisophthalonitrile | Garden fungicide[1670] |
| Captafol fungicide | Chemical manufacture[1671] |
| Tibutyl tin oxide | Carpet fungicide[1672] |
| Acrylate adhesives (cyanoacrylate and methacrylate—"crazy glue," "super glue") | Dental workers[1673] and other occupations[1674, 1675] |
| Ammonia | Silver polishing[1676] |
| Polyester | Spray painting[1677] |
| Polypropylene | Plastic bag manufacture[1678] |
| Polyfunctional aziridine | Paint manufacture[1679] |
| Metabisulfite | Food processing[1680] |

a specific IgE response (positive result on RAST) to the occupational agent. Cigarette smokers appear to have a markedly increased risk for sensitization to IgE-inducing agents;[1068, 1069] in one study of such workers exposed to platinum salts, the relative risk was 5.[1070]

The prevalence of allergic occupational asthma in occupations at risk is approximately 20%, a figure similar to that for atopy in the general population.[1071, 1072] This suggests that after intense and prolonged exposure to aeroallergens, most atopic persons will develop manifestations of allergic airway disease. Moreover, some occupational allergens appear to be particularly capable of eliciting an IgE response, even in nonatopic persons; for example, as many as 66% of workers exposed to *Bacillus subtilis* enzymes in the detergent industry develop asthma.[1073, 1074] Some allergens may be encountered in occupational and nonoccupational settings. Between 1981 and 1986, at least 12 outbreaks of asthma occurred in the city of Barcelona. The recognition that the majority of affected persons lived close to the harbor led to a search for the responsible agent, which was eventually proved to be soybeans, which were periodically unloaded at one of the docks.[1075] Although dockworkers were preferentially affected, the "epidemic" spread into the adjoining area of the city, and in this sense it does not fit the strict diagnostic criteria for occupational asthma.

**Animal Products.** Up to 30% of exposed workers develop specific IgE responses to proteins from the fur or urine of rats, mice, guinea pigs, or rabbits. Symptoms begin within 4 years of initial exposure; conjunctivitis and rhinitis commonly precede the onset of bronchoconstriction.[1076] HLA-B14 and -DR4 have been associated with an increased risk of sensitization to some of these animals.[1077] Seafood exposure has emerged as an important cause of occupational asthma.[1078] Exposed workers include fishers, processing plant personnel, and cooks; recreational anglers exposed to live bait fish are also at risk.[1079] Agents that have been shown to be associated with asthma include snow and king crabs, prawns, squid, oysters, trout, and dried or processed fishmeal.[1078]

**Grain Dust.** A small percentage of atopic workers develop IgE-mediated acute and delayed airway responses to specific antigens in grain dust, including those related to mites and weevils, and to the specific grains themselves.[1080] It is of interest that the incidence of atopy in grain elevator workers is less than in the general population, presumably because persons who have atopy, asthma, and increased nonspecific airway responsiveness avoid or drop out of that particular workforce.[1081, 1082] However, pre-employment respiratory symptoms, positive allergy skin test results, and increased NSBR are significantly associated with the development of work-related respiratory complaints in seasonal grain handlers.[1083]

Chronic exposure to grain dust may result in persistent functional derangement. For example, in one study of 587 grain elevator workers, 288 had respiratory symptoms and 102 showed significant impairment of lung function.[1084] Exposure of 22 of the 102 patients to grain dust was associated with an immediate and/or late response typical of an IgE-mediated allergic airway reaction in 6; the remaining 16 exhibited more fixed airway obstruction, presumably representing a form of industrial bronchitis or COPD. This form

of occupational airway disease is discussed in more detail in Chapter 55 (*see* page 2175).

About 5% to 20% of bakers develop allergy manifested by rhinitis and/or asthma.[1072] Unlike the situation in grain workers, specific allergy to cereal grains (wheat, rye, barley, oats, and triticale) can be detected by skin tests and RAST in the vast majority of affected persons. Sensitivity to cereals, including rice, can also be seen in people who cook at home.[1085] Rarely, persons who are allergic to flour show cross-reacting sensitization to bananas.[1086]

**Latex.** There has been a substantial increase in the prevalence of allergic skin and airway sensitivity to latex among workers involved in the manufacture and inspection of latex products and among health care workers and patients who use latex gloves or are exposed to latex products.[1087–1093] The reactions can range from mild urticaria to life-threatening anaphylaxis.[1094] In one large study of 2,062 employees in a general hospital in Canada, latex allergy documented by skin testing was present in 12%;[1095] predictors of sensitization included atopy and the presence of work-related symptoms. In another investigation of 100 patients who had spina bifida, latex allergy was identified in 29%;[1096] an association was found between sensitization and the number of medical procedures (operations, bladder catheterizations, and cystoscopies) that the patients had undergone.

The increase in latex sensitivity appears to be at least partly related to the switch from talc to cornstarch as the most commonly used lubricant in the gloves; although cornstarch is not more efficient than talc in binding latex allergens, it may remain airborne longer and thus more easily reach the lower respiratory tract.[1097] However, there also appears to be an increase in the prevalence of latex allergy in the general population; for example, in one study of 1,000 blood donors (in which health care workers were excluded), 6.4% had positive tests for anti–latex IgE antibodies.[1098] It is possible that this general increase in sensitivity is related to higher levels of airborne latex allergens derived from automobile tire debris.[1099, 1100] It is of interest that some affected persons show cross-reactivity to allergens derived from fruits such as bananas, avocados, kiwi, plums, peaches, figs, and chestnuts,[673, 1101–1104] and some cross-reactivity between latex antibodies and ragweed and pollen allergens has also been documented.[1105]

Latex allergy can be diagnosed with high sensitivity and specificity using skin tests or a measure of latex-specific IgE in the serum.[1106] Cornstarch used in surgical gloves can also elicit an allergic response by itself,[1107] as occurred in two nurses who experienced anaphylaxis on this basis.[1108]

**Miscellaneous Substances.** Allergic sensitization to the high-molecular-weight laxative psyllium is another cause of occupational asthma and anaphylaxis in health care workers.[1109, 1110] One nurse suffered mild recurrent rhinitis while preparing the medication for patients but experienced severe life-threatening anaphylaxis when she ingested some herself.[1111] Of 193 workers in chronic care institutions, 5% showed a positive skin test to psyllium and 12% had circulating specific IgE.[1112] Workers who prepare these medications are also at risk. In a study of 125 pharmaceutical workers who prepared psyllium from *Ispaghula* husks and the laxative senna from senna seeds, 8% were allergic to psyllium and 15% were allergic to senna; four cases of definite occupational asthma were identified.[1113] In another study, 48 of

92 exposed pharmaceutical factory workers developed respiratory, eye, or skin symptoms during exposure to *Ispaghula*.[1114]

In one study of 14 workers who had long-term exposure to pancreatic extracts in the pharmaceutical industry, three patterns of response were distinguished:[1115] all showed positive immediate skin tests to pancreatic extracts, and some had positive inhalation challenges; 2 of the 14 had documented extrinsic allergic alveolitis, and 7 had clinical signs suggestive of emphysema. Although it was possible that the last named was related to enzymatic elastolytic destruction, there was no documentation of loss of lung recoil or pathologic confirmation of emphysema.

### Possible Allergic Bronchoconstriction

The list of low-molecular-weight (less than 1,000) substances that can induce asthma in exposed workers is constantly increasing (*see* Table 54–1). Many features are present in this form of industrial asthma that suggest an allergic mechanism: (1) only about 5% of exposed persons develop asthma, and the occurrence of sensitivity is not strictly dose-dependent—both factors that argue against a direct toxic or pharmacologic effect; (2) after a latent period, sensitization increases with the duration of exposure, as in proven allergic airway syndromes; (3) exposure to a minute concentration of the offending agent results in classic immediate and/or late bronchoconstrictive responses, the latter being followed by a prolonged increase in NSBH; (4) hapten-specific IgE is present in some cases, with tissue and blood eosinophilia present in many;[16, 1116] and (5) activated T cells and eosinophils are present in the airway walls of affected persons.[1117]

Despite these observations, a number of other features argue against classic type I or III allergy as the cause of these syndromes, including (1) the absence of positive skin responses and specific IgE or IgG in many patients, (2) the presence of specific IgE and IgG in asymptomatic workers, (3) no difference in the prevalence of sensitization between atopic and nonatopic persons, and (4) the fact that cigarette smokers are less likely to develop sensitivity, the exact opposite of allergic bronchoconstriction associated with high-molecular-weight allergens.[1068]

**Plicatic Acid.** This substance is a component of western red cedar *(Thuja plicata)* and is the best studied in this category. A case has also been reported of a sawmill worker who was sensitive to eastern white cedar *(Thuja occidentalis)* and who showed cross-reactivity to western red cedar; eastern white cedar contains approximately half the plicatic acid present in the western red variety.[1118] The clinical, epidemiologic, and pathophysiologic features of the syndrome associated with exposure to this agent have been most clearly documented in cedar sawmill workers.[1119–1123] Approximately 4% of such workers develop sensitivity to plicatic acid over an exposure period ranging from months to years. There are no clinical or historical characteristics, including the presence or absence of atopy, that permit prediction of which workers will be affected. Specific IgE antibody to plicatic acid–human serum albumin conjugate is found in approximately 40% of patients tested. In one study of 185 patients, inhalation provocation testing showed isolated immediate airway reactions in 7%, isolated late reactions in 44%, and dual reactions in 49%.[1119] Patients who

have a dual response have significantly more severe asthma, associated with a lower baseline $FEF_{25-75}$ and a greater degree of NSBH.[1124] The degree of NSBR can predict the response to plicatic acid, and NSBR is increased in severity following development of a late response to western red cedar.[1118, 1125] Symptoms of cough and dyspnea can be insidious in onset and predominantly nocturnal, presumably as a result of the delayed response, making diagnosis difficult. Both symptoms and pulmonary function abnormalities increase with the duration and intensity of exposure.[1126]

The prognosis for recovery following the development of western red cedar sensitivity is similar to that for other low-molecular-weight agents.[1127, 1128] Approximately 60% of sensitive persons have persistent symptoms 4 years after cessation of exposure; those whose symptoms are of longer duration prior to diagnosis and whose pulmonary function is worse at diagnosis are less likely to recover completely.[1119, 1120, 1127, 1129, 1130] The $PC_{20}$ for methacholine at the time of diagnosis is predictive of outcome, and workers who show no improvement also have persisting NSBH.[1127, 1130]

**Anhydrides.** The anhydrides are used in the production of epoxy resins, plastics, and adhesives. Exposure to these agents can cause one of four clinical syndromes: (1) a simple irritant response, (2) asthma and rhinitis, (3) delayed airway obstruction accompanied by systemic symptoms, and (4) rarely, alveolar hemorrhage and anemia.[1131–1133] Immunoglobulins directed against anhydride–protein conjugates have been implicated in the pathogenesis of the asthma–rhinitis syndrome (IgE) and the late systemic response (IgG).[1134–1136] Risk factors for the development of sensitivity include the level of exposure and the development of specific IgE or IgG.[1137] A reduction in exposure levels in the workplace results in a decreased incidence of the late IgG-mediated syndrome but not of the IgE response.[1138] Sensitization has been associated with HLA-DR3.[1139] The prognosis of anhydride-related asthma appears to be better than isocyanate- or plicatic acid–induced asthma; in one study of 11 patients, there were no residual pulmonary function abnormalities or symptoms 1 year after removal from exposure.[1140]

**Isocyanates.** These substances are used as hardeners in paint, varnish, molds, polyurethane foam, adhesives, and plastics. Exposure to them, particularly to toluene diisocyanate (TDI), is the most common cause of occupational asthma. The risk to exposed workers is substantial; up to 20% develop airway sensitivity.[16, 1141, 1142] TDI, hexamethylene diisocyanate (HDI), or diphenylmethane diisocyanate (MDI) hypersensitivity can cause persistent asthma despite removal from the occupational source.[1141, 1143, 1144] The clinical, epidemiologic, and pathophysiologic features are similar to those of plicatic acid sensitivity, although a nonspecific irritant reaction, RADS, and extrinsic allergic alveolitis have also been reported.[1145–1148] The prognosis for recovery appears to be somewhat worse than disease caused by plicatic acid,[1149] and several fatal cases have been reported.[1150, 1151] The pathologic changes in the airway mucosa of patients who have TDI-related asthma have been studied in autopsy and biopsy material and have been found to be similar to those in extrinsic asthma.[1151, 1152] Despite evidence for permanent and severe damage in some cases, examination of serial biopsy specimens has shown that removal from exposure can result in reversal of the pathologic abnormalities.[1153]

An isolated negative methacholine challenge for NSBH does not exclude the presence of TDI hypersensitivity, because NSBR decreases after an affected person leaves the workplace.[1154] As with plicatic acid, a delayed response is associated with a prolonged increase in NSBR.[392, 1155, 1241] In one study of 114 patients who had TDI-induced asthma, challenge with the agent was followed by an isolated immediate response in 24 patients, a dual response in 40, and an isolated late response in 50;[1156] the patients who had the dual response had a longer history of symptoms and more severe airway obstruction prior to challenge. In another study, both the delayed response and the increased NSBR were shown to be blocked by high doses of oral prednisone.[1157] Animal models have been used to study the mechanism of the enhanced nonspecific response: in guinea pigs, TDI causes severe airway inflammation and epithelial damage and can increase the sensitivity and maximal response of the trachealis muscle.[1158, 1159]

Sensitivity to isocyanates is associated with the *HLA-DQB1\*0503* allele and the allelic combination *DQB1\*0201/0301*. In addition, the allele *DQB1\*0501* and the haplotype *DQA1\*0101-DQB1\*0501-DR1* have been found to be more prevalent in exposed but healthy persons, suggesting a protective effect.[1160–1163] The results of another study suggest that an amino acid substitution in the DQB1 antigen may be directly involved in the pathogenesis.[1164]

**Metals.** Of the metals and metal salts that induce asthma, platinum is the best documented; there is strong evidence that the reaction is IgE-mediated[1165] and is related to the intensity of exposure and to cigarette smoking.[1166] Cobalt sensitivity also seems to be related to allergen-specific IgE.[1167] The mechanism and prevalence of asthma caused by zinc, nickel, chromium, and aluminum have been less well established.[1168–1175] Some aluminum workers develop chronic air-flow obstruction; although the condition is often called "potroom asthma," in most cases it appears to be another example of occupational COPD.[1176]

**Miscellaneous Substances.** Although formaldehyde was first reported as a cause of occupational asthma in 1939, its importance as a sensitizer is unclear;[1177] in one investigation of 28 patients who complained of respiratory symptoms related to exposure, only 3 had definite immediate responses, late responses, or both.[1177, 1178] Urea formaldehyde used as an insulator or binder in particle board has been reported to cause asthma.[1179, 1180] In addition to its use as a tissue fixative, glutaraldehyde is employed in the processing of x-ray films and in the cleaning of endoscopes; asthma has been reported in workers exposed to the substance in all of these settings.[1181, 1182]

The existence of "meat wrappers' asthma," thought to be caused by the cutting of polyvinylchloride film on a hot wire, is questionable; several investigators have failed to show objective evidence of airway narrowing in exposed workers, despite ocular and bronchial symptoms.[1183, 1184] In one case, bronchial challenge was positive in a person whose symptoms were related to a shrink-wrapping process that employed polyethylene rather than polyvinylchloride.[1185]

Although the soldering agent colophony, a product of pine resin, has been used for over 100 years, asthma secondary to exposure was not recognized until 1977.[1186–1188] It is now recognized that the substance is a relatively common cause of both occupational asthma and contact dermatitis.[1189, 1190] In one retrospective study, many workers who left an electronics factory for respiratory health reasons had been exposed to solder flux—an illustration of how workers can self-select prior to diagnosis or medical intervention.[1191] Solder fluxes that do not contain colophony also have been reported to cause asthma.[1192]

### Diagnosis

The diagnosis of occupational asthma requires the demonstration that the patient's symptoms are caused by asthma and are related to the work environment. As with nonoccupational asthma, the diagnosis is established by a combination of clinical history, allergy skin tests, routine pulmonary function tests, bronchodilator response testing, and tests of NSBR. Although these tests are helpful, they may not be sufficient to provide a definitive diagnosis in some patients. In these persons, challenge with the suspected agent is required for confirmation. Documentation that the asthma is caused by work- or hobby-related exposure requires a high index of suspicion. A carefully taken occupational history should be obtained from all patients who have adult-onset asthma; it is worth emphasizing that in some cases occupational exposure can also exacerbate pre-existing asthma. Six major categories of exposure should be considered in taking a history: (1) animals, shellfish, fish, or arthropods; (2) wood, plants, and vegetables; (3) enzymes and pharmaceutical agents; (4) chemicals (including solder fluxes and dyes); (5) metals; and (6) dusts, fumes, and gases.[1059] Although substances associated with dental work do not fit easily into any of these categories, it should be remembered that dentists and dental technicians are at risk for occupational asthma and other respiratory diseases.[1193]

Because most respirologists are not experienced in the assessment of occupational hazards, it may be appropriate to consult an expert in occupational health or a public health authority if it is unclear whether an occupational exposure is involved.[1059] This may be especially helpful if symptoms develop during or immediately after exposure to a specific agent, or if there is a high incidence of respiratory complaints in similarly exposed workers. However, symptoms can begin after working hours or can be solely nocturnal. Patients should be questioned concerning remission of their symptoms during weekends and holidays and exacerbation on return to work. Although almost one half of patients who have occupational asthma develop symptoms in the first 2 years of exposure, it should be remembered that symptoms first occur after 10 years of exposure in about 20% of patients.[1194, 1195]

The documentation of positive results on skin testing with a battery of allergens proves atopy and makes it more likely that a patient will experience symptoms in response to high-molecular-weight agents that stimulate IgE production. A positive result on a skin test or RAST with a known occupational sensitizer is very suggestive of occupational asthma; however, skin test results can be positive in workers who are asymptomatic, especially those exposed to low-molecular-weight substances. In persons who are exposed to platinum salts, laboratory animals, acid anhydrides, or insects, a positive result on skin testing coupled with a clear history of work-related asthma is often sufficient for diagnosis.[1058]

Patients who have occupational asthma frequently manifest normal lung function at the time of presentation, and it may be necessary to document functional impairment related to work exposure.[1196] Recognized patterns of derangement include a greater than 20% decline in PEFR or FEV$_1$ over a work shift and a progressive decline in flow rates over the work week with improvement on weekends.[1197–1199] Because of the potential for delayed responses, 24-hour records of PEFR using portable peak flow meters may be helpful.[16, 1198]

When first seen by the physician, the majority of patients manifest NSBR, although its absence does not exclude the diagnosis of occupational asthma.[397, 398] Besides helping to confirm the diagnosis, serial tests of NSBR can help document that the asthma is work related.[16, 1200, 1201] An increase in NSBR during a period of exposure and a decrease during absence from work provide strong evidence for occupational sensitivity. Tests of NSBR can also help to predict the severity of the response to a challenge with a specific sensitizing agent.[1202] Although both peak flow monitoring and serial measures of NSBR are useful in establishing a diagnosis, they are not as specific or sensitive as inhalational challenge with the offending substance.[1200, 1203, 1204]

A significant airway response to a specific challenge remains the most definitive means of establishing a causal relationship, provided that a nonspecific irritant response can be ruled out. However, such bronchial provocation testing with suspected specific occupational agents need not be carried out in all patients to prove the diagnosis and should not be undertaken lightly. The tests can cause severe systemic reactions and even anaphylaxis. A detailed review of methodology and safety has been published.[1205] Challenges should be performed by experienced personnel in a setting where resuscitation facilities are available and where the patient can be closely observed.[16] Besides the danger of a severe immediate response, there is the possibility of delayed and prolonged effects from a single exposure; a delayed response is especially common following exposure to the low-molecular-weight agents, which can precipitate recurrent nocturnal asthma following a single exposure.[1206] It has been suggested that challenge should be undertaken only to prove a new occupational sensitizer, to determine the specific agent in a complex exposure, or for medicolegal purposes.[16]

### Nonspecific Occupational Bronchoconstriction

Patients who have asthma that is unrelated to a specific occupational exposure can suffer episodic exacerbation of their symptoms when exposed to a variety of irritants in the workplace. As a result of NSBH, asthmatic workers exposed to nonspecific stimuli such as cold dry air and gaseous or particulate industrial pollutants will develop work-related airway narrowing. Although the term "reflex" implies involvement of a vagal reflex arc, this may not be important in these nonspecific responses; in fact, "nonspecific (irritant or reflex) occupational bronchoconstriction" might be a better term. Because the reactions are no more than aggravations of pre-existing asthma, we and others believe that affected persons should not be considered to have occupational asthma.[16]

### Reactive Airways Dysfunction Syndrome

Acute exposure to a high concentration of certain gases, vapors, and smoke can produce severe bronchial and bronchiolar injury that causes narrowing and hyper-responsiveness of airways in the exposed worker.[16, 1207–1209] This condition, which has been called *reactive airways dysfunction syndrome* (RADS), develops following a single or repeated exposure to a variety of substances (Table 54–3), including hydrogen sulfide, ammonia, diethylene diamine, chlorine, toxic fumes from plastics and acetic acid,[1210] and smoke from several types of materials.[1208, 1211] Although exposure to aerosols and fumes in swine confinement buildings is most likely to produce a form of organic dust toxic syndrome (ODTS) that may progress to fixed air-flow obstruction (occupational COPD), the levels of toxic fumes in swine confinement buildings can be very high, and a case of RADS has been described in this setting.[1212] In high concentrations, isocyanate fumes may cause RADS rather than the more usual form of delayed occupational asthma.[1148]

Although most cases develop in the workplace, the syndrome can also occur following environmental exposure, as exemplified by reports of the condition in policemen after exposure to roadside fumes from truck accidents[1213] and in children exposed to a high concentration of chlorine in a swimming pool;[1214] we have also seen one patient in whom

### Table 54–3. CAUSES OF REACTIVE AIRWAYS DYSFUNCTION SYNDROME

| AGENT | OCCUPATION/EXPOSURE | SELECTED REFERENCE(S) |
|---|---|---|
| Isocyanates | Plumbers | 1681 |
| Ethylene oxide | | 1682 |
| Diethylaminoethanol and diethylene diamine | | 1683 |
| Metal fumes | Welding | 1684 |
| Sodium hypochlorite and hydrochloric acid | | 1685 |
| Pesticide (metam sodium) | Derailed tank car | 1686 |
| Acetic acid | | 1210, 1687 |
| Chlorine | Household cleaning products, paper mills and pulp mills, swimming pool workers | 1688 1689, 1690 |
| Sulfur dioxide | | |
| Ammonia | | |
| Hydrogen sulfide | Oil industry | |
| Smoke | From a variety of materials | 1208, 1211 |
| Bromine and hydrobromic acid | Disinfectant in hot tub | 1691 |

it developed as a result of combustion of a plastic endotracheal tube during laser surgery. RADS differs from the immunologic forms of occupational asthma, in part by the minimal or absent latency between exposure and symptoms. Airway obstruction typically develops within 24 hours of exposure, and some degree of obstruction and exaggerated nonspecific airway responsiveness persist for months. Slow resolution usually, but not invariably,[1215, 1216] follows. Patients often show a greater degree of fixed air-flow obstruction than is seen in those who have other forms of occupational asthma—a finding that has been attributed to an increased amount of submucosal fibrous tissue.[1217] In the acute stage, RADS is characterized pathologically by sloughing of the respiratory epithelium and replacement by a fibrinohemorrhagic exudate.[1218, 1219] The mechanism by which a single exposure causes prolonged sequelae is unknown; however, evidence of epithelial regeneration and airway wall inflammation can be detected by endobronchial biopsy in patients and in experimental animals in the absence of the basement membrane or smooth muscle changes of asthma.[1208, 1219, 1220]

### Miscellaneous Occupational Airway Disorders

Some occupations involve exposure to substances that are thought to cause a direct, nonidiosyncratic airway effect in a dose-dependent fashion in all or most exposed workers.[16] The most common substances implicated in this type of reaction are cotton dust (byssinosis), grain dust (grain fever), and the noxious aerosols generated in livestock confinement buildings.[1221, 1222] A similar syndrome has also been described in factory workers exposed to the output from a contaminated humidifier.[1223, 1224] The common pathogenetic link in these disorders may be the presence of bacterial endotoxin in the dust or aerosol. Endotoxin has also been hypothesized to be responsible for pulmonary dysfunction developing in workers in a fiberglass wool manufacturing plant.[1225]

These disorders are referred to collectively as *organic dust toxic syndrome* (ODTS) and are discussed in detail in Chapter 59 (*see* page 2379). Such disorders should not be called "occupational asthma": although some affected workers clearly develop reversible airway obstruction, they fail to manifest the eosinophilia and diurnal lability of expiratory flow that are characteristic of asthma due to other causes.[1226] In addition, because fixed air-flow obstruction can develop in workers after prolonged exposure, these conditions are more correctly designated industrial COPD; their long-term effects on lung function are discussed in greater detail in Chapter 55 (*see* page 2174).[1227, 1228]

Byssinosis is a chronic airway disease that occurs in textile workers exposed to the dust of cotton, flax, hemp, and jute. In its early stages, it is characterized by acute dyspnea, cough, and wheeze on Monday mornings following a weekend away from the workplace; the symptoms decrease during the work week, despite continued exposure. The incidence and severity of symptoms and functional impairment are proportional to the exposure, in both duration and intensity.[16, 1229] The magnitude of the response to acute exposure in the workplace correlates with the long-term loss of lung function as measured by annual decline in $FEV_1$.[1230] Bronchoconstriction can develop in normal persons in response to an aerosol of cotton bract extract, the degree of

bronchoconstriction possibly being related to nonspecific airway responsiveness.[1231, 1232]

The two most widely investigated theories of the pathogenesis are related to the presence of a histamine-releasing substance or endotoxin in the cotton.[16, 1233, 1234] Although histamine release by cotton has been demonstrated *in vitro* and blood levels of histamine increase in affected persons during Monday morning attacks, the bulk of evidence supports endotoxin as the offending substance.[1235] Cotton dust is contaminated by endotoxin-containing bacteria, and the magnitude of a worker's airway response to exposure correlates more closely with levels of endotoxin in the dust than with the concentration of dust.[1234, 1236] Endotoxin can activate complement *in vitro* and in guinea pigs can produce an acute airway response with subsequent tachyphylaxis similar to the Monday morning phenomenon in human beings.[1237, 1238] There is no evidence to support the presence of specific IgE- or IgG-mediated immunologic responses in the development of byssinosis.

A pharmacologic mechanism is probably responsible for the acute "asthma" described in workers spraying organophosphate insecticides; these agents act as anticholinesterases, allowing an exaggerated effect of vagal stimulation.[16] However, persistent asthma has also been reported after exposure to organophosphates, suggesting that additional pathogenetic mechanisms may be involved in some cases.[1239] The single-celled flagellated sea algae that contribute to "red tide" (*Ptychodiscus brevis*) can become airborne in ocean spray; the algal toxin can cause bronchoconstriction in exposed persons by direct acetylcholine release from cholinergic nerve endings.[1240] As discussed previously, most evidence supports an allergic (or at least idiosyncratic) mechanism in the production of isocyanate-induced asthma;[1115, 1241] however, it is possible that pharmacologic dose-dependent inhibition of various biologic enzymes and receptors (including beta agonist receptors) might contribute to the airway response.[16, 1116, 1242]

## RADIOLOGIC MANIFESTATIONS

The most common radiographic abnormalities in patients who have asthma are bronchial wall thickening and hyperinflation; less frequent manifestations include peripheral oligemia, increased central lung markings, and prominence of the hila.[1243–1247] The prevalence of these abnormalities is influenced by several factors, including age at onset and severity of asthma, and the presence of other disease or complications of asthma.[1244, 1245, 1248–1250] The influence of age at onset on the presence or absence of radiographic abnormalities was assessed in one investigation of 117 patients older than 15 years of age;[1248] radiographic abnormalities were identified in 31% of the patients whose asthma had its onset before the age of 15 years but in none of those in whom it occurred after 30.

The incidence of radiographic abnormalities is also affected by disease severity. In a study of 58 patients ranging in age from 10 to 69 years (mean age 33 years) in whom the asthma was categorized as "severe," evidence of pulmonary overinflation was detected in 42 (73%).[1251] In this report, the author drew attention to the rapidity with which signs of overinflation can disappear following appropriate therapy, sometimes in as short a time as 24 hours.[1251]

In the presence of acute severe asthma or during a prolonged, intractable attack, the most characteristic radiographic signs are pulmonary hyperinflation and expiratory air trapping (Fig. 54–12). The former is manifested by increase in the depth of the retrosternal space and in lung height and flattening of the diaphragm (Fig. 54–13). In one investigation of 12 asthmatic patients in whom the presence of hyperinflation was assessed by the subjective evaluation of chest radiographs as well as planimetric measurement, the latter studies revealed a mean increase in TLC of 0.46 liter during acute exacerbation;[1250] the only subjective radiographic variable that allowed reliable distinction of acute exacerbation from recovery was an increase in lung height.

Cardiac size is almost invariably normal, although the long, narrow cardiac silhouette commonly seen in patients who have emphysema is occasionally observed in those who have asthma. Prominence of the main pulmonary artery and its hilar branches with rapid tapering is probably indicative of transient precapillary pulmonary arterial hypertension secondary to hypoxia and occurs in approximately 10% of patients (Fig. 54–14).[1252] Abnormal vascular patterns include diffuse narrowing and blood flow redistribution into the upper lobes, the latter in the absence of other signs of postcapillary hypertension, and paucity of vessels in the outer 2 to 4 cm of the lungs (Fig. 54–15). This "subpleural oligemia" is especially evident when accompanied by an increased prominence of the hilar and mid-lung vessels and is reversible with treatment.

The prevalence of bronchial wall thickening in chronic asthma was assessed in one investigation of 57 nonsmoking patients with disease of variable severity.[1244] The clinical severity of asthma was assessed using a scoring system that graded the disease from mild (score of 1) to incapacitating (score of 5).[1253] Bronchial wall thickening was evident on the chest radiograph in 22% of patients who had grade 1 asthma, 26% who had grade 2, 35% who had grade 3, and 46% who had grade 4 or 5.

The thickening occurs in both segmental and subsegmental bronchi and can be seen either as ring shadows when viewed end on or as "tramline" opacities when viewed *en face*. Smaller bronchi measuring 3 to 5 mm in diameter, normally invisible on conventional chest radiographs, may

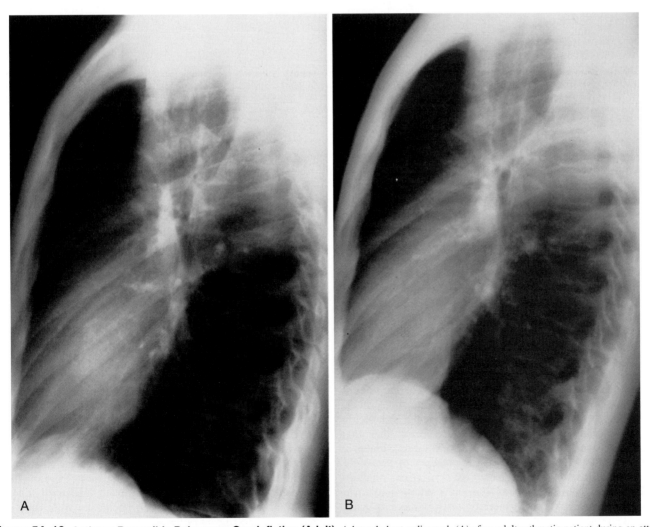

**Figure 54–12. Asthma: Reversible Pulmonary Overinflation (Adult).** A lateral chest radiograph *(A)* of an adult asthmatic patient during an attack of severe bronchospasm reveals a low position and flat configuration of the diaphragm, indicating severe pulmonary overinflation. Approximately 1 year later during a remission *(B)*, lung volume had returned to normal. Note that the curvature of the sternum and thoracic spine did not change, because these structures do not participate in acute hyperinflation in the adult.

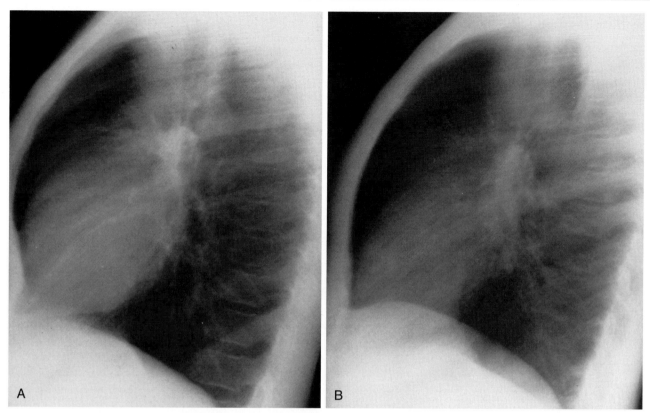

**Figure 54–13. Asthma: Reversible Pulmonary Overinflation (Adolescent).** A lateral chest radiograph *(A)* of a young asthmatic patient during an episode of severe, acute bronchospasm reveals an increase in the volume of the retrosternal and retrocardiac spaces, flattening of the diaphragm, anterior bowing of the sternum, and a slight kyphosis. Following therapy four days later *(B)* the abnormal findings have cleared except for persistence of an increased retrocardiac space. Note that hyperinflation tends to affect the skeleton to a greater extent in the young patient than in the adult, presumably as a result of more pliable cartilaginous and bony structures.

be identified (Fig. 54–16). These findings probably represent intramural and peribronchial thickening caused by inflammation or fibrosis or both. Although the thickening is usually permanent, it may decrease or disappear entirely following treatment (Fig. 54–17).

Despite the observations just outlined, the chest radiograph has a limited role in the diagnosis of asthma. It is often normal, even during an acute attack; moreover, when it is abnormal, the findings are nonspecific. There are two main indications for chest radiography in these patients: (1) to exclude other conditions that cause wheezing throughout the chest, particularly emphysema, congestive heart failure, and obstruction of the trachea or major bronchi; and (2) to identify complications such as pneumothorax. Several studies have been carried out to evaluate the efficacy of radiographic examination in asthmatic patients, and the conclusions are not by any means unanimous. In one study of 117 adults admitted to the hospital with severe acute asthma, the investigators found radiographic abnormalities other than those directly related to asthma that affected management in 10 patients (9%);[1254] in 9 of these, the presence of consolidation or atelectasis was not detected on clinical examination. In this series, overinflation was a common finding and correlated significantly with tachycardia, pulsus paradoxus, and a decrease in FEV$_1$; bronchial wall thickening was also frequent. In another investigation, 528 chest radiographs from 122 adults were reviewed; each film represented a separate acute asthmatic attack.[1254a] Only 2.2% of the radiographs

revealed parenchymal opacities, atelectasis, pneumothorax, or pneumomediastinum (pulmonary overinflation was not included as an abnormal finding). In one study of 75 children and young adults who were admitted to the hospital for acute exacerbations, a pattern of inversion of pulmonary artery blood flow was seen in those who had more severe symptoms and functional impairment;[1255] the authors suggested that acute right ventricular dilatation restricted left ventricular filling, resulting in an elevation of pulmonary venous pressure.

In another retrospective study of chest radiographs obtained in 135 of 695 patients who presented in the emergency room with asthma, 19 (14%) showed abnormalities that could have altered the management of the patient.[1256] (Obviously, the 135 patients who had radiographs had been selected from among the 695 cases; however, it is not clear which clinical features increased the index of suspicion that led to the performance of radiography). In another investigation of adult asthmatic patients admitted to the hospital for exacerbations of asthma, chest radiographs revealed some abnormality in 50% of patients;[1257] in 5% the abnormality resulted in a change in management strategy. In a third, retrospective investigation of 1,016 adults admitted to the hospital with acute asthma, radiographic findings were classified into the following groups:[1245] (1) normal: 536 patients (53%); (2) features compatible with obstructive lung disease: 323 patients (32%); (3) complications of asthma, including infection, atelectasis, pneumomediastinum, and pneumotho-

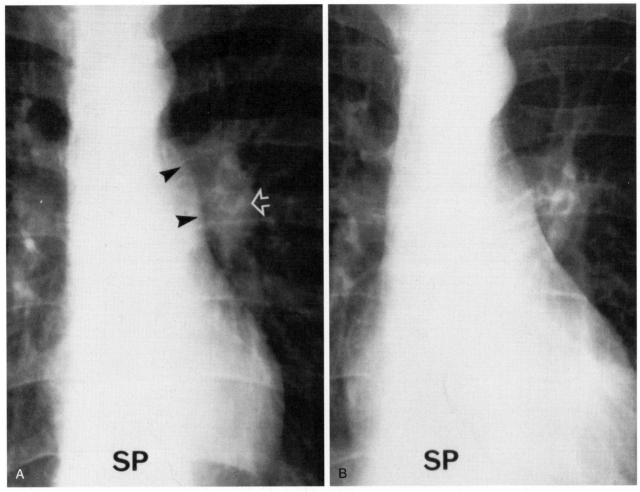

**Figure 54–14. Asthma: Reversible Precapillary Pulmonary Hypertension.** A detail view of the heart and left hilum from a posteroanterior radiograph *(A)* reveals enlargement of the main pulmonary artery *(arrowheads)* and left interlobar artery *(open arrow)*, consistent with the presence of pulmonary arterial hypertension. At the time of this study, the patient, a young man, was experiencing a severe attack of acute bronchospasm. Approximately 2 years later during a period of remission, a repeat radiograph *(B)* demonstrates a return to normal of the configuration of the main and interlobar arteries. Note that the heart has increased in size during this interval, presumably reflecting the high transpulmonary pressure that existed during the acute attack and the consequent reduction in venous return.

rax: 83 patients (8%); and (4) important incidental findings including tuberculosis, heart failure, and pulmonary neoplasm: 68 cases (7%). Therefore, approximately 15% of patients presenting with symptoms severe enough to require hospital admission had clinically significant radiographic abnormalities. The authors concluded, and we concur, that admission chest radiography is indicated in adults presenting with severe asthma.

High-resolution computed tomography (HRCT) has allowed visualization of airways in asthmatic patients in much greater detail than plain radiography and has made possible the investigation of the site, magnitude, and distribution of airway narrowing *in vivo* (Fig. 54–18). In addition to providing more accurate and detailed images, the digital nature of the data from which the CT image is generated allows a quantitative approach to the analysis of airway dimensions. The most common abnormalities seen on HRCT are bronchial wall thickening, narrowing of the bronchial lumen, bronchial dilatation (bronchiectasis), patchy areas of decreased attenuation and vascularity, and air trapping.[1244, 1258–1261] The distribution of bronchial abnormalities is often heterogeneous; some airways have normal thickness and

diameter, while others have thick walls and are narrowed or dilated. As with the findings on the chest radiograph, the prevalence of HRCT abnormalities increases with increased severity of symptoms.[1244, 1261] Considerable variation exists, however, in the reported frequency and patterns of abnormality. This variation is related to a variety of factors, including differences in technique, data analysis, diagnostic criteria, and patient selection (e.g., smokers or nonsmokers).

Window level, window width, the size of the field of view (FOV), and the reconstruction algorithm affect the quality of the CT image and the accuracy of airway lumen and wall dimensions (*see* Chapter 12). The window level has been shown to be especially important in quantitative studies of airway wall dimensions. The results of studies examining the relationship between window level and airway measurements have shown that airway wall thickness measurements are greater, and lumen areas less, when images are photographed at lower (more negative) window levels.[1262, 1263] In some studies, window levels and widths have been adjusted to make airways easier to visualize, and measurements made on the resulting images. For example, in one investigation the window level was adjusted to find

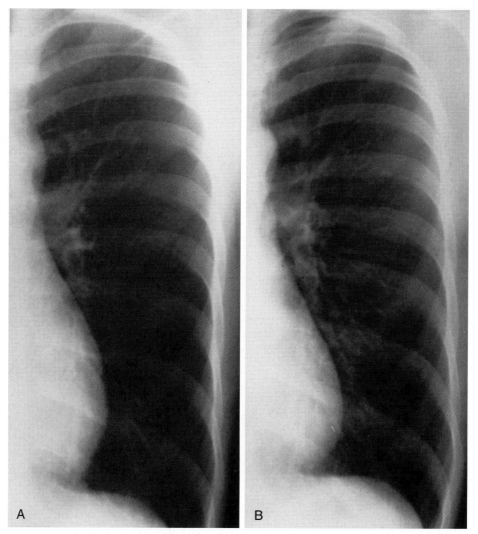

**Figure 54–15. Asthma: Peripheral Oligemia.** A detail view of the left lung from a posteroanterior chest radiograph *(A)* of a young man during an episode of acute bronchospasm reveals moderate hyperinflation. The vasculature in the outer 2 to 3 cm of lung is inconspicuous and barely visible, creating a subpleural shell of oligemic lung. A repeat study 1 year later during remission *(B)* shows less hyperinflation; the pulmonary vessels now taper normally, and most are visible well into the lung periphery.

the lowest value at which the airway wall appeared to be an unbroken ring, at which point the settings were used to make measurements;[1264] during these adjustments, the authors found that the lumen of some airways disappeared completely, suggesting that the window level chosen may have resulted in overestimation of airway wall thickness and underestimation of airway lumen area. The same investigators used different window levels in the same and different patients; because they did not make any comparison with a known standard, these results are not anatomically accurate. A number of investigators have used phantom airways in an attempt to determine the window levels and widths that would provide the most accurate measurements; on the basis of the results, it is now accepted that a window level of $-450$ HU is ideal.[1262, 1263] The optimal window width for measurements of bronchial wall thickness is 1,000 to 1,400 HU. In a study of inflation-fixed lungs, window widths narrower than 1,000 HU were shown to lead to substantial magnification of bronchial wall thickness, whereas a window width of 1,500 HU resulted in slight underestimation.[1263a] Several investigators have shown that at the appropriate window level and width, the smallest airways on which reasonably accurate measurements of lumen diameter can be made are between 1.5 and 2 mm in diameter.[1244, 1265, 1266]

HRCT scans have been used to compare airway dimensions before and after an intervention such as the administration of a bronchoconstricting agonist; in these situations, the lung sections imaged before and after the intervention have been matched on the basis of anatomic features such as vascular or bronchial bifurcations, fissures, and mediastinal structures. The ability to match the levels pre- and post-intervention has been greatly aided by the development of volumetric or spiral CT. With the latter technique, data from a large portion of lung can be acquired during a single breath-hold while collimation remains at 1 mm. Lung volume influences airway wall and lumen dimensions;[1267] thus, if the intervention itself has the capacity to alter lung volume, changes in airway dimensions might not represent a primary effect. In an attempt to avoid this artifact, some investigators have used a spirometer in the CT suite in an attempt to ensure that lung volumes are comparable before and after a bronchoconstricting stimulus.[1260]

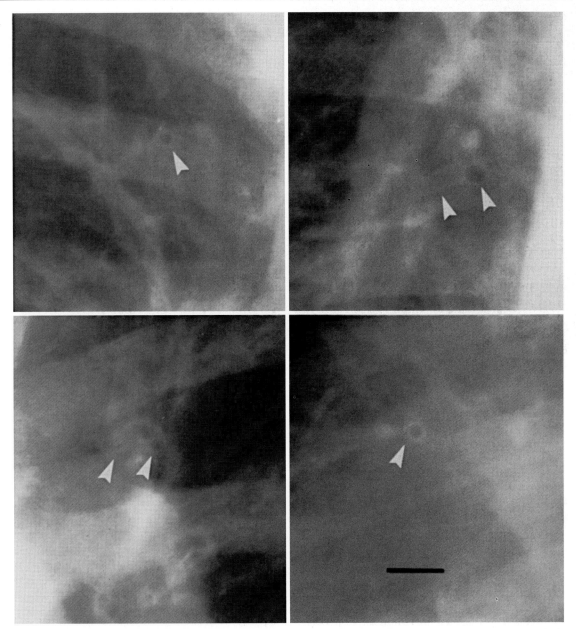

**Figure 54–16. Asthma: Bronchial Wall Thickening.** Detail views from four areas of the lungs from posteroanterior and lateral chest radiographs reveal thick-walled airways measuring 3 to 5 mm in diameter that are not normally visible *(arrowheads)*. The bar represents 1 cm. The patient was a young boy with atopic asthma.

To date, only one study has reported on the use of quantitative HRCT techniques to examine the effects of airway smooth muscle contraction on normal and asthmatic human airways.[1260] In this study, investigators found that airways narrowed throughout the bronchial tree after nebulized methacholine challenge, although the percent narrowing was greater in the intermediate-sized airways (2 to 4 mm in diameter). The magnitude and distribution of airway narrowing were not different in the asthmatics and the normal people, although the concentration of methacholine in the aerosol administered to the normal people was about 25-fold greater than that administered to the asthmatics. A puzzling finding of this study was that airway wall area decreased during airway narrowing in the normal persons but not in the asthmatics; this difference was significant in airways less than 6 mm in initial diameter.

A number of investigators have described, although not quantified, the HRCT findings in asthmatic patients.[1244, 1258, 1261, 1268–1270] The results of these studies are based on subjective assessment of the CT findings interpreted by radiologists blinded to the clinical status of the patients. In one investigation, bronchial wall thickening was present in 44 of 48 (92%) asthmatic patients, compared with 5 to 27 (19%) healthy persons *(see* Fig. 54–18).[1258] In a second investigation, bronchial thickening was seen in 44% of HRCT scans from 39 asthmatic patients, compared with only 4% of scans from 14 normal persons.[1261] In a third investigation, bronchial wall thickening was reported in 16 of 17 asthmatic patients who had clinical evidence of allergic bronchopulmonary aspergillosis and in 9 of 11 asthmatic persons who did not.[1271] The asthmatic airway wall thickening may not be reversible, at least in the short term; for example, in an

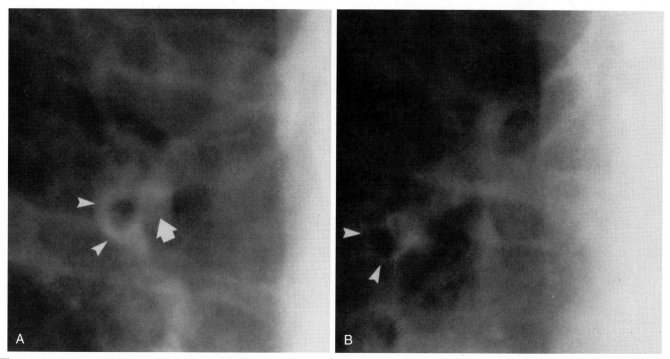

**Figure 54–17. Asthma: Reversibility of Bronchial Wall Thickening.** A detail view of the right hilar region from a posteroanterior chest *(A)* shows a moderately thickened wall of the anterior segmental bronchus of the upper lobe *(arrowheads)*, adjacent to its companion artery *(closed arrow)*. Approximately 1 year later *(B)*, the bronchial wall was almost normal in thickness *(arrowheads)*. The patient was a young woman who was hospitalized during a particularly severe episode of bronchospasm at the time of the radiograph *(A)*, whereas in *B* she was in remission.

investigation of 10 patients who underwent scanning during an acute attack and then 2 weeks later after receiving an intensive course of corticosteroid therapy, no change in wall dimensions was evident.[1244]

Airway narrowing in asthmatics can also be estimated on HRCT by assessment of the distribution of lumen areas in randomly selected airways. For example, in one investigation, the authors demonstrated that the frequency distribution of airway lumen areas was shifted to the left (a preponderance of smaller lumen sizes) in asthmatic patients compared with age-matched normal people.[1260] Another method of measuring airway lumen area is to compare it to that of the accompanying blood vessel and calculate a ratio, as is done for the detection of bronchiectasis. In one investigation in which this was performed, the mean inner bronchial-to-arterial diameter ratio in asthmatics who had a normal $FEV_1$ or a moderately reduced $FEV_1$ (greater than 60% of predicted) was 0.60 ± 0.16 or 0.60 ± 0.18, respectively, and was not significantly different from that in normal persons (ratio of 0.65 ± 0.16).[1261] In asthmatic patients whose $FEV_1$ was less than 60% of predicted, the mean ratio (0.48 ± 0.11) was significantly lower than that in normal persons. In this study, there was no difference in the ratios measured in different lobes or segments. Patients who have moderate or severe asthma have a greater airway wall thickness to outer bronchial diameter (T/D) ratio and a greater percentage of wall area (defined as [wall area/total airway area] × 100) than patients who have mild asthma or normal individuals.[1270a]

Airways can also be excessively dilated in asthmatic patients, as assessed by measurement of the arterial-to-bronchial diameter ratio (Fig. 54–19).[1261, 1258, 1270–1272] The reported prevalence of bronchial dilatation in asthmatic patients who

do not have clinical evidence of allergic bronchopulmonary aspergillosis ranges between 18% and 77% in these studies and is significantly higher than in appropriate control subjects. For example, in one of these studies, 36% of all airways examined from 48 asthmatic patients had bronchial dilatation (defined as an internal diameter greater than that of the accompanying artery);[1258] 77% had at least one dilated bronchus. (However, bronchial dilatation was also found in 19% of all airways examined in 27 healthy persons, and 59% of the subjects had at least one dilated bronchus.) In another study, bronchial dilatation was observed in 31% of CT scans in 39 asthmatic patients, compared with 4% of CT scans in 14 normal persons.[1261]

The significance of bronchial dilatation in asthmatic patients is uncertain. The fact that about 5% to 20% of airways are bigger than the accompanying artery in healthy persons[1261, 1258] illustrates that there is a wide normal variation in this ratio.[1273] There is also significant heterogeneity between airways in their degree of dilatation or narrowing in the same person. This heterogeneity could be between parallel airways, or it could be serially distributed along the airway. An alternative explanation for airway dilatation is a narrowing of the accompanying artery resulting in an apparent increase in the bronchial diameter. Pulmonary arteries are reactive to changes in alveolar oxygen tension, and an increased bronchial-to-arterial diameter ratio has been observed in HRCT studies performed at altitude compared with those performed at sea level, presumably owing to the reduced ambient oxygen tension at altitude.[1274]

Other findings on HRCT in asthmatic patients include localized areas of low attenuation and vascularity and air trapping (Fig. 54–20).[1247, 1261] These are the result of abnormalities of ventilation-perfusion distribution that are com-

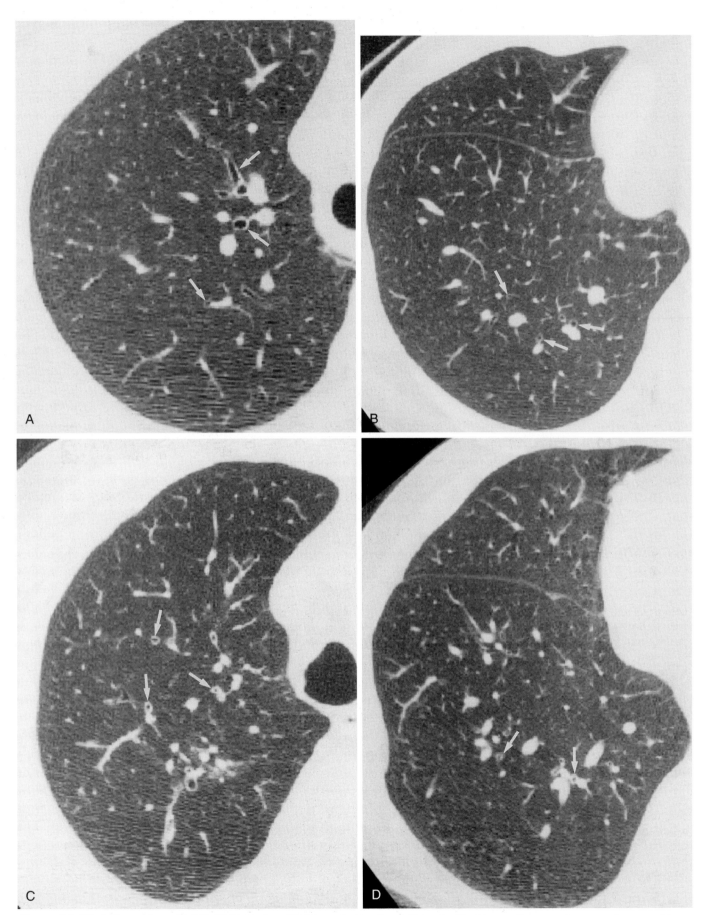

**Figure 54–18. Asthma: Bronchial Wall Thickening.** HRCT scan images *(A* and *B)* in a healthy 34-year-old woman show normal upper and lower lobe bronchi *(arrows)*. HRCT scans in a patient who has chronic asthma *(C* and *D)* demonstrate thickening of the bronchial walls *(arrows)*. Decreased diameter of the lumen of several bronchi is also evident, particularly in the right lower lobe.

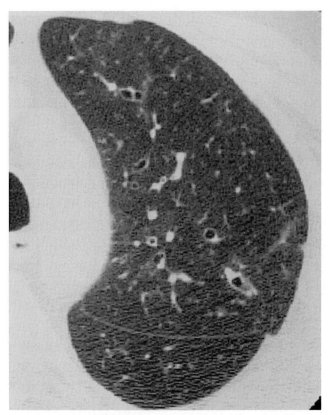

**Figure 54–19. Asthma: Bronchial Dilation.** An HRCT scan in a 57-year-old man with chronic asthma demonstrates left upper lobe bronchiectasis. The patient was a nonsmoker who did not have a history of recurrent infections.

mon in asthma, even during clinically stable periods, and have been well described by scintigraphy (Fig. 54–21).[1275–1278] In one investigation, air trapping was demonstrated on expiratory HRCT in approximately 50% of 39 asthmatic patients, compared with 14% of 14 normal persons;[1261] air trapping was seen in 45% of asthmatic patients who had an $FEV_1$ of >80% predicted, 50% of those who had an $FEV_1$ between 60% and 79% predicted, and 67% of those who had an $FEV_1$ less than 60% predicted.

In another investigation, the percent of the pixels in a CT slice that had an attenuation less than −900 HU were calculated;[1259] the slices were obtained at the level of the aortic arch and immediately cephalad to the diaphragm. The authors scanned 18 asthmatic patients and 22 normal persons at both full inspiration and full expiration using 1.5-mm and 10-mm scan collimation. Significantly more extensive low-attenuation areas were found in the diaphragmatic 1.5-mm slice on expiratory scans in the asthmatics (10 ± 1.44%) than in the normal control subjects (1 ± 3%). The percentages of low-attenuation areas were less in the 10-mm slices but were still significantly different; however, the differences between asthmatics and normals disappeared on the inspiratory scans. The asthmatics were older than the normal controls (mean age 54 years versus 32 years), which may have biased the data; results of previous CT studies (performed at near full inspiration) show that low-attenuation regions on CT, defined by a density mask of −950 HU, are more extensive with increasing age.[1279] However, the absence of a difference in mean attenuation density on inspiratory scans strongly suggests that there was little or no emphysema in the asthmatics and that gas trapping caused by airway closure was the cause of the differences.

Another group of investigators has examined the extent of "emphysema" using 10-mm slice thickness and a visual scoring system.[1249] In this study, they compared 10 chronic nonsmoking asthmatic patients whose mean TLC was 109% predicted with age- and sex-matched smokers whose mean TLC was 105% predicted. A median of 1% (range 0 to 4%) of lung was affected by "emphysema" in asthmatics, and a median of 10% (range 1 to 60%) was affected in the smokers. Another group of investigators performed measurements of lung attenuation at FRC and RV in 15 patients with asthma and 6 healthy control subjects before and after bronchial provocation with methacholine and after reversal of provocation with albuterol.[1279a] After methacholine, patients with asthma showed a 20% to 36% decrease in $FEV_1$ and significant decreases in the median and lower 10th percentile regions of the attenuation values at both FRC and RV. Control subjects showed a decrease of less than 10% in $FEV_1$ and no significant change in the lung attenuation values. After albuterol, the $FEV_1$ and attenuation values of the asthmatic patients returned to baseline levels.

## CLINICAL MANIFESTATIONS

The diagnosis of asthma is based largely on a history of periodic paroxysms of dyspnea, usually at rest as well as on exertion, interspersed with intervals of complete or nearly complete remission. Some patients have a more chronic form of the disease characterized by more persistent symptoms; however, periodic exacerbation and remission occur in almost all cases. Cough can be a prominent symptom, and nonsmoking patients who have asthma can fulfill the diagnostic criteria for chronic bronchitis.[1280] The diagnosis is strengthened by a history of eczema or hay fever or by a family history of allergic phenomena.

Meticulous inquiry into circumstances initiating attacks, although time-consuming, undoubtedly constitutes the most important diagnostic procedure and is vital in directing management. If the patient is a child, questioning should be directed toward the possible association of ingestion of a particular food or drink with the onset of attacks. Seasonal occurrence is of importance in suggesting either pollen sensitivity or allergic asthma precipitated by insects. Careful inquiry should be made into possible antigens in the home, especially those from domestic pets, cockroaches, and bedding or carpets, which can harbor house dust mites. The patient may have recognized an association between the onset of symptoms and exposure to a dusty environment at the workplace. A history of drug intake should be looked for; specifically, the patient should be questioned about the use of beta blockers, ASA, and ACE inhibitors. Exercise may be the only apparent provoking factor; in such circumstances, the presence of the disease may go unrecognized if clinical examination and pulmonary function tests are not performed at appropriate times.[1281] When a history of exercise-induced attacks is elicited, it should be determined if the prior ingestion of any particular food precipitates the attacks.[796]

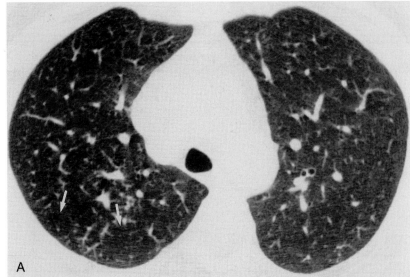

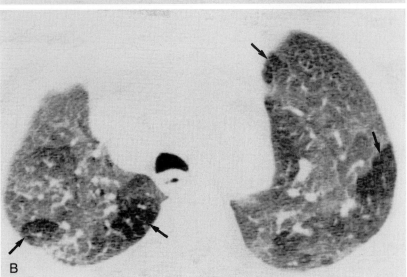

**Figure 54–20. Asthma: Air Trapping.** HRCT performed at end-inspiration *(A)* shows subtle localized areas of decreased attenuation and vascularity *(arrows)*. HRCT performed at the end of maximal expiration *(B)* shows several bilateral areas of air trapping *(arrows)*. The patient was a 45-year-old lifelong nonsmoker who had chronic asthma.

The patient should be questioned as to whether there is an association between the onset of asthmatic attacks and infections of the upper or lower respiratory tract, with particular emphasis on the occurrence of postnasal drip and facial pain, which suggest the presence of sinusitis. Additional historical features of importance include a prior history of rhinitis, eczema, or anaphylaxis and symptoms suggestive of GER. An attempt should be made to correlate the onset of attacks with emotional disturbance; if the patient is a child, this should include interview of the parents. Finally, the patient should be questioned as to the relationship between onset of attacks and exposure to cold air or to irritating dusts, fumes, or odors and the effects of changing temperature and humidity.

In both atopic and nonatopic patients, the original asthmatic episode commonly is termed "acute bronchitis," with or without fever or upper respiratory symptoms. In this situation, the diagnosis of asthma may not be suspected, particularly in elderly patients, who are more prone to chronic bronchitis;[1282] in such patients, wheezing and paroxysmal nocturnal dyspnea often are attributed to irreversible obstructive airway disease or left ventricular failure.[1283]

In the majority of patients, the onset of an attack of asthma is heralded by an unproductive cough and wheeze, and only subsequently do the sensations of suffocation and tightness in the chest develop. The onset of dyspnea seldom is abrupt. The severity of airway narrowing that is required to cause dyspnea varies widely.[1284] Paroxysms occur most commonly at night; when they are severe, the patient may feel obliged to sit on the edge of the bed or to stagger to the window in the vain hope of obtaining more oxygen. Cough (with normal pulmonary function) is the sole presenting symptom in some patients *(see* farther on). Nocturnal breathlessness is a common symptom, and careful history taking may be necessary to distinguish asthma from paroxysmal nocturnal dyspnea of cardiac origin.

Physical findings include tachypnea, hyper-resonance on percussion, inspiratory and expiratory rhonchi and wheezes, decreased breath sounds, and prolonged expiration. In very severe attacks, wheezing may not be apparent, the clinical picture being one of air hunger; in such circumstances, there is use of accessory muscles of respiration, diminished breath sounds without rhonchi, pulsus paradoxus, and often cyanosis.[1285, 1286] The correlation between physical

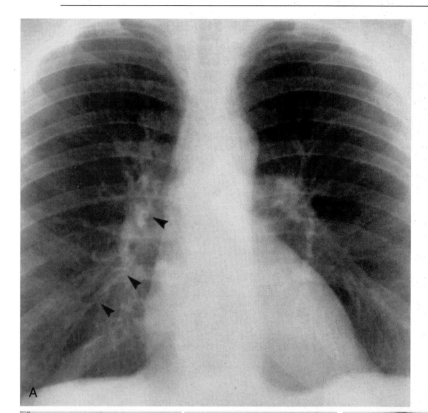

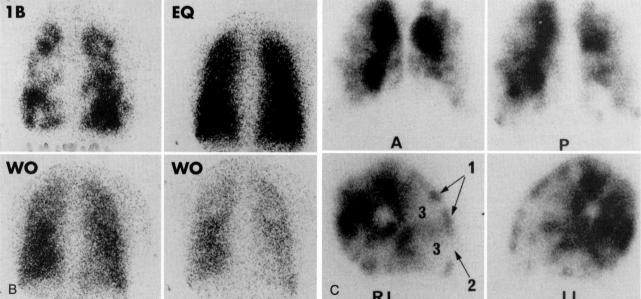

**Figure 54–21. Asthma: Ventilation-Perfusion Abnormalities.** A posteroanterior chest radiograph *(A)* is normal except for mild overinflation and bronchial wall thickening *(arrowheads)*. A ventilation lung scintigram *(B)* reveals unequal deposition of the radioisotope in the central parenchyma on the initial breath (IB), with relative sparing peripherally; equilibration (EQ) was eventually achieved centrally and peripherally, although air trapping occurred in both areas during the washout (WO) phase. A perfusion scan *(C)* in anterior (A), posterior (P), right lateral (RL), and left lateral (LL) positions demonstrates deficits in the perfusion pattern in the lower lobes and posterior parts of the upper lobes. Note the rim of maintained perfusion in the cortex (1) that alternates with adjacent regions of cortical hypoperfusion (2); in both instances, the proximal medulla (3) is focally underperfused. The presence of maintained perfusion adjacent to contiguous medullary hypoperfusion on a scintigram is designated the "stripe sign"; its identification effectively excludes thromboembolic disease as the cause of the oligemia.

findings suggestive of asthma and the severity of airway obstruction as measured objectively is not close. Although it has been reported that the $FEV_1$ can be roughly estimated with a combination of auscultation and palpation of the accessory muscles,[1287, 1288] appropriate assessment of asthma severity requires objective measurement of maximal expiratory flow.

An abnormal degree of pulsus paradoxus has been correlated with severity of asthma.[1289–1291] On inspiration, the systolic arterial pressure in normal persons decreases by up to 5 mm Hg, whereas in patients who have asthma the pressure may drop by 10 mm Hg or more. This is probably the result of increased negative intrathoracic pressure secondary to airway obstruction.[1292] The negative swings in intrathoracic pressure can decrease systolic pressure by at least two mechanisms: (1) the increased right ventricular volume caused by the negative pressure may result in a leftward shift of the interventricular septum, leading to interference with left ventricular diastolic filling; and (2) the negative intrathoracic pressure acts as an afterload on the left ventricle because of the communication between the ventricle and the great vessels outside the thorax, which are not exposed to the negative pressure.[1293]

Although some patients who come to hospital emergency rooms present with attacks of asthma that develop over a period of hours, most have had progressive symptoms over days to weeks, often with a more rapid deterioration during the previous 24 hours.[1294] Younger, atopic persons are more likely to present with exacerbations of rapid onset.[1295] Occasionally, the onset is so insidious that the diagnosis is not considered, particularly in elderly smokers.[1296] In fact, the diagnosis of asthma in the elderly can be especially challenging. Although the disease is often considered to be a disease of the young, it is common in older persons, and it is in the older age group that the highest incidence of death from asthma has been reported.[1297] Such persons may present in an atypical fashion because of poor perception of dyspnea and more prominent cough;[1298] in fact, they are often considered to have COPD, emphysema, or congestive heart failure.[1296] When there is diagnostic uncertainty, a 2-week course of oral corticosteroid is a good means of determining the magnitude of the reversible component of airway obstruction.[1297]

Patients who have acute severe asthma may be too dyspneic or exhausted to speak and may be stuporous or even comatose as a result of hypoxemia, hypercarbia, and (rarely) water intoxication (*see* farther on); they commonly manifest tachycardia (heart rate greater than 130) and pronounced pulsus paradoxus. As a result of airway obstruction and exhaustion, they can exhibit such severe restriction of air flow that wheezing is absent and breath sounds are barely discernible.[1299, 1300] In a small subset of patients with very severe asthma, the disease appears to be steroid-resistant.[1301] These persons do not improve significantly after a 14-day course of oral steroids, and their peripheral eosinophilia is also resistant to suppression by steroids. It appears that the genesis of corticosteroid-resistant asthma involves an acquired resistance of T cells to glucocorticoid regulation of cytokine secretion.[1302, 1303] Although in a small subset of patients the disease is truely steroid-resistant, many patients who appear to respond poorly to steroid therapy have significant ongoing exposure to allergen, are noncompliant, or are administering inhaled medication innappropriately.

A number of algorithms have been designed in an attempt to assess asthma severity in order to provide prognostic information and guide therapy.[1304–1307] Physical examination is unreliable,[1308] and no single symptom or test can be used to judge severity. In addition, the available algorithms do not allow clear separation of the underlying severity of the disease from the effectiveness of therapy. One severity schema, which was proposed by the Global Initiative for Asthma (GINA), is shown in Table 54–4.[1309]

### Diurnal Variation and Nocturnal Asthma

Both normal individuals and asthmatic patients show a circadian rhythm in airway caliber, as measured by PEF or $FEV_1$,[1310] although the diurnal variation is much more pronounced in the latter group; the lowest values for expiratory flow are recorded in the early hours of the morning (2 to 4 A.M.).[1311, 1312] The magnitude of within-day variation in $FEV_1$ or PEFR correlates with nonspecific airway responsiveness; although it is less sensitive than the latter, it has been suggested as an alternative or additional diagnostic test for asthma.[1313]

The most prominent clinical manifestation related to

### Table 54–4. CLINICAL FEATURES OF ASTHMA SEVERITY

| | |
|---|---|
| Intermittent | Intermittent symptoms <1 time per week |
| | Brief exacerbations (from a few hours to a few days) |
| | Nighttime asthma symptoms <2 times a month |
| | Asymptomatic and normal lung function between exacerbations |
| | PEF or $FEV_1$: >80% of predicted; variability <20% |
| Mild persistent | Symptoms >1 time a week but <1 time per day |
| | Exacerbations may affect activity and sleep |
| | Nighttime asthma symptoms >2 times a month |
| | PEF or $FEV_1$: >80% of predicted; variability 20–30% |
| Moderate persistent | Symptoms daily |
| | Exacerbations affect activity and sleep |
| | Nighttime asthma symptoms >1 time per week |
| | Daily use of inhaled short-acting beta$_2$ agonists |
| | PEF or $FEV_1$: >60% to <80% of predicted; variability >30% |
| Severe persistent | Continuous symptoms |
| | Frequent exacerbations |
| | Frequent nighttime asthma symptoms |
| | Physical activities limited by asthma symptoms |
| | PEF or $FEV_1$: <60% of predicted; variability >30% |

From Lenfant C, Khalaev N: Global initiative for asthma. *In* Global Strategy for Asthma Management and Prevention. NIH publication No. 95-3659. NHLBI/WHO Workshop Report 1:1, 1995.

diurnal variation are the symptoms of nocturnal asthma, which are in turn associated with the phenomenon of "morning dipping" in expiratory flow.[1314] Although an early-morning exacerbation in asthmatic symptoms was described in 1698 by Sir John Floyer,[1315] interest in the phenomenon has been rekindled because of demonstration of the severe obstruction that can be associated with the symptoms in some patients. Asthmatic patients show a circadian rhythm in airway responsiveness,[1316] plasma epinephrine, cortisol, cyclic adenosine monophosphate (cAMP), and histamine.[1317] There also appears to be a nocturnal increase in inflammatory markers in BAL fluid; in one study, patients who had at least a 20% decrease in $FEV_1$ between 4 P.M. and 4 A.M. showed increased eosinophils and neutrophils in BAL fluid.[1318] Nocturnal worsening of airway inflammation has been confirmed in additional studies.[1319–1321]

Despite many investigations, the precise mechanisms by which nocturnal asthma and airway inflammation occur remain unclear. Rarely, the nocturnal asthma can be attributed to the development of hypersensitivity to antigens in bedding material, such as silkworm contamination of silk-filled bed quilts.[1322] The initial suggestion that exposure to the house dust mite was the inciting mechanism[674] is an unlikely sole explanation, because some nonatopic persons also demonstrate the phenomenon. Other mechanisms that have been suggested include (1) a circadian rhythm in autonomic parasympathetic tone, (2) nocturnal down-regulation of beta-adrenergic receptors, (3) gastroesophageal reflux, (4) decreased functional residual capacity (FRC) during recumbency, (5) nocturnal airway wall edema causing an uncoupling of airway parenchymal interdependence, (6) decreased nocturnal mucociliary clearance, (7) nocturnal airway cooling, (8) sleep itself, (9) a variation in circulating cAMP, corticosteroid, or catecholamine secretion, and (10) fluctuating endorphin levels.[1323–1329]

Some of these proposed mechanisms are in fact highly unlikely. Sleep itself is not a necessary factor because the obstruction develops, albeit somewhat less severely, when nocturnal sleep is prevented.[1330, 1331] The phenomenon is not related to either apneic episodes during sleep or any sleep state,[1332] although the bronchoconstriction can be more severe during rapid eye movement (REM) sleep.[1333] Infusion of corticosteroids to block the normal early-morning dip in circulating levels and administration of naloxone to prevent variation in endorphin levels are ineffective in prevention.[1325, 1334]

It is most likely that nocturnal airway obstruction is caused by a complex interaction of several of these factors.[1335] The decrease in circulating catecholamines may be especially important: there is a decrease in circulating epinephrine secretion that is related in time to the nocturnal decrease in PEFR.[1324, 1336, 1337] Decreased catecholamine levels would allow increased smooth muscle shortening and possibly an increase in mast cell mediator release and worsening inflammation.[1324]

### Cough

The presence of the isolated symptom of persistent cough is a frequent reason for referring a patient to a respiratory specialist (*see* page 380).[1338, 1339] It may occur either with or without sputum production and is often nocturnal. Because it may be the sole or initial presenting symptom in patients who have asthma,[1283, 1340, 1341] and because asthma is a common disease, many such referral cases ultimately prove to be related to asthma. For example, in one study of 182 patients who presented with unexplained cough and who were evaluated over a mean follow-up period of 4.4 years, 29 (16%) had asthma.[1342] Patients in whom asthma is the underlying cause of cough almost invariably have an increase in nonspecific airway responsiveness, and their cough responds to treatment of the asthma. Measurement of the total eosinophil count may be a useful screening technique to identify patients in whom asthma is the underlying cause of coughing.[1342, 1343] A condition of chronic cough associated with eosinophilic bronchitis and responsive to inhaled steroids may occur without bronchial hyper-responsiveness or wheeze.[1344]

Coughing is thought to be initiated by stimulation of airway epithelial irritant receptors. Although these are the same receptors that mediate reflex bronchoconstriction, the ability of some stimuli to initiate coughing and bronchoconstriction is clearly unrelated. The inhalation of hypo-osmolar and hyperosmolar aerosols causes both coughing and bronchoconstriction in asthmatic patients.[1345, 1346] The bronchoconstriction appears to be an effect of the abnormal osmolarity alone, but coughing is related to the ion content of the aerosol; lack of a permeant ion such as chloride or bromide causes coughing irrespective of the osmolarity of the solution.[1345] Nebulized hypo-osmolar and hyperosmolar solutions of citric acid cause coughing even if the bronchoconstriction is blocked, although both inhaled beta agonist and anticholinergic agents decrease the severity of the coughing.[1345, 1347] Inhaled local anesthetic attenuates the coughing but not the

bronchoconstriction associated with hypo-osmolar aerosols.[1348]

A cough threshold can be measured by administering progressively increasing concentrations of citric acid aerosol and noting the lowest concentration that reproducibly causes coughing.[1349] A wide variability exists in the cough threshold among normal persons;[1350] asthmatic patients do not have a lower threshold for provoked coughing paralleling the increased tendency of their airways to undergo bronchoconstriction. It has been suggested that postnasal drip can cause persistent coughing in some asthmatic patients and that pharyngeal inflammation can contribute to upper airway obstruction in these patients.[1351] Before cough is attributed to asthma, it is important to rule out postnasal drip secondary to sinusitis, GER, and the ingestion of an ACE inhibitor.[1338]

## LABORATORY FINDINGS

The sputum expectorated by patients experiencing an attack of asthma characteristically contains numerous eosinophils and, in some cases, Charcot-Leyden crystals. It should be emphasized, however, that sputum eosinophilia is not diagnostic of asthma.[1352] When infection is superimposed, as is often the case, the sputum becomes mucopurulent and, rarely, blood-streaked. Recently, the cytologic and chemical changes in the sputum of asthmatics have been systematically explored as means of assessing the severity of airway inflammation, and rigorous standards of analysis have been proposed.[1353, 1354] The combination of sputum eosinophil count and a measure of the level of eosinophil cationic protein (ECP) has been shown to be a more sensitive and specific means of distinguishing between asthmatic patients and normal individuals than measurement of these parameters in the peripheral blood.[1355] Sequential monitoring of ECP, IL-5, and fibrinogen in addition to eosinophils has proved useful in following the course of airway inflammation during acute exacerbations of asthma and for assessing the response to therapy.[1356]

The white blood cell count usually is normal or slightly elevated. It should be remembered, however, that leukocytosis can also be caused by therapy: adrenergic agonists cause demargination of neutrophils, and corticosteroids increase their production in bone marrow.[1357] Eosinophils usually do not exceed 10% but may constitute up to 35% of the total white cell count. In a comparative study of 40 children with bronchiectasis and 43 with asthma, significant peripheral eosinophilia was found in none of the former but in 37 (86%) of the latter;[1358] its degree was unrelated to the severity of the asthma, and it was often present between attacks.

The serum level of several enzymes is not uncommonly increased. High levels of serum aspartate transaminase (AST), lactate dehydrogenase (LDH), and creatine kinase (CK) usually are attributed to tissue hypoxemia, although it has been suggested that excessive muscular activity is responsible for the increases in CK.[1359] One group of investigators found that isoenzyme pattern was largely an increase in $LDH_3$ and $LDH_5$, the former being derived from the lung and the latter from the liver.[1360] Serum alpha$_1$-antitrypsin levels have been found to be significantly higher in patients who have intrinsic asthma than in those who have extrinsic disease or in healthy persons.[1361] Elevated levels of antidiuretic hormone (ADH) have been found during episodes of acute severe asthma.[1362–1364] The production of this substance is controlled by volume receptors located in the left atrium, by pressor receptors in the carotid body, and by osmoreceptors in the hypothalamus. The decreased pulmonary blood flow in asthma may stimulate atrial volume receptors—a possibility that should not be overlooked in planning fluid therapy if water intoxication is to be avoided.[1362] Such intoxication could contribute to an altered state of consciousness in some patients in status asthmaticus.[1363, 1364]

Allergy skin tests may be useful in confirming the culpability of a specific allergen suspected by the patient or to identify exposure to allergens that are not suspected, such as house dust mite, or identified by the patient, such as cat dander. When the clinical situation suggests sensitivity to a specific allergen, confirmation may be obtained by RAST assay for a specific IgE antibody in the serum.[613, 641]

A more reliable method of identifying suspected antigens is bronchial (inhalational) provocation testing.[658, 1365] This is rarely done except for the confirmation of sensitization to an occupational allergen. When skin test results are positive, the inhaled allergen should be well diluted and initially administered in small amounts. This method of testing may elicit immediate or delayed reactions that should be documented objectively by spirographic recordings made before and at intervals after the administration of the extract. Allergens that may be employed for such inhalation testing include not only organic molecules but also gases, vapors, and fumes.[658, 1365] The delayed reactions may occur alone or in combination with an antecedent immediate reaction (dual reaction).[658] As discussed previously, nonspecific inhalation challenge with histamine or methacholine is an important diagnostic technique in some patients and may have value in monitoring the response to long-term therapy.

Electrocardiographic changes may occur during episodes of asthma and, in patients who were previously healthy, may be associated with severe air-flow obstruction.[1366–1368] Sinus tachycardia is almost invariable; right axis deviation, clockwise rotation of the heart, right ventricular hypertrophy, right atrial P waves, and ST-segment or T-wave abnormalities may also be seen. These changes are closely associated with hypoxemia but not necessarily with pulmonary hypertension.[1290, 1366] Although pulmonary artery pressure may not be greatly elevated relative to atmospheric pressure, the transmural pulmonary artery pressure (pulmonary artery–pleural pressure) may be markedly increased as a result of the more negative swings in pleural pressure. This is because it is the difference between the intravascular or intracardiac pressure and the surrounding pleural pressure that determines the load on the right ventricle.[1368a]

## PULMONARY FUNCTION TESTS

As might be expected, aberrations in pulmonary function vary, depending largely upon whether the asthma is in remission or exacerbation and, if the latter, upon the severity of the attack. Many patients whose asthma is in remission have normal pulmonary function;[1369–1371] in fact, values may be normal even when auscultation reveals wheezing.[1371] Even when maximal expiratory flows and volumes are within the normal predicted range, inhalation of a bronchodilator can result in a greater than 15% increase in $FEV_1$ or forced vital capacity (FVC). On the other hand, pulmonary function test results in symptom-free patients are not always normal;[7] for example, both increased airway resistance and impaired distribution of inspired gas have been well documented during symptom-free periods.[8] These observations should not be surprising, because the relationship between symptoms and function depends on the patient's ability to detect airway obstruction, and some patients are unable to sense the presence of severe airway obstruction ($FEV_1$ less than 50% predicted) after methacholine inhalation.[1372] Symptom-free adults who had asthma in childhood often manifest residual abnormalities of pulmonary function.[1373]

When the $FEV_1$ is completely normal, sophisticated tests of small airways function may still reveal abnormalities.[1369, 1374, 1375] For example, reversible abnormalities of small airways have been identified during the hay fever season in patients who have allergic rhinitis but who have no pulmonary symptoms.[1376] In addition to the fact that patients who have allergic rhinitis can have increased nonspecific airway responsiveness, these data suggest that subclinical airway disease may be present in these persons.

Whatever the pathogenesis of airway narrowing, the resulting increase in resistance leads to decreased flow, hyperinflation, gas trapping, and, ultimately, an increase in the work of breathing. There has been much interest in determining which airways are the primary site of the increased resistance. The density dependence of maximal expiratory flow is frequently used to try to separate large central from small peripheral airway narrowing; to the extent that this test is reliable, it appears that both central and peripheral airways may be narrowed in patients who have asthma.[1377–1381] Decreased density dependence of maximal expiratory flow, suggesting predominant small airway obstruction, occurs in older patients who have a long history of asthma,[1382] in asthmatics who smoke,[1383] and in patients who have a late allergic response to antigen challenge.[1384] Despite these observations, the demonstration that density dependence may be an unreliable method of detecting the site of obstruction leaves open the question of which airways are involved in asthma. In one study in which the site of airway narrowing was visualized using HRCT after methacholine challenge, all airways were affected, although the maximal narrowing was in airways 2 to 4 mm in diameter.[1385] Peripheral airway resistance has been shown to be increased in patients who have mild disease using direct measurement via a bronchoscopic technique.[1386]

Airway narrowing, irrespective of site, is most easily detected by measurements of maximal expiratory flow, derived from either volume-time or flow-volume plots.[1387, 1388] Maximal expiratory flow can be decreased as a result of one or more of several mechanisms, including decreased lung elastic recoil, increased air-flow resistance, and increased compressibility of airways; in asthmatic patients, the first of these is usually relatively well preserved, while the last two have been shown to be important mechanisms.[1389]

In addition to decreasing flow during an asthmatic attack, airway narrowing results in gas trapping manifested by an increase in residual volume (RV) and the RV/TLC ratio and by a decrease in vital capacity (VC).[1390–1393] The increase in RV is probably related to closure of the narrowed peripheral airways.[1389, 1394] The increase in airway resistance is also associated with an increase in FRC.[1387, 1395] In normal persons, FRC during tidal breathing is determined by the balance between the outward elastic recoil of the chest wall and the inward recoil of the lung. An increase in FRC could result from loss of lung recoil or from persistent inspiratory muscle activity during expiration; the latter has been shown to contribute to the increase in FRC that occurs during pharmacologically induced bronchoconstriction.[1396, 1397] An additional mechanism for hyperinflation during an asthmatic attack is a dynamic resetting of FRC secondary to the prolonged expiratory phase of the respiratory cycle.[1398] Active laryngeal narrowing, by further slowing expiration, could contribute to hyperinflation.[1399] The hyperinflation associated with induced asthma is caused predominantly by an increased volume of the rib cage rather than of the abdominal compartment.[1400, 1401]

The hyperinflation associated with asthma and other obstructive pulmonary diseases is associated with advantages and disadvantages.[1398] By increasing lung recoil, it dilates the intraparenchymal airways and provides a load that impedes airway smooth muscle shortening;[404, 1402] in addition, it can improve the distribution of ventilation and prevent the phenomenon of tidal expiratory flow occurring on the maximal expiratory flow-volume curve.[1398] On the other hand, hyperinflation increases the inspiratory muscles' work of breathing and places them on an inefficient part of their length-tension curve. Increased resistive work is normally considered the major load applied to inspiratory muscles in asthma; however, elastic work has been shown to be more important in experimental studies.[1403] Although hyperinflation decreases resistive work by dilating the airways, it increases the inspiratory muscle elastic work by moving the lung and chest wall to a less compliant portion of their pressure-volume curves. Hyperinflation leads to inspiratory muscle shortening; because inspiratory muscles show a classic length-tension relationship, they are less able to develop tension at short lengths. Hyperinflation can also uncouple the parallel arrangement between the crural and costal portions of the diaphragm, forcing the two parts to contract in series; such an arrangement is less able to handle increased loads.[1398]

Although there is no question that RV and FRC increase with exacerbations of asthma, the existence of changes in TLC is more controversial. In some patients, an increase in TLC can be demonstrated during an asthmatic attack, followed by a return toward normal during recovery.[1395, 1404] Part of the apparent increase may have been an artifact secondary to an overestimation of TLC when measured plethysmographically in the presence of obstruction. The acute changes in TLC that have been reported following induced bronchoconstriction in asthmatic patients can almost certainly be explained by such errors in the plethysmographic method.[1405–1409] However, increases in TLC have also been observed when TLC was measured using the helium dilution technique, and in one study a radiographic assessment of TLC made during an acute attack of asthma was significantly higher than in the same patients following recovery, indicating that acute changes in TLC can be real.[1410]

TLC is determined by a balance between the elastic recoil of the lung and chest wall and the strength and shortening ability of the inspiratory muscles. An increase in TLC in acute asthma could be caused by a reversible decrease in lung elastic recoil.[1411] It is also possible that breathing at high lung volumes for prolonged periods may alter surface or tissue forces, as has been shown in a few normal subjects.[1412, 1413] Alternatively, there could be adaptive changes in the inspiratory muscles that allow greater-than-normal shortening. In a study of the long-term effect of asthma on TLC, 10 patients in whom the disease had its onset before the age of 8 years were compared with 8 patients in whom it began after the age of 18 years.[1414] Even during a period of remission, TLC was found to be significantly higher in the 10 early-onset patients, and measurement of the pressure-volume curves of their lungs indicated loss of elastic recoil; the patients who had late-onset disease had normal values of TLC.

As an asthmatic episode resolves, there is improvement in expiratory flow and VC and a decrease in FRC and RV. A decrease in symptoms may accompany the return of lung volumes to normal before changes in $FEV_1$ are observed, presumably as a result of the reversal of hyperinflation and gas trapping.[1402] Flow rates measured at low lung volumes ($FEF_{25-75}$, $\dot{V}max_{25}$, $\dot{V}max_{50}$) may take longer to improve or may never return to normal predicted values.[1390]

The steady-state diffusing capacity of the lungs ($DLCO_{SS}$) is normal in the majority of patients,[1387] although it may undergo progressive decline in the presence of severe obstruction.[1390, 1392, 1415] By contrast, the single-breath diffusing capacity ($DLCO_{SB}$) is often elevated during an asthma attack:[1415–1417] In one study of 163 asthmatic children in whom the mean $FEF_{25-75}$ was 55% of predicted, $DLCO_{SB}$ averaged $120 \pm 18\%$ of predicted.[1418] In another investigation of 80 stable asthmatic patients, the $DLCO_{SB}$ was significantly increased at $117 \pm 17\%$ of predicted.[1419] In the latter group, the increased $DLCO_{SB}$ was associated with a more uniform gravitational distribution of perfusion. A possible explanation for this apparent paradox is an increase in pulmonary capillary blood volume as a result of the more negative inspiratory intrathoracic pressure secondary to obstruction of the airways and/or a small increase in pulmonary artery pressure that lessens the gravitational gradient.[1419] $DLCO_{SB}$ increased by an average of 18% in 10 normal persons breathing through an inspiratory resistance and decreased appreciably after bronchodilatation in 31 asthmatic patients.[1418]

An alternative explanation for the apparent increase in $DLCO_{SB}$ during an asthma attack has been suggested.[1420] In measuring $DLCO_{SB}$, it is sometimes assumed that carbon monoxide (CO) uptake occurs only during breath-holding, whereas in fact some CO is taken up during inspiration and expiration; in the presence of air-flow obstruction, the inspiratory and expiratory times are prolonged, thus increasing CO uptake and resulting in a falsely elevated value for $DLCO_{SB}$.

Most patients who have asthma have some degree of hypoxemia, whereas hypocapnia is observed during all but the most severe attacks. Gas exchange may be impaired in symptom-free patients who have asthma.[1421, 1422] The hypoxemia is the result of ventilation-perfusion ($\dot{V}/\dot{Q}$) mismatching,[1421, 1423–1427] which in some cases is caused by a closing volume above FRC.[1375] In one study of 113 asthmatic children in remission, the $PaO_2$ was less than 90% of the normal predicted value in 71%.[1423] In asymptomatic asthmatic subjects who were studied by the multiple inert gas technique, the $\dot{V}/\dot{Q}$ distribution showed no shunt;[1424] however, there was a bimodal distribution of V̇/Q̇ ratios, one compartment having very low values, possibly as a result of collateral ventilation of lung regions in which the airways were completely occluded but collaterally ventilated. Inhalation of a beta-adrenergic bronchodilator increased the perfusion to the low V̇/Q̇ region and lowered the arterial $Po_2$, suggesting pharmacologic reversal of hypoxic vasoconstriction in these regions.[1424] Similarly, administration of 100% $O_2$ increases V̇/Q̇ maldistribution, presumably by the same mechanism.[1428]

As airway obstruction increases in severity and the lungs become hyperinflated during an attack of asthma, V̇/Q̇ maldistribution worsens and hypoxemia increases.[1392, 1429] In one study of 101 patients who had exacerbations of extrinsic asthma, 91 had some degree of hypoxemia, 73 had hypocapnia and respiratory alkalosis, and only 10, who had very severe airway obstruction, had hypercapnia.[1430] Hypoxemia is almost always observed in acute asthmatic attacks; however, the reported incidence of hypercapnia varies, being as high as 50% of patients in some studies.[1431, 1432] Although severe derangements in gas exchange and acid-base balance identify patients who have severe airway obstruction, it is important to remember that normal or mildly abnormal values may also be seen in this clinical situation.

Multiple inert gas studies in stable asthmatic patients frequently show a bimodal distribution of V̇/Q̇ ratios, with an increase in low V̇/Q̇ areas. There is variation in the degree of abnormality in V̇/Q̇ distribution with time, a feature that correlates with changes in arterial $Po_2$. In patients who have severe acute asthma and require mechanical ventilation, the pattern of V̇/Q̇ distribution is similar, although a larger fraction of perfusion is related to lower V̇/Q̇ areas.[1433]

Respiratory alkalosis is the only acid-base disturbance seen during mild asthmatic attacks; however, metabolic and mixed acidosis can occur during severe exacerbations. In one study of 103 patients in status asthmaticus, 23 were hypocapnic, 26 were eucapnic, 25 had a metabolic acidosis, and 14 had a mixed acidosis.[1434] The 38% incidence of some degree of metabolic acidosis in this series is surprising; however, blood lactic acid levels were increased, and it is possible that anaerobic glycolysis in the failing respiratory muscles was the source of the lactate. In another study of 109 adults, approximately 17% of 164 episodes of acute asthma were associated with metabolic acidosis.[1435] In some patients, the acidosis is not caused by excessive lactate levels but is of the non–anion-gap type.[1436] Lactic acidosis in severe asthma also may be related to high-dose parenteral $beta_2$ agonist therapy.[1437]

The relationship between changes in $Pao_2$ and $FEV_1$ is not clear; some investigators have found that the two vary directly,[1387, 1438, 1439] while others have noted a poor correlation.[1440] Treatment can improve $Pao_2$ without producing a simultaneous increase in expiratory flow.[1441] In one study in which V̇/Q̇ distribution (as measured by the multiple inert gas technique) and maximal expiratory flow were measured before and after exercise-induced bronchoconstriction, no correlation was found between the decrease in $FEV_1$ and the V̇/Q̇ maldistribution.[1442] On the other hand, in another investigation in children, arterial oxygen saturation measured using a pulse oximeter at the time of presentation for acute severe asthma was shown to be a predictor of outcome and response to therapy.[1443] When comparable degrees of

obstruction (as reflected in decreased SGaw) were induced by inhaled methacholine and antigen, the antigen challenge was associated with more severe hypoxemia, suggesting more peripheral airway obstruction.[1444] The discrepancy between measures of air-flow obstruction and gas exchange was illustrated in another study in which no clear relationship was found between decreased $FEV_1$ and V̇/Q̇ mismatch, as assessed by the multiple inert gas technique, after antigen challenge.[1445]

In acute prolonged attacks, the $Pao_2$ often drops below 60 mm Hg,[1290, 1299] the $FEV_1$ becomes less than 1, and the peak flow decreases to less than 60 liters/minute.[1299, 1440] As the severity and duration of obstruction increase, patients become exhausted, their respiratory muscles fatigue, and hypercapnia ensues.[1392, 1429, 1446] Unlike in COPD, hypercapnia in asthma is never a steady-state situation; the measured partial pressure of carbon dioxide ($Pco_2$) generally decreases in response to therapy or rises steeply within minutes or hours. Patients in whom such increases are noted should be under constant surveillance.[1447] Occasionally, patients who do not have severe bronchoconstriction have $CO_2$ retention,[1448–1450] probably as a result of hyposensitivity of the respiratory center. As patients recover from severe acute attacks, the ventilatory response to $CO_2$ returns to normal in the majority; however, some of those who present with hypercapnia fail to show improvement.[1448]

### Control of Breathing

Most asthmatic patients appear to have normal or enhanced respiratory drive. Unlike that in patients who have COPD, the ventilatory response to hypoxia and hypercapnia is normal despite alterations in baseline lung function. In fact, when more precise measurements of neural drive are employed—e.g., mouth occlusion pressure at 100 milliseconds ($PM_{0.1}$) or mean inspiratory flow ($VT/TI$)—asthmatic patients have increased respiratory drive at any given $Pao_2$ or $Paco_2$.[1451–1454] The preserved or increased drive to breathe observed in asthma has been attributed to either rapid fluctuations in respiratory impedance that prevent adaptive changes or increased stimulation of irritant receptors secondary to the chronic mucosal inflammation.[1451] Irritant receptor stimulation can increase respiratory drive even if reflex bronchoconstriction is blocked.[1453] It is likely that stimulation of afferent nerves from inspiratory muscles (muscle spindles and stretch receptors) is also an important input that maintains respiratory drive under load.[1455]

The preservation of drive to breathe in asthmatic patients has both beneficial and adverse effects. The normal drive is associated with an ability to detect and respond to increased loads on the respiratory system;[1456, 1457] at comparable loads (as determined by severity of obstruction), hypercapnic respiratory failure is much less likely to develop in patients who have asthma than in those who have COPD. Unfortunately, the ability to perceive an increased respiratory impedance appears to be coupled to the sensation of dyspnea, and most asthmatic patients experience more respiratory distress for a given degree of obstruction than patients who have COPD. This heightened sensation of dyspnea may be related to the rapidity of onset of the air-flow obstruction.[1458] An impaired perception of obstruction and decreased dyspnea may be a risk factor for the development of life-threatening asthma.[1459] During REM sleep, asthmatic patients may experience a decrease in intercostal muscle activity that results in paradoxical chest wall movement.[1460, 1461]

## PROGNOSIS AND NATURAL HISTORY

### Complications

Complications of asthma are much more common in children than in adults and consist of pneumonia, atelectasis, mucoid impaction and mucous plugging, pneumomediastinum, and (rarely) arterial air embolism. Lower respiratory tract viral infection occurs more frequently and tends to be more severe among asthmatic patients than in the population at large.[1462] Atelectasis occurs predominantly in children and is the result of mucous plugging or mucoid impaction.[1463–1465] Although radiographically demonstrable atelectasis occurs very uncommonly in adult asthmatic patients (and then usually in association with mucoid impaction), it is probable that mucous plugging of smaller bronchi and bronchioles occurs much more frequently than is recognized. In such circumstances, it is assumed that pulmonary collapse distal to the obstructed airway is prevented by collateral ventilation.

Pneumomediastinum is an uncommon complication of asthma, and as with the more common complications, it occurs predominantly in children.[1464, 1466, 1467] The sudden onset of chest pain suggests the diagnosis.[1468] In patients who have a chest tube inserted for pneumothorax and in whom the ipsilateral lung fails to re-expand, obstruction of central airways by impacted mucus should be suspected.[1469] In older children[1467] and in adults,[1470] subcutaneous "emphysema" should be easily recognizable clinically. A precordial "click" or "crunch" synchronous with the heartbeat (Hamman's sign) suggests the presence of pneumomediastinum; however, this also occurs in association with pneumothorax and elevation of the left hemidiaphragm as a result of gas in the gastric fundus. Occasionally, air dissects along pulmonary vessels through the pericardial reflection, resulting in pneumopericardium.[1471] A single case has been reported of sudden death in status asthmaticus from arterial air embolism.[1472]

In asthmatic patients who require mechanical ventilation during an acute attack, systemic hypotension and barotrauma can occur secondary to dynamic hyperinflation.[1473–1475] Mechanically ventilated patients can also develop profound muscle weakness, a complication that can prolong the necessary duration of ventilation and hospitalization. Several factors may contribute to this complication, including (1) a skeletal muscle myopathic process that involves the respiratory muscles and is related to the high doses of corticosteroids that these patients receive, (2) an abnormality at the level of the neuromuscular junction that appears to relate to the use of neuromuscular-blocking agents,[1476–1478] and (3) skeletal muscle damage secondary to a high dose of parenteral beta$_2$ agonists.[1479] The dose and duration of neuromuscular blocker and steroid therapy have been shown to be independent predictors of the development of muscle weakness.[1480, 1481] There is also an inverse relationship between respiratory and peripheral muscle strength and systemic corticosteroid dosage in chronic asthma.[1482]

### Recovery from Acute Asthmatic Episodes

Predicting the need for hospitalization and the rapidity of recovery from acute episodes of asthma has received considerable attention.[1483–1486] The requirement for hospitalization and a slow (days to weeks) symptomatic and functional recovery in asthmatic patients are associated with several factors, including age greater than 40 years, nonatopic disease, a longer duration of symptoms prior to admission, poor long-term control of symptoms, and the use of maintenance corticosteroids.[1484] The rapidity with which flow rates improve during the first 6 hours can also be used to predict a patient's recovery time.[1487] In one retrospective study, a scoring system based on pulse rate, respiratory rate, pulsus paradoxus, PEFR, the use of accessory muscles, and the severity of dyspnea and wheeze was 90% effective in predicting the need for hospitalization and the relapse rate following discharge from the emergency department;[1486] however, application of the same scoring system prospectively to 114 acutely ill asthmatic patients failed to predict the need for admission or the likelihood of relapse.[1485]

Approximately 40% of asthmatics who require mechanical ventilation are extubated within 24 hours and 70% within 72 hours.[1473] The mortality among asthmatic patients who require mechanical ventilation during an acute attack averages 13%, with wide variability between studies; causes of death include anoxic encephalopathy, barotrauma, and intensive care unit complications such as gastrointestinal hemorrhage and sepsis.[1473, 1488] The rapidity of recovery from episodes of acute severe disease is influenced by the development of respiratory muscle weakness. In a multicenter study of 121 asthmatic patients who underwent mechanical ventilation for a near-fatal attack, the subsequent mortality from asthma was 10% at 1 year, 14% at 2 years, and 23% at 3 years;[1489] older age was the most significant risk factor for subsequent death. These results graphically illustrate why a near-fatal asthma attack is an important predictor of subsequent mortality.

### Remissions

Studies in children have shown that a number of factors are associated with a poor long-term prognosis, including early onset of symptoms, multiple attacks in the initial year, clinical and physiologic evidence of persisting airway obstruction, pulmonary hyperinflation, chest deformity, and impairment of growth.[654, 1490–1492] Morbidity has been reported to be greater in poorer families, suggesting unequal access to therapy.[1493]

Airway hyper-responsiveness is associated with lower-than-normal increments in lung function during growth and persistent asthma. A multivariate analysis in 200 children showed that skin test sensitivity to house dust mite, molds, pollen, and milk proteins was associated with a significant risk for persistent asthma.[1494] The prognosis in patients whose asthmatic attacks are intermittent[1495] and who show evidence for lability of expiratory flow[1496] is considerably better than in those whose symptoms are continuous and whose obstruction is relatively fixed. In this context, it is noteworthy that intermittent asthma usually has its onset before the age of 16 years, whereas persistent airway obstruction usually begins later in life. Associated bronchitis worsens the prognosis significantly and is more common in patients who have continuous asthma.

Studies of asthmatic children support the high incidence of remission; 90% of 449 patients whose asthma had its onset before the age of 14 years were assessed 20 years later, and only 30% still suffered from the disease.[1498, 1499] In another study, 70% of children who had had a diagnosis of asthma were in apparent remission by the age of 10 years, while 30% continued to have asthmatic episodes.[29] Almost 60% of children who "wheeze" before the age of 3 years are asymptomatic by age 6.[72] The remissions that occur in some patients during childhood may be related to the heterogeneity of underlying mechanisms that lead to asthma. A subset of infants who are diagnosed as having asthma have transient early wheezing associated with maternal smoking during gestation and reduced postnatal lung function; these children do not show evidence of atopy and tend to be asymptomatic by age 6. It is likely that their "asthma" is the result of viral respiratory infection superimposed on anatomically smaller airways. The children who develop persistent asthma start with normal lung function but develop atopy and eventually airway hyper-responsiveness.[72, 91] In an 8-year follow-up study of 2,289 children who were aged 6 to 8 years when first seen, active and passive cigarette smoking, lower socioeconomic status, number of children and of furry pets in the household, and use of gas cookers were associated with persistent symptoms.[1497]

The remissions experienced later in life by adolescents and young adults may not be permanent. In a 14-year follow-up of 441 children, the cumulative prevalence of asthma increased until the age of 7 years and then progressively decreased until the age of 17 to 18 years, at which time 70% were considered "cured" (no symptoms or treatment for 1 year); however, subsequent "relapses" occurred, so that at an average age of 26 years, only 57% were still "cured."[1500] Additional relapses tend to occur with increasing age. The risk also appears to be increased in those who smoke cigarettes.[1501] Remissions during adolescence do not seem to be directly related to the onset of puberty.[73] Previously asthmatic children retain a high prevalence of airway hyper-responsiveness and positive results on allergy skin tests, although they are less atopic and have less airway hyper-responsiveness than currently asthmatic children.[1502] Similarly, asymptomatic adults who have a history of asthma show persistence of airway hyper-responsiveness.[1503]

The increased recognition that extrinsic asthma has its origins in infancy has led to the hypothesis that institution of preventive strategies early in life could have a lasting beneficial effect, decreasing the later development of allergy and asthma.[1504] This concept of a developmental "window" of increased susceptibility is supported by the observation that month of birth is a determinant of sensitization to certain seasonal environmental allergens[1505] and of the later development of asthma.[1504] Preventive interventions have included decreased exposure to intrauterine and environmental tobacco smoke, encouragement of breast feeding, avoidance of known potent food allergens, extermination of house dust mite, and the use of mattress covers.[1504] In one prospective study, a cohort of infants at risk of allergic disease (i.e., two first-degree relatives had atopy) were randomized to a primary prevention or control group;[1506–1508] a significant decrease in the prevalence of positive results on allergy skin tests and a trend for a reduction in allergic disease including asthma and eczema were evident at 1, 2, and 4 years of follow-up. Another preventive hypothesis that is being tested is the early and aggressive use of inhaled corticosteroids.[1509] It is too early to say whether these strategies will have long-term beneficial effects.

Although a characteristic feature of asthma is some degree of reversibility of the air-flow obstruction, it is clear that long-standing asthma can lead to a relatively fixed narrowing; for example, in one study of 89 patients who had the disease for a mean of 22 years, persistent functional impairment was present despite prolonged aggressive therapy with bronchodilators and corticosteroids.[1510] An 18-year follow-up case-control study of 92 asthmatic patients showed an accelerated age-related decline in $FEV_1$,[1511] an observation confirmed in other studies.[1512] The fixed component of airway narrowing in long-standing asthma is probably related to airway wall fibrosis.[200, 1513, 1514] This hypothesis is supported by functional studies showing that the airways of asthmatic patients are less distensible than those of normal subjects.[9, 199]

### Mortality

Death from asthma occurs predominantly in adults 40 to 60 years of age[1515] and in children under the age of 2 years. In 1980, death rates from asthma in patients aged 5 to 34 years ranged from 0.2 per 100,000 in the United States to 3 per 100,000 in New Zealand.[31] Since that time, the death rate in New Zealand has fallen dramatically (to about 0.5 per 100,000 persons aged 5 to 34 in 1994), while it has increased slowly and steadily in most other countries, including Canada, Australia,[1516] England and Wales,[1517] Germany, Japan,[1518] and the United States (to about 0.4 per 100,000 persons aged 5 to 34 in 1994).[1519–1524] Asthma death rates in Australia have been intermediate between those of New Zealand and those of Europe and North America; they appeared to peak at about 1.5 per 100,000 population (ages 5 to 34) and have subsequently decreased in parallel with the decline in New Zealand.[1525] It is most unlikely that these changes or the large variation between countries can be attributed to the unreliability of death certificate reporting, because in this age group, asthma is unlikely to be confused with COPD; nor is it likely that the changes can be explained by changes in disease coding.[1523, 1526]

During the years 1959 to 1966, an unexpected increase in mortality attributed to asthma was observed in the United Kingdom, New Zealand, and Australia, affecting patients aged 5 to 34 years, particularly those between 10 and 19.[1527–1531] The transient increase in mortality was initially attributed to the potent nonselective beta-adrenergic aerosol bronchodilators used during that period;[1528–1531] however, retrospective analysis has not completely supported this explanation.[1532, 1533] Investigations into the circumstances surrounding the deaths identified a number of risk factors, including a long history of asthma, previous hospital admissions for severe asthma, widely varying flow rates, delayed perception of the severity of the final attack, and under-use of corticosteroids.[1534]

After 1966, death rates in the countries in which the mortality rates had increased returned to "pre-epidemic" levels, but by 1977 they had increased again in New

Zealand.[1535, 1536] Death rates for Maoris (19 in 1,000 deaths) and Polynesians (9 in 1,000) were significantly higher than for patients of European origin (5 in 1,000), but the death rate for the latter group was three times higher than that in the United Kingdom. The age at the time of death was bimodally distributed, with a peak near 20 and another near 65 years. Seventy per cent of deaths occurred between 8:00 P.M. and 8:00 A.M., and more than half the people died at home. No single cause for the increase was identified, although risk factors were similar to those observed in the previous studies, including under-use of corticosteroids.[1535–1537]

Concern that this second "epidemic" of asthma deaths was also related to therapy was increased by the results of three case-control studies suggesting that the deaths were associated with the introduction of the potent beta$_2$-adrenergic agonist fenoterol in a high-dose formulation.[1538–1540] The results of another investigation have shown that fenoterol use constitutes a risk for near-fatal asthma as well.[1541] A number of other investigations have provided additional support for the hypothesis. For example, in a double-blind cross-over study, the regular use of fenoterol (two puffs 4 times a day) had a detrimental effect on asthma control as compared with the use of a beta$_2$ agonist on an as-needed, or "rescue," basis.[1542] In a retrospective study of asthma deaths and near-deaths in Saskatchewan, Canada, excessive use of fenoterol and salbutamol was associated with increased fatal or near-fatal asthma even after correction for potential confounding factors.[1543–1545] Despite these observations, the authors of a meta-analysis of beta agonist use and death from asthma concluded that although there was a significant relationship, the effect was very small and potentially confounded.[1546] In addition, the most recent comparison of as-needed and regular beta$_2$ agonist use showed minimal differences in 255 patients with mild asthma who were studied in a parallel-group, double-blind, 16-week trial;[1547] those receiving regular beta$_2$-agonist therapy showed only a slightly increased peak flow variability and airway responsiveness compared with the as-needed group.

It is biologically plausible that chronic use of beta agonists could have detrimental effects in asthma.[1548] Chronic administration of the drug leads to down-regulation of expression of beta$_2$ receptors on airway smooth muscle and other cells and induces changes in beta$_2$-adrenergic signal transduction pathways.[1539, 1549, 1550] In fact, even a 1-week course of regular beta$_2$-agonist therapy results in functional down-regulation of beta$_2$ receptors, as evidenced by a reduction in the protective effect of an acute dose of salbutamol against bronchoconstriction induced by methacholine, adenosine, and antigen.[1540, 1551] NSBH has also been shown to increase after chronic administration of beta agonists,[1552] and beta$_2$ agonists have the potential to increase the production of IgE.[1553] In addition to these direct adverse effects, excess reliance on bronchodilators may lead to delay in seeking more appropriate care, increasing the risk of severe and even fatal attacks. The clinical and experimental studies that showed a link between the regular use of short-acting beta agonists, worsening of asthma control, and increased mortality, combined with the potential biologic explanations for such a detrimental effect, engendered caution among clinicians when ultra-long-acting beta agonists (salmeterol and formoterol) were introduced. However, prospective investigations have not shown detrimental effects of their chronic use.[1554] In fact, the results of some studies suggest a long-term beneficial effect of salmeterol when combined with inhaled corticosteroids on quality of life, asthma symptoms, and need for use of relief medication.[1555, 1556]

Racial and ethnic differences in asthma mortality rates have been well-documented; for example, in the United States, age-adjusted mortality in African Americans increased from 1.5 per 100,000 in 1978 to 3.7 in 1994, while over the same time period the rates in whites increased from 0.5 to 1.2.[1524] A similar discrepancy exists for asthma death rates between the white and colored populations of South Africa.[1557] Rates are also higher in Americans of Hispanic origin.[1558] Asthma prevalence, morbidity, and mortality are also higher in large American cities.[1559] It is likely that all or a major part of these differences are related to adverse environmental influences and limited access to adequate medical care in the financially disadvantaged ethnic groups.

Patients who have life-threatening asthma have usually had symptoms of increasing severity over a period of days,[1560] although rapid deterioration may be seen. In one study, 8 of 26 patients deteriorated rapidly over a period of minutes to hours; in 3 of these, the attack was triggered by ASA.[1561] In a 2-year study of asthma deaths in New Zealand, 11 occurred in children aged 0 to 14 years;[1562] 7 of the children died in less than 3 hours from the onset of their final attack, and all died outside the hospital. The factors that appeared to increase the risk of death in these children were similar to those described for adults. In a case-control study of asthma deaths in the 8- to 18-year-old age group, increased asthma symptoms in the week preceding death, a decrease in prednisone dosage, conflict between physician and parent, and a disregard of asthmatic symptoms were all factors that were associated with an increased risk of death.[1563] In another case-control study, hospitalized patients who died of asthma were shown to have had inadequate management, including the inappropriate use of sedatives, inadequate steroid and beta-adrenergic dosages, excessive theophylline dosage, and a failure to institute mechanical ventilation in a timely fashion.[1564] Over-reliance on the home use of nebulized bronchodilators may also be a contributing cause.[1565]

It is unclear whether the increased asthma mortality that has been observed worldwide is the result of an increase in severity or is simply a reflection of the increased prevalence.[1522] The trends in asthma mortality, like those in prevalence, are disturbing and puzzling. They have occurred over a period when our understanding of the basic pathophysiologic mechanisms responsible for asthma has increased enormously and during which we have seen the development of a variety of effective pharmacologic therapies. In New Zealand, where the biggest increases occurred, the changes have been attributed to socioeconomic factors such as increasing barriers to primary health care and poverty, in addition to over-reliance on the use of potent bronchodilator medications, which delays the seeking of more appropriate therapy.[1526] The subsequent dramatic decline in mortality is believed to be secondary to widespread physician and patient education, the implementation of guidelines, and the substantial increase in the use of inhaled corticosteroids.[1526]

The factors that contribute to an increased risk of fatal asthma can be divided into those related to the physician, the patient, and the environment.[1566] Among the first of these are failure of the physician to objectively evaluate the severity of an acute attack of asthma by measuring expiratory flow rates, failure to prescribe appropriate anti-inflammatory therapy, and failure to educate the patient about appropriate avoidance strategies for important triggering factors.[1567] One method to detect patient-related factors is to study patients who have survived a near-fatal asthma attack; such patients have a decreased perception of dyspnea in comparison with that in patients who have equal degrees of obstruction but have no history of near-fatal asthma attacks.[1568, 1569] Additional patient factors are poor compliance, lower socioeconomic status, and a prior history of a severe asthma attack requiring mechanical ventilation.[1570–1572] Measures of airway responsiveness may be predictive of risk for severe, potentially fatal attacks; patients who have had life-threatening attacks are very sensitive to histamine, with characteristically steep dose-response curves.[1573] The most important environmental factor is probably inhalation of high concentrations of potent aeroallergens; for example, in one case-control study from the Midwestern United States, exposure to *Alternaria alternata* in the fall months was shown to be a risk factor for fatal and near-fatal disease.[1574] The dust from soybeans has also been associated with an outbreak of asthma deaths in the port city of Barcelona.[1575]

# REFERENCES

1. Scadding JG: Definition and the clinical categories of asthma. *In* Clark TJH, Godfrey S (eds): Asthma. 2nd ed. London, Chapman and Hall, 1983, pp 1–11.
2. American Thoracic Society: Chronic bronchitis, asthma, and pulmonary emphysema. Am Rev Respir Dis 85:762, 1962.
3. Matthys H: Definition and assessment of asthma. Lung 168:51, 1990.
4. Global Initiative for Asthma: Global strategy for asthma management and prevention. NHLBI/WHO Workshop Report. NIH publication No. 95-3659. Bethesda, MD, National Institutes of Health, National Heart, Lung, and Blood Institute, 1995.
5. Woolcock AJ: Definitions and clinical classification. *In* Barnes PJ, Grunstein MM, Leff AR, et al (eds): Asthma. Vol. 1. Philadelphia, Lippincott-Raven, 1997, p 27.
6. Scadding JG: Asthma and bronchial reactivity. BMJ Clin Res Ed 294:1115, 1987.
7. Mok JYQ, Simpson H: Pulmonary function in severe chronic asthma in children during apparent clinical remission. Eur J Respir Dis 64:487, 1983.
8. Bates DV: Impairment of respiratory function in bronchial asthma. Clin Sci 11:203, 1952.
9. Wilson JW, Li X, Pain MC: The lack of distensibility of asthmatic airways. Am Rev Respir Dis 148:806, 1993.
10. Report of the Committee on Emphysema, American College of Chest Physicians: Criteria for the assessment of reversibility in airway obstruction. Chest 65:552, 1974.
11. Marsh G, Meyers A, Bias B: The epidemiology and genetics of atopic allergy. N Engl J Med 305:1551, 1981.
12. Smith JM: Prevalence and natural history of asthma in schoolchildren. BMJ 1:711, 1961.
13. Beall GN, Heiner DC, Tashkin DP, et al: Asthma: New ideas about an old disease. Ann Intern Med 78:405, 1973.
14. Falliers CJ, Cardoso RR de, Bare HN, et al: Discordant allergic manifestation in monozygotic twins: Genetic identity vs. clinical, physiologic, and biochemical differences. J Allergy 47:207, 1971.
15. Hopp RJ, Bewtra AK, Watt GD, et al: Genetic analysis of allergic disease in twins. J Allerg Clin Immunol 73:265, 1984.
16. Chan-Yeung M, Lam S: State of the art: Occupational asthma. Am Rev Respir Dis 133:686, 1986.
17. Szczeklik A, Nizankowska E, Serafin A, et al: Autoimmune phenomena in bronchial asthma with special reference to aspirin intolerance. Am J Respir Crit Care Med 152:1753, 1995.
18. Inouye T, Tarlo S, Broder I, et al: Severity of asthma in skin test–negative and skin test–positive patients. J Allergy Clin Immunol 75:313, 1985.
19. Pirson F, Charpin D, Sansonetti M, et al: Is intrinsic asthma a hereditary disease? Allergy 46:367, 1991.
20. Sibbald B, Turner Warick M: Factors influencing the prevalence of asthma among first degree relatives of extrinsic and intrinsic asthmatics. Thorax 34:322, 1979.
21. Kroegel C, Jäger L, Walker C. Is there a place for instrisic asthma as a distinct immunopathological entity? Eur Respir J 10:513, 1997.
22. Kroegel C, Jäger L, Walker C: Is there a place for intrinsic asthma as a distinct immunopathological entity? Eur Respir J 10:513, 1997.
23. Walker C, Bode E, Boer L, et al: Allergic and non-allergic asthmatics have distinct patterns of T cell activation and cytokine production in peripheral blood and BAL. Am Rev Respir Dis 146:109, 1992.
24. Tang MLK, Coleman J, Kemp AS: Interleukin-4 and interferon gamma production in atopic and nonatopic children with asthma. Clin Exp Allergy 25:515, 1995.
25. Humbert M, Durham SR, Ying S, et al: IL-4 and IL-5 mRNA and protein in bronchial biopsies from patients with atopic and nonatopic asthma: Evidence against "intrinsic" asthma being a distinct immunopathologic entity. Am J Respir Crit Care Med 154:1497, 1996.
26. Sears MR: Risk factors: Immunoglobulin E and atopy. Asthma 1:71, 1997.
27. Burrows B, Martinez FD, Halonen M, et al: Association of asthma with serum IgE levels and skin test reactivity to allergens. N Engl J Med 320:271, 1989.
28. McFadden ER: Pathogenesis of asthma. J Allergy Clin Immunol 73:413, 1984.
29. Williams E, McNicol KN: Prevalence, natural history, and relationship of wheezy bronchitis and asthma in children. An epidemiological study. BMJ 4:321, 1969.
30. von Mutius E, Weiland SK, Fritzsch C, et al: Increasing prevalence of hay fever and atopy among children in Leipzig, East Germany. Lancet 351:862, 1998.
31. Woolcock AJ: Worldwide differences in asthma prevalence and mortality: Why is asthma mortality so low in the U.S.A.? Chest 90:40S, 1986.
32. Peat JK, van den Berg RH, Green WF, et al: Changing prevalence of asthma in Australian children. BMJ 308:1591, 1994.
33. Rona RJ, Chinn S, Burney PGJ: Trends in the prevalence of asthma in Scottish and English primary school children 1982–1992. Thorax 50:992, 1995.
34. Crockett A, Cranston J, Alpers J: The changing prevalence of asthmalike symptoms in South Australian rural schoolchildren. J Pediatr Child Health 31:213, 1995.
35. Toelle BG, Peat JK, van den Berg RH, et al: Comparison of three definitions of asthma: A longitudinal perspective. J Asthma 34:161, 1997.
36. Jarvis D, Lai E, Luczynska C, et al: Prevalence of asthma and asthmalike symptoms in young adults living in three East Anglian towns. Br J Gen Pract 44:493, 1994.
37. Cullen KJ: Climate and chest disorders in school children. BMJ 4:65, 1972.
38. Cookson JB, Makoni G: Prevalence of asthma in Rhodesian Africans. Thorax 35:833, 1980.
39. Ross I: Bronchial asthma in Malaysia. Br J Dis Chest 78:369, 1984.
40. Salome CM, Woolcock AJ: Ethnic differences. *In* Barnes PJ, Grunstein MM, Leff AR, et al (eds): Asthma. Vol. 1. Philadelphia, Lippincott-Raven, 1997, p 63.
41. Crane J, Lewis S, Slater T, et al: The self reported prevalence of asthma symptoms among New Zealanders. N Z Med J 107:417, 1994.
42. Gold DR, Rotnitzky A, Damokosh AI, et al: Race and gender differences in respiratory illness prevalence and their relationship to environmental exposures in children 7 to 14 years of age. Am Rev Respir Dis 148:10, 1993.
43. Ng TP, Hui KP, Tan WC: Prevalence of asthma and risk factors among Chinese, Malay and Indian adults in Singapore. Thorax 49:347, 1994.
44. Lai CK, Douglass C, Ho SS, et al: Asthma epidemiology in the Far East. Clin Exp Allergy 26:5, 1996.
45. von Mutius E, Martinez FD, Fritzsch C, et al: Prevalence of asthma and atopy in two areas of West Germany and East Germany. Am J Respir Crit Care Med 149:358, 1994.
46. Wichmann HE: Possible explanation for the different trends of asthma and allergy in East and West Germany. Clin Exp Allergy 26:621, 1996.
47. Trepka MJ, Heinrich J, Wichmann HE: The epidemiology of atopic diseases in Germany: An East-West comparison. Rev Environ Health 11:119, 1996.
48. IgE, parasites and allergy (editorial). Lancet 1:894, 1976.
49. Carswell F, Meakins RH, Harland PSEG: Parasites and asthma in Tanzanian children. Lancet 2:706, 1976.
50. Lynch NR, Hagel I, Perez M, et al: Effect of antihelmintic treatment on the allergic reactivity of children in a tropical slum. J Allergy Clin Immunol 92:404, 1993.
51. Woolcock AJ, Colman MH, Jones MW: Atopy and bronchial reactivity in Australian and Malaysian populations. Clin Allergy 8:155, 1978.
52. Woolcock AJ, Green W, Alpers MP: Asthma in a rural highland area of Papua New Guinea. Am Rev Respir Dis 123:565, 1981.
53. Woolcock AJ, Dowse GK, Temple K, et al: The prevalence of asthma in the South-Fore people of Papua New Guinea. A method for field studies of bronchial reactivity. Eur J Respir Dis 64:571, 1983.
54. Dowse GK, Smith D, Turner KJ, et al: Prevalence and features of asthma in a sample survey of urban Goroka, Papua New Guinea. Clin Allergy 15:429, 1985.
55. Turner KJ, Stewart GA, Woolcock AJ, et al: Relationship between mite densities and the prevalence of asthma: Comparative studies in two populations in the Eastern Highlands of Papua New Guinea. Clin Allergy 18:331, 1988.
56. Weiss ST, Sparrow D, O'Connor GT: The interrelationship among allergy, airways responsiveness, and asthma. J Asthma 30:329, 1993.
57. Halken S, Høst A, Nilsson L, Taudorf E: Passive smoking as a risk factor for development of obstructive respiratory disease and allergic sensitization. Allergy 50:97, 1995.
58. Landau LI: Bronchiolitis and asthma: Are they related? Thorax 49:293, 1994.
59. Settipane RJ, Hagy GW, Settipane GA: Long-term risk factors for developing asthma and allergic rhinitis: A 23-year follow-up study of college students. Allergy Proc 15:21, 1994.
60. Sears MR, Burrows B, Flannery EM, et al: Gender and allergen related risks for development of hay fever and asthma. Clin Exp Allergy 23:941, 1993.
61. Corne J, Smith S, Schreiber J, Holgate ST: Prevalence of atopy in asthma. Lancet 344:344, 1994.
62. Gergen PJ, Turkeltaub PC: The association of individual allergen reactivity with respiratory disease in a national sample: Data from the second National Health and Nutritional Examination Survey, 1976–1980 (NHANES II). J Allergy Clin Immunol 90:579, 1992.
63. Sporik R, Holgate ST, Platts-Mills TAE, Cogswell JJ: Exposure to house dust mite allergen (Der P 1) and development of asthma in childhood. N Engl J Med 323:502, 1990.
64. Burrows B, Sears MR, Flannery EM, Holdaway MD: Relations of bronchial responsiveness to allergy skin test reactivity, lung function, respiratory symptoms, and diagnoses in thirteen-year-old New Zealand children. J Allerg Clin Immunol 95:548, 1995.
65. Sears MR, Burrows B, Flannery EM, et al: Relation between airway responsiveness and serum IgE in children with asthma and in apparently normal children. N Engl J Med 325:1067, 1991.
66. Weiss ST: The role of eosinophils in the pathogenesis of asthma. Curr Opin Immunol 6:860, 1994.
67. Wartenberg D, Ehrlich R, Lilienfeld D: Environmental tobacco smoke and childhood asthma: Comparing exposure metrics using probability plots. Environ Res 64:122, 1994.
68. Cook DG, Strachan DP: Parental smoking and prevalence of respiratory symptoms and asthma in school age children. Thorax 52:1081, 1997.
69. Weiss ST: Smoking and asthma. Compr Ther 20:606, 1994.
70. Murray M, Webb MSC, O'Callaghan C: Respiratory status and allergy after bronchiolitis. Arch Dis Child 67:482, 1992.
71. Martinez FD: Risk factors, development and natural history. Asthma 1:121, 1997.

72. Martinez FG, Wright AL, Taussig LM, et al: Asthma and wheezing in the first six years of life. N Engl J Med 332:122, 1995.
73. Zannolli R, Morgese G: Does puberty interfere with asthma? Med Hypotheses 48:27, 1997.
74. Skobeloff EM, Spivey WH, St Clair SS, Schoffstal JM: The influence of age and sex on asthma admissions. JAMA 268:3437, 1992.
75. Ford RM: Aetiology of asthma: A review of 11,551 cases (1958–1968). Med J Aust 1:628, 1969.
76. Sears MR: Descriptive epidemiology of asthma. Lancet 350:SII1, 1997.
77. Burney PGJ: Epidemiologic trends. Asthma 1:35, 1997.
78. Woolcock AJ, Peat JK: Evidence for the increase in asthma world-wide. Ciba Found Symp 206:122, 1997.
79. Skonsberg O, Clench-Aas J, Leegaard J, et al: Prevalence of bronchial asthma in school children in Oslo, Norway. Comparison of data obtained in 1993 and 1981. Allergy 50:806, 1995.
80. Magnus P, Kongerud J, Bakke JV: Do we have an asthma epidemic? Tidsskr Nor Laegeforen 111:972, 1991.
81. Ciba Foundation Symposium 206. The rising trends in asthma. Chichester, John Wiley & Sons, 1997.
82. Seaton A, Godden DJ, Brown K: Increase in asthma: A more toxic environment or a more susceptible population? Thorax 49:171, 1994.
83. Woolcock AJ, Peat JK, Trevillion LM: Is the increase in asthma prevalence linked to increase in allergen load? Allergy 50:935, 1995.
84. Bolton-Smith C, Smith WCS, Woodward M, Tunstall-Pedoe H: Nutrient intakes of different social class groups: Results from the Scottish Heart Health Study (SHHS). Br J Nutr 65:321, 1991.
85. Greene LS: Asthma and oxidant stress: Nutritional, environmental, and genetic risk factors. J Am Coll Nutr 14:317, 1995.
86. Becklake MR, Ernst P: Environmental factors. Lancet 350:SII10, 1997.
87. Shirakawa T, Enomoto T, Shimazu S, Hopkin JM: The inverse association between tuberculin responses and atopic disorder. Science 275:77, 1997.
88. Shaheen SO, Aaby P, Hall AJ, et al: Measles and atopy in Guinea-Bissau. Lancet 347:1792, 1996.
89. Serfafini U: Do infections protect against asthma and atopy? Allergy 52:955, 1997.
90. Strachan DP: Hay fever, hygiene and household size. BMJ 299:1259, 1989.
91. von Mutius E: Progression of allergy and asthma through childhood to adolescence. Thorax 51:S3, 1996.
92. Sandford A, Weir T, Paré PD: The genetics of asthma. Am J Respir Crit Care Med 153:1749, 1996.
93. Martinez FD: Complexities of the genetics of asthma. Am J Respir Crit Care Med 156:S117, 1997.
94. Dewar JC, Wheatley AP: The heritability of allergic disease. In Hall IP (ed): Genetics of Asthma and Atopy. Vol 33. Basel, Karger, 1996, pp 4–34.
95. Sibbald B, Rink E, D'Souza M: Is the prevalence of atopy increasing? Br J Gen Pract 40:338, 1990.
96. Barbee RA, Kaltenborn W, Lebowitz MD, Burrows B: Longitudinal changes in allergen skin test reactivity in a community population sample. J Allergy Clin Immunol 7:16, 1987.
97. Lander ES, Schork NJ: Genetic dissection of complex traits. Science 265:2037, 1994.
98. Greally M, Jagoe WS, Greally J: The genetics of asthma. Irish Med J 75:403, 1982.
99. Dold S, Wjst M, von Mutius E, et al: Genetic risk for asthma, allergic rhinitis, and atopic dermatitis. Arch Dis Child 67:1018, 1992.
100. Van Arsdel PP, Motulsky AG: Frequency and heritability of asthma and allergic rhinitis in college students. Acta Genet 9:101, 1959.
101. Longo G, Strinati R, Poli F, Fumi F: Genetic factors in non-specific bronchial hyperreactivity. Am J Dis Child 141:331, 1987.
102. Hanson B, McGue M, Roitman-Johnson B, et al: Atopic disease and immunoglobulin E in twins reared apart and together. Am J Hum Genet 48:873, 1991.
102a. Townley RG, Bewtra AK, Nair NM, et al: Methacholine inhalation challenge studies. J Allergy Clin Immunol 64:569, 1979.
103. Edfors-Lubx ML: Allergy in 7000 twin pairs. Acta Allergol 26:249, 1971.
104. Tang MLK, Kemp AS, Thorburn J, Hill DJ: Reduced interferon-γ in neonates and subsequent atopy. Lancet 344:983, 1994.
105. Sibbald B, Turner-Warwick M: Factors influencing the prevalence of asthma in first degree relatives of extrinsic and intrinsic asthmatics. Thorax 34:332, 1979.
106. Burrows B, Sears MR, Flannery EM, et al: Relationships of bronchial responsiveness assessed by methacholine to serum IgE, lung function, symptoms, and diagnoses in 11-year-old New Zealand children. J Allergy Clin Immunol 90:376, 1992.
107. Townley RG, Guirgis H, Bewtra A, et al: IgE levels and methacholine inhalation responses in monozygous and dizygous twins. J Allergy Clin Immunol 57:227, 1976.
108. Konig P, Godfrey S: Exercise-induced bronchial lability in monozygotic and dizygotic twins. J Allergy Clin Immunol 54:280, 1974.
109. Ericsson CH, Svartengren M, Mossberg B, et al: Bronchial reactivity and allergy-promoting factors in monozygotic twins discordant for allergic rhinitis. Ann Allergy 67:53, 1991.
110. Svartengren M, Ericsson CH, Mossberg B, Camner P: Bronchial reactivity and atopy in asthma-discordant monozygotic twins. Ann Allergy 64:124, 1990.
111. Collaborative study on the genetics of Asthma. Nat Genet 15:389, 1997.
112. Daniels SE, Bhatttacharrya S, James A, et al: A genome-wide search for quantitative trait loci underlying asthma. Nature 383:247, 1996.

113. Cookson WOCM, Sharp PA, Faux JA, Hopkin JM: Linkage between immunoglobulin E responses underlying asthma and rhinitis and chromosome 11q. Lancet 1:1292, 1989.
114. Sandford AJ, Shirakawa T, Moffatt MF, et al: Localisation of atopy and β subunit of high-affinity IgE receptor (FcεRI) on chromosome 11q. Lancet 341:332, 1993.
115. Collee JM, ten Kate LP, de Vries HG, et al: Allele sharing on chromosome 11q13 in sibs with asthma and atopy. Lancet 342:936, 1993.
116. Shirakawa T, Hashimoto T, Furuyama J, Morimoto K: Linkage between severe atopy and chromosome 11q13 in Japanese families. Clin Genet 46:228, 1994.
117. Hizawa N, Yamaguchi E, Furuya K, et al: Association between high serum total IgE levels and D11S97 on chromosome 11q13 in Japanese subjects. J Med Genet 32:363, 1995.
118. van Herwerden L, Harrap SB, Wong ZYH, et al: Linkage of high-affinity IgE receptor gene with bronchial hyperreactivity, even in absence of atopy. Lancet 346:1262, 1995.
119. Meyers DA, Postma DS, Panhuysen CIM, et al: Evidence for a locus regulating total serum IgE levels mapping to chromosome 5. Genomics 23:464, 1994.
120. Marsh DG, Neely JD, Breazeale DR, et al: Linkage analysis of IL4 and other chromosome 5q31.1 markers and total serum immunoglobulin E concentrations. Science 264:1152, 1994.
121. Amelung PJ, Bleecker ER, Postma DS, et al: A locus regulating bronchial hyperresponsiveness maps to chromosome 5q. Am J Resp Crit Care Med 151:A341, 1995.
122. Moffatt MF, Hill MR, Cornelis F, et al: Genetic linkage of T-cell receptor a/d complex to specific IgE responses. Lancet 343:1597, 1994.
123. Howell WM, Holgate ST: Human leukocyte antigen genes and allergic disease. Monogr Allergy 33:53, 1996.
124. Verhoef A, Higgins JA, Thorpe CJ, et al: Clonal analysis of the atopic immune response to the group 2 allergen of Dermatophagoides spp.: Identification of HLA-DR and -DQ restricted T cell epitopes. Int Immunol 5:1589, 1993.
125. Marsh DG, Huang SK: Molecular genetics of human immune responsiveness to pollen allergens. Clin Exp Allergy 21(suppl 1):168, 1991.
126. Tautz C, Rihs H-P, Thiele A, et al: Association of class II sequences encoding DR1 and DQ5 specificities with hypersensitivity to chironomid allergen Chi t I. J Allergy Clin Immunol 93:918, 1994.
127. Caraballo L, Marrugo J, Jimenez S, et al: Frequency of DPB1*0401 is significantly decreased in patients with allergic asthma in a mulatto population. Hum Immunol 32:157, 1991.
128. Hsieh K-H, Shieh C-C, Hsieh R-P, Liu W-J: Association of HLA-DQw2 with Chinese childhood asthma. Tissue Antigens 38:181, 1991.
129. Turner MW, Brostoff J, Wells RS, et al: HLA in eczema and hayfever. Clin Exp Immunol 27:43, 1997.
130. Marsh DG, Meyers DA, Freidhoff LR, et al: Association of HLA phenotypes A1, B8, Dw3 and A3, B7, Dw2 with allergy. Int Arch Allergy Appl Immunol 66(suppl):48, 1981.
131. Ostergaard PA, Ericksen J: Association between HLA-A1/B8 in children with extrinsic asthma and IgA deficiency. Eur J Pediatr 131:263, 1979.
132. Rachelefsky G, Park MS, Siegel S, et al: Strong association between B-lymphocyte group-2 specificity and asthma. Lancet 2:1042, 1976.
133. Thurton CWG, Morris L, Buckingham JA, et al: Histocompatibility antigens in asthma: Population and family studies. Thorax 34:670, 1979.
134. Tiwari JL, Terasaki PI: HLA and Disease Associations. New York, Springer-Verlag, 1985.
135. Candore G, Colucci AT, Modica MA, Caruso C: HLA-B8,DR3 T cell impairment is completely restored by in vitro treatment with interleukin-2. Immunopharmacol Immunotoxicol 13:551, 1991.
136. Modica MA, Zambito AM, Candore G, Caruso C: Markers of T lymphocyte activation in HLA-B8,DR3–positive individuals. Immunobiology 181:257, 1990.
137. Del Prete G: Human Th1 and Th2 lymphocytes: Their role in the pathophysiology of atopy. Allergy 47:450, 1992.
138. Szentivanyi A: The β-adrenergic theory of the atopic abnormality in bronchial asthma. J Allergy 42:203, 1968.
139. Reihsaus E, Innis M, MacIntyre N, Liggett SB: Mutations in the gene encoding for the β2-adrenergic receptor in normal and asthmatic subjects. Am J Respir Cell Mol Biol 8:334, 1993.
140. Weir TD, Malleck N, Sandford AJ, et al: Genetic polymorphisms of the beta2-adrenergic receptor in fatal and near-fatal asthma. Am J Respir Crit Care Med 158:787, 1998.
141. Turki J, Pak J, Green SA, et al: Genetic polymorphisms of the β2-adrenergic receptor in nocturnal and nonnocturnal asthma. J Clin Invest 95:1635, 1995.
142. Martinez FD, Graves PE, Baldini M, et al: Association between genetic polymorphisms of the beta (2)-adrenoceptor and response to albuterol in children with and without a history of wheezing. J Clin Invest 100:3184, 1997.
143. Green SA, Turki J, Innis M, Liggett SB: Amino-terminal polymorphisms of the human β2-adrenergic receptor impart distinct agonist-promoted regulatory properties. Biochemistry 33:9414, 1994.
144. Tan S, Hall IP, Dewar J, et al: Association between beta(2)-adrenoceptor polymorphism and susceptibility to bronchodilator desensitisation in moderately severe stable asthmatics. Lancet 350:995, 1997.
145. Hall IP: Beta2-adrenoceptor polymorphisms and asthma. Monogr Allergy 33:153, 1996.
146. Bai TR: Abnormalities in airway smooth muscle in fatal asthma. Am Rev Respir Dis 141:552, 1990.

147. Whicker SD, Armour CL, Black JL: Responsiveness of bronchial smooth muscle from asthmatic patients to relaxant and contractile agonists. Pulmonary Pharmacol 1:25, 1988.

148. Hall IP, Wheatley A, Wilding P, Liggett SB: Association of Glu 27 β₂-adrenoceptor polymorphism with lower airway reactivity in asthmatic subjects. Lancet 345:1213, 1995.

149. Katz RM, Lieberman J, Siegel SC: Alpha-1-antitrypsin levels and prevalence of Pi variant phenotypes in asthmatic children. J Allergy Clin Immunol 57:41, 1976.

150. Hyde JS, Werner P, Kumar CM, Moore BS: Protease inhibitor variants in children and young adults with chronic asthma. Ann Allergy 43:8, 1979.

151. Hoffman JJML, Kramps JA, Dijkman JH: Intermediate α₁-antitrypsin deficiency in atopic allergy. Clin Allergy 11:555, 1981.

152. Lieberman J, Colp C: A role for intermediate heterozygous alpha-1-antitrypsin deficiency in obstructive lung disease. Chest 98:522, 1990.

153. Gaillard MC, Kilroe-Smith TA, Nogueira C, et al: Alpha-1-protease inhibitor in bronchial asthma: Phenotypes and biochemical characteristics. Am Rev Respir Dis 145:1311, 1992.

154. Townley RG, Southard JG, Radford P, et al: Association of MS Pi phenotype with airway hyperresponsiveness. Chest 98:594, 1990.

155. Lindmark B, Svenonius E, Eriksson S: Heterozygous α₁-antichymotrypsin and PiZ α₁-antitrypsin deficiency. Prevalence and clinical spectrum in asthmatic children. Allergy 45:197, 1990.

156. Benessiano J, Crestani B, Mestari F, et al: High frequency of a deletion polymorphism of the angiotensin-converting enzyme gene in asthma. J Allergy Clin Immunol 99:53, 1997.

157. Moffatt MR, Cookson WO: Tumor necrosis factor haplotypes and asthma. Hum Mol Genet 6:551, 1997.

158. Campbell DA, Wa E Li Kam, Britton J, et al: Polymorphism at the tumour necrosis factor locus and asthma. Monogr Allergy 33:125, 1996.

159. Rosenwasser LJ, Borish L: Genetics of atopy and asthma: the rationale behind promoter-based candidate gene studies (IL-4 and IL-10). Am J Respir Crit Care Med 156:S152, 1997.

160. Warner JO, Norman AP, Soothill JF: Cystic fibrosis heterozygosity in the pathogenesis of allergy. Lancet 1:990, 1976.

161. Gyukovits K, Markus V, Bittera I: Cystic-fibrosis heterozygosity in childhood bronchial asthma. Lancet 1:203, 1977.

162. Davies PB: Autonomic and airway reactivity in obligate heterozygotes for cystic fibrosis. Am Rev Respir Dis 129:911, 1984.

163. Counahan R, Mearns MB: Prevalence of atopy and exercise-induced bronchial lability in relatives of patients with cystic fibrosis. Arch Dis Child 50:477, 1975.

164. Davies PB, Byard PJ: Heterozygotes for cystic fibrosis: Models for study of airway and autonomic reactivity. J Appl Physiol 66:2124, 1989.

165. Schroeder SA, Gaughan DM, Swift M: Protection against bronchial asthma by CFTR ΔF508 mutation: A heterozygote advantage in cystic fibrosis. Nat Med 1:703, 1995.

166. Glynn AA, Michaels L: Bronchial biopsy in chronic bronchitis and asthma. Thorax 15:142, 1960.

167. Laitinen LA, Heino M, Laitinen A, et al: Damage of the airway epithelium and bronchial reactivity in patients with asthma. Am Rev Respir Dis 131:599, 1985.

168. Sanerkin NG, Evans MD: The sputum in bronchial asthma: pathognomonic patterns. J Pathol Bacteriol 89:535, 1965.

169. Cutz E, Levison H, Cooper DM: Ultrastructure of airways in children with asthma. Histopathology 2:407, 1978.

170. Kuwano K, Bosken CH, Paré PD, et al: Small airways dimensions in asthma and in chronic obstructive pulmonary disease. Am Rev Respir Dis 148:1220, 1993.

171. Carroll N, Elliot J, Morton A, James A: The structure of large and small airways in nonfatal and fatal asthma. Am Rev Respir Dis 147:405, 1993.

172. Laitinen LA, Laitinen A, Haahtela T: Airway mucosal inflammation even in patients with newly diagnosed asthma. Am Rev Respir Dis 147:697, 1993.

173. Behrens BL, Clark RA, Presley DM, et al: Comparison of the evolving histopathology of early and late cutaneous and asthmatic responses in rabbits after a single antigen challenge. Lab Invest 56:101, 1987.

174. Dunnill MS: The pathology of asthma, with special reference to changes in the bronchial mucosa. J Clin Pathol 13:27, 1960.

175. Naylor B: The shedding of the mucosa of the bronchial tree in asthma. Thorax 17:69, 1962.

176. Sakula A: Charcot-Leyden crystals and Curschmann spirals in asthmatic sputum. Thorax 41:503, 1986.

177. Kupper T, Spies S, Wehle K, et al: Detection of Charcot-Leyden crystals by fluorescence microscopy of Papanicolaou-stained smears of sputum, bronchoalveolar lavage fluid, and bronchial secretions. Cytopathology 5:262, 1994.

178. Naylor B: Curschmann's spirals in pleural and peritoneal effusions. Acta Cytol 34:474, 1990.

179. Walker KR, Fullmer CD: Progress report on study of respiratory spirals. Acta Cytol 14:396, 1970.

180. Aikawa T, Shimura S, Sasaki H, et al: Marked goblet cell hyperplasia with mucus accumulation in the airways of patients who died of severe acute asthma attack. Chest 101:916, 1992.

181. Montefort S, Roberts JA, Beasley R, et al: The site of disruption of the bronchial epithelium in asthmatic and non-asthmatic subjects. Thorax 47:499, 1992.

182. Laitinen LA, Heino M, Laitinen A, et al: Damage of the airway epithelium and bronchial reactivity in patients with asthma. Am Rev Respir Dis 131:599, 1985.

183. Montefort S, Herbert CA, Robinson C, Holgate ST: The bronchial epithelium as a target for inflammatory attack in asthma. Clin Exp Allergy 22:511, 1992.

184. Persson CGA: Plasma exudation. Asthma 1:917, 1997.

185. Bai A, Eidelman DH, Hogg JC, et al: Proposed nomenclature for quantifying subdivisions of the bronchial wall. J Appl Physiol 77:1011, 1994.

186. Huber HL, Koessler KK: The pathology of bronchial asthma. Arch Intern Med 30:689, 1992.

187. Houston JC, de Nevasquez S, Trounce JR: A clinical and pathological study of fatal cases of status asthmaticus. Thorax 8:207, 1953.

188. James AL, Hogg JC, Dunn LA, Paré PD: The use of internal perimeter to compare airway size and to calculate smooth muscle shortening. Am Rev Respir Dis 138:136, 1988.

189. James AL, Paré PD, Hogg JC: Effects of lung volume, bronchoconstriction, and cigarette smoke on morphometric airways dimensions. J Appl Physiol 64:913, 1988.

190. James AL, Paré PD, Hogg JC: The mechanics of airway narrowing in asthma. Am Rev Respir Dis 139:242, 1989.

191. Bosken CH, Wiggs BR, Paré PD, Hogg JC: Small airway dimensions in smokers with obstruction to airflow. Am Rev Respir Dis 142:563–70, 1990.

192. Sobonya RE: Concise clinical study. Quantitative structural alterations in long-standing allergic asthma. Am Rev Respir Dis 130:289, 1984.

193. Martinez-Hernandez A, Amenta PS: The basement membrane in pathology. Lab Invest 48:656, 1983.

194. Roche WR, Beasley R, Williams JH, Holgate ST: Subepithelial fibrosis in the bronchi of asthmatics. Lancet 1:520, 1989.

195. Gabbrielli S, Di Lollo S, Stanflin N, et al: Myofibroblast and elastic and collagen fiber hyperplasia in the bronchial mucosa: A possible basis for the progressive irreversibility of airway obstruction in chronic asthma. Pathologica 86:157, 1994.

196. Brewster CEP, Howarth PH, Djukanovic R, et al: Myofibroblasts and subepithelial fibrosis in bronchial asthma. Am J Respir Cell Mol Biol 3:507, 1990.

197. Boulet LP, Boulet M, Laviolette M, et al: Airway inflammation after removal from the casual agent in occupational asthma due to high and low molecular weight agents. Eur Respir J 7:1567, 1994.

198. Saetta M, Maestrelli P, Turato G, et al: Airway wall remodelling after cessation of exposure to isocyanates in sensitized asthmatic subjects. Am J Respir Crit Care Med 151:489, 1995.

199. Colebatch HJH, Greaves IA, Ng CKY: Pulmonary mechanics in diagnosis. In de Kock MA, Nadel JA, Lewis CM (eds): Mechanics of Airway Obstruction in Human Respiratory Disease. Cape Town, AA Balkema, 1979.

200. Harkonen E, Virtanen I, Linnala A, et al: Modulation of fibronectin and tenascin production in human bronchial epithelial cells by inflammatory cytokines in vitro. Am J Respir Cell Mol Biol 13:109, 1995.

201. Roberts C: Asthma as a fibrotic disease. Chest 107:S111, 1995.

202. Paré PD, Bai TR, Roberts CR: The structural and functional consequences of chronic allergic inflammation of the airways. Ciba Found Symp 206:71, 1997.

203. Aubert J-D, Dalal BI, Bai TR, et al: Transforming growth factor-β gene expression in human airways. Thorax 49:225, 1994.

204. Aubert J-D: Platelet-derived growth factor and its receptor in lungs from patients with asthma and chronic airflow obstruction. Am J Physiol 266:L655, 1994.

205. Bousquet J, Chanez P, Lacoste JY, et al: Asthma: A disease remodelling the airways. Allergy 47:3, 1992.

206. Bramley AJ, Roberts CR, Schellenberg RR: Collagenase increases shortening of human bronchial smooth muscle in vitro treatment causes increased contractility of human bronchial smooth muscle in vitro. Am J Respir Crit Care Med 152:1513, 1995.

207. Bramley AM, Thomson RJ, Roberts CR, Schellenberg RR: Hypothesis: Excessive bronchoconstriction in asthma is due to decreased airway elastance. Eur Respir J 7:337, 1994.

208. Shale DJ, Lane DJ, Fisher CWS, et al: Endobronchial polyp in an asthmatic subject. Thorax 38:75, 1983.

209. Dunnill MS, Massarella GR, Anderson JA: A comparison of the quantitative anatomy of the bronchi in normal subjects, in status asthmaticus, in chronic bronchitis, and in emphysema. Thorax 24:176, 1969.

210. Sobonya RE: Quantitative structural alterations in long-standing allergic asthma. Am Rev Respir Dis 130:289, 1984.

211. Hossain S: Quantitative measurement of bronchial muscle in man with asthma. Am Rev Respir Dis 107:99, 1973.

212. James AL, Paré PD, Hogg JC: The mechanics of airway narrowing in asthma. Am Rev Respir Dis 132:242, 1985.

213. Dube J, Chakir J, Laviolette M, et al: In vitro procollagen synthesis and proliferative phenotype of bronchial fibroblasts from normal and asthmatic subjects. Lab Invest 78:297, 1998.

214. Heard BE, Hossain S: Hyperplasia of bronchial muscle in asthma. J Pathol 110:319, 1973.

215. Ebina M, Takahashi T, Chiba T, Motomiya M: Cellular hypertrophy and hyperplasia of airway smooth muscles underlying bronchial asthma. A 3-D morphometric study. Am Rev Respir Dis 48:720, 1993.

216. Ebina M, Yaegashi H, Chiba R, et al: Hyperreactive site in the airway tree of asthmatic patients revealed by thickening of bronchial muscles. Am Rev Respir Dis 141:1327, 1990.

217. Thomson RJ, Bramley AM, Schellenberg RR: Airway muscle stereology: implications for increased shortening in asthma. Am J Respir Crit Care Med 154:749, 1996.

218. Carroll NG, Cooke C, James AL: Bronchial blood vessel dimensions in asthma. Am J Respir Crit Care Med 155:689, 1997.

219. Saetta M, Di Stefano A, Rosina C, et al: Quantitative structural analysis of peripheral airways and arteries in sudden fatal asthma. Am Rev Respir Dis 143:138, 1991.

220. Sur S, Crotty TB, Kephart GM, et al: Sudden-onset fatal asthma: A distinct entity with few eosinophils and relatively more neutrophils in the airway submucosa? Am Rev Respir Dis 148:713, 1993.

221. Guerzon M, Paré PD, Michoud M, et al: The number and distribution of mast cells in monkey lungs. Am Rev Respir Dis 119:59, 1979.

222. Connell JT: Asthmatic deaths. Role of the mast cell. JAMA 215:769, 1971.

223. Hogg JC: The pathophysiology of asthma. Chest 82:85, 1982.

224. Leff A: Pathophysiology of asthmatic bronchoconstriction. Chest 82:135, 1982.

225. Jeffrey PK, Godfrey RW, Adelroth E, et al: Effects of treatment on airway inflammation and thickening of basement membrane reticular collagen in asthma. Am Rev Respir Dis 145:890, 1992.

226. Barnes PJ: Cytokines as mediators of chronic asthma. Am J Respir Crit Care Med 150:S43, 1994.

227. Cousins DJ, Staynov DZ, Lee TH: Regulation of cytokine genes implicated in asthma and atopy. Monogr Allergy 33:138, 1996.

228. Robinson DS, Durham SR, Kay AB: Cytokines. 3. Cytokines in asthma. Thorax 48:845, 1993.

229. Osler W: The Principles and Practice of Medicine. 1892, p 497.

230. Barnes PJ. Pathophysiology of asthma. Br J Clin Pharmacol 42:3, 1996.

231. Goldstein RA, Paul WE, Metcalfe DD, et al: Asthma. Ann Intern Med 121:698, 1994.

232. Pilewski JM, Albelda SM: Cell adhesion molecules in asthma: Homing, activation, and airway remodeling. Am J Respir Cell Mol Biol 12:1, 1995.

233. Bloemen PG, Henricks PA, Nijkamp FP: Cell adhesion molecules and asthma. Clin Exp Allergy 27:128, 1997.

234. Goldring K, Warner JA: Cell matrix interactions in asthma. Clin Exp Allergy 27:22, 1997.

235. Kay AB: T cells as orchestrators of the asthmatic response. Ciba Found Symp 206:56, 1997.

236. Kline JN, Hunninghake GW: T-lymphocyte dysregulation in asthma. Proc Soc Exp Biol Med 207:243, 1994.

237. Corrigan CJ, Kay AB: T-cell/eosinophil interactions in the induction of asthma. Eur Respir J Suppl 22:72S, 1996.

238. Denburg JA, Inman MD, Leber B, et al: The role of the bone marrow in allergy and asthma. Allergy 51:141, 1996.

239. Simon HU, Blaser K: Inhibition of programmed eosinophil death: A key pathogenic event for eosinophilia? Immunol Today 16:53, 1995.

240. Wasserman SI: Mast cells and airway inflammation in asthma. Am J Respir Crit Care Med 150:S39, 1994.

241. Rossi GL, Olivieri D: Does the mast cell still have a key role in asthma? Chest 112:523, 1997.

242. de Pater-Huijsen FL, Pompen M, Jansen HM, Out TA: Products from mast cells influence T lymphocyte proliferation and cytokine production—relevant to allergic asthma? Immunol Lett 57:47, 1997.

243. Kay AB: Basic mechanisms in allergic asthma. Eur J Respir Dis 63:9, 1982.

244. Knol EF, Mul FP, Lie WJ, et al: The role of basophils in allergic disease. Eur Respir J Suppl 22:126S, 1996.

245. Findlay SR, Lichtenstein LM: Basophil "releasability" in patients with asthma. Am Rev Respir dis 122:53, 1980.

246. Gaddy JN, Busse WW: Enhanced IgE-dependent basophil histamine release and airway reactivity in asthma. Am Rev Respir Dis 134:969, 1986.

247. Marone G, Poto S, Celestino D, Bonini S: Human basophil releasability. III. Genetic control of human basophil releasability. J Immunol 137:3588, 1986.

248. Leff AR: Inflammatory mediation of airway hyperresponsiveness by peripheral blood granulocytes. The case for the eosinophil. Chest 106:1202, 1994.

249. Djukanovic R, Roche WR, Wilson JW, et al: Mucosal inflammation in asthma. Am Rev Respir Dis 142:434, 1997.

250. Dahl R, Venge P: Role of the eosinophil in bronchial asthma. Eur J Respir Dis 63:23, 1982.

251. Taniguchi WJ, Mita W, Saito H: Increased generation of leukotriene $C_4$ from eosinophils in asthmatic patients. Allergy 40:571, 1985.

252. Ayars GH, Altman LC, Gleich GJ: Eosinophil and eosinophil granule-mediated pneumocyte injury. J Allergy Clin Immunol 76:595, 1985.

253. Frigas E, Loegering DA, Solley GO, et al: Elevated levels of the eosinophil granule major basic protein in the sputum of patients with bronchial asthma. Mayo Clin Proc 56:345, 1981.

254. Diaz P, Galleguillos FR, Gonzalez MC, et al: Bronchoalveolar lavage in asthma—the effect of disodium cromoglycate (Cromolyn) on leukocyte counts, immunoglobulins, and complement. J Allergy Clin Immunol 74:41, 1984.

255. Dahl R, Venge P, Olsson I: Variations of blood eosinophils and eosinophil cationic protein in serum in patients with bronchial asthma, studies during inhalation challenge test. Allergy 33:211, 1978.

256. Busse WW, Nagata M, Sedgwick JB: Characteristics of airway eosinophils. Eur Respir J Suppl 22:132s, 1996.

257. Kay AB, Barata L, Meng Q, et al: Eosinophils and eosinophil-associated cytokines in allergic inflammation. Int Arch Allergy Immunol 113:196, 1997.

258. Gleich GJ, Fryer AD, Jacoby DB: Eosinophil granule proteins and bronchial hyperactivity. *In* Holgate ST, Austen K, Lichtenstein LM, et al (eds): Asthma: Physiology, Immunopharmacology, and Treatment. London, 1993, pp 119–129.

259. Gundel RH, Letts LG, Gleich GJ: Human eosinophil major basic protein induces airway constriction and airway hyperresponsiveness in primates. J Clin Invest 87:1470, 1991.

260. Gleich GJ, Jacoby DB, Fryer AD: Eosinophil-associated inflammation in bronchial asthma: A connection to the nervous system. Int Arch Allergy Immunol 107:205, 1995.

261. Evans CM, Fryer AD, Jacoby DB, et al: Pretreatment with antibody to eosinophil major basic protein prevents hyperresponsiveness by protecting neuronal M2 muscarinic receptors in antigen-challenged guinea pigs. J Clin Invest 100:2254, 1997.

262. Joseph M, Tonnel AB, Jorfier G, et al: Involvement of immunoglobulin E in the secretory processes of alveolar macrophages from asthmatic subjects. J Clin Invest 71:221, 1983.

263. Aubas P, Cosso B, Godard P, et al: Decreased suppressor cell activity of alveolar macrophages in bronchial asthma. Am Rev Respir Dis 130:875, 1984.

264. Arnoux B, Joseph M, Simoes MH, et al: Antigenic release of paf-acether and beta-glucuronidase from alveolar macrophages of asthmatics. Bull Eur Physiopathol Respir 23:119, 1987.

265. Schulman ES, Liu MC, Proud D, et al: Human lung macrophages induce histamine release from basophils and mast cells. Am Rev Respir Dis 131:230, 1985.

266. Martin TR, Altman LC, Albert RK, et al: Leukotriene-$B_4$ production by the human alveolar macrophage—a potential mechanism for amplifying inflammation in the lung. Am Rev Respir Dis 129:106, 1984.

267. Lane SJ, Sousa AR, Lee TH: The role of the macrophage in asthma. Allergy 49:201, 1994.

268. Holt P: Dendritic cell population in the lung and airway wall. Asthma 1:453, 1997.

269. Lambrecht BN, Pauwels RA, Bullock GR: The dendritic cell: Its potent role in the respiratory immune response. Cell Biol Int 20:111, 1996.

270. Gosset P, Jeannin P, Lassalle P, et al: The role of endothelial cells in asthma. Asthma 1:507, 1997.

271. Polito AJ, Proud D: Epithelial cells as inflammatory cells. Asthma 1:491, 1997.

272. Sime PJ, Tremblay GM, Xing Z, et al: Interstitial and bronchial fibroblasts. Asthma 1:475, 1997.

273. Widdicombe JG: Reflex control of tracheobronchial smooth muscle in experimental and human asthma. *In* Austen KF, Lichtenstein LM (eds): Asthma—Physiology, Immunopharmacology, and Treatment. Vol. II. New York, Academic Press, 1977, p 225.

274. Hogan MB, Greenberger PA: Histamine. Asthma 1:537, 1997.

275. Allen DH, Mathison DA, Wagner PD, et al: Mediator release during antigen inhalation in experimental asthma in dogs. Am Rev Respir Dis 111:148, 1975.

276. Polosa R, Djukanovic R, Rajakulasingam K, et al: Skin responses to bradykinin, kallidin, and [desArg9]-bradykinin in nonatopic and atopic volunteers. J Allergy Clin Immunol 92:683, 1993.

277. Kuna P, Reddigari SR, Schall TJ, et al: Characterization of the human basophil response to cytokines, growth factors, and histamine-releasing factors of the intercrine/chemokine family. J Immunol 150:1932, 1993.

278. Kang B, Townley RG, Lee CK, et al: Bronchial reactivity to histamine before and after sodium cromoglycate in bronchial asthma. BMJ 1:867, 1976.

279. Bleecker ER, Cotton DJ, Fischer SP, et al: The mechanism of rapid, shallow breathing after inhaling histamine aerosol in exercising dogs. Am Rev Respir Dis 114:909, 1976.

280. Guz A: Control of ventilation in man with special reference to abnormalities in asthma. *In* Austen KF, Lichtenstein LM (eds): Asthma—Physiology, Immunopharmacology and Treatment. Vol II. New York, Academic Press, 1977, p 211.

281. Long WM, Sprung CL, El Fawal H, et al: Effects of histamine on bronchial artery blood flow and bronchomotor tone. J Appl Physiol 59:254, 1985.

282. Beer J, Osband E, McCaffrey P, et al: Abnormal histamine-induced suppressor-cell function in atopic subjects. N Engl J Med 306:454, 1982.

283. White J, Eiser NM: The role of histamine and its receptors in the pathogenesis of asthma. Br J Dis Chest 77:215, 1983.

284. Popa VT: Effect of an $H_1$ blocker, chlorpheniramine, on inhalation tests with histamine and allergen in allergic asthma. Chest 78:442, 1980.

285. Samuelsson B: Leukotrienes: Mediators of immediate hypersensitivity. Science 220:568, 1983.

286. Murphy RC, Hammarstrom S, Samuelsson B: Leukotriene C: A slow-reacting substance from murine mastocytoma cells. Proc Natl Acad Sci U S A 76:427, 1979.

287. Robinson C, Holgate S: New perspectives on the putative role of eicosanoids in airway hyperresponsiveness. J Allergy Clin Immunol 76:140, 1985.

288. Lewis RA, Robin JL: Arachidonic acid derivatives as mediators of asthma. J Allergy Clin Immunol 76:259, 1985.

289. Adelroth E, Morris MM, Hargreave FE, et al: Airway responsiveness to leukotrienes C4 and D4 and to methacholine in patients with asthma and normal controls. N Engl J Med 315:480, 1986.

290. Lewis RA: A presumptive role for leukotrienes in obstructive airways diseases. Chest 88:98S, 1985.

291. Smith LJ, Greenberger PA, Patterson R, et al: The effect of inhaled leukotriene-D4 in humans. Am Rev Respir Dis 131:368, 1985.

292. Griffin M, Weiss JW, Leitch AG, et al: Effects of leukotriene D on the airways in asthma. N Engl J Med 308:436, 1983.

293. Barnes NC, Piper PJ, Costello JF: Comparative effects of inhaled leukotriene $C_4$ and histamine in normal human subjects. Thorax 39:500, 1984.

294. Creticos PS, Peters SP, Adkinson NF Jr, et al: Peptide leukotriene release after antigen challenge in patients sensitive to ragweed. N Engl J Med 310:1626, 1984.

295. Manning PJ, Rokach J, Malo JL, et al: Urinary leukotriene E4 levels during early and late asthmatic responses. J Allergy Clin Immunol 86:211, 1990.

296. MacGlashan DW, Schleimer RP, Peters SP, et al: Generation of leukotrienes by purified human lung mast cells. J Clin Invest 70:747, 1982.

297. Smith CM, Christie PE, Hawksworth, RJ, et al: Urinary leukotriene-E4 levels after allergen and exercise challenge in bronchial asthma. Am Rev Respir Dis 144:1411, 1991.

298. Drazen JM, O'Brien J, Sparrow D, et al: Recovery of leukotriene E4 from the urine of patients with airway obstruction. Am Rev Respir Dis 146:104, 1992.

299. Knapp HR, Sladek D, Fitzgerald GA: Increased excretion of leukotriene-E4 during aspirin-induced asthma. J Lab Clin Med 119:48, 1992.

300. Israel E, Fischer AR, Rosenberg MA, et al: The pivotal role of 5-lipoxygenase products in the reaction of aspirin-sensitive asthmatics to aspirin. Am Rev Respir Dis 148:1447, 1993.

301. Nasser SM, Patel M, Bell GS, Lee TH: The effect of aspirin desensitization on urinary leukotriene E4 concentrations in aspirin-sensitive asthma. Am J Respir Crit Care Med 151:1326, 1995.

302. Fischer AR, Drazen JM: Leukotrienes. In Barnes PJ, Grunstein MM, Leff AR, et al (eds): Asthma. Vol. 1. Philadelphia, Lippincott-Raven, 1997, p 547.

303. O'Byrne PM: Leukotrienes in the pathogenesis of asthma. Chest 111:27S, 1997.

304. O'Byrne PM: Cyclooxygenase products. In Barnes PJ, Grunstein MM, Leff AR, et al (eds): Asthma. Vol. 1. Philadelphia, Lippincott-Raven, 1997, p 559.

305. O'Byrne PM: Eicosanoids and asthma. Ann N Y Acad Sci 744:251, 1994.

306. Dvornik DM: Tissue selective inhibition of prostaglandin biosynthesis by etodolac. J Rheumatol Suppl 47:40, 1997.

307. Pairet M, Engelhardt G: Distinct isoforms (COX-1 and COX-2) of cyclooxygenase: Possible physiological and therapeutic implications. Fundam Clin Pharmacol 10:1, 1996.

308. Walters EH, Davies BH: Dual effect of prostaglandin $E_2$ on normal airways smooth muscle *in vivo*. Thorax 37:918, 1982.

309. Mathé AA, Hedqvist P: Effect of prostaglandins $F_2$ alpha and $E_2$ on airway conductance in healthy subjects and asthmatic patients. Am Rev Respir Dis 111:313, 1975.

310. Cuthbert MF: Effect on airways resistance of prostaglandin $E_1$ given by aerosol to healthy and asthmatic volunteers. BMJ 4:723, 1969.

311. Smith AP, Cuthbert MF: Antagonistic action of aerosols of prostaglandins $F_{2\alpha}$ and $E_2$ on bronchial muscle tone in man. BMJ 3:212, 1972.

312. Mathé AA, Hedqvist P, Holmgren A, et al: Bronchial hyperreactivity to prostaglandin $F_{2\alpha}$ and histamine in patients with asthma. BMJ 1:193, 1973.

313. Fish HE, Newball HH, Norman PS, et al: Novel effects of $PGF_2$ on airway function in asthmatic subjects. J Appl Physiol 54:105, 1983.

314. Fish JE, Jameson LS, Albright A, et al: Modulation of the bronchomotor effects of chemical mediators by prostaglandin-$F_2$-alpha in asthmatic subjects. Am Rev Respir Dis 130:571, 1985.

315. Weir EK, Greer BE, Smith SC, et al: Bronchoconstriction and pulmonary hypertension during abortion induced by 15-methyl-prostaglandin $F_2$-alpha and histamine in patients with asthma. Am J Med 60:556, 1976.

316. Hardy CC, Robinson C, Tattersfield AE, et al: The bronchoconstrictor effect of inhaled prostaglandin $D_2$ in normal and asthmatic men. N Engl J Med 311:209, 1984.

317. Austen KF, Orange RP: Bronchial asthma: The possible role of the chemical mediators of immediate hypersensitivity in the pathogenesis of subacute chronic disease. Am Rev Respir Dis 112:423, 1975.

318. Green K, Hedqvist P, Svanborg N: Increased plasma levels of 15-keto-13,14-dihydro-prostaglandin $F_{2\alpha}$ after allergen-provoked asthma in man. Lancet 2:1419, 1974.

319. Patel KR: Atropine, sodium cromoglycate, and thymoxamine in $PGF_{2\alpha}$-induced bronchoconstriction in extrinsic asthma. BMJ 2:360, 1975.

320. Fish JE, Ankin MG, Adkinson NF, et al: Indomethacin modification of immediate-type immunologic airway responses in allergic asthmatic and non-asthmatic subjects: Evidence for altered arachidonic acid metabolism in asthma. Am Rev Respir Dis 123:609, 1981.

321. Wilson BA, Bar-Or O, O'Byrne PM: The effects of indomethacin on refractoriness following exercise both with and without a bronchoconstrictor response. Eur Respir J 7:2174, 1994.

322. Schall TJ, Bacon KB, Gleich GJ: Chemokines, leukocyte trafficking, and inflammation. Curr Opin Immunol 6:865, 1994.

323. Lukacs NW, Strieter RM, Chensue SW, Kunkel SL: Activation and regulation of chemokines in allergic airway inflammation. J Leukoc Biol 59:13, 1996.

324. Chung KF: Chemokines. In Barnes PJ, Grunstein MM, Leff AR, et al (eds): Asthma. Vol. 1. Philadelphia, Lippincott-Raven, 1997, p 673.

325. Lamkhioued B, Renzi PM, Abi-Younes S, et al: Increased expression of eotaxin in bronchoalveolar lavage and airways of asthmatics contributes to the chemotaxis of eosinophils to the site of inflammation. J Immunol 159:4593, 1997.

326. Teran LM, Campos MG, Begishvilli BT, et al: Identification of neutrophil chemotactic factors in bronchoalveolar lavage fluid of asthmatic patients. Clin Exp Allergy 27:396, 1997.

327. Morley J, Sanjar S, Page C: The platelet in asthma. Lancet 2:1142, 1984.

328. Basran GS, Page CP, Paul W, et al: Platelet-activating factor: A possible mediator of the dual response to allergen? Clin Allergy 14:75, 1984.

329. Kurosawa M, Yamshita T, Kurimoto F: Increased levels of blood platelet-activating factor in bronchial asthmatic patients with active symptoms. Allergy 49:60, 1994.

330. Cuss FM, Dixon CM, Barnes PJ: Effects of inhaled platelet-activating factor on pulmonary function and bronchial responsiveness in man. Lancet 2:189, 1986.

331. Bochner BS, Undem BJ, Lichtenstein LM: Immunological aspects of allergic asthma. Annu Rev Immunol 12:295, 1994.

332. Barnes PJ: Asthma as an axon reflex. Lancet 1:242, 1986.

333. Ollerenshaw S, Jarvis D, Woolcock A, et al: Absence of immunoreactive vasoactive intestinal polypeptide in tissue from the lungs of patients with asthma. New Engl J Med 320:1244, 1989.

334. Ollerenshaw SL, Jarvis D, Sullivan CE, Woolcock AJ: Substance P immunoreactive nerves in airways from asthmatics and nonasthmatics. Eur Respir J 4:673, 1991.

335. Lilly CM, Bai TR, Shore SA, et al: Neuropeptide content of lungs from asthmatic and nonasthmatic patients. Am J Respir Crit Care Med 151:548, 1995.

336. Nieber K, Baumgarten CR, Rathsack R, et al: Substance P and β-endorphin-like immunoreactivity in lavage fluids of subjects with and without allergic asthma. J Allergy Clin Immunol 90:646, 1992.

337. Crimi N, Palermo F, Oliveri R, et al: Inhibition of neutral endopeptidase potentiates bronchoconstriction induced by neurokinin A in asthmatic patients. Clin Exp Allergy 24:115, 1994.

338. Fuller RW, Dixon CMS, Barnes PJ: Bronchoconstrictor response to inhaled capsaicin in humans. J Appl Physiol 58:1080, 1985.

339. Curran AD: The role of nitric oxide in the development of asthma. Int Arch Allergy Immunol 111:1, 1996.

340. Barnes PJ, Kharitonov SA: Exhaled nitric oxide in monitoring asthma. Drugs Today 33:715, 1997.

341. Barnes PJ, Liew FY: Nitric oxide and asthmatic inflammation. Immunol Today 16:128, 1995.

342. Persson MG, Zetterstrom O, Agrenius V, et al: Single-breath nitric oxide measurements in asthmatic patients and smokers. Lancet 343:146, 1994.

343. Hay DWP, Henry PJ, Goldie RG: Is endothelin-1 a mediator in asthma? Pulmonary perspective. Am J Respir Crit Care Med 154:1594, 1996.

344. Howarth PH, Redington AE, Springall DR, et al: Epithelially derived endothelin and nitric oxide in asthma. Int Arch Allergy Immunol 107:228, 1995.

345. Kraft M, Beam WR, Wenzel SE, et al: Blood and bronchoalveolar lavage endothelin-1 levels in nocturnal asthma. Am J Respir Crit Care Med 149:946, 1994.

346. Redington AE, Springall DR, Ghatei MA, et al: Endothelin in bronchoalveolar lavage fluid and its relation to airflow obstruction in asthma. Am J Respir Crit Care Med 151:1034, 1995.

347. Trifilieff A, Da Silva A, Gies JP: Kinins and respiratory tract diseases. Eur Respir J 6:576, 1993.

348. Fuller RW, Dixon CM, Cuss FM, et al: Bradykinin-induced bronchoconstriction in humans. Mode of action. Am Rev Respir Dis 135:176, 1987.

349. Newball HH, Berninger RW, Talamo RC, et al: Anaphylactic release of a basophil kallikrein-like activity. 1. Purification and characterization. J Clin Invest 64:457, 1979.

350. Newball HH, Talamo RC, Lichtenstein LM: Anaphylactic release of a basophil kallikrein-like activity: A mediator of immediate hypersensitivity reactions. J Clin Invest 64:466, 1979.

351. Millar EA, Angus RM, Hulks G, et al: Activity of the renin-angiotensin system in acute severe asthma and the effect of angiotensin II on lung function. Thorax 49:492, 1994.

352. Glovsky MM, Nagata S, Schellenberg RR, et al: Are products of complement activation $C_{3a}$ and $C_{5a}$ relevant factors in bronchial asthma? Chest 87:169S, 1985.

353. Stevens WJ, Bridts CH: IgG-containing and IgE-containing circulating immune complexes in patients with asthma and rhinitis. J Allergy Clin Immunol 73:276, 1984.

354. Stewart RM, Weir EK, Montgomery MR, et al: Hydrogen peroxide contracts airway smooth muscle: A possible endogenous mechanism. Respir Physiol 45:333, 1981.

355. Jarjour NN, Calhoun WJ: Enhanced production of oxygen radicals in asthma. J Lab Clin Med 123:131, 1994.

356. Heilpern S, Rebuck AS: Effect of disodium cromoglycate (Intal) on sputum protein composition. Thorax 27:726, 1972.

357. Brogan TD, Ryley HC, Neale L, et al: Soluble proteins of bronchopulmonary secretions from patients with cystic fibrosis, asthma, and bronchitis. Thorax 30:72, 1975.

358. Lopez-Vidriero MT, Reid L: Chemical markers of mucus and serum glycoproteins and their relation to viscosity in mucoid and purulent sputum from various hypersecretory diseases. Am Rev Respir Dis 117:465, 1978.

359. Wanner A, Salathe M, O'Riordan TG: Mucociliary clearance in the airways. Am J Respir Crit Care Med 154:1868, 1996.

360. Shelhamer J, Kaliner M: Editorial: Respiratory mucus production in asthma. Clin Respir Physiol 21:301, 1985.

361. O'Riordan TG, Zwang J, Smaldone GC: Mucociliary clearance in adult asthma. Am Rev Respir Dis 146:598, 1992.

362. Bateman JRM, Pavia D, Sheahan NF, et al: Impaired tracheobronchial clearance in patients with mild stable asthma. Thorax 38:463, 1983.

363. Pavis D, Bateman JRM, Sheahan NF, et al: Tracheobronchial mucociliary clearance in asthma: Impairment during remission. Thorax 40:171, 1985.

364. Wanner A: Alteration of tracheal mucociliary transport in airway disease. Effect of pharmacologic agents. Chest 80(6 Suppl):867, 1981.

365. Messina MS, O'Riordan TG, Smaldone GC: Changes in mucociliary clearance during acute exacerbations of asthma. Am Rev Respir Dis 143:993, 1991.

366. Agnew JE, Bateman JR, Sheahan NF, et al: Effect of oral corticosteroids on

mucus clearance by cough and mucociliary transport in stable asthma. Bull Eur Physiopathol Respir 19:37, 1983.

367. Wanner A: Allergic mucociliary dysfunction. J Allergy Clin Immunol 72:347, 1983.

368. Mezey RJ, Cohn MA, Fernandez RJ, et al: Mucociliary transport in allergic patients with antigen-induced bronchospasm. Am Rev Respir Dis 118:677, 1978.

369. Weissberger D, Oliver W, Abraham WM, et al: Impaired tracheal mucus transport in allergic bronchoconstriction: Effect of terbutaline pretreatment. J Allergy Clin Immunol 67:357, 1981.

370. Maurer DR, Sielczak M, Oliver W Jr, et al: Role of ciliary motility in acute allergic mucociliary dysfunction. J Appl Physiol 52:1018, 1982.

371. Ahmed T, Greenblatt DW, Birch S, et al: Abnormal mucociliary transport in allergic patients with antigen-induced bronchospasm. Role of slow-reacting substance of anaphylaxis. Am Rev Respir Dis 124:110, 1981.

372. Nieminen MM, Moilanen EK, Nyholm JEJ, et al: Platelet-activating factor impairs mucociliary transport and increases plasma leukotriene B4 in man. Eur Respir J 4:551, 1991.

373. Phipps RJ, Denas SM, Wanner A: Antigen stimulates glycoprotein secretion and alters ion fluxes in sheep trachea. J Appl Physiol 55:1593, 1983.

374. Allegra L, Abraham WM, Chapman GA, et al: Duration of mucociliary dysfunction following antigen challenge. J Appl Physiol 55:726, 1983.

375. Dulfano MJ, Luk CK: Sputum and ciliary inhibition in asthma. Thorax 37:646, 1982.

376. Dolovich J, Hargreave FE, O'Byrne P, et al: Asthma terminology: Troubles in wordland. Am Rev Respir Dis 134:1102, 1986.

377. Orehek J: Asthma without airway hyperreactivity: Fact or artifact? Eur J Respir Dis 63:1, 1982.

378. Boushey HA, Holtzman MJ, Shuler JR, et al: State of the art: Bronchial hyperreactivity. Am Rev Respir Dis 121:389, 1980.

379. Simonsson BG: Airway hyperreactivity: Definition and short review. Eur J Respir Dis Suppl 131:9, 1983.

380. Hargreave FE, Woolcock AJ (eds): Airway Responsiveness—Measurement and Interpretation. Mississauga, Ontario, Astra Mississauga, 1985.

381. Mann JS, Cushley MJ, Holgate ST: Adenosine-induced bronchoconstriction in asthma—role of parasympathetic stimulation and adrenergic inhibition. Am Rev Respir Dis 132:1, 1985.

382. Borum P: Nasal methacholine challenge—test for the measurement of nasal reactivity. J Allergy Clin Immunol 63:253, 1979.

383. Druce HM, Wright RH, Kossoff D, et al: Cholinergic nasal hyperreactivity in atopic subjects. J Allergy Clin Immunol 76:445, 1985.

384. Douglas JS, Ridgway R, Brink C: Airway responses of the guinea pig in vivo and in vitro. J Pharmacol Exp Ther 202:116, 1977.

385. Snapper JR, Drazen JM, Loring SH, et al: Distribution of pulmonary responsiveness to aerosol histamine in dogs. J Appl Physiol 44:738, 1978.

386. Habib MP, Paré PD, Engel LA: Variability of airway responses to inhaled histamine in normal subjects. J Appl Physiol 47:51, 1979.

387. Hirshman CA, Malley A, Downes H: Basenji-Greyhound dog model of asthma: Reactivity to *Ascaris suum*, citric acid and methaeboline. J Appl Physiol 49:953, 1980.

388. Pauwels R, Van der Straeten M, Weyne J, et al: Genetic factors in non-specific bronchial reactivity in rats. Eur J Respir Dis 66:98, 1985.

389. Simonsson BG: Airway hyperreactivity. Definition and short review. *In* Simonsson BG (ed): Airway hyperreactivity. Eur J Respir Dis 64(Suppl 131):9, 1983.

390. Zamel N, Leroux M, Vanderdoelen JL: Airway responses to inhaled methacholine in healthy nonsmoking twins. J Appl Physiol 56:936, 1984.

391. Halperin SA, Eggleston PA, Beasley P, et al: Exacerbation of asthma in adults during experimental rhinovirus infection. Am Rev Respir Dis 132:976, 1985.

392. Boushey HA, Holtzman MJ: Experimental airway inflammation and hyperreactivity—searching for cells and mediators. Am Rev Respir Dis 131:312, 1985.

393. Mapp CE, Polato R, Maestrelli P, et al: Time course of the increase in airway responsiveness associated with late asthmatic reactions to toluene di-isocyanate in sensitized subjects. J Allergy Clin Immunol 75:568, 1985.

394. Lam S, Wong R, Yeung M: Nonspecific bronchial reactivity in occupational asthma. J Allergy Clin Immunol 1979:613, 28.

395. Ramsdale EH, Morris MM, Roberts RS, et al: Asymptomatic bronchial hyperresponsiveness in rhinitis. J Allergy Clin Immunol 75:573, 1985.

396. Stevens VJ, Vermeire PA: Bronchial responsiveness to histamine and allergy in patients with asthma, rhinitis, cough. Eur J Respir Dis 61:203, 1980.

397. Banks DE, Barkman HW Jr, Butcher BT, et al: Absence of hyperresponsiveness to methacholine in a worker with methylene diphenyl diisocyanate (MDI)-induced asthma. Chest 89:389, 1986.

398. Staunescu DC, Frans A: Bronchial asthma without increased airway reactivity. Eur J Respir Dis 63:5, 1982.

399. Hargreave FE, Ramsdale EH, Pugsley SO: Occupational asthma without bronchial hyperresponsiveness. Am Rev Respir Dis 130:513, 1984.

400. Giffon E, Orehek J, Vervloet D, et al: Asthma without airway hyperresponsiveness to carbachol. Eur J Respir Dis 70:229, 1987.

401. Bechtel JJ, Starr T, Dantzker DR, et al: Airway hyperreactivity in patients with sarcoidosis. Am Rev Resp Dis 124:759, 1981.

402. Olafsson M, Simonsson BG, Hansson SB: Bronchial reactivity in patients with recent pulmonary sarcoidosis. Thorax 40:51, 1985.

403. Freedman PM, Ault B: Bronchial hyperreactivity to methacholine in farmer's lung disease. J Allergy Clin Immunol 67:59, 1981.

404. Mönkäre S, Haahtela T, Ikonen M, et al: Bronchial hyperreactivity to inhaled histamine in patients with farmer's lung. Lung 159:145, 1981.

405. Mönkäre S: Clinical aspects of farmer's lung: Airway reactivity, treatment and prognosis. Eur J Respir Dis 65:1, 1984.

406. Ramsdell JW, Nachtwey FJ, Moser KM, et al: Bronchial hyperreactivity in chronic obstructive bronchitis. Am Rev Respir Dis 126:829, 1982.

407. Yan K, Salome CM, Woolcock AJ, et al: Prevalence and nature of bronchial hyperresponsiveness in subjects with chronic obstructive pulmonary disease. Am Rev Respir Dis 132:27, 1985.

408. Bahous J, Cartier A, Ouimet G, et al: Nonallergic bronchial hyperexcitability in chronic bronchitis. Am Rev Respir Dis 129:216, 1984.

409. Woolcock AJ, Peat JK, Salome CN, et al: Prevalence of bronchial hyperresponsiveness and asthma in a rural adult population. Thorax 42:361, 1987.

410. Britton WJ, Woolcock AJ, Peat JK, et al: Prevalence of bronchial hyperresponsiveness in children: The relationship between asthma and skin reactivity to allergens in two communities. Int J Epidemiol 15:202, 1986.

411. Weiss ST, Tager IB, Weiss JW, et al: Airway responsiveness in a population sample of adults and children. Am Rev Respir Dis 129:898, 1984.

412. Mortagy AK, Howell JB, Waters WE: Respiratory symptoms and bronchial reactivity: Identification of a syndrome and its relation to asthma. BMJ 293:525, 1986.

413. Fish JE, Ankin MG, Kelly JF, et al: Regulation of bronchomotor tone by lung inflation in asthmatic and nonasthmatic subjects. J Appl Physiol 50:1079, 1981.

414. Orehek J: The concept of airway "sensitivity" and "reactivity." Eur J Respir Dis 64(Suppl 131):27, 1983.

415. Michoud MC, Lelorier J, Amyot R: Factors modulating the individual variability of airway responsiveness to histamine. The influence of $H_1$ and $H_2$ receptors. Bull Eur Physiopathol Respir 17:807, 1981.

416. Woolcock AJ, Salome CM, Yan K: The shape of the dose-response curve to histamine in asthmatic and normal subjects. Am Rev Respir Dis 130:71, 1984.

417. Sterk P, Daniel E, Zamel N, et al: Limited maximal airway narrowing in nonasthmatic subjects—role of neural control and prostaglandin in release. Am Rev Respir Dis 132:865, 1985.

418. Michoud MC, Lelorier J, Amyot R: Factors modulating the individual variability of airway responsiveness to histamine. The influence of $H_1$ and $H_2$ receptors. Bull Eur Physiopath Respir 17:807, 1981.

419. Woolcock AJ, Salome CM, Yan K: The shape of the dose-response curve to histamine in asthmatic and normal subjects. Am Rev Respir Dis 130:71, 1984.

420. Sterk P, Daniel E, Zamel N, et al: Limited maximal airway narrowing in nonasthmatic subjects—role of neural control and prostaglandin in release. Am Rev Respir Dis 132:865, 1985.

421. Cockcroft DW, Berscheid BA: Slope of the dose-response curve: Usefulness in assessing bronchial responses to inhaled histamine. Thorax 38:55, 1983.

422. Malo J, Cartier A, Pineau L, et al: Slope of the dose-response curve to inhaled histamine and methacholine and PC20 in subjects with symptoms of airway hyperexcitability and in normal subjects. Am Rev Respir Dis 132:644, 1985.

423. Beaupré A, Malo JL: Histamine dose-response curves in asthma: Relevance of the distinction between PC20 and reactivity in characterising the clinical state. Thorax 36:731, 1981.

424. Orehek J, Gayrard P, Smith AP, et al: Airway response to carbachol in normal and asthmatic subjects. Am Rev Respir Dis 115:937, 1977.

425. O'Connor G, Sparrow D, Taylor D, et al: Analysis of dose-response curves to methacholine. An approach suitable for population studies. Am Rev Respir Dis 136:1412, 1987.

426. Salome CM, Schoeffel RE, Woolcock AJ: Comparison of bronchial reactivity to histamine and methacholine in asthmatics. Clin Allergy 10:541, 1980.

427. Juniper EF, Frith PA, Dunnett C, et al: Reproducibility and comparison of response to inhaled histamine and methacholine. Thorax 33:705, 1978.

428. Juniper EF, Frith PA, Hargreave FE: Airway responsiveness to histamine and methacholine—relationship to minimum treatment to control symptoms of asthma. Thorax 36:575, 1981.

429. Thomson NC, O'Byrne PM, Hargreave FE: Prolonged asthmatic responses to inhaled methacholine. J Allergy Clin Immunol 71:357, 1983.

430. Madsen F, Rathlou NHH, Frolund L, et al: Short and long term reproducibility of responsiveness to inhaled histamine: Rt compared to $FEV_1$ as measurement of response to challenge. Eur J Respir Dis 67:193, 1985.

431. Ryan G, Dolovich MB, Roberts RS, et al: Standardization of inhalation provocation tests: Two techniques of aerosol generation and inhalation compared. Am Rev Respir Dis 123:195, 1981.

432. Ruffin RE, Alpers JH, Crockett AJ, et al: Repeated histamine inhalation tests in asthmatic patients. J Allergy Clin Immunol 67:285, 1981.

433. Ten Velde GPM, Kreukniet J: The histamine inhalation provocation test and its reproducibility. Respiration 45:131, 1984.

434. Löwhagen O, Lindholm NB: Short-term and long-term variation in bronchial response to histamine in asthmatic patients. Eur J Respir Dis 64:466, 1983.

435. Juniper EF, Frith PA, Hargreave FE: Long-term stability of bronchial responsiveness to histamine. Thorax 37:288, 1982.

436. Anderson RC, Cuff MT, Frith PA, et al: Bronchial responsiveness to inhaled histamine and exercise. J Allergy Clin Immunol 63:315, 1979.

437. O'Byrne PM, Ryan G, Morris M, et al: Asthma induced by cold air and its relation to non-specific bronchial responsiveness to methacholine. Am Rev Respir Dis 125:281, 1982.

438. Aquilina AT: Comparison of airway reactivity induced by histamine, methacholine and isocapnic hyperventilation in normal and asthmatic subjects. Thorax 38:766, 1983.

439. Anderson SD, Schoeffel RE, Finney M: Evaluation of ultrasonically nebulized solutions for provocation testing in patients with asthma. Thorax 38:284, 1983.

440. Ryan G, Latimer KM, Dolovich J, et al: Bronchial responsiveness to histamine: Relationship to diurnal variation of peak flow rate, improvement after bronchodilator, and airway calibre. Thorax 37:423, 1982.

441. Khoo KT, Connolly CK: A comparison of three methods of measuring broncholability in asthmatics, bronchitic cigarette smokers and normal subjects. Respiration 45:219, 1984.

442. Hopp R, Bewtra A, Nair N, et al: The effect of age on methacholine response. J Allergy Clin Immunol 76:609, 1985.

443. Zamel N: Threshold of airway response to inhaled methacholine in healthy men and women. J Appl Physiol 56:129, 1984.

444. Moreno RH, Hogg JC, Paré PD: Mechanism of airway narrowing. Am Rev Respir Dis 133:1171, 1986.

445. Rubinfield AR, Pain MCF: Relationship between bronchial reactivity, airway caliber, and severity of asthma. Am Rev Respir Dis 115:381, 1977.

446. Ulrik CS: Bronchial responsiveness to inhaled histamine in both adults with intrinsic and extrinsic asthma: The importance of prechallenge forced expiratory volume in one (1) second. J Allergy Clin Immunol 1:120, 1993.

447. Cockcroft D: Airway hyperresponsiveness. *In* Barnes PJ, Grunstein MM, Leff AR, et al (eds): Asthma. Vol. 1. Philadelphia, Lippincott-Raven, 1997, p 1253.

448. Wiggs BR, Bosken C, Paré PD, et al: A model of airway narrowing in asthma and in chronic obstructive pulmonary disease. Am Rev Respir Dis 145:251, 1992.

449. Folkow B: The haemodynamic consequences of adoptive structural changes of the vessels in hypertension. Clin Sci 41:1, 1971.

450. Lambert RK, Wiggs BR, Kuwano K, et al: Functional significance of increased airway smooth muscle in asthma and COPD. J Appl Physiol 74:2771, 1993.

451. Karnovsky MJ, Edelman ER: Heparin/heparan sulphate regulation of vascular smooth muscle cell behavior. *In* Page C, Black J (eds): Airways and Vascular Remodeling. Cambridge, Academic Press, 1994.

452. Lambert RK. Role of bronchial basement membrane in airway collapse. J Appl Physiol 71:666, 1991.

453. Lambert RK, Codd SL, Alley MR, Pack RJ: Physical determinants of bronchial mucosal foldng. J Appl Physiol 77:1206, 1994.

454. Wiggs BR, Hrousis CA, Drazen JM, Kamm RD: On the mechanism of mucosal folding in normal and asthmatic airways. J Appl Physiol 83:1814, 1997.

455. Chung KF, Snashall PD: Effect of prior bronchoconstriction on the airway response in normal subjects. Thorax 39:40, 1984.

456. Ruffin RE, Dolovich MB, Wolff RK, et al: The effects of preferential deposition of histamine in the human airway. Am Rev Respir Dis 117:485, 1978.

457. Smaldone GC, Messina MS: Flow limitation, cough, and patterns of aerosol deposition in humans. J Appl Physiol 59:515, 1985.

458. Bates JH: Stochastic model of the pulmonary airway tree and its implications for bronchial responsiveness. J Appl Physiol 75:2493, 1993.

459. Hounam RF, Morgan A: Particle deposition. *In* Brain JD, Proctor DF, Reid LM (eds): Respiratory Defense Mechanisms, Part I. New York, Marcel Dekker, 1977, p 125.

460. Bourbeau J, Delfino R, Ernst P: Tracheal size is a determinant of the bronchoconstrictive response to inhaled methacholine. Eur Respir J 6:991, 1993.

461. Hogg JC: Bronchial mucosal permeability and its relationship to airways hyperreactivity. J Allergy Clin Immunol 67:421, 1981.

462. Laitinen LA, Heino M, Laitinen A, et al: Damage of the airway epithelium and bronchial reactivity in patients with asthma. Am Rev Respir Dis 131:599, 1985.

463. Laitinen LA, Haahtela T, Kava T, et al: Non-specific bronchial reactivity and ultrastructure of the airway epithelium in patients with sarcoidosis and allergic alveolitis. *In* Simonsson BG (ed): Airway hyperreactivity. Eur J Respir Dis 64(Suppl 131):267, 1983.

464. Dusser DJ, Collignon MA, Stanislas-Leguern G: Respiratory clearance of $^{99m}$Tc-DTPA and pulmonary involvement in sarcoidosis. Am Rev Respir Dis 134:493, 1986.

465. Hulbert WM, McLean T, Hogg JC: The effect of acute airway inflammation on bronchial reactivity in guinea pigs. Am Rev Respir Dis 132:7, 1985.

466. Boucher RC, Paré PD, Hogg JC: Relationship between airway hyperreactivity and permeability in *Ascaris*-sensitive monkeys. J Allergy Clin Immunol 64:197, 1979.

467. Elwood RK, Kennedy S, Belzberg A, et al: Respiratory mucosal permeability in asthma. Am Rev Respir Dis 128:523, 1983.

468. O'Byrne PM, Dolovich M, Dirks R, et al: Lung epithelial permeability: Relation to nonspecific airway responsiveness. J Appl Physiol 57:77, 1984.

469. el Donno M, Chetta A, Foresi A, et al: Lung epithelial permeability and bronchial responsiveness in subjects with stable asthma. Chest 111:1255, 1997.

470. Lemarchand P, Chinet T, Collignon MA, et al: Bronchial clearance of DTPA is increased in acute asthma but not in chronic asthma. Am Rev Respir Dis 145:147, 1992.

471. Borland C, Chamberlain A, Barber B, et al: Pulmonary epithelial permeability after inhaling saline, distilled water "fog" and cold air. Chest 87:373, 1985.

472. Higenbottam T, Borland C, Barber B, et al: Pulmonary epithelial permeability after inhaled distilled water "fog." Chest 87:156S, 1985.

473. Roehrs JD, Rogers WR, Johanson WG Jr: Bronchial reactivity to inhaled methacholine in cigarette-smoking baboons. J Appl Physiol 50:754, 1981.

474. King M, Kelly S, Cosio M: Alteration of airway reactivity by mucus. Respir Physiol 62:47, 1985.

475. Kelly L, Kolbe J, Mitzner W, et al: Bronchial blood flow affects recovery from contriction in dog lung periphery. J Appl Physiol 60:1954, 1986.

476. Michoud MC, Paré PD, Boucher R, et al: Airway responses to histamine and methacholine in *Ascaris suum*–allergic rhesus monkeys. J Appl Physiol 45:846, 1978.

477. Vidruk EH, Hahn HL, Nadel JA, et al: Mechanisms by which histamine stimulates rapidly adapting receptors in dog lungs. J Appl Physiol 43:397, 1977.

478. Palmer JB, Cuss FM, Warren JB, et al: Effect of infused vasoactive intestinal peptide on airway function in normal subjects. Thorax 41:663, 1986.

478a. Palmer JB, Cuss FM, Barnes PJ: VIP and PHM and their role in nonadrenergic inhibitory responses in isolated human airways. J Appl Physiol 61:1322, 1986.

479. Lundberg JM, Saria A: Bronchial smooth muscle contraction induced by stimulation of capsaicin-sensitive sensory neurons. Acta Physiol Scand 116:473, 1982.

480. Lundberg JM, Saria A: Capsaicin-induced desensitization of airway mucosa to cigarette smoke, mechanical, and chemical irritants. Nature 302:251, 1983.

481. Martin JG, Collier B: Acetylcholine release from canine isolated airway is not modulated by norepinephrine. J Appl Physiol 61:1025, 1986.

482. Tanaka DT, Grunstein MM: Effect of substance-P on neurally mediated contraction of rabbit airway smooth muscle. J Appl Physiol 60:458, 1986.

483. Barnes PJ, Basbaum CB, Nadel JA: Autoradiographic localization of autonomic receptors in airway smooth muscle: Marked differences between large and small airways. Am Rev Respir Dis 127:758, 1983.

484. Douglas NJ, Sudlow MF, Flenley DC: Effect of an inhaled atropine-like agent on normal airway function. J Appl Physiol 46:256, 1979.

485. Holtzman MJ, Sheller JR, Dimeo MA, et al: Effect of ganglionic blockade on bronchial reactivity in atopic subjects. Am Rev Respir Dis 122:17, 1980.

486. Sheppard D, Epstein J, Skoogh BE, et al: Variable inhibition of histamine-induced bronchoconstriction by atropine in subjects with asthma. J Allergy Clin Immunol 73:82, 1984.

487. O'Byrne PM, Thomson NC, Latimer KM, et al: The effect of inhaled hexamethonium bromide and atropine sulphate on airway responsiveness to histamine. J Allergy Clin Immunol 76:97, 1985.

488. Boulet LP, Latimer KM, Roberts RS, et al: The effects of atropine on allergen-induced increases in bronchial responsiveness to histamine. Am Rev Respir Dis 130:368, 1984.

489. Kallenbach JM, Webster T, Dowdeswell R, et al: Reflex heart rate control in asthma: Evidence of parasympathetic overactivity. Chest 87:644, 1985.

490. Sturani C, Sturani A, Tosi I: Parasympathetic activity assessed by diving reflex and by airway response to methacholine in bronchial asthma and rhinitis. Respiration 48:321, 1985.

491. Costello RW, Fryer AD: Cholinergic mechanisms in asthma. Asthma 1:965, 1997.

492. Fryer AD, Wills-Karp M: Dysfunction of M2 muscarinic receptors in pulmonary parasympathetic nerves after antigen challenge in guinea-pigs. J Appl Physiol 71:2255, 1991.

493. Okayama M, Shen T, Midorikawa J, et al: Effect of pilocarpine on propranolol-induced bronchoconstriction in asthma. Am J Respir Crit Care Med 149:76, 1994.

494. Aizawa H, Matsuzaki Y, Ishibashi M, et al: A possible role of nonadrenergic inhibitory nervous system in airway hyperreactivity. Respir Physiol 50:187, 1982.

495. Matsumoto N, Inoue H, Ichinose M, et al: Effective sites by sympathetic beta-adrenergic and vagal nonadrenergic inhibitory stimulation in constricted airways. Am Rev Respir Dis 132:1113, 1985.

496. Taylor SM, Paré PD, Armour CL, et al: Airway reactivity in chronic obstructive pulmonary disease—failure of in vivo methacholine responsiveness to correlate with cholinergic, adrenergic, or nonadrenergic responses in vitro. Am Rev Respir Dis 132:30, 1985.

497. Taylor SM, Paré PD, Schellenberg R: Cholinergic and nonadrenergic mechanisms in human and guinea pig airways. J Appl Physiol 56:958, 1984.

498. Michoud MC, Amyot R, Jeanneret-Grosjean A, et al: Reflex decrease of histamine-induced bronchoconstriction after laryngeal stimulation in humans. Am Rev Respir Dis 136:618, 1987.

499. Michoud MC, Jeanneret-Grosjean A, Cohen A, Amyot R: Reflex decrease of histamine-induced bronchoconstriction after laryngeal stimulation in asthmatic patients. Am Rev Respir Dis 138:1548, 1988.

500. Lammers J-W, Minette M, McCusker M, et al: Non-adrenergic bronchodilator mechanisms in normal human subjects *in vivo*. J Appl Physiol 64:1817, 1988.

501. Diamond L, Szarek JL, Gillespie MN, et al: In vivo bronchodilator activity of vasoactive intestinal peptide in the cat. Am Rev Respir Dis 28:827, 1983.

502. Barnes PJ, Dixon CMS: The effect of inhaled vasoactive intestinal peptide on bronchial reactivity to histamine in humans. Am Rev Respir Dis 130:162, 1984.

503. Barnes PJ: The third nervous system in the lung: Physiology and clinical perspectives (editorial). Thorax 39:561, 1984.

504. Bai TR, Bramley AM. Effect of an inhibitor of nitric oxide synthase on neural relaxation of human bronchi. Am J Physiol 8:L425, 1993.

505. Ellis JL, Undem BJ: Inhibition by L-NG-nitro-L-arginine of nonadrenergic inhibitory responses in isolated central and peripheral airways. Am Rev Respir Dis 146:1543, 1992.

506. Richardson JB: Nerve supply to the lungs. Am Rev Respir Dis 119:785, 1979.

507. Carstairs JR, Nimmo AJ, Barnes PJ: Auto-radiographic visualization of beta-adrenoceptor subtypes in human lung. Am Rev Respir Dis 132:541, 1985.

508. Carstairs JR, Nimmo AJ, Barnes PJ: Auto-radiographic localization of beta-adrenoceptors in human lung. Eur J Pharmacol 105:189, 1984.

509. Szentivanyi A: The beta-adrenergic theory of the atopic abnormality in bronchial asthma. J Allergy 42:203, 1968.

510. Shelhamer JH, Marom Z, Kaliner M: Abnormal beta-adrenergic responsiveness in allergic subjects. 2. The role of selective beta 2-adrenergic hyporeactivity. J Allergy Clin Immunol 71:57, 1983.

511. Parker CW, Smith JW: Alterations in cyclic adenosine monophosphate metabolism in human bronchial asthma. I: Leukocyte responsiveness to beta-adrenergic agents. J Clin Invest 52:48, 1973.

512. Brooks SM, McGowan K, Altenau P: Relationship between beta-adrenergic binding in lymphocyte and severity of disease in asthma. Chest 75:232, 1979.

513. Kariman K: Beta-adrenergic receptor binding in lymphocytes from patients with asthma. Lung 158:41, 1980.

514. Brooks SM, McGowan K, Bernstein IL, et al: Relationship between numbers of beta-adrenergic receptors in lymphocytes and disease severity in asthma. J Allergy Clin Immunol 63:401, 1979.

515. Goldie RG, Spina D, Henry PJ, et al: In vitro responsiveness of human asthmatic bronchus to carbachol, histamine, beta-adrenoceptor agonists and theophylline. Br J Clin Pharmacol 22:669, 1986.

516. Cerrina J, Le Roy Laurdie M, Labat C, et al: Comparison of human bronchial muscle responses to histamine in vivo with histamine and isoproterenol agonists in vitro. Am Rev Respir Dis 134:57, 1986.

517. Patterson JW, Lulich KM, Golpie RG: The role of beta-adrenoceptors in bronchial hyperreactivity. *In* Morley J (ed): Bronchial Hyperreactivity. Sydney, Academic Press, 1982, p 19.

518. Galant SP, Duriseti L, Underwood S, et al: Decreased beta-adrenergic receptors on polymorphonuclear leukocytes after adrenergic therapy. N Engl J Med 299:933, 1978.

519. Galant SP, Duriseti L, Underwood S, et al: Beta-adrenergic receptors of polymorphonuclear particulates in bronchial asthma. J Clin Invest 65:577, 1980.

520. Busse WW, Bush RK, Cooper W: Granulocyte response in vitro to isoproterenol, histamine, and prostaglandin E₁ during treatment with beta-adrenergic aerosols in asthma. Am Rev Respir Dis 120:377, 1979.

521. Conolly ME, Tashkin DP, Hui KKP, et al: Selective subsensitization of beta-adrenergic receptors in central airways of asthmatics and normal subjects during long-term therapy with inhaled salbutamol. J Allergy Clin Immunol 70:423, 1982.

522. Tashkin DP, Conolly ME, Deutsch RI, et al: Subsensitization of beta-adrenoceptors in airways and lymphocytes of healthy and asthmatic subjects. Am Rev Respir Dis 125:185, 1982.

523. Guillot C, Fornaris M, Badier M, et al: Spontaneous and provoked resistance to isoproterenol in isolated human bronchi. J Allergy Clin Immunol 74:713, 1984.

524. Bruynzeel PLB: Changes in the β-adrenergic system due to β-adrenergic therapy: Clinical consequences. Eur J Respir Dis 135(Suppl 65):62, 1984.

525. Meurs H, Köeter GH, de Vries K, et al: Dynamics of the lymphocyte beta-adrenoceptor system in patients with allergic bronchial asthma. Eur J Respir Dis 135(Suppl 65):47, 1984.

526. Meurs H, Köeter GH, de Vries K, et al: The beta-adrenergic system and allergic bronchial asthma changes in lymphocyte beta-adrenergic receptor number and adenylate cyclase activity after an allergen-induced asthmatic attack. J Allergy Clin Immunol 70:272, 1982.

527. Bai TR, Mak JC, Barnes PJ: A comparison of beta-adrenergic receptors and in vitro relaxant responses to isoproterenol in asthmatic airway smooth muscle. Am J Respir Cell Mol Biol 6:647, 1992.

528. Kiyingi KS, Anderson SD, Temple DM, et al: Beta-adrenoceptor blockade with propranolol and bronchial responsiveness to a number of bronchial provocation tests in non-asthmatic subjects. Eur J Respir Dis 66:256, 1985.

529. Zaid G, Beall GN: Bronchial response to beta-adrenergic blockade. N Engl J Med 275:580, 1966.

530. Orehek J, Gayrard P, Grimaud C, et al: Effect of beta-adrenergic blockade on bronchial sensitivity to inhaled acetylcholine in normal subjects. J Allergy Clin Immunol 55:164, 1975.

531. Kiyingi KS, Anderson SD, Temple DM, et al: Beta-adrenoceptor blockade with propranolol and bronchial responsiveness to a number of bronchial provocation tests in non-asthmatic subjects. Eur J Respir Dis 66:256, 1985.

532. Langer I: The bronchoconstrictor action of propranolol aerosol in asthmatic subjects. J Physiol (Lond) 190:41, 1967.

533. Grieco MH, Pierson RN: Mechanism of bronchoconstriction due to beta-adrenergic blockade. J Allergy Clin Immunol 48:143, 1971.

534. Richardson PS, Sterling GM: Effects of beta-adrenergic receptor blockade on airway conductance and lung volume in normal and asthmatic subjects. BMJ 3:143, 1969.

535. Diggory P, Heyworth P, Chau G, et al: Unsuspected bronchospasm in association with topical timolol—a common problem in elderly people: Can we easily identify those affected and do cardioselective agents lead to improvement? Age Ageing 23:17, 1994.

536. Ind PW, Dixon CMS, Fuller RW, Barnes PJ: Anticholinergic blockade of beta blocker–induced bronchoconstriction. Am Rev Respir Dis 138:1390, 1989.

537. Barnes PJ: Endogenous plasma adrenaline in asthma. Eur J Respir Dis 64:559, 1983.

538. Gouge SF, Daniels DJ, Smith CE: Exacerbation of asthma after pyridostigmine during Operation Desert Storm. Mil Med 159:108, 1994.

539. Warren JB, Keynes RJ, Brown MJ, et al: Blunted sympathoadrenal response to exercise in asthmatic subjects. Br J Dis Chest 76:147, 1982.

540. Barnes PJ, Brown MJ, Silverman M, et al: Circulating catecholamines in exercise- and hyperventilation-induced asthma. Thorax 36:435, 1981.

541. Sands MF, Douglas FL, Green J, et al: Homeostatic regulation of bronchomotor tone by sympathetic activation during bronchoconstriction in normal and asthmatic humans. Am Rev Respir Dis 132:993, 1985.

542. Barnes PJ: Adrenergic receptors of normal and asthmatic airways. Eur J Respir Dis 135(Suppl 65):62, 1984.

543. Kneussl MP, Richardson JB: Alpha-adrenergic receptors in human and canine tracheal and bronchial smooth muscle. J Appl Physiol 45:307, 1978.

544. Thomson NC, Daniel EE, Hargreave FE: Role of smooth muscle alpha-1-receptors in nonspecific bronchial responsiveness in asthma. Am Rev Respir Dis 126:521, 1982.

545. Black JL, Salome CM, Yan N, et al: Comparison between airways response to an alpha adrenoceptor and histamine in asthmatic and non-asthmatic subjects. Br J Clin Pharmacol 14:464, 1982.

546. Black JL, Salome C, Yan N, et al: The action of prazosin and propylene glycol on methoxamine-induced bronchoconstriction in asthmatic subjects. Br J Clin Pharmacol 18:349, 1984.

547. Black J, Vincenc K, Salome C: Inhibition of methoxamine-induced bronchoconstriction by ipratropium bromide and disodium cromoglycate in asthmatic subjects. Br J Clin Pharmacol 20:41, 1985.

548. Henderson WR, Shelhamer JH, Reingold DB, et al: Alpha-adrenergic hyperresponsiveness in asthma: Analysis of vascular and pupillary responses. N Engl J Med 300:642, 1979.

549. Davis PB: Pupillary responses and airway reactivity in asthma. J Allergy Clin Immunol 77:667, 1986.

550. Utting JA: Alpha-adrenergic blockade in severe asthma. Br J Dis Chest 73:317, 1979.

551. Jenkins C, Breslin ABX, Marlin GE: The role of alpha-adrenoceptors and beta-adrenoceptors in airway hyperresponsiveness to histamine. J Allergy Clin Immunol 75:364, 1985.

552. Barnes PJ, Wilson NM, Vickers H: Prazosin, an alpha-1-adrenoceptor antagonist, partially inhibits exercise-induced asthma. J Allergy Clin Immunol 68:411, 1981.

553. Walden SM, Bleecker ER, Chahal K, et al: Effect of alpha-adrenergic blockade on exercise-induced asthma and conditioned cold air. Am Rev Respir Dis 130:357, 1984.

554. Eiser NM: Hyperreactivity. Its relationship to histamine receptors. Eur J Respir Dis 64(Suppl 131):99, 1983.

555. Smith AP, Dunlop LS: In vitro evidence of H₂ receptors in human bronchus and their role in allergic bronchospasm. Br J Dis Chest 74:314, 1980.

556. Thomson NC, Kerr JW: Effect of inhaled H₁ and H₂ receptor antagonists in normal and asthmatic subjects. Thorax 35:428, 1980.

557. White J, Smith AP, Leopold D, et al: Effects of H₂ antagonists in asthma. Br J Chest 74:315, 1980.

558. Nogrady SG, Bevan C: H₂-receptor blockade and bronchial hyperreactivity to histamine in asthma. Thorax 36:268, 1981.

559. Tashkin PD, Ungerer R, Wolfe R, et al: Effect of orally administered cimetidine on histamine- and antigen-induced bronchospasm in subjects with asthma. Am Rev Respir Dis 125:691, 1982.

560. Nathan RA, Segall N, Glover GC, et al: The effects of H₁ and H₂ antihistamines on histamine inhalation challenges in asthmatic patients. Am Rev Respir Dis 120:1251, 1979.

561. Lichtenstein LM, Gillespie F: Inhibition of histamine release by histamine controlled by H₂ receptors. Nature 244:287, 1973.

562. Kaliner M: Human lung tissue and anaphylaxis: The effects of histamine on the immunologic release of mediators. Am Rev Respir Dis 118:1015, 1978.

563. Eiser NM, Guz A, Mills J, et al: Effect of H₁ and H₂ receptor antagonists on antigen bronchial challenge. Thorax 33:534, 1978.

564. Anderson KE: Airway hyperreactivity, smooth muscle and calcium. Eur J Respir Dis 64(Suppl 131):49, 1983.

565. Fleming WW, McPhillips JJ, Westfall DP: Post-junctional supersensitivity and subsensitivity of excitable tissue to drugs. Ergeb Physiol 68:55, 1968.

566. Barnes PJ: Calcium-channel blockers and asthma. Thorax 38:481, 1983.

567. Daniel EE, Davis C, Jones T, et al: Control of airway smooth muscle. *In* Hargreave FE (ed): Airway Reactivity: Mechanisms and Clinical Relevance. Mississauga, Ontario, Astra Mississauga, 1980, p 80.

568. Liu Y, Sasaki H, Ishii M, et al: Effect of circadian rhythm on bronchomotor tone after deep inspiration in normal and in asthmatic subjects. Am Rev Respir Dis 132:278, 1985.

569. Antonissen LA, Mitchell RW, Kroeger EA, et al: Mechanical alterations of airway smooth muscle in a canine asthmatic model. J Appl Physiol 46:681, 1979.

570. Schellenberg RR, Paré PD, Hards J, Ishida K: Smooth muscle mechanics: Implications for airway hyperresponsiveness. Int Arch Allergy Appl Immunol 94:291, 1991.

571. de Jongste JC, Mons H, Bonata IL, Kerrebijn KF: In vitro responses of airways from an asthmatic patient. Eur J Resp Dis 71:23, 1987.

572. Bai TR: Abnormalities in airway smooth muscle in fatal asthma. Am Rev Respir Dis 141:552, 1990.

573. Coflesky JT, Jones RC, Reid LM, Evans JN: Mechanical properties and structure of isolated pulmonary arteries remodeled by chronic hyperoxia. Am Rev Respir Dis 136:388, 1987.

574. Karnovsky MJ, Edelman ER: Heparin/heparan sulphate regulation of vascular smooth muscle cell behavior. *In* Page C, Black J (eds): Airways and Vascular Remodelling. Cambridge, Academic Press, 1994.

575. Vincenc KS, Black JL, Yan K, et al: Comparison of in vivo and in vitro responses to histamine in human airways. Am Rev Respir Dis 128:875, 1983.

576. Armour CL, Lazar NM, Schellenberg RR, et al: A comparison of in vivo and in vitro human airway reactivity to histamine. Am Rev Respir Dis 129:907, 1984.

577. Roberts J, Raeburn D, Rodger I, et al: Comparison of in vivo airway responsiveness and in vitro smooth muscle sensitivity to methacholine in man. Thorax 39:837, 1984.

578. Roberts JA, Rodger IW, Thomson NC: Airway responsiveness to histamine in man: Effect of atropine on in vivo and in vitro comparison. Thorax 40:261, 1985.

579. Whicker SD, Armour CL, Black JL: Responsiveness of bronchial smooth muscle from asthmatic patients to relaxant and contractile agonists. Pulm Pharmacol 1:25, 1988.

580. Skloot G, Permutt S, Togias A: Airway hyperresponsiveness in asthma: A problem of limited smooth muscle relaxation. J Clin Invest 96:2393, 1995.

581. Chetta A, Foresi A, Garavaldi G, et al: Evaluation of bronchial responsiveness by pharmacological challenges in asthma. Inhaled propranolol in comparison with histamine and methacholine. Respiration 54(Suppl 1):84, 1988.

582. Lim TK, Pride NB, Ingram JRJ: Effects of volume history during spontaneous and acutely induced air-flow obstruction in asthma. Am Rev Respir Dis 135:591, 1987.

583. Pellegrino RV, Brusasco V: Maximal bronchoconstriction in humans. Relationship to deep inhalation and airway sensitivity. Am J Respir Crit Care Med 153:115, 1996.

584. Wheatley JR, Pare PD, Engel LA: Reversibility of induced bronchoconstriction by deep inspiration in asthmatic and normal subjects. Eur Respir J 2:331, 1989.

585. Colebatch HJ, Finucane KE, Smith MM: Pulmonary conductance and elastic recoil relationships in asthma and emphysema. J Appl Physiol 34:143, 1973.

586. Green M, Mead J: Time dependence of flow-volume curves. J Appl Physiol 37:793, 1974.

587. Fish, JE, MG Ankin, JF Kelly, VI Peterman: Regulation of bronchomotor tone by lung inflation in asthmatic and nonasthmatic subjects. J Appl Physiol 50:1079, 1981.

588. Fredberg J, Jones K, Nathan M, et al: Friction in airway smooth muscle: Mechanism, latch and implications in asthma. J Appl Physiol 81:2704, 1996.

589. Paré P, Wiggs B, James A, et al: The comparative mechanics and morphology of airways in asthma and in chronic obstructive pulmonary disease. Am Rev Respir Dis 143:1189, 1991.

590. Macklem PT: A theoretical analysis of the effect of airway smooth muscle load on airway narrowing. Am J Resp Crit Care Med 153:83, 1996.

591. Ingram RH Jr: Relationships among airway-parenchymal interactions, lung responsiveness, and inflammation in asthma. Giles F. Filley Lecture. Chest 107:148S, 1995.

592. Stephens NL, Van Niekerk W: Isometric and isotonic contractions in airway smooth muscle. Can J Physiol Pharmacol 55:833, 1977.

593. Stephens NL, Kroeger E, Media JA: Force-velocity characteristics of respiratory airway smooth muscle. J Appl Physiol 26:285, 1969.

594. Stephens NL, Mitchell RW, Antonissen A, et al: Airway smooth muscle: Physiologic properties and metabolism. *In* Hargreave FE (ed): Airway Reactivity: Mechanisms and Clinical Relevance. Mississauga, Ontario, Astra Mississauga, 1980, p 110.

594a. Moore BJ, Hilliam CC, Verburgt LM, et al: Shape and position of the complete dose-response curve for inhaled metacholine in normal subjects. Am J Respir Crit Care Med 154:642, 1996.

595. Macklem PT: Bronchial hyporesponsiveness. Chest 87:158S, 1985.

596. De Kock MA: Functional anatomy of the trachea and main bronchi. *In* De Kock MA, Nadel JA, Lewis CM (eds): Mechanisms of Airway Obstruction in Human Respiratory Disease. Capetown, South African Medical Research Council, 1979, p 49.

597. Martin JG, Dong-Jie D, Macklem PT: Effects of lung volume on methacholine-induced bronchoconstriction in normal subjects. Am Rev Respir Dis 133:A15, 1986.

598. Thurlbeck WM, Pun R, Toth J, et al: Bronchial cartilage in chronic obstructive lung disease. Am Rev Respir Dis 109:73, 1974.

599. Bramley AM, Thomson RJ, Roberts CR, Schellenberg RR: Hypothesis: Excessive bronchoconstriction in asthma is due to decreased airway elastance. Eur Respir J 7:337, 1994.

600. Bramley AM, Roberts CR, Schellenberg RR: Collagenase increases shortening of human bronchial smooth muscle in vitro. Am J Respir Crit Care Med 152:1513, 1995.

601. Paré PD, Roberts CR, Bai TR, et al: The functional consequences of airway remodeling in asthma. Monaldi Arch Chest Dis 52:589, 1997.

602. Holtzman MJ: Inflammation of the airway epithelium and the development of airway hyperresponsiveness. *In* Herzog H, Perruchoud AP (eds): Asthma and Bronchial Hyperreactivity. Basel, Karger, 1984, p 165.

603. Cockcroft DW, Ruffin RE, Dolovich J, et al: Allergen-induced increase in non-allergic bronchial reactivity. Clin Allergy 7:503, 1977.

604. Altounyan REC: Changes in histamine and atropine. Responsiveness as a guide to diagnosis and evaluation of therapy in obstructive airways disease. *In* Pepys J, Frankland AW (eds): Disodium Cromoglycate in Allergic Airways Disease. London, Butterworths, 1970, p 47.

605. Bar-Sela S, Schleuter DP, Kitt SR, et al: Antigen-induced enhancement of bronchial reactivity. Chest 88:114, 1985.

606. Black J, Schoeffel R, Sundrum R, et al: Increased responsiveness to methacholine and histamine after challenge with ultrasonically nebulised water in asthmatic subjects. Thorax 40:427, 1985.

607. Smith CM, Anderson SD, Black JL: Methacholine responsiveness increases after ultrasonically nebulized water but not after ultrasonically nebulized hypertonic saline in patients with asthma. J Allergy Clin Immunol 79:85, 1987.

608. Cartier A, Thomson NC, Frith PA, et al: Allergen-induced increase in bronchial responsiveness to histamine—relationship to the late asthmatic response and change in airway caliber. J Allergy Clin Immunol 70:170, 1982.

609. Boulet LP, Cartier A, Thomson NC, et al: Asthma and increases in nonallergic bronchial responsiveness from seasonal pollen exposure. J Allergy Clin Immunol 71:399, 1983.

610. Machado L: Increased bronchial hypersensitivity after early and late bronchial reactions provoked by allergen inhalation. Allergy 40:580, 1985.

611. Durham SR, Craddock CF, Cookson WD, et al: Increases in airway responsiveness to histamine precede allergen-induced late asthmatic responses. J Allergy Clin Immunol 82:764, 1988.

611a. Sotomayor H, Badier M, Vervloet D, et al: Seasonal increase of carbachol airway responsiveness in patients allergic to grass pollen—reversal by corticosteroids. Am Rev Respir Dis 130:56, 1984.

612. van der Heide S, de Monchy JG, de Vries K, et al: Seasonal variation in airway hyperresponsiveness and natural exposure to house dust mite allergens in patients with asthma. J Allergy Clin Immunol 93:470, 1994.

613. Cartier A, L'Archeveque J, Malo JL: Exposure to a sensitizing occupational agent can cause a long-lasting increase in bronchial responsiveness to histamine in the absence of significant changes in airway caliber. J Allergy Clin Immunol 78:1185, 1986.

614. Fabbri LM, Di Giacomo R, Dal Vecchio L, et al: Prednisone, indomethacin and airway responsiveness in toluene diisocyanate–sensitized subjects. Bull Eur Physiopathol Respir 21:421, 1985.

615. Dolovich J, Hargreave F: The asthma syndrome—inciters, inducers and host characteristics. Thorax 36:641, 1981.

616. Nadel JA: Inflammation and asthma. J Allergy Clin Immunol 73(Suppl):651, 1984.

617. Wills-Karp M: Smooth muscle as a direct or indirect target accounting for bronchopulmonary hyperresponsiveness. Res Immunol 148:59, 1997.

618. Gavett SH, O'Hearn DJ, Karp CL, et al: Interleukin-4 receptor blockade prevents airway responses induced by antigen challenge in mice. Am J Physiol 272:L253, 1997.

619. Watson N, Bodtke K, Coleman RA, et al: Role of IgE in hyperresponsiveness induced by passive sensitization of human airways. Am J Respir Crit Care Med 155:839, 1997.

620. Black JL, Marathon R, Armour CL, Johnson PRA: Sensitization alters contractile responses and calcium influx in human airway smooth muscle. J Allergy Clin Immunol 84:440, 1989.

621. Ben-Jebria A, Marthan R, Rossetti M, Savineau JP: Effect of passive sensitization on the mechanical activity of human isolated bronchial smooth muscle induced by substance P, neurokinin A and VIP. Br J Pharmacol 109:131, 1993.

622. Smith L, McFadden ER Jr: Bronchial hyperreactivity revisited. Ann Allergy Asthma Immunol 74:454; quiz 469, 1995.

623. Haley KJ, Drazen JM: Inflammation and airway function in asthma: What you see is not necessarily what you get. Am J Resp Crit Care Med 157:1, 1998.

624. Crimi E, Spanevello A, Neri M, et al: Dissociation between airway inflammation and airway hyperresponsiveness in allergic asthma. Am J Crit Care Med 157:4, 1998.

625. Killian D, Cockcroft DW, Hargreave FE, et al: Factors in allergen-induced asthma: Relevance of the intensity of the airways allergic reaction and nonspecific bronchial reactivity. Clin Allergy 6:219, 1976.

626. Cockcroft DW, Ruffin RE, Frith PA, et al: Determinants of allergen-induced asthma: Dose of allergen, circulating IgE antibody concentration, and bronchial responsiveness to inhaled histamine. Am Rev Respir Dis 120:1053, 1979.

627. Neijens HJ, Degenhart HC, Raatgeep HC, et al: Study on the significance of bronchial hyperreactivity in the bronchial obstruction after inhalation of cat dander allergen. J Allergy Clin Immunol 64:507, 1979.

628. Nathan RA, Kinsman RA, Spector SL, et al: Relationship between airways response to allergens and nonspecific bronchial reactivity. J Allergy Clin Immunol 64:491, 1979.

629. Stuckey MS, Witt CS, Schmitt LH, et al: Histamine sensitivity influences reactivity to allergens. J Allergy Clin Immunol 373:75, 1985.

630. Pauwels R: Mediators and non-specific bronchial hyperreactivity. Eur J Respir Dis 64:95, 1983.

631. Schlueter DP, Soto RJ, Baretta ED, et al: Airway response to hair spray in normal subjects and subjects with hyperreactive airways. Chest 75:544, 1979.

632. Smith P, Stitik F, Smith J, et al: Tantalum inhalation and airway responses. Thorax 34:486, 1979.

633. Hargreave FE, Ryan G, Thomson NC, et al: Bronchial responsiveness to histamine or methacholine in asthma: Measurement and clinical significance. Eur J Respir Dis 63:79, 1982.

634. Hargreave FE, Ramsdale H, Dolovich J: Measurement of airway responsiveness in clinical practice. *In* Hargreave FE, Woolcock AJ (eds): Airway Responsiveness: Measurement and Interpretation. Mississauga, Ontario, Astra Mississauga, 1985, p 122.

635. Jansen DF, Timens W, Kraan J, et al: (A)symptomatic bronchial hyper-responsiveness and asthma. Respir Med 91:121, 1997.

636. Woolcock AJ: Tests of airway responsiveness in epidemiology. *In* Hargreave FE, Woolcock AJ (eds): Airway Responsiveness: Measurement and Interpretation. Mississauga, Ontario, Astra Mississauga, 1985, p 136.

637. Woolcock AJ, Yan K, Salome CM: Effect of therapy on bronchial hyperresponsiveness in the long-term management of asthma. Clin Allergy 18:165, 1988.

638. Plaschke P, Bake B: Pronounced bronchial hyper-responsiveness and asthma severity. Clin Physiol 14:197, 1994.

639. Chan-Yeung M, Lam S, Tse KS: Measurement of airway responsiveness in occupational asthma. *In* Hargreave FE, Woolcock AJ (eds): Airway Responsiveness: Measurement and Interpretation. Mississauga, Ontario, Astra Mississauga, 1985, p 129.

640. Prieto L, Berto JM, Lopez M, Peris A: Modifications of PC20 and maximal degree of airway narrowing to methacholine after pollen season in pollen sensitive asthmatic patients. Clin Exp Allergy 23:172, 1993.

641. Wide L, Bennich H, Johansson SGO: Diagnosis of allergy by an in-vitro test for allergen antibodies. Lancet 2:1105, 1967.

642. Wanner A, Russi E, Brodnan J, et al: Prolonged bronchial obstruction after a single antigen challenge in ragweed asthma. J Allergy Clin Immunol 76:177, 1985.

643. Cockcroft DW, Hoeppner VH, Werner GD: Recurrent nocturnal asthma after bronchoprovocation with western red cedar sawdust: Association with acute increases in nonallergic bronchial responsiveness. Clin Allergy 14:61, 1984.

644. Kaliner M: Hypotheses on the contribution of late-phase allergic responses to the understanding and treatment of allergic disease. J Allergy Clin Immunol 73:311, 1984.

645. Durham SR, Lee TH, Cromwell O, et al: Immunologic studies in allergen-induced late-phase asthmatic reactions. J Allergy Clin Immunol 74:49, 1984.

646. Machado L, Stalenheim G, Malmberg P: Early and late allergic bronchial reactions: Physiological characteristics. Clin Allergy 16:111, 1986.

647. Gleich GJ: The late phase of the immunoglobulin-E–mediated reaction—a link between anaphylaxis and common allergic disease. J Allergy Clin Immunol 70:160, 1982.

648. Lam S, LeRiche J, Phillips D, et al: Cellular and protein changes in bronchial lavage fluid after late asthmatic reaction in patients with red cedar asthma. J Allergy Clin Immunol 80:44, 1987.

649. Hogg JC: The pathology of asthma. Chest 87:152S, 1985.

650. Joseph M, Gounni AS, Kusnierz JP, et al: Expression and functions of the high-affinity IgE receptor on human platelets and megakaryocyte precursors. Eur J Immunol 27:2212, 1997.

651. Gounni AS, Lamkhioued B, Ochiai K, et al: High-affinity IgE receptor on eosinophils is involved in defence against parasites. Nature 367:183, 1994.

652. Truong MJ, Liu FT, Capron M: Human granulocytes express functional IgE-binding molecules, Mac-2/epsilon. Ann N Y Acad Sci 725:234, 1994.

653. Turner-Warwick M: Advances in asthma: Hypersensitivity mechanisms. BMJ 4:355, 1969.

654. Warren CPW, Tse KS: Serum and sputum immunoglobulin E levels in respiratory diseases in adults. Can Med Assoc J 110:425, 1974.

655. McNichol KN, Williams HE: Spectrum of asthma in children. 2. Allergic components Br Med J 4:12, 1973.

656. Palmer LJ, Paré PD, Faux JA, et al: Fc epsilon R1-beta polymorphism and total serum IgE levels in endemically parasitized Australian Aborigines. Am J Hum Genet 61:182, 1997.

657. Barbee RA, Halonen M, Lebowitz M, et al: Distribution of IgE in a community population sample—correlations with age, sex, and allergen skin test reactivity. J Allergy Clin Immunol 68:106, 1981.

658. Pepys J, Hutchcroft BJ: Bronchial provocation tests in etiologic diagnosis and analysis of asthma. Am Rev Respir Dis 112:829, 1975.

659. Bryant DH: Role of IgG in human asthma. In Austen KF, Lichtenstein LM (eds): Asthma—Physiology, Immunopharmacology and Treatment. Vol. II. New York, Academic Press, 1977, p 315.

660. Barbee RA, Lebowitz MD, Thompson HC, et al: Immediate skin-test reactivity in a general population sample. Ann Intern Med 84:129, 1976.

661. Hagy GW, Settipane GA: Bronchial asthma, allergic rhinitis, and allergy skin tests among college students. J Allergy 44:323, 1969.

662. Curran WS, Goldman G: The incidence of immediately reacting allergy skin tests in a "normal" adult population. Ann Intern Med 55:777, 1961.

663. Buisseret PD: Seasonal allergic symptoms due to fungal spores. BMJ 2:507, 1976.

664. Chatterjee J, Hargreave FE: Atmospheric pollen and fungal spores in Hamilton in 1972 estimated by the Hirst automatic volumetric spore trap. Can Med Assoc J 110:659, 1974.

665. Ordman D: Seasonal respiratory allergy in Windhoek: The pollen and fungus factors. S Afr Med J 44:250, 1970.

666. Kabe J, Aoki Y, Ishizaki T, et al: Relationship of dermal and pulmonary sensitivity to extracts of Candida albicans. Am Rev Respir Dis 104:348, 1971.

667. Pepys J, Faux JA, Longbottom JO, et al: Candida albicans precipitins in respiratory disease in man. J Allergy 41:305, 1968.

668. Rosenberg GL, Rosenthal RR, Norman PS: Inhalation challenge with ragweed pollen in ragweed-sensitive asthmatics. J Allergy Clin Immunol 71:302, 1983.

669. Knox RB: Grass pollen, thunderstorms and asthma. Clin Exp Allergy 23:354, 1993.

670. Salvaggio J, Aukrust L: Mold-induced asthma. J Allergy Clin Immunol 68:327, 1981.

671. Platts-Mills TAE, Sporik RB, Chapman MD, Heymann PW: The role of indoor allergens in asthma. Allergy 50:5, 1995.

672. Sporik R, Ingram JM, Price W, et al: Association of asthma with serum IgE and skin-test reactivity to allergens among children living at high altitude: Tickling the dragon's breath. Am J Respir Crit Care Med (in press).

673. Tauer-Reich I, Fruhmann G, Czuppon AB, et al: Allergens causing bird fancier's asthma. Allergy 49:448, 1994.

674. Maunsell K, Wraith DG, Cunnington AM: Mites and house-dust allergy in bronchial asthma. Lancet 1:1267, 1968.

675. Mites and asthma. Lancet 1:1295, 1968.

676. Gaddie J, Skinner C, Palmer KNV: Hyposensitization with house dust mite vaccine in bronchial asthma. BMJ 2:561, 1976.

677. Blythe ME, Al Ubaydi F, Williams JD, et al: Study of dust mites in three Birmingham hospitals. BMJ 1:62, 1975.

678. Mumcuoglu KY, Abed Y, Armenios B, et al: Asthma in Gaza refugee camp children and its relationship with house dust mites. Ann Allergy 72:163, 1994.

679. Charpin D, Birnbaum J, Haddi E, et al: Altitude and allergy to house dust mites: A paradigm of the influence of environmental exposure on allergic sensitization. Am Rev Respir Dis 143:983, 1991.

680. Peat JK, Britton WJ, Salome CM, Woolcock AJ: Bronchial hyperresponsiveness in two populations of Australian school children. Clin Allergy 17:297, 1987.

681. Brown H, Morrow, Filer JL: Role of mites in allergy to house dust. BMJ 3:646, 1968.

682. Pepys J, Chan M, Hargreave FE: Mites and house-dust allergy. Lancet 1:1270, 1968.

683. Pauli G, Bessot JC, Hirth C, et al: Dissociation of house dust allergies—a comparison between skin tests, inhalation tests, specific IgE and basophil histamine release measurements. J Allergy Clin Immunol 63:245, 1979.

684. Squillace SP, Sporik RB, Rakes G, et al: Sensitization to dust mites as a dominant risk factor for asthma among adolescents living in central Virginia. Multiple regression analysis of a population-based study. Am J Respir Crit Care Med 156:1760, 1997.

685. Rosenstreich DL, Eggleston P, Kattan M, et al: The role of cockroach allergy and exposure to cockroach allergen in causing morbidity among inner-city children with asthma. N Engl J Med 336:1356, 1997.

686. Kern RA: Asthma due to sensitization to a mushroom fly (Aphiochaeta agarici). J Allergy 9:604, 1938.

687. Truitt GW: The mushroom fly as a cause of bronchial asthma. Ann Allergy 9:513, 1951.

688. Young E, Pattel S, Stoneham M, et al: The prevalence of reaction to food additives in a survey population. J R Coll Physicians Lond 21:241, 1987.

689. Warner JO: Food intolerance and asthma. Clin Exp Allergy 25:29, 1995.

690. Bock SA, Sampson HA: Food allergy in infancy. Pediatr Clin North Am 41:1047, 1994.

691. Licorish K, Novey HS, Kozak P, et al: Role of Alternaria and Penicillium spores in the pathogenesis of asthma. J Allergy Clin Immunol 76:819, 1985.

692. Kraske GK, Shinaberger JH, Klaustermeyer WB: Severe hypersensitivity reaction during hemodialysis. Ann Allergy Asthma Immunol 78:217, 1997.

693. Purello D'Ambrosio F, Savica V, Gangemi S, et al: Ethylene oxide allergy in dialysis patients. Nephrol Dial Transplant 12:1461, 1997.

693a. Wooding LG, Teuber SS, Gershwin ME: Latex allergy. Compr Ther 22:384, 1996.

694. Lewis PJ, Austen KF: Fatal systemic anaphylaxis in man. N Engl J Med 270:597, 1964.

695. Hanashiro PK, Weil MH: Anaphylactic shock in man. Report of two cases with detailed hemodynamic and metabolic studies. Arch Intern Med 119:129, 1967.

696. Parker CW: Drug therapy: Drug allergy (third of three parts). N Engl J Med 292:957, 1975.

697. Barr SE: Allergy to Hymenoptera stings. JAMA 228:718, 1974.

698. Welch H, Lewis CN, Weinstein HI, et al: Severe reactions to antibiotics: A nationwide survey. Antibiot Med Clin Ther 4:800, 1957.

699. Bernstein IL, Ausdenmoore RW: Iatrogenic bronchospasm occurring during clinical trials of a new mucolytic agent, acetylcysteine. Dis Chest 46:469, 1964.

700. Raskin P: Bronchospasm after inhalation of pancreatic dornase. Am Rev Respir Dis 98:697, 1968.

701. Miller WC, Awe R: Effect of nebulized lidocaine on reactive airways. Am Rev Respir Dis 111:739, 1975.

702. Sheffer AL, Rocklin RE, Goetzl EJ: Immunologic components of hypersensitivity reactions to cromolyn sodium. N Engl J Med 293:1220, 1975.

703. Peterson IA, Grant IWB, Crompton GK: Severe bronchoconstriction provoked by sodium cromoglycate. BMJ 2:916, 1976.

703a. Bryant DH, Pepys J: Bronchial reactions to aerosol inhalant vehicle. BMJ 1:1319, 1976.

704. Bryant DH, Pepys J: Bronchial reactions to aerosol inhalant vehicle. BMJ 1:1319, 1976.

705. Austen KF: Current concepts: Systemic anaphylaxis in the human being. N Engl J Med 291:661, 1974.

706. Routledge RC, De Kretser DMH, Wadsworth LD: Severe anaphylaxis due to passive sensitization by donor blood. BMJ 1:434, 1976.

707. Ramirez MA: Horse asthma following blood transfusion. Report of a case. JAMA 73:984, 1919.

708. Spector SL: Update on exercise-induced asthma. Ann Allergy 71:571, 1993.

709. Weiler JM: Exercise-induced asthma: A practical guide to definitions, diagnosis, prevalence, and treatment. Allergy Asthma Proc 17:315, 1996.

710. McFadden ER Jr, Gilbert IA: Exercise-induced asthma. N Engl J Med 330:1362, 1994.

711. McFadden ER Jr: Exercise-induced airway obstruction. Clin Chest Med 16:671, 1995.

712. Anderson SD: Exercise-induced asthma. In Middelton E, Reed CE, Ellis EF (eds): Allergy: Principles and Practice. St. Louis, CV Mosby, 1986.

713. Lockhart A, Régnard J, Dessanges JF, et al: State of the art: Exercise- and hyperventilation-induced asthma. Bull Eur Physiopathol Res 21:399, 1985.

714. Custovic A, Arifhodzic N, Robinson A, Woodcock A: Exercise testing revisited. The response to exercise in normal and atopic children. Chest 105:1127, 1994.

715. Beck KC, Offord KP, Scanlon PD: Bronchoconstriction occurring during exercise in asthmatic subjects. Am J Respir Crit Care Med 149:352, 1994.

716. Brudno DS, Wagner JM, Rupp NT: Length of postexercise assessment in the determination of exercise-induced bronchospasm. Ann Allergy 73:227, 1994.

717. Blackie SP, Hilliam C, Village R, Paré PD: The time course of bronchoconstric-

tion in asthmatics during and after isocapnic hyperventilation. Am Rev Respir Dis 142:1133, 1990.

718. Lee TH, Anderson SD: Editorial: Heterogeneity of mechanisms in exercise-induced asthma. Thorax 40:481, 1985.

719. Koh YY, Lim HS, Min KU: Airway responsiveness to allergen is increased 24 hours after exercise challenge. J Allergy Clin Immunol 94:507, 1994.

720. Cypcar D, Lemanske RF Jr: Asthma and exercise. Clin Chest Med 15:351, 1994.

721. Mansfield L, McDonnell J, Morgan W, et al: Airway response in asthmatic children during and after exercise. Respiration 38:135, 1979.

722. Stirling DR, Cotton DJ, Graham BL, et al: Characteristics of airway tone during exercise in patients with asthma. J Appl Physiol 54:934, 1983.

723. McFadden ER, Soter NA, Ingram RH: Magnitude and site of airway response to exercise in asthmatics in relation to arterial histamine levels. J Allergy Clin Immunol 66:472, 1980.

724. Neijens HJ, Gargani G, Kralingen A, et al: Central versus peripheral airway obstruction in bronchial responsiveness due to exercise. Eur J Respir Dis 63:105, 1982.

725. McFadden ER Jr, Ingram RH Jr: Large and small airway effects with exercise and other bronchoconstrictor stimuli. Eur J Respir Dis 63:99, 1982.

726. Spiro SG, Bierman CW, Petheram IS: Reproducibility of flow rates measured with low density gas mixtures in exercise-induced bronchospasm. Thorax 36:852, 1981.

727. Voy RO: The U.S. Olympic Committee experience with exercise-induced bronchospasm, 1984. Med Sci Sports Exerc 18:328, 1986.

728. Weiler JM, Metzger WJ, Donnelly AL, et al: Prevalence of bronchial hyperresponsiveness in highly trained athletes. Chest 90:23, 1986.

729. Mannix ET, Farber MO, Palange P, et al: Exercise-induced asthma in figure skaters. Chest 109:312, 1996.

730. Voy RO: The U.S. Olympic Committee experience with exercise-induced bronchospasm. Med Sci Sports Exerc 18:328, 1986.

731. Larsson K, Ohlsen P, Larsson T, et al: High prevalence of asthma in cross country skiers. BMJ 307:1326, 1993.

732. Potts J: Factors associated with respiratory problems in swimmers. Sports Med 21:256, 1996.

733. Warren JB, Jennings SJ, Clark TJH: Effect of adrenergic and vagal blockade on the normal human airway response to exercise. Clin Sci 66:79, 1984.

734. Jain AK, Walia V, Khanna SP, et al: Effect of exercise on pulmonary function tests in normal first degree relations of asthmatic subjects. Indian J Chest Dis Allied Sci 33:73, 1991.

735. König P, Godfrey S: Prevalence of exercise-induced bronchial lability in families of children with asthma. Arch Dis Child 48:513, 1973.

736. Neijens HJ, Wesselius T, Kerrebijn KF: Exercise-induced bronchoconstriction as an expression of bronchial hyperreactivity—a study of its mechanisms in children. Thorax 36:517, 1981.

737. Weiss JW, Rossing TH, McFadden ER, et al: Relationship between bronchial responsiveness to hyperventilation with cold and methacholine in asthma. J Allergy Clin Immunol 72:140, 1983.

738. Hodgson WC, Cotton DJ, Warner GD, et al: Relationship between bronchial response to respiratory heat exchange and nonspecific airways reactivity in asthmatic patients. Chest 85:465, 1984.

739. O'Byrne PM, Ryan G, Morris M, et al: Asthma induced by cold air and its relation to nonspecific bronchial responsiveness to methacholine. Am Rev Respir Dis 125:281, 1982.

740. Mellis CM, Kattan M, Keens TG, et al: Comparative study of histamine and exercise challenges in asthmatic children. Am Rev Respir Dis 117:911, 1978.

741. Chatham M, Bleecker ER, Smith PL, et al: A comparison of histamine, methacholine, and exercise on airway reactivity in normal and asthmatic subjects. Am Rev Respir Dis 126:235, 1982.

742. Banner AS, Green J, O'Connor M: Relation of respiratory water loss to coughing after exercise. N Engl J Med 311:883, 1984.

743. Banner AS, Chausow A, Green J: The tussive effect of hyperpnea with cold air. Am Rev Respir Dis 131:362, 1985.

744. Chen WY, Horton DJ, Souhrada JF: Respiratory heat and water loss and exercise-induced asthma. Physiologist 19:152, 1976.

745. Chen WY, Horton DJ: Heat and water loss from the airways and exercise-induced asthma. Respiration 34:305, 1977.

746. Strauss RH, McFadden ER, Ingram RH: Enhancement of exercise-induced asthma by cold air. N Engl J Med 297:743, 1977.

747. Strauss RH, McFadden ER, Ingram RH, et al: Influence of heat and humidity on airway obstruction induced by exercise in asthma. J Clin Invest 61:433, 1978.

748. Deal EC Jr, McFadden ER Jr, Ingram RH Jr, et al: Role of respiratory heat exchange in production of exercise-induced asthma. J Appl Physiol 46:467, 1979.

749. Deal EC, McFadden ER, Ingram RH, et al: Hyperpnea and heat flux: Initial reaction sequence in exercise-induced asthma. J Appl Physiol 46:476, 1979.

750. Zeballos RJ, Shturman-Ellstein R, McNally JF Jr, et al: The role of hyperventilation in exercise-induced bronchoconstriction. Am Rev Respir Dis 118:877, 1978.

751. Tweeddale PM, Godden DJ, Grant IWB: Hyperventilation or exercise to induce asthma? Thorax 36:596, 1981.

752. Nisar M, Spence DP, West D, et al: A mask to modify inspired air temperature and humidity and its effect on exercise induced asthma. Thorax 47:446, 1992.

753. Vecchiet L, Flacco L, Marini I, et al: Effects of cold stimulus of the chest wall on bronchial resistance. Respiration 47:253, 1985.

754. Horton DJ, Chen WY: Effects of breathing warm humidified air on bronchoconstriction induced by body cooling and by inhalation of methacholine. Chest 75:24, 1979.

755. Wilson NM, Dixon C, Silverman M: Increased bronchial responsiveness caused by ingestion of ice. Eur J Respir Dis 66:25, 1985.

756. Smith CM, Anderson SD: Hyperosmolarity as the stimulus to asthma induced by hyperventilation? J Allergy Clin Immunol 77:729, 1986.

757. Kivity S, Souhrada JP, Melzer E: A dose-response-like relationship between minute ventilation and exercise-induced bronchoconstriction in young asthmatic patients. Eur J Respir Dis 61:342, 1980.

758. Mahler DA, Loke J: Lung function after marathon running at warm and cold ambient temperatures. Am Rev Respir Dis 124:154, 1981.

759. McFadden ER, Ingram RH: Exercise-induced airway obstruction. Annu Rev Physiol 45:453, 1983.

760. McFadden ER, Denison DM, Waller JF, et al: Direct recordings of the temperatures in the tracheobronchial tree in normal man. J Clin Invest 69:700, 1982.

761. Baile EM, Dahlby RW, Wiggs BR, et al: Role of tracheal and bronchial circulation in respiratory heat exchange. J Appl Physiol 58:217, 1985.

762. McFadden ER Jr: Respiratory heat and water exchange: Physiological and clinical implications. J Appl Physiol 54:331, 1983.

763. Deal EC, McFadden ER, Ingram RH Jr, et al: Esophageal temperature during exercise in asthmatic and nonasthmatic subjects. J Appl Physiol 46:484, 1979.

764. McFadden ER Jr, Pichurko BM, Bowman HF, et al: Thermal mapping of the airways in humans. J Appl Physiol 58:564, 1985.

765. McFadden ER, Ingram RJ Jr: Exercise-induced asthma: Observations on the initiating stimulus. N Engl J Med 301:763, 1979.

766. Anderson SD, Shoeffel RE, Follet R, et al: Sensitivity to heat and water loss at rest and during exercise in asthmatic patients. Eur J Respir Dis 63:459, 1982.

767. Shturman-Ellstein R, Zeballos RJ, Buckley JM, et al: The beneficial effect of nasal breathing on exercise-induced bronchoconstriction. Am Rev Respir Dis 118:65, 1978.

768. Griffin MP, McFadden ER, Ingram RH: Airway cooling in asthmatic and nonasthmatic subjects during nasal and oral breathing. J Allergy Clin Immunol 69:354, 1982.

769. Anderson SD: Is there a unifying hypothesis for exercise-induced asthma? J Allergy Clin Immunol 73(Suppl):660, 1984.

770. Hahn A, Anderson SD, Norton AR, et al: A reinterpretation of the effect of temperature and water content of the inspired air in exercise-induced asthma. Am Rev Respir Dis 130:575, 1985.

771. Sheppard D, Eschenbacher WL: Respiratory water loss as a stimulus to exercise-induced bronchoconstriction. J Allergy Clin Immunol 73(Suppl):640, 1984.

772. Eschenbacher W, Sheppard D: Respiratory heat loss is not the sole stimulus for bronchoconstriction induced by isocapnic hyperpnea with dry air. Am Rev Respir Dis 131:894, 1985.

773. Argyros GJ, Phillips YY, Rayburn DB, et al: Water loss without heat flux in exercise-induced bronchospasm. Am Rev Respir Dis 147:1419, 1993.

774. Schoeffel RE, Anderson SD, Altounyan REC: Bronchial hyperreactivity in response to inhalation of ultrasonically nebulized solutions of distilled water and saline. BMJ 283:1285, 1981.

775. Elwood RK, Hogg JC, Paré PD: Airway responses to osmolar challenge in asthma. Am Rev Respir Dis 125:61A, 1982.

776. Makker HK, Holgate ST: Relation of the hypertonic saline responsiveness of the airways to exercise-induced asthma symptom severity and to histamine or methacholine reactivity. Thorax 48:142, 1993.

777. Makker HK, Walls AF, Goulding D, et al: Airway effects with local challenge with hypertonic saline in exercise-induced asthma. Am J Respir Crit Care Med 149:1012, 1994.

778. Finney MJB, Anderson SD, Black JL: The effect of non-isotonic solutions on human isolated airway smooth muscle. Respir Physiol 69:277, 1987.

779. Deal EC, Wasserman SI, Soter NA, et al: Evaluation of role played by mediators of immediate hypersensitivity in exercise-induced asthma. J Clin Invest 65:659, 1980.

780. Lee TH, Nagakura T, Cromwell O, et al: Neutrophil chemotactic activity and histamine in atopic and nonatopic subjects after exercise-induced asthma. Am Rev Respir Dis 129:409, 1984.

781. Anderson SD, Bye PTP, Shoeffel RE, et al: Arterial plasma histamine levels at rest, and during and after exercise in patients with asthma—effects of terbutaline aerosol. Thorax 36:259, 1981.

782. Venge P, Henriksen J, Dahl R, Hakansson L: Exercise-induced asthma and the generation of neutrophil chemotactic activity. J Allergy Clin Immunol 85:498, 1990.

783. Lee TH, Brown MJ, Navy L, et al: Exercise-induced release of histamine and neutrophil chemotactic factor in atopic asthmatics. J Allergy Clin Immunol 70:73, 1982.

784. Lee TH, Nagakura T, Papageorgiou N, et al: Special problems—mediators in exercise-induced asthma. J Allergy Clin Immunol 73(Suppl):634, 1984.

785. Nagakura T, Lee TH, Assoufi BK, et al: Neutrophil chemotactic factor in exercise-induced and hyperventilation-induced asthma. Am Rev Respir Dis 128:294, 1983.

786. Nagy L: Serum neutrophil chemotactic activity and exercise-induced asthma. Eur J Respir Dis 64:161, 1983.

787. O'Byrne PM: Exercise-induced bronchoconstriction: Elucidating the roles of leukotrienes and prostaglandins. Pharmacotherapy 17:31S, 1997.

788. Finnerty JP, Twentyman OP, Harris A, et al: Effect of GR32191, a potent thromboxane receptor antagonist, on exercise-induced bronchoconstriction in asthma. Thorax 46:190, 1991.

789. Johnson CE, Belfield PW, Davis S, et al: Platelet activation during exercise-induced asthma: Effect of prophylaxis with cromoglycate and salbutamol. Thorax 41:290, 1986.

790. Findlay SR, Dvorak AM, Kagey-Sobotka A, et al: Hyperosmolar triggering of histamine release from human basophils. J Clin Invest 67:1604, 1981.

791. Flint KC, Hudspith BN, Leung KBP, et al: The hyperosmolar release of histamine from bronchoalveolar mast cells and its inhibition by sodium cromoglycate. Thorax 40:717, 1985.

792. Rimmer J, Bryant DH: Effect of hypo- and hyper-osmolarity on basophil histamine release. Clin Allergy 16:221, 1986.

793. Sheffer AL, Soter ER, McFadden ER, et al: Exercise-induced anaphylaxis—a distinct form of physical allergy. J Allergy Clin Immunol 71:311, 1983.

794. Sheffer AL, Tong AKF, Murphy GF, et al: Exercise-induced anaphylaxis—a serious form of physical allergy associated with mast cell degranulation. J Allergy Clin Immunol 75:479, 1985.

795. Moneret-Vautrin DA, Kanny G: Food-induced anaphylaxis. A new French multicenter study. Bull Acad Natl Med 179:161, 1995.

796. Wade JD, Liang MH, Sheffer AL: Exercise-induced anaphylaxis: Epidemiologic observations. Prog Clin Biol Res 297:175, 1989.

797. Caffarelli C, Cavagni G, Giordano S, et al: Reduced pulmonary function in multiple food-induced, exercise-related episodes of anaphylaxis. J Allergy Clin Immunol 98:762, 1996.

798. Kidd JM, Cohen SH, Sosman AJ, et al: Food-dependent exercise-induced anaphylaxis. J Allergy Clin Immunol 71:407, 1983.

799. Soter NA, Wasserman SI, Austen FK, et al: Release of mast-cell mediators and alterations in lung function in patients with cholinergic urticaria. N Engl J Med 302:604, 1980.

800. Kahn RC: Humidification of the airways: Adequate for function and integrity? Chest 84:510, 1983.

801. Jarjour NN, Calhoun WJ: Exercise-induced asthma is not associated with mast cell activation or airway inflammation. J Allergy Clin Immunol 89:60, 1992.

802. Broide DH, Eisman S, Ramsdell JW, et al: Airway levels of mast cell–derived mediators in exercise-induced asthma. Am Rev Respir Dis 141:563, 1990.

803. Crimi E, Balbo A, Milanese M, et al: Airway inflammation and occurrence of delayed bronchoconstriction in exercise-induced asthma. Am Rev Respir Dis 146:507, 1992.

804. Ahmed T, Garrigo J, Danta I: Preventing bronchoconstriction in exercise-induced asthma with inhaled heparin. N Engl J Med 329:90, 1993.

805. Fanta CH, McFadden ER Jr, Ingram RH Jr: Effects of cromolyn sodium on the response to respiratory heat loss in normal subjects. Am Rev Respir Dis 123:161, 1981.

806. Jones RM, Horn CR, Lee DV, et al: Bronchodilator effects of disodium cromoglycate in exercise-induced bronchoconstriction. Br J Dis Chest 77:362, 1983.

807. Breslin FJ, McFadden ER, Ingram RH Jr: The effects of cromolyn sodium on the airway responses to hyperpnea and cold air in asthma. Am Rev Respir Dis 122:11, 1980.

808. Makker HK, Lau LC, Thomson HW, et al: The protective effect of inhaled leukotriene D4 receptor antagonist ICI 204,219 against exercise-induced asthma. Am Rev Respir Dis 147:1413, 1993.

809. McNally JF Jr, Enright P, Hirsch JE, et al: The attenuation of exercise-induced bronchoconstriction by oropharyngeal anaesthesia. Am Rev Respir Dis 119:247, 1979.

810. Enright PL, McNally JF, Souhrada JF: Effect of lidocaine on the ventilatory and airway responses to exercise in asthmatics. Am Rev Respir Dis 122:823, 1980.

811. Fanta H, Ingram RH Jr, McFadden ER Jr: A reassessment of the effects of oropharyngeal anaesthesia in exercise-induced asthma. Am Rev Respir Dis 122:381, 1980.

812. Griffin MP, McFadden ER, Ingram RH, et al: Controlled analysis of the effects of inhaled lignocaine in exercise-induced asthma. Thorax 37:741, 1982.

813. de Gouw HW, Diamant Z, Kuijpers EA, et al: Role of neutral endopeptidase in exercise-induced bronchoconstriction in asthmatic subjects. J Appl Physiol 81:673, 1996.

814. Deal EC, McFadden ER Jr, Ingram RH, et al: Effects of atropine on potentiation of exercise-induced bronchospasm by cold air. J Appl Physiol 45:238, 1978.

815. Griffin MP, Fung KF, Ingram RH Jr, et al: Dose-response effects of atropine on thermal stimulus-response relationships in asthma. J Appl Physiol 53:1576, 1982.

816. O'Byrne PM, Thomson NC, Morris M, et al: The protective effect of inhaled chlorpheniramine and atropine on bronchoconstriction stimulated by airway cooling. Am Rev Respir Dis 128:611, 1983.

817. Makker HK, Holgate ST: The contribution of neurogenic reflexes to hypertonic saline–induced bronchoconstriction in asthma. J Allergy Clin Immunol 92:82, 1993.

818. Chen WY, Brenner AM, Weiser PC, et al: Atropine- and exercise-induced bronchoconstriction. Chest 79:651, 1981.

819. Sheppard D, Epstein J, Holtzman MJ, et al: Effect of route of atropine delivery on bronchospasm from cold air and methacholine. J Appl Physiol 54:130, 1983.

820. Wilson NM, Barnes PJ, Vickers H, et al: Hyperventilation-induced asthma: Evidence for two mechanisms. Thorax 37:657, 1982.

821. McFadden ER, Lenner KAM, Strohl KP: Post-exertion at airway rewarming and thermally induced asthma: New insights into pathophysiology and possible pathogenesis. J Clin Invest 78:18, 1986.

822. McFadden ER Jr: Hypothesis: Exercise-induced asthma as a vascular phenomenon. Lancet 335:880, 1990.

823. Tsai CL, Saidel GM, McFadden ER Jr, Fouke JM: Radial heat and water transport across the airway wall. J Appl Physiol 69:222, 1990.

824. Gilbert IA, McFadden ER Jr: Airway cooling and rewarming. The second reaction sequence in exercise-induced asthma. J Clin Invest 90:699, 1992.

825. Freed AN: Models and mechanisms of exercise-induced asthma. Eur Respir J 8:1770, 1995.

826. Edmunds AT, Tooley W, Godfrey S: The refractory period after exercise-induced asthma. Its duration and relation to the severity of exercise. Am Rev Respir Dis 117:247, 1978.

827. Rosenthal RR, Laube BL, Hood DB, Norman PS: Analysis of refractory period after exercise and eucapnic voluntary hyperventilation challenge. Am Rev Respir Dis 141:368, 1990.

828. Nowak D, Kuziek G, Jorres R, Magnussen H: Comparison of refractoriness after exercise- and hyperventilation-induced asthma. Lung 169:57, 1991.

829. Haas F, Levin N, Pasierski S, et al: Reduced hyperpnea-induced bronchospasm following repeated cold air challenge. J Appl Physiol 61:210, 1986.

830. Weiler-Ravell D, Godfrey S: Do exercise-induced and antigen-induced asthma utilize the same pathways? Antigen provocation in patients rendered refractory to exercise-induced asthma. J Allergy Clin Immunol 67:391, 1981.

831. Rosenthal RR, Laube B, Jaeger JJ: Methacholine sensitivity is unchanged during the refractory period following an exercise or isocapnic challenge. Am Rev Respir Dis 129:A250, 1984.

832. Hahn AG, Nogrady SG, Tumulty D, et al: Histamine reactivity during the refractory period after exercise-induced asthma. Thorax 39:919, 1984.

833. Belcher NG, Murdoch R, Dalton N, et al: Circulating concentrations of histamine, neutrophil chemotactic activity, and catecholamines during the refractory period in exercise-induced asthma. J Allergy Clin Immunol 81:100, 1988.

834. Anderson SD, Schoeffel RE: Respiratory heat and water loss during exercise in patients with asthma—effect of repeated exercise challenge. Eur J Respir Dis 63:472, 1982.

835. Ben-Dov I, Gur I, Bar-Yishay E, et al: Refractory period following induced asthma: Contributions of exercise and isocapnic hyperventilation. Thorax 38:849, 1983.

836. Satake T, Kato M, Takagi K, et al: Role of prostaglandins in exercise-induced asthma. Adv Physiol Sci 10:369, 1981.

837. O'Byrne PM, Jones GL: The effect of indomethacin on exercise-induced bronchoconstriction and refractoriness after exercise. Am Rev Respir Dis 134:69, 1986.

838. Manning PJ, Watson RM, O'Bryan PM: Exercise-induced refractoriness in asthmatic subjects involves leukotriene and prostaglandin interdependent mechanisms. Am Rev Respir Dis 148:950, 1993.

839. Pavord I, Lazarowicz H, Inchley D, et al: Cross refractoriness between sodium metabisulphite and exercise-induced asthma. Thorax 49:245, 1994.

840. Ben-Dov I, Bar-Yishay E, Godfrey S: Refractory period after exercise-induced asthma is unexplained by respiratory heat loss. Am Rev Respir Dis 125:530, 1982.

841. Bar-Yishay E, Godfrey S: Mechanisms of exercise-induced asthma. Lung 162:195, 1984.

842. Hahn A, Nogrady S, Burton G, et al: Absence of refractoriness in asthmatic subjects after exercise with warm, humid inspirate. Thorax 40:418, 1985.

843. Tam E, Geffroy B, Myers D, et al: Effect of eucapnic hypoxia on bronchomotor tone and on the bronchomotor response to dry air in asthmatic subjects. Am Rev Respir Dis 132:690, 1985.

844. Schiffman PL, Ryan A, Whipp BJ, et al: Hyperoxic attenuation of exercise-induced bronchospasm in asthmatics. J Clin Invest 63:30, 1979.

845. Resnick AD, Deal EC, Ingram RH, et al: A critical assessment of the mechanism by which hyperoxia attenuates exercise-induced asthma. J Clin Invest 64:541, 1979.

846. Bierman C, Spiro S, Petheram I: Characterization of the late response in exercise-induced asthma. J Allergy Clin Immunol 74:701, 1984.

847. Rubinstein I, Levison H, Slutsky AS, et al: Immediate and delayed bronchoconstriction after exercise in patients with asthma. N Engl J Med 317:482, 1987.

848. Varga EM, Eber E, Zach MS: Cold air challenge for measuring airway reactivity in children: Lack of a late asthmatic reaction. Lung 168:267, 1990.

849. Verhoeff NP, Speelberg B, van den Berg NJ, et al: Real and pseudo late asthmatic reactions after submaximal exercise challenge in patients with bronchial asthma. A new definition for late asthmatic responses after exercise challenge. Chest 98:1194, 1990.

850. Hofstra WB, Sterk PJ, Neijens HJ, et al: Occurrence of a late response to exercise in asthmatic children: Multiple regression approach using time-matched baseline and histamine control days. Eur Respir J 9:1348, 1996.

851. Iikura Y, Inui H, Nagakura T, et al: Factors predisposing to exercise-induced late asthmatic responses. J Allergy Clin Immunol 75:285, 1985.

852. Boulet LP, Legris C, Turcotte H: Prevalence and characteristics of late asthmatic responses to exercise in an adult population. J Allergy Clin Immunol 77:163A, 1986.

853. Boulet LP, Legris C, Turcotte H: Bronchial responsiveness to histamine after repeated exercise-induced bronchospasm. Respiration 52:237, 1987.

854. Boner AL, Sette L, Piacentini G, et al: Exercise-induced biphasic responses and methacholine reactivity in asthma. Ann Allergy 65:284, 1990.

855. Hall WJ, Hall CB: Alterations in pulmonary function following respiratory viral infection. Chest 76:458, 1979.

856. Hall WJ, Hall CB, Speers DM: Respiratory syncytial virus infection in adults. Clinical, virologic, and serial pulmonary function studies. Ann Intern Med 88:203, 1978.

857. O'Connor SA, Jones DP, Collinsa JV, et al: Changes in pulmonary function after naturally acquired respiratory infection in normal persons. Am Rev Respir Dis 120:1087, 1979.

858. Little JW, Hall WJ, Douglas RG Jr, et al: Airway hyperreactivity and peripheral airway dysfunction in influenza A infection. Am Rev Respir Dis 118:295, 1978.

859. Aquilina AT, Hall WJ, Douglas RG Jr, et al: Airway reactivity in subjects with viral upper respiratory tract infections: The effects of exercise and cold air. Am Rev Respir Dis 122:3, 1980.

860. Laitinen LA, Elkin RB, Empey DW, et al: Bronchial hyperresponsiveness in normal subjects during attenuated influenza virus infection. Am Rev Respir Dis 143:358, 1991.

861. Hafermann DR, Cissik JH, Byrd RB, et al: Effects of influenza vaccination on the peripheral airways of healthy human volunteers. Chest 75:468, 1979.

862. Banks J, Bevan C, Fennerty A, et al: Association between rise in antibodies and increase in airway sensitivity after intramuscular injection of killed influenza virus in asthmatic patients. Eur J Respir Dis 66:268, 1985.

863. DeJongste JC, Degenhart HJ, Neijens HJ, et al: Bronchial responsiveness and leucocyte reactivity after influenza vaccine in asthmatic patients. Eur J Respir Dis 65:196, 1984.

864. Jenkins CR, Breslin ABX: Upper respiratory tract infections and airway reactivity in normal and asthmatic subjects. Am Rev Respir Dis 130:879, 1984.

865. Sterk PJ: Virus-induced airway hyperresponsiveness in man. Eur Respir J 6:894, 1993.

866. Hegele RG, Hayashi S, Hogg JC, Paré PD: Mechanisms of airway narrowing and hyperresponsiveness in viral respiratory tract infections. Am J Respir Crit Care Med 151:1659, discussion 1664, 1995.

867. Pattemore PK, Johnston SL, Bardin PG: Viruses as precipitants of asthma symptoms. I. Epidemiology. Clin Exp Allergy 22:325, 1992.

868. Hudgel DW, Langston L, Selner JC, et al: Viral and bacterial infections in adults with chronic asthma. Am Rev Respir Dis 120:393, 1979.

869. Lambert HP, Stern H: Infective factors in exacerbations of bronchitis and asthma. BMJ 3:323, 1972.

870. Minor TE, Dick EC, DeMeo AN, et al: Viruses as precipitants of asthma attacks in children. JAMA 227:292, 1974.

871. Clarke CW: Relationship of bacterial and viral infections to exacerbations of asthma. Thorax 34:344, 1979.

872. Seggev JS, Lis I, Siman-Tov R, et al: *Mycoplasma pneumoniae* is a frequent cause of exacerbation of bronchial asthma in adults. Ann Allergy 57:263, 1986.

873. Bardin PG, Fraenkel DJ, Sanderson G, et al: Amplified rhinovirus colds in atopic subjects. Clin Exp Allergy 24:457, 1994.

874. Johnston SL, Pattemore PK, Sanderson G, et al: The relationship between upper respiratory infections and hospital admissions for asthma: A time-trend analysis. Am J Respir Crit Care Med 154:654, 1996.

875. Kava T: Effect of respiratory infections on exacerbation of asthma in adult patients. A six-month follow-up. Allergy 41:556, 1986.

876. Davies RJ, Holford-Strevens VC, Wells ID, et al: Bacterial precipitins and their immunoglobulin class in atopic asthma, non-atopic asthma, and chronic bronchitis. Thorax 31:419, 1976.

877. Bardin PG, Johnston SL, Pattemore PK: Viruses as precipitants of asthma symptoms. II. Physiology and mechanisms. Clin Exp Allergy 22:809, 1992.

878. Corne JM, Holgate ST: Mechanisms of virus-induced exacerbations of asthma. Thorax 52:380, 1997.

879. Johnston SL: Natural and experimental rhinovirus infections of the lower respiratory tract. Am J Respir Crit Care Med 152:S46, 1995.

880. Gern JE, Busse WW: The effects of rhinovirus infections on allergic airway responses. Am J Respir Crit Care Med 152:S40, 1995.

881. Martinez FD, Wright AL, Taussig LM, et al: Asthma and wheezing in the first six years of life. N Engl J Med 332:133, 1995.

882. Openshaw PJM, O'Donnell R: Asthma and the common cold: Can viruses imitate worms? Thorax 49:101, 1994.

883. Kolnaar BG, van Lier A, van den Bosch WJ, et al: Asthma in adolescents and young adults: Relationship with early childhood respiratory morbidity. Br J Gen Pract 44:73, 1994.

884. Korppi M, Reijonen T, Pysa L, Juntunen-Backman K: A 2- to 3-year outcome after bronchiolitis. Am J Dis Child 147:628, 1993.

885. Osundwa VM, Dawod ST, Ehlayel M: Recurrent wheezing in children with respiratory syncytial virus (RSV) bronchiolitis in Qatar. Eur J Pediatr 152: 1001, 1993.

886. Priftis D, Everard M, Milner AD: Outcome of severe acute bronchiolitis needing mechanical ventilation. Lancet 335:607, 1990.

887. Similä S, Linna O, Lanning P, et al: Chronic lung damage caused by adenovirus type 7: A 10 year follow-up study. Chest 80:127, 1981.

888. Wohl M, Chernick V: State of the art: Bronchiolitis. Am Rev Respir Dis 118:759, 1978.

889. Welliver RC: RSV and chronic asthma. Lancet 34:789, 1995.

890. Korppi M, Kuikka L, Reijonen T, et al: Bronchial asthma and hyperreactivity after early childhood bronchiolitis or pneumonia. Arch Pediatr Adolesc Med 148:1079, 1994.

891. Noble V, Murray M, Webb MS, et al: Respiratory status and allergy nine to 10 years after acute bronchiolitis. Arch Dis Child 76:315, 1997.

892. Pifferi M, Bertelloni C, Viegi G, et al: Airway response to a bronchodilator in healthy parents of infants with bronchiolitis. Chest 105:706, 1994.

893. Sigurs N, Bjarnason R, Sigurbergsson F, et al: Asthma and immunoglobulin E antibodies after respiratory syncytial virus bronchiolitis: A prospective cohort study with matched controls. Pediatrics 95:500, 1995.

894. Welliver RC, Duffy L: The relationship of RSV-specific immunoglobulin E antibody responses in infancy, recurrent wheezing and pulmonary function at age 7–8 years. Pediatr Pulmonol 15:19, 1993.

895. Dakhama A, Vitalis TZ, Hegele RG: Persistence of respiratory syncytial virus (RSV) infection and development of RSV-specific IgG1 response in a guinea-pig model of acute bronchiolitis. Eur Respir J 10:20, 1997.

896. Vitalis TZ, Keicho N, Itabashi S, et al: A model of latent adenovirus 5 infection in the guinea pig *(Cavia porcellus)*. Am J Respir Cell Mol Biol 14:225, 1997.

897. Stevenson DD, Mathison DA, Tan EM, et al: Provoking factors in bronchial asthma. Arch Intern Med 135:777, 1975.

898. Giraldo B, Blumenthal MN, Spink WW: Aspirin intolerance in asthma, a clinical and immunological study. Ann Intern Med 71:479, 1969.

899. Settipane GA, Chafee FH, Klein DK: Aspirin intolerance. 2. A prospective study of an atopic and normal population. J Allergy Clin Immunol 53:200, 1974.

900. Slepian IK, Mathews KP, McLean JA: Aspirin-sensitive asthma. Chest 87:386, 1985.

901. Ogino S, Harada T, Okawachi I, et al: Aspirin-induced asthma and nasal polyps. Acta Otolaryngol Suppl (Stockh) 430:21, 1986.

902. Grzelewska-Rzymowska I, Bogucki A, Szmidt M, et al: Migraine in aspirin-sensitive asthmatics. Allergol Immunopathol (Madr) 13:13, 1985.

903. Szczeklik A: Mechanism of aspirin-induced asthma. Allergy 52:613, 1997.

904. Weltman JK, Szaro RP, Settipane GA: An analysis of the role of IgE in intolerance to aspirin and tartrazine. Allergy 33:273, 1978.

905. Pleskow WW, Stevenson DD, Mathison DA, et al: Aspirin-sensitive rhinosinusitis/asthma—spectrum of adverse reactions to aspirin. J Allergy Clin Immunol 71:574, 1983.

906. Picado C, Castillo JA, Montserrat JM, Augusti-Vidal A: Aspirin-intolerance as a precipitating factor of life-threatening attacks of asthma requiring mechanical ventilation. Eur Respir J 2:127, 1989.

907. Marquette CH, Salnier F, Leroy O, et al: Long-term study prognosis for near-fatal asthma. Am Rev Respir Dis 146:76, 1992.

908. Parker CW: Aspirin-sensitive asthma. *In* Austen KF, Lichtenstein LM (eds): Asthma—Physiology, Immunopharmacology and Treatment. Vol II. New York, Academic Press, 1977, p 301.

909. Hollingsworth HM, Center DM: Neutrophil chemotactic factor (NCF) in aspirin-induced bronchospasm. Chest 87:167S, 1985.

910. Hollingsworth HM, Downing ET, et al: Identification and characterization of neutrophil chemotactic activity in aspirin-induced asthma. Am Rev Respir Dis 130:373, 1984.

911. Martelli NA, Usandivaras G: Inhibition of aspirin-induced bronchoconstriction by sodium cromoglycate inhalation. Thorax 32:684, 1977.

912. Martelli NA: Bronchial and intravenous provocation tests with indomethacin in aspirin-sensitive asthmatics. Am Rev Respir Dis 120:1073, 1979.

913. Herbert WG, Scopelitis E: Ketorolac-precipitated asthma. South Med J 87:282, 1994.

914. Craig T, Richerson HB, Moeckli J: Problem drugs for the patient with asthma. Compr Ther 22:339, 1996.

915. Settipane RA, Schrank PJ, Simon RA, et al: Prevalence of cross-sensitivity with acetaminophen in aspirin-sensitive asthmatic subjects. J Allergy Clin Immunol 96:480, 1995.

916. Park HS, Lim YS, Suh JE, et al: Sodium salicylate sensitivity in an asthmatic patient with aspirin sensitivity. J Korean Med Sci 6:113, 1991.

917. Bianco S, Robuschi M, Petrigni G, et al: Efficacy and tolerability of nimesulide in asthmatic patients intolerant to aspirin. Drugs 46(Suppl 1):115, 1993.

918. Lee TH: Mechanism of aspirin sensitivity. Am Rev Resour Dis 145:34, 1992.

919. Szczeklik A, Grylglewski RJ, Czerniawska-Mysik G: Relationship of inhibition of prostaglandin biosynthesis by analgesics to asthma attacks in aspirin-sensitive patients. BMJ 1:67, 1975.

920. Kumlin M, Dahlen B, Bjorck T, et al: Urinary excretion of leukotriene E4 and 11-dehydro-thromboxane B2 in response to bronchial provocations with allergen, aspirin, leukotriene D4, and histamine in asthmatics. Am Rev Respir Dis 146:96, 1992.

921. Sladek K, Dworski R, Soja J, et al: Eicosanoids in bronchoalveolar lavage fluid of aspirin-intolerant patients with asthma after aspirin challenge. Am J Respir Crit Care Med 149:940, 1994.

922. Dahlen B, Margolskee DJ, Zetterstrm O, Dahlen S-E: Effect of the leukotriene receptor antagonist MK-0679 on baseline pulmonary function in aspirin sensitive asthmatic subjects. Thorax 48:1205, 1993.

923. Yamamoto H, Nagata M, Kuramitsu K, et al: Inhibition of analgesic-induced asthma by leukotriene receptor antagonist ONO-1078. Am J Respir Crit Care Med 150:254, 1994.

924. Mullarkey MF, Thomas PS, Hansen JA, et al: Association of aspirin-sensitive asthma with HLA-DQw2. Am Rev Respir Dis 133:261, 1986.

925. Lympany PA, Welsh KI, Christie PE, et al: An analysis with sequence-specific oligonucleotide probes of the association between aspirin-induced asthma and antigens of the HLA system. J Allergy Clin Immunol 92:114, 1993.

926. Perichon B, Krishnamoorthy R: Asthma and HLA system. Allerg Immunol (Paris) 23:301, 1991.

927. Dekker JW, Nizankowska E, Schmitz-Schumann M, et al: Aspirin-induced asthma and HLA-DRB1 and HLA-DPB1 genotypes. Clin Exp Allergy 27:574, 1997.

928. Dajani BM, Sliman NA, Shubair KS, et al: Bronchospasm caused by intravenous hydrocortisone sodium succinate (Solu-Cortef) in aspirin-sensitive patients. J Allergy Clin Immunol 68:201, 1981.

929. Szczeklik A, Nizankowska E, Czerniawska-Mysik G, et al: Hydrocortisone and airflow impairment in aspirin-induced asthma. J Allergy Clin Immunol 76:530, 1985.

930. Feigenbaum BA, Stevenson DD, Simon RA: Hydrocortisone sodium succinate does not cross-react with aspirin in aspirin-sensitive patients with asthma. J Allergy Clin Immunol 96:545, 1995.

931. Imokawa S, Sato A, Taniguchi M, et al: Lipoxygenase inhibitor–provoked acute asthma in a patient with asthma relieved by aspirin. Ann Allergy Asthma Immunol 75:112, 1995.

932. Ayres JG, Miles JF: Oesophageal reflux and asthma. Eur Respir J 9:107, 1996.

933. Harding SM, Richeter JE: Gastroesophageal reflux disease and asthma. Semin Gastrointestinal Dis 3:139, 1992.

934. Sontag SJ, Schnell TG, Miller TQ, et al: Prevalence of esophagitis in asthmatics. Gut 33:872, 1992.

935. Allen CJ, Newhouse MT: Gastroesophageal reflux and chronic respiratory disease. Am Rev Respir Dis 129:645, 1984.

936. Boyle JT, Tuchman DN, Altschuler SM, et al: Mechanisms for the association of gastroesophageal reflux and bronchospasm. Am Rev Respir Dis 131:S16, 1985.

937. Ducoloné A, Vandevenne A, Jouin H, et al: Gastroesophageal reflux in patients with asthma and chronic bronchitis. Am Rev Respir Dis 135:327, 1987.

938. Jack CIA, Calverley PMA, Donelly RJ, et al: Simultaneous tracheal and oesophageal pH measurements in asthmatic patients with gastro-oesophageal reflux. Thorax 50:201, 1995.

939. Perpiña M, Ponce J, Marco V, et al: The prevalence of asymptomatic gastroesophageal reflux in bronchial asthma and in non-asthmatic individuals. Eur J Respir Dis 64:582, 1983.

940. Ekström T, Tibbling L: Gastro-oesophageal reflux and triggering of bronchial asthma: A negative report. Eur J Respir Dis 71:177, 1987.

941. Spaulding HS, Mansfield LE, Stein MR, et al: Further investigation of the association between gastroesophageal reflux and bronchoconstriction. J Allergy Clin Immunol 69:516, 1982.

942. Davis RS, Larsen GL, Grunstein MM: Respiratory response to intraesophageal acid infusion in asthmatic children during sleep. J Allergy Clin Immunol 72:393, 1983.

943. Andersen LI, Schmidt A, Bundgaard A: Pulmonary function and acid application in the esophagus. Chest 90:358, 1986.

944. Perpiña M, Pellicer C, Marco V, et al: The significance of the reflex bronchoconstriction provoked by gastroesophageal reflux in bronchial asthma. Eur J Respir Dis 66:91, 1985.

945. Wright RA, Millar SA, Corsello BF: Acid-induced esophago-bronchial-cardiac reflexes in humans. Gastroenterology 99:71, 1990.

946. Schan CA, Harding SM, Haile JM, et al: Gastroesophageal reflux–induced bronchoconstriction. An intraesophageal acid infusion study using state-of-the-art technology. Chest 106:731, 1994.

947. Nelson HS: Gastroesophageal reflux and pulmonary disease. J Allergy Clin Immunol 73:547, 1984.

948. Tan WC, Martin RJ, Pandey R, Ballard RD: Effects of spontaneous and simulated gastroesophageal reflux on sleeping asthmatics. Am Rev Respir Dis 141:1394, 1990.

949. Herve P, Denjean A, Jian R, et al: Intraesophageal perfusion of acid increases the bronchomotor response to methacholine and to isocapnic hyperventilation in asthmatic subjects. Am Rev Respir Dis 134:986, 1986.

950. Goodall RJR, Earis JE, Cooper DN, et al: Relationship between asthma and gastro-oesophageal reflux. Thorax 36:116, 1981.

951. Simpson WG: Gastroesophageal reflux disease and asthma. Diagnosis and management. Arch Intern Med 155:798, 1995.

951a. Sontag S, O'Connell S, Greenlee H, et al: Is gastroesophageal reflux a factor in some asthmatics? Am J Gastroenterol 82:119, 1987.

952. Miles JF, Noble K, Mathews HR, et al: Gastroesophageal reflux in patients with brittle asthma. Thorax 48:1055, 1993.

953. Moote W, Lloyd DA, McCourtie DR: Increase in gastroesophageal reflux during methacholine-induced bronchospasm. J Allergy Clin Immunol 78:619, 1986.

954. Spector S, Luparello TJ, Kopetzky MT, et al: Response of asthmatics to methacholine and suggestion. Am Rev Respir Dis 113:43, 1976.

955. Wright GLT: Asthma and the emotions: Aetiology and treatment. Med J Aust 1:961, 1965.

956. Horton DJ, Suda WL, Kinsman RA, et al: Bronchoconstrictive suggestion in asthma: A role for airways hyperreactivity and emotions. Am Rev Respir Dis 117:1029, 1978.

957. Lewis RA, Lewis MN, Tattersfield AE: Asthma induced by suggestion—is it due to airway cooling? Am Rev Respir Dis 129:691, 1984.

958. Demeter SL, Cordasco EM: Hyperventilation syndrome and asthma. Am J Med 81:989, 1986.

959. Busse WW, Kiecolt-Glaser JK, Coe C, et al: NHLBI Workshop summary. Stress and asthma. Am J Respir Crit Care Med 151:249, 1995.

960. Ostro BD, Lipsett MJ, Mann JK, et al: Indoor air pollution and asthma. Am J Respir Crit Care Med 149:1400, 1994.

961. Bates DV: The effects of air pollution on children. Environ Health Perspect 103:49, 1995.

961a. Bates DV, Sizto R: A study of hospital admissions and air pollutants in Southern Ontario. In Lee SD, Schneider T, Grant LD, et al (eds): Aerosols. Chelsea, MI, Lewis Publishers, 1986.

962. Ussetti P, Roca J, Agusti AGN, et al: Another asthma outbreak in Barcelona. Role of oxides of nitrogen. Lancet 1:156, 1984.

962a. Chapman RS, Calafiore DC, Hasselblad V: Prevalence of persistent cough and phlegm in young adults in relation to long-term ambient sulfur oxide exposure. Am Rev Respir Dis 132:261, 1985.

963. Avol E, Linn W, Shamoo D, et al: Respiratory effects of photochemical oxidant air pollution in exercising adolescents. Am Rev Respir Dis 132:619, 1985.

964. Hazucha MJ, Ginsberg JF, McDonnell WF, et al: Effects of 0.1 ppm nitrogen dioxide on airways of normal and asthmatic subjects. J Appl Physiol 54:730, 1983.

965. Schoettlin CE, Landau E: Air pollution and asthmatic attacks in the Los Angeles area. Public Health Rep 76:545, 1961.

966. Lewis R, Gilkeson M, McCaldin RO: Air pollution and New Orleans asthma. Public Health Rep 77:947, 1962.

967. Weill H, Ziskind MM, Derbes V, et al: Further observations on New Orleans asthma. Arch Environ Health 8:184, 1964.

968. Weill H, Ziskind MM, Dickerson RC, et al: Epidemic asthma in New Orleans. JAMA 190:811, 1964.

969. Smith RBW, Kolb EJ, Phelps HW, et al: Tokyo-Yokohama asthma. An area specific air pollution disease. Arch Environ Health 8:805, 1964.

970. Phelps HW, Koike S: Tokyo-Yokohama asthma. The rapid development of respiratory distress presumably due to air pollution. Am Rev Respir Dis 86:55, 1962.

971. Bates DV: Observations on asthma. Environ Health Perspect 103:243, 1995.

972. Bates DV, Baker-Anderson M, Sizto R: Asthma attack periodicity: A study of hospital emergency visits in Vancouver. Environ Res 51:51, 1990.

973. Hill DJ, Smart IJ, Knox RB: Childhood asthma and grass pollen aerobiology in Melbourne. Med J Aust 1:426, 1979.

974. Barnes PJ: Air pollution and asthma. Postgrad Med J 70:319, 1994.

975. Newman-Taylor A: Environmental determinants of asthma. Lancet 345:296, 1995.

976. Peden DB: Mechanisms of pollution-induced airway disease: In vivo studies. Allergy 52:37, 1997.

977. Casillas AM, Nel AE: An update on the immunopathogenesis of asthma as an inflammatory disease enhanced by environmental pollutants. Allergy Asthma Proc 18:227, 1997.

978. Molfino NA, Wright SC, Katz I, et al: Effect of low concentrations of ozone on inhaled allergen responses in asthmatic subjects. Lancet 338:199, 1991.

979. Koenig JQ, Pierson WE, Horike M, et al: Bronchoconstrictor responses to sulfur dioxide or sulfur dioxide plus sodium chloride droplets in allergic, nonasthmatic adolescents. J Allergy Clin Immunol 69:339, 1982.

980. Jaeger MJ, Tribble D, Wittig HJ: Effect of 0.5 ppm sulfur dioxide on the respiratory function of normal and asthmatic subjects. Lung 156:119, 1979.

981. Folinsbee LJ, Bedi JF, Horvath SM: Pulmonary response to threshold levels of sulfur dioxide (1.0 ppm) and ozone (0.3 ppm). J Appl Physiol 58:1783, 1985.

982. Snashall PD, Baldwin C: Mechanisms of sulphur dioxide–induced bronchoconstriction in normal and asthmatic man. Thorax 37:118, 1982.

983. Sheppard D, Saisho AK, Nadel JA, et al: Exercise increases sulfur dioxide–induced bronchoconstriction in asthmatic subjects. Am Rev Respir Dis 123:486, 1981.

984. Bethel RA, Epstein J, Sheppard D, et al: Sulfur dioxide–induced bronchoconstriction in freely breathing, exercising, asthmatic subjects. Am Rev Respir Dis 128:987, 1983.

985. Sheppard D, Wong WS, Uehara CF, et al: Lower threshold and greater bronchomotor responsiveness of asthmatic subjects to sulfur dioxide. Am Rev Respir Dis 122:873, 1980.

986. Roger LJ, Kehrl HR, Hazucha M, et al: Bronchoconstriction in asthmatics exposed to sulfur dioxide during repeated exercise. J Appl Physiol 59:784, 1985.

987. Linn WS, Venet TG, Shamoo DA, et al: Respiratory effects of sulfur dioxide in heavily exercising asthmatics—a dose-response study. Am Rev Respir Dis 127:278, 1983.

988. Kehrl HR, Roger LJ, Hazucha MJ, et al: Differing response of asthmatics to sulfur dioxide exposure with continuous and intermittent exercise. Am Rev Respir Dis 135:350, 1987.

989. Sheppard D, Nadel JA, Boushey HA: Effect of the oronasal breathing route on sulfur dioxide–induced bronchoconstriction in exercising asthmatic subjects. Am Rev Respir Dis 125:627, 1982.

990. Bethel RA, Erle DJ, Epstein J, et al: Effect of exercise rate and route of inhalation on sulfur dioxide–induced bronchoconstriction in asthmatic subjects. Am Rev Respir Dis 128:592, 1983.

991. Magnussen H, Jorres R, Wagner HM, von Nieding G: Relationship between the airway response to inhaled sulfur dioxide, isocapnic hyperventilation, and histamine in asthmatic subjects. Int Arch Occup Environ Health 62:485, 1990.

992. Sheppard D, Eschenbacher WL, Boushey HA, et al: Magnitude of the interaction between the bronchomotor effects of sulfur dioxide and those of dry (cold) air. Am Rev Respir Dis 130:52, 1984.

993. Bethel RA, Sheppard D, Epstein J, et al: Interaction of sulphur dioxide and dry cold air causing bronchoconstriction in asthmatic subjects. J Appl Physiol 57:419, 1984.

994. Linn WS, Shamoo DA, Anderson KR, et al: Effects of heat and humidity on the responses of exercising asthmatics to sulfur dioxide exposure. Am Rev Respir Dis 131:221, 1985.

995. Kulle TJ, Sauder LR, Hebel JR, et al: Ozone response relationships in healthy nonsmokers. Am Rev Respir Dis 132:36, 1985.

996. Linn WS, Buckley RD, Spier CE, et al: Health effects of ozone exposure in asthmatics. Am Rev Respir Dis 117:835, 1978.

997. Lauritzen SK, Adams WC: Ozone inhalation effects consequent to continuous exercise in females: Comparison to males. J Appl Physiol 59:1601, 1985.

998. McDonnell W, Chapman R, Leigh M, et al: Respiratory responses of vigorously

exercising children to 0.12 ppm ozone exposure. Am Rev Respir Dis 132:875, 1985.

999. Hackney JD, Linn WS, Mohler JG, et al: Experimental studies on human health effects of air pollutants. II. Four-hour exposure to ozone alone and in combinations with other pollutant gases. Arch Environ Health 30:379, 1975.

1000. Bates DV, Ball GM, Burnham CD, et al: Short-term effects of ozone on the lung. J Appl Physiol 32:176, 1972.

1001. Hazucha M, Silverman F, Parent C, et al: Pulmonary function in a man after short-term exposure to ozone. Arch Environ Health 27:183, 1973.

1002. Hackney JD, Linn WS, Law DC, et al: Experimental studies on human health effects of air pollutants. III. Two-hour exposure to ozone and in combination with other pollutant gases. Arch Environ Health 30:385, 1975.

1003. Hackney JD, Linn WS, Buckley RD, et al: Scientific communications. Experimental studies on human health effects of air pollutants. I. Design considerations. Arch Environ Health 30:373, 1975.

1004. Kerr HD, Kulle TJ, McIlhany ML, et al: Effects of ozone on pulmonary function in normal subjects. An environmental-chamber study. Am Rev Respir Dis 111:763, 1975.

1005. Kagawa J, Toyama T: Effects of ozone and brief exercise on specific airway conductance in man. Arch Environ Health 30:36, 1975.

1006. Golden JA, Nadel JA, Boushey HA: Bronchial hyperirritability in healthy subjects after exposure to ozone. Am Rev Respir Dis 118:287, 1978.

1007. Holtzman MJ, Cunningham JH, Sheller JR, et al: Effect of ozone on bronchial reactivity in atopic and nonatopic subjects. Am Rev Respir Dis 120:1059, 1979.

1008. Holtzman MJ, Fabbri LM, O'Byrne PM, et al: Importance of airway inflammation for hyperresponsiveness induced by ozone. Am Rev Respir Dis 127:686, 1983.

1009. O'Byrne PM, Walters EH, Gold BD, et al: Neutrophil depletion inhibits airway hyperresponsiveness induced by ozone exposure. Am Rev Respir Dis 130:214, 1984.

1010. O'Byrne PM, Walters EH, Alzawa H, et al: Indomethacin inhibits the airway hyperresponsiveness but not the neutrophil influx induced by ozone in dogs. Am Rev Respir Dis 130:220, 1984.

1011. Fabbri LM, Aizawa H, Alpert SE, et al: Airway hyperresponsiveness and changes in cell counts in bronchoalveolar lavage after ozone exposure in dogs. Am Rev Respir Dis 129:288, 1984.

1012. McBride DE, Koenig JQ, Luchtel DL, et al: Inflammatory effects of ozone in the upper airways of subjects with asthma. Am J Respir Crit Care Med 149:1192, 1994.

1013. Forastiere F, Corbo GM, Pistelli R, et al: Bronchial responsiveness in children living in areas with different air pollution levels. Arch Environ Health 49:111, 1994.

1014. Bauer MA, Utell MJ, Morrow PE, et al: Inhalation of 0.30 ppm nitrogen dioxide potentiates exercise-induced bronchospasm in asthmatics. Am Rev Respir Dis 134:1203, 1986.

1015. Bylin G, Lindvall T, Rehn T, et al: Effects of short-term exposure to ambient nitrogen dioxide concentrations on human bronchial reactivity and lung function. Eur J Respir Dis 66:205, 1985.

1016. Parham WM, Shepard RH, Norman PS, et al: Analysis of time course and magnitude of lung inflation effects on airway tone—relation to airway reactivity. Am Rev Respir Dis 128:240, 1983.

1017. Berry RB, Pai UP, Fairshter RD: Effect of age on changes in flow rates and airway conductance after a deep breath. J Appl Physiol 68:635, 1990.

1018. Orehek J, Charpin D, Velardocchio JM, et al: Bronchomotor effect of bronchoconstriction-induced deep inspirations in asthmatics. Am Rev Respir Dis 121:297, 1980.

1019. Fish JE, Kehoe TJ, Cugell DW: Effect of deep inspiration on maximum expiratory flow rates in asthmatic subjects. Respiration 36:57, 1978.

1020. Zamel N, Hughes D, Levison H, et al: Partial and complete maximum expiratory flow-volume curves in asthmatic patients with spontaneous bronchospasm. Chest 83:35, 1983.

1021. Pliss LB, Ingenito EP, Ingram RH Jr: Responsiveness, inflammation, and effects of deep breaths on obstruction in mild asthma. J Appl Physiol 66:2298, 1989.

1022. Lim TK, Ang SM, Rossing TH, et al: The effects of deep inhalation on maximal expiratory flow during intensive treatment of spontaneous asthmatic episodes. Am Rev Respir Dis 140:340, 1989.

1023. Beaupré A, Badier M, Delpierre S, et al: Airways response of asthmatics to carbachol and to deep inspiration. Eur J Respir Dis 64:108, 1983.

1024. Brusasco V, Rocchi D: Effects of volume history and time dependence of flow-volume curves on assessment of bronchial response to inhaled methacholine in normals. Respiration 41:106, 1981.

1025. Beaupré A, Orehek J: Factors influencing the bronchodilator effect of a deep inspiration in asthmatic patients with provoked bronchoconstriction. Thorax 37:124, 1982.

1026. Hida W, Arai M, Shindoh C, et al: Effect of inspiratory flow rate on bronchomotor tone in normal and asthmatic subjects. Thorax 39:86, 1984.

1027. Day A, Zamel N: Failure of cholinergic blockade to prevent bronchodilatation following deep inspiration. J Appl Physiol 58:1449, 1985.

1028. Burns CB, Taylor WR, Ingram RH Jr: Effects of deep inhalation in asthma: Relative airway and parenchymal hysteresis. J Appl Physiol 59:1590, 1985.

1029. Mitchell RW, Rabe KF, Magnussen H, Leff AR: Passive sensitization of human airways induces myogenic contractile responses in vitro. J Appl Physiol 83:1276, 1997.

1030. Genton C, Frei PC, Pécoud A: Value of oral provocation tests to aspirin and food additives in the routine investigation of asthma and chronic urticaria. J Allergy Clin Immunol 76:40, 1985.

1031. Bush RK, Taylor SL, Holden K, et al: Prevalence of sensitivity to sulfiting agents in asthmatic patients. Am J Med 81:816, 1986.

1032. Stevenson DD, Simon RA: Sensitivity to ingested metabisulfites in asthmatic subjects. J Allergy Clin Immunol 68:26, 1981.

1033. Dahl R, Henriksen JM, Harving H: Red wine asthma: A controlled challenge study. J Allergy Clin Immunol 78:1126, 1986.

1034. Koepke JW, Christopher KL, Chai H, et al: Dose-dependent bronchospasm from sulfites in isoetharine. JAMA 251:2982, 1984.

1035. Allen DH, Delohery J, Baker G: Monosodium L-glutamate–induced asthma. J Allergy Clin Immunol 80:530, 1987.

1036. Ayres JG, Clark TJH: Alcoholic drinks and asthma—a survey. Br J Dis Chest 77:370, 1983.

1037. Shimoda T, Kohno S, Takao A, et al: Investigation of the mechanism of alcohol-induced bronchial asthma. J Allergy Clin Immunol 97:74, 1996.

1038. Gong H, Tashkin DP, Calvarese BM: Alcohol-induced bronchospasm in an asthmatic patient—pharmacologic evaluation of the mechanism. Chest 80:167, 1981.

1039. Geppert EF, Boushey HA: An investigation of the mechanism of ethanol-induced bronchoconstriction. Am Rev Respir Dis 118:135, 1978.

1040. Wantke F, Gotz M, Jarisch R: The red wine provocation tests: Intolerance to histamine as a model for food intolerance. Allergy Proc 15:27, 1994.

1041. Kaufman J, Schmitt S, Barnard J, et al: Angiotensin-converting enzyme inhibitors in patients with bronchial responsiveness and asthma. Chest 101:922, 1992.

1042. Lunde H, Hedner T, Samuelsson O, et al: Dyspnoea, asthma, and bronchospasm in relation to treatment with angiotensin-converting enzyme inhibitor. BMJ 308:18, 1994.

1043. Lang DM, Alpern MB, Visintainer PF, et al: Elevated risk of anaphylactoid reaction from radiographic contrast media is associated with both beta-blocker exposure and cardiovascular disorders. Arch Intern Med 153:2033, 1993.

1044. Louie S, Krzanowski JJ Jr, Bukantz SC, et al: Effects of ergometrine on airway smooth muscle contractile responses. Clin Allergy 15:173, 1985.

1045. Shim C, Williams MH Jr: Effect of odors in asthma. Am J Med 80:18, 1986.

1046. Millqvist E, Lowhagen O: Placebo-controlled challenges with perfume in patients with asthma-like symptoms. Allergy 51:434, 1996.

1047. Kumar P, Caradonna-Graham VM, Gupta S, et al: Inhalation challenge effects of perfume scent strips in patients with asthma. Ann Allergy Asthma Immunol 75:429, 1995.

1048. Dahms TE, Bolin JF, Slavin RG: Passive smoking—effects on bronchial asthma. Chest 80:530, 1981.

1049. Murray AB, Harrison BJ: The effect of cigarette smoke from the mother on bronchial responsiveness and severity of symptoms in children with asthma. J Allergy Clin Immunol 77:575, 1986.

1050. Higenbottam TW, Feyeraband C, Clark TJH: Cigarette smoking in asthma. Br J Dis Chest 74:279, 1980.

1051. Gibbs C, Coutts II, Lock R, et al: Premenstrual exacerbation of asthma. Thorax 39:833, 1984.

1052. Hanley SP: Asthma variation with menstruation. Br J Dis Chest 75:306, 1981.

1053. Eliasson O, Scherzer HH, DeGraff AC Jr: Morbidity in asthma in relation to the menstrual cycle. J Allergy Clin Immunol 77:87, 1986.

1054. Chandler MH, Schuldheisz S, Phillips BA, Muse KN: Premenstrual asthma: The effect of estrogen on symptoms, pulmonary function, and beta-2 receptors. Pharmacotherapy 17:224, 1997.

1055. Beynon HL, Garbett ND, Barnes PJ: Severe premenstrual exacerbations of asthma: Effect of intramuscular progesterone. Lancet 2:370, 1988.

1056. Kraft M, Maritin RJ: Nocturnal asthma. In Barnes PJ, Grunstein MM, Leff AR, Woolcock AJ (eds): Asthma. Vol 2. Philadelphia, Lippincott-Raven, 1997, pp 2005–2024.

1057. Packe GE, Ayres JG: Asthma outbreak during a thunderstorm. Lancet 2:199, 1985.

1058. Venables KM, Chan-Yeung M: Occupational asthma. Lancet 349:1465, 1997.

1059. Chan-Yeung M, Malo J-L: Aetiological agents in occupational asthma. Eur Respir J 7:346, 1994.

1060. Newman LS: Occupational asthma. Diagnosis, management and prevention. Clin Chest Med 16:621, 1995.

1061. Bernstein DI: Allergic reactions to workplace allergens. JAMA 278:1907, 1997.

1062. de la Hoz RE, Young RO, Pedersen DH: Exposure to potential occupational asthmogens: Prevalence data from the National Occupational Exposure Survey. Am J Ind Med 31:195, 1997.

1063. Lagier F, Cartier A, Malo JL: Statistiques medico-legales sur l'asthme professionel au Quebec de 1986 a 1988: Medico-legal statistics on occupational asthma in Quebec between 1986 and 1988. Rev Mal Respir 7:337, 1990.

1064. Meredith SK, Taylor VM, McDonald JC: Occupational respiratory disease in the United Kingdom 1989. A report to the British Thoracic Society and the Society of Occupational Medicine by the SWORD project group. Br J Ind Med 48:292, 1991.

1065. Contreras G, Rousseau R, Chan-Yeung M: Short-report: occupational respiratory diseases in British Columbia. Occup Environ Med 51:710, 1994.

1066. Musk AW, Venables KM, Crook B, et al: Respiratory symptoms, lung function and sensitisation to flour in a British bakery. Br J Ind Med 46:636, 1989.

1067. Juniper CP, How MJ, Goodwin BFG, Kinshott AK: Bacillus subtilis enzymes: A seven (7)-year clinical, epidemiological and immunological study of an industrial allergen. J Soc Occup Med 27:3, 1977.

1068. Chan-Yeung M: Occupational asthma. Chest 98:124S, 1994.

1069. McSharry C, Anderson K, McKay IC, et al: The IgE and IgG antibody responses to aerosols of Nephrops norvegicus (prawn) antigens: The association with clinical hypersensitivity and with cigarette smoking. Clin Exp Immunol 97:499, 1994.

1070. Venables KM, Dally MB, Nunn AJ, et al: Smoking and occupational allergy in workers in a platinum refinery. BMJ 299:939, 1989.

1071. Cartier A, Malo JL, Forest F, et al: Occupational asthma in snow crab–processing workers. J Allergy Clin Immunol 74:261, 1984.

1072. Thiel H, Ulmer WNT: Baker's asthma: Development and possibility of treatment. Chest 78:S400, 1980.

1073. Mitchell CA, Gandevia B: Respiratory symptoms and skin test sensitivity in works exposed to proteolytic enzyme in detergent industry. Am Rev Respir Dis 104:1, 1971.

1074. Franz T, McMurran KD, Brooks S, et al: Clinical immunologic and physiologic observations in factory workers exposed to *B. subtilis* enzyme dust. J Allergy 42:170, 1971.

1075. Anto JM, Sunyer J, Newman Taylor AJ: Comparison of soybean epidemic asthma and occupational asthma. Thorax 51:743, 1996.

1076. Agrup G, Belin L, Sjöstedt L, et al: Allergy to laboratory animals in laboratory technicians and animal keepers. Br J Ind Med 43:192, 1986.

1077. Low B, Sjostedt L, Willers L: Laboratory animal allergy: Possible association with HLA B15 and DR4. Tissue Antigens 31:224, 1988.

1078. Malo JL, Cartier A: Occupational reactions in the seafood industry. Clin Rev Allergy 11:223, 1993.

1079. Siracusa A, Bettini P, Bacoccoli R, et al: Asthma caused by live fish bait. J Allergy Clin Immunol 93:424, 1994.

1080. Belin L: Hyperreactivity in clinical practice—induction by occupational factors. Eur J Respir Dis 64(Suppl 131):285, 1983.

1081. Broder I, Mintz S, Hutcheon M: Comparison of respiratory variables in grain elevator workers and civic outside workers of Thunder Bay, Canada. Am Rev Respir Dis 119:193, 1979.

1082. Mink JT, Gerrard JW, Cockcroft DW, et al: Increased bronchial reactivity to inhaled histamine in nonsmoking grain workers with normal lung function. Chest 77:28, 1980.

1083. Cookson WO, Ryan G, MacDonald S, et al: Atopy, non-allergic bronchial reactivity, and past history as determinants of work related symptoms in seasonal grain handlers. Br J Ind Med 43:396, 1986.

1084. Chan-Yeung M, Wong R, Maclean L: Respiratory abnormalities among grain elevator workers. Chest 75:461, 1979.

1085. Lezaun A, Igea JM, Quirce S, et al: Asthma and contact urticaria caused by rice in a housewife. Allergy 49:92, 1994.

1086. Savonius B, Kanerva L: Anaphylaxis caused by banana. Allergy 48:215, 1993.

1087. Hunt LW, Fransway AF, Reed CE, et al: An epidemic of occupational allergy to latex involving health care workers. J Occup Environ Med 37:1204, 1995.

1088. Pisati G, Baruffini A, Bernabeo F, Stanizzi R: Bronchial provocation testing in the diagnosis of occupational asthma due to latex surgical gloves. Europ Respir J 7:332, 1994.

1089. Vandenplas O: Occupational asthma caused by natural rubber latex. Eur Respir J 8:1957, 1995.

1090. Tarlo SM, Wong L, Roos J, Booth N: Occupational asthma caused by latex in a surgical glove manufacturing plant. J Allergy Clin Immunol 85:626, 1990.

1091. Santos R, Hernandez-Ayup S, Galache P, et al: Severe latex allergy after a vaginal examination during labor: A case report. Am J Obstet Gynecol 177:1543, 1997.

1092. Lebenbom-Mansour MH, Oesterle JR, Ownby DR, et al: The incidence of latex sensitivity in ambulatory surgical patients: A correlation of historical factors with positive serum immunoglobin E levels. Anesth Analg 85:44, 1997.

1093. Woods JA, Lambert S, Platts-Mills TA, et al: Natural rubber latex allergy: Spectrum, diagnostic approach, and therapy. J Emerg Med 15:71, 1997.

1094. Ho A, Chan H, Tse KS, Chan-Yeung M: Occupational asthma due to latex in health care workers. Thorax 51:1280, 1996.

1095. Liss GM, Sussman GL, Deal K, et al: Latex allergy: Epidemiological study of 1351 hospital workers. Occup Environ Med 54:335, 1997.

1096. Nieto A, Estornell F, Mazon A, et al: Allergy to latex in spina bifida: A multivariate study of associated factors in 100 consecutive patients. J Allergy Clin Immunol 98:501, 1996.

1097. Lundberg M, Wrangsjo K, Johansson SG: Latex allergy from glove powder—an unintended risk with the switch from talc to cornstarch? Allergy 52:1222, 1997.

1098. Ownby DR, Ownby HE, McCullough J, Shafer AW: The prevalence of anti–latex IgE antibodies in 1000 volunteer blood donors. J Allergy Clin Immunol 97:1188, 1996.

1099. Miguel AG, Cass GR, Weiss J, Glovsky MM: Latex allergens in tire dust and airborne particles. Environ Health Perspect 104:1180, 1996.

1100. Williams PB, Buhr MP, Weber RW, et al: Latex allergen in respirable particulate air pollution. J Allergy Clin Immunol 95:88, 1995.

1101. Caruso B, Caputo M, Senna G, Andri L: Immunoblotting study of specific antibody patterns against latex and banana. Allergie et Immunol (Paris) 25:187, 1993.

1102. Freeman GL: Cooccurrence of latex and fruit allergies. Allergy Asthma Proc 18:85, 1997.

1103. Weiss SJ, Halsey JF: A nurse with anaphylaxis to stone fruits and latex sensitivity: Potential diagnostic difficulties to consider. Ann Allergy Asthma Immunol 77:504, 1996.

1104. Diez-Gomez ML, Quirce S, Aragoneses E, Cuevas M: Asthma caused by *Ficus benjamina* latex: Evidence of cross-reactivity with fig fruit and papain. Ann Allergy Asthma Immunol 80:24, 1998.

1105. Fuchs T, Spitzauer S, Vente C, et al: Natural latex, grass pollen, and weed pollen share IgE epitopes. J Allergy Clin Immunol 100:356, 1997.

1106. Ebo DG, Stevens WJ, Bridts CH, De Clerck LS: Latex-specific IgE, skin testing, and lymphocyte transformation to latex in latex allergy. J Allergy Clin Immunol 100:618, 1997.

1107. Crippa M, Pasolini G: Allergic reactions due to glove-lubricant powder in health-care workers. Int Arch Occup Environ Health 70:399, 1997.

1108. Seggev JS, Mawhinney TP, Yunginger JW, Braun SR: Anaphylaxis due to cornstarch in surgical glove powder. Ann Allergy 65:152, 1990.

1109. Malo JL, Cartier A, L'Archeveque J, et al: Prevalence of occupational asthma and immunologic sensitization to psyllium among health personnel in chronic care hospitals. Am Rev Respir Dis 42:1359, 1990.

1110. Sussman GL, Dorian W: Psyllium anaphylaxis. Allergy Proc 11:241, 1990.

1111. Vaswani SK, Hamilton RG, Valentine MD, Adkinson NF Jr: Psyllium laxative–induced anaphylaxis, asthma, and rhinitis. Allergy 51:266, 1996.

1112. Malo JL, Cartier A, Ghezzo H, et al: Prevalence of occupational asthma and immunologic sensitization to psyllium among health personnel in chronic care hospitals. Am Rev Respir Dis 142:1359, 1990.

1113. Marks GB, Salome CM, Woolcock AJ: Asthma and allergy associated with occupational exposure to ispaghula and senna products in a pharmaceutical work force. Am Rev Respir Dis 144:1065, 1991.

1114. McConnochie K, Edwards JH, Fifield R: Ispaghula sensitization in workers manufacturing a bulk laxative. Clin Exp Allergy 20:199, 1990.

1115. Wiessman KJ, Baur X: Occupational lung disease following long-term inhalation of pancreatic extracts. Eur J Respir Dis 66:13, 1985.

1116. Bernstein IL: Isocyanate-induced pulmonary diseases: A current perspective. J Allergy Clin Immunol 70:24, 1982.

1117. Mapp CE, Saetta M, Maestreeli P, et al: Mechanisms and pathology of occupational asthma. Eur Respir J 7:544, 1994.

1118. Cartier A, Chan N, Malo JL, et al: Occupational asthma caused by eastern white cedar (*Thuja occidentalis*) with demonstration that plicatic acid is present in this wood dust and is the causal agent. J Allergy Clin Immunol 77:639, 1984.

1119. Lam S, Tan F, Chan H, et al: Relationship between types of asthmatic reaction, nonspecific bronchial reactivity, and specific IgE antibodies in patients with red cedar asthma. J Allergy Clin Immunol 72:134, 1983.

1120. Chan-Yeung M: Immunologic and nonimmunologic mechanisms in asthma due to western red cedar (*Thuja plicata*). J Allergy Clin Immunol 70:32, 1982.

1121. Chan-Yeung M: Fate of occupational asthma: A follow-up study of patients with occupational asthma due to western red cedar (*Thuja plicata*). Am Rev Respir Dis 116:1023, 1977.

1122. Chan-yeung M, Vedal S, Kus J, et al: Symptoms, pulmonary function and bronchial hyperreactivity in western red cedar workers compared to those in office workers. Am Rev Respir Dis 130:1038, 1984.

1123. Vedal S, Chan-Yeung M, Enarson DA, et al: Plicatic acid–specific IgE and nonspecific bronchial hyperresponsiveness in western red-cedar workers. Allergy Clin Immunol 78:1103, 1986.

1124. Paggiaro PL, Chan-Yeung M: Pattern of specific airway response in asthma due to western red cedar (*Thuja plicata*): Relationship with length of exposure and lung function measurements. Clin Allergy 17:333, 1987.

1125. Cockcroft DW, Cotton DJ, Mink JT: Nonspecific bronchial hyperreactivity after exposure to western red cedar. Am Rev Respir Dis 119:505, 1979.

1126. Vedal S, Chan-Yeung M, Enarson D, et al: Symptoms and pulmonary function in western red cedar workers related to duration of employment and dust exposure. Arch Environ Health 41:179, 1986.

1127. Chan-Yeung M, Grzybowski S: Prognosis in occupational asthma (editorial). Thorax 40:241, 1985.

1128. Venables KM, Topping MD, Nunn AJ, et al: Immunologic and functional consequences of chemical (tetrachlorophthalic anhydride)-induced asthma after four years of avoidance of exposure. J Allergy Clin Immunol 80:212, 1987.

1129. Hudson P, Cartier A, Pineau L, et al: Follow-up of occupational asthma caused by crab and various agents. J Allergy Clin Immunol 76:682, 1985.

1130. Chan-Yeung M, MacLean L, Paggiaro PL: Follow-up study of 232 patients with occupational asthma caused by western red cedar (*Thuja plicata*). J Allergy Clin Immunol 79:792, 1987.

1131. Bardana EJ Jr, Andrasch RH: Occupational asthma secondary to low molecular weight agents used in the plastic and resin industries. Eur J Respir Dis 64:241, 1983.

1132. Baur X, Czuppon AB, Rauluk I, et al: A clinical and immunological study on 92 workers occupationally exposed to anhydrides. Int Arch Occup Environ Health 67:395, 1995.

1133. Gannon PF, Sherwood Burge P, Hewlett C, Tee RD: Haemolytic anaemia in a case of occupational asthma due to maleic anhydride. Br J Ind Med 49:142, 1992.

1134. Zeiss CR, Wolkonsky P, Pruzansky JJ, et al: Clinical and immunologic evaluation of trimellitic anhydride workers in multiple industrial settings. J Allergy Clin Immunol 70:15, 1982.

1135. Bernstein DI, Zeiss CR, Wolkonsky P, et al: The relationship of total serum IgE and blocking antibody in trimellitic anhydride–induced occupational asthma. J Allergy Clin Immunol 72:714, 1983.

1136. Moller DR, Gallagher JS, Bernstein DI, et al: Detection of IgE-mediated respiratory sensitization in workers exposed to hexahydrophthalic anhydride. J Allergy Clin Immunol 75:663, 1985.

1137. Grammer LC, Shaughnessy MA, Lowenthal M, Yarnold PR: Risk factors for immunologically mediated respiratory disease from hexahydrophthalic anhydride. J Occup Med 36:642, 1994.

1138. Bernstein DI, Roach DE, McGrath KG, et al: The relationship of airborne trimellitic anhydride concentrations to trimellitic anhydride–induced symptoms and immune responses. J Allergy Clin Immunol 72:709, 1983.

1139. Young RP, Barker RD, Pile KD, et al: The association of HLRA-dr3 with specific IgE to inhaled acid anhydrides. Am J Respir Crit Care Med 151:219, 1995.

1140. Grammer LC, Shaughnessy MA, Hogan MB, et al: Study of employees with anhydride-induced respiratory disease after removal from exposure. J Occup Environ Med 37:820, 1995.

1141. Baur X: Occupational asthma due to isocyanates. Lung 174:23, 1996.

1142. Bernstein JA: Overview of diisocyanate occupational asthma. Toxicology 111:181, 1996.

1143. Moller DR, McKay RT, Bernstein IL, et al: Persistent airways disease caused by toluene diisocyanate. Am Rev Respir Dis 134:175, 1986.

1144. Moller DR, Brooks SM, McKay RT, et al: Chronic asthma due to toluene diisocyanate. Chest 90:494, 1986.

1145. Zeiss CR, Kanellakes TM, Bellone JD, et al: Immunoglobulin E–mediated asthma and hypersensitivity pneumonitis with precipitating anti-hapten antibodies due to diphenylmethane diisocyanate (Mdi) exposure. J Allergy Clin Immunol 65:346, 1980.

1146. Fink JN, Schlueter DP: Bathtub refinisher's lung: An unusual response to toluene diisocyanate. Am Rev Respir Dis 118:955, 1978.

1147. Vandenplas O, Malo J-L, Saetta M, et al: Occupational asthma and extrinsic alveolitis due to isocyanates: Current status and perspectives. Br J Ind Med 50:213, 1993.

1148. Lemiere C, Malo JL, Boulet LP, Boulet M: Reactive airways dysfunction syndrome induced by exposure to a mixture containing isocyanate: Functional and histopathologic behaviour. Allergy 51:262, 1996.

1149. Paggiaro Pl, Vagaggini B, Bacci E, et al: Prognosis of occupational asthma. Eur Respir J 7:761, 1994.

1150. Carino M, Aliani M, Licitra C, et al: Death due to asthma at workplace in a diphenylmethane diisocyanate–sensitized subject. Respiration 64:111, 1997.

1151. Fabbri LM, Saetta M, Picotti G, Mapp CE: Late asthmatic reactions, airway inflammation and chronic asthma in toluene-diisocyanate–sensitized subjects. Respiration 58:18, 1991.

1152. Saetta M, Di Stefano A, Maestrelli P, et al: Airway mucosal inflammation in occupational asthma induced by toluene diisocyanate. Am Rev Respir Dis 145:160, 1992.

1153. Saetta M, Maestrelli P, Turato G, et al: Airway wall remodeling after cessation of exposure to isocyanates in sensitized asthmatic subjects. Am J Respir Crit Care Med 151:489, 1995.

1154. Mapp CE, Dal Vecchio L, Boschetto P, et al: Toluene diisocyanate–induced asthma without airway hyperresponsiveness. Eur J Respir Dis 68:89, 1986.

1155. Vandenplas O, Delwiche JP, Jamart J, et al: Increase in non-specific bronchial hyperresponsiveness as an early marker of bronchial response to occupational agents during specific inhalation challenges. Thorax 51:472, 1996.

1156. Paggiaro PL, Innocenti A, Bacci E, et al: Specific bronchial reactivity to toluene diisocyanate: Relationship with baseline clinical findings. Thorax 41:279, 1986.

1157. Fabbri LM, Chiesura-Corona P, Delvecchio L, et al: Prednisone inhibits late asthmatic reactions and the associated increase in airway responsiveness induced by toluene-diisocyanate in sensitized subjects. Am Rev Respir Dis 132:1010, 1985.

1158. McKay RT, Brooks SM: Hyperreactive airway smooth muscle responsiveness after inhalation of toluene diisocyanate vapors. Am Rev Respir Dis 129:296, 1984.

1159. Gordon T, Sheppard D, McDonald DM, et al: Airway hyperresponsiveness and inflammation induced by toluene diisocyanate in guinea pigs. Am Rev Respir Dis 132:1106, 1985.

1160. Bignon JS, Aron Y, Ju LY, et al: HLA class II alleles in isocyanate-induced asthma. Am J Respir Crit Care Med 149:71, 1994.

1161. Rihs HP, Barbalho-Krolls T, Huber H, et al: No evidence for the influence of HLA class II in alleles in isocyanate-induced asthma. Am J Ind Med 32:522, 1997.

1162. Mapp Ce, Saetta M, Maestrelli P, et al: Low molecular weight pollutants and asthma: Pathogenetic mechanisms and genetic factors. Eur Respir J 7:1559, 1994.

1163. Balboni A, Baricordi OR, Fabbri LM, et al: Association between toluene diisocyanate–induced asthma and DQB1 markers: A possible role for aspartic acid at position 57. Eur Respir J 9:207, 1996.

1164. Mapp CE: Occupational asthma: Interactions between genetic factors and adverse environment? Med Lav 85:187, 1994.

1165. Pepys J, Pickering CAC, Hughes EG: Asthma due to inhaled chemical agents: Complex salts of platinum. Clin Allergy 2:391, 1972.

1166. Calverley AE, Rees D, Dowdeswell RJ, et al: Platinum salt sensitivity in refinery workers: Incidence and effects of smoking and exposure. Occup Environ Med 52:661, 1995.

1167. Kusaka Y, Iki M, Kumagai S, Goto S: Epidemiological study of hard metal asthma. Occup Environ Med 53:188, 1996.

1168. Bright P, Burge PS, O'Hickey SP, et al: Occupational asthma due to chrome and nickel electroplating. Thorax 52:28, 1997.

1169. Malo JL, Cartier A, Dolovich J: Occupational asthma due to zinc. Eur Respir J 6:447, 1993.

1170. Simonsson BG, Sjoberg A, Rolf C, et al: Acute and long-term airway hyperreactivity in alumin-salt–exposed workers with nocturnal asthma. Eur J Respir Dis 66:105, 1985.

1171. Field GB: Pulmonary function in aluminum smelters. Thorax 39:743, 1984.

1172. Malo JL, Cartier A, Doepner M, et al: Occupational asthma caused by nickel sulfate. J Allergy Clin Immunol 69:55, 1982.

1173. Metals and the lung (editorial). Lancet 2:903, 1984.

1174. Sprince NL, Chamberlin RI, Hales CA, et al: Respiratory disease in tungsten carbide production workers. Chest 86:549, 1984.

1175. Gheysens B, Auwerx J, Van den Eeckhout A, et al: Cobalt-induced bronchial asthma in diamond polishers. Chest 88:740, 1985.

1176. Desjardins A, Bergeron JP, Ghezzo H, et al: Aluminium potroom asthma confirmed by monitoring of forced expiratory volume in one second. Am J Respir Crit Care Med 150:1714, 1994.

1177. Burge PS, Harries MG, Lam WK, et al: Occupational asthma due to formaldehyde. Thorax 40:255, 1985.

1178. Frigas E, Filley W, Reed C: Bronchial challenge with formaldehyde gas: Lack of bronchoconstriction in 13 patients suspected of having formaldehyde-induced asthma. Mayo Clin Proc 59:295, 1984.

1179. Frigas E, Filley WV, Reed CE: Asthma induced by dust from urea-formaldehyde foam insulating material. Chest 79:706, 1981.

1180. Cockcroft DW, Hoeppner VH, Colovich J: Occupational asthma caused by cedar urea formaldehyde particle board. Chest 82:49, 1982.

1181. Gannon PF, Bright P, Campbell M, et al: Occupational asthma due to glutaraldehyde and formaldehyde in endoscopy and x-ray departments. Thorax 50:156, 1995.

1182. Chan-Yeung M, McMurren T, Catonio-Begley F, Lam S: Occupational asthma in a technologist exposed to glutaraldehyde. J Allergy Clin Immunol 91:974, 1993.

1183. Krumpe PE, Finley TN, Martinez NN: The search for expiratory obstruction in meat wrappers studied on the job. Am Rev Respir Dis 119:611, 1979.

1184. Eisen EA, Hegman DH, Smith TJ: Across-shift changes in the pulmonary function of meat-wrappers and other workers in the retail food industry. Scand J Work Environ Health 11:21, 1985.

1185. Gannon PF, Burge PS, Benfield GF: Occupational asthma due to polyethylene shrink wrapping (paper wrapper's asthma). Thorax 47:759, 1992.

1186. Perks WH, Burge PS, Pepys J, et al: Respiratory disease in an electronics factory. Br J Dis Chest 72:257, 1978.

1187. Burge PS, Perks W, O'Brien IM, et al: Occupational asthma in an electronics factory. Thorax 34:13, 1979.

1188. Ozhiganoua VN, Ivanoua IS, Dueva LA: Bronchial asthma in radio equipment assemblers. Sov Med 4:139, 1977.

1189. Keira T, Aizawa Y, Karube H, et al: Adverse effects of colophony. Ind Health 35:1, 1997.

1190. Sadhra S, Foulds IS, Gray CN, et al: Colophony—uses, health effects, airborne measurement and analysis. Ann Occup Hyg 38:385, 1994.

1191. Perks WH, Burge PS, Rehahn M, et al: Work-related respiratory disease in employees leaving an electronics factory. Thorax 34:19, 1979.

1192. Convery RP, Ward RJ, Hendrick DJ: Occupational asthma due to a widely used soft solder flux not containing colophony. Eur Respir J 10:238, 1997.

1193. Choudat D: Occupational lung diseases among dental technicians. Tuber Lung Dis 75:99, 1994.

1194. Chan-Yeung M, Malo JL: Occupational asthma. N Engl J Med 333:107, 1995.

1195. Malo JL, Ghezzo H, D'Aquino C, et al: Natural history of occupational asthma: Relevance of type of agent and other factors in the rate of development of symptoms in affected subjects. J Allergy Clin Immunol 90:937, 1992.

1196. Bright P, Burge PS: Occupational lung disease? 8. The diagnosis of occupational asthma from serial measurements of lung function at and away from work. Thorax 51:857, 1996.

1197. Burge SP, Perks WH, O'Brien IM, et al: Occupational asthma in an electronics factory: A case control study to evaluate aetiological factors. Thorax 34:300, 1979.

1198. Burge SP, O'Brien IM, Harries MG: Peak flow rate records in the diagnosis of occupational asthma due to colophony. Thorax 34:308, 1979.

1199. Burge SP, O'Brien IM, Harries MG: Peak flow rate records in the diagnosis of occupational asthma due to isocyanates. Thorax 34:317, 1979.

1200. Ulrik CS, Backer V, Skov PG: Usefulness of repeated measurements of bronchial hyperresponsiveness for the diagnosis of occupational asthma. J Asthma 31:35, 1994.

1201. Vandenplas O, Delwiche JP, Jamart J, Van de Weyer R: Increase in non-specific bronchial hyperresponsiveness as an early marker of bronchial response to occupational agents during specific inhalation challenges. Thorax 51:472, 1996.

1202. Lam S, Tan F, Chan H, et al: Relationship between types of asthmatic reaction, non-specific bronchial reactivity and specific IgE antibodies in patients with red cedar asthma. J Allergy Clin Immunol 72:134, 1983.

1203. Perrin B, Lagier F, L'Archeveque J, et al: Occupational asthma: Validity of monitoring of peak expiratory flow rates and non-allergic bronchial responsiveness as compared to specific inhalation challenge. Eur Respir J 5:40, 1992.

1204. Merget R, Reineke M, Rueckmann A, et al: Nonspecific and specific bronchial responsiveness in occupational asthma caused by platinum salts after allergen avoidance. Am J Respir Crit Care Med 150:1146, 1994.

1205. Vandenplas O, Malo J-L: Inhalation challenges with agents causing occupational asthma. Eur Respir J 10:2612, 1997.

1206. Cockcroft DW, Hoeppner VH, Werner GD: Recurrent nocturnal asthma after bronchoprovocation with western red cedar sawdust: Association with acute increase in non-allergic bronchial responsiveness. Clin Allergy 14:61, 1984.

1207. Gandevia B: Occupational asthma. Med J Aust 2:332, 1970.

1208. Brooks SM, Weiss MA, Bernstein IL: Reactive airways dysfunction syndrome (RADS): Persistent asthma syndrome after high level irritant exposures. Chest 88:376, 1985.

1209. Lemiere C, Malo JL, Gautrin D: Nonsensitizing causes of occupational asthma. Med Clin North Am 80:749, 1996.

1210. Kern DG: Outbreak of the reactive airways of dysfunction syndrome after a spill of glacial acetic acid. Am Rev Respir Dis 144:1058, 1991.

1211. Chan-Yeung M, Lam S, Kennedy S, Frew A: Persistent asthma after repeated exposure to high concentrations of gases in pulpmills. Am J Respir Crit Care Med 149:1676, 1994.

1212. Cormier Y, Coll B, Laviolette M, Boulet LP: Reactive airways dysfunction syndrome (RADS) following exposure to toxic gases of a swine confinement building. Eur Respir J 9:1090, 1996.

1213. Promisloff RA, Lenchner GS, Phan A, Cichelli AV: Reactive airway dysfunction syndrome in three police officers following a roadside chemical spill. Chest 98:928, 1990.

1214. Mustchin CP, Pickering CAC: "Coughing water": Bronchial hyperreactivity induced by swimming in a chlorinated pool. Thorax 34:682, 1979.

1215. Moore BB, Sherman M: Chronic reactive airway disease following acute chlorine gas exposure in an asymptomatic atopic patient. Chest 100:855, 1991.

1216. Piirila PL, Nordman H, Korhonen OS, Winblad I: A thirteen-year follow-up of respiratory effects of acute exposure to sulfur dioxide. Scand J Work Environ Health 22:191, 1996.

1217. Gautrin D, Boulct LP, Boutet M, et al: Is reactive airways dysfunction syndrome (RADS) a variant of occupational asthma? J Allergy Clin Immunol 93:12, 1994.

1218. Lemiere C, Malo JL, Boutet M: Reactive airways dysfunction syndrome due to chlorine: Sequential bronchial biopsies and functional assessment. Eur Respir J 10:241, 1997.

1219. Demnati R, Fraser R, Ghezzo H, et al: Time-course of functional and pathological changes after a single high acute inhalation of chlorine in rats. Eur Respir J 11:922, 1998.

1220. Meggs WJ, Elsheik T, Metzger WJ, et al: Nasal pathology and ultrastructure in patients with chronic airway inflammation (RADS and RUDS) following an irritant exposure. J Toxicol Clin Toxicol 34:383, 1996.

1221. Cormier Y, Boulet LP, Bedard G, Tremblay G: Respiratory health of workers exposed to swine confinement buildings only or to both swine confinement buildings and dairy barns. Scand J Work Environ Health 17:269, 1991.

1222. Choudat D, Goehen M, Korobaeff M, et al: Respiratory symptoms and bronchial reactivity among pig and dairy farmers. Scand J Work Environ Health 20:45, 1994.

1223. Hendrick DJ: Editorial: Contaminated humidifiers and the lung. Thorax 40:244, 1985.

1224. Burge PS, Finnegan M, Horsfield N, et al: Occupational asthma in a factory with a contaminated humidifier. Thorax 40:248, 1985.

1225. Milton DK, Wypij D, Kriebel D, et al: Endotoxin exposure-response in a fiberglass manufacturing facility. Am J Ind Med 29:3, 1996.

1226. Cinkotai FF, Sharpe TC, Gibbs ACC: Circadian rhythms in peak expiratory flow rate in workers exposed to cotton dust. Thorax 39:759, 1984.

1227. Tockman MS, Baser M: Is cotton dust exposure associated with chronic effects? Am Rev Respir Dis 130:1, 1984.

1228. Schachter EN, Maunder LR, Beck GJ: The pattern of lung function abnormalities in cotton textile workers. Am Rev Respir Dis 129:523, 1984.

1229. Beck GJ, Schacter EN, Maunder LR: The relationship of respiratory symptoms and lung function loss in cotton textile workers. Am Rev Respir Dis 130:6, 1984.

1230. Glindmeyer HW, Lefante JJ, Jones RN, et al: Cotton dust and across-shift change in $FEV_1$ as predictors of annual change in $FEV_1$. Am J Respir Crit Care Med 149:584, 1994.

1231. Schachter EN, Brown S, Zuskin E, et al: Airway reactivity in cotton bract–induced bronchospasm. Am Res Respir Dis 123:273, 1981.

1232. Schachter EN, Zuskin E, Buck MG, et al: Airway reactivity and cotton bract–induced bronchial obstruction. Chest 87:51, 1986.

1233. Edwards JH, Alzubaidy TS, Altikriti R, et al: Byssinosis: Inhalation challenge with polyphenol. Chest 85:215, 1984.

1234. Rylander R, Haglind P, Lundholm M: Endotoxin in cotton dust and respiratory function decrement among cotton workers in an experimental cardroom. Am Rev Respir Dis 131:209, 1985.

1235. Rylander R: Health effects of cotton dust exposures. Am J Ind Med 17:39, 1990.

1236. Castellan RM, Olenchock SA, Hankinson JL, et al: Acute bronchoconstriction induced by cotton dust: Dose-related response to endotoxin and other dust factors. Ann Intern Med 101:159, 1984.

1237. Wilson MR, Sehul A, Ory R, et al: Activation of the alternative complement pathway by extracts of cotton dust. Clin Allergy 10:303, 1980.

1238. Pernis B, Vigliani EC, Cavagna C, et al: The role of bacterial endotoxins on occupational diseases caused by inhaling vegetable dusts. Br J Ind Med 18:120, 1961.

1239. Deschamps D, Questel F, Baud FJ, et al: Persistent asthma after acute inhalation of organophosphate insecticide (letter). Lancet 344:1712, 1994.

1240. Asai S, Krzanowski JJ, Anderson WH, et al: Effects of the toxin of red tide, *Ptychodiscus brevis*, on canine tracheal smooth muscle—a possible new asthma-triggering mechanism. J Allergy Clin Immunol 69:418, 1982.

1241. Chester EH, Martinez-Catinchi FL, Schwartz HJ, et al: Patterns of airway reactivity to asthma produced by exposure to toluene di-isocyanate. Chest 75:229, 1979.

1242. McKay RT, Brooks SM: Effects of toluene diisocyanate on beta-adrenergic receptor function—biochemical and physiologic studies. Am Rev Respir Dis 128:50, 1983.

1243. Hodson ME, Simon G, Batten JC: Radiology of uncomplicated asthma. Thorax 29:296, 1974.

1244. Paganin F, Trussard V, Seneterre E, et al: Chest radiography and high resolution computed tomography of the lungs in asthma. Am Rev Respir Dis 146:1084, 1992.

1245. Pickup CM, Nee PA, Randall PE: Radiographic features in 1016 adults admitted to hospital with acute asthma. J Accid Emerg Med 11:234, 1994.

1246. Webb WR: Radiology of obstructive pulmonary disease. Am J Roentgenol 169:637, 1997.

1247. Lynch DA: Imaging of asthma and allergic bronchopulmonary mycosis. Radiol Clin North Am 36:129, 1998.

1248. Hodson ME, Simon G, Batten JC: Radiology of uncomplicated asthma. Thorax 29:296, 1974.

1249. Kinsella MM, Müller NL, Staples C, et al: Hyperinflation in asthma and emphysema. Assessment by pulmonary function testing and computed tomography. Chest 94:286, 1988.

1250. Blackie SP, Al-Majed S, Staples CA, et al: Changes in total lung capacity during acute spontaneous asthma. Am Rev Respir Dis 142:79, 1990.

1251. Rebuck AS: Radiological aspects of severe asthma. Australas Radiol 14:264, 1970.

1252. Genereux GP: Radiology and pulmonary immunopathologic lung disease. *In* Steiner, RE (ed): Recent Advances in Radiology and Medical Imaging. New York, Churchill Livingstone, 1983, pp 213–240.

1253. Bousquet J, Chanez P, Lacoste JY, et al: Eosinophilic inflammation in asthma. N Engl J Med 323:1033, 1990.

1254. Petheram IS, Kerr IH, Collins JV: Value of chest radiographs in severe acute asthma. Clin Radiol 32:281, 1981.

1254a. Zieverink SE, Harper AP, Holden RW, et al: Emergency room radiography of asthma: An efficacy study. Radiology 145:27, 1982.

1255. Joorabchi B, Hammoude E, Khalid MA: Radiographic inversion of pulmonary blood flow in acute asthma. Clin Pediatrics 33:286, 1994.

1256. Dalton AM: A review of radiological abnormalities in 135 patients presenting with acute asthma. Arch Emerg Med 8:36, 1991.

1257. Rossi OV, Lahde S, Laitinen J, Huhti E: Contribution of chest and paranasal sinus radiographs to the management of acute asthma. Int Arch Allergy Immunol 105:96, 1994.

1258. Lynch DA, Newell JD, Tschomper BA, et al: Uncomplicated asthma in adults: Comparison of CT appearance of the lungs in asthmatic and healthy subjects. Radiology 188:829, 1993.

1259. Newman KB, Lynch DA, Newman LS, et al: Quantitative computed tomography detects air trapping due to asthma. Chest 106:105, 1994.

1260. Okazawa M, Müller NL, McNamara AE, et al: Human airway narrowing measured using high resolution computed tomography. Am J Respir Crit Care Med 154:1557, 1996.

1261. Park CS, Müller NL, Worthy SA, et al: Airway obstruction in asthmatic and healthy individuals: Inspiratory and expiratory thin-section CT findings. Radiology 203:361, 1997.

1262. Webb WR, Gamsu G, Wall SD, et al: CT of a bronchial phantom: Factors affecting appearance and size measurements. Invest Radiol 19:394, 1984.

1263. McNamara AE, Müller NL, Okazawa M, et al: Airway narrowing in excised canine lungs measured by high-resolution computed tomography. J Appl Physiol 73:307, 1992.

1263a. Bankier AA, Fleischmann D, Mallek R, et al: Bronchial wall thickness: Appropriate window settings for thin-section CT and radiologic-anatomic correlation. Radiology 199:831, 1996.

1264. Senéterre E, Paganin F, Bruel JM, et al: Measurement of the internal size of bronchi using high-resolution computed tomography (HRCT). Eur Respir J 7:596, 1994.

1265. Amirav I, Kramer S, Grunstein M, Hoffman E: Assessment of methacholine-induced airway constriction with ultrafast high-resolution computed tomography. J Appl Physiol 75:2239, 1993.

1266. Herold C, Brown R, Mitzner W, et al: Assessment of pulmonary airway reactivity with high-resolution CT. Radiology 181:369, 1991.

1267. Brown R, Mitzner W: Effect of lung inflation and airway muscle tone on airway diameter in vivo. J Appl Physiol 79:1581, 1996.

1268. Arakawa H, Webb WR: Air trapping on expiratory high-resolution CT scans in the absence of inspiratory scan abnormalities: Correlation with pulmonary function tests and differential diagnosis. Am J Roentgenol 170:1349, 1998.

1269. Grenier P, Mourey-Gerosa I, Benali K, et al: Abnormalities of the airways and lung parenchyma in asthmatics: CT observations in 50 patients and inter- and intraobserver variability. Eur Radiol 6:199, 1996.

1270. Paganin F, Senéterre E, Chanez P, et al: Computed tomography of the lungs in asthma: Influence of disease severity and etiology. Am J Respir Crit Care Med 153:110, 1996.

1270a. Awadh N, Müller NL, Park CS, et al: Airway wall thickness in patients with near fatal asthma and control groups: Assessment with high resolution computed tomographic scanning. Thorax 53:248, 1998.

1271. Angus P, Davies M-I, Cowan M, et al: Computed tomographic scanning of the lung in patients with allergic bronchopulmonary aspergillosis and in asthmatic patients with a positive skin test to *Aspergillus fumigatus*. Thorax 49:586, 1994.

1272. Neeld D, Goodman L, Gurney J, et al: J. Computerized tomography in the evaluation of allergic bronchopulmonary aspergillosis. Am Rev Respir Dis 142:1200, 1990.

1273. Kim S, Im J, Kim I, et al: Normal bronchial and pulmonary arterial diameters measured by thing section CT. J Comp Assist Tomog 19:365, 1995.

1274. Kim J, Müller NL, Park CS, et al: Broncho-arterial ratio on thin-section CT: Comparison between high altitude and sea level. J Comput Assist Tomogr 21:306, 1997.

1275. Wagner PD, Hedenstierna G, Bylin G: Ventilation-perfusion inequality in chronic asthma. Am Rev Respir Dis 136:605, 1987.

1276. Ferrer A, Roca J, Wagner PM, et al: Airway obstruction and ventilation-perfusion relationships in acute severe asthma. Am Rev Respir Dis 147:579, 1993.

1277. Blair DN, Coppage L, Shaw C: Medical imaging in asthma. J Thorac Imag 1:23, 1986.

1278. Sostman HD, Gottschalk AG: The stripe sign: A new sign for diagnosis of nonembolic defects on pulmonary perfusion scintigraphy. Radiology 142:737, 1982.

1279. Gevenois P, Scillia P, de Maertelaer V, et al: The effects of age, sex, lung size, and hyperinflation on CT lung densitometry. Am J Roentgenol 167:1169, 1996.

1279a. Goldin JG, McNitt-Gray MF, Sorenson SM, et al: Airway hyperreactivity: Assessment with helical thin-section CT. Radiology 208:321, 1998.

1280. Simonsson BG: Chronic cough and expectoration in patients with asthma and in patients with alpha$_1$-antitrypsin deficiency. Eur J Respir Dis 118:123, 1982.

1281. Fitch KD, Godfrey S: Asthma and athletic performance. JAMA 236:152, 1976.

1282. Lee HY, Stretton TB: Asthma in the elderly. BMJ 4:93, 1972.

1283. McFadden ER Jr: Exertional dyspnea and cough as prelude to acute attacks of bronchial asthma. N Engl J Med 292:555, 1975.

1284. Baumann UA, Haerdi E, Keller R: Relations between clinical signs and lung function in bronchial asthma: How is acute bronchial obstruction reflected in dyspnoea and wheezing? Respiration 50:294, 1986.

1285. McFadden ER Jr, Kiser R, de Groot WJ: Acute bronchial asthma: Relations between clinical and physiologic manifestations. N Engl J Med 288:221, 1973.

1286. Spirometry in asthma (editorial). N Engl J Med 288:262, 1973.

1287. Pratter MR, Hingston DM, Irwin RS: Diagnosis of bronchial asthma by clinical evaluation: An unreliable method. Chest 84:42, 1983.

1288. Pardee NE, Winterbauer RH, Morgan EH, et al: Combinations of 4 physical signs as indicators of ventilatory abnormality in obstructive pulmonary syndromes. Chest 77:354, 1980.

1289. Knowles GK, Clark TJH: Pulsus paradoxus as a valuable sign indicating severity of asthma. Lancet 2:1356, 1973.

1290. Rebuck AS, Reed J: Assessment and management of severe asthma. Am J Med 51:788, 1971.

1291. Rebuck AS, Pengally LD: Development of pulsus paradoxus in the presence of airways obstruction. N Engl J Med 288:66, 1973.

1292. Galant SP, Groncy CE, Shaw KC: The value of pulsus paradoxus in assessing the child with status asthmaticus. Pediatrics 61:46, 1978.

1293. McGregor M: Current concepts: Pulsus paradoxus. N Engl J Med 301:480, 1979.

1294. Bellamy D, Collins JV: "Acute" asthma in adults. Thorax 34:36, 1979.

1295. Arnold AG, Lane DJ, Zapata E: The speed of onset and severity of acute severe asthma. Br J Dis Chest 76:157, 1982.

1296. Stellman JL, Spicer JE, Clayton RM: Morbidity from chronic asthma. Thorax 37:218, 1982.

1297. Jack CI, Lye M: Asthma in the elderly patient. Gerontology 42:61, 1996.

1298. Dow L: The diagnosis of asthma in older people. Clin Exp Allergy 24:156, 1994.

1299. Senior RM, Lefrak RS, Korenblat PE: Status asthmaticus. JAMA 231:1277, 1972.

1300. Treatment of status asthmaticus. BMJ 4:563, 1972.

1301. Szefler SJ, Leung DY: Glucocorticoid-resistant asthma: Pathogenesis and clinical implications for management. Eur Respir J 10:1640, 1997.

1302. Corrigan CJ: Glucocorticoid-resistant asthma. T-lymphocyte defects. Am J Respir Crit Care Med 154:S53, 1996.

1303. Vrugt B, Djukanovic R, Bron A, Aalbers R: New insights into the pathogenesis of severe corticosteroid-dependent asthma. J Allergy Clin Immunol 98:S22, S33, 1996.

1304. Woolcock AJ: Assessment of asthma severity. In Barnes PJ, Grunstein MM, Leff AR, Woolcock AJ (eds): Asthma. Vol 2. Philadelphia, Lippincott-Raven, 1997, pp 1499–1503.

1305. Guidelines on the management of asthma. British Thoracic Society. Thorax 48:S1, 1993.

1306. Guidelines for the diagnosis and management of bronchial asthma. Committee on the Definition, Treatment, and Management of Bronchial Asthma. Japanese Society for Allergology. Allergy 27:1, 1995.

1307. Woolcock AJ, Jenkins CR: Management guidelines. In Barnes PJ, Grunstein MM, Leff AR, Woolcock AJ (eds): Asthma. Vol 2. Philadelphia, Lippincott-Raven, 1997, pp 1819–1830.

1308. O'Connor GT, Weiss ST: Clinical and symptom measures. Am J Respir Crit Care Med. 149:S21, S29, 1994.

1309. Lenfant C, Khaltaev N, Global Initiative for Asthma: In Global strategy for asthma management and prevention. NHLBI/WHO Workshop Report 1:1, 1995.

1310. Troyanov S, Chezzo H, Cartier A, Malo JL: Comparison of circadian variations using FEV$_1$ and peak expiratory flow rates among normal and asthmatic subjects. Thorax 49:775, 1994.

1311. Todisco T, Grassi V, Sorbini C: Circadian rhythms of respiratory functions in asthmatics. Respiration 40:128, 1980.

1312. Connolly CK: Diurnal rhythms in airway obstruction. Br J Dis Chest 73:357, 1979.

1313. Bahous J, Cartier A, Malo JL: Monitoring of peak expiratory flow rates in subjects with mild airway hyperexcitability. Bull Eur Physiol Respir 21:25, 1985.

1314. Turner-Warwick M: On observing patterns of airflow obstruction in chronic asthma. Br J Dis Chest 71:73, 1977.

1315. Sakula A: Sir John Floyer's "A Treatise of the Asthma" (1698). Thorax 39:248, 1984.

1316. Oosterhoff Y, Koeter GH, De Monchy JG, et al: Circadian variation in airway responsiveness to methacholine, propranolol, and AMP in atopic asthmatic subjects. Am Rev Respir Dis 147:512, 1993.

1317. Barnes P, Fitzgerald G, Brown M, et al: Nocturnal asthma and changes in circulating epinephrine, histamine and cortisol. N Engl J Med 303:263, 1980.

1318. Martin RJ, Cicutto LC, Smith HR, et al: Airways inflammation in nocturnal asthma. Am Rev Respir Dis 143:351, 1991.

1319. Jarjour NN, Calhoun WJ, Busse WW: Enhanced metabolism of oxygen radicals in nocturnal asthma. Am Rev Respir Dis 146:905, 1992.

1320. Kraft M, Djukanovic R, Wilson S, et al: Alveolar tissue inflammation in asthma. Am J Respir Crit Care Med 154:1505, 1996.

1321. Oosterhoff Y, Timens W, Postma DS: The role of airway inflammation in the pathophysiology of nocturnal asthma. Clin Exp Allergy 25:915, 1995.

1322. Johansson SG, Wuthrich B, Zortea-Caflish C: Nightly asthma caused by allergens in silk-filled bed quilts: Clinical and immunologic studies. J Allergy Clin Immunol 75:452, 1985.

1323. Jönsson E, Mossberg B: Impairment of ventilatory function by supine posture in asthma. Eur J Respir Dis 65:496, 1984.

1324. Bush RK: Nocturnal asthma: Mechanisms and the role of theophylline in treatment. Postgrad Med J 67(Suppl 4):S20, 1991.

1325. Al-Damluji S, Thompson PJ, Citron KM, et al: Effect of naloxone on circadian rhythm in lung function. Thorax 38:914, 1983.

1326. Szefler SJ, Ando R, Cicutto LC, et al: Plasma histamine, epinephrine, cortisol, and leukocyte beta-adrenergic receptors in nocturnal asthma. Clin Pharmacol Ther 49:59, 1991.

1327. Pak J, Martin RJ, Irvin CG: Uncoupling of the airways and parenchyma in subjects with nocturnal asthma. Am Rev Respir Dis 145:A595, 1992.

1328. Martin RJ, Pak J, Irvin CG: Effect of lung volume maintenance during sleep in nocturnal asthma. J Appl Physiol 75:1467, 1993.

1329. Ballard RD, Pak J, White DP: Influence of posture and sustained loss of lung volume on pulmonary function in awake asthmatic subjects. Am Rev Respir Dis 144:499, 1991.

1330. Hetzel MR, Clark TJH: Does sleep cause nocturnal asthma? Thorax 34:749, 1979.

1331. Catterall JR, Rhind GB, Stewart IC, et al: Effect of sleep deprivation on overnight bronchoconstriction in nocturnal asthma. Thorax 41:676, 1986.

1332. Montplaisir J, Walsh J, Malo JL: Nocturnal asthma—features of attacks, sleep and breathing patterns. Am Rev Respir Dis 125:18, 1982.

1333. Shapiro CM, Catterall JR, Montgomery I, et al: Do asthmatics suffer bronchoconstriction during rapid eye movement sleep? BMJ 292:1161, 1986.

1334. Soutar CA, Costello J, Ijaduola O, et al: Nocturnal and morning asthma: Relationship to plasma corticosteroids and response to cortical infusion. Thorax 30:436, 1975.

1335. Martin RJ: Nocturnal asthma. Ann Allergy 72:5, 1994.

1336. Soutar CA, Carruthers M, Pickering CAC: Nocturnal asthma and urinary adrenaline and noradrenaline excretion. Thorax 32:677, 1977.

1337. Bates ME, Clayton M, Calhoun W, et al: Relationship of plasma epinephrine and circulating eosinophils to nocturnal asthma. Am J Respir Crit Care Med 149:667, 1994.

1338. Chung KF, Lalloo UG: Diagnosis and management of chronic persistent dry cough. Postgrad Med J 72:594, 1996.

1339. Lalloo UG, Barnes PJ, Fan Chung D: Pathophysiology and clinical presentation of cough. J Allergy Clin Immunol 98:S91, 1996.

1340. Corrao WM, Braman SS, Irwin RS: Chronic cough as the sole presenting manifestation of bronchial asthma. N Engl J Med 300:633, 1979.

1341. Poe RH, Israel RH, Utell MJ, et al: Chronic cough—bronchoscopy or pulmonary function testing? Am Rev Respir Dis 126:160, 1982.

1342. Puolijoki H, Lahdensuo A: Chronic cough as a risk indicator of bronchopulmonary disease. Eur J Respir Dis 71:77, 1987.

1343. Cohen RM, Grant W, Lieberman P, et al: The use of methacholine inhalation, methacholine skin testing, distilled water inhalation challenge and eosinophil counts in the evaluation of patients presenting with cough and/or nonwheezing dyspnea. Ann Allergy 56:308, 1986.

1344. Gibson PG, Dolovich J, Denburgh J, et al: Chronic cough: Eosinophilic bronchitis without asthma. Lancet 1:1246, 1989.

1345. Eschenbacher WL, Boushey HA, Sheppard D: Alteration in osmolarity of inhaled aerosols causes bronchoconstriction and cough, but absence of a permeant anion causes cough alone. Am Rev Respir Dis 129:211, 1984.

1346. Higenbottam T: Cough induced by changes of ionic composition of airway surface liquid. Bull Eur Physiol Respir 20:553, 1985.

1347. Pounsford J, Birch M, Saunders K: Effect of bronchodilators on the cough response to inhaled citric acid in normal and asthmatic subjects. Thorax 40:662, 1985.

1348. Sheppard D, Rizk NW, Boushey HA, et al: Mechanism of cough and bronchoconstriction induced by distilled water aerosol. Am Rev Respir Dis 127:691, 1983.

1349. Arnup NE, Fleetham JA: Cough threshold: Variation within a normal population and relationship to bronchial reactivity. Am Rev Respir Dis 123:A129, 1981.

1350. Pounsford J, Saunders K: Diurnal variation and adaptation of the cough response to citric acid in normal subjects. Thorax 40:657, 1985.

1351. Irwin RS, Pratter MR, Holland PS, et al: Postnasal drip causes cough and is associated with reversible upper airway obstruction. Chest 85:346, 1984.

1352. O'Connell JM, Baird LI, Campbell AH: Sputum eosinophilia in chronic bronchitis and asthma. Respiration 35:65, 1978.

1353. Pavord ID, Pizzichini MM, Pizzichini E, Hargreave FE: The use of induced sputum to investigate airway inflammation. Thorax 52:498, 1997.

1354. Pizzichini E, Pizzichini MM, Efthimiadis A, et al: Indices of airway inflammation in induced sputum: Reproducibility and validity of cell and fluid-phase measurements. Am J Respir Crit Care Med 154:308, 1996.

1355. Pizzichini E, Pizzichini MM, Efthimiadis A, et al: Measuring airway inflammation in asthma: Eosinophils and eosinophilic cationic protein in induced sputum compared with peripheral blood. J Allergy Clin Immunol 99:539, 1997.

1356. Pizzichini MM, Pizzichini E, Clelland L, et al: Sputum in severe exacerbations of asthma: Kinetics of inflammatory indices after prednisone treatment. Am J Respir Crit Care Med 155:1501, 1997.

1357. Lemanske RF Jr, Busse WW: Asthma. JAMA 278:1855, 1997.

1358. Strang LB: Eosinophilia in children with asthma and bronchiectasis. BMJ 1:167, 1960.

1359. Karetzky MS: Blood studies in untreated patients with acute asthma. Am Rev Respir Dis 112:607, 1975.

1360. Usher DJ, Shepherd RJ, Deegan T: Serum lactate dehydrogenase isoenzyme activities in patients with asthma. Thorax 29:685, 1976.

1361. Szczeklik A, Turowska B, Czerniawska-Mysik G, et al: Serum alpha$_1$-antitrypsin in bronchial asthma. Am Rev Respir Dis 109:487, 1974.

1362. Singleton R, Moel DI, Cohn RA: Preliminary observation of impaired water excretion in treated status asthmaticus. Am J Dis Child 140:59, 1986.

1363. Baker JW, Yerger S, Segar WE: Elevated plasma antidiuretic hormone levels in status asthmaticus. Mayo Clin Proc 51:31, 1976.

1364. Benfield GFA, Odoherty K, Davies BH: Status asthmaticus and the syndrome of inappropriate secretion of antidiuretic hormone. Thorax 37:147, 1982.

1365. Pepys J: Current concepts: Inhalation challenge tests in asthma. N Engl J Med 293:758, 1975.

1366. Gunstone RF: Right heart pressures in bronchial asthma. Thorax 26:39, 1971.

1367. Ahonen A: Analysis of the changes in ECG during status asthmaticus. Respiration 37:85, 1979.

1368. Gelb AF, Lyons HA, Fairshter RD, et al: P-pulmonale in status asthmaticus. J Allergy Clin Immunol 64:18, 1979.

1368a. Cassidy SS, Mitchell JH: Effects of positive pressure breathing on right and left ventricular preload and afterload. Fed Proc 40:2178, 1981.

1369. Woolcock AJ, Vincent NJ, Macklem PT: Frequency dependence of compliance as a test for obstruction in the small airways. J Clin Invest 48:1097, 1969.

1370. Orzalesi MM, Cook CD, Hart MC: Pulmonary function in symptom-free asthmatic patients. Acta Paediatr Scand 53:401, 1964.

1371. Burrows D, Penman RWB: Prognosis of the eczema-asthma syndrome. BMJ 2:825, 1960.

1372. Rubinfeld AR, Pain MCF: Perception of asthma. Lancet 1:882, 1976.

1373. Jones RHT, Jones RS: Ventilatory capacity in young adults with a history of asthma in childhood. BMJ 2:976, 1966.

1374. Hill DJ, Landau LI, Phelan PD: Small airway disease in asymptomatic asthmatic adolescents. Am Rev Respir Dis 106:873, 1972.

1375. McCarthy D, Milic-Emili J: Closing volume in asymptomatic asthma. Am Rev Respir Dis 107:559, 1973.

1376. Morgan EJ, Hall DR: Abnormalities of lung function in hay fever. Thorax 31:80, 1976.

1377. Loke J, Ganeshananthan M, Palm CR, et al: Site of airway obstruction in asymptomatic asthmatic children. Lung 159:35, 1981.

1378. Fairshter RD, Wilson AF: Relationship between the site of airflow limitation and localization of the bronchodilator response in asthma. Am Rev Respir Dis 122:27, 1980.

1379. Despas PJ, Leroux M, Macklem PT: Site of airway obstruction in asthma as determined by measuring maximal expiratory flow breathing air and a helium-oxygen mixture. J Clin Invest 51:3235, 1972.

1380. Chan-Yeung M, Abboud R, Tsao MS, et al: Effect of helium on maximal expiratory flow in patients with asthma before and during induced bronchoconstriction. Am Rev Respir Dis 113:433, 1976.

1381. Benatar SR, Clark TJR, Cochrane GM: Clinical relevance of the flow rate response to low density gas breathing in asthmatics. Am Rev Respir Dis 111:126, 1975.

1382. Partridge MR, Saunders KB: The site of airflow limitation in asthma—the effect of time, acute exacerbations of disease and clinical features. Br J Dis Chest 75:263, 1981.

1383. Antic R, Macklem PT: Influence of clinical factors on the site of airways obstruction in asthma. Am Rev Respir Dis 114:851, 1976.

1384. Metzger WJ, Nugent K, Richerson HB: Site of airflow obstruction during early and late phase asthmatic responses to allergen bronchoprovocation. Chest 88:369, 1985.

1385. Okazawa M, Muller N, McNamara AE, et al: Human airway narrowing measured using high resolution computed tomography. Am J Respir Crit Care Med 54:1557, 1996.

1386. Wagner EM, Liu MC, Weinmann GG, et al: Peripheral lung resistance in normal and asthmatic subjects. Am Rev Respir Dis 141:584, 1990.

1387. Meisner P, Hugh-Jones P: Pulmonary function in bronchial asthma. Br Med J 1:470, 1968.

1388. Olive JT Jr, Hyatt RE: Maximal expiratory flow and total respiratory resistance during induced bronchoconstriction in asthmatic subjects. Am Rev Respir Dis 106:366, 1972.

1389. Clark TJH, Godfrey S, Pride NB: Physiology. In Clark TJH, Godfrey S (eds): Asthma. London, Chapman and Hall, 1983, p 12.

1390. Wang T-R, Levison H: Pulmonary function in children with asthma at acute attack and symptom-free status. Am Rev Respir Dis 99:719, 1969.

1391. Blackhall MI, Jones RS: Lung volume and its subdivisions in normal and asthmatic males. Thorax 28:89, 1973.

1392. Palmer KNV, Kelman GR: A comparison of pulmonary function in extrinsic and intrinsic bronchial asthma. Am Rev Respir Dis 107:940, 1973.

1393. Mayfield JD, Paez PN, Nicholson DP: Static and dynamic lung volumes and ventilation-perfusion abnormality in adult asthma. Thorax 26:591, 1971.

1394. Pedersen OF, Thiessen B, Naeraa N, et al: Factors determining residual volume in normal and asthmatic subjects. Eur J Respir Dis 65:99, 1984.

1395. Woolcock AJ, Read J: Lung volumes in exacerbations of asthma. Am J Med 41:259, 1966.

1396. Martin J, Powell E, Shore S, et al: The role of respiratory muscles in the hyperinflation of bronchial asthma. Am Rev Respir Dis 121:441, 1980.

1397. Müller N, Bryan AC, Zamel N: Tonic inspiratory muscle activity as a cause of hyperinflation in asthma. J Appl Physiol 50:279, 1981.

1398. Macklem PT: Hyperinflation (editorial). Am Rev Respir Dis 129:1, 1984.

1399. Collett PW, Brancatisano T, Engel LA: Changes in the glottic aperture during bronchial asthma. Am Rev Respir Dis 128:719, 1983.

1400. Ringel ER, Loring SH, McFadden ER, et al: Chest wall configurational changes before and during acute obstructive episodes in asthma. Am Rev Respir Dis 128:607, 1983.

1401. Lennox S, Mengeot PM, Martin JG: The contributions of rib cage and abdominal displacements to the hyperinflation of acute bronchospasm. Am Rev Respir Dis 132:679, 1985.

1402. Woolcock AJ, Read J: Improvement in bronchial asthma not reflected in forced expiratory volume. Lancet 2:1323, 1965.

1403. Martin JG, Shore SA, Engel LA: Mechanical load and inspiratory muscle action during induced asthma. Am Rev Respir Dis 128:455, 1983.

1404. Woolcock AJ, Rebuck AS, Cade JF, et al: Lung volume changes in asthma measured concurrently by two methods. Am Rev Respir Dis 104:703, 1971.

1405. Shore S, Miolic-Emili J, Martin JG: Reassessment of body plethysmographic technique for the measurement of thoracic gas volume in asthmatics. Am Rev Respir Dis 126:515, 1982.

1406. Stanescu DC, Rodenstein D, Cauberghs M, et al: Failure of body plethysmography in bronchial asthma. J Appl Physiol 52:939, 1982.

1407. Rodenstein D, Stanescu DC: Elastic properties of the lung in acute induced asthma. J Appl Physiol 54:152, 1983.

1408. Kirby JG, Juniper EF, Hargreave FE, et al: Total lung capacity does not change during methacholine-stimulated airway narrowing. J Appl Physiol 61:2144, 1986.

1409. Brown R, Ingram RH, McFadden ER: Problems in the plethysmographic assessment of changes in total lung capacity in asthma. Am Rev Respir Dis 118:685, 1978.

1410. Blackie SP, Al-Majed S, Staples CA, et al: Changes in total lung capacity during acute spontaneous asthma. Am Rev Respir Dis 142:79, 1990.

1411. Woolcock AJ, Read J: The static elastic properties of the lungs in asthma. Am Rev Respir Dis 98:788, 1968.

1412. Holmes PW, Campbell AH, Barter CE: Acute changes of lung volumes and lung mechanics in asthma and in normal subjects. Thorax 33:394, 1978.

1413. Hillman DR, Finucane KE: The effect of hyperinflation on lung elasticity in healthy subjects. Respir Physiol 54:295, 1983.

1414. Greaves IA, Colebatch HJ: Large lungs after childhood asthma: A consequence of enlarged air spaces. Aust N Z J Med 15:427, 1985.

1415. Ohman JL Jr, Schmidt-Nowara W, Lawrence M, et al: The diffusing capacity in asthma. Effect of airflow obstruction. Am Rev Respir Dis 107:932, 1973.

1416. Lawther PJ, Brooks AG, Waller RE: Respiratory function measurements in a cohort of medical students. Thorax 25:172, 1970.

1417. Ogilvie CM: Pulmonary function in asthma. BMJ 1:768, 1968.

1418. Keens TG, Mansell A, Krastins IRB, et al: Evaluation of the single-breath diffusing capacity in asthma and cystic fibrosis. Chest 76:41, 1979.

1419. Collard P, Njinou B, Nejadnik B, et al: Single-breath diffusing capacity for carbon monoxide in stable asthma. Chest 105:1426, 1994.

1420. Graham BL, Mink JT, Cotton DJ, et al: Overestimation of the single-breath carbon monoxide diffusing capacity in patients with air-flow obstruction. Am Rev Respir Dis 129:403, 1984.

1421. Levine G, Housley E, MacLeod P, et al: Gas exchange abnormalities in mild bronchitis and asymptomatic asthma. N Engl J Med 282:1277, 1970.

1422. Palmer KNV, Kelman GR: Pulmonary function in asthmatic patients in remission. BMJ 1:485, 1975.

1423. Wolf B, Gaultier C, Lopez C, et al: Hypoxemia in attack-free asthmatic children: Relationship with lung volumes and lung mechanics. Bull Eur Physiopathol Respir 19:471, 1983.

1424. Wagner PD, Dantzker DB, Iacovoni VE, et al: Ventilation-perfusion inequality in asymptomatic asthma. Am Rev Respir Dis 118:511, 1978.

1425. Graff-Lonnevig V, Bevegard S, Eriksson BO: Ventilation and pulmonary gas exchange at rest and during exercise in boys with bronchial asthma. Eur J Respir Dis 61:357, 1980.

1426. Wagner PD, Hedenstierna G, Bylin G: Ventilation-perfusion inequality in chronic asthma. Am Rev Respir Dis 136:605, 1987.

1427. Roca J, Ramis L, Rodriguez-Roison R, et al: Serial relationships between ventilation-perfusion inequality and spirometry in acute severe asthma requiring hospitalization. Am Rev Respir Dis 137:1055, 1988.

1428. Corte P, Young IH: Ventilation-perfusion relationships in symptomatic asthma; response to oxygen and clemastine. Chest 88:167, 1985.

1429. Palmer KNV, Diament ML: Dynamic and static lung volumes and blood-gas tensions in bronchial asthma. Lancet 1:591, 1969.

1430. McFadden ER Jr, Lyons HA: Arterial blood-gas tension in asthma. N Engl J Med 278:1027, 1968.
1431. Tai E, Read J: Blood-gas tensions in bronchial asthma. Lancet 1:644, 1967.
1432. Simpson H, Forfar JO, Grubb DJ: Arterial blood gas tensions and pH in acute asthma in childhood. BMJ 3:460, 1968.
1433. Rodriguez-Roison R, Ballester E, Roca J, et al: Mechanisms of hypoxemia in patients with status asthmaticus requiring mechanical ventilation. Am Rev Respir Dis 139:732, 1989.
1434. Roncoroni AJ, Adrogué HJA, De Obrutsky CW, et al: Metabolic acidosis in status asthmaticus. Respiration 33:85, 1976.
1435. Alberts WM, Williams JH, Ramsdell JW: Metabolic acidosis as a presenting feature in acute asthma. Ann Allergy 57:107, 1986.
1436. Okrent DG, Tessler S, Twersky RA, et al: Metabolic acidosis not due to lactic acidosis in patients with severe acute asthma. Crit Care Med 15:1098, 1987.
1437. O'Connell MB, Ibere C: Continuous intravenous terbutaline infusions for adult patients with status asthmaticus. Ann Allergy 64:213, 1990.
1438. Rees HA, Millar JS, Donald KW: A study of the clinical course and arterial blood gas tensions of patients in status asthmaticus. Q Med J 37:541, 1968.
1439. Palmer KNV, Diament ML: Relative contributions of obstructive and restrictive ventilatory impairment in the production of hypoxaemia and hypercapnia in chronic bronchitis. Lancet 1:1233, 1968.
1440. Banner AS, Shah RS, Addington WW: Rapid prediction of need for hospitalization in acute asthma. JAMA 235:1337, 1976.
1441. Stanescu DC, Teculescu DB: Pulmonary function in status asthmaticus: Effect of therapy. Thorax 25:581, 1970.
1442. Young IH, Corte P, Schoeffel RE: Pattern and time course of ventilation-perfusion inequality in excercise-induced asthma. Am Rev Respir Dis 125:304, 1982.
1443. Geelhoed GC, Landau LI, Le Souef PN: Evaluation of SaO₂ as a predictor of outcome in 280 children presenting with acute asthma. Ann Emerg Med 23:1236, 1994.
1444. Olgiati R, Birch S, Rao A, et al: Differential effects of methacholine and antigen challenge on gas exchange in allergic subjects. J Allergy Clin Immunol 67:325, 1981.
1445. Lagerstrand L, Larsson K, Ihre E, et al: Pulmonary gas exchange response following allergen challenge in patients with allergic asthma. Eur Respir J 5:1176, 1992.
1446. Wilson AF, Suprenant EL, Beall GN, et al: The significance of regional pulmonary function changes in bronchial asthma. Am J Med 48:416, 1970.
1447. Mountain RD, Sahn SA: Clinical features and outcome in patients with acute asthma presenting with hypercapnia. Am Rev Respir Dis 138:535, 1988.
1448. Rebuck AS, Read J: Patterns of ventilatory response to carbon dioxide during recovery from severe asthma. Clin Sci 41:13, 1971.
1449. Hudgel DW, Weil JV: Depression of hypoxic and hypercapnic ventilatory drives in severe asthma. Chest 68:493, 1975.
1450. Hudgel DW, Weil JV: Asthma associated with decreased hypoxia. Ann Intern Med 80:622, 1974.
1451. Kelsen SG, Fleegler B, Altose MD: The respiratory neuromuscular response to hypoxia, hypercapnia and obstruction to airflow in asthma. Am Rev Respir Dis 120:517, 1979.
1452. Zackon H, Despas PJ, Anthonisen NR: Occlusion pressure responses in asthma and chronic obstructive lung disease. Am Rev Respir Dis 114:917, 1976.
1453. Pack AI, Hertz BC, Ledlie JF, et al: Reflex effects of aerosolized histamine on phrenic nerve activity. J Clin Invest 70:424, 1982.
1454. Kassabian J, Miller KD, Lavietes MH: Respiratory center output and ventilatory timing in patients with acute airway (asthma) and alveolar (pneumonia) disease. Chest 81:536, 1982.
1455. Chapman KR, Rebuck AS: Inspiratory and expiratory resistive loading as a model of dyspnea in asthma. Respiration 44:425, 1983.
1456. Burki NK, Mitchell K, Chaudhary BA, et al: The ability of asthmatics to detect added resistive loads. Am Rev Respir Dis 117:71, 1978.
1457. Gottfried SB, Altose MD, Kelsen SG, et al: Perception of changes in airflow resistance in obstructive pulmonary disorders. Am Rev Respir Dis 124:566, 1981.
1458. Turcotte H, Tahan M, Leblanc P, Boulet LP: Perception of acute or progressive resisitive loads in normal and asthmatic subjects. Respiration 60:203, 1993.
1459. Kikuchi Y, Okabe S, Tamura G, et al: Chemosensitivity and perception of dyspnea in patients with a history of near-fatal asthma. N Engl J Med 330:1383, 1994.
1460. Issa FG, Sullivan CE: Respiratory muscle activity and thoracoabdominal motion during acute episodes of asthma during sleep. Am Rev Respir Dis 132:999, 1985.
1461. Tabachnick E, Müller NL, Levison H, et al: Chest wall mechanics and pattern of breathing during sleep in asthmatic adolescents. Am Rev Respir Dis 124:269, 1981.
1462. Bendkowski B: Asian influenza (1957) in allergic patients. BMJ 2:1314, 1958.
1463. Luhr J: Atelectasis in bronchial asthma during childhood. Nord Med 60:1198, 1958.
1464. Eggleston PA, Ward BH, Pierson WE, et al: Radiographic abnormalities in acute asthma in children. Pediatrics 54:442, 1974.
1465. Lecks HI, Whitney T, Wood D, et al: Newer concepts in occurrence of segmental atelectasis in acute bronchial asthma and status asthmaticus in children. J Asthma Res 4:65, 1966.
1466. Bierman CW: Pneumomediastinum and pneumothorax complicating asthma in children. Am J Dis Child 114:42, 1967.
1467. Ozonoff MB: Pneumomediastinum associated with asthma and pneumonia in children. J Roentgenol 95:112, 1965.
1468. Dattwyler RJ, Goldman MA, Bloch KJ: Pneumomediastinum as a complication of asthma in teenage and young adult patients. J Allergy Clin Immunol 63:412, 1979.
1469. Lewis M, Kallenbach J, Zaltzman M, et al: Acute respiratory failure in a young asthmatic patient. Chest 84:733, 1983.
1470. D'Assumpcao C, Smith WG: Spontaneous mediastinal and subcutaneous emphysema complicating bronchial asthma. Med J Aust 1:328, 1967.
1471. Toledo TM, Moore WL, Nash DA, et al: Spontaneous pneumopericardium in acute asthma. Case report and review of the literature. Chest 62:118, 1972.
1472. Segal AJ, Wasserman M: Arterial air embolism: A cause of sudden death in status asthmaticus. Radiology 99:271, 1971.
1473. Leatherman J: Life-threatening asthma. Clin Chest Med 15:453, 1994.
1474. Tuxen DV, Lane S: The effects of ventilatory pattern on hyperinflation, airway pressures, and circulation in mechanical ventilation of patients with severe airflow obstruction. Am Rev Respir Dis 136:872, 1987.
1475. Tuxen DV, Williams TJ, Scheinkestel CD: Use of a measurement of pulmonary hyperinflation to control the level of mechanical ventilation in patients with acute severe asthma. Am Rev Respir Dis 145:1136, 1992.
1476. Nates JL, Cooper DJ, Day B, Tuxen DV: Acute weakness syndromes in critically ill patients—a reappraisal. Anaesth Intensive Care 25:502, 1997.
1477. Leatherman JW, Fluegel WL, David WS, et al: Muscle weakness in mechanically ventilated patients with severe asthma. Am J Respir Crit Care Med 153:1686, 1996.
1478. Tousignant CP, Bevan DR, Eisen AA, et al: Acute quadriparesis in an asthmatic treated with atracurium. Can J Anaesth 42:224, 1995.
1479. Sykes AP, Lawson N, Finnegan JA, Ayres JG: Creatine kinase activity in patients with brittle asthma treated with long term subcutaneous terbutaline. Thorax 46:580, 1991.
1480. Douglass JA, Tuxen DV, Horne M, et al: Myopathy in severe asthma. Am Rev Respir Dis 146:517, 1992.
1481. Awadh N, Al-mane F, D'yachkova Y, et al: Myopathy following mechanical ventilation for acute severe asthma: The role of muscle relaxants and corticosteroids. Submitted to Chest.
1482. Decramer M, Lacquet LM, Fagard R, Rogiers P: Corticosteroids contribute to muscle weakness in chronic airflow obstruction. Am J Respir Crit Care Med 150:11, 1994.
1483. Smith AP: Patterns of recovery from acute severe asthma. Br J Dis Chest 75:132, 1981.
1484. Jenkins PF, Benfield GFA, Smith AP: Predicting recovery from acute severe asthma. Thorax 36:835, 1981.
1485. Centor RM, Yarbrough B, Wood JP: Inability to predict relapse in acute asthma. N Engl J Med 310:577, 1984.
1486. Fischl MA, Pitchenik A, Gardner LB: An index predicting relapse and need for hospitalization in patients with acute bronchial asthma. N Engl J Med 305:783, 1981.
1487. Benfield GFA, Smith AP: Predicting rapid and slow response to treatment in acute severe asthma. Br J Dis Chest 77:249, 1983.
1488. Williams Tj, Tuxen DV, Scheinkestel CD: Risk factors for morbidity in mechanically ventilated patients with acute severe asthma. Am Rev Respir Dis 146:607, 1992.
1489. Marquette CH, Saulnier F, Leroy O, et al: Long-term prognosis of near-fatal asthma. A six (6)-year follow-up study of 145 asthmatic patients who underwent mechanical ventilation for a near-fatal attack of asthma. Am Rev Respir Dis 146:76, 1992.
1490. McNichol KN, Williams HE: Spectrum of asthma in children. I. Clinical and physiological components. BMJ 4:7, 1973.
1491. Roorda RJ: Prognostic factors for the outcome of childhood asthma in adolescence. Thorax 51:S7, 1996.
1492. Jenkins MA, Hopper JL, Bowes G, et al: Factors in childhood as predictors of asthma in adult life. BMJ 309:90, 1994.
1493. Strachan DP, Anderson HR, Limb ES, et al: A national survey of asthma prevalence, severity and treatment in Great Britain. Arch Dis Child 30:174, 1994.
1494. Mazon A, Nieto A, Javier Nieto F, et al: Prognostic factors in childhood asthma: A logistic regression analysis. Ann Allergy 72:455, 1994.
1495. Ogilvie AG: Asthma: A study in prognosis of 1,000 patients. Thorax 17:183, 1962.
1496. Blackhall MI: Effect of age on fixed and labile components of airway resistance in asthma. Thorax 26:325, 1971.
1497. Withers NJ, Low L, Holgate ST, et al: The natural history of respiratory symptoms in a cohort of adolescents. Am J Respir Crit Care Med 158:352, 1998.
1498. Rackemann FN, Edwards MC: Asthma in children. A follow-up study of 688 patients after an interval of twenty years. N Engl J Med 246:815, 1952.
1499. Rackemann FN, Edwards MC: Asthma in children. A follow-up study of 688 patients after an interval of twenty years (concluded). N Engl J Med 246:858, 1952.
1500. Cserhati E, Mezei G, Kelemen J: Late prognosis of bronchial asthma in children. Respiration 46:160, 1984.
1501. Strachan D, Gerritsen J: Long-term outcome of early childhood wheezing: Population data. Eur Respir J Suppl 21:42S, 1996.
1502. Radford PJ, Hopp RJ, Biven RE, et al: Longitudinal changes in bronchial hyperresponsiveness in asthmatic and previous asthmatic children. Chest 101:624, 1992.

1503. Boulet LP, Turcotte H, Brochu A: Persistence of airway obstruction and hyper-responsiveness in subjects with asthma remission. Chest 105:1024, 1994.

1504. Hide DW: Strategies for the prevention of atopic asthma. Pediatr Allergy Immunol 7:117, 1996.

1505. Eriksson NE, Holmen A: Skin prick tests with standardized extracts of inhalant allergens in 7099 adult patients with asthma or rhinitis: Cross-sensitizations and relationships to age, sex, month of birth and year of testing. J Invest Allergol Clin Immunol 6:36, 1996.

1506. Arshad SH, Matthews S, Gant C, Hide DW: Effect of allergen avoidance on development of allergic disorders in infancy. Lancelot 339:1493, 1992.

1507. Hide DW, Matthews S, Matthews L, et al: Effect of allergen avoidance in infancy on allergic manifestations at age two years. J Allergy Clin Immunol 93:842, 1994.

1508. Hide DW, Matthews S, Tariq S, Arshad SH: Allergen avoidance in infancy and allergy at four years of age. Allergy 51:89, 1996.

1509. van Essen-Zandvliet EE, Hughes MD, Waalkens HJ, et al: Remission of childhood asthma after long-term treatment with an inhaled corticosteroid (budesonide): Can it be achieved? Eur Respir J 7:63, 1994.

1510. Brown PJ, Greville HW, Finucane KE: Asthma and irreversible airflow obstruction. Thorax 39:131, 1984.

1511. Peat JK, Woolcock AJ, Cullen K: Rate of decline of lung function in subjects with asthma. Eur J Respir Dis 70:171, 1986.

1512. Ulrik CS, Lange P: Decline of lung function in adults with bronchial asthma. Am J Respir Crit Care 150:629, 1994.

1513. Gauldie J, Jordana M, Cox G, et al: Fibroblasts and other structural cells in airway inflammation. Am Rev Respir Dis 145:S14, 1992.

1514. Boulet LP, Chakir J, Dube J, et al: Airway inflammation and structural changes in airway hyperresponsiveness and asthma: And overview. Can Respir J 5:16, 1998.

1515. Alexander HL: A historical account of death from asthma. J Allergy 34:305, 1963.

1516. Jenkins MA, Hurley SF, Jolley DJ, et al: Trends in Australian mortality of asthma, 1979–1985. Med J Aust 149:620, 1988.

1517. Burney PG: Asthma mortality in England and Wales: Evidence for a further increase, 1974–84. Lancet 2:323, 1986.

1518. Nakamura Y, Lbarthe DR: Secular trends in mortality from asthma in Japan, 1979–1988: Comparison with the United States. Int J Epidemiol 23:143, 1994.

1519. Paulozzi LJ, Coleman JJ, Buist AS: A recent increase in asthma mortality in the northwestern United States. Ann Allergy 56:392, 1986.

1520. Evans R, Mullally DI, Wilson RW, et al: National trends in the morbidity and mortality of asthma in the U.S. Prevalence, hospitalization and death from asthma over two decades: 1965–1984. Chest 91 (Suppl 6):65S, 1987.

1521. Sly RM: Mortality from asthma, 1979–1984. J Allergy Clin Immunol 82:705, 1988.

1522. Beasley R, Pearce N, Crane J: International trends in asthma mortality. Ciba Found Symp 206:140, 1997.

1523. Crane J, Pearce NE, Burgess CD, Beasley R: Asthma deaths. Asthma 1:49, 1997.

1524. Sly RM, O'Donnell R: Stabilization of asthma mortality. Ann Allergy Asthma Immunol 78:347, 1997.

1525. Sly RM: Changing asthma mortality. Ann Allergy 73:259, 1994.

1526. Garrett J, Kolbe J, Richards G, et al: Major reduction in asthma morbidity and continued reduction in asthma mortality in New Zealand: What lessons have been learned? Thorax 50:303, 1995.

1527. Stolley PD: Asthma mortality. Why the United States was spared an epidemic of deaths due to asthma. Am Rev Respir Dis 105:883, 1972.

1528. Speizer FE, Doll R: A century of asthma deaths in young people. BMJ 3:245, 1968.

1529. Speizer FE, Doll R, Heaf P: Observations on recent increase in mortality from asthma. BMJ 1:335, 1968.

1530. Speizer FE, Doll R, Heaf P, et al: Investigation into use of drugs preceding death from asthma. BMJ 1:339, 1968.

1531. Asthma deaths: A question answered. BMJ 4:443, 1972.

1532. Stableforth DE: Death from asthma. Thorax 38:801, 1983.

1533. Stewart CJ, Nunn AJ: Are asthma mortality rates changing? Br J Dis Chest 79:229, 1985.

1534. Bateman JRM, Clarke SW: Sudden death in asthma. Thorax 34:40, 1979.

1535. Sears MR, Rea HH, Beaglehole R, et al: Asthma mortality in New Zealand: A two year national study. N Z Med J 98:271, 1985.

1536. Sutherland DC, Beaglehole R, Fenwick J, et al: Death from asthma in Auckland: Circumstances and validation of causes. N Z Med J 97:845, 1984.

1537. Sears MR: Why are deaths from asthma increasing? Eur J Respir Dis 147(Suppl):175, 1984.

1538. Crane J, Pearce N, Flatt A, et al: Prescribed fenoterol and death from asthma in New Zealand, 1981–83: Case control study. Lancet 39:917, 1989.

1539. Fenoterol and death from asthma in New Zealand, 1977–1981: A new case control design. J Clin Res Pharmacoepidemiol 4:142, 1990.

1540. Grainger J, Woodman K, Pearce N, et al: Prescribed fenoterol and death from asthma in New Zealand 1981–7: A further case-control study. Thorax 46:105, 1991.

1541. Burgess C, Pearce N, Thiruchelvam R, et al: Prescribed drug therapy and near-fatal asthma attacks. Eur Resp J 7:498, 1994.

1542. Sears MR, Taylor DR, Print CC, et al: Regular inhaled β-agonist treatment in bronchial asthma. Lancet 336:1391, 1990.

1543. Spitzer WO, Suissa S, Ernst P, et al: Asthma death and near-fatal asthma in relation to β-agonist use. N Engl J Med 326:501, 1992.

1544. Suissa S, Ernst P, Spitzer WO: Beta-agonist use and death from asthma (letter). JAMA 271:821, 1994.

1545. Suissa S, Ernst P, Boivin JF, et al: A cohort analysis of excess mortality in asthma and the use of inhaled beta-agonists. Am J Respir Crit Care Med 149:604, 1994.

1546. Mullen ML, Mullen B, Carey M: The association between β-agonist use and death from asthma. A meta-analytic integration of case-control studies. JAMA 270:1842, 1993.

1547. Drazen JM, Israel E, Boushey HA, et al: Comparison of regularly scheduled with as-needed use of albuterol in mild asthma. N Engl J Med 335:841, 1996.

1548. Bai TR: β₂ adrenergic receptors in asthma: A current perspective. Lung 170:125, 1992.

1549. Brink C: Tolerance of guinea pig airway muscle preparations to relaxant agonists induced by chronic exposure to isoprenaline in vivo. Br J Pharmacol 73:13, 1981.

1550. Whicker SD, Black JL: β-receptor desensitization in human airway tissue preparations. Am Rev Respir Dis 143:A429, 1991.

1551. Giannini D, Carletti A, Dente FL, et al: Tolerance to the protective effect of salmeterol on allergen challenge. Chest 110:1452, 1996.

1552. Kozlik-Feldmann R, von Berg A, Berdel D, Reinhardt D: Long-term effects of formoterol and salbutamol on bronchial hyperreactivity and beta-adrenoceptor density on lymphocytes in children with bronchial asthma. Eur J Med Res 1:465, 1996.

1553. Fedyk ER, Adawi A, Looney RJ, Phipps RP: Regulation of IgE and cytokine production by cAMP: Implications for extrinsic asthma. Clin Immunol Immunopathol 81:101, 1996.

1554. Taylor DR, Sears MR, Cockcroft DW: The beta-agonist controversy. Med Clin North Am 80:719, 1996.

1555. Woolcock A, Lundback BO, Ringdal N, Jacques LA: Comparison of addition of salmeterol to inhaled steroids with doubling of the dose of inhaled steroids. Am J Respir Crit Care Med 153:1481, 1996.

1556. D'Alonzo GE, Nathan RA, Henochowicz S, et al: Salmeterol xinafoate as maintenance therapy compared with albuterol in patients with asthma. JAMA 271:1412, 1994.

1557. Ehrlich RI, Bourne DE: Asthma deaths among coloured and white South Africans: 1962 to 1988. Respir Med 88:195, 1994.

1558. Carter-Pokras OD, Gergen PJ: Reported asthma among Puerto Rican, Mexican-American and Cuban children, 1982–1984. Am J Public Health 83:580, 1994.

1559. Lang DM: Trends in U.S. asthma mortality: Good news and bad news (editorial: comment). Ann Allergy Asthma Immunol 78:333, 1997.

1560. McFadden ER Jr, Warren EL: Observations on asthma mortality. Ann Intern Med 127:142, 1997.

1561. Picado C, Montserrat JM, Roca J, et al: Mechanical ventilation in severe exacerbation of asthma. Study of 26 cases with six deaths. Eur J Respir Dis 64:102, 1983.

1562. Sears MR, Rea HH, Fenwick J: Deaths from asthma in New Zealand. Arch Dis Child 61:6, 1986.

1563. Strunk RC, Mrazek DA, Fuhrmann GS, et al: Physiologic and psychological characteristics associated with deaths due to asthma in childhood. A case-controlled study. JAMA 254:1193, 1985.

1564. Eason J, Markowe HL: Controlled investigation of deaths from asthma in hospitals in the North East Thames region. BMJ 294:1255, 1987.

1565. Sears MR, Rea HH, Fenwick J, et al: 75 deaths in asthmatics prescribed home nebulizers. BMJ 294:477, 1987.

1566. FitzGerald JM, Macklem PT: Fatal asthma. Annu Rev Med 47:161, 1996.

1567. Rea HH, Sears MR, Beaglehole R, et al: Lessons from the national asthma mortality study: Circumstances surrounding death. N Z Med J 100:10, 1987.

1568. Kikuchi Y, Okabe S, Tamra G, et al: Chemosensitivity and perception of dyspnea in patients with a history of near fatal asthma. N Engl J Med 330:1329, 1994.

1569. Gibson GJ: Perception, personality, and respiratory control in life-threatening asthma. Thorax 50 (Suppl 1):S2, 1995.

1570. Boulet LP, Chapman K, Green L, FitzGerald JM: Asthma education. Chest 106:184S, 1994.

1571. Car W, Zeitel L, Weiss K: Variations in asthma hospitalizations and deaths in New York City. Am J Public Health 82:59, 1994.

1572. Turner MO, Crump S, Contreras GR, et al: A prospective evaluation of risk factors for near-fatal asthma: Clinical characteristics. Am J Respir Crit Care Med 149:514A, 1994.

1573. Pouw EM, Koeter GH, de Monchy JG, et al: Clinical assessment after a life-threatening attack of asthma; the role of bronchial hyperreactivity. Eur Respir J 3:861, 1990.

1574. O'Hallaren NT, Yuninger JW, Offoert KP, et al: Exposure to an aero-allergen as a possible precipitating factor in respiratory arrest in young patients with asthma. N Engl J Med 324:285, 1991.

1575. Anto JM, Sunyer J, Rodriguez-Roisin R, et al: Community outbreaks of asthma associated with inhalation of soybean dust. N Engl J Med 320:502, 1989.

1576. Petry RW, Voss MJ, Kroutil LA, et al: Monkey dander asthma. J Allergy Clin Immunol 75:268, 1985.

1577. Jimenez Gomez I, Anton E, Picans I, Jerez J, Obispo T. Occupational asthma caused by mink urine. Allergy. 51:364–5, 1996.

1578. Bernaola G, Echechipia S, Urrutia I, Fernandez E, Audicana M, Fernandez de Corres L. Occupational asthma and rhinoconjunctivitis from inhalation of dried cow's milk caused by sensitization to alpha-lactalbumin. Allergy. 49:189–91, 1994.

1579. Ylonen J, Mantyjarvi R, Taivainen A, Virtanen T. IgG and IgE antibody responses to cow dander and urine in farmers with cow-induced asthma. Clin Exp Allergy. 22:83–90, 1992.

1580. Brennan NJ. Pig Butcher's asthma: case report and review of the literature. Irsih Med J. 78:321–322, 1985.

1581. Armentia A, Martin-Santos J, Subiza J, et al. Occupational asthma due to frogs. Ann Allergy. 60:209–210, 1988.

1582. Bar-Sela S, Teichtahl H, Lutsky I. Occupational asthma in poultry workers. J allergy Clin Immunol. 73:271–275, 1984.

1583. Olaguibel JM, Hernandez D, Morales P, Peris A, Basina A. Occupational asthma caused by inhalation of casein. Allergy 45:306–308, 1990.

1584. Lusky I, Teichtahl H, Bar-Sela S: Occupational asthma due to poultry mites. J Allergy Clin Immunol 73:56, 1984.

1585. Burge SB, Hendy M, Hodgson ES: Occupational asthma, rhinitis, and dermatitis due to tetrazene in a detonator manufacturer. Thorax 39:470, 1984.

1586. Van Hage-Hamsten HI, Johansson SS, Höglund S, et al: Storage site allergy is common in a farming population. Clin Allergy 15:555, 1985.

1587. Spieksma FT, Vooren PH, Kramps JA, et al: Respiratory allergy to laboratory fruit flies (*Drosophila melanogaster*). J Allergy Clin Immunol 77:108, 1986.

1588. Kino T, Oshima S: Allergy to insects in Japan. 1. Reaginic sensitivity to moth and butterfly in patients with bronchial asthma. J Allergy Clin Immunol 61:10, 1978.

1589. Kaufman GL, Baldo BA, Tovey ER, et al: Inhalant allergy following occupational exposure to blowflies. Clin Allergy 16:65, 1986.

1590. Gold B, Mathews K, Burge H: Occupational asthma caused by sewer flies. Am Rev Respir Dis 131:949, 1985.

1591. Ostrom NK, Swanson MC, Agarwal MK, et al: Occupational allergy to honeybee-body dust in a honey-processing plant. J Allergy Clin Immunol 77:736, 1986.

1592. Prichard M, Turner KJ: Acute hypersensitivity to ingested processed pollen. Aust N Z J Med 15:346, 1985.

1593. Quirce S, Cuevas M, Olaguibel JM, Tabar AI. Occupational asthma and immunologic responses induced by inhaled carmine among employees at a factory making natural dyes. J Allergy Clin Immunol 93 (1 Pt):44–52, 1994.

1594. Delgado J, Gomez E, Palma JL, Gonzalez J, Monteserin FJ, Martinez A, Martinez J. Occupational rhinoconjuctivitis and asthma caused by *Tetranychus urticae* (red spider mite). A case report. Clin Exp Allergy 24:477–80, 1994.

1595. Lugo G, Cipolla C, Bonfiglioli R, Sassi C, Maini S, Cancellieri MP, Raffi GB, Pisi E. A new risk of ocupational disease: allergic asthma and rhinoconjunctivitis in persons working with beneficial arthropods. Preliminary data. Int Arch Occup Environ Health 65:291, 1994.

1596. Kaufman GL, Gandevia BH, Bellas TE, Tovey ER, Baldo BA. Occupational allergy in an entomological research centre. I. Clinical aspects of reaction to the sheep blowfly (*Lucilia cuprina*). Br J Ind Med. 46:473–478, 1989.

1597. Meister W. Professional asthma owing to Daphnia allergy. Allerg Immunol (Leipz). 24:191–193, 1978.

1598. Michel FB, Guin JJ, Seignalet C, et al. Allergie à Panonychus ulmi (Koch). Rev Fr Allergol. 17:93–97, 1977.

1599. Spieksma FTM, Vooren Ph, Kramps JA, Dijkman JH. Respiratory allergy to laboratory fruit flies (*Drosophila melanogaster*). J Allergy Clin Immunol. 77:108–113, 1986.

1600. Wittich FW. Allergic rhinitis and asthma due to sensitization to the Mexican bean weevil (*Zabrotes subfastiatus* boh.). J Allergy. 12:42–45, 1940.

1601. Malo J-L, Cartier A, Ghezzo H, et al: Patterns of improvement in spirometry, bronchial hyperresponsiveness, and specific IgE antibody levels after cessation of exposure in occupational asthma caused by snow-crab processing. Am Rev Respir Dis 138:807, 1988.

1602. Prichard MG, Ryan G, Walsh BJ, et al: Skin test and RAST responses to wheat and common allergens and respiratory disease in bakers. Clin Allergy 15:203, 1985.

1603. Osterman K, Johansson SGO, Zetterström O: Diagnostic tests in allergy to green coffee. Allergy 40:336, 1985.

1604. Karr RM, Lehrer SB, Butcher BT, et al: Coffee workers asthma—a clinical appraisal using radioallergosorbent test. J Allergy Clin Immunol 62:143, 1978.

1605. Topping MD, Henderson TRS, Luczynska CM, et al: Castor bean allergy among workers in the felt industry. Allergy 37:603, 1982.

1606. Davison AG, Britton MG, Forrester JA, et al: Asthma in merchant seamen and laboratory workers caused by allergy to castor beans: Analysis of allergens. Clin Allergy 13:553, 1983.

1607. Twiggs JT, Yunginger JW, Agarwal MK, et al: Occupational asthma in a florist caused by the dried plant, baby's breath. J Allergy Clin Immunol 69:49, 1982.

1608. Falleroni AE, Zeiss CR, Levitz D: Occupational asthma secondary to inhalation of garlic dust. J Allergy Clin Immunol 68:156, 1981.

1609. Lybarger JA, Gallagher JS, Pulver SW: Occupational asthma induced by inhalation and ingestion of garlic. J Allergy Clin Immunol 69:448, 1982.

1610. van Toorenenbergen AW, Dieges PH: Immunoglobulin E antibodies against coriander and other spices. J Allergy Clin Immunol 76:477, 1985.

1611. Davidson AE, Passero MA, Settipane GA. Buckwheat-induced anaphylaxis: a case report. Annals of Allergy. 69:439–40, 1992.

1612. Perfetti L, Lehrer SB, McCants M, Malo JL. Occupational asthma caused by cacao. Allergy. 52:778–80, 1997.

1613. Cohen AJ, Forse MS, Tarlo SM. Occupational asthma caused by pectin inhalation during the manufacture of jam. Chest. 103:309–11, 1993.

1614. Shirai T, Sato A, Hara Y. Epigallocatechin gallate. The major causative agent of green tea-induced asthma. Chest. 106:1801–5, 1994.

1615. Lavaud F, Perdu D, Prevost A, Vallerand H, Cossart C, Passemsard F. Bakers's asthma related to soybean lecithin exposure. Allergy. 49:159–62, 1994.

1616. Subiza J, Subiza JL, Escribano PM, Hinojosa M, Garcia R, Jerez M, Subiza E. Occupational asthma caused by Brazil ginseng dust. J Allergy Clin Immunol 88:731, 1991.

1617. Cartier A, Malo JL, Pineau L, et al: Occupational asthma due to pepsin. J Allergy Clin Immunol 73:574, 1984.

1618. Muir DC, Verrall AB, Julian JA, Millman JM, Beaudin MA, Dolovich J. Occupational sensitization to lactase. Am J Ind Med 31:570, 1997.

1619. Lemiere C, Cartier A, Dolovich J, Malo JL. Isolated late asthmatic reaction after exposure to a high-molecular-weight occupational agent, subtilisin. Chest 110:823, 1996.

1620. Joliat TL, Weber RW. Occupational asthma and rhinoconjunctivitis from inhalation of crystalline bovine serum albumin powder. Ann Allergy 66:301, 1991.

1621. Marks GB, Salome CM, Woolcock AJ. Asthma and allergy associated with occupational exposure to ispaghula and senna products in a pharmaceutical work force. Am Rev Respir Dis 144:1065, 1991.

1622. Lambourn EM, Hayes JP, McAllister WA, Taylor A J. Occupational asthma due to EPO 60. Br J Ind Med 49:294, 1992.

1623. Kleine-Tebbe J, Wahl R, Dierks K, Kunkel G. IgE-mediated inhalant allergy against human corticotropin-releasing hormone. Int Arch Allergy Appl Immunol 95:309, 1991.

1624. Losada E, Hinojosa M, Moneo I, et al: Occupational asthma caused by cellulase. J Allergy Clin Immunol 77:635, 1986.

1625. Piirila P, Estlander T, Hytonen M, Keskinen H, Tupasela O, Tuppurainen M. Rhinitis caused by ninhydrin develops into occupational asthma. Eur Respir J 10:1918, 1997.

1626. Moller DR, Gallagher JS, Bernstein DI, et al: Detection of IgE-mediated respiratory sensitization in workers exposed to hexahydrophthalic anhydride. J Allergy Clin Immunol 75:663, 1985.

1627. Meadway J: Asthma and atopy in workers with an epoxy adhesive. Br J Dis Chest 74:149, 1980.

1628. Howe W, Venables KM, Topping MD, et al: Tetrachlorophthalic anhydride asthma—Evidence for specific IgE antibody. J Allergy Clin Immunol 71:5, 1983.

1629. Harries MG, Sherwood Burge P, et al: Isocyanate asthma: Respiratory symptoms due to 1,5-naphthylene di-isocyanate. Thorax 34:762, 1979.

1630. Tse KS, Johnson A, Chan H, et al: A study of serum antibody activity in workers with occupational exposure to diphenylmethane diisocyanate. Allergy 40:314, 1985.

1631. Butcher BT, Karr RM, O'Neill CE, et al: Inhalation challenge and pharmacologic studies of toluene diisocyanate (TDI)-sensitive work. J Allergy Clin Immunol 64:146, 1979.

1632. Zammit-Tabona M, Sherkin M, Kijek K, et al: Asthma caused by diphenylmethane diisocyanate in foundry workers—clinical, bronchial provocation, and immunologic studies. Am Rev Respir Dis 128:226, 1983.

1633. Venables KM, Dally MB, Burge PS, et al: Occupational asthma in a steel coating plant. Br J Intern Med 42:517, 1985.

1634. Alexandersson R, Gustafsson P, Hedenstierna G, et al: Exposure to naphthalene-diisocyanate in a rubber plant: Symptoms and lung function. Arch Environ Health 41:85, 1986.

1635. Bush RK, Yunginger JW, Reed CE: Asthma due to African zebra wood (*Microberlinia*) dust. Am Rev Respir Dis 117:601, 1978.

1636. Lung disease in dental laboratory technicians. Lancet 1:1200, 1985.

1637. Sorić M, Godnić-Cyar J, Gomzi M, et al: The role of atopy in potroom workers' asthma. Am J Intern Med 9:239, 1986.

1638. Gheysens B, Auwerx J, Van den Eeckhout A, et al: Cobalt-induced bronchial asthma in diamond polishers. Chest 88:740, 1985.

1639. Ulinski S, Palczynski C, Gorski P. Occupational rhinitis and bronchial asthma due to morphine: evidence from inhalational and nasal challenges. Allergy. 51:914–8, 1996.

1640. Perrin B, Malo JL, Cartier A, et al: Occupational asthma in a pharmaceutical worker exposed to hydralazine. Thorax 45:980, 1990.

1641. Seaton A. Ipecacuanha asthma: an old lesson. Thorax 45:974, 1990.

1642. Agius RM, Davison AG, Hawkins ER, et al: Occupational asthma in salbutamol process workers. Occup Environ Med 51:397, 1994.

1643. Stenton SC, Dennis JH, Hendrick DJ. Occupational asthma due to ceftazidime. Eur Respir J 8:1421, 1995.

1644. Moscato G, Galdi E, Scibilia J, et al: Occupational asthma, rhinitis and urticaria due to piperacillin sodium in a pharmaceutical worker. Eur Respir J 8:467, 1995.

1645. Lundgren R, Soderberg M, Rosenhall L, et al: Development of increased airway responsiveness in two nurses performing methacholine and histamine challenge tests. Allergy 47:188, 1992.

1646. Savonius B, Keskinen H, Tuppurainen M, et al: Occupational asthma caused by ethanolamines. Allergy 49:877, 1994.

1647. Blainey AD, Ollier S, Cundell D, et al: Occupational asthma in a hairdressing salon. Thorax 41:42, 1986.

1648. Parra FM, Igea JM, Quirce S, et al: Occupational asthma in a hairdresser caused by persulphate salts. Allergy 47:656, 1992.

1649. Ng TP, Lee HS, Lee FY, et al: Occupational asthma due to ethylene diamine. Ann Acad Med Singapore 20:399, 1991.

1650. Malo JL, Pineau L, Cartier A: Occupational asthma due to azobisformamide. Clin Allergy 15:261, 1985.

1651. Graham VAL, Coe MJS, Davies RJ: Occupational asthma after exposure to a diazonium salt. Thorax 36:950, 1981.

1652. Corrado OJ, Osman J, Davies RJ: Asthma and rhinitis after exposure to glutaraldehyde in endoscopy units. Hum Toxicol 5:325, 1986.

1653. Cockcroft DW, Cartier A, Jones G, et al: Asthma caused by occupational exposure to a furan-based binder system. J Allergy Clin Immunol 66:458, 1980.

1654. Baser ME, Tockman MS, Kennedy TP: Pulmonary function and respiratory symptoms in polyvinylchloride fabrication workers. Am Rev Respir Dis 131:203, 1985.

1655. Robertson AS, Weir DC, Burge PS: Occupational asthma due to oil mists. Thorax 43:200, 1988.

1656. Choudat D, Neukirch F, Brochard P, et al: Allergy and occupational exposure to hydroquinone and to methionine. Br J Ind Med 45:376, 1988.

1657. Musk AW, Peach S, Ryan G: Occupational asthma in a mineral analysis laboratory. Br J Ind Med 45:381, 1988.

1658. Bourke SJ, Convery RP, Stenton SC, et al: Occupational asthma in an isothiazolinone manufacturing plant. Thorax 52:746, 1997.

1659. Piirila P, Estlander T, Keskinen H, et al: Occupational asthma caused by triglycidyl isocyanurate (TGIC). Clin Exp Allergy 27:510, 1997.

1660. Moscato G, Omodeo P, Dellabianca A, et al: Occupational asthma and rhinitis caused by 1,2-benzisothiazolin-3-one in a chemical worker. Occup Med 47:249, 1997.

1661. Burge PS, Richardson MN: Occupational asthma due to indirect exposure to lauryl dimethyl benzyl ammonium chloride used in a floor cleaner. Thorax 49:842, 1994.

1662. Ferguson H, Thomas KE, Ollier S, et al: Bronchial provocation testing of sodium isononanoyl oxybenzene sulphonate. Hum Exp Toxicol 9:83, 1990.

1663. Hayes JP, Lambourn L, Hopkirk JA, et al: Occupational asthma due to styrene. Thorax 46:396, 1991.

1664. Nilsson R, Nordlinder R, Wass U, et al: Asthma, rhinitis, and dermatitis in workers exposed to reactive dyes. Br J Ind Med 50:65, 1993.

1665. Romano C, Sulotto F, Pavan I, et al: A new case of occupational asthma from reactive dyes with severe anaphylactic response to the specific challenge. Am J Ind Med 21:209, 1992.

1666. Miller ME, Lummus ZL, Bernstein DI: Occupational asthma caused by FD&C blue dye no. 2. Allergy Asthma Proc 17:31, 1996.

1667. Bernstein JA, Stauder T, Bernstein DI, et al: A combined respiratory and cutaneous hypersensitivity syndrome induced by work exposure to quaternary amines. J Allergy Clin Immunol 94:257, 1994.

1668. Ng TP, Lee HS, Malik MA, et al: Asthma in chemical workers exposed to aliphatic polyamines. Occup Med 45:45, 1995.

1669. Aleva RM, Aalbers R, Koeter GH, et al: Occupational asthma caused by a hardener containing an aliphatic and a cycloaliphatic diamine. Am Rev Respir Dis 45:1217, 1992.

1670. Honda I, Kohrogi H, Ando M, et al: Occupational asthma induced by the fungicide tetrachloroisophthalonitrile. Thorax 47:760, 1992.

1671. Royce S, Wald P, Sheppard D, et al: Occupational asthma in a pesticides manufacturing worker. Chest 103:295, 1993.

1672. Shelton D, Urch B, Tarlo SM: Occupational asthma induced by a carpet fungicide—tributyl tin oxide. J Allergy Clin Immunol 90:274, 1992.

1673. Lozewicz S, Davison AG, Hopkirk A, et al: Occupational asthma due to methyl methacrylate and cyanoacrylates. Thorax 40:836, 1985.

1674. Savonius B, Keskinen H, Tuppurainen M, et al: Occupational respiratory disease caused by acrylates. Clin Exp Allergy 23:416, 1993.

1675. Chan CC, Cheong TH, Lee HS, et al: Case of occupational asthma due to glue containing cyanoacrylate. Ann Acad Med Singapore 23:731, 1994.

1676. Lee HS, Chan CC, Tan KT, et al: Burnisher's asthma—a case due to ammonia from silverware polishing. Singapore Med J 34:565, 1993.

1677. Cartier A, Vandenplas O, Grammer LC, et al: Respiratory and systemic reaction following exposure to heated electrostatic polyester paint. Eur Respir J 7:608, 1994.

1678. Malo JL, Cartier A, Pineault L, et al: Occupational asthma due to heated polypropylene. Eur Respir J 7:415, 1994.

1679. Kanerva L, Keskinen H, Autio P, et al: Occupational respiratory and skin sensitization caused by polyfunctional aziridine hardener. Clin Exp Allergy 25:432, 1995.

1680. Malo JL, Cartier A, Desjardins A: Occupational asthma caused by dry metabisulphite. Thorax 50:585; discussion 589, 1995.

1681. Palczynski C, Jakubowski J, Gorski P: Reactive airways dysfunction syndrome. International J Occup Med Environ Health 7:113, 1994.

1682. Deschamps D, Rosenberg N, Soler P, et al: Persistent asthma after accidental exposure to ethylene oxide. Br J Ind Med 49:523, 1992.

1683. Gadon ME, Melius JM, McDonald GJ, et al: New-onset asthma after exposure to the steam system additive 2-diethylaminoethanol. A descriptive study. J Occup Med 36:623, 1994.

1684. Langley RL: Fume fever and reactive airways dysfunction syndrome in a welder. South Med J 84:1034, 1991.

1685. Deschamps D, Soler P, Rosenberg N, et al: Persistent asthma after inhalation of a mixture of sodium hypochlorite and hydrochloric acid. Chest 105:1895, 1994.

1686. Cone JE, Wugofski L, Balmes JR, et al: Persistent respiratory health effects after a metam sodium pesticide spill. Chest 106:500, 1994.

1687. Rajan KG, Davies BH: Reversible airways obstruction and interstitial pneumonitis due to acetic acid. Br J Ind Med 46:67, 1989.

1688. Murphy D, Fairman R, Lapp NL, et al: Severe airways disease due to the inhalation of fumes from cleaning agents. Chest 69:372, 1976.

1689. Kennedy SM, Enarson DA, Janssen RG, et al: Lung health consequences of reported accidental chlorine gas exposures among pulpmill workers. Am Rev Respir Dis 143:74, 1991.

1690. Henneberger PK, Ferris BG Jr, Sheehe PR: Accidental gassing incidents and the pulmonary function of pulp mill workers. Am Rev Respir Dis 148:63, 1993.

1691. Burns MJ, Linden CH: Another hot tub hazard. Toxicity secondary to bromine and hydrobromic acid exposure. Chest 111:816, 1997.

# Chronic Obstructive Pulmonary Disease

Chronic respiratory disease related to cigarette smoking has had an enormous impact on society in this century. Between 1950 and 1970, the death rates for obstructive respiratory disease doubled every 5 years.[1] In the United States, the age-adjusted mortality plateaued for men between 1979 and 1993 but increased 126% for women.[2, 3] These increases are particularly striking, considering the overall decline in death rates and in deaths from heart disease over the same time period.[4] In the United States, chronic obstructive pulmonary disease (COPD) represents the fifth most important cause of death, killing more Americans than does diabetes mellitus.[5] Worldwide, COPD has been ranked as the 12th leading cause of disability-adjusted life years and has been projected to increase to the 5th most important contributor by 2020.[6] As might be expected from these figures, COPD also has an important economic impact: there is good evidence that it constitutes one of the most important causes of work incapacity and restricted activity in both the United States and the United Kingdom.[7]

The definition of "chronic obstructive lung disease" remains controversial. In earlier editions of this book, chronic bronchitis and emphysema were discussed separately, because each was thought to contribute to the development of COPD. Although chronic bronchitis is a clinical diagnosis based on excessive mucus secretion, it was believed that mucus hypersecretion was associated with airway narrowing in some patients. However, the results of the classic follow-up study by Peto and associates suggested that there was little, if any, connection between coughing and sputum production and the eventual development of air-flow obstruction.[8] In this investigation, 2,718 men were studied by questionnaire and spirometry over a 20-year period. During this time, there were 104 deaths from respiratory failure and 103 from pulmonary carcinoma. When adjusted for the initial value for the forced expiratory volume in 1 second (FEV$_1$), the clinical diagnosis of chronic bronchitis had no predictive value for death from COPD and only a weak predictive value for carcinoma. Stated simply, patients were just as likely to die from COPD whether or not they coughed and expectorated. On the other hand, initial FEV$_1$ values had a powerful predictive value for mortality; an initial FEV$_1$ two standard deviations below predicted normal was associated with a 52-fold risk of death from COPD, and a value between one and two standard deviations below normal was accompanied by a 20-fold increased risk (Fig. 55–1).

In another long-term follow-up study of men and women who smoked, initial values for the ratio of FEV$_1$ to forced vital capacity (FVC) (FEV$_1$/FVC) and for the mean forced expiratory flow at mid-FVC (FEF$_{25-75}$) were found to be the best predictors of longitudinal decline in lung function in men.[9] The results of these studies have been challenged by those of a large study from Denmark comprising 13,756 men and women and spanning a period of 10 years, during which there were 2,288 deaths;[10] although the initial FEV$_1$ value was the most powerful predictor of death from obstructive lung disease, mucus hypersecretion was also a significant predictor and interacted with obstruction. Subsequent analyses of this cohort have confirmed that a clinical diagnosis of chronic bronchitis contributes to the predicted rate of decline in FEV$_1$ and to the risk for hospitalization and death from COPD.[11, 12] Despite these results we believe that chronic bronchitis should not be considered a part of the definition of COPD, because it can occur in the absence of airway obstruction.

Moreover, it is clear that chronic air-flow obstruction can develop in persons who never fulfill the criteria for chronic bronchitis; similarly, chronic cough and phlegm can persist for years without the development of air-flow obstruction. To further confuse matters, some patients develop significant emphysema with only minor degrees of air-flow obstruction[13] while others experience symptomatic air-flow obstruction in the absence of emphysema or loss of elastic recoil, suggesting that intrinsic airway narrowing is an important factor in some patients.[14]

The terminology of the latter form of disease has been the subject of some controversy.[15–19] One suggestion is that the term "chronic bronchitis" should be reserved for patients who have mucus hypersecretion and air-flow obstruction;[20] however, this leaves patients who have air-flow obstruction but no cough or phlegm production, and those who have cough and phlegm but no obstruction, without a diagnostic category. The division into chronic "simple" and "obstructive" forms of bronchitis is also unsatisfactory, because it is the bronchioles that are the main site of obstruction. "Small airway disease" was first suggested as the name for a specific clinical syndrome but does not communicate the basic functional derangement of obstruction.[21] "Chronic obstructive bronchiolitis" is perhaps the best descriptive label but could be confused with other specific and nonspecific forms

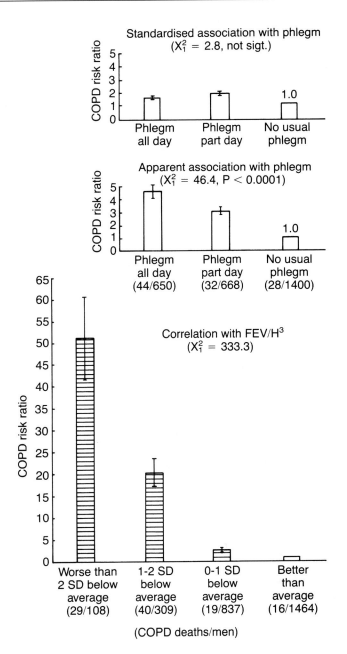

**Figure 55–1. Risk Factors for the Development of Chronic Obstructive Pulmonary Disease (COPD).** In a study of almost 3,000 men followed for 20 or more years to determine which factors predisposed to death from chronic obstructive pulmonary disease, the results as depicted in this graph showed that chronic cough and sputum production (standardized association with phlegm) did not increase risk but that the initial value for forced expiratory flow was strongly associated with subsequent death from COPD. Men in whom the initial FEV$_1$ was two standard deviations or more below the average value had a risk for death from COPD 52 times greater than those in whom the FEV$_1$ was equal to the average. (From Peto R, Speizer FE, Cochrane AL, et al: Am Rev Respir Dis 128:491, 1983.)

of bronchiolitis (*see* Chapter 58). The problems with precise definition have led to the suggestion that a term such as "chronic obstructive lung disease" (COLD), "chronic obstructive pulmonary disease" (COPD), or "chronic airflow obstruction" (CAO) be used to describe the disease in this group of patients.[16] Hypothesizing that asthma, emphysema, and chronic bronchitis are varied host manifestations of a single underlying disorder characterized by nonspecific bronchial hyper-responsiveness and atopy, a group of Dutch investigators has suggested combining these disorders under the term "chronic nonspecific lung disease" (CNSLD); however, this designation has not been generally applied.[22, 23] For the purposes of this text, the following definitions apply; they are similar to those suggested in an American Thoracic Society (ATS) statement on standards for the diagnosis of patients who have COPD.[24]

**Chronic Bronchitis.** In clinical practice, the diagnosis of chronic bronchitis is based on a history of excessive expectoration of mucus. Because standardization of the quantity of mucus produced is necessary in order to compare populations, quantitative (and somewhat arbitrary) estimates have been incorporated into the clinical definition—for example, one popular definition states that "expectoration must occur on most days during at least 3 consecutive months for not less than 2 consecutive years."[25] These criteria exclude patients who have a chronic dry cough, although direct questioning of many of these will elicit a history of expectoration of small amounts of sputum on arising in the morning or of swallowing of bronchial secretions. Questionnaires to be administered by interviewers have been developed by workers at the National Heart and Lung Institute (NHLI) and the British Medical Research Council (BMRC) for epidemiologic studies. Responses to these two questionnaires reveal very similar results and are reproducible. Slight modifications have been suggested for completion of the questionnaire without the use of an interviewer.[26]

All other causes of chronic coughing and expectoration must be eliminated before a diagnosis of chronic bronchitis is made clinically. In some cases, it may be difficult or impossible to differentiate the disease from asthma; however, the fact that asthma is characterized by airway narrowing that is relatively rapidly reversible either spontaneously or with treatment is of value in the differential diagnosis in the majority of patients. The term *asthmatic bronchitis* has been used to describe patients who fulfill the diagnostic criteria for both conditions.

Because the definition of chronic bronchitis given previously does not include air-flow obstruction,[27] and because chronic coughing and sputum production are not necessarily associated with the development of air-flow obstruction, the clinical usefulness of this diagnosis is limited. Clearly, the term *bronchitis* also implies airway inflammation, and in fact, the bronchial mucosa of patients who have chronic expectoration of mucus does show a more prominent cellular inflammatory infiltrate than that in the mucosa of smokers who do not have chronic cough and sputum production;[28, 29] however, the significance of this finding is uncertain.

**Emphysema.** Emphysema can be defined as abnormal permanent enlargement of air spaces distal to the terminal bronchioles, accompanied by destruction of their walls, without obvious fibrosis.[30] Inclusion of the last proviso is somewhat controversial, because it excludes irregular emphysema and some cases of paraseptal emphysema from the definition, and because centrilobular emphysema is commonly associated with microscopic foci of fibrosis. Irregular emphysema and paraseptal emphysema are often associated with local-

ized pulmonary injury such as pneumonia or with a chronic pulmonary disease such as sarcoidosis or silicosis; because the air-space enlargement in such cases is focal, an effect on pulmonary function is typically absent or minimal, and these conditions are not included under the "COPD umbrella."[17] Nevertheless, from a descriptive point of view, we believe it is appropriate to consider them as variants of emphysema. For the purposes of definition, it is also important to note that simple air-space enlargement can occur without tissue destruction, such as in Down's syndrome; such enlargement is not considered to be a form of emphysema.

Although strictly speaking, emphysema can be diagnosed only pathologically, certain alterations in pulmonary function and certain radiologic features allow its detection *in vivo* and an estimation of its severity. The use of CT in particular has allowed a fairly precise quantification of the extent of emphysema, although this modality is insensitive to minor degrees of alveolar destruction. In general, emphysema is accompanied by a loss of lung elastic recoil, which is thought to cause air-flow obstruction, hyperinflation, and gas trapping; however, as discussed farther on, loss of recoil can occur in the absence of emphysema.

**Chronic Obstructive Pulmonary Disease.** The diagnosis of chronic bronchitis is made on the basis of clinical history and emphysema on the basis of morphology. Although many patients who have COPD suffer from one or both of these disorders, COPD is characterized solely by functional abnormalities. It has been defined as "persistent, largely irreversible airway obstruction in which the underlying pathophysiology is not precisely known,"[16] or "a chronic, slowly progressive airway obstructive disorder resulting from some combination of pulmonary emphysema and irreversible reduction in the caliber of small airways in the lung."[31] To retain any usefulness, the term should exclude specific well-defined entities characterized by persistent obstruction, such as asthma, bronchiectasis, bronchiolitis, and cystic fibrosis.

Because irreversible airway obstruction cannot be easily attributed solely to loss of elastic recoil or airway narrowing in the vast majority of patients, use of the term *COPD* or its synonyms has increased. In fact, a combination of intrinsic airway narrowing and loss of lung elasticity coexists in most patients who have COPD. Synonyms for COPD include COLD, CAO, and chronic air-flow limitation (CAL). Although the first two are acceptable, CAL is misleading because it suggests that air-flow limitation is unique to this entity. In fact, everyone has maximal expiratory air-flow limitation; it is the severity of the limitation that is abnormal in COPD.

In the following pages, the epidemiology, etiology, pathogenesis, pathology, and clinical manifestations of COPD, rather than the separate entities of chronic bronchitis and emphysema, are discussed. When possible, the mechanisms and consequences of airway obstruction caused by intrinsic airway narrowing and those resulting from loss of elastic recoil are separated; we recognize that in many patients, separation is not possible. Because COPD, as defined, is characterized in functional terms and because the chest radiograph and CT scan reveal gross morphology, the approach taken in the radiology section is of necessity different; here, the characteristics of chronic bronchitis and emphysema are considered separately.

## EPIDEMIOLOGY

The confusion in terminology has led to difficulty in defining the incidence of COPD. In Great Britain, the combination of chronic cough and expectoration, dyspnea, and airflow obstruction was traditionally labeled "chronic bronchitis,"[32] whereas in North America, the tendency was to refer to this constellation of symptoms and functional impairment as "emphysema." Prior to the general acceptance of standard definitions and of the classification of COPD proposed in the CIBA symposium in 1952,[27] the use of these different terms gave the false impression that the death rate from so-called chronic bronchitis in England and Wales was approximately 40 times that in the United States.[33] In fact, subsequent epidemiologic studies showed that the incidence of the disease in England and Wales is very similar to that in the United States.[34] Misclassification of patients still occurs not infrequently. In a community study of 351 patients who received a new diagnosis of asthma, chronic bronchitis, or emphysema over an 8-year period, 45% had a prior or concomitant diagnosis of another obstructive pulmonary disease;[35] older men were more likely to be labeled with a diagnosis of emphysema, and younger women were more often called asthmatic.

Many of the studies of prevalence and incidence include patients who have a clinical diagnosis of chronic bronchitis based on cough and expectoration. However, because chronic bronchitis is not invariably associated with obstruction and because COPD can develop without cough and expectoration, many of these studies are of questionable significance. In the late 1980s, between 15% and 20% of middle-aged British men and 8% to 9% of women reported persistent cough and phlegm production.[36] The prevalence of these symptoms has been decreasing progressively in the United Kingdom and the United States in proportion to the decline in cigarette smoking. In a random sample of over 9,000 individuals from the United Kingdom conducted at approximately the same time as the previously mentioned study, approximately 10% of men and women had spirometric values two or more standard deviations below values predicted on the basis of age and height;[18] the percentage of abnormal values increased with increasing age.

Despite a change in the International Classification of Disease (ICD) coding of respiratory disease in 1978, the time trends in reported mortality rates for chronic lung diseases probably accurately reflect changes in the prevalence of COPD. In the United Kingdom, age-adjusted mortality rates for chronic respiratory diseases declined between the 1970s and 1990s in men, and between the 1950s and 1960s in women, although the rates in women may now be increasing again. In one study, the rate of decline was thought to be faster than can be explained by the decrease in cigarette smoking, suggesting that other factors may be affecting this relationship.[37] In Australia, age-adjusted mortality rates decreased about 5% between 1964 and 1990 in men;[38] however, over the same time period, there was a 2.6-fold increase among women. Similar decreases in men and increases in women have been reported for death from emphysema in the United States.[3] There is substantial variation both within and between countries in the rates of mortality from COPD that cannot be explained by differences in cigarette smoking or disease classification.[39–41]

Men have a significantly increased risk for the development of COPD,[42] a difference for which cigarette consumption is a major responsible factor.[43] However, retrospective and prospective studies designed to analyze risk factors for the development of COPD show that men are at increased risk even when adjustment is made for the amount smoked.[9, 44–49] Additional factors that could contribute to the gender differences include occupational pollution and method of cigarette smoking. For example, a propensity for the development of COPD is seen in cigarette smokers who have the habit of retaining the cigarette in the mouth between puffs[50] and in those who extinguish and re-light cigarettes,[51] behavioral characteristics that are more common in men. The results of studies comparing the natural history in men and in women have shown that the disease is more rapidly progressive and more severe in men.[9, 52–54]

COPD is generally more severe in white than in nonwhite cigarette smokers, a difference that cannot be explained by the amount or duration of cigarette smoking or by whether or not smoke is inhaled.[55, 56] Individuals of African American heritage also have been reported to be less susceptible than other ethnic groups to the emphysema-producing effect of cigarette smoking.[57] Alcoholics[58] and patients who have coronary artery disease[59] are particularly prone to the development of COPD, a propensity that is attributable to excessive cigarette smoking in the latter group but not in the former. Patients who have COPD are more likely than those in control groups to have a family history of respiratory disease, a hereditary tendency that is stronger in women than in men.[52, 60]

## ETIOLOGY AND PATHOGENESIS

There is abundant evidence that several etiologic factors are involved in the development of COPD. Clinical and epidemiologic studies have focused on the contributions of cigarette smoke (active and passive), air pollution (occupational or urban), infection (especially during childhood), climate, heredity, socioeconomic status, atopy, nonspecific airway hyper-responsiveness, diet, and nutrition.[61] Cigarette smoking is by far the most important of these factors; in fact, many of the others simply represent modifiers of the host response to cigarette smoke. Despite these observations, it has been estimated that only 10% to 20% of chronic heavy smokers will ever develop symptomatic COPD;[62, 63] thus, it is clear that factors other than cigarette smoking are involved in many cases.

One way to test for factors that increase the risk of the development of symptomatic COPD is to measure longitudinal declines in $FEV_1$ over a period of years in large population groups, and to determine which features characterize those patients who have an accelerated decline in lung function.[49, 64, 65] After the age of approximately 30 years, healthy nonsmokers show a nearly linear yearly decline in $FEV_1$ of between 10 and 35 ml, occurring predominantly as a result of a decrease in lung elastic recoil. Smokers show an exaggerated decline (30 to 70 ml/year), the rate increasing with the intensity of cigarette smoking.[9, 65, 66] In a 15-year study of 2,406 Belgian Air Force personnel, the rate of yearly decline in $FEV_1$ allowed the prediction that 4% of heavy smokers and 0.5% of nonsmokers would develop an $FEV_1$ of less than 1.2 liters by the age of 65.[66]

The other major predictor of the rapid deterioration in lung function observed in longitudinal studies is the state of function at the beginning of the study:[66, 67] patients who have lower $FEV_1$ values to begin with show more rapid deterioration, even when adjustment is made for amount smoked and other potential risk factors. Just as the "rich get richer," the obstructed become more obstructed! This important phenomenon, called the "horse race effect," simply states that individuals whose lung function is impaired for any reason are at increased risk for the development of symptomatic COPD (Fig. 55–2).

### Tobacco Smoke

As indicated, cigarette smoking is by far the most important contributor to the development of chronic bronchitis and COPD. Although the conditions do occur in nonsmokers,[68] they do so rarely.[57–59, 69–71] Comparative studies of the prevalence of coughing and expectoration in adult cigarette smokers and nonsmokers have shown a remarkable predominance among the former,[72] the prevalence rates in pipe and cigar smokers lying somewhere in between.[73–76] The symptoms of chronic cough and phlegm production can develop soon after commencement of the smoking habit, although symptomatic air-flow obstruction usually does not become apparent until after 20 or 30 years of smoking or after the age of 50.[77]

Comparison of expiratory flow rates in smokers and nonsmokers has revealed an increase in airway obstruction in the former,[78–82] with the dose-response relationship between the degree of impairment of air flow and the amount smoked being statistically significant.[46, 83–86] The duration and intensity of smoking are of equal importance in calculating a dose-response relationship; these factors can be combined into a single index by calculating the pack-years (packs of 20 cigarettes/day $\times$ years smoked).[86] In large cross-sectional population studies, an influence of smoking on lung function can be detected as early as 20 years of age;[86] in one longitudinal study of children and adolescents, smoking diminished the rate of increase in expiratory air flow that normally occurs with growth.[87] Smoking cessation is usually associated with some improvement in lung function, and the symptoms of coughing and sputum expectoration often disappear completely; although the improvement in function may be small, the rate of annual decline in lung function diminishes or returns to a normal rate of decline. For reasons that are unclear, individuals who stop smoking and then restart have steeper rates of decline in lung function than those who continue the smoking habit uninterrupted.[88] The initial benefit of smoking cessation is influenced by age and gender; in one study, women showed a mean increase in $FEV_1$ of 4.3% and 2.5% at ages 20 and 80 years, respectively, while men improved only 1.2% at age 20 and showed no improvement at age 80.[89]

Pipe smokers tend to avoid pulmonary inhalation of smoke by closing off the oropharyngeal isthmus; smoke is puffed into the mouth and then exhaled through the mouth and nose.[90] Despite the lack of pulmonary smoke inhalation, both pipe and cigar smokers are also at risk of developing and dying of COPD, although less so than cigarette smokers.[91] The relative risk is more pronounced for those who switch from cigarettes to a pipe or cigars, because they inhale the smoke to a greater extent than do pipe and cigar smokers who have never smoked cigarettes.[92]

Besides the total number of cigarettes smoked, the pattern of smoke inhalation can influence the total dose and the distribution within the lungs of the toxic gases and particles. Pulmonary symptoms and, to some extent, lung function correlate with the individual patient's subjective assessment of the depth of smoke inhalation.[93] The breathing pattern and "inhaled puff volume" can be measured during smoking using the respiratory inductive plethysmograph;[94] with this device, it has been shown that there is wide variability in the depth and speed of inhalation and in the breath-hold time following inhalation.[95, 96] Slow, deep inhalation of smoke followed by breath-holding increases alveolar deposition of smoke and could favor the development of emphysema, whereas rapid, shallow inspiratory puffs without breath-holding encourage airway deposition and could result in inflammation and airway narrowing. The pattern of cigarette smoke exhalation can also influence the deposition of particles; coughing or flow-limited expiration tends to cause the accumulation of inhaled particles at the flow-limiting sites in central airways, presumably as a result of the increase in regional turbulence that develops.[97] A central location of particulate accumulation could explain the large airway changes of COPD and the tendency for pulmonary carcinoma to occur in these airways. In fact, it is possible that there is a vicious cycle in which air-flow obstruction results in more flow-limited breathing and thus in more localized particle deposition.

Tobacco smoke is a complex mixture of more than 100 volatile and particulate chemical substances, and it is not known which of the components are responsible for the development of chronic bronchitis or COPD. Although smoking cigarettes that have low tar content is associated with a decrease in the symptoms of chronic bronchitis,[98] the

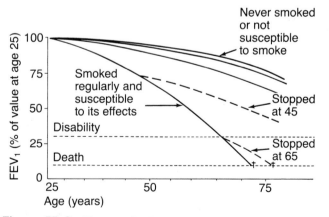

**Figure 55–2. Changes in FEV₁ with Aging.** This figure shows the percentage change in $FEV_1$ versus age for smokers and nonsmokers. Nonsmokers show a gradual decline in $FEV_1$ with age, and smokers who are not susceptible to the effects of cigarette smoke show a similar although somewhat accelerated decline. Individuals who are susceptible to cigarette smoke and who smoke regularly demonstrate an accelerated decline in $FEV_1$, which increases in rapidity with increasing age ("horse race effect"). Smoking cessation returns the rate of decline to that observed in the nonsmoking or nonsusceptible population. (From Peto R, Speizer FE, Cochrane AL, et al: Am Rev Respir Dis 128:491, 1983.)

evidence that they decrease the incidence of COPD or its rate of progression is less compelling.[31, 99] Similarly, the use of cigarette filters was found to be unimportant in one cross-sectional study.[86] Despite these observations, the results of one study suggested that fewer deaths could be ascribed to emphysema among smokers of low-tar than among smokers of medium- and high-tar cigarettes.[100] Some individuals develop immediate-type hypersensitivity to raw tobacco antigens; however, the sensitivity shows no correlation with symptoms of COPD, and it is unlikely that allergy to cigarette smoke is an important factor in the pathogenesis of COPD.[101, 102]

In addition to irreversible airway obstruction, transitory bronchoconstriction[103–110] and nonuniform distribution of ventilation[107, 108] have been described during the act of cigarette smoking. In one study of the acute effects of cigarette smoking, heavy smokers tended to show more pronounced acute bronchoconstriction than that noted among light smokers or nonsmokers.[103] Despite these observations, there is no known relationship between this acute effect of cigarette smoking and the long-term deleterious effects.

Considerable interest has been shown in establishing whether the level of pre-existing nonspecific bronchial responsiveness (NSBR) is a determinant of the long-term response to cigarette smoking (*see* farther on); the antithesis, i.e., the effect of smoking on NSBR, has also been addressed. Although some young and middle-aged chronic asymptomatic smokers manifest significantly increased airway responsiveness,[111–113] acute smoking (four cigarettes) has no effect on NSBR.[114] The combination of smoking and atopy, manifested by allergic rhinitis, is additive in inducing hyper-responsiveness.[115]

Although personal cigarette smoking is certainly the most important risk factor in the development of COPD, the possible harmful effects of passive or side-stream smoking—i.e., environmental tobacco smoke (ETS)—have also received considerable attention.[116, 117] Although the exposure is small compared with that experienced by "mainstream" smokers, nonsmoking persons who are in the same room or house as a smoker can show pulmonary deposition of smoke particles as well as increased blood levels of nicotine and carboxyhemoglobin.[118, 119] Infants and children living in the same household as parents or siblings who smoke are especially vulnerable to the effects of passive smoking. The results of several epidemiologic studies have shown an increased incidence of respiratory illness and functional impairment in such persons, the effect being greater with maternal than with paternal smoking.[116, 120–123] For example, in one study, it was shown that exposure to cigarette smoke during the first years of life doubled the infant's risk of pneumonia or "bronchitis";[124] however, it is possible that this association could have resulted from an increased incidence of infection in the parents and cross-infection between members of the family. Irrespective of the causality of the relationship, these early pulmonary insults may predispose to the later development of COPD.

Normal lung growth and development can be also be affected in infants who have been passively exposed to cigarette smoke; for example, in one longitudinal study of lung function in children, maternal smoking was associated with an increase in $FEV_1$ 7% less than that expected over a 7-year period.[125] The effect on adults is less clear, although

in some studies, individuals passively exposed to cigarette smoke have shown a slight but significant decrease in maximal expiratory flow.[126, 127] In one study of 3,914 adults who had never smoked cigarettes, exposure to ETS as a child and as an adult was associated with a relative risk of 1.7 for the development of symptomatic air-flow obstruction.[128] Although the magnitude of the risk associated with passive cigarette smoking is small in cross-sectional studies, extended longitudinal follow-up studies will be necessary to quantify the ultimate impact, because slight changes in lung structure and function in children may predispose to later disease.[116, 117] As predicted by the "horse race effect," a decrease in expiratory flow at an early age will contribute to a more rapid subsequent decline in function, so that any small changes in "starting lung function" may be crucial.

### Air Pollution

The relationship between COPD and the breathing of polluted air has been investigated with reference to both urban atmospheric pollution and specific occupational exposure. There is no doubt that certain chemical fumes and dusts, if present in sufficient concentration, can cause acute and chronic airway damage and obstruction; however, except in heavily polluted regions and with certain industrial exposures, the effects are minor compared with the influence of cigarette smoking.[129] It is also possible that short-term increases in the levels of pollutants can precipitate exacerbations of air-flow obstruction in persons who have established disease.

#### Environmental and Domestic Air Pollution

The chemicals responsible for urban air pollution can be divided into two major categories: (1) reducing agents, consisting mainly of carbonaceous particulate matter, measured as PM10 (particulate matter < 10 μm in diameter) and sulfur dioxide ($SO_2$); and (2) oxidizing substances, including the hydrocarbons, oxides of nitrogen, products of photochemical reactions, such as ozone ($O_3$), aldehydes, and peroxyacetylnitrate, and other organic nitrates.

Although there is little evidence that urban air pollution by itself can cause clinically significant airway obstruction,[130, 131] the data suggest that it plays a significant additive role with cigarette smoke in the development of COPD[132, 133] and may contribute to the progression of disability in patients already affected. The effects of low concentrations of $SO_2$, nitrogen dioxide ($NO_2$), and $O_3$ on lung function in normal individuals are discussed in the section on environmental provocation of asthma (*see* page 2114); acute exposure to these substances, especially when accompanied by exercise, results in transient pulmonary function abnormalities and, in some patients, prolonged enhancement of NSBR. In patients who have COPD, exposure causes a similar transient impairment of lung function,[134–136] and it is probable that multiple repeated exposures, especially if combined with cigarette smoking, can cause permanent derangement.

The results of many studies have provided support for this hypothesis. In one investigation from Milan, Italy, in which four urban regions were compared, a correlation was found between $SO_2$ levels in the atmosphere, carboxyhemoglobin levels, and nonspecific airway responsiveness in both smokers and nonsmokers.[137] The results of several epidemiologic studies have revealed a higher incidence of chronic bronchitis and COPD among urban dwellers; although other factors may be involved, this association is likely to be at least partly related to air pollution in the cities.[138–141] A 7-year study of an adult population in Berlin, New Hampshire, revealed a decrease in the prevalence of chronic bronchitis and COPD coincident with a decrease in air pollution;[7, 142, 143] the improvement was noted even after the effects of aging and a change in cigarette smoking habits were taken into account.[142] The results of another study showed significant impairment of pulmonary function in a large group of residents in the highly polluted Tokyo and Yokohama regions of Japan compared with that in residents of an area that had less atmospheric pollution.[144] The relative importance of urban air quality and cigarette smoking was evaluated with respect to annual rate of decline in $FEV_1$ in one study in the Los Angeles area of California; the urban region that had the highest levels of sulfates was associated with a significantly increased rate of decline in $FEV_1$, which in men was 70% of that attributed to cigarette smoking.[145] Histologic abnormalities similar to those seen in cigarette smokers have also been found in individuals exposed to polluted air for a long period of time.[145a]

Children, in whom the lungs are still growing, may be particularly vulnerable to the effects of air pollution. The incidence of lower respiratory tract infections is higher in children who live in environments that have high levels of air pollution,[146, 147] and childhood infection is especially likely to impair subsequent lung function (*see* farther on). Domestic air pollution may also have an important deleterious effect on children's lungs. The use of natural gas in home cooking also is associated with an increase in the incidence of childhood respiratory illness and pulmonary dysfunction, independent of the effects of parental smoking.[148, 149] Fires that are used indoors for domestic cooking are another source of residential air pollution; for example, in rural Nepal, where indoor wood and dung fires are common, a very high incidence of obstructive lung disease, emphysema, and cor pulmonale has been observed in both men and women.[150, 151] In India, women who use biomass fuels for cooking have been found to have worse lung function than those who use liquefied petroleum gas or kerosene.[152] Although cigarette smoking is relatively uncommon among women in Mexico and Colombia, they are heavily exposed to this biomass smoke; careful case-control studies have shown a significant risk for symptoms and obstructive pulmonary function associated with such exposure.[153, 154] Similarly, an increased incidence of "simple" chronic bronchitis has been reported in women who live in igloos and tents in which there is heavy smoke pollution.[155, 156] Additional potential sources of air pollution in the home include house dust, hair sprays, insecticides, and soap powders. In a survey carried out in rural Western Australia, exposure to these substances was thought to play a role in the development of COPD.[157]

A sudden increase in the amount of air pollution, such as occurs with smog, can result in increased morbidity and mortality in patients who have established COPD.[158–160] In addition to these more dramatic associations, sophisticated time series analyses have shown significant relationships between hospital admission and emergency room visit rates for COPD and atmospheric levels of $SO_2$, $O_3$, and PM10.[161–164] Of interest, there is often a delay of a day or more between the peak levels of the pollutant and the increased symptoms. The concentrations that provoke the increased morbidity are below those suggested as acceptable lower limits in some countries.[161]

### Occupational Dust and Fume Exposure

There have been many attempts to relate occupational dust and/or fume exposure to the development of COPD. Unfortunately, the results of most studies are difficult to interpret because of the presence of other accepted or suspected etiologic factors (e.g., cigarette smoke). Interpretive errors can also occur in cross-sectional studies as a result of the tendency of workers to move to different jobs within the occupational environment, particularly when those who take another job are physically fit and those who remain are disabled,[165, 166] or when affected individuals drop out of the workforce.[167] Longitudinal studies of the rate of decline of lung function in exposed workers, corrected for potential confounding risk factors, constitute an acceptable standard means of assessment but take many years to complete.[168] Another confounding factor is the difficulty in distinguishing between individuals who have occupational asthma in response to specific sensitizing agents and those who have fixed air-flow obstruction.[168, 169]

Despite these difficulties, a number of investigators have concluded that there is unequivocal evidence for a significant effect of dust on lung function in some occupations.[20, 168] In one study of 8,515 adults from the midwestern and eastern United States, in which adjustment was made for smoking habits, age, gender, and city of residence, individuals who had been exposed to dust, gases, and fumes showed a significantly increased incidence of respiratory symptoms and air-flow obstruction ($FEV_1/FVC < 0.6$).[170] In another investigation from Norway, a history of having worked in an occupation that involved exposure to quartz, metal gases, aluminum dust, welding, or asbestos resulted in odds ratios for the presence of air-flow obstruction ($FEV_1/FVC < 70\%$ and $FEV_1 < 80\%$ of predicted) of between 2.3 and 2.7.[171] An increased annual rate of decline in $FEV_1$ has also been seen in workers exposed to inorganic dusts (coal and hard rock miners, foundry workers, metal workers), fumes (chemical workers, welders), organic dusts (cotton, grain), and smoke.[20, 168, 172–176] Although there is controversy over the relative importance of smoking and exposure to dust in the workplace,[129] it is likely that when smokers work with noxious respiratory agents, COPD occurs with unusual frequency and/or severity.

Exposure to dusts that are known to produce fibrotic pneumoconioses can result in air-flow obstruction, the severity of which is not necessarily related to the extent of fibrosis. The variation in pathologic response to single agents may be related to particle size and deposition pattern;[177] for example, larger particles tend to impact on airways and cause air-flow obstruction, whereas smaller particles reach alveolar air spaces, where they induce fibrosis, leading to a restrictive ventilatory defect. In a 9-year longitudinal study of U.S. coal miners, the deleterious effect of dust exposure was found to be about a third to a half as important as that of smoking.[173] The authors of a meta-analysis found that coal mining and, to a greater extent, gold mining were associated with excess morbidity due to COPD.[178] When the data are adjusted for the amount of smoking, coal miners and gold miners show more severe emphysema at autopsy than do nonexposed workers;[20, 179–181] to the extent that emphysema is associated with air-flow obstruction, this supports an independent effect of inorganic dust inhalation on airway function. In another study of coal miners, the extent of emphysema correlated most closely with the coal content of the lungs, while the silica content was positively associated with the extent of fibrosis.[182] When emphysema is quantified either at autopsy or by CT scanning, nonsmokers who have silicosis without progressive massive fibrosis do not have emphysema, although they may have air-flow obstruction.[183, 184] Although exposure to asbestos dust is associated with abnormalities of small airway function,[185] smoking is substantially more important to the development of significant symptomatic obstruction.[186, 187] However, it is worth noting that the prevalence of emphysema as assessed by CT scan is twice as high in workers who have early asbestosis (54%) than in asbestos workers who do not have fibrotic lung disease;[188] it is likely that emphysema in these patients contributes to the severity of air-flow obstruction.

Exposure to cadmium in the workplace is unusual among occupational exposures in that it appears to lead to COPD by causing emphysema,[189] sometimes rapidly progressive.[190] The mechanism by which exposure to the metal leads to emphysema is unclear. Although cadmium chloride does not appear to cause destruction of lung elastin,[191] it does selectively inhibit fibroblast proliferation and production of procollagen.[192] Cadmium is also an important contaminant of tobacco and may play a role in cigarette smoking–related emphysema.

There is an increasing list of occupations associated with exposure to organic dusts that can affect pulmonary function and lead to the development of COPD; implicated substances include cotton, grain, cork, wood, and the dust, aerosol, and fumes that are generated in slaughterhouses and livestock confinement buildings.[168, 193–197] The airway disease associated with chronic exposure to cotton dust is called byssinosis and is described in more detail in Chapter 54 (*see* page 2124). Although some individuals who are exposed to organic dusts develop reversible air-flow obstruction (see discussion of occupational asthma in Chapter 54, page 2117) others suffer an insidious progression of fixed air-flow obstruction.[168, 198, 199] The acute changes in lung function that occur during one work shift are predictive of the rate of decline in lung function in exposed workers in longitudinal studies.[200, 201] The acute response to these organic dusts has been called "organic dust toxic syndrome" (ODTS) and is discussed in Chapter 59 (*see* page 2379) In most of these occupations, endotoxin in the dust is believed to be an important pathogenetic constituent; endotoxin can stimulate an acute inflammatory reaction in the airway via release of tumor necrosis factor, interleukins IL-1 and IL-6, and other cytokines.[196]

Grain dust is a mixture of insects, fungi, bacteria, silicates, herbicides, pesticides, and mammalian debris, extracts of which can release histamine and activate complement.[202] Because of the complex composition of grain dust, it is not surprising that a number of syndromes and mechanisms are associated with dust exposure. Both workers and nonworkers who are exposed experimentally to grain dust can develop a

syndrome called grain fever, consisting of elevated temperature, flushing, headache, chest tightness, cough, dyspnea, an elevated white blood cell count, and a reduction in maximal expiratory flow.[203, 204] Workers can also develop leukocytosis and a significant decrease in maximal expiratory flow over a working shift.[205] There is no evidence of an immunologic mechanism in the development of these acute responses, and as in other organic dust disorders, endotoxin within the dust is probably the major pathogenetic factor.

Although exposure to grain dust can cause immediate allergic responses in a small number of individuals, it more often leads to persistent airway obstruction. For example, in one study of 587 grain elevator workers, 288 had respiratory symptoms and 102 showed significant impairment of lung function.[206] Exposure of 22 of the 102 patients to grain dust was associated with an immediate and/or late response typical of an IgE-mediated allergic airway reaction in 6; the remaining 16 exhibited more fixed airway obstruction, presumably representing a form of industrial bronchitis or COPD. The incidence of cough, sputum production, wheeze, and air-flow obstruction is also higher in grain-exposed than in nonexposed workers, as is a more rapid rate of decline in $FEV_1$.[207–211] Grain workers who have symptoms and pulmonary function deficits are also more likely to show increased NSBR; however, this probably represents a consequence of their impairment rather than a predisposing factor.[211–213]

Workers who are exposed to swine in buildings in which animals are confined in high density commonly have respiratory symptoms, bronchial hyper-responsiveness, and abnormalities of lung function (*see* page 2379).[214, 215] Such pulmonary disease does not appear to be the result of allergic sensitization to swine antigens but is instead related to a lower airway inflammatory response caused by the toxic effects of inhaled endotoxin, aerosolized disinfectants, and ammonia.[216–218] In one longitudinal study, exposure was associated with an accelerated decline in lung function,[219] suggesting that the condition is a form of occupational COPD similar to that related to cotton (byssinosis) and grain dust.

A 5-year study of 168 firefighters and 1,474 control subjects revealed a significant acceleration in the rate of decline in $FEV_1$ in the firefighters when age, smoking history, and initial lung function were taken into account.[220] However, not all studies have revealed abnormal lung function in firefighters (*see* Chapter 62). Chemicals such as toluene diisocyanate (TDI), which can cause occupational asthma, can also produce a nonidiosyncratic acceleration of functional deterioration in occupationally exposed workers, both smokers and nonsmokers.[172]

Chronic air-flow obstruction can also result from heavy and prolonged marijuana[221, 222] and opium[223] smoking; the latter has been accompanied by emphysema and pleuropulmonary fibrosis and the former by airway inflammation similar to that seen in tobacco cigarette smokers.[223a]

### Infection

Of the variety of possible relationships between lower respiratory tract infection and COPD, the following are the most important:

• Infection during childhood may increase the subsequent risk of COPD by affecting lung function, lung growth, or pulmonary defense mechanisms.

- Respiratory infection in patients who have established COPD may accelerate subsequent functional deterioration.
- Established COPD may increase the incidence and severity of respiratory infection.

The results of retrospective studies have provided fairly conclusive evidence that lower respiratory tract infection in children is a significant risk factor for the subsequent development of COPD during adulthood.[224–228] Childhood "bronchitis," especially before the age of 2 years, is associated with persistently abnormal lung function and thus represents an important risk factor.[229–231] In one remarkable study, objective evidence of a lower respiratory tract infection was associated with significant impairment of lung function 60 to 70 years later![232]

The question remains as to whether childhood infection is a marker of susceptibility to respiratory illness or is the initiating insult that causes the subsequent development of symptomatic airway obstruction.[233] Possible mechanisms by which the interaction may occur include (1) a direct effect of lower respiratory infection on the maximal achieved lung function or on the rate of decline in lung function, (2) reverse causation, in which children predisposed to the later development of COPD have increased susceptibility to infection, and (3) an increased susceptibility to both lower respiratory infections and the development of COPD as a result of common host or environmental factors.[228] The results of some longitudinal studies in infants support a contribution of the second of these mechanisms;[234–237] in all of these studies, measures of lung function impairment in early infancy predicted later development of lower respiratory tract infection associated with wheezing. The biologic basis for this association is uncertain. However, it is possible that individuals who have congenitally smaller airways are more likely to develop symptoms during viral infection and that the same anatomic variation may predispose such individuals to the later development of excessive airway narrowing in response to cigarette smoke.[228] In support of this hypothesis are the observations that low birth weight has an independent effect in predicting impairment in adult lung function[238] and that patients who have pulmonary hypoplasia may present with ventilatory failure in adulthood.[239]

The interrelationships among infection, inhalation of pollutants, and host defense mechanisms are complex. Exposure to atmospheric or residential air pollution (including ETS) not only is associated with an increased incidence of childhood viral respiratory infections[146, 147, 240] but also appears to have an independent detrimental effect on lung function.[116, 120, 235] In addition, pollutants may interfere with macrophage efficiency, thus increasing susceptibility to infection.[44, 241] Another mechanism by which viral infection could lead to later COPD is via the development of latent infection.[242, 243] This hypothesis is based on studies using the polymerase chain reaction (PCR) and immunohistochemistry[243, 244] in which portions of the adenoviral genome and viral proteins have been shown to be present in the lung tissue of patients who have COPD. The fact that certain adenoviral genes are detectable and others are not suggests that parts of the viral genome may be incorporated into the human genome. Proteins produced by these genes, such as the proinflammatory molecule E1A, can alter the phenotype of airway epithelial cells and could enhance the subsequent inflammatory response to cigarette smoke.[245]

As indicated previously, childhood respiratory infection could exert a long-term effect by producing slight functional impairment, which later predisposes to accelerated deterioration. In a study of 96 children 9 years after recovery from croup, a significant decrease in vital capacity and maximal expiratory flow rates and an increase in the ratio of residual volume to total lung capacity (RV/TLC) and in NSBR were observed in comparison to age-matched control subjects.[246] The results of one investigation showed the regional death rate from COPD in England and Wales to be strongly related to the infant mortality from bronchitis and pneumonia in the same geographic regions approximately 30 years earlier;[247] statistical analysis suggested that lower respiratory tract infection during early childhood was as important as cigarette smoking in influencing the geographic distribution of the COPD.

It has been proposed that a lack of secretory immunoglobulin A (IgA) is common in patients who have chronic bronchitis and may predispose to infection and obstruction.[248] However, the results of a number of studies have shown that levels of both secretory IgA (measured in saliva or in nasal or bronchial secretions) and serum IgA are within normal limits in the great majority of patients who have COPD.[249–253] There is also no evidence for an impaired inflammatory response as a risk factor for COPD. Qualitative and quantitative cytologic and bacteriologic studies of the sputum of 60 patients during an acute exacerbation of COPD showed a normal pattern of neutrophil increase during the infection and the appearance of macrophages after the infection.[254] In another study of 100 patients who had COPD, normal cutaneous delayed hypersensitivity and phagocytic intracellular killing activity were demonstrated;[255] however, there was a significant impairment in the ability of peripheral leukocytes to reduce nitroblue tetrazolium. High levels of mucus antibodies have been demonstrated in patients who have chronic bronchitis, a finding that may simply reflect the presence of chronic infection and impaired mucociliary clearance that would permit abnormal reabsorption of mucus antigens.[256]

Although airway function worsens acutely during intercurrent viral and bacterial respiratory infections in patients who have pre-existing COPD, whether these infections produce permanent functional impairment and accelerate the natural course of the disease has not been established. Physiologic studies of airway function in normal individuals who have naturally occurring[257–261] or experimentally induced[262] viral infection have shown changes indicative of reversible airway obstruction and impaired gas exchange;[263] however, it is possible that similar insults can cause a progression of irreversible airway obstruction in some patients who have COPD.[264] Smokers have been shown to be more susceptible than nonsmokers to the long-term sequelae of *Mycoplasma pneumoniae* infection.[263] However, in a long-term study designed to assess the influence of *Haemophilus influenzae* infection on airway obstruction, the development of obstruction was correlated with smoking habits but not with the infection itself.[265] Despite a severe decline in pulmonary function during respiratory infections, most patients who have COPD improve to their pre-exacerbation status after resolution of the infection, although irreversible deficits develop in some.[266]

Infection results in acute episodes or exacerbations of

COPD in which there is symptomatic and physiologic deterioration. The sputum often becomes purulent,[267] cultures usually growing *H. influenzae* and sometimes *Streptococcus pneumoniae*;[42, 268–271] antibodies to these organisms are found in the serum of many of these patients.[265, 272, 273] Despite these observations indicating primary infection, it is likely that bacteria are more often secondary invaders following an acute viral infection of the lower respiratory tract. Viral infection is responsible for the majority of clinical exacerbations in patients who have COPD.[274–283] In one third to two thirds of such exacerbations, viruses and, less commonly, *M. pneumoniae* and *Chlamydia pneumoniae* have been isolated, or their presence has been demonstrated serologically.[282–284b] Evidence for such infection is found far less frequently during periods of remission.[282, 283] The rhinoviruses and myxoviruses—the latter particularly during epidemics—appear to be especially common.[274, 280, 282, 283] Series differences in the percentage of acute episodes in which a specific virus is identified may depend on the means by which the organisms are identified or on variation in the accepted definition of what constitutes an exacerbation. Another significant factor appears to be exposure of the adult who has chronic bronchitis to schoolchildren in the family; for example, in one study of six families, a specific virus was associated with acute exacerbations of COPD in 60% of affected adults who were exposed to schoolchildren but in only 29% of those in households without schoolchildren.[281]

It is also possible that chronic tuberculosis may produce airway obstruction. In one study of 1,043 patients who had this infection, the data suggested that smoking and tuberculosis had an additive effect in producing airway obstruction.[285]

### Climate

Patients who have COPD often relate exacerbations of their disease to climatic factors, particularly variations in humidity and temperature. There are also seasonal variations in morbidity from obstructive lung disease that are incompletely explained by known risk factors.[286] It is possible that the effect of high humidity relates to the high level of air pollution that in many geographic areas accompanies humid weather. In temperate climates, excessive air dryness during cold weather, particularly in apartments, seems to aggravate symptoms, and the use of a humidifier usually results in a decrease in cough and greater ease of expectoration. In one study, fluid deprivation for 16 hours in humid heat resulted in dehydration and a significant decrease in $FEV_1$, not only in patients who had obstructive airway disease but also in normal individuals.[287] In patients who have established COPD, both exposure of the facial skin to and inhalation of cold dry air cause bronchoconstriction.[288] The number of emergency clinic visits by patients who have COPD has also been found to be increased with the onset of cold weather;[289] although this may be attributable to breathing cold air, the excessive dryness created by indoor heating or the inhalation of dust from convection currents around radiators may be at least as important.

In a study of 60,000 London Transport employees that extended over 5 years, absence from work for 4 or more days attributed to "bronchitis" was closely associated with the number and density of foggy days.[290] In another survey

of a large group of patients in which data were obtained from diaries, it was concluded that although exacerbations of COPD tended to occur with changing weather, air pollution rather than the weather itself was responsible for these episodes.[160] Climate similarly may alter the clinical presentation of COPD; for example, it has been reported that in the warm, dry air of Tucson, Arizona, chronic cough is frequently nonproductive.[291]

Some patients who have COPD appear to be abnormally sensitive to the inhalation of cold air.[292, 293] The degree of bronchoconstriction following cold air inhalation correlates with the magnitude of bronchodilation that occurs following inhalation of aerosol beta-adrenergic agonist[294] and with nonspecific responsiveness to methacholine.[295] Asthmatic patients with comparable starting values of $FEV_1$ develop more severe obstruction after breathing cold or dry air, suggesting that the mechanism of hyper-responsiveness is different in the two conditions.[295]

### Heredity

Evidence that genetic susceptibility is a major risk factor for COPD includes the following:[296, 297]

- an increased incidence of COPD or chronic bronchitis in relatives of cases compared with relatives of controls[298–305]
- the presence of significant correlations in lung function between parents and children and between siblings who have COPD, and of higher correlations between parents and children or between siblings than between spouses[300, 306–308]
- a decreased prevalence of disease or less similarity in lung function with increased genetic distance[298, 309, 310]
- the presence of a greater concordance of disease and similarity in lung function in monozygotic than in dizygotic twins[309, 311–316]

Although the results of many studies show an aggregation of COPD in families, there is no clear mendelian pattern of inheritance. In addition, the effects of a shared environment cannot be excluded; for example, it is possible that parental smoking could be a contributing factor to an offspring's decreased lung function. Nevertheless, the evidence suggests that the increased prevalence of COPD in relatives of affected individuals compared with that in relatives of normal individuals cannot be explained by differences in other known risk factors. Twin studies in particular support a large genetic contribution to the variability in lung function and to susceptibility to the effects of cigarette smoking. For example, in one investigation of monozygotic and dizygotic twins, susceptibility of one monozygotic twin to the effects of cigarette smoke meant that both twins who smoked developed reductions in lung function;[313] by contrast, other monozygotic twin pairs appeared to be nonsusceptible and, despite similar degrees of smoking intensity, maintained normal lung function. This concordance of changes in lung function with similar degrees of smoking intensity was not seen in dizygotic twins.

The association of extremely low levels of alpha$_1$ globulin with an increased prevalence of emphysema and air-flow obstruction was the first specific genetic abnormality shown to be a risk factor for COPD, and a deficiency of alpha$_1$-antitrypsin (alpha$_1$-antiprotease; *see* page 2231) remains the most clearly defined and well-studied genetic risk factor for COPD. Homozygous alpha$_1$-antiprotease inhibitor deficiency (PiZZ) is associated with a 30-fold increased risk for the development of symptomatic COPD; however, it accounts for less than 1% of cases, because the frequency of the genetic defect is only 1 in 2,000 to 1 in 4,000.[317] Although heterozygous deficiency (PiMZ) is associated with serum alpha$_1$-antiprotease levels that are approximately 60% of normal, because it occurs more frequently (1 in 100 to 4 in 100), an increased risk in such individuals could explain a greater familial tendency for the development of COPD. Two types of cross-sectional studies have been used to address this hypothesis: (1) the prevalence of intermediate deficiency in a population of patients who have COPD has been compared with that in a matched population of individuals who do not have COPD; and (2) the prevalence of COPD in a population of patients who have intermediate deficiency has been compared with that in a population of individuals who have normal serum antiprotease levels and phenotypes. The second type of study is generally considered superior but is more difficult to perform. Numerous studies of both types have been carried out (*see* page 2231),[297] the bulk of evidence supporting the thesis that intermediate deficiency is a risk factor.

Following the description of the association between emphysema and alpha$_1$-antiprotease inhibitor deficiency, it was hypothesized that other inherited markers or deficiencies would be discovered to explain the genetic tendency for the development of COPD.[318] Many genes and gene products have been tested for potential involvement in the pathogenesis of COPD (Table 55–1); unfortunately, progress in identifying such genes has been modest. In the vast majority of cases, the underlying defect that constitutes the genetic predisposition for the development of COPD is unknown.

### Alpha$_1$-Antichymotrypsin

Like alpha$_1$-antiprotease inhibitor, alpha$_1$-antichymotrypsin (alpha$_1$-ACT) is a serum protease inhibitor and acute phase reactant. It is synthesized by hepatocytes and alveolar macrophages[319] and is known to inhibit pancreatic chymotrypsin, neutrophil cathepsin G, mast cell chymase, and the production of neutrophil superoxide.[320] Alpha$_1$-ACT deficiency has a prevalence of approximately 1% in the Swedish population. Hereditary deficiency has been shown to be

associated with an autosomal dominant inheritance pattern.[321, 322]

No consistent clinical phenotype is associated with the deficiency; however, an increased prevalence has been reported in patients who have childhood asthma[323] and COPD.[324, 325] In two studies, affected patients had increased values of RV and RV/TLC[321, 322] Two point mutations in the alpha$_1$-ACT gene have been associated with decreased alpha$_1$-ACT serum concentrations and COPD; one such mutation was found in 4 of 100 unrelated patients who had COPD and none of 100 controls in a German population;[324] all 4 had serum alpha$_1$-ACT concentrations approximately 60% of normal and alpha$_1$-antiprotease inhibitor levels within the normal range. However, the prevalence of this mutation may vary in different populations, because it was not detected in 102 Russian COPD patients[326] or in 169 patients who had COPD in a Canadian study.[327]

A second mutation was reported in 3 of 200 unrelated COPD patients and none of 100 controls;[325] the mean alpha$_1$-ACT serum level in the heterozygotes was 80% of normal, and the mutant protein had defective function and an altered pattern on isoelectric focusing. One of the heterozygotes belonged to a family in which 3 members were affected with severe early-onset COPD.

### Cystic Fibrosis Transmembrane Regulator

Conceivably, individuals who are heterozygous for an abnormal cystic fibrosis transmembrane regulator gene *(CFTR)* could have altered airway water and ion regulation and altered mucociliary clearance in response to airway irritants. However, comparisons of parents of patients who have cystic fibrosis (obligate heterozygotes for a *CFTR* mutation) with unaffected individuals have not revealed any significant differences in lung function or history of asthma or chronic bronchitis.[328–331] However, heterozygotes have been shown to have increased bronchial reactivity to methacholine[332] and an increased incidence of wheeze accompanied by decreased FEV$_1$ and FEF$_{25-75}$.[333] Because *CFTR* has been identified as the gene responsible for cystic fibrosis, a number of studies have been designed to determine if heterozygosity for its mutations increases the risk for COPD; although some weak associations have been reported, the overall results suggest that such mutations are unlikely to make a significant contribution to the pathogenesis of COPD.[334–339]

### Vitamin D–Binding Protein

Vitamin D–binding protein (VDBP) is a 55-kilodalton (kDa) protein secreted by the liver that is able to bind extracellular actin and endotoxin in addition to vitamin D. It also enhances the chemotactic activity of C5a and C5a des-Arg for neutrophils by one to two orders of magnitude[340] and can act as a macrophage-activating factor.[341] Numerous isoforms of VDBP have been identified by isoelectric focusing. Two common substitutions in exon 11 of the gene result in three possible isoforms, termed 1F, 1S, and 2. The last of these has been shown by three groups of investigators to protect against the development of COPD, with odds ratios between 0.7 and 0.2.[302, 342, 343] It has been speculated that the

### Table 55–1. GENES IMPLICATED IN PATHOGENESIS OF CHRONIC OBSTRUCTIVE PULMONARY DISEASE

Alpha$_1$-antitrypsin
Alpha$_1$-antichymotrypsin
Cystic fibrosis transmembrane regulator
Vitamin D–binding protein
Alpha$_2$-macroglobulin
Cytochrome P-4501A1
ABH secretor, Lewis and ABO blood groups
HLA
Immunoglobulin deficiency
Extracellular superoxide dismutase[1315, 1316]
Secretory leukocyte proteinase inhibitor (SLPI)[1317]
Cathepsin G[1318]

mechanism underlying this association is defective chemotactic or macrophage activation capability in the 2 isoform.[343]

### Alpha$_2$-Macroglobulin

Alpha$_2$-macroglobulin is a broad-spectrum serum protease inhibitor that is synthesized by hepatocytes, alveolar macrophages,[344] and lung fibroblasts.[345] The substance is thought to have a protective role in the lung. Although its large size (725 kDa) prevents significant transport from blood to the alveolar interstitium or air space, increased vascular permeability during inflammation could allow it to enter the interstitial space.[346] An increase in alpha$_2$-macroglobulin levels can be detected in the sputum of patients who have acute chest infections.[347] Elevated levels also have been reported in the serum of patients who have alpha$_1$-antiprotease inhibitor deficiency, irrespective of the presence or absence of COPD;[348, 349] such an elevation is not seen in patients who have emphysema unrelated to alpha$_1$-antiprotease inhibitor deficiency and may reflect an attempt to compensate for deficiency of this enzyme.

Hereditary deficiency of alpha$_2$-macroglobulin is rare; however, occasional patients have been identified in whom the mechanism of transmission was shown to be autosomal dominant.[350, 351] Although symptoms suggestive of respiratory disease were not found in these individuals, it is possible they were not old enough to have developed COPD; in addition, neither study included the results of pulmonary function tests or smoking histories. A mutation of the gene has been reported in a single 42-year-old patient who had alpha$_2$-macroglobulin serum levels 50% of normal and severe COPD;[352] chronic pulmonary disease had been present since childhood. Unfortunately, smoking history was again not reported. Complete lack of alpha$_2$-macroglobulin has not been described and may be incompatible with life.

### Cytochrome P-4501A1, Microsomal Epoxide Hydrolase, and Glutathione S-Transferase

Cytochrome P-4501A1 is an enzyme that metabolizes exogenous compounds to a form that enables them to be excreted in the urine or bile. It is found throughout the lung and may play a role in the activation of procarcinogens to their carcinogenic forms; the enzyme is produced by the *CYP1A1* gene, and mutations at this locus have been associated with pulmonary carcinoma.[353] In one study, the prevalence of a mutation in exon 7 of *CYP1A1* that increases the activity of the enzyme was also found to be associated with an increased risk for centrilobular emphysema.[354]

There are also variable forms of the microsomal epoxide hydrolase enzyme, which is responsible for first-pass metabolism of a variety of xenobiotics; in one study, the slow-activity form of the enzyme was found to be significantly more prevalent in patients who had COPD and in those who had emphysema (odds ratios of 4.1 and 5.0, respectively).[355] A deletion polymorphism in the glutathione S-transferase gene has been shown to be weakly protective for the development of emphysema in smokers;[356] it is possible that this effect may be related to an alteration in removal of oxygen radicals (*see* further on).

### Blood Group Antigens

The association of COPD with the ABO, secretor, and Lewis genes has been the focus of several studies. The ABO locus on chromosome 9 determines the activity of a glycosyltransferase, which converts glycoprotein H into the A or B antigens, thus determining blood type. Both an association between the A blood group and COPD[357] and an accelerated decline in lung function in a 5-year longitudinal study[358] have been reported. However, in another study, the investigators found that individuals who had blood group A had a smaller decline in lung function than that observed in individuals with other blood groups.[359] The results of several other studies have failed to confirm any association of ABO alleles and pulmonary function.[315, 360, 361]

Approximately 80% of the population secretes ABO antigens into saliva, plasma, and respiratory tract secretions. The ability to do this is determined by the secretor locus on chromosome 19q and is inherited as an autosomal dominant trait. The relation between impaired lung function and secretion of these antigens is controversial; some investigators have found evidence for an association[342, 362] and others have not.[360, 361, 363] The Lewis blood group has also been investigated as a possible risk factor for air-flow obstruction.[364] In white populations, about 90% of the individuals have the dominant *Le* allele and produce Lewis a substance. Individuals who are secretors convert this to Lewis b substance and therefore have both a and b substances in their serum; Lewis-positive nonsecretors have only the a substance in their serum. A significant increase in air-flow obstruction has been reported in Lewis-negative individuals (relative risk 7.2).[364] The authors of this report suggested that it is the presence of b substance rather than secretor status that protects against air-flow obstruction. In one study, blood group O individuals who are either Lewis-negative or nonsecretors have been found to have impaired lung function and a higher prevalence of wheezing and asthma;[365] individuals who were both Lewis-negative and nonsecretors had very low values for indices of lung function. Lewis-positive secretors were found to have lower lung function if they had blood group A compared with group O.

The reason for the association of ABO, Lewis, and secretor genes with COPD remains unclear; however, it may be related to their role in the adhesion of infectious agents.[366] Recurrent respiratory infections, especially in childhood, are known to be a risk factor for COPD, and particular alleles of these blood groups may increase susceptibility to infection.

### Human Leukocyte Antigen Locus

Associations between the human leukocyte antigen (HLA) class I genes and COPD have been investigated in a study of heavy smokers who had high FEV$_1$ values and never-smokers who had low values;[367] a significant decrease in the expected frequency of the *HLA-Bw16 allele* (odds ratio = 0.2) and a significant increase in the expected frequency of the HLA-B7 antigen (odds ratio = 3.8) were observed in the latter group. It is not clear whether these associations are related to variations in the HLA alleles themselves or to susceptibility genes linked with the HLA alleles.

### Immunoglobulin Deficiency

Patients who have IgA deficiency, either alone or in combination with IgG deficiency, are known to have recurrent respiratory infections.[368] Such individuals have also been reported to have abnormal lung function;[369, 370] selective IgA deficiency was also associated with COPD in a large three-generation pedigree.[371]

### Connective Tissue Proteins

Several hereditary diseases of connective tissue, including cutis laxa,[372–374] Marfan's syndrome,[375, 376] and Ehlers-Danlos syndrome,[377] have been associated with the development of emphysema (*see* page 676). Some have been associated with an abnormality of a specific connective tissue protein[375] caused by abnormalities in the corresponding gene.

### *Socioeconomic Factors, Diet, and Nutrition*

An increased risk for the development of COPD in individuals of lower socioeconomic status has been shown in a number of epidemiologic studies. This socioeconomic factor is difficult to separate from related factors such as smoking habits, industrial exposure, passive smoking, diet, and childhood infection;[148] however, careful analysis has shown an independent effect on symptoms and ventilatory function.[18]

A number of mechanisms have been investigated to explain the effect of socioeconomic status on pulmonary function. In Great Britain, people who live in homes without central heating have significantly worse lung function; because central heating is more common in the homes of the well-off, this could be one explanation for the effect.[378, 379] However, it cannot represent the sole factor, because central heating is either universal or unnecessary in North America, where a socioeconomic risk factor also exists.[380] Alcohol consumption is also related to socioeconomic status. In one large cross-sectional study, it was associated with lower values of $FEV_1$;[380] however, when data were corrected for smoking, age, gender, and socioeconomic status, the effect was not significant. In fact, in one autopsy study, the incidence of centrilobular emphysema was lower in individuals with a history of excessive consumption of alcohol, even after correction for age and smoking history.[381]

Other possible mechanisms to explain the socioeconomic effect include crowded living conditions, which in turn increase the incidence of respiratory infections, and nutritional status. As mentioned previously, birth weight and weight at 1 year of age are significant risk factors for later COPD and may be surrogate markers for socioeconomic-related differences in nutritional status.[238] A similar interaction could underlie the relationship that has been observed between dietary and plasma levels of vitamin C (ascorbic acid) and physician-diagnosed chronic bronchitis.[382] Another dietary modifier of risk for COPD appears to be the protection provided by consumption of fish containing the polyunsaturated fatty acids eicosapentaenoic acid and docosahexaenoic acid. These substances act as competitive inhibitors of arachidonic acid metabolism and down-regulate the endogenous production of proinflammatory prostaglandins and leukotrienes.[383] In one study of 8,960 former or current smokers,

the odds ratios for chronic bronchitis, emphysema, and COPD were 0.66, 0.31, and 0.50, respectively, among individuals in the quartile for highest consumption of these fatty acids.[384] Nutritional status as judged by body mass index is a predictor of survival in patients who have established COPD; however, it is unclear that this represents a causal relationship.[385]

### *Atopy and Nonspecific Bronchial Hyper-responsiveness: The Dutch Hypothesis*

In the 1960s, a group of Dutch investigators proposed that patients who have an inherited tendency for atopy and increased nonspecific bronchial responsiveness (NSBR) have a higher risk of developing asthma or irreversible air-flow obstruction, the ultimate phenotype depending primarily on exogenous environmental factors.[386, 387] This so-called "Dutch hypothesis" has not been refuted; in fact, data are accumulating to support it.[22] It is not clear exactly how atopy and bronchial hyper-responsiveness could cause COPD; however, it is possible that repeated episodes of acute bronchoconstriction related to smoke inhalation lead to fixed narrowing in individuals who have hyper-responsive airways. Alternatively, the association may be related to an exaggerated inflammatory response to smoke in atopic individuals.[388]

The results of a number of studies have supported the association of nonspecific bronchial hyper-responsiveness (NSBH) and lower maximal values of $FEV_1$ in early adulthood,[389] as well as a more rapid annual decline in $FEV_1$.[390–396] Interpretation of these studies is potentially confounded by the established relationship between the degree of NSBR and the initial $FEV_1$ value in COPD. In asthmatic patients, bronchial hyper-responsiveness can occur in the presence of normal baseline measurements of lung function; however, in patients who have COPD it is associated with, and to some extent caused by, abnormal "prechallenge" lung function.[397–402] Because an initial $FEV_1$ value less than normal is a known risk factor for the development of COPD, the relationship between NSBH and a decline in $FEV_1$ could be spurious.[387, 403] For example, in a 3-year study of 985 patients who had COPD, the rate of decline in $FEV_1$ was negatively related to the initial bronchodilator response;[404] to the extent that bronchodilator response reflects NSBH, this observation argues against a relationship. On the other hand, the results of a large cross-sectional analysis of a random population of 1,905 individuals supported a relationship between NSBH and pulmonary symptoms: even when cigarette smoking was controlled for, individuals who had increased bronchial responsiveness to histamine were significantly more likely to have symptoms of obstructive airway disease.[405]

The most powerful evidence in support of NSBH as an independent risk factor for COPD comes from the large American Lung Health Study in which approximately 6,000 smokers who had mild air-flow obstruction were followed for 5 years with yearly measurements of $FEV_1$.[406] The results showed that airway reactivity to methacholine as measured by the dose-response slope was an important predictor of progression of airway obstruction independent of the baseline level of obstruction.[407] Individuals who have NSBH not only are more likely to develop symptoms and functional deterioration but are also less likely to have remission of these symptoms occurring either spontaneously or after smoking cessation.[408]

Additional support for the Dutch hypothesis is derived from population studies in which a positive relationship has been shown between decreased FEV$_1$ levels and skin test responses to allergens, blood and sputum eosinophilia, and elevated serum IgE levels.[409–413] Relatives of patients who have COPD also have increased blood levels of IgE.[414] Serum levels of IgE normally decline after 15 years of age but tend to remain elevated in smokers, even in the absence of skin test responsiveness; smoking cessation is accompanied by a decline in IgE levels to their normal range. Although it is uncertain what antigens stimulate the increased IgE in smokers, in one study of 30 smokers and 30 nonsmokers, 11 of the former and only 2 of the latter had specific IgE directed against *S. pneumoniae,* an organism commonly recovered from the respiratory tract of smokers who have chronic bronchitis;[415] this suggests that the elevated IgE levels in smokers are at least partly attributable to specific antibody directed against microorganisms that infect the airways.

It is unlikely that the increased IgE level represents antibody production in response to components of tobacco; however, it could be a consequence of increased respiratory mucosal permeability or smoke-induced modulation of the numbers or function of helper or suppressor T lymphocytes.[412, 416] In support of the former mechanism are data derived from studies of rats, in which cigarette smoke exposure has been found to increase the likelihood of sensitization to inhaled but not to injected antigens.[417] Evidence in support of the latter supposition comes from studies that show an increased ratio of CD4$^+$/CD8$^+$ lymphocytes and an increase in IL-4 secretion by lymphocytes in the blood of smokers.[418, 419] Although it is clear that smoking increases serum IgE, it is less certain that the magnitude of the increase is a predictor of the rate of decline in FEV$_1$ in individual smokers.[420] In some cross-sectional and longitudinal studies, the predictive value of serum IgE levels is lost when correction is made for the influence of asthma and cigarette smoking,[421–423] or when asthmatic individuals are excluded from the analysis.[424] However, in other investigations, increased IgE levels appear to be an independent contributor to COPD risk. In one study of 1,533 individuals followed for 20 years, an elevated total serum IgE level was modestly predictive of the development of air-flow obstruction, even after correction for asthma and cigarette smoking.[425] Both smoking status and a raised total IgE level were significantly associated with a reduced FEV$_1$/FVC value in another study of 324 elderly individuals.[426]

Another explanation for the relationship between atopy, NSBH, and the development of COPD is based on the interpretation of longitudinal studies of cohorts in Chicago and Arizona.[31, 427] According to this, there are at least two groups of patients who have chronic air-flow obstruction. One group is composed of individuals who have many of the characteristics of asthma, including atopy, episodic bronchoconstriction, and a slow decline in lung function. The other, larger group of patients is composed of those who tend to be heavy smokers, have no evidence of atopy, experience the insidious onset of dyspnea, and have decreased diffusing capacity and radiographic evidence of emphysema.

### Mucus and Mucociliary Clearance in Chronic Bronchitis and Chronic Obstructive Pulmonary Disease

Biochemical analysis of the sputum of patients who have chronic bronchitis shows an increased concentration of serum proteins and glycoproteins, indicating the presence of a serum transudate.[428] In the presence of infectious exacerbations, the concentration of these serum proteins is increased further and is accompanied by a decreased concentration of secretory IgA, indicating increased epithelial permeability or impaired epithelial secretion, or both.[429] An alteration in the visco-elastic properties of mucus also occurs in patients who have chronic bronchitis.[430] However, measurements of viscosity and elasticity *in vitro* do not invariably correlate well with measurements of mucus transport rate; for example, no correlation was found between sputum visco-elasticity and ciliary or cough clearance in one investigation.[431] In another study, both *in vivo* clearance and *in vitro* transport of sputum on a frog palate were found to be significantly related.[432]

The effect of cigarette smoking on mucociliary clearance has been examined in individuals who do not have symptoms of chronic bronchitis.[433, 434] In a study in which mucociliary clearance and aerosol deposition were compared in 30 asymptomatic smokers who had small airway dysfunction (selected on the basis of an abnormal closing volume and isoflow volume) and in 20 nonsmokers who did not have evidence of small airway dysfunction, delayed peripheral lung clearance and increased heterogeneity in the deposition of radioaerosol were observed in the smokers, suggesting nonuniform distribution of ventilation.[435] In another study in which the tracheal mucus velocity technique was used to compare central airway clearance in several groups of subjects, mucus velocity was decreased in older nonsmokers compared with young nonsmokers, and central mucus velocity was significantly impaired in young smokers who manifested no evidence of small airway disease;[436] ex-smokers showed some improvement in mucociliary clearance but not to normal levels. Patients who had chronic bronchitis, with or without airway obstruction, showed marked reduction in tracheal mucus velocity.

In patients who have COPD, the relationship between the amount smoked and decreased expiratory flow rates is closer than that between the smoking history and impairment of mucociliary clearance, suggesting that there is considerable interindividual variation in the effect of smoke on mucociliary clearance.[437] In patients who have similar smoking histories and similar degrees of air-flow obstruction, those who have pulmonary carcinoma show more severe impairment of mucociliary clearance rates.[438]

The magnitude of the impairment of mucociliary clearance in smokers and patients who have COPD is dependent on the measurement technique that is employed. For example, when patients who have air-flow obstruction and normal individuals are compared, studies of central airway clearance show a less marked decrease in clearance, whereas more significant differences are noted when whole-lung studies are performed using measurement of radioaerosol clearance or techniques that encourage peripheral deposition.[439] This difference probably results from the finding of more central deposition in the obstructed patients, a confounding variable that biases results toward enhanced mucociliary clearance in these patients. Cough appears to be a more important and effective mechanism of mucociliary clearance in patients who have chronic bronchitis than in normal individuals[440] and careful control of cough frequency is important in the study of mucociliary clearance in patients who have obstructive airway disease.[441, 442]

The precise mechanism by which cigarette smoking and chronic bronchitis impair mucociliary clearance is unclear and probably multifactorial. Anatomic factors are probably involved: patients who have chronic bronchitis have an increased number of ultrastructurally abnormal cilia,[443, 444] as well as replacement of ciliated cells by goblet cells and metaplastic squamous cells. In addition, the simple increase in the quantity of secreted mucus could disrupt the clearance mechanism. The results of one *in vitro* study showed that the particulate fraction of cigarette smoke can acutely decrease the electrical potential difference across dog tracheal epithelium and impair ion transport;[445] such impairment could cause a reduction in the volume of sol-phase secretions, resulting in an imbalance between mucus and sol-phase constituents and impaired clearance.

The importance of increased mucus production and impaired mucociliary clearance in the pathogenesis of the airway obstruction associated with smoking is an interesting and difficult problem to address. The existence of patients who have the dyskinetic cilia syndrome (*see* page 2281) allows a comparison of airway function in patients who have an isolated clearance defect and in those who have mucus hypersecretion as well. In one investigation in which mucociliary clearance and airway function were compared in patients who had ciliary dyskinesia, chronic bronchitis, cystic fibrosis, or emphysema secondary to homozygous alpha$_1$-antiprotease inhibitor deficiency, patients in the first group showed marked impairment of mucociliary clearance as evidenced by 92% retention of a radioaerosol 2 hours after inhalation (the normal value is less than 35%).[446] Patients who had COPD caused by smoking had less severe impairment of clearance, retention amounting to 65% at 2 hours; patients who had cystic fibrosis also had less abnormal clearance rates than those seen in individuals in the ciliary dyskinesia group, although pulmonary function was significantly more impaired. Patients who had alpha$_1$-antiprotease inhibitor deficiency showed no abnormality of mucociliary clearance, although they manifested marked air-flow obstruction. The investigators concluded that impaired mucociliary clearance may be a contributing mechanism in the production of obstruction in patients who have COPD, but that it is not the primary underlying cause. Most patients who have ciliary dyskinesia develop mild chronic airway obstruction by the age of 25 to 40 years, indicating that severe dysfunction of mucociliary clearance can cause obstructive pulmonary disease.

In patients who have COPD, tracheobronchial clearance of technetium-labeled particles is enhanced by the inhalation of hypertonic saline aerosol[447] and by parenteral administration of beta-adrenergic agonists.[448]

### Pathogenesis of Emphysema

It is now widely accepted that an imbalance between elastolytic and antielastolytic factors within the lung is the fundamental pathogenetic abnormality in emphysema.[449–451] The many factors that influence this dynamic balance are shown in Figure 55–3. The neutrophil is probably the most important source of elastase in emphysema. Human neutrophil elastase is a glycoprotein with a molecular mass of 22 to 35 kDa that is stored in azurophilic granules and is released following stimulation with chemotactic agents and during phagocytosis. Besides elastin and collagen, it degrades a broad spectrum of proteins, including fibronectin, immunoglobulins, complement components, clotting factors, and the glycoproteins that make up the interstitial connective tissue of the lung. Other proteinases and elastases may also play a role in the pathogenesis of emphysema.[452] Both alveolar and interstitial macrophages contain a variety of metalloproteinases (MMPs) that have elastase and collagenase activity; because these cells are significantly increased in number in smokers, these enzymes must be considered as potential culprits. In fact, increased levels of MMPs have been detected in the bronchoalveolar lavage (BAL) fluid of patients who have emphysema.[453–455]

Lung elastin is normally protected from excessive elastolytic damage by alpha$_1$-protease inhibitor (alpha$_1$-PI)—i.e., alpha$_1$-antiprotease—and other circulating and locally produced antiproteinases. Alpha$_1$-PI is a 54 kDa glycoprotein that is synthesized in the liver and circulates in the blood. On serum protein electrophoresis it migrates with the alpha globulin band—hence its name; in fact, alpha$_1$-PI makes up the majority of the protein content of the alpha$_1$ band (normal = 0.18 to 0.20 g/liter). The level and electrophoretic mobility of alpha$_1$-PI is determined by variations in genotype that alter the phenotype of the protein; and as discussed farther on (*see* page 2231), more than 60 of these variants exist. Most of the phenotypes are associated with normal blood levels of alpha$_1$-PI; however, patients who have the phenotypes ZZ, SZ, and SS can have very low levels of alpha$_1$ globulin (10% or less), and those who have the heterozygous phenotypes MZ and MS can have a mild to moderate decrease (60% to 80% of normal). Alpha$_1$-PI completely blocks the action of neutrophil elastase at equivalent molar concentrations by acting like a substrate for the enzyme and forming a stable complex with it; it is less effective against the MMP, which it only partly inhibits. Neutrophil and macrophage elastases can also be inhibited by a 720 kDa circulating alpha$_2$-macroglobulin; however, the large molecular weight prevents escape of this substance from the vasculature, and because the site of elastolytic damage is the interstitial space, alpha$_2$-macroglobulin is not believed to be of major importance in the pathogenesis of emphysema.[456]

Another potentially important antiproteinase is bronchial mucus proteinase inhibitor, a 12-kDa protein that is also known as antileukoproteinase or secretory leukocyte proteinase inhibitor (SLPI). SLPI is produced by airway epithelial cells and can inhibit neutrophil elastase even after it has bound to elastin.[457] The large airways contain relatively high concentrations of SLPI, and SLPI possesses certain physical properties that allow it to function as the principal antiproteinase at this site.[458–460] In theory, a defect in the metabolism of SLPI could predispose affected individuals to the development of emphysema and COPD; however, no genetic variants of SLPI that decrease its levels or impair its function have been identified. In one investigation of 114 individuals who had various alpha$_1$-antitrypsin genotypes and 10 patients who had early-onset COPD and no evidence of alpha$_1$-antitrypsin deficiency, no mutations were discov-

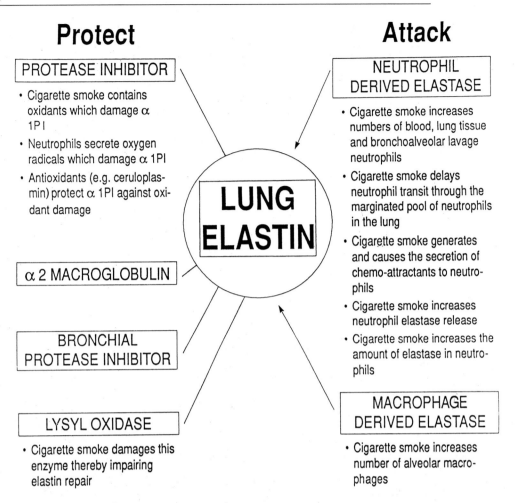

**Figure 55–3. Pathogenesis of Emphysema.** Cigarette smoke interacts with the proteolysis-antiproteolysis balance at a number of sites. The overall effect is to promote increased breakdown of elastin and to interfere with repair.

**Protect**

PROTEASE INHIBITOR

- Cigarette smoke contains oxidants which damage α 1PI
- Neutrophils secrete oxygen radicals which damage α 1PI
- Antioxidants (e.g. ceruloplasmin) protect α 1PI against oxidant damage

α 2 MACROGLOBULIN

BRONCHIAL PROTEASE INHIBITOR

LYSYL OXIDASE

- Cigarette smoke damages this enzyme thereby impairing elastin repair

LUNG ELASTIN

**Attack**

NEUTROPHIL DERIVED ELASTASE

- Cigarette smoke increases numbers of blood, lung tissue and bronchoalveolar lavage neutrophils
- Cigarette smoke delays neutrophil transit through the marginated pool of neutrophils in the lung
- Cigarette smoke generates and causes the secretion of chemo-attractants to neutrophils
- Cigarette smoke increases neutrophil elastase release
- Cigarette smoke increases the amount of elastase in neutrophils

MACROPHAGE DERIVED ELASTASE

- Cigarette smoke increases number of alveolar macrophages

ered for polymorphisms in exons 2, 3, and 4 of the SLPI gene, suggesting that structural alterations in the protein do not play a major role in the pathogenesis of COPD.[461]

The lung possesses the enzymatic capacity to replace and repair damaged structural proteins, and there is normally a slow turnover of elastin and collagen. Such synthesis and repair necessitate the presence of the enzyme lysyl oxidase, which catalyzes the cross-linking of collagen and elastin. In animals, beta-aminopropionitrite blocks lysyl oxidase and exaggerates the effects of elastase (*see* farther on). Cigarette smoke not only blunts the increase in lysyl oxidase that normally follows elastolytic injury[450] but also increases the number of circulating and pulmonary neutrophils.[462–465] There is also a significant relationship between white blood cell count and lung function irrespective of smoking habit. In one study of smokers, former smokers, and nonsmokers, an inverse relationship was found between white blood cell count and the $FEV_1$.[463] Persons who have higher white blood cell counts have been found to show a more rapid decline in $FEV_1$ over a 10-year follow-up period.[462] Interestingly, a higher white blood cell count and a lower $FEV_1$ were both found to be significant predictors of mortality in a longitudinal follow-up study of a North American cohort.[466] In an animal model, chronic exposure to cigarette smoke increases the leukocyte count and the size of the mitotic and postmitotic pools of granulocytes in the bone marrow, as well as reducing the maturation time of polymorphonuclear cells.[467] In addition to increased leukocytes, the blood of smokers

contains higher-than-normal amounts of acute phase–reactive proteins including ninth component of complement, ceruloplasmin, and alpha₁-PI. These data support the concept that smoke induces a chronic low-grade inflammatory reaction.[468] The increased number of pulmonary neutrophils in smokers has been demonstrated in both BAL fluid[465, 469] and lung tissue,[464] although in one study there was no correlation between lavage and tissue neutrophils.[470]

The dynamics of neutrophil transit through the lung are of considerable interest and potential importance in the pathogenesis of emphysema.[471, 472] A pool of marginated leukocytes two to three times the number of neutrophils in the circulating blood is normally present in the human lung. The vast majority of these marginated cells are located within the pulmonary capillaries; these turn over slowly with the circulating pool. *In vivo* studies have shown that approximately 20% of labeled leukocytes are retained within the lung's marginating pool in a single pass through the pulmonary circulation.[473] The delay in leukocyte passage through the lung is partly a mechanical effect related to discrepancies in capillary segment diameter and to the size and deformability of leukocytes.[471] Regional blood flow and transit time are also involved: in regions where blood flow is high and transit time relatively fast, such as at the lung base, neutrophil delay is less.[474] The delayed transit of white blood cells through the upper lung regions could explain the upper lobe predominance of centrilobular emphysema.

Cigarette smoking acutely decreases the deformability

of neutrophils, an effect that is mediated by an oxidant action on the microfilament-actin component of the cytoskeleton.[475, 476] The longer a neutrophil remains in the pulmonary microvasculature, the more likely it is to interact with chemotactic or activating stimuli that could result in adherence, migration into the interstitium, and release of elastase. The acute inhalation of cigarette smoke increases the pulmonary sequestration of leukocytes by delaying their transit through the lung.[477]

Cigarette smoke causes an increase in the peripheral blood neutrophil count and a marked increase in pulmonary neutrophils. The mechanism by which the bone marrow is stimulated by cigarette smoking is unclear. It has been suggested that alveolar macrophages release cytokines, such as granulocyte-macrophage colony–stimulating factor (GM-CSF), during their ingestion of particles.[478] The attraction of neutrophils to the lung is easier to explain; cigarette smoke can act directly as a chemoattractant for inflammatory cells and can also increase the migration of leukocytes from the vascular space to the interstitium by stimulating the release of chemotactic factors from alveolar macrophages and airway epithelial cells.[479, 480] Smoke has been shown in *in vitro* studies to activate complement and generate C5a, an extremely potent chemotactic substance.[469, 481] Evidence for complement activation is more apparent in smokers who have more severe abnormalities of lung function and worse emphysema.[482] Collagen and elastin breakdown products may attract inflammatory cells to the site of injury, initiating a vicious circle.[450] Cigarette smoke has also been shown to enhance neutrophil adhesion to the endothelium.[483] Patients who have COPD have decreased levels of a chemotactic factor inactivator, which could also increase the extravasation of activated leukocytes.[484]

In addition to attracting neutrophils, cigarette smoke can cause the release of elastase from neutrophils; it may stimulate neutrophils to actively secrete elastase or may simply damage the cell membrane, thereby releasing the enzyme.[485] A number of investigators have shown that the amount of neutrophil elastase per cell is increased in smokers who have airway obstruction;[486–488] however, whether it is the smoking that increases the levels is unclear. The peripheral neutrophils of smokers also show a higher-than-normal content of myeloperoxidase, an enzyme that can oxidatively inactivate alpha$_1$-PI.[489] Cigarette smokers exhibit greatly increased numbers of alveolar macrophages[490–492] in which metabolic[460] and elastolytic[491, 493] activity is increased. When stimulated, peripheral blood leukocytes of smokers who have air-flow obstruction accumulate greater amounts of intracellular and extracellular oxidants than do the cells of smokers who do not have air-flow obstruction.[494]

Besides increasing the number and elastolytic capacity of inflammatory cells, cigarette smoke can tip the balance toward elastolysis by interfering with the ability of alpha$_1$-PI to inhibit the elastase that is released.[458] The active site on alpha$_1$-PI is a methionine-serine bond at position 358; it is susceptible to oxidant damage, which results in a complete block of the ability of alpha$_1$-PI to inhibit elastase.[495] The gas phase of cigarette smoke is a rich source of oxidizing agents; it has been estimated that one puff of cigarette smoke contains more than 10$^{14}$ free radicals.[496] Nitric oxide (NO) is also present in cigarette smoke at concentrations of 500 to 1000 parts per million (ppm), and it can quickly react with

superoxide anion to form the cytotoxic peroxynitrate radical.[497] These reactive molecules can impair alpha$_1$-PI by inhibiting its ability to bind and inactivate proteinases,[498, 499] can cause damage and fragmentation of lung elastin and collagen, and can interfere with elastin synthesis and repair.[500, 501] Activated neutrophils and macrophages also release oxygen radicals that may have a similar effect; because there is about a 10-fold increase in pulmonary leukocytes and a 2- to 4-fold increase in alveolar macrophages in smokers, the oxidant burden is considerable.[502]

The increased free radical formation in smokers is accompanied by a decrease in circulating and intrapulmonary antioxidant capacity. Among the depleted antioxidant molecules in plasma are ascorbic acid, alpha tocopherol, vitamin E, and beta carotene;[502] a decreased amount of glutathione is also seen in alveolar macrophages. Evidence for increased oxidative stress in smokers is supported by the finding of elevated levels of lipid peroxides in the plasma.[503] A relative inability to scavenge oxygen radicals may be a risk factor for elastolytic lung injury; in one study, the antioxidant activity of plasma was found to be deficient in individuals who had a family history of lung disease, and there was a significant relationship between antioxidant activity and FEV$_1$/FVC.[504]

It has been difficult to show that alpha$_1$-PI activity is decreased in the serum of smokers. Alpha$_1$-PI content and activity must be separately measured to show that there is a decrease in the active form. In some studies, circulating alpha$_1$-PI activity has been found to be reduced, whereas in others, it is normal.[505–508] Acute heavy cigarette smoking causes a transient decrease in the antielastase capacity of circulating alpha$_1$-PI[509] and an increase in the blood levels of elastase.[510]

The concentration of oxidizing substances in the lung is likely to be much higher in the interstitium, where levels of smoke constituents and numbers of activated leukocytes are greatest. Because this is the site of elastase-induced injury,[511] it is here that inactivation of alpha$_1$-PI would have the most harmful effect; studies of sputum and BAL fluid show that there is inactivation or impaired function of alpha$_1$-PI in the lungs of smokers, especially those who have obstructive lung disease.[512–515] Ceruloplasmin is an important circulating antioxidant and can theoretically protect alpha$_1$-PI from oxidative damage. Ceruloplasmin has been detected in the BAL fluid of both smokers and nonsmokers;[516] although smokers had higher levels, it was less active as an antioxidant. Oxidative damage induced by smoke may also impair the antielastase activity of the low-molecular-weight SLPI.[517]

Additional evidence to support the proteolytic mechanism for the pathogenesis of emphysema comes from quantitative studies of the total amount of lung tissue and of elastin in emphysematous lungs. The amount of lung tissue can be estimated using CT; in severe emphysema, total tissue mass is significantly reduced compared with that of nonemphysematous or mildly emphysematous lungs. There is also decreased lung elastin content, as measured by an assay for desmosine.[518] Evidence of elastin degradation can be assessed by measuring breakdown products of elastin in the blood and urine. In one study employing an immunoassay for soluble elastin fragments in plasma, levels in emphysematous patients were approximately 25 times higher than those in normal nonsmokers;[519] there were also significant correlations between loss of lung recoil, CT estimates of emphysema severity, and plasma levels of the fragments. However, these results were not confirmed in another investigation.[520] Desmosine and isodesmosine are elastin-specific cross-linking molecules that are excreted in the urine. In a 12-year study of smokers who had a rapid or a slow decline in $FEV_1$, there was a significantly higher (30%) level of urinary desmosine in the rapid-decline group.[521] Similarly, urinary elastin degradation products were higher in smokers than in nonsmokers and higher still in smokers who had COPD in a cross-sectional study.[522] Abnormalities of elastic tissue structure have also been found in the lungs of patients who have panlobular or centrilobular emphysema on both light and electron microscopic examination.[523]

Although the total elastin content of the lung appears to decrease during the development of emphysema, there is evidence that the amount of collagen is actually increased. One group of investigators measured the hydroxyproline content of the lung per unit volume of distended lung or per unit surface area of alveolar wall;[524] the collagen content was increased in the lungs of the patients who had emphysema but not in those of smokers who did not have emphysema. It was increased the most in the lungs that had panlobular emphysema.

Although the bulk of the experimental and clinical evidence supports an imbalance in the relationship between antiproteolytic and proteolytic factors as crucial in the genesis of emphysema, there is still no explanation for why only a subset of smokers develops symptomatic emphysema. In particular, no differences in the content or releasibility of proteolytic enzymes have been demonstrated between smokers who do or do not have emphysema.[525]

### Experimental Emphysema

Emphysema can be produced in animals by increasing proteolysis in the lung or by interfering with the synthesis and turnover of protein.

**Protease-Induced Emphysema.** A variety of proteolytic enzymes has been used to produce emphysema in different animal species. In the initial studies, the disease was produced in rats by repeated intratracheal instillation of papain, a proteinase derived from the fruit of the papaw tree (*Carica papaya*).[526] It has subsequently been administered intratracheally or by aerosol in dogs, hamsters, and rabbits.[527–539] The resulting emphysema is usually mild, unless excessive exposure causes pulmonary hemorrhage. Pancreatic elastase,[540, 541] homogenates of polymorphonuclear leukocytes and macrophages, and purified human neutrophil elastase also have been shown to cause morphologic and physiologic changes comparable to those of human emphysema.[537, 542–547] When administered via the airway, elastase is far more effective than when injected intravenously, presumably because antiproteinases inactivate the enzyme in the latter situation. Physical exercise or mechanical ventilation following administration of elastase does not increase its effect.[548, 549] The emphysema that results from exogenous elastase is more severe if blood levels of antiproteinase are decreased,[550] but its development is completely inhibited or attenuated if alpha$_1$-PI, SLPI, or a synthetic elastase inhibitor is administered before elastase.[533, 539, 551–555]

A single dose of intratracheal elastase can cause progressive elastolytic damage; in dogs, elastin-derived peptide fragments can be detected in the blood for 40 days after the administration of a single dose.[556] It is possible that elastase is taken up by macrophages and then slowly released, accounting for its prolonged action.[450] Human neutrophil elastase also stimulates secretory cell metaplasia in hamsters, and this is also blocked by alpha$_1$-PI.[557] In a rat model of emphysema produced by intratracheal administration of porcine pancreatic elastase, morphologic examination and scanning electron microscopy revealed sheets of elastin to be disrupted and associated with multiple fenestrations, while there was a marked increase in thickness and a disorganization of the collagen fiber network;[558] a similar pattern of thickened and disorganized collagen fibrils was observed in emphysematous human lungs. Similarly, in a guinea pig model of emphysema caused by chronic exposure to cigarette smoke, there was evidence for an increased content of lung collagen as well as an increased collagenolytic capacity.[559] As mentioned previously, increased collagen content has been reported in the lungs of individuals who had centrilobular or panlobular emphysema.[524]

In an experiment in dogs, repeated intravenous injection of bacterial endotoxin over 17 weeks was shown to cause sequestration of neutrophils in the pulmonary vasculature and mild emphysema (increased mean linear intercept and loss of lung recoil).[560] Endotoxin injected intravenously into monkeys also causes alveolar disruption;[561] daily injections of endotoxin were associated with a transient but profound reduction in the number of circulating leukocytes, presumably as a result of pulmonary sequestration. These observations offer important support for the proteolysis-antiproteolysis theory of the pathogenesis of emphysema, because they show that an imbalance in favor of elastolysis may occur when neutrophils are activated and sequestered within the lung. A similar mechanism could explain the predominant lower zonal emphysema that develops in drug abusers who repeatedly inject talc-containing medications intravenously.[562]

The ability to induce overexpression of certain genes using transgenic technology and to disable their function using "knock-outs" has opened up a new area of study of the pathogenesis of emphysema.[563] In mice, the transgenic overexpression of human collagenase (MMP-1) leads to an emphysema-like lung lesion,[564] and a mouse in which the macrophage elastase gene (MMP-12) was "knocked out" failed to develop emphysema when exposed to cigarette smoke.[565] Although it has generally been assumed that alveolar destruction is an irreversible process, a recent study in rats showed that treatment with retinoic acid may be able to cause re-alveolarization of lung previously made emphysematous using elastase.[566]

**Lathyrogen-Induced Emphysema.** Cross-linking between collagen fibers is necessary for normal connective tissue synthesis and repair. Defective bonding between collagen and elastin occurs in animals fed the seed of *Lathyrus odoratus*,[567] and a substance that interferes with the bonding process is therefore called a lathyrogen. Lysyl oxidase is the enzyme that catalyzes the cross-linking; a well-investigated lathyrogen that inhibits it is beta-aminopropionitrile. Administration of the latter substance to neonatal rats results in the development of large alveoli and increased lung compliance.[568] Moreover, when it is administered at the same time as when elastase is given, it causes more severe emphysema than when elastase is given alone.[450] Lysyl oxidase is dependent on minute concentrations of copper as a cofactor for its action, and it has been shown that copper-deficient rats[569] and pigs[570] develop larger air spaces and greater loss of lung elasticity than do animals that have normal copper levels. In one cross-sectional population study of 397 men, there was a significant relationship in nonsmokers between $FEV_1$ and the copper content of drinking water.[571] Defective bonding between collagen and elastin is believed to be the underlying mechanism for the inherited emphysema-like changes found in the lungs of the "blotchy mouse."[572, 573]

**Cadmium-Induced Emphysema.** Cadmium chloride in aerosol form has been reported to produce centrilobular emphysema in rats[574] and hamsters,[450] whereas it causes extensive fibrosis, irregular emphysema, and pulmonary overinflation in guinea pigs;[575] beta-aminopropionitrile enhances emphysema formation in hamsters.[450] Human contact with cadmium can be associated with ingestion of food, particularly seafood, or inhalation of environmental pollutants and cigarette smoke. It has been shown that about 70% of the cadmium content of cigarette tobacco passes into the smoke. Cadmium is stored in the liver; in one study, patients who had COPD were found to have a mean liver cadmium content more than three times that found in a control group, a level that may simply reflect the influence of cigarette smoking and air pollution.[576]

**Other Models of Emphysema.** A morphologic and physiologic state simulating emphysema can be produced in animals by continuous exposure to moderately increased levels of $NO_2$.[545, 577–579] Although such animals can live a normal life span, at autopsy they have voluminous lungs with a large functional residual capacity (FRC), obliteration of terminal bronchioles, and distention and loss of alveoli.[579] Emphysema-like changes can also be produced in the lungs of certain animal species by chronic exposure to phosgene and cigarette smoke.[545]

## PATHOLOGIC CHARACTERISTICS

Although many investigators have carried out traditional descriptive pathologic studies of the morphologic abnormalities in COPD,[579a] our understanding of the clinical significance of their findings has been greatly advanced by investigations in which pulmonary function and structure have been compared. This is particularly so for studies in which morphometric measurements of the extent of pathologic change and the relative volume or area of various tissues and airspaces have been obtained. Clinical specimens in which such studies correlating morphology and function have been performed are of three major types:

1. Lungs that have been examined after death from patients who have undergone pulmonary function tests during life. A potential disadvantage of such studies is that terminal events and a prolonged time interval between assessment of function and death can make the pathologic findings unrepresentative of the morphologic abnormalities existing at the time the function studies were performed.

2. Lungs excised at autopsy in which certain function tests have been performed before fixation and pathologic examination. Although this permits close association in time between lung structure and function, there are potential errors in extrapolating the function of excised lungs to the *in vivo* state.

3. Lungs excised surgically from patients in which function has been measured immediately preoperatively. Although this is perhaps the most accurate method, potential methodologic limitations include inadequacy of sampling (resulting from the ability to examine only one lung or lobe and from a nonuniform distribution of pathologic abnormalities) and inaccuracy related to the influence of the underlying lesion responsible for the resection.

Because the vast majority of patients who have chronic air-flow obstruction have abnormalities in both the conducting airways and the lung parenchyma, it is artificial to discuss the pathology of chronic bronchitis and emphysema separately. Consequently, in this section we describe the pathologic characteristics of the large airways, small airways, and lung parenchyma, recognizing that the changes in individual patients may be located predominantly in one of these sites.

### Trachea and Bronchi

Abnormalities of the trachea and major bronchi are common in COPD and involve virtually all tissue components, including the surface epithelium, tracheobronchial glands, muscularis mucosa, connective tissue of the lamina propria and submucosa, and cartilage. Changes in the tracheobronchial glands have probably been the subject of greatest attention. Reid was the first to quantify the changes and correlate them with the clinical syndrome of excessive cough and mucus expectoration.[580] The yardstick that she suggested for the assessment of the presence and severity of gland hypertrophy consists of the ratio of the width of a mucous gland to the width of the adjacent bronchial wall measured from the airway epithelial basement membrane to the inner edge of the perichondrium (Fig. 55–4). Although many investigators have demonstrated reasonable correlation between this measurement (known as the Reid index) and the presence and severity of mucus hypersecretion,[580–583] others have shown that the correlation is better with morphometric estimates of the absolute area or volume of mucous glands.[584–586]

In fact, there is very little practical diagnostic value in the assessment of tracheobronchial gland enlargement. Although very high and very low values for the Reid index predict the presence or absence of chronic bronchitis with reasonable accuracy, intermediate values (which are found in the majority of both normal individuals and those with chronic bronchitis) possess virtually no predictive value for the presence of chronic cough and phlegm production.[587–590] Second, and perhaps more important, measurements of bronchial gland hypertrophy generally do not correlate with the severity of airway obstruction.[584, 591]

The increase in size of tracheobronchial glands is sometimes apparent by simple observation of histologic sections of airways from patients who have chronic bronchitis (*see* Fig. 55–4). The increase is probably related more to hyperplasia than to hypertrophy.[592] The ratio of mucous cells to

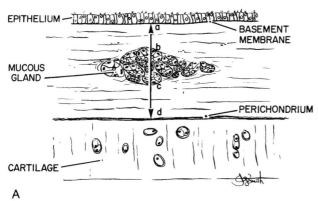

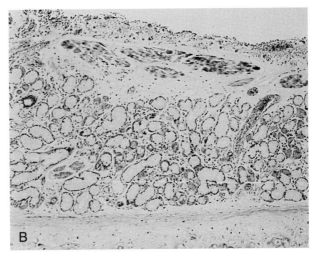

**Figure 55–4. Bronchial Gland Hypertrophy and the Reid Index.** A diagrammatic representation of a bronchial wall *(A)* shows the measurements by which the Reid index is calculated: the maximum thickness of a bronchial gland internal to the cartilage (b to c) is divided by the distance from the basement membrane to the inner perichondrium (a to d). A section of segmental bronchus *(B)* from a patient who had chronic productive cough shows diffuse glandular hypertrophy, the Reid index being approximately 0.6. (*A* is from Thurbeck WM: Chronic Airflow Obstruction in Lung Disease. Philadelphia, WB Saunders Co, 1976, p 33.)

serous cells within the gland is also increased in some cases. The openings of the bronchial gland ducts into the airway lumen may be plugged with mucus and are often dilated,[593] presumably reflecting the increase in volume of secretion; the latter abnormality has been appreciated on bronchograms as small depressions or diverticula on the airway luminal surface and on scanning electron micrographs (Fig. 55–5). It has also been suggested that some diverticula are related to loss of subepithelial connective tissue and herniation of airway mucosa between smooth muscle bundles.[593]

The quantity of bronchial cartilage has been found to be decreased in patients who have COPD in some[594–598] but not all[590, 599, 600] investigations. The most severe deficiency has been seen in the segmental and subsegmental airways; generally, the changes have been more apparent in the lower than in the upper lobes. In both normal individuals and patients who have COPD, maximal forced expiratory maneuvers result in flow-limiting collapse of segments of central cartilaginous airways.[601, 602] Because cartilage provides an important contribution to the relative incompressibility of these airways, its deficiency might be expected to result in more prominent collapse. Although some studies of the relationship between pressure and cross-sectional area of the trachea in patients who have COPD have shown increased "compliance,"[603] suggesting that the loss observed histologically possesses a functional counterpart, the results of one systematic study in 72 patients who underwent lobectomy or pneumonectomy showed no relationship between the amount of cartilage in bronchi and measures of maximal expiratory flow.[604, 605]

The pathogenesis of the cartilage abnormality is unclear. In experimental animals, damage to cartilage by proteolytic enzymes results in air-flow obstruction unaccompanied by changes in lung elastic recoil or in dimensions of small airways.[233, 606, 607] Thus, it is possible that the chronic airway inflammation associated with COPD causes proteolytic damage to structural proteins in the large airways; to the extent that such damage increases the collapsibility of the large airways, maximal expiratory flow will be decreased. It has

also been suggested that deficiency of airway elastic tissue may be caused by the same mechanism and can have the same functional consequences.[608]

The amount of smooth muscle in the bronchial wall of patients who have chronic bronchitis has been found to be increased by some investigators[609–611] but to be normal by others.[612] The relationship between such an increase and the presence of airway hyper-responsiveness or variability of severity of air-flow obstruction in COPD patients is not clear. One investigator found an increase in the number of small nerve twigs as well as an increase in the size of larger nerve branches in the proximal bronchi of patients who had COPD.[613]

Chronic inflammatory cells, especially lymphocytes, are typically increased in number in the tracheobronchial wall. In one study, cough and sputum expectoration were shown to correlate more closely with the number of such inflammatory cells than with gland volume, suggesting that inflammation of large airway mucosa and glands may be important in the pathogenesis of mucus production.[614]

Epithelial changes in the trachea and major bronchi are common in patients who have COPD and include hyperplasia of goblet and basal cells and squamous metaplasia, sometimes associated with dysplasia.[615, 616] Although such changes are not likely to contribute directly to airway obstruction, they may interfere with mucociliary clearance.

### Bronchioles

The demonstration by Hogg and associates that airways smaller than 2 to 3 mm in internal diameter are the major site of increase in resistance to air flow in lungs removed at autopsy from patients who had obstructive lung disease resulted in the focus of increased attention on these airways.[617] The peripheral location of increased airway resistance in patients who have COPD has been confirmed *in vivo* using micromanometer-tipped catheters introduced into the peripheral airways.[618] Although the exact mechanism for the increase in resistance is incompletely understood, it ap-

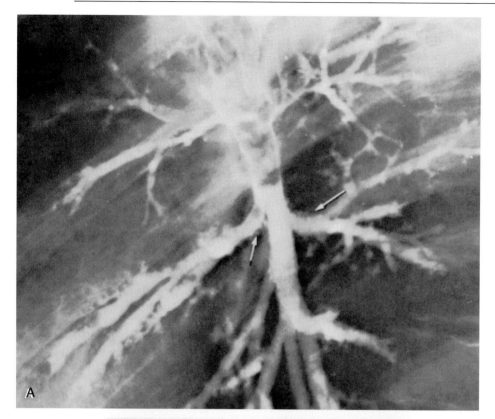

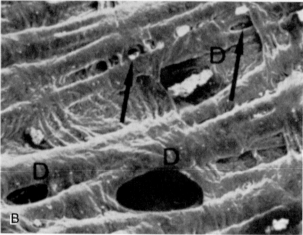

**Figure 55–5. Bronchial Wall Diverticula in Chronic Obstructive Pulmonary Disease: Bronchographic and Scanning Micrographic Appearance.** A lateral projection of the major and segmental bronchi from a right bronchogram *(A)* shows filling of several outpouchings or diverticula on the inferior aspect of the middle lobe bronchus and the upper surface of the superior segmental bronchus of the lower lobe *(arrows)*. Many of the segmental bronchi have lost their normal tapering, suggesting cylindrical bronchiectasis. A scanning electron micrograph *(B)* from a 64-year-old smoker shows several small *(arrows)* and large (D) diverticula. (*B,* ×34.) (*B* is from Wang N-S, Ling W-L: Hum Pathol 8:304, 1977.)

pears to be related to one or more of several abnormalities, including[619]

- a loss of elastic recoil in the peribronchiolar alveolar interstitial tissue
- a loss of the alveolar attachments to the outer wall of the small airways; a significant relationship exists between the number of such attachments and the results of tests of airflow obstruction in human lungs at autopsy,[620] and the alveolar attachments also show enlarged fenestrae in individuals who have decreased expiratory flow, suggesting that elastolytic disruption of the supportive framework of the small airways results from "spill-over" of the inflammatory process to adjacent alveolar walls[621]
- an abnormality of bronchiolar surface–active lipids, resulting in an alteration of the relationship between pressure and cross-sectional area in much the same way as the

change in the pressure-volume curve of the lung occurs in the presence of pulmonary edema
- chronic inflammation and fibrosis of the airway wall* (Fig. 55–6), resulting in a thickening of the wall at the expense of the lumen; serial reconstruction of the membranous bronchioles in patients who have emphysema has shown that there are localized areas of bronchiolar stenosis in addition to diffuse narrowing[622]
- competition for space between the terminal bronchiole and the dilated air spaces in foci of centrilobular emphysema[623]

---

*The term "small airway disease" has been used not only to describe these pathologic abnormalities but also to refer to a distinct clinical presentation that is seen in a small number of patients who have a "specific" clinical-radiologic-pathologic form of COPD.[21, 625] We believe that the use of the term in the latter context should be abandoned, to prevent confusion. Disease of the small airways is one of the abnormalities that leads to airway obstruction in COPD; it is not a disease in its own right.

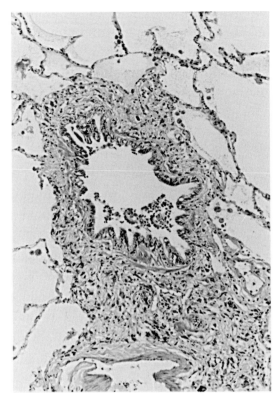

**Figure 55–6. Chronic Obstructive Pulmonary Disease: Bronchiolar Narrowing.** A section of a membranous bronchiole shows a moderate degree of mural thickening, predominantly the result of a mononuclear inflammatory infiltrate and fibrosis. The lumen is partly filled with macrophages and neutrophils.

- accumulation of mucus in the airway lumen secondary to goblet cell hyperplasia and impaired mucociliary clearance

The severity of different aspects of the inflammatory reaction in membranous bronchioles can be measured using a semiquantitative grading schema.[626] With this system, bronchioles are examined microscopically and the following pathologic features assessed: inflammatory cell infiltration, hyperplasia of goblet cells, squamous metaplasia, fibrosis, smooth muscle hyperplasia, and pigment deposition. The system has been modified for the respiratory bronchioles by omitting the categories of squamous cell metaplasia and goblet cell hyperplasia and including the accumulation of intraluminal macrophages.[627] Grading is performed by comparing the light microscopic appearance of individual membranous and respiratory bronchioles with a set of "standard" micrographs and assigning a grade of 0 to 3 on the basis of increasing severity of the abnormality.[628] The total score for an individual patient is the observed score expressed as a percentage of the highest possible score (3 multiplied by the number of airways examined). Scores for each component of the inflammatory response are assigned, and a total pathology score is calculated as the sum of the component scores. Separate scores for membranous and respiratory bronchioles are determined. There are no "normal" values; however, the system provides a method of ranking individual lungs for the severity of the different pathologic changes and of comparing calculated ranks with altered pulmonary function.

More quantitative morphometric estimates of airway changes can also be used, such as measurements of the number of inflammatory cells per mm² of airway wall,[629] the thickness of the airway wall,[630] the ratio of airway size to the size of the accompanying pulmonary artery,[631] and the number of airways per unit lung area or volume.[632] These measurements are more difficult to make and more time-consuming than is use of the grading system, and for the most part the correlations between them and the more subjective assessment of structural damage have been close.[629, 633–635]

When the lungs of smokers are compared with those of nonsmokers at autopsy, the former show narrowing and inflammatory changes in membranous and respiratory bronchioles;[636] the airway narrowing is correlated with decreased maximal expiratory flow and increased total airway resistance.[637, 638] There have been a number of attempts to show a correlation between the so-called tests of small airway function—closing capacity, $\Delta N_2$/liter, $FEF_{25-75}$, $\dot{V}max$ on helium/oxygen ($He/O_2$), and the volume of isoflow on $He/O_2$ and air—and specific pathologic changes. The rationale behind these studies was the hope that these tests could detect pathologic changes in small airways at a potentially reversible stage before fibrosis and obliteration occurred.

The majority of these studies have shown that closing volume, closing capacity, $\Delta N_2$/liter, and maximal flows at low lung volumes do in fact correlate with the quantitative measurements and semiquantitative estimates of peripheral airway pathology.[633, 639–644] In patients who have an $FEV_1$ value within the normal range but who have significant abnormalities of small airways as demonstrated by these tests, an inflammatory cell infiltrate and goblet cell metaplasia are particularly evident.[643, 645] In some studies, decreased expiratory flows are associated with a decrease in the amount of muscle in peripheral airways, suggesting that there may be smooth muscle atrophy rather than hypertrophy;[643, 646] however, an association of air-flow obstruction and increased bronchiolar muscle has been found in smokers in other studies.[611] Theoretically, the density dependence of maximal expiratory flow and the volume of isoflow on air and $He/O_2$ flow-volume curves should be tests of peripheral airway function; however, attempts to correlate abnormalities in these tests with pathologic changes in the peripheral airways have been disappointing.[640, 647] Many individuals show well-preserved density dependence despite a substantial decrease in maximal expiratory flow and severe inflammation of small airways,[647] perhaps because flow-limiting segments remain in central airways despite the increase in peripheral airway resistance.

A number of investigators have found an association between the severity of small airway changes and the presence and degree of emphysema,[634, 648, 649] leading to the hypothesis that the inflammation that results in thickening and narrowing of the small airways also causes destruction of alveolar walls.[634] However, many patients who have airway obstruction and small airway abnormalities on histologic examination have no emphysema. In addition, membranous and respiratory bronchiolar inflammation is significantly worse in the lower lobes, while centrilobular emphysema is invariably more severe in the upper lobes.[650–652]

Airway remodeling occurs in COPD as well as in asthma. As discussed in greater detail elsewhere, the bronchiolar wall can be divided into three compartments: (1) an inner wall, consisting of epithelium, basement membrane, lamina propria, and submucosa; (2) an outer wall, consisting of the connective tissue between the muscle layer and the surrounding parenchyma (the adventitia); and (3) the smooth muscle layer.[653] By using the basement membrane length in an individual airway as a yardstick of airway size, the area occupied by the tissue in the different compartments can be quantified and different subject groups can be compared.[654, 655] The results of several such studies have shown that all components of the airway wall are thickened in smokers who develop COPD compared with those in smokers who do not.[611, 656] For example, in one study of 30 smokers who had COPD (mean $FEV_1/FVC$ 55% predicted) and 30 smokers who did not have air-flow obstruction (mean $FEV_1/FVC$ 77% predicted), 200 airways, 90% of which were membranous bronchioles, were examined in each group;[656] the mean measured luminal diameter in the unobstructed group was 0.81 mm, and in the obstructed group, 0.70 mm ($P < 0.05$). The regression lines relating wall thickness to basement membrane length showed that the airways in the obstructed lungs were thicker throughout the airway size range that was measured. The muscle, epithelium, and connective tissue all were significantly increased in thickness in the obstructed lungs. In addition, the wall thickness correlated significantly with the semiquantitative pathology score ($r = 0.61$). Similar findings were reported in a study of 72 smokers who had variable degrees of air-flow obstruction;[401] the airway wall thickness was also found to be related to airway responsiveness after correction for baseline $FEV_1$ and lung elastic recoil.

A relationship between airway wall thickness and airway hyper-responsiveness has also been reported by another group of investigators, especially in the subgroup of COPD patients who have centrilobular as opposed to panlobular emphysema.[657] Mucosal thickening in bronchi correlates with the thickening in bronchioles and with measures of airway obstruction.[304] In addition, the peribronchiolar fibrous tissue can extend into the perivascular space and could contribute to pulmonary hypertension in COPD.[658]

The nature of the cellular infiltrate in the inflamed airways in COPD can be characterized more precisely by immunohistochemical examination. In one study, the cell types in 10 smokers who had air-flow obstruction were compared with those in 10 smokers who did not;[659] the only significant difference between the groups was an increase in the number of B lymphocytes in the adventitia of the obstructed lungs. In another investigation of airway structure

and function, the bronchodilator response in patients who had COPD was related to the extent of eosinophil infiltration in the inflamed bronchioles.[660] In smokers who develop air-flow obstruction, there is a disproportionate hyperplasia of pulmonary neuroendocrine cells; it it possible that this is a marker for the susceptible smoker rather than a secondary phenomenon.[661–663]

### The Lung Parenchyma

The characteristic pathologic abnormality of the lung parenchyma in COPD is emphysema, which can be defined simply as the presence of enlarged air spaces secondary to destruction of alveolar walls.* Depending on the predominant site of such destruction within the acinus, several morphologic subtypes of emphysema can be identified. As described in Chapter 1, the acinus consists of all tissue distal to the terminal bronchiole, comprising three or more generations of respiratory bronchioles, followed by alveolar ducts, alveolar sacs, and alveoli (Fig. 55–7). Predominant involvement of the proximal or distal acinar tissue is referred to as proximal acinar (centrilobular) or distal acinar (paraseptal) emphysema, respectively; involvement of the entire acinus is termed panacinar (panlobular) emphysema. Emphysema that cannot be localized to a particular site within the acinus is termed irregular (scar or cicatricial) emphysema. These anatomic distinctions have both functional and pathogenic associations. For example, selective involvement of the proximal acinus causes a greater degree of loss of function than when destruction takes place predominantly in the alveolar sacs and alveoli. In addition, it has been suggested that the pathogenesis of centrilobular emphysema is related to the interaction of airway hyper-responsiveness and airborne toxins, while that of panlobular emphysema is related to a deficiency of blood-borne protective mechanisms.[665]

In everyday practice, the presence and severity of emphysema are usually assessed pathologically on gross specimens with the naked eye; such assessment can be facilitated by impregnating lung slices with barium and viewing them in water with a dissecting microscope[666] and by the use of a standardized series of photographs.[667] A number of techniques also have been proposed to quantify and characterize emphysema microscopically. The measurement of Lm—the

---

*A diffuse, relatively homogeneous enlargement of air spaces in excess of the dimensions predicted on the basis of age but without destruction of alveolar walls has been called "senile" emphysema.[664]

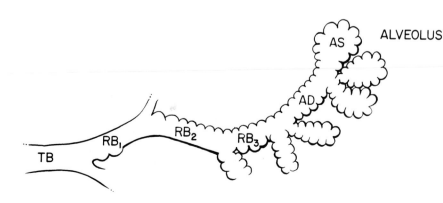

**ALVEOLUS**

**Figure 55–7. Component Parts of the Acinus.** This diagrammatic representation of the acinus shows a terminal bronchiole (TB), respiratory bronchioles of the first ($RB_1$), second ($RB_2$), and third ($RB_3$) orders, an alveolar duct (AD), and an alveolar sac (AS). The acinus is that part of the lung distal to a terminal bronchiole. (From Thurlbeck WM: Chronic Airflow Obstruction in Lung Disease. Philadelphia, WB Saunders Co, 1976, p 15.)

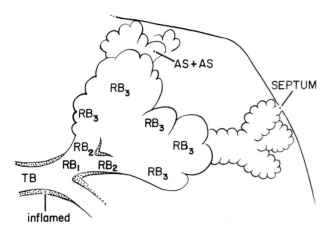

**Figure 55–8. Centrilobular Emphysema.** In centrilobular (proximal acinar) emphysema, respiratory bronchioles are predominantly involved. See Figure 55–7 for abbreviations. (From Thurlbeck WM: Chronic Airflow Obstruction in Lung Disease. Philadelphia, WB Saunders Co, 1976, p 15.)

average distance (mean length) between alveolar walls—is relatively simple but is influenced by the degree of inflation of the lung. Calculation of air-space wall surface area per unit volume is more sensitive in detecting abnormalities, especially in the diffuse air-space enlargement of panlobular emphysema.[668, 669] Using microscopic criteria, centrilobular and panlobular emphysema can be differentiated and correlated with changes in airway function and lung recoil. Centrilobular emphysema is associated with small airway inflammatory changes, while panlobular emphysema is more closely related to loss of lung elasticity.[670, 671]

### Proximal Acinar (Centrilobular) Emphysema

As indicated previously, proximal acinar emphysema is primarily related to destruction of parenchymal tissue in the region of the proximal respiratory bronchioles (Fig. 55–8). Although the term "centrilobular" is frequently used to refer to this pathologic feature, the fact that each secondary lobule

contains multiple acini means that disease characteristically occurs in several foci instead of being located precisely in the center of the lobule (Fig. 55–9). The term "centriacinar" has also been used to describe this form of emphysema; however, the central portion of the acinus is composed predominantly of alveolar ducts and is not affected until disease is relatively advanced.[672] For these reasons, the use of "centriacinar" or "centrilobular" to describe this form of emphysema is somewhat inaccurate. In order to obviate this inexactitude, Thurlbeck proposed that the more descriptive term "proximal acinar emphysema" be used instead;[672, 673] however, because of its widespread use, *centrilobular emphysema* (CLE) is used throughout this text.

CLE is found predominantly in cigarette smokers and is the most common form of clinically and functionally significant emphysema. The pathology of its earliest stage has not been well established. Examination of corrosion models of human lungs obtained post mortem has shown slight enlargement of alveoli in the acinus and loss of alveoli arising from respiratory bronchioles.[674] The earliest lesion may be fenestrae that can be seen by electron microscopy in the alveolar walls adjacent to small airways (Fig. 55–10);[621, 675] theoretically, increase in size and number of these fenestrae results in their coalescence, so that eventually the alveolar wall disappears. The results of morphometric studies have shown that the number of alveolar walls attached to the small airways decreases in emphysema, supporting this concept. Both normal and abnormal alveolar attachments to the external perimeter of small airways can be quantified, and their numbers have been shown to correlate with semiquantitative measures of airway inflammation and with measures of lung recoil.[676–678] These early morphologic abnormalities can occur in the absence of the gross pathologic changes of emphysema. The reason for the localization of early disease to parenchyma around respiratory bronchioles is also not certain, but may reflect the "spillover" into this site of inflammatory cells centered on these airways.[620, 679]

Another method which has been proposed to detect

**Figure 55–9. Centrilobular Emphysema: Anatomic Location within the Lobule.** A cut section of lung parenchyma reveals multiple foci of emphysema distributed in a patchy fashion; most are associated with anthracotic pigment. The parenchyma adjacent to the interlobular septa *(arrows)* is essentially normal. The emphysematous spaces clearly are not limited to the central portion of the lobule but rather are scattered within it in a distribution corresponding approximately to the location of the proximal respiratory bronchioles. (The specimen was inflated with polyethylene glycol and air-dried.) (Bar = 8 mm.)

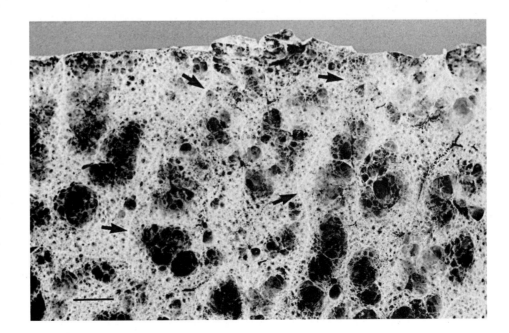

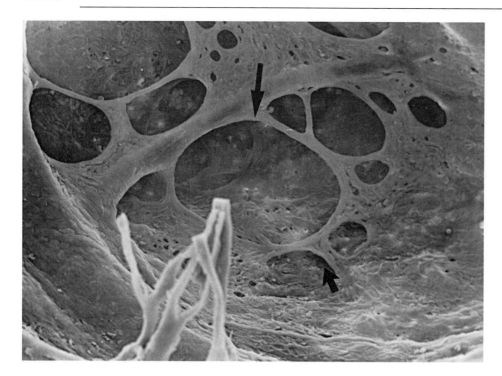

**Figure 55–10. Alveolar Wall Fenestrae.** A scanning electron micrograph of an alveolar wall shows multiple small *(short arrow)* and large *(long arrow)* fenestrae. (Courtesy of Dr. N.-S. Wang, McGill University, Montreal.)

alveolar wall disruption is the measurement of a "destructive index" (DI).[680] This is determined using a point-count system to calculate the percentage of destroyed space as a fraction of the total alveolar and duct space. The measure is abnormal in smokers before there is a significant increase in mean linear intercept and thus may be a more sensitive indicator of early emphysema.[681] One group of investigators found DI and a measure of the decrease in volume density of alveolar tissue to correlate inversely with the number of neutrophils and directly with the number of lymphocytes in the alveolar region, suggesting that cell-mediated immunity may be important in tissue destruction.[682, 711]

With progression of the disease, pathologic abnormalities become more clearly evident. The earliest light microscopic change is dilation of respiratory bronchioles accompanied by loss of adjacent alveolar septa (Fig. 55–11). As the disease progresses, several respiratory bronchioles become confluent, creating an enlarged space supplied by a terminal bronchiole proximally and leading to relatively normal alveolar tissue.[683–685] At this stage, the disease is clearly visible grossly as multiple, regularly spaced foci of tissue loss. Because of the association of CLE with cigarette smoking, there is usually prominent deposition of anthracotic pigment in the emphysematous foci, resulting in a distinctive black and gray ("checkerboard") appearance (Fig. 55–12).

With further progression, the relatively discrete foci of mild disease become confluent, so that an entire lobule or even whole segments of lung parenchyma are eventually affected (Fig. 55–13). Although completely empty spaces several centimeters in diameter can be formed in this way, blood vessels or fine strands of residual lung parenchyma often traverse the emphysematous spaces. At this stage, it may be difficult to distinguish centrilobular from panlobular emphysema; however, except in the most advanced cases, the former typically affects the parenchyma unevenly, so that areas showing early changes diagnostic of the condition

can usually be found. This variable severity is most obvious during examination of whole-lung slices, in which the disease can be seen to show considerable upper zonal predominance, particularly affecting the apical and posterior segments of the upper lobes and the superior segment of the lower lobes (Fig. 55–14).[684, 686–688] A variety of factors theoretically contribute to this zonal predilection:[689]

- Underperfusion of upper lobes relative to their ventilation, leading to a relative undersupply of blood-derived antiprotease
- Slower transit time of leukocytes through the upper lobes than through the lower lobes, allowing a longer time for the leukocyte elastase to be released
- Preferential deposition of particulate material in the upper lobes despite the gradient in ventilation distribution, perhaps because the caliber of airways is greater and the linear velocity of air flow is less than in the lower lobes; these differences can result in deeper penetration of inhaled particles in the upper lobes
- Less effective clearance of inhaled material from the upper lobes
- Increased mechanical stress on the alveolar walls in nondependent lung regions as a result of more negative pleural pressure and relative hyperinflation, making disruption of elastic fibers more likely

### Panacinar (Panlobular) Emphysema

Panlobular emphysema (PLE) has also been called "unselective" because the acinus and secondary lobules are involved diffusely, rather than selectively as is the case in proximal and distal acinar disease (Figs. 55–15 and 55–16). As with CLE, the initial morphologic changes have been poorly documented. Examination of thick sections of lung has shown abnormal fenestrations approximately 20 μm in

*Text continued on page 2196*

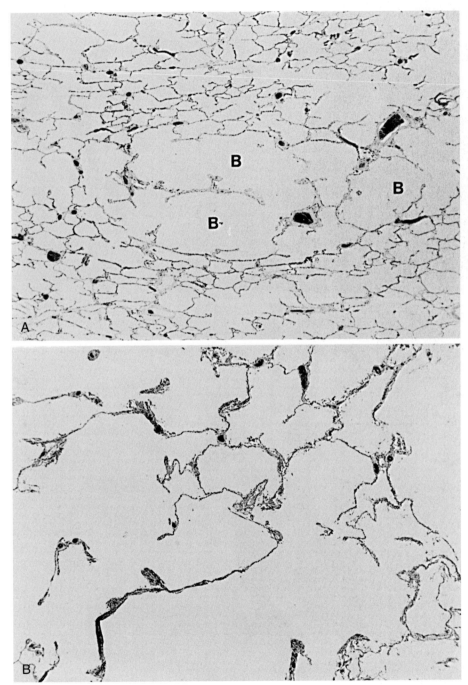

**Figure 55–11. Centrilobular Emphysema: Comparison of Mild and Severe.** A section of lung parenchyma *(A)* reveals early centrilobular emphysema; note the slight dilation of respiratory bronchioles (B) associated with blunting and loss of alveolar septa. The adjacent parenchyma is normal. A section of lung parenchyma *(B)* photographed at the same magnification as in *A* shows advanced emphysema, almost no normal alveolar air spaces being identifiable. *(A, B,* ×25.)

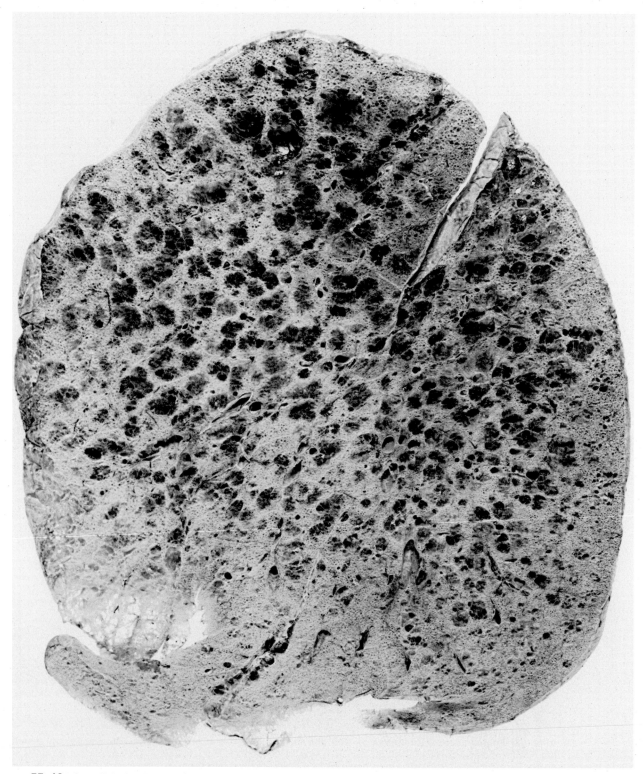

**Figure 55–12. Centrilobular Emphysema: Moderate.** A sagittal slice of left lung in its midportion shows numerous fairly discrete foci of emphysema. Each focus appears black as a result of the deposition of anthracotic pigment, resulting in contrast with the adjacent unaffected lung and a characteristic "checkerboard" appearance. Note the gradient in severity of emphysema from apex to base. (The specimen was inflated with polyethylene glycol and air-dried.)

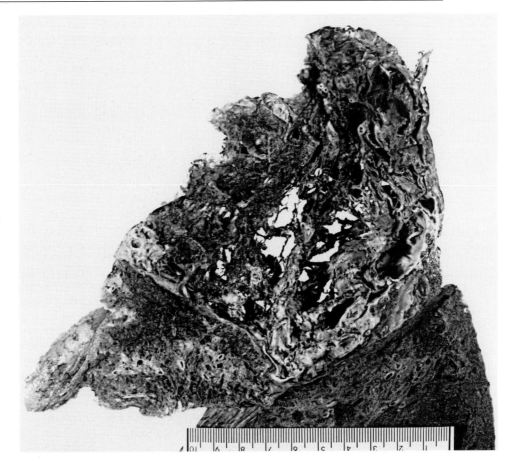

**Figure 55–13. Centrilobular Emphysema: Severe.** A magnified view of a slice of the right lung that had been inflated and fixed with formalin shows extensive loss of tissue in the upper lobe. The lack of tissue is responsible for the characteristic wrinkled appearance of the cut surface.

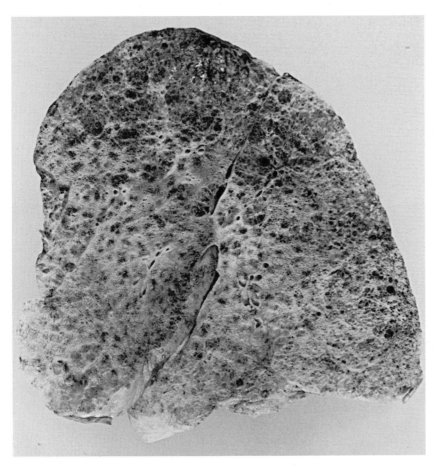

**Figure 55–14. Centrilobular Emphysema: Upper Zone Predominance.** A slice of right lung shows moderately advanced centrilobular emphysema. The tendency to greater involvement of the apex of the upper lobe and superior segment of the lower lobe is clearly evident. (The specimen was inflated with polyethylene glycol and air-dried.)

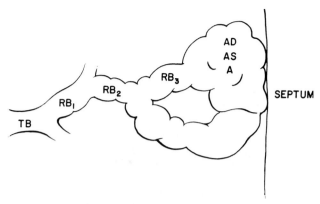

**Figure 55–15. Panacinar Emphysema.** In panacinar emphysema, the enlargement and destruction of air spaces involve the acinus more or less uniformly. A, alveolus; *see* Figure 55–7 for other abbreviations. (From Thurlbeck WM: Chronic Airflow Obstruction in Lung Disease. Philadelphia, WB Saunders Co, 1976, p 15.)

diameter in the walls of the dilated alveoli.[690] As with CLE, it is possible that they represent the initial abnormality. It has been suggested by some authors that the earliest abnormality is dilation of alveolar ducts.[691, 692]

Macroscopically, mild to moderate PLE is subtle and is best seen by examination of barium-impregnated slices through the dissecting microscope. On lung slices, the loss of parenchymal tissue may be evidenced only by curling of the pleura into the adjacent lung and by the projection of bronchovascular bundles above the cut surface (Fig. 55–17). In severe disease, affected parenchyma may consist of no more than large air spaces through which strands of tissue and blood vessels pass like struts ("cotton-candy" lung). The disease characteristically shows a predilection for the lower lobes and anterior lung zones, a feature that may be manifested in whole excised lungs by the presence of basal bullae (Fig. 55–18).[684, 686, 693] In some cases, PLE is associated with CLE, in which circumstance the lower lobe predominance may be less obvious.

PLE is characteristically seen in association with alpha$_1$-antiprotease inhibitor deficiency; for unknown reasons, it is also seen in patients who have emphysema secondary to intravenous talcosis (*see* page 1857). Although PLE is often associated with cigarette smoking, such exposure may be absent or minimal, resulting in relatively little deposition of anthracotic pigment. In fact, PLE is the form of the disease most often seen in nonsmokers.[694, 695]

### Distal Acinar (Paraseptal) Emphysema

Distal acinar (paraseptal) emphysema selectively involves the alveolar ducts and sacs in the peripheral portion of the acinus (Fig. 55–19). Grossly, it is usually focal and consists of small emphysematous spaces in a more or less continuous zone of variable length located in the periphery of the lung adjacent to the pleura or interlobular septa (Fig. 55–20). In some cases, there is an increase in collagen in the vicinity of the emphysema, suggesting that it is caused by a localized inflammatory process (possibly infectious pneumonia in which there have been both tissue destruction and secondary fibrosis). Bullae may develop from coalescence of distended, destroyed alveoli. Distal acinar emphysema is not uncommonly identified if specifically searched for in autopsy specimens; however, it is limited in extent in the vast majority of cases and, with the exception of the occasional occurrence of spontaneous pneumothorax, gives rise to no symptoms.

### Irregular Emphysema

As the name suggests, irregular emphysema shows no consistent relationship to any portion of the acinus (Fig. 55–21). It is always associated with fibrosis; thus, according to some definitions it should not even be classified as emphysema.[696] As with some cases of paraseptal emphysema, the association of irregular emphysema with fibrosis suggests a relationship with inflammation (Fig. 55–22). In some instances, such as remote foci of granulomatous inflammation,

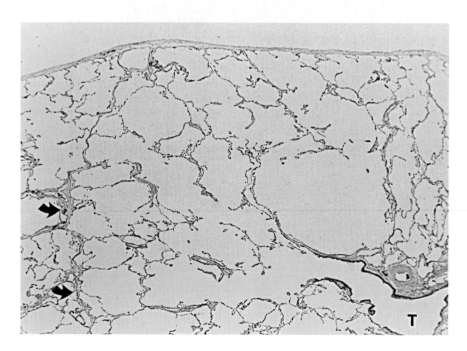

**Figure 55–16. Panacinar Emphysema.** This section from a 52-year-old man who had alpha$_1$-antiprotease inhibitor deficiency shows more or less diffuse air-space enlargement and loss of alveolar septa involving all the tissue between the pleura, interlobular septum *(arrows)*, and a terminal bronchiole (T). (×16.)

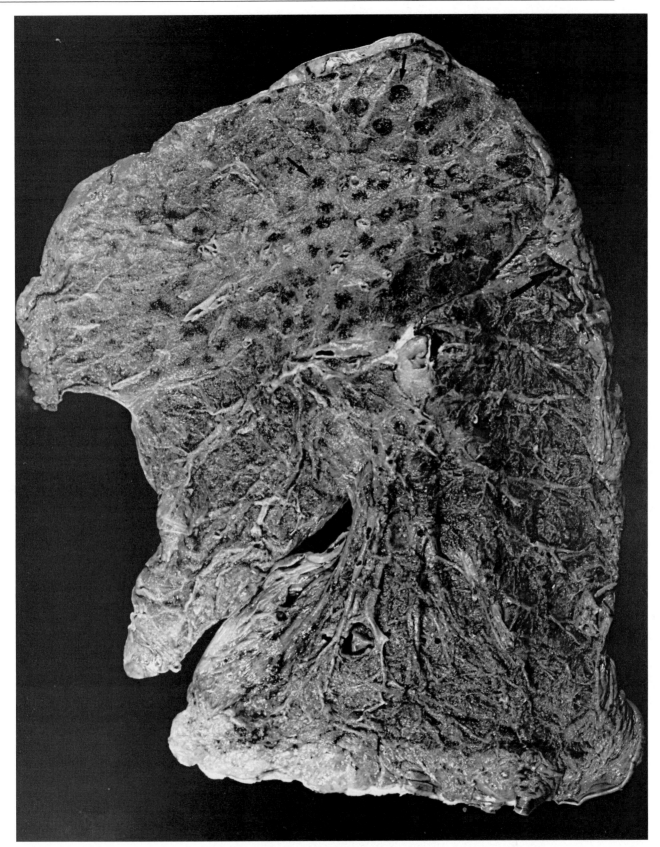

**Figure 55–17. Emphysema: Mixed Centrilobular and Panacinar (Alpha₁-Antiprotease Inhibitor Deficiency).** A sagittal slice of the left lung near the hilum shows patchy foci of parenchymal destruction associated with anthracotic pigment deposition in the apical portion of the upper lobe *(short arrows),* representing mild centrilobular emphysema. The lingula and lower lobe show a more severe and more diffuse loss of tissue, manifested by the inward-folding pleura in the superior segment *(long arrow)* and the prominent bronchovascular bundles. The patient was a 52-year-old man who had alpha₁-antiprotease inhibitor deficiency and a 35-pack-year smoking history. The specimen was inflated and fixed with formalin.

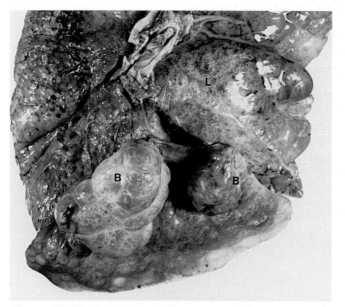

**Figure 55–18. Panacinar Emphysema: Basal Bulla Formation.**
The medial aspect of a left lower lobe shows two bullae (B), the larger approximately 5 cm in maximum dimension. The surface of the lingula (L) has a bubbly appearance, reflecting the presence of abundant air and insufflated formalin in the absence of lung parenchyma.

this association is clearly evident; in others, it can only be assumed. Because of its association with scars, irregular emphysema is probably the most common form seen pathologically; usually, however, it is limited in extent and results in no functional or clinical abnormalities.

### Structure-Function Correlation in Emphysema

The association of emphysema and air-flow obstruction is thought to be caused by a loss of lung elasticity. Because maximal expiratory flow is dependent on lung elastic recoil

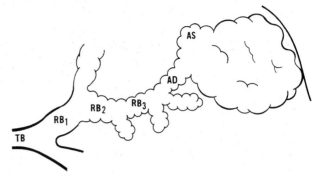

**Figure 55–19. Paraseptal Emphysema.** In paraseptal (distal acinar) emphysema, the peripheral part of the acinus (alveolar ducts and sacs) is predominantly involved. *See* Figure 55–7 for abbreviations. (From Thurlbeck WM: Chronic Airflow Obstruction in Lung Disease. Philadelphia, WB Saunders Co, 1976, p 16.)

as well as on airway size and collapsibility, and because emphysema is often associated with a loss of normal elasticity, it has come to be accepted that emphysema causes loss of lung elasticity and that this is the cause of the decreased expiratory flow. However, it is clear that loss of lung elasticity can occur in the absence of obvious emphysema.[697, 698] These observations have led to the idea that loss of lung elasticity and emphysema may be essentially unrelated.[699, 700] Our understanding of the inconsistent relationship between emphysema and loss of elasticity comes from studies of structure and function: lung elasticity is assessed by measuring the elastic recoil pressures at fixed percentages of total lung volume or by characterizing the shape of the entire pressure-volume curve with an exponential constant (K) (*see* Fig. 17–5, page 411). Although the lungs of patients who have morphologically documented emphysema tend to have increased values for K and low lung recoil pressures,[697, 701–703] these findings are by no means universal.

Studies of lung pressure–volume behavior and its rela-

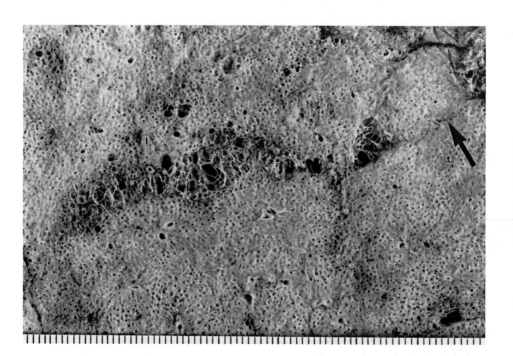

**Figure 55–20. Paraseptal Emphysema.** A magnified view of an upper lobe lung slice reveals a well-delimited zone of emphysema in a linear pattern contiguous with an interlobular septum *(arrow)* immediately under the pleura. The adjacent lung parenchyma is normal. The linearity and proximity to the septum indicate the paraseptal nature of the emphysema.

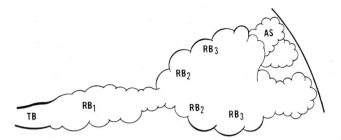

**Figure 55–21. Irregular Emphysema.** In irregular emphysema, the acinus is irregularly involved. This form is often accompanied by scarring in the lung. *See* Figure 55–7 for abbreviations. (From Thurlbeck WM: *Chronic Airflow Obstruction in Lung Disease.* Philadelphia, WB Saunders Company, 1976, p 17.)

tionship to lung structure in a variety of animal species have shown that the shape of the pressure-volume curve is strongly influenced by the average size (Lm) of the air spaces contributing to the expired volume.[704] Species that have small alveoli (i.e., small Lm) have relatively stiff lungs (low K), whereas those that have large alveoli have relatively compliant lungs (high K).

There is also an association between K and Lm in human lungs examined at autopsy.[705, 706] The pressure-volume curve reflects the mean alveolar size of the air spaces that contribute to the expirate. In lungs removed at autopsy, the pressure-volume curve for centrilobular emphysematous spaces has been characterized radiographically using lead dust to outline the spaces (Fig. 55–23).[707] The results showed that these spaces do not contribute much to the total expired volume and that their pressure-volume behavior demonstrates less compliance than that of the lungs in which the spaces were found; in fact, the compliance was even less than that of normal lungs. The loss of elasticity and increased compliance found in the lungs of patients who have emphysema must therefore reflect the pressure-volume behavior of air spaces other than those affected by CLE. In one study in which preoperative lung pressure–volume curves were compared with postoperative morphology, the shape of the pressure-volume curve was found to correlate with the average size of air spaces (Lm) located away from centrilobular emphysematous areas in the excised lobes and lungs;[697] K correlated with Lm irrespective of the presence of emphysematous spaces.

The sequence of events in the development of COPD and emphysema probably begins with the simultaneous development of inflammatory changes in the small airways and adjacent alveolar septa. The inflammation results in narrowing of the lumen of the small airways, accentuated by the loss of alveolar attachments. As individual alveolar walls are disrupted, alveoli coalesce, and the average size of air spaces increases, resulting in a loss of elasticity (increased K) and an increase in TLC.[708] If the destruction of alveolar walls progresses, the enlarged air spaces coalesce to form visible centrilobular emphysematous areas; however, as the disease advances, these spaces contribute less to the expired air volume and to the pressure-volume characteristics of the lungs and more to the "trapped gas." Both the intrinsic narrowing of airways and the loss of elasticity contribute to the obstruction to air flow; even in the absence of detectable emphysema, both mechanisms may be important.[697]

### Vascular and Cardiac Abnormalities

The increased vascular resistance seen in some patients who have emphysema is related to a combination of loss of vascular bed,[709] hypoxia-induced vascular smooth muscle contraction, and narrowing of small intrapulmonary vessels caused by thickening of their walls and loss of parenchymal support.[710] The earliest vascular lesion may be intimal thickening,[710] which progresses as air flow becomes more limited.[712, 713] Smokers and patients who have mild air-flow obstruction have an increased number of small muscular arteries and an increased thickness of the intima and media of pulmonary vessels,[649, 714, 715] changes that correlate with the severity of small airway inflammation and the extent of emphysema.[649, 716, 717] In advanced COPD and emphysema, there may be a marked increase in the extent of anastomosis between the bronchial arteries and the pulmonary circulation.[718, 719]

## RADIOLOGIC MANIFESTATIONS

As discussed previously (*see* page 2168), chronic bronchitis is defined clinically, emphysema pathologically, and COPD functionally. As diagnostic tools that reveal predominantly morphologic abnormalities, the chest radiograph and the CT scan can demonstrate abnormalities attributable to chronic bronchitis or emphysema but can disclose variations caused by COPD only by inference. In the following pages, therefore, only the first two disease entities are addressed.

### Chronic Bronchitis

The radiographic manifestations of uncomplicated chronic bronchitis are poorly documented, because correlation of radiographic findings with pathologic specimens has generally not been performed, and because investigators have not systematically excluded patients who have emphysema. The principal abnormalities are bronchial wall thickening and an increase in lung markings, sometimes referred to as the "dirty chest."[720–724]

Bronchial wall thickening may be seen end-on as ring shadows or *en face* as tubular shadows ("tram tracks").[721, 723] In one investigation of approximately 300 men, including approximately equal numbers of normal individuals and patients who had chronic bronchitis, emphasis was placed on assessing the thickness of bronchial walls visualized end-on in the parahilar zones.[723] These airways, which were identified in roughly 80% of both groups, represent branches of the anterior or posterior segmental bronchi of the upper lobes, or the superior segmental bronchi of the lower lobes (Fig. 55–24). They range in diameter from approximately 3 to 7 mm and thus represent different stages in bronchial subdivision. Thickening of their walls can usually be easily identified (Fig. 55–25). On the basis of subjectively assessed bronchial wall thickness, 54 of 81 (67%) patients who had chronic bronchitis were interpreted as having increased wall thickness, compared with 34 of 81 (42%) normal individuals. Objective measurements showed a mean ratio of wall thickness to outer bronchial diameter of 0.36 ± 0.08 in patients who had chronic bronchitis compared with 0.32 ± 0.08 in normal individuals. Step-wise discriminant analysis showed

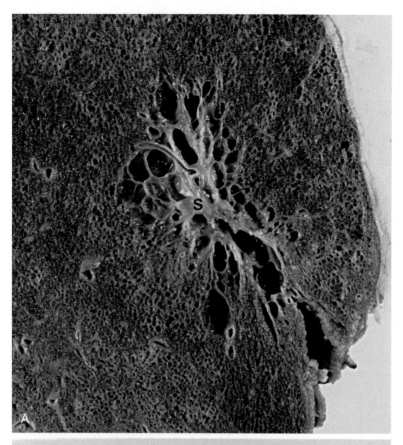

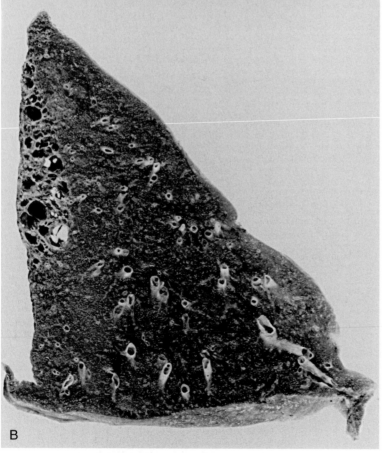

**Figure 55–22. Irregular Emphysema.** A magnified slice of lung parenchyma *(A)* reveals a small scar (S) surrounded by irregularly shaped emphysematous spaces. The cause of the disease was not determined. A section of the lower lobe from another patient *(B),* shows a well-defined zone of emphysema in the posterior subpleural region. The remaining lung parenchyma is normal. Note that the tissue between the emphysematous spaces is thickened as a result of fibrosis. Both the fibrous tissue and the location suggest that the emphysema is the result of remote pneumonia.

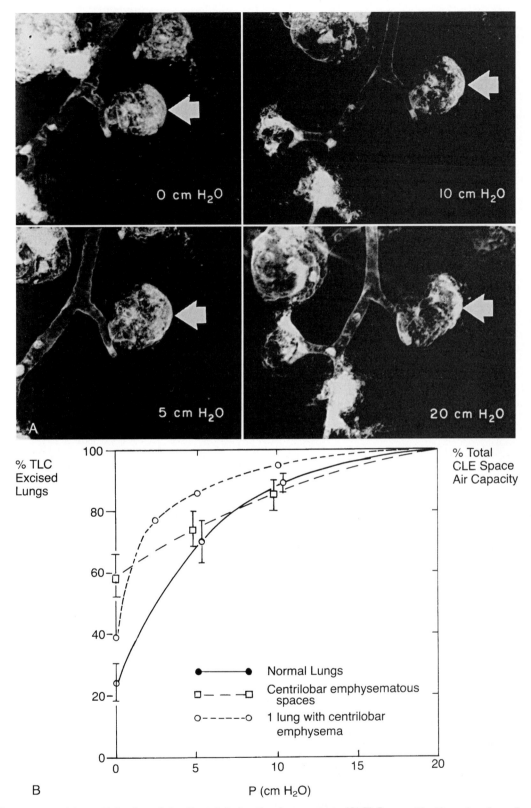

**Figure 55–23. Pressure-Volume Behavior of the Centrilobular Emphysematous (CLE) Space.** The illustration shows four radiographs *(A)* of a CLE space whose wall has been coated with insufflated lead *(arrow).* At increasing transpulmonary pressures of 0, 5, 10, and 20 cm $H_2O$, the volume of the space changes little despite large changes in transpulmonary pressure. In *B,* pressure-volume curves are shown for normal lung, a lung with centrilobular emphysema, and a CLE space. Volume is expressed as per cent of volume at total lung capacity (TLC). Although the whole lung with emphysema shows a decrease in lung elastic recoil at most lung volumes, the shape of the pressure-volume curve for the CLE space is flat with apparent decrease in compliance. (From Hogg JC, Nepszy SJ, Macklem PT, et al: J Clin Invest 48:1306, 1969.)

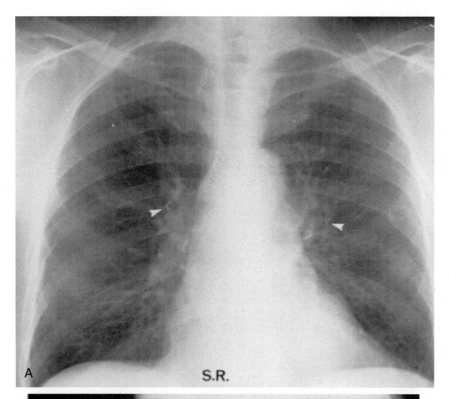

S.R.

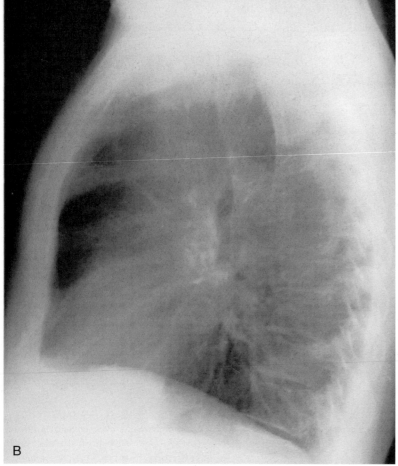

**Figure 55–24. Chronic Bronchitis.** A poster-oanterior chest radiograph demonstrates thickened bronchial walls viewed end-on in the right and left upper lobes *(arrowheads).* Lung volume, vasculature, and cardiac size are normal. These features are compatible with chronic bronchitis. The patient was a 58-year-old man who had a 15-year history of chronic productive cough.

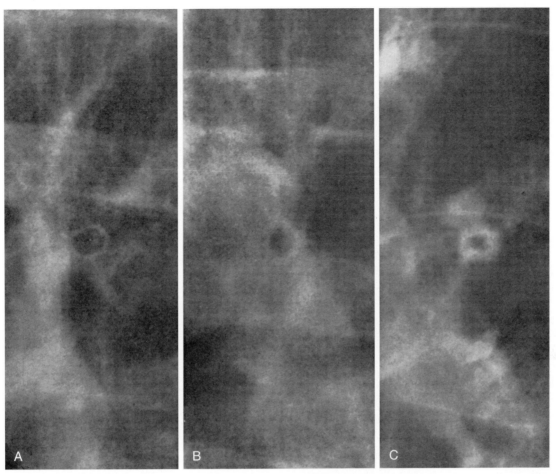

**Figure 55–25. Bronchial Wall Thickening as Assessed from Parahilar Bronchi Viewed End-on.** Views of the left parahilar zone from posteroanterior chest radiographs from three different patients show a normal bronchus *(A),* a bronchus with moderate wall thickening *(B),* and a bronchus with marked wall thickening *(C). (A, B,* and *C* are from Fraser RG, Fraser RS, Renner JW, et al. Radiology 120:1, 1976.)

that the median estimate of bronchial wall thickness was of some value in differentiating normal individuals from patients who had chronic bronchitis; however, the presence of thickening could not be used as an absolute criterion for the presence of chronic bronchitis, nor could its absence be construed as evidence against that diagnosis.[723] Parallel-line shadows ("tram tracks") are seldom seen on the radiograph of normal individuals; this finding has been considered to be present with increased frequency in patients who have chronic bronchitis by some investigators[721] but has not been considered to be a feature of the disease by others.[720, 725]

The term *prominent lung markings* ("dirty chest") refers to a general accentuation of linear markings throughout the lungs associated with loss of definition of vascular margins.[726] The abnormality was observed in 18% of 119 patients who had chronic bronchitis in one study.[721] The increased markings in chronic bronchitis presumably result from increase in lung density secondary to accumulation of inflammatory cells and fibrous tissue in the airway walls.[726]

Limited information is available from HRCT in chronic bronchitis. In one investigation of 175 healthy adults, including 98 current smokers, 26 ex-smokers, and 51 nonsmokers, no evidence of bronchial wall thickening was found on radiographs from any of the subjects;[727] however, on HRCT scans, it was considered to be present in 32 (33%) of the

smokers, 4 (16%) of the ex-smokers, and 9 (18%) nonsmokers. As a group, patients who had bronchial wall thickening had significantly lower mid-expiratory flow rates ($\dot{V}max_{50}$) and were more likely to have chronic cough and sputum production. As with other airway diseases, chronic bronchitis may result in air trapping. In one investigation of 20 patients who had emphysema, 20 who had chronic bronchitis, and 20 healthy individuals, spirometrically triggered CT images at 90% of vital capacity showed similar mean lung attenuation for patients who had chronic bronchitis and for normal individuals, and decreased attenuation in patients with emphysema.[728] At 10% of vital capacity, patients who had chronic bronchitis and those who had emphysema had lower mean lung attenuation than that in the normal individuals. As the authors pointed out, however, the study was based on "relatively extreme selection criteria" and included only patients who had chronic bronchitis and an $FEV_1$ of less than 70% of predicted; therefore, the results may not be applicable to patients who have less severe air-flow obstruction.

In summary, chronic bronchitis is not a radiologic diagnosis. Although changes may be observed on the radiograph or HRCT scan suggesting that bronchitis is present, it is inappropriate for the radiologist to do other than indicate that the findings are compatible with that diagnosis.

## Emphysema

The radiographic abnormalities in emphysema reflect the presence of lung destruction, secondary alterations in the vascular pattern, and increased lung volume. Direct signs of emphysema, such as bullae and irregular areas of radiolucency related to tissue loss, can be seen on the chest radiograph in some patients (Fig. 55–26).[726, 729, 730] Bullae may be single or multiple (*see* also page 2236). Their walls are usually of no more than hairline thickness, so that it may be difficult to distinguish them from uninvolved parenchyma. In fact, large bullae can be observed pathologically that are invisible on the chest radiograph, even in retrospect;[731] such bullae are usually situated anteriorly or posteriorly, where their presence is masked by normal lung, or in the subpleural zone, where the absence of visible blood vessels prevents appreciation of vascular distortion (Fig. 55–27).[731]

In the majority of cases, the radiographic findings reflect secondary alterations in the vascular pattern and the presence of overinflation (Fig. 55–28).[729, 730, 732, 733] Vascular

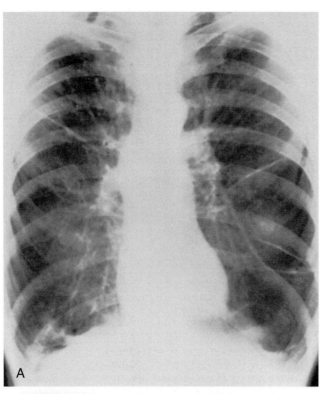

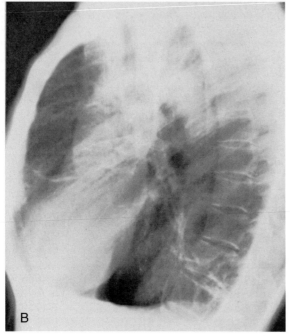

**Figure 55–26. Emphysema Associated with Bullae.** Posteroanterior *(A)* and lateral *(B)* chest radiographs from a 43-year-old woman reveal severe overinflation of both lungs. The diaphragm is low and its superior surface concave. Note the prominent costophrenic muscle slips. The retrosternal air space is deepened. Numerous bullae are present in both lower lung zones, particularly the left. The peripheral vasculature of the lungs is severely diminished, but there is no evidence of pulmonary arterial hypertension. (It is probable that the upper lung zones are less severely involved than the lower, permitting redistribution of blood flow and minimizing the risk of development of hypertension.)

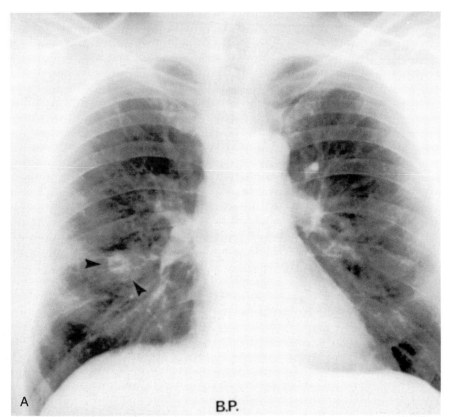

**Figure 55–27. Diffuse Emphysema Associated with Only Mild Overinflation.** Posteroanterior *(A)* and lateral *(B)* chest radiographs reveal a mass *(arrowheads)* in the lateral segment of the middle lobe, subsequently proved to be a primary adenocarcinoma. Lung volume is only mildly increased, as evidenced by the lateral projection. Apart from focal areas of oligemia (e.g., the right base and right upper lobe) and a curvilinear displacement of some vessels, the radiographic appearance of the pulmonary vasculature is within normal limits.

*Illustration continued on following page*

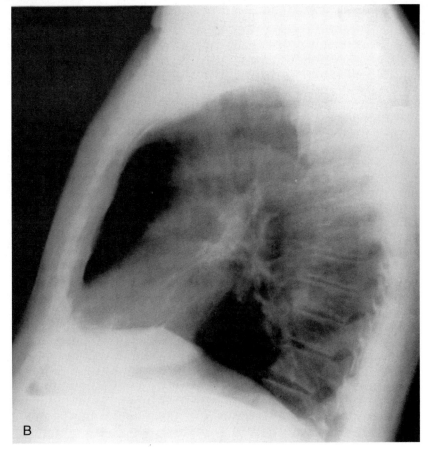

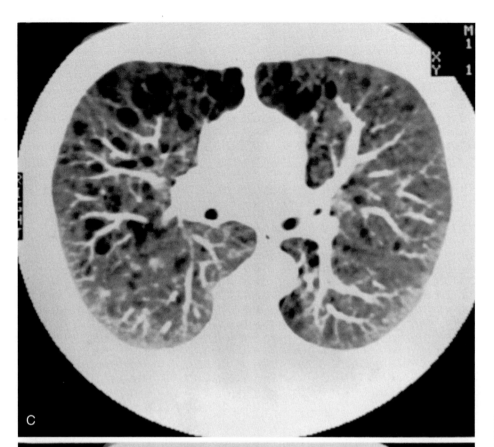

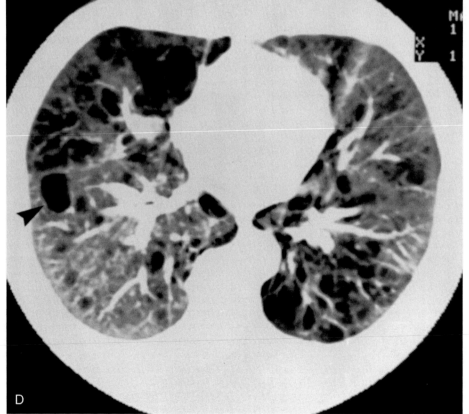

**Figure 55–27** *Continued.* Conventional 10-mm-collimation CT scans *(C* and *D)* demonstrate extensive emphysema with bullae *(arrowheads).* The patient was a 60-year-old man.

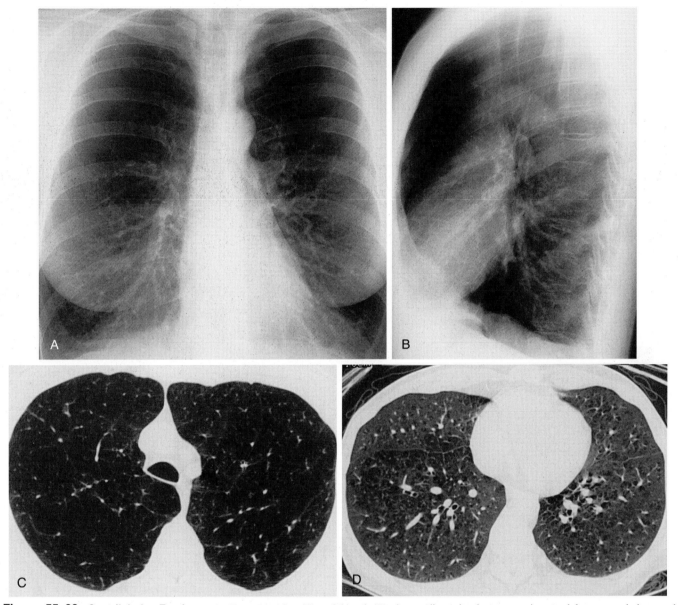

**Figure 55–28. Centrilobular Emphysema.** Posteroanterior *(A)* and lateral *(B)* chest radiographs demonstrate increased lucency and decreased vascularity in the upper lobes, marked overinflation with flattening of the diaphragm, and increase in the retrosternal air space. An HRCT scan through the upper lobes *(C)* demonstrates severe emphysema; a scan at a more caudad level *(D)* demonstrates relatively mild centrilobular emphysema. The patient was a 49-year-old smoker.

abnormalities related to emphysema include local avascular areas, distortion of the vessels, increased branching angles and loss of normal sinuosity of vessels, decrease in the peripheral vascular markings, and enlargement of the main pulmonary arteries (Fig. 55–29).[731, 734, 735] Diminution in the caliber of the pulmonary vessels, with increased rapidity of tapering distally, has a relatively high specificity for the diagnosis of emphysema;[725, 731] however, it has a sensitivity of only 15% for the detection of mild to moderate disease and 40% for the detection of severe involvement.[734] Although localized avascular areas, narrowing of mid-lung vessels, and an enlarged pulmonary arterial trunk have also been shown to be significantly associated with the extent of emphysema observed pathologically, these parameters are inferior to the presence of overinflation.[736]

The most reliable sign of overinflation is flattening of the diaphragmatic domes (*see* Fig. 55–28).[729, 730, 737] When the configuration of the diaphragm is concave superiorly, the presence of emphysema is virtually certain in adults (*see* Fig. 55–26). The diaphragm is considered flattened when the highest level of the diaphragmatic contour is less than 1.5 cm above a line connecting the costophrenic and vertebrophrenic junctions on the posteroanterior radiograph or a line connecting the sternophrenic and posterior costophrenic angles on the lateral view, or when the sternodiaphragmatic angle on the lateral radiograph is 90 degrees or greater.[726, 729, 730] In one investigation, a flattened diaphragm on the posteroanterior chest radiograph was present in 94% of patients who had severe emphysema, 76% of those who had moderate emphysema, and 21% of those who had mild emphysema;[737] only 4% of patients without emphysema showed the abnormality.

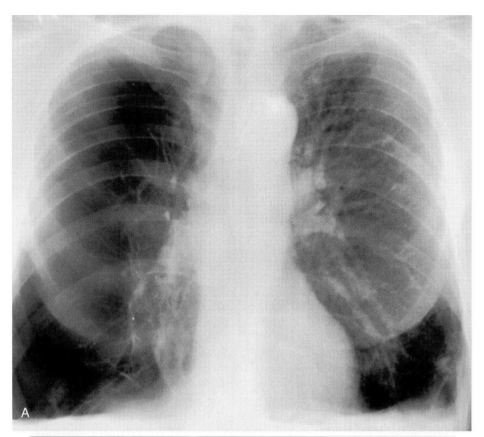

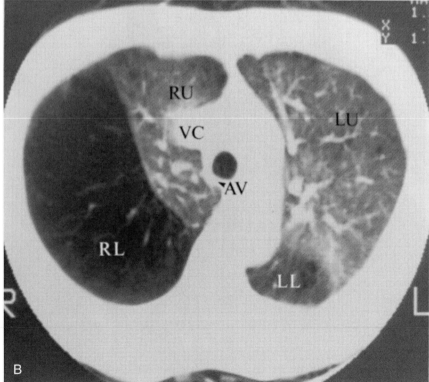

**Figure 55–29. Severe Local Emphysema.** A posteroanterior chest radiograph *(A)* demonstrates marked oligemia and overinflation of the right lung and base of the left lower lobe. The appearance of the right lung could conceivably be caused by a giant bulla. The left hilum is enlarged whereas the right hilum is small and displaced inferiorly. A CT scan *(B)* through the upper lobes at the level of the azygos vein arch (AV) shows severe overinflation and oligemia of the right lower lobe (RL); note that thin attenuated vessels can be identified throughout the distended lobe, inicating diffuse emphysema rather than a bulla. Similar but much less pronounced changes are present in the left lower lobe (LL). The right upper lobe (RU) is compressed and displaced anteromedially. The vasculature in the left upper lobe (LU) is dilated, and there is a diffuse increase in CT density of the parenchyma.

Other helpful signs of overinflation include an increase in the retrosternal air space, an increase in lung height, and a low position (depression) of the diaphragm. The retrosternal air space is the space between the anterior margin of the ascending aorta and the sternum. It is considered to be increased when the horizontal distance between the sternum and the most anterior margin of the ascending aorta is greater than 2.5 cm.[729, 730] The lung height is considered increased when it measures 30 cm or more from the dome of the right hemidiaphragm to the tubercle of the first rib.[738] The identification of the dome of the right hemidiaphragm at or below the anterior end of the seventh rib is also suggestive of hyperinflation;[739, 740] however, this finding has a low sensitivity[741] and is less helpful in diagnosis than is a change in contour.[729, 730]

The greatest diagnostic accuracy on the radiograph is obtained by using a combination of findings. For example, in one investigation, a combination of hyperinflation and vascular changes allowed the correct diagnosis of emphysema in 29 (97%) of 30 autopsy-proven cases in which the patients had been symptomatic, as well as 8 (47%) of 17 autopsy-proven cases involving asymptomatic individuals.[733] In another investigation, the presence of emphysema was assessed in 60 patients (33 who had emphysema and 27 normal controls) using the following radiographic criteria: (1) depression or flattening of the diaphragm on the postero-anterior radiograph, (2) irregular radiolucency of the lungs, (3) increased retrosternal space on the lateral radiograph, and (4) flattening of the diaphragm on the lateral radiograph. At least two of the four criteria had to be present for a diagnosis of emphysema. Using these criteria, all 14 symptomatic and 13 of 19 (68%) asymptomatic patients who had emphysema were correctly diagnosed;[729] no false-positive diagnoses were made. Based on these and other data,[731, 742] it can be calculated that the presence of two or more of the four radiographic features just listed usually requires a pathologic emphysema score (obtained by the panel grading method) of 30 out of 100 or greater.[743]

Pulmonary arterial hypertension secondary to emphysema usually is easily recognizable by a combination of a deficiency in the peripheral vasculature and an increase in the size of the hilar pulmonary arteries. In cases in which previous chest films are available for comparison, the latter should be readily apparent; when no previous films exist, a diameter of the right interlobar artery exceeding 16 mm should be regarded as convincing evidence of pulmonary arterial hypertension. Peripheral arterial deficiency often is localized to certain areas of the lungs, vessels elsewhere being of normal or even increased caliber. In such cases, the hilar arteries are usually of normal size, suggesting that the relatively uninvolved portions of the lungs are the sites of redistributed blood flow, thus—at least temporarily—delaying the development of pulmonary arterial hypertension. In cases of general arterial deficiency, in which redistribution of blood flow to normal regions is impossible, the development of hypertension is manifested by an increase in the size of the hilar arteries and a greater discrepancy in the caliber of central and peripheral vessels (Fig. 55–30).

### Computed Tomography

On CT scans, emphysema is characterized by the presence of areas of abnormally low attenuation, usually without

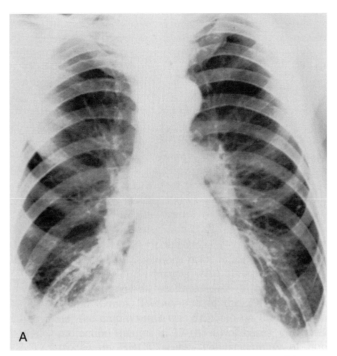

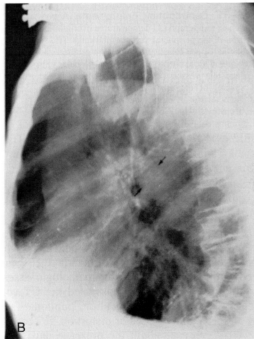

**Figure 55–30. Emphysema with Pulmonary Arterial Hypertension.** Posteroanterior *(A)* and lateral *(B)* chest radiographs reveal severe overinflation of both lungs as evidenced by marked flattening of the diaphragm (seen to best advantage in lateral projection) and increase in the depth of the retrosternal air space. The lungs are oligemic, arterial deficiency being more apparent in the upper two thirds than in the bases. The hilar pulmonary arteries are moderately enlarged and taper rapidly distally. In lateral projection, note the shadow of the dilated descending branch of the left pulmonary artery *(arrow)*. Despite the evidence of severe pulmonary arterial hypertension, the heart is only slightly enlarged. The patient was a 71-year-old man.

visible walls (Fig. 55–31);[743–747] occasionally, walls 1 mm or less may be seen. On HRCT scans, vessels can be seen within the areas of low attenuation.[748] Several groups of investigators have shown that CT, particularly HRCT, findings correlate closely with the presence and severity of

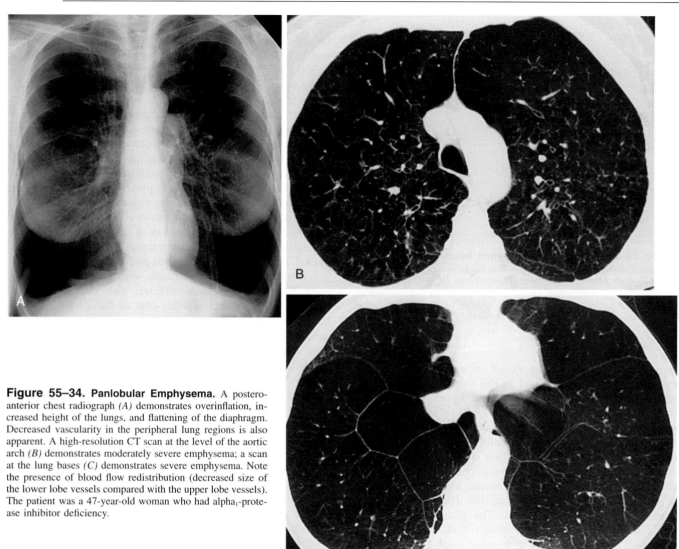

**Figure 55–34. Panlobular Emphysema.** A postero-anterior chest radiograph *(A)* demonstrates overinflation, increased height of the lungs, and flattening of the diaphragm. Decreased vascularity in the peripheral lung regions is also apparent. A high-resolution CT scan at the level of the aortic arch *(B)* demonstrates moderately severe emphysema; a scan at the lung bases *(C)* demonstrates severe emphysema. Note the presence of blood flow redistribution (decreased size of the lower lobe vessels compared with the upper lobe vessels). The patient was a 47-year-old woman who had alpha$_1$-protease inhibitor deficiency.

attenuation and a paucity of vessels *(see* Fig. 55–34).[743, 744, 752, 765] Severe panlobular emphysema leads to diffuse low attenuation and paucity of vascular markings; although these features allow ready identification of advanced disease, mild or moderately severe disease may be difficult to distinguish from normal parenchyma.[745, 752] In one investigation of 10 patients who had panlobular emphysema, the correlation with pathologic findings using the panel grading method was 0.90 for conventional CT and 0.96 for HRCT;[752] however, the extent of emphysema was consistently underestimated, although less so on HRCT scans than on conventional CT scans. Furthermore, the diagnosis was missed in three patients on conventional CT scans and in two patients on HRCT scans. In another investigation of 17 patients who had moderate to severe panlobular emphysema associated with alpha$_1$-antiprotease inhibitor deficiency, all patients were found to have areas of low attenuation corresponding to parenchymal destruction and reduced vascularity.[765] Bulla formation was seen in 7 of 17 patients. The emphysema could be seen to involve all lung zones on the chest radiographs and HRCT scans, with only a slight lower lung zone predominance.

Bronchiectasis may also be seen on CT scans from patients who have panlobular emphysema. For example, it was identified in 6 of the 17 patients (35%) in the study just cited.[765] In another investigation of 14 patients who had alpha$_1$-antitrypsin deficiency, 6 (43%) had evidence of bronchiectasis on CT scans, including 2 who had cystic bronchiectasis.[766] Patients who had bronchiectasis had significantly higher infection rates than patients without bronchiectasis. Occasionally, bronchiectasis is present prior to the development of emphysema.[767, 768]

Paraseptal (distal acinar) emphysema is characterized on CT scans by the presence of areas of low attenuation in the subpleural lung regions separated by intact interlobular septa (Fig. 55–35).[743, 744] Because centrilobular emphysema and paraseptal emphysema produce localized areas of low attenuation, they are easier to recognize on CT scans than is panlobular disease.[743, 745, 752]

### Objective Quantification of Emphysema

The extent of emphysema can be assessed objectively by CT using a computer program that quantifies the volume

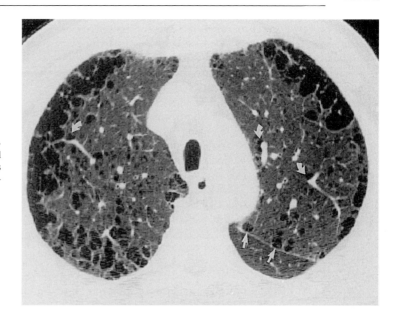

**Figure 55–35. Paraseptal Emphysema.** An HRCT scan demonstrates emphysema, predominantly in subpleural distribution and focally along the interlobar fissure *(straight arrow)* and vessels *(curved arrows).* The appearance is characteristic of paraseptal (distal acinar) emphysema.

of lung that has abnormally low attenuation values (Fig. 55–36).[754–756, 769, 770] One such program involves the use of a "density mask," which highlights areas of attenuation below a given threshold. One group of investigators compared "density mask" estimates with the visual assessment of emphysema in 28 patients who underwent conventional CT prior to lung resection for tumor.[754] The pathologic score was obtained using a modification of the panel grading system; according

to this, 7 patients had no emphysema and 21 had emphysema scores ranging from 5 to 100. In each patient, a single representative CT scan was compared with the corresponding pathologic specimen. The investigators assessed the accuracy of density masks, highlighting all voxels with attenuation values less than −920, −910, and −900 HU. Correlation between the three different density mask scores and the pathologic assessment of emphysema was good (all r > 0.83, P <

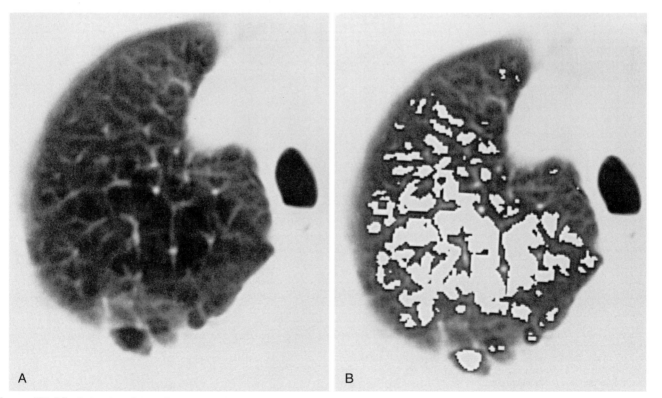

**Figure 55–36. Objective Quantification of Emphysema.** A view of the right upper lobe from a conventional CT scan *(A)* demonstrates the presence of emphysema. Using a computer program ("density mask"), all voxels below a given threshold are automatically highlighted *(B)*. The highlighted areas correspond to voxels with attenuation values less than −910 HU. The CT program automatically quantifies the volume of lung that contains areas with attenuation below the given threshold as well as the volume of the remaining lung.

0.001). The best correlations were observed when all voxels with attenuation values between −910 and −1024 HU were highlighted. The correlation between the mean density mask score and the pathologic score for emphysema was 0.89. By comparison, the correlation between the mean of visual scores by two independent observers and the pathologic score for emphysema was 0.90. There was excellent correlation between the extent of emphysema assessed using the density mask at −910 HU and the subjective assessment of extent of emphysema (r = 0.95). When the density mask at −910 HU was used, three cases with emphysema scores of 10 were missed, and emphysema was diagnosed in one normal lung; by comparison, two independent chest radiologists on two separate occasions missed two cases of emphysema with pathologic scores of 10. The first observer missed one additional case, and the second observer missed four additional cases with pathologic scores ranging from 5 to 20.[754]

Spiral CT allows rapid quantification of the volume of lung involved with emphysema.[771, 772] The use of predetermined threshold attenuation values with this technique enables display of the distribution of emphysema in multiple planes and in three dimensions (Fig. 55–37).[771, 772]

The optimal threshold for the assessment of the presence of emphysema depends on the slice thickness and on whether the CT scan is obtained at end-inspiration or at end-expiration. One group of investigators performed HRCT using 1-mm collimation at 1-cm intervals prior to surgery in 63 patients.[755] They measured the relative areas associated with attenuation values lower than eight thresholds ranging from −900 to −970 HU and compared the results with those obtained from the corresponding pathologic specimens cut in the same plane as that used for the HRCT scans. The optimal threshold value for objective quantification of emphysema on HRCT scans was −950 HU; using this threshold value, there was no significant difference between the extent of emphysema as assessed by HRCT or by morphometry. Subsequently, the same group demonstrated that inspiratory HRCT scans obtained using −950 HU as the threshold correlate best with the macroscopic extent of emphysema.[756] They also showed that HRCT scans obtained at the end of maximal expiration correlate better with measurements of air-flow obstruction than do inspiratory HRCT scans, a finding that may reflect the presence of airway disease in addition to emphysema.[772a] The correlation between inspiratory HRCT scans (threshold value −950 HU) and vital capacity and $FEV_1$ (% of predicted) were −0.24 and −0.50, respectively, compared with −0.48 and −0.68, respectively, for expiratory HRCT scans (threshold value −910 HU).

Lung density as measured by CT is affected by many variables, including patient size, location of the areas of emphysema, depth of inspiration, type of CT scanner, collimation, kilovoltage, and reconstruction algorithm.[754, 773] In spite of these limitations, objective assessment of emphysema using a threshold CT attenuation value has been shown to correlate closely with the visual assessment of emphysema[754] and with the pathologic extent of emphysema.[754–757]

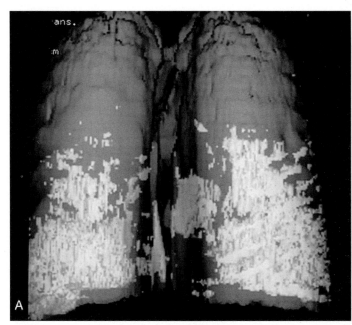

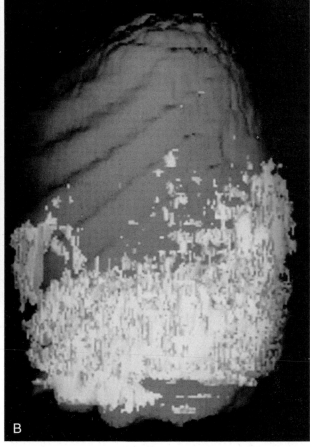

**Figure 55–37. Objective Quantification of Panacinar Emphysema.** Posterior *(A)* and left lateral *(B)* three-dimensional reconstruction images from a spiral CT study show the areas of emphysema highlighted in white and normal lung tissue as areas of gray. The emphysema involves almost exclusively the lower lung zones. The areas that are highlighted have attenuation values equal or less than −910 HU. (Courtesy Dr. Ella Kazerooni, University of Michigan Medical Center, Ann Arbor, MI.)

CT also allows measurement of overall lung volumes.[774–778] In one investigation of 85 patients, including 60 who had emphysema, there was good correlation between lung volumes determined using conventional CT and the FRC as determined by plethysmography (r = 0.79).[776] As the authors pointed out, the CT lung volumes correlate better with FRC than with TLC, because the CT scans are obtained while the patient is supine, usually following a normal inspiratory effort, whereas plethysmographic lung volumes are determined with the patient in the sitting position.[776]

Lung volume and thoracic dimensions can also be measured using single breath-hold magnetic resonance (MR) imaging.[778] In one investigation in which measurements of lung volume obtained using spiral CT and single breath-hold MR imaging and TLC obtained using plethysmography were compared in 15 patients who had severe emphysema, good correlation was found between the CT-determined lung volume and TLC (r = 0.87) and between the MR imaging–determined lung volume and TLC (r = 0.71).[778] The mean lung volumes (L) were 6.71 ± 1.04 for CT, 7.00 ± 1.13 for MR, and 8.12 ± 1.47 for plethysmographic TLC.

The main advantage of CT over MR imaging and plethysmography is in the assessment of the volume of lung involved with emphysema and regional changes in lung volume after lung volume reduction surgery or bullectomy. Techniques for objective measurement of lung volume on chest radiography are discussed in Chapter 13 (*see* page 308). Decreases in lung volume and changes in thoracic dimensions after lung volume reduction surgery have been measured using chest radiography,[779] CT,[777, 778, 780] and MR imaging;[778] measurements of changes in lung volume after surgery using these various techniques have been shown to correlate closely with the decrease in lung volumes as determined by plethysmography.

## CLINICAL MANIFESTATIONS

Patients who have COPD complain of cough, sputum expectoration, and dyspnea. In over 75% of cases, either cough antedates the onset of dyspnea or the two symptoms appear simultaneously; in one study of 175 patients, shortness of breath preceded the onset of cough in only 22%.[781] The majority of patients who complain of cough and expectoration have mucoid sputum that is only periodically yellow or green. In the absence of other signs of acute infection, hemoptysis is very uncommon, and its presence should stimulate a careful search for other causes, particularly pulmonary carcinoma. In temperate climates, most patients attest to an increased frequency of respiratory infections during the winter, and such episodes may increase the severity of dyspnea. Most patients are heavy smokers;[782, 783] however, the number of years and the intensity of smoking do not correlate closely with the frequency and duration of coughing, the volume of sputum expectoration,[783] or the degree of pulmonary dysfunction.[782]

When COPD is mild or moderate in severity, dyspnea occurs only on exertion; as the disease worsens, however, dyspnea is precipitated by less and less effort and in the terminal stages may be present at rest. In patients who have severe COPD, the severity of dyspnea can be influenced by posture; in one study, patients who had $FEV_1$ values less than 20% of predicted were more short of breath when they were standing or sitting erect than when they were supine or sitting leaning forward.[784] The influence of posture on the mechanical advantage of the diaphragm and the intercostal inspiratory muscles is the likely explanation for this effect. Dyspnea induced by the upright posture and relieved by recumbency is termed "platypnea" and can also occur after pneumonectomy or following pulmonary thromboemboli.[785] In the latter conditions, it may be associated with orthodeoxia (a decrease in arterial saturation produced by the upright posture).[785] Conversely, patients who have COPD may complain of orthopnea (increased dyspnea in the supine posture), in which circumstance accompanying left heart failure should be excluded. The assumption of the recumbent posture can be associated with either an improvement or deterioration in arterial $PO_2$; there are no clinical or physiologic features that allow prediction of which will occur in an individual patient.[786] In normal individuals in the decubitus position, the majority of ventilation goes to the dependent lung; however, in some patients who have COPD, ventilation is predominantly distributed to the nondependent lung,[787] presumably because of airway closure in the dependent lung.

The dyspnea of COPD is not closely related to abnormalities of arterial blood gases, a dissociation that is highlighted by the clinical separation of patients who have emphysema into "pink puffers" (type A) and "blue bloaters" (type B).[788, 789] The former tend to be thinner, do not have clinical signs of cor pulmonale or right heart failure, are relatively well oxygenated, do not have hypercapnia, and complain of severe dyspnea. "Blue bloaters," on the other hand, have peripheral edema caused by right heart failure, more severe hypoxemia and hypercapnia, and less dyspnea. Although the great majority of patients who have COPD cannot be placed precisely into one of these categories, the concept that there is a spectrum of clinical presentations is valuable. The physiologic and clinical responses to a given degree of air-flow obstruction differ in different people, part of the variation probably being the result of differences in the responsiveness of the respiratory center to hypoxia and hypercapnia. There is an extremely wide range of responsiveness to hypoxia and hypercapnia in the general population (*see* page 417), and it is likely that individuals who have well-developed ventilatory responsiveness will show preservation of blood gas values at the expense of increased respiratory effort when disease does develop; conversely, those who have relatively blunted respiratory center responsiveness may hypoventilate, thus allowing $PaO_2$ to fall further and $PCO_2$ to rise higher. This biologic variation may, in part, explain the variable clinical picture in patients who have COPD.

In many patients who have only chronic cough and sputum expectoration, physical examination of the chest usually reveals no abnormalities, at least during quiet breathing. However, at maximal expiration or during rapid deep breathing, expiratory wheezes are audible in most.[790] In one study of 83 patients who had COPD, the presence of wheeze did not relate to the severity of obstruction, so that the significance of this physical finding during forced expiration is dubious;[791] however, during quiet expiration, wheeze did correlate with a decrease in $FEV_1$ and with the magnitude of response to bronchodilators. Rhonchi usually are more numerous in patients who complain of shortness of breath on exertion; they are commonly present during both inspiration and expiration.

When emphysema becomes widespread, it gives rise to physical signs attributable to the combination of airway obstruction, bullae, and pulmonary overinflation. The most characteristic of these signs is decreased intensity of breath sounds, usually described incorrectly as a reduction in "air entry." Expiration becomes prolonged; this can be timed by the examiner while listening through a stethoscope placed over the patient's trachea during a maximal expiration from TLC. Whereas expiration takes less than 4 seconds in normal individuals, it may take several times longer in patients who have emphysema.[783, 792] Loss of parenchymal elasticity results in wide fluctuations in intrapleural pressure that may be manifested clinically by intercostal and supraclavicular indrawing during inspiration and jugular venous distention during expiration.

When lung volumes are markedly increased and the thoracic cage is fixed in an inspiratory position, the physical signs are characteristic: The chest becomes barrel-shaped, and the thoracic kyphosis may be considerably increased; the shoulders are raised, and the chest tends to move *en bloc,* often with contraction of the accessory muscles of respiration in the neck.[793] A decrease in length of the trachea that is palpable above the sternal notch has been described in such patients;[792] "tracheal descent" has been noted during inspiration and ascribed to downward pull of the depressed diaphragm and to overinflation of the lungs.

Flattening of the diaphragm is believed to be responsible for a paradoxical inward movement of the lower thoracic costal margins during inspiration (Hoover's sign).[794] When anterior and posterior movements of the chest and abdomen are recorded separately on electromagnetic ventilation monitors, asynchronous breathing movements can be detected in some patients who have advanced COPD and indicate an extremely poor prognosis.[795, 796] Paradoxical abdominal motion at rest is a sign of inspiratory muscle fatigue or recruitment of expiratory muscles and is seen only in patients who have severe disease. Pulmonary overinflation may be evidenced by increased resonance of the percussion note, although this may be difficult to evaluate in obese or muscular patients. None of the many physical signs seen in patients who have COPD correlate with airway conductance except forced expiratory time.[797]

Clinical assessment is a relatively inexact method of detecting and quantifying pulmonary hypertension, right ventricular hypertrophy, and right heart failure in patients who have COPD.[798] Examination of the heart may be difficult, because separation of the heart from the anterior chest wall by overinflated lung results in varying degrees of faintness of heart sounds; in some cases, auscultation of the heart can be performed satisfactorily only when the stethoscope is placed over the epigastrium. Assessment of jugular venous pressure is also difficult because of wide swings in intrathoracic pressure, and peripheral edema may be due to other causes. The detection of a right ventricular parasternal heave or of tricuspid insufficiency is helpful if either is present, but these are infrequent findings. Accentuation of the second heart sound is not a sensitive indicator of pulmonary hypertension in COPD.[798]

Patients who have advanced COPD tend to have a low body mass index.[799, 800] The decreased body weight is related to the severity of the airway obstruction and blood gas abnormalities and has been attributed to both increased caloric use and decreased caloric intake.[801–803] However, in one study, dietary caloric intakes were similar in a group of underweight COPD patients and in age-matched controls, and the weight loss was explained on the basis of a hypermetabolic state and increased plasma catecholamine levels.[804] Nutritional supplements in malnourished patients who have COPD can increase body weight and inspiratory muscle strength but do not improve ventilation.[805]

## LABORATORY FINDINGS

Secondary polycythemia develops in some patients who have COPD and chronic hypoxemia. Among patients who have similar degrees of hypoxemia, hemoglobin and hematocrit levels tend to be normal or low in COPD patients who live at sea level,[806] whereas levels in otherwise normal individuals who live at high altitudes tend to be elevated; however, an increased red cell volume is masked by a proportional increase in plasma volume in some patients in the former group. In such cases, demonstration of the absolute degree of polycythemia requires direct measurement of blood volume.[807, 808] Increased carboxyhemoglobin levels can also contribute to the development of polycythemia. In one study of 47 patients who had hypoxemia (mean $PaO_2 = 52$ mm Hg), the increased red blood cell mass correlated with carboxyhemoglobin levels;[809] oxygen therapy corrected the polycythemia only in those patients who discontinued smoking and thus diminished their carboxyhemoglobin levels.

In some patients who have COPD and chronic hypoxemia, the red cell mass fails to increase.[808] In one study, this failure could not be attributed to decreased erythropoietin production and was assumed to be the result of a bone marrow defect.[808] A delay in complete incorporation of radioactive iron into the erythrocytes of patients who have COPD has been found to be proportional to the degree of associated hypoxemia;[807] because parenterally administered iron increases the red cell mass,[810] it is possible that the physiologic response to lack of oxygen may be limited by the availability of iron for hemoglobin synthesis. In patients who have secondary polycythemia, nocturnal arterial oxygen desaturation is more severe than in patients who have similar degrees of obstruction in whom daytime arterial $PO_2$ values are identical but polycythemia is absent.[811] Administration of continuous oxygen to patients who have polycythemia results in a decrease in hematocrit values.[812] In addition, a decrease in the hematocrit level following venisection is associated with an improvement in arterial blood gas values, presumably owing to decreased blood viscosity and improved cardiac output.[813]

Patients who have COPD manifest impaired water handling and electrolyte exchange.[814, 815] In one study, patients who received a standard water load excreted only half the amount excreted by normal controls over a four-hour period;[814] water excretion was inversely proportional to the arterial $PaCO_2$. The abnormalities in water excretion may not be directly related to hypercapnia, because acute hypercapnia (increase in $PaCO_2$ from 36 to 52 mm Hg) in ventilated patients has not been found to cause any change in plasma atrial natriuretic peptide, renin, angiotensin II, aldosterone, or vasopressin.[816] However, renal excretion is impaired during respiratory failure and usually improves during recovery. In a study of the effects of hypoxia, hyperoxia, and hypercapnia on patients in respiratory failure, urine flow and kidney function decreased when $PaO_2$ was raised;[817] when $PaO_2$ was lowered, renal function improved. However, function deteriorated abruptly when hypoxia became severe ($PaO_2$ <40 mm Hg). The level of $PaCO_2$ had no measurable effect until it reached 65 mm Hg, at which point renal function abruptly decreased. The results of this study reflect the response of the kidney to blood gas changes over relatively short periods of time, and it is questionable whether they can be extrapolated to more protracted exposures in patients who have respiratory failure.[818]

Potassium depletion can be a major complication of both acute[819] and chronic[820] respiratory failure. The ion tends to move from tissue cells to plasma, and although serum potassium values may be normal, total exchangeable potassium may be greatly reduced.[820] Diuretics and corticosteroid therapy may add to the deficiency, and when elimination of $CO_2$ is excessive, hypokalemic hypochloremic alkalosis may develop. Abrupt decreases in $PaCO_2$ may increase renal potassium loss and contribute to potassium depletion.[821]

## PULMONARY HEMODYNAMICS AND CARDIAC FUNCTION

Pulmonary arterial hypertension, right ventricular hypertrophy (cor pulmonale), and right ventricular failure are serious complications of severe COPD.[713, 798, 822] Strictly speaking, the term *cor pulmonale* can be applied only when there is evidence for right ventricular hypertrophy secondary to lung disease; however, in practice, the term is often used to characterize a clinical syndrome of peripheral edema, jugular venous distention, and hepatic engorgement secondary to right ventricular failure.[798]

The pulmonary hypertension that leads to cor pulmonale and right heart failure in COPD is the result of several mechanisms, including hypoxic vasoconstriction of the muscular pulmonary arteries, a loss of pulmonary capillary bed, a decrease in pulmonary vascular compliance,[823] and vascular wall remodeling. Pharmacologic factors may also be involved. One important agent that contributes to the normally low pulmonary vascular resistance is nitric oxide (NO); in COPD, the endothelial production of NO appears to be decreased.[824] In addition, circulating levels of the powerful pulmonary vasoconstrictor endothelin-1 have been found by one group of investigators to be increased in patients who have emphysema and pulmonary hypertension.[825]

With mild to moderate grades of COPD ($FEV_1$ of 40% to 80% predicted), the pulmonary artery pressure (Ppa) is usually normal at rest but increases with moderate exercise.[714] In the presence of severe COPD ($FEV_1$ < 40% of predicted), pulmonary hypertension is usually present at rest (mean Ppa > 20 mm Hg) and undergoes a disproportionate increase during mild exercise[826–828] or with exposure to cold;[829] its severity correlates with the degree of arterial desaturation and arterial $PCO_2$.[830]

Exacerbations of COPD are associated with acute worsening of pulmonary hypertension, although the Ppa usually returns to pre-exacerbation levels following treatment.[830, 831] During exacerbations, the pulmonary hypertension is relatively refractory to the correction of hypoxemia, suggesting that mechanisms other than hypoxic vasoconstriction are important in this setting.[832] Although the development of peripheral edema in patients who have established COPD is usually an indication of right-sided heart failure, some patients who develop this complication do not show hemodynamic deterioration, in which case the mechanism for the edema is unclear.[833]

Pulmonary artery pressure can also increase acutely during the episodes of hypoxemia that occur during sleep, and it has been suggested that recurrent nocturnal pulmonary hypertension can eventually result in pathologic changes in pulmonary vessels and fixed hypertension.[834, 835] However, in one study of 94 patients with COPD who did not have obstructive sleep apnea, Ppa was not correlated with the degree and duration of oxygen desaturation during sleep.[836] Oral and parenteral smooth muscle–relaxing drugs cause a decrease in Ppa, but not to normal levels.[837, 838]

In the absence of therapy, the pulmonary hypertension in patients who have COPD progresses slowly but inexorably,[831] the increase in Ppa over time correlating with a decrease in $FEV_1$ and $PaO_2$;[839, 840] this increase can be prevented by chronic $O_2$ therapy.[841, 842] In one study,[842] 16 patients who had severe COPD ($FEV_1$ = 0.9 liter) were followed for 47 months prior to and 31 months after the institution of long-term $O_2$ therapy. During the period before $O_2$ therapy, mean Ppa increased from 23 to 28 mm Hg and $PaO_2$ decreased from 59 to 50 mm Hg; during the 31 months following the institution of $O_2$ therapy, Ppa decreased from 28 to 24 mm Hg and $PaO_2$ remained stable at 50 mm Hg (all measurements were made during the breathing of room air). Nocturnal $O_2$ therapy may be particularly beneficial in preventing the progression of pulmonary hypertension.[843] In patients who have COPD, the long-term response of the pulmonary vasculature to the breathing of an enriched oxygen mixture can be predicted by measuring changes in Ppa during a 24-hour period of $O_2$ administration. In one study of 43 patients, 25 showed a decrease greater than 5 mm Hg in Ppa after breathing 28% $O_2$ for 24 hours;[844] these individuals showed significantly improved survival after 1, 2, and 3 years of chronic low-flow $O_2$ therapy, in comparison with those who did not show an acute decrease in Ppa.

Although there is a relationship between arterial desaturation and pulmonary hypertension, there is also significant interindividual variation. Patients who have COPD can be divided into two groups on the basis of the change in the ratio of physiologic dead space to tidal volume ($V_T/V_D$)[845] and their pulmonary arterial pressure during oxygen breathing.[846] Approximately two thirds show an increase in dead space while breathing oxygen, and it has been suggested that these individuals respond to hypoxemia with pulmonary vasoconstriction; when oxygen is administered, hypoxic vasoconstriction is abolished and blood flow to poorly ventilated areas of the lungs increases, with a resultant increase in $V_D/V_T$. In other words, in "vascular responders," perfusion remains relatively well matched to ventilation, and blood gas tensions are preserved at the expense of an increase in pulmonary vascular resistance and an increased load on the right side of the heart. By contrast, hypoxic vasoconstriction and pulmonary hypertension do not develop in "vascular nonresponders," although for a given degree of pulmonary disease, blood gas values are worse. Vascular nonresponsiveness can have a beneficial effect on patient survival, suggesting that it is not the abnormal blood gas level *per se* but the patient response to the hypoxemia that is detrimental to survival.[846a]

Because of the deficiencies of clinical examination in detecting pulmonary artery hypertension in patients who have COPD (*see* page 2216), and because Ppa is such a good predictor of prognosis in these individuals, a number of attempts have been made to develop noninvasive methods to estimate it. Although the size of the right descending pulmonary artery[847] and the hilar-cardiothoracic ratio[848] on plain chest radiographs are reasonably sensitive in detecting the presence of pulmonary arterial hypertension, they give no indication of its severity. Echocardiographic estimates of systolic and diastolic pulmonary artery diameters[849] and the time interval between tricuspid valve closure and pulmonic valve opening[850] have both been shown to correlate with Ppa.

A number of variables derived from continuous-wave or pulsed Doppler echocardiography also can be employed to determine right ventricular peak systolic pressure, which can be used as an estimate of Ppa.[851–853] Although the increase in retrosternal air in COPD patients whose lungs are hyperinflated can hamper accurate echocardiographic assessment, adequate examinations can be accomplished in up to 80% of patients.[854] The use of the tricuspid regurgitant jet is probably the most accurate; although its successful use is dependent on the presence of at least a small amount of tricuspid valve regurgitation, such regurgitation occurs in the majority of patients who have COPD.[855] In one study of 100 patients who had pulmonary hypertension secondary to COPD, echocardiographic assessment was useful for estimation of Ppa in 30;[851] in these patients, the correlation with mean Ppa was 0.73. In another investigation, pulsed Doppler echocardiography was successful in 60 of 66 (91%) patients;[856] "latent" pulmonary hypertension, which was revealed only during an exercise test, was also accompanied by significant changes in Doppler findings. Correlations between echocardiographic and cardiac catheterization estimates of Ppa as high as 0.98 have been reported in selected patients.[857] The accuracy of noninvasive techniques to measure Ppa is discussed in more detail in Chapter 50 (*see* page 1886).

Prolonged pulmonary hypertension causes right ventricular hypertrophy and, ultimately, right ventricular failure. Right ventricular hypertrophy can be diagnosed by electrocardiography and echocardiography. The electrocardiogram (ECG) may be perfectly normal in patients who have COPD despite the development of increased pulmonary vascular resistance on exercise; however, as airway obstruction becomes more severe, signs of right axis deviation develop, with large S waves and diphasic T waves over the left precordium beyond the $V_2$ position. These changes correlate best with total pulmonary vascular resistance.[858] As $FEV_1$/FVC decreases further, there is an increased frequency of P waves greater than 2.0 mm, P axis greater than +75 degrees, S waves greater than 5 mm in leads $V_5$ and $V_6$, and QRS axis greater than +75 degrees.[859] An R/S ratio of less than 1.0 in lead $V_6$ is also good evidence for right ventricular hypertrophy. In a study of 71 patients in whom ECG changes during life were correlated with right ventricular mass at

autopsy, 30 had definite and 3 probable right ventricular hypertrophy, 20 had normal ventricular weight, and 18 had left ventricular hypertrophy.[860] Four criteria were found to be the most reliable indicators of right ventricular hypertrophy: an S1, Q3 pattern; right axis deviation of +110 degrees or more; an S1, S2, S3 pattern; and an R/S ratio in $V_6$ of 1.0 or less.[860]

Right ventricular function can be assessed by measuring right ventricular ejection fraction with single-pass[861] or gated equilibration radionuclide techniques,[862, 863] or more invasively using a thermistor-tipped volumetric pulmonary artery catheter.[864] The normal right ventricle ejects approximately 55% of its end-diastolic blood volume with each cardiac contraction. Severe COPD is associated with a significant decrease in this value,[862, 865] a close relationship existing between the increase in Ppa and the decrease in ejection fraction.[866] In patients who have COPD, exercise does not normally increase right ventricular ejection fraction,[867] although in one study, exercise in the presence of supplemental oxygen was associated with improved right ventricular function.[861] In a study of 15 patients who had COPD, the assessment of right ventricular function with single-photon emission computed tomography (SPECT) using thallium 201 to measure myocardial perfusion was complementary to the measurement of right ventricular ejection fraction in the identification of the presence of cor pulmonale.[868] MR imaging is at present probably the standard modality for measuring right ventricular mass; however, although it has the advantage of avoiding exposure to radiation, it is time-consuming and expensive.[869]

Most investigators have shown that left ventricular function as assessed by ejection fraction (LVEF) is relatively normal in patients who have COPD, although dysfunction may be observed when cor pulmonale and right ventricular failure have developed.[862, 865, 870] In one study of 100 patients and no evidence of ischemic, hypertensive or valvular heart disease, the mean LVEF was 52th ± 11%, versus 61th ± 8% in normal individuals;[822] only one patient who had COPD had an LVEF less than 30%. There is more convincing evidence that left ventricular function is impaired during exercise in COPD.[871] At autopsy, left ventricular hypertrophy is present in up to 30% of patients who have COPD;[872, 873] in most cases, however, it can be attributed to concomitant hypertensive or arteriosclerotic heart disease.[874] As right ventricular hypertrophy increases, the interventricular septum thickens; when this is associated with right ventricular dilation and leftward shift of the septum, this may decrease the diastolic compliance of the left ventricle.[875–877]

Reduced left ventricular compliance may explain the results of studies in which mild elevation in pulmonary arterial wedge pressure and left ventricular end-diastolic pressure have been found in some patients who have COPD.[714] However, measurement of pulmonary arterial wedge pressure may not be a reliable indicator of left ventricular end-diastolic pressure in patients who have COPD. This is certainly the case if the catheter is wedged in an area of Zone II blood flow conditions; however, even in Zone III, the pulmonary artery wedge pressure may overestimate end-diastolic pressure.

Chronic cor pulmonale may be associated with cardiac arrhythmias, as was the case in 33 of 70 patients in one series[878] and in 47 of 102 patients in another.[879] In one study of 35 hospitalized patients in whom ECGs were recorded continuously for 72 hours, arrhythmias were identified in 31 (89%); 20 were sufficiently severe to require therapy.[880] Supraventricular arrhythmias were found to be slightly more common than ventricular, the most frequent being atrial and multifocal tachycardia; ventricular arrhythmias were often preceded by premature ventricular contractions or supraventricular arrhythmias and were associated with a poor prognosis. Seventy per cent of the patients who had ventricular arrhythmia died during their hospital stay, and none survived to the end of the 2.5-year study period.

Prognosis is significantly related to the pulmonary hemodynamic and right ventricular consequences of COPD.[881] In one investigation of 50 patients who had COPD, cardiovascular function was evaluated by catheterization when the clinical condition was stable; survival was inversely related to pulmonary vascular resistance.[882] Two different patterns of cardiovascular abnormality were found in patients who had high vascular resistance. One consisted of low cardiac output, relatively normal blood gas levels, and near-normal resting pulmonary arterial pressure—an "emphysematous" type of COPD. The second pattern consisted of a well-maintained cardiac output with more severe pulmonary hypertension and blood gas abnormalities; this was found in a group of patients judged clinically to have a predominantly "bronchitic" type of disease. Patients in the first group were unlikely to be diagnosed clinically as having cor pulmonale, because cardiomegaly, chronic congestive heart failure, and ECG evidence of right ventricular hypertrophy were relatively infrequent; by contrast, patients in the second group more regularly presented with the classic clinical and ECG features of pulmonary heart disease.

## RESPIRATORY MUSCLE FUNCTION

Inspiratory muscle fatigue may be the final common pathway that causes ventilatory failure in patients who have COPD. A number of factors can adversely influence respiratory muscle performance in these patients:

- The muscles must work against an increased load as a result of increased pulmonary resistance.
- The muscles are at a mechanical disadvantage because of pulmonary hyperinflation; in the presence of hyperinflation, the muscle fibers become shorter than the optimal length at which overlap of actin and myosin filaments permits maximal force generation for a given neural input and oxygen consumption.[883]
- By changing the geometry of the thoracic cage and its relationship to the inspiratory muscles, hyperinflation adds to the inefficient action of the muscles.
- Patients tend to be malnourished, resulting in impairment of muscle strength and endurance.
- With the development of cor pulmonale and right ventricular failure, cardiac output decreases, creating the potential for inadequate inspiratory muscle blood flow to meet increased demands.

Theoretically, it might be expected that patients who have COPD would develop increased strength of the inspiratory muscles as a result of hypertrophy, because these are continuously working against an increased impedance; in

fact, the data suggest that they undergo atrophy. At autopsy, diaphragmatic weight in patients who had emphysema is decreased rather than increased.[884] Part of this decrease may be the result of general malnutrition, because in the general population, body weight is significantly related to diaphragmatic weight at autopsy; however, in patients who had emphysema, the decrease in diaphragmatic weight is out of proportion to the decrease in body weight.[884]

Muscle fibers from various respiratory muscles have been studied in COPD patients who had lung resection for pulmonary carcinoma. When compared with normal individuals, patients had atrophy of type 1 and type 2 muscle fibers in the costal portion of the diaphragm and the intercostal muscles;[885] the degree of muscle fiber atrophy was significantly related to the severity of preoperative air-flow obstruction and to body weight as a percent predicted ideal body weight.[885, 886] In addition, there was a lower level of oxidative enzymes in the diaphragm of patients who had COPD.[887] In hamsters that have elastase-induced emphysema, the diaphragm shortens because of loss of sarcomeres; however, it also thickens, so that total diaphragmatic weight and strength are unchanged.[888, 889]

Inspiratory muscle strength can be assessed by measuring maximal inspiratory mouth pressure (PImax), and the diaphragm itself can be specifically assessed by measuring maximal transdiaphragmatic pressure (Pdi Max). In children who have obstructive pulmonary disease (mainly that due to cystic fibrosis), PImax is decreased when measured at FRC; this effect is evidently caused mainly by the mechanical disadvantage resulting from hyperinflation, because performance of the test at predicted normal FRC produces normal results.[890] In adults who have COPD, however, the decrease in strength appears to be more than can be accounted for by the mechanical disadvantage alone.[891, 892]

The decreased inspiratory strength and increased load put the inspiratory muscles of patients who have COPD at risk of developing fatigue, defined as the inability of a muscle to generate the maximal force of which it is usually capable, despite maximal effort. In most skeletal muscles, fatigue develops when a muscle is used repetitively to generate greater than 15% to 20% of its maximal force. The respiratory muscles are relatively fatigue-resistant, because with each breath they can develop up to 40% of their maximal force (PI/PImax = 40%) virtually indefinitely.[893] However, when pressures in excess of 40% of maximal are generated with each breath, fatigue eventually develops; the greater the percentage of maximum generated with each breath, the faster the onset of fatigue. The development of fatigue can also be altered by the breathing pattern; the longer the inspiratory phase of the respiratory cycle (duty cycle), the lower the pressure that can be generated indefinitely.

The development of inspiratory muscle fatigue can be predicted by measuring the tension-time index, which is the product of the duty cycle—inspiratory time/total respiratory cycle time (TI/Ttot)—and the inspiratory pressure (PI) expressed as a percentage of the maximal inspiratory pressure (PI/PImax); a tension-time index greater than 0.15 will result in fatigue. Patients who have COPD breathe using a higher-than-normal tension-time index, both because PI is increased secondary to the increased impedance of the lung and because PImax is decreased as a result of muscle atrophy and mechanical disadvantage. In one study of 20 patients who had COPD, the tension-time index of the diaphragm during tidal breathing at rest averaged 0.05 (range 0.01 to 0.12); when the tension-time index was increased to more than 0.15 by prolonging the inspiratory duration, electromyographic indicators of diaphragmatic fatigue developed.[894] Although the tension-time index may not be above the critical value of 0.15 during resting tidal breathing, the reserve for increase in force generation is reduced in patients who have COPD (threefold) compared with normal individuals (eightfold). Besides tension and duty cycle, the work performed by the inspiratory muscles is also a determinant of fatigue; for the same tension and duty cycle, a muscle that contracts and shortens consumes more oxygen than does the same muscle contracting isometrically.[895, 896]

The diagnosis of respiratory muscle fatigue in patients who have COPD can be made by showing an inability to generate previously achievable pressures using voluntary contraction or bilateral phrenic nerve stimulation.[897] In addition, there is a shift in the frequency distribution of the electromyogram (EMG) signals in a muscle that is performing potentially fatiguing tasks.[893]

In patients who have COPD, inspiratory muscle fatigue develops during exercise and, unlike in normal individuals, is probably a major determinant of maximal exercise performance.[898, 899] The fatigue can be delayed and exercise endurance increased by the administration of supplemental oxygen. The beneficial effect of $O_2$ is chiefly the result of a decrease in ventilation at any level of exercise; however, it may also derive from a direct effect on muscle performance.[898] In patients who have COPD, inspiratory muscle strength and endurance can be improved by specific training programs;[900, 901] in addition, their capacity to exercise can be augmented.[902, 903] The results of these studies suggest that despite the increased impedance to breathing, inspiratory muscle weakness and atrophy may develop in some patients as a result of relative disuse. It is possible that dyspnea causes some patients to avoid exercise, with resulting respiratory muscle deconditioning, thus initiating a vicious circle. In patients who have COPD, inspiratory rib cage muscles make an increasing contribution to total inspiratory pressure during exercise.[904]

Although muscle fatigue is usually considered to be an unsteady state, the concept of chronic respiratory muscle fatigue has been suggested to occur in patients who have COPD and chronic ventilatory failure. The basis for this concept was derived from studies that showed an improvement in muscle and lung function and a decrease in dyspnea in hypercapnic patients by resting respiratory muscles with ventilatory support overnight.[893] Despite this theoretical benefit, the results of one controlled trial have proved negative: 184 patients who had severe COPD were randomized to a home negative-pressure ventilator designed to achieve nocturnal respiratory muscle rest or to a placebo device; there was no difference in the primary outcome measure, the 6-minute walk test, after a 12-week period.[905]

If chronic inspiratory muscle fatigue does exist, patients who have COPD would not derive benefit from inspiratory muscle training. The link between inspiratory muscle fatigue and ventilatory respiratory failure in COPD has also led to the suggestion that inspiratory muscle dysfunction is a risk factor for death.[906]

## PULMONARY FUNCTION TESTS

Although the basic pathophysiologic processes that contribute to the development of COPD are varied, the functional abnormalities that they cause are similar. Certain pulmonary function tests help to predict which pathologic process is predominant in an individual patient; however, the most important applications of such tests lie in detecting the presence of disease (preferably at an early stage) and in following its progression. Although symptomatic COPD develops in only a proportion of smokers, these individuals can be identified long before the development of symptoms, because the disease follows an insidiously progressive course for years prior to clinical presentation.[907] Smoking cessation in such individuals results in some functional improvement but, more important, causes a normalization in the rate of age-related decline of lung function.[406, 908] Thus, COPD can be prevented, but only if it is recognized at an early stage by pulmonary function testing. In addition to aiding in the recognition of disease, pulmonary function studies help to quantify the degree of functional impairment in individual patients and are useful in research studies of the natural history and pathogenesis of COPD.

### Small Airway Tests

As previously indicated, the demonstration by Hogg and colleagues in 1968 that airways smaller than 3 mm in internal diameter were the most important site of increase in resistance in patients who have established airway disease led to the development of tests to detect abnormalities of small airway function.[617, 909–911] Presumably, a test that could detect abnormal function in the airways prior to the onset of a decrease in $FEV_1$ would allow the identification of a subset of smokers who had preclinical COPD and were therefore at risk for the development of symptomatic disease. Intensive smoking cessation campaigns directed at such individuals could be expected to have a more important preventive effect than a program targeting all smokers.

The so-called small airway tests that were developed included the measurement of the frequency dependence of dynamic compliance (Cdyn), the single-breath nitrogen washout ($\Delta N_2$/liter, closing volume and closing capacity), the density dependence of maximal expiratory flow, and flows at low lung volumes ($FEF_{25-75}$ and the instantaneous forced expiratory flow rates at 50% and 25%, respectively, of vital capacity—i.e., $\dot{V}max_{50}$ and $\dot{V}max_{25}$). Other than the $FEF_{25-75}$ and the $\dot{V}max_{25}$ and $\dot{V}max_{50}$, which are measured on spirometric tracings and flow-volume curves, respectively, these tests are no longer performed on a routine or even an experimental basis; we therefore include only a brief description of each.

Frequency dependence of Cdyn is a decrease in compliance with increasing frequency of breathing. In normal individuals, dynamic compliance remains constant as frequency of breathing increases up to 60 to 90 breaths per minute. Cdyn decreases as frequency increases if there are substantially different time constants in peripheral parallel lung units. In the presence of patchy small airway narrowing, Cdyn would be expected to decrease with increasing respiratory frequency; in fact, some smokers who do not have a significant decrease in maximal expiratory flow do show frequency dependence of Cdyn.[912]

Because it is the small airways that close at low lung volumes,[913] the single-breath nitrogen washout test (closing volume and closing capacity) is theoretically an attractive test for the detection of early abnormalities in COPD. The single-breath test also gives a measure of the evenness of lung emptying. The slope of the alveolar plateau (phase 3) would be flat if all lung units emptied homogenously; sequential emptying of units would occur if there were regional differences in small airway resistance and air-space compliance. Both closing volume and the slope of phase 3 are abnormal in some smokers;[909] moreover, these derangements have good correlation with pathologic abnormalities in membranous and respiratory bronchioles.[626, 627] These tests of small airway function may be abnormal even when the decrease in maximal expiratory flow is caused by loss of lung elasticity.[914]

Density dependence of maximal expiratory flow should theoretically decrease in patients who have small airway narrowing because the equal pressure point moves from large to small airways where the flow regime is more closely laminar rather than turbulent. However, in practice, the density dependence of maximal expiratory flow has not proved to be an effective screening test; in addition, it does not appear to relate to pathologic abnormalities in small airways.[915] In patients who have established COPD and definite bronchiolar pathology, density dependence may be preserved, possibly because flow-limiting segments remain in central airways despite the increase in peripheral resistance. In addition, the test has a large coefficient of variation when repeated on the same subject.[916] The results of animal studies have also put into question the usefulness of density dependence in identifying the site of flow limitation.[917, 918]

Decreased expiratory flow at low lung volumes should also reflect small airway narrowing. During most of the $FEV_1$ maneuver, flow either is not limited or is limited at choke points in central airways; because the equal-pressure point and choke points move outward in the lung at low lung volumes, flow at these volumes ($\dot{V}max50$, $\dot{V}max25$, $FEF_{25-75}$) is influenced to a greater extent by narrowing at these sites.

The basic premise behind the hypothesis that small airway tests will predict later decline in $FEV_1$ is that they are more sensitive than simple spirometry; however, there is now considerable evidence that this is incorrect. Small airway resistance probably contributes more to total pulmonary resistance than was originally believed (50% rather than 10 to 20%).[919] It has been shown that changes in $FEV_1$ and $FEV_1/FVC$ parallel those in the small airway tests,[920–922] and although the absolute changes in $FEV_1$ may be less than those in small airway test values, they are of equal or greater significance because the coefficients of variation of $FEV_1$ and FVC are much smaller. The results of longitudinal studies have, in general, not confirmed the hypothesis that abnormalities in small airway tests will predict longitudinal decline in $FEV_1$.[923, 924] Alteration in the forced expiratory spirogram occurs in young smokers and probably identifies those at risk.[925] Because spirometry is easier and cheaper to perform, it will probably remain the most valuable test in the clinical management and epidemiologic investigation of patients who have COPD.[926]

## Maximal Expiratory Flow

Expiratory flow can be measured as peak flow (PEFR), flow in the first second of a forced vital capacity maneuver ($FEV_1$), average flow over the middle half of the forced expired volume ($FEF_{25-75}$, formerly called the maximal midexpiratory flow rate [MMEF]), or instantaneous flow rates at different percentages of the FVC ($\dot{V}max_{50}$, $\dot{V}max_{25}$). All of these measures are decreased in patients who have COPD. The $FEV_1$ has the advantage of being the most reproducible in a given individual and there is little evidence that $FEF_{25-75}$, $\dot{V}max_{50}$, or $\dot{V}max_{25}$ is more sensitive in detecting the early stages of the disease.[927, 928] There is a wide range of values within the normal population for these tests; however, the range is narrowed by expressing forced expiratory flow as a percentage of FVC ($FEV_1/FVC\%$). $FEV_1$ and $FEV_1/FVC$ are lower in patients who have COPD if they breath-hold at TLC before performing the maximal expiratory effort; this phenomenon is also seen in normal individuals and is probably caused by a decline in lung recoil during the deep inspiration.[929]

Examination of a flow-volume curve provides additional information in a patient who has air-flow obstruction. If the decreased flow is caused by upper airway obstruction, the shape of the expiratory and inspiratory curves will be characteristic (*see* page 2027). It has been suggested that the shape of the expiratory flow-volume curve can be helpful in determining whether the obstruction is caused by emphysema or asthma.[930] In one study, the ratio of maximal flow at 50% of FVC to specific airway conductance during quiet breathing was useful in this discrimination.[931] The patients who had COPD had a lower ratio than those who had asthma, suggesting a disproportionate dynamic narrowing of the airways during forced expiration. The ratio of forced expiratory flow to forced inspiratory flow at isovolume has also been suggested as a measure that can be used to distinguish emphysema from diseases that cause intrinsic airway narrowing, the hypothesis being that patients who have emphysema will show disproportionate expiratory obstruction as a result of dynamic airway collapse.[932]

With the development of obstructive pulmonary disease, forced expiratory flow decreases over the entire vital capacity range, and the effort-independent portion of the curve becomes more curvilinear than normal and is convex (lowered toward the volume axis) (Fig. 55–38).[933] The decrease

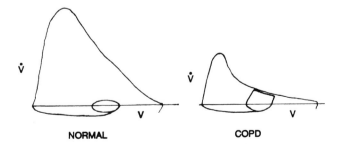

**Figure 55–38. Flow-Volume Curve in a Normal Individual and a Patient with Severe Chronic Obstructive Pulmonary Disease (COPD).** A normal tidal flow-volume ($\dot{V}$-V) loop and a complete maximal expiratory flow-volume curve show that during tidal breathing, the patient with COPD achieves maximal expiratory flow. There is considerable reserve for increased expiratory flow in the normal person.

in maximal expiratory flow that characterizes COPD is the result of increased airway resistance and loss of lung elastic recoil.[934] Although it has been clearly established that the bronchioles are the major site of the increased resistance, there is also evidence that excessive large airway collapsibility contributes to expiratory air-flow limitation.

Expiratory air-flow limitation occurs during forced expiration when pleural pressure exceeds intra-airway pressure, causing narrowing of the tracheobronchial tree downstream (mouthward) from the equal-pressure point.[934–937] The site of this narrowing has been assessed using measurements of bronchial pressure, with and without radiographic measurements of bronchial caliber.[601, 602, 938] In normal individuals, all bronchi undergo roughly the same reduction in caliber during forced expiration, from a maximum at the height of inspiration to a minimum at the end of expiration (Fig. 55–39). By contrast, in patients who have COPD, forced expiration causes a disproportionate collapse of the large proximal bronchi, particularly the large bronchi of the lower lobes (Fig. 55–40). In one study, airway caliber reduction at this location averaged 67%, compared with 49% in normal individuals.[939] The importance of peripheral airway obstruction and excessive central airway collapsibility in COPD has been confirmed using dynamic measurements of intrabronchial pressure during forced expiration.[602]

Figure 55–41 depicts simultaneous measurements of bronchial pressures and dimensions (obtained at cinebronchography) during a single forced inspiration and expiration in a normal individual and in a patient who had COPD. Several alterations are apparent in the recordings of the patient:

- Inspiratory flow is mildly reduced and expiratory flow is markedly reduced, despite the fact that the pressure producing the flow (alveolar pressure) is almost the same as in the normal individual (i.e., resistance is much greater).
- The lower lobe bronchus collapses so much during forced

expiration that its caliber becomes less than that of the distal segmental bronchi.
- The lower lobe bronchus collapses simultaneously with an abrupt decrease in the expiratory flow.
- The decrease in pressure across the lower lobe bronchus during expiration amounts to almost the total pressure drop from alveolus to mouth (whereas in the normal individual it represents only a relatively small proportion).
- During inspiration, the lower lobe bronchus no longer obstructs flow, and all obstruction is in the small airways.

These results suggest that in some patients who have COPD, there are two levels of obstruction: one in the small airways and the other in the central bronchi, the latter being present only during forced expiration under circumstances of dynamic compression. Although the excessive central airway collapsibility in COPD is partly related to a larger transmural pressure difference secondary to the peripheral airway obstruction, there is evidence that the lobar bronchi are also excessively compliant as a result of structural changes in their walls, such as atrophy of the cartilage plates.[596–598, 940]

The relative contribution of loss of elastic recoil and increased resistance to flow through airways upstream from the flow-limiting segments can be determined by plotting maximal flow against static recoil pressure; the slope of this relationship represents upstream conductance. If a decrease in flow is related entirely to loss of elasticity, the slope of the maximal flow–static recoil plot will be normal; however, when airway narrowing is the cause, the slope is decreased (increased upstream resistance). In most patients who have COPD, the loss of flow is related to a combination of loss of recoil and airway narrowing.[932, 941, 942]

Patients who have COPD can show a substantial increase in forced expiratory flow following inhalation of a bronchodilator. In one 3-year study, the mean increase in $FEV_1$ following inhaled beta-adrenergic agonist was 15%;[943] nearly a third of the patients showed an increase greater

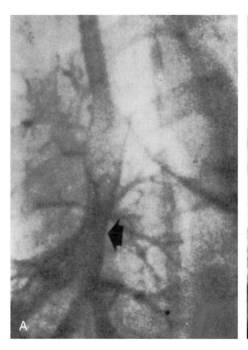
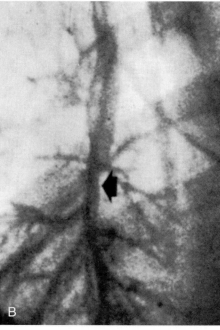

**Figure 55–39. Bronchial Dynamics in a Normal Individual.** Selected frames from cinestrips of a right bronchogram of a normal individual. The frame on the left *(A)* shows maximal caliber on full inspiration, and that on the right *(B),* minimal caliber on forced expiration. The lower lobe bronchus is indicated by *arrows.* Note the roughly proportional reduction in caliber of all airways on expiration. Compare with Figure 55–40. (*A* and *B* reprinted from Fraser RG, Macklem PT: Frontiers of Pulmonary Radiology. New York, Grune & Stratton, Inc, 1969, p 76, with permission of the authors and publishers.)

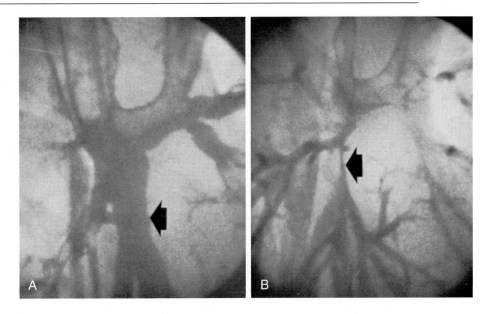

**Figure 55–40. Bronchial Dynamics in Emphysema.** Selected frames from a cinebronchogram of a patient with advanced emphysema reveal a normal configuration and caliber of the central bronchi at total lung capacity *(A)*. During forced expiration *(B)*, the lower lobe bronchus *(arrow)* collapsed abruptly, reducing its caliber from 11 to 1.5 mm. *(A* and *B* reprinted from Fraser RG, Macklem PT: Frontiers of Pulmonary Radiology. New York, Grune & Stratton, Inc, 1969, p 76, with permission of the authors and publishers.)

than 20%. Although the percentage increase in $FEV_1$ was substantial, the absolute increase was small (0.15 liter, or 5% of predicted normal). The percentage increase in $FEV_1$ was inversely related to the initial $FEV_1$ expressed as a percentage of predicted; in other words, patients in whom the air-flow obstruction was more severe showed a greater percentage increase in $FEV_1$ than that seen in those who had lesser degrees of obstruction. This is mainly a mathematical

artifact, however, because the absolute increase in $FEV_1$ was less in patients who had the worst air-flow obstruction. The results of this study show that patients who have asthma or COPD cannot be easily distinguished by their response to inhaled bronchodilator, especially if the response is measured as a relative change in flow. Some patients who have COPD also show substantial improvement in function following a course of oral corticosteroid therapy[944, 945] and, like

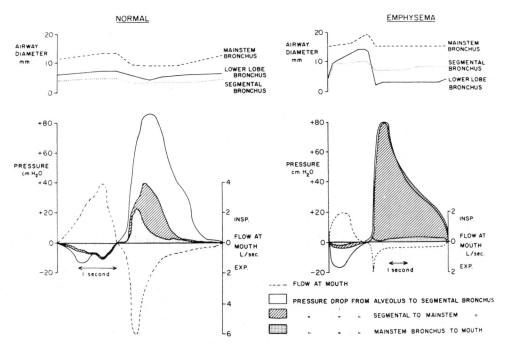

**Figure 55–41. Simultaneous Measurements of Bronchial Pressures and Dimensions in a Normal Individual and a Patient with Emphysema.** Alveolar pressure, bronchial pressure, flow at the mouth, and airway diameters in a normal individual *(left)* and a patient with emphysema *(right)* during a single forced inspiration and expiration. These tracings were obtained with two bronchial pressure catheters in place, one immediately proximal and one immediately distal to the lower lobe bronchus. The two lower graphs show recordings of flow at the mouth *(dotted line)*, alveolar pressure, and the two bronchial pressures during inspiration and during forced expiration. Simultaneous measurements of bronchial diameters of the main, lower lobe, and segmental bronchi are shown above. The clear area represents decrease in pressure from the alveolus to the segmental bronchus; the shaded area is the decrease from the segmental bronchus through the lower lobe bronchus to the main bronchus; and the dotted area is the increase in pressure from the main bronchus to the mouth. See text for description. (Reprinted from Fraser RG, Macklem PT: Frontiers of Pulmonary Radiology. New York, Grune & Stratton, Inc, 1969, p 76, with permission of the authors and publishers.)

asthmatic patients, can show substantial diurnal variation in expiratory flow[946, 947] and a decrease in expiratory flow rates coincident with beta-blocker therapy.[948]

In one investigation of eight nonallergic patients who had COPD, the circadian change in $FEV_1$ was $27 \pm 2\%$, compared with $7 \pm 1\%$ in eight age- and sex-matched control subjects.[949] The lowest values were recorded at night; in the patients, these values were associated with evidence of increased vagal tone and decreased catecholamine secretion, suggesting that an imbalance in autonomic nervous system activity may be responsible.

Middle-aged smokers who have relatively normal expiratory flow can exhibit substantial abnormalities of the distribution of inspired gas,[950, 951] although the significance of the maldistribution in terms of the progression of obstruction is unknown. The results of some studies have shown that ventilation maldistribution correlates with tests of small airway function,[950] whereas other studies have shown poor correlation.[951] Patients who have COPD show increased airway and pulmonary resistance.[952, 953] Airway resistance can increase paradoxically following a deep inspiration, although to a lesser degree than is seen in some asthmatic patients.[952] The forced oscillation technique allows the measurement of resistance over a wide range of frequencies. An increased frequency dependence of resistance measured in the 8- to 24-Hz range has been reported in patients who have mild airflow obstruction.[954] Theoretically, the increase in pulmonary resistance in patients who have COPD could be expected to be associated with a decrease in the density dependence of resistance, because the site of increased resistance is small airways. However, in a study of 40 patients who had mild to moderate COPD such a decrease was not found in those who had increased resistance;[955] a concomitant narrowing of the upper airway could explain these results. It has been shown that there is both inspiratory and expiratory narrowing of the larynx in patients who have COPD and that the narrowing correlates with severity of lower airway obstruction as measured by $FEV_1$;[956] because the flow regimen across the larynx is density-dependent, the increased upper airway resistance could mask a decrease in density dependence of lower airway resistance.

### Lung Volumes

The initial alteration in lung volumes in patients who have COPD is an increase in residual volume (RV).[957] As the disease worsens, RV increases further and encroaches on vital capacity; FRC and TLC also increase. The early change in RV is probably related to premature airway closure at the lung bases, as has been demonstrated in otherwise asymptomatic young (24 years of age) smokers.[958] In normal individuals and in patients who have mild COPD, there is no difference between the values for slow and forced expiratory vital capacity, or between inspiratory and expiratory vital capacity; when obstruction becomes more severe, the FVC can decrease disproportionately,[959, 960] perhaps as a result of dynamic compression and closure of airways as well as time-dependent and volume-history dependent changes in airway caliber. Vital capacity can decrease substantially in patients who have COPD when they assume the supine posture; in one study of 30 patients, the mean decrease was 11%.[946]

The increase in FRC is caused by at least two mechanisms, the first being decreased elastic recoil. Since FRC is determined by the static balance between the outward recoil of the chest wall and the inward recoil of the lung, loss of lung elasticity can occur with the development of COPD such that the volume at equilibration increases toward the relaxed position of the chest wall (about 70% of TLC).

A second mechanism is dynamic hyperinflation as a result of an increased expiratory resistance and a prolonged expiratory phase of the respiratory cycle.[958, 961] Patients who have COPD may expire along their maximal expiratory flow-volume curve and inspire before the lung and chest wall reach their static equilibrium volume and while alveolar pressure is still positive.[961–963] This phenomenon, which has been called "auto-PEEP" (i.e., auto–positive end-expiratory pressure) or "intrinsic PEEP," has a number of important physiologic consequences. The increased intrathoracic pressure can adversely affect venous return to the right side of the heart, and the hyperinflation puts the inspiratory muscles both at a mechanical disadvantage and at a shorter-than-optimal length on their length-tension curve. On the positive side, the hyperinflation dilates intraparenchymal airways and decreases the resistive work of breathing. The detection of flow limitation occurring during tidal breathing can be accomplished by applying a negative pressure at the airway during expiration and comparing the flow-volume curve of the ensuing expiration with that of the preceding control breath.[964]

Although the prolonged expiration and "intrinsic PEEP" are caused primarily by increased resistance in the lower tracheobronchial tree, there is evidence that glottic narrowing may also contribute. As mentioned previously, glottic narrowing occurs on expiration in patients who have COPD,[956] and expiratory resistive loading results in active laryngeal narrowing in normal individuals.[965] The former phenomenon may be analogous to pursed-lip breathing, acting to control expiratory flow and prevent lower airway collapse. However, the importance to dynamic hyperinflation of obstruction in the lower tracheobronchial tree was illustrated in one study in which FRC decreased after inhaled bronchodilators only in COPD patients who were expiring along their maximal flow-volume curve during tidal breathing.[966] When normal individuals change from an erect or sitting to supine or lateral decubitus position, FRC decreases by about 30% and 15%, respectively;[967] however, when patients who have COPD change position, there is no change in FRC.

TLC is determined by the balance between the ability of the inspiratory muscles to shorten and the inward recoil of lung and chest wall. The increase in TLC in patients who have COPD is thought to be caused by a decrease in the inward elastic recoil of the lung. It is also possible that adaptive changes may occur in the inspiratory muscles as a consequence of chronic hyperinflation, which would allow greater shortening. Such an adaptive response to chronic hyperinflation has been demonstrated in the diaphragm of hamsters that had experimental emphysema;[968] the entire diaphragm shortened as a result of a drop-out of sarcomeres, resulting in a relative preservation of the length-tension relationship of individual sarcomeres. There is evidence for a similar adaptive response in humans who have COPD and hyperinflation.[883]

Although it is clear that TLC increases with the development of COPD, the magnitude of the increase is controversial. The two most frequently employed methods to determine TLC—the helium dilution technique and body plethysmography—are both subject to error in patients who have COPD. The former tends to underestimate thoracic gas volume to the extent that inspired gas fails to equilibrate with intrathoracic gas beyond obstructed airways;[969, 970] by contrast, the plethysmographic technique tends to overestimate thoracic gas volume, because changes in mouth pressure during panting may be less than the simultaneous changes in the alveolar pressure.[971] Esophageal pressure more accurately reflects alveolar pressure and gives a closer estimate of true TLC.[969, 972] Because the underestimation of the measurement of alveolar pressure by mouth pressure is frequency-dependent, the simplest way to overcome the potential error in the plethysmographic measurement of TLC is to limit the panting frequency to 1 Hz or less;[973, 974] with this precaution, the plethysmographic method provides the most accurate measurements.

The changes in lung distensibility that occur in COPD are also reflected by an alteration in the shape and position of the lung pressure-volume curve. The maximal elastic recoil pressure at TLC and recoil pressures at various percentages of TLC decrease with increasing age;[975–977] in smokers, this decrease occurs at an accelerated rate.[978, 979] Unfortunately, there is a large range of normal values for absolute elastic recoil pressures, creating difficulty in designating abnormality in an individual patient. A narrower range of normality can be achieved by describing the entire pressure-volume curve of the lungs using an exponential equation:

$$V = A - Be^{-kp}$$

where V = lung volume, A = theoretical maximal lung volume at infinite transpulmonary pressure, B = the lung volume at zero transpulmonary pressure, P = transpulmonary pressure, and k = a constant that describes the shape of the exponential relationship between pressure and volume.[975]

As discussed in Chapter 17 (see page 411), an increase in k reflects a loss of lung recoil and a shift in the pressure-volume curve upward and to the left. k increases with age in nonsmoking men and women,[975] and the increase is greater in smokers.[978] Although k has been correlated with the presence of emphysema in some studies,[706, 980] it probably more accurately reflects the mean size of the air spaces that contribute to expired volume.[705] In smokers who have no emphysema, an increase in k correlates with an increase in TLC and a decrease in diffusing capacity divided by alveolar volume.[978, 981] In one study of lungs obtained at autopsy, k was found to correlate with $\Delta N_2$/liter, suggesting that it reflects not only increased lung distensibility but also an increased variation in the distensibility of different lung units.[982]

Although surface forces are the main contributor to the shape of the pressure-volume curve, there is evidence that parenchymal smooth muscle contraction can also affect recoil. Inhalation of a beta$_2$-agonist results in a leftward shift of the pressure-volume curve (> 1.5 cm $H_2O$);[983] acute smoking cessation causes a similar decrease in recoil pressure without a decrease in maximal expiratory flow, suggesting that one or more components of cigarette smoke

cause contraction of parenchymal and airway smooth muscle.[984]

### Arterial Blood Gases

Arterial blood gas tensions are commonly disturbed in patients who have COPD; the more severe the disease, the more likely that hypoxemia and hypercapnia will be present.[733] Episodes of arterial desaturation occur in patients who have COPD during sleep and during activities of daily living;[985] they are particularly likely to occur in association with infectious exacerbations. Air travel also can be associated with significant arterial oxygen desaturation in patients who have COPD;[986] cabin pressure in commercial jet airliners is maintained between 690 and 560 mm Hg, which is equivalent to the barometric pressure at altitudes between 900 and 2,400 meters.[986]

The arterial hypoxemia is a result of alveolar hypoventilation and ventilation-perfusion mismatching. On the basis of the multiple inert gas technique, three patterns of ventilation-perfusion mismatch have been recognized:[987, 988] (1) in about 50% of patients, there is an increase in ventilation to high $\dot{V}A/\dot{Q}$ areas with no shunt or low $\dot{V}A/\dot{Q}$ regions; (2) in 20% of patients, there is an increase in perfusion to low $\dot{V}A/\dot{Q}$ regions with no shunt and no high $\dot{V}A/\dot{Q}$ regions; and (3) in the remaining 30%, there is an increase in both the high and low $\dot{V}A/\dot{Q}$ regions.

It has been suggested that the high $\dot{V}A/\dot{Q}$ regions represent areas in which elastolysis has caused high compliance, but in which perfusion is low as a result of capillary bed destruction.[987] Some investigators have found this pattern of gas exchange to be more common in the type A ("pink puffer") COPD patient;[987] they have suggested that the low $\dot{V}A/\dot{Q}$ regions are units that have obstructed airways that are ventilated via collateral channels. An increase in the low $\dot{V}A/\dot{Q}$ regions tended to be more common in the type B ("blue bloater") patient. The high $\dot{V}A/\dot{Q}$ regions correspond to areas of emphysema on CT scans, whereas the low $\dot{V}A/\dot{Q}$ regions presumably represent areas of peripheral airway narrowing or obliteration.[989] Intrapulmonary right-to-left shunting and diffusion impairment do not contribute to the gas exchange abnormalities seen in COPD patients at rest.[987, 988]

The uneven distribution of inspired gas can be demonstrated by the single-breath $O_2$ test,[990] the multiple-breath $N_2$ washout,[991] or the closed-circuit He method (which is also used to measure FRC and RV).[992, 993] The time taken for the inhaled He to be equilibrated in the lung is termed the *mixing efficiency.* In the early stages of COPD, this may be normal as measured by the He technique, although more refined techniques, particularly those using radioactive xenon, frequently show regional inequalities of ventilation and perfusion.[994–996] Disturbances in the $\dot{V}A/\dot{Q}$ ratios can also be detected by measurement of the physiologic dead space or the ratio of dead space to tidal volume.[997–999] One consequence of the development of emphysema is a lowering of the resistance to collateral flow. In one study, collateral resistance was estimated by the rapidity of equilibration of inhaled He distal to an airway obstructed with a balloon catheter;[1000] the rate of rise in He was 10 times faster beyond the obstructed airway in 6 patients who had emphysema than in 12 normal individuals.

In COPD of mild to moderate severity, hypoxemia typically occurs without hypercapnia. Although the $\dot{V}_A/\dot{Q}$ inequality impairs both the uptake of $O_2$ and the elimination of $CO_2$, the tendency for elevation of $Pa_{CO_2}$ is overcome by an increase in alveolar ventilation to well-perfused units; however, the increase in ventilation cannot correct the hypoxemia because of the alinear shape of the $O_2$ dissociation curve (*see* page 110). When COPD becomes severe, $CO_2$ retention eventually occurs as total alveolar ventilation decreases and is accompanied by more severe hypoxemia. The relative contributions of $\dot{V}_A/\dot{Q}$ mismatch and alveolar hypoventilation to the observed hypoxemia can be determined by calculating the $P_{(A-a)O_2}$ (*see* page 112). The strong correlation between decreased $Pa_{O_2}$ and increased $Pa_{CO_2}$ in patients who have COPD indicates that alveolar hypoventilation contributes significantly to the hypoxemia.[1001] However, an increase in arterial $P_{CO_2}$ does not occur until the $FEV_1$ is less than approximately 1.2 liters. The presence of hypercapnia in a patient who has an $FEV_1$ greater than 1.5 liters should raise the possibility of an abnormality in the central control of ventilation.

Blood gas tensions deteriorate during exacerbations of COPD.[1002] Although viral or bacterial respiratory tract infections are frequently implicated as the cause of such episodes, this cannot be proved in many instances. Exacerbations are frequently associated with right-sided heart failure and fluid overload, which could in themselves impair arterial blood gas tensions. Cardiac output can influence arterial blood gases by changing the mixed venous tensions of $O_2$ and $CO_2$. Given a certain disturbance of $\dot{V}_A/\dot{Q}$ matching and a fixed metabolic rate, mixed venous $P_{O_2}$ will fall and mixed venous $P_{CO_2}$ will rise as cardiac output decreases. The changes in mixed venous gas tensions will be reflected in arterial gas tensions. The development of right-sided heart failure and decreased cardiac output will therefore worsen arterial blood gas levels, other things being equal.[1003] The fluid retention associated with episodes of right-sided heart failure could also contribute to worsening gas exchange by causing interstitial pulmonary edema and more severe $\dot{V}_A/\dot{Q}$ mismatch.[1002, 1004] One group of investigators measured ventilation-perfusion distributions in 13 patients who were hospitalized for acute exacerbations of COPD and again approximately 1 month after discharge during a stable period.[1005] Although shunting was not detected, there was a widening of $\dot{V}_A/\dot{Q}$ distribution, occurring mainly as a result of an increase in perfusion to poorly ventilated regions; a decrease in mixed venous arterial saturation also contributed to the increased hypoxemia.

Although hypercapnia does not develop in patients who have COPD until the $FEV_1$ has fallen to below approximately 1.2 liters, the correlation between $FEV_1$ and $Pa_{CO_2}$ below that threshold is poor;[1006, 1007] for example, patients who have an $FEV_1$ of 0.6 liter can have either a normal $Pa_{CO_2}$ or chronic hypercapnia. Stable patients who have chronic hypercapnia can reduce arterial $P_{CO_2}$ to normal levels by voluntary hyperventilation.

Genetic differences in respiratory drive are a major contributor to the variable response to airway obstruction. The adult offspring of patients who have COPD and hypercapnia show depressed ventilatory responses to hypoxia and hypercapnia compared with the responses in the offspring of patients with equal degrees of obstruction who do not have

hypercapnia.[1008–1010] Patients who have COPD and hypercapnia also show an abnormally small increase in minute ventilation when exposed to hypoxic or hypercapnic gas mixtures; however, this cannot be interpreted as decreased drive, because it could be explained by increased respiratory system impedance (increased resistance and decreased dynamic compliance) in the presence of normal drive. The measurement of mouth pressure achieved after 0.1 second of an occluded inspiratory effort (P0.1) during a hypoxic or hypercapnic challenge provides a better estimate of drive;[1011] because there is no flow or volume change during the obstructed breath, the pressure is not influenced by the mechanics of the respiratory system, although it is influenced by the mechanical advantage of the inspiratory muscles. Because the patient does not realize that the breath has been obstructed within the 0.1-second period, a voluntary response to the obstruction is also not a problem. Another way to assess central respiratory drive in patients who have air-flow obstruction is to correct the ventilatory response to hypoxia and hypercapnia by taking into account the maximal voluntary ventilation.[1012]

When respiratory drive is assessed using the P0.1 or the corrected ventilatory response, patients who have COPD and $CO_2$ retention still exhibit decreased drive in comparison with normal individuals.[1013, 1014] This is in contrast to individuals who have asthma, in whom respiratory drive is increased. It is likely that the hypoventilation is related partly to genetic factors that influence ventilatory control and partly to an acquired tolerance to the stimulatory effects of hypoxia and hypercapnia.[1014] Although it has been suggested that endogenous endorphin secretion could depress respiratory drive and mediate the tolerance to elevated $P_{CO_2}$, the results of experiments designed to test this hypothesis have been predominantly negative.[1015–1017] Increased buffering capacity of the cerebrospinal fluid also does not account for the depressed ventilatory response.[1018]

Although P0.1 is a better measurement of respiratory drive in patients who have COPD than is ventilation, it too can be influenced by respiratory mechanics. In one study, a more precise estimate of neural drive to the diaphragm was measured using needle EMG recordings from individual diaphragmatic motor units;[1019] during quiet breathing, patients who had COPD (mean $FEV_1$ of 0.82 liter) had a 70% increase in neural input to the diaphragm. Patients who have COPD and hypercapnia may have impaired load detection: in one study of eight patients who were challenged with an external resistive-load or methacholine-induced bronchoconstriction, the resulting decrease in tidal volume and increase in $P_{CO_2}$ were related to the acuity with which the patients could perceive changes in intrathoracic pressure.[1020] The ability to recognize and respond to added resistive and elastic loads is impaired in patients who have COPD; this fault may be related to increased endorphin secretion, as suggested by the finding that naloxone increases the compensatory response to added resistance.[1015, 1021]

Patients who have COPD and hypercapnia also appear to have an altered ventilatory pattern that may contribute to the $CO_2$ retention,[1006, 1007, 1022] respiratory rates being more rapid and tidal volumes smaller than in patients who have equal degrees of obstruction and who do not have hypercapnia. This pattern of rapid shallow breathing does not decrease minute ventilation, but because dead space remains constant and $V_T$ decreases, the ratio $V_D/V_T$ increases, resulting in a decrease in alveolar ventilation. This inefficient breathing pattern may be caused in part by excessive stimulation of respiratory epithelial irritant receptors. Rapid shallow breathing is also stimulated by inhalation of histamine and methacholine;[1023, 1024] inhalation of an aerosol of local anesthetic causes an increase in $V_T$ and a decrease in respiratory frequency in these patients.[1025, 1026] Rapid shallow breathing occurs in patients during "acute-on-chronic" hypercapnic exacerbations of their air-flow obstruction;[1011] it is possible that airway inflammation and inflammatory mediator release during the acute episode stimulate irritant receptors, thus altering the ventilatory pattern and contributing to the abnormalities of arterial blood gases. It is also conceivable that respiratory muscle fatigue contributes to the altered breathing pattern. In stable patients who have severe COPD, hypercapnia and rapid shallow breathing are related to inspiratory muscle strength.[1027]

The depressed ventilatory response to hypoxia and hypercapnia in COPD does not improve during prolonged home $O_2$ therapy,[1028] but the oxygen has a beneficial effect by decreasing dyspnea. The dyspnea experienced by patients who have COPD is caused not by the alteration in blood gas tensions but by the increased effort needed to maintain ventilation.[1029]

### The Effects of Sleep

Sleep has profound effects on ventilatory control and arterial blood gases in patients who have COPD and is frequently associated with a worsening of hypoxemia and hypercapnia.[1030, 1031] When $PaO_2$ values fall low enough to reach the steep portion of the $O_2$ dissociation curve, the decrease in arterial saturation may be considerable. Patients who have COPD have poor-quality sleep as a result of decreased total sleep time, increased sleep stage shifts, and increased arousal frequency.[1032, 1033] If such patients are not identified on the basis of increased daytime somnolence,[1034] the frequency of apneic episodes is not increased in comparison with that in the normal population.[1032, 1034] However, despite the lack of frank apneas, many patients manifest episodic arterial desaturation during sleep, the severity being greater in "blue bloaters" than in "pink puffers."[1034] The desaturation is also more severe during rapid eye movement (REM) sleep than during slow-wave sleep and appears to be related to periods of hypoventilation, or "hypopneas."[1035] REM sleep can be divided into two stages: (1) so-called *phasic REM*, during which there are rapid eye movements, myoclonic twitches, and an alteration in breathing pattern; and (2) *tonic REM*, during which there is generalized muscular atonia. It has been shown that the most significant desaturation occurs in association with the altered breathing pattern at the onset of phasic REM.[1036]

More severe desaturation probably develops in "blue bloaters" because they are more hypoxic to begin with and because any additional hypoventilation moves oxygen saturation levels onto the steep descending portion of the $O_2$ dissociation curve.[1034] It has also been suggested that sleep desaturation is a factor that predisposes patients to the development of a clinical picture of "blue bloating";[1037] however, it is more likely that the excessive nocturnal desaturation is secondary to the pre-existing hypoventilation. The associa-

tion of hypercapnia during the day and oxygen desaturation during sleep was examined in one study of COPD patients who took part in a nocturnal $O_2$ therapy trial;[1038] patients who had higher daytime arterial $PCO_2$ values were found to develop nocturnal oxygen desaturation that was significantly worse than that in patients who had normal daytime arterial $PCO_2$ values, even though the two groups showed similar values for $FEV_1$. In another study of 94 patients who had COPD, daytime hypercapnia was the only significant independent predictor of the degree of nocturnal oxygen desaturation.[836]

The hypocapnic episodes during sleep could be caused by decreased central ventilatory drive or by increased respiratory system impedance. In a study in which respiratory effort was assessed by measuring intrathoracic esophageal pressure swings during hypopnea, the swings were decreased in approximately half of the patients and increased in the remainder.[1039] In fact, individual patients can manifest hypopneic episodes during both increased and decreased pressure swings.[1040] In another investigation, the response of upper airway resistance to $CO_2$ breathing during sleep was compared in normal individuals and in patients who had COPD; the resistance failed to decrease as much during hypercapnia in the COPD patients, explaining, in part, their diminished ventilatory response.[1041] The magnitude of sleep desaturation is inversely related to daytime arterial saturation and to the ventilatory response to hypoxia and hypercapnia during wakefulness.[1042] Episodes of nocturnal desaturation are associated with a worsening of pulmonary hypertension; although nocturnal $O_2$ administration does not prevent hypopnea, it does block the pulmonary vascular response.[1043] COPD is not associated with an increase in the incidence of obstructive apnea, but because both are relatively common chronic disorders, their simultaneous occurrence is not infrequent.[1044]

The effect on sleep quality of $O_2$ administration is controversial. In one study, $O_2$ therapy was found to improve sleep quality,[1033] but in another there was no reduction in the number of arousals or increase in total sleep time despite correction of desaturation with supplemental $O_2$;[1032] the investigators in the latter study suggested that it may be the increased arterial $PCO_2$ that disturbs sleep in these individuals. In another study of patients who had severe but stable COPD, supplemental $O_2$ did not significantly increase nocturnal $CO_2$.[1045]

### The Effects of Exercise

Exercise can also influence arterial blood gas tensions; in some patients, exercise induces pronounced arterial desaturation and hypercapnia, whereas in others, gas exchange is improved.[1046–1048] Although some investigators have found it difficult to predict which patients will improve and which will deteriorate,[1049] others have reported that patients in whom desaturation occurs during exercise have significantly worse air-flow obstruction, a lower diffusing capacity,[1050] a higher $V_D/V_T$, and a lower $V_T$.[1051, 1052] Supplemental $O_2$ improves maximal work performance and endurance in patients who have COPD,[1053, 1054] mainly by decreasing the level of ventilation for any given workload[1055] and, possibly, by causing bronchodilation and a decrease in airway resistance.[1053] A large carbohydrate meal immediately before exercise decreases exercise capacity by transiently increasing $CO_2$ production.[1056, 1057] Metabolism of carbohydrate occurs with a respiratory quotient of 1.0 (one molecule of $CO_2$ produced for each molecule of $O_2$ consumed), whereas fat metabolism and protein metabolism both produce less $CO_2$ for a similar caloric output (respiratory quotients of 0.8 and 0.7, respectively). However, this phenomenon is rarely of clinical importance unless a patient who has fixed ventilation (ventilatory support) is given a large carbohydrate load.

During exercise, patients who have COPD show a normal relationship between cardiac output and total body oxygen consumption,[1058] suggesting that circulatory factors do not contribute to exercise limitation; in fact, such limitation is chiefly related to a diminished ventilatory capacity. The ventilatory requirement for any given work output is also increased because the wasted ventilation fraction of each breath is larger (increased $V_D/V_T$) and because the $O_2$ uptake per breath is decreased owing to hypoxemia.[1059] In addition, the high $O_2$ consumption by respiratory muscles working against abnormal loads may divert $O_2$ away from other exercising muscles.[1058] Despite the limits to breathing, the ventilatory response during exercise was the best predictor of the maximal oxygen consumption ($V_{O_2}$max) in one group of patients.[1060]

Even during maximal exercise, normal individuals do not achieve the level of ventilation of which they are capable, leaving considerable ventilatory reserve. By contrast, patients who have COPD usually stop exercising at or very close to their maximal achievable ventilation; this level can be predicted from combined measurements of $FEV_1$ and inspiratory muscle strength.[1061, 1062] The accuracy of prediction of exercise limitation is increased by measuring patients' ability to increase expiratory flow beyond the envelope of the flow-volume curve and to resist dynamic hyperinflation.[1063] The symptom that stops patients who have COPD from exercising further is dyspnea, a sensation that probably originates in respiratory muscle afferent receptors. Dyspnea is related to the ratio of the force-generating and -shortening ability of inspiratory muscles to the force and shortening required for a given ventilatory level. It can occur because the force-generating ability is reduced (respiratory muscle weakness), because the force requirements of ventilation are increased (increased impedance), or as a result of a combination of these factors. In COPD, the force requirements are increased because of increased airway resistance, and the force-generating ability is decreased because of hyperinflation and (in severe disease) malnutrition.[1064, 1065]

During exercise, patients who have severe COPD can manifest paradoxical motion of the rib cage and abdomen[1066] and can recruit expiratory muscles;[1067] abdominal expiratory muscle contraction can passively stretch the relaxed diaphragm during exhalation, and the subsequent sudden relaxation of those muscles allows a passive inspiratory diaphragmatic movement.[1067] Malnourished patients who have COPD have significantly lower exercise and muscle aerobic capacity; the high dead-space ventilation and high oxygen cost of breathing in these patients may contribute to weight loss.[1068, 1069]

### Acid-Base Balance

Measurement of arterial pH, hydrogen ion concentration, and bicarbonate provides important information about the acid-base status of patients who have COPD. When an excess of $CO_2$ is compensated for by an increase in bicarbonate, it can be reliably concluded that the respiratory failure is not of acute onset; patients who have this finding show a greater efficiency in buffering acute changes in levels of $CO_2$.[1070] An arterial pH within or above the normal range is unusual in uncomplicated respiratory acidosis and suggests concomitant metabolic alkalosis, usually secondary to the use of diuretics. Alternatively, during acute exacerbations of COPD, there may be "relative hyperventilation," the $P_{CO_2}$ decreasing as a result of increased drive but not reaching normal levels. Such an "acute respiratory alkalosis" superimposed on chronic respiratory acidosis can mimic other complex acid-base disturbances.

An elevated $P_{CO_2}$ associated with a normal or only slightly raised bicarbonate level suggests that the hypoventilation and respiratory acidosis are of recent onset. However, this conclusion is not justified if there is coexisting metabolic acidosis that has depressed the bicarbonate level. Even when there is severe hypoxemia, anaerobic metabolism does not result in the formation of lactic acid and metabolic acidosis unless there is an associated systemic circulatory disorder that causes inadequate tissue perfusion.[1071] In any assessment of arterial blood gas abnormalities and their relationship to neurologic symptoms and signs, it must be remembered that gas tensions and acid-base balance in the cerebrospinal fluid are different from those in the arterial blood and more correctly reflect the environment of the respiratory center.[1072, 1073]

### The Effects of Therapy

The hypoxemia of COPD is easily corrected by increasing the concentration of inspired oxygen; however, such an increase also causes a variable increase in arterial $P_{CO_2}$, both in the stable state[1074] and (especially) during episodes of acute ventilatory respiratory failure.[1075, 1076] The administration of supplemental $O_2$ causes a decrease in minute ventilation ($\dot{V}_E$). Traditionally, it has been assumed that the rise in $P_{CO_2}$ is secondary to this decrease. The accepted dogma has been that patients who have COPD and chronic $CO_2$ retention have depressed ventilatory drive in response to $CO_2$ and rely on hypoxic stimulation to maintain a given level of ventilation; administration of supplemental $O_2$ decreases the hypoxic drive, resulting in a further decrease in $\dot{V}_E$ and hypercapnia. However, the results of some studies have challenged this hypothesis.[1074, 1075, 1077] An alternative explanation is that $O_2$ administration worsens the matching of ventilation and perfusion, increases $V_D/V_T$, and causes a decrease in alveolar ventilation for a given $\dot{V}_E$. Oxygen widens the dispersion of the $\dot{V}_A/\dot{Q}$ by increasing the perfusion to poorly ventilated lung regions, presumably by blocking hypoxic vasoconstriction in these areas.[1077, 1078] Support for this mechanism is derived from observations that supplemental $O_2$ results in only a transient decrease in $\dot{V}_E$ in some patients who have COPD, whereas the increase in $Pa_{CO_2}$ is persistent.

Inhaled nitric oxide (NO) at a concentration of 40 ppm,[1079] but not 15 ppm,[1060] also worsens $\dot{V}_A/\dot{Q}$ matching at rest by the same mechanism. On the other hand, NO has a beneficial effect on hemodynamics and gas exchange during exercise. At 40 ppm, NO attenuated the increase in Ppa and the decrease in Pao$_2$ by increasing blood flow to normal $\dot{V}A/$ $\dot{Q}$ regions;[1080] presumably, during exercise, NO is preferentially distributed to well-ventilated regions with normal $\dot{V}A/$ $\dot{Q}$ ratios. Interestingly, NO at 40 ppm had no effect on respiratory resistance in either normal individuals or COPD patients, suggesting that vascular smooth muscle is more sensitive to the relaxant effects of NO than is airway smooth muscle.[1081] Concentrations of exhaled NO are normal or depressed in patients who have COPD, which is in contrast to the elevated levels in patients who have bronchiectasis and asthma.[1082]

The administration of aerosol or intravenous bronchodilators may be followed by changes in ventilation-perfusion matching in patients who have COPD.[1083–1085] The change in Pao$_2$ varies from patient to patient, depending on the bronchodilator used, its dose and method of administration, and the length of time elapsed between its administration and the measurement of arterial blood gases.[1083] Arterial Po$_2$ usually falls in response to aerosolized beta-adrenergic drugs.[1085, 1086]

### Diffusing Capacity

The single-breath diffusing capacity (DLCO$_{SB}$) of persons who smoke cigarettes is lower than that of age-matched nonsmokers, even in the absence of other evidence of lung dysfunction. Part of the decrease is caused by elevated blood carboxyhemoglobin levels; however, even after correction for the back-pressure of carbon monoxide (CO), individuals who smoke have lower values of DLCO$_{SB}$.[1087] DLCO$_{SB}$ decreases significantly during acute smoking, an effect that may be related to an acute reduction in pulmonary capillary blood volume;[1088] it returns toward normal within a week of smoking cessation.[1089] The DLCO$_{SB}$ increases when normal individuals assume the supine from the sitting position, presumably because pulmonary capillary blood volume increases; however, such a change in posture by cigarette smokers does not cause the same increase in diffusing capacity, suggesting the possibility of impaired pulmonary vascular distensibility.[1087] The results of a study of 1,174 individuals enrolled in the Tucson Epidemiological Study showed a significant decrease in DLCO$_{SB}$ and DLCO$_{SB}$/VA as a function of FEV$_1$/FVC, after exclusion of patients who had a diagnosis of asthma.[1090] Asthmatic patients tend to have increased values for DLCO$_{SB}$, but in those without asthma, reduced FEV$_1$/FVC was associated with reduced DLCO$_{SB}$, suggesting undiagnosed emphysema. The single-breath diffusing capacity can be overestimated in patients who have advanced COPD.[1091] Standard techniques to measure DLCO$_{SB}$ assume that the CO uptake occurs only during the breath-hold time; however, CO is also taken up during the inspiratory and expiratory phases of the test, and because patients who have COPD have prolonged inspiratory and expiratory times, more CO can be absorbed and DLCO$_{SB}$ overestimated. A three-equation method to calculate DLCO$_{SB}$ that accounts for CO uptake during inspiration and expiration has been developed and validated.[1092–1094]

The diffusing capacity measured by both the single-breath and the steady-state CO methods is usually reduced in patients who have COPD. There is reasonably close correlation between severely reduced diffusing capacity during life and the finding of extensive emphysema at autopsy[733]

or on CT.[1095] Even patients who have relatively normal lung volumes and airway resistance have been shown to have significantly reduced DLCO$_{SB}$, a reduction that has been correlated with the extent of emphysema found in lobectomy specimens. Some authors consider the diffusing capacity to be of differential diagnostic value in patients who have COPD, a reduction indicating emphysema and normal values indicating intrinsic airway narrowing.[1096, 1097] However, it should be appreciated that emphysema of mild to moderate severity can be observed at autopsy in patients who have had normal diffusing capacity during life.[733, 981] The reduction in diffusing capacity in COPD is the result of a decrease in the membrane component, a reduction in capillary blood volume, and mismatch of ventilation and perfusion;[1098] limitation of diffusion in the gas phase of the emphysematous spaces may also contribute.[1099, 1100] A degree of reduction of DLCO$_{SB}$ in COPD has been found to predict future decline in FEV$_1$[1101] and survival in a home O$_2$ therapy program.[1102]

### Effect of Smoking Cessation on Lung Function

Smoking cessation results in an acute decrease in lung elastic recoil[1103, 1104] but a sustained increase in maximal flow and volumes.[1104, 1105] Although the improvement in function is slight and rarely returns values to predicted normal, smoking cessation also decreases the annual rate of decline in lung function (Fig. 55–42).[406, 1106, 1107] The improvement in flow rates and in values for tests of small airway function (closing capacity and $\Delta N_2$/liter) begins as early as 1 week following cessation and continues for 6 to 8 months.[1105, 1108] Nonspecific airway responsiveness to inhaled methacholine, which may be increased in smokers, also returns toward normal with cessation of smoking.[1108]

## PROGNOSIS AND NATURAL HISTORY

Over a period of years, most patients who have COPD experience slow but inexorable worsening of symptoms and

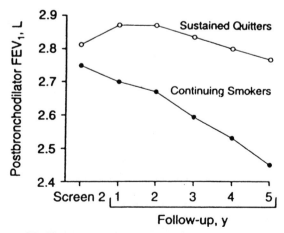

**Figure 55–42. Chronic Obstructive Pulmonary Disease: Effect of Smoking Cessation.** The graph shows the mean decline in FEV$_1$ expressed in liters in the approximately 2,000 persons who stopped smoking for a period of 5 years in the Lung Health Study plotted versus the decline in FEV$_1$ in approximately 4,000 persons who continued to smoke. It is clear that smoking cessation causes a small initial improvement in lung function and then a substantial moderation in the rate of decline.

progressive impairment of pulmonary function.[1109] In the National Institutes of Health (NIH) Lung Health Study of 6,000 individuals, of whom 4,000 continued to smoke throughout the 5-year study period, the mean rate of decline in lung function in the smokers was about 65 ml/year, which was significantly faster than in those who stopped smoking, about 35 ml/year (*see* Fig. 55–42).[406] Follow-up studies of patients seeking medical help may not accurately reflect the prognosis for COPD in the general population;[907, 1110] however, when ventilatory impairment becomes sufficiently severe to result in dyspnea, progression to severe disability can be expected within 6 to 10 years.[907, 1111] In addition, although a gradual decline terminating in respiratory failure and death seems virtually inevitable once the patient who has COPD seeks medical aid because of dyspnea, life span has been greatly prolonged with modern methods of management. In one study, 64 patients who had hypercapnia survived for a period of 2 to 15 years.[1112]

When disease is advanced, repeated episodes of acute-on-chronic respiratory failure may occur; approximately 75% of these patients survive such crises,[1113, 1114] although 50% die within 1 year[1113] and 70% within 2 years of the initial episode.[1114] The prediction of survival during episodes of acute-on-chronic respiratory failure was studied in 733 patients using the APACHE III database;[1115, 1116] 51% of the patients required mechanical ventilation within 24 hours of admission, and the mean duration of intubation was 7.5 days. The overall hospital mortality was 33%; features that were associated with significantly improved survival included younger age, better premorbid quality of life, higher mental status and blood pressure, and lower heart rate, creatinine, white blood cell count, and plasma glucose. Patients who had sepsis or pneumonia had a significantly higher mortality than those in whom the exacerbation was a postoperative complication (44% versus 26%). A logistic regression model based on the APACHE III variables correctly predicted hospital outcomes in 78% of patients. In the SUPPORT study (Study to Understand Prognoses and Preferences for Outcomes and Risks of Treatment), 1,016 adults admitted to a hospital for exacerbations of COPD were followed during and for at least 6 months after hospital discharge.[1117] The in-hospital mortality was only 11%; however, the 6-month, 1-year, and 2-year mortality was 33%, 43%, and 49%, respectively.

When cor pulmonale develops in the course of COPD, the prognosis is extremely poor, although therapeutic innovations have brought about some improvements. In 1954, one third of patients died during the first episode of right-sided heart failure; of the remainder, the mean interval from the time of the first attack to death was 18 months. By contrast, between 1967 and 1969, the mean survival time of patients who had disease of similar severity was approximately 31 months.[1118] Although the outlook has continued to improve since that time, a review of several more recent studies showed that when patients who have COPD develop peripheral edema secondary to right-sided heart failure, the 5-year survival rate is about 30%.[798]

A variety of additional (albeit not necessarily independent) variables have been found to be associated with prognosis. In the state of Colorado, the mortality rate standardized for age rises with increasing altitude, presumably because the lower barometric pressure induces more severe hypoxemia.[1119] Clinical factors that aid in prognostication include age, pulmonary artery pressure (Ppa), post-bronchodilator $FEV_1$ (% of predicted), and percentage of ideal body weight.[1120] In a long-term follow-up study of 175 patients who had COPD, Ppa, $FEV_1$, and $PaCO_2$ were equally effective in predicting survival.[1121] If Ppa was less than 20 mm Hg at the beginning of the study, the 5-year survival averaged 72%, compared with 49% for patients in whom the Ppa was greater than 20 mm Hg; $PaCO_2$ levels above 45 mm Hg were associated with 45% 5-year survival, whereas 70% of patients who had a $PaCO_2$ in the normal range survived 5 years. Age, initial $FEV_1$ value, and the presence of cor pulmonale were the best predictors of mortality in a 15-year study of 200 American patients who had COPD.[1122] In other longitudinal studies, the yearly increase in Ppa and pulmonary vascular resistance, the absence of an increase in $PaO_2$ with exercise, and the presence of electrocardiographic evidence of right ventricular hypertrophy were also predictive of decreased survival.[1123–1126] In patients who have similar physiologic derangements, individuality inventory testing suggests that the outlook is worse in those who have greater psychologic distress and difficulty in coping.[1127] Prognosis is improved by smoking cessation and by participation in comprehensive pulmonary rehabilitation programs.[1120]

Long-term supplemental $O_2$ also increases the survival time of patients who have advanced COPD.[1128, 1129] The beneficial effect of $O_2$ is proportional to the hours per day it is used; in one study, for example, patients who received $O_2$ for 19 hours or more survived significantly longer than those who received $O_2$ for 12 or 15 hours per day.[1128] The exact mechanism by which $O_2$ therapy prolongs survival is not clear; in one study, lung function did not show improvement in the patients who received supplemental $O_2$, and Ppa did not decrease significantly, although the increase in Ppa was less than would have been expected without $O_2$.[1130] Prevention of severe oxygen desaturation during sleep may decrease cardiac irritability, a possible contributing factor to the beneficial effects of $O_2$.[1131] Retrospective follow-up suggests that those who benefit the most are women[1132] and patients who have lower baseline $PaO_2$ (< 49 mm Hg) and higher baseline Ppa (> 29 mm Hg).[1133]

Despite the foregoing, the use of uncontrolled $O_2$ therapy for respiratory failure in patients who have severe COPD can cause serious complications. A high concentration of inspired alveolar oxygen can cause worsening of hypercapnia by interfering with hypoxic vasoconstriction, increasing "physiologic" dead space, and depressing minute ventilation.[1074, 1075] An abrupt and sometimes catastrophic rise in $PCO_2$ can result in coma and death, especially in patients experiencing acute-on-chronic exacerbations of COPD.[819, 1134, 1135]

The cause of death in end-stage COPD is variable; in one retrospective review of patients enrolled in a long-term $O_2$ therapy program, death was attributed to acute-on-chronic respiratory failure in 38%, heart failure in 13%, pulmonary infection in 11%, pulmonary thromboembolism in 10%, cardiac arrhythmia in 8%, and pulmonary carcinoma in 7%.[1136]

Advanced COPD has a profoundly negative impact on quality of life. Several groups of investigators have developed and validated COPD-specific quality of life questionnaires.[1137–1140] These allow the health effects of COPD to be compared with those of other chronic diseases, and such instruments are being used with increasing frequency to assess disability and response to therapy in COPD, rather than relying on purely physiologic measures. Lung transplantation and lung volume reduction surgery are being offered with increasing frequency to patients who have end-stage COPD.[1141] The clinical challenge is to select the patients who will benefit the most from these procedures.[1142–1144]

## ALPHA₁-PROTEASE INHIBITOR DEFICIENCY

The association of alpha₁-antitrypsin deficiency and emphysema was first described by Eriksson in 1964[318] and has subsequently been confirmed by many other investigators.[1145] Approximately 90% of the antiproteolytic activity in serum is associated with the alpha₁ globulin fraction, and only 10% with alpha₂ globulin.[1146] The initial studies used trypsin as the proteolytic enzyme; as a result, the inhibitor in the alpha₁ band became known as "alpha₁-antitrypsin." In fact, this substance is able to inhibit a wide variety of proteases and is therefore more correctly termed "alpha₁-protease inhibitor," "alpha₁-proteinase inhibitor," or "alpha₁-antiprotease." We prefer to use the term *alpha₁-protease inhibitor* (alpha₁-PI) and to refer to the deficiency as *alpha₁-PI deficiency*.

Human plasma contains at least six proteolytic inhibitors, the predominant one being alpha₁-PI.[1147] As a group, they have a regulatory function in maintaining the equilibrium between coagulation and fibrinolysis and in the liberation of kinins. Alpha₁-PI has been shown to inhibit a number of proteolytic enzymes, including trypsin, chymotrypsin, elastase, collagenase, urokinase, plasmin, thrombin, kallikrein, and leukocyte and bacterial proteases.[1145, 1148, 1149]

Quantitative analysis of alpha₁-PI requires measurement of its inhibitory capacity or determination of its amount in the serum by immunoassay.[1145, 1150, 1151] Because the substance can be inactivated without changing its immunologic characteristics, the former measure is more accurate. Deficiency of alpha₁-PI in homozygotes can be suspected when the alpha₁ globulin fraction is 0.2 gm/dl or less on serum electrophoresis; however, this method is not reliable in screening to identify heterozygotes.[1146] Serum trypsin inhibitory capacity is 0.85 unit or more in normal individuals, 0.4 to 0.85 unit in heterozygotes, and less than 0.4 unit in homozygotes who have severe deficiency. Employing an immuno-based nephelometric method, normal values for serum concentrations of alpha₁-PI are between 0.93 and 1.77 gm/liter and values less than 0.30 gm/liter represent severe deficiency; values can also be expressed as $\mu$mol/liter, the lower limit of normal being about 11 $\mu$mol/liter).[1152] However, because of the well-documented overlap of serum concentrations of alpha₁-PI, particularly between normal individuals and patients in the intermediate range, protease inhibitor (Pi) phenotyping or genotyping is necessary for the recognition of heterozygotes.[1150, 1153, 1154]

Alpha₁-PI is an acute phase–reactant protein, the serum levels of which may rise in the presence of inflammation (infectious or noninfectious), pregnancy, or malignant disease; following the administration of estrogens; or postoperatively.[1146, 1155] Serum levels are also higher in individuals who are cigarette smokers or who are exposed to high concentrations of dust.[1156] In any of these circumstances,

heterozygotes may show an increase in serum concentration of alpha₁-PI to normal values; similarly, severe infections in homozygous ZZ individuals are occasionally associated with an elevation of values to intermediate levels.[1157] In certain infections, notably those caused by some species of *Pseudomonas* and by *Proteus mirabilis*, an alpha₁-PI inactivator is produced that permits uninhibited destruction of lung tissue by proteolytic enzymes.[1158] At the other extreme, *S. pneumoniae* contains a potent inhibitor of elastase; this finding may explain the lack of lung destruction with this infection despite the presence of enormous numbers of activated neutrophils.[450]

Alpha₁-PI is produced in large amounts by the liver and to a lesser extent by alveolar macrophages and peripheral blood monocytes.[1159] It is a very polymorphic protein; over 70 variants have been identified[1160] using crossed electrophoresis[1161] and isoelectric focusing.[1162] A monoclonal antibody that is specific for the protein with the single amino acid substitution of 342 Lys (PiZ) has also been developed.[1163] The Z variant of alpha₁-PI has deficient antiproteolytic function; more important, it is improperly processed in the rough endoplasmic reticulum and aggregates within the cell. Large amounts of the Z variant of the alpha₁-PI protein accumulate in hepatocytes, where they can be seen histologically and are associated with the development of hepatic disease (*see* further on).[1164]

### PI Phenotypes

In his original investigations, Eriksson showed that alpha₁-PI levels in deficient patients (homozygotes) were about 20% of normal, whereas levels in carriers (heterozygotes) were about 60% of normal.[318] The results of subsequent studies in families of patients who have alpha₁-PI deficiency suggest that this distribution can be explained on the basis of the autosomal recessive mode of inheritance of the disorder; carriers have two codominant genes, one contributing about 50% and the other about 10% of the total alpha₁-PI concentration. This theory readily explains the trimodal distribution of alpha₁-PI concentrations, whereby (1) deficient individuals possess two genes, each of which is responsible for 10% of normal concentration, for a total of 20%; (2) carriers possess one deficient (10%) and one normal (50%) gene, for a total of 60% of normal concentration; and (3) normal individuals possess two normal genes, each of which contributes 50% for a total of 100% of the alpha₁-PI concentration.[1165]

By far the commonest codominant allele determining structure and serum concentrations of alpha₁-PI is the gene *PiM*, which has been found in homozygotes (*MM*) in over 90% of the populations of Oslo and St. Louis,[1166, 1167] in 88% of New York State inhabitants,[1168] and in 87% of the populations of northern Ireland[1169] and Montreal.[1170] *PiMM* is associated with normal quantitative determinations of alpha₁-PI. Other alleles, designated *PiS, PiF, PiI, PiX, PiP, PiZ*, and so on, occur far less frequently. In most series, the major antiprotease variants other than *MM* have been found to be *MS, MZ, FM, IM, SS, SZ,* and *ZZ,* each ranging in frequency from 6% to less than 0.1%.[1167–1169]

### The PiZZ Phenotype

The gene *PiZ* in the homozygous state (*ZZ*) is associated with an increased frequency of pulmonary emphysema.

Individuals with the PiZZ phenotype have a clearly accelerated rate of decline in lung function even in the absence of smoking;[1171, 1172] however, smokers comprise the majority of individuals in whom symptomatic airflow obstruction develops at a younger age.[1173, 1174] This phenotype also is associated with the lowest serum concentration of alpha$_1$-PI (excluding that in the rare *Pi^null* homozygotes) and the lowest total serum antiprotease activity (amounting to only 20% of normal).[1175] It is found once in every 1,500 to 5,000 live births[1176-1179] and has been identified in 1% to 10% of patients who have clinically diagnosed emphysema.[1180-1183] It is particularly prevalent in patients less than 45 years of age whose chest radiographs manifest a predominantly basal distribution of emphysema. It has been estimated that patients who have homozygous alpha$_1$-PI deficiency have a 50%[1184] to 80%[1185] chance of developing emphysema.

As indicated previously, cigarette smoking plays an important role in the production of emphysema in patients who have alpha$_1$-PI deficiency.[1186] Symptoms of dyspnea and evidence of air-flow obstruction bring smokers who have alpha$_1$-PI deficiency to medical attention in the third and fourth decades of life, whereas nonsmokers may not present until the sixth or seventh decade.[1187-1189] In one 13-year study of 69 individuals who had the PiZZ phenotype, the rate of decrease in FEV$_1$ was 80 ml per year for nonsmokers and 317 ml per year for smokers.[1188] Despite this, there is wide variability in the degree of dysfunction in smokers and nonsmokers of the same age, and advanced disease has been described in nonsmokers[1190] and in children.[1191]

It is believed that the abnormal gene for alpha$_1$-PI deficiency derives from northern and central European countries. Low antiprotease levels have been found in up to 10% of individuals who have northern, central, or western European background. Antiprotease deficiency is much less common (about 2% of the population) in Italians, Jews, Mexicans, and African Americans.[1192, 1193] In one study of 2,285 blood donors in St. Louis, phenotyping revealed the major antiprotease variants only 40% as often in blacks as in the balance of the study group.[1167] In another study of 1,841 Californian high school students, heterozygous and homozygous deficiency states were detected in 3% of white individuals but in none of 461 people of Mexican origin or of other races.[1194] Prevalence studies of phenotypes must be interpreted with care. In Tucson, Arizona, a prevalence rate for severe deficiency (PiZZ or PiSZ) of 1 in 368 was found in 2,944 individuals.[1148] In keeping with the prevalence of ZZ and SZ phenotypes in the American population at large, a rate of 1 in 676 would have been predicted for white Americans. This discrepancy suggests that patients who have severe deficiency may move to Arizona.

The PiZ variant of alpha$_1$-PI has a polypeptide core similar to that in the normal type PiM; however, it is deficient in the carbohydrate component, sialic acid,[1148, 1195] and its secretion is blocked in hepatocytes.[1195-1197] The PiZ antiprotease has a lysine substituted for the normal glutamic acid at the 342 position. The glutamic acid residue is the site of sialic acid attachment, and it is the failure of sialization that causes abnormal folding of the protein and the defective secretion.[1198] In PiS phenotypes, a valine residue replaces glutamic acid.[1148, 1199] Interestingly, the development of emphysema has been described in the recessively inherited disorder of sialic acid metabolism called Salla disease,

which has been linked to a locus on chromosome 6q;[1200, 1200a] the exact pathogenic mechanism for the development of emphysema in this rare defect and its possible association with alpha$_1$-PI deficiency remain unclear.

In PiZZ homozygotes, the protein folds abnormally and is therefore retained in the endoplasmic reticulum of the hepatocytes resulting in the presence of globular PAS-positive, diastase-resistant intracytoplasmic inclusion bodies.[1195-1197] The main component of this inclusion material has been shown to be a protein of approximately the same molecular size as that of serum alpha$_1$-PI and with similar immunologic properties;[1201] however, chemical analysis has revealed a total absence of sialic acid.[1195, 1201] It is unclear why only a subset of affected individuals develop hepatic manifestations of the disorder.[1202] The presence of the globules can be associated with several manifestations of hepatic disease, including cholestasis, hepatitis, and cirrhosis; however, alpha$_1$-PI deficiency is a relatively rare cause of these abnormalities compared with other conditions such as primary biliary cirrhosis and chronic active hepatitis. In fact, high levels of antiproteolytic enzyme are found in the serum in the latter condition, presumably reflecting the inflammatory process.[1203] Occasionally, cirrhosis and emphysema coexist.[1191, 1204, 1205] Some cases of cirrhosis are complicated by hepatoma.[1205-1207]

### Other PI Variants

Heterozygotes who have a *PiM* gene combined with a *PiZ* gene (*MZ*) or a *PiS* gene (*MS*) may show alpha$_1$-PI activity and concentration in the intermediate or low normal range.[1208] Rarely, emphysema has been described in patients showing Pi variants other than PiZZ. PiSZ has been associated with alpha$_1$-PI levels as low as those seen in PiZZ patients;[1193] in one study of 25 such patients, emphysema was present only in those who smoked.[1209] Fifty-nine PiSZ patients have been identified among the 1,129 individuals who are being followed in the U.S. alpha$_1$-PI Deficiency Registry.[1210] Overall air-flow obstruction is less common and milder among the PiSZ than among the PiZZ patients.

A genotype designated as *PiM$_{Duarte}$*[1211] and a "null gene" for alpha$_1$-PI[1212] have been described, both of which lead to severe deficiency in homozygotes. In contrast to the Z variant, the M$_{Duarte}$ variant has normal mobility on acid-starch electrophoresis and therefore, in the heterozygous state with the normal M form, cannot be distinguished by phenotyping procedures. Similarly, when intermediate antiprotease deficiency is found in the presence of a normal phenotypic pattern, the patient may have inherited one null gene for alpha$_1$-PI.[1213] Rare cases have been described in which serum alpha$_1$-PI has been completely absent ("null" homozygotes), accompanied by an absence of liver globules, a combination that may represent complete deletion of the gene for alpha$_1$-PI synthesis.[1148, 1214] Severe emphysema develops more rapidly in these patients than in those who have the PiZZ variant, suggesting that even 20% of the normal plasma concentration of alpha$_1$-PI can provide some protection to the lungs.[1200, 1214]

The vast majority of patients who develop symptomatic COPD and emphysema have the *PiMM* genotype and normal levels of alpha$_1$-PI. There are subtypes of the PiMM phenotype (e.g., M1, M2, M3) that can be recognized using isoelectric focusing, and it has been suggested that M1M2 and M2M2 types exhibit a higher incidence of COPD.[1215] With the exception of those who have the $M_{Duarte}$ variant,[1211] patients who have other Pi variants do not have intracytoplasmic PAS-staining globules in their hepatocytes. The mechanism or mechanisms responsible for reduced alpha$_1$-PI serum concentration in patients who have variants other than PiZZ are unknown.

Two groups have reported an association between a mutation in the 3′ region of the alpha$_1$-PI gene and COPD.[1216–1218] The incidence of heterozygosity for the mutation in a group of patients who had COPD or pulmonary emphysema was reported to be 15% or 18%, respectively, compared with 5% in healthy controls. In addition, a family has been identified in which the mutation segregated with COPD and, in homozygotes, was associated with the onset of symptoms at a younger age.[1218] Another study in which the mutation frequency was compared in smokers who did and in those who did not develop COPD has not confirmed an increased risk associated with this mutation.[1219]

Because the 3′ mutation occurs in a region of the gene that is believed to bind to transcription factors, it has been suggested that the 3′ mutation may affect the regulation of alpha$_1$-PI gene expression.[1217, 1220] As indicated previously, alpha$_1$-PI is an acute phase protein whose serum concentration increases two- to threefold during inflammation.[1221] Presumably, the acute phase response has evolved to attenuate the proteolytic tissue destruction that occurs at sites of acute injury. A deficient acute phase increase in alpha$_1$-PI levels following viral or bacterial respiratory infections could exaggerate the proteolytic destruction of lung tissue that accompanies the release of neutrophil elastase and other enzymes. Despite this hypothesis, a study of the acute phase increase in alpha$_1$-PI levels following open-heart surgery showed no difference in the rise in alpha$_1$-PI levels in individuals who had the 3′ mutation compared with normal people;[1222] interestingly, individuals who were heterozygous for the *Z* and *S* alleles did show a decreased acute phase augmentation of the alpha$_1$-PI levels, suggesting that this mechanism may be important in these individuals. Alveolar macrophages and pulmonary interstitial macrophages are both capable of producing alpha$_1$-PI.[1222a] If the alpha$_1$-PI gene expression in these cells is influenced by the mutation, then a disturbance of the proteolytic-antiproteolytic balance could also develop within the microenvironment of the inflamed lung.

### Clinical and Functional Manifestations of Severe Alpha$_1$-Protease Inhibitor Deficiency

In the vast majority of smokers who have COPD, airway obstruction relates to a combination of loss of lung elasticity and airway narrowing; it is difficult to separate the relative contribution of each of these mechanisms in individual patients. The existence of nonsmoking patients who have severe antiprotease deficiency should permit the study of a pure form of elastolytic lung injury unadulterated by the airway inflammation and narrowing associated with cigarette smoke. Studies of asymptomatic individuals who have severe alpha$_1$-PI deficiency have revealed a pattern that is believed to represent early emphysema,[1223–1225] the major abnormalities being a loss of lung elastic recoil and a redistribution of blood flow characterized by a loss of the normal perfusion gradient from apex to base. At this stage, the patient may show hyperinflation without evidence of airway obstruction, at least as measured by routine methods.

When symptoms develop in patients who have the PiZZ phenotype, pulmonary function testing reveals a decreased $FEV_1$, $FEV_1/FVC$, and $DL_{CO}/V_A$.[1226] The relative contribution of loss of lung recoil and airway narrowing to decreased expiratory flow can be determined by plotting maximal flow against recoil pressure at isovolume points (Fig. 55–43). In most patients who have homozygous alpha$_1$-PI deficiency, the decreased flow can be attributed to loss of elasticity; in some, however, there also appears to be an element of increased upstream resistance.[1227] When symptoms are severe, the disturbances of pulmonary function are similar to those in "ordinary" emphysema.[1228] Of some interest is the fact that the incidence of chronic cough and sputum production is increased in patients who have alpha$_1$-PI deficiency, irrespective of their smoking history;[1187, 1229] this clinical manifestation could be related to an increased susceptibility to pulmonary infection. There is considerable evidence for

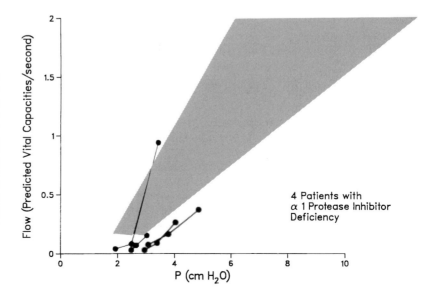

**Figure 55–43. Maximal Flow-Static Recoil Plots in Four Patients with Alpha$_1$-Protease Inhibitor Deficiency.** Maximal expiratory flow can be limited because of a decrease in lung elastic recoil or an increase in upstream resistance. In patients with relatively pure emphysema, such as occurs in alpha$_1$-protease inhibitor deficiency, maximal expiratory flow is limited primarily by a loss of lung elastic recoil. This can be appreciated by plotting maximal flow expressed as per cent predicted vital capacity per second versus lung elastic recoil derived from a static pressure-volume curve of the lung. In this diagram, plots from four patients with homozygous deficiency show that the slope of the maximal flow–recoil plot is normal and that maximal flow is limited because of a loss of recoil.

an increased risk for the development of bronchiectasis in patients who have severe alpha$_1$-PI deficiency; in fact, occasional patients present with features suggesting this abnormality.[1230, 1230a, 1231] There is also some evidence for an increased propensity to develop asthma in deficient individuals.[1232]

The impact of the introduction of replacement therapy with alpha$_1$-PI purified from human blood has been difficult to assess, because a randomized controlled trial has not been attempted.[1152] Instead, registries of deficient patients have been established, and the natural history of the disease is being studied in patients who receive therapy compared with historical controls and individuals who do not receive therapy for a variety of reasons.[1233–1236] One interesting finding is the observation that survival is different in index cases (mean 49 years) from that in family members (mean 69 years) who have comparable levels of alpha$_1$-PI.[1237] The difference cannot be explained by differences in cigarette smoking, suggesting that additional environmental or genetic factors or both are important.[605] Follow-up studies from a Danish registry indicate that the 2-year survival rate in untreated patients is nearly 100% when FEV$_1$ is greater than 33% of predicted but is only 50% at an FEV$_1$ of 15%.[1235] A longitudinal decline in lung density as assessed using CT has been reported in patients who have alpha$_1$-PI deficiency;[1238] this may serve as a practical means of following the response to therapy.

### COPD in Intermediate Alpha$_1$-Protease Inhibitor Deficiency

Two types of study have been employed in an attempt to identify an increased risk for COPD in the relatively common *MS* and *MZ* genotypes. In case-control studies, the prevalence of alpha$_1$-PI genotypes in individuals who have the clinical features of COPD is compared with that in people who do not have air-flow obstruction and who are matched as closely as possible for other potential predictors of COPD. In general, the results of these studies have shown the odds ratio for COPD in *MZ* individuals to be significantly increased (between 1.5 and 5.0, depending on the study).[1239–1245] The prevalence of the *MZ* variant in the case populations ranges between 3.9% and 14.2%, whereas in the controls it varies between 1.0% and 5.3%.

Investigators have also assessed the risk of the *MZ* genotype by studying lung function in the general population.[1246–1253] In these studies, a population sample is phenotyped for alpha$_1$-PI variants, and the prevalence of COPD in those with the MZ phenotype is compared with the prevalence in those with the MM phenotype. Many of these studies have been based on small numbers of patients and have had insufficient power to detect an affect of the MZ or MS phenotype. However, most of the larger studies have shown no significant difference in respiratory symptoms or pulmonary function in the MZ individuals compared with those who are MM. In theory, population-based studies designed to examine the predictive value of a genotype are superior to case-control methods, because there is less chance of a systematic bias. However, in COPD, in which an environmental factor (i.e., cigarette smoking) plays an important role, population studies may have insufficient sensitivity to detect a factor that increases risk only slightly.

For example, in one study of 143 MZ and 143 MM individuals drawn from a population of over 10,000 people, no difference in lung function was found between the two groups;[1253] however, only 37% of the subjects were current smokers, 35% had never smoked, and 60% were less than 54 years of age.

Differences between MZ and MM individuals have been demonstrated in some studies; for example, one group of investigators found an increased prevalence of COPD in MZ heterozygotes who had smoked but no difference in the incidence of COPD between MM and MZ nonsmokers.[1254] In other studies, MZ individuals have been shown to have greater loss of elastic recoil,[1255] significantly lower expiratory flow rates (even in the absence of smoking),[1256] and more rapid decline in lung function over a long period of follow-up.[303, 1257]

## BULLOUS DISEASE OF THE LUNGS

A bulla can be defined as a sharply demarcated, air-containing space 1 cm or more in diameter that possesses a smooth wall 1 mm or less in thickness. The space may be unilocular or separated into several compartments by thin septa. The walls are formed by pleura, connective tissue septa, or compressed lung parenchyma. The lesion may arise *de novo*, in which case the surrounding lung tissue is normal; however, it occurs more commonly in association with other disease, usually emphysema or remote infection. Although the term "pneumatocele" is sometimes used as a synonym for bulla, in our opinion use of this word should be restricted to a thin-walled, gas-filled space within the lung that develops in association with acute pneumonia (*see* page 508).

It is useful and traditional to divide patients who have bullous disease of the lungs into two groups: those who have COPD and those judged to have normal pulmonary parenchyma between the bullae and who thus are free of airway obstruction (primary bullous disease).[1258–1262] A familial occurrence has been reported in patients who have the latter form.[1263, 1264] The incidence of bullae is increased in patients who have connective tissue diseases such as Marfan's syndrome[1265] and Ehlers-Danlos syndrome.[1266]

### Pathologic Characteristics

Bullae have traditionally been divided into three morphologic types.[1267] Type 1 lesions originate in a subpleural location or in the vicinity of parenchymal scars. They are commonly located in the apex of an upper lobe or along the costophrenic rim of the middle lobe and lingula. Each bulla characteristically has a narrow neck and usually contains only gas, without evidence of alveolar remnants or blood vessels. When seen in an excised lung, such a bulla appears as a spherical sac projecting above the pleural surface (Fig. 55–44); of necessity, it extends into the contiguous lung *in vivo*, compressing the parenchyma and causing some degree of atelectasis. Multiple bullae may be seen to extend in rows beneath the pleura, in some cases coalescing to form large air spaces that may be visible radiographically. It is possible that this type is related pathogenetically to paraseptal emphysema.[1259, 1260]

Type 2 bullae are also superficial in location but have

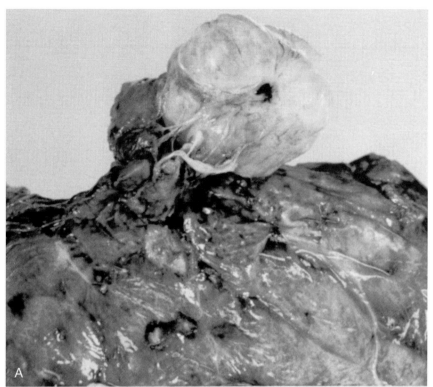

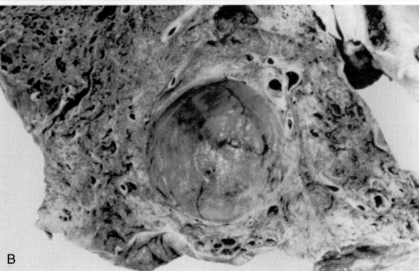

**Figure 55–44. Bullae.** A discrete narrow-necked bulla *(A)* is present on the apical aspect of the upper lobe. The basal portion of the lower lobe from another patient *(B)* shows a spherical, smooth-walled bulla projecting into the lung parenchyma (the other half of the bulla extended to the lateral pleural surface). The remainder of the lung parenchyma shows moderate emphysema.

a very broad neck. They may occur anywhere over the lung surface but most often develop over the anterior edge of the upper and middle lobes or lingula and over the diaphragmatic surface. In contrast to type 1 lesions, this variety characteristically contains blood vessels and strands of partially destroyed lung, indicating that it probably represents a localized exaggeration of generalized emphysema. Although any of the three types of bullae can rupture and cause pneumothorax, the most common to do so is type 2; for example, in one study of 54 resected bullae associated with spontaneous pneumothorax, 65% were of this type.[1268]

Type 3 bullae lie within the lung substance (Fig. 55–45) but are otherwise similar to the type 2 variety and commonly contain strands of partially destroyed lung and intact blood vessels. They appear to affect both upper and lower lobes

equally. Although a type 3 bulla usually represents an exaggerated form of generalized emphysema, it occasionally develops in its absence, in which case it probably represents the residuum of a lung abscess.

An unusual abnormality termed *placentoid bullous lesion* has been described in several otherwise healthy young adults.[1269] Pathologically, the lesion has a somewhat spongy, cystic structure that resembles the normal placenta or the placenta complicated by hydatidiform mole. Histologic examination has shown the spongy appearance to be related to the presence of papillary structures that have an edematous or fibrotic core, resembling placental villi. Otherwise typical bullae or panlobular emphysema have been present elsewhere in the lung in some patients. Although the fundamental nature of the lesion is uncertain, it has been speculated

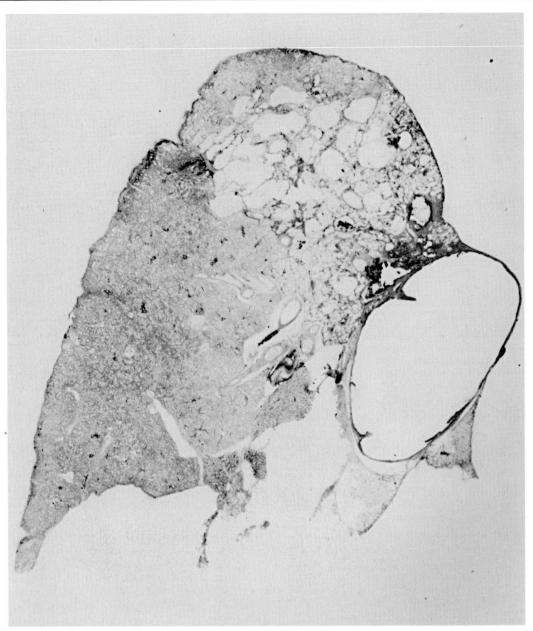

**Figure 55–45. Centrilobular Emphysema with Bulla Formation.** A paper mounted slice of a left lung cut in the sagittal plane shows moderately severe centrilobular emphysema in the central portion of the upper lobe and a large bulla in the lingula.

that it may represent the effect on a bulla of lung torsion with subsequent lymphatic obstruction and lymphangiectasis.[1269]

### Radiologic Manifestations

Bullae are manifested on the chest radiograph as thin-walled, sharply demarcated areas of avascularity (Fig. 55–46). The walls are characteristically apparent as hairline shadows; however, because bullae are most often located at or near the lung surface, only a portion of the wall is usually visible (Fig. 55–47). A location within the substance of the lung renders identification much more difficult, and even peripheral bullae may be missed on the radiograph.[732, 1270] Bullae are evident much more commonly in the upper lobes than elsewhere, particularly in asymptomatic individuals;[1259, 1260] however, in patients who have widespread em-

physema, there is only a slight predilection for bullae in the upper lobes.[1267]

As might be expected, CT allows greatly improved visibility of a bulla identified on the radiograph and may reveal bullae not even suspected (*see* Fig. 55–47).[744, 1270] It is particularly valuable in defining the anatomy of bullae and in determining the extent of emphysema or parenchymal compression of adjacent lung tissue.[1270–1274] In one investigation of nine patients who had bullae that occupied at least one third of a hemithorax, eight were smokers and one was a lifelong nonsmoker.[1273] The bullae ranged in diameter from 1 to 20 cm (Fig. 55–48). In all patients, the lesions were predominantly subpleural in distribution; intraparenchymal bullae, present in seven patients, were less than 3 cm in diameter. The predominant abnormality on HRCT was paraseptal emphysema, although eight of the nine patients had

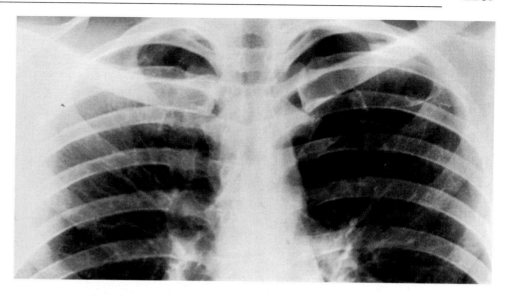

**Figure 55–46. Multiple Bullae in Otherwise Normal Lung.** A view of the upper half of the thorax from a posteroanterior radiograph reveals numerous curved hairline shadows in the upper portion of the left lung representing the walls of multiple large bullae. A single bulla is present in the right paramediastinal area.

evidence of mild to moderately severe centrilobular emphysema.

Bullae may be large enough to compress the adjacent lung parenchyma; although compression is usually relatively mild,[1273] it may result in sufficient atelectasis to appear as a mass-like opacity (Fig. 55–49). In one investigation of 11 patients who had such opacities, the areas of atelectasis involved mainly the upper lobes;[1274] smaller foci of atelectasis were present in the remaining lobes. Re-expansion of the atelectatic lung with resolution of the mass-like appearance occurred in seven of the eight patients who underwent resection of bullae. CT also allows assessment of the volume of the bullae at both total lung capacity and residual volume. In one investigation of 43 patients, bullae were found to contribute little to expired lung volume;[1270] RV/TLC for the bullae averaged approximately 90%, whereas total lung RV/TLC was approximately 60%. The majority of bullae decrease in size between CT scans performed at end-inspiration and scans performed at the end of maximal expiration; occasionally they may remain unchanged in size.[1275]

Rarely, bullae disappear as a result of secondary infection[1259, 1261, 1276–1278] or because of inflammatory stenosis of its subtending airway.[770] However, in many cases they enlarge progressively (Fig. 55–50) and may come to occupy most of a lung (Fig. 55–51). In one investigation of 49 patients for whom serial radiographs were available for 1 to more than 10 years, the lesions consistently enlarged;[1259] some increased slowly and continuously, whereas others remained constant in size for several years and then, for no obvious reason, enlarged. In many cases, bullae were apparent radiographically for many years before the onset of symptoms; this has been our experience also.

Infection usually is manifested radiologically by a fluid level within the bulla,[1261, 1276, 1277] with or without evidence of pneumonitis in the surrounding lung parenchyma. Occasionally, fluid accumulation is caused by hemorrhage,[1279] a complication that may be suspected when there is an accompanying drop in hemoglobin level; rarely, hemorrhage may be severe enough to necessitate emergency surgery.[1280] In one patient who had emphysema and *Aspergillus fumigatus* infection and who presented with massive hemoptysis, pulmonary angiography demonstrated a large pulmonary artery pseudoaneurysm.[1281] Although the development of an air-fluid level within a bulla is usually indicative of infection, it also may be the result of carcinoma.[1282]

Because bullae commonly do not produce any symptoms, their presence may become evident only when chest radiography is carried out during investigation of acute lower respiratory tract infection. In such circumstances, the radiographic appearance may be misinterpreted as a lung cavity secondary to abscess formation; differentiation is aided by the fact that most patients who have infected bullae are much less ill than those who have acute lung abscess. In addition, infected bullae usually have much thinner walls (Fig. 55–52), are surrounded by lesser degrees of pneumonitis, and contain much less fluid than cavitated lung abscesses.[1283–1285] Complete clearing of fluid from an infected bulla may be protracted, in one series averaging about 6 weeks.[1286]

Spontaneous pneumothorax commonly occurs in association with localized areas of emphysema or bullae affecting the lung apices. In one investigation of 116 patients who had surgically treated pneumothorax, 69 had parenchymal abnormalities identified on the radiograph;[1287] the most common findings consisted of apical bullae (seen in 51 patients), apical scarring (in 17), and diffuse emphysema (in 9). In fact, bullae and localized areas of emphysema not apparent on the radiograph can be seen on the CT scan in over 80% of patients who have spontaneous pneumothorax.[1288–1290] For example, in one investigation of 35 patients who had this abnormality, bullae or smaller localized areas of emphysema were identified on the CT scan in 31 (89%) and on the radiograph in only 11 (31%);[1288] in all of these patients, the chest radiograph had been initially interpreted as showing no parenchymal abnormalities. In another investigation of 27 nonsmoking patients who had spontaneous pneumothorax, 21 (81%) had localized bullae or smaller areas of emphysema visible on the CT scan;[1290] focal areas of emphysema were identified at surgery in three additional patients. In none of these patients were the parenchymal abnormalities visible on the chest radiograph. Rarely, pneumothorax is associated with large bullae involving the lower lobes.[1263]

When spontaneous pneumothorax develops in association with bullae, it may be much more easily identified when

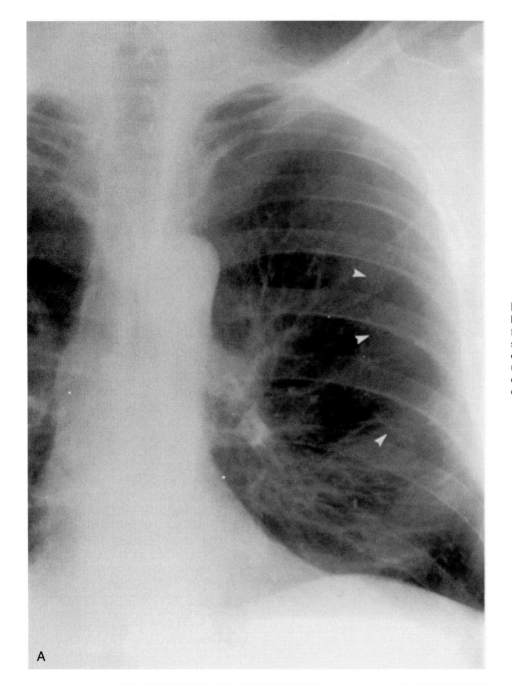

**Figure 55–47. Bullae and Paraseptal Emphysema.** A detail view of the left lung from a posteroanterior chest radiograph *(A)* shows curvilinear hairline-thick subpleural opacities *(arrowheads)* in the middle and upper parts of the lung. There is no evidence of pulmonary overinflation or generalized oligemia.

**Figure 55–47** *Continued.* HRCT scans through the mid-trachea *(B)* and carina *(C)* show multiple small foci of emphysema *(arrowheads)* widely dispersed throughout the upper lobes. A number of bullae *(open arrows)* are also evident in the subpleural parenchyma of the upper and lower lobes; on the left, interlobular septa (IS) partition the bullae into prominent arcades. These latter findings are characteristic of paraseptal emphysema. The patient was a middle-aged man who had mild dyspnea.

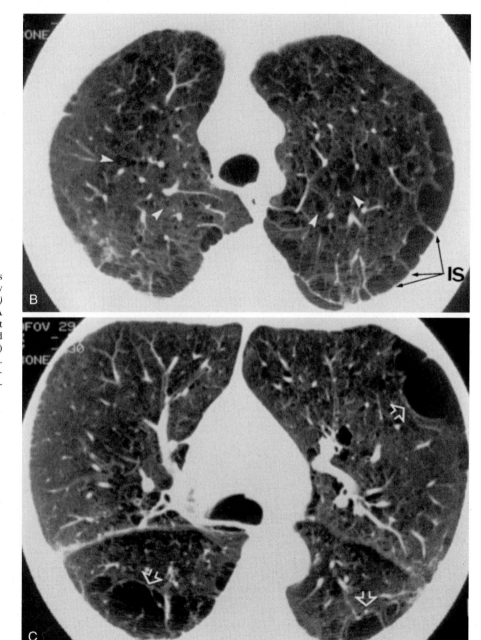

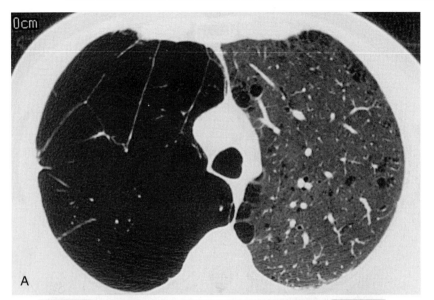

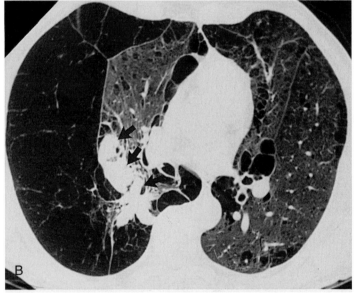

**Figure 55–48. Asymmetric Bullous Lung Disease.** An HRCT scan through the upper lobes *(A)* demonstrates replacement of the parenchyma on the right side by large bullae, associated with a shift of the mediastinum to the left. Mild emphysema is present in the left upper lobe. An HRCT scan obtained at a more caudad level *(B)* demonstrates compressive atelectasis *(arrows)* in the right middle and lower lobes and a shift of the mediastinum to the left. The patient was a 68-year-old smoker.

the lung is collapsed than when it is fully inflated; this improved visibility results from the tendency of bullae to remain air-containing while the surrounding lung collapses. Sometimes, the distinction of spontaneous pneumothorax from large bullae occupying much of the volume of one lung can be difficult (Fig. 55–53); in such circumstances, CT can be helpful in clarifying the diagnosis.[1291]

### Clinical Manifestations

Primary bullous disease characteristically is unassociated with symptoms or signs and causes minimal or no abnormality in pulmonary function. Sometimes patients complain of dyspnea on exertion[1262, 1292] or, rarely, present with severe pulmonary insufficiency and cor pulmonale;[1293] in such cases, the lung function impairment may be the result of concomitant COPD.[1261] As discussed previously, a bulla occasionally ruptures and causes pneumothorax. Enlargement occurring as a result of decreased ambient pressure in an airliner can cause air emboli and sudden death.[1294]

### Pulmonary Function Tests

In patients who have primary bullous disease, the vital capacity usually is within normal range, although FRC and RV may be increased, especially if they are measured by the body plethysmograph. (Because the small necks of many bullae permit very slow distribution of inspired gas, results obtained with inert gas techniques may be misleading.) Mixing efficiency may be severely impaired. Flow rates and diffusing capacity are normal or near normal, although diffusion may be affected if adjacent lung parenchyma is severely compressed. Blood gas measurements typically are normal at rest but may reveal hypoxemia during exercise.[1260, 1261] Results of bronchospirometry in patients who have unilateral bullae have shown decreased vital capacity and minute volume of ventilation in the involved lung;[1295] however, the most striking interlung difference occurs in the distribution of inert gas, which is impaired on the affected side as a result of poor ventilation of the bullae.[1259] Bullae rarely contribute significantly to dead space ventilation because they are so poorly ventilated.[1296] In primary bullous disease,

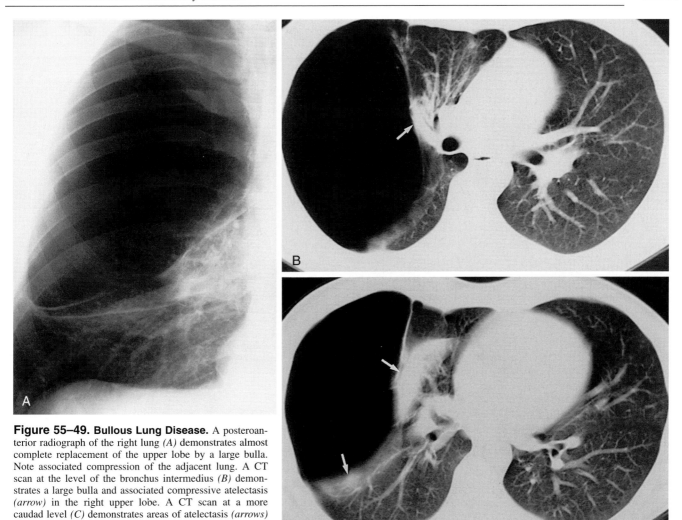

**Figure 55–49. Bullous Lung Disease.** A posteroanterior radiograph of the right lung *(A)* demonstrates almost complete replacement of the upper lobe by a large bulla. Note associated compression of the adjacent lung. A CT scan at the level of the bronchus intermedius *(B)* demonstrates a large bulla and associated compressive atelectasis *(arrow)* in the right upper lobe. A CT scan at a more caudad level *(C)* demonstrates areas of atelectasis *(arrows)* in the right middle and lower lobes; the left lung is normal. The patient was a 32-year-old man.

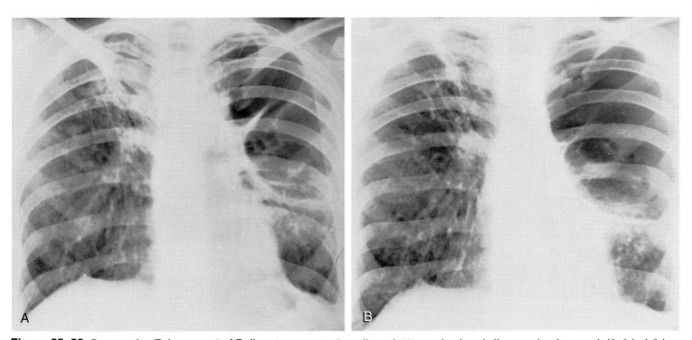

**Figure 55–50. Progressive Enlargement of Bullae.** A posteroanterior radiograph *(A)* reveals a large bulla occupying the upper half of the left lung. The extensive bilateral parenchymal disease is the result of chronic tuberculosis. Approximately 1 year later *(B)*, the bulla has increased considerably in size.

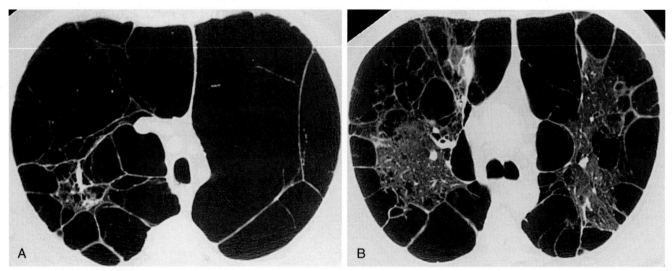

**Figure 55–51. Severe Bullous Lung Disease.** HRCT scans *(A* and *B)* demonstrate almost complete replacement of the upper lobes by numerous large bullae. The patient was a 57-year-old man who was a heavy smoker.

airway resistance is usually within normal limits at high lung volumes but may be increased at low lung volumes as a result of the reduction in elastic recoil.[1297]

The rationale for bullectomy lies in the potential for healthy lung to expand and fill the space occupied by the bullae and in the expected postoperative increase in elastic recoil pressure that reduces the tendency for airways to collapse on expiration.[1298] In the great majority of patients who have primary bullous disease, there is no clinical disability and therefore surgery is not indicated. However, when bullae are large, surgical removal using video-assisted thora-

coscopy[1299] or via standard thoracotomy may be necessary; in such circumstances, pulmonary function studies carried out before and after surgery have revealed significant improvement.[1260, 1261, 1300, 1301]

Bullae that occur in a background of COPD are associated with similar changes in pulmonary function to those that occur in patients who have COPD without bullae. Pulmonary function studies reveal a decrease in the vital capacity; an increase in FRC and RV; an increased, normal, or decreased TLC; impaired mixing efficiency; reduction in flow rates; decreased diffusing capacity at rest and during exercise; and

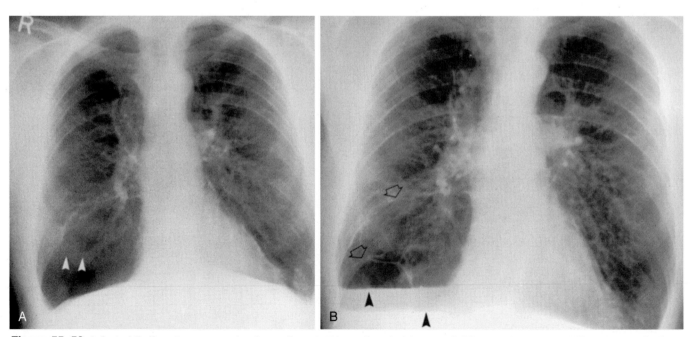

**Figure 55–52. Infected Bullae.** A posteroanterior chest radiograph *(A)* reveals typical features of diffuse emphysema. In addition, the supradiaphragmatic portion of the right lower lobe is severely oligemic, and there is displacement of vessels upward, backward, and laterally by one or more large bullae; a faint curvilinear opacity may represent the wall of a bulla *(arrowheads)*. A chest radiograph obtained three months later *(B)* demonstrates two long fluid levels *(arrowheads)* in adjacent bullae. Note that the walls of the bullae are more clearly outlined *(open arrows)*, presumably as a result of thickening of adjacent tissue by an inflammatory reaction. The fluid levels regressed very slowly over a period of 6 weeks.

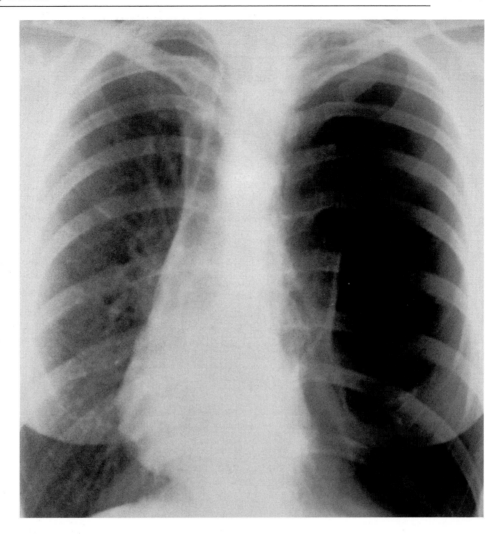

**Figure 55–53. Large Bulla Simulating Pneumothorax.** A posteroanterior chest radiograph demonstrates a severely overinflated and almost totally oligemic left hemithorax. A small amount of distorted and compressed left lung parenchyma can be seen contiguous with the heart border. The mediastinum is displaced to the right. The vasculature of the right lung is within normal limits. The patient was an asymptomatic middle-aged woman.

(usually) hypoxemia and hypercarbia. In one study, cardiac catheterization revealed a rise in Ppa with exercise in all cases.[1260] This contrasts with the findings in primary disease, in which normal Ppa values have been recorded at rest and during exercise. In patients who have both bullae and COPD, surgical intervention is not nearly as successful as in patients who have primary bullous disease; nevertheless, some patients improve clinically and show better gas exchange and lung elastic recoil postoperatively,[1295, 1296, 1298, 1302] particularly when the bullae are large.[1302, 1303]

## MISCELLANEOUS CAUSES OF EMPHYSEMA

Unilateral or lobar emphysema (unilateral hyperlucent lung) is one of the very few "diseases" whose name derives entirely from the manifestations it produces radiographically—a state in which the density of one lung (sometimes only one lobe or both lower lobes) is markedly less than the density of the other. The condition was originally described by Swyer and James.[1304–1306] The underlying pathogenetic mechanism is bronchiolitis (*see* page 2337).

Patients who have intravenous talcosis may present with obstructive lung disease, in which case the chest radiograph and CT scan characteristically show lower lobe emphysema with variable upper lobe fibrosis (*see* page 1858). For unknown reasons, the emphysema is typically panlobular in type. The pathogenesis of the disease is related to injection of a variety of drugs, most of which have talc as a "filler."[1307, 1308] Panlobular emphysema has also been associated with hypocomplementemic urticarial vasculitis.[1309, 1310] Although almost all affected patients have been smokers, the severity of the associated lung disease has been out of proportion to what might be expected with the degree of cigarette smoking, suggesting that the obstructive disease is directly related to the presence of hypocomplementemic urticarial vasculitis. Despite the documentation of normal or elevated levels of alpha$_1$-PI in most patients,[1311] it has been suggested that the underlying pathologic abnormality is panlobular emphysema.[1309, 1312]

Findings suggestive of emphysema have been reported with surprising frequency in relatively young patients who have human immunodeficiency virus infection in the absence of other risk factors, suggesting that the process may be a direct manifestation of the viral infection.[1313, 1314]

# REFERENCES

1. Burrows B: Foreword, symposium on chronic respiratory disease. Med Clin North Am 57:545, 1973.
2. Mannino DM, Brown C, Giovino GA: Obstructive lung disease deaths in the United States from 1979 through 1993. An analysis using multiple-cause mortality data. Am J Respir Crit Care Med 156:814, 1997.
3. Riggs JE. Longitudinal Gompertzian analysis of emphysema mortality in the US, 1962–1987: The differing basis for evolving mortality patterns in men and women. Mech Ageing Dev 64:161, 1992.
4. Wise RA: Changing smoking patterns and mortality from chronic obstructive pulmonary disease. Prev Med 26:418, 1997.
5. Deaths from chronic obstructive pulmonary disease in the United States, 1987. Stat Bull Metrop Insur Co 71:20, 1990.
6. Murray CJL, Lopez AD: Global mortality, disability, and the contribution of risk factors—global burden of disease study. Lancet 349:1436, 1997.
7. Ferris B Jr: Chronic bronchitis and emphysema: Classification and epidemiology. Med Clin North Am 57:637, 1973.
8. Peto R, Speizer FE, Cochrane AL, et al: The relevance in adults of air-flow obstruction, but not of mucus hypersection, to mortality from chronic lung disease—results from 20 years of prospective observation. Am Rev Respir Dis 128:491, 1983.
9. Burrows B, Knudson RJ, Camilli AE, et al: The "horse-racing effect" and predicting decline in forced expiratory volume in one second from screening spirometry. Am Rev Respir Dis 135:788, 1987.
10. Lange P, Nyboe J, Appleyard M, et al: Relation of ventilatory impairment and of chronic mucus hypersecretion to mortality from obstructive lung disease and from all causes. Thorax 45:579, 1990.
11. Prescott E, Lange P, Vestbo J: Chronic mucus hypersecretion in COPD and death from pulmonary infection. Eur Respir J 8:1333, 1995.
12. Vestbo J, Prescott E, Lange P: Association of chronic mucus hypersecretion with $FEV_1$ decline and chronic obstructive pulmonary disease morbidity. Copenhagen City Heart Study Group. Am J Respir Crit Care Med 153:1530, 1996.
13. Hogg JC, Wright JL, Wiggs BR, et al: Lung structure and function in cigarette smokers. Thorax 49:473, 1994.
14. Gelb AF, Schein M, Kuei J, et al: Limited contribution of emphysema in advanced chronic obstructive pulmonary disease. Am Rev Respir Dis 147:1157, 1993.
15. Turner-Warwick M: Some clinical problems in patients with airways obstruction. Chest 82(Suppl):3, 1982.
16. Fletcher CM, Pride NB: Definitions of emphysema, chronic bronchitis, asthma, and airflow obstruction: 25 years on from the CIBA symposium (editorial). Thorax 39:81, 1984.
17. Snider GL: What's in a name? Names, definitions, descriptions, and diagnostic criteria of diseases, with emphasis on chronic obstructive pulmonary disease. Respiration 62:297, 1995.
18. Strachan DP: Epidemiology: A British prospective. In Calverley P, Pride N (eds): Chronic Obstructive Pulmonary Disease. London, Chapman & Hall, 1995, pp 47–68.
19. Snider GL: What's in a name? Names, definitions, descriptions, and diagnostic criteria of diseases, with emphasis on chronic obstructive pulmonary disease. Respiration 62:297, 1995.
20. Becklake MR: Chronic airflow limitation: Its relationship to work in dusty occupations. Chest 88:608, 1985.
21. Macklem PT, Thurlbeck WM, Fraser RG, et al: Chronic obstructive disease of small airways. Ann Intern Med 74:167, 1971.
22. Sluiter HJ, Koeter GH, de Monchy JG, et al: The Dutch hypothesis (chronic non-specific lung disease) revisited. Eur Respir J 4:479, 1991.
23. Sterk PJ: Farewell to "CARA"? (editorial). Neth J Med 45:139, 1994.
24. ATS standards for the diagnosis and care of patients with chronic obstructive pulmonary disease. Am J Respir Crit Care Med 152(Suppl):77, 1995.
25. American Thoracic Society (Statement by Committee on Diagnostic Standards for Nontuberculous Respiratory Diseases): Definitions and classification of chronic bronchitis, asthma, and pulmonary emphysema. Am Rev Respir Dis 85:762, 1962.
26. Lebowitz MD, Burrows B: Comparison of questionnaires: The BMRC and NHLI respiratory questionnaires and a new self-completion questionnaire. Am Rev Respir Dis 113:627, 1976.
27. Report of the conclusions of a Ciba Guest Symposium: Terminology, definitions and classification of chronic pulmonary emphysema and related conditions. Thorax 14:286, 1959.
28. Jeffrey PK: Morphology of the airway wall in asthma and in chronic obstructive pulmonary disease. Am Rev Respir Dis 143:1152, 1991.
29. Mullen JB, Wright JL, Wiggs BR, et al: Structure of central airways in current smokers and ex-smokers with and without mucus hypersecretion: Relationship to lung function. Thorax 42:843, 1987.
30. Snider GL, Kleinerman JL, Thurlbeck WM, et al: The definition of emphysema—report of a National Heart, Lung, and Blood Institute Division of Lung Diseases Workshop. Am Rev Respir Dis 132:182, 1985.
31. Pride NB, Burrows B: Development of impaired lung function: Natural history and risk factors. In Calverley P, Pride N (eds): Chronic Obstructive Pulmonary Disease. London, Chapman & Hall, 1995, pp 69–91.
32. Oswald NC: Chronic bronchitis and emphysema: A symposium II. Clinical aspects of chronic bronchitis. Br J Radiol 32:289, 1959.
33. Fletcher CM: Chronic bronchitis. Its prevalence, nature, and pathogenesis. Am Rev Respir Dis 80:483, 1959.
34. Reid DD, Anderson DO, Ferris BG, et al: An Anglo-American comparison of the prevalence of bronchitis. BMJ 2:1487, 1964.
35. Dodge R, Cline MG, Burrows B: Comparisons of asthma, emphysema, and chronic bronchitis diagnoses in a general population sample. Am Rev Respir Dis 133:981, 1986.
36. Cullinan P: Persistent cough and phlegm: Prevalence and clinical characteristics in south-east England. Respir Med 86:143, 1992.
37. Lee PN, Fry JS, Forey BA: Trends in lung cancer, chronic obstructive lung disease, and emphysema death rates for England and Wales 1941–85 and their relation to trends in cigarette smoking. Thorax 45:657, 1990.
38. Crockett AJ, Cranston JM, Moss JR, Alpers JH: Trends in chronic obstructive pulmonary disease mortality in Australia. Med J Aust 161:600, 1994.
39. Cooreman J, Thom TJ, Higgins MW: Mortality from chronic obstructive pulmonary diseases and asthma in France, 1969–1983. Comparisons with the United States and Canada. Chest 97:213, 1990.
40. Barker DJP, Osmond C: Childhood respiratory infection and chronic bronchitis in England and Wales. BMJ 293:1271, 1986.
41. Brown CA, Crombie IK, Tunstall-Pedoe H: Failure of cigarette smoking to explain international differences in mortality from chronic obstructive pulmonary disease. J Epidemiol Community Health 48:134, 1994.
42. Menkes HA, Cohen BH, Beaty TH, et al: Risk factors, pulmonary function, and mortality. Prog Clin Biol Res 147:501, 1984.
43. College of General Practitioners: Chronic bronchitis in Great Britain. A national survey carried out by the Respiratory Diseases Study Group of the College of General Practitioners. BMJ 2:973, 1961.
44. Tager I, Speizer FE: Role of infection in chronic bronchitis. N Engl J Med 292:563, 1975.
45. Zuskin E, Valie F: Effect of short term cigarette smoking on simple tests of ventilatory capacity in medical students. Am Rev Respir Dis 110:198, 1974.
46. Grimes CA, Hanes B: Influence of cigarette smoking on the spirometric evaluation of employees of a large insurance company. Am Rev Respir Dis 108:273, 1973.
47. Higgins MW, Keller JB, Becker M, et al: An index of risk for obstructive airway disease. Am Rev Respir Dis 125:144, 1982.
48. Higgins MW, Keller JB, Landis JR, et al: Risk of chronic obstructive pulmonary disease—collaborative assessment of the validity of the Tecumseh Index of Risk. Am Rev Respir Dis 130:380, 1984.
49. Sherrill DL, Lebowitz MD, Burrows B: Epidemiology of chronic obstructive pulmonary disease. Clin Chest Med 11:375, 1990.
50. Rimington J: Chronic bronchitis: Method of cigarette smoking. BMJ 1:776, 1973.
51. Rimington J: Cigarette smoker's bronchitis: The effect of relighting. BMJ 2:591, 1974.
52. Webster JR Jr, Kettel LJ, Moran F, et al: Chronic obstructive pulmonary disease. A comparison between men and women. Am Rev Respir Dis 98:1021, 1968.
53. Oswald NC, Medvei VC, Waller RE: Chronic bronchitis: A 10-year follow-up. Thorax 22:279, 1967.
54. Fletcher CM, Elmes PC, Fairbairn AS, et al: The significance of respiratory symptoms and the diagnosis of chronic bronchitis in a working population. BMJ 2:257, 1959.
55. Seltzer CC, Siegelaub AB, Friedman GD, et al: Differences in pulmonary function related to smoking habits and race. Am Rev Respir Dis 110:598, 1974.
56. Gillum RF: Chronic obstructive pulmonary disease in blacks and whites: Mortality and morbidity. J Natl Med Assoc 82:417, 1990.
57. Miller GJ: Cigarette smoking and irreversible airways obstruction in the West Indies. Thorax 29:495, 1974.
58. Emirgil C, Sobol BJ, Heymann B, et al: Pulmonary function in alcoholics. Am J Med 57:69, 1974.
59. Sobol BJ, Herbert WH, Emirgil C: The high incidence of pulmonary functional abnormalities in patients with coronary artery disease. Chest 65:148, 1974.
60. Burrows B, Niden AH, Barclay WR, et al: Chronic obstructive lung disease. 1. Clinical and physiologic findings in 175 patients and their relationship to age and sex. Am Rev Respir Dis 91:521, 1965.
61. Silverman EK, Speizer FE: Risk factors for the development of chronic obstructive pulmonary disease. Med Clin North Am 80:501, 1996.
62. Fletcher C, Peto R, Tinker C, Speizer FE: The Natural History of Chronic Bronchitis: An Eight Year Follow-up Study of Working Men in London. Oxford, Oxford University Press, 1976.
63. Bascom R: Differential susceptibility to tobacco smoke: Possible mechanisms. Pharmacogenetics 1:102, 1991.
64. Sherrill DL, Lebowitz MD, Knudson RJ, Burrows B: Longitudinal methods for describing the relationship between pulmonary function, respiratory symptoms and smoking in elderly subjects: The Tucson Study. Eur Respir J 6:342, 1993.
65. Kerstjens HA, Rijcken B, Schouten JP, Postma DS: Decline of $FEV_1$ by age and smoking status: Facts, figures, and fallacies. Thorax 52:820, 1997.
66. Clément J, Van de Woestijne KP: Rapidly decreasing forced expiratory volume in one second or vital capacity and development of chronic airflow obstruction. Am Rev Respir Dis 125:553, 1982.
67. Beaty TH, Menkes HA, Cohen BH, et al: Risk factors associated with longitudinal change in pulmonary function. Am Rev Respir Dis 129:660, 1984.

68. Whittemore AS, Perlin SA, Di Ciccio Y: Chronic obstructive pulmonary disease in lifelong nonsmokers: Results from NHANES. Am J Public Health 85:702, 1995.
69. Cullen KJ, Stenhouse NS, Welborn TA, et al: Chronic respiratory disease in a rural community. Lancet 2:657, 1968.
70. Dysinger PW, Lemon FR, Crenshaw GL, et al: Pulmonary emphysema in a non-smoking population. Dis Chest 43:17, 1963.
71. Payne M, Kjelsberg M: Respiratory symptoms, lung function, and smoking habits in an adult population. Am J Public Health 54:261, 1964.
72. Thurlbeck WM: Chronic Airflow Obstruction in Lung Disease. Major Problems in Pathology. Vol 5. Philadelphia, WB Saunders, 1976.
73. Boucot KR, Cooper DA, Weiss W: Smoking and the health of older men. 1. Smoking and chronic cough. Arch Environ Health 4:59, 1962.
74. Wynder EL, Lemon FR, Mantel N: Epidemiology of persistent cough. Am Rev Respir Dis 91:679, 1965.
75. Peters GA, Miller RD: Effect of smoking on asthma and emphysema. Mayo Clin Proc 35:353, 1960.
76. Anderson DO, Ferris BG Jr: Role of tobacco smoking in the causation of chronic respiratory disease. N Engl J Med 267:787, 1962.
77. Mueller RE, Keble DL, Plummer J, et al: The prevalence of chronic bronchitis, chronic airway obstruction, and respiratory symptoms in a Colorado city. Am Rev Respir Dis 103:209, 1971.
78. Brinkman GL, Coates EO Jr: The effect of bronchitis, smoking, and occupation on ventilation. Am Rev Respir Dis 87:684, 1963.
79. Barker GS: Lung function in elderly male heavy smokers and nonsmokers. Am Rev Respir Dis 91:409, 1965.
80. Wilson RH, Meador RS, Jay BE, et al: The pulmonary pathologic physiology of persons who smoke cigarettes. N Engl J Med 262:956, 1960.
81. Sharp JT, Paul O, Lepper MH, et al: Prevalence of chronic bronchitis in an American male urban industrial population. Am Rev Respir Dis 91:510, 1965.
82. Bower G: Respiratory symptoms and ventilatory function in 172 adults employed in a bank. Am Rev Respir Dis 83:684, 1961.
83. Weiss W, Boucot KR, Cooper DA, et al: Smoking and the health of older men. II. Smoking and ventilatory function. Arch Environ Health 7:538, 1963.
84. Larson RK: The chronic effect of cigarette smoking on pulmonary ventilation. Am Rev Respir Dis 88:630, 1963.
85. Franklin W, Lowell FC: Unrecognized airway obstruction associated with smoking: A probable forerunner of obstructive pulmonary emphysema. Ann Intern Med 54:379, 1961.
86. Beck GJ, Doyle CA, Schachter EN, et al: Smoking and lung function. Am Rev Respir Dis 123:149, 1981.
87. Tager IB, Muñoz A, Rosner B, et al: Effect of cigarette smoking on the pulmonary function of children and adolescents. Am Rev Respir Dis 131:752, 1985.
88. Sherrill DL, Enright P, Cline M, et al: Rates of decline in lung function among subjects who restart cigarette smoking. Chest 109:1001, 1996.
89. Sherrill DL, Holberg CJ, Enright PL, et al: Longitudinal analysis of the effects of smoking onset and cessation on pulmonary function. Am J Respir Crit Care Med 149:591, 1994.
90. Rodenstein D, Stănescu D: Pattern of inhalation of tobacco smoke in pipe, cigarette, and never smokers. Am Rev Respir Dis 132:628, 1985.
91. Lange P, Nyboe J, Appleyard M, et al: Relationship of the type of tobacco and inhalation pattern to pulmonary and total mortality. Eur Respir J 5:1111, 1992.
92. Wald NJ, Watt HC: Prospective study of effect of switching from cigarettes to pipes or cigars on mortality from three smoking-related diseases. BMJ 314:1860, 1997.
93. Paoletti P, Camilli AE, Holberg CJ, et al: Respiratory effects in relation to estimated tar exposure from current and cumulative cigarette consumption. Chest 88:849, 1985.
94. Tobin MJ, Sackner MA: Monitoring smoking patterns of low and high tar cigarettes with inductive plethysmography. Am Rev Respir Dis 126:258, 1982.
95. Medici TC, Unger S, Ruegger M, et al: Smoking pattern of smokers with and without tobacco smoke–related lung diseases. Am Rev Respir Dis 131:385, 1985.
96. Taylor DR, Reid WD, Paré PD, et al: Cigarette smoke inhalation patterns and bronchial reactivity. Thorax 43:65, 1988.
97. Smaldone GC, Messina MS: Enhancement of particle deposition by flow-limiting segments in humans. J Appl Physiol 49:509, 1985.
98. Schenker MV, Samet JM, Speizer FE: Effect of cigarette tar content and smoking habits on respiratory symptoms in women. Am Rev Respir Dis 125:684, 1982.
99. Sparrow D, Stefos T, Bossé R, et al: The relationship of tar content to decline in pulmonary function in cigarette smokers. Am Rev Respir Dis 127:56, 1983.
100. Lee PN, Garfinkel L: Mortality and type of cigarette smoked. J Epidemiol Community Health 35:16, 1981.
101. Lehrer SB, Barbandi F, Taylor JP, et al: Tobacco smoke sensitivity—is there an immunologic basis? J Allergy Clin Immunol 240:73, 1984.
102. Lehrer SB, Wilson MR, Salvaggio JE, et al: Immunogenic properties of tobacco smoke. J Allergy Clin Immunol 62:368, 1978.
103. Guyatt AR, Berry G, Alpers JH, et al: Relationship of airway conductance and its immediate change on smoking to smoking habits and symptoms of chronic bronchitis. Am Rev Respir Dis 101:44, 1970.
104. Nadel JA, Comroe JH Jr: Acute effects of inhalation of cigarette smoke on airway conductance. J Appl Physiol 16:713, 1961.
105. Sterling GM: Mechanism of bronchoconstriction caused by cigarette smoking. BMJ 3:275, 1967.
106. Costello JF, Sudlow MF, Douglas NJ, et al: Acute effects of smoking tobacco and a tobacco substitute on lung function in man. Lancet 2:678, 1975.
107. McCarthy DS, Craig DB, Cherniack RM: The effect of acute, intensive cigarette smoking on maximal expiratory flows and the single-breath nitrogen washout trace. Am Rev Respir Dis 113:301, 1976.
108. Chiang ST, Wang BC: Acute effects of cigarette smoking on pulmonary function. Am Rev Respir Dis 101:860, 1970.
109. Higenbottam T, Hamilton D, Feyerband C, et al: Acute effects of smoking a single cigarette on the airway resistance and the maximal and partial forced expiratory flow volume curves. Br J Dis Chest 74:37, 1980.
110. Taveira DA, Silva AM, Hamosh P: Airways response to inhaled tobacco smoke: Time course, dose dependence and effect of volume history. Respiration 41:96, 1981.
111. Malo JL, Filiatrault S, Martin RR, et al: Bronchial responsiveness to inhaled methacholine in young asymptomatic smokers. J Appl Physiol 52:1464, 1982.
112. Taylor RG, Clarke SW: Bronchial reactivity to histamine in young male smokers. Eur J Respir Dis 66:320, 1985.
113. Kabiraj MU, Simonsson BG, Groth S, et al: Bronchial reactivity, smoking, and alpha₁-antitrypsin: A population-based study of middle-aged men. Am Rev Respir Dis 126:864, 1982.
114. McIntyre EL, Ruffin RE, Alpers JH, et al: Lack of short-term effects of cigarette smoking on bronchial sensitivity to histamine and methacholine. Eur J Respir Dis 63:535, 1982.
115. Buczko GB, Zamel N: Combined effect of cigarette smoking and allergic rhinitis on airway responsiveness to inhaled methacholine. Am Rev Respir Dis 129:15, 1984.
116. Weiss ST, Tager IB, Schenker M, et al: The health effects of involuntary smoking. Am Rev Respir Dis 128:933, 1983.
117. Bake B: Effects in humans. Does environmental tobacco smoke affect lung function? In Rylander R, Peterson Y, Snella M-C (eds): Environmental tobacco smoke. Report from a workshop on effects and exposure levels, Geneva, Switzerland. March 15–17, 1983, Eur J Respir Dis 65(Suppl 133):85, 1984.
118. Hiller FC, McCusker KT, Mazumder MK, et al: Deposition of sidestream cigarette smoke in the human respiratory tract. Am Rev Respir Dis 125:405, 1982.
119. Jarvis MJ, Russell MAH, Feyerabend C, et al: Absorption of nicotine and carbon monoxide from passive smoking under natural conditions of exposure. Thorax 31:829, 1983.
120. Tashkin DP, Clark VA, Simmons M, et al: The UCLA population studies of chronic obstructive respiratory disease: Relationship between parental smoking and children's lung function. Am Rev Respir Dis 129:891, 1984.
121. Weiss ST, Taher IB, Speizer FE, et al: Passive smoking: Its relationship to respiratory symptoms, pulmonary function and nonspecific bronchial responsiveness. Chest 84:651, 1983.
122. Burchfiel CM, Higgins MW, Keller JB, et al: Passive smoking in childhood. Respiratory conditions and pulmonary function in Tecumseh, Michigan. Am Rev Respir Dis 133:966, 1986.
123. Tsimoyianis GV, Jacobson MS, Feldman JG: Reduction in pulmonary function and increased frequency of cough associated with passive smoking in teenage athletes. Pediatrics 80:32, 1987.
124. Colley JRT, Holland WW, Corkhill RT: Influence of passive smoking and parental phlegm on pneumonia and bronchitis in early childhood. Lancet 2:1031, 1974.
125. Tager B, Weiss T, Muñoz A, et al: Longitudinal study of the effects of maternal smoking on pulmonary function in children. N Engl J Med 309:699, 1983.
126. Comstock GW, Meyer MB, Helsing KJ, et al: Respiratory effects of household exposures to tobacco smoke and gas cooking. Am Rev Respir Dis 124:143, 1981.
127. White RW, Froeb F: Small airways dysfunction in nonsmokers chronically exposed to tobacco smoke. N Engl J Med 302:720, 1980.
128. Robbins AS, Abbey DE, Lebowitz MD: Passive smoking and chronic respiratory disease symptoms in non-smoking adults. Int J Epidemiol 22:809, 1993.
129. Morgan WKC: On dust, disability and death (editorial). Am Rev Respir Dis 134:639, 1986.
130. Cohen CA, Hudson AR, Clausen JL, et al: Respiratory symptoms, spirometry, and oxidant air pollution in nonsmoking adults. Am Rev Respir Dis 105:251, 1972.
131. Zepletal A, Jech J, Paul T, et al: Pulmonary function studies in children living in an air-polluted area. Am Rev Respir Dis 107:400, 1973.
132. Lambert PM, Reid DD: Smoking, air pollution, and bronchitis in Britain. Lancet 1:853, 1970.
133. Van der Lende R, Rijcken B: Longitudinal versus cross-sectional studies in measuring effect of smoking, air pollution and hyperreactivity on VC and FEV₁. Bull Eur Physiopathol Respir 19:85, 1983.
134. Solic J, Hazucha J, Bromberg A, et al: The acute effects of 0.2 ppm ozone in patients with chronic obstructive pulmonary disease. Am Rev Respir Dis 125:664, 1982.
135. Linn S, Fischer D, Medway A, et al: Short-term respiratory effects of 0.12 ppm ozone exposure in volunteers with chronic obstructive pulmonary disease. Am Rev Respir Dis 125:658, 1982.
136. Kehrl HR, Hazucha MJ, Solic JJ, et al: Responses of subjects with chronic obstructive pulmonary disease after exposures to 0.3 ppm ozone. Am Rev Respir Dis 131:719, 1985.
137. Clini V, Pozzi G, Ferrara A, et al: Bronchial hyperreactivity and arterial carboxyhemoglobin as detectors of air pollution in Milan: A study on normal subjects. Respiration 47:1, 1985.

138. Oshima Y, Ishizaki T, Miyamoto T, et al: Air pollution and respiratory diseases in the Tokyo-Yokohama area. Am Rev Respir Dis 90:572, 1964.

139. Dohan FC, Taylor EW: Air pollution and respiratory disease. A preliminary report. Am J Med Sci 240:337, 1960.

140. Holland WW, Reid DD: The urban factor in chronic bronchitis. Lancet 1:445, 1965.

141. Tzonou A, Maragoudakis G, Trichopoulos D, et al: Urban living, tobacco smoking, and chronic obstructive pulmonary disease: A study in Athens. Epidemiology 3:57, 1992.

142. Ferris BG Jr, Higgins ITT, Higgins MW, et al: Chronic nonspecific respiratory disease in Berlin, New Hampshire, 1961 to 1967. A follow-up study. Am Rev Respir Dis 107:110, 1973.

143. Ferris BG Jr, Higgins ITT, Higgins MW, et al: Chronic nonspecific respiratory disease, Berlin, New Hampshire, 1961–1967: A cross-sectional study. Am Rev Respir Dis 104:232, 1971.

144. Smith RBW, Kolb EJ, Phelps HW, et al: Tokyo-Yokohama asthma: An area-specific air pollution disease. Arch Environ Health 8:805, 1964.

145. Tashkin DP, Detels R, Simmons M, et al: The UCLA population studies of chronic obstructive respiratory disease: XI. Impact of air pollution and smoking on annual change in forced expiratory volume in one second. Am J Respir Crit Care Med 149:1209, 1994.

145a. Souza MB, Saldiva PHN, Pope CA III, et al: Respiratory changes due to long-term exposure to urban levels of air pollution. A histopathologic study in humans. Chest 113:1312, 1998.

146. Douglas JWB, Waller RE: Air pollution and respiratory infection in children. Br J Prev Soc Med 20:1, 1966.

147. Lunn JE, Knowelden J, Handyside AJ: Patterns of respiratory illness in Sheffield infant schoolchildren. Br J Prev Soc Med 21:7, 1967.

148. Ware JH, Dockery DW, Spiro A, et al: Passive smoking, gas cooking and respiratory health of children living in 6 cities. Am Rev Respir Dis 129:366, 1984.

149. Ekwo EE, Weinberger MM, Lachenbruch PA, et al: Relationship of parental smoking and gas cooking to respiratory disease in children. Chest 662:84, 1983.

150. Pandey MR: Prevalence of chronic bronchitis in a rural community of the hill region of Nepal. Thorax 39:331, 1984.

151. Pandey MR: Domestic smoke pollution and chronic bronchitis in a rural community of the hill region of Nepal. Thorax 39:337, 1984.

152. Behera D, Jindal SK, Malhotra HS: Ventilatory function in non-smoking rural Indian women using different cooking fuels. Respiration 61:89, 1994.

153. Perez-Padilla R, Regalado J, Vedal S, et al: Exposure to biomass smoke and chronic airway disease in Mexican women. A case-control study. Am J Respir Crit Care Med 154:701, 1996.

154. Dennis RJ, Maldonado D, Norman S, et al: Woodsmoke exposure and risk for obstructive airways disease among women. Chest 109:115, 1996.

155. Woolcock AJ, Blackburn CRB, Freeman MH, et al: Studies of chronic (nontuberculous) lung disease in New Guinea populations. The nature of the disease. Am Rev Respir Dis 102:575, 1970.

156. Jones HL Jr: COPD in women in developing countries. Chest 65:704, 1974.

157. Cullen KJ, Elder J, Adams AR, et al: Additional factors in chronic bronchitis. BMJ 1:394, 1970.

158. Bates DV: Air pollutants and the human lung. The James Waring Memorial Lecture. Am Rev Respir Dis 105:1, 1972.

159. Lebowitz MD, Bendheim P, Cristea G, et al: The effect of air pollution and weather on lung function in exercising children and adolescents. Am Rev Respir Dis 109:262, 1974.

160. Lawther PJ, Waller RE, Henderson M: Air pollution and exacerbations of bronchitis. Thorax 25:525, 1970.

161. Ponka A, Virtanen M: Chronic bronchitis, emphysema, and low-level air pollution in Helsinki, 1987–1989. Environ Res 65:207, 1994.

162. Sunyer J, Saez M, Murillo, et al: Air pollution and emergency room admissions for chronic obstructive pulmonary disease: A 5-year study. Am J Epidemiol 137:701, 1993.

163. Moolgavkar SH, Luebeck EG, Anderson EL: Air pollution and hospital admissions for respiratory causes in Minneapolis–St. Paul and Birmingham. Epidemiology 8:364, 1997.

164. Anderson HR, Spix C, Medina S, et al: Air pollution and daily admissions for chronic obstructive pulmonary disease in 6 European cities: Results from the APHEA project. Eur Respir J 10:1064, 1997.

165. Medical Research Council: Chronic bronchitis and occupation. M.R.C. report. BMJ 1:101, 1966.

166. Lane RE: Chronic bronchitis and occupation. Br J Tuberc 52:11, 1958.

167. McDonald JC: Epidemiology. *In* Weill H, Turner-Warwick M (eds): Occupational Lung Diseases: Research Approaches and Methods. New York, Marcel Dekker, 1981, p 373.

168. Hendrick DJ: Occupational and chronic obstructive pulmonary disease (COPD). Thorax 51:947, 1996.

169. Dosman JA, Kania J, Cockcroft DW: Occupational obstructive disorders: Nonspecific airways obstruction and occupational asthma. Med Clin North Am 74:823, 1990.

170. Korn RJ, Dockery DW, Speizer FE, et al: Occupational exposures and chronic respiratory symptoms. A population-based study. Am Rev Respir Dis 136:298, 1987.

171. Bakke S, Baste V, Hanoa R, Gulsvik A: Prevalence of obstructive lung disease in a general population: Relation to occupational title and exposure to some airborne agents. Thorax 46:863, 1991.

172. Diem JE, Jones RN, Hendrick DJ, et al: Five year longitudinal study of workers employed in a new toluene diisocyanate manufacturing plant. Am Rev Respir Dis 126:420, 1982.

173. Attfield MD: Longitudinal decline in $FEV_1$ in United States coalminers. Thorax 40:132, 1985.

174. Soutar CA, Hurley JF: Relation between dust exposure and lung function in miners and ex-miners. Br J Ind Med 43:307, 1986.

175. Rylander R: Organic dusts—from knowledge to prevention. Scand J Work Environ Health 20:116, 1994.

176. Cotes JE, Feinmann EL, Male VJ, et al: Respiratory symptoms and impairment in shipyard welders and caulker/burners. Br J Ind Med 46:292, 1989.

177. Morgan WKC: Industrial bronchitis. Br J Ind Med 35:285, 1978.

178. Oxman AD, Muir DC, Shannon HS, et al: Occupational dust exposure and chronic obstructive pulmonary disease. A systematic overview of the evidence. Am Rev Respir Dis 148:38, 1993.

179. Ruckley VA, Gauld SJ, Chapman JS, et al: Emphysema and dust exposure in a group of coal workers. Am Rev Respir Dis 129:528, 1984.

180. Becklake MR, Irwig L, Kielkowski D, et al: The predictors of emphysema in South African gold miners. Am Rev Respir Dis 135:1234, 1987.

181. Hnizdo E, Sluis-Cremer GK, Abramowitz JA: Emphysema type in relation to silica dust exposure in South African gold miners. Am Rev Respir Dis 143:1241, 1991.

182. Leigh J, Driscoll TR, Cole BD, et al: Quantitative relation between emphysema and lung mineral content in coalworkers. Occup Environ Med 51:400, 1994.

183. Kinsella M, Muller N, Vedal S, et al: Emphysema in silicosis. A comparison of smokers with nonsmokers using pulmonary function testing and computed tomography. Am Rev Respir Dis 141:1497, 1990.

184. Hnizdo E, Sluis-Cremer GK, Baskind E, Murray J: Emphysema and airway obstruction in non-smoking South African gold miners with long exposure to silica dust. Occup Environ Med 51:557, 1994.

185. Cohen BM, Adasczik A, Cohen EM, et al: Small airways changes in workers exposed to asbestos. Respiration 45:296, 1984.

186. Sue D, Oren A, Hansen J, et al: Lung function and exercise performance in smoking and non-smoking asbestos-exposed workers. Am Rev Respir Dis 132:612, 1985.

187. Bégin R, Boileau R, Péloquin S: Asbestos exposure, cigarette smoking, and airflow limitation in long-term Canadian chrysotile miners and millers. Am J Ind Med 11:55, 1987.

188. Bégin R, Filion R, Ostiguy G: Emphysema in silica- and asbestos-exposed workers seeking compensation. Chest 108:647, 1995.

189. Davison AG, Fayers PM, Newman Taylor AJ, et al: Cadmium fume inhalation and emphysema. Lancet 1:663, 1988.

190. Leduc D, de Francquen P, Jacobovitz D, et al: Association of cadmium exposure with rapidly progressive emphysema in a smoker. Thorax 48:570, 1993.

191. Snider GL, Lucey EC, Faris B, et al: Cadmium chloride–induced air-space enlargement with interstitial pulmonary fibrosis is not associated with destruction of lung elastin. Implications for the pathogenesis of human emphysema. Am Rev Respir Dis 137:918, 1988.

192. Chambers RC, McAnulty RJ, Shock A, et al: Cadmium selectively inhibits fibroblast procollagen production and proliferation. Am J Physiol 267:L300, 1994.

193. Chan-Yeung M, Wong R, MacLean L, et al: Respiratory survey of workers in a pulp and paper mill in Powell River, British Columbia. Am Rev Respir Dis 122:249, 1980.

194. Alegre J, Morell F, Cobo E: Respiratory symptoms and pulmonary function of workers exposed to cork dust, toluene diisocyanate and conidia. Scand J Work Environ Health 16:175, 1990.

195. Zejda JE, Dosman JA: Respiratory disorders in agriculture. Tuber Lung Dis 74:74, 1993.

196. Von Essen S: The role of endotoxin in grain dust exposure and airway obstruction. Curr Opin Pulm Med 3:198, 1997.

197. Hagmar L, Schutz A, Hallberg T, Sjoholm A: Health effects of exposure to endotoxins and organic dust in poultry slaughter-house workers. Int Arch Occup Environ Health 62:159, 1990.

198. Tockman MS, Baser M: Is cotton dust exposure associated with chronic effects? Am Rev Respir Dis 130:1, 1984.

199. Schachter EN, Maunder LR, Beck GJ: The pattern of lung function abnormalities in cotton textile workers. Am Rev Respir Dis 129:523, 1984.

200. Glindmeyer HW, Lefante JJ, Jones RN, et al: Cotton dust and across-shift change in $FEV_1$ as predictors of annual change in $FEV_1$. Am J Respir Crit Care Med 149:584, 1994.

201. Becklake MR: Relationship of acute obstructive airway change to chronic (fixed) obstruction. Thorax 50(Suppl):S16, 1995.

202. Chan-Yeung M, Lam S: State of the art: Occupational asthma. Am Rev Respir Dis 133:686, 1986.

203. Dopico GA, Flaherty D, Bhansali P, et al: Grain fever syndrome induced by inhalation of airborne grain dust. J Allergy Clin Immunol 69:435, 1982.

204. Cockcroft AE, McDermott M, Edwards JH, et al: Grain exposure symptoms and lung function. Eur J Respir Dis 64:189, 1983.

205. doPico GA, Reddan W, Anderson S, et al: Acute effects of grain dust exposure during a work shift. Am Rev Respir Dis 128:399, 1983.

206. Chan-Yeung M, Wong R, Maclean L: Respiratory abnormalities among grain elevator workers. Chest 75:461, 1979.

207. Dosman JA, Graham BL, Cotton DJ: Chronic bronchitis and exposure to cereal grain dust (editorial). Am Rev Respir Dis 120:477, 1979.

208. Cotton DJ, Graham BL, Li KYR, et al: Effects of smoking and occupational exposure on peripheral airway function in young cereal grain workers. Am Rev Respir Dis 126:660, 1982.
209. Tabona M, Chan-Yeung M, Enarson D, et al: Host factors affecting longitudinal decline in lung spirometry among grain elevator workers. Chest 85:782, 1984.
210. Yach D, Myers J, Bradshaw D, et al: A respiratory epidemiologic survey of grain mill workers in Cape-Town, South Africa. Am Rev Respir Dis 131:505, 1985.
211. Enarson DA, Vedal S, Chan-Yeung M: Rapid decline in FEV$_1$ in grain handlers—relation to level of dust exposure. Am Rev Respir Dis 132:814, 1985.
212. Mink JT, Gerrard JW, Cockcroft DW, et al: Increased bronchial reactivity to inhaled histamine in nonsmoking grain workers with normal lung function. Chest 77:28, 1980.
213. Enarson DA, Chan-Yeung M, Tabona M, et al: Predictors of bronchial hyperexcitability in grain handlers. Chest 87:452, 1985.
214. Cormier Y, Boulet LP, Bedard G, Tremblay G: Respiratory health of workers exposed to swine confinement buildings only or to both swine confinement buildings and dairy barns. Scand J Work Environ Health 17:269, 1991.
215. Choudat D, Goehen M, Korobaeff M, et al: Respiratory symptoms and bronchial reactivity among pig and dairy farmers. Scand J Work Environ Health 20:45, 1994.
216. Vogelzang PF, van der Gulden JW, Preller L, et al: Bronchial hyperresponsiveness and exposure in pig farmers. Int Arch Occup Environ Health 70:327, 1997.
217. Cormier Y, Duchaine C, Israel-Assayag E, et al: Effects of repeated swine building exposures on normal naive subjects. Eur Respir J 10:516, 1997.
218. Preller L, Doekes G, Heederik D, et al: Disinfectant use as a risk factor for atopic sensitization and symptoms consistent with asthma: An epidemiological study. Eur Respir J 9:1407, 1996.
219. Senthielselvan A, Dosman JA, Kirychuk SP, et al: Accelerated lung function decline in swine confinement workers. Chest 111:1733, 1997.
220. Sparrow D, Bossé R, Rosner B, et al: The effect of occupational exposure on pulmonary function. Am Rev Respir Dis 125:319, 1982.
221. Tashkin DP, Shapiro BJ, Lee YE, et al: Subacute effects of heavy marihuana smoking on pulmonary function in healthy men. N Engl J Med 294:125, 1976.
222. Tashkin DP, Coulson AH, Clark VA, et al: Respiratory symptoms and lung function in habitual heavy smokers of marijuana alone, smokers of marijuana and tobacco, smokers of tobacco alone, and nonsmokers. Am Rev Respir Dis 135:209, 1987.
223. DaCosta JL, Tock EPC, Boey HK: Lung disease with chronic obstruction in opium smokers in Singapore. Thorax 26:555, 1971.
223a. Roth MD, Arora A, Barsky SH, et al: Airway inflammation in young marijuana and tobacco smokers. Am J Respir Crit Care Med 157:928, 1998.
224. Colley JRT, Reid DD: Urban and social origins of childhood bronchitis in England and Wales. BMJ 2:213, 1970.
225. Colley JRT, Douglas JWB, Reid DD: Respiratory disease in young adults: Influence of early childhood lower respiratory tract illness, social class, air pollution, and smoking. BMJ 3:195, 1973.
226. Cederlöf R, Edfors ML, Friberg L, et al: Hereditary factors, "spontaneous cough" and "smoker's cough." A study of 7,800 twin-pairs with the aid of mailed questionnaires. Arch Environ Health 14:401, 1967.
227. Britten N, Davies JM, Colley JR: Early respiratory experience and subsequent cough and peak expiratory flow rate in 36 year old men and women. BMJ 294:1317, 1987.
228. Britton J, Martinez FD: The relationship of childhood respiratory infection to growth and decline in lung function. Am J Respir Crit Care Med 154(Suppl):240, 1996.
229. Boule M, Gaultier C, Tournier G, et al: Lung function in children with recurrent bronchitis. Respiration 38:127, 1979.
230. Woolcock AJ, Leeder SR, Peat JK, et al: The influence of lower respiratory illness in infancy and childhood and subsequent cigarette smoking on lung function in Sydney school children. Am Rev Respir Dis 120:5, 1979.
231. Woolcock A, Peat J, Leeder S, et al: The development of lung function in Sydney children: Effects of respiratory illness and smoking. A ten year study. Eur J Respir Dis 65:1, 1985.
232. Shaheen SO, Barker DJ, Holgate ST: Do lower respiratory tract infections in early childhood cause chronic obstructive pulmonary disease? Am J Respir Crit Care Med 151:1649, 1995.
233. Hallett WY: Infection: The real culprit in chronic bronchitis and emphysema? Med Clin North Am 57:735, 1973.
234. Martinez RD, Morgan WJ, Wright AL, et al. Diminished lung function as a predisposing factor for wheezing respiratory illness in infants. N Engl J Med 319:1112, 1988.
235. Tager IB, Hanrahan JP, Tosteson TD, et al: Lung function, pre- and post-natal smoke exposure, and wheezing in the first year of life. Am Rev Respir Dis 147:811, 1993.
236. Young S, O'Keeffe PT, Arnott J, Landau LI: Lung function, airway responsiveness, and respiratory symptoms before and after bronchiolitis. Arch Dis Child 72:16, 1995.
237. Martinez FD, Wright AL, Taussig LM, et al: Asthma and wheezing in the first six years of life. N Engl J Med 332:133, 1995.
238. Barker DJ, Godfrey KM, Fall C, et al: Relation of birth weight and childhood respiratory infection to adult lung function and death from chronic obstructive airways disease. BMJ 303:671, 1991.
239. Mas A, Mirapeix RM, Domingo C, et al: Pulmonary hypoplasia presented in adulthood as a chronic respiratory failure: Report of two cases. Embryology, clinical symptoms and diagnostic procedures. Respiration 64:240, 1997.
240. Holland WW: Beginnings of bronchitis. Thorax 37:401, 1982.
241. Hallett WY: Infection: The real culprit in chronic bronchitis and emphysema? Med Clin North Am 57:735, 1973.
242. Hegele RG, Hayashi S, Hogg JC, Paré PD: Mechanisms of airway narrowing and hyperresponsiveness in viral respiratory tract infections. Am J Respir Crit Care Med 151:1659, 1995.
243. Matsuse T, Hayashi S, Kuwano K, et al: Latent adenoviral infection in the pathogenesis of chronic airways obstruction. Am Rev Respir Dis 146:177, 1992.
244. Elliott WM, Hayashi S, Hogg JC: Immunodetection of adenoviral E1A proteins in human lung tissue. Am J Respir Cell Mol Biol 12:642, 1995.
245. Keicho N, Elliott WM, Hogg JC, Hayashi S. Adenovirus E1A gene dysregulates ICAM-1 expression in transformed pulmonary epithelial cells. Am J Respir Cell Mol Biol 16:23, 1997.
246. Gurwitz D, Corey M, Levison H, et al: Pulmonary function and bronchial reactivity in children after croup. Am Rev Respir Dis 122:95, 1980.
247. Barker DJ, Osmond C: Childhood respiratory infection and adult chronic bronchitis in England and Wales. BMJ 293:1271, 1986.
248. Medici TC, Buergi H: The role of immunoglobulin A in endogenous bronchial defense mechanisms in chronic bronchitis. Am Rev Respir Dis 103:784, 1971.
249. Lewis DM, Lapp N, Burrell R: Quantitation of secretory immunoglobulin A in chronic pulmonary disease. Am Rev Respir Dis 101:55, 1970.
250. Siegler DIM, Citron KM: Serum and parotid salivary IgA in chronic bronchitis and asthma. Thorax 29:313, 1974.
251. Falk GA, Okinaka AJ, Siskind GW: Immunoglobulins in the bronchial washings of patients with chronic obstructive pulmonary disease. Am Rev Respir Dis 105:14, 1972.
252. Orfanakis MG, Smith CB, Klauber MR, et al: Factors related to serum and secretory immunoglobulin concentrations in patients with chronic obstructive pulmonary disease. Am Rev Respir Dis 107:728, 1973.
253. Gump DW, Christmas WA, Forsyth BR, et al: Serum and secretory antibodies in patients with chronic bronchitis. Arch Intern Med 132:847, 1973.
254. Medici TC, Chodosh S: Sputum cell dynamics in bacterial exacerbations of chronic bronchial disease. Arch Intern Med 129:597, 1972.
255. Ritts RE, Miller RD, LeDuc PV, et al: Phagocytosis and cutaneous delayed hypersensitivity in patients with chronic obstructive pulmonary disease. Chest 69:474, 1976.
256. Massala C, Amendolea MA, Bonini S: Mucus antibodies in pulmonary tuberculosis and chronic obstructive lung disease. Lancet 2:821, 1976.
257. Picken JJ, Niewoehner DE, Chester EH: Prolonged effects of viral infections of the upper respiratory tract upon small airways. Am J Med 52:738, 1972.
258. Fridy WW Jr, Ingram RH Jr, Hierholzer JC, et al: Airway function during mild viral respiratory illness. Ann Intern Med 80:150, 1974.
259. Hall WJ, Hall CB, Speers DM: Respiratory syncytial virus infection in adults. Clinical, virologic, and serial pulmonary function studies. Ann Intern Med 88:203, 1978.
260. O'Connor SA, Jones DP, Collinsa JV, et al: Changes in pulmonary function after naturally acquired respiratory infection in normal persons. Am Rev Respir Dis 120:1087, 1979.
261. Little JW, Hall WJ, Douglas RG Jr, et al: Airway hyperreactivity and peripheral airway dysfunction in influenza A infection. Am Rev Respir Dis 118:295, 1978.
262. Blair HT, Greenberg SB, Stevens PM, et al: Effects of rhinovirus infection on pulmonary function of healthy human volunteers. Am Rev Respir Dis 114:95, 1976.
263. McFarlane JT, Morris MJ: Abnormalities in lung function following clinical recovery from *Mycoplasma pneumoniae* pneumonia. Eur J Respir Dis 63:337, 1982.
264. Macklem PT: Obstruction in small airways. Am J Med 52:721, 1972.
265. May JR, Peto R, Tinker CM, et al: A study of *Haemophilus influenzae* precipitins in the serum of working men in relation to smoking habits, bronchial infection, and airway obstruction. Am Rev Respir Dis 108:460, 1973.
266. Bates DV: The fate of the chronic bronchitic: A report of the ten-year follow-up in the Canadian Department of Veterans' Affairs coordinated study of chronic bronchitis. Am Rev Respir Dis 108:1043, 1973.
267. Fisher M, Akhtar AJ, Calder MA, et al: Pilot study of factors associated with exacerbations in chronic bronchitis. BMJ 4:187, 1969.
268. Burns MW, May JR: *Haemophilus influenzae* precipitins in the serum of patients with chronic bronchial disorders. Lancet 1:354, 1967.
269. May JR, Delves DM: The survival of *Haemophilus influenzae* and pneumococci in specimens of sputum sent to the laboratory by post. J Clin Pathol 17:254, 1964.
270. May JR, May DS: Bacteriology of sputum in chronic bronchitis. Tubercle 44:162, 1963.
271. Jenne JW, MacDonald FM, Lapinski EM, et al: The course of chronic *Haemophilus* bronchitis treated with massive doses of penicillin combined with streptomycin. Am Rev Respir Dis 101:907, 1970.
272. Reichek N, Lewin EB, Rhoden DL, et al: Antibody responses to bacterial antigens during exacerbations of chronic bronchitis. Am Rev Respir Dis 101:238, 1970.
273. Smith CB, Golden CA, Kanner RE, et al: *Haemophilus influenzae* and *Haemophilus parainfluenzae* in chronic obstructive pulmonary disease. Lancet 1:1253, 1976.
274. McNamara MJ, Phillips IA, Williams OB: Viral and *Mycoplasma pneumoniae* infections in exacerbations of chronic lung disease. Am Rev Respir Dis 100:19, 1969.
275. Sommerville RG: Respiratory syncytial virus in acute exacerbations of chronic bronchitis. Lancet 2:1247, 1963.

276. Stark JE, Heath RB, Curwen MP: Infection with influenza and parainfluenza viruses in chronic bronchitis. Thorax 20:124, 1965.

277. Ross CAC, McMichael S, Eadie MB, et al: Infective agents and chronic bronchitis. Thorax 21:461, 1966.

278. Eadie MB, Stott EJ, Grist NR: Virological studies in chronic bronchitis. BMJ 2:671, 1966.

279. Stenhouse AC: Viral antibody levels and clinical status in acute exacerbations of chronic bronchitis: A controlled prospective study. BMJ 3:287, 1968.

280. Grist NR: Group discussion: Virus infections in chronic bronchitis. 1. In acute exacerbations. *In* Tyrrell DAJ (ed): College of Pathologists, Acute Respiratory Diseases. Symposium organized by the College of Pathologists, London, February 1968. J Clin Pathol 21(Suppl 2):98, 1968.

281. Stern H: Group discussion: Virus infections in chronic bronchitis. A family study. *In* Tyrrell DAJ (ed): College of Pathologists, Acute Respiratory Diseases. Symposium organized by the College of Pathologists, London, February 1968. J Clin Pathol 21(Suppl 2):99, 1968.

282. Lamy ME, Pouthier-Simon F, Debacker-Willame E: Respiratory viral infections in hospital patients with chronic bronchitis. Chest 63:336, 1973.

283. Gump DW, Phillips CA, Forsyth BR, et al: Role of infection in chronic bronchitis. Am Rev Respir Dis 113:465, 1976.

284. Carilli AD, Gohd RS, Gordon W: A virologic study of chronic bronchitis. N Engl J Med 270:123, 1964.

284a. Von Hertzen L, Alakarppa H, Koskinen R, et al: *Chlamydia pneumoniae* infection in patients with chronic obstructive pulmonary disease. Epidemiol Infect 118:155, 1997.

284b. Von Hertzen L, Isoaho R, Leinonen M, et al: *Chlamydia pneumoniae* antibodies in chronic obstructive pulmonary disease. Int J Epidemiol 25:658, 1996.

285. Snider GL, Doctor L, Demas TA, et al: Obstructive airway disease in patients with treated pulmonary tuberculosis. Am Rev Respir Dis 103:625, 1971.

286. Osborne ML, Vollmer WM, Buist AS: Periodicity of asthma, emphysema, and chronic bronchitis in a northwest health maintenance organization. Chest 110:1458, 1996.

287. Govindaraj M: The effect of dehydration on the ventilatory capacity in normal subjects. Am Rev Respir Dis 105:842, 1972.

288. Koskela HO, Koskela AK, Tukiaineu HO: Bronchoconstriction due to cold weather in COPD. The roles of direct airway effects and cutaneous reflex mechanisms. Chest 110:632, 1996.

289. Greenburg L, Field F, Reed JI, et al: Asthma and temperature change. An epidemiological study of emergency clinic visits for asthma in three large New York hospitals. Arch Environ Health 8:642, 1964.

290. Cornwall CJ, Raffle PAB: Bronchitis—sickness absence in London transport. Br J Ind Med 18:24, 1961.

291. Burrows B, Lebowitz MD: Characteristics of chronic bronchitis in a warm, dry region. Am Rev Respir Dis 112:365, 1975.

292. Wells RE Jr, Walker JEC, Hickler RB: Effects of cold air on respiratory airflow resistance in patients with respiratory-tract disease. N Engl J Med 263:268, 1960.

293. Hsieh Y-C, Frayser R, Ross JC: The effect of cold-air inhalation on ventilation in normal subjects and in patients with chronic obstructive pulmonary disease. Am Rev Respir Dis 98:613, 1968.

294. Arnup ME, Mendella LA, Anthonisen NR, et al: Effects of cold air hyperpnea in patients with chronic obstructive lung disease. Am Rev Respir Dis 128:236, 1983.

295. Ramsdale E, Roberts R, Morris M, et al: Differences in responsiveness to hyperventilation and methacholine in asthma and chronic bronchitis. Thorax 40:422, 1985.

296. Tockman MS, Khoury MJ, Cohen BH: The epidemiology of COPD. *In* Lefant C (ed): Lung Biology in Health and Disease. Chronic Obstructive Disease. New York, Marcel Dekker, 1985, p 43.

297. Sandford AJ, Weir TD, Paré PD: Genetic risk factors for chronic obstructive pulmonary disease. Eur Respir J 10:1380, 1997.

298. Tager I, Tishler PV, Rosner B, et al: Studies of the familial aggregation of chronic bronchitis and obstructive airways disease. Int J Epidemiol 7:55, 1978.

299. Khoury MJ, Beaty TH, Newill CA, et al: Genetic-environmental interactions in chronic airways obstruction. Int J Epidemiol 15:65, 1986.

300. Higgins M, Keller J: Familial occurrence of chronic respiratory disease and familial resemblance in ventilatory capacity. J Chron Dis 28:239, 1975.

301. Speizer FE, Rosner B, Tager I: Familial aggregation of chronic respiratory disease: Use of national health interview survey data for specific hypothesis testing. Int J Epidemiol 5:167, 1976.

302. Kueppers F, Miller RD, Gordon H, et al: Familial prevalence of chronic obstructive pulmonary disease in a matched pair study. Am J Med 63:336, 1977.

303. Madison R, Zelman R, Mittman C: Inherited risk factors for chronic lung disease. Chest 77(Suppl 2):255, 1980.

304. Larson RK, Barman ML, Kueppers F, Fudenberg HH: Genetic and environmental determinants of chronic obstructive pulmonary disease. Ann Intern Med 72:627, 1970.

305. Cohen BH, Diamond EL, Graves CG, et al: A common familial component in lung cancer and chronic obstructive pulmonary disease. Lancet 2:523, 1977.

306. Tager IB, Rosner B, Tishler PV, et al: Household aggregation of pulmonary function and chronic bronchitis. Am Rev Respir Dis 114:485, 1976.

307. Kauffmann F, Tager IB, Muñoz A, Speizer FE: Familial factors related to lung function in children aged 6–10 years. Am J Epidemiol 129:1289, 1989.

308. Devor EJ, Crawford MH: Family resemblance for normal pulmonary function. Ann Hum Biol 11:439, 1984.

309. Redline S, Tishler PV, Rosner B, et al: Genotypic and phenotypic similarities in pulmonary function among family members of adult monozygotic and dizygotic twins. Am J Epidemiol 129:827, 1989.

310. Silverman EK, Chapman HA, Drazen JM, et al: Genetic epidemiology of severe, early-onset chronic obstructive pulmonary disease. Risk to relatives for airflow obstruction and chronic bronchitis. Am J Respir Crit Care Med 157:1770, 1998.

311. Zamel N, Webster P, Lorimer E, et al: Environment versus genetics in determining bronchial susceptibility to cigarette smoking. Chest 80(Suppl):57, 1981.

312. Redline S, Tishler PV, Lewitter FI, et al: Assessment of genetic and nongenetic influences on pulmonary function: A twin study. Am Rev Respir Dis 135:217, 1987.

313. Webster PM, Lorimer EG, Man SFP, et al: Pulmonary function in identical twins: Comparison of nonsmokers and smokers. Am Rev Respir Dis 119:223, 1979.

314. Hankins D, Drage C, Zamel N, Kronenberg R: Pulmonary function in identical twins raised apart. Am Rev Respir Dis 125:119, 1982.

315. Hubert HB, Fabsitz RR, Feinleib M, Gwinn C: Genetic and environmental influences on pulmonary function in adult twins. Am Rev Respir Dis 125:409, 1982.

316. Man SFP, Zamel N: Genetic influences on normal variability of maximum expiratory flow-volume curves. J Appl Physiol 41:874, 1976.

317. Lilienfeld AM, Lilienfeld D: Foundations of Epidemiology, 2nd ed. New York, Oxford University Press, 1980, pp 346–347.

318. Eriksson S: Pulmonary emphysema and alpha$_1$-antitrypsin deficiency. Acta Med Scand 175:197, 1964.

319. Burnett D, McGillivray DH, Stockley RA: Evidence that alveolar macrophages can synthesize and secrete alpha$_1$-antichymotrypsin. Am Rev Respir Dis 129:473, 1984.

320. Kilpatrick L, Johnson JL, Nickbarg EB, et al: Inhibition of human neutrophil superoxide generation by alpha$_1$-antichymotrypsin. J Immunol 146:2388, 1991.

321. Eriksson S, Lindmark B, Lilja H: Familial alpha$_1$-antichymotrypsin deficiency. Acta Med Scand 220:447, 1986.

322. Lindmark BE, Arborelius M, Eriksson SG: Pulmonary function in middle-aged women with heterozygous deficiency of the serine protease inhibitor alpha$_1$-antichymotrypsin. Am Rev Respir Dis 141:884, 1990.

323. Lindmark B, Svenonius E, Eriksson S: Heterozygous alpha$_1$-antichymotrypsin and PiZ alpha$_1$-antitrypsin deficiency. Prevalence and clinical spectrum in asthmatic children. Allergy 45:197, 1990.

324. Poller W, Faber J-B, Scholz S, et al: Mis-sense mutation of alpha$_1$-antichymotrypsin gene associated with chronic lung disease. Lancet 339:1538, 1992.

325. Poller W, Faber J-P, Weidinger S, et al: A leucine-to-proline substitution causes a defective alpha$_1$-antichymotrypsin allele associated with familial obstructive lung disease. Genomics 17:740, 1993.

326. Samilchuk EI, Chuchalin AG: Mis-sense mutation of alpha$_1$-antichymotrypsin gene and chronic lung disease. Lancet 342:624, 1993.

327. Sandford AJ, Chagani T, Weir TD, Paré PD: Alpha$_1$-antichymotrypsin mutations in patients with chronic obstructive pulmonary disease. Dis Markers 13:257, 1998.

328. Anderson CM, Freeman M, Allan J, Hubbard L: Observations on (i) sweat sodium levels in relation to chronic respiratory disease in adults and (ii) the incidence of respiratory and other disease in parents and siblings of patients with fibrocystic disease of the pancreas. Med J Aust 1:965, 1962.

329. Orzaleski MM, Kohner D, Cook CD, Shwachman H: Anamnesis. Sweat electrolyte and pulmonary function studies in parents of patients with cystic fibrosis of the pancreas. Acta Paediatr 52:267, 1963.

330. Batten J, Muir D, Simon G, Cedric C: The prevalence of respiratory disease in heterozygotes for the gene for fibrocystic disease of the pancreas. Lancet 1:1348, 1963.

331. Hallett WY, Knudson AG, Massey FJ: Absence of detrimental effect of the carrier state for the cystic fibrosis gene. Am Rev Respir Dis 90:714, 1965.

332. Davies PB: Autonomic and airway reactivity in obligate heterozygotes for cystic fibrosis. Am Rev Respir Dis 129:911, 1984.

333. Davis PB, Vargo K: Pulmonary abnormalities in obligate heterozygotes for cystic fibrosis. Thorax 42:120, 1987.

334. Dumur V, Lafitte J-J, Gervais R, et al: Abnormal distribution of cystic fibrosis δF$_{508}$ allele in adults with chronic bronchial hypersecretion. Lancet 335:1340, 1990.

335. Gervais R, Lafitte J-J, Dumur V, et al: Roussel P. 1993. Sweat chloride and δF508 mutation in chronic bronchitis or bronchiectasis. Lancet 342:997, 1993.

336. Artlich A, Boysen A, Bunge S, et al: Common CFTR mutations are not likely to predispose to chronic bronchitis in northern Germany. Hum Genet 95:226, 1995.

337. Entzian P, Müller E, Boysen A, et al: Frequency of common cystic fibrosis gene mutations in chronic bronchitis patients. Scand J Lab Invest 55:263, 1995.

338. Pignatti PF, Bombieri C, Marigo C, et al: Increased incidence of cystic fibrosis gene mutations in adults with disseminated bronchiectasis. Hum Mol Genet 4:635, 1995.

339. Gasparini P, Savoia A, Luisetti M, et al: The cystic fibrosis gene is not likely to be involved in chronic obstructive pulmonary disease. Am J Respir Cell Mol Biol 2:297, 1990.

340. Kew RR, Webster RO: Gc-globulin (vitamin D–binding protein) enhances the neutrophil chemotactic activity of C5a and C5a desArg. J Clin Invest 82:364, 1988.

341. Yamamoto N, Homma S: Vitamin D–binding protein (group-specific compo-

nent) is a precursor for the macrophage-activating signal factor from lysophosphatidylcholine-treated lymphocytes. Proc Natl Acad Sci U S A 88:8539, 1991.

342. Horne SL, Cockcroft DW, Dosman JA: Possible protective effect against chronic obstructive airways disease by the GC 2 allele. Hum Hered 40:173, 1990.

343. Schellenberg D, Paré PD, Weir TD, et al: Vitamin D–binding protein variants and the risk of COPD. Am J Respir Crit Care Med 157:957, 1998.

344. White R, Janoff A, Godfrey HP: Secretion of alpha-2-macroglobulin by alveolar macrophages. Lung 158:9, 1980.

345. Mosher DF, Wing WA: Synthesis and secretion of alpha₂-macroglobulin by cultured human fibroblasts. J Exp Med 143:462, 1976.

346. Böhm N, Shah I, Totovi̇f V, Karitzky D: Combined alpha₁-antitrypsin and alpha₂-macroglobulin deficiency syndrome: Light microscopic evidence of collagenolytic, elastolytic and myolytic tissue lesions. Path Res Prac 168:17, 1980.

347. Burnett D, Stockley RA: Serum and sputum alpha₂-macroglobulin in patients with chronic obstructive airways disease. Thorax 36:512, 1981.

348. Brissenden JE, Cox DW: alpha₂-macroglobulin in patients with obstructive lung disease, with and without alpha₁-antitrypsin deficiency. Clin Chim Acta 128:241, 1983.

349. Ganrot PO, Laurell CB, Eriksson S: Obstructive lung disease and trypsin inhibitors in alpha₁-antitrypsin deficiency. Scand J Clin Lab Invest 19:205, 1967.

350. Bergqvist D, Nilsson IM: Hereditary alpha₂-macroglobulin deficiency. Scand J Haematol 23:433, 1979.

351. Stenbjerg S: Inherited alpha₂-macroglobulin deficiency. Thrombosis Res 22:491, 1981.

352. Poller W, Barth J, Voss B: Detection of an alteration of the alpha₂-macroglobulin gene in a patient with chronic lung disease and serum alpha₂-macroglobulin deficiency. Hum Genet 83:93, 1989.

353. Drakoulis N, Cascorbi I, Brockmöller J, et al: Polymorphisms in the human CYP1A1 gene as susceptibility factors for lung cancer: Exon-7 mutation (4889 A to G), and a T to C mutation in the 3′-flanking region. Clin Invest 72:240, 1994.

354. Cantlay AM, Lamb D, Gillooly M, et al: Association between the CYP1A1 gene polymorphism and susceptibility to emphysema and lung cancer. J Clin Pathol Mol Pathol 48:M210, 1995.

355. Smith CAD, Harrison DJ: Association between polymorphism in gene for microsomal epoxide hydrolase and susceptibility to emphysema. Lancet 350:630, 1997.

356. Harrison DJ, Cantlay AM, Rae F, et al: Frequency of glutathione S-transferase M1 deletion in smokers with emphysema and lung cancer. Hum Exp Toxicol 16:356, 1997.

357. Cohen BH, Ball WC, Brashears S, et al: Risk factors in chronic obstructive pulmonary disease (COPD). Am J Epidemiol 105:223, 1977.

358. Beatty TH, Menkes HA, Cohen BH, Newill CA: Risk factors associated with longitudinal change in pulmonary function. Am Rev Respir Dis 129:660, 1984.

359. Krzyzanowski M, Jedrychowski W, Wysocki M: Factors associated with change in ventilatory function and the development of chronic obstructive pulmonary disease in a 13-year follow-up of the Cracow study. Am Rev Respir Dis 134:1011, 1986.

360. Higgins MW, Keller JB, Becker M, et al: An index of risk for obstructive airways disease. Am Rev Respir Dis 125:144, 1982.

361. Vestbo J, Hein HO, Suadicani P, et al: Genetic markers for chronic bronchitis and peak expiratory flow in the Copenhagen Male Study. Dan Med Bull 40:378, 1993.

362. Cohen BH, Bias WB, Chase GA, et al: Is ABH nonsecretor status a risk factor for obstructive lung disease? Am J Epidemiol 111:285, 1980.

363. Abboud RT, Yu P, Chan-Yeung M, Tan F: Lack of relationship between ABH secretor status and lung function in pulp mill workers. Am Rev Respir Dis 126:1089, 1982.

364. Horne SL, Cockcroft DW, Lovegrove A, Dosman JA: ABO, Lewis and secretor status and relative incidence of airflow obstruction. Dis Markers 3:55, 1985.

365. Kauffmann F, Frette C, Pham Q-T, et al: Associations of blood group–related antigens to FEV₁, wheezing and asthma. Am J Respir Crit Care Med 153:76, 1996.

366. Raza MW, Blackwell CC, Molyneaux P, et al: Association between secretor status and respiratory viral illness. BMJ 303:815, 1991.

367. Kauffmann F, Kleisbauer J-P, Cambon-de-Mouzon A, et al: Genetic markers in chronic air-flow limitation: A genetic epidemiologic study. Am Rev Respir Dis 127:263, 1983.

368. Oxelius VA, Laurell AB, Lindquist B, et al: IgG subclasses in selective IgA deficiency. N Engl J Med 304:1476, 1981.

369. Björkander J, Bake B, Oxelius VA, Hanson LA: Impaired lung function in patients with IgA deficiency and low levels of IgG2 or IgG3. N Engl J Med 313:720, 1985.

370. O'Keefe S, Gzel A, Drury R, et al: Immunoglobulin G subclasses and spirometry in patients with chronic obstructive pulmonary disease. Eur Respir J 4:932, 1991.

371. Webb DR, Condemi JJ: Selective immunoglobulin A deficiency and chronic obstructive lung disease. Ann Intern Med 80:618, 1974.

372. Meine F, Grossman H, Forman W, et al: The radiographic findings in congenital cutis laxa. Radiology 113:687, 1974.

373. Lally JF, Gohel VK, Dalinka MK, et al: The roentgenographic manifestations of cutis laxa (generalized elastolysis). Radiology 113:605, 1974.

374. Bonneau D, Huret JL, Godeau G, et al: Recurrent ctb(7)(q31.3) and possible laminin involvement in a neonatal cutis laxa with a Marfan phenotype. Hum Genet 87:317, 1991.

375. Ramirez F: Fibrillin mutations in Marfan syndrome and related phenotypes. Curr Opin Genet Devel 6:309, 1996.

376. Wood JR, Bellamy D, Child AH, et al: Pulmonary disease in patients with Marfan syndrome. Thorax 39:780, 1984.

377. Maeda T, Suzuki Y, Haeno S, et al: Ehlers-Danlos syndrome and congenital heart anomalies. Intern Med 35:200, 1996.

378. Rasmussen FV: Associations between housing conditions, smoking habits and ventilatory lung function in men with clean jobs. Br J Dis Chest 72:261, 1978.

379. Rasmussen FV, Borchsenius L, Winslow JB, et al: Associations between housing conditions, smoking habits and ventilatory lung function in men with clean jobs. Scand J Respir Dis 59:264, 1978.

380. Cohen BH, Celentano DD, Chase GA, et al: Alcohol consumption and airways obstruction. Am Rev Respir Dis 121:205, 1980.

381. Pratt PC, Vollmer RT: The beneficial effect of alcohol consumption on the prevalence and extent of centrilobular emphysema. Chest 85:372, 1984.

382. Schwartz J, Weiss ST: Dietary factors and their relation to respiratory symptoms. Am J Epidemiol 132:67, 1990.

383. Britton J: Dietary fish oil and airways obstruction. Thorax 50(Suppl):11, 1995.

384. Shahar E, Folsom AR, Melnick SL, et al: Dietary n-3 polyunsaturated fatty acids and smoking-related chronic obstructive pulmonary disease. Atherosclerosis Risk in Communities Study Investigators. N Engl J Med 331:228, 1994.

385. Gray-Donald K, Gibbons L, Shapiro SH, et al: Nutritional status and mortality in chronic obstructive pulmonary disease. Am J Respir Crit Care Med 153:961, 1996.

386. Pride NB: Which smokers develop progressive airflow obstruction. Eur J Respir Dis 64(Suppl 126):79, 1983.

387. Weiss ST, Speizer FE: Increased levels of airways responsiveness as a risk factor for development of chronic obstructive lung disease: What are the issues? Chest 86:3, 1984.

388. de Jong JW, Koeter GH, Postma DS: The significance of airway responsiveness in the onset and evolution of chronic obstructive pulmonary disease. Clin Exp Allergy 27:1114, 1997.

389. Rijcken B, Weiss ST: Longitudinal analyses of airway responsiveness and pulmonary function decline. Am J Respir Crit Care Med 154(Suppl):246, 1996.

390. Barter CE, Campbell AH: Relationship of constitutional factors and cigarette smoking to decrease in one second forced expiratory volume. Am Rev Respir Dis 113:305, 1976.

391. Taylor RG, Joyce H, Gross E, et al: Bronchial reactivity to inhaled histamine and annual rate of decline in FEV₁ in male smokers and ex-smokers. Thorax 40:9, 1985.

392. Kanner RE: The relationship between airways responsiveness and chronic airflow limitation. Chest 86:54, 1984.

393. Postma DS, de Vries K, Koeter GH, et al: Independent influence of reversibility of air-flow obstruction and nonspecific hyperreactivity on the long-term course of lung function in chronic air-flow obstruction. Am Rev Respir Dis 134:276, 1986.

394. Rijcken B, Schouten JP, Xu X, et al: Airway hyperresponsiveness to histamine associated with accelerated decline in FEV₁. Am J Respir Crit Care Med 151:1377, 1995.

395. Frew AJ, Kennedy SM, Chan-Yeung M: Methacholine responsiveness, smoking, and atopy as risk factors for accelerated FEV₁ decline in male working populations. Am Rev Respir Dis 146:878, 1992.

396. O'Connor GT, Sparrow D, Weiss ST: A prospective longitudinal study of methacholine airway responsiveness as a predictor of pulmonary-function decline: The Normative Aging Study. Am J Respir Crit Care Med 152:87, 1995.

397. Ramsdell JW, Nachtwey FJ, Moser KM, et al: Bronchial hyperreactivity in chronic obstructive bronchitis. Am Rev Respir Dis 126:829, 1982.

398. Yan K, Salome CM, Woolcock AJ, et al: Prevalence and nature of bronchial hyperresponsiveness in subjects with chronic obstructive pulmonary disease. Am Rev Respir Dis 132:27, 1985.

399. Bahous A, Cartier A, Ouimet G, et al: Nonallergic bronchial hyperexcitability in chronic bronchitis. Am Rev Respir Dis 129:216, 1984.

400. Ulrik CS, Backer V: Longitudinal determinants of bronchial responsiveness to inhaled histamine. Chest 113:973, 1998.

401. Riess A, Wiggs B, Verburgt L, et al: Morphologic determinants of airway responsiveness in chronic smokers. Am J Respir Crit Care Med 154:1444, 1996.

402. Sterk PJ: The determinants of the severity of acute airway narrowing in asthma and COPD. Respir Med 86:391, 1992.

403. Paré PD, Armour C, Taylor S, et al: Airway hyperreactivity in COPD: Cause or effect? An *in vivo, in vitro* comparison. Chest 91:405, 1987.

404. Anthonisen NR, Wright EC, Hodgkin JE: Prognosis in chronic obstructive pulmonary disease. Am Rev Respir Dis 133:14, 1986.

405. Rijcken B, Schouten JP, Weiss ST, et al: The relationship of nonspecific bronchial responsiveness to respiratory symptoms in a random population sample. Am Rev Respir Dis 136:62, 1987.

406. Anthonisen NR, Connett JE, Kiley JP, et al: Effects of smoking intervention and the use of an inhaled anticholinergic bronchodilator on the rate of decline of FEV₁. The Lung Health Study. JAMA 272:1497, 1994.

407. Tashkin DP, Altose MD, Connett JE, et al: Methacholine reactivity predicts changes in lung function over time in smokers with early chronic obstructive pulmonary disease. The Lung Health Study Research Group. Am J Respir Crit Care Med 153:1802, 1996.

408. Xu X, Rijcken B, Schouten JP, Weiss ST: Airways responsiveness and development and remission of chronic respiratory symptoms in adults. Lancet 350:1431, 1997.

409. Taylor RG, Gross E, Joyce H, et al: Smoking, allergy, and the differential white blood cell count. Thorax 40:17, 1985.
410. Burrows B, Lebowitz MD, Barbee RA, et al: Interactions of smoking and immunologic factors in relation to airways obstruction. Chest 84:657, 1983.
411. Burrows B, Hasan FM, Barbee RA, et al: Epidemiologic observations on eosinophilia and its relation to respiratory disorders. Am Rev Respir Dis 122:709, 1980.
412. Casterline CL: Interaction of immunoglobulin E and cigarette smoke: Predisposition to symptomatic lung disease? Chest 84:652, 1983.
413. Frette C, Annesi I, Korobaeff M, et al: Blood eosinophilia and $FEV_1$. Cross-sectional and longitudinal analyses. Am Rev Respir Dis 143:987, 1991.
414. Pauwels R, Van Der Straeten M: Total serum IgE levels in normals and patients with chronic non-specific lung diseases. Allergy 33:254, 1978.
415. Bloom JW, Halonen M, Dunn AM, et al: Pneumococcus-specific immunoglobulin E in cigarette smokers. Clin Allergy 16:25, 1986.
416. Burrows B, Halonen M, Barbee RA, et al: The relationship of serum immunoglobulin-E to cigarette smoking. Am Rev Respir Dis 124:523, 1981.
417. Zetterstrom O, Nordvall SL, Bjorksten B, et al: Increased IgE antibody responses in rats exposed to tobacco smoke. J Allergy Clin Immunol 75:594, 1985.
418. Tollerud DJ, Clark JW, Morris-Brown L, et al: The effects of cigarette smoking on T cell subsets. Am Rev Respir Dis 139:1446, 1989.
419. Byron KA, Varigos GA, Wootton AM: Interleukin-4 production is increased in cigarette smokers. Clin Exp Immunol 95:333, 1994.
420. Villar MT, Holgate ST: IgE, smoking and lung function (editorial). Clin Exp Allergy 25:206, 1995.
421. Burrow B, Knudson RJ, Cline MG, Lebowitz MD: A re-examination of risk factors for ventilatory impairment. Am Rev Respir Dis 138:829, 1988.
422. Parker DR, O'Connor GT, Sparrow D, et al: The relationship of nonspecific airway responsiveness and atopy to the rate of decline of lung function. Am Rev Respir Dis 141:589, 1990.
423. Taylor RG, Joyce H, Gross E, et al: Bronchial reactivity to inhaled histamine and annual rate of decline in $FEV_1$ in male smokers and ex-smokers. Thorax 40:9, 1985.
424. O'Connor GT, Sparrow D, Segal M, Weiss ST: Risk factors for ventilatory impairment among middle-aged and elderly men. The Normative Aging Study. Chest 103:376, 1993.
425. Sherrill DL, Lebowitz MD, Halonen M, et al: Longitudinal evaluation of the association between pulmonary function and total serum IgE. Am J Respir Crit Care Med 152:98, 1995.
426. Dow L, Coggon D, Campbell MJ, et al: The interaction between immunoglobulin E and smoking in airflow obstruction in the elderly. Am Rev Respir Dis 146:402, 1992.
427. Burrows B: Epidemiologic evidence for different types of chronic airflow obstruction. Am Rev Respir Dis 143:1452, 1991.
428. Lopez-Vidriero MT, Reid L: Chemical markers of mucous and serum glycoproteins and their relation to viscosity in mucoid and purulent sputum from various hypersecretory diseases. Am Rev Respir Dis 117:465, 1978.
429. Girard F, Puchelle E, Aug F, et al: Protein evolution in bronchial secretions during an episode of superinfection in chronic bronchitis. Bull Eur Physiopathol Respir 15:513, 1979.
430. Puchelle E, Zahm J-M, Aug F: Viscoelasticity, protein content and ciliary transport rate of sputum in patients with recurrent and chronic bronchitis. Biorheology 18:659, 1981.
431. Hasani A, Pavia D, Agnew JE, Clarke SW: Regional lung clearance during cough and forced expiration technique (FET): Effects of flow and viscoelasticity. Thorax 49:557, 1994.
432. Puchelle E, Zahm JM, Girard F, et al: Mucociliary transport in vivo and in vitro. Relations to sputum properties in chronic bronchitis. Eur J Respir Dis 61:254, 1980.
433. Foster WM, Langenback E, Bergofsky E, et al: Disassociation in the mucociliary function of central and peripheral airways of asymptomatic smokers. Am Rev Respir Dis 132:633, 1985.
434. Wanner A, Salathe M, O'Riordan TG: Mucociliary clearance in the airways. Am J Respir Crit Care Med 154:1868, 1996.
435. Weiss T, Dorow P, Felix R: Regional mucociliary removal of inhaled particles in smokers with small airways disease. Respiration 44:338, 1983.
436. Goodman RM, Yergin BM, Landa JF, et al: Relationship of smoking history and pulmonary function tests to tracheal mucus velocity in non-smokers, young smokers, ex-smokers and patients with chronic bronchitis. Am Rev Respir Dis 117:205, 1978.
437. Agnew JE, Little F, Pavia D, et al: Mucus clearance from the airways in chronic bronchitis: Smokers and ex-smokers. Bull Eur Physiopathol Respir 18:473, 1982.
438. Matthys H, Vastag E, Kohler D, et al: Mucociliary clearance in patients with chronic bronchitis and bronchial carcinoma. Respiration 44:329, 1983.
439. Svartengren K, Ericsson CH, Svartengren M, et al: Deposition and clearance in large and small airways in chronic bronchitis. Exp Lung Res 22:555, 1996.
440. Lauque D, Aug F, Puchelle E, et al: Efficiency of mucociliary clearance and cough in bronchitis. Bull Eur Physiopathol Respir 20:145, 1985.
441. Yeates DB: The role of mucociliary transport in the pathogenesis of chronic obstructive pulmonary disease. *In* Chantler EEN, Elder JB, Elstein M (eds): Mucus in Health and Disease. No 2. Advances in Experimental Medicine and Biology. New York, Plenum Press, 1982, p 411.
442. Oldenburg FA Jr, Dolovich MD, Montgomery JM, et al: Effects of postural drainage, exercise and cough on mucus clearance in chronic bronchitis. Am Rev Respir Dis 120:739, 1979.
443. Lungarella G, Fonzi L, Ermini G, et al: Abnormalities of bronchial cilia in patients with chronic bronchitis. Lung 161:147, 1983.
444. Verra F, Escudier E, Lebargy F, et al: Ciliary abnormalities in bronchial epithelium of smokers, ex-smokers, and nonsmokers. Am J Respir Crit Care Med 151:630, 1995.
445. Welsh JM: Cigarette smoke inhibition of ion transport in canine tracheal epithelium. J Clin Invest 71:1615, 1983.
446. Mossberg B, Camner P: Impaired mucociliary transport as a pathogenetic factor in obstructive pulmonary diseases. Chest 77:265, 1980.
447. Pavia D, Thomson ML, Clarke SW: Enhanced clearance of secretions from the human lung after the administration of hypertonic saline aerosol. Am Rev Respir Dis 117:199, 1978.
448. Mossberg B, Strandbert K, Camner P: Stimulatory effect of beta-adrenergic drugs on mucociliary transport. Scand J Respir Dis 101(Suppl):71, 1977.
449. Janoff A: Elastase in tissue injury. Annu Rev Med 36:207, 1985.
450. Janoff A: Elastases and emphysema—current assessment of the protease-antiprotease hypothesis. Am Rev Respir Dis 132:417, 1985.
451. Snider GL: The pathogenesis of emphysema—20 years of progress. Am Rev Respir Dis 124:321, 1981.
452. Shapiro SD: Mighty mice: Transgenic technology "knocks out" questions of matrix metalloproteinase function. Matrix Biol 15:527, 1997.
453. Finlay GA, Russell KJ, McMahon KJ, et al: Elevated levels of matrix metalloproteinases in bronchoalveolar lavage fluid of emphysematous patients. Thorax 52:502, 1997.
454. Finlay GA, LR OD, Russell KJ, EM DA, Masterson JB, et al: Matrix metalloproteinase expression and production by alveolar macrophages in emphysema. Am J Respir Crit Care Med 156:240, 1997.
455. Muley T, Wiebel M, Schulz V, Ebert W: Elastinolytic activity of alveolar macrophages in smoking-associated pulmonary emphysema. Clin Investig 72:269, 1994.
456. Gadek JE, Fells GA, Zimmerman RL, et al: Antielastases of the human alveolar structures—implications for the protease-antiprotease theory of emphysema. J Clin Invest 68:889, 1981.
457. Sallenave J-M, Shulmann J, Crossley J, et al: Regulation of secretory leukocyte proteinase inhibitor (SLPI) and elastase-specific inhibitor (ESI/Elafin) in human airway epithelial airway cells by cytokines and neutrophilic enzymes. Am J Respir Cell Mol Biol 11:733, 1994.
458. Evans MD, Pryor WA: Cigarette smoking, emphysema, and damage to alpha$_1$-proteinase inhibitor. Am J Physiol 266:L593, 1994.
459. Hoidal JR, Niewoehner DE: Pathogenesis of emphysema. Chest 83:679, 1983.
460. Kuhn C, Senior RM: The role of elastases in the development of emphysema. Lung 155:185, 1978.
461. Abe T, Kobayashi N, Yoshimura K, et al: Expression of the secretory leukoprotease inhibitor gene in epithelial cells. J Clin Invest 87:2207, 1991.
462. Sparrow D, Glynn RJ, Cohen M, et al: The relationship of the peripheral leukocyte count and cigarette smoking to pulmonary function among adult men. Chest 86:383, 1984.
463. Chan Yeung M, Buncio AD: Leukocyte count, smoking and lung function. Am J Med 76:31, 1984.
464. Ludwig P, Schwartz B, Hoidal J, et al: Cigarette smoking causes accumulation of polymorphonuclear leukocytes in alveolar septum. Am Rev Respir Dis 131:828, 1985.
465. Martin T, Raghu G, Maunder R, et al: The effects of chronic bronchitis and chronic airflow obstruction on lung cell populations recovered by bronchoalveolar lavage. Am Rev Respir Dis 132:254, 1985.
466. Weiss ST, Segal MR, Sparrow D, Wager C: Relation of $FEV_1$ and peripheral blood leukocyte count to total mortality. The normative aging study. Am J Epidemiol 142:493, 1995.
467. Terashima T, Wiggs B, English D, et al: The effect of cigarette smoking on the bone marrow. Am J Respir Crit Care Med 15:1021, 1997.
468. Bridges RB, Wyatt RJ, Rehm SR: Effects of smoking on inflammatory mediators and their relationship to pulmonary dysfunction. Eur J Respir Dis 146(Suppl):145, 1986.
469. Hunninghake GW, Crystal RG: Cigarette smoking and lung destruction—accumulation of neutrophils in the lungs of cigarette smokers. Am Rev Respir Dis 128:833, 1983.
470. Hobson JE, Wright JL, Wiggs BR, et al: Comparison of the cell content of lung lavage fluid with the presence of emphysema and peripheral airways inflammation in resected lungs. Respiration 50:1, 1986.
471. Hogg JC: Neutrophil kinetics and lung injury. Physiol Rev 67:1249, 1987.
472. Selby C, Drost E, Gillooly M, Cameron E, Lamb D and MacNee W. Neutrophil sequestration in lungs removed at surgery. The effect of microscopic emphysema. Am J Respir Crit Care Med 149:1526, 1994.
473. Muir AL, Cruz M, Martin BA, et al: Leukocyte kinetics in the human lung. Role of exercise and catecholamines. J Appl Physiol 57:711, 1984.
474. Hogg JC, Martin BA, Lee S, et al: Regional differences in erythrocyte transit in normal. J Appl Physiol 59:1266, 1985.
475. Drost EM, Selby C, Lannan S, et al: Changes in neutrophil deformability following in vitro smoke exposure: Mechanism and protection. Am J Respir Cell Mol Biol 6:287, 1993.
476. Drost EM, Selby C, Bridgeman MME, MacNee W: Decreased deformability after acute cigarette smoking in humans. Am Rev Respir Dis 148:1277, 1993.
477. MacNee W, Wiggs B, Belzberg AS, Hogg JC: The effects of cigarette smoking on neutrophil kinetics in human lungs. N Engl J Med 321:924, 1989.

478. Hogg JC: The traffic of polymorphonuclear leukocytes through pulmonary microvessels in health and disease. Felix Fleischner Lecture. Am J Roentgenol 163:769, 1994.

479. Hunninghake GW, Crysal RG. Cigarette smoking and lung destruction: Accumulation of neutrophils in the lungs of cigarette smokers. Am Rev Respir Dis 128:833, 1983.

480. Shoji S, Ertl RF, Koyama S, et al: Cigarette smoke stimulates release of neutrophil chemotactic activity from cultured bovine bronchial epithelial cells. Clin Sci 88:337, 1995.

481. Kew RR, Ghebrehiwet B, Janoff A, et al: Cigarette smoke can activate the alternative pathway of complement in vitro by modifying the third component of complement. J Clin Invest 75:1000, 1985.

482. Kosmas EN, Zorpidou D, Vassilareas V, et al: Decreased C4 complement component serum levels correlate with the degree of emphysema in patients with chronic bronchitis. Chest 112:341, 1997.

483. Klut ME, Doerschuk CM, Hogg JC, et al: Activation of neutrophils within pulmonary microvessels of rabbits exposed to cigarette smoke. Am J Respir Cell Mol Biol 9:82, 1993.

484. Lam S, Chan-Yeung M, Abboud R, et al: Interrelationships between serum chemotactic factor inactivator, alpha₁-antitrypsin deficiency and chronic obstructive lung disease. Am Rev Respir Dis 121:507, 1980.

485. Blue M-L, Janoff A: Possible mechanisms of emphysema in cigarette smokers. Release of elastase from human polymorphonuclear leukocytes by cigarette smoke condensate in vitro. Am Rev Respir Dis 117:317, 1978.

486. Rodriguez JR, Seals JE, Radin A, et al: Neutrophil lysosomal elastase activity in normal subjects and in patients with chronic obstructive pulmonary disease. Am Rev Respir Dis 119:409, 1979.

487. Abboud RT, Rushton J-M, Grzybowski S, et al: Interrelationships between neutrophil elastase, serum alpha₁-antitrypsin, lung function, and chest radiography in patients with chronic airflow obstruction. Am Rev Respir Dis 120:31, 1979.

488. Kramps JA, Bakker W, Dijkman JH, et al: A matched-pair study of the leukocyte elastase–like activity in normal persons and in emphysematous patients with and without alpha₁-antitrypsin deficiency. Am Rev Respir Dis 121:253, 1980.

489. Bridges RB, Wyatt RJ, Rehm SR: Effect of smoking on peripheral blood leukocytes and serum antiproteases. Eur J Respir Dis 139(Suppl):24, 1985.

490. Finley TN, Swenson EW, Curran WS, et al: Bronchopulmonary lavage in normal subjects and patients with obstructive lung disease. Ann Intern Med 66:651, 1967.

491. Harris JO, Olsen GN, Castle JR, et al: Comparison of proteolytic enzyme activity in pulmonary alveolar macrophages and blood leukocytes in smokers and nonsmokers. Am Rev Respir Dis 111:579, 1975.

492. Harris JO, Swenson EW, Johnson JE III: Human alveolar macrophages: Comparison of phagocytic ability, glucose utilization, and ultrastructure in smokers and nonsmokers. J Clin Invest 49:2086, 1970.

493. Reilly JJ Jr, Chen P, Sailor LZ, et al: Cigarette smoking induces an elastolytic cysteine proteinase in macrophages distinct from cathepsin L. Am J Physiol 261:L41, 1991.

494. Richards GA, Theron AJ, Van Der Merwe CA, et al: Spirometric abnormalities in young smokers correlate with increased chemiluminescence responses of activated blood phagocytes. Am Rev Respir Dis 139:181, 1989.

495. Cohen AB: The effects in vivo and in vitro of oxidative damage to purified alpha₁-antitrypsin and to the enzyme-inhibiting activity of plasma. Am Rev Respir Dis 119:953, 1979.

496. Pryor WA, Stone K: Oxidants in cigarette smoke: Radicals, hydrogen peroxide, peroxynitrate and peroxynitrite. Ann N Y Acad Sci 686:12, 1993.

497. Padmaja S, Huie RE: The reaction of nitric oxide with organic peroxyl radicals. Biochem Biophys Res Commun 195:539, 1993.

498. Carp H, Janoff A: Possible mechanisms of emphysema in smokers: In vitro suppression of serum elastase–inhibitory capacity by fresh cigarette smoke and its prevention by antioxidants. Am Rev Respir Dis 118:617, 1978.

499. Janoff A, Dearing R: Alpha₁-proteinase inhibitor is more sensitive to inactivation by cigarette smoke than is leukocyte elastase. Am Rev Respir Dis 126:691, 1982.

500. Cantin A, Crystal RG: Oxidants, antioxidants and the pathogenesis of emphysema. Eur J Respir Dis 66(Suppl 139):7, 1985.

501. Laurent P, Janoff A, Dagan HM: Cigarette smoke blocks cross-linking of elastin in vitro. Am Rev Respir Dis 127:189, 1983.

502. Rahman I, MacNee W: Role of oxidants/antioxidants in smoking-induced lung diseases. Free Radic Biol Med 21:669, 1996.

503. al Senaidy AM, al Zahrany YA, al Faqeeh MB: Effects of smoking on serum levels of lipid peroxides and essential fat-soluble antioxidants. Nutr Health 12:55, 1997.

504. Taylor JC, Madison R, Kosinska D: Is antioxidant deficiency related to chronic obstructive pulmonary disease? Am Rev Respir Dis 134:285, 1986.

505. Lellouch J, Claude JR, Martin JP, et al: Smoking does not reduce the functional activity of serum alpha₁ proteinase inhibitor—an epidemiologic study of 719 healthy men. Am Rev Respir Dis 132:818, 1985.

506. Chowdhury P, Bone RC, Louria DB, et al: Effect of cigarette smoke on human serum trypsin inhibitory capacity and antitrypsin concentrations. Am Rev Respir Dis 126:177, 1982.

507. Martin WJ II, Taylor JC: Abnormal interaction of alpha₁-antitrypsin and leukocyte elastolytic activity in patients with chronic obstructive pulmonary disease. Am Rev Respir Dis 120:411, 1979.

508. Binder R, Stone RJ, Calore JD, et al: Serum antielastase and neutrophil elastase levels in PiM phenotype cigarette smokers with airflow obstruction. Respiration 47:267, 1985.

509. Fera T, Abboud RT, Johal SS, et al: Effect of smoking on functional activity of plasma alpha₁-protease inhibitor. Chest 91:346, 1987.

510. Abboud RT, Fera T, Johal S, et al: Effects of smoking on plasma neutrophil elastase levels. J Lab Clin Med 108:294, 1986.

511. Damiano VV, Tsang A, Kucich U, et al: Immunolocalization of elastase in human emphysematous lungs. J Clin Invest 78:482, 1986.

512. Stockley RA, Burnett D: Alpha₁-antitrypsin and leukocyte elastase in infected and noninfected sputum. Am Rev Respir Dis 120:1081, 1979.

513. Abboud RT, Fera T, Richter A, et al: Acute effect of smoking on the functional activity of alpha₁-protease inhibitor in bronchoalveolar lavage fluid. Am Rev Respir Dis 131:79, 1985.

514. Ogushi F, Hubbard RC, Vogelmeier C, et al: Risk factors for emphysema. Cigarette smoking is associated with a reduction in the association rate constant of lung alpha₁-antitrypsin for neutrophil elastase. J Clin Invest 87:1060, 1991.

515. Fujita J, Nelson NL, Daughton DM, et al: Evaluation of elastase and antielastase balance in patients with chronic bronchitis and pulmonary emphysema. Am Rev Respir Dis 142:57, 1990.

516. Galdston M, Levytska V, Schwartz MS, et al: Ceruloplasmin: Serum concentration and impaired antioxidant activity in cigarette smokers, and ability to prevent suppression of elastase inhibitory capacity of alpha₁-protease inhibitor. Am Rev Respir Dis 129:258, 1984.

517. Rasche B, Hochstrasser K, Albrecht GJ, et al: An elastase-specific inhibitor from human bronchial mucus. Respiration 44:397, 1983.

518. Cardoso WV, Sekhon HS, Hyde DM, Thurlbeck WM: Collagen and elastin in human pulmonary emphysema. Am Rev Respir Dis 147:975, 1993.

519. Dillon TJ, Walsh RL, Scicchitano R, et al: Plasma elastin–derived peptide levels in normal adults, children, and emphysematous subjects. Physiologic and computed tomographic scan correlates. Am Rev Respir Dis 146:1143, 1992.

520. Frette C, Jacob MP, Defouilloy C, et al: Lack of a relationship of elastin peptide level to emphysema assessed by CT scans. Am J Respir Crit Care Med 153:1544, 1996.

521. Gottlieb DJ, Stone PJ, Sparrow D, et al: Urinary desmosine excretion in smokers with and without rapid decline of lung function: The Normative Aging Study. Am J Respir Crit Care Med 154:1290, 1996.

522. Stone PJ, Gottlieb DJ, O'Connor GT, et al: Elastin and collagen degradation products in urine of smokers with and without chronic obstructive pulmonary disease. Am J Respir Crit Care Med 151:952, 1995.

523. Fukuda Y, Masuda Y, Ishizaki M, et al: Morphogenesis of abnormal elastic fibers in lungs of patients with panacinar and centriacinar emphysema. Hum Pathol 20:652, 1989.

524. Lang MR, Fiaux GW, Gillooly M, et al: Collagen content of alveolar wall tissue in emphysematous and nonemphysematous lungs. Thorax 49:319, 1994.

525. Renkema TE, Postma DS, Noordhoek JA, et al: In vitro release of neutrophil elastase, myeloperoxidase and beta-glucuronidase in patients with emphysema and healthy subjects. Eur Respir J 4:1237, 1991.

526. Gross P, Pfitzer EA, Tolker E, et al: Experimental emphysema: Its production with papain in normal and silicotic rats. Arch Environ Health 11:50, 1965.

527. Rubin LJ, Windberg P, Taylor W, Heatfield B: Pulmonary vascular structural and functional changes in papain-induced emphysema in dogs. Am Rev Respir Dis 136:704, 1987.

528. Mink SN: Expiratory flow limitation and the response to breathing a helium-oxygen gas mixture in a canine model of pulmonary emphysema. J Clin Invest 73:1321, 1984.

529. Marco V, Meranze DR, Bentivoglio LG, et al: Papain-induced experimental emphysema in the dog. Fed Proc 28:526, 1969.

530. Pushpakom R, Hogg JC, Woolcock AJ, et al: Experimental papain-induced emphysema in dogs. Am Rev Respir Dis 102:778, 1970.

531. Kilburn KH, Dowell AR, Pratt PC: Morphological and biochemical assessment of papain-induced emphysema. Arch Intern Med 127:884, 1971.

532. Goldring IP, Park SS, Greenberg L, et al: Sequential anatomic changes in lungs exposed to papain and other proteolytic enzymes. In Mittman C (ed): Pulmonary Emphysema and Proteolysis. New York, Academic Press, 1972, p 389.

533. Kleinerman J, Rynbrandt DJ: Papain-induced emphysema in hamsters: The effect of agents that increase serum alpha₁-antitrypsin. In Mittman C (ed): Pulmonary Emphysema and Proteolysis. New York, Academic Press, 1972, p 421.

534. Harley RA: Pulmonary vascular changes in experimental papain emphysema. In Mittman C (ed): Pulmonary Emphysema and Proteolysis. New York, Academic Press, 1972, p 449.

535. Caldwell EJ: The physiologic and anatomic effects of papain on the rabbit lung. In Mittman C (ed): Pulmonary Emphysema and Proteolysis. New York, Academic Press, 1972, p 487.

536. Johanson WG Jr, Reynolds RC, Scott TC, et al: Connective tissue damage in emphysema. An electron microscopic study of papain-induced emphysema in rats. Am Rev Respir Dis 107:589, 1973.

537. Weinbaum G, Marco V, Ikeda T, et al: Enzymatic production of experimental emphysema in the dog. Route of exposure. Am Rev Respir Dis 109:351, 1974.

538. Snider GL, Hayes JA, Franzblau C, et al: Relationship between elastolytic activity and experimental emphysema-inducing properties of papain preparations. Am Rev Respir Dis 110:254, 1974.

539. Martorana PA, Share NN: Effect of human alpha₁-antitrypsin on papain-induced emphysema in the hamster. Am Rev Respir Dis 113:607, 1976.

540. Karlinsky JB, Catanese A, Honeychurch C, et al: In vitro effects of elastase and collagenase on mechanical properties of hamster lungs. Chest 69:275, 1976.

541. Karlinsky JB, Snider GL, Franzblau C, et al: In vitro effects of elastase and collagenase on mechanical properties of hamster lungs. Am Rev Respir Dis 113:769, 1976.

542. Marco V, Mass B, Meranze DR, et al: Induction of experimental emphysema in dogs using leukocyte homogenates. Am Rev Respir Dis 104:595, 1971.

543. Kimbel P, Mass B, Ikeda T, et al: Emphysema in dogs induced by leukocyte contents. *In* Mittman C (ed): Pulmonary Emphysema and Proteolysis. New York, Academic Press, 1972, p 411.

544. Mass B, Ikeda T, Meranze DR, et al: Induction of experimental emphysema. Cellular and species specificity. Am Rev Respir Dis 106:384, 1974.

545. Karlinsky JB, Snider GL: State of the art: Animal models of emphysema. Am Rev Respir Dis 117:1109, 1978.

546. Senior RM, Tegner H, Kuhn C, et al: The induction of pulmonary emphysema with human leukocyte elastase. Am Rev Respir Dis 116:469, 1977.

547. Hyman AL, Spannhake EW, Kadowitz RJ, et al: Physiologic and morphologic observations of the effects of intravenous elastase on the lung. Am Rev Respir Dis 117:97, 1978.

548. Martorana AP, Schaper J, Van Even P, et al: The effect of physical exercise on elastase-induced emphysema in hamsters. Am Rev Respir Dis 120:1209, 1979.

549. Polzin JK, Napier JS, Taylor JC, et al: Effect of elastase and ventilation on elastic recoil of excised dog lungs. Am Rev Respir Dis 119:377, 1979.

550. Blackwood RA, Correta JM, Manol I, et al: Alpha₁-antitrypsin deficiency and increased susceptibility to elastase-induced experimental emphysema in a rat model. Am Rev Respir Dis 120:1375, 1979.

551. Martorana PA, Richard JW, McKeel NW, et al: Inhibition of papain-induced emphysema in the hamster by human alpha₁-antitrypsin. Can J Physiol Pharmacol 52:758, 1974.

552. Kaplan PD, Kuhn C, Pierce JA: The induction of emphysema with elastase. I. The evolution of the lesion and the influence of serum. J Lab Clin Med 82:349, 1973.

553. Tarján E, Petö L, Appel J, et al: Prevention of elastase-induced emphysema by aerosol administration of a specific synthetic elastase inhibitor. Eur J Respir Dis 64:442, 1983.

554. Gudapaty SR, Liener IE, Hoidal JR, et al: The prevention of elastase-induced emphysema in hamsters by the intratracheal administration of a synthetic elastase inhibitor bound to albumin microspheres. Am Rev Respir Dis 159:132, 1985.

555. Rudolphus A, Kramps JA, Dijkman JH: Effect of human antileucoprotease on experimental emphysema. Eur Respir J 4:31, 1991.

556. Kucich U, Christner P, Weinbaum G, et al: Immunologic identification of elastin-derived peptides in the serums of dogs with experimental emphysema. Am Rev Respir Dis 122:461, 1980.

557. Stone PJ, Lucey EC, Virca GD, et al: Alpha₁-protease inhibitor moderates human neutrophil elastase–induced emphysema and secretory cell metaplasia in hamsters. Eur Respir J 3:673, 1990.

558. Finlay GA, O'Donnell MD, O'Connor CM, et al: Elastin and collagen remodeling in emphysema. A scanning electron microscopy study. Am J Pathol 149:1405, 1996.

559. Selman M, Montano M, Ramos C, Vanda B, et al: Tobacco smoke–induced lung emphysema in guinea pigs is associated with increased interstitial collagenase. Am J Physiol 271:L734, 1996.

560. Guenter CA, Coalson JJ, Jacques J, et al: Emphysema associated with intravascular leukocyte sequestration: Comparison with papain-induced emphysema. Am Rev Respir Dis 123:79, 1981.

561. Wittels EH, Coalson JJ, Welch MH, et al: Pulmonary intravascular leukocyte sequestration. A potential mechanism of lung injury. Am Rev Respir Dis 109:502, 1974.

562. Paré JP, Cote G, Fraser RS: Long term follow-up of drug abusers with intravenous talcosis. Am Rev Respir Dis 139:233, 1989.

563. Shapiro SD: The pathogenesis of emphysema: The elastase:antielastase hypothesis 30 years later. Proc Assoc Am Physicians 107:346, 1995.

564. D'Armiento J, Dalal SS, Okada Y, et al: Collagenase expression in the lungs of transgeneic mice causes pulmonary emphysema. Cell 71:955, 1992.

565. Hautamaki RD, Kobayashi DK, Senior RM, Shapiro SD: Requirement for macrophage elastase for cigarette smoke–induced emphysema in mice. Science 277:2002, 1997.

566. Massaro GD, Massaro D: Retinoic acid treatment abrogates elastase-induced pulmonary emphysema in rats. Nature Med 3:675, 1997.

567. McKusick VA: Heritable Disorders of Connective Tissue. 4th ed. St. Louis, CV Mosby, 1972, p 187.

568. Kida K, Thurlbeck WM: Lack of recovery of lung structure and function after the administration of beta aminoproprionitrile in the postnatal period. Am Rev Respir Dis 122:467, 1980.

569. O'Dell BL, Kilburn KH, McKenzie WN, et al: The lung of the copper-deficient rat. Am J Pathol 91:413, 1978.

570. Soskel NT, Watanabe S, Hammond E, et al: A copper-deficient, zinc-supplemented diet produces emphysema in pigs. Am Rev Respir Dis 126:316, 1982.

571. Sparrow D, Silkert JE, Weiss ST, et al: The relationship of pulmonary function to copper concentrations in drinking water. Am Rev Respir Dis 126:312, 1982.

572. Tetley TD, Phillips GJ, Guz A, Fox B: The blotchy mouse, lung desmosine, and emphysema. Ann N Y Acad Sci 624:358, 1991.

573. Fisk DE, Kuhn C: Emphysema-like changes in the lungs of the blotchy mouse. Am Rev Respir Dis 113:787, 1976.

574. Snider GL, Hayes JA, Korthy AL, et al: Centrilobular emphysema experimentally induced by cadmium chloride aerosol. Am Rev Respir Dis 108:40, 1973.

575. Thurlbeck WM, Foley FD: Experimental pulmonary emphysema: The effect of intratracheal injection of cadmium chloride solution in the guinea pig. Am J Pathol 42:431, 1963.

576. Lewis GP, Lyle H, Miller S: Association between elevated hepatic water-soluble protein-bound cadmium levels and chronic bronchitis and/or emphysema. Lancet 2:1330, 1969.

577. Freeman G, Haydon GB: Emphysema after low-level exposure to NO₂. Arch Environ Health 8:125, 1964.

578. Freeman G, Crane SC, Stephens RJ, et al: Pathogenesis of the nitrogen dioxide–induced lesion in the rat lung: A review and presentation of new observations. Am Rev Respir Dis 98:429, 1968.

579. Freeman G, Crane SC, Furiosi NJ, et al: Covert reduction in ventilatory surface in rats during prolonged exposure to subacute nitrogen dioxide. Am Rev Respir Dis 106:563, 1972.

579a. Jeffery PK: Structural and inflammatory changes in COPD: A comparison with asthma. Thorax 53:129, 1998.

580. Reid L: Measurement of the bronchial mucous gland layer: A diagnostic yardstick in chronic bronchitis. Thorax 15:132, 1960.

581. Thurlbeck WM, Angus GE: The variation of Reid index measurements within the major bronchial tree. Am Rev Respir Dis 95:551, 1967.

582. Hayes JA: Distribution of bronchial gland measurements in a Jamaican population. Thorax 24:619, 1969.

583. Scott KWM: An autopsy study of bronchial mucous gland hypertrophy in Glasgow. Am Rev Respir Dis 107:239, 1973.

584. Jamal K, Cooney TP, Fleetham JA, et al: Chronic bronchitis—correlation of morphologic findings to sputum production and flow rates. Am Rev Respir Dis 129:719, 1984.

585. Mitchell RS, Stanford RE, Johnson JM, et al: The morphologic features of the bronchi, bronchioles, and alveoli in chronic airway obstruction: A clinicopathologic study. Am Rev Respir Dis 114:137, 1976.

586. Oberholzer M, Dalquen P, Wyss M, et al: The applicability of the gland/wall ratio (Reid index) to clinicopathological correlation studies. Thorax 33:779, 1978.

587. Saetta M, Di Stefano A, Maestrelli P, et al: Structural aspects of airway inflammation in COPD. Monaldi Arch Chest Dis 49(3 Suppl 1):43, 1994.

588. Mitchell RS, Ryan SF, Petty TL, et al: The significance of morphologic chronic hyperplastic bronchitis. Am Rev Respir Dis 93:720, 1966.

589. Thurlbeck WM, Angus GE: A distribution curve for chronic bronchitis. Thorax 19:436, 1964.

590. Takizawa T, Thurlbeck WM: A comparative study of four methods of assessing the morphologic changes in chronic bronchitis. Am Rev Respir Dis 103:774, 1971.

591. Martin CJ, Katsura S, Cochran TH: The relationship of chronic bronchitis to the diffuse obstructive pulmonary syndrome. Am Rev Respir Dis 102:362, 1970.

592. Douglas AN: Quantitative study of bronchial mucous gland enlargement. Thorax 35:198, 1980.

593. Wang NS, Ying WL: Morphogenesis of human bronchial diverticulum. A scanning electron microscopic study. Chest 69:201, 1976.

594. Nagai A, West W, Paul J, et al: The National Institutes of Health Intermittent Positive-Pressure Breathing Trial—Pathology Studies. 1. Interrelationship between morphologic lesions. Am Rev Respir Dis 132:937, 1985.

595. Tandon MK, Campbell AH: Bronchial cartilage in chronic bronchitis. Thorax 24:607, 1969.

596. Thurlbeck WM, Pun R, Toth J, et al: Bronchial cartilage in chronic obstructive lung disease. Am Rev Respir Dis 109:73, 1974.

597. Maisel JC, Silvers GW, Mitchell RS, et al: Bronchial atrophy and dynamic expiratory collapse. Am Rev Respir Dis 98:988, 1968.

598. Maisel JC, Silvers GW, George MS, et al: The significance of bronchial atrophy. Am J Pathol 67:371, 1972.

599. Restrepo GL, Heard BE: Air trapping in chronic bronchitis and emphysema. Measurements of the bronchial cartilage. Am Rev Respir Dis 90:395, 1964.

600. Linhartova A, Anderson AE, Foraker AG: Site predilection of airway inflammation by emphysema type. Arch Pathol Lab Med 108:662, 1984.

601. Macklem PT, Fraser RG, Brown WG: Bronchial pressure measurements in emphysema and bronchitis. J Clin Invest 44:897, 1965.

602. Macklem PT, Wilson NJ: Measurement of intrabronchial pressure in man. J Appl Physiol 20:653, 1965.

603. Baier H, Zarzecki S, Wanner A, et al: Influence of lung inflation on the cross-sectional area of central airways in normals and in patients with lung disease. Respiration 41:145, 1981.

604. Tiddens HA, Paré PD, Hogg JC, et al: Cartilaginous airway dimensions and airflow obstruction in human lungs. Am J Respir Crit Care Med 152:260, 1995.

605. Tiddens HA, Bogaard JM, de Jongste JC, et al: Physiological and morphological determinants of maximal expiratory flow in chronic obstructive lung disease. Eur Respir J 9:1785, 1996.

606. Caldwell EJ, Fry DL: Pulmonary mechanics in the rabbit. J Appl Physiol 27:280, 1969.

607. McCormack G, Moreno R, Hogg JC, et al: Lung mechanics in papain-treated rabbits. J Appl Physiol 60:242, 1986.

608. Bowen JH, Woodard BH, Pratt PC: Bronchial collapse in obstructive lung disease. Chest 80:510, 1981.

609. Hossain S, Heard BE: Hyperplasia of bronchial muscle in chronic bronchitis. J Pathol 101:171, 1970.

610. Carlile A, Edwards C: Structural variation in the named bronchi of the left lung. A morphometric study. Br J Dis Chest 77:344, 1983.
611. Kuwano K, Bosken CH, Paré PD, et al: Small airways dimensions in asthma and in chronic obstructive pulmonary disease. Am Rev Respir Dis 148:1220, 1993.
612. Dunnill MS, Massarella GR, Anderson JA: A comparison of the quantitative anatomy of the bronchi in normal subjects, in status asthmaticus, in chronic bronchitis, and in emphysema. Thorax 24:176, 1969.
613. Edwards C: Bronchial nerves in chronic obstructive airways disease: A preliminary report. J Pathol 159:287, 1989.
614. Mullen JBM, Wright JL, Wiggs BR, et al: Reassessment of inflammation of airways in chronic bronchitis. BMJ 291:1235, 1985.
615. Ellefsen P, Tos M: Goblet cells in the human trachea. Quantitative studies of a pathological biopsy material. Arch Otolaryngol 95:547, 1972.
616. Reid L: Bronchial mucus production in health and disease. *In* Liebow AA, Smith DE (eds): International Academy of Pathology Monographs in Pathology. Vol 8: The Lung. Baltimore, Williams & Wilkins, 1968, pp 87–108.
617. Hogg JC, Macklem PT, Thurlbeck WM: Site and nature of airway obstruction in chronic obstructive lung disease. N Engl J Med 278:1355, 1968.
618. Yanai M, Sekizawa K, Ohrui T, et al: Site of airway obstruction in pulmonary disease: Direct measurement of intrabronchial pressure. J Appl Physiol 72:1016, 1992.
619. Hogg JC: Airway pathology of functional significance in chronic bronchitis and chronic obstructive airway disease. Agents Actions Suppl 30:11, 1990.
620. Petty TL, Silvers GW, Stanford RE, et al: Radial traction and small airway disease in excised human lungs. Am Rev Respir Dis 133:132, 1986.
621. Cosio MG, Shiner RJ, Saetta M, et al: Alveolar fenestrae in smokers: Relationship with light microscopic and functional abnormalities. Am Rev Respir Dis 133:126, 1986.
622. Verbeken EK, Cauberghs M, Lauweryns JM, van de Woestijne KP: Anatomy of membranous bronchioles in normal, senile and emphysematous human lungs. J Appl Physiol 77:1875, 1994.
623. Verbeken EK, Cauberghs M, van de Woestijne KP: Membranous bronchioles and connective tissue network of normal and emphysematous lungs. J Appl Physiol 81:2468, 1996.
624. Scott KWM, Steiner GM: Postmortem assessment of chronic airways obstruction by tantalum bronchography. Thorax 30:405, 1975.
625. Thurlbeck WM: The pathology of small airways in chronic airflow limitation. Eur J Respir Dis 63:9, 1982.
626. Cosio MG, Ghezzo H, Hogg JC, et al: The relations between structural changes in small airways and pulmonary function tests. N Engl J Med 298:1277, 1977.
627. Wright JL, Lawson LM, Paré PD, et al: The detection of small airways disease. Am Rev Respir Dis 129:989, 1984.
628. Wright JL, Cosio M, Wiggs BJ, et al: A morphologic grading scheme for membranous and respiratory bronchioles. Arch Pathol Lab Med 109:163, 1985.
629. Wright JL, Paré PD, Nelems JM, et al: The nature of peripheral airway inflammations in emphysema (abstract). Fed Proc 39:332, 1980.
630. Wright JL, Hobson J, Wiggs BR, et al: Effect of cigarette smoke on structure of the small airways. Lung 165:91, 1987.
631. Berend N, Woolcock AJ, Marlin GK: The relationship between bronchial and arterial diameters in normal human lungs. Thorax 34:354, 1979.
632. Matsuba K, Thurlbeck WM: Disease of the small airways in chronic bronchitis. Am Rev Respir Dis 107:552, 1973.
633. Berend N, Wright JL, Thurlbeck WM, et al: Small airways disease—reproducibility of measurements and correlation with lung function. Chest 79:263, 1981.
634. Petty TL, Silvers GW, Stanford RE, et al: Small airway disease is associated with elastic recoil changes in excised human lungs. Am Rev Respir Dis 130:42, 1984.
635. Adesina AM, Vallyathan V, McQuillen EN, et al: Bronchiolar inflammation and fibrosis associated with smoking. A morphologic cross-sectional population analysis. Am Rev Respir Dis 143:144, 1991.
636. Cosio MG, Hale KA, Niewoehner DE, et al: Morphologic and morphometric effects of prolonged cigarette smoking on the small airways. Am Rev Respir Dis 122:265, 1980.
637. Niewoehner DE, Knoke JD, Kleinerman J, et al: Peripheral airways as a determinant of ventilatory function in the human lung. J Clin Invest 60:139, 1970.
638. Niewoehner DE, Kleinerman J: Morphologic basis of pulmonary resistance in the human lung and effects of aging. J Appl Physiol 36:412, 1974.
639. Salmon RB, Saidel GM, Inkley SR, et al: Relationship of ventilation inhomogeneity to morphologic variables in excised human lungs. Am Rev Respir Dis 126:686, 1982.
640. Berend N, Thurlbeck WM: Correlations of maximum expiratory flow with small airway dimensions and pathology. J Appl Physiol 52:346, 1982.
641. Petty TL, Silvers G, Stanford RE, et al: Small airway pathology is related to increased closing capacity and abnormal slope of phase III in excised lungs. Am Rev Respir Dis 121:449, 1980.
642. Berend N, Woolcock AJ, Marlin GE, et al: Correlation between the function and structure of the lung in smokers. Am Rev Respir Dis 119:695, 1979.
643. Wright JL, Lawson LM, Paré PD, et al: The detection of small airways disease. Am Rev Respir Dis 129:989, 1984.
644. Petty TL, Silvers GW, Stanford RE, et al: Small airway dimension and size distribution in human lungs with an increased closing capacity. Am Rev Respir Dis 125:535, 1982.
645. Berend N, Skoog C, Thurlbeck WM, et al: Single-breath nitrogen test in excised human lungs. J Appl Physiol 51:1568, 1981.
646. Nagai A, West W, Thurlbeck WM, et al: The National Institutes of Health Intermittent Positive-Pressure Breathing Trial—Pathology Studies. 2. Correlation between morphologic findings, clinical findings, and evidence of expiratory air-flow obstruction. Am Rev Respir Dis 132:946, 1985.
647. Paré PD, Brooks LA, Coppin CA, et al: Density-dependence of maximal expiratory flow and its correlation with small airway disease in smokers. Am Rev Respir Dis 131:521, 1985.
648. Linhartová A, Anderson AE: Small airways in severe panlobular emphysema—mural thickening and premature closure. Am Rev Respir Dis 127:42, 1983.
649. Hale KA, Ewing SL, Gosnell BA, et al: Lung disease in long-term cigarette smokers with and without chronic air-flow obstruction. Am Rev Respir Dis 130:716, 1984.
650. Berend N: Lobar distribution of bronchiolar inflammation in emphysema. Am Rev Respir Dis 124:218, 1981.
651. Wright JL, Wiggs BJ, Hogg JC, et al: Airway disease in upper and lower lobes in lungs of patients with and without emphysema. Thorax 282:39, 1984.
652. Saito K, Thurlbeck WM: Measurement of emphysema in autopsy lungs, with emphasis on interlobar differences. Am J Respir Crit Care Med 151:1373, 1995.
653. Bai A, Eidelman DH, Hogg JC, et al: Proposed nomenclature for quantifying subdivisions of the bronchial wall. J Appl Physiol 77:1011, 1994.
654. James AL, Hogg JC, Dunn LA, Paré PD: The use of internal perimeter to compare airway size and to calculate smooth muscle shortening. Am Rev Respir Dis 138:136, 1988.
655. James AL, Paré PD, Hogg JC: Effects of lung volume, bronchoconstriction, and cigarette smoke on morphometric airways dimensions. J Appl Physiol 64:913, 1988.
656. Bosken CH, Wiggs BR, Paré PD, Hogg JC: Small airway dimensions in smokers with obstruction to airflow. Am Rev Respir Dis 142:563, 1990.
657. Finkelstein R, Ma HD, Ghezzo H, et al: Morphometry of small airways in smokers and its relationship to emphysema type and hyperresponsiveness. Am J Respir Crit Care Med 152:267, 1995.
658. Andoh Y, Shimura S, Aikawa T, et al: Perivascular fibrosis of muscular pulmonary arteries in chronic obstructive pulmonary disease. Chest 102:1645, 1992.
659. Bosken CH, Hards J, Gatter K, Hogg JC: Characterization of the inflammatory reaction in the peripheral airways of cigarette smokers using immunocytochemistry. Am Rev Respir Dis 145:911, 1992.
660. Nagai A, Thurlbeck WM, Konno K: Responsiveness and variability of airflow obstruction in chronic obstructive pulmonary disease. Clinicopathologic correlative studies. Am J Respir Crit Care Med 151:635, 1995.
661. Aguayo SM: Determinants of susceptibility to cigarette smoke. Potential roles for neuroendocrine cells and neuropeptides in airway inflammation, airway wall remodeling, and chronic airflow obstruction. Am J Respir Crit Care Med 149:1692, 1994.
662. Aguayo SM: Neuroendocrine cells and airway wall remodelling in chronic airflow obstruction: A perspective. Monaldi Arch Chest Dis 49:243, 1994.
663. Finkelstein R, Fraser RS, Ghezzo H, Cosio MG: Alveolar inflammation and its relation to emphysema in smokers. Am J Respir Crit Care Med 152:1666, 1995.
664. Wright JL: Emphysema: Concepts under change—a pathologist's perspective. Mod Pathol 8:873, 1995.
665. Saetta M, Finkelstein R, Cosio MG: Morphological and cellular basis for airflow limitation in smokers. Eur Respir J 7:1505, 1994.
666. Heard BE: A pathological study of emphysema of the lungs with chronic bronchitis. Thorax 13:136, 1958.
667. Thurlbeck WM, Dunnill MS, Hartung W, et al: A comparison of three methods of measuring emphysema. Hum Pathol 1:215, 1970.
668. McLean A, Warren PM, Gillooly M, et al: Microscopic and macroscopic measurements of emphysema: relation to carbon monoxide gas transfer. Thorax 47:144, 1992.
669. Gillooly M, Lamb D: Airspace size in lungs of lifelong non-smokers: Effect of age and sex. Thorax 48:39, 1993.
670. Kim WD, Eidelman DH, Izquierdo JL, et al: Centrilobular and panlobular emphysema in smokers. Two distinct morphologic and functional entities. Am Rev Respir Dis 144:1385, 1991.
671. Saetta M, Kim WD, Izquierdo JL, et al: Extent of centrilobular and panacinar emphysema in smokers' lungs: Pathological and mechanical implications. Eur Respir J 7:664, 1994.
672. Thurlbeck WM: Chronic Airflow Obstruction in Lung Disease. Philadelphia, WB Saunders, 1976.
673. Thurlbeck WM: The pathobiology and epidemiology of human emphysema. J Toxicol Environ Health 13:323, 1984.
674. Pump KK: The pattern of development of emphysema in the human lung. Am Rev Respir Dis 108:610, 1973.
675. Linhartová A: Lesions in resected lung parenchyma with regard to possible initial phase of pulmonary emphysema. An ultrastructural study. Pathol Res Pract 181:71, 1986.
676. Saetta M, Ghezzo H, et al: Loss of alveolar attachments in smokers. A morphometric correlate of lung function impairment. Am Rev Respir Dis 132:894, 1985.
677. Nagai A, Yamawaki I, Takazawa T, Thurlbeck WM: Alveolar attachments in emphysema of human lungs. Am Rev Respir Dis 144:888, 1991.
678. Willems LN, Kramps J, Stijnen T, et al: Relation between small airways disease and parenchymal destruction in surgical lung specimens. Thorax 45:89, 1990.
679. Saetta M, Finkelstein R, Cosio MG: Morphological and cellular basis for airflow limitation in smokers. Eur Respir J 7:1505, 1994.

680. Saetta M, Shiner RJ, Angus GE, et al: Destructive index: A measurement of lung parenchymal destruction in smokers. Am Rev Respir Dis 131:764, 1985.
681. Eidelman DH, Ghezzo H, Kim WD, Cosio MG: The destructive index and early lung destruction in smokers. Am Rev Respir Dis 144:156, 1991.
682. Eidelman D, Saetta MP, Ghezzo H, et al: Cellularity of the alveolar walls in smokers and its relation to alveolar destruction. Functional implications. Am Rev Respir Dis 141:1547, 1990.
683. McLean KH: The histology of generalized pulmonary emphysema. I. The genesis of the early centrolobular lesion: Focal emphysema. Australas Ann Med 6:124, 1957.
684. Thurlbeck WM: Chronic obstructive lung disease. Pathol Annu 3:367, 1968.
685. Leopold JG, Gough J: The centrilobular form of hypertrophic emphysema and its relation to chronic bronchitis. Thorax 12:219, 1957.
686. Anderson AE Jr, Foraker AG: Centrilobular emphysema and panlobular emphysema: Two different diseases. Thorax 28:547, 1973.
687. Sweet HC, Wyatt JP, Fritsch AJ, et al: Panlobular and centrilobular emphysema. Correlation of clinical findings with pathologic patterns. Ann Intern Med 55:565, 1961.
688. Snider GL, Brody JS, Doctor L: Subclinical pulmonary emphysema. Incidence and anatomic features. Am Rev Respir Dis 85:666, 1962.
689. Cockcroft DW, Horne SL: Localization of emphysema within the lung. Chest 82:483, 1982.
690. Boren HG: Alveolar fenestrae. Relationship to the pathology and pathogenesis of pulmonary emphysema. Am Rev Respir Dis 85:328, 1962.
691. Thurlbeck WM: Pulmonary emphysema. Am J Med Sci 246:332, 1963.
692. Horsfield K, Cumming G, Hicken P: A morphologic study of airway disease using bronchial casts. Am Rev Respir Dis 93:900, 1966.
693. Thurlbeck WM: The incidence of pulmonary emphysema with observations on the relative incidence and spatial distribution of various types of emphysema. Am Rev Respir Dis 87:206, 1963.
694. Anderson AE Jr, Furlaneto JA, Foraker AG: Bronchopulmonary derangements in nonsmokers. Am Rev Respir Dis 101:518, 1970.
695. Sutinen S, Vaajalahti P, Pääkkö P, et al: Prevalence, severity and types of pulmonary emphysema in a population of deaths in a Finnish city. Correlation with age, sex and smoking. Scand J Respir Dis 59:101, 1978.
696. Snider GL, Kleinerman JL, Thurlbeck WM, et al: The definition of emphysema. Report of a National Heart, Lung, and Blood Institute Division of Lung Diseases Workshop. Am Rev Respir Dis 132:182, 1985.
697. Osborne S, Hogg JC, Wright JL, et al: Exponential analysis of the pressure-volume curve: Correlation with mean linear intercept and emphysema in human lungs. Am Rev Respir Dis 137:1083, 1988.
698. Thurlbeck WM: Post-mortem lung volumes. Thorax 34:735, 1979.
699. Thurlbeck WM: Smoking, airflow limitation and the pulmonary circulation. Am Rev Respir Dis 122:183, 1980.
700. Thurlbeck WM: Aspects of chronic airflow obstruction. Chest 72:341, 1977.
701. Berend N, Thurlbeck WM: Exponential analysis of pressure-volume relationship in excised human lungs. J Appl Physiol 52:838, 1982.
702. Petty TL, Silvers GW, Stanford RE, et al: Functional correlations with mild and moderate emphysema in excised human lungs. Am Rev Respir Dis 124:700, 1981.
703. Silvers GW, Petty TL, Stanford RE, et al: Elastic recoil changes in early emphysema. Thorax 35:490, 1980.
704. Haber PS, Colebatch HJH, Ng CKY, et al: Alveolar size as a determinant of pulmonary distensibility in mammalian lungs. J Appl Physiol 54:837, 1983.
705. Greaves IA, Colebatch HJH: Elastic behaviour and structure of normal and emphysematous lungs post-mortem. Am Rev Respir Dis 121:127, 1980.
706. Verbeken EK, Cauberghs M, Mertens I, et al: The senile lung. Comparison with normal and emphysematous lungs. 2. Functional aspects. Chest 101:800, 1992.
707. Hogg JC, Nepszy SJ, Macklem PT, et al: Elastic properties of the centrilobular emphysematous space. J Clin Invest 48:1306, 1969.
708. Colebatch HJH, Greaves IA: Chronic airflow obstruction. Evolution of disordered function in cigarette smokers. Med J Aust 142:607, 1985.
709. Reid JA, Heard BE: The capillary network of normal and emphysematous human lungs studied by injections of India ink. Thorax 18:201, 1963.
710. Fernie JM, McLean A, Lamb D: Significant intimal abnormalities in muscular pulmonary arteries of patients with early obstructive lung disease. J Clin Pathol 41:730, 1988.
711. Finkelstein R, Fraser RS, Ghezzo H, Cosio MG: Alveolar inflammation and its relation to emphysema in smokers. Am J Respir Crit Care Med 152:1666, 1995.
712. Weitzenblum E: The pulmonary circulation and the heart in chronic lung disease. Monaldi Arch Chest Dis 49:231, 1994.
713. Wilkinson M, Langhorn CA, Heath D, et al: A pathophysiological study of 10 cases of hypoxic cor pulmonale. Q J Med 66:65, 1988.
714. Wright JL, Lawson L, Paré PD, et al: The structure and function of the pulmonary vasculature in mild chronic obstructive pulmonary disease—the effect of oxygen and exercise. Am Rev Respir Dis 128:702, 1983.
715. Hale KA, Niewoehner DE, Cosio MG, et al: Morphologic changes in the muscular pulmonary arteries: Relationship to cigarette smoking, airway disease and emphysema. Am Rev Resp Dis 122:273, 1980.
716. Scott KWM: Quantitation of thick-walled peripheral lung vessels in chronic airway obstruction. Thorax 31:315, 1976.
717. Magee F, Wright JL, Wiggs BR, et al: Pulmonary vascular structure and function in chronic obstructive pulmonary disease. Thorax 43:183, 1988.
718. Cudkowicz L, Armstrong JB: The bronchial arteries in pulmonary emphysema. Thorax 8:46, 1953.
719. Jacobson G, Turner AF, Balchum O, et al: Pulmonary arteriovenous shunts in emphysema demonstrated by wedge arteriography. Am J Roentgenol 93:868, 1965.
720. Simon G, Galbraith HJB: Radiology of chronic bronchitis. Lancet 265:850, 1953.
721. Bates DV, Gordon CA, Paul GI, et al: Chronic bronchitis: Report on the third and fourth stages of the co-ordinated study of chronic bronchitis in the Department of Veterans Affairs, Canada. Med Serv J Can 22:5, 1966.
722. Simon G: Chronic bronchitis and emphysema: A symposium. III. Pathological findings and radiological changes in chronic bronchitis and emphysema. (b) Radiological changes in chronic bronchitis. Br J Radiol 32:292, 1959.
723. Fraser RG, Fraser RS, Renner JW, et al: The roentgenologic diagnosis of chronic bronchitis. A reassessment with emphasis on parahilar bronchi seen end-on. Radiology 120:1, 1976.
724. Webb WR: Radiology of obstructive pulmonary disease. Am J Roentgenol 169:637, 1997.
725. Simon G: Principles of Chest X-Ray Diagnosis. 3rd ed. London, Butterworth, 1971.
726. Takasugi JE, Godwin JD: Radiology of chronic obstructive pulmonary disease. Radiol Clin North Am 36:29, 1998.
727. Remy-Jardin M, Remy J, Boulenguez C, et al: Morphologic effects of cigarette smoking on airways and pulmonary parenchyma in healthy adult volunteers: CT evaluation and correlation with pulmonary function tests. Radiology 186:107, 1993.
728. Lamers RJ, Thelissen GR, Kessels A, et al: Chronic obstructive pulmonary disease: evaluation with spirometrically controlled CT lung densitometry. Radiology 193:109, 1994.
729. Sutinen S, Christoforidis AJ, Klugh GA, et al: Roentgenologic criteria for the recognition of non-symptomatic pulmonary emphysema: Correlation between roentgenologic findings and pulmonary pathology. Am Rev Respir Dis 91:69, 1965.
730. Pratt PC: Role of conventional chest radiography in diagnosis and exclusion of emphysema. Am J Med 82:998, 1987.
731. Laws JW, Heard BE: Emphysema and the chest film: A retrospective radiological and pathological study. Br J Radiol 35:750, 1962.
732. Simon G: Radiology and emphysema. Clin Radiol 15:293, 1964.
733. Thurlbeck WM, Henderson JA, Fraser RG, et al: Chronic obstructive lung disease. A comparison between clinical, roentgenologic, functional and morphological criteria in chronic bronchitis, emphysema, asthma and bronchiectasis. Medicine 49:81, 1970.
734. Thurlbeck WM, Simon G: Radiographic appearance of the chest in emphysema. Am J Roentgenol 130:429, 1978.
735. Miniati M, Filippi E, Falaschi F, et al: Radiologic evaluation of emphysema in patients with chronic obstructive pulmonary disease. Am J Respir Crit Care Med 151:1359, 1995.
736. Katsura S, Martin CJ: The roentgenologic diagnosis of anatomic emphysema. Am Rev Respir Dis 96:700, 1967.
737. Nicklaus TM, Stowell DW, Christiansen WR, et al: The accuracy of the roentgenologic diagnosis of chronic pulmonary emphysema. Am Rev Respir Dis 93:889, 1966.
738. Reich SB, Weinshelbaum A, Yee J: Correlation of radiographic measurements and pulmonary function tests in chronic obstructive pulmonary disease. Am J Roentgenol 144:695, 1985.
739. Burki NK: Conventional chest films can identify air flow obstruction. Chest 93:675, 1988.
740. Thurlbeck WM, Simon G: Radiographic appearance of the chest in emphysema. Am J Roentgenol 130:429, 1978.
741. Pratt PC: Chest radiographs cannot identify airflow obstruction (letter). Chest 93:1120, 1988.
742. Lohela P, Sutinen S, Pääkkö P, et al: Diagnosis of emphysema on chest radiographs. Fortschr Geb Rontgenstr Nuklearmed Erganzungsband 141:395, 1984.
743. Thurlbeck WM, Müller NL: Emphysema: Definition, imaging, and quantification. Am J Roentgenol 163:1017, 1994.
744. Austin JHM, Müller NL, Friedman PJ, et al: Glossary of terms for CT of the lungs: Recommendations of the Nomenclature Committee of the Fleischner Society. Radiology 200:327, 1996.
745. Miller RR, Müller N, Vedal S, et al: Limitations of computed tomography in the assessment of emphysema. Am Rev Respir Dis 139:980, 1989.
746. Webb WR, Stein MG, Finkbeiner WE, et al: Normal and diseased isolated lungs: High-resolution CT. Radiology 166:81, 1988.
747. Itoh H, Murata K, Konishi J, et al: Diffuse lung disease: Pathologic basis for the high-resolution computed tomography findings. J Thorac Imaging 8:176, 1993.
748. Bonelli FS, Hartman TE, Swensen SJ, et al: Accuracy of high-resolution CT in diagnosing lung diseases. Am J Roentgenol 170:1507, 1998.
749. Foster WL Jr, Pratt PC, Roggli VL, et al: Centrilobular emphysema: CT-pathologic correlation. Radiology 159:27, 1986.
750. Bergin C, Müller NL, Nichols DM, et al: The diagnosis of emphysema: A computed tomographic–pathologic correlation. Am Rev Respir Dis 133:541, 1986.
751. Hruban RH, Meziane MA, Zerhouni EA, et al: High resolution computed tomography of inflation-fixed lungs: Pathologic-radiologic correlation of centrilobular emphysema. Am Rev Respir Dis 136:935, 1987.
752. Spouge D, Mayo JR, Cardoso W, Müller NL: Panacinar emphysema: CT and pathologic findings. J Comput Assist Tomogr 17:710, 1993.

753. Kuwano K, Matsuba K, Ikeda T, et al: The diagnosis of mild emphysema: Correlation of computed tomography and pathologic scores. Am Rev Respir Dis 141:169, 1990.

754. Müller NL, Miller RR, Abboud RT: "Density mask": An objective method to quantitate emphysema using computed tomography. Chest 94:782, 1988.

755. Gevenois PA, de Maertelaer V, de Vuyst P, et al: Comparison of computed density and macroscopic morphometry in pulmonary emphysema. Am J Respir Crit Care Med 152:653, 1995.

756. Gevenois PA, de Vuyst P, Sy M, et al: Pulmonary emphysema: Quantitative CT during expiration. Radiology 199:825, 1996.

757. Gevenois PA, Koob MC, Jacobovitz D, et al: Whole lung sections for CT-pathologic correlations: Modified Gough-Wentworth technique. Invest Radiol 28:242, 1993.

758. Remy-Jardin M, Remy J, Gosselin B, et al: Sliding thin slab, minimum intensity projection technique in the diagnosis of emphysema: Histopathologic-CT correlation. Radiology 200:665, 1996.

759. Bergin CJ, Müller NL, Miller RR: CT in the qualitative assessment of emphysema. J Thorac Imaging 1:94, 1986.

760. Napel S, Rubin GD, Jeffrey RB: STS-MIP: A new reconstruction technique for CT of the chest. J Comput Assist Tomogr 17:832, 1993.

761. Murata K, Itoh H, Todo G, et al: Centrilobular lesions of the lung: Demonstration by high-resolution CT and pathologic correlation. Radiology 161:641, 1986.

762. Welch MH, Reinecke ME, Hammarsten JF, et al: Antitrypsin deficiency in pulmonary disease: The significance of intermediate levels. Ann Intern Med 71:533, 1969.

763. Bell RS: The radiographic manifestations of alpha-1 antitrypsin deficiency. An important recognizable pattern of chronic obstructive pulmonary disease (COPD). Radiology 95:19, 1970.

764. Rosen RA, Dalinka MK, Gralino BJ Jr, et al: The roentgenographic findings in alpha-1 antitrypsin deficiency (AAD). Radiology 95:25, 1970.

765. Guest PJ, Hansell DM: High resolution computed tomography (HRCT) in emphysema associated with alpha-1-antitrypsin deficiency. Clin Radiol 45:260, 1992.

766. King MA, Stone JA, Diaz PT, et al: $\alpha_1$-antitrypsin deficiency: Evaluation of bronchiectasis with CT. Radiology 199:137, 1996.

767. Shin MS, Ho KJ: Bronchiectasis in patients with $\alpha_1$-antitrypsin deficiency: A rare occurrence? Chest 104:1384, 1993.

768. Jones DK, Godden D, Cavanagh P: Alpha-1-antitrypsin deficiency presenting as bronchiectasis. Br J Dis Chest 79:301, 1985.

769. Gould GA, MacNee W, McLean A, et al: CT measurements of lung density in life can quantitate distal airspace enlargement—an essential defining feature of human emphysema. Am Rev Respir Dis 137:380, 1988.

770. Sakai N, Michima M, Nishimura K, et al: An automated method to assess the distribution of low attenuation areas on chest CT scans in chronic pulmonary emphysema patients. Chest 106:1319, 1994.

771. Kazerooni EA, Whyte RI, Flint A, et al: Imaging of emphysema and lung volume reduction surgery. RadioGraphics 17:1023, 1997.

772. Mergo PJ, Williams WF, Gonzalez-Rothi R, et al: Three-dimensional volumetric assessment of abnormally low attenuation of the lung from routine helical CT: Inspiratory and expiratory quantification. Am J Roentgenol 170:1355, 1998.

772a. Müller NL, Thurlbeck WM: Thin-section CT, emphysema, air trapping and airway obstruction. Radiology 199:621, 1996.

773. Zerhouni EA, Boukadoum M, Siddiky MA, et al: A standard phantom for quantitative CT analysis of pulmonary nodules. Radiology 149:767, 1983.

774. Hoffman EA, Sinak LJ, Robb RA, et al: Noninvasive quantitative imaging of shape and volume of lungs. J Appl Physiol 54:1414, 1983.

775. Denison DM, Morgan MDL, Miller AB: Estimation of regional gas and tissue volumes of the lung in supine man using computed tomography. Thorax 41:620, 1986.

776. Kinsella M, Müller NL, Abboud RT, et al: Quantitation of emphysema by computed tomography using a "density mask" program and correlation with pulmonary function tests. Chest 97:315, 1990.

777. Bae KT, Slone RM, Gierada DS, et al: Patients with emphysema: Quantitative CT analysis before and after lung volume reduction surgery. Work in progress. Radiology 203:705, 1997.

778. Gierada DS, Hakimian S, Slone RM: MR analysis of lung volume and thoracic dimensions in patients with emphysema before and after lung volume reduction surgery. Am J Roentgenol 170:707, 1998.

779. Takasugi JE, Wood DE, Godwin JD, et al: Lung-volume reduction surgery for diffuse emphysema: Radiologic assessment of changes in thoracic dimensions. J Thorac Imaging 13:36, 1998.

780. Holbert JM, Brown ML, Sciurba FC, et al: Changes in lung volume and volume of emphysema after unilateral lung reduction surgery: Analysis with CT lung densitometry. Radiology 201:793, 1996.

781. Burrows B, Niden AH, Barclay WR, et al: Chronic obstructive lung disease. II. Relationship of clinical and physiologic findings to the severity of airways obstruction. Am Rev Respir Dis 92:665, 1965.

782. Kass I, O'Brien LE, Zamel N, et al: Lack of correlation between clinical background and pulmonary function tests in patients with chronic obstructive pulmonary diseases. A retrospective study of 140 cases. Am Rev Respir Dis 107:64, 1973.

783. Miller RD, Hepper NGG, Kueppers F, et al: Host factors in chronic obstructive pulmonary disease in an upper Midwest rural community: Design, case selection and clinical characteristics in a matched pair study. Mayo Clin Proc 51:709, 1976.

784. Sharp JT, Drutz WS, Moisan T, et al: Postural relief of dyspnea in severe chronic obstructive pulmonary disease. Am Rev Respir Dis 122:201, 1980.

785. Seward JB, Hayes DL, Smith HC, et al: Platypnea-orthodeoxia: Clinical profile, diagnostic workup, management, and report of seven cases. Mayo Clin Proc 59:221, 1984.

786. Minh VD, Chun D, Fairshter RD, et al: Supine change in arterial oxygenation in patients with chronic obstructive pulmonary disease. Am Rev Respir Dis 133:820, 1986.

787. Shim C, Chun KJ, Williams MH Jr, et al: Positional effects on distribution of ventilation in chronic obstructive pulmonary disease. Ann Intern Med 105:346, 1986.

788. Dornhorst AD: Respiratory insufficiency. Lancet 1:1185, 1955.

789. Burrows B, Fletcher CM, Heard BE, et al: The emphysematous and bronchial types of chronic airways obstruction. Lancet 1:830, 1966.

790. Marks A: Chronic bronchitis and emphysema: Clinical diagnosis and evaluation. Med Clin North Am 57:707, 1973.

791. Marini JJ, Pierson DJ, Hudson LD, et al: The significance of wheezing in chronic airflow obstruction. Am Rev Respir Dis 120:1069, 1979.

792. Campbell EJM: Physical signs of diffuse airways obstruction and lung distention. Thorax 24:1, 1969.

793. Christie RV: Emphysema of the lungs. BMJ 1:105, 1944.

794. Hoover CF: Definitive percussion and inspection in estimating size and contour of heart. JAMA 75:1626, 1920.

795. Ashutosh K, Gilbert R, Auchincloss JH Jr, et al: Asynchronous breathing movements in patients with chronic obstructive pulmonary disease. Chest 67:553, 1975.

796. Sharp JT, Goldberg NB, Druz WS, et al: Thoracoabdominal motion in chronic obstructive pulmonary disease. Am Rev Respir Dis 115:47, 1977.

797. Godfrey S, Edwards RHT, Campbell EJM, et al: Clinical and physiological associations of some physical signs observed in patients with chronic airways obstruction. Thorax 25:285, 1970.

798. MacNee W: Pathophysiology of cor pulmonale in chronic obstructive pulmonary disease. Part I. Am J Respir Crit Care Med 150:833, 1994.

799. Openbrier DR, Irwin MM, Rogers RM, et al: Nutritional status and lung function in patients with emphysema and chronic bronchitis. Chest 83:17, 1983.

800. Boushy SF, Adhikari PK, Sakamoto A, et al: Factors affecting prognosis in emphysema. Dis Chest 45:402, 1964.

801. Braun SR, Keim NL, Dixon RM, et al: The prevalence and determinants of nutritional changes in chronic obstructive pulmonary disease. Chest 86:558, 1984.

802. Goldstein SA, Thomashow B, Askanazi J: Functional changes during nutritional repletion in patients with lung disease. Clin Chest Med 7:141, 1986.

803. Goldstein S, Askanazi J, Weissman C, et al: Energy expenditure in patients with chronic obstructive pulmonary disease. Chest 91:222, 1987.

804. Hofford JM, Milakofsky L, Vogel WH, et al: The nutritional status in advanced emphysema associated with chronic bronchitis. A study of amino acid and catecholamine levels. Am Rev Respir Dis 141:902, 1990.

805. Wilson DO, Rogers RM, Sanders MH, et al: Nutritional intervention in malnourished patients with emphysema. Am Rev Respir Dis 134:672, 1986.

806. Vanier T, Dulfano MJ, Wu C, et al: Emphysema, hypoxia and the polycythemic response. N Engl J Med 269:169, 1963.

807. Lertzman M, Israels LG, Cherniack RM: Erythropoiesis and ferrokinetics in chronic respiratory disease. Ann Intern Med 56:821, 1962.

808. Gallo RC, Fraimow W, Cathcart RT, et al: Erythropoietic response in chronic pulmonary disease. Arch Intern Med 113:559, 1964.

809. Calverley MA, Leggett RJ, McElderry L, et al: Cigarette smoking and secondary polycythemia in hypoxic cor pulmonale. Am Rev Respir Dis 125:507, 1982.

810. Fielding J, Zorab PA: Polycythaemia and iron deficiency in pulmonary "emphysema." Lancet 2:284, 1964.

811. Wedzicha JA, Cotes PM, Empey DW, et al: Serum immunoreactive erythropoietin in hypoxic lung disease with and without polycythaemia. Clin Sci 69:413, 1985.

812. Chamberlain DA, Millard FJC: The treatment of polycythaemia secondary to hypoxic lung disease by continuous oxygen administration. Q J Med 32:341, 1963.

813. Patakas DA, Christaki PI, Louridas GE, et al: Control of breathing in patients with chronic obstructive lung diseases and secondary polycythemia after venesection. Respiration 49:257, 1986.

814. White RJ, Woodings DF: Impaired water handling in chronic airways disease. BMJ 2:561, 1971.

815. Telfer N, Weiner JM, Merrill Q: Distribution of sodium and potassium in chronic obstructive pulmonary disease. Am Rev Respir Dis 111:166, 1975.

816. Chabot F, Mertes PM, Delorme N, et al: Effect of acute hypercapnia on alpha atrial natriuretic peptide, renin, angiotensin II, aldosterone, and vasopressin plasma levels in patients with COPD. Chest 107:780, 1995.

817. Kilburn KH, Dowell AR: Renal function in respiratory failure. Arch Intern Med 127:754, 1971.

818. Renal function in respiratory failure (editorial). JAMA 216:131, 1971.

819. Filley GF: Acid regulation and $CO_2$ retention. Chest 58:417, 1970.

820. Schloerb PR, King CR, Kerby G, Ruth WE: Potassium depletion in patients with chronic respiratory failure. Am Rev Respir Dis 102:53, 1970.

821. Turino GM, Goldring RM, Heinemann HO: Renal response to mechanical ventilation in patients with chronic hypercapnia. Am J Med 56:151, 1974.

822. MacNee W: Pathophysiology of cor pulmonale in chronic obstructive pulmonary disease. Part II. Am J Respir Crit Care Med 150:1158, 1994.

823. Schrijen F, Urtiaga B: Pulmonary blood volume in chronic lung disease—changes with legs raised and during exercise. Chest 81:544, 1982.

824. Din-Xuan AT, Higenbottam TW, Clelland CA, et al: Impairment of endothelium-dependent pulmonary artery relaxation in chronic obstructive lung disease. N Engl J Med 324:1539, 1991.

825. Yamakami T, Taguchi O, Gabazza EC, et al: Arterial endothelin-1 level in pulmonary emphysema and interstitial lung disease. Relation with pulmonary hypertension during exercise. Eur Respir J 10:2055, 1997.

826. Albert RK, Muramoto A, Caldwell J, et al: Increases in intrathoracic pressure do not explain the rise in left ventricular end-diastolic pressure that occurs during exercise in patients with chronic obstructive pulmonary disease. Am Rev Respir Dis 132:623, 1985.

827. Light RW, Mintz HM, Linden GS, et al: Hemodynamics of patients with severe chronic obstructive pulmonary disease during progressive upright exercise. Am Rev Respir Dis 130:391, 1984.

828. Oswald-Mammosser M, Apprill M, Bachez P, et al: Pulmonary hemodynamics in chronic obstructive pulmonary disease of the emphysematous type. Respiration 58:304, 1991.

829. Bedu M, Giraldo H, Janicot H, et al: Interaction between cold and hypoxia on pulmonary circulation in COPD. Am J Respir Crit Care Med 153:1242, 1996.

830. Weitzenblum E, Hirth C, Parini JP, et al: Clinical, functional and pulmonary hemodynamic course of patients with chronic obstructive pulmonary disease followed-up over 3 years. Respiration 36:1, 1978.

831. Weitzenblum E, Jezek V: Evolution of pulmonary hypertension in chronic respiratory disease. Bull Eur Physiopathol Respir 20:73, 1985.

832. Degaute JP, Domenighetti G, Naeije R, et al: Oxygen delivery in acute exacerbation of chronic obstructive pulmonary disease—effects of controlled oxygen therapy. Am Rev Respir Dis 124:26, 1981.

833. Weitzenblum E, Apprill M, Oswald M, et al: Pulmonary hemodynamics in patients with chronic obstructive pulmonary disease before and during an episode of peripheral edema. Chest 105:1377, 1994.

834. Block AJ, Boysen PG, Wynne JW, et al: The origins of cor pulmonale—a hypothesis. Chest 75:109, 1979.

835. Midgren B, White T, Petersson K, et al: Nocturnal hypoxaemia and cor pulmonale in severe chronic lung disease. Bull Eur Physiopathol Respir 21:527, 1985.

836. Chaouat A, Weitzenblum E, Kessler R, et al: Sleep-related $O_2$ desaturation and daytime pulmonary haemodynamics in COPD patients with mild hypoxaemia. Eur Respir J 10:1730, 1997.

837. Sturani C, Bassein L, Schiavina M, et al: Oral nifedipine in chronic cor pulmonale secondary to severe chronic obstructive pulmonary disease (COPD). Chest 84:135, 1983.

838. Naeije R, Mélot C, Mols P, et al: Reduction in pulmonary hypertension by prostaglandin-$E_1$ in decompensated chronic obstructive pulmonary disease. Am Rev Respir Dis 125:1, 1982.

839. Weitzenblum E, Loiseau A, Hirth C, et al: Course of pulmonary hemodynamics in patients with chronic obstructive pulmonary disease. Chest 75:656, 1979.

840. Schrijen F, Uffholtz H, Polu JM, et al: Pulmonary and systemic hemodynamic evolution in chronic bronchitis. Am Rev Respir Dis 117:25, 1978.

841. Gluskowski J, Jedrzejewska-Makowska M, Hawrylkiewicz I, et al: Effects of prolonged oxygen therapy on pulmonary hypertension and blood viscosity in patients with advanced cor pulmonale. Respiration 44:177, 1983.

842. Weitzenblum E, Sautegeau A, Ehrhart M, et al: Long-term oxygen therapy can reverse the progression of pulmonary hypertension in patients with chronic obstructive pulmonary disease. Am Rev Respir Dis 131:493, 1985.

843. Fletcher EC, Levin DC: Cardiopulmonary hemodynamics during sleep in subjects with chronic obstructive pulmonary disease. Chest 85:6, 1984.

844. Ashutosh K, Dunsky M: Noninvasive tests for responsiveness of pulmonary hypertension to oxygen. Prediction of survival in patients with chronic obstructive lung disease and cor pulmonale. Chest 92:393, 1987.

845. Lindsay DA, Read J: Pulmonary vascular responsiveness in the prognosis of chronic obstructive lung disease. Am Rev Respir Dis 105:242, 1972.

846. Rebuck AS, Vandenberg RA: The relationship between pulmonary arterial pressure and physiologic dead space in patients with obstructive lung disease. Am Rev Respir Dis 107:423, 1973.

846a. Read J: The lungs and circulation in chronic pulmonary disease. J R Coll Physicians Lond 5:221, 1971.

847. Matthay RA, Schwarz MI, Ellis JH, et al: Pulmonary artery hypertension in chronic obstructive pulmonary disease: chest radiographic assessment. Invest Radiol 16:95, 1981.

848. Chetty KG, Brown SE, Light RW: Identification of pulmonary hypertension in chronic obstructive pulmonary disease from routine chest radiographs. Am Rev Respir Dis 126:338, 1982.

849. Soroldoni M, Ferrarini F, Biffi E, et al: M-mode subxiphoid echocardiography in assessing pulmonary hypertension. Its usefulness in chronic obstructive pulmonary disease. Respiration 47:164, 1985.

850. Williams IP, Boyd MJ, Humberstone AM, et al: Pulmonary arterial hypertension and emphysema. Br J Dis Chest 78:211, 1984.

851. Tramarin R, Torbicki A, Marchandise B, et al: Doppler echocardiographic evaluation of pulmonary artery pressure in chronic obstructive pulmonary disease. A European multicentre study. Working Group on Noninvasive Evaluation of Pulmonary Artery Pressure. Eur Heart J 12:103, 1991.

852. Burghuber OC, Brunner CH, Schenk P, Weissel M: Pulsed Doppler echocardiography to assess pulmonary artery hypertension in chronic obstructive pulmonary disease. Monaldi Arch Chest Dis 48:121, 1993.

853. Brecker SJ, Xiao HB, Stojnic BB, et al: Assessment of the peak tricuspid regurgitant velocity from the dynamics of retrograde flow. Int J Cardiol 34:267, 1992.

854. Marchandise B, De Bruyne B, Delaunois L, Kremer R: Non-invasive prediction of pulmonary hypertension in chronic obstructive pulmonary disease by echocardiography. Chest 91:361, 1987.

855. Morrison DA, Ovitt T, Hammermeister KE: Functional tricuspid regurgitation and right ventricular dysfunction in pulmonary hypertension. Am J Cardiol 62:108, 1988.

856. Migueres M, Escamilla R, Coca F, et al: Pulsed Doppler echocardiography in the diagnosis of pulmonary hypertension in COPD. Chest 98:280, 1990.

857. Schiller NB, Sahn DJ: Pulmonary pressure measurement by Doppler and two-dimensional echocardiography in adult and pediatric populations. In Weir EK, Archer SL, Reeves JT (eds): The Diagnosis and Treatment of Pulmonary Hypertension. New York, Futura Publishing, 1992, pp 41–59.

858. Taha RA, Boushy SF, Thompson HK Jr, et al: The electrocardiogram in chronic obstructive pulmonary disease. Am Rev Respir Dis 107:1067, 1973.

859. Tandon MK: Correlations of electrocardiographic features with airway obstruction in chronic bronchitis. Chest 63:146, 1973.

860. Murphy ML, Hutcheson F: The electrocardiographic diagnosis of right ventricular hypertrophy in chronic obstructive pulmonary disease. Chest 65:622, 1974.

861. Olvey SK, Reduto LA, Stevens PM, et al: First pass radionuclide assessment of right and left ventricular ejection fraction in chronic pulmonary disease—effect of oxygen upon exercise response. Chest 78:4, 1980.

862. MacNee W, Morgan A, Wathen C, et al: Right ventricular performance during exercise in chronic obstructive pulmonary disease: The effects of oxygen. Respiration 48:206, 1985.

863. Takao M, Miyahara Y, Shinboku H, et al: Noninvasive assessment of right heart function by $^{81m}$Kr equilibrium radionuclide ventriculography in chronic pulmonary disease. Chest 109:67, 1996.

864. Keller CA, Ohar J, Ruppel G, et al: Right ventricular function in patients with severe COPD evaluated for lung transplantation. Lung Transplant Group. Chest 107:1510, 1995.

865. Macnee W, Xue QF, Hannan WJ, et al: Assessment by radionuclide angiography of right and left ventricular function in chronic bronchitis and emphysema. Thorax 38:494, 1983.

866. Burghuber O, Bergmann H, Silberbauer K, et al: Right ventricular performance in chronic air flow obstruction. Respiration 45:124, 1984.

867. Mahler D, Brent B, Loke J, et al: Right ventricular performance and central circulatory hemodynamics during upright exercise in patients with chronic obstructive pulmonary disease. Am Rev Respir Dis 130:722, 1984.

868. Yamaoka S, Yonekura Y, Koide H, et al: Noninvasive method to assess cor pulmonale in patients with chronic obstructive pulmonary disease. Chest 92:10, 1987.

869. Turnbull LW, Ridgeway JP, Biernacki W, et al: Assessment of the right ventricle by magnetic resonance imaging in chronic obstructive lung disease. Thorax 45:597, 1990.

870. Seibold H, Roth U, Lippert R, et al: Left heart function in chronic obstructive lung disease. Klin Wochenschr 64:433, 1986.

871. MacNee W, Morgan AD, Wathen CG, et al: Right ventricular performance during exercise in chronic obstructive pulmonary disease. Respiration 48:206, 1985.

872. Kohama A, Tanouchi J, Masatsugu H, et al: Pathologic involvement of the left ventricle in chronic cor pulmonale. Chest 98:794, 1990.

873. Edwards CW: Left ventricular hypertrophy in emphysema. Thorax 29:75, 1974.

874. Murphy ML, Adamson J, Hutcheson F: Left ventricular hypertrophy in patients with chronic bronchitis and emphysema. Ann Intern Med 81:307, 1974.

875. Jardin F, Gueret P, Prost JF, et al: Two-dimensional echocardiographic assessment of left ventricular function in chronic obstructive pulmonary disease. Am Rev Respir Dis 129:135, 1984.

876. Roux JJ, Deveze JL, Escojido H, et al: Left ventricular function in chronic obstructive pulmonary disease after decompensation. Respiration 38:43, 1979.

877. Vonk Noordegraaf A, Marcus JT, Roseboom B, et al: The effect of right ventricular hypertrophy on left ventricular ejection fraction in pulmonary emphysema. Chest 112:640, 1997.

878. Hudson LD, Kurt TL, Petty TL, et al: Arrhythmias associated with acute respiratory failure in patients with chronic airway obstruction. Chest 63:661, 1973.

879. Corazzo LJ, Pastor BH: Cardiac arrhythmias in chronic cor pulmonale. N Engl J Med 259:862, 1958.

880. Holford FD, Mithoefer JC: Cardiac arrhythmias in hospitalized patients with chronic obstructive pulmonary disease. Am Rev Respir Dis 108:879, 1973.

881. Bishop JM, Cross KW: Physiological variables and mortality in patients with various categories of chronic respiratory disease. Bull Eur Physiopathol Respir 20:495, 1985.

882. Burrows B, Kettel LJ, Niden AH, et al: Patterns of cardiovascular dysfunction in chronic obstructive lung disease. N Engl J Med 286:912, 1972.

883. De Troyer A: Effect of hyperinflation on the diaphragm. Eur Respir J 10:708, 1997.

884. Thurlbeck WM: Diaphragm and body weight in emphysema. Thorax 33:483, 1978.

885. Sánchez J, Medrano G, Debesse B, et al: Muscle fibre types in costal and crural diaphragm in normal men and in patients with moderate chronic respiratory disease. Clin Resir Physiol 21:351, 1985.

886. Campbell JA, Hughes RL, Saghal V, et al: Alterations in intercostal muscle morphology and biochemistry in patients with obstructive lung disease. Am Rev Respir Dis 122:679, 1980.

887. Sánchez J, Bastien C, Medrano G, et al: Metabolic enzymatic activities in the diaphragm of normal men and patients with moderate chronic obstructive pulmonary disease. Bull Eur Physiopathol Respir 20:535, 1985.

888. Kelsen SG, Wolanski T, Supinski GS, et al: The effect of elastase-induced emphysema on diaphragmatic muscle structure in hamsters. Am Rev Respir Dis 127:330, 1983.

889. Supinski GS, Kelsen SG: Effect of elastase-induced emphysema on the force-generating ability of the diaphragm. J Clin Invest 70:978, 1982.

890. Gaultier C, Boulé M, Tourmier G, et al: Inspiratory force reserve of the respiratory muscles in children with chronic obstructive pulmonary disease. Am Rev Respir Dis 132:811, 1985.

891. Rochester DF, Braun NMT: Determinants of maximal inspiratory pressure in chronic obstructive pulmonary disease. Am Rev Respir Dis 132:42, 1985.

892. Polkey MI, Kyroussis D, Hamnegard CH, et al: Diaphragm strength in chronic obstructive pulmonary disease. Am J Respir Crit Care Med 154:1310, 1996.

893. Grassino A, Macklem PT: Respiratory muscle fatigue and ventilatory failure. Annu Rev Med 35:625, 1984.

894. Bellemare F, Grassino A: Force reserve of the diaphragm in patients with chronic obstructive pulmonary disease. J Appl Physiol 55:8, 1983.

895. Dodd DF, Kelly S, Collett PW, et al: Pressure-time product, work rate, and endurance during resistive breathing in humans. J Appl Physiol 64:1397, 1988.

896. Collett PW, Perry C, Engel L: Pressure-time product, flow, and O$_2$ cost of resistive breathing in humans. J Appl Physiol 58:1263, 1965.

897. Aubier M, Murciano D, Lecocguic Y, et al: Bilateral phrenic stimulation: A simple technique to assess diaphragmatic fatigue in humans. J Appl Physiol 58:58, 1985.

898. Bye P, Esau S, Levy R, et al: Ventilatory muscle function during exercise in air and oxygen in patients with chronic air-flow limitation. Am Rev Respir Dis 236:132, 1985.

899. Wilson SH, Cooke NT, Moxham J, et al: Sternomastoid muscle function and fatigue in normal subjects and in patients with chronic obstructive pulmonary disease. Am Rev Respir Dis 129:460, 1984.

900. Aldrich TK: The application of muscle endurance training techniques to the respiratory muscles in COPD. Lung 163:15, 1985.

901. Belman MJ, Mittman C (with the technical assistance of Robert Weir): Ventilatory muscle training improves exercise capacity in chronic obstructive pulmonary disease. Am Rev Respir Dis 121:273, 1980.

902. Pardy RL, Rivington RN, Despas PJ, et al: The effects of inspiratory muscle training on exercise performance in chronic airflow limitation. Am Rev Respir Dis 123:426, 1981.

903. Pardy RL, Rivington RN, Despas PJ, et al: Inspiratory muscle training compared with physiotherapy in chronic airflow limitation. Am Rev Respir Dis 123:421, 1981.

904. Yan S, Kaminski D, Sliwinski P: Inspiratory muscle mechanics of patients with chronic obstructive pulmonary disease during incremental exercise. Am J Respir Crit Care Med 156:807, 1997.

905. Shapiro SH, Ernst P, Gray-Donald K, et al: Effect of negative pressure ventilation in severe chronic obstructive pulmonary disease. Lancet 340:1425, 1992.

906. Siwinski P, Macklem PT: Inspiratory muscle dysfunction as a cause of death in COPD patients. Monaldi Arch Chest Dis 52:380, 1997.

907. Burrows B, Earle RH: Course and prognosis of chronic obstructive lung disease. A prospective study of 200 patients. N Engl J Med 280:397, 1969.

908. Camilli AE, Burrows B, Knudson RJ, et al: Longitudinal changes in forced expiratory volume in one second in adults: Effect of smoking and smoking cessation. Am Rev Respir Dis 135:794, 1987.

909. Buist AS, Ghezzo H, Anthonisen NR, et al: Relationship between the single-breath N$_2$ test and age, sex and smoking habit in three North American cities. Am Rev Respir Dis 120:305, 1979.

910. Becklake MR, Leclerc M, Strobach H, et al: The N$_2$ closing volume test in population studies: Sources of variation and reproducibility. Am Rev Respir Dis 111:141, 1975.

911. Becklake MR, Permutt S: Evaluation of tests of lung function for "screening" for early detection of chronic obstructive lung disease. In Macklem PT, Permutt S (eds): The Lung in the Transition Between Health and Disease. New York, Marcel Dekker, 1979, p 345.

912. Martin PR, Lindsay D, Despas P, et al: The early detection of airway obstruction. Am Rev Respir Dis 111:119, 1975.

913. Murtagh PS, Proctor DF, Permutt S, et al: Bronchial closure with mechoyl in excised dog lobes. J Appl Physiol 31:409, 1971.

914. Demedts M, Cosemans J, De Roo M, et al: Emphysema with minor airway obstruction and abnormal tests of small airway disease. Respiration 35:148, 1978.

915. Paré PD, Brooks LA, Coppin CA, et al: Density dependence of maximal expiratory flow and its correlation with small airway disease in smokers. Am Rev Resp Dis 131:521, 1985.

916. Rossoff LJ, Csima A, Zamel N, et al: Reproducibility of maximum expiratory flow in severe chronic obstructive pulmonary disease. Bull Eur Physiopathol Respir 15:1129, 1979.

917. Jadue C, Greville H, Coalson JJ, et al: Forced expiration and HeO$_2$ response in canine peripheral airway obstruction. J Appl Physiol 58:1788, 1985.

918. Mink SN: Expiratory flow limitation and the response to breathing a helium-oxygen gas mixture in a canine model of pulmonary emphysema. J Clin Invest 73:1321, 1984.

919. Van de Woestijne KP: Are the small airways really quiet? Eur J Respir Dis 63:19, 1982.

920. Detels R, Tashkin DP, Simmons MS, et al: The UCLA population studies of chronic obstructive respiratory disease. 5. Agreement and disagreement of tests in identifying abnormal lung function. Chest 82:630, 1982.

921. Dosman JA, Cotton DJ, Graham BL, et al: Sensitivity and specificity of early diagnostic tests of lung function in smokers. Chest 79:6, 1981.

922. Nemery B, Moavero NE, Brasseur L, et al: Significance of small airway tests in middle-aged smokers. Am Rev Respir Dis 124:232, 1981.

923. Olofsson J, Bake B, Svardsudd K, et al: The single breath N$_2$-test predicts the rate of decline in FEV$_1$. Eur J Respir Dis 69:46, 1986.

924. Buist AS, Vollmer WM, Johnson LR, et al: Does the single-breath test identify the susceptible individual? Chest 85:105, 1984.

925. Walter S, Nancy NR, Collier CR, et al: Changes in the forced expiratory spirogram in young male smokers. Am Rev Respir Dis 119:717, 1979.

926. Solomon DA: Clinical significance of pulmonary function tests: Are small airways tests helpful in the detection of early airflow obstruction? Chest 74:567, 1978.

927. Bake B: Is maximum mid-expiratory flow rate sensitive to small airways obstruction? Eur J Respir Dis 62:150, 1981.

928. Marrero O, Beck GJ, Schachier EN: Discriminating power of measurements from maximum expiratory flow-volume curves. Respiration 49:263, 1986.

929. Koulouris NG, Rapakoulias P, Rassidakis A, et al: Dependence of forced vital capacity manoeuvre on time course of preceding inspiration in patients with restrictive lung disease. Eur Respir J 10:2366, 1997.

930. Herzog H, Keller R, Perruchoud A, et al: The combined flow-volume pressure-resistance diagram for classification of airways obstruction. In DeKock MA, Nadel JA, Lewis CM (eds): Mechanisms of Airways Obstruction in Human Respiratory Disease. Cape Town, AA Balkema, 1979, p 333.

931. Mellisant CF, Van Noord JA, Van de Woestijne KP, Demedts M: Comparison of dynamic lung function indices during forced and quiet breathing in upper airway obstruction, asthma, and emphysema. Chest 98:77, 1990.

932. Colebatch HJH, Greaves IA: Chronic airflow obstruction. Evolution of disordered function in cigarette smokers. Med J Aust 142:607, 1985.

933. Hyatt RE, Rodarte JR: Changes in lung mechanics. In Macklem PT, Permutt S (eds): The Lung in the Transition Between Health and Disease. New York, Marcel Dekker, 1979, p 73.

934. Mead J, Turner JM, Macklem PT, et al: Significance of relationship between lung recoil and maximum expiratory flow. J Appl Physiol 22:95, 1967.

935. Fry DL, Hyatt RE: Pulmonary mechanics. A unified analysis of the relationship between pressure, volume and gas flow in the lungs of normal and diseased human subjects. Am J Med 29:672, 1960.

936. Dayman H: Expiratory spirogram. Am Rev Respir Dis 83:842, 1961.

937. Dekker E, Defarges JG, Heemstra H: Direct measurement of intrabronchial pressure; its application to location of check-valve mechanism. J Appl Physiol 13:35, 1958.

938. Fraser RG, Macklen PT, Brown WG: Airway dynamics in bronchiectasis: A combined cinefluorographic-manometric study. Am J Roentgenol 93:821, 1965.

939. Fraser RG, Macklem PT: Bronchial dynamics in health and obstructive airway disease: Physiology and roentgenology. In Simon M, Potchen EJ, LeMay M (eds): Frontiers of Chest Radiology. New York, Grune & Stratton, 1969, p 76.

940. Wright RR: Bronchial atrophy and collapse in chronic obstructive pulmonary emphysema. Am J Pathol 37:63, 1960.

941. Paré PD, Coppin CA, Brooks LA, et al: Upstream resistance in COPD patients with emphysema and small airway inflammation (abstract). Am Rev Respir Dis 127:256, 1983.

942. Paré PD, Hogg JC: Lung structure-function relationships. In Calverley P, Pride N (eds): Chronic Obstructive Pulmonary Disease. London, Chapman & Hall, 1995, pp 33.

943. Anthonisen NR, Wright EC: Bronchodilator response in chronic obstructive pulmonary disease. Am Rev Respir Dis 133:814, 1986.

944. Wardman AG, Binns V, Clayden AD, et al: The diagnosis and treatment of adults with obstructive airways disease in general practice. Br J Dis Chest 80:19, 1986.

945. Kerstjens HA, Brand PL, Quanjer PH, et al: Variability of bronchodilator response and effects of inhaled corticosteroid treatment in obstructive airways disease. Dutch CNSLD Study Group. Thorax 48:722, 1993.

946. Dawkins KD, Muers MF: Diurnal variation in airflow obstruction in chronic bronchitis. Thorax 36:618, 1981.

947. Ramsdale EH, Morris MM, Hargreave FE: Interpretation of the variability of peak flow rates in chronic bronchitis. Thorax 41:771, 1986.

948. Chester EJ, Schwartz HJ, Fleming GM, et al: Adverse effect of propranolol on airway function in nonasthmatic chronic obstructive lung disease. Chest 79:540, 1981.

949. Postma DS, Keyzer JJ, Koëter GH, et al: Influence of the parasympathetic and sympathetic nervous system on nocturnal bronchial obstruction. Clin Sci 69:251, 1985.

950. Emmett PC, Love RG, Hannan WJ, et al: The relationship between the pulmonary distribution of inhaled fine aerosols and tests of small airway function. Bull Eur Physiopathol Respir 20:325, 1984.

951. Barter SJ, Cunningham DA, Lavender JP, et al: Abnormal ventilation scans in middle-aged smokers—comparison with tests of overall lung function. Am Rev Respir Dis 132:148, 1985.

952. Fairshter RD: Airway hysteresis in normal subjects and individuals with chronic airflow obstruction. J Appl Physiol 48:1505, 1985.

953. Guillemi S, Wright JL, Hogg JC, et al: Density dependence of pulmonary resistance: Correlation with small airway pathology. Eur Respir J (5):789, 1995.

954. Clément J, Làndsér FJ, Van de Woestijne KP, et al: Total resistance and reactance in patients with respiratory complaints with and without airways obstruction. Chest 83:215, 1983.

955. Guillemi S, Wright JL, Hogg JC, et al: Density dependence of pulmonary resistance: Correlation with airway pathology. Eur Respir J 8:789, 1995.

956. Higenbottam T, Payne J: Glottis narrowing in lung disease. Am Rev Respir Dis 125:746, 1982.

957. Hogg JC, Wright JL, Paré PD, et al: Airway disease: Evolution, pathology, and recognition. Med J Aust 142:605, 1985.

958. York EL, Jones RL: Effects of smoking on regional residual volume in young adults. Chest 79:12, 1981.

959. Hughes JA, Hutchison DCS: Errors in the estimation of vital capacity from expiratory flow-volume curves in pulmonary emphysema. Br J Dis Chest 76:279, 1982.

960. Brusasco V, Pellegrino R, Rodarte JR: Vital capacities in acute and chronic airway obstruction: Dependence on flow and volume histories. Eur Respir J 10:1316, 1997.

961. Fleury B, Murciano D, Talamo C, et al: Work of breathing in patients with chronic obstructive pulmonary disease in acute respiratory failure. Am Rev Respir Dis 131:822, 1985.

962. Purro A, Appendini L, Patessio A, et al: Static intrinsic PEEP in COPD patients during spontaneous breathing. Am J Respir Crit Care Med 157:1044, 1998.

963. Morris MJ, Madgwick RG, Lane DJ: Difference between functional residual capacity and elastic equilibrium volume in patients with chronic obstructive pulmonary disease. Thorax 51:415, 1996.

964. Koulouris NG, Dimopoulou I, Valta P, et al: Detection of expiratory flow limitation during exercise in COPD patients. J Appl Physiol 82:723, 1997.

965. Brancatisano TP, Dodd DS, Collett PW, et al: Effect of expiratory loading on glottic dimensions in humans. J Appl Physiol 58:605, 1985.

966. Pellegrino R, Brusasco V: Lung hyperinflation and flow limitation in chronic airway obstruction. Eur Respir J 10:543, 1997.

967. Marini JJ, Tyler ML, Hudson LD, et al: Influence of head-dependent positions on lung volume and oxygen saturation in chronic air-flow obstruction. Am Rev Respir Dis 129:101, 1984.

968. Farkas GA, Roussos CH: Adaptability of the hamster diaphragm to exercise and/or emphysema. J Appl Physiol 53:1263, 1982.

969. Paré PD, Coppin CA: Errors in the measurement of total lung capacity in patients with chronic obstructive pulmonary disease. Thorax 38:468, 1983.

970. Burns CB, Scheinhorn DJ: Evaluation of single-breath helium dilution total lung capacity in obstructive lung disease. Am Rev Respir Dis 130:580, 1985.

971. Rodenstein DO, Stănescu DC: Reassessment of lung volume measurement by helium dilution and by body plethysmography in chronic air-flow obstruction. Am Rev Respir Dis 126:1040, 1982.

972. Piquet J, Harf A, Lorino H, et al: Lung volume measurements by plethysmography in chronic obstructive pulmonary disease. Influence of the panting pattern. Bull Eur Physiopathol Respir 20:31, 1985.

973. Bégin P, Peslin R: Influence of panting frequency on thoracic gas volume measurements in chronic obstructive pulmonary disease. Am Rev Respir Dis 130:121, 1984.

974. Rodenstein DO, Stănescu DC: Frequency dependence of plethysmographic volume in healthy and asthmatic subjects. J Appl Physiol 54:159, 1983.

975. Colebatch HJH, Greaves IA, Ng CKY, et al: Exponential analysis of elastic recoil and aging in healthy males and females. J Appl Physiol 47:683, 1979.

976. Gibson GJ, Pride NB, Davis J, et al: Exponential description of the static pressure-volume curve of normal and diseased lungs. Am Rev Respir Dis 120:799, 1979.

977. Knudson RJ, Kaltenborn WT: Evaluation of lung elastic recoil by exponential curve analysis. Respir Physiol 46:29, 1981.

978. Colebatch HJH, Greaves IA, Ng CKY, et al: Pulmonary distensibility and ventilatory function in smokers. Bull Eur Physiopathol Respir 21:439, 1985.

979. Corbin RP, Loveland M, Martin RR, et al: A four-year follow-up study of lung mechanics in smokers. Am Rev Respir Dis 120:293, 1979.

980. Paré PD, Brooks LA, Bates J, et al: Exponential analysis of the lung pressure-volume curve as a predictor of pulmonary emphysema. Am Rev Respir Dis 126:54, 1982.

981. Knudson RJ, Bloom JW, Knudson DE, et al: Subclinical effects of smoking. Chest 86:20, 1984.

982. Berend N, Glanville AR, Grunstein MM, et al: Determinants of the slope of phase III of the single breath nitrogen test. Bull Eur Physiopathol Respir 20:521, 1985.

983. De Troyer A, Yernault JC, Rodenstein D, et al: Influence of beta₂-agonist aerosols on pressure-volume characteristics of the lungs. Am Rev Respir Dis 118:987, 1978.

984. Zamel N, Webster PM: Improved expiratory air flow dynamics with smoking cessation. Bull Eur Physiopathol Respir 20:19, 1984.

985. Soguel Schenkel N, Burdet L, de Muralt B, Fitting JW: Oxygen saturation during daily activities in chronic obstructive pulmonary disease. Eur Respir J 9:2584, 1996.

986. Schwartz JS, Bencowitz HZ, Moser KM, et al: Air travel hypoxemia with chronic obstructive pulmonary disease. Ann Intern Med 100:473, 1984.

987. Wagner PD, Dantzker DR, Dueck R, et al: Ventilation-perfusion inequality in chronic obstructive pulmonary disease. J Clin Invest 59:203, 1977.

988. Marthan R, Castaing Y, Manier G, et al: Gas exchange alterations in patients with chronic obstructive lung disease. Chest 87:470, 1985.

989. Yamaguchi K, Mori M, Kawai A, et al: Inhomogeneities of ventilation and the diffusing capacity to perfusion in various chronic lung diseases. Am J Respir Crit Care Med 156:86, 1997.

990. Comroe JH Jr, Fowler WS: Lung function studies. VI. Detection of uneven alveolar ventilation during a single breath of oxygen. Am J Med 10:408, 1951.

991. Darling RC, Cournand A, Mansfield JS, et al: Studies on the intrapulmonary mixture of gases. I. Nitrogen elimination from blood and body tissues during high oxygen breathing. J Clin Invest 19:591, 1940.

992. Meneely GR, Kaltreider NL: The volume of the lung determined by helium dilution. Description of the method and comparison with other procedures. J Clin Invest 28:129, 1949.

993. Bates DV, Christie RV: Intrapulmonary mixing of helium in health and in emphysema. Clin Sci 9:17, 1950.

994. Anthonisen NR, Bass H, Heckscher T, et al: Recent observation on the measurement of regional $\dot{V}/\dot{Q}$ ratios in chronic lung disease. J Nucl Biol Med 11:73, 1967.

995. Bentivoglio LG, Beerel F, Stewart PB, et al: Studies of regional ventilation and perfusion in pulmonary emphysema using xenon 133. Am Rev Respir Dis 88:315, 1963.

996. Dore EK, Poe ND, Ellestad MH, et al: Lung perfusion and inhalation scanning in pulmonary emphysema. Am J Roentgenol 104:770, 1968.

997. Pontoppidan H, Hedley-Whyte J, Bendixen HH, et al: Ventilation and oxygen requirements during prolonged artificial ventilation in patients with respiratory failure. N Engl J Med 273:401, 1965.

998. Kamat SR, Dulfano MJ, Segal MS: The effects of intermittent positive pressure breathing (IPPB/I) with compressed air in patients with severe chronic nonspecific obstructive pulmonary disease. Am Rev Respir Dis 86:360, 1962.

999. Torres G, Lyons HA, Emerson P: The effects of intermittent positive pressure breathing on the intrapulmonary distribution of inspired air. Am J Med 29:946, 1960.

1000. Morrell NW, Wignall BK, Biggs T, Seed WA: Collateral ventilation and gas exchange in emphysema. Am J Respir Crit Care Med 150:635, 1994.

1001. Palmer KNV, Diament ML: Relative contributions of obstructive and restrictive ventilatory impairment in the production of hypoxaemia and hypercapnia in chronic bronchitis. Lancet 1:1233, 1968.

1002. Gertz I: Blood volume and arterial blood gases in patients with chronic obstructive lung disease during and after acute respiratory failure. Scand J Respir Dis 60:6, 1979.

1003. Mithoefer JC, Ramirez C, Cook W, et al: The effect of mixed venous oxygenation on arterial blood chronic obstructive pulmonary disease. The basis for a classification. Am Rev Respir Dis 117:259, 1978.

1004. Paré PD, Brooks LA, Baile EM, et al: The effect of systemic venous hypertension on pulmonary function and lung water. J Appl Physiol 51:592, 1981.

1005. Barbera JA, Roca J, Ferrer A, et al: Mechanisms of worsening gas exchange during acute exacerbations of chronic obstructive pulmonary disease. Eur Respir J 10:1285, 1997.

1006. Parot S, Saunier C, Schrijen F, et al: Concomitant changes in function tests, breathing pattern and $Pa_{CO_2}$ in patients with chronic obstructive pulmonary disease. Bull Eur Physiopathol Respir 18:145, 1982.

1007. Parot S, Miara B, Milic-Emili J, et al: Hypoxemia, hypercapnia and breathing pattern in patients with chronic obstructive pulmonary disease. Am Rev Respir Dis 126:822, 1982.

1008. Mountain R, Zwillich C, Weil J, et al: Hypoventilation in obstructive lung disease: The role of familial factors. N Engl J Med 298:521, 1978.

1009. Kawakami Y, Irie T, Kishi F, et al: Familial aggregation of abnormal ventilatory control and pulmonary function in chronic obstructive pulmonary disease. Eur J Respir Dis 62:56, 1981.

1010. Kawakami Y, Irie T, Shida A, et al: Familial factors affecting arterial blood gas values and respiratory chemosensitivity in chronic obstructive pulmonary disease. Am Rev Respir Dis 125:420, 1982.

1011. Milic-Emili J: Recent advances in clinical assessment of control of breathing. Lung 160:1, 1982.

1012. Fahey PJ, Hyde RW: "Won't breathe" vs "Can't breathe": Detection of depressed ventilatory drive in patients with obstructive pulmonary disease. Chest 84:19, 1983.

1013. Bradley CA, Fleetham JA, Anthonisen NR, et al: Ventilatory control in patients with hypoxemia due to obstructive lung disease. Am Rev Respir Dis 120:21, 1979.

1014. Hedemark LL, Kronenberg RS: Chemical regulation of respiration. Chest 82:488, 1982.

1015. Santiago TV, Remolina C, Scoles V III, et al: Endorphins and the control of breathing: Ability of naloxone to restore flow-resistive load compensation in chronic obstructive pulmonary disease. N Engl J Med 304:1190, 1981.

1016. Tobin MJ, Jenouri G, Sackner MA, et al: Effect of naloxone on breathing pattern in patients with chronic obstructive pulmonary disease with and without hypercapnia. Respiration 44:419, 1983.

1017. Montserrat JM, Ballester E, Sopeña JJ, et al: Effect of naloxone on arterial gases in chronically obstructed patients with acute respiratory failure. Eur J Respir Dis 66:77, 1985.

1018. Flenley DC, Franklin DH, Millar JS, et al: The hypoxic drive to breathing in chronic bronchitis and emphysema. Clin Sci 38:503, 1970.

1019. De Troyer A, Leeper JB, McKenzie DK, Gandevia SC: Neural drive to the diaphragm in patients with severe COPD. Am J Respir Crit Care Med 155:1335, 1997.

1020. Oliven A, Kelsen SG, Deal EC Jr, et al: Respiratory pressure sensation. Relationship to changes in breathing pattern and $P_{CO_2}$ during acute increase in airway resistance in patients with chronic obstructive pulmonary disease. Am Rev Respir Dis 132:1214, 1985.

1021. Gottfried SB, Redline S, Altose MD, et al: Respiratory sensation in chronic obstructive pulmonary disease. Am Rev Respir Dis 132:954, 1985.

1022. Loveridge B, West P, Anthonisen N, et al: Breathing patterns in patients with chronic obstructive pulmonary disease. Am Rev Respir Dis 130:730, 1984.

1023. Pardy RL, Rivington RN, Milic-Emili J, et al: Control of breathing in chronic obstructive pulmonary disease—the effect of histamine inhalation. Am Rev Respir Dis 125:6, 1982.

1024. Oliven A, Cherniack NS, Deal EC, et al: The effects of acute bronchoconstriction on respiratory activity in patients with chronic obstructive pulmonary disease. Am Rev Respir Dis 131:236, 1985.

1025. Fennerty AG, Banks J, Bevan C, et al: Role of airway receptors in the breathing pattern of patients with chronic obstructive lung disease. Thorax 40:268, 1985.

1026. Muriciano D, Aubier M, Viau F, et al: Effects of airway anesthesia on pattern of breathing and blood gases in patients with chronic obstructive pulmonary disease during acute respiratory failure. Am Rev Respir Dis 126:113, 1982.

1027. Gorini M, Misuri G, Corrado A, et al: Breathing pattern and carbon dioxide retention in severe chronic obstructive pulmonary disease. Thorax 51:677, 1996.

1028. Fleetham JA, Bradley CA, Kryger MH, et al: The effect of low flow oxygen therapy on the chemical control of ventilation in patients with hypoxemic COPD. Am Rev Respir Dis 122:833, 1980.

1029. Burki NK: Breathlessness and mouth occlusion pressure in patients with chronic obstruction of the airways. Chest 76:527, 1979.

1030. Koo KW, Sax DS, Snider GL: Arterial blood gases and pH during sleep in chronic obstructive pulmonary disease. Am J Med 58:663, 1975.

1031. Flick MR, Block AJ: Continuous in-vivo monitoring of arterial oxygenation in chronic obstructive lung disease. Ann Intern Med 86:725, 1977.

1032. Fleetham J, West P, Mezon B, et al: Sleep, arousals, and oxygen desaturation in chronic obstructive pulmonary disease—the effect of oxygen therapy. Am Rev Respir Dis 126:429, 1982.

1033. Calverley PMA, Brezinova V, Douglas NJ, et al: The effect of oxygenation on sleep quality in chronic bronchitis and emphysema. Am Rev Respir Dis 126:206, 1982.

1034. Guilleminault C, Cummiskey J, Motta J, et al: Chronic obstructive airflow disease and sleep studies. Am Rev Respir Dis 122:397, 1980.

1035. Douglas NJ, Calverley PMA, Leggett RJE, et al: Transient hypoxemia during sleep in chronic bronchitis and emphysema. Lancet 1:1, 1979.

1036. George CF, West P, Kryger MH: Oxygenation and breathing pattern during phasic and tonic REM in patients with chronic obstructive pulmonary disease. Sleep 10:234, 1987.

1037. DeMarco FJ, Wynne JW, Block AJ, et al: Oxygen desaturation during sleep as a determinant of the "blue and bloated" syndrome. Chest 79:621, 1981.

1038. Perez-Padilla R, Conway W, Roth T, et al: Hypercapnia and sleep $O_2$ desaturation in chronic obstructive pulmonary disease. Sleep 10:216, 1987.

1039. Arand DL, McGinty DJ, Littner MR, et al: Respiratory patterns associated with hemoglobin desaturation during sleep in chronic obstructive pulmonary disease. Chest 80:183, 1981.

1040. Littner MR, McGinty DJ, Arand DL, et al: Determinants of oxygen desaturation in the course of ventilation during sleep in chronic obstructive pulmonary disease. Am Rev Respir Dis 122:849, 1980.

1041. Meurice JC, Marc I, Series F: Influence of sleep on ventilatory and upper airway response to $CO_2$ in normal subjects and patients with COPD. Am J Respir Crit Care Med 152:1620, 1995.

1042. Tatsumi K, Kimura H, Kunitomo F, et al: Sleep arterial oxygen desaturation and chemical control of breathing during wakefulness in COPD. Chest 90:68, 1986.

1043. Boysen PG, Block AJ, Wynne JW, et al: Nocturnal pulmonary hypertension in patients with chronic obstructive pulmonary disease. Chest 76:536, 1979.

1044. Weitzenblum E, Chaouat A, Charpentier C, et al: Sleep-related hypoxaemia in chronic obstructive pulmonary disease: Causes, consequences and treatment. Respiration 64:187, 1997.

1045. Goldstein RS, Ramcharan V, Bowes G, et al: Effect of supplemental nocturnal oxygen on gas exchange in patients with severe obstructive lung disease. N Engl J Med 310:425, 1984.

1046. Minh VD, Lee HM, Dolan GF, et al: Hypoxemia during exercise in patients with chronic obstructive pulmonary disease. Am Rev Respir Dis 120:787, 1979.

1047. Raffestin B, Escourrou P, Legrand A, et al: Circulatory transport of oxygen in patients with chronic airflow obstruction exercising maximally. Am Rev Respir Dis 125:426, 1982.

1048. Stewart RI, Lewis CM: Arterial oxygenation and oxygen transport during exercise in patients with chronic obstructive pulmonary disease. Respiration 49:161, 1986.

1049. Bellone A, Frisinghelli A, Pozzi et al: Exercise-induced hypoxaemia in emphysematous type chronic obstructive pulmonary disease. Monaldi Arch Chest Dis 51:117, 1996.

1050. Owens G, Rogers R, Pennock B, et al: The diffusing capacity as a predictor of arterial oxygen desaturation during exercise in patients with chronic obstructive pulmonary disease. N Engl J Med 310:1218, 1984.

1051. Van Meerhaeghe A, Sergysels R: Control of breathing during exercise in patients with chronic airflow limitation with or without hypercapnia. Chest 84:565, 1983.

1052. Giminez M, Servera E, Candina R, et al: Hypercapnia during maximal exercise in patients with chronic airflow obstruction. Bull Eur Physiopathol Respir 20:113, 1985.

1053. Scano G, van Meerhaeghe A, Willeput R, et al: Effect of oxygen on breathing during exercise in patients with chronic obstructive lung disease. Eur J Respir Dis 63:23, 1982.

1054. Bradley BL, Garner AE, Billiu D, et al: Oxygen-assisted exercise in chronic obstructive lung disease. The effect on exercise capacity and arterial blood gas tensions. Am Rev Respir Dis 118:239, 1978.

1055. Stein DA, Bradley BL, Miller WC, et al: Mechanism of oxygen effects on exercise in patients with chronic obstructive pulmonary disease. Chest 81:6, 1982.

1056. Brown SE, Wiener S, Brown RA, et al: Exercise performance following a carbohydrate load in chronic airflow obstruction. J Appl Physiol 58:1340, 1985.

1057. Brown SE, Nagendran RC, McHugh JW, et al: Effects of a large carbohydrate load on walking performance in chronic air-flow obstruction. Am Rev Respir Dis 132:960, 1985.

1058. Lockhart A: Exercise-limiting factors in chronic obstructive lung diseases. Bull Eur Physiopathol Respir 15:305, 1979.

1059. Brown HV, Wasserman K: Exercise performance in chronic obstructive pulmonary disease. Med Clin North Am 65:525, 1981.

1060. Moinard J, Manier G, Pillet O, Castaing Y: Effect of inhaled nitric oxide on hemodynamics and VA/Q inequalities in patients with chronic obstructive pulmonary disease. Am J Respir Crit Care Med 149:1482, 1994.

1061. Dillard T, Piantadosi S, Rajagopal K, et al: Prediction of ventilation at maximal exercise in chronic airflow obstruction. Am Rev Respir Dis 143:230, 1985.

1062. Montes de Oca M, Rassulo J, Celli BR: Respiratory muscle and cardiopulmonary function during exercise in very severe COPD. Am J Respir Crit Care Med 154:1284, 1996.

1063. Bauerle O, Chrusch CA, Younes M: Mechanisms by which COPD affects exercise tolerance. Am J Respir Crit Care Med 157:57, 1998.

1064. Killian KJ, Jones NL: The use of exercise testing and other methods in the investigation of dyspnea. Clin Chest Med 5:99, 1984.

1065. Ferrari K, Goti P, Misuri G, et al: Chronic exertional dyspnea and respiratory muscle function in patients with chronic obstructive pulmonary disease. Lung 175:311, 1997.

1066. Delgado HR, Braun SR, Skatrud JB, et al: Chest wall and abdominal motion during exercise in patients with chronic obstructive pulmonary disease. Am Rev Respir Dis 126:200, 1982.

1067. Dodd DS, Brancatisano T, Engel LA, et al: Chest wall mechanics during exercise in patients with severe chronic air-flow obstruction. Am Rev Respir Dis 129:33, 1984.

1068. Palange P, Forte S, Felli A, et al: Nutritional state and exercise tolerance in patients with COPD. Chest 107:1206, 1995.

1069. Jounieaux V, Mayeux I: Oxygen cost of breathing in patients with emphysema or chronic bronchitis in acute respiratory failure. Am J Respir Crit Care Med 152:2181, 1995.

1070. Ingram RH Jr, Miller RB, Tate LA: Acid-base response to acute carbon dioxide changes in chronic obstructive pulmonary disease. Am Rev Respir Dis 108:225, 1973.

1071. Eldridge F: Blood lactate and pyruvate in pulmonary insufficiency. N Engl J Med 274:878, 1966.

1072. Merwath CR, Sieker HO, Manfredi F: Acid-base relations between blood and cerebrospinal fluid in normal subjects and patients with respiratory insufficiency. N Engl J Med 265:310, 1961.

1073. Dunkin RS, Bondurant S: The determinants of cerebrospinal fluid $Po_2$. The effects of oxygen and carbon dioxide breathing in patients with chronic lung disease. Ann Intern Med 64:71, 1966.

1074. Sassoon CSH, Hassell KT, Mahutte CK, et al: Hyperoxic-induced hypercapnia in stable chronic obstructive pulmonary disease. Am Rev Respir Dis 135:907, 1987.

1075. Aubier M, Murciano D, Milic-Emili J, et al: Effects of the administration of $O_2$ on ventilation and blood gases in patients with chronic obstructive pulmonary disease during acute respiratory failure. Am Rev Respir Dis 122:747, 1980.

1076. Aubier M, Murciano D, Fournier M, et al: Central respiratory drive in acute respiratory failure of patients with chronic obstructive pulmonary disease. Am Rev Respir Dis 122:191, 1980.

1077. Guenard H, Verhas M, Todd-Prokopek A, et al: Effects of oxygen breathing on regional distribution of ventilation and perfusion in hypoxemic patients with chronic lung disease. Am Rev Respir Dis 125:12, 1982.

1078. Lee J, Read J: Effect of oxygen breathing on distribution of pulmonary blood flow in chronic obstructive lung disease. Am Rev Respir Dis 96:1173, 1967.

1079. Barbera JA, Roger N, Roca J, et al: Worsening of pulmonary gas exchange with nitric oxide inhalation in chronic obstructive pulmonary disease. Lancet 347:436, 1996.

1080. Roger N, Barbera JA, Roca J, et al: Nitric oxide inhalation during exercise in chronic obstructive pulmonary disease. Am J Respir Crit Care Med 156:800, 1997.

1081. Roger N, Barbera JA, Farre R, et al: Effect of nitric oxide inhalation on respiratory system resistance in chronic obstructive pulmonary disease. Eur Respir J 9:190, 1996.

1082. Barbera JA: Nitric oxide in chronic obstructive pulmonary disease. Monaldi Arch Chest Dis 51:528, 1996.

1083. Stone DJ, Zaldivar C, Keltz H: The effects of very low doses of nebulized isoproterenol, nebulized saline, and intravenous isoproterenol on blood gases in patients with chronic bronchitis. Am Rev Respir Dis 101:511, 1970.

1084. Pflug AE, Cheney FW Jr, Butler J: The effects of an ultrasonic aerosol on pulmonary mechanics and arterial blood gases in patients with chronic bronchitis. Am Rev Respir Dis 101:710, 1970.

1085. Rao S, Wilson DB, Brooks RC, et al: Acute effects of nebulization of *N*-acetylcysteine on pulmonary mechanics and gas exchange. Am Rev Respir Dis 102:17, 1970.

1086. Stone DJ, Keltz H, Samortin T, et al: The effect of β-adrenergic inhibition on respiratory gas exchange and lung function. Am Rev Respir Dis 103:503, 1971.

1087. Miller A, Thornton JC, Warshaw R, et al: Single breath diffusing capacity in a representative sample of the population of Michigan, a large industrial state—predicted values, lower limits of normal, and frequencies of abnormality by smoking history. Am Rev Respir Dis 127:270, 1983.

1088. Sansores RH, Paré PD, Abboud RT: Acute effect of cigarette smoking on the carbon monoxide diffusing capacity of the lung. Am Rev Respir Dis 146:951, 1992.

1089. Sansores RH, Paré P, Abboud RT: Effect of smoking cessation on pulmonary carbon monoxide diffusing capacity and capillary blood volume. Am Rev Respir Dis 146:959, 1992.

1090. Knudson RJ, Kaltenborn WT, Burrows B: Single breath carbon monoxide transfer factor in different forms of chronic airflow obstruction in a general population sample. Thorax 45:514, 1990.

1091. Graham BL, Mink JT, Cotton DJ, et al: Overestimation of the single-breath carbon monoxide diffusing capacity in patients with air-flow obstruction. Am Rev Respir Dis 129:403, 1984.

1092. Cotton DJ, Soparkar GR, Grahan BL: Diffusing capacity in the clinical assessment of chronic airflow limitation. Med Clin North Am 80:549, 1996.

1093. Graham BL, Mink JT, Cotton DJ: Reproducibility of three equation diffusing capacity (Dlcosb), mixing efficiency (Emix) and normalized phase three helium slope (SN) in normal subjects (abstract). Am J Respir Crit Care Med 151:A786, 1995.

1094. Soparkar GR, Mink JT, Graham BL, et al: Measurement of temporal changes in Dlcosb-3EQ from small alveolar samples in normal subjects. J Appl Physiol 76:1494, 1994.

1095. Gould GA, Redpath AT, Ryan M, et al: Lung CT density correlates with measurements of airflow limitation and the diffusing capacity. Eur Respir J 4:141, 1991.

1096. Burrows B, Fletcher CM, Heard BE, et al: Emphysematous and bronchial types of chronic airways obstruction: Clinicopathological study of patients in London and Chicago. Lancet 1:830, 1966.

1097. Gonzalez E, Weill H, Ziskind MM, et al: The value of the single breath diffusing capacity in separating chronic bronchitis from pulmonary emphysema. Dis Chest 53:229, 1968.

1098. Morrison NJ, Abboud RT, Müller NL, et al: Pulmonary capillary blood volume in emphysema. Am Rev Respir Dis 141:53, 1990.

1099. Georg J, Lassen NA, Millemgaard K, et al: Diffusion in the gas phase of the lungs in normal and emphysematous subjects. Clin Sci 29:525, 1965.

1100. Williams MH Jr, Park SS: Diffusion of gases within the lungs of patients with chronic obstructive pulmonary disease. Am Rev Respir Dis 98:210, 1968.

1101. Cauberghs M, Clement J, Van de Woestijne KP: Functional alterations accompanying a rapid decline in ventilatory function. Am Rev Respir Dis 147:379, 1993.

1102. Dubois P, Machiels J, Smeets F, et al: CO transfer capacity as a determining factor of survival for severe hypoxaemic COPD patients under long-term oxygen therapy. Eur Respir J 3:1042, 1990.

1103. Michaels R, Sigurdson M, Thurlbeck S, et al: Elastic recoil of the lung in cigarette smokers: The effect of nebulized bronchodilator and cessation of smoking. Am Rev Respir Dis 119:707, 1979.

1104. Zamel N, Leroux M, Ramcharan V, et al: Decrease in lung recoil pressure after cessation of smoking. Am Rev Respir Dis 119:205, 1979.

1105. Buist AS, Nagy JM, Sexton GJ, et al: The effect of smoking cessation on pulmonary function. A 30-month follow-up of two smoking cessation clinics. Am Rev Respir Dis 120:953, 1979.

1106. Bossé R, Sparrow D, Rose CL, et al: Longitudinal effect of age and smoking cessation on pulmonary function. Am Rev Respir Dis 123:378, 1981.

1107. Tashkin D, Clark V, Coulson A, et al: The UCLA population studies of chronic obstructive respiratory disease. VIII. Effects of smoking cessation on lung function—a prospective study of a free-living population. Am Rev Respir Dis 130:707, 1984.

1108. Simonsson BG, Rolf C: Bronchial reactivity to methacholine in ten nonobstructive heavy smokers before and up to one year after cessation of smoking. Eur J Respir Dis 63:526, 1982.

1109. Bates DV: The J. Burns Amberson Lecture. The fate of the chronic bronchitic: A report of the ten-year follow-up in the Canadian Department of Veterans' Affairs coordinated study of chronic bronchitis. Am Rev Respir Dis 108:1043, 1973.

1110. Mitchell RS: Outlook in emphysema and chronic bronchitis. N Engl J Med 280:445, 1969.

1111. Jones NL, Burrows B, Fletcher CM: Serial studies of 100 patients with chronic airway obstruction in London and Chicago. Thorax 22:327, 1967.

1112. Vandenbergh E, Clement J, de Woestijne KP: Course and prognosis of patients with advanced chronic obstructive pulmonary disease. Evaluation by means of functional indices. Am J Med 55:736, 1973.

1113. Burk RH, George RB: Acute respiratory failure in chronic obstructive pulmonary disease. Arch Intern Med 132:865, 1973.

1114. Moser KM, Shibel EM, Beamon AJ: Acute respiratory failure in obstructive lung disease. JAMA 225:705, 1973.

1115. Knaus WA, Wagner DP, Draper EA, et al: The APACHE III prognostic system: Risk prediction of hospital mortality for critically ill hospitalized adults. Chest 100:1619, 1991.

1116. Sun X, Muir J-F, Kakim RB, Knaus WA: Prognosis of acute respiratory failure in patients with chronic obstructive pulmonary disease. *In* Enfant C (ed): Lung Biology in Health and Disease. Acute Respiratory Failure in Chronic Obstructive Pulmonary Disease. New York, Marcel Dekker, 1996.

1117. Connors AF Jr, Dawson NV, Thomas C, et al: Outcomes following acute exacerbation of severe chronic obstructive lung disease. The SUPPORT investigators (Study to Understand Prognoses and Preferences for Outcomes and Risks of Treatments). Am J Respir Crit Care Med 154:959, 1996.

1118. Ude AC, Howard P: Controlled oxygen therapy and pulmonary heart failure. Thorax 26:572, 1971.

1119. Moore LG, Rohr AL, Maisenback JK, et al: Emphysema mortality is increased in Colorado residents at high altitude. Am Rev Respir Dis 126:225, 1982.

1120. Hodgkin JE: Prognosis in chronic obstructive pulmonary disease. Clin Chest Med 11:555, 1990.

1121. Weitzenblum E, Hirth C, Ducolone A, et al: Prognostic value of pulmonary artery pressure in chronic obstructive pulmonary disease. Thorax 36:752, 1981.

1122. Traver GA, Cline MG, Burrows B, et al: Predictors of mortality in chronic obstructive pulmonary disease. A 15-year follow-up study. Am Rev Respir Dis 119:895, 1979.

1123. Finlay M, Middleton HC, Peake MD, et al: Cardiac output, pulmonary hypertension, hypoxemia and survival in patients with chronic obstructive airways disease. Eur J Respir Dis 64:252, 1983.

1124. Kawakami Y, Terai T, Yamamoto H, et al: Exercise and oxygen inhalation in relation to prognosis of chronic obstructive pulmonary disease. Chest 81:182, 1982.

1125. Kok-Jensen A, Ebbehoj K: Prognosis of chronic obstructive lung disease in relation to radiology and electrocardiogram. Scand J Respir Dis 58:304, 1977.

1126. Postma DS, Burema J, Gimeno F, et al: Prognosis in severe chronic obstructive pulmonary disease. Am Rev Respir Dis 119:356, 1979.

1127. Ashutosh K, Haldipur C, Boucher ML: Clinical and personality profiles and survival in patients with COPD. Chest 111:95, 1997.

1128. Nocturnal Oxygen Therapy Trial Group: Continuous or nocturnal oxygen therapy in hypoxemic chronic obstructive lung disease. Ann Intern Med 93:391, 1980.

1129. Medical Research Council Working Party: Long term domiciliary oxygen therapy in chronic hypoxic cor pulmonale complicating chronic bronchitis and emphysema. Lancet 1:681, 1981.

1130. Timms RM, Khaja FU, Williams GW: The nocturnal oxygen therapy trial group. Hemodynamic response to oxygen therapy in chronic obstructive pulmonary disease. Ann Intern Med 102:29, 1985.

1131. Flick MR, Block AJ: Nocturnal vs diurnal cardiac arrhythmias in patients with chronic obstructive pulmonary disease. Chest 75:8, 1979.

1132. Strom K: Survival of patients with chronic obstructive pulmonary disease receiving long-term domiciliary oxygen therapy. Am Rev Respir Dis 147:585, 1993.

1133. MacNee W: Predictors of survival in patients treated with long-term oxygen therapy. Respiration 59:5, 1992.

1134. Arnold WH Jr, Grant JL: Oxygen-induced hypoventilation. Am Rev Respir Dis 95:255, 1967.

1135. McNicol MW, Campbell EJM: Severity of respiratory failure. Arterial blood-gases in untreated patients. Lancet 1:336, 1965.

1136. Zielinski J, MacNee W, Wedzicha A, et al: Causes of death in patients with COPD and chronic respiratory failure. Monaldi Arch Chest Dis 52:43, 1997.

1137. Ketelaars CA, Schlosser MA, Mostert R, et al: Determinants of health-related quality of life in patients with chronic obstructive pulmonary disease. Thorax 51:39, 1996.

1138. Guyatt GH, Townsend M, Keller J, et al: Measuring functional status in chronic lung disease: conclusions from a randomized control trial. Respir Med 83:293, 1989.

1139. Ferrer M, Alonso J, Morera J, et al: Chronic obstructive pulmonary disease stage and health-related quality of life. The Quality of Life of Chronic Obstructive Pulmonary Disease Study Group. Ann Intern Med 127:1072, 1997.

1140. Harper R, Brazier JE, Waterhouse JC, et al: Comparison of outcome measures for patients with chronic obstructive pulmonary disease (COPD) in an outpatient setting. Thorax 52:879, 1997.

1141. Sciurba FC, Rogers RM: Lung reduction surgery for emphysema. Curr Opin Pulm Med 2:97, 1996.

1142. McKenna RJ Jr, Brenner M, Fischel RJ, et al: Patient selection criteria for lung volume reduction surgery. J Thorac Cardiovasc Surg 114:957, 1997.

1143. Keller CA, Ruppel G, Hibbett A, et al: Thoracoscopic lung volume reduction surgery reduces dyspnea and improves exercise capacity in patients with emphysema. Am J Respir Crit Care Med 156:60, 1997.

1144. Hoppin FG Jr: Theoretical basis for improvement following reduction pneumoplasty in emphysema. Am J Respir Crit Care Med 155:520, 1997.

1145. Ad Hoc Committee to Review Antitrypsin Methods: Statement on methods for detecting alpha₁-antitrypsin abnormalities. *In* Mittman C (ed): Pulmonary Emphysema and Proteolysis. New York, Academic Press, 1972, p 141.

1146. Lieberman J: Alpha₁-antitrypsin deficiency. Med Clin North Am 57:691, 1973.

1147. Heimburger N: Introductory remarks. Proteinase inhibition in human serum. Identification, concentration, chemical properties, enzymatic specificity. *In* Mittman C (ed): Pulmonary Emphysema and Proteolysis. New York, Academic Press, 1972, p 307.

1148. Morse JO: Alpha₁-antitrypsin deficiency. N Engl J Med 299:1045, 1978.

1149. Geratz JD: Specific low-molecular-weight inhibitors of trypsin. Their structure, activity relationships, and possible clinical uses. *In* Mittman C (ed): Pulmonary Emphysema and Proteolysis. New York, Academic Press, 1972, p 325.

1150. Talamo RC, Langley CE, Hyslop NE Jr: A comparison of functional and immunochemical measurements of serum alpha$_1$-antitrypsin. *In* Mittman C (ed): Pulmonary Emphysema and Proteolysis. New York, Academic Press, 1972, p 167.

1151. Laurell CB: Antigen-antibody crossed electrophoresis. Anal Biochem 10:358, 1965.

1152. Wiedemann HP, Stoller JK: Lung disease due to alpha$_1$-antitrypsin deficiency. Curr Opin Pulm Med 2:155, 1996.

1153. Talamo RC, Langley CE, Levine BW, et al: Genetic vs. quantitative analysis of serum alpha$_1$-antitrypsin. N Engl J Med 287:1067, 1972.

1154. Pierce JA: More on antitrypsin (editorial). N Engl J Med 287:1095, 1972.

1155. Ihrig J, Kleinerman J, Rynbrandt DJ: Serum antitrypsins in animals: Studies of species variations, components, and the influence of certain irritants. Am Rev Respir Dis 103:377, 1971.

1156. Ashley MJ, Corey P, Chan-Yeung M, et al: Smoking, dust exposure and serum alpha$_1$-antitrypsin. Am Rev Respir Dis 121:783, 1980.

1157. Laurell CB: Variation of the alpha$_1$-antitrypsin level of plasma. *In* Mittman C (ed): Pulmonary Emphysema and Proteolysis. New York, Academic Press, 1972, p 161.

1158. Moskowitz RW, Heinrich G: Bacterial inactivation of human serum alpha$_1$-antitrypsin: A possible factor in the pathogenesis of pulmonary disease related to antitrypsin deficiency states. *In* Mittman C (ed): Pulmonary Emphysema and Proteolysis. New York, Academic Press, 1972, p 261.

1159. Mornex J-F, Chytil-Weir A, Martinet Y, et al: Expression of the alpha-1-antitrypsin gene in mononuclear phagocytes of normal and alpha-1-antitrypsin deficient individuals. J Clin Invest 77:1952, 1986.

1160. Cox DW, Johnson AM, Fagerhol MK: Report of nomenclature meeting for alpha$_1$-antitrypsin. Hum Genet 53:429, 1980.

1161. Fagerhol MK, Laurell CB: The Pi system—inherited variants of serum alpha$_1$ antitrypsin. Prog Med Genet 7:96, 1970.

1162. Allen RC, Harley RA, Talamo RC: A new method for determination of alpha-1-antitrypsin phenotypes using isoelectric focusing on polyacrylamide gel slabs. Am J Clin Pathol 62:732, 1974.

1163. Zegers HM, Claassen E, Gerritse K, et al: Detection of genetic variants of alpha$_1$-antitrypsin with site-specific monoclonal antibodies. Clin Chem 37:1606, 1991.

1164. Birrer P, McElvaney NG, Chang-Stroman LM, Crystal RG: Alpha$_1$-antitrypsin deficiency and liver disease. J Inher Metab Dis 14:512, 1991.

1165. Fagerhol MK: Genetics of a Pi System. *In* Mittman C (ed): Pulmonary Emphysema and Proteolysis. New York, Academic Press, 1972, p 123.

1166. Fagerhol MK: Serum Pi types in Norwegians. Acta Pathol Microbiol Scand 70:421, 1967.

1167. Pierce JA, Eradio B, Dew TA: Antitrypsin phenotypes in St. Louis. JAMA 231:609, 1975.

1168. Webb DR, Hyde RW, Schwartz RH, et al: Serum alpha$_1$-antitrypsin variants, prevalence and clinical spirometry. Am Rev Respir Dis 108:918, 1973.

1169. Cole RB, Nevin NC, Blundell G, et al: Relation of alpha$_1$-antitrypsin phenotype to the performance of pulmonary function tests and to the prevalence of respiratory illness in a working population. Thorax 31:149, 1976.

1170. Talamo RC, Thurlbeck WM: Alpha$_1$-antitrypsin Pi types in postmortem blood. Am Rev Respir Dis 112:201, 1975.

1171. Black LF, Kueppers F: Alpha$_1$-antitrypsin deficiency in non-smokers. Am Rev Respir Dis 117:421, 1978.

1172. Janus ED, Phillips NT, Carrell RW: Smoking, lung function and alpha$_1$-antitrypsin deficiency. Lancet 1:152, 1985.

1173. Brantley ML, Paul LD, Miller BH, et al: Clinical features and history of the destructive lung disease associated with alpha$_1$-antitrypsin deficiency of adults with pulmonary symptoms. Am Rev Respir Dis 138:327, 1988.

1174. Tobin MJ, Cook PJL, Hutchinson DCS: Alpha$_1$-antitrypsin deficiency: The clinical and physiological features of pulmonary emphysema in subjects homozygous for P$_i$ type Z: A survey by the British Thoracic Association. Br J Dis Chest 77:14, 1983.

1175. Falk GA, Briscoe WA: Alpha$_1$-antitrypsin deficiency in chronic obstructive pulmonary disease. Ann Intern Med 72:430, 1970.

1176. Alper CA: Deficiency of alpha$_1$-antitrypsin. Ann Intern Med 78:298, 1973.

1177. Buist AS, Adams BE, Azzam AH, et al: Pulmonary function in young children with alpha$_1$-antitrypsin deficiency: Comparison with matched control subjects. Am Rev Respir Dis 122:817, 1980.

1178. Sveger T: Liver disease in alpha$_1$-antitrypsin deficiency detected by screening of 200,000 infants. N Engl J Med 294:1316, 1976.

1179. O'Brien ML, Buist NRM, Murphey WH: Neonatal screening for alpha$_1$-antitrypsin deficiency. J Pediatr 92:1006, 1978.

1180. Jones MC, Thomas GO: Alpha$_1$-antitrypsin deficiency and pulmonary emphysema. Thorax 26:652, 1971.

1181. Enzyme deficiency and emphysema. BMJ 3:655, 1971.

1182. Falk GA, Briscoe WA: Alpha$_1$-antitrypsin deficiency in chronic obstructive pulmonary disease. Ann Intern Med 72:430, 1970.

1183. Hutchison DCS, Cook PJL, Barter CE, et al: Pulmonary emphysema and alpha$_1$-antitrypsin deficiency. BMJ 1:689, 1971.

1184. Alpha$_1$-antitrypsin deficiency and liver disease in childhood. BMJ 1:758, 1973.

1185. Kueppers F, Black LF: Alpha$_1$-antitrypsin and its deficiency. Am Rev Respir Dis 110:176, 1974.

1186. Tobin MJ, Cook PJL, Hutchison DCS, et al: Alpha$_1$-antitrypsin deficiency—the clinical and physiological features of pulmonary emphysema in subjects homozygous for Pi-type-Z—a survey by the British Thoracic Association. Br J Dis Chest 77:14, 1983.

1187. Black LF, Kueppers F: Alpha$_1$-antitrypsin deficiency in nonsmokers. Am Rev Respir Dis 117:421, 1978.

1188. Janus ED, Phillips NT, Carrell RW, et al: Smoking, lung function and alpha$_1$-antitrypsin deficiency. Lancet 1:152, 1985.

1189. Brantly ML, Paul LD, Miller BH, et al: Clinical features and history of the destructive lung disease associated with alpha$_1$-antitrypsin deficiency of adults with pulmonary symptoms. Am Rev Respir Dis 138:327, 1988.

1190. Mittman C, Lieberman J, Marasso F, et al: Smoking and chronic obstructive lung disease in alpha$_1$-antitrypsin deficiency. Chest 60:214, 1971.

1191. Glasgow JFT, Lynch MJ, Hercz A, et al: Alpha$_1$-antitrypsin deficiency in association with both cirrhosis and chronic obstructive lung disease in two sibs. Am J Med 54:181, 1973.

1192. Mittman C: Summary of symposium on pulmonary emphysema and proteolysis. Am Rev Respir Dis 105:430, 1972.

1193. Fagerhol MK: The incidence of alpha$_1$-antitrypsin variants in chronic obstructive pulmonary disease. *In* Mittman C (ed): Pulmonary Emphysema and Proteolysis. New York, Academic Press, 1972, p 51.

1194. Lieberman J, Gaidulis L, Roberts L: Racial distribution of alpha$_1$-antitrypsin variants among junior high school students. Am Rev Respir Dis 114:1194, 1976.

1195. Jeppsson JO, Larsson C, Eriksson S: Characterization of alpha$_1$-antitrypsin in the inclusion bodies from the liver in alpha$_1$-antitrypsin deficiency. N Engl J Med 293:576, 1975.

1196. Lieberman J: Heat lability of alpha$_1$-antitrypsin variants. Chest 64:579, 1973.

1197. Lieberman J, Mittman C, Gordon HW: Alpha$_1$-antitrypsin in the livers of patients with emphysema. Science 175:63, 1972.

1198. Yu MH, Lee KN, Kim J: The Z type variation of human alpha$_1$-antitrypsin causes a protein folding defect. Nat Struct Biol 2:363, 1995.

1199. Curiel DT, Chytil A, Courtney M, Crystal RG: Serum alpha$_1$-antitrypsin deficiency associated with the common S-type (Glu264—Val) mutation results from intracellular degradation of alpha$_1$-antitrypsin prior to secretion. J Biol Chem 264:10477, 1989.

1200. Pääkö P, Ryhänen L, Rantala H, et al: Pulmonary emphysema in a nonsmoking patient with Salla disease. Am Rev Respir Dis 135:979, 1987.

1200a. Schleutker J, Laine AP, Haataja L, et al: Linkage disequilibrium utilized to establish a refined genetic position of the Salla disease locus on 6q14–q15. Genomics 27:286, 1995.

1201. Eriksson S, Larsson C: Purification and partial characterization of PAS-positive inclusion bodies from the liver in alpha$_1$-antitrypsin deficiency. N Engl J Med 292:176, 1975.

1202. Perlmutter DH: Alpha-1-antitrypsin deficiency: biochemistry and clinical manifestations. Ann Med 28:385, 1996.

1203. Kueppers F, Dickson ER, Summerskill WHJ: Alpha$_1$-antitrypsin phenotypes in chronic active liver disease and primary biliary cirrhosis. Mayo Clin Proc 51:286, 1976.

1204. Donlan CJ Jr, Ross DG, Golembieski M, et al: Pulmonary emphysema and liver disease. JAMA 232:1147, 1975.

1205. Triger DR, Millward-Sadler GH, Czaykowski AA, et al: Alpha$_1$-antitrypsin deficiency and liver disease in adults. Q J Med 45:351, 1976.

1206. Lieberman J: Emphysema, cirrhosis, and hepatoma with alpha$_1$-antitrypsin deficiency. Ann Intern Med 81:850, 1974.

1207. Elzouki AN, Eriksson S: Risk of hepatobiliary disease in adults with severe alpha$_1$-antitrypsin deficiency (PiZZ): Is chronic viral hepatitis B or C an additional risk factor for cirrhosis and hepatocellular carcinoma? Eur J Gastroenterol Hepatol 8:989, 1996.

1208. Lieberman J, Gaidulis L, Garoutte B, et al: Identification and characteristics of the common alpha$_1$-antitrypsin phenotypes. Chest 62:557, 1972.

1209. Hutchison DC, Tobin MJ, Cook PJL, et al: Alpha$_1$-antitrypsin deficiency—clinical and physiological features in heterozygotes of Pi type SZ. A survey by the British Thoracic Association. Br J Dis Chest 77:28, 1983.

1210. Turino GM, Barker AF, Brantly ML, et al: Clinical features of individuals with PI*SZ phenotype of alpha$_1$-antitrypsin deficiency. Alpha$_1$-Antitrypsin Deficiency Registry Study Group. Am J Respir Crit Care Med 154:1718, 1996.

1211. Lieberman J, Gaidulus L, Klotz SD: A new deficient variant of alpha$_1$-antitrypsin (M$_{duarte}$). Inability to detect the heterozygous state by antitrypsin phenotyping. Am Rev Respir Dis 113:31, 1976.

1212. Cox DW, Levison H: Emphysema of early onset associated with a complete deficiency of alpha$_1$-antitrypsin (null homozygotes). Am Rev Respir Dis 137:371, 1988.

1213. Lieberman J, Gaidulis L, Schleissner PJA: Intermediate alpha$_1$-antitrypsin deficiency from a null gene (M phenotypes). Chest 70:532, 1976.

1214. Cook L, Janus ED, Brenton S, et al: Absence of alpha-1-antitrypsin (Pi Null Bellingham) and the early onset of emphysema. Aust N Z J Med 24:263, 1994.

1215. Bencze K, Sabatke L, Fruhmann G, et al: Alpha$_1$-antitrypsin—the PIMM subtypes—do they play a role in development of chronic obstructive pulmonary diseases. Chest 77:761, 1980.

1216. Kalsheker NA, Hodgson IJ, Watkins GL, et al: Deoxyribonucleic acid (DNA) polymorphism of the alpha$_1$-antitrypsin gene in chronic lung disease. Br Med J 294:1511, 1987.

1217. Kalsheker NA, Watkins GL, Hill S, et al: Independent mutations in the flanking sequence of the alpha$_1$-antitrypsin gene are associated with chronic obstructive airways disease. Disease Markers 8:151, 1990.

1218. Poller W, Meison C, Olek K: DNA polymorphisms of the alpha$_1$-antitrypsin gene region in patients with chronic obstructive pulmonary disease. Eur J Clin Invest 20:1, 1990.

1219. Sandford AJ, Spinelli JJ, Weir TD, Paré PD: Mutation in the 3′ region of the

# *Bronchiectasis and Other Bronchial Abnormalities*

## BRONCHIECTASIS

### General Features

Bronchiectasis is best defined as irreversible dilation of a portion of the bronchial tree. As such, it is a relatively common pathologic or HRCT finding that occurs in association with many conditions (Table 56–1). Although it has decreased in importance as a clinically significant affliction—particularly one requiring surgical resection—since the advent of antibiotic therapy,[1, 2] the abnormality has nevertheless engendered a resurgence of interest as a result of several factors: (1) Advances in medical therapy have led to relatively prolonged survival in patients who have cystic fibrosis, ciliary dyskinetic syndromes, and some immune deficiency syndromes, increasing the pool of patients with these disorders in the population; (2) recurrent bacterial infection, *Pneumocystis carinii* pneumonia, and tuberculosis in human immunodeficiency virus (HIV)–infected subjects can lead to the rapid development of bronchiectasis;[3] (3) the condition has been recognized as an important complication of heart, lung,[4] and bone marrow[5] transplantation; and (4) advances in radiologic imaging have made the recognition of relatively minor degrees of bronchiectasis much easier.[6] The increased ability to detect bronchiectasis by HRCT means that the spectrum of clinical manifestations associated with the diagnosis has been broadened, and it is now recognized that it may be seen in asymptomatic individuals or in patients who complain only of mild cough unassociated with copious production of purulent sputum. As a result, bronchiectasis detected solely by HRCT is now associated with a number of conditions, such as rheumatoid disease and obliterative bronchiolitis, that were not previously associated with the condition.

The most important cause of clinically significant bronchiectasis in North America and Europe today is cystic fibrosis (*see* page 2298). In areas of the world where this disease is rare and in "developing" societies in which the incidence of serious childhood infection is still appreciable, postinfective bronchiectasis is still of great significance. Hereditary immunologic and structural abnormalities are also important: In one study of 4,000 children referred for respiratory disease to a tertiary center, 41 (1%) had chronic bronchiectasis not related to cystic fibrosis;[6a] 6 of these (15%) had a congenital malformation as a risk factor, 7 (17%) had primary ciliary dyskinesia, 11 (27%) had an immunologic abnormality, 2 (5%) had aspirated, and 15 (36%) had no accepted risk factor. Bronchiectasis has been the subject of a number of reviews.[7–10a]

### Etiology and Pathogenesis

The three most important mechanisms that contribute to the pathogenesis of bronchiectasis are infection, airway obstruction, and peribronchial fibrosis. In some cases, all three mechanisms are involved; in others, one is the principal or sole pathogenetic process. Although bronchial infection is present in many patients at some point in the disease, the extent to which it is a cause or an effect of the bronchiectasis is not always clear.

The role of inflammation as a critical factor in the pathogenesis of bronchiectasis has been emphasized increasingly[11, 12] and is discussed in detail in the section on pathogenesis in cystic fibrosis (*see* page 2301). In this condition and in other forms of bronchiectasis, increased levels of the powerful leukocyte chemoattractant interleukin-8 and other proinflammatory cytokines, such as tumor necrosis factor-α and interleukin-1,[13] are found in high concentrations in the sputum.[14] The cytokines are produced by both damaged airway epithelial cells and inflammatory cells in the airway wall; by attracting more inflammatory cells, they perpetuate

## Table 56–1. CLASSIFICATION AND CAUSES OF BRONCHIECTASIS

| General Category | Specific Examples | Selected References |
|---|---|---|
| Inherited cellular or molecular defects | Cystic fibrosis | |
| | Homozygous; occasionally heterozygosity for function-alterating mutations in the CFTR protein | 296 |
| | Alpha$_1$-antitrypsin deficiency | |
| Dyskinetic cilia syndromes | Kartagener's syndrome | |
| Inherited or acquired deficiency in host defense | X-linked agammaglobulinemia | |
| | Selective IgG deficiency | |
| | Common variable immunodeficiency | |
| | Selective IgA, IgM, or IgE deficiency | |
| | Nezelof's syndrome | 297 |
| | Chronic granulomatous disease of childhood | |
| | Rare lymphocyte syndrome (TAP2 gene mutation) | 298 |
| | HIV infection | |
| Congenital abnormalities of bronchial or vascular structure | Absent or defective cartilage (Williams-Campbell syndrome) | |
| | Intraluminal webs | |
| | Tracheal bronchus | 32 |
| | Mounier-Kuhn syndrome | |
| | Bronchial atresia | |
| | Unilateral pulmonary artery agenesis | 45 |
| | Pulmonary sequestration | |
| | Bronchogenic cyst | 299 |
| Acquired bronchial obstruction | | |
| Intraluminal obstruction | Neoplasm | |
| | Foreign body | |
| | Broncholith | |
| | Papillomatosis | 300 |
| External compression | Lymph node enlargement | |
| | Neoplasm | |
| | Pulmonary artery band migration | 301 |
| Infection | | |
| Bacteria | *Staphylococcus aureus* | |
| | *Streptococcus pneumoniae* | 10a |
| | *Klebsiella pneumoniae* | |
| | *Mycobacterium tuberculosis* | |
| | *Mycobacterium avium-intracellulare* | |
| | *Mycoplasma pneumoniae* | |
| | *Bordetella* sp. | |
| Viral infections | Human papillomavirus | 302 |
| | Latent adenovirus infection | 46 |
| | Influenza virus | |
| | Herpes simplex | |
| | Measles virus | |
| Fungi | *Histoplasma capsulatum* | |
| | *Pneumocystis carinii* | 10a |
| Post-toxic bronchitis or pneumonitis | Ammonia inhalation | |
| | Smoke inhalation | 51 |
| | Gastric acid aspiration | |
| | Mineral oil aspiration | 53 |
| | Paraquat ingestion | 57 |
| | Acrolein ingestion | 56 |
| Parenchymal fibrosis | Chronic tuberculosis | |
| | Sarcoidosis | |
| Immunologic abnormality | Allergic bronchopulmonary aspergillosis | |
| | Lung allograft rejection | 4 |
| | Graft-versus-host disease post bone marrow transplant | 5 |
| | Rheumatoid disease | |
| | Sjögren's syndrome | |
| | Inflammatory bowel disease | 335, 336 |
| Miscellaneous | Yellow nail syndrome | 30 |
| | Young's syndrome | |
| | Dyskeratosis congenita | |

HIV, human immunodeficiency virus.

the response. The inflammatory cells release a variety of proteolytic enzymes, including collagenases[15, 16] and elastase,[17, 18] that locally produced or serum-derived antiproteases are insufficient to neutralize.[19] The balance between these proteolytic and antiproteolytic forces is important in determining the development and degree of airway damage; this is exemplified by alpha$_1$-antitrypsin deficiency, in which an endogenous lack of antiprotease activity is presumably responsible for the development of bronchiectasis as well as emphysema.[20–22] The detection of increased amounts of epithelial cell cytoskeletal protein cytokeratin 19 in bronchoalveolar lavage fluid provides evidence that the proteases actually cause epithelial cell disruption.[23] Airway epithelial cells and macrophages respond to the chronic inflammation by increasing expression of nitric oxide synthase,[24] and it has been suggested that measurement of expired nitric oxide may be useful as a marker of disease activity.[25]

Once airway damage has occurred and bronchiectasis is established, it is common for certain strains of microorganisms to colonize the dilated airways. In addition, some of the conditions associated with bronchiectasis, such as cystic fibrosis and dyskinetic cilia syndrome, are characterized by abnormal mucociliary clearance, and it is possible that this deficiency itself predisposes to local airway colonization. *Pseudomonas aeruginosa* is particularly important in this regard; as assessed by HRCT, its presence is associated with more extensive disease as well as thicker, more dilated airways.[26, 27] *Branhamella catarrhalis* has also been increasingly recognized as an important lower respiratory tract pathogen in bronchiectasis.[28] Whatever the pathogenesis of the colonization, it is likely that the chronic inflammatory reaction to the organisms results in progressive bronchial wall damage and dilation; this can cause an even greater deficiency of mucociliary clearance,[71] establishing a vicious cycle and ever-increasing bronchiectasis.[29] It is possible that a similar scenario contributes to the bronchiectasis associated with Young's syndrome, dyskeratosis congenita,[30] and Sjögren's syndrome.

It is likely that retained secretions also cause some degree of airway dilation.[31] The most common example of this process is acquired airway obstruction, either partial or complete.[32, 33] The pathogenesis of the airway dilation in this situation is probably a combination of several mechanisms, including distention by mucus, impaired clearance leading to bronchial infection, and atelectasis of the parenchyma distal to the obstruction with transmission of radial traction to the peripheral airways. Retained secretions also may be important in the pathogenesis of Williams-Campbell syndrome, a congenital form of bronchiectasis in which the underlying abnormality is a deficiency in the amount of airway cartilage (*see* page 2285). Abnormal bronchial wall structure is also likely responsible for the bronchiectasis associated with a tracheal bronchus[34] and the Mounier-Kuhn syndrome (*see* page 2285).[35]

By predisposing to bronchial infection or colonization, immunologic deficiency states such as hypogammaglobulinemia and chronic granulomatous disease of childhood may act by the same mechanism as impaired mucociliary clearance. Both generalized and specific gamma globulin deficiency syndromes increase risk for bronchiectasis. In the generalized forms (e.g., X-linked agammaglobulinemia and common variable immunodeficiency), HRCT can be used to detect pulmonary involvement early in the course of disease,[36] and appropriate replacement therapy can retard its progression significantly.[37] Patients who have X-linked agammaglobulinemia develop bronchiectasis at a younger age than those with common variable immunodeficiency.[38] Approximately 40% of the latter patients, but not patients with X-linked disease, show mediastinal lymphadenopathy on HRCT.[38] The risk for bronchiectasis is also increased in patients who have severe selective IgA deficiency,[39] IgE deficiency (Job's syndrome),[40] and, to a lesser extent, selective deficiency of a specific IgG subclass (*see* page 725).[41, 42]

It has been suggested that bronchiectasis secondary to childhood measles and pertussis pneumonia is also caused by a vicious cycle, initiated by damage to the airway wall and a local impairment of bacterial clearance that causes an increased susceptibility to colonization.[29] Perhaps in the same category is the bronchiectasis associated with Swyer-James syndrome,[43] the pathogenesis almost certainly relating to acute bronchiolitis in infancy or childhood (*see* page 2337). Although it is possible that some cases of pulmonary artery hypoplasia associated with bronchiectasis are acquired and possess a pathogenesis similar or identical to that of Swyer-James syndrome,[44] congenital bronchiectasis can certainly accompany unilateral agenesis of a pulmonary artery.[45] Latent infection by viruses such as adenovirus resulting in ongoing inflammation and progressive airway damage is another mechanism that has been suggested to explain the long delay that may occur between childhood pneumonia and the presentation of bronchiectasis during adolescence or adulthood.[46]

The pathogenesis of the bronchiectasis that occurs after necrotizing pneumonia is most likely related to several mechanisms, including airway damage, parenchymal fibrosis, and a reservoir of organisms that colonizes residual cavities. Recurrent bacterial bronchitis and pneumonia as well as infections by opportunistic organisms are presumably related to the bronchiectasis that is being increasingly recognized as a complication of HIV infection.[47–49] The bronchiectasis that develops after the inhalation of various fumes or gases such as ammonia[50] or smoke[51] or after aspiration of oily substances[52, 53] or liquid gastric contents (especially in heroin addicts)[54, 55] is also likely related to airway damage and chronic bacterial colonization.

The bronchiectasis that has been reported after acute pneumonitis secondary to ingestion of acrolein[56] or paraquat[57] as well as that which occurs in patients who have postprimary tuberculosis or some interstitial lung diseases, such as sarcoidosis,[58] is of a somewhat different pathogenesis. In these conditions, the parenchyma appears to be the primary site of disease, fibrosis resulting in retraction and secondary bronchial dilation (*traction bronchiectasis*).

The bronchiectasis in allergic bronchopulmonary aspergillosis, lung allograft rejection, and the graft-versus-host reaction after bone marrow transplantation appears to be a consequence of immunologically mediated airway inflammation. A similar process also may be responsible for the bronchiectasis and bronchiolitis associated with rheumatoid disease,[59] ulcerative colitis,[60–62] Felty's syndrome,[63] and Sjögren's syndrome.[64] The advent of HRCT for the noninvasive diagnosis of bronchiectasis has revealed a much higher prevalence of bronchiectasis in patients who have rheumatoid disease than was formerly appreciated.[65, 66] For example, in one study of 88 randomly selected patients who had rheumatoid disease, 30% had HRCT evidence of bronchiectasis;[67] 22% had pulmonary nodules, 17% had subpleural micronodules and pseudoplaques, 14% had ground-glass opacities, and 10% had honeycombing. Of the 39 patients who had chronic respiratory symptoms, 69% had abnormalities on HRCT (however, 29% of those without symptoms also had abnormalities).

The results of reports of the temporal relationship between the development of rheumatoid disease and bronchiectasis are contradictory. For example, in one study of 23 patients, arthritis predated the recognition of bronchiectasis in 18 (74%).[68] In a case-control study in which the clinical and laboratory features of 32 patients who had the combination of rheumatoid arthritis and bronchiectasis were compared with those of 32 patients who did not have bronchiectasis, the bronchiectasis preceded the arthritis in 30 (94%);[69] the results also showed that the presence of bronchiectasis was not associated with a more aggressive form of arthritis. In another study, bronchiectasis antedated joint disease in 12 of 14 patients (86%).[66] Certain HLA-DQ variants appear to predispose to the complication.[70]

Bronchiectasis is bilateral in approximately 50% of patients and in the great majority affects the basal segments of the lower lobes.[72] Occasionally, it is isolated to a specific lobe or segment.[73] In about 10% of cases, the middle lobe or lingula is affected without concomitant involvement of the ipsilateral lower lobe (*middle lobe syndrome*). Although

complete or partial obstruction of the middle lobe or lingular bronchus plays a causative role in some cases, it is uncommonly found at bronchoscopy or on pathologic examination;[74] the pathogenesis of the disease in these cases is uncertain.

### Pathologic Characteristics

On the basis of the results of a study of 45 lobes removed because of bronchiectasis in which the pathologic and bronchographic findings were correlated, the disease has been classified morphologically into three groups.[75]

**Group I: Cylindrical Bronchiectasis.** The bronchi are of regular outline and not greatly increased in diameter distally; their lumens tend to end squarely and abruptly (Fig. 56–1). Although patent anatomically, the smaller bronchi and bronchioles are plugged with thick, purulent material. The number of subdivisions of the bronchial tree from the main bronchus to the periphery is slightly decreased (16 subdivisions compared with 17 to 20 normally).

**Group II: Varicose Bronchiectasis.** In this group, the degree of dilation is somewhat greater than that in Group I, and local constrictions cause an irregularity of outline that resembles varicose veins. There is also much more obliteration of peripheral bronchi than in Group I; some bronchi can be seen to terminate abruptly in fibrous tissue that continues as a discrete cord toward the periphery of the lung. The average number of patent bronchial subdivisions was 4 bron-

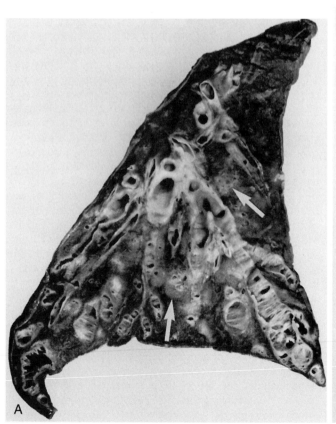
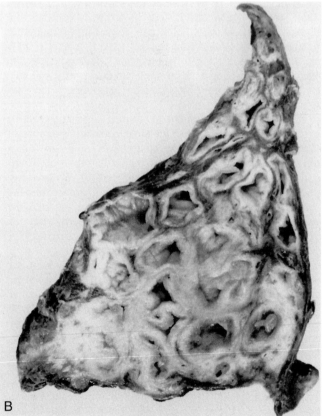

**Figure 56–1. Bronchiectasis.** Illustrated are the cut sections of lower lobes from two patients who had bronchiectasis, that in *A* showing mild ("cylindrical") bronchiectasis and that in *B*, severe ("saccular" or "cystic") disease. Although much of the parenchyma in *A* is normal, focal areas of organizing pneumonia are apparent *(arrows)*. This process is advanced in *B*, there being almost no evidence of residual normal parenchyma.

chographically, 6.5 macroscopically, and 8 microscopically (compared with 17 to 20 normally).

**Group III: Saccular (Cystic) Bronchiectasis.** In this group, bronchial dilation increases progressively toward the periphery (*see* Fig. 56–1), at which point the airways have a ballooned appearance. The maximal number of subdivisions that could be counted by any technique was five. No remnants of the peripheral bronchial tree could be shown to be directly continuous with the dilated bronchi. Rarely, a localized focus of saccular bronchiectasis becomes filled with inspissated mucus, forming a mucocele (Fig. 56–2).

Bronchiectasis often varies considerably in severity between different lobes and even between different segments in the same lobe. Occasionally, severe ectasia is identified in one segment and the remaining lung is apparently normal (Fig. 56–3). In such cases, examination of the airways proximal to the ectatic bronchi may reveal the cause of the ectasia, usually a neoplasm such as squamous cell carcinoma (Fig. 56–4) or carcinoid tumor; rarely a benign cause, such as fibrous stricture or broncholithiasis, is identified. The localization of the bronchiectasis as well as the presence and nature of associated parenchymal disease also may be important clues to its cause and pathogenesis. For example, bronchiectasis that is restricted to the posterior segment of an upper lobe is most likely the result of tuberculosis (Fig. 56–5), whereas disease that is intimately associated with parenchymal fibrosis (Fig. 56–6) is likely secondary to the fibrosis itself (traction bronchiectasis). It is important to remember, however, that parenchymal fibrosis may also be

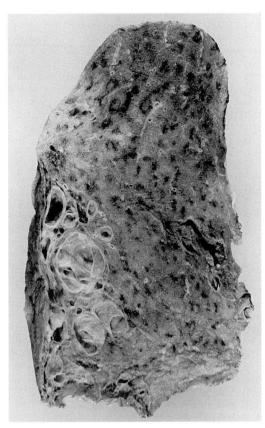

**Figure 56–3. Cystic Bronchiectasis.** A slice of left lower lobe shows bronchiectasis with a prominent "saccular" component in the posterior basal segment; the remaining lower lobe and upper lobe bronchi appear normal. The etiology was not determined but was presumed to be postinfective.

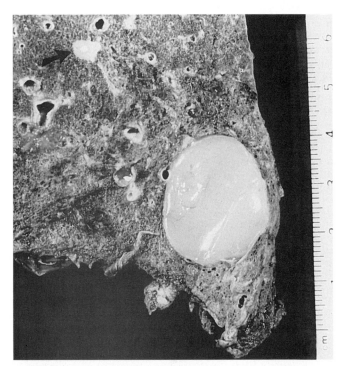

**Figure 56–2. Localized Bronchiectasis with Mucocele Formation.** A magnified view of the posterior basal portion of the right lower lobe shows a well-circumscribed nodular collection of mucus, shown on additional sectioning to be within an ectatic bronchus. The adjacent lung is fibrotic and contains a small, healed granuloma *(arrow)*; histologic examination showed it to contain *Histoplasma capsulatum*. Focal stenosis of the airway wall, possibly secondary to histoplasmosis, was evident about 1 cm proximal to the mucocele.

the result of organized pneumonia occurring as a *result* of infection experienced by patients who have bronchiectasis (*see* Fig. 56–1). In fact, the combination of parenchymal fibrosis and bronchiectasis may lead to diagnostic confusion in some cases, particularly with respect to distinguishing cyst formation (honeycombing) in idiopathic pulmonary fibrosis from ectatic airways (Fig. 56–7); however, the latter can usually be identified by their elongated appearance in at least some areas and by a greater prominence in the central rather than the peripheral lung.

In addition to luminal dilation, microscopic examination often shows the bronchial wall to be irregular in shape. Fibrosis and chronic inflammation, frequently with lymphoid follicle formation (Fig. 56–8), are almost invariable.[76] Foci of neuroendocrine cell hyperplasia (tumorlets) are not uncommon in the affected airways or adjacent pulmonary parenchyma.[77] The pulmonary parenchyma frequently shows evidence of recent or remote pneumonia, atelectasis, and obstructive pneumonitis. Chronic inflammation and fibrosis (either in the wall or lumen, or both) are also common in membranous bronchioles (Fig. 56–9) and are important in causing air-flow obstruction. The bronchial artery circulation is typically markedly increased;[78] bronchial wall ulceration with disruption of bronchial arteries secondary to focal infection is considered to be the pathogenesis of the hemorrhage that so often complicates the disease.

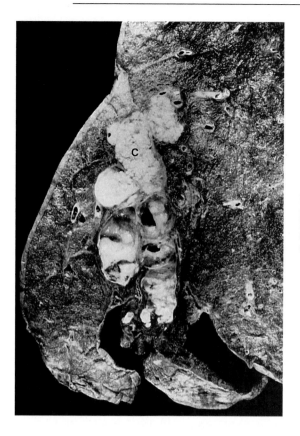

**Figure 56–4. Bronchiectasis Secondary to Airway Obstruction.** The posterior portion of this lower lobe shows a carcinoma completely occluding a subsegmental bronchus (C). Two distal airway branches are markedly ectatic and partially filled with mucus. The carcinoma is obvious in this case; however, it is occasionally very small and only evident following careful dissection of airways proximal to the ectasia.

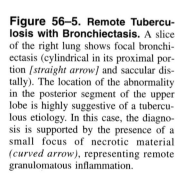

**Figure 56–5. Remote Tuberculosis with Bronchiectasis.** A slice of the right lung shows focal bronchiectasis (cylindrical in its proximal portion _[straight arrow]_ and saccular distally). The location of the abnormality in the posterior segment of the upper lobe is highly suggestive of a tuberculous etiology. In this case, the diagnosis is supported by the presence of a small focus of necrotic material _(curved arrow)_, representing remote granulomatous inflammation.

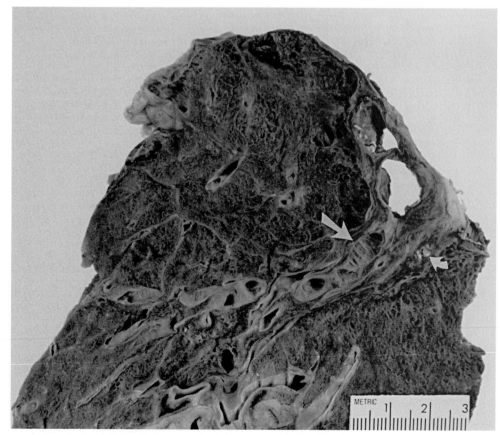

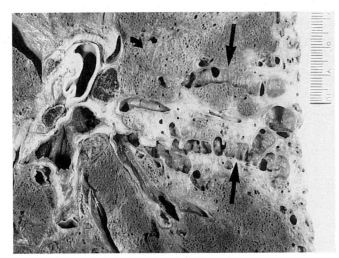

**Figure 56–6. Traction Bronchiectasis in Idiopathic Pulmonary Fibrosis.** A magnified view of the midportion of an upper lobe shows patchy fibrosis, most marked in the parenchyma adjacent to the pleura and one bronchus; it is relatively mild elsewhere *(curved arrow)*. Two bronchi show a mild to moderate degree of cylindrical bronchiectasis *(straight arrows)*.

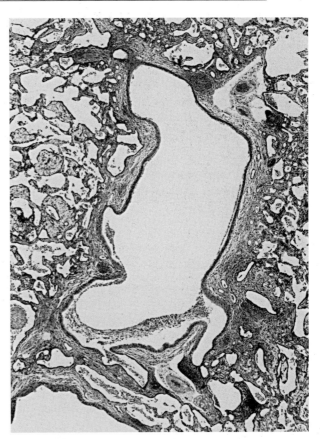

**Figure 56–8. Bronchiectasis: Histologic Appearance.** A section of a mildly dilated bronchus shows the airway to have an irregular contour. The wall is fibrotic and shows chronic inflammation, focally with lymphoid follicle formation. The adjacent parenchyma shows fibrosis and patchy inflammation.

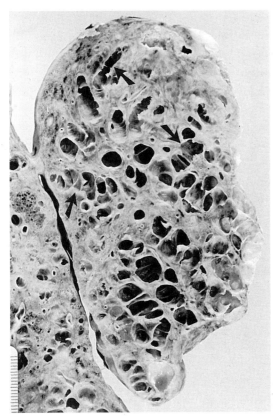

**Figure 56–7. Traction Bronchiectasis Associated with Pulmonary Fibrosis.** A slice of the left upper lobe shows extensive fibrosis and the presence of multiple cystic spaces, at first glance somewhat resembling the "honeycomb" lung of idiopathic pulmonary fibrosis. However, the central rather than peripheral location of the "cysts" and their linear appearance in several areas *(arrows)* indicate that they are in fact ectatic bronchi. The right lung and the left lower lobe (a portion of which is illustrated) also showed patchy fibrosis but only focal, mild bronchiectasis. The etiology of the bronchiectasis was not determined.

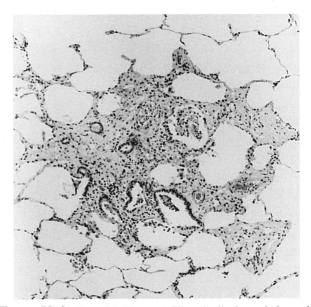

**Figure 56–9. Bronchiolitis and Fibrosis in Association with Bronchiectasis.** The section shows an irregular focus of fibrosis associated with scattered mononuclear inflammatory cells. Several spaces lined by bronchiolar type epithelium are evident; however, none can be definitely identified as the original bronchiolar lumen. This appearance is characteristic of bronchiolar injury distal to ectatic bronchi.

### Radiologic Manifestations

#### Radiography

A variety of radiographic abnormalities characterize bronchiectasis, including the following:[6, 79–82]

1. Parallel line opacities (*tram tracks*), representing thickened bronchial walls (Fig. 56–10).

2. Tubular opacities, representing mucus-filled bronchi (Fig. 56–11).

3. Ring opacities or cystic spaces measuring up to 2 cm in diameter and sometimes containing air-fluid levels (Fig. 56–12), usually localized but rarely associated with destruction of an entire lung.[83]

4. Increase in size and loss of definition of the pulmonary markings in specific segmental areas of the lungs (Fig. 56–13), a change that has been shown to be the result of peribronchial fibrosis and (to a lesser extent) retained secretions.[79, 80]

5. Crowding of the pulmonary vascular markings, indicating the almost invariable loss of volume associated with the condition (Fig. 56–14); such atelectasis is usually caused by mucus obstruction of peripheral rather than central bronchi.[79, 80]

6. Evidence of oligemia as a result of reduction in pulmonary artery perfusion, a finding usually noted in more severe disease.

7. Signs of compensatory overinflation of the remainder of the lung (*see* Fig. 56–14).

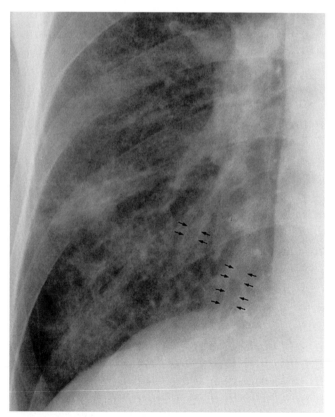

**Figure 56–10. Bronchiectasis with Tram Tracks.** A view of the right lower chest from a posteroanterior radiograph in a 46-year-old man who had chronic productive cough demonstrates parallel line opacities (tram tracks) *(arrows)* as a result of thickened dilated bronchi. The diagnosis of bronchiectasis was confirmed on HRCT.

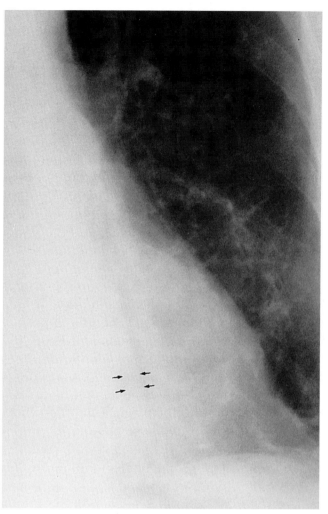

**Figure 56–11. Mucus-Filled Ectatic Bronchi.** A view of the left lower chest from a posteroanterior radiograph in a 69-year-old man shows left lower lobe atelectasis and decreased vascularity. A tubular structure is identified *(arrows)* that does not have the normal tapering and branching pattern expected from a pulmonary vessel. HRCT showed left lower lobe bronchiectasis with mucus-filled bronchi.

Because of the greater prevalence of severe disease in the past, radiographs of patients who had bronchiectasis were usually abnormal and often allowed a confident diagnosis of the condition; for example, in a review of 112 patients published in 1955, only 7% had normal chest radiographs.[80] As a result of a decrease in the number of patients who have severe disease (at least in "developed" countries) and the availability of HRCT to identify cases of relatively mild bronchiectasis, more recent studies have shown that the radiograph is often normal or shows nonspecific findings.[6, 84] The most illustrative findings in this regard are derived from a prospective study of 84 patients who were suspected of having bronchiectasis on the basis of clinical manifestations.[82] Thirty-seven patients had normal radiographs; on HRCT, 32 had normal findings and 5 (14%) had cylindrical bronchiectasis. Of the 47 patients who had abnormal radiographs, 36 (77%) had bronchiectasis at HRCT, and 11 (23%) had normal findings. Thus, the sensitivity of the chest radiograph in this study was 88% (41 of 46 cases of bronchiecta-

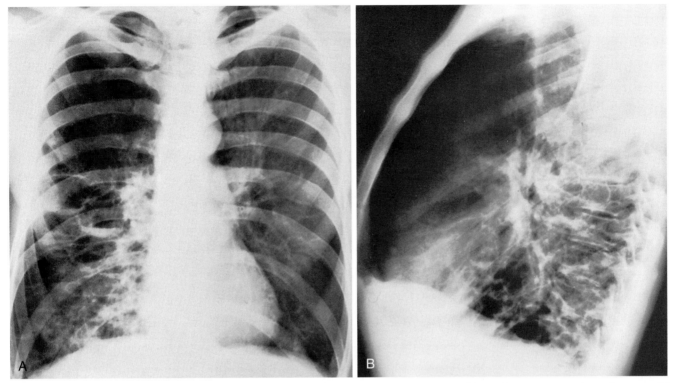

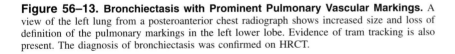

**Figure 56–12. Cystic Bronchiectasis.** Posteroanterior *(A)* and lateral *(B)* radiographs of a 38-year-old man demonstrate extensive replacement of the right lower lobe by multiple thin-walled cysts, many of which contain air-fluid levels. The left lung is normal; the right upper and middle lobes show severe oligemia.

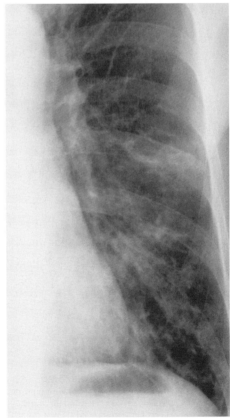

**Figure 56–13. Bronchiectasis with Prominent Pulmonary Vascular Markings.** A view of the left lung from a posteroanterior chest radiograph shows increased size and loss of definition of the pulmonary markings in the left lower lobe. Evidence of tram tracking is also present. The diagnosis of bronchiectasis was confirmed on HRCT.

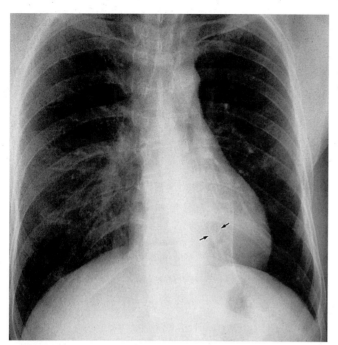

**Figure 56–14. Bronchiectasis with Left Lower Lobe Atelectasis.** A posteroanterior chest radiograph in a 27-year-old man demonstrates left lower lobe atelectasis. Ectatic thick-walled bronchi *(arrows)* can be seen within the atelectatic lobe. Note the compensatory overinflation of the left upper lobe.

sis diagnosed by HRCT), and the specificity was 74%. There was a significant correlation between the severity of abnormalities seen on the chest radiograph and the severity of bronchiectasis at HRCT ($r = 0.62$).

### Computed Tomography

On the basis of the results of the previously mentioned study and other investigations, it is now generally accepted that HRCT is the imaging modality of choice to establish

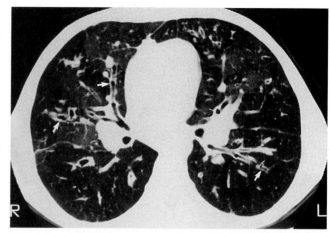

**Figure 56–16. Bronchiectasis with Lack of Bronchial Tapering.** An HRCT scan demonstrates lack of tapering *(arrows)* and thickening of the walls of bronchi in the right middle and left lower lobes. Ectatic bronchi are also evident in cross-section (signet-ring sign). The patient was a 15-year-old boy who had cystic fibrosis.

the presence of bronchiectasis and to determine its precise extent. Characteristic findings include the following:[86–90]

1. An internal bronchial diameter greater than that of the adjacent pulmonary artery (Fig. 56–15).

2. Lack of bronchial tapering, defined as a bronchus that has the same diameter as its parent branch for a distance of more than 2 cm (Fig. 56–16).

3. Visualization of bronchi within 1 cm of the costal pleura (Fig. 56–17).

4. Visualization of bronchi abutting the mediastinal pleura (*see* Fig. 56–17).

5. Bronchial wall thickening (*see* Figs. 56–15 to 56–17).

The HRCT appearance of ectatic bronchi varies depending on the type of bronchiectasis and on the orientation of the

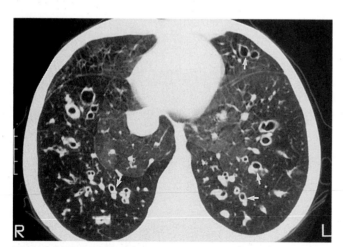

**Figure 56–15. Bronchiectasis with Signet-Ring Sign.** An HRCT scan demonstrates numerous bronchi with an internal diameter greater than that of the adjacent pulmonary artery (signet-ring sign) in the lower lobes and lingula *(arrows)*. The patient was a 15-year-old boy who had cystic fibrosis.

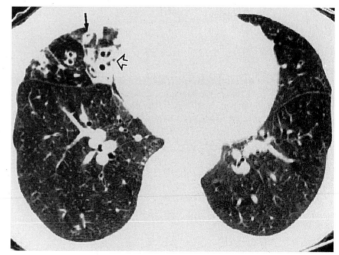

**Figure 56–17. Bronchiectasis.** An HRCT scan in a 50-year-old woman who had bronchiectasis demonstrates bronchi within 1 cm of the costal pleura *(straight arrow)* and abutting the mediastinal pleura *(open arrow)*. The bronchiectasis was presumed to be the result of previous tuberculosis.

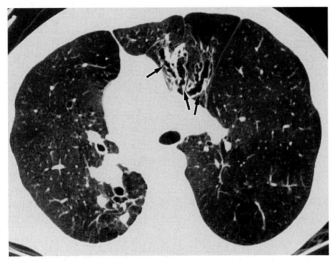

**Figure 56–18. Varicose Bronchiectasis.** An HRCT scan demonstrates ectatic bronchi that have an undulating wall *(arrows)* characteristic of varicose bronchiectasis. Bronchiectasis is also evident in the right lung. The patient was a 46-year-old man who had long-standing central bronchiectasis as a result of allergic bronchopulmonary aspergillosis.

airways relative to the plane of the HRCT scan. For example, in cylindrical bronchiectasis, bronchi coursing horizontally are visualized as parallel lines ("tram tracks") *(see* Fig. 56–16), whereas vertically oriented bronchi appear as circular lucencies larger than the diameter of the adjacent pulmonary artery, resulting in a "signet-ring" appearance *(see* Fig. 56–15).[90, 91] Varicose bronchiectasis is characterized by the presence of nonuniform bronchial dilation (Fig. 56–18), whereas cystic bronchiectasis results in a cluster of thin-walled cystic spaces often containing air-fluid levels (Fig. 56–19). HRCT allows ready distinction of cylindrical from cystic bronchiectasis; however, distinction of varicose from cystic bronchiectasis is often difficult,[86] unless the affected bronchus courses in the same horizontal plane as the CT section. The size of the ectatic bronchi decreases on end-

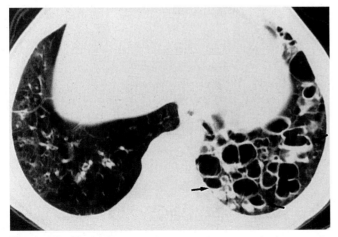

**Figure 56–19. Cystic Bronchiectasis.** An HRCT scan demonstrates thin-walled cystic spaces throughout the left lower lobe and lingula; several have air-fluid levels *(arrows).* Mild bronchiectasis is present in the right lower lobe. The patient was a 32-year-old man who had bronchiectasis following childhood viral infection.

expiratory as compared with end-inspiratory HRCT scans;[91a] occasionally, they collapse completely because of their increased compliance.[10a]

Several groups have assessed the accuracy of HRCT in the diagnosis of bronchiectasis.[86–89, 92] In one study of 36 patients who had a characteristic clinical history or radiographic findings, bronchography was performed in 44 lungs and the results used as the gold standard;[86] the sensitivity of HRCT was found to be 96% and the specificity 93%. Close analysis of the results showed that HRCT and bronchography were normal in 15 patients and demonstrated a similar presence and extent of bronchiectasis in 25. In two cases, bronchiectasis was better seen on HRCT than on bronchography; in one, bronchography demonstrated cylindrical bronchiectasis when HRCT was normal, and in another, HRCT showed cylindrical bronchiectasis, whereas bronchography, in retrospect, had been misinterpreted as negative.[86] In a second investigation in which HRCT was compared with bronchography in 259 segmental bronchi from 70 lobes of 27 lungs, HRCT was positive in 87 of 89 segmental bronchi shown to have bronchiectasis at bronchography (sensitivity, 98%) and negative in 169 of 170 segmental bronchi without bronchiectasis (specificity, 99%).[87] In a third investigation in which the results of preoperative HRCT scans were compared with the pathologic findings in 47 lobes from 22 patients who had undergone surgical resection, abnormalities were detected on HRCT in all lobes;[88] however, bronchiectasis was clearly identified on HRCT in only 41 of the 47 (87%). Three of the remaining six cases had extensive consolidation but no evidence of bronchial dilation on HRCT; in two cases, focal mucoid impaction was misinterpreted as a lung nodule, and in one case, focal cystic bronchiectasis containing a mycetoma was misinterpreted as a cavitating carcinoma.

Thus, although HRCT allows confident diagnosis of the presence and extent of bronchiectasis in the majority of patients, as with most other diseases, it is not 100% sensitive and specific, and several limitations of the technique need to be recognized.[88, 89, 93]

1. There is a normal variability in the bronchoarterial diameter ratio depending on the population being assessed, the altitude at which the examination is performed, and the window levels and window widths at which scans are photographed. In a study done in Denver (altitude 1,600 m), 16 of 27 (59%) normal subjects had at least one bronchus with an internal diameter greater than that of the adjacent pulmonary artery.[93] In a subsequent investigation, bronchoarterial diameter ratios at altitude were found to be significantly greater than those at sea level, presumably as a result of hypoxic vasoconstriction.[94] In this study, 9 of 17 (57%) normal subjects living at altitude and only 2 of 16 (12%) normal subjects living at sea level had at least one bronchus that had an internal diameter equal to or greater than that of the adjacent pulmonary artery on HRCT images photographed at a window level of −450 HU. At a window level of −700 HU, only 2 of 17 (12%) normal subjects living at altitude and none of those living at sea level had bronchoarterial ratios equal to or greater than 1. These results illustrate the important influence of the HRCT window level in the assessment of bronchial and arterial diameters and thus the diagnosis of bronchiectasis.

The analysis in the last-named study was based on

careful measurement of the diameters of the bronchi and pulmonary artery using a Vernier caliper. The authors pointed out that subjective visual assessment tends to overestimate the internal diameter of the bronchus relative to that of the pulmonary artery.[94] In a study performed at sea level and based on subjective assessment, bronchoarterial diameter ratios greater than 1 were identified in 21% of 26 normal controls and in 95% of 59 patients who had bronchiectasis.[89] In this and other[93] studies, no normal individual had a bronchoarterial diameter ratio equal to or greater than 1.5. Therefore, a bronchoarterial diameter ratio can be considered a reliable sign of bronchiectasis by itself only when it is at least 1.5; when it is greater than 1 and less than 1.5, it must be present in several airways or associated with other findings, such as bronchial wall thickening and lack of bronchial tapering, or both.[89, 93] Care should be taken to assess the smallest cross-sectional airway diameter, to avoid making comparisons near bifurcations of bronchi or vessels (because the two may not divide at the same level), and not to overcall bronchiectasis in areas that have decreased vessel size as a result of local vasoconstriction. Because of the difficulty in appreciating the presence of bronchial or vascular bifurcation, the diagnosis of cylindrical bronchiectasis should be made only when bronchial dilation is seen on more than one computed tomographic level.

2. Visualization of peripheral bronchi is more specific in the diagnosis of bronchiectasis than increased bronchoarterial diameter ratios but has a slightly lower sensitivity. For example, in one study of 26 normal subjects, none had bronchi visualized within 1 cm of the costal pleura or abutting the mediastinal pleura.[89] Of 49 patients who had bronchiectasis, bronchi were visualized within 1 cm of the costal pleura in 81% and abutting the mediastinal pleura in 53%.

3. Bronchial wall thickening on HRCT is fairly common in bronchiectasis; for example, in one investigation of 47 lobes in which there was surgically proven disease, it was considered to be present in 32 (68%).[88] The abnormality is a nonspecific finding, however, that may also be seen in other conditions, particularly asthma,[93, 94] and in asymptomatic smokers.[95] Although measurements of normal bronchial wall thickness have been published, in clinical practice the analysis is based on subjective assessment.[86, 88, 90] Such estimates are influenced by the window level and width at which the HRCT images are photographed.[96, 97] Optimal assessment is obtained using a window level of −700 HU and a width of 1,000 HU; higher window levels are too dark,[98] and other window widths, particularly those less than 1,000 HU, lead to substantial artifactual wall thickening.[97]

4. Bronchi that course obliquely, such as the segmental bronchi of the middle lobe and lingula, are not optimally visualized on routine cross-sectional CT images. Visualization of these bronchi can be optimized by using oblique HRCT scans obtained by angling the CT gantry 20 degrees cranially.[99]

5. Bronchi filled with secretions are visualized as tubular or branching structures when they course horizontally or as nodules when they are oriented perpendicular to the plane of section (Fig. 56–20). They can usually be recognized by careful analysis of adjacent HRCT sections. Mucoceles, however, may be confused with a pulmonary tumor.[88]

6. In patients who have parenchymal consolidation or atelectasis, ectatic bronchi filled with secretions or blood may not be apparent on HRCT.[88] More commonly, bronchi are air filled and dilated because of a local increase in lung elastic recoil. This reversible bronchial dilation is particularly frequent in the resolving phase of acute pneumonia.[100, 101] With complete resolution of the pneumonia, the dilation gradually disappears, although it may take as long as 3 to 4 months before the normal dimensions of the bronchial tree can be appreciated. Because of this, an interval of 3 to 6 months should be allowed to elapse after acute pneumonia before a definitive diagnosis of bronchiectasis is made on HRCT.

7. Cardiac and respiratory motion may lead to suboptimal bronchial visualization; the resultant image artefacts can obscure the features of bronchiectasis or may result in

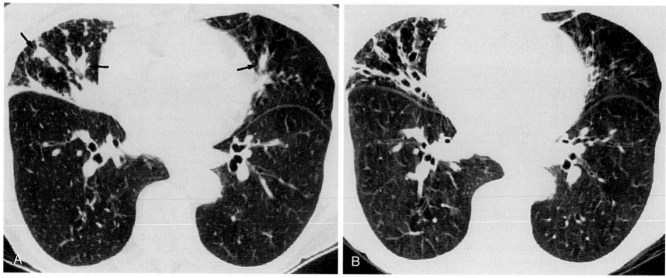

**Figure 56–20. Mucus-Filled Bronchi.** An HRCT scan *(A)* demonstrates tubular and nodular *(arrows)* opacities in the right middle lobe and lingula. A scan performed following expectoration of the mucus *(B)* shows that the opacities represented ectatic bronchi filled with secretions. The patient was an 80-year-old woman who had bronchiectasis as a result of previous tuberculosis.

changes that mimic bronchiectasis.[102] Such motion artefacts can be minimized by using short scan times (≤1 second).

As a result of the considerations listed previously, the recommended HRCT technique for the assessment of potential of bronchiectasis consists of 1- to 2-mm collimation scans at 10-mm intervals through the chest photographed using a window level of −700 HU and a window width of 1,000 HU. It has also been suggested that improved visualization may be obtained by using thin-section spiral CT. In one investigation of 50 consecutive patients who had clinical symptoms suggestive of bronchiectasis, HRCT was performed at 10-mm intervals, and spiral CT was carried out using 3-mm collimation volumetric scanning during a 24-second breath hold.[103] Bronchiectasis was noted in 22 patients on HRCT compared with 26 on spiral CT (including all those in whom it was identified on HRCT). HRCT showed evidence of bronchiectasis in 77 segments, whereas spiral CT documented it in 90. The radiation dose delivered using spiral CT was 3.5 times greater, however, than that delivered using HRCT. On the basis of these observations, the authors recommended that spiral CT be used in patients in whom there is high clinical suspicion of bronchiectasis and questionable findings on HRCT. Use of thicker sections (e.g., 4- to 5-mm collimation scans) results in a slight decrease in sensitivity compared with HRCT,[82, 104] whereas the use of 10-mm collimation scans decreases the sensitivity to about 60%.[105, 106]

In addition to bronchiectasis itself, a number of other abnormalities are seen with increased frequency in patients who have the disease, including areas of decreased lung attenuation and perfusion, tracheomegaly, and mediastinal lymph node enlargement (Fig. 56–21). In one investigation of 70 patients who had chronic purulent sputum production and in whom HRCT scans were obtained at full inspiration and at end expiration, bronchiectasis was identified in approximately 52% of lobes.[107] Areas of decreased attenuation were identified on HRCT performed at end inspiration in 20% of lobes and on expiratory scans in 34%. These areas were more prevalent in lobes that had bronchiectasis, and their extent correlated with the extent and severity of bronchiectasis; specifically, they were most prevalent in lobes that had extensive or widespread cystic bronchiectasis. Areas of decreased attenuation were also seen in lobes without overt bronchiectasis. Multiple regression analysis demonstrated that the extent of areas that had decreased attenuation was inversely related to the forced expiratory volume in 1 second ($FEV_1$) ($r = -0.57$) and $FEV_1$/forced vital capacity (FVC) ($r = -0.49$) and correlated positively with the residual volume (RV) ($r = 0.49$). The degree of attenuation was also independently and positively related to the extent and severity of bronchiectasis but was unrelated to age, smoking history, clinical evidence of asthma, age at onset of sputum production, or presence of an underlying cause. In another investigation, in which HRCT scans were compared with the pathologic findings in 47 lobes that had been resected for complications of bronchiectasis, areas of decreased attenuation were identified in 21 of the lobes (45%);[88] these areas were seen only in patients who had bronchiolitis in association with bronchiectasis.

Lymph node enlargement is seen relatively commonly on CT in patients who have bronchiectasis, particularly when it is associated with cystic fibrosis. In one investigation, it was detected in 12 of 42 (29%) patients who had bronchiectasis.[108] In a review of the radiographic findings in 48 adult patients who had cystic fibrosis, lymph node enlargement was found in 25 (52%), hilar in 22 (46%), and mediastinal in 21 (44%).[109] The lymphadenopathy was chronic and slowly progressive in all patients, and in no case did it resolve. Hypertrophied bronchial arteries result in tubular or nodular areas of soft tissue attenuation around the central airways and in the mediastinum;[109a] their vascular nature can be recognized readily following intravenous administration of contrast.

### Bronchography

For a long time, bronchography was the radiologic gold standard for the demonstration of the presence and extent of bronchiectasis, allowing accurate assessment of cylindrical (Fig. 56–22), varicose (Fig. 56–23), and cystic (Fig. 56–24) disease. Because of the risks of allergic reaction to the bronchographic medium—ranging from bronchospasm to iodism to anaphylaxis and death—and the temporary impairment of ventilation and gas exchange, the procedure has been replaced by HRCT. It has been suggested, however, that selective bronchography performed through the fiberoptic bronchoscope and using an iso-osmolar, nonionic contrast medium, might be helpful in selected cases.[110, 111] (A dimeric contrast medium is required because monomeric nonionic agents at iso-osmolar concentrations do not provide sufficient iodine concentration.) This procedure appears to be well tolerated, although some patients develop headaches, nausea, and flushing.[112] The technique should be reserved for patients who have recurrent hemoptysis and in whom the HRCT scan result is normal or shows questionable abnormalities.[113]

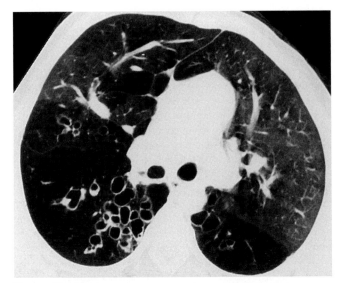

**Figure 56–21. Cystic Bronchiectasis.** An HRCT scan demonstrates cystic bronchiectasis in the right lower and left lower lobes and, to a lesser extent, in the right upper lobe. The areas of bronchiectasis are associated with marked decrease in attenuation and vascularity, presumed to be due to obliterative bronchiolitis. The patient was a 32-year-old man who had long-standing bronchiectasis following childhood viral infection.

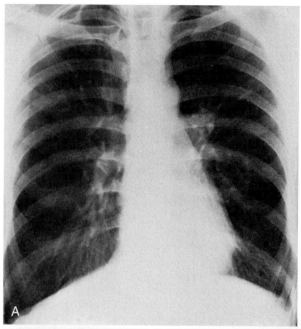

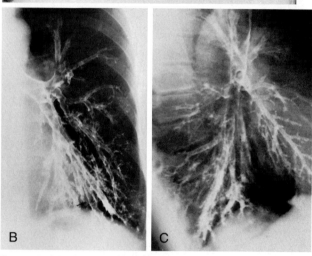

**Figure 56–22. Cylindrical Bronchiectasis.** A posteroanterior radiograph *(A)* demonstrates slight elevation of the left hemidiaphragm, chiefly in its posterior portion (see *C*). The linear markings in the basal segments of the left lower lobe are more prominent than normal and have lost their sharp definition; they are slightly crowded. Elsewhere, the lungs appear normal. A left bronchogram in posteroanterior *(B)* and lateral *(C)* projections reveals uniform dilation of all basal bronchi of the left lower lobe; prominent transverse striations are present in the lateral basal bronchus *(arrow)*. All bronchiectatic segments end abruptly, and there is little or no peripheral filling. The remainder of the bronchial tree is normal. In lateral projection, note the crowding of the bronchiectatic segments and the elevation of the posterior portion of the hemidiaphragm, both findings indicating moderate loss of volume. This 31-year-old man had a history of productive cough dating from an attack of whooping cough and bronchopneumonia as a child; pulmonary function study results were normal.

## Clinical Manifestations

As indicated previously, many patients who have bronchiectasis have no symptoms referable to the bronchiectasis itself and therefore are not included in clinical series describing symptoms and signs. When present, the main symptoms are cough and expectoration of purulent sputum; hemoptysis and recurrent fever are less common. Chest pain is not infrequently experienced over the area of bronchiectasis; for example, in one study of 80 patients, it was present in 18 (23%).[114]

The quantity of sputum varies with the severity of the disease. Some patients become aware of purulent expectoration only after respiratory infections (which tend to be frequent). Postinfective bronchiectasis often presents as a pediatric disease, the history commonly dating from early childhood; for example, in one series of 116 patients, 50% gave a history indicating the onset of symptoms before the third birthday.[72] In a majority of cases, a history can be elicited of pneumonia developing as a complication of measles, whooping cough, or some other contagious disease of childhood. For example, in one study of 123 adult patients (mean age, 57 ± 17 years) who had well-documented disease, 86 (70%) had a history of a potentially causative event, most often pneumonia.[115] Hemoptysis occurs in about 50% of older patients but is relatively rare in children. If the disease is widespread, the patient may complain of shortness of breath.

Persistent crackles localized to the area of major involvement are detectable in about 70% of cases.[115] If the bronchiectasis is associated with significant airway obstruction, diffuse or localized wheezing may be audible.[115] Two groups have suggested that analysis of the timing and wave form of crackles may aid in differentiating bronchiectasis from other respiratory disorders.[116, 117]

The most common extrathoracic manifestation is finger clubbing, seen in about one third of cases;[72] brain abscess,[118] amyloidosis,[119] and neuropathy have also been reported.[120] Patients may show evidence of a systemic inflammatory response, as evidenced by decreased body weight and serum albumin and increased total serum globulin, alpha₁-antitrypsin, and white blood cell count.[121] Rarely, the disease is complicated by a systemic vasculitis syndrome associated with purpuric skin lesions and elevated levels of circulating immune complexes[122] and requiring immunosuppressive therapy;[123, 124] in some patients, this has been associated with crescentic glomerulonephritis and increased levels of antineutrophil cytoplasmic antibody.[125, 126]

### Pulmonary Function Studies

There is no specific pattern of pulmonary function abnormality, although a combination of obstruction and restriction should raise suspicion of the disease. Patients who have radiographically localized disease suffer little or no functional impairment. In one study of 123 patients, 66 (54%) showed an obstructive pattern;[115] as might be expected, the degree of obstruction was greater among patients who had smoked cigarettes. In the presence of appreciable atelectasis, the abnormality of function may be restrictive, with a decrease in vital capacity (VC), functional residual capacity (FRC), and total lung capacity (TLC). In more diffuse disease, the pattern is similar to that of obstructive disease, with proportionally greater decrease in the timed VC and, in many cases, impairment of gas mixing, an increase in the FRC, and a reduction of diffusing capacity.[127]

In one study of 50 patients who had bronchiectasis (excluding forms associated with tuberculosis or hypogammaglobulinemia), the predominant functional abnormality consisted of air-flow obstruction unaccompanied by hyperinflation;[128] values of individual tests were 83%, 150%, and

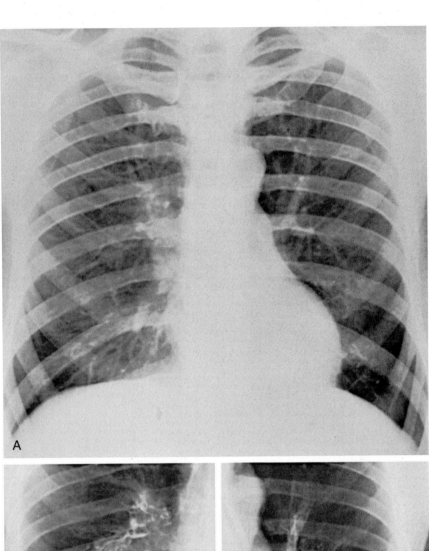

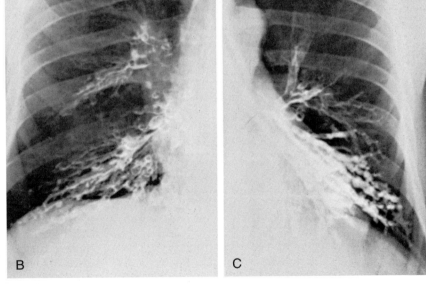

**Figure 56–23. Varicose Bronchiectasis.** A posteroanterior radiograph *(A)* of this 38-year-old man shows a rather subtle change in the size of the vascular markings throughout the lungs, the upper lobe vessels being somewhat larger than normal and the lower lobe vessels being comparatively inconspicuous. Right *(B)* and left *(C)* bronchograms reveal extensive dilation of all basal bronchi of the lower lobes and of the right middle lobe; the dilation is not uniform, as in Figure 56–22, but is characterized by numerous local constrictions that give the bronchi a configuration resembling varicose veins. There is a notable absence of peripheral filling. This patient gave a history of the accidental ingestion of camphorated oil 1 year previously and had had productive cough ever since.

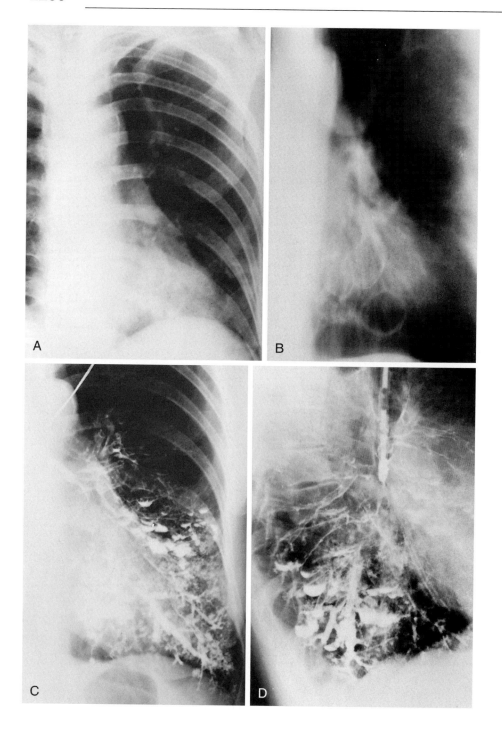

**Figure 56–24. Cystic Bronchiectasis.** A view of the left hemithorax from a posteroanterior radiograph *(A)* reveals several well-defined cystic spaces measuring almost 3 cm in diameter in the lower portion of the left lung, seen to better advantage on an anteroposterior tomogram *(B)*; several patchy shadows of increased opacity are scattered throughout much of the left lower lobe. Posteroanterior *(C)* and lateral *(D)* projections of a left bronchogram reveal numerous cystic spaces containing contrast material, in many areas presenting as fluid levels. The patient was a 46-year-old woman.

90% predicted for VC, RV, and diffusing capacity of the lungs for carbon monoxide (DLCO) (corrected for alveolar volume). In 35 of the 50 patients, $FEV_1$ was less than 80% of predicted, and in 34, the $FEV_1$/FVC ratio was less than 70%. Of the 29 patients in whom the $FEV_1$ was greater than 1.5 liters, an inhalation dose-response curve for methacholine showed that the provocative concentration producing a 20% decrease in $FEV_1$ ($PC_{20}$) was less than 16 mg/ml in 20 (69%). Because there was a significant relationship between $PC_{20}$ and the prechallenge $FEV_1$, these results suggest that the airway hyperresponsiveness was a consequence of the airway disease. Lung function is worse and its rate of decline faster in patients who are chronically infected with *P. aerugi-*

*nosa* as opposed to other organisms; however, it is unclear whether this is a cause-and-effect relationship.[129]

The degree of air-flow obstruction may be quite variable, either spontaneously or after treatment with inhaled bronchodilator. In a study of 85 Chinese patients who had diffuse or localized disease and no evidence of cystic fibrosis, 23 (27%) had significant air-flow reversibility;[130] in these individuals, increased airway responsiveness to methacholine, increased eosinophils, a higher prevalence of atopy, and elevated serum IgE levels suggested an asthmatic component to their disease. In another investigation of 47 patients, bronchial hyperresponsiveness to inhaled methacholine ($PC_{20}$ < 8 mg/ml) was present in 21 of the 47 patients (45%) in whom it was measured and was related to the asthmatic features as well as to baseline $FEV_1$.[131] The degree of lung function impairment is also related to indices of ongoing airway inflammation, such as the presence of sputum eosinophils, higher peripheral leukocyte count, and increased sputum elastolytic activity.[132]

In a study of distribution and clearance of tagged radioactive aerosol particles 2 μm in diameter in 14 patients who had bronchiectasis, particles were found to be deposited in central bronchi and were cleared more slowly than normal.[133] The central deposition was attributed to increased turbulence in obstructed larger airways, permitting impaction by inertia; the impaired clearance was similar to that seen in simple bronchitis and was ascribed to damage to the mucociliary apparatus. The considerable impairment in tracheobronchial clearance that occurs in patients who have bronchiectasis has been confirmed in additional studies.[134]

### Prognosis and Natural History

A number of investigators have shown that bronchiectasis is progressive in some patients, either after pulmonary resection for localized postinfective bronchiectasis or in patients who have not undergone resectional surgery.[72, 135, 136] Despite the occurrence of such progressive disease, the prognosis has improved considerably in the last 50 years. In a 1940 report based on a follow-up of 400 patients, 92% of the deaths were directly attributed to the bronchiectasis, and about 70% of the patients died before the age of 40 years.[137] By contrast, in a 1969 report of a 12-year follow-up of 62 patients, only 50% of the deaths that occurred were attributed to bronchiectasis or its complications;[138] the average age at death was 55 years, and only two patients died who were under the age of 40. In a third study in 1974 in which the results of surgical and medical management were reviewed for 393 patients who were followed over a period up to 15 years, only 9% died.[139] Finally, in a 1981 review of 116 patients, the reported mortality rate was 19% during a 14-year follow-up period, the mean age at death being 54 years.[140]

### Specific Causes of Bronchiectasis

#### Dyskinetic Cilia Syndrome

The syndrome of situs inversus, paranasal sinusitis, and bronchiectasis was first reported by Siewert in 1904, but acquired its eponym somewhat later after Kartagener described it in detail.[141] Since that time, it has become clear that other abnormalities are occasionally associated with the classic triad, including transposition of the great vessels,[142] trilocular or bilocular heart, pyloric stenosis, urethral meatus on the ventral ridge of the glans penis,[143] and postcricoid web (Paterson-Brown-Kelly syndrome).[144] Because of the presence of these congenital anomalies and of the familial association of the disorder in some cases,[145] a hereditary abnormality was assumed to be the cause. The precise nature of the defect, however, eluded recognition until 1975, when two subjects were described who had Kartagener's syndrome accompanied by immotile spermatozoa and cilia.[146] The authors of this report were the first to suggest that the immotile cilia were the underlying abnormality responsible for the classic features of the disease.

Since that time, numerous reports have appeared confirming the presence of abnormalities of ciliary structure and function in patients with the syndrome.[147, 148] The identification of these abnormalities as the cause of the condition initially led to the use of the more descriptive term *immotile cilia syndrome* in place of Kartagener's syndrome. It has since become clear that most patients with the disease possess cilia that do move, although the motion is invariably uncoordinated and ineffective.[149, 150] It has thus been suggested that the condition be termed *dyskinetic cilia syndrome* or *primary ciliary dyskinesia*. In support of this concept is the observation of a variant of dyskinetic cilia syndrome in which the cilia were ultrastructurally normal but showed a "trembling" hypermotility.[151] Some investigators have even suggested that microscopic examination and quantification of the frequency and pattern of ciliary beating from mucosal biopsy specimens is a more effective means of establishing a diagnosis than is electron microscopy.[152]

The incidence of dyskinetic cilia syndrome in whites is estimated to be between 1 in 12,500[153] to 40,000.[143] These estimates are less than the figures reported for the Japanese population,[154] a difference that has been attributed to a greater prevalence of consanguinity in marriage among the Japanese. The proportion of cases of bronchiectasis that are attributed to dyskinetic cilia syndrome has been reported to be higher in North Africans (36%) than in Europeans (4%).[155] A report of three Maori who had abnormal ciliary ultrastructure and bronchiectasis suggested that the high incidence of bronchiectasis in Polynesians could be related to ciliary dyskinesia;[156] however, the results of a larger study indicated that these individuals did not fit the pattern of most patients who have dyskinetic cilia syndrome, including the absence of situs inversus.[157, 158] It has been suggested that the ciliary defects described in these patients may be acquired rather than congenital.[159–161] A similar conclusion was reached in a study of Canadian First Nations children, who also have a high prevalence of bronchiectasis.[162]

The mode of inheritance of dyskinetic cilia syndrome best fits with an autosomal recessive pattern.[154, 163–165] The variety of ultrastructural defects associated with the clinical syndrome suggests considerable genetic heterogeneity.[166] In addition, patients have been described who have classic Kartagener's syndrome and abnormal airway ciliary ultrastructure but normal spermatozoa[167–169] or who have sterility associated with ultrastructural abnormalities of sperm but normal respiratory ciliary structure and function,[170] indicating that discordance in phenotypic presentation can occur. Dyskinetic cilia syndrome has also been reported in association with Marfan's syndrome,[171] polysplenia,[172] hepatic steatosis,[173] hydrocephalus,[174] and Usher's syndrome (an autosomal recessive disease characterized by congenital sensorineural deafness, vestibular dysfunction, and retinitis pigmentosa).[175]

The structure and function of the normal cilium are complex and have been reviewed previously (*see* Chapter 1, page 6). Briefly, each cilium contains an axoneme consisting of two central microtubules surrounded by nine peripheral pairs of microtubules. The peripheral and central microtubules are joined by radial spokes, and the peripheral microtubules connect to each other by inner and outer dynein arms; the latter are believed to be the site of energy conversion leading to ciliary movement. Ultrastructural abnormalities in each of these components have been identified in patients who have dyskinetic cilia syndrome (Fig. 56–25), including a lack of outer dynein arms, absent or short radial spokes,[172] deficient central sheath, absent or defective inner dynein arms,[176] absent central microtubules, disorientation of the central tubules,[177] transposition of peripheral microtubules,[178, 179] and supernumerary microtubules;[180] the most

common of these is a lack of dynein arms. A combination of structural defects is often present.[181] In some patients, the abnormality is in the basal bodies rather than the cilium itself.[182] Classic Kartagener's syndrome and severe childhood bronchiectasis have also been reported in patients who have ultrastructurally normal cilia;[183] in some of these individuals, disease has been attributed to abnormally long cilia;[184] in others, it is possible that the structural defect develops later in life or that a functional defect can occur

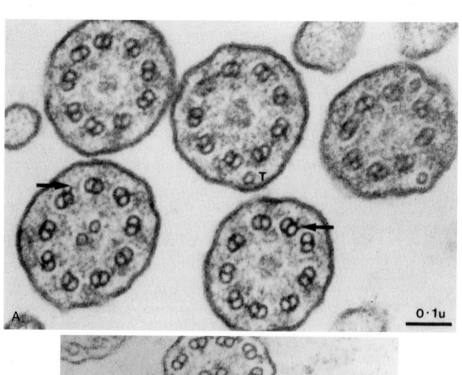

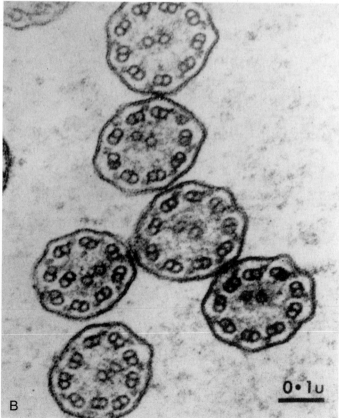

**Figure 56–25. Ciliary Abnormalities in Dyskinetic Cilia Syndrome.** A cross-section of a group of cilia and microvilli *(A)* shows that most of the outer ciliary doublets lack dynein arms, although occasional partial arms are present *(arrows).* The central tubules are also absent in four of the cilia; supernumerary single tubules (T) are occasionally present. (Original magnification, ×130,000.) (From Wakefield St J, Waite D: Mucociliary transport and ultrastructural abnormalities in Polynesian bronchiectasis. Am Rev Respir Dis 121:1003, 1980.) A cross-section of cilia from another patient *(B)* shows the absence of inner dynein arms. (Original magnification, ×100,000.) (From Neustein HG, Nickerson B, O'Neal M: Kartagener's syndrome with absence of inner dynein arms of respiratory cilia. Am Rev Respir Dis 122:979, 1980.)

without morphologic abnormalities.[185–187] A classification system for the various disorders of ciliary motility has been proposed (*see* Table 56–1).[172]

Structural and functional defects of cilia can be acquired rather than congenital,[188, 189] and it has occasionally proved difficult to distinguish the two in single biopsy specimens of nasal or bronchial mucosa.[190, 191] Such abnormalities are not uncommon, having been described in a high proportion of cigarette smokers,[192–195] in individuals with chronic bronchitis and influenza or other viral infection,[147, 196] and in some apparently normal individuals who manifest neither acute nor chronic respiratory disease.[194, 196–198] Derangements include compound cilia (showing partial or multiple complete axonemes within a single cell membrane), internalized cilia (projecting into cytoplasmic cavities in the cell apex rather than into the airway), cilia with disorganized axonemes, changes in the ciliary membrane or amount of cytoplasm, transposition of microtubules,[194] radial spoke defects,[194] flaccid cilia,[147] and a variety of microtubular abnormalities.[196–198] In one study, patients who had chronic upper respiratory infection unrelated to dyskinetic cilia syndrome showed a high prevalence of ciliary disorientation;[189] this abnormality correlated more closely with decreased mucociliary clearance than did ciliary beat frequency. (Ciliary disorientation in the absence of any other structural defect, however, can also be an inherited cause of dyskinetic cilia syndrome.[199])

Despite these observations, differentiation between acquired and congenital defects should usually be straightforward if sufficient cilia are examined, the characteristic feature of the former being the polymorphic nature of the structural changes.[195, 200] A quantitative study of ciliary beat frequency, beat pattern, and ultrastructure was conducted in a large group of normal subjects, patients with atopic rhinitis, asymptomatic smokers, patients with pulmonary disease not related to dyskinetic cilia syndrome, and patients with dyskinetic cilia syndrome.[200] About 5% of the cilia from normal subjects and patients with non–dyskinetic cilia syndrome pulmonary disease had abnormal ciliary structure, whereas 30% to 95% of cilia from patients with dyskinetic cilia syndrome were structurally abnormal; beat frequency and pattern of ciliary motion were obviously different in the latter group. In another study, patients who had dyskinetic cilia syndrome were distinguishable from those with acquired abnormalities on the basis of lower ciliary beat frequency, greater ciliary disorientation, and a significantly higher incidence of peripheral to central tubule defects.[201] In patients who have dyskinetic cilia syndrome, there is a good correlation between abnormalities of nasal and bronchial ciliary structure, supporting the practice of using less invasive nasal sampling as the diagnostic test.[202]

The abnormalities identified in ciliary microtubular structure may represent only part of a generalized disease process. Thus, presumably reflecting the necessity of microtubules for phagocytic cell motility, leukocyte chemotaxis and phagocytosis appear to be mildly impaired in patients who have dyskinetic cilia syndrome; for example, polymorphonuclear leukocytes show an excessive rambling and circuitous movement when placed on a flat surface.[203–205] Although the bactericidal activity of the neutrophils is normal, it is possible that the decreased motility and phagocytosis

could contribute to the increased frequency of pulmonary infections to which these patients are subject.

The radiographic manifestations of dyskinetic cilia syndrome have been described in a study of 30 patients, 15 of each sex.[206] Ages ranged from newborn to 26 years. Radiographic abnormalities were evident in all patients, including bronchial wall thickening, hyperinflation, segmental atelectasis or consolidation, and segmental bronchiectasis. Except for the presence of situs inversus (Fig. 56–26), which is present in about half the patients,[206] the radiologic features are not specific and resemble those of bronchiectasis from a variety of other causes. Although the bronchiectasis can be widespread on HRCT, it involves predominantly or exclusively the lower lobes in approximately 50% of patients.[206a]

Clinically, individuals who have full-blown dyskinetic cilia syndrome have chronic rhinitis, sinusitis, otitis, recurrent bronchitis, bronchiectasis, male sterility, corneal abnormalities, and a poor sense of smell. To make a diagnosis, it is recommended that patients must have a history of chronic bronchial infection and rhinitis from early childhood, combined with one or more of the following features:[147] (1) situs inversus or dextrocardia in the patient or a sibling, (2) living but immotile spermatozoa, (3) tracheobronchial clearance that is absent or nearly so, and (4) cilia that have ultrastructural defects characteristic of the syndrome. The association of otitis with the lower respiratory tract symptoms is a consistent feature and should alert one to the possibility of a ciliary defect.[207]

The decrease in airway mucociliary clearance in patients who have dyskinetic cilia syndrome is profound and is greater than that seen in individuals who have advanced cystic fibrosis, bronchiectasis of other cause, chronic obstructive pulmonary disease, or asthma.[208–210] Despite this, severe air-flow obstruction does not develop, suggesting that impaired mucociliary clearance may contribute to the production of obstructive airway disease but is not of major importance.[208] Early in the course of the disease, patients have a pattern of functional abnormalities consistent with small airway dysfunction and increased bronchial responsiveness to methacholine; however, one group of patients followed over a period of 4 to 14 years showed a remarkably stable pattern of mild obstruction.[211, 212]

### Young's Syndrome

Young's syndrome (obstructive azoospermia) is characterized by infertility related to mechanical obstruction of the genital tract accompanied by sinusitis and bronchiectasis.[213, 214] The combination of infertility and sinopulmonary infections may suggest a diagnosis of cystic fibrosis or dyskinetic cilia syndrome.[215, 216] In fact, some mutations in the CFTR gene are associated with congenital bilateral absence of the vas deferens (CBAVD),[217] and CFTR mutations have been reported in almost 50% of men with obstructive azoospermia of unknown cause.[218] Although these observations raise the possibility that Young's syndrome, CBAVD, and cystic fibrosis may have a similar genetic basis, one group showed that 12 patients who had an obstructed urogenital tract with an anatomically intact vas deferens and bronchiectasis had no CFTR mutations,[214] suggesting that Young's syndrome and CBAVD are different clinical entities. It is likely, however, that previously reported series of pa-

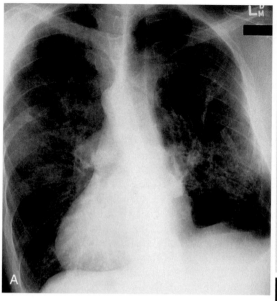

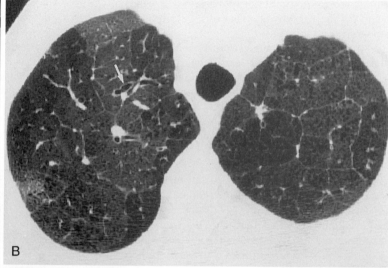

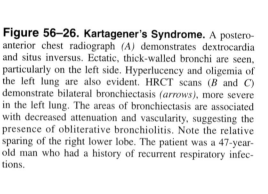

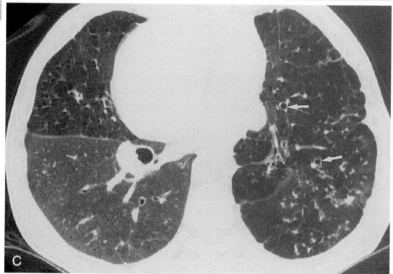

**Figure 56–26. Kartagener's Syndrome.** A postero-anterior chest radiograph *(A)* demonstrates dextrocardia and situs inversus. Ectatic, thick-walled bronchi are seen, particularly on the left side. Hyperlucency and oligemia of the left lung are also evident. HRCT scans *(B* and *C)* demonstrate bilateral bronchiectasis *(arrows)*, more severe in the left lung. The areas of bronchiectasis are associated with decreased attenuation and vascularity, suggesting the presence of obliterative bronchiolitis. Note the relative sparing of the right lower lobe. The patient was a 47-year-old man who had a history of recurrent respiratory infections.

tients who had Young's syndrome included some patients who would now be considered to have cystic fibrosis. A familial disorder characterized by oligospermia, impaired spermatic motility, bronchiectasis, and normal ciliary ultrastructure has also been reported.[219]

It has been hypothesized that simple epididymal obstruction is not the only cause of the azoospermia seen in patients who have Young's syndrome because surgical correction is relatively ineffective in restoring fertility. The results of an epidemiologic study from the United Kingdom suggest that some cases may be caused by mercurous chloride, which was formally used in teething powders and worm medication in that country;[220] the incidence of the syndrome fell from 50% of 227 patients who had epididymal obstruction in men born before 1955 (when the use of these compounds was discontinued) to 17% of 47 similarly obstructed patients born since that time. The latter value is similar to that in another review of 102 patients who had obstructive azoospermia, of whom 23% were considered to have Young's syndrome.[221] The syndrome has been reported rarely in some other parts of the world, such as Japan.[222]

In one study of 14 patients who had Young's syndrome

and 14 age-matched, smoking-matched control subjects, a significant decrease in mucociliary clearance and slight but definite abnormalities of pulmonary function were found in the patients.[223] Despite this, no abnormalities of airway mucus, ciliary beating, or ciliary structure have been described to explain the functional defect.[224]

### Syndrome of Yellow Nails, Lymphedema, Pleural Effusion, and Bronchiectasis

A syndrome of yellow nails and lymphedema was first described in 1964;[225] pleural effusion was later added as a frequent feature of the disease (Fig. 56–27).[226] Some physicians restrict the diagnosis to patients who have the complete triad, whereas others accept any two characteristics. Typically the nails grow slowly, are yellowish green in color, and are thickened and excessively curved from side to side; they have a tendency to become infected.[227, 228]

In one review of 97 patients, lymphedema was first identified in neonates or in patients as old as 65 years;[229] the median age at onset was 40 years. Eighty-nine per cent of the patients had yellow nails, 80% had lymphedema of

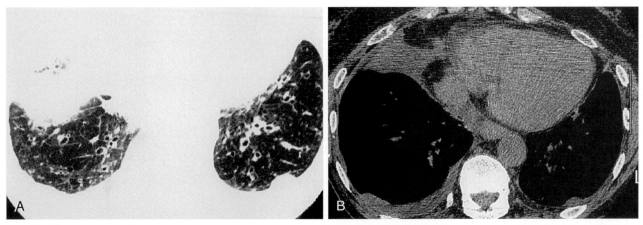

**Figure 56–27. Yellow Nail Syndrome.** An HRCT scan *(A)* demonstrates bronchiectasis involving the basal segments of the lower lobes. Soft tissue windows *(B)* show small bilateral pleural effusions and mild pleural thickening. The patient was a 75-year-old woman who presented with yellow nails, lymphedema, and bilateral pleural effusions several years previously. She had undergone pleurodesis for recurrent large pleural effusions.

varying severity, and 36% had pleural effusion. In 29% of patients, the initial symptom was related to pleural effusion. Patients often give a history of recurrent attacks of bronchitis and may have chronic sinusitis, bronchiectasis, and recurrent pneumonia. Of 12 patients reported from the Mayo Clinic, 8 had recurrent pleural effusion, and 5 had bronchiectasis;[230] in this series, the first manifestation of the syndrome was either lymphedema or yellow nails, pleural effusion appearing somewhat later in all cases. In two other series, bronchiectasis and yellow nails were reported as developing simultaneously in three patients aged 10, 18, and 20 years, lymphedema becoming manifest somewhat later in each patient.[231, 232] Rarely, edema is the predominant manifestation, as in one case in which chylous ascites developed in association with diffuse lymphangiectasia involving the whole small bowel.[233]

The lymphedema results from hypoplasia (sometimes atresia) of the lymphatics, defects that can be demonstrated by peripheral lymphangiography.[227] It is often mild and usually affects the lower extremities; sometimes, other areas, such as the breast[231] or face,[234] are involved. The pleural and, occasionally, pericardial fluid is characteristically an exudate and may be chylous.[235] Light and electron microscopy shows dilation of both visceral and parietal pleural lymphatics associated with perilymphatic inflammation; the pleural fluid characteristically contains a high percentage of lymphocytes.[236]

The pathogenesis of the bronchiectasis is unknown, although it is frequently associated with sinusitis, suggesting a generalized respiratory mucosal abnormality.[230] In one patient, the bronchiectasis was confined to the upper lobes.[237] As with bronchiectasis associated with other abnormalities, HRCT has been successfully employed to identify the presence and extent of airway abnormality.[238]

The syndrome has been reported in association with a variety of other diseases, including immunologic deficiency in siblings,[230] thyroid disease, hypogammaglobulinemia in various forms, the nephrotic syndrome, a transient decrease in circulating B lymphocytes,[238a] and protein-losing enteropathy.[229, 239] One case of obstructive sleep apnea has been reported in which the authors suggested that edema of the pharynx and palate contributed to the upper airway obstruction.[240]

### Williams-Campbell Syndrome

As indicated previously, Williams-Campbell syndrome is a congenital form of bronchiectasis in which the pathophysiologic mechanism is believed to be a deficiency in the amount of airway cartilage. The condition was first described in 1960;[241] since that time, additional groups of cases, some showing a familial clustering[242, 243] or associated with congenital abnormalities,[243a] have been reported.[244] Pathologic examination of the airways in some of these cases has shown a symmetric deficiency in airway cartilage involving the tracheobronchial tree distal to segmental bronchi;[241, 244a] however, there is evidence that larger airways may also be involved.[244b]

HRCT findings are characteristic and consist of cystic bronchiectasis limited to the fourth-, fifth-, and sixth-generation bronchi (i.e., distal to the first-generation segmental bronchi).[245–247a] Expiratory HRCT shows collapse of the bronchi and distal air trapping.[245] This combination of findings is virtually diagnostic of the syndrome.[245] Affected individuals usually present in infancy with repeated chest infections and evidence of bronchiectasis; the clinical course may be one of rapid deterioration or prolonged survival.

### Mounier-Kuhn Syndrome

The Mounier-Kuhn syndrome is a congenital abnormality characterized by atrophy or absence of elastic fibers and thinning of the smooth muscle layer in the trachea and main bronchi. These airways are thus flaccid and markedly dilated on inspiration and collapsible on expiration. A broad spectrum of functional impairment has been associated with the syndrome, ranging from minimal disease with preservation of function to severe bronchiectasis, emphysema, and pulmonary fibrosis.

The syndrome can be diagnosed from the plain radiograph by measuring the transverse and sagittal diameters of the trachea and main bronchi (Fig. 56–28). For women, it can be considered to be present when transverse and sagittal diameters of the trachea exceed 21 and 23 mm, respectively, and the diameters of the right and left main bronchi exceed 19.8 and 17.4 mm; for men, the corresponding figures are 25 and 27 mm for the transverse and sagittal diameters of

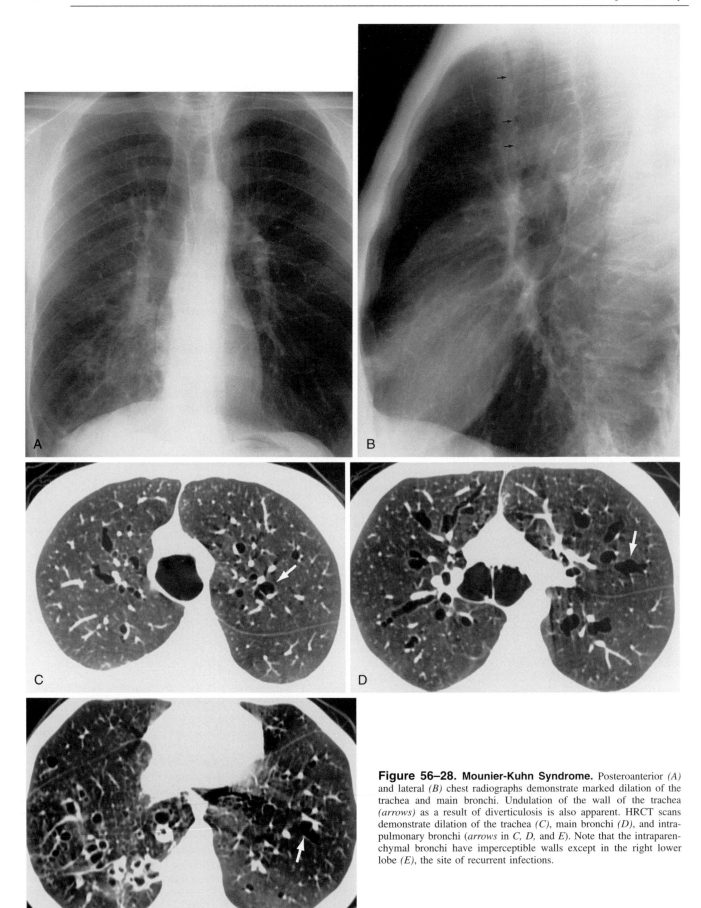

**Figure 56–28. Mounier-Kuhn Syndrome.** Posteroanterior *(A)* and lateral *(B)* chest radiographs demonstrate marked dilation of the trachea and main bronchi. Undulation of the wall of the trachea *(arrows)* as a result of diverticulosis is also apparent. HRCT scans demonstrate dilation of the trachea *(C)*, main bronchi *(D)*, and intrapulmonary bronchi *(arrows in C, D,* and *E)*. Note that the intraparenchymal bronchi have imperceptible walls except in the right lower lobe *(E)*, the site of recurrent infections.

the trachea and 21.1 and 18.4 mm for the diameters of the right and left main bronchi.[35] Dilation of the trachea and bronchi and undulation of the wall as a result of tracheal and bronchial diverticulae are well seen on both conventional CT and HRCT.[248–251] CT performed at end expiration may also show complete collapse of the trachea and main bronchi.[250–252] HRCT is particularly helpful in demonstrating the presence of associated bronchiectasis;[249, 251] less commonly, it reveals diffuse dilation of thin-walled intraparenchymal bronchi (*see* Fig. 56–28).[251]

## BRONCHOLITHIASIS

The term *broncholithiasis* is used to denote the presence of calcified or ossified material within the lumen of the tracheobronchial tree. Theoretically, this material can originate in several ways:[253] (1) aspiration of bone or *in situ* calcification of aspirated foreign material that has impacted within the bronchial wall; (2) erosion of calcified or ossified bronchial cartilage plates into the airway wall and eventual extrusion into the lumen; (3) migration to a bronchus of calcified material from a distant site, such as a pleural plaque[254] or the kidney (via a nephrobronchial fistula);[255] and (4) erosion and extrusion of calcified necrotic material from a bronchopulmonary lymph node into the bronchial lumen. The last-named is by far the most common of these mechanisms. It is usually associated with long-standing foci of necrotizing granulomatous lymphadenitis; any organism leading to such inflammation, including *Mycobacterium tuberculosis*, *Histoplasma capsulatum*, *Coccidioides immitis*, and a variety of others,[256] can theoretically cause the complication. In North America, the most common agent is probably *H. capsulatum*, a feature most likely related to the high incidence of lymphadenitis in endemic areas.[257, 258] Despite the fact that it is the most frequent pathogenetic mechanism, the incidence of broncholithiasis complicating granulomatous infection is undoubtedly quite low.[259]

Broncholiths are variable in size, ranging from less than 1 mm to exceptional examples weighing 139 gm.[260] They are usually irregular in shape, may have a granular or smooth surface (Fig. 56–29), and often possess spurlike projections or sharp edges. It has been hypothesized that repeated physical impingement of these hard projections on the bronchial wall during the respiratory cycle is responsible for the erosion of calcified material within lymph nodes into the airway lumen.[254] The effects of broncholithiasis are variable and depend on the size and degree of calcification of the stone. Those that contain relatively little calcium may disintegrate easily and be manifested by recurrent lithoptysis with or without hemoptysis. By contrast, stones that are heavily calcified or ossified are less likely to break up and can cause occlusion with distal bronchiectasis and obstructive pneumonitis.

Histologic examination of broncholiths typically shows amorphous, sometimes laminated necrotic material with extensive dystrophic calcification (Fig. 56–30); bone is seen

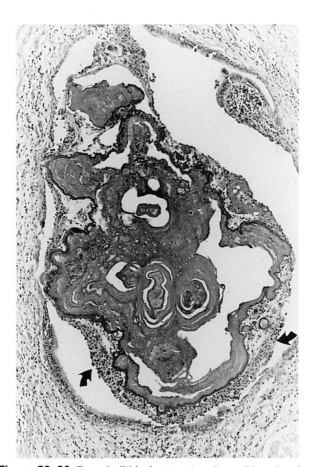

**Figure 56–30. Broncholithiasis.** A section of a small bronchus shows the lumen to be almost completely filled by an irregularly shaped, laminated concretion of heavily calcified material. An acute inflammatory exudate surrounds the material focally *(arrows)*; the airway wall shows fibrosis and chronic inflammation. The affected airway was approximately 5 mm in diameter. Incidental finding in a pneumonectomy specimen removed for carcinoma. The cause of the "stone" was not apparent.

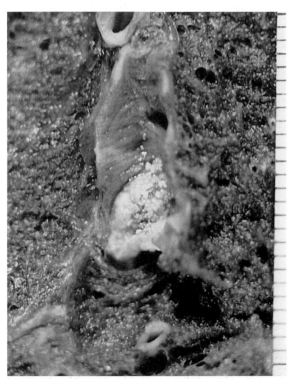

**Figure 56–29. Broncholithiasis.** A magnified view of a small bronchus shows it to be occluded by a finely granular white concretion, which was very hard. Typical features of chronic (inactive) fibrocaseous tuberculosis were present elsewhere in the lobe.

occasionally. Organisms may be identified within the material with appropriate special stains.[256, 260] The adjacent bronchial wall is invariably inflamed and may be ulcerated; in the latter situation, an acute inflammatory exudate is present within the airway lumen and may contain fragments of the broncholith (Fig. 56–31). It has been suggested that focal pigmented scars in the bronchial mucosa that are occasionally found incidentally at autopsy may represent the site of a prior broncholith that had perforated the airway.[258]

Radiographic manifestations of broncholithiasis include change of position or disappearance of a calcific focus on serial radiographs or development of airway obstruction, resulting in lobar or segmental atelectasis, mucoid impaction, or expiratory air trapping.[261–263] Although a specific diagnosis can seldom be made on the plain chest radiograph, broncholiths can usually be readily identified on CT (Fig. 56–32).[264–267] Relatively thin sections (≤5 mm) are required to determine accurately the exact location of the calcification within the bronchus;[267] thicker sections result in volume averaging of the broncholith, bronchus, and surrounding tissues.

In one study of 15 patients who had broncholithiasis proved by bronchoscopy, surgery, or lithoptysis, all had calcified nodes on CT.[267] In the 10 patients in whom the calcified material ultimately was proven to be endobronchial,

6 were interpreted as being endobronchial on CT and 4 to be peribronchial. In one case, involvement of a subsegmental bronchus was not evident on 10-mm-thick sections but could be clearly seen on 5-mm thick sections. Broncholiths were identified on bronchoscopy in only 5 of the 15 cases. Other findings included atelectasis in 11 patients, obstructive pneumonitis in 4, and bronchiectasis in 4. The authors concluded that broncholithiasis can be strongly suggested on CT when there is a calcified lymph node that is either endobronchial or peribronchial and is associated with findings of bronchial obstruction, such as atelectasis, obstructive pneumonitis, or bronchiectasis.

The most prominent symptom is cough, which is usually nonproductive of sputum but frequently associated with hemoptysis. Less commonly, the presence of secondary infection causes pain, chills, and fever. A history of prior expectoration of calcified material (lithoptysis) is not uncommon, as in 44 of 99 patients in one series.[253] In most instances, this history probably represents gradual disintegration and expectoration of a single mass of calcified material. Rarely, gradual dissolution and expectoration of a broncholith results in disappearance of symptoms, as illustrated by one patient whose left vocal cord paralysis disappeared after expectoration of calcified material.[268]

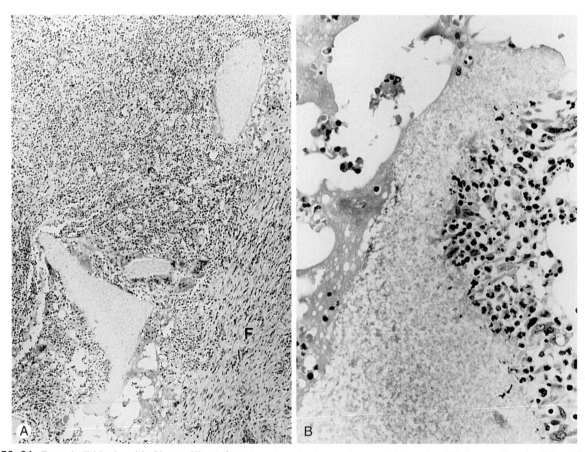

**Figure 56–31. Broncholithiasis with Airway Ulceration.** A section of a large subsegmental bronchus *(A)* shows a fibrosis of its wall (F) and an acute inflammatory exudate within its lumen (the epithelium has been destroyed). Several finely granular fragments of a broncholith can be seen in the exudate (magnified in *B*). The patient was a middle-aged man who presented with hemoptysis and an ill-defined upper lobe opacity on the chest radiograph; lobectomy was performed for a presumed diagnosis of carcinoma. Silver stain of the broncholith fragments revealed fungi consistent with *Histoplasma capsulatum.*

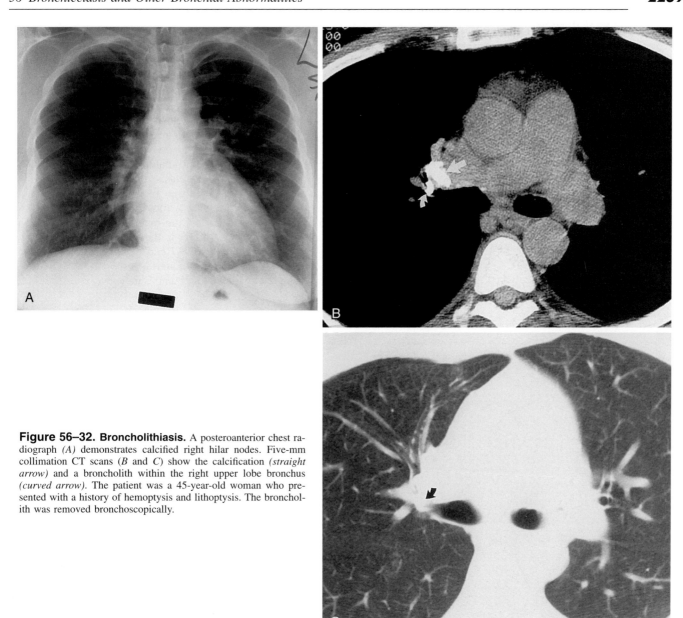

**Figure 56–32. Broncholithiasis.** A posteroanterior chest radiograph *(A)* demonstrates calcified right hilar nodes. Five-mm collimation CT scans *(B* and *C)* show the calcification *(straight arrow)* and a broncholith within the right upper lobe bronchus *(curved arrow).* The patient was a 45-year-old woman who presented with a history of hemoptysis and lithoptysis. The broncholith was removed bronchoscopically.

## BRONCHIAL FISTULAS

Bronchial fistulas can be established with many structures, both within the thorax and outside it (Table 56–2). The principal underlying causes are infection and carcinoma; either may originate in the lung or in the organ with which the fistula is associated. Trauma, other noninfectious inflammatory processes, and foreign bodies (either aspirated or introduced for therapeutic or diagnostic purposes) are occasional causes.

The most common form is probably bronchopleural fistula, usually after lobectomy or pneumonectomy for pulmonary carcinoma.[269] The origin of such fistulas is almost always the bronchial stump; dehiscence of sutures related to surgical technique, infection, or the formation of friable granulation tissue at the anastomotic site are the cause of the stump disruption in most cases. In one review of 256 consecutive patients who underwent pneumonectomy (of

whom 8 [3%]) developed fistulas), the most important risk factor for fistula formation was the development of a postsurgical pulmonary complication necessitating ventilation.[270] Dehiscence usually occurs soon after the surgery; almost all cases develop within 90 days.[269] Rupture, however, has been reported months after aspergillus colonization of the stump[271] and, in one patient, after intubation of the stump 9 years after right pneumonectomy.[272]

Radiographic manifestations of bronchopleural fistulas after lobectomy or pneumonectomy include an increase in the amount of gas in the pleural or pneumonectomy space, lack of normal shift of the mediastinum, or reappearance of gas in a previously fluid-filled hemithorax.[273–275] Peripheral airway bronchopleural fistulas can present radiographically as persistent pneumothorax, tension pneumothorax, or hydropneumothorax.[273, 274] CT often allows direct visualization and localization of the fistula as well as assessment of the underlying cause.[275, 276] For example, in one investigation

## Table 56–2. BRONCHIAL FISTULAS

| Site | Cause | Selected References |
|---|---|---|
| **Nonvascular Intrathoracic Structures** | | |
| Esophagus | | — |
|   Congenital | | 280, 281 |
|   Acquired | Carcinoma of lung or esophagus | 303 |
| | Foreign body aspiration | 304 |
| | Esophageal diverticulum | 279 |
| | Iatrogenic perforation | 305 |
| | Crohn's disease | 306 |
| | Tuberculosis | 307, 308 |
| | Bronchial artery embolization | 309, 310 |
| Mediastinum | Pulmonary carcinoma | — |
| | Pulmonary abscess | — |
| | Mediastinitis | 311 |
| | Bronchogenic cyst | 312 |
| Pleura | Pulmonary carcinoma | 277 |
| | Acute pneumonia/pulmonary abscess | 277 |
| | Septic pulmonary embolism | 313 |
| | Tuberculosis | 277, 314 |
| | Penetrating or blunt trauma | 276, 277 |
| | Radiation | 315 |
| | Postpneumonectomy/lobectomy | 270 |
| | Aspirated foreign material | 316 |
| **Intrathoracic Vessels and the Heart** | | |
| Aorta | Aneurysm | 283 |
| | Postpneumonectomy | 317 |
| | Postvascular surgery | 318 |
| Pulmonary artery | Pulmonary carcinoma | — |
| | Postpneumonectomy/lobectomy | — |
| Superior vena cava | Venous catheter | 319, 320 |
| Heart | Ventricular aneurysm | 321 |
| | Implantable defibrillator patch | 322 |
| **Abdominal Organs** | | |
| Colon | Crohn's disease | 287, 323 |
| | Abdominal sepsis and subphrenic abscess | 286 |
| | Carcinoma of colon | 324 |
| | Tuberculosis | 325 |
| Stomach | | 326 |
| Small intestine | | 327 |
| Liver and biliary tract | | |
| | Cholecystitis and cholelithiasis; choledocholithiasis | 288, 289 |
| | Trauma | 328 |
| | Hydatid disease | 329 |
| | Amebiasis | 330 |
| Pancreas | Trauma | 331 |
| | Acute pancreatitis | — |
| Kidney | Calculus-associated pyelonephritis, primary perinephric abscess, tuberculosis | 332, 333 |
| **Miscellaneous** | | |
| Hand | Extension of subcutaneous mycetoma | 334 |

of 20 patients who had bronchopleural fistulas involving segmental bronchi or more distal airways, the fistula was identified on CT in 10.[276] Five of the 10 had acute bacterial pneumonia with peripheral areas of necrosis or abscess formation that contained fluid and air bubbles that were shown on CT to communicate directly with the pleural space; 4 had ectatic peripheral airways that communicated with the pleural space. In the remaining patient, the communication was between peripheral air spaces within a bronchioloalveolar cell carcinoma and the pleural space.

HRCT is superior to conventional CT in the demonstration of bronchopleural fistulas.[275, 276] The optimal technique consists of volumetric spiral CT imaging using HRCT technique (1- to 2-mm collimation scans) through the areas of parenchymal abnormality. Three-dimensional reconstruction of the data allows display of the entire course of the fistula.[275, 277]

There are many causes of bronchoesophageal fistulas (*see* Table 56–2).[278] The diagnosis is often suggested by the presence of concomitant esophageal and pulmonary disease; however, congenital bronchoesophageal fistulas can present in adults,[279] in which case the presence of the esophageal abnormality is often not immediately apparent (*see* page 627). In one report of seven such patients, the chief pre-

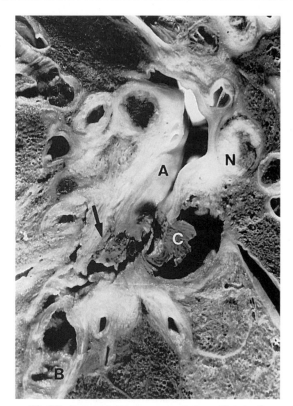

**Figure 56–33. Bronchial-Pulmonary Artery Fistula Secondary to Pulmonary Carcinoma.** A magnified view of a slice of left lung near the hilum shows the smooth intimal surface of the lower lobe pulmonary artery (A). More distally, the surface is discolored and appears necrotic *(arrow)*. A blood clot is also present outside the vessel wall in a small cavity (C). Carcinoma can be seen in the peribronchial tissue and in a perivascular lymph node (N). It originated in the lower lobe bronchus, a segmental branch of which is evident at the bottom *(B)*. The endobronchial carcinoma could only be seen on the reverse side of the lung slice and is not illustrated here; it involved the airway lumen, the peribronchovascular interstitial tissue, and lymph node as shown. It had also extended into the pulmonary artery at the site indicated by the *arrow*. The patient was a 55-year-old man who presented with massive hemoptysis.

senting symptoms were recurrent bouts of coughing after drinking and hemoptysis;[280] in most cases, the duration of symptoms exceeded 15 years. The esophageal opening of these congenital fistulas is most often in its lower third; segmental, main, or lobar bronchi can be affected. The diagnosis of a bronchoesophageal fistula is suggested by the identification of foreign material in respiratory tract secretions or pleural fluid on microscopic examination[281] or by the presence of an amylase concentration higher than that of the blood as a result of contamination by saliva; it can usually be confirmed by esophagography.

As might be expected, fistulas with intrathoracic vessels typically present as hemoptysis, sometimes dramatic and fatal. The latter course, however, is not always seen; for example, in one review of 145 patients who underwent repair of descending thoracic and thoracoabdominal aortic aneurysms, the 1-year mortality of the 8 who presented with hemoptysis secondary to an aortobronchial fistula was 13%, a value similar to that of those who did not have fistulas.[282] The majority of aortobronchial fistulas probably develop during acute aneurysm formation (e.g., in association with trauma or dissection); however, communication can occur

months or years after initial aneurysm formation.[283] The most common vessel involved in bronchovascular fistulas is probably the pulmonary artery, the most frequent causes being lung abscess and carcinoma (Fig. 56–33). Local bronchial infection—typically at the anastomotic site and often with *Aspergillus* species—is sometimes the cause in lung transplant recipients.[284]

The formation of bronchial fistulas with intra-abdominal organs is rare. Colobronchial fistulas develop most often in association with abdominal sepsis and subphrenic abscess;[285] primary colonic carcinoma and Crohn's disease are less frequent causes.[286, 287] The complication may be manifested by the expectoration of malodorous or frankly feculent material; barium enema is diagnostic but can result in exacerbation of lung disease by introducing a bolus of fecal material into the lung.[285] Expectorated bile (biliptysis) is a clue to the presence of a biliary tract fistula;[288, 289] the diagnosis can be confirmed using transhepatic cholangiography, endoscopic retrograde cholangiopancreatography, or radionuclide (HIDA) scanning.[274]

## MISCELLANEOUS BRONCHIAL ABNORMALITIES

*Toxic epidermal necrolysis* (TEN) is an uncommon disorder characterized by a diffuse erythematous skin rash that is followed by the formation of large bullae; separation of

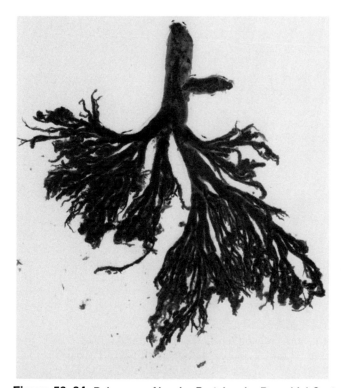

**Figure 56–34. Pulmonary Alveolar Proteinosis: Bronchial Cast Formation.** Illustrated is a cast of the right lower lobe bronchial tree that was expectorated by a 57-year-old woman who gave a 5-year history of dyspnea and episodes of expectoration of bronchial casts similar to the one illustrated. Open lung biopsy showed the characteristic pathologic changes of pulmonary alveolar proteinosis. Despite repeated bronchoalveolar lavage, her symptoms progressed and she died of respiratory failure 1 year later. (Courtesy of Dr. R. Chapela and Dr. R. Sansores, National Respiratory Disease Institute of Mexico.)

necrotic epidermis results in an appearance resembling burned skin (hence the synonym *scalded skin syndrome*). The abnormality is usually a complication of staphylococcal infection or a drug reaction. Tracheobronchial involvement is probably more common than is generally appreciated. In one prospective review of 41 consecutive patients who had TEN, clinical features of chest involvement were specifically investigated, and chest radiography and arterial blood gas analysis were routinely performed;[290] 10 patients were found to have evidence of respiratory tract involvement during the acute disease (dyspnea in 10, mucus hypersecretion in 7, and hypoxemia [$PaO_2 = 59 \pm 8$ mm Hg] in 10). Radiograph results were normal in 8 of the 10 patients and showed "interstitial infiltrates" in 2. Bronchoscopy demonstrated sloughing of bronchial epithelium in the proximal airways in all 10 patients. Such sloughing has been found by other investigators to be associated with severe airway obstruction.[291] Mucosal vesicles may also be seen at bronchoscopy.[292]

The term *plastic bronchitis* refers to the expectoration of material that takes the form of a cast of the bronchial tree.[293] The abnormality can be seen in association with several diseases, including allergic bronchopulmonary aspergillosis (probably the most common cause), cystic fibrosis, bronchiectasis of varied causes, acute or chronic pneumonia,[293a] alveolar proteinosis (Fig. 56–34), and airway lymphoid hyperplasia;[294] occasionally, no underlying cause can be identified.[293] The casts usually correspond to only a few segmental and subsegmental bronchi; however, they may correspond to the major portion of an entire lobe. The composition and morphology of the casts depends on the underlying cause; a classification into two general types—inflammatory and acellular—has been proposed.[293a]

*Obliterative bronchitis* is an uncommon abnormality that is analogous to obliterative bronchiolitis and, in fact, is most often seen in association with it. As such, it is most common in patients who have received lung or heart-lung transplants; in these situations, it is usually a minor component of the airway disease and probably contributes little to clinical and functional abnormalities. Rarely, the process appears to affect the bronchi predominantly.[295]

# REFERENCES

1. Glauser EM, Cook CD, Harris GBC: Bronchiectasis: A review of 187 cases in children with follow-up pulmonary function studies in 58. Acta Paediatr Scand 165(Suppl):1, 1966.
2. Sanderson JM, Kennedy MCS, Johnson MF, et al: Bronchiectasis: Results of surgical and conservative management (a review of 393 cases). Thorax 29:407, 1974.
3. Bard M, Couderc LJ, Saimot AG, et al: Accelerated obstructive pulmonary disease in HIV infected patients with bronchiectasis. Eur Respir J 11:771, 1998.
4. Loubeyre P, Revel D, Delignette A, et al: Bronchiectasis detected with thin-section CT as a predictor of chronic lung allograft rejection. Radiology 194:213, 1995.
5. Morehead RS: Bronchiectasis in bone marrow transplantation. Thorax 52:390, 1997.
6. Smith IE, Flower CDR: Review article: Imaging in bronchiectasis. Br J Radiol 69:589, 1996
6a. Nikolazik WH, Warner JO: Aetiology of chronic suppurative lung disease. Arch Dis Child 70:141, 1994.
7. Barker AF: Bronchiectasis. Semin Thorac Cardiovasc Surg 7:112, 1995.
8. Barker AF, Bardana EJ: Bronchiectasis: Update of an orphan disease. Am Rev Respir Dis 137:969, 1988.
9. Trucksis M, Swartz MN: Bronchiectasis: A current view. Top Infect Dis 11:170, 1991.
10. Wescott JL: Bronchiectasis: Imaging in diffuse lung disease. Radiol Clin North Am 29:1031, 1991.
10a. McGuinness G, Naidich DP: Bronchiectasis: CT/clinical correlations. Semin Ultrasound CT MRI 16:395, 1995.
11. Nicotra MB: Bronchiectasis. Semin Respir Infect 9:31, 1994.
12. Eller J, Lapa E, Silva JR, et al: Cells and cytokines in chronic bronchial infection. Ann N Y Acad Sci 725:331, 1994.
13. Pang G, Ortega M, Zighang R, et al: Autocrine modulation of IL-8 production by sputum neutrophils in chronic bronchial sepsis. Am J Respir Crit Care Med 155:726, 1997.
14. Richman-Eisenstat JB, Jorens PG, Hebert CA, et al: Interleukin-8: An important chemoattractant in sputum of patients with chronic inflammatory airway diseases. Am J Physiol 264:L413, 1993.
15. Sepper R, Konttinen YT, Ding Y, et al: Human neutrophil collagenase (MMP-8), identified in bronchiectasis BAL fluid, correlates with severity of disease. Chest 107:1641, 1995.
16. Sepper R, Konttinen YT, Sorsa T, et al: Gelatinolytic and type IV collagenolytic activity in bronchiectasis. Chest 106:11299, 1994.
17. Fahy JV, Schuster A, Ueki I, et al: Mucus hypersecretion in bronchiectasis: The role of neutrophil proteases. Am Rev Respir Dis 146:1430, 1992.
18. Lloberes P, Montserrat E, Montserrat JM, et al: Sputum sol phase proteins and elastase activity in patients with clinically stable bronchiectasis. Thorax 47:88, 1992.
19. Sepper R, Konttinen YT, Ingman T, et al: Presence, activities, and molecular forms of cathepsin G, elastase, and alpha 1-antitrypsin, and alpha 1-antichymotrypsin in bronchiectasis. J Clin Immunol 15:27, 1995.
20. Rodriguez-Cintron W, Guntupalli K, Fraire AE: Bronchiectasis and homozygous (P1ZZ) alpha 1-antitrypsin deficiency in a young man. Thorax 50:424, 1995.
21. King MA, Stone JA, Diaz PT, et al: Alpha 1-antitrypsin deficiency: Evaluation of bronchiectasis with CT. Radiology 199:137, 1996.
22. Shin MS, Ho KJ: Bronchiectasis in patients with alpha 1-antitrypsin deficiency: A rare occurrence? Chest 104:1384–1386, 1993.
23. Nakamura H, Abe S, Shibata Y, et al: Elevated levels of cytokeratin 19 in the bronchoalveolar lavage fluid of patients with chronic airway inflammatory diseases—a specific marker for bronchial epithelial injury. Am J Respir Crit Care Med 155:1217, 1997.
24. Tracey WR, Xue C, Klinghofer V, et al: Immunochemical detection of inducible NO synthase in human lung. Am J Physiol 266:L722, 1994.
25. Kharitonov SA, Wells AU, O'Connor BJ, et al: Elevated levels of exhaled nitric oxide in bronchiectasis. Am J Respir Crit Care Med 151:1889, 1995.
26. Miszkiel KA, Wells AU, Rubens MB, et al: Effects of airway infection by Pseudomonas aeruginosa: A computed tomographic study. Thorax 52:260, 1997.
27. Nagaki M, Shimura S, Tanno Y, et al: Role of chronic Pseudomonas aeruginosa infection in the development of bronchiectasis. Chest 102:1464, 1992.
28. Klingman KL, Pye A, Murphy TF, et al: Dynamics of respiratory tract colonization by Branhamella catarrhalis in bronchiectasis. Am J Respir Crit Care Med 152:1072, 1995.
29. Cole PJ: Inflammation: A two-edged sword—the model of bronchiectasis. Eur J Respir Dis 69(Suppl 147):6, 1986.
30. Verra F, Kouzan S, Saiag P, et al: Bronchoalveolar disease in dyskeratosis congenita. Eur Respir J 5:497, 1992.
31. Croxatto OC, Lanari A: Pathogenesis of bronchiectasis: Experimental study and anatomic findings. J Thorac Surg 27:51, 1954.
32. Lewiston NJ: Bronchiectasis in childhood. Pediatr Clin North Am 31:865, 1984.
33. Box K, Derr KM, Jeffrey RR, et al: Endobronchial lipoma associated with lobar bronchiectasis. Respir Med 85:71, 1991.
34. Vignale L, Parentini GC: Tracheal bronchus associated with bronchiectasis. Panminerva Med 34:96, 1992.
35. Woodring JH, Howard RS 2d, Rehm SR: Congenital tracheobronchomegaly

(Mounier-Kuhn syndrome): A report of 10 cases and review of the literature. J Thorac Imag 6:1, 1991.
36. Curtin JJ, Webster AD, Farrant J, et al: Bronchiectasis in hypogammaglobulinaemia—a computed tomography assessment. Clin Radiol 44:82, 1991.
37. Sweinberg SK, Wodell RA, Grodofsky MP, et al: Retrospective analysis of the incidence of pulmonary disease in hypogammaglobulinemia. J Allergy Clin Immunol 88:96, 1991.
38. Curtin JJ, Murray JG, Apthorp LA, et al: Mediastinal lymph node enlargement and splenomegaly in primary hypogammaglobulinaemia. Clin Radiol 50:489, 1995.
39. Gomez-Carrasco JA, Barrera-Gomez MJ, Garcia-Mourino V, et al: Selective and partial IgA deficiency in an adolescent male with bronchiectasis. Allergol Immunopathol 22:261, 1994.
40. Lui RC, Inculet RI: Job's syndrome: A rare cause of recurrent lung abscess in childhood. Ann Thorac Surg 50:992, 1990.
41. De Gracia J, Rodrigo MJ, Morell F, et al: IgG subclass deficiencies associated with bronchiectasis. Am J Respir Crit Care Med 153:650, 1996.
42. Feldman J, Weltman M, Wadee A, et al: A study of immunoglobulin G subclass levels in black and white patients with various forms of obstructive lung disease. S Afr Med J 83:9, 1993.
43. Salmanzadeh A, Pomeranz SJ, Ramsingh PS: Ventilation-perfusion scintigraphic correlation with multimodality imaging in a proven case of Swyer-James (Macleod's) syndrome. Clin Nucl Med 22:115, 1997.
44. Steinberg I, Lyons HA: Ipsilateral hypoplasia of a pulmonary artery in advanced bronchiectasis. Am J Roentgenol 101:939, 1967.
45. Bouros D, Paré P, Panagou P, et al: The varied manifestation of pulmonary artery agenesis in adulthood. Chest 108:670, 1995.
46. Bateman ED, Hayashi S, Kuwano K, et al: Latent adenoviral infection in follicular bronchiectasis. Am J Respir Crit Care Med 151:170, 1995.
47. Holmes AH, Trotman-Dickenson B, Edwards A, et al: Bronchiectasis in HIV disease. J Med 85:875, 1992.
48. Verghese A, Al-Samman M, Nabhan D, et al: Bacterial bronchitis and bronchiectasis in human immunodeficiency virus infection. Arch Intern Med 154:2086, 1994.
49. McGuinness G, Naidich DP, Garay S, et al: AIDS associated bronchiectasis: CT features. J Comput Assist Tomogr 17:260, 1993.
50. Hoeffler HB, Schweppe HI, Greenberg SD: Bronchiectasis following pulmonary ammonia burn. Arch Pathol Lab Med 106:686, 1982.
51. Tasaka S, Kanazawa M, Mori M, et al: Long-term course of bronchiectasis and bronchiolitis obliterans as late complication of smoke inhalation. Respiration 62:40, 1995.
52. Dossing M, Khan JH: Nasal or oral oil application on infants: A possible risk factor for adult bronchiectasis. Eur J Epidemiol 11:141, 1995.
53. Annobil SH, Morad NA, Kameswaran M, et al: Bronchiectasis due to lipid aspiration in childhood: Clinical and pathological correlates. Ann Trop Paediatr 16:19–25, 1996.
54. Landau LI, Phelan PD, Williams HE: Ventilatory mechanics in patients with bronchiectasis starting in childhood. Thorax 29:304, 1974.
55. Banner AS, Muthuswamy P, Shah RS, et al: Bronchiectasis following heroin-induced pulmonary edema—rapid clearing of pulmonary infiltrates. Chest 69:552, 1976.
56. Mahut B, Delacourt C, de Blic J, et al: Bronchiectasis in a child after acrolein inhalation. Chest 104:1286, 1993.
57. Lee SH, Lee KS, Ahn JM, et al: Paraquat poisoning of the lung: Thin-section CT findings. Radiology 195:271, 1995.
58. Udwadia ZF, Pilling JR, Jenkins PF, et al: Bronchoscopic and bronchographic findings in 12 patients with sarcoidosis and severe or progressive airways obstruction. Thorax 45:272, 1990.
59. Takanami I, Imamuma T, Yamamoto Y, et al: Bronchiectasis complicating rheumatoid arthritis. Respir Med 89:453, 1995.
60. Gabazza EC, Taguchi O, Yamakami T, et al: Bronchopulmonary disease in ulcerative colitis. Intern Med 31:1155, 1992.
61. Garg K, Lynch DA, Newell JD: Inflammatory airways disease in ulcerative colitis: CT and high-resolution CT features. J Thorac Imaging 8:159, 1993.
62. Gionchetti P, Schiavina M, Campieri M, et al: Bronchopulmonary involvement in ulcerative colitis. J Clin Gastroenterol 12:647, 1990.
63. Quantrill SJ, Mahmoud K: Bronchiectasis and Felty's syndrome. Respir Med 90:249, 1996.
64. Robinson DA, Meyer CF: Primary Sjögren's syndrome associated with recurrent sinopulmonary infections and bronchiectasis. J Allergy Clin Immunol 94:263, 1994.
65. Hassan WU, Keaney NP, Holland CD, et al: High resolution computed tomography of the lung in lifelong non-smoking patients with rheumatoid arthritis. Ann Rheum Dis 54:308, 1995.
66. Despaux J, Polio JC, Toussirot E, et al: Rheumatoid arthritis and bronchiectasis: A retrospective study of fourteen cases. Rev Rhum Engl Ed 63:801, 1996.
67. Cortet B, Flipo RM, Remy-Jardin M, et al: Use of high resolution computed tomography of the lungs in patients with rheumatoid arthritis. Ann Rheum Dis 54:815, 1995.
68. Shadick NA, Fanta CH, Weinblatt ME, et al: Bronchiectasis: A late feature of severe rheumatoid arthritis. Medicine 73:161, 1994.

69. McMahon MJ, Swinson DR, Shettar S, et al: Bronchiectasis and rheumatoid arthritis: A clinical study. Ann Rheum Dis 53:482, 1993.

70. Hillarby MC, McMahon MJ, Grennan DM, et al: HLA associations in subjects with rheumatoid arthritis and bronchiectasis but not with other pulmonary complications of rheumatoid disease. Br J Rheumatol 32:794, 1993.

71. Veale D, Rodgers AD, Griffiths CJ, et al: Variability in ciliary beat frequency in normal subjects and in patients with bronchiectasis. Thorax 48:1018, 1993.

72. Clark NS: Bronchiectasis in childhood. BMJ 1:80, 1963.

73. Hessén I: Bronchiectasis of the apical segment of the lower lobe. Acta Radiol 48:7, 1957.

74. Kwon KY, Myers JL, Swensen SJ, et al: Middle lobe syndrome: A clinicopathological study of 21 patients. Hum Pathol 26:302, 1995.

75. Reid L: Reduction in bronchial subdivision in bronchiectasis. Thorax 5:233, 1950.

76. Whitwell F: A study of the pathology and pathogenesis of bronchiectasis. Thorax 7:213, 1952.

77. Cunningham GJ, Nassau E, Walter JB: The frequency of tumour-like formations in bronchiectatic lungs. Thorax 13:64, 1958.

78. Cudkowicz L: Bronchiectasis and bronchial artery circulation. *In* Moser KM (ed): Pulmonary Vascular Diseases. Lung Biology in Health and Disease Series. Vol 14. New York, Marcel Dekker, 1979, p 165.

79. Gudbjerg CE: Bronchiectasis: Radiological diagnosis and prognosis after operative treatment. Acta Radiol (Suppl):143, 1957.

80. Gudbjerg CE: Roentgenologic diagnosis of bronchiectasis: An analysis of 112 cases. Acta Radiol 43:209, 1955.

81. Munro NC, Han LY, Currie DC, et al: Radiologic evidence of progression of bronchiectasis. Respir Med 86:397, 1992.

82. van der Bruggen-Bogaarts BAHA, van der Bruggen HMJG, van Waes PFGM, et al: Screening for bronchiectasis: A comparative study between chest radiography and high-resolution CT. Chest 109:608, 1996.

83. Bateson EM, Woo-Ming M: Destroyed lung: A report of cases in West Indians and Australian aborigines. Clin Radiol 27:223, 1976.

84. Currie DC, Cooke JC, Morgan AD, et al: Interpretation of bronchograms and chest radiographs in patients with chronic sputum production. Thorax 42:278, 1987.

85. Silverman PM, Godwin JD: CT/bronchographic correlations in bronchiectasis. J Comput Assist Tomogr 11:52, 1987.

86. Grenier P, Maurice F, Musset D, et al: Bronchiectasis: Assessment by thin-section CT. Radiology 161:95, 1986.

87. Young K, Aspestrand F, Kolbenstvedt A: High-resoltuion CT and bronchography in the assessment of bronchiectasis. Acta Radiol 32:439, 1991.

88. Kang EY, Miller RR, Müller NL: Bronchiectasis: Comparison of preoperative thin-section CT and pathologic findings in resected specimens. Radiology 195:649, 1995.

89. Kim JS, Müller NL, Park CS, et al: Cylindrical bronchiectasis: Diagnostic findings on thin-section CT. Am J Roentgenol 168:751, 1997.

90. McGuinness G, Naidich DP, Leitman BS, et al: Pictorial essay: Bronchiectasis: CT evaluation. Am J Roentgenol 160:253, 1995.

91. Naidich DP, McCauley DI, Khouri NF, et al: Computed tomography of bronchiectasis. J Comput Assist Tomogr 6:437, 1982.

91a. Worthy SA, Brown MJ, Müller NL: Technical note: Cystic air spaces in the lung: Change in size on expiratory high-resolution CT in 23 patients. Clin Radiol 53:515, 1998.

92. Giron J, Skaff F, Maubon A, et al: The value of thin-section CT scans in the diagnosis and staging of bronchiectasis: Comparison with bronchography in a series of fifty-four patients. Ann Radiol 31:25, 1988.

93. Lynch DA, Newell JD, Tschomper BA, et al: Uncomplicated asthma in adults: Comparison of CT appearance of the lungs in asthmatic and healthy subjects. Radiology 188:829, 1993.

94. Park CS, Müller NL, Worthy SA, et al: Airway obstruction in asthmatic and healthy individuals: Inspiratory and expiratory thin-section CT findings. Radiology 203:361, 1997.

95. Remy-Jardin M, Remy J, Boulenguez C, et al: Morphologic effects of cigarette smoking on airways and pulmonary parenchyma in healthy adult volunteers: CT evaluation and correlation with pulmonary function tests. Radiology 186:107, 1993.

96. McNamara AE, Müller NL, Okazawa M, et al: Airway narrowing in excised canine lungs measured by high-resolution computed tomography. J Appl Physiol 73:307, 1992.

97. Bankier AA, Fleischmann D, Mallek R, et al: Bronchial wall thickness: Appropriate window settings for thin-section CT and radiologic-anatomic correlation. Radiology 199:831, 1996.

98. Müller NL, Miller RR: Diseases of the bronchioles: CT and histopathologic findings. Radiology 196:3, 1995.

99. Remy-Jardin M, Remy J: Comparison of vertical and oblique CT in evaluation of bronchial tree. J Comput Assist Tomogr 12:956, 1988.

100. Pontius JR, Jacobs LG: The reversal of advanced bronchiectasis. Radiology 68:204, 1957.

101. Nelson SW, Christoforidis A: Reversible bronchiectasis. Radiology 71:375, 1958.

102. Tarver RD, Conces DJ, Godwin JD: Motion artifacts on CT simulate bronchiectasis. Am J Roentgenol 151:1117, 1988.

103. Lucidarme O, Grenier P, Coche E, et al: Bronchiectasis: Comparative assessment with thin-section CT and helical CT. Radiology 200:673, 1996.

104. Joharjy IA, Bashi SA, Adbullah AK: Value of medium-thickness CT in the diagnosis of bronchiectasis. Am J Roentgenol 149:1133, 1987.

105. Müller NL, Bergin CJ, Ostrow DN, et al: Role of computed tomography in the recognition of bronchiectasis. Am J Roentgenol 143:971, 1984.

106. Silverman PM, Godwin DJ: CT-bronchographic correlations in bronchiectasis. J Comput Assist Tomogr 11:52, 1987.

107. Hansell DM, Wells AU, Rubens MB, et al: Bronchiectasis: Functional significance of areas of decreased attenuation at expiratory CT. Radiology 193:369, 1994.

108. Thomas RD, Blaquiere RM: Reactive mediastinal lymphadenopathy in bronchiectasis assessed by CT. Acta Radiol 34:489, 1993.

109. Don CJ, Dales RE, Desmarais RL, et al: The radiographic prevalence of hilar and mediastinal adenopathy in adult cystic fibrosis. Can Assoc Radiol J 48:265, 1997.

109a. Song J-W, Im J-G, Shim Y-S, et al: Hypertrophied bronchial artery at thin-section CT in patients with bronchiectasis: Correlation with CT angiographic findings. Radiology 208:187, 1998.

110. Morcos SK, Baudouin SV, Anderson PB, et al: Iotrolan in selective bronchography via the fiberoptic bronchoscope. Br J Radiol 62:383, 1989.

111. Morcos SK, Anderson PB, Kennedy A: Bronchography with iotrolan 300 via the flexible bronchoscope in the evaluation of focal lung opacity. J Bronchol 1:112, 1994.

112. Morcos SK, Anderson PB, Baudouin SV, et al. Suitability of and tolerance to iotrolan 300 in bronchography via the fiberoptic bronchoscope. Thorax 45:628, 1990.

113. Naidich DP, Harkin TJ: Airways and lung: CT versus bronchography through the fiberoptic bronchoscope. Radiology 200:613, 1996.

114. Munro NC, Currie DC, Garbet ND, et al: Chest pain in chronic sputum production: A neglected symptom. Respir Med 83:339, 1989.

115. Nicotra MB, Rivera M, Dale AM, et al: Clinical, pathophysiologic, and microbiologic characterization of bronchiectasis in an aging cohort. Chest 108:955, 1995.

116. Celebi G, Kalayci T, Aysan T, et al: Application of multivariate linear discriminant analysis to lung sounds in some pulmonary diseases. Monaldi Arch Chest Dis 51:42, 1996.

117. Sovijarvi AR, Piirila P, Luukkonen R: Separation of pulmonary disorders with two-dimensional discriminant analysis of crackles. Clin Physiol 16:171, 1996.

118. Leibovitch G, Maaravi Y, Shalev O: Multiple brain abscesses caused by *Streptococcus bovis*. J Infect 23:195, 1991.

119. Goldsmith DJ, Roberts IS, Short CD, et al: Complete clinical remission and subsequent relapse of bronchiectasis-related (AA) amyloid induced nephrotic syndrome. Nephron 74:572, 1996.

120. Caughey JE, Wilson RF, Borrie J: Peripheral neuropathy (peripheral neuritis) with bronchiectasis. Thorax 13:59, 1958.

121. Tanaka E, Tada K, Amitani R, et al: Systemic hypersensitivity vasculitis associated with bronchiectasis. Chest 102:647, 1992.

122. Hilton AM, Hasleton PS, Bradlow A, et al: Cutaneous vasculitis and immune complexes in severe bronchiectasis. Thorax 39:185, 1984.

123. Tanaka E, Tada K, Amitani R, et al: Systemic hypersensitivity vasculitis associated with bronchiectasis. Chest 102:647, 1992.

124. In B, McAteer JA, Gardiner PV, et al: Chronic suppurative lung disease with associated vasculitis. Postgrad Med J 71:24, 1995.

125. Sitara D, Hoffbrand BI: Chronic bronchial suppuration and antineutrophil cytoplasmic antibody (ANCA) positive systemic vasculitis. Postgrad Med J 66:669, 1990.

126. McKane WS, Velasco N, Farrington K: ANCA-positive crescentic glomerulonephritis in chronic bronchiectasis. Nephrol Dial Transplant 10:1447, 1995.

127. Cherniack N, Vosti KL, Saxton GA, et al: Pulmonary function tests in fifty patients with bronchiectasis. J Lab Clin Med 53:693, 1959.

128. Bahous J, Cartier A, Pineau L, et al: Pulmonary function tests and airway responsiveness to methacholine in chronic bronchiectasis of the adult. Bull Eur Physiopathol Respir 20:375, 1984.

129. Evans SA, Turner SM, Bosch BJ, et al: Lung function in bronchiectasis: The influence of *Pseudomonas aeruginosa*. Eur Respir J 9:1601, 1996.

130. Ip MS, So SY, Lam WK, et al: High prevalence of asthma in patients with bronchiectasis in Hong Kong. Eur Respir J 5:418, 1992.

131. Ip M, Lam WK, So SY, et al: Analysis of factors associated with bronchial hyperreactivity to methacholine in bronchiectasis. Lung 169:43, 1991.

132. Ip M, Lauder IJ, Wong WY, et al: Multivariate analysis of factors affecting pulmonary function in bronchiectasis. Respiration 60:45, 1993.

133. Lourenco RV, Loddenkemper R, Carton RW: Patterns of distribution and clearance of aerosols in patients with bronchiectasis. Am Rev Respir Dis 106:857, 1972.

134. Currie DC, Pavia D, Agnew JE, et al: Impaired tracheobronchial clearance in bronchiectasis. Thorax 42:126, 1987.

135. Helm WH, Thompson VC: The long-term results of resection for bronchiectasis. QJM 27:353, 1958.

136. Avery ME, Riley MC, Weiss A: The course of bronchiectasis in childhood. Bull Hopkins Hosp 109:20, 1961.

137. Perry KMA, King DS: Bronchiectasis—a study of prognosis based on a follow-up of 400 patients. Am Rev Tuberc 41:531, 1940.

138. Konietzko NFJ, Carton RW, Leroy EP: Causes of death in patients with bronchiectasis. Am Rev Respir Dis 100:852, 1969.

139. Sanderson JM, Kennedy MCS, Johnson MF, et al: Bronchiectasis: Results of surgical and conservative management: A review of 393 cases. Thorax 29:407, 1974.

140. Ellis DA, Thornley PE, Wightman AJ, et al: Present outlook in bronchiectasis: Clinical and social study and review of factors influencing prognosis. Thorax 31:659, 1981.

141. Kartagener M: Zur Pathogenese der bronchiektasien; bronchiektasien bei situs viscerum inversus. Beitr Klin Tuberk 83:489, 1933.
142. Solomon MH, Winn KJ, White RD, et al: Kartagener's syndrome with corrected transposition—conducting system studies and coronary arterial occlusion complicating valvular replacement. Chest 69:677, 1976.
143. Holmes LB, Blennerhassett JB, Austen KF: A reappraisal of Kartagener's syndrome. Am J Med Sci 255:13, 1968.
144. Todd NW Jr, Yodaiken RE: A patient with Kartagener and Paterson-Brown-Kelly syndromes. JAMA 234:1248, 1975.
145. Overholt EL, Bauman DF: Variants of Kartagener's syndrome in the same family. Ann Intern Med 48:574, 1958.
146. Camner P, Mossberg B, Afzelius BA: Evidence for congenitally nonfunctioning cilia in the tracheobronchial tract in two subjects. Am Rev Respir Dis 112:807, 1975.
147. Afzelius BA: Immotile-cilia syndrome and ciliary abnormalities induced by infection and injury. Am Rev Respir Dis 124:107, 1981.
148. Schidlow DV: Primary ciliary dyskinesia (the immotile cilia syndrome). Ann Allergy 73:457, 1994.
149. Pedersen M, Mygind N: Ciliary motility in the "immotile cilia syndrome": First results of microphoto-oscillographic studies. Br J Dis Chest 74:239, 1980.
150. Rossman CM, Forrest JB, Lee RMKW: The dyskinetic cilia syndrome—abnormal ciliary motility in association with abnormal ciliary ultrastructure. Chest 80:860, 1981.
151. Pedersen M: Specific types of abnormal ciliary motility in Kartagener's syndrome and analogous respiratory disorders: A quantified microphoto-oscillographic investigation of 27 patients. Eur J Respir Dis 127:78, 1983.
152. van der Baan S, Veerman AJ, Wulffraat N, et al: Primary ciliary dyskinesia: Ciliary activity. Acta Otolaryngol 102:274, 1986.
153. Kroon AA, Heij JM, Kuijper WA, et al: Function and morphology of respiratory cilia in situs inversus. Clin Otolaryngol 16:294, 1991.
154. Katsuhara K, Kawamoto S, Wakabayashi T, et al: Situs inversus totalis and Kartagener's syndrome in a Japanese population. Chest 61:56, 1972.
155. Verra F, Escudier E, Bignon J, et al: Inherited factors in diffuse bronchiectasis in the adult: A prospective study. Eur Respir J 4:937, 1991.
156. Waite D, Wakefield SJ, Steele R, et al: Cilia and sperm tail abnormalities in Polynesian bronchiectatics. Lancet 2:132, 1978.
157. Wakefield SJ, Waite D: Abnormal cilia in Polynesians with bronchiectasis. Am Rev Respir Dis 121:1003, 1980.
158. Waite DA, Wakefield SJ, Mackay JB, et al: Mucociliary transport and ultrastructural abnormalities in Polynesian bronchiectasis. Chest 80:896, 1981.
159. Fox B, Bull T: Abnormal cilia in Polynesians with bronchiectasis (letter to editor). Am Rev Respir Dis 123:142, 1981.
160. Clarke SW, Lopez-Vidriero MT, Pavia D, et al: Abnormal cilia in Polynesians with bronchiectasis (letter to editor). Am Rev Respir Dis 123:141, 1981.
161. Waite DA, Wakefield SJ, Moriarty KM, et al: Polynesian bronchiectasis. Eur J Respir Dis 127:31, 1983.
162. Rubin BK, Kumar V: Chronic lung disease in Canadian aboriginal children is not caused by abnormal cilia. Can Respir J 4:211, 1997.
163. Moreno A, Murphy EA: Inheritance of Kartagener syndrome. Am J Hum Genet 8:305, 1981.
164. Rott HD: Genetics of Kartagener's syndrome. Eur J Respir Dis 127:1, 1983.
165. Sturgess JM, Thompson MW, Czegledy-Nagy E, et al: Genetic aspects of immotile cilia syndrome. Am J Med Genet 25:149, 1986.
166. Chao J, Turner JA, Sturgess JM, et al: Genetic heterogeneity of dynein-deficiency in cilia from patients with respiratory disease. Am Rev Respir Dis 126:302, 1982.
167. Jonsson MS, McCormick JR, Gillies CG, et al: Kartagener's syndrome with motile spermatozoa. N Engl J Med 307:1131, 1982.
168. Matwijiw I, Thliveris JA, Faiman C: Aplasia of nasal cilia with situs inversus, azoospermia and normal sperm flagella: A unique variant of the immotile cilia syndrome. J Urol 137:522, 1987.
169. Munro NC, Currie DC, Lindsay KS, et al: Fertility in men with primary ciliary dyskinesia presenting with respiratory infection. Thorax 49:684–687, 1994.
170. Moryan A, Guay AT, Kurtz S, et al: Familial ciliary dyskinesis: A cause of infertility without respiratory disease. Fertil Steril 44:539, 1985.
171. Ras GJ, Van Wyk CJ: Primary ciliary dyskinesia in association with Marfan's syndrome: A case report. S Afr Med J 64:212, 1983.
172. Sturgess JM, Chao J, Wong J, et al: Cilia with defective radial spokes: A cause of human respiratory disease. N Engl J Med 300:53, 1979.
173. Paolucci F, Cinti S, Cangiotti A, et al: Steatosis associated with immotile cilia syndrome: An unrecognized relationship? J Hepatol 14:317, 1992.
174. De Santi MM, Magni A, Valletta EA, et al: Hydrocephalus, bronchiectasis, and ciliary aplasia. Arch Dis Child 65:543, 1990.
175. Bonneau D, Raymond F, Kremer C, et al: Usher syndrome type I associated with bronchiectasis and immotile nasal cilia in two brothers. J Med Genet 30:2534, 1993.
176. Wilton LJ, Teichtahl H, Temple-Smith PD, et al: Kartagener's syndrome with motile cilia and immotile spermatozoa: Axonemal ultrastructure and function. Am Rev Respir Dis 134:1233, 1986.
177. Rutman A, Cullinan P, Woodhead M, et al: Ciliary disorientation: A possible variant of primary ciliary dyskinesia. Thorax 48:770, 1993.
178. Sturgess JM, Chao J, Turner JAP, et al: Transposition of ciliary microtubules: Another cause of impaired ciliary motility. N Engl J Med 303:318, 1980.
179. Moreau MF, Chretien MF, Dubin J, et al: Transposed ciliary microtubules in Kartagener's syndrome: A case report with electron microscopy of bronchial and nasal brushings. Acta Cytol 29:248, 1985.
180. Antonelli M, Modesti A, Quattrucci S, et al: Supernumerary microtubules in the cilia of two siblings causing "immotile cilia syndrome." Eur J Respir Dis 64:607, 1983.
181. Min Y-G, Shin J-S, Choi S-H, et al: Primary ciliary dyskinesia: Ultrastructural defects and clinical features. Rhinology 33:189, 1995.
182. Lungarella G, De Santi MM, Palatresi R, et al: Ultrastructural observations on basal apparatus of respiratory cilia in immotile cilia syndrome. Eur J Respir Dis 66:165, 1985.
183. Afzelius BA, Gargani G, Romano C: Abnormal length of cilia as a possible cause of defective mucociliary clearance. Eur J Respir Dis 66:173, 1985.
184. Niggemann B, Muller A, Nolte A, et al: Abnormal length of cilia—a cause of primary ciliary dyskinesia—a case report. Eur J Pediatr 151:73, 1992.
185. Herzon FS, Murphy S: Normal ciliary ultrastructure in children with Kartagener's syndrome. Ann Otol 89:81, 1980.
186. Greenstone MA, Dewar A, Cole PJ: Ciliary dyskinesia with normal ultrastructure. Thorax 38:875, 1983.
187. Escudier E, Escalier D, Homasson JP, et al: Unexpectedly normal cilia and spermatozoa in an infertile man with Kartagener's syndrome. Eur J Respir Dis 70:180, 1987.
188. Gonzalez S, von Bassewitz DB, Grundmann E, et al: Atypical cilia in hyperplastic, metaplastic, and dysplastic human bronchial mucosa. Ultrastruct Pathol 8:345, 1985.
189. Rayner CF, Rutman A, Dewar A, et al: Ciliary disorientation in patients with chronic upper respiratory tract inflammation. Am J Respir Crit Care Med 151:800–804, 1995.
190. Robson AM, Smallman LA, Gregory J, et al: Ciliary ultrastructure in nasal brushings. Cytopathology 4:149, 1993.
191. Lee RMKW, Rossman CM, O'Brodovich H, et al: Ciliary defects associated with the development of bronchopulmonary dysplasia—ciliary motility and ultrastructure. Am Rev Respir Dis 129:190, 1984.
192. McDowell EM, Barrett LA, Harris CC, et al: Abnormal cilia in human bronchial epithelium. Arch Pathol Lab Med 100:429, 1976.
193. Ailsby RL, Ghadially FN: Atypical cilia in human bronchial mucosa. J Pathol 109:75, 1973.
194. Smallman LA, Gregory J: Ultrastructural abnormalities of cilia in the human respiratory tract. Hum Pathol 17:848, 1986.
195. Verra F, Escudier E, Lebargy F, et al: Ciliary abnormalities in bronchial epithelium of smokers, ex-smokers, and non-smokers. Am J Respir Crit Care Med 151:630, 1995.
196. Lungarella G, Fonzi L, Ermini G: Abnormalities of bronchial cilia in patients with chronic bronchitis: An ultrastructural and quantitative analysis. Lung 161:147, 1983.
197. Wisseman CL, Simel DL, Spock A, et al: The prevalence of abnormal cilia in normal pediatric lungs. Arch Pathol Lab Med 105:552, 1981.
198. Fox B, Bull TB, Makey AR, et al: The significance of ultrastructural abnormalities of human cilia. Chest 80:796, 1981.
199. Rayner CF, Rutman A, Dewar A, et al: Ciliary disorientation alone as a cause of primary ciliary dyskinesia syndrome. Am J Respir Crit Care Med 153:1123, 1996.
200. Rossman CM, Lee RMKW, Forrest JB, et al: Nasal ciliary ultrastructure and function in patients with primary ciliary dyskinesia compared with that in normal subjects and in subjects with various respiratory diseases. Am Rev Respir Dis 129:161, 1984.
201. de Iongh RU, Rutland J: Ciliary defects in healthy subjects, bronchiectasis, and primary ciliary dyskinesia. Am J Respir Crit Care Med 151:1559, 1995.
202. Verra F, Fleury-Feith J, Boucherat M, et al: Do nasal ciliary changes reflect bronchial changes? An ultrastructural study. Am Rev Respir Dis 147:908, 1993.
203. Englander LL, Malech HL: Abnormal movement of polymorphonuclear neutrophils in the immotile cilia syndrome: Cinemicrographic analysis. Exp Cell Res 135:468, 1981.
204. Valerius NH, Knudsen BB, Pedersen M, et al: Defective neutrophil motility in patients with primary ciliary dyskinesia. Eur J Clin Invest 13:489, 1983.
205. Afzelius BA, Ewetz L, Palmblad J, et al: Structure and function of neutrophil leukocytes from patients with the immotile-cilia syndrome. Acta Med Scand 208:145, 1980.
206. Nadel HR, Stringer DA, Levison H, et al: The immotile cilia syndrome: Radiological manifestations. Radiology 154:651, 1985.
206a. Reiff DB, Wells AU, Carr DH, et al: CT findings in bronchiectasis: Limited value in distinguishing between idiopathic and specific types. Am J Roentgenol 165:261, 1995.
207. Turner JAP, Corkey CW, Lee JY, et al: Clinical expressions of immotile cilia syndrome. Pediatrics 67:805, 1981.
208. Mossberg B, Camner P: Impaired mucociliary transport as a pathogenetic factor in obstructive pulmonary diseases. Chest 77:265, 1980.
209. Kollberg H, Mossberg B, Afzelius BA, et al: Cystic fibrosis compared with the immotile-cilia syndrome: A study of mucociliary clearance, ciliary ultrastructure, clinical picture and ventilatory function. Scand J Respir Dis 59:297, 1978.
210. Camner P, Mossberg B, Afzelius BA, et al: Measurements of tracheobronchial clearance in patients with immotile-cilia syndrome and its value in differential diagnosis. Eur J Respir Dis 127:57, 1983.
211. Evander E, Arborelius M Jr, Johnson B, et al: Lung function and bronchial reactivity in six patients with immotile cilia syndrome. Eur J Respir Dis 127:137, 1983.
212. Corkey CW, Levison H, Turner JA, et al: The immotile cilia syndrome: A longitudinal study. Am Rev Respir Dis 124:544, 1981.

213. Handelsman DJ, Conway AJ, Boylan LM, et al: Young's syndrome: Obstructive azoospermia and chronic sinopulmonary infections. N Engl J Med 310:3, 1984.

214. Le Lannou D, Jezequel P, Blayau M, et al: Obstructive azoospermia with agenesis of vas deferens or with bronchiectasia (Young's syndrome): A genetic approach. Hum Reprod 10:338, 1995.

215. Schanker HM, Rajfer J, Saxon A: Recurrent respiratory disease, azoospermia, and nasal polyposis: A syndrome that mimics cystic fibrosis and immotile cilia syndrome. Arch Intern Med 145:2201, 1985.

216. Hughes TM, Skolnick JL, Belker AM: Young's syndrome: An often unrecognized correctable cause of obstructive azoospermia. J Urol 137:1238, 1987.

217. Oates RD, Amos JA: The genetic basis of congenital bilateral absence of the vas deferens and cystic fibrosis. J Androl 15:1–8, 1994.

218. Jarvi K, Zielenski J, Wilschanski M, et al: Cystic fibrosis transmembrane conductance regulator and obstructive azoospermia. Lancet 345:1578, 1995.

219. Davis PB, Hubbard VS, Garvin AJ: Bronchiectasis and oligospermia: Two families. Thorax 40:376, 1985.

220. Hendry WF, A'Hern RP, Cole PJ: Was Young's syndrome caused by exposure to mercury in childhood? BMJ 307:1579, 1993.

221. Jequier AM: Obstructive azoospermia: A study of 102 patients. Clin Reprod Fertil 3:21, 1985.

222. Hasegawa A, Ohe M, Yamazaki K, et al: A rare case of Young's syndrome in Japan. Intern Med 33:649, 1994.

223. Pavia D, Agnew JE, Bateman JRM: Lung mucociliary clearance in patients with Young's syndrome. Chest 80:892, 1981.

224. de Iongh R, Ing A, Rutland J: Mucociliary function, ciliary ultrastructure, and ciliary orientation in Young's syndrome. Thorax 47:184, 1992.

225. Samman PD, White WF: The "yellow nail" syndrome. Br J Dermatol 76:153, 1964.

226. Emerson PA: Yellow nails, lymphedema, and pleural effusion. Thorax 21:247, 1966.

227. Yellow nails (editorial). Lancet 1:1492, 1973.

228. Leading article: Yellow nails and oedema. BMJ 4:130, 1972.

229. Nordkild P, Kormann-Andersen H, Struve-Christensen E: Yellow nail syndrome: The triad of yellow nails, lymphedema and pleural effusions. Acta Med Scand 219:221, 1986.

230. Hiller E, Rosenow EC III, Olsen AM: Pulmonary manifestations of the yellow nail syndrome. Chest 61:452, 1972.

231. Bowers D: Unequal breasts, yellow nails, bronchiectasis and lymphedema. Can Med Assoc J 100:437, 1969.

232. Dilley JJ, Kierland RR, Randall RV, et al: Primary lymphedema associated with yellow nails and pleural effusions. JAMA 204:670, 1968.

233. Malek NP, Ocran K, Tietge UJ, et al: A case of the yellow nail syndrome associated with massive chylous ascites, pleural and pericardial effusions. Z Gastroenterol 34:763, 1996.

234. Hassard AD, Martin J, Ross J: Yellow nail syndrome and chronic sinusitus. J Otolaryngol 13:318, 1984.

235. Morandi U, Golinelli M, Brandi L, et al: "Yellow nail syndrome" associated with chronic recurrent pericardial and pleural effusions. Eur J Cardiothorac Surg 9:42, 1995.

236. Solal-Celigny P, Cormier Y, Fournier M: The yellow nail syndrome—light and electron microscopic aspects of the pleura. Arch Pathol Lab Med 107:183, 1983.

237. McNicholas WT, Quigley C, Fitzgerald MX: Upper lobe bronchiectasis in the yellow nail syndrome: Report of a case. Ir J Med Sci 153:394, 1984.

238. Wiggins J, Strickland B, Chung KF: Detection of bronchiectasis by high-resolution computed tomography in the yellow nail syndrome. Clin Radiol 43:377, 1991.

238a. Parry CM, Powell RJ, Johnston IDA: Yellow nails, bronchiectasis and low circulating B cells. Respir Med 88:475, 1994.

239. Battaglia A, Di Ricco G, Mariani G, et al: Pleural effusion and recurrent bronchopneumonia with lymphedema, yellow nails and protein-losing enteropathy. Eur J Respir Dis 66:65, 1985.

240. Knuckles MLF, Hodge SJ, Roy TM, et al: Yellow nail syndrome in association with sleep apnea. Int J Dermatol 25:588, 1986.

241. Williams H, Campbell P: Generalized bronchiectasis associated with deficiency of cartilage in the bronchial tree. Arch Dis Child 35:182, 1960.

242. Wayne KS, Taussig LM: Probable familial congenital bronchiectasis due to cartilage deficiency (Williams-Campbell syndrome). Am Rev Respir Dis 114:15, 1976.

243. Jones VF, Eid NS, Franco SM, et al: Familial congenital bronchiectasis: Williams-Campbell syndrome. Pediatr Pulmonol 16:263, 1993.

243a. Lee P, Bush A, Warner JO: Left bronchial isomerism associated with bronchomalacia, presenting with intractable wheeze. Thorax 46:459, 1991.

244. Williams HE, Landau LI, Phelan PD: Generalized bronchiectasis due to extensive deficiency of bronchial cartilage. Arch Dis Child 47:423, 1972.

244a. Mitchell RE, Bury RG: Congenital bronchiectasis due to deficiency of bronchial cartilage (Williams-Campbell syndrome): A case report. J Pediatr 87:230, 1975.

244b. Palmer SM Jr, Layish DT, Kussin PS, et al: Lung transplantation for Williams-Campbell syndrome. Chest 113:534, 1998.

245. Kaneko K, Kudo S, Tashiro M, et al: Case report: Computed tomography findings in Williams-Campbell syndrome. J Thorac Imaging 6:11, 1991.

246. Watanabe Y, Nishiyama H, Kanayama H, et al: Case report: Congenital bronchiectasis due to cartilage deficiency: CT demonstration. J Comput Assist Tomogr 11:701, 1987.

247. Hartman TE, Primack SL, Lee KS, et al: CT of bronchial and bronchiolar diseases. Radiographics 14:991, 1994.

247a. McAdams HP, Erasmus J: Chest case of the day: Williams-Campbell syndrome. Am J Roentgenol 165:190, 1995.

248. Dunne MG, Reiner B: CT features of tracheobronchomegaly. J Comput Assist Tomogr 12:388, 1988.

249. Shin MS, Jackson RM, Ho KJ: Tracheobronchomegaly (Mounier-Kuhn syndrome): CT diagnosis. Am J Roentgenol 150:777, 1988.

250. Doyle AJ: Demonstration on computed tomography of tracheomalacia in tracheobronchomegaly (Mounier-Kuhn syndrome). Br J Radiol 62:176, 1989.

251. Kwong JS, Müller NL, Miller RR: Diseases of the trachea and main-stem bronchi: correlation of CT with pathologic findings. Radiographics 12:645, 1992.

252. Goh RH, Dobranowski J, Kahana L, et al: Case report: Dynamic computed tomography evaluation of tracheobronchomegaly. Can Assoc Radiol J 46:212, 1995.

253. Moersch HJ, Schmidt HW: Broncholithiasis. Ann Otol 68:548, 1959.

254. Uragoda CG: Broncholithiasis secondary to intrapleural calcification. BMJ 2:1635, 1966.

255. Gordonson J, Sargent EN: Nephrobroncholithiasis: Report of a case secondary to renal lithiasis with a nephrobronchial fistula. Am J Roentgenol 110:701, 1970.

256. Weed LA, Andersen HA: Etiology of broncholithiasis. Dis Chest 37:270, 1960.

257. Straub M, Schwarz J: The healed primary complex in histoplasmosis. Am J Clin Pathol 25:727, 1955.

258. Hotchi M, Schwarz J: Etiology of pigmented scars in the bronchial mucosa. Am J Clin Pathol 58:654, 1972.

259. Schmidt HW, Clagett OT, McDonald JR: Broncholithiasis. J Thorac Surg 19:226, 1950.

260. Bhagavan BS, Rao DRG, Weinberg T: Histoplasmosis producing broncholithiasis. Arch Pathol 91:577, 1971.

261. Vix VA: Radiographic manifestations of broncholithiasis. Radiology 128:295, 1978.

262. Gurney JW, Conces DJ Jr: Pulmonary histoplasmosis. Radiology 199:297, 1996.

263. Conces DJ Jr: Histoplasmosis. Semin Roentgenol 1:14, 1996.

264. Kowal LE, Goodman LR, Zarro VJ, et al: CT diagnosis of broncholithiasis. J Comput Assist Tomogr 7:321, 1983.

265. Shin MS, Ho KJ: Broncholithiasis: Its detection by computed tomography in patients with recurrent hemoptysis of unknown etiology. J Comput Tomogr 7:189, 1983.

266. Adler O, Peleg H: Computed tomography in the diagnosis of broncholithiasis. Eur J Radiol 7:211, 1987.

267. Conces DJ, Tarver RD, Vix VA: Broncholithiasis: CT features in 15 patients. Am J Roentgenol 157:249, 1991.

268. Unfug HV: Vocal-cord paralysis from calcified hilar lymph node cured by spontaneous broncholithoptysis. N Engl J Med 272:527, 1965.

269. Hollaus PH, Lax F, el-Nashef BB, et al: Natural history of bronchopleural fistula after pneumonectomy: A review of 96 cases. Ann Thorac Surg 63:1391, 1997.

270. Wright CD, Wain JC, Mathisen DJ, et al: Postpneumonectomy bronchopleural fistula after sutured bronchial closure: Incidence, risk factors, and management. J Thorac Cardiovasc Surg 112:1367, 1996.

271. Parry MF, Coughlin FR, Zambetti FX: Aspergillus empyema. Chest 81:768, 1982.

272. Epstein SK, Gottlieb DJ, Faling LJ: Bronchial stump disruption following inadvertent right mainstem intubation 9 years after pneumonectomy. Am J Emerg Med 11:47, 1993.

273. Lauckner ME, Beggs I, Armstrong RF: The radiological characteristics of bronchopleural fistula following pneumonectomy. Anaesthesia 38:452, 1983.

274. Powner DJ, Bierman MI: Thoracic and extrathoracic bronchial fistulas. Chest 100:480, 1991.

275. Stern EJ, Sun H, Haramati LB: Peripheral bronchopleural fistulas: CT imaging features. Am J Roentgenol 167:117, 1996.

276. Westcott JL, Volpe JP: Peripheral bronchopleural fistula: CT evaluation in 20 patients with pneumonia, empyema, or postoperative air leak. Radiology 196:175, 1995.

277. Vogel N, Wolcke B, Kauczor HU, et al: Detection of a bronchopleural fistula with spiral CT and 3D reconstruction. Aktuelle Radiol 5:176, 1995.

278. Gerzic Z, Rakic S, Randjelovic T: Acquired benign esophagorespiratory fistula: Report of 16 consecutive cases. Ann Thorac Surg 50:724, 1990.

279. Kim JH, Park KH, Sung SW, et al: Congenital bronchoesophageal fistulas in adult patients. Ann Thorac Surg 60:151, 1995.

280. Azoulay D, Regnard JF, Magdeleinat P, et al: Congenital respiratory-esophageal fistula in the adult: Report of nine cases and review of the literature. J Thorac Cardiovasc Surg 104:381, 1992.

281. Eriksen KR: Oesophageal fistula diagnosed by microscopic examination of pleural fluid. Acta Chir Scand 128:771, 1964.

282. von Segesser LK, Tkebuchava T, Niederhauser U, et al: Aortobronchial and aortoesophageal fistulas as risk factors in surgery of descending thoracic aortic aneurysms. Eur J Cardiothorac Surg 12:195, 1997.

283. Fernandez Gonzalez AL, Montero JA, Luna D, et al: Aortobronchial fistula secondary to chronic post-traumatic thoracic aneurysm. Tex Heart Inst J 23:174, 1996.

284. Kessler R, Massard G, Warter A, et al: Bronchial-pulmonary artery fistula after unilateral lung transplantation: A case report. J Heart Lung Transplant 16:674, 1997.

285. Ashley S, Corlett SK, Windle R, et al: Colobronchial fistula: A late complication of appendicitis. Thorax 43:420, 1988.

286. Savage PJ, Donovan WM, Kilgore TL: Colobronchial fistula in a patient with carcinoma of the colon. South Med J 75:246, 1982.

287. Mera A, Sugimoto M, Fukuda K, et al: Crohn's disease associated with colobronchial fistula. Intern Med 35:957, 1996.
288. Moreira VF, Arocena C, Cruz F, et al: Bronchobiliary fistula secondary to biliary lithiasis: Treatment by endoscopic sphincterotomy. Dig Dis Sci 39:1994, 1994.
289. Koch KA, Crump JM, Monteiro CB: A case of biliptysis. J Clin Gastroenterol 20:49, 1995.
290. Lebargy F, Wolkenstein P, Gisselbrecht M, et al: Pulmonary complications in toxic epidermal necrolysis: A prospective clinical study. Intensive Care Med 23:1237, 1997.
291. Dasgupta A, O'Malley J, Mallya R, et al: Bronchial obstruction due to respiratory mucosal sloughing in toxic epidermal necrolysis. Thorax 49:935, 1994.
292. Kamata T, Sakamaki F, Fujita H, et al: Toxic epidermal necrolysis with tracheobronchial and pulmonary complications. Intern Med 33:252, 1994.
293. Jett JR, Tazelaar HD, Keim LW, et al: Plastic bronchitis: An old disease revisited. Mayo Clin Proc 66:305, 1991.
293a. Seear M, Hui H, Magee F, et al: Bronchial casts in children: A proposed classification based on nine cases and a review of the literature. Am J Respir Crit Care Med 155:364, 1997.
294. Wiggins J, Sheffield E, Jeffery PK, et al: Bronchial casts associated with hilar lymphatic and pulmonary lymphoid abnormalities. Thorax 44:226, 1989.
295. Kargi HA, Kuhn C: Bronchiolitis obliterans: Unilateral fibrous obliteration of the lumen of bronchi with atelectasis. Chest 93:1107, 1988.
296. Pignatti PF, Bombieri C, Marigo C, et al: Increased incidence of cystic fibrosis gene mutations in adults with disseminated bronchiectasis. Hum Mol Genet 4:635, 1995.
297. Novis BH, Gilinsky NH, Wright JP, et al: Plasma cell infiltration of the small intestine, recurrent pulmonary infections, and cellular immunodeficiency (Nezelof's syndrome). Am J Gastroenterol 80:891, 1985.
298. Donato L, de la Salle H, Hanau D, et al: Association of HLA class I antigen deficiency related to a TAP2 gene mutation with familial bronchiectasis. J Pediatr 127:895, 1995.
299. Kitano Y, Iwanaka T, Tsuchida Y, et al: Esophageal duplication cyst associated with pulmonary cystic malformations. J Pediatr Surg 30:1724, 1995.
300. Williams SD, Jamieson DH, Prescott CA: Clinical and radiological features in three cases of pulmonary involvement from recurrent respiratory papillomatosis. Int J Pediatr Otorhinolaryngol 30:71, 1994.
301. Parry RL, Gordon S, Sherman NJ: Pulmonary artery band migration producing endobronchial obstruction. J Pediatr Surg 32:48, 1997.
302. Katial RK, Ranlett R, Whitlock WL: Human papillomavirus associated with solitary squamous papilloma complicated by bronchiectasis and bronchial stenosis. Chest 106:1887, 1994.
303. Burt M, Diehl W, Martini N, et al: Malignant esophagorespiratory fistula: Management options and survival. Ann Thorac Surg 52:1222, 1991.
304. Taha AS, Nakshabendi I, Russell RI: Vocal cord paralysis and oesophago-broncho-aortic fistula complicating foreign body–induced oesophageal perforation. Postgrad Med J 68:277, 1992.
305. Meysman M, Noppen M, Delvaux G, et al: Broncho-mediastinal fistula following perforation of the oesophagus. Respirology 1:217, 1996.
306. Steel A, Dyer NH, Mattews HR: Cervical Crohn's disease with esophagopulmonary fistula. Postgrad Med J 64:706, 1988.
307. Schafer H, Ewig S, Hasper E, et al: Bronchopulmonary infection with *Mycobacterium malmoense* presenting as a bronchoesophageal fistula. Tuber Lung Dis 77:287, 1996.
308. Bhatia R, Mitra DK, Mukherjee S, et al: Bronchoesophageal fistula of tuberculous origin in a child. Pediatr Radiol 22:154, 1992.
309. Hsu HK, Su JM: Giant bronchoesophageal fistula: A rare complication of bronchial artery embolization. Ann Thorac Surg 60:1797, 1995.
310. Munk PL, Morris DC, Nelems B: Left main bronchial-esophageal fistula: A complication of bronchial artery embolization. Cardiovasc Intervent Radiol 13:95, 1990.
311. Van Straalen HC, Jansveld KA, Michels LF, et al: Mediastinitis with fistula formation to the left main bronchus: A complication of wisdom tooth extraction. Chest 106:623, 1994.
312. De Nunzio MC, Evans AJ: Case report: The computed tomographic features of mediastinal bronchogenic cyst rupture into the bronchial tree. Br J Radiol 67:589, 1994.
313. MacMillan JC, Milstein SH, Samson PC: Clinical spectrum of septic pulmonary embolism and infarction. J Thorac Cardiovasc Surg 75:670, 1978.
314. Hulnick DH, Naidich DP, McCauley, et al: Pleural tuberculosis evaluated by computed tomography. Radiology 149:759, 1983.
315. Frytak S, Lee RE, Pairolero PC, et al: Necrotic lung and bronchopleural fistula as complications of therapy in lung cancer. Cancer Invest 6:139, 1988.
316. Pneumocutaneous fistula secondary to aspiration of grass (letter). J Pediatr 82:737, 1973.
317. Hoff SJ, Johnson JE, Frist WH: Aortobronchial fistula after unilateral lung transplantation. Ann Thorac Surg 56:1402, 1993.
318. Caes F, Taeymans Y, Van Nooten G: Aortobronchial fistula: A late complication of coarctation repair by patch aortoplasty. Thorac Cardiovasc Surg 41:80, 1993.
319. Winkler TR, Hanlin RJ, Hinke TD, et al: Unusual cause of hemoptysis: Hickman-induced cavabronchial fistula. Chest 102:1285, 1992.
320. Lipton ME: Case report: Venobronchial fistula—an unusual chest radiograph presentation of a central venous line complication. Clin Radiol 44:283, 1991.
321. Camero LG, Cushing FR: False left ventricular aneurysm with ventriculo-bronchial fistula and massive haemoptysis. Scand Cardiovasc J 31:117, 1997.
322. Verheyden CN, Price L, Lynch DJ, et al: Implantable cardioverter defibrillator patch erosion presenting as hemoptysis. Cardiovasc Electrophysiol 5:961, 1994.
323. Domej W, Kullnig P, Petritsch W, et al: Colobronchial fistula: A rare complication of Crohn's colitis. Am Rev Respir Dis 142:1225, 1990.
324. Hines DR, Granson PA, Taylor RL: Colo-pleuro-bronchial fistula due to carcinoma of the colon. Ann Thorac Surg 2:594, 1966.
325. Crotis TJ, Dalrymple JD, Buhrumann JR: Tuberculous bronchocolic fistula. S Afr Med J 54:795, 1978.
326. Murray DJ: A sudden increase in expired nitrogen: Diagnosis and management of a bronchial-gastric fistula. Anesthesiology 88:539, 1998.
327. Finkelstein R, Small D: Jejunobronchial fistula: Case report and brief discussion of the literature. Mayo Clin Proc 69:1082, 1994.
328. Oparah SS, Mandal AK: Traumatic thoracobiliary (pleurobiliary and bronchobiliary) fistulas: Clinical and review study. J Trauma 18:539, 1978.
329. Borrie J, Shaw JHF: Hepatobronchial fistula caused by hydatid disease: The Dunedin experience 1952–79. Thorax 36:25, 1981.
330. Roy DC, Ravindran P, Padmanabhan R: Bronchobiliary fistula secondary to amebic liver abscess. Chest 62:523, 1972.
331. Cox CL Jr, Anderson JN, Guest JL Jr: Bronchopancreatic fistula following traumatic rupture of the diaphragm. JAMA 237:1461, 1977.
332. Caberwal D, Katz J, Reid R, et al: A case of nephrobronchial and colobronchial fistula presenting as lung abscess. J Urol 117:371, 1977.
333. Nadler RB, Naughton CK, Figenshau RS: Nephro-bronchial fistula. J Urol 154:518, 1995.
334. Fishal AH, Sharfi AR, Sheik HE, et al: Internal fistula formation: An unusual complication of mycetoma. Trans R Soc Trop Med Hyg 90:550, 1996.
335. Spira A, Grossman R, Balter M: Large airway disease associated with inflammatory bowel disease. Chest 113:1723, 1998.
336. Stockley RA: Commentary: Bronchiectasis and inflammatory bowel disease. Thorax 53:526, 1998.

# Cystic Fibrosis

Cystic fibrosis (CF) is a hereditary disease of mendelian recessive transmission also known as *mucoviscidosis* or *cystic fibrosis of the pancreas*. The fundamental abnormality consists of the production of abnormal secretions from a variety of exocrine glands, including the salivary and sweat glands and those of the pancreas, large bowel, and tracheobronchial tree. With the first description of the latter abnormalities by di Sant'Agnese in 1953,[1] the designation cystic fibrosis became generally accepted and that of mucoviscidosis largely discarded. The major clinical manifestations are obstructive pulmonary disease, which is found in varying degrees of severity in almost all patients, and pancreatic insufficiency (present in 80% to 90%).[2, 3] Although a family history may suggest the diagnosis, confirmation requires the demonstration of elevated levels of sodium and chloride in sweat or the determination of homozygosity for a mutant genotype.

## EPIDEMIOLOGY

CF is the most common lethal genetically transmitted disease among whites; the estimated incidence in this group is about 1 case per 2,000 to 3,500 live births.[4, 5] The incidence is as high as 1 per 500 in Scotland.[6] There is no sex predominance. The disease is uncommon in nonwhites; its incidence among African Americans is 1 in 17,000 and among North American Indians and Asians 1 in 90,000.[4] Asians who have CF may have a more severe clinical course than matched white controls.[7] Although CF is most often identified during infancy or childhood, a significant number of cases are first recognized in adolescents or adults;[8] in 80%, the diagnosis is made before the age of 5 years and in 10% during adolescence.[4, 9] As discussed farther on, the variability in the age of onset and in the rapidity of disease progression in CF is related, in part, to the type of mutation in the cystic fibrosis transmembrane conductance regulator (CFTR) gene; patients who have mild disease and are diagnosed in adulthood are more likely to have one of the rare mutations that have less effect on the protein's function.[10]

## ETIOLOGY AND PATHOGENESIS

### Genetic Factors

As indicated, CF is a hereditary disease transmitted as an autosomal recessive trait. The responsible gene was identified in 1989[11–13] and is located on the long arm of chromosome 7.[14] The protein product of the gene (CFTR) contains 1,480 amino acids and has two transmembrane-spanning domains and two intracellular nucleotide-binding domains. It functions as a cyclic adenosine monophosphate (cAMP)–regulated chloride channel in the apical membrane of airway epithelial cells, tracheobronchial gland cells (principally serous cells),[15–17] and (in the fetus) type II pneumocytes.[18, 19] At these sites, it is involved in chloride and water transport from the cells into the lumen of the airways.

The most common mutation associated with gene dysfunction is a three base-pair deletion, which causes loss of the amino acid phenylalanine at position 508 of the protein. This mutation, termed ΔF508, accounts for about 70% of the mutant alleles on the CFTR gene; however, more than 550 additional mutations have been identified that can result in the CF phenotype.[20] The prevalence of the ΔF508 mutation varies greatly among different populations, ranging, for example, from only 20% in Ashkenazi Jews[21] to as high as 90% in a sample of the general population of Denmark.[22] Sixty per cent of mutant chromosomes in affected Ashkenazi Jews carry a nonsense mutation (W1282X).[23] In Spain, there is marked heterogeneity for CFTR mutations; about 75 different mutations need to be screened to detect 90% of the cases of CF.[24] About 50% of patients are homozygous for the ΔF508 mutation; of the remaining genotypes, most are

ΔF508 in combination with 1 of about 10 other relatively common mutations.

About 1 in 20 to 25 whites is heterozygous for one of the abnormal CF genes. No clinical characteristics have been demonstrated that identify these individuals because they do not express the disease and generally are unaware that they are carriers unless they have children with CF.[25] Each clinically unaffected brother or sister of a patient with CF has a two thirds chance of being a carrier. If a carrier of one mutant gene produces children with someone who is also heterozygous for a mutant gene, each pregnancy has a 25% risk of resulting in a child with the disease. If one parent has no familial history of CF and the other parent has the disease, there is a 1 in 40 chance of their child being affected.[25]

Because effective genetic counseling is dependent on identifying heterozygous carriers and on prenatal detection of affected homozygotes, considerable research has been carried out to develop tests for heterozygosity. Fortunately, the discovery of the gene and the specific mutations that alter it has allowed the carrier state to be recognized by genotyping (using the polymerase chain reaction) in most affected families. Prenatal screening is also possible by genotyping of DNA in cells obtained by amniocentesis or chorionic villus aspiration.[26]

The observation that so many different mutations of the CFTR gene can lead to CF, and that the mutations cause abnormal function of the protein by different mechanisms, has led to a search for possible genotype-phenotype associations. The phenotypic variations that have been examined include the magnitude of sweat chloride elevation, the presence and degree of pancreatic insufficiency, and the severity and age of onset of pulmonary disease. It was known even before the discovery of the CFTR gene that the severity of pancreatic dysfunction varied between affected families, suggesting genetic heterogeneity.[27] Most homozygous mutations, including the nonsense, splice-variant, frame-shift, and deletion forms, result in pancreatic insufficiency; however, some of the mis-sense mutations that cause only a dysfunctional membrane protein can be associated with mild disease and adequate pancreatic function.[28] A number of mutant variants have also been associated with mild lung disease or late-onset pulmonary involvement.[29–31] Despite these examples, marked variation in pancreatic and pulmonary disease severity can be seen in affected siblings who share the same CFTR genotype, so that other genetic or environmental factors must influence these manifestations.[32, 33]

Mutations of the CFTR gene have been classified into five categories:[34] class 1 mutations, such as premature-stop codons, in which no protein is produced (null mutations); class 2, in which most of the protein does not reach the cell membrane (e.g., ΔF508); class 3, in which the protein fails to respond to cAMP; class 4, associated with production of a protein that has a reduced response to cAMP; and class 5, in which there is a decreased production of a normally functioning chloride channel. Sweat chloride levels are increased with all classes of mutation; however, some class 4 mutations are associated with levels that overlap the normal range (e.g., A455E),[35] even if only one of the patient's chromosomes produces the less dysfunctional protein (e.g., the genotype: ΔF508-R117H).[34] Some classes of mutation affect all of the functions of CFTR, whereas others impair its ability to act as a chloride channel but not its activity as a regulator of other ion channels.[36]

Since class 1 mutations cause the most significant biochemical defect, it might be predicted that they would be associated with the most severe clinical manifestations; the observation that this is not necessarily the case again illustrates that other, as yet unidentified, genetic or environmental factors influence the natural history of the disease.[37] Patients homozygous for the ΔF508 mutation generally have an earlier onset of pulmonary disease and are more likely to have pancreatic dysfunction than heterozygotes.[38, 39] The second most common mutation in Dutch families (A455E) is associated with a later age of onset, less pancreatic insufficiency, a lower incidence of diabetes, and less abnormal lung function.[40] Genotype has a strong influence on the age at diagnosis of CF. In one study of 143 adult patients, clinical characteristics and genotype were compared in those diagnosed before the age of 16 years (mean age at diagnosis, 4.6 years = early diagnosis) with those diagnosed after age 16 (mean age at diagnosis, 28 years = late diagnosis);[41] the late diagnosis group had better pulmonary function, less pancreatic insufficiency (12% versus 81%) and less colonization with *Pseudomonas aeruginosa* (24% versus 70%). None of the late diagnosis group, but 58% of the early diagnosis group, was homozygous for ΔF508.

Mutations in the CFTR gene are also associated with reproductive tract abnormalities in men. About 80% of men who have congenital bilateral absence of the vas deferens (CBAVD) have mutations of the CFTR gene; especially frequent is a 5-thymidine variant (IV 58-5T) in the eighth intron, which causes defective splicing of exon 9.[42] CFTR mutations have also been reported in 47% of men who have obstructive azoospermia of unknown etiology.[43] Although this result suggests that Young's syndrome (obstructive azoospermia and bronchiectasis), CBAVD, and CF may have a similar genetic basis, the authors of another study of 12 patients who were obstructed but had an anatomically intact vas deferens and chronic suppurative lung disease found no CFTR mutations,[44] implying that Young's syndrome and CBAVD are different clinical entities.

## Fluid and Electrolyte Secretion

Spurred by research on CF and the discovery that CFTR is a chloride channel, much has been learned about normal and abnormal human airway ion transport.[45, 46] The details of airway fluid transport and mucociliary clearance are discussed in more depth in Chapters 1 and 3 (*see* pages 60 and 127). Briefly, the traditional concept is that the airway surface liquid consists of two phases: a periciliary sol layer and a discrete mucous layer. The airway epithelium adjusts the height of the sol layer by secreting or absorbing water to optimize contact of the cilia with the more rigid mucous layer, thus facilitating mucociliary clearance from the respiratory tract. Water transport is primarily controlled by an $Na^+,K^+$-ATPase pump located on the basal lateral surface of the airway epithelial cells. This pump generates an electrochemical gradient that produces a potential difference across the epithelium. The gradient causes a net movement of $Na^+$ from the lumen into the cell; water and $Cl^-$ follow the $Na^+$ passively through paracellular pathways and across a number of apical Cl$^-$ channels, one of which is CFTR. There are conflicting reports about the composition of the airway surface liquid in patients who have CF. In one study of adult patients, no differences from normal were detected for Na$^+$, Cl$^-$, or osmolarity;[47] however, in an investigation of the lower airway secretions of infants who had CF before the development of respiratory tract infection, lower than normal chloride levels were identified.[48]

Patients who have CF have a marked increase in the electrical potential difference across their nasal and tracheobronchial epithelium compared with controls or their heterozygous relatives.[49] The abnormally high membrane potential is also present in the cultured respiratory epithelial cells of these patients[51] but not in cells from individuals who have bronchiectasis unassociated with CF. Because the drug amiloride decreases the transepithelial electrical difference in patients who have CF and selectively inhibits sodium transport across airway epithelium, it has been suggested that the defect is related to excessive transmucosal transport of sodium followed by dehydration of airway secretions. Although it is now clear that the increased sodium absorption is secondary to the defect in a chloride channel (CFTR), the use of nebulized amiloride can reduce mucous viscosity and increase mucociliary clearance and has been suggested as a rational approach to drug therapy.[52]

The CFTR protein forms a transmembrane chloride channel that is located at the apical surface of airway epithelial and mucosal gland cells. Although usually closed, the channel opens and permits chloride transport when an intracytoplasmic regulatory region of the protein is phosphorylated by the action of intracellular cAMP.[53] The mutations that cause CF all affect the function of CFTR, although the manner in which they do so is different for different mutations. The $\Delta$F508 mutant protein actually can function as a chloride channel; however, the mutation results in abnormal protein folding, so that it is not correctly processed in the endoplasmic reticulum and is prematurely degraded before it can make its way to the cell membrane. Some nonsense mutations prevent the CFTR protein from being made at all (e.g., a premature-stop codon); others involve a single amino acid substitution (mis-sense mutation) that results in a protein that does not function properly being inserted into the cell membrane. Additional variants include frame-shift and splice defects, which cause an altered messenger RNA sequence and result in abnormal protein length or function.[23, 53]

Although it is now certain that CFTR acts as a chloride channel, some of the abnormalities of epithelial fluid and electrolyte balance in CF, such as the excessive sodium absorption by CF epithelium, are hard to explain simply on the basis of a defective chloride channel. In fact, the simple paradigm that failure of chloride and water secretion causes abnormally viscous airway secretions, leading to impaired mucociliary clearance and therefore increased susceptibility to respiratory tract infection, does not explain all the physiologic and clinical data. This raises the possibility that CFTR may have additional functions. For example, there is evidence that it may act as a regulator of potassium channels or alternate chloride channels;[36] the results of one study support the hypothesis that CFTR also functions as a cAMP-dependent regulator of airway sodium transport.[54]

Another possible function of CFTR is as an ion channel involved in pH adjustment within intracellular organelles.

An acid pH is required for appropriate protein sialylation, a defect that might lead to altered surface proteins on respiratory epithelial cells, which could in turn result in an increased binding affinity for bacteria such as *P. aeruginosa*.[55] In support of this hypothesis are the results of one study in which airway epithelial cells from CF patients showed greater binding of *P. aeruginosa* and *Staphylococcus aureus* than control epithelia; transfection of the cells with the normal CFTR gene reversed this difference.[56] The results of additional studies suggest that defective CFTR somehow alters the ability of the lower respiratory tract to clear certain microorganisms, particularly *P. aeruginosa*. CF epithelial cells show enhanced bacterial adhesion,[56] decreased bacterial uptake,[57] and decreased activity of an as yet unidentified substance that kills bacteria.[58] The putative bactericidal factor is secreted by normal and CF airway epithelial cells but requires a low cationic medium to function; the high surface NaCl concentration believed to be present in CF secretions apparently inactivates the factor.[58] In another study of cultured human airway epithelial cells expressing the $\Delta$F508 mutant CFTR, cells were defective in uptake of *P. aeruginosa* compared with cells expressing the normal protein.[57]

It is also possible that structural alterations in airway epithelial tight junctions may contribute to abnormal fluid and electrolyte transfer. Freeze-fracture studies of epithelial cells from patients who have CF have shown an increase in isolated intercellular junctional elements as well as basal extension of junctions at the apicolateral aspect of the cells.[59, 60] Although these changes are probably secondary to chronic airway inflammation rather than an intrinsic defect, it has been hypothesized that they may act to increase the resistance to flow of fluid and ions across the epithelium.[59]

The abnormal secretion of electrolytes associated with mutations in CFTR varies from one exocrine gland to another. Pancreatic secretions are severely deficient in electrolytes, particularly bicarbonate. Saliva from parotid, submaxillary, and sublingual glands contains normal amounts of sodium and chloride; however, secretion from minor salivary glands, similar to that of sweat glands, shows an excess of these electrolytes.[2, 61, 62] Submaxillary saliva has a high concentration of calcium.[63] The sweat of patients who have CF contains elevated concentrations of sodium and chloride and, to a lesser extent, potassium. The primary secretions in sweat glands are normally isotonic but become hypotonic in their ducts as a result of the reabsorption of sodium in excess of water.[2] The determination of sodium and chloride concentrations in sweat is a basic requirement for the diagnosis of CF (*see* farther on).

Although earlier attempts to produce a mouse model of CF led to early lethal gastrointestinal disease, more recent experiments have led to a transgenic mouse that shows mucus retention and an impaired capacity to clear *S. aureus* and *Burkholderia cepacia*.[64] No therapy, other than limited attempts at gene replacement,[65] has been developed to specifically correct the abnormal chloride transport. However, knowledge of the gene's function has led to some alternate therapeutic approaches, including the combined administration by aerosol of an epithelial sodium-channel blocker, amiloride, and of a nucleotide agonist, uridine 5' triphosphate, which stimulates chloride transport by alternate pathways.[66, 67]

## Mucoprotein Secretion and Mucociliary Clearance

The abnormal rheologic properties of exocrine gland secretions in CF and the important role played by these abnormal secretions in the pathophysiology of the disease have resulted in considerable attention being directed to an examination of their biochemical makeup. A number of organic substances present in exocrine secretions could play a role in the formation of the thick, tenacious material that obstructs the various body conducting systems. In the lung, most interest has centered around the mucous glycoproteins that are secreted in increased amounts in CF and are capable of forming visco-elastic gels. Unfortunately, many of the methods of measuring the physical properties of sputum are unreliable; in CF, there is the additional complicating factor of infection, which is almost certainly a secondary phenomenon. Nasal and tracheobronchial mucous glycoproteins contain a higher than normal content of sulfate, which may be a determinant of physical properties.[2] One group of investigators has shown that the lipid content of CF airway secretions is increased.[68]

In patients who have CF and air-flow obstruction, impaired mucociliary clearance is an almost invariable feature. In one study of 14 adult patients, in which the Teflon disk method was used to measure the rate of mucociliary clearance from the central airways, clearance was shown to be markedly depressed (2.6 mm/min compared with a normal value of 20 mm/min).[69] Within this small group of patients, most of whom had severe air-flow obstruction, there was no correlation between tracheal mucous velocity and abnormalities of pulmonary function. Despite the marked decrease in clearance, the rate was doubled by inhalation of terbutaline, a beta-adrenergic agonist.[70] In another study, patients who had CF were divided into groups on the basis of their tracheal mucociliary clearance rates;[71] a substantial number had normal mucociliary clearance, and these tended to be the ones without air-flow obstruction. Those who had the slowest clearance also had the lowest Shwachman-Kulczycki scores,* the worst blood gases, and the most severe expiratory air-flow obstruction.

In an attempt to explain the altered clearance of secretions in patients with CF, their sputum has been examined for its biochemical and visco-elastic characteristics. When sputum samples from such patients and from those with chronic bronchitis, bronchiectasis, or asthma were matched for purulence, that from the CF group was shown to have higher levels of serum glycoproteins, suggesting increased serum transudation in these patients.[72] The visco-elastic properties of sputum from CF patients have also been studied using a magnetic oscillatory microrheometer; although there was no characteristic abnormality, markedly purulent sputum had higher elasticity and viscosity and a lower viscosity-to-elasticity ratio.[73] The rate of transport of mucus from patients with CF on the isolated frog palate was less than would be predicted from its visco-elastic properties, suggesting the possibility of an inhibitory factor in the sputum. Despite these observations, the investigators concluded that CF mucus is probably normal except for the effects of purulence.[73] This conclusion is supported by a study in which the muco-

ciliary transport rates of sputum samples from patients (measured using a frog palate assay technique) correlated with scores of clinical severity and evidence of superinfection.[74]

Part of the increased sputum viscosity in CF is the result of the breakdown of inflammatory cells, which leads to an increase in sputum DNA content. The long DNA molecules intertwine with mucous glycoproteins, increasing the rigidity of the gel. The contribution of DNA to sputum viscosity in CF has been addressed by the development of aerosolized therapy with human recombinant deoxyribonuclease I (rhDNase), the naturally occurring enzyme responsible for DNA degradation. *In vitro*, rhDNase can decrease the viscosity of purulent sputum; moreover, it has been shown in clinical trials to result in modest improvement in lung function.[75, 76]

There may also be acquired abnormalities of ciliary function in CF that contribute to the impairment in clearance of secretions. Using an *in vitro* assay, one group showed that sputum from patients who had bronchiectasis caused a significant decrease in ciliary beat frequency;[77] this inhibiting effect was attenuated by $\alpha_1$-antiprotease inhibitor, suggesting that it was mediated by a protease. In support of this concept are the results of another study that showed that ciliary function was inhibited by neutrophil elastase (NE), levels of which are markedly increased in the airway secretions of CF patients.[78] The beat frequency of nasal cilia in patients who have CF is normal, although nasal clearance of mucus is decreased, suggesting an alteration in the coupling of cilia and mucus.[79] Ultrastructural examination of respiratory cilia in CF patients shows nonspecific changes.[80, 81]

## Infection and Inflammation

Respiratory infection by bacteria such as *S. aureus, P. aeruginosa,* and *B. cepacia* appears to play a major role in the pathogenesis of CF.[82] Chronic "colonization" of the airways by mucoid, alginate-producing variants of *P. aeruginosa* is recognized as a major cause of pulmonary deterioration.[83] An increase in the incidence of *B. cepacia* colonization has also been documented; the presence of this organism is associated with more rapid deterioration.[84, 85] A correlation exists between the severity of the pulmonary disease and the frequency with which these bacteria are isolated.[86] The fact that bacteria such as *P. aeruginosa* and *B. cepacia* can be continuously cultured from the lung of some CF patients, even during relatively asymptomatic periods, has led to the concept that their airways are colonized rather than infected with these organisms. However, infection is a more appropriate term because the increased levels of cytokines and proteases that can be detected in sputum and bronchoalveolar lavage fluid are indicative of ongoing inflammation associated with tissue destruction.[87]

Humoral immunologic host defense mechanisms are not impaired, and the administration of bacterial or viral antigen results in the development of specific antibodies.[88–91] In fact, immunoglobulin levels are often increased, presumably in response to chronic infection. Moreover, the serum level of antibody against strains of *P. aeruginosa* correlates with decline in lung function, and it has been suggested that the intensity of the humoral immune response is related to the degree of pulmonary damage.[92] Although abnormalities

---

*The Shwachman-Kulczycki score is a grading system for CF severity based on clinical, functional, and radiographic features.

of macrophage[93] and lymphocyte[94] function have been reported in patients who have CF, they almost certainly represent a secondary effect rather than a cause of the increased susceptibility to pulmonary infection.

Local defenses against a variety of bacteria are defective because of reduced mucociliary transport. In addition, there are specific abnormalities that predispose patients with CF to infection by certain bacterial species. Serum from CF patients who are colonized by *P. aeruginosa* specifically inhibits the phagocytosis of this organism by alveolar macrophages.[95] A similar phenomenon occurs in non-CF patients who are chronically colonized with *P. aeruginosa*.[96] The ability of the serum from these patients to inhibit opsonization and phagocytosis of this organism is caused by a shift in the immunoglobulin G (IgG) subclasses of antibody to the lipopolysaccharide antigens of *P. aeruginosa*:[96, 97] chronically colonized patients show an increase in the level of IgG2 relative to the other IgG subclasses, and the *opsonic index* (the ratio of IgG3 and IgG1 to IgG2 and IgG4) is inverted—that is, (IgG3 + IgG1)/(IgG2 + IgG4) is less than 1 rather than greater than 1.[96] There is also evidence that bacterial strains that become colonizers may be "selected" for their ability to adhere to the airway epithelium.[97a]

The emergence of *B. cepacia* as an opportunist pathogen in CF is providing an increased challenge in patient care. The organism is associated with several problems: (1) innate multiresistance to antimicrobial agents (e.g., in the Brompton hospital in London, England, about 5% of patients with CF were colonized with *B. cepacia,* and 68% of the organisms showed initial multidrug resistance);[98] (2) evidence for person-to-person transmission of epidemic strains through nosocomial or social contacts; and (3) cepacia syndrome, a fulminating, potentially fatal pneumonia that occurs in up to 20% of colonized patients.[99] In some studies, DNA fingerprinting has shown that certain epidemic strains of the organism are widespread, suggesting that stringent methods should be adopted to prevent person-to-person spread among CF patients;[100] however, some investigators have found person-to-person spread among patients attending the same CF clinic to be unusual.[101]

Patients who have CF have been shown to have circulating immune complexes in their blood.[102] With the exception of the episodic inflammatory arthritis and erythema that occasionally develop,[103, 104] the presence and level of these complexes do not correlate specifically with any particular clinical feature;[102, 105] however, high levels appear to be associated with a worse prognosis.[105, 106] For example, in a 5-year prospective study of 139 CF patients, the presence of circulating immune complexes was associated with a 31% death rate, whereas in a group without detectable immune complexes, there were no deaths.[106] It is unknown whether the elevated immune complexes are related to bacterial antibodies; however, in one study, increased serum antibodies to *P. aeruginosa* lipopolysaccharide and endotoxin A were correlated with both the level of circulating immune complexes and the degree of complement activation, and the combination was associated with a worse prognosis.[107]

There is increasing evidence that a major factor in the pathogenesis of pulmonary disease in CF is the exuberant host response to infection. The inflammatory reaction leads to a chronic destructive process that obstructs the airways, gradually causing widespread bronchiectasis, decreased pulmonary gas exchange, hyperinflation, and ultimately respiratory failure.[108, 109] The airway inflammation in CF is characterized by massive influx of polymorphonuclear leukocytes (PMNs), which can represent as many as 95% of the cell population in epithelial lining fluid (less than 5% of cells recovered with bronchoalveolar lavage in normal adults are PMNs).[110] PMNs are attracted to the airway by chemotactic factors produced by microorganisms as well as by chemoattractant cytokines synthesized and released from airway tissue cells and from the inflammatory cells. Bronchoalveolar lavage fluid from CF patients contains high concentrations of a variety of proinflammatory cytokines including interleukin (IL)-1, IL-6, IL-8, and tumor necrosis factor.[111, 112]

PMNs contain a battery of proteolytic enzymes, including elastase and collagenase. NE is an extremely potent proteolytic enzyme that has diverse functions within the tracheobronchial tree, all of which, if unchecked, could contribute to the pathogenesis of the airway disease.[113] There is evidence that the level of NE in airway secretions is associated with pulmonary disease. A number of investigators have demonstrated strikingly elevated levels of NE in CF sputum and in airway fluid obtained at bronchoscopy; moreover, the levels correlate with overall clinical severity and measures of pulmonary dysfunction.[114] In addition, NE is increased in airway fluid during exacerbations of pulmonary disease, and plasma levels of elastase-antiprotease complexes rise during disease exacerbations and fall during subsequent therapy.[115]

There are several mechanisms by which excessive NE could contribute to pulmonary disease progression in CF:

1. It is, in itself, an extremely potent mucus secretagogue for airway epithelial cells and submucosal glands.[116]

2. It is capable of hydrolyzing all of the major connective tissue proteins that make up the lung matrix.[110] Destruction of the airway walls is a prominent feature of the airways in CF, and there is evidence of increased elastin degradation, as detected by higher than normal levels of desmosines (elastin breakdown products) in the urine of patients with CF.[117]

3. NE can also perpetuate airway inflammation by establishing a positive feedback loop. It stimulates the production of IL-8 from airway epithelial cells and the release of leukotriene B4 (LTB-4) from lung macrophages.[118] IL-8 and LTB-4, both powerful chemoattractants, are present in physiologically significant amounts in the airway fluid of patients who have CF.[119, 120] The cysteinyl leukotrienes LTC4, LTD4, and LTE4 have also been detected in increased amounts in the sputum of children who have CF.[121] There is a clear association between the content of IL-8 and active NE levels in the bronchoalveolar lavage fluid.[122]

4. NE can also potentiate CF airway disease by interfering with the host's resistance to bacteria. The adherence of *P. aeruginosa* organisms to the respiratory tract epithelium is enhanced after proteolytic removal of fibronectin from cell surfaces.[123]

Alpha₁-antitrypsin ($\alpha_1$-AT) protects against excessive elastase-induced lung destruction during pulmonary bacterial infection. Plasma $\alpha_1$-AT is increased in CF patients compared with controls, suggesting that there are homeostatic mechanisms that attempt to compensate for the increased elastase load.[124] However, the massive PMN infiltration and the accompanying NE release that occur in response to pulmonary infection overwhelms the protective capacity of this antiprotease. In fact, it has been estimated that the molar concentration of NE in CF sputum is 12 times greater than that of $\alpha_1$-AT.[114] In addition, much of the $\alpha_1$-AT that is present is inactivated by NE and, to a lesser extent, by the elastase produced by bacterial pathogens.[125] The imbalance between the levels of NE and antielastase develops early in the course of disease; in one study, 20 of 27 children, including 2 of 4 1-year-olds, showed an increased number of PMNs in epithelial lining fluid and evidence for complexed or degraded $\alpha_1$-AT protein.[126]

There is some evidence that inflammation can occur in the airways of CF patients at an early age, even before there is evidence of bacterial infection.[127, 128] In one investigation of bronchoalveolar lavage fluid from 16 infants who had CF (mean age, younger than 9 months) and 11 control infants, the former showed high levels of neutrophils, NE, and IL-8;[127] in 7 of the infants, these markers of inflammation were found without microbiologic evidence of infection. However, the results of a more recent study suggest that cellular or molecular markers of inflammation are found only during or after respiratory infection.[129]

## PATHOLOGIC CHARACTERISTICS

Most pathologic studies of neonates or infants who have died of CF have shown essentially normal lungs. For example, in two studies of such individuals who died of meconium ileus at birth or before 3 weeks of age, there was little or no pulmonary structural abnormality or mucous gland hypertrophy.[130, 131] In another investigation of infants younger than 4 months of age, both with and without a history of meconium ileus or pulmonary infection, no differences from control measurements were found in tracheal gland and submucosal area or in tracheal airway diameter;[132] only tracheal gland acinar diameter was significantly increased in the CF patients compared with controls.

In contrast to these rather minor abnormalities, older patients who die of the disease invariably show pulmonary changes pathologically, including airway plugging by mucopurulent debris, bronchiectasis, bronchial wall thickening, acute and organizing pneumonia (often with abscess formation), bronchiolar fibrosis or dilation, and focal areas of atelectasis and overinflation[133] (Fig. 57–1). Focal emphysema can also be seen but is rarely appreciable, except in patients who reach adulthood;[134, 135] occasionally, bullae and blebs are present.[136] Interstitial pneumonitis is seen occasionally.[137] All these changes are variable in severity and patchy in distribution; however, there is a tendency to more marked involvement of the upper lobes.[138]

As might be expected from the discussion of disease pathogenesis, the most prominent changes are centered

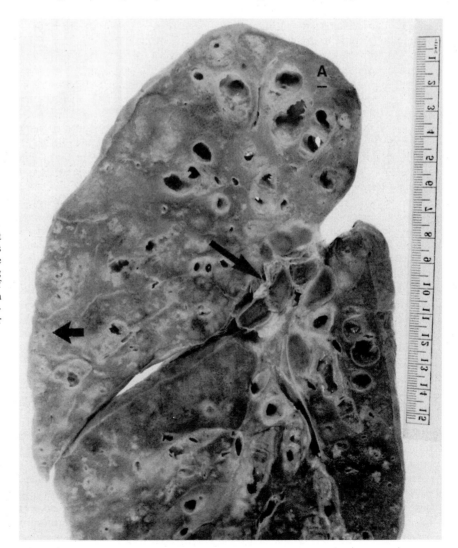

**Figure 57–1. Cystic Fibrosis.** A slice of the left lung from a 23-year-old man with cystic fibrosis shows variably severe bronchiectasis, worse in the apicoposterior segment *(A)*. Extensive organizing pneumonia in the same region and multiple foci of acute bronchopneumonia, most marked in the lingula *(short arrow)*, are present. Note the hyperplastic peribronchial lymph nodes at the junction of the upper and lower lobes *(long arrow)*.

around the airways. Bronchi may show cylindrical, varicose, or saccular dilation, the latter sometimes appearing as large, irregularly shaped, cystlike spaces[136] (Fig. 57–2). Histologic examination typically reveals marked chronic inflammation of the bronchial wall, partial or complete luminal occlusion by purulent material, focal epithelial ulceration, and cartilage destruction (Fig. 57–3).[138a] Detailed morphometric measurements made on the airways of patients with advanced CF obtained at autopsy or at the time of transplantation have shown marked thickening of all layers of the airway wall (epithelium, lamina reticularis, smooth muscle, and adventitia), findings that are similar to those reported in fatal asthma.[139] As with bronchi, bronchioles may be dilated and filled with mucopurulent debris; often, however, there is significant narrowing or obliteration as a result of fibrosis[135, 140] (Fig. 57–4). Foci of acute or organizing bronchiolitis are common (Fig. 57–5) and presumably represent the precursors of this narrowing. There is immunohistochemical evidence that *P. aeruginosa* may be localized in these dam-

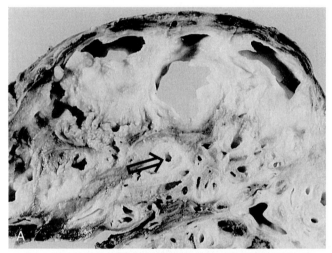

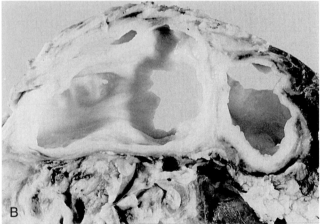

**Figure 57–2. Cystic Fibrosis: Apical "Cysts."** Magnified views of the front *(A)* and back *(B)* aspects of a single slice of lung taken from the midportion of an autopsy specimen showing elongated cystic spaces that have thick fibrous walls. Examination of contiguous slices showed the cysts to be interconnected and continuous proximally with a subsegmental bronchus. Histologic examination showed cartilage in the walls of some cystic spaces. The appearance thus suggests that the spaces are at least partly the result of bronchiectasis. Note also the marked bronchial wall thickening in *A (arrow)*.

aged airways[141] (although some investigators have found the highest bacterial concentration in large airways).[142]

Most patients who die from CF manifest right ventricular hypertrophy at autopsy; for example, 30 of 36 patients in one study showed evidence of hypertrophy, and the remaining 6 patients showed some degree of hypertrophy of pulmonary artery muscle unassociated with right ventricular hypertrophy.[143] The authors of this study found that right ventricular hypertrophy was rarely recognized clinically, presumably because the pulmonary manifestations overshadowed the cardiac ones. Smaller arteries that normally develop in postnatal life were reduced in number in all cases, an abnormality that was most apparent in those lung zones that were most severely damaged and presumably hypoxic.[143]

## RADIOLOGIC MANIFESTATIONS

The earliest manifestations of CF on the chest radiograph consist of round or poorly defined linear opacities measuring 3 to 5 mm in diameter and located within 2 to 3 cm of the pleura;[144, 145] thickened bronchial walls without bronchial dilation, mild hyperinflation, and hilar lymph node enlargement are seen less commonly.[144] The thickened bronchial walls are usually seen as ring shadows.[144] A common but nonspecific early finding is a distinctly outlined orifice of the right upper lobe bronchus on the lateral chest radiograph, a feature that was identified in 90% of CF patients in one study (compared with 25% of patients who had asthma and 18% of controls).[146]

Progression of disease is characterized by increases in bronchial diameter, bronchial wall thickness, lung volume, and the number and size of peripheral nodular opacities and by the development of mucoid impaction and focal areas of consolidation[144] (Fig. 57–6). Bronchiectasis, bronchial wall thickening, and mucous plugging are particularly frequent and are evident on the radiograph in 90% to 100% of adult patients[144, 148, 151] (Fig. 57–7). Bronchiectasis—identified as parallel lines or as ring shadows larger than the accompanying pulmonary artery—is usually widespread on the radiograph but tends to affect mainly the upper lobes.[144, 149] When filled with secretions or inspissated mucus, these bronchi are seen as nodular, finger-like or branching, bandlike opacities[150, 151] (Fig. 57–8). Cystic spaces are seen in about 25% to 30% of adult patients, particularly in the upper lobes (Fig. 57–9), representing either cystic bronchiectasis, bullae, or acute or healed abscesses.[136, 151, 152] Hyperinflation is seen in about 80% of adults patients and tends to involve mainly the lower lobes.[144]

Recurrent foci of consolidation occur in most patients, and lobar or segmental atelectasis occurs in about 50%.[144, 151] In one study of 50 patients in which serial films obtained over a 1- to 5-year or longer period were reviewed, lobar atelectasis was detected in 16 and segmental atelectasis in 12;[144] the former affected the right upper lobe in about 45% of cases, the left upper lobe in 35% of cases, and the right middle lobe in 20% of cases. Other radiographic manifestations include enlarged hila,[144] tracheal dilation,[153] pneumothorax, and pneumomediastinum.[151] Hilar enlargement may be due to lymph node enlargement, seen in 30% to 50% of adult patients,[151, 154] or dilation of the central pulmonary arteries secondary to pulmonary arterial hypertension.[151] Me-

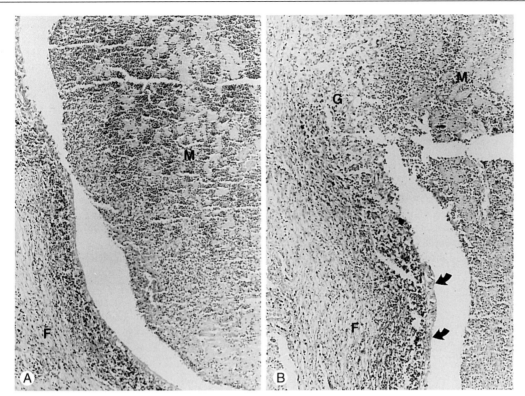

**Figure 57–3. Cystic Fibrosis: Bronchial Wall Inflammation.** Sections show two views of a dilated bronchus. In both, the lumen is almost completely filled by abundant mucopurulent material (M), and the wall shows chronic inflammation and fibrosis (F). The epithelium in *B* is focally ulcerated (residual epithelium is indicated by *arrows*) and replaced by a layer of granulation tissue (G).

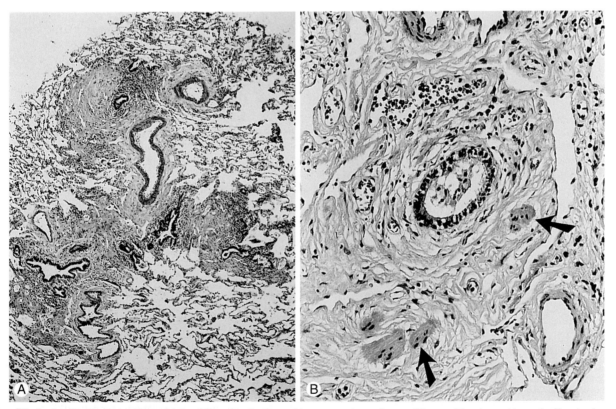

**Figure 57–4. Cystic Fibrosis: Bronchiolar Fibrosis.** Sections of lung parenchyma from a 22-year-old patient with cystic fibrosis show severe fibrosis of the peribronchiolar interstitium and the bronchiolar mucosa (the latter illustrated by the increase in tissue between the epithelium and muscularis (*arrows* in *B*).

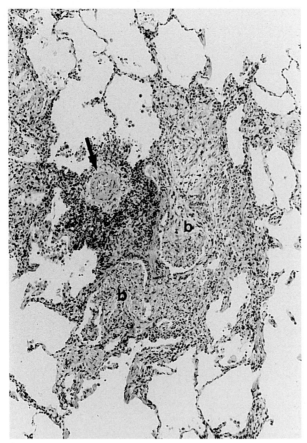

**Figure 57–5. Cystic Fibrosis: Organizing Bronchiolitis.** The section shows two small bronchioles (b) whose lumina are both occluded by plugs of fibroblastic tissue. The adjacent lung parenchyma shows mild interstitial fibrosis. The pulmonary artery accompanying the bronchioles *(arrow)* shows marked medial thickening, suggesting hypertension.

diastinal lymph node enlargement is also commonly seen on both radiographs and CT.[151, 154] For example, in one study of 48 adults, CT showed hilar lymphadenopathy in 46% and mediastinal lymphadenopathy in 44%; the latter most commonly involved the paratracheal, aortopulmonary window, and subcarinal regions.[154] Patients with lymphadenopathy had more severe pulmonary involvement (as assessed by the Brasfield scoring system) than patients without lymphadenopathy.[154]

Chest radiographic abnormalities have been incorporated into a number of semiquantitative clinical scoring schemes that are believed to be of value in predicting prognosis and directing therapy.[155] The Brasfield system is a 25-point score based on a 0 to 4 grading of air trapping, linear markings, nodular cystic lesions, large lesions (atelectasis or consolidation), and general severity (an extra point is given for cardiomegaly or evidence for pulmonary hypertension). This system has been used extensively and shows good interobserver reproducibility and correlation with abnormalities of pulmonary function.[156–159] In one review, 3,038 chest radiographs were obtained from 230 patients aged 3 days to 50 years and scored using the Brasfield system.[147] The scores from all the patients were plotted against age, and a single age-based severity curve was derived in which the mean scores, 95% confidence limits, and percentiles could be appreciated. The rate in decline of Brasfield points was slightly

less than 1% per year. Additional radiographic scoring systems include the National Institutes of Health chest radiographic score,[160] which has operating characteristics similar to the Brasfield system;[161] the Chrispin and Norman system;[162] and the Northern score,[163] which can be performed on a posteroanterior radiograph.

As discussed in Chapter 56, HRCT has become the diagnostic method of choice for the detection of bronchiectasis; in patients who have CF, the added anatomic detail afforded by this imaging modality can be striking. HRCT is particularly useful for identifying early involvement of peripheral airways, manifested by small nodular opacities in the center of secondary lobules anatomically remote from areas affected by bronchiectasis *(see Fig. 57–8)*. This "tree-in-bud" pattern corresponds to branching bronchioles whose walls are thickened by fibrous tissue and inflammatory cells and whose lumens are filled with secretions.[164–166] The other feature of small airway involvement in CF that can be appreciated using HRCT is a mosaic pattern of attenuation, with areas of decreased attenuation often in a lobular distribution *(see Fig. 57–9)*. Correlation of HRCT and pathologic findings in three patients undergoing lung transplantation has shown that this pattern is caused by the presence of obliterative bronchiolitis.[166] The decreased attenuation is secondary to lobular hypoperfusion or gas trapping. The presence of such gas trapping is best appreciated on images obtained after expiration to residual volume.[167]

HRCT is clearly more sensitive than radiography in detecting mild disease in CF (Fig. 57–10).[50, 168, 168a, 168b] For example, in one study of 38 adult patients who had mild disease who were examined with both methods, mild bronchiectasis was detected in 23 of the patients by HRCT but in only 4 by radiography.[168] HRCT has also been shown to reveal additional abnormalities not visible on conventional chest radiographs, particularly mucoid impaction.[169] A detailed scoring system for pulmonary abnormalities detected on HRCT has been proposed that involves a 0 to 2 or 0 to 3 score for the presence and extent of bronchiectasis, peribronchial thickening, mucous plugging, atelectasis or consolidation, and cystic or emphysematous changes.[170] It is also based on a 25-point system and can be interchanged with the Brasfield scoring method.

Patients with CF may have pulmonary exacerbation, that is, acute worsening of cough and sputum production, without any change in the pattern or extent of parenchymal abnormalities on the radiograph.[171] Similarly, there is usually no change in the pattern of findings on HRCT during an acute exacerbation, although the extent of abnormalities is increased.[172] In a prospective study of 19 adult patients who underwent HRCT after the onset of an exacerbation and who had follow-up HRCT after 2 weeks of hospitalization with treatment, the only finding limited to the time of the exacerbation was the presence of air-fluid levels in bronchiectatic cavities; however, this abnormality was seen in only 2 of the 19 patients.[172] Findings that improved with therapy included centrilobular nodules, mucous plugging, peribronchial thickening, and air-fluid levels; bronchiectasis and mosaic perfusion were not reversible.

Although the bronchiectasis in CF tends to be most severe in the upper lobes,[149, 151] in most adult patients, it is widespread;[173] occasionally, it is limited to the upper or middle lobes[173] or is asymmetric in distribution *(see Fig.*

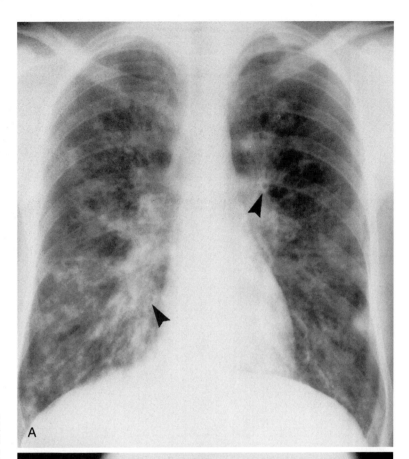

**Figure 57–6. Cystic Fibrosis.** Posteroanterior *(A)* and lateral *(B)* chest radiographs demonstrate diffuse bronchial wall thickening *(arrowheads)*, peribronchial thickening, diffuse small patchy opacities, and areas of inhomogeneous air-space consolidation. Note the remarkable thickening of the posterior wall of the bronchus intermedius (IS). The lungs are moderately overinflated. Both hila are enlarged, almost certainly as a result of lymph node enlargement rather than pulmonary arterial hypertension. The patient was a 24-year-old man.

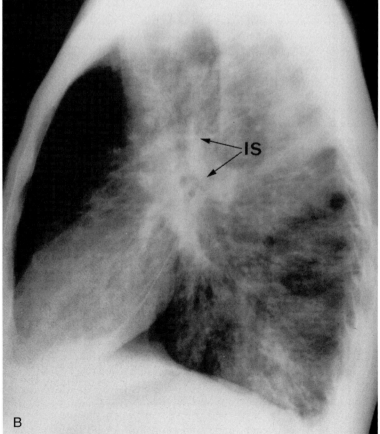

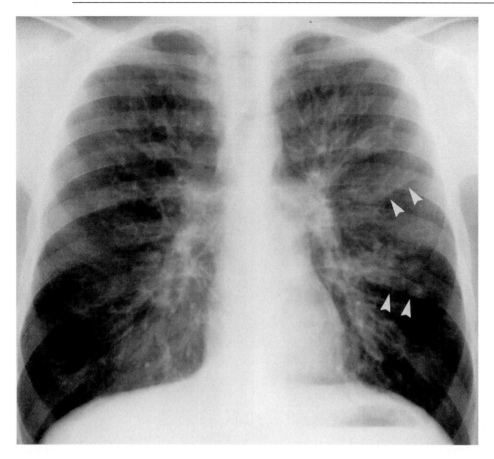

**Figure 57–7. Cystic Fibrosis.** A posteroanterior chest radiograph reveals diffuse bronchial wall thickening and moderate hyperinflation. Several dilated thick-walled bronchi are visible *(arrowheads)*, now air containing but probably the site of mucous plugs that have been recently expectorated. Note the prominent rim of subpleural oligemia in both lungs, indicating diminished blood flow to the lung periphery. The patient was a 19-year-old man who reported that he occasionally coughed up "ropey" material.

57–10). This predominant upper lobe distribution is distinct from that seen in patients who have impaired mucociliary clearance, hypogammaglobulinemia, and idiopathic bronchiectasis, which tend to have a lower lobe predominance.[173] However, by itself, distribution of bronchiectasis is of limited value in the differential diagnosis of the etiology in any individual patient;[173] for example, in the absence of appropriate history, one group of investigators found that the correct diagnosis of CF was suggested in adult patients only 50% of the time.[174] The differential diagnosis includes severe asthma, especially when complicated by allergic bronchopulmonary aspergillosis and mucous plugging, and other causes of diffuse bronchiectasis, such as the dyskinetic cilia syndromes and hypogammaglobulinemia.[173, 175]

In a study in which magnetic resonance (MR) imaging and conventional radiographs were compared for the detection of thoracic abnormalities, the former proved superior in revealing hilar and mediastinal node enlargement and in distinguishing nodes from prominent hilar vessels.[176] However, because of the superior spatial resolution of HRCT, MR imaging plays a limited, if any, role in the assessment of these patients.

## CLINICAL MANIFESTATIONS

### The Lungs

Involvement of the lungs is manifested clinically principally by recurrent chest infections associated with wheezing,

dyspnea, productive cough, and hemoptysis. Malnutrition and protein depletion are also consequences of recurrent lung infection, which can in turn accelerate the course of pulmonary disease.[177, 178] As discussed previously, infection is predominantly caused by bacteria, although viruses, mycoplasma, and fungi are occasionally responsible. The most common organisms are *P. aeruginosa* of the mucoid and nonmucoid types, *S. aureus*, and *Haemophilus influenzae*; sputum culture shows good correlation with cultures obtained by quantitative culture of distal airway secretions.[179] The isolation of gram-negative bacilli other than *P. aeruginosa* from the tracheobronchial tree has increased in recent years;[85] the presence of *B. cepacia* in particular is associated with the terminal stages of the disease.

The role of nonbacterial infection in respiratory exacerbations of CF has been studied less than bacterial infection. Acute deterioration can occur during episodes of influenza A, a potentially preventable viral infection.[180] Allergic bronchopulmonary aspergillosis occurs in 5% to 10% of patients and can be associated with an accelerated decline in lung function if unrecognized and untreated (*see* farther on);[181, 182] aspergillomas and invasive fungal infections have been reported less frequently.[183, 184] Although nontuberculous mycobacteria have been cultured from respiratory tract secretions in 10% to 15% of reported cases, definitive evidence of a pathogenic effect is uncommon (*see* page 850).[185, 185a]

Hemoptysis is a common complication.[186] Although usually small in amount, it is occasionally massive, and fatality as a direct result of bleeding is not uncommon. The hemoptysis is usually related to the extensive angiogenesis

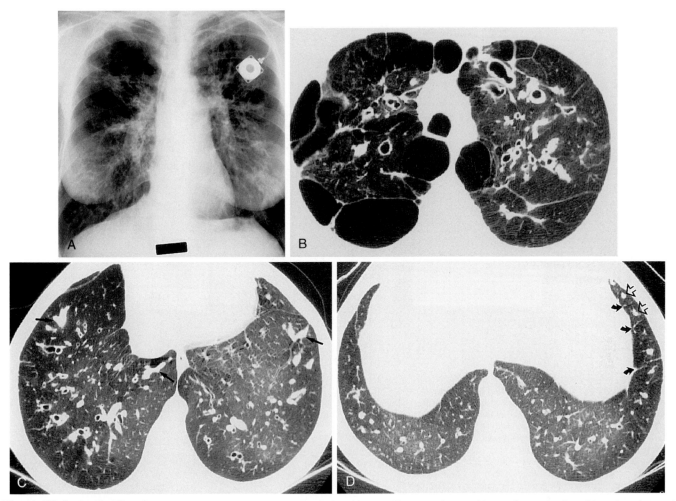

**Figure 57–8. Cystic Fibrosis.** A posteroanterior chest radiograph *(A)* in a 39-year-old woman shows evidence of extensive bronchiectasis and several large bullae, particularly in the right upper lobe. An HRCT scan at the level of the upper lobes *(B)* also demonstrates bullae, more severe on the right, and widespread bronchiectasis. A scan at the level of the lower lung zones *(C)* demonstrates less severe bronchiectasis, branching opacities representing mucoid impaction *(straight arrows)*, and areas of decreased attenuation and vascularity, particularly in the dependent lung regions and in the medial segment of the right lower lobe. A third scan at a more caudad level *(D)* demonstrates centrilobular nodular opacities *(open arrows)* measuring 3 to 5 mm in diameter and representing dilated fluid-filled bronchioles. Decreased attenuation and vascularity within the secondary lobules demarcated by interlobular septa *(curved arrows)* can also be identified.

that affects the bronchial microvasculature in bronchiectasis; sometimes it is the result of large bronchial artery–pulmonary artery fistulas.[187, 188] Bronchoscopy may be useful in identifying the bleeding site in such cases; although bronchial arteriography may do the same, its main role is to identify a route for therapeutic embolization.[186] Respiratory insufficiency develops frequently in the later stages of the disease. Ventilation-perfusion inequality is worsened by acute infectious episodes and may be associated with reversible cardiac decompensation. Eventually, persistent pulmonary arterial hypertension and cor pulmonale develop in many patients. Pneumothorax is common and frequently recurrent;[189, 190] it was observed in 7 of 49 patients in one series.[191]

There is a higher incidence of atopy and asthma among patients who have CF than among the general population.[192–194] Many patients show type I and type III hypersensitivity reactions to a variety of antigens, including food, bacteria, fungi, human body tissues, and other allergens.[195] One group of investigators measured serum IgE and IgG levels, peripheral eosinophil counts, nonspecific bronchial

responsiveness, and skin test responses to a variety of allergens in 25 patients with CF and 25 age-matched controls.[193] The CF patients manifested significantly higher serum IgG and IgE levels, higher eosinophil counts, and greater airway responsiveness than did the controls; 81% showed positive skin test responses, compared with 36% of the controls. Similarly, the patients had more atopic symptoms, and 76% of them had a positive family history of atopy, as compared with 25% of the controls. In another study of 100 patients who had CF, 46% were found to be atopic—22% with asthma and 24% with allergic rhinitis.[194] Atopy and allergic symptoms are not associated with earlier age of onset, more severe symptoms, more rapid pulmonary function deterioration, or worse survival rates.[196, 197]

Allergic pulmonary disease is also manifested by an increased prevalence of allergic bronchopulmonary aspergillosis. The frequency with which IgE antibodies and serum precipitins to *Aspergillus* species and *Candida albicans* have been identified is higher in patients with CF than in those with bronchial asthma.[91, 198, 199] In one study in which 100 unselected CF patients were screened for features of allergic

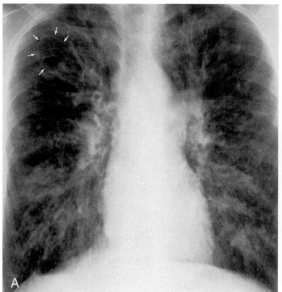

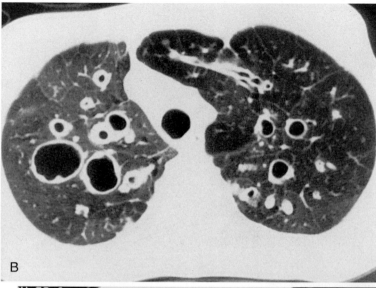

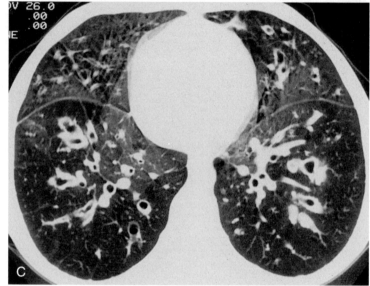

**Figure 57–9. Cystic Fibrosis.** A posteroanterior chest radiograph *(A)* shows marked bronchial wall thickening and extensive bronchiectasis. A large cystic lesion is present in the right upper lobe *(arrows)*. An HRCT scan *(B)* at the level of the upper lobes demonstrates cystic bronchiectasis. A scan at the level of the lower lung zones *(C)* also demonstrates widespread bronchiectasis, although the bronchial dilation is less marked than that in the upper lobes. Areas of low attenuation and decreased vascularity are also evident. After double-lung transplantation, pathologic evaluation demonstrated severe obliterative bronchiolitis involving mainly the lower lobes in a distribution similar to that of the areas of decreased attenuation on HRCT.

bronchopulmonary aspergillosis, the early skin test response was positive in 53% and the late in 21%.[194] Serum precipitins against *Aspergillus fumigatus* were detected in 51% of patients, and serum IgE levels were significantly increased in 21%. Using a combination of a positive immediate skin test, positive precipitins, and a history of transient pulmonary opacities, 10% of the 100 patients were judged to have allergic bronchopulmonary aspergillosis. There is evidence that the increased incidence of atopy in patients with CF is not secondary to bronchiectasis itself; in a study of 23 patients in whom bronchiectasis was unrelated to CF, there was no increase in the incidence of skin test responsiveness, eosinophilia, or elevated blood levels of IgE.[200]

Physical findings in adult patients with CF are typical of bronchiectasis and obstructive airway disease. Coarse crackles may be localized but are often diffuse; generalized wheezing should suggest the possibility of asthma. Patients are more subject to asthma than the average individual, so that it is important to measure flow rates before and after use of a bronchodilator to recognize a reversible component to the obstruction. Finger clubbing is an almost invariable

sign in patients who have advanced disease, and hypertrophic pulmonary osteoarthropathy has been reported.[201] In one study of 300 patients, 15% complained of long bone or joint pain typical of hypertrophic pulmonary osteoarthropathy;[202] about 80% manifested radiographic evidence of periostitis. The latter group had more severe pulmonary disease. Patients with clubbing and skeletal changes have been reported to have increased blood levels of prostaglandins E and $F_{2\alpha}$.[203]

### Genitourinary Tract

Reproductive failure in males is usually the result of absence of the vas deferens.[204] In a 1972 survey of 105 CF centers, normal fertility was found in only 2% to 3% of affected men;[205] women with CF are also relatively infertile, the probable cause being abnormal cervical mucus. The latter does not hydrate normally at midcycle and contains only 80% water, whereas about 95% hydration appears to be necessary for normal sperm migration.[206] Intrauterine in-

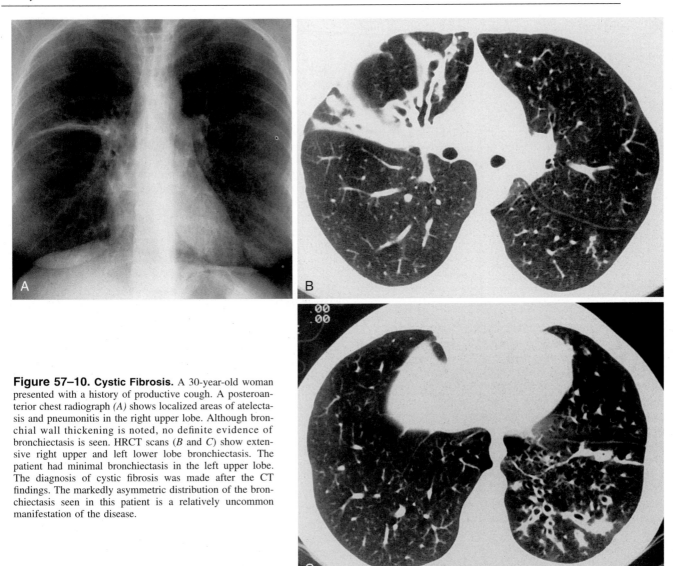

**Figure 57–10. Cystic Fibrosis.** A 30-year-old woman presented with a history of productive cough. A posteroanterior chest radiograph *(A)* shows localized areas of atelectasis and pneumonitis in the right upper lobe. Although bronchial wall thickening is noted, no definite evidence of bronchiectasis is seen. HRCT scans *(B* and *C)* show extensive right upper and left lower lobe bronchiectasis. The patient had minimal bronchiectasis in the left upper lobe. The diagnosis of cystic fibrosis was made after the CT findings. The markedly asymmetric distribution of the bronchiectasis seen in this patient is a relatively uncommon manifestation of the disease.

semination results in normal pregnancy. Pregnancy does not appear to have adverse effects in women who have mild to moderately severe disease.[206–208]

### Gastrointestinal Tract

About 10% to 15% of neonates who have CF develop intestinal obstruction as a result of meconium ileus; surgical therapy is sometimes required. Abnormal intestinal mucoproteins and an excess of tenacious intestinal mucus are presumably responsible for the obstruction. *Meconium ileus equivalent* and *distal intestinal obstruction syndrome* are terms used to describe intestinal obstruction that occurs after the neonatal period.[209] The defect in fluid and electrolyte secretion in the crypt epithelial cells likely plays an important role in the formation of the viscous luminal contents; pancreatic insufficiency also contributes. Abrupt discontinuation of pancreatic enzyme therapy may precipitate acute intestinal obstruction in children and adults.[210] These meconium masses tend to develop in the terminal ileum and may

be discovered on routine physical examination; usually, they are mobile and nontender. The clinical presentation is of colicky abdominal pain, vomiting, constipation, and abdominal distention. Radiographs of the abdomen may show evidence of small bowel obstruction. The differential diagnosis includes volvulus, intussusception, serosal adhesions related to previous surgery, and fibrosing colonopathy (colonic strictures believed to be related to high-strength pancreatic enzyme therapy).[210–212] Although the occurrence of meconium ileus in neonates is associated with a worse long-term prognosis than when it manifests at a later age, successful treatment is commonly followed by prolonged survival.[213]

Esophageal dysfunction and gastroesophageal reflux occur with increased frequency, especially in patients who have impaired pulmonary function; the mechanism responsible for this increased prevalence is unclear.[214] Rectal prolapse occurs in as many as 20% of untreated CF patients younger than 5 years of age; in one series of 386 patients, it was observed in 87 (23%).[215] In this study, the abnormality was the presenting complaint in 16 patients; in 3 patients, it occurred 7 to 10 years before the diagnosis of CF was recognized. Patients with CF also have an increased prevalence of inguinal hernia, Crohn's disease, celiac disease, and adenocarcinoma of the digestive tract.[210]

## Liver and Biliary Tract

Hepatic involvement is manifested by steatosis and focal biliary cirrhosis. The latter is characteristic of CF and is present in 25% to 30% of patients. Most are asymptomatic;[216] however, symptomatic disease manifested by ascites, peripheral edema, or hematemesis (secondary to portal hypertension) is seen in 2% to 5%. The gallbladder is abnormal in up to one third of patients;[217] abnormalities include nonfunctioning gallbladder (30%), microgallbladder (10% to 30%), and gallstones (5% to 30%).[218]

## Pancreas

In most patients, pancreatic dysfunction is secondary to a deficiency of enzymes as a result of duct obstruction by mucoid secretions and exocrine atrophy. Such pancreatic insufficiency occurs in about 90% of patients who have CF and is related to the genotype. Specific genotypes are consistently associated with either pancreatic insufficiency or adequate pancreatic function, but not with both.[28] The enzyme deficiency results in poor digestion, particularly of fat, so that patients characteristically have bulky, greasy, foul-smelling stools. Associated complications include failure to thrive and vitamin deficiencies. The disease can be mistaken for that seen in the Shwachman-Diamond syndrome, a rare disease characterized by metaphyseal chondrodysplasia, neutropenia, and pancreatic exocrine insufficiency.[219, 220] Laboratory findings of pancreatic insufficiency are described farther on.

Uncommonly, pancreatic involvement is manifested by recurrent attacks of acute pancreatitis; rarely, this is the initial presentation in young adults.[221] The incidence of symptomatic glucose intolerance is estimated to be at least 1%, two or three times higher than that in the general population younger than 25 years of age.[2] In older patients, the incidence of diabetes may be as high as 8%,[222] and it is becoming an increasingly important part of the burden of illness with increasing duration of life.[223]

## Miscellaneous Abnormalities

Although radiographic opacification of the *paranasal sinuses* due to chronic sinusitis and polyposis is almost universal in patients with CF, symptoms are said to be uncommon. However, complaints of frontal headache and nasal obstruction can often be elicited with directed questioning.[224, 225] Episodic *arthropathy* has been reported in some children and appears to be associated with high levels of circulating immune complexes.[37] This complication occurs even more frequently in adults, in whom it has been associated with increased levels of antibodies directed against bacterial heat shock proteins.[226] Rarely, *dermatitis* secondary to nutritional deficiency of zinc, protein, and es-

sential fatty acids is the presenting manifestation.[227] *Osteoporosis* is seen in some patients.

The number of reported cases of *amyloidosis* associated with CF has risen dramatically since the original description of this association in 1977;[228] the complication probably reflects greater longevity associated with current therapy, since all reported cases have been in adolescents and young adults. In a retrospective autopsy study of 33 clinically documented patients with CF who were at least 15 years of age at the time of death, one group of investigators found 11 with amyloid deposits in multiple organs;[229] however, this relatively high incidence was not found in another review of 23 patients in whom no evidence of amyloidosis was found.[230] The spleen, liver, and kidneys are most commonly affected, the lung only rarely. In most cases, symptoms related to amyloid deposition are absent; nephrotic syndrome has been reported rarely.[231]

## DIAGNOSIS AND LABORATORY FINDINGS

### The Sweat Test

Although the diagnosis of CF may be suggested by family history, persistent respiratory disease, or clinical evidence of pancreatic insufficiency, confirmation requires a positive sweat test. Genotyping is an alternative method of diagnosis; however, the large number of uncommon mutations that can lead to CF make it difficult to provide a routine screen that is comprehensive enough to rival the sensitivity of sweat testing. Determination of electrolyte concentration in sweat is subject to considerable error, and a laboratory with a sufficient volume of tests as well as experienced technicians is essential for reliable analysis. As an example of potential error, about half of the patients referred to one large CF center with positive sweat tests were found on repeat analysis to have values within normal limits.[2]

Both the method of sample collection and the analysis of electrolyte concentrations are important. Direct-reading skin electrodes are useful only for screening. The most generally accepted method is pilocarpine iontophoresis sweat collection, with chemical analysis of ionic composition.[232] Employing this method, one group showed a reasonably clear differentiation of controls from patients with the disease, although a few (generally adults in the 40- to 70-year-old range) fell into a "gray" area.[233] As mentioned previously, certain class 4 and 5 mutations that cause lesser degrees of CFTR dysfunction may show sweat chloride values in the normal range.[34, 35] With this method, the amount of sweat collected should never weigh less than 50 mg and ideally should be more than 100 mg. False-positive results may occur in patients who have adrenal insufficiency, glucose-6-phosphate deficiency, glycogen storage disease, diabetes, hypothyroidism, nephrogenic diabetes insipidus, and ectodermal dysplasia.[2, 4, 233]

Values for sodium and chloride concentrations in sweat increase with advancing age.[233] Sweat electrolyte testing is not reliable in newborn infants. In children, a chloride concentration of 60 mEq/L or higher indicates the presence of CF; a value of 50 mEq/L requires repeating. Because healthy normal adults may have values above 60 mEq/L, a diagnosis of CF should not be made at this level in the absence of an appropriate clinical history and unless repeated values of sodium and chloride are at or above this level.[3, 25] With a cut-off of 40 mEq/L, the measurement of sweat chloride levels results in a 100% sensitivity and 93% specificity for the diagnosis of CF.[234] However, the absolute level of sweat chloride does not provide a prognostic index of disease severity.[235]

A number of alternate diagnostic techniques have been developed, including one in which sweat osmolarity can be measured on as little as 10 μl of sweat[234, 236] and another in which nail clippings are analyzed for increased chloride content by x-ray microanalysis;[237] like many other tests for CF, however, their sensitivity has not been evaluated using the standard sweat chloride as a gold standard.

Although there may be a slight increase in the incidence of respiratory infections in siblings of patients with CF,[238] there is no convincing evidence of an increase in chronic respiratory disease in heterozygous parents.[238–241] Studies in which sweat electrolyte levels have been determined in heterozygotes and controls have revealed no significant differences.[239, 240] Original reports that patients with COPD possess higher than normal sweat electrolyte levels[242–245] have not been substantiated;[238, 246, 247] however, it remains theoretically possible that heterozygosity for a mutant CFTR gene could increase the risk of the development of COPD in heavy smokers.[248]

### Genetic Testing

Incorporation of molecular biologic techniques into a rapid, cost-efficient, and specific diagnostic test for most CF genotypes is now possible using the multiplex polymerase chain reaction.[249] This technologic development has allowed the implementation of population screening for heterozygote carriers of the CFTR mutations. Because the gene was cloned in 1989, there have been a number of trials of population screening that have been recently reviewed.[250] Of the two models tested to date—screening during pregnancy and screening of young adults in the reproductive age range—the former appears to be the most efficient and acceptable alternative. Prenatal diagnosis using polymerase chain reaction is also possible on cells obtained at amniocentesis or chorionic villus sampling between 11 and 18 weeks of pregnancy. Fetal cells have been recovered from the coelomic cavity at 7 to 12 weeks' gestation (colocentesis); if this technique proves safe, it could provide the earliest method to establish the diagnosis in utero.[26]

### Tests of Pancreatic Function

Pancreatic insufficiency can be demonstrated by the finding of unsplit fat globules and undigested meat fibers on smears of stool, by measuring the chymotrypsin content of stool, or by the determination of bicarbonate and enzyme content of aspirated duodenal secretions following stimulation with secretin and pancreozymin.[2] The identification of increased levels of albumin in meconium[251] and of bile acids in stool[252] are two other tests that have proved useful for some investigators. The measurement of serum immunoreactive pancreatic lipase and trypsinogen has been evaluated as a simple test of pancreatic function.[253–255] In one study, serum trypsinogen levels were measured in 381 patients who had CF and in 99 controls;[253] 314 of the patients had pancreatic dysfunction as evidenced by abnormal pancreatic stimulation tests or steatorrhea documented by fecal fat balance studies, or both. In patients younger than 2 years who had steatorrhea, serum trypsinogen levels were significantly elevated, but in those older than 6 years, malabsorption was associated with significantly lower blood levels. This age-related decline in blood enzyme levels has been confirmed by others.[254, 255] Ultrasonic examination of the pancreas is effective in the detection of structural abnormalities; however, these are not closely correlated with functional status.[256, 257]

### Pulmonary Function Tests

Tests of pulmonary function can now be performed on infants who have CF using the new technique of thoracic squeeze and measurement of expiratory flow. With this method, abnormal function has been found in affected infants even before the development of signs and symptoms.[258] Most investigators have found that the various tests that measure small airway function are the most sensitive means of detecting pulmonary involvement.[259–261] Early impairment of intrapulmonary gas mixing has also been reported.[262–264] As the disease progresses, vital capacity diminishes and residual volume increases, the latter sometimes to four or five times predicted normal, with a resultant increase in total thoracic gas volume.[261, 265, 266] $FEV_1$ values fall, and $D_{LCO}$ may decrease.[259] Dynamic hyperinflation occurs during exercise in severely obstructed patients, contributing to the increased work of breathing and the sensation of dyspnea.[267] Patients who have a low diffusing capacity tend to show arterial desaturation when they exercise.[267]

A nebulized bronchodilator produces less response in patients with CF than in those with asthma.[268] In some patients, bronchodilators may have a detrimental effect, perhaps by increasing large airway collapsibility;[269] as in patients with COPD, an anticholinergic bronchodilator may be more effective than a beta-adrenergic agent.[270] Some loss of lung recoil has been demonstrated by measurements of lung pressure-volume curves in children and young adults;[271] however, the major factor reducing expiratory flow appears to be airway obstruction.[272] Patients with advanced disease may also manifest abnormal collapse of large airways on expiration.[273]

Hypoxemia is present in some patients and hypercapnia in a minority. The impairment in gas exchange is the result of shunt and $\dot{V}/\dot{Q}$ inequality.[274] In one study in which the multiple inert gas technique was used to assess the gas exchange abnormalities in six adult patients, the arterial hypoxemia was explained equally by shunt and areas of low $\dot{V}/\dot{Q}$ ratios.[275] Extensive studies of respiratory center control and of the mechanics of ventilation have been reported in children.[276] The ratio of physiologic dead space to tidal volume increases, as does the alveolar-arterial oxygen difference.[259]

Episodes of arterial desaturation occur during sleep, the largest decrease occurring during rapid-eye-movement sleep.[277, 278] The desaturation is the result of a decrease in ventilation and worsening gas exchange. The former is in turn caused by a fall in tidal volume with no change in frequency and can be as profound as 50% during rapid-eye-movement sleep. The hypoventilation is not associated with overt central or obstructive apnea.[279] Part of the decrease during sleep is related to postural hypoxemia caused by a decrease in functional residual capacity in the supine position.[277, 280] In one group of 33 patients, the change from a sitting to a supine position caused a mean decrease in $P_{O_2}$ of $6.5 \pm 6.8$ mm Hg, accompanied by trivial changes in arterial $P_{CO_2}$.[280] Nocturnal hypoxemia could play an important role in contributing to pulmonary hypertension and cor pulmonale in advanced disease.[279] Ventilatory response to inspired carbon dioxide is impaired in proportion to the degree of airway obstruction.[281]

The demonstration that inspiratory muscle weakness and fatigue can play a role in the respiratory failure of COPD has resulted in considerable study of inspiratory muscle strength in patients with CF.[282–284] Although some investigators report a decrease in respiratory muscle strength in malnourished patients,[282] others have found normal strength despite hyperinflation and malnutrition[283–285] and have suggested that the chronic increase in the work of breathing in these patients may have a training effect.

In a follow-up study of 132 patients with CF in whom pulmonary function changes were documented over periods ranging from 4 to 7 years, considerable variation was found in the rate of change in flow rates and forced vital capacity, the general pattern being consistent with a model of exponential decline.[286] During the follow-up period, the pulmonary function of 33 patients (25%) remained stable or improved, possibly reflecting a mild form of pulmonary disease or efficacy of therapy. In this study, progress of the disease resulted in a rate of decline in pulmonary function values that was steeper in female than in male patients. In another investigation of 366 patients, the rate of decline in lung function was accelerated among those who had pancreatic insufficiency or were homozygous for ΔF508.[287] Passive cigarette smoke exposure in the home appears to accelerate the loss of lung function in children with CF; in one study, the $FEV_1$ of exposed children was 4% less than that in an unexposed group for every 10 cigarettes smoked in the household per day.[288]

In an attempt to determine the degree of correlation between radiographic changes and pulmonary function, 69 patients with CF had measurements of vital capacity, maximal midexpiratory flow rate, diffusing capacity, arterial blood gases, and dead space–to–tidal volume ratio as an index of ventilation-perfusion imbalance.[289] Chest radiographs were assessed independently for air trapping, bronchial wall thickening, cyst formation, retained secretions, and extent of the disease. Overall, the correlation between abnormalities in pulmonary function and radiographically detectable pulmonary disease was excellent. In another correlative study designed to determine the usefulness of computer-assisted ventilation-perfusion scanning in the analysis of regional pulmonary function in patients with CF, ventilation-perfusion scintiphotographs were obtained of 25 children and adolescents aged 8 months to 17 years and compared with chest radiographs.[290] Ventilation-perfusion ratio gradients were reversed in patients with predominantly upper-zone disease, and regional ventilation-perfusion ratios were uneven in distribution. The magnitude and location of the abnormalities on the scans correlated well with radiographic scores. The investigators concluded that quantitative assessment of regional ventilation and perfusion is a useful technique for assessing severity of pulmonary disease in CF. In a more recent study, heterogeneity of ventilation distribution judged by radionuclide ventilation scans was shown to correlate well with measures of lung function.[291]

Exercise capacity in patients who have CF is reduced as a result of both pulmonary and nutritional factors: lung disease has an effect by limiting maximal achievable ventilation, and malnutrition causes a loss of muscle mass and strength. The associated reduction in everyday activities may result in peripheral muscle deconditioning.[292] It has been suggested that improving the nutritional status of patients who have CF may prevent decreases in activity levels and quality of life.[293] Interestingly, patients who have CF and decreased body mass and peripheral muscle strength may have relatively preserved respiratory muscle strength, possibly as a result of a selective "training stimulus" from chronic lung disease.[294]

## PROGNOSIS AND NATURAL HISTORY

As a result of improved medical care, chiefly through antibiotic therapy, life expectancy has increased dramatically during the past few decades.[295–297] Whereas the survival rate for patients older than 17 years used to be about 5%,[298, 299] it had increased to greater than 50% by the 1970s;[2, 25] for infants born today in the United Kingdom, the predicted mean life expectancy is 40 years.[300]

The prognosis varies in different countries; for example, in a comparative study, the death rates in England and Wales were found to be two times higher than those in Victoria, Australia;[301] in England and Wales, a child had an 80% chance of surviving to 9 years of age, whereas in Victoria, there was an 80% chance of surviving to 20 years of age. The death rates in Australia were similar to those in North America, whereas those in New Zealand were closer to those in England and Wales.[302] This regional difference was attributed to the practice in Australia and North America of managing patients in centralized specialist centers.[301] In the United States, survival is influenced by the insurance status of the patients; in one study of 189 individuals with CF who were born between 1955 and 1970, median survival was 6.1 years for those without health insurance and 20.5 years for those with Medicaid or private insurance.[303] Prognosis also relates to the age at diagnosis. In one study, the clinical course of 40 patients diagnosed as having CF by a neonatal screening test was compared with that of 56 patients born before the institution of the screening procedure;[304] the average number of hospitalization days during the first 2 years of life was approximately 4 in the former group and 27 in the latter. Although this difference is partly the result of the earlier diagnosis of mild cases, it also relates to the institution of appropriate preventative and therapeutic measures early in the course of the disease. In another investigation, the clinical course of 19 patients detected during a screening program was compared with that of 30 patients detected clinically during the same time period;[305] the patients detected by screening showed improved survival, a greater increase in body weight, and a lesser decrease in $FEV_1$

percentage predicted over the first 12 years of life. Mass screening for CF could now be accomplished relatively easily by using genotyping at birth. The results of these studies suggest that such an approach may be an appropriate and cost-effective method to improve both survival and quality of life.[306]

Scoring of abnormalities on the chest radiograph has been used both to define patient groups and to predict survival. Based on the 25-point Brasfield system (the highest rating being given for a perfectly normal chest radiograph), 535 patients were divided into two groups according to the radiographic scores designated during the first year of treatment.[307] Patients in whom the degree of pulmonary involvement was sufficiently reversible to return to near normal, as evidenced by a score of 19 or more points, were placed in group I. Those who showed no improvement or never achieved a score higher than 18 points were placed in group II. Follow-up studies revealed decidedly different survival rates for the two groups: only 13 of 280 patients (5%) in group I died during an 18-year-period, compared with 106 of 255 patients (41%) in group II. Undoubtedly, this improved prognosis can be explained at least partly by earlier recognition of the disease and by the detection of milder cases. A variety of lung function tests have also been used to predict prognosis. In one study of 92 patients, progressive maximal exercise test results were found to be no more informative in predicting survival over a 5-year follow-up than $FEV_1$.[308]

Infants who have severe pancreatic insufficiency usually die of meconium ileus, whereas children and young adults die of respiratory failure, cor pulmonale, pneumonia, or, occasionally, massive hemoptysis. In patients who live to the age of 18 years, subsequent survival is best predicted from clinical features.[309] Nutritional status is one of the most important of these.[310, 311] The development of pulmonary hypertension and cor pulmonale is associated with a poor prognosis; most patients die within 2 years of the appearance of the latter complication.[312] Low body weight and *B. cepacia* colonization of the tracheobronchial tree have also been identified as negative prognostic indicators.[309] In one case-control study, 124 patients colonized by *B. cepacia* were matched with 124 noncolonized controls for age and sex.[313]

Thirty-two of the colonized patients died in the first year of follow-up, as opposed to 8 of the control patients; there were no differences in mortality in the second year of follow-up. Although some of the differences in mortality could be related to pre-existing lung function (the colonized patients had worse pulmonary function before colonization), the infections also appeared to have an additional negative effect because the annual rate of decline in the colonized survivors was more rapid than in the noncolonized patients.

*P. aeruginosa* colonization has a less dramatic effect on survival and lung function. In one study of 895 patients attending a pediatric CF clinic, the prevalence of *P. aeruginosa* colonization over a 13-year period was 82%;[314] patients who developed colonization in their first year of life had a 10-year survival rate (85%), similar to that of those colonized between the ages of 1 and 7 years (87%) or those colonized after 7 years of age (78%). By the age of 7 years, the $FEV_1$ percentage predicted was 10% lower in those colonized by *P. aeruginosa* than that in noncolonized patients. The results of one retrospective study suggested that early, focal chest radiographic abnormalities may be associated with a poorer outcome.[315]

In one investigation of 142 patients, the clinical evaluation at age 18 was used to determine prognostic factors. The evaluation was based on the Shwachman-Kulczycki scoring system,[316] a chest radiographic scoring system, pulmonary function tests, height-adjusted weight, sputum bacteriologic results, number of previous hospitalizations, age at onset of clubbing, and frequency of complications. A stepwise logistic regression analysis identified the Shwachman-Kulczycki score as the best predictor. A score of 30 to 49 predicted an average survival of 5 years beyond age 18, whereas a score of 65 to 75 predicted an additional 12 years of life.

With the development of programs for lung transplantation, the survival in advanced CF is being extended even longer (*see* Chapter 45). However, the results of a recent review suggest that patients face significant obstacles to the success of transplantation, including airway colonization with gram-negative organisms, pancreatic insufficiency, glucose intolerance, and osteoporosis. The survival rate after transplantation is about 60% to 85% at 1 year and 50% to 70% at 2 years.[317–319]

# REFERENCES

1. di Sant'Agnese PA, Darling RC, Perera GA, et al: Abnormal electrolyte composition of sweat in cystic fibrosis of the pancreas: Clinical significance and relationship to the disease. Pediatrics 12:549, 1953.
2. Wood RE, Boat TF, Doershuk CF: Cystic fibrosis. Am Rev Respir Dis 113:833, 1976.
3. Addington WW, Cugell DW, Zelkowitz PS, et al: Cystic fibrosis of the pancreas: A comparison of the pulmonary manifestations in children and young adults. Chest 59:306, 1971.
4. Rosenstein BJ, Langbaum TS, Metz SJ, et al: Cystic fibrosis: Diagnostic considerations. Johns Hopkins Med J 150:113, 1982.
5. Bye MR, Ewig JM, Quittell LM: Cystic fibrosis. Lung 172:251, 1994.
6. FitzSimmons SC: The changing epidemiology of cystic fibrosis. J Pediatr 122:1, 1993.
7. Bowler IM, Estlin EJ, Littlewood JM: Cystic fibrosis in Asians. Arch Dis Child 68:120, 1993.
8. Hunt B, Geddes DM: Newly diagnosed cystic fibrosis in middle and later life. Thorax 40:23, 1985.
9. Fitzpatrick SB, Rosenstein BJ, Langbaum TS, et al: Diagnosis of cystic fibrosis during adolescence. J Adolesc Health Care 7:38, 1986.
10. Rosenstein BJ, Levine J, Langbaum TS, et al: Cystic fibrosis in adults: Delayed diagnosis in three siblings. South Med J 79:319, 1986.
11. Kerem B, Rommens JM, Buchanan JA, et al: Identification of the cystic fibrosis gene: Genetic analysis. Science 245:1073, 1989.
12. Riordan JR, Rommens JM, Kerem B, et al: Identification of the cystic fibrosis gene: Cloning and characterization of complementary DNA. Science 245:1066, 1989.
13. Rommens JM, Iannuzzi MC, Kerem B, et al: Identification of the cystic fibrosis gene: Chromosome walking and jumping. Science 245:1059, 1989.
14. Zielenski J, Rozmahel R, Bozon D, et al: Genomic DNA sequence of the cystic fibrosis transmembrane conductance regulator (CFTR) gene. Genomics 10:214, 1991.
15. Dalemans W, Barbry P, Champigny G, et al: Altered chloride ion channel kinetics associated with the delta F508 cystic fibrosis mutation. Nature 354:526, 1991.
16. Tsui LC: Probing the basic defect in cystic fibrosis. Curr Opin Genet Dev 1:4, 1991.
17. Engelhart JF, Yankaskas JR, Ernst SA, et al: Submucosal glands are the predominant site of CFTR expression in the human bronchus. Nature Genet 2:240, 1992.
18. McCray PB Jr, Wohlford-Lenane CL, Snyder JM: Localization of cystic fibrosis transmembrane conductance regulator mRNA in human fetal lung tissue by in situ hybridization. J Clin Invest 90:619, 1992.
19. McCray PB Jr, Bettencourt JD, Bastacky J, et al: Expression of CFTR and a cAMP-stimulated chloride secretory current in cultured human fetal alveolar epithelial cells. Am J Respir Cell Mol Biol 9:578, 1993.
20. Zielenski J, Tsui LC: Cystic fibrosis: Genotypic and phenotypic variations. Ann Rev Genet 29:777, 1995.
21. Shoshani T, Augarten A, Gazit E, et al: Association of a nonsense mutation (w1282X), the most common mutation in the Ashkenazi Jewish cystic fibrosis patients in Israel, with presentation of severe disease. Am J Hum Genet 50:222, 1992.
22. The Cystic Fibrosis Genetic Analysis Consortium: Worldwide survey of the F508 mutation: Report from the Cystic Fibrosis Genetic Analysis Consortium. Am J Hum Genet 47:354, 1990.
23. Tsui L-C: The cystic fibrosis transmembrane conductance regulator gene. Am J Respir Crit Care Med 151:S47, 1995.
24. Casals T, Ramos MD, Gimenez J, et al: High heterogeneity for cystic fibrosis in Spanish families: 75 mutations account for 90-percent of chromosomes. Hum Genet 101:365, 1997.
25. Bowman BH, Mangos JA: Current concepts in genetics: Cystic fibrosis. N Engl J Med 294:937, 1976.
26. Findlay I, Atkinson G, Chambers M, et al: Rapid genetic diagnosis at 7–9 weeks gestation: Diagnosis of sex, single gene defects and DNA fingerprint from coelomic samples. Hum Reprod 11:2548, 1996.
27. Corey M, Durie D, Moore G, et al: Familial concordance of pancreatic function in cystic fibrosis. J Pediatr 115:274, 1989.
28. Kristidis P, Bozon D, Corey M, et al: Genetic determination of exocrine pancreatic function in cystic fibrosis. Am J Hum Genet 50:1178, 1992.
29. Cutting GR, Kasch LM, Tsui L-C, et al: Two patients with cystic fibrosis, nonsense mutations in each cystic fibrosis gene, and mild pulmonary disease. N Engl J Med 323:1685, 1996.
30. al-Jader LN, Meredith AL, Ryley HC, et al: Severity of chest disease in cystic fibrosis patients in relation to their genotypes. J Med Genet 29:883, 1992.
31. Santamaria F, Salvatore D, Castiglione O, et al: Lung involvement, the delta F508 mutation and DNA haplotype analysis in cystic fibrosis. Hum Genet 88:639, 1992.
32. Kiesewetter S, Macek M Jr, Davis C, et al: A mutation in CFTR produces different phenotypes depending on chromosomal background. Nature Genet 5:274, 1993.
33. Estivill X, Ortigosa L, Perez-Frias J, et al: Clinical characteristics of 16 cystic fibrosis patients with the missense mutation R334W, a pancreatic insufficiency mutation with variable age of onset and interfamilial clinical differences. Hum Genet 95:331, 1995.
34. Wilschanski M, Zielenski J, Markiewicz D, et al: Correlation of sweat chloride concentration with classes of the cystic fibrosis transmembrane conductance regulator gene mutations. J Pediatr 127:705, 1995.
35. Gan KH, Veeze HJ, van den Ouweland AM, et al: A cystic fibrosis mutation associated with mild lung disease. N Engl J Med 333:95, 1995.
36. Fulmer SB, Schwiebrt EM, Morales MM, et al: Two cystic fibrosis transmembrane conductance regulator mutations have different effects on both pulmonary phenotype and regulation of outwardly rectified chloride currents. Proc Natl Acad Sci U S A 92:6832, 1995.
37. Wulffraat NM, de Graeff-Meeder ER, Rijkers GT, et al: Prevalence of circulating immune complexes in patients with cystic fibrosis and arthritis. J Pediatr 125:374, 1994.
38. Kerem E, Corey M, Kerem BS, et al: The relation between genotype and phenotype in cystic fibrosis: Analysis of the most common mutation (delta F508). N Engl J Med 323:1517, 1990.
39. Mohon RT, Wagener JS, Abman SH, et al: Relationship of genotype to early pulmonary function in infants with cystic fibrosis identified through neonatal screening. J Pediatr 122:550, 1993.
40. Gan KH, Veeze HJ, van den Ouweland AM, et al: A cystic fibrosis mutation associated with mild lung disease. N Engl J Med. 333:95, 1995.
41. Gan KH, Geus WP, Bakker W, et al: Genetic and clinical features of patients with cystic fibrosis diagnosed after the age of 16 years. Thorax 50:1301, 1995.
42. Oates RD, Amos JA: The genetic basis of congenital bilateral absence of the vas deferens and cystic fibrosis. J Androl 15:1, 1994.
43. Jarvi K, Zielenski J, Wilschanski M, et al: Cystic fibrosis transmembrane conductance regulator and obstructive azoospermia. Lancet 345:1578, 1995.
44. Le Lannou D, Jezequel P, Blayau M, et al: Obstructive azoospermia with agenesis of vas deferens or with bronchiectasia (Young's syndrome): A genetic approach. Hum Reprod 10:338, 1995.
45. Boucher RC: Human airway ion transport: Part 1. Am J Respir Crit Care Med 150:271, 1994.
46. Boucher RC: Human airway ion transport: Part 2. Am J Respir Crit Care Med 150:581, 1994.
47. Knowles MR, Robinson JM, Wood RE et al: Ion composition of airway surface liquid of patients with cystic fibrosis as compared with normal and disease-control subjects. J Clin Invest 100:2588, 1997.
48. Hull J, Skinner W, Robertson C: Elemental content of airway surface liquid from infants with cystic fibrosis. Am J Respir Crit Care Med 157:10, 1998.
49. Knowles M, Gatzy J, Boucher R, et al: Increased bioelectric potential difference across respiratory epithelia in cystic fibrosis. N Engl J Med 305:1489, 1981.
50. Taccone A, Romano L, Marzoli A, et al: High-resolution computed tomography in cystic fibrosis. Eur J Radiol 15:125, 1992.
51. Yankaskas JR, Cotton CU, Knowles MR, et al: Culture of human nasal epithelial cells on collagen matrix supports: A comparison of bioelectric properties of normal and cystic fibrosis epithelia. Am Rev Respir Dis 132:1281, 1985.
52. Tomkiewicz RP, App EM, Zayas JG, et al: Amiloride inhalation therapy in cystic fibrosis: Influence on ion content, hydration and rheology of sputum. Am J Respir Dis 148:1002, 1993.
53. Welsh MJ, Smith AE: Cystic fibrosis. Sci Am 273:52, 1995.
54. Stutts MJ, Canessa CM, Olsen JC, et al: CFTR as a cAMP-dependent regulator of sodium channels. Science 269:847, 1995.
55. Barasch J, al-Awqati Q: Defective acidification of the biosynthetic pathway in cystic fibrosis. J Cell Sci Suppl 17:229, 1993.
56. Imundo L, Barasch J, Prince A, et al: Cystic fibrosis epithelial cells have a receptor for pathogenic bacteria on their apical surface. Proc Natl Acad Sci U S A 92:3019, 1995.
57. Pier GB, Grout M, Zaidi TS, et al: Role of mutant CFTR in hypersusceptibility of cystic fibrosis patients to lung infections. Science 271:64, 1996.
58. Smith JJ, Travis SM, Greenberg EP, et al: Cystic fibrosis airway epithelia fail to kill bacteria because of abnormal airway surface fluid. Cell 85:229, 1996.
59. Godfrey RWA, Severs NJ, Jeffery PK: Structural alterations of airway epithelial tight junctions in cystic fibrosis: Comparison of transplant and postmortem tissue. Am J Respir Cell Mol Biol 9:148, 1993.
60. Carson JL, Collier AM, Gambling TM, et al: Ultrastructure of airway epithelial cell membranes among patients with cystic fibrosis. Hum Pathol 21:640, 1990.
61. di Sant'Agnese PA, Davis PB: Research in cystic fibrosis (third of three parts). N Engl J Med 295:597, 1976.
62. Wiesmann UN, Boat TF, di Sant'Agnese PA: Flow-rates and electrolytes in minor-salivary-gland saliva in normal subjects and patients with cystic fibrosis. Lancet 2:510, 1972.
63. Warton KL, Blomfield J: Hydroxyapatite in the pathogenesis of cystic fibrosis. BMJ 3:570, 1971.
64. Davidson DJ, Dorin JR, McLachlan G, et al: Lung disease in the cystic fibrosis mouse exposed to bacterial pathogens. Nature Genet 9:351, 1995.
65. Crystal RG, McElvaney NG, Rosenfeld MA, et al: Administration of an adenovirus containing the human CFTR cDNA to the respiratory tract of individuals with cystic fibrosis. Nature Genet 8:42, 1994.
66. Bennett WD, Olivier KN, Zeman KL, et al: Effect of uridine 5'-triphosphate plus amiloride on mucociliary clearance in adult cystic fibrosis. Am J Respir Crit Care Med 153:1796, 1996.
67. Olivier KN, Bennett WD, Hohneker KW, et al: Acute safety and effects on

mucociliary clearance of aerosolized uridine 5′-triphosphate ± amiloride in normal human adults. Am J Respir Crit Care Med 154:217, 1996.

68. Sahu S, Lynn WS: Lipid composition of airway secretions from patients with asthma and patients with cystic fibrosis. Am Rev Respir Dis 115:233, 1977.

69. Wanner A: Alteration of tracheal mucociliary transport in airway disease: Effect of pharmacologic agents. Chest 80(6 Suppl):867, 1981.

70. Wood RE, Wanner A, Hirsch J, et al: Tracheal mucociliary transport in patients with cystic fibrosis and its stimulation by terbutaline. Am Rev Respir Dis 111:733, 1975.

71. Yeates DB, Sturgess JM, Kahn SR, et al: Mucociliary transport in trachea of patients with cystic fibrosis. Arch Dis Child 51:28, 1976.

72. Lopez-Vidriero MT, Reid L: Chemical markers of mucous and serum glycoproteins and their relation to viscosity in mucoid and purulent sputum from various hypersecretory diseases. Am Rev Respir Dis 117:465, 1978.

73. King M: Is cystic fibrosis mucus abnormal? Pediatr Res 15:120, 1981.

74. Puchelle E, Jacquot J, Beck G, et al: Rheological and transport properties of airway secretions in cystic fibrosis: Relationships with the degree of infection and severity of the disease. Eur J Clin Invest 15:389, 1985.

75. Fuchs HJ, Borowitz DS, Christiansen DH, et al: Effect of aerosolized recombinant human DNase on exacerbations of respiratory fibrosis. N J Med 331:637, 1994.

76. Laube BL, Auci RM, Shields DE, et al: Effect of rhDNase on airflow obstruction and mucociliary clearance in cystic fibrosis. Am J Respir Crit Care Med 153:752, 1996.

77. Smallman LA, Hill SL, Stockley RA: Reduction of ciliary beat frequency in vitro by sputum from patients with bronchiectasis: A serine proteinase effect. Thorax 39:663, 1984.

78. O'Connor CM, Gaffney K, Keane J, et al: Alpha 1-proteinase inhibitor, elastase activity, and lung disease severity in cystic fibrosis. Am Rev Respir Dis 148:1665, 1993.

79. Rutland J, Cole PJ: Nasal mucociliary clearance and ciliary beat frequency in cystic fibrosis compared with sinusitis and bronchiectasis. Thorax 36:654, 1981.

80. Katz SM, Holsclaw DS Jr: Ultrastructural features of respiratory cilia in cystic fibrosis. Am J Clin Pathol 73:682, 1980.

81. Armengot M, Escribano A, Carda C, et al: Nasal mucociliary transport and ciliary ultrastructure in cystic fibrosis. A comparative study with healthy volunteers. Int J Pediatr Otorhinolaryngol 40:27, 1997.

82. Govan JRW, Deretic V: Microbial pathogenesis in cystic fibrosis: Mucoid *Pseudomonas aeruginosa*. Microbiol Rev 60:539, 1996.

83. Govan JR, Nelson JW: Microbiology of lung infection in cystic fibrosis. BMJ 48:912, 1992.

84. Thomassen MJ, Demko CA, Klinger JD, et al: *Pseudomonas cepacia* colonization among patients with cystic fibrosis: A new opportunist. Am Rev Respir Dis 131:791, 1985.

85. Klinger JD, Thomassen MJ: Occurrence and antimicrobial susceptibility of gramnegative nonfermentative bacilli in cystic fibrosis patients. Diagn Microbiol Infect Dis 3:149, 1985.

86. Bruns WT, Brown BA: L forms in patients with cystic fibrosis. Am Rev Respir Dis 101:935, 1970.

87. Cantin A: Cystic fibrosis lung inflammation: Early sustained and severe. Am J Respir Crit Care Med 151:939, 1995

88. di Sant'Agnese PA, Talamo RC: Pathogenesis and physiopathology of cystic fibrosis of the pancreas (concluded). N Engl J Med 277:1399, 1967.

89. di Sant'Agnese PA, Talamo RC: Pathogenesis and physiopathology of cystic fibrosis of the pancreas (continued). N Engl J Med 277:1344, 1967.

90. di Sant'Agnese PA, Talamo RC: Pathogenesis and physiopathology of cystic fibrosis of the pancreas. Fibrocystic disease of the pancreas (mucoviscidosis). N Engl J Med 277:1287, 1967.

91. Mearns M, Longbottom J, Batten J: Precipitating antibodies to *Aspergillus fumigatus* in cystic fibrosis. Lancet 1:538, 1967.

92. Winnie GB, Cowan RG: Respiratory tract colonization with *Pseudomonas aeruginosa* in cystic fibrosis: Correlations between anti-*Pseudomonas aeruginosa* antibody levels and pulmonary function. Pediatr Pulmonol 10:92, 1992.

93. Wilson GB, Fudenberg HH: Does a primary host defense abnormality involving monocytes-macrophages underlie the pathogenesis of lung disease in cystic fibrosis? Med Hypotheses 8:527, 1982.

94. Ravia Y, Avivi L, Goldman B, et al: Differences between cystic fibrosis and normal cells in the degree of satellite association. Hum Genet 71:294, 1985.

95. Shryock TR, Mollé JS, Klinger JD, et al: Association with phagocytic inhibition G antibody subclass levels in serum from patients with cystic fibrosis. J Clin Microbiol 23:513, 1986.

96. Fick RB Jr, Olchowski J, Squier SU, et al: Immunoglobulin-G subclasses in cystic fibrosis: IgG2 response to *Pseudomonas aeruginosa* lipopolysaccharide. Am Rev Respir Dis 133:418, 1986.

97. Moss RB, Hsu YP, Sullivan MM, et al: Altered antibody isotype in cystic fibrosis: Possible role in opsonic deficiency. Pediatr Res 20:453, 1986.

97a. Schwab UE, Wold AE, Carson JL, et al: Increased adherence of *Staphylococcus aureus* from cystic fibrosis lungs to airway epithelial cells. Am Rev Respir Dis 148:365, 1993.

98. Taylor RF, Gaya H, Hodson ME: *Pseudomonas cepacia:* Pulmonary infection in patients with cystic fibrosis. Respir Med 87:187, 1993.

99. Govan JRW, Hughes JE, Vandamme P: *Burkholderia cepacia,* taxonomic and ecological issues. J Med Microbiol 45:395, 1996.

100. Mahenthiralingam E, Campbell ME, Henry DA, et al: Epidemiology of *Burkholderia cepacia* infection in patients with cystic fibrosis: Analysis by randomly amplified polymorphic DNA fingerprinting. J Clin Microbiol 34:2914, 1996.

101. Ryley HC, Ojeniyi B, Hoiby N, et al: Lack of evidence of nosocomial cross-infection by *Burkholderia cepacia* among Danish cystic fibrosis patients. Eur J Clin Microbiol Infect Dis 15:755, 1996.

102. Hodson ME, Beldon I, Batten JC, et al: Circulating immune complexes in patients with cystic fibrosis in relation to clinical features. Clin Allergy 15:363, 1985.

103. Rush PJ, Shore A, Coblentz C, et al: The musculoskeletal manifestations of cystic fibrosis. Semin Arthritis Rheum 15:213, 1986.

104. Dinwiddie R, Crawford O: Recent advances in cystic fibrosis research. J R Soc Med 86:7, 1993

105. Disis ML, McDonald TL, Colombo JL, et al: Circulating immune complexes in cystic fibrosis and their correlation to clinical parameters. Pediatr Res 20:385, 1986.

106. Wisnieski JJ, Todd EW, Fuller RK, et al: Immune complexes and complement abnormalities in patients with cystic fibrosis: Increased mortality associated with circulating immune complexes and decreased function of the alternative complement pathway. Am Rev Respir Dis 132:770, 1985.

107. Moss RB, Hsu YP, Lewiston NJ, et al: Association of systemic immune complexes, complement activation, and antibodies to *Pseudomonas aeruginosa* lipopolysaccharide and exotoxin A with mortality in cystic fibrosis. Am Rev Respir Dis 133:648, 1986.

108. Zach MS: Lung disease in cystic fibrosis—an updated concept. Pediatr Pulmonol 8:188, 1990.

109. Elborn JS, Shale DJ: Lung injury in cystic fibrosis. Thorax 45:970, 1990.

110. Allen DA: Opportunities for the use of aerosolized α-1-antitrypsin for the treatment of cystic fibrosis. Chest 110:S256, 1996.

111. Kronborg G, Hansen MB, Svenson M, et al: Cytokines in sputum and serum from patients with cystic fibrosis and chronic *Pseudomonas aeruginosa* infection as markers of destructive inflammation in the lungs. Pediatr Pulmonol 15:292, 1993.

112. Bonfield TL, Panuska JR, Konstan MW, et al: Inflammatory cytokines in cystic fibrosis lungs. Am J Respir Crit Care Med 152:2111, 1995.

113. Döring G: The role of neutrophil elastase in chronic inflammation. Am J Respir Crit Care Med 150:S114, 1994.

114. O'Connor CM, Gaffney K, Keane J, et al: Alpha 1-proteinase inhibitor, elastase activity, and lung disease severity in cystic fibrosis. Am Rev Respir Dis 148:1665, 1993.

115. Suter S, Schaad UB, Tegner H, et al: Levels of fire granulocyte elastase in bronchial secretions from patients with cystic fibrosis: Effect of antimicrobial treatment against *Pseudomonas aeruginosa*. J Infect Dis 153:902, 1986.

116. Nadel JA: Protease actions on airway secretions: Relevance to cystic fibrosis. Ann N Y Acad Sci 642:286, 1991.

117. Stone PJ, Konstan MW, Berger M, et al: Elastin and collagen degradation products in urine of patients with cystic fibrosis. Am J Respir Crit Care Med 152:157, 1995.

118. Konstan MW, Walenga RW, Hilliard KA, et al: Leukotriene B4 is markedly elevated in the epithelial lining fluid of patients with cystic fibrosis. Am Rev Respir Dis 148:896, 1993.

119. Hubbard RC, Fells G, Gadek J, et al: Neutrophil accumulation in the lung in α1-antitrypsin deficiency: Spontaneous release of leukotriene B4 by alveolar macrophages. J Clin Invest 88:901, 1991.

120. Nakamura H, Yoshimura K, McElvaney NG, et al: Neutrophil elastase in respiratory epithelial lining fluid of individuals with cystic fibrosis induces interleukin-8 gene expression in a human bronchial epithelial cell line. J Clin Invest 89:1478, 1992.

121. Spencer DA, Sampson AP, Green CP, et al: Sputum cysteinyl-leukotriene levels correlate with the severity of pulmonary disease in children with cystic fibrosis. Pediatr Pulmonol 12:90, 1992.

122. McElvaney NG, Nakamura H, Birrer P, et al: Modulation of airway inflammation in cystic fibrosis: In vivo suppression of interleukin-8 levels on the respiratory epithelial surface by aerosolization of recombinant secretory leukoprotease inhibitor. J Clin Invest 90:1296, 1992.

123. Plotkowski MC, Veck G, Tournier JM, et al: Adherence of *Pseudomonas aeruginosa* to respiratory epithelium and the effect of leucocyte elastase. J Med Microbiol 30:285, 1989.

124. Cantin AM, Lafrenaye S, Begin RO: Antineutrophil elastase activity in cystic fibrosis serum. Pediatr Pulmonol 11:249, 1991.

125. Suter S, Chevallier I: Proteolytic inactivation of α-1-antiprotease inhibitor in infected bronchial secretions from patients with cystic fibrosis. Eur Respir J 4:40, 1991.

126. Birrer P, McElvaney NG, Rudeberg A, et al: Protease-antiprotease imbalance in the lungs of children with cystic fibrosis. Am J Respir Crit Care Med 150:207, 1994.

127. Konstan MW, Hilliard KA, Norvell TM, et al: Bronchoalveolar lavage findings in cystic fibrosis patients with stable, clinically mild disease suggest ongoing infection and inflammation. Am J Respir Cit Care Med 150:448, 1994.

128. Khan TZ, Wagener JS, Bost T, et al: Early pulmonary inflammation in infants with cystic fibrosis. Am J Respir Crit Care Med 151:1075, 1994.

129. Armstrong DS, Grimwood K, Carlin JB: Lower airway inflammation in infants and young children with cystic fibrosis. Am J Respir Crit Care Med 156:1197, 1997.

130. Kraemer R: Onset of pulmonary involvement in cystic fibrosis. Eur J Pediatr 139:239, 1982.

131. Chow CW, Landau LI, Taussig LM, et al: Bronchial mucous glands in the newborn with cystic fibrosis. Eur J Paediatr 139:240, 1982.

132. Ogrinc G, Kampalath B, Tomashefski JF: Destruction and loss of bronchial cartilage in cystic fibrosis. Hum Pathol 29:65, 1998.

133. Vawter GF, Shwachman H: Cystic fibrosis in adults: An autopsy study. In Sommers SC, Rosen PP (eds): Pathology Annual. Part 2. Vol 14. New York, Appleton-Century-Crofts, 1979, p 357.

134. Wentworth P, Gough J, Wentworth JE: Pulmonary changes and cor pulmonale in mucoviscidosis. Thorax 23:582, 1968.

135. Sobonya RE, Taussig LM: Quantitative aspects of lung pathology in cystic fibrosis. Am Rev Respir Dis 134:290, 1986.

136. Tomashefski JF Jr, Bruce M, Stern RC, et al: Pulmonary air cysts in cystic fibrosis: Relation of pathologic features to radiologic findings and history of pneumothorax. Hum Pathol 16:253, 1985.

137. Tomashefski JF Jr, Konstan MW, Bruce MC, et al: The pathologic characteristics of interstitial pneumonia in cystic fibrosis: A retrospective autopsy study. Am J Clin Pathol 91:522, 1989.

138. Tomashefski JF, Bruce M, Goldberg HI, et al: Regional distribution of macroscopic lung disease in cystic fibrosis. Am Rev Respir Dis 133:535, 1986.

138a. Sturgess J, Imrie J: Quantitative evaluation of the development of tracheal submucosal glands in infants with cystic fibrosis and control infants. Am J Pathol 106:303, 1982.

139. Tiddens HAWM, Koopman LP, Lambert RK, et al: personal communication.

140. Esterly JR, Oppenheimer EH: Cystic fibrosis of the pancreas: Structural changes in peripheral airways. Thorax 23:670, 1968.

141. Baltimore RS, Christie CDC, Smith GJW: Immunohistopathologic localization of *Pseudomonas aeruginosa* in lungs from patients with cystic fibrosis: Implications for the pathogenesis of progressive lung deterioration. Am Rev Respir Dis 140:1650, 1989.

142. Potts SB, Roggli VL, Spock A: Immunohistologic quantification of *Pseudomonas aeruginosa* in the tracheobronchial tree from patients with cystic fibrosis. Pediatr Pathol Lab Med 15:707, 1995.

143. Ryland D, Reid L: The pulmonary circulation in cystic fibrosis. Thorax 30:285, 1975.

144. Friedman PJ, Harwood IR, Ellenbogen PH: Pulmonary cystic fibrosis in the adult: Early and late radiologic findings with pathologic correlation. Am J Roentgenol 136:1131, 1981.

145. Mitchell-Heggs P, Mearns M, Batten JC: Cystic fibrosis in adolescents and adults. Q J Med 179:v9, 1976.

146. Reinig JW, Sanchez FW, Thomason DM, et al: The distinctly visible right upper lobe bronchus on the lateral chest: A clue to adolescent cystic fibrosis. Pediatr Radiol 15:222, 1985.

147. Cleveland RH, Neish AS, Zurakowski D, et al: Cystic fibrosis: a system for assessing and predicting progression. Am J Roentgenol 170:1067, 1998.

148. Grum, CM, Lynch JP: Chest radiographic findings in cystic fibrosis. Semin Respir Infect 7:193, 1992.

149. Wood BP: Cystic fibrosis: 1997. Radiology 204:1, 1997.

150. Waring WW, Brunt CH, Hilman BC: Mucoid impaction of the bronchi in cystic fibrosis. Pediatrics 39:166, 1967.

151. Friedman PJ: Chest radiographic findings in the adult with cystic fibrosis. Semin Roentgenol 22:114, 1987.

152. Grum CM, Lynch JP III: Chest radiographic findings in cystic fibrosis. Semin Respir Infect 7:193, 1992.

153. Griscom NT, Vawter GF, Stigol LC: Radiologic and pathologic abnormalities of the trachea in older patients with cystic fibrosis. Am J Roentgenol 148:691, 1987.

154. Don CJ, Dales RE, Desmarais RL, et al: The radiographic prevalence of hilar and mediastinal adenopathy in adult cystic fibrosis. Can Assoc Radiol J 48:265, 1997.

155. Shale DJ: Chest radiology in cystic fibrosis: Is scoring useful? Thorax 49:847, 1994.

156. Lewiston N, Moss R, Hindi R, et al: Interobserver variance in clinical scoring for cystic fibrosis. Chest 91:879, 1987.

157. O'Laoide, RM, Fahy J, Coffey M, et al: A chest radiograph scoring system in adult cystic fibrosis: Correlation with pulmonary function. Clin Radiol 43:308, 1991.

158. Rosenberg SM, Howatt WF, Grum CM: Spirometry and chest roentgenographic appearance in adults with cystic fibrosis. Chest 101:961, 1992.

159. Borgo G, Cabrini G, Mastella G, et al: Phenotypic intrafamilial heterogeneity in cystic fibrosis. Clin Genet 44:48, 1993.

160. Taussig LM, Kattwinkel J, Friedwald WT, et al: A new prognostic score and clinical evaluation system for cystic fibrosis. J Pediatr 82:380, 1973.

161. Sawyer SM, Carlin JB, DeCampo M, et al: Critical evaluation of three chest radiographic scores in cystic fibrosis. Thorax 49:863, 1994.

162. Crispin A, Norman A: The systematic evaluation of the chest radiograph in cystic fibrosis. Pediatr Radiol 2:101, 1974.

163. Conway SP, Pond MN, Bowler I, et al: The chest radiograph in cystic fibrosis: A new scoring system compared with the Chrispin-Norman and Brasfield scores. Thorax 49:860, 1994.

164. Murata K, Itoh H, Todo G: Centrilobular lesions of the lung: Demonstrated by high-resolution CT and pathologic correlation. Radiology 161:641, 1986.

165. Friedman PJ: Radiology of the airways with emphasis on the small airways. J Thorac Imaging 1:7, 1986.

165a. Müller NL, Miller RR: Diseases of the bronchioles: CT and histopathologic findings. Radiology 196:3, 1995.

166. Kang EY, Miller RR, Müller NL: Bronchiectasis: Comparison of preoperative thin-section CT and pathologic findings in resected specimens. Radiology 195:649, 1995.

167. Stern EJ, Frank MS: Small airway disease of the lungs: Findings at expiratory CT. Am J Roentgenol 147:670, 1986.

168. Santis G, Hodson ME, Strickland B: High-resolution computed tomography in adult cystic fibrosis patients with mild lung disease. Clin Radiol 44:20, 1991.

168a. Hansell DM, Strickland B: High-resolution computed tomography in pulmonary cystic fibrosis. Br J Radiol 62:1, 1989.

168b. Lynch DA, Brasch RC, Hardy KA, et al: Pediatric pulmonary disease: Assessment with high-resolution ultrafast CT. Radiology 176:243, 1990.

169. Jacobsen LE, Houston CS, Habbick BF, et al: Cystic fibrosis: A comparison of computed tomography and plain chest radiographs. J Can Assoc Rad 37:17, 1986.

170. Bhalla M, Turcios N, Aponte N, et al: Cystic fibrosis: Scoring system with thin section CT. Radiology 179:783, 1991.

171. Greene KE, Takasugi JE, Godwin JD, et al: Radiographic changes in acute exacerbations of cystic fibrosis in adults: A pilot study. Am J Roentgenol 163:557, 1994.

172. Shah RM, Sexauer W, Ostrum BJ, et al: High-resolution CT in the acute exacerbation of cystic fibrosis: Evaluation of acute findings, reversibility of those findings, and clinical correlation. Am J Roentgenol 169:375, 1997.

173. Reiff DB, Wells AU, Carr DH, et al: CT findings in bronchiectasis: limited value in distinguishing between idiopathic and specific types. Am J Roentgenol 165:261, 1995.

174. Amorosa JK, Laraya-Cuasay LR, Sohn L, et al: Radiologic diagnosis of cystic fibrosis in adults and children. Acad Radiol 2:222, 1995.

175. Shah RM, Friedman AC, Ostrum BJ, et al: Pulmonary complications of cystic fibrosis in adults. Crit Rev Diagn Imaging 36:441, 1995.

176. Fiel SB, Friedman AC, Caroline DF, et al: Magnetic resonance imaging in young adults with cystic fibrosis. Chest 91:181, 1987.

177. Shepherd RW, Holt TL, Thomas BJ, et al: Nutritional rehabilitation in cystic fibrosis: Controlled studies of effects on nutritional growth retardation, body protein turnover, and course of pulmonary disease. J Pediatr 109:788, 1986.

178. Holt TL, Ward LC, Francis PJ, et al: Whole body protein turnover in malnourished cystic fibrosis patients and its relationship to pulmonary disease. Am J Clin Nutr 41:1061, 1985.

179. Gilljam H, Malmborg AS, Strandvik B: Conformity of bacterial growth in sputum and contamination free endobronchial samples in patients with cystic fibrosis. Thorax 41:641, 1986.

180. Conway SP, Simmonds EJ, Littlewood JM: Acute severe deterioration in cystic fibrosis associated with influenza A virus infection. Thorax 47:112, 1992.

181. Simmonds EJ, Littlewood JM, Evans EG: Cystic fibrosis and allergic bronchopulmonary aspergillosis. Arch Dis Child 65:507, 1990.

182. Knutsen A, Slavin RG: Allergic bronchopulmonary mycosis complicating cystic fibrosis. Semin Respir Infect 7:179, 1992.

183. Logan M, McLoughlin R, Gibney RG: Aspergilloma complicating cystic fibrosis. Am J Radiol 161:674, 1993

184. Grahame-Clarke CNE, Roberts CM, Empey DW: Chronic necrotizing pulmonary aspergillosis and pulmonary phycomycosis in cystic fibrosis. Respir Med 88:465, 1994.

185. Tomashefski JF Jr, Stern RC, Demko CA, et al: Nontuberculosis mycobacteria in cystic fibrosis: An autopsy study. Am J Respir Crit Care Med 154:523, 1996.

185a. Olivier KN, Yankaskas JR, Knowles MR: Nontuberculous mycobacterial pulmonary disease in cystic fibrosis. Semin Respir Infect 11:272, 1996.

186. Cipolli M, Perini S, Valletta EA, et al: Bronchial artery embolization in the management of hemoptysis in cystic fibrosis. Pediatr Pulmonol 19:344, 1995

187. Holsclaw DS, Grand RJ, Shwachman H: Massive hemoptysis in cystic fibrosis. J Pediatr 76:829, 1970.

188. Leading Article: Haemoptysis in cystic fibrosis. BMJ 4:702, 1970.

189. Boat TF, di Sant'Agnese PA, Warwick WJ, et al: Pneumothorax in cystic fibrosis. JAMA 209:1498, 1969.

190. McLaughlin FJ, Matthews WJ, Strieder DJ, et al: Pneumothorax in cystic fibrosis: Management and outcome. J Pediatr 100:863, 1982.

191. Mitchell-Heggs PF, Batten JC: Pleurectomy for spontaneous pneumothorax in cystic fibrosis. Thorax 25:165, 1970.

192. Wönne R, Hoffmann D, Posselt HG, et al: Bronchial allergy in cystic fibrosis. Clin Allergy 15:455, 1985.

193. Tobin MJ, Maguire O, Reen D, et al: Atopy and bronchial reactivity in older patients with cystic fibrosis. Thorax 35:807, 1980.

194. Laufer P, Fink JN, Bruns WT, et al: Allergic bronchopulmonary aspergillosis in cystic fibrosis. J Allerg Clin Immunol 73:44, 1984.

195. McFarlane H, Holzel A, Brenchley P, et al: Immune complexes in cystic fibrosis. BMJ 1:423, 1975.

196. Wilmott RW, Tyson SL, Matthew DJ, et al: Cystic fibrosis survival rates: The influences of allergy and *Pseudomonas aeruginosa*. Am J Dis Child 139:669, 1985.

197. Pitcher-Wilmott RW, Levinsky RJ, Gordon I, et al: Pseudomonas infection, allergy, and cystic fibrosis. Arch Dis Child 57:582, 1982.

198. Galant SP, Rucker RW, Groncy CE, et al: Incidence of serum antibodies to several *Aspergillus* species and to *Candida albicans* in cystic fibrosis. Am Rev Respir Dis 114:325, 1976.

199. Zeaske R, Burns WT, Fink JN, et al: Immune responses to *Aspergillus* in cystic fibrosis. J Allergy Clin Immunol 82:73, 1988.

200. Murphy MB, Reen DJ, Fitzgerald MX: Atopy, immunological changes and respiratory function in bronchiectasis. Thorax 39:179, 1984.

201. Matthay MA, Matthay RA, Mills DM, et al: Hypertrophic osteoarthropathy in adults with cystic fibrosis. Thorax 31:572, 1976.

202. Cohen AM, Yulish BS, Wasser KB, et al: Evaluation of pulmonary hypertrophic osteoarthropathy in cystic fibrosis. A comprehensive study. Am J Dis Child 140:74, 1986.

203. Lemen RJ, Gates AJ, Mathe AA, et al: Relationships among digital clubbing, disease severity, and serum prostaglandins F2alpha and E concentrations in cystic fibrosis patients. Am Rev Respir Dis 117:639, 1978.
204. Kaplan E, Shwachman H, Perlmutter AD, et al: Reproductive failure in males with cystic fibrosis. N Engl J Med 279:65, 1968.
205. Taussig LM, Lobeck CC, di Sant'Agnese PA, et al: Fertility in males with cystic fibrosis. N Engl J Med 287:586, 1972.
206. Kredentser JV, Pokrant C, McCoshen JA, et al: Intrauterine insemination for infertility due to cystic fibrosis. Fertil Steril 45:425, 1986.
207. Palmer J, Dillon-Baker C, Tecklin JS, et al: Pregnancy in patients with cystic fibrosis. Ann Intern Med 99:596, 1983.
208. Seale TW, Flux M, Rennert OM, et al: Reproductive defects in patients of both sexes with cystic fibrosis: A review. Ann Clin Lab Sci 15:152, 1985.
209. Hodson ME, Mearns MB, Batten JC: Meconium ileus equivalent in adults with cystic fibrosis of pancreas: A report of six cases. BMJ 2:790, 1976.
210. Chaun H, Davidson GF, Wong LTK: Gastrointestinal manifestations of cystic fibrosis. B C Med J 35:26, 1993.
211. Agrons GA, Corse WR, Markowitz RI, et al: Gastrointestinal manifestations of cystic fibrosis: Radiologic-pathologic correlation. Radiographics 16:871, 1996.
212. Lloyd-Still JD: Cystic fibrosis and colonic strictures: A new "iatrogenic" disease. J Clin Gastroenterol 21:2, 1995.
213. Schwachman H: Meconium ileus: Ten patients over 28 years of age. J Pediatr Surg 18:570, 1983.
214. Gustafsson PM, Fransson SG, Kjellman NI, Tibbling L: Gastro-oesophageal reflux and severity of pulmonary disease in cystic fibrosis. Scand J Gastroenterol 26:449, 1991.
215. Kulczycki LL, Shwachman H: Studies in cystic fibrosis of the pancreas: Occurrence of rectal prolapse. N Engl J Med 259:409, 1958.
216. Colombo C, Apostolo MG, Assaisso M, et al: Liver disease in cystic fibrosis. Neth J Med 41:119, 1992.
217. Park RTW, Grand RJ: Gastrointestinal manifestations of cystic fibrosis. Gastroenterology 81:1143, 1981.
218. Jebbink MC, Heijerman HG, Masclee AA, et al: Gallbladder disease in cystic fibrosis. Neth J Med 41:123, 1992.
219. Lozada-Munoz L, Aliaga MD: Shwachman-Diamond syndrome: The clinical imitator of cystic fibrosis. Puerto Rico Health Sci J 14:275, 1995.
220. Berrocal T, Simon MJ, al-Assir I, et al: Shwachman-Diamond syndrome: Clinical, radiological and sonographic aspects. Pediatr Radiol 25:289, 1995.
221. Masaryk TJ, Achkar E: Pancreatitis as initial presentation of cystic fibrosis in young adults: A report of two cases. Dig Dis Sci 28:874, 1983.
222. Abdul-Karim FW, Dahms BB, Velasco ME, et al: Islets of Langerhans in adolescents and adults with cystic fibrosis: A quantitative study. Arch Pathol Lab Med 110:602, 1986.
223. Lanng S: Diabetes mellitus in cystic fibrosis. Eur J Gastroenterol Hepatol 8:744, 1996.
224. Nishioka GJ, Cok PR: Paranasal sinus disease in patients with cystic fibrosis. Otolaryngol Clin North Am 29:193, 1996.
225. Gentile VG, Isaacson G: Patterns of sinusitis in cystic fibrosis. Laryngoscope 106:1005, 1996.
226. al-Shamma MR, McSharry C, McLeod K: Role of heat shock proteins in the pathogenesis of cystic fibrosis arthritis. Thorax 52:1056, 1997.
227. Darmstadt GL, Schmidt CP, Wechsler DS, et al: Dermatitis as a presenting sign of cystic fibrosis. Arch Dermatol 128:1358, 1992.
228. Ristow SC, Condemi JJ, Stuard ID, et al: Systemic amyloidosis in cystic fibrosis. Am J Dis Child 131:886, 1977.
229. McGlennen RC, Burke BA, Dehner LP: Systemic amyloidosis complicating cystic fibrosis. A retrospective pathologic study. Arch Pathol Lab Med 10:879, 1986.
230. Travis WD, Castile R, Vawter G, et al: Secondary (AA) amyloidosis in cystic fibrosis. A report of three cases. Am J Clin Pathol 85:419, 1986.
231. Gaffney K, Gibbons D, Keogh B, et al: Amyloidosis complicating cystic fibrosis. Thorax 48:949, 1993.
232. Gibson LE, Cooke RE: A test for concentration of electrolytes in sweat in cystic fibrosis of the pancreas utilizing pilocarpine by iontophoresis. Pediatrics 23:545, 1959.
233. Jones JD, Steige H, Logan GB: Variations of sweat sodium values in children and adults with cystic fibrosis and other diseases. Mayo Clin Proc 45:768, 1970.
234. Warwick WJ, Huang NN, Waring WW, et al: Evaluation of a cystic fibrosis screening system incorporating a miniature sweat stimulator and disposable chloride sensor. Clin Chem 32:850, 1986.
235. Corkey CW, Corey M, Gaskin K, et al: Prognostic value of sweat-chloride levels in cystic fibrosis: A negative report. Eur J Respir Dis 64:434, 1983.
236. Franck J, Shmerling DH: The use of sweat osmolarity in the diagnosis of cystic fibrosis. Helv Pediatr Acta 39:347, 1984.
237. Chapman AL, Fegley B, Cho CT, et al: X-ray microanalysis of chloride in nails from cystic fibrosis and control patients. Eur J Respir Dis 66:218, 1985.
238. Anderson CM, Freeman M, Allan J, et al: Observations on (i) sweat sodium levels in relation to chronic respiratory disease in adults and (ii) the incidence of respiratory and other disease in parents and siblings of patients with fibrocystic disease of the pancreas. Med J Aust 1:965, 1962.
239. Hallett WY, Knudson AG Jr, Massey FJ Jr: Absence of detrimental effect of the carrier state for the cystic fibrosis gene. Am Rev Respir Dis 92:714, 1965.
240. Orzalesi MM, Kohner D, Cook CD, et al: Anamnesis, sweat electrolyte and pulmonary function studies in parents of patients with cystic fibrosis of the pancreas. Acta Paediatr 52:267, 1963.
241. Batten J, Muir D, Simon G, et al: The prevalence of respiratory disease in heterozygotes for the gene for fibrocystic disease of the pancreas. Lancet 1:1348, 1963.
242. Karlish AJ, Tárnoky AL: Mucoviscidosis and chronic lung disease in adults. Am Rev Respir Dis 88:810, 1963.
243. Coates EO Jr, Brinkman GL: Sweat chloride in patients with chronic bronchial disease and its relation to mucoviscidosis (cystic fibrosis). Am Rev Respir Dis 87:673, 1963.
244. Bernard E, Israel L, Debris MM: Chronic bronchitis and mucoviscidosis. Am Rev Respir Dis 85:22, 1962.
245. Wood JA, Fishman AP, Reemtsma K, et al: A comparison of sweat chlorides and intestinal fat absorption in chronic obstructive pulmonary emphysema and fibrocystic disease of the pancreas. N Engl J Med 260:951, 1959.
246. Muir D, Batten J, Simon G: Mucoviscidosis and adult chronic bronchitis: Their possible relationship. Lancet 1:181, 1962.
247. Sekelj P, Belmonte M, Rasmussen K: Survey of electrolytes of unstimulated sweat from the hand in normal and diseased adults. Am Rev Respir Dis 108:603, 1973.
248. Luisetti M, Pignatti PF: The search for susceptibility genes of COPD. Monaldi Arch Chest Dis 50:28, 1995.
249. Kant JA, Mifflin TE, McGlennen R, et al: Molecular diagnosis of cystic fibrosis. Clin Lab Med 15:877, 1995.
250. Brock DJ: Population screening for cystic fibrosis. Curr Opin Pediatr 8:635, 1996.
251. Stephan U, Busch EW, Kollberg H, et al: Cystic fibrosis detection by means of a test-strip. Pediatrics 55:35, 1975.
252. Weber AM, Roy CC, Morin CL, et al: Malabsorption of bile acids in children with cystic fibrosis. N Engl J Med 289:1001, 1973.
253. Durie PR, Forstner GG, Gaskin KJ, et al: Age-related alterations of immunoreactive pancreatic cationic trypsinogen in sera from cystic fibrosis patients with and without pancreatic insufficiency. Pediatr Res 20:209, 1986.
254. Cleghorn G, Benjamin L, Corey M, et al: Serum immunoreactive pancreatic lipase and cationic trypsinogen for the assessment of exocrine pancreatic function in older patients with cystic fibrosis. Pediatrics 77:301, 1986.
255. Bollbach R, Becker M, Rotthauwe HW, et al: Serum immunoreactive trypsin and pancreatic lipase in cystic fibrosis. Eur J Pediatr 144:167, 1985.
256. Swobodnik W, Wolf A, Wechsler JG, et al: Ultrasound characteristics of the pancreas in children with cystic fibrosis. J Clin Ultrasound 13:469, 1985.
257. Graham N, Manhire AR, Stead RJ, et al: Cystic fibrosis: Ultrasonographic findings in the pancreas and hepatobiliary system correlated with clinical data and pathology. Clin Radiol 36:199, 1985.
258. Tepper RS, Montgomery GL, Ackerman V, et al: Longitudinal evaluation of pulmonary function in infants and very young children with cystic fibrosis. Pediatr Pulmonol 16:96, 1993.
259. Featherby EA, Weng T-R, Crozier DN, et al: Dynamic and static lung volumes, blood gas tensions, and diffusing capacity in patients with cystic fibrosis. Am Rev Respir Dis 102:737, 1970.
260. Neuburger N, Levison H, Kruger B: Transit time analysis of the forced expiratory vital capacity in cystic fibrosis. Am Rev Respir Dis 114:753, 1976.
261. Landau LI, Phelan PD: The spectrum of cystic fibrosis: A study of pulmonary mechanics in 46 patients. Am Rev Respir Dis 108:593, 1973.
262. Harrison GM, Vallbona C, Murray J: Quantitative studies of intrapulmonary gas mixing and distribution in children with cystic fibrosis. Am J Dis Child 100:530, 1960.
263. DeMuth GR, Howatt W, Talner N: Intrapulmonary gas distribution in cystic fibrosis. Am J Dis Child 100:582, 1960.
264. DeMuth GR, Howatt WF, Talner NS: Intrapulmonary gas distribution in cystic fibrosis. Am J Dis Child 103:129, 1962.
265. Beier FR, Renzetti AD Jr, Mitchell M, et al: Pulmonary pathophysiology in cystic fibrosis. Am Rev Respir Dis 94:430, 1966.
266. Tomashefski JF, Christoforidis AJ, Abdullah AK: Cystic fibrosis in young adults: An overlooked diagnosis with emphasis on pulmonary function and radiological patterns. Chest 57:28, 1970.
267. Lebecque P, Lapierre JG, Lamarre A, et al: Diffusion capacity and oxygen desaturation effects on exercise in patients with cystic fibrosis. Chest 91:693, 1987.
268. Chang N, Levison H: The effect of a nebulized bronchodilator administered with or without intermittent positive pressure breathing on ventilatory function in children with cystic fibrosis and asthma. Am Rev Respir Dis 106:867, 1972.
269. Zach MS, Oberwaldner B, Forche G, et al: Bronchodilators increase airway instability in cystic fibrosis. Am Rev Respir Dis 131:537, 1985.
270. Larsen GL, Barron RJ, Cotton EK, et al: A comparative study of inhaled atropine sulfate and isoproterenol hydrochloride in cystic fibrosis. Am Rev Respir Dis 119:399, 1979.
271. Zapletal A, Desmond KJ, Demizio D, et al: Lung recoil and the determination of airflow limitation in cystic fibrosis and asthma. Pediatr Pulmonol 15:13, 1993.
272. Mansell A, Dubrawsky C, Levison H, et al: Lung elastic recoil in cystic fibrosis. Am Rev Respir Dis 109:190, 1974.
273. Landau LI, Taussig LM, Macklem PT, et al: Contribution of inhomogeneity of lung units to the maximal expiratory flow-volume curve in children with asthma and cystic fibrosis. Am Rev Respir Dis 111:725, 1975.
274. Coates AL, Boyce P, Shaw DG, et al: Relationship between the chest radiograph, regional lung function studies, exercise tolerance, and clinical condition in cystic fibrosis. Arch Dis Child 56:106, 1981.
275. Dantzker DR, Patten GA, Bower JS, et al: Gas exchange at rest and during exercise in adults with cystic fibrosis. Am Rev Respir Dis 125:400, 1982.

276. Coates AL, Desmond KJ, Milic-Emili J, et al: Ventilation, respiratory center output, and contribution of the rib cage and abdominal components to ventilation during CO2 rebreathing in children with cystic fibrosis. Am Rev Respir Dis 124:526, 1981.

277. Muller NL, Francis PW, Gurwitz D, et al: Mechanism of hemoglobin desaturation during rapid-eye-movement sleep in normal subjects and patients with cystic fibrosis. Am Rev Respir Dis 121:463, 1980.

278. Tepper RS, Skatrud JB, Dempsey JA, et al: Ventilation and oxygenation changes during sleep in cystic fibrosis. Chest 84:388, 1983.

279. Ruzica J, Fitzpatrick MF: Obstructive lung disease and sleep. Obstruct Lung Dis 80(Pt. 2):821, 1996.

280. Stokes DC, Wohl ME, Khaw KT, et al: Postural hypoxemia in cystic fibrosis. Chest 87:785, 1985.

281. Lwin N, Giammona ST: Ventilatory responses to inspired CO2 in patients with cystic fibrosis. Chest 61:206, 1972.

282. Szeinberg A, England S, Mindorff C, et al: Maximal inspiratory and expiratory pressures are reduced in hyperinflated, malnourished, young adult male patients with cystic fibrosis. Am Rev Respir Dis 132:766, 1985.

283. Marks J, Pasterkamp H, Tal A, et al: Relationship between respiratory muscle strength, nutritional status, and lung volume in cystic fibrosis and asthma. Am Rev Respir Dis 133:414, 1986.

284. O'Neill S, Leahy F, Pasterkamp H, et al: The effects of chronic hyperinflation, nutritional status, and posture on respiratory muscle strength in cystic fibrosis. Am Rev Respir Dis 128:1051, 1983.

285. Lands L, Desmond KJ, Demizio D, et al: The effects of nutritional status and hyperinflation on respiratory muscle strength in children and young adults. Am Rev Respir Dis 141:1506, 1990.

286. Corey M, Levison H, Crozier D: Five-to-seven years course of pulmonary function in cystic fibrosis. Am Rev Respir Dis 114:1085, 1976.

287. Corey M, Edwards L, Levison H, et al: Longitudinal analysis of pulmonary function decline in patients with cystic fibrosis. J Pediatr 131:809, 1997.

288. Smyth A, O'Hea U, Williams G, et al: Passive smoking and impaired lung function in cystic fibrosis. Arch Dis Child 71:353, 1994.

289. Reilly BJ, Featherby EA, Weng T-R, et al: The correlation of radiological changes with pulmonary function in cystic fibrosis. Radiology 98:281, 1971.

290. Alderson PO, Secker-Walker RH, Strominger DB, et al: Quantitative assessment of regional ventilation and perfusion in children with cystic fibrosis. Radiology 111:151, 1974.

291. Kuni CC, Budd JR, Regelmann WE, et al: Comparison of Tc-99m DTPA aerosol ventilation studies with pulmonary function testing in cystic fibrosis. Clin Nucl Med 18:15, 1993.

292. Lands LC, Heigenhauser GJ, Jones NL: Analysis of factors limiting maximal exercise performance in cystic fibrosis. Clin Sci 83:391, 1992.

293. Boucher GP, Lands LC, Hay JA, Hornby L: Activity levels and the relationship to lung function and nutritional status in children with cystic fibrosis. Am J Phys Med Rehabil 76:311, 1997.

294. Lands LC, Heigenhauser GJ, Jones NL: Respiratory and peripheral muscle function in cystic fibrosis. Am Rev Respir Dis 147:865, 1993.

295. Wilmott RW, Tyson SL, Dinwiddie R, et al: Survival rates in cystic fibrosis. Arch Dis Child 58:835, 1983.

296. Berkin KE, Alcock SR, Stack BH, et al: Cystic fibrosis: A review of 26 adolescent and adult patients. Eur J Respir Dis 67:103, 1985.

297. Dodge JA, Morison S, Lewis PA, et al: Incidence, population, and survival of cystic fibrosis in the UK, 1968–95. Arch Dis Child 77:493, 1997.

298. Brusilow SW: Cystic fibrosis in adults. Annu Rev Med 21:99, 1970.

299. Shwachman H, Kulczycki LL, Khaw K-T: Studies in cystic fibrosis: A report on sixty-five patients over 17 years of age. Pediatrics 36:689, 1965.

300. Elborn JS, Shale DJ, Britton JR: Cystic fibrosis: Current survival and population estimates to the year 2000. Thorax 46:881, 1991.

301. Phelan P, Hey E: Cystic fibrosis mortality in England and Wales and in Victoria, Australia 1976–1980. Arch Dis Child 59:71, 1984.

302. Wesley AW, Stewart AW: Cystic fibrosis in New Zealand: Incidence and mortality. N Z Med J 98:321, 1985.

303. Blumenfeld A, Slaugenhaupt SA, Axelrod FB, et al: Localization of the gene for familial dysautonomia on chromosome 9 and definition of DNA markers for genetic diagnosis. Nature Genet 4:160, 1993.

304. Wilcken B, Chalmers G: Reduced morbidity in patients with cystic fibrosis detected by neonatal screening. Lancet 2(8468):1319, 1985.

305. Dankert-Roelse JE, te Meerman GJ: Long term prognosis of patients with cystic fibrosis in relation to early detection by neonatal screening and treatment in a cystic fibrosis centre. Thorax 50:712, 1995.

306. Dodge JA: Determinants of pancreatic and pulmonary status of cystic fibrosis. Lancet 337:54, 1991.

307. Doershuk CF, Matthews LW, Tucker AS, et al: Evaluation of a prophylactic and therapeutic program for patients with cystic fibrosis. Pediatrics 36:675, 1965.

308. Moorcroft AJ, Dodd ME, Webb AK: Exercise testing and prognosis in adult cystic fibrosis. Thorax 52:291, 1997.

309. Huang NN, Schidlow DV, Szatrowski TH, et al: Clinical features, survival rate, and prognostic factors in young adults with cystic fibrosis. Am J Med 82:871, 1987.

310. Roulet M: Protein-energy malnutrition in cystic fibrosis patients. Acta Paediatr Suppl 395:43, 1994.

311. Bakker W: Nutritional state and lung disease in cystic fibrosis. Neth J Med 41:130, 1992.

312. Penketh ARL, Wise A, Mearns MB, et al: Cystic fibrosis in adolescent and adults. Thorax 42:526, 1987.

313. Lewin LO, Byard PJ, Davis PB: Effect of *Pseudomonas cepacia* colonization on survival and pulmonary function of cystic fibrosis patients. J Clin Epidemiol 43:125, 1990.

314. Kerem E, Corey M, Gold R, et al: Pulmonary function and clinical course in patients with cystic fibrosis after pulmonary colonization with *Pseudomonas aeruginosa*. J Pediatr 116:714, 1990.

315. Mukhopadhyay S, Kirby ML, Duncan AW, et al: Early focal abnormalities on chest radiographs and respiratory prognosis in children with cystic fibrosis. Br J Radiol 69:122, 1996.

316. Schwachman H, Kulczycki LL: Long term study of one hundred and five patients with cystic fibrosis. Am J Dis Child 96:6, 1958.

317. Rayan PJ, Stableforth DE: Referral for lung transplantation: Experience of a Birmingham Adult Cystic Fibrosis Centre between 1987 and 1994. Thorax 51:302, 1996.

318. Stillwell PC, Mallory GB: Pediatric lung transplantation. Clin Chest Med 18:405, 1997.

319. Mendeloff EN, Huddleston CB, Mallory GB, et al: Pediatric and adult lung transplantation for cystic fibrosis. J Thorac Cardiovasc Surg 115:404, 1998.

# CHAPTER 58

# *Bronchiolitis*

## CLASSIFICATION AND PATHOLOGIC CHARACTERISTICS

A variety of pulmonary diseases are characterized predominantly by inflammation of membranous and respiratory bronchioles. Such bronchiolitis can be classified in two ways: (1) according to its proved or presumed etiology or the pulmonary or systemic diseases with which it is often associated (Table 58–1); and (2) according to its histologic features (Table 58–2). A variety of conceptual and nosologic problems exist with both of these classification schemes. This has come about in part because the terms applied to the histologic reaction patterns associated with bronchiolitis have also been used to describe presumed pathophysiologic mechanisms and specific disease entities. Although there is some correspondence among these three, the same term has sometimes been used to mean different things by different authors, and multiple terms have been used to describe one disease process. For example, the terms *obliterative*

*bronchiolitis* and *bronchiolitis obliterans organizing pneumonia* (BOOP) have similar names and some shared pathologic features but significantly different radiographic and clinical features.

To confuse matters even further, there is not always a one-to-one relationship between a particular histologic pattern and a specific disease entity or process. For example, bronchiolitis associated with rheumatoid disease may be manifested histologically by obliterative bronchiolitis, follicular bronchiolitis, or BOOP, each of which is associated with a fairly characteristic constellation of clinical and radiologic features. On the other hand, obliterative bronchiolitis is a characteristic feature of some cases of bone marrow and lung transplantation and of connective tissue disease. As a result of these problems in terminology as well as the real variation in pathologic, clinical, and radiologic features, it is difficult to establish a single all-encompassing classification of bronchiolitis.

Although an etiologic classification is useful for reminding the physician when to suspect the presence of bronchiolitis, in our opinion, the more convenient scheme is based on the histologic characteristics for two important reasons: (1) the histologic patterns of bronchiolitis generally show a better correlation with the clinical and radiologic manifestations of disease than the various etiologies, and (2) the histologic classification shows better correlation with the natural history of disease and the response to therapy. For example, BOOP or follicular bronchiolitis in rheumatoid disease can be expected to respond favorably to corticosteroid therapy, whereas obliterative bronchiolitis usually progresses inexorably to respiratory failure despite treatment.

The classification scheme presented in Table 58–2 is based on a consideration of two pathologic processes: inflammation and fibrosis. The first is related simply to the traditional separation of inflammation into acute and chronic reactions, the former characterized by an exudate of fluid and neutrophils and, frequently, by tissue necrosis and the latter by tissue infiltration by mononuclear cells. From this perspective, bronchiolitis can be subdivided into acute and chronic forms. The first of these is typically associated with processes that cause bronchiolar injury over a short period of time, such as viral infection (Fig. 58–1) or the inhalation of toxic gases. The second is typically associated with more prolonged injury and may itself have a variety of pathologic forms. Some of these variants are histologically distinctive and have thus been described by specific terms, such as *respiratory bronchiolitis, follicular bronchiolitis,* and *diffuse panbronchiolitis* (DPB). The histologic categorization of

## Table 58–1. ETIOLOGIC AGENTS AND CLINICAL CONDITIONS ASSOCIATED WITH BRONCHIOLITIS

### INHALATION OF GASES, FUMES, AND DUSTS

Toxic fumes
Cigarette smoke
Irritant gases ($NO_2$, $SO_2$, ammonia, chlorine, phosgene, HCl)
Mineral dust fumes (e.g., from welding)
Mineral dust particles (e.g., asbestos, silica)
Grain dust

### INFECTION

*Viruses*

Respiratory syncytial virus
Parainfluenza viruses (types 1 and 3)
Adenoviruses (especially types 3, 7, and 21)
Influenza
Rhinovirus
Paramyxoviruses (measles or mumps)
Varicella zoster virus
Cytomegalovirus
Human immunodeficiency virus (HIV)[235]

*Fungi*

*Aspergillus* species[237]
*Pneumocystis carinii*

*Bacteria*

*Bordetella pertussis*

*Parasites*

Malaria
*Cryptosporidium* species
Microsporidia *(Encephalitozoon hellem)*[236]

*Miscellaneous Organisms*

*Mycoplasma pneumoniae*
*Chlamydia* species

### DRUGS AND CHEMICALS

Hexamethonium
L-Tryptophan
Busulphan
Bleomycin
Methotrexate
Lomustine
Penicillamine
Gold
Free-base cocaine
Sulfasalazine
Naproxen
Amiodarone
Amphotericin B
Acebutolol
Sulindac
Paraquat
*Sauropus androgynus*[242]

### IMMUNOLOGIC DISEASE

*Organ Transplantation*

Bone marrow
Heart-lung
Lung

*Connective Tissue Disease*

Rheumatoid arthritis
Systemic lupus erythematosus
Dermatomyositis
Sjögren's syndrome
Eosinophilic fasciitis
Progressive systemic sclerosis
Mixed connective tissue disease
Polymyalgia rheumatica

*Miscellaneous Immunologic Conditions*

Idiopathic pulmonary fibrosis
Extrinsic allergic alveolitis
Acute and chronic eosinophilic pneumonia[238]
Wegener's granulomatosis
Behçet's disease
Chronic thyroiditis
Ulcerative colitis[239]
Primary biliary cirrhosis[240]

### NEOPLASIA

Carcinoid tumor[241]

### MISCELLANEOUS CONDITIONS

Irradiation
Aspiration[3]

Modified from King TE: Overview of bronchiolitis. Clin Chest Med 14:607, 1993; Costabel U, Guzman J, Teschler H: Bronchiolitis obliterans with organizing pneumonia: Outcome. Thorax 50:559, 1995; and Yousem SA: Small airway disease. Pathol Annu 26:109, 1991.

## Table 58–2. BRONCHIOLITIS: PATHOLOGIC CLASSIFICATION WITH CORRESPONDING CLINICAL, FUNCTIONAL, AND RADIOLOGIC FEATURES

| FORMS OF BRONCHIOLITIS | HISTOLOGIC CHARACTERISTICS | CLINICAL FEATURES | FUNCTIONAL FEATURES | RADIOGRAPHIC FEATURES | HRCT FEATURES |
|---|---|---|---|---|---|
| **Acute bronchiolitis** | Predominantly acute but also chronic inflammation associated with epithelial necrosis and a variable degree of inflammation in the adjacent lung parenchyma | Characteristic of infection (particularly viruses and *Mycoplasma pneumoniae*). Also seen as an early reaction following inhalation of toxic fumes or gases. | Obstruction and hyperinflation | Reticulonodular opacities | Centrilobular nodules and branching lines; patchy or diffuse distribution. |
| **Chronic bronchiolitis** | Chronic inflammation (variable numbers of lymphocytes, plasma cells, and histiocytes) and fibrosis. The epithelium may be metaplastic (goblet cells), and there may be increased smooth muscle. Several relatively specific clinicopathologic variants can be seen. | This pattern is the major pathologic finding in the membranous bronchioles of cigarette smokers. It can also be seen following chronic irritation of the airways caused by a variety of inhaled substances (e.g., grain dust and some minerals) and in bronchiectasis and extrinsic allergic alveolitis. | Along with loss of lung elastic recoil, this is the cause of airflow obstruction in chronic obstructive pulmonary disease. | Reticulonodular opacities | Centrilobular nodules |
| Respiratory bronchiolitis | Accumulation of macrophages within membranous and respiratory bronchioles accompanied by a variable degree of lymphocyte infiltration and fibrosis in the bronchiolar wall and peribronchiolar interstitium | This is the earliest lesion seen in cigarette smokers. Patients are usually young and asymptomatic. When dyspnea is associated with radiographic abnormalities and restrictive lung function, the abnormality has been termed *respiratory bronchiolitis–associated interstitial pneumonia* (possibly representing an early manifestation of desquamative interstitial pneumonitis). | May be associated with a mild obstructive pattern or, in some patients, restrictive changes | Ground-glass opacities | Ground-glass attenuation and poorly defined centrilobular nodular opacities; upper lobe predominance |
| Follicular bronchiolitis | Abundant lymphoid tissue, frequently with prominent germinal centers, situated in the walls of bronchioles and, to some extent, bronchi | Most often described in association with rheumatoid arthritis but may be seen in immunodeficiency syndromes and hypersensitivity reactions | Restrictive or obstructive functional abnormality | Reticulonodular opacities | Centrilobular nodules and branching lines |
| Diffuse panbronchiolitis | Mural and intraluminal infiltrates of acute and chronic inflammatory cells. The lesions are centered predominantly on respiratory bronchioles and are associated with a striking accumulation of foamy macrophages within the airway wall and adjacent parenchyma. | Typically seen in patients from Japan and South East Asia | Associated with the progressive development of an obstructive ventilatory defect | Reticulonodular opacities | Centrilobular nodules and branching lines; bronchiolectasis, bronchiectasis, diffuse distribution |

*Table continued on following page*

**Table 58–2. BRONCHIOLITIS: PATHOLOGIC CLASSIFICATION WITH CORRESPONDING CLINICAL, FUNCTIONAL, AND RADIOLOGIC FEATURES** *Continued*

| FORMS OF BRONCHIOLITIS | HISTOLOGIC CHARACTERISTICS | CLINICAL FEATURES | FUNCTIONAL FEATURES | RADIOGRAPHIC FEATURES | HRCT FEATURES |
|---|---|---|---|---|---|
| **Obliterative bronchiolitis** | Fibrous tissue predominantly between the muscularis mucosa and epithelium of membranous bronchioles resulting in more or less concentric airway narrowing. An inflammatory cell infiltrate and fibrosis in the submucosa are variable in intensity but often mild. | Characteristically seen in bone marrow and lung transplant recipients and in some connective tissue diseases (particularly rheumatoid disease) | Progressive airflow obstruction, hyperinflation, and ventilatory respiratory failure | Hyperinflation and peripheral areas of vascular attenuation | Low attenuation and mosaic attenuation; air trapping on expiratory HRCT |
| **Bronchiolitis obliterans organizing pneumonia (BOOP)** | Focal necrosis of the respiratory bronchiolar and alveolar duct epithelium associated with partial or complete air-space occlusion by fibroblast (myofibroblast) proliferation. Mild to moderate interstitial pneumonitis and air-space fibrosis in adjacent parenchyma. | The lesion is most often of unknown etiology, but may occur in association with many causes, including connective tissue diseases, viral and bacterial pneumonia, drugs, aspiration, and airway obstruction. | Restrictive pattern | Patchy, usually bilateral air-space consolidation | Multifocal consolidation, often predominantly peribronchial or subpleural; ground-glass opacities |

these conditions clearly depends on the availability of tissue; however, the clinical and radiologic features associated with specific histologic patterns are often sufficiently characteristic to permit a strong presumptive diagnosis.

In addition to these relatively distinctive patterns of chronic bronchiolitis, nonspecific chronic bronchiolitis characterized by infiltration of the bronchiolar wall by lymphocytes, plasma cells, and histiocytes, accompanied by a variable degree of fibrosis, can be encountered in a variety of situations, including chronic obstructive pulmonary disease[1] (Fig. 58–2), bronchiectasis (Fig. 58–3), lung transplantation (in which it has sometimes been designated lymphocytic bronchiolitis[2]), aspiration of oral or gastric secretions (Fig. 58–4) (a situation that may be associated with foreign body giant cells histologically and with bronchorrhea and wheeze clinically),[3] and chronic inhalation of organic and inorganic dusts[4, 5] (Fig. 58–5). As is evident from this list, the pathogenesis of bronchiolitis in these conditions is varied.

A cause for chronic bronchiolitis is not always apparent, as was shown in one study of four women between the ages of 37 and 59 years who had evidence of airway obstruction on pulmonary function testing but had no history of cigarette smoking, connective tissue disease, significant occupational or environmental dust exposure, bronchiectasis, emphysema, or asthma.[6] Radiograph results were normal or nearly normal; HRCT scan findings were normal in two patients and showed minimal centrilobular thickening in one and diffuse airway dilation in the other. Histologic examination of lung biopsy specimens showed mild thickening of bronchiolar walls, predominantly as a result of an increase in fibrous tissue and muscle. The investigators suggested that the com-

bination of clinical and pathologic findings be designated "cryptogenic constrictive bronchiolitis."[6] It is possible that this represents an early stage of obliterative bronchiolitis.

The term *small airways disease* has also been used to refer to an apparently distinct form of chronic bronchiolitis. In the original report of this "condition," seven patients were described who had air-flow obstruction but no evidence of emphysema and a diffuse reticular or reticulonodular pattern on chest radiography. Histologic examination showed a variable degree of chronic bronchiolar inflammation and mucous plugging.[7] Several of the patients had extensive bronchiectasis at autopsy, and it is possible that the bronchiolar abnormalities represented no more than the reaction seen in the distal airways of patients with this condition; other patients were cigarette smokers, raising the possibility that the bronchiolar disease was related to this agent. Few workers have subsequently investigated the abnormality.[8, 9] In one report of nine patients thought to correspond clinically and functionally to those in the initial report of small airways disease, histologic examination of open-lung biopsy specimens also showed fibrosis and nonspecific chronic inflammation of bronchiolar walls.[9] Patients again had a varied clinical picture; although bronchiectasis was not documented in any, four were smokers, two were ex-smokers, and three were nonsmokers. The authors of this study thought that the abnormality most likely represented a nonspecific reaction to several insults rather than a distinct clinicopathologic entity and suggested that the term "chronic transmural bronchiolitis" was a more appropriate designation. Although we concur with this basic interpretation, we feel that the terms *small airways disease* and *chronic transmural bronchiolitis*

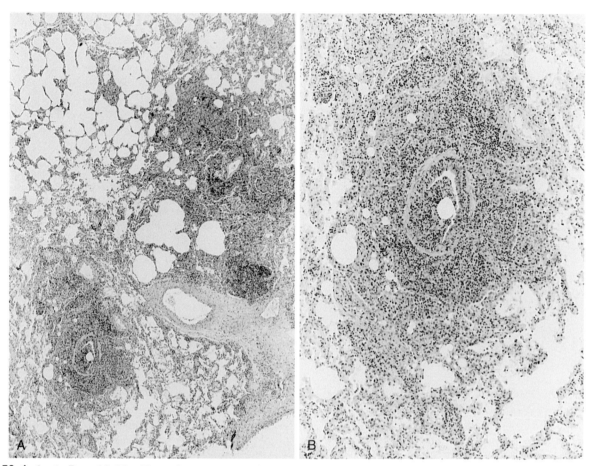

**Figure 58–1. Acute Bronchiolitis: *Mycoplasma pneumoniae.*** Sections from an open-lung biopsy of a 32-year-old man *(A)* show several foci of inflammation centered on membranous bronchioles. A magnified view of one focus *(B)* shows marked inflammation somewhat obscuring the airway wall and lumen and extending into the adjacent alveoli. Both neutrophilic and lymphocytic components were evident at higher magnification.

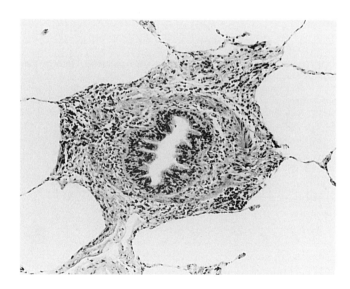

**Figure 58–2. Chronic Bronchiolitis Associated with Tobacco Smoke.** The wall of this small membranous bronchiole is moderately thickened by fibrous tissue and an infiltrate of mononuclear inflammatory cells (predominantly lymphocytes). The abnormality is common in cigarette smokers, in whom it is often associated with functional evidence of airway obstruction.

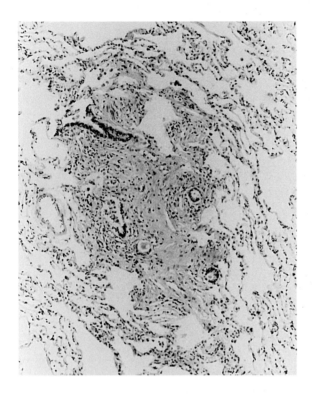

**Figure 58–3. Chronic Bronchiolitis Secondary to Bronchiectasis.** The section shows a focus of fibrous tissue associated with several variably sized lumens lined by bronchiolar-type epithelium. A mild inflammatory infiltrate (predominantly lymphocytes) is present. The original airway lumen is difficult to identify with certainty. The appearance is characteristic of healed bronchiolar injury associated with bronchiectasis but can also be seen after bronchiolitis of other etiologies.

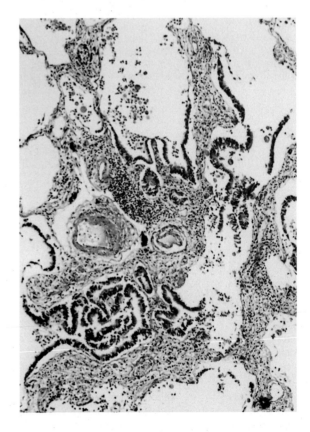

**Figure 58–4. Bronchiolitis Caused by Aspirated Gastric Contents.** A section of a small membranous bronchiole shows distortion and moderately severe fibrosis and chronic inflammation. The bronchiolar epithelium extends into the adjacent parenchyma, which is also emphysematous. Multiple foci of fibrosis and inactive granulomas, some containing foreign material, were present elsewhere in the lung parenchyma. (*A*, ×120; *B*, ×70.)

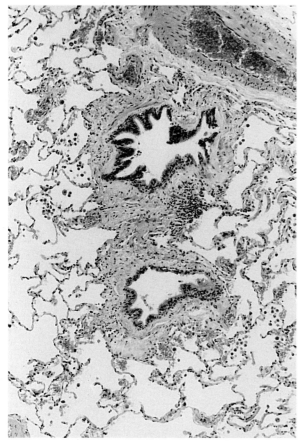

**Figure 58–5. Asbestos-Related Peribronchiolar Fibrosis.** The section shows two membranous bronchioles with walls that are moderately thickened, predominantly as a result of an increase in collagen in the peribronchiolar interstitial tissue; mild chronic inflammation is also evident focally. The patient was a 60-year-old man who had pulmonary carcinoma; he had worked in various jobs for an asbestos mining company. There was no evidence of parenchymal interstitial fibrosis.

only add to semantic confusion and should not be used to refer to a separate diagnostic category of bronchiolitis.

Although there is some degree of overlap with the acute and chronic forms of bronchiolitis as described previously, bronchiolitis can also be subdivided histologically into two forms on the basis of the pattern of fibrosis (Fig. 58–6). The first, which we prefer to call *obliterative bronchiolitis* but which has also been termed *constrictive bronchiolitis*, is characterized by a proliferation of fibrous tissue predominantly between the epithelium and the muscularis mucosa; the proliferation results in a more or less concentric narrowing of the airway lumen, which in its most extreme form, results in complete obliteration. Although fibrous tissue can also be seen in the submucosal and peribronchial tissue, it is typically a relatively minor factor in causing airway narrowing.[10] The epithelium overlying the abnormal fibrous tissue may be flattened or metaplastic but is usually intact (i.e., without evidence of ulceration). By contrast, the epithelium in cases of the second form of bronchiolitis is invariably absent, at least focally. Granulation tissue or plugs of fibroblastic tissue extend from these areas of epithelial damage into the airway lumen, resulting in partial or, occasionally, complete obstruction. Although this histologic pattern

may be the only abnormality seen in the lung, in most cases, it is associated with a similar epithelial injury and fibroblastic reaction in the adjacent parenchyma. Thus, for practical purposes, the bronchiolitis occurs in association with pneumonitis; as a result, the term *bronchiolitis obliterans organizing pneumonia* is frequently used to describe this form of disease.[11, 12] (Although we and others believe the term *cryptogenic organizing pneumonia* is a more appropriate label for the abnormality,[13–15] because of the widespread use of the former term, we continue to use it in this text.)

## RADIOLOGIC MANIFESTATIONS

The radiographic features of bronchiolitis are highly variable and are related to a number of factors, including the extent of airway involvement, the chronicity of the disorder, and the presence or absence of underlying parenchymal abnormality. The radiographic abnormalities are essentially limited to two patterns: hyperinflation and peripheral attenuation of vascular markings (Fig. 58–7), associated with obliterative bronchiolitis, and air-space consolidation in BOOP[12, 16, 17] (Fig. 58–8). The degree of reproducibility in the detection of hyperinflation, peribronchial wall thickening, perihilar linear opacities, atelectasis, and consolidation were compared in one study of 40 cases of bronchiolitis. There was considerable interobserver and intraobserver variability in interpretation of the radiographs; the finding of hyperinflation was most reproducible.[18] The interpretation is strongly influenced by the clinical information provided to the radiologist; if bronchiolitis is mentioned on the requisition, features of bronchiolitis are reported even on radiographs with normal findings.[19] In another study, there was no correlation between the clinical severity of the bronchiolitis and the degree of radiologic change.[20] The anatomic detail that can be revealed using HRCT allows an appreciation of greater radiologic variability; in fact, a number of radiologic and pathologic correlative studies have demonstrated that HRCT can suggest the predominant histologic pattern of bronchiolitis.[21, 22, 22a] Because of this ability, HRCT is clearly the radiologic method of choice for investigating a patient suspected on clinical or radiographic grounds of having bronchiolitis.

As the previous discussion implies, a number of patterns can be seen on HRCT in patients who have bronchiolitis; these include centrilobular nodules and branching lines, areas of decreased attenuation, air-space consolidation, and ground-glass attenuation. Thickening of the bronchiolar wall or filling of dilated bronchioles with granulation tissue, mucus, or pus results in a pattern of small centrilobular nodules and branching lines. These abnormalities represent enlarged bronchioles coursing perpendicular and parallel to the CT plane of section. This pattern is characteristic of acute infectious bronchiolitis; in some cases, it is accompanied by scattered areas of ground-glass attenuation or consolidation[22] (Fig. 58–9). A similar CT appearance can be seen in immunocompromised patients who develop acute *Aspergillus* bronchiolitis[23] (Fig. 58–10) or endobronchial spread of tuberculosis.[23a] A pattern of centrilobular nodules and branching lines ("tree-in-bud") is also seen in DPB.[24–26] Small centrilobular nodules reflecting bronchiolar inflammation and wall

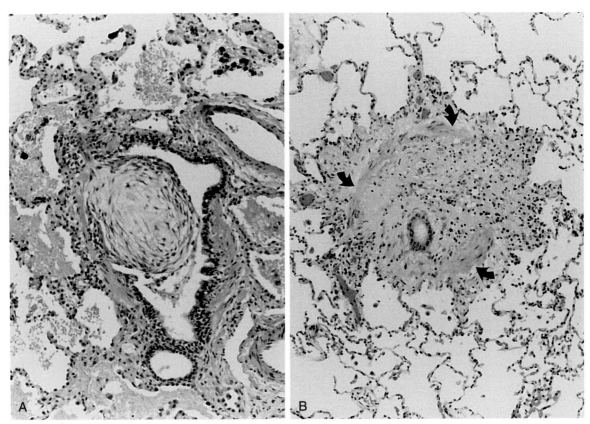

**Figure 58–6. Bronchiolitis with Fibrosis.** Sections of membranous bronchioles from two patients show two major histologic patterns of bronchiolar fibrosis. In *A*, a plug of fibroblastic tissue partially occludes the airway lumen. The epithelium is absent where the fibrous tissue is in contact with the airway wall, suggesting that the latter represents organization of an exudate secondary to epithelial ulceration. The patient had experienced an episode of presumed bacterial pneumonia about 1 month before death. This pattern of fibrosis is usually seen in association with similar plugs of fibroblastic tissue in alveolar air spaces, in which case the abnormality is termed *bronchiolitis obliterans organizing pneumonia.* In *B*, the airway lumen is markedly narrowed by fibrous tissue that more or less completely surrounds intact epithelium (residual muscularis mucosa is indicated by *arrows*). The patient had long-standing rheumatoid disease and had developed progressive dyspnea associated with obstructive lung function.

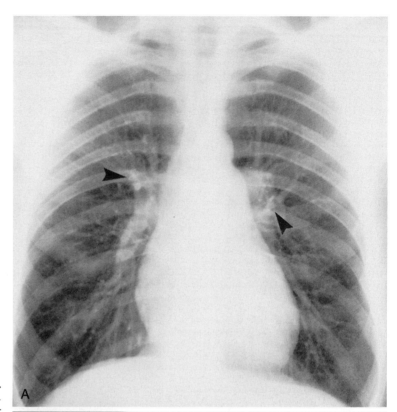

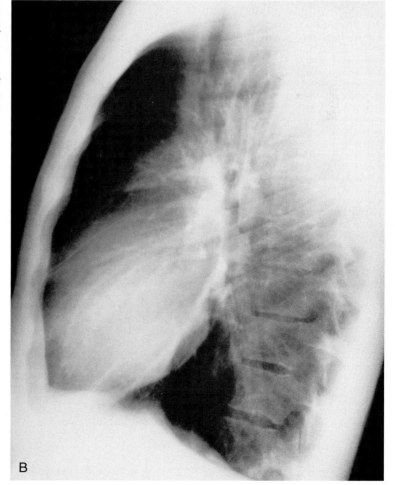

**Figure 58–7. Obliterative Bronchiolitis of Unknown Etiology.** Posteroanterior *(A)* and lateral *(B)* chest radiographs demonstrate pulmonary overinflation. The vasculature in the lower lung zones appears somewhat attenuated and in the upper lung zones more prominent than normal, indicating recruitment. When these changes are considered in conjunction with prominence of the main pulmonary artery and probable right ventricular enlargement, the findings are consistent with pulmonary arterial hypertension. Bronchial walls are thickened *(arrowheads)*. Histologic examination of the lungs at autopsy showed typical changes of obliterative bronchiolitis and pulmonary artery hypertension. The patient was a young man who presented with progressive dyspnea and right-sided heart failure.

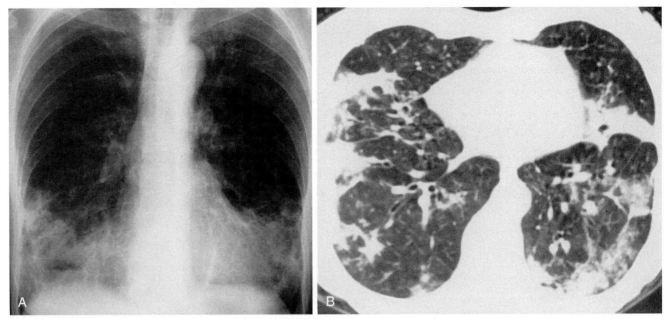

**Figure 58–8. Bronchiolitis Obliterans Organizing Pneumonia (BOOP).** A posteroanterior chest radiograph *(A)* in a 64-year-old woman demonstrates bilateral areas of consolidation involving the lower lung zones. A CT scan *(B)* demonstrates the predominantly peribronchial and subpleural distribution of the areas of consolidation. The diagnosis of idiopathic BOOP was confirmed by open biopsy.

thickening can sometimes be seen in patients who have diseases that affect the larger airways, such as asthma, chronic obstructive pulmonary disease, and bronchiectasis.[27, 28] The centrilobular nodules in infectious bronchiolitis and panbronchiolitis usually have well-defined, sharp margins,[22, 25, 28] whereas those seen in patients who have respiratory bronchiolitis typically have poorly defined margins[22, 29, 30] (Fig. 58–11).

A heterogeneous pattern of attenuation (mosaic attenua-

tion) consisting of areas of decreased density and vascularity is characteristic of obliterative bronchiolitis (Fig. 58–12).[17, 31, 32, 32a] The variation in attenuation of individual lobules is accentuated when images are obtained after the patient exhales to residual volume[32a, 33, 34, 34a] (Fig. 58–13). This pattern is presumed to be caused by heterogeneity of airway involvement resulting in patchy airway closure. The areas of decreased attenuation are the result of airway closure (causing air trapping) and local hypoxemia (causing pulmonary arte-

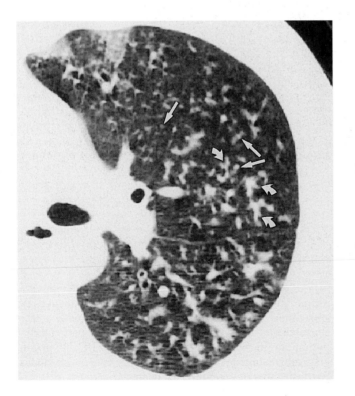

**Figure 58–9. Bronchiolitis Related to *Mycoplasma pneumoniae.*** A view of the left upper lung from an HRCT scan demonstrates small centrilobular nodules *(straight arrows)* and branching linear opacities *(curved arrows)* ("tree-in-bud" pattern). Localized areas of ground-glass attenuation are also evident anteriorly. Open-lung biopsy demonstrated an exquisitely bronchiolocentric process with inflammation of the bronchiolar wall and the presence of intraluminal exudate. Serologic tests were positive for *M. pneumoniae.* (From Müller NL, Miller RR: Diseases of the bronchioles: CT and histopathologic findings. Radiology 196:3, 1995.)

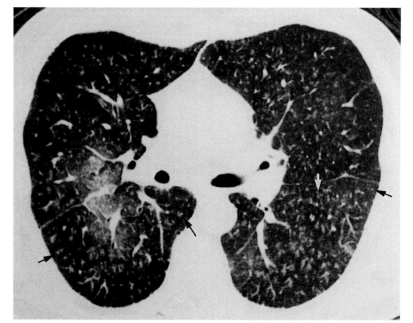

**Figure 58–10. Bronchiolitis Related to *Aspergillus* Species.** An HRCT scan demonstrates bilateral centrilobular nodular and branching opacities *(arrows)*. Also noted is a focal area of ground-glass attenuation in the right lung. The diagnosis of *Aspergillus* bronchiolitis and early bronchopneumonia was confirmed by open-lung biopsy. The patient was a 52-year-old man who had leukemia.

rial vasoconstriction). The increased attenuation is caused by redistribution of blood flow to the relatively normal lung. Small, focal areas of low attenuation, as well as small areas of air trapping, can also be seen in healthy subjects.[32, 35, 36]

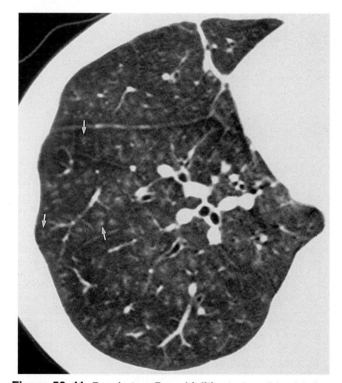

**Figure 58–11. Respiratory Bronchiolitis.** A view of the right lower lung from an HRCT scan demonstrates poorly defined centrilobular nodular opacities *(arrows)* and localized areas of ground-glass attenuation. The diagnosis of respiratory bronchiolitis was confirmed by transbronchial biopsy. The patient was a 54-year-old heavy smoker who subsequently stopped the habit; a follow-up CT scan performed 5 years later was normal. (Courtesy of Dr. Takeshi Johkoh, Osaka University Medical School, Osaka, Japan.)

Although these can affect one or several lobules at various sites, they are most commonly seen in the superior segments of the lower lobes and near the tip of the lingula. Usually, they involve less than 25% of the cross-sectional area of one lung at one scan level.[35] Mosaic attenuation and air trapping can be considered abnormal when they affect a volume of lung equal to or greater than a pulmonary segment and are not limited to the superior segment of the lower lobe or the lingula tip.[32, 36] Mosaic attenuation and air trapping are seen on HRCT in patients who have obliterative bronchiolitis regardless of etiology,[17, 22, 32, 37] extrinsic allergic alveolitis,[38, 39] asthma,[36, 39a, 39b] and bronchiectasis.[27, 39c] It should be remembered, however, that similar findings are occasionally seen in patients who have pulmonary vascular abnormalities, particularly hypertension secondary to chronic thromboembolism.[39d]

Unilateral or bilateral areas of consolidation are characteristic of BOOP (Fig. 58–14). The consolidation is often patchy; although it may have a random distribution, in about 50% of cases, it affects mainly the peribronchial or subpleural lung regions.[40, 41] The consolidation reflects the presence of organizing pneumonia. Centrilobular nodular opacities may reflect the presence of intrabronchiolar granulation tissue polyps or peribronchiolar consolidation. Focal areas of consolidation can also be seen in association with centrilobular nodular and branching linear opacities in infectious bronchiolitis and bronchopneumonia.[22, 23]

Ground-glass attenuation can be seen in association with respiratory bronchiolitis,[22, 29, 30] respiratory bronchiolitis with interstitial lung disease,[22, 42] and BOOP.[40, 41] In respiratory bronchiolitis, the abnormality is bilateral, may be diffuse or patchy in distribution, and tends to involve predominantly or exclusively the upper lung zones.[29, 30] Ground-glass attenuation is also often seen in association with areas of consolidation in BOOP.[40, 41, 43] Occasionally, particularly in immunocompromised patients who have BOOP, ground-glass attenuation is the only abnormality evident on HRCT.[41] Extrinsic allergic alveolitis is characterized on HRCT by

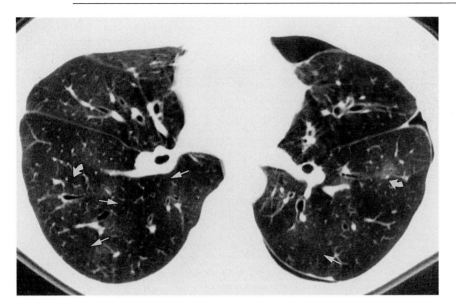

**Figure 58–12. Obliterative Bronchiolitis.**
HRCT demonstrates localized areas of decreased attenuation *(straight arrows)* and areas of slightly increased attenuation *(curved arrows)*, a pattern known as *mosaic attenuation.* Note the greater number and size of vessels within the areas that have increased attenuation. The patient was a 29-year-old woman who developed bronchiolitis as a result of chronic graft-versus-host disease. Incidental note is made of a small left pneumothorax.

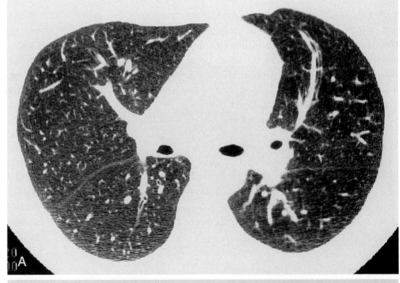

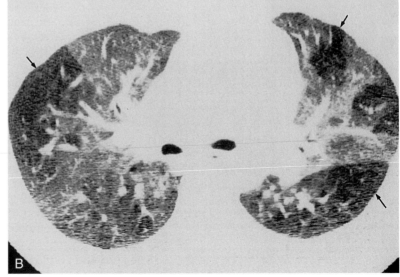

**Figure 58–13. Obliterative Bronchiolitis: Value of Expiratory HRCT.** A 32-year-old woman demonstrated progressive shortness of breath and airway obstruction 1 year after bone marrow transplantation. Inspiratory HRCT *(A)* shows questionable localized areas of low attenuation. HRCT performed at end expiration *(B)* demonstrates several areas of air trapping *(arrows)*. These can be readily distinguished from the normal increased attenuation seen at end expiration in the normal lung. (From Worthy SL, Müller NL: Small airways disease. Radiol Clin North Am 36:163, 1998.)

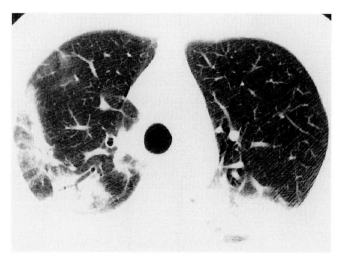

**Figure 58–14. Bronchiolitis Obliterans Organizing Pneumonia (BOOP).** HRCT at the level of the aortic arch shows bilateral areas of consolidation in a predominantly subpleural and peribronchial distribution. The patient was a 46-year-old man who had idiopathic BOOP diagnosed at video-assisted thoracoscopic biopsy. (From Worthy SL, Müller NL: Small airways disease. Radiol Clin North Am 36:163, 1998.)

the presence of poorly defined centrilobular opacities and extensive bilateral areas of ground-glass attenuation. Localized areas of low attenuation also have been observed in 50% to 70% of patients[38, 39] (Fig. 58–15). These areas have been confirmed to represent air trapping on expiratory CT scan[39] and to correlate with both an increase in residual volume and the residual volume–to–total lung capacity (TLC) ratio;[38] they are presumed to be secondary to bronchiolitis.[38]

## SPECIFIC CLINICOPATHOLOGIC FORMS OF BRONCHIOLITIS

The following includes a discussion of the features of the different etiologies and forms of bronchiolitis according to the classifications shown in Tables 58–1 and 58–2;[44, 45] additional details of some of the conditions are provided in appropriate sections of the book.

### Acute Bronchiolitis

#### Acute Infectious Bronchiolitis

Acute bronchiolitis is characteristically the result of infection by organisms such as viruses, *Mycoplasma pneumoniae,* and *Chlamydia* species. Symptomatic viral infection of the small airways is most common and most severe in children younger than 3 years; males are more often affected than females.[46–48] Although it is likely that the trachea and large bronchi are also involved in most cases, it is the involvement of the small airways that is responsible for most of the morbidity. The incidence of infectious bronchiolitis is as high as 10 per 100 children per year in the first year of life in the United States.[49, 50] In a prospective study of 253 healthy infants in Australia, the disease was recognized in 7% during the first 2 years of life;[51] 1% required hospitaliza-

tion. In infants, the most common etiologic agents are the respiratory syncytial virus (RSV), the adenoviruses (types 3, 7, and 21), rhinovirus, and parainfluenza virus (especially type 3). *Chlamydia* species and *M. pneumoniae* are also responsible for some cases.

The organisms can be cultured from respiratory tract secretions or detected using antibodies or the polymerase chain reaction (PCR). Although the responsible organism is not identified in many cases, the use of powerful new molecular biology diagnostic tests has the potential to increase diagnostic yields; for example, in one study of 152 nasopharyngeal aspirates from patients who had bronchiolitis, PCR-based techniques were able to detect *Chlamydia pneumoniae* in 1.3% and *Chlamydia trachomatis* in 17%.[52]

Details of the epidemiologic and clinical features of viral respiratory tract infection in general and bronchiolitis in particular are given in Chapter 29; however, a few general comments are in order at this point. Infection by viruses and organisms such as *Chlamydia* and *Mycoplasma* species can vary in severity from a mild upper respiratory tract infection to croup, tracheobronchitis, bronchiolitis, and pneumonia. The morbidity and mortality rates vary considerably with different organisms; for example, about 1% of patients with proven RSV bronchiolitis die,[46] whereas in some series in which infection has been caused by a variety of organisms, the death rate has been much higher (e.g., 5.5% of 1,230 patients in one review[53]). Most deaths occur in infants younger than 6 months of age and in patients who have congenital anomalies. Additional risk factors for severe or fatal bronchiolitis include bronchopulmonary dysplasia, prematurity, and immunodeficiency.[54, 55] Breastfeeding affords a protective benefit,[56, 57] whereas antenatal maternal cigarette smoking, passive postnatal smoke exposure, and short gestation increase the incidence of bronchiolitis.[54, 58] Children from homes that are at a lower socioeconomic level are also more likely to have bronchiolitis that requires admission to hospital.[59]

Histologic examination of the airways of patients who have infectious bronchiolitis usually shows necrosis of the respiratory epithelium and a mixed lymphocytic and neutrophilic peribronchial and intraepithelial infiltrate (*see* Fig. 58–1). Some degree of accompanying interstitial pneumonitis is frequently seen, accompanied by a variable degree of atelectasis and hyperinflation.[49] In more long-standing cases, evidence of epithelial regeneration may be present. Sometimes (particularly following adenovirus infection), bronchiolectasis, obliterative bronchiolitis, and bronchiectasis remain as sequelae and are associated with the Swyer-James syndrome (*see* farther on).[60, 61] Although intraepithelial viral replication and subsequent epithelial cell lysis is the likely explanation for these pathologic findings in most cases, there is evidence that the immune response, especially in cases of RSV infection, may play a role in the pathogenesis.[49]

The radiographic findings of viral and mycoplasmal bronchiolitis consist of hyperinflation, reticulonodular opacities, and patchy areas of consolidation and atelectasis[62–64] (Fig. 58–16). Hyperinflation is particularly common in children younger than 2 years; it occurs less often in children between the ages of 3 and 5 and is uncommon in older patients.[65] Pathologic correlation shows these patterns to be related to peribronchiolitis and to small focal areas of atelectasis and pneumonitis.[22, 66] Cases of bronchiolitis associated

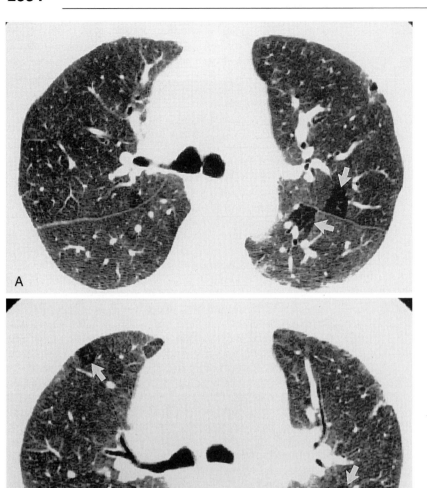

A

B

**Figure 58–15. Extrinsic Allergic Alveolitis.** HRCT obtained at end inspiration *(A)* shows bilateral areas of ground-glass attenuation and focal areas of decreased attenuation and decreased vascularity *(arrows)*. The areas of decreased attenuation have a configuration and size that correspond to a secondary pulmonary lobule. HRCT obtained at end expiration *(B)* shows air trapping *(arrows)*. The latter is presumably related to bronchiolitis, whereas the areas of ground-glass attenuation reflect the presence of alveolitis.

with adenovirus and influenza virus often have more extensive radiographic changes than those caused by RSV.[67] Mycoplasma may cause a radiographic pattern indistinguishable from that of viral pneumonia.[68] The findings consist of a reticular, nodular (Fig. 58–17), or reticulonodular pattern followed by patchy areas of consolidation.[68, 69] HRCT may demonstrate centrilobular nodules or branching lines, which reflect the presence of bronchiolitis (*see* Fig. 58–9), and focal areas of consolidation.

The clinical manifestations in infants typically begin with symptoms of an upper respiratory tract infection, which is followed 2 to 3 days later by the abrupt onset of dyspnea, tachypnea (respiratory rates between 50 and 80 breaths per minute), fever, cyanosis, and often severe prostration.[70] Physical signs include widespread low- and high-pitched wheezes, fine and coarse crackles, and evidence of hyperinflation. In previously healthy infants, the usual course of the disease consists of 2 or 3 days of severe symptoms followed by progressive recovery. About 2% to 5% of hospitalized infants develop severe gas exchange abnormalities and ventilatory respiratory failure. Functional residual capacity is in-

creased during the acute episode and returns to normal with resolution.[71] Pulse oximetry and the presence of crackles and cyanosis on clinical examination most closely predict the severity of the subsequent clinical course.[72]

The relative importance of edema, inflammatory cell infiltration, and airway smooth muscle contraction to the airway narrowing of bronchiolitis is controversial.[73] Acute administration of a beta₂-adrenergic agonist has been found to have a beneficial effect;[74] however, adrenaline, which has both beta₂ and alpha effects, appears to be superior, perhaps because it constricts dilated bronchial microvessels.[75] The relationship between bronchiolitis and recurrent wheeze and the development of asthma is controversial and is discussed further on page 2111.

Adults are probably infected with respiratory tract viruses as often as infants, but in otherwise healthy individuals, the consequences of infection are usually much less severe; however, extensive inflammation of the small bronchioles can be a potentially fatal complication.[76] Adults may be spared the severe symptoms characteristic of the infection in infants because their small airways contribute less to total

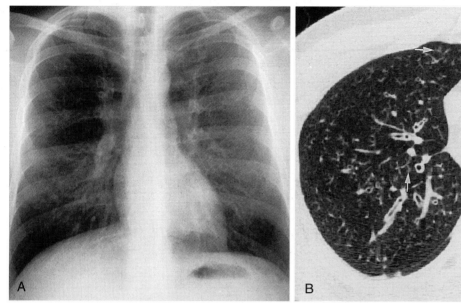

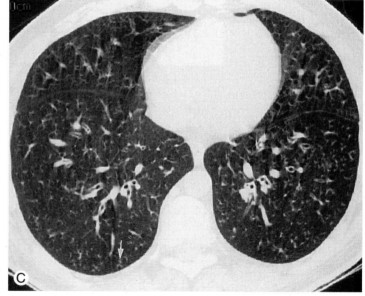

**Figure 58–16. Acute Bronchiolitis Related to *Mycoplasma pneumoniae.*** A 32-year-old man presented with fever, dry cough, and rapidly progressive shortness of breath. A postero-anterior chest radiograph *(A)* demonstrates bronchial wall thickening, increased lung volumes, and poorly defined small parenchymal opacities. An HRCT scan through the upper lobes *(B)* confirms the presence of extensive bronchial wall thickening and demonstrates centrilobular nodular and branching linear opacities *(arrows)*. Also noted are localized areas of decreased attenuation and vascularity, presumably secondary to bronchiolar obstruction. HRCT at a more caudad level *(C)* shows similar findings. Serologic tests were positive for *M. pneumoniae.*

pulmonary resistance;[77] in a morphologic-physiologic correlative study, the resistance of the peripheral airways of children younger than 5 years was found to be relatively high compared with that of older children and adults, making the former group particularly susceptible to bronchiolar infection.[77]

### Bronchiolitis Related to Toxic Gases, Fumes, and Dusts

A variety of inorganic and organic agents can cause inhalational lung injury; bronchiolitis may be the major manifestation or a minor component of such injury.[78] Acute exposure to smoke,[79] $SO_2$, the oxides of nitrogen, and a variety of other gases and fumes can cause bronchiolitis that is associated with severe air-flow obstruction. Symptoms of cough and dyspnea appear minutes or hours after exposure and may be accompanied by the development of pulmonary edema within 4 to 24 hours. The pathologic changes at this stage consist mainly of necrosis of bronchiolar epithelium

associated with an acute inflammatory exudate.[80] If patients survive this acute disease, a delayed second phase may occur within 2 to 5 weeks. This is characterized clinically by increased obstruction, fever, chills, cough, dyspnea, and cyanosis;[81–83] corresponding pathologic findings are predominantly those of obliterative bronchiolitis.[84] When the concentrations of gases or fumes are not so high, acute symptoms may be minimal, and there can be a symptom-free period before the second phase begins.

During a fire, a large number of potentially injurious chemicals may be generated, depending on what is burning. Wood and wood products are associated with carbon monoxide, oxides of nitrogen, acetaldehyde, and formaldehyde; plastics with carbon monoxide, hydrogen chloride, and phosgene; and silk, nylon, and wool with ammonia and hydrogen cyanide.[78] Hydrogen chloride, phosgene, $NO_2$, $SO_2$, and ammonia react with water to produce strong acids and alkalis that damage the epithelium. Smoke-induced injury also acts by oxygen radical formation. Long-term exposure to lower

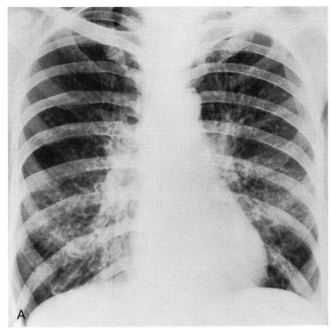

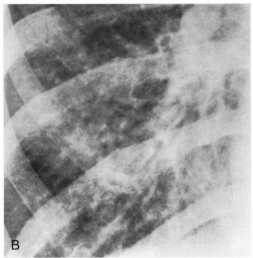

**Figure 58–17. Acute Bronchiolitis Related to *Mycoplasma pneumoniae.*** A posteroanterior radiograph *(A)* shows an extensive, coarse reticulonodular pattern throughout both lungs associated with moderate pulmonary overinflation. The pattern is well seen in a magnified view of the lower portion of the right lung *(B)*. This 70-year-old man was admitted to the hospital with an acute respiratory illness; pulmonary function studies revealed changes consistent with extensive obstruction of small airways. *Mycoplasma* species infection was confirmed.

levels of the products of combustion may lead to more chronic bronchiolar inflammation and progressive air-flow obstruction, as is seen in professional firefighters.[85]

Bronchiolitis is a prominent component of extrinsic allergic alveolitis[86, 87] and is also the probable cause of the obstructive ventilatory defect seen in workers chronically exposed to grain dust.[88] Exposure to a variety of organic substances containing microorganisms may also result in organic dust toxic syndrome.[89] Clinical manifestations of this condition include cough, fever, and myalgia.[90, 91] Pathologically, it is characterized by a mononuclear inflammatory infiltrate within the walls of respiratory bronchioles. Although the pathogenesis is not known, it has been hypothe-

sized that it is caused by high concentrations of endotoxin in the dust; a similar mechanism may underlie the symptoms of obstructive lung function and bronchiolitis experienced by workers in the poultry and swine confinement industries (*see* page 2379).[92–95]

### Chronic Bronchiolitis

#### *Bronchiolitis Associated with Connective Tissue Disease*

Bronchiolitis is an occasional complication of a number of connective tissue diseases (*see* Table 58–1), particularly rheumatoid disease (*see* page 1445).[96–103] In the latter condition, it may take a variety of forms, including obliterative bronchiolitis, follicular bronchiolitis,[104] lymphocytic bronchiolitis, BOOP,[105] and (rarely) DPB;[106] chronic bronchiolitis also may be seen as a result of bronchiectasis. The obliterative form may be more frequent in patients with rheumatoid disease who have been treated with penicillamine[107] or gold.[108] However, despite the widespread use of penicillamine in progressive systemic sclerosis, no cases of bronchiolitis have been reported,[103] suggesting that it is the underlying connective tissue disease rather than the drug that is responsible. BOOP is more common in rheumatoid disease than is interstitial pneumonitis.[109] In Sjögren's syndrome, lymphocytic or follicular bronchiolitis is the most frequently encountered form; in affected individuals, it may be part of a more generalized process of lymphocytic interstitial pneumonitis.[103] Abnormalities of lung function are dependent on the predominant pathologic changes that are present; in obliterative bronchiolitis, there is severe airway obstruction unassociated with evidence of loss of lung recoil or impaired diffusion.[110, 111]

#### *Obliterative Bronchiolitis Associated with Organ Transplantation*

Obliterative bronchiolitis is an important complication of bone marrow, lung, and heart-lung transplantation (*see* pages 1728 and 1707).[112, 113] It is a relatively uncommon complication of the first of these, seen in 5% or less of patients who receive allogenic transplants;[114] however, it has been reported in up to 70% of lung transplant recipients and has been the cause of death of more than half of the affected individuals.[115–118] Most patients present with a history of cough and progressive breathlessness. Lung function testing reveals progressive air-flow obstruction.[119, 120]

The pathogenesis of the bronchiolitis in these patients is varied. Although obliterative bronchiolitis in heart-lung transplant recipients is almost invariably a manifestation of rejection,[121] two cases have been described in which infection with the normally harmless commensal organism *Corynebacterium pseudodiphtheriticum* was implicated in the pathogenesis.[122] Coexistent cytomegalovirus infection likely accelerates the course of bronchiolitis in lung transplant recipients.[123] Most patients who have obliterative bronchiolitis in the setting of bone marrow transplantation have evidence of chronic graft-versus-host disease (GVHD) elsewhere in the body, and it has been suggested that the bronchiolitis may represent a primary manifestation of this process in the lungs.[124–127] However, the variability of bronchoalveolar lavage (BAL) fluid findings in obliterative bronchiolitis (at times lymphocyte predominant, which is characteristic of GVHD, and at times neutrophil predominant)[128] and its demonstration in the absence of GVHD in some series[129] suggest that the pathogenesis is more complicated and, perhaps, multifactorial.

### Swyer-James Syndrome

Swyer-James syndrome is an uncommon abnormality characterized radiographically by a hyperlucent lobe or lung and functionally by normal or reduced volume during inspiration and air trapping during expiration.[130] The condition has also been termed *Macleod's syndrome*,[131] *unilateral* or *lobar emphysema,* and *unilateral hyperlucent lung.* As some of these terms suggest, the abnormality has been considered by some to represent a variant of emphysema. However, it is now clear that the hyperlucency of the affected lung or lobe is primarily the result of decreased pulmonary blood volume secondary to bronchiolar obliteration rather than of destruction of pulmonary parenchyma; as a result, we prefer to include a discussion of the syndrome in a chapter on bronchiolitis. Unfortunately, use of the terms *unilateral emphysema* and *unilateral hyperlucent lung* has also directed attention to a single radiographic feature of a disease that in fact has a variety of modes of expression. For example, the condition may occur in various anatomic distributions, including one segment,[132] one lobe, two lobes in the right lung, and the lower lobe of one lung and the upper lobe of the other. Other disease entities, such as proximal interruption of a pulmonary artery and massive thromboembolism, can cause unilateral hyperlucency and decreased lung volume;[133] however, in contrast to Swyer-James syndrome, these conditions are not associated with air trapping.

### Pathogenesis

There is substantial evidence that the syndrome is initiated by viral bronchiolitis. In many cases, the disease is recognized (or at least suspected) in childhood when chest radiography is carried out in the investigation of repeated respiratory infections. In others, the condition does not become apparent until adulthood on the basis of a screening chest radiograph of a completely asymptomatic patient. Inquiry in these cases often reveals a history of acute lower respiratory tract infection, generally during childhood.[134–137] For example, a baseline normal chest radiograph was obtained in one child shortly before the development of an adenoviral pneumonia; after resolution of the pneumonia, the affected lung was hyperlucent, and on subsequent follow-up, it was of reduced volume and exhibited gas trapping and bronchographic evidence of bronchiectasis.[138] In another report, all of six children who developed the syndrome had definite or highly suggestive evidence of previous adenoviral pneumonia[139] (Fig. 58–18).

Most cases of Swyer-James syndrome, therefore, probably begin as an acute bronchiolitis that progresses to fibrous obliteration of the airway lumen; the peripheral parenchyma is largely unaffected and remains inflated because of collateral ventilation with resulting air trapping. Destructive changes characteristic of emphysema also supervene in some cases.[140] The pathogenesis of this complication is unclear;

however, it is conceivable that infection persists in some cases, with consequent elastolysis from phagocytic proteases. In a recent study, analysis of cells obtained by BAL from two patients showed an increased number of CD8+ T cells (T-suppressor cytotoxic), suggesting to the authors that there was an ongoing active process.[141]

### Pathologic Characteristics

There have been few descriptions of the pathologic characteristics of Swyer-James syndrome. Specimens that have been examined have shown bronchitis, bronchiectasis, chronic bronchiolitis, obliterative bronchiolitis, and a variable degree of destruction of lung parenchyma.[130, 142–144] Focal anthracosis, which is almost invariable in adult lungs with centrilobular emphysema, is typically absent in affected lungs, probably because of the young age at which the condition is usually acquired and the reduction in ventilation that characterizes the disease.

### Radiologic Manifestations

The radiographic manifestations usually are easily recognized and are virtually pathognomonic. A posteroanterior radiograph of the chest exposed at TLC reveals a remarkable difference in the radiolucency of the two lungs (or of the affected and unaffected lobes), caused not by a relative increase in air in the affected lung but by decreased perfusion. The peripheral pulmonary markings are diminutive as a result of vascular narrowing and attenuation. The ipsilateral hilum also is diminutive but is present, a feature of value in the differentiation from proximal interruption of a pulmonary artery (pulmonary artery agenesis). In radiographs exposed at TLC, the volume of the affected lung (or lobe) either is comparable to that of the normal contralateral lung or is reduced (Fig. 58–19); it is seldom, if ever, increased. The volume of the affected lung depends to a large extent on the age of the patient at the time of the infectious insult: the younger the patient at the time of the bronchiolitis or pneumonia, the smaller the fully developed lung, presumably because the insult retards further maturation.[142, 145] However, the volume probably relates also to the presence of focal atelectasis and fibrosis.[140]

One of the characteristic radiologic features of Swyer-James syndrome—in fact, a *sine qua non* for diagnosis—is the presence of air trapping during expiration (*see* Fig. 58–19). This is a reflection of airway obstruction and is extremely valuable in differentiating the syndrome from other conditions that may give rise to unilateral or lobar hyperlucency. Because the contralateral lung is normal, expiration (particularly if rapid) causes the mediastinum to swing abruptly toward the normal lung; in addition, excursion of the hemidiaphragms is markedly asymmetric because it is severely diminished on the affected side. Radiographs exposed at residual volume also accentuate the disparity in radiolucency of the two lungs; the density of the normal lung is much greater. This is related to the fact that the normal lung contains less air and, perhaps more important, to the fact that its blood flow is virtually the total output of the right ventricle. Pulmonary angiography outlines clearly the diminutive hilar vessels on the affected side and the much narrowed, attenuated arteries coursing through the

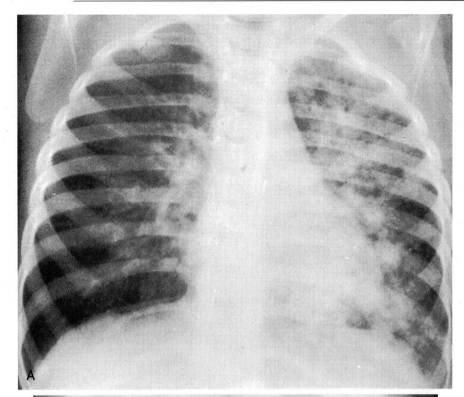

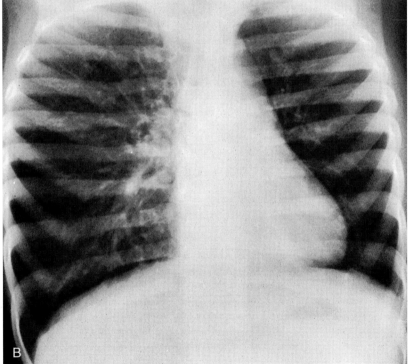

**Figure 58–18. Swyer-James Syndrome.**
This girl was first seen at the Winnipeg Children's Hospital at the age of 17 months with a history of recent onset of cough and fever. A chest radiograph *(A)* reveals patchy pneumonia involving the left lung and the medial third of the right lung. The etiology was not established at that time, although several months later, titers of 1:32 to adenovirus were found on two occasions, suggesting that this may have been the responsible organism. Three and one half years after the initial episode, a chest radiograph *(B)* reveals marked asymmetry in density of the two lungs, the left being relatively radiolucent and showing a sparsity of vascular markings; it is also considerably smaller than the right.

radiolucent lung (*see* Fig. 58–18). The findings on pulmonary angiography can be misleading; unless the contrast medium is injected directly into the affected pulmonary artery, this vessel may not be opacified, creating the erroneous impression that the abnormality may represent proximal interruption of the pulmonary artery.[136] However, pulmonary arteriography is now seldom indicated in the investigation of these patients because inspiratory and expiratory radiographs and CT or spiral CT angiography are usually sufficient for diagnosis.[22, 146–149]

In one study of nine patients who had Swyer-James syndrome, 8- to 10-mm collimation CT scans were compared with bronchography (seven) and angiography (five).[148] Eight of the nine affected lungs had decreased attenuation on CT; the other was small but had normal attenuation. Air trapping was present in all cases; on the expiratory CT scan, there

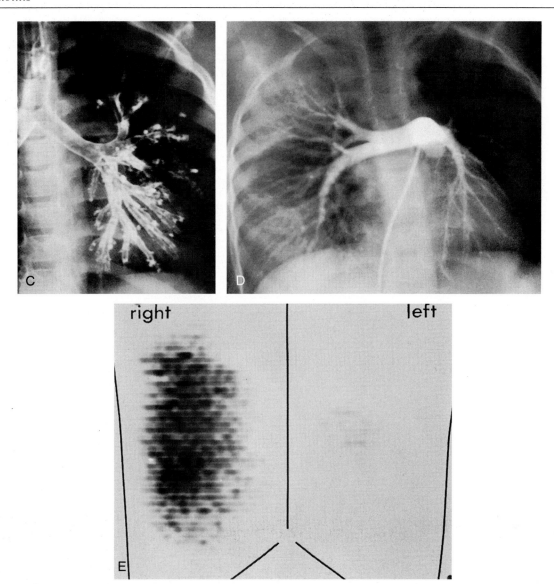

**Figure 58–18** *Continued.* A left bronchogram *(C)* demonstrates general slight dilation of all segmental bronchi, each bronchus terminating abruptly in a squared or truncated ending. The appearance is highly suggestive of obliterative bronchiolitis and mild cylindrical bronchiectasis. A pulmonary angiogram *(D)* reveals marked disparity in the perfusion of the two lungs, with most of the contrast medium passing to the right. Decreased perfusion is also evident in the scan in *E.* (Courtesy of Dr. R. I. Macpherson.)

was no appreciable change in the volume of the affected lung, whereas the normal lung decreased in volume. All nine patients had evidence of bronchiectasis and decreased size of the pulmonary vessels (Fig. 58–20). The CT findings were similar to those seen at bronchography and arteriography. In another study of eight patients (of whom seven had HRCT 1.5- to 2-mm collimation scans and one conventional CT), seven had unilateral hyperlucent lung on the radiograph and one had asymmetric areas of hyperlucency.[149] On CT scans, five patients demonstrated bilateral areas of decreased attenuation, and five had areas of normal attenuation within the hyperlucent lung, indicating that the process was much more heterogeneous than previously suspected. Air trapping within the hyperlucent lung was confirmed with the expiratory CT scan in five patients. Bronchiectasis was seen in only three of the eight patients.

Ventilation-perfusion lung scans may provide useful information in selected cases.[150, 151] In one review of 607 perfusion lung scans performed over a 1-year period, 13 revealed total absence of perfusion of one lung. Only one of these was due to the Swyer-James syndrome; the remainder were the result of pulmonary thromboembolism, parenchymal lung disease, pulmonary carcinoma, congenital heart disease, and pneumonectomy. Radionuclide $\dot{V}/\dot{Q}$ scans may reveal additional areas of involvement, as in a patient in whom an area of diminished perfusion was detected in the contralateral lung, which did not appear hyperlucent on a conventional chest radiograph.[152] Ventilation-perfusion lung imaging is preferable to perfusion scanning alone because the latter does not exclude purely vascular abnormalities, such as thromboembolism.[153] Selective bronchial arteriography and bronchial arterial lung scans have revealed extensive systemic hypervascularity and increased perfusion of the hyperlucent lung.[154] The diminutive pulmonary artery to an affected lung can be detected by echocardiography.[155]

Although not performed nowadays, a characteristic de-

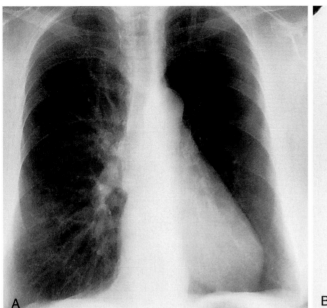

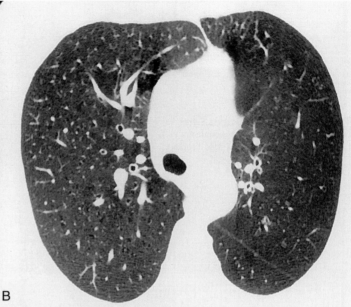

**Figure 58–19. Swyer-James Syndrome.** A posteroanterior chest radiograph *(A)* shows increased radiolucency and decreased vascularity and size of the left lung. An HRCT scan *(B)* at end inspiration confirms the radiographic findings. The left lung is decreased in volume and is associated with shift of the mediastinum and of the anterior junction line to the left. HRCT performed at end expiration *(C)* reveals air trapping in the left lung, associated with shift of the mediastinum and of the junction line to the midline. The patient was a 61-year-old woman.

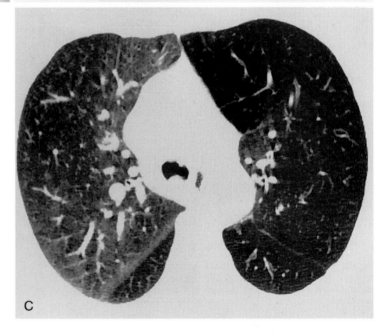

formity of the bronchial tree was identified in early bronchographic studies.[130, 136, 144, 145] The segmental bronchi are irregularly dilated and end abruptly in squared or tapered terminations in the vicinity of the fifth- or sixth-generation divisions *(see* Fig. 58–18). Filling of peripheral bronchiolar radicals is notable by its absence, even with repeated deep breaths. Cinebronchographic examination of the patient illustrated in Figure 58–21 revealed disproportionate collapse of the lower lobe bronchus on forced expiration and cough, with reduction in caliber from 11 mm at TLC to 1.5 mm at residual volume.

Although a number of conditions can manifest with a radiographic appearance similar to that of Swyer-James syndrome, in only one is there a serious potential difficulty. A partly obstructing lesion situated within a main bronchus can create a triad of radiographic signs that are indistinguishable—a smaller than normal lung volume, air

trapping on expiration, and diffuse oligemia as a result of hypoxic vasoconstriction *(see* Fig. 58–20). As a consequence, in any patient presenting with these signs, the presence of a lesion within the ipsilateral main bronchus must be excluded before a diagnosis of Swyer-James syndrome is accepted; the easiest way to accomplish this is by bronchoscopy, although spiral CT is probably just as effective (Fig. 58–22). Other conditions that give rise to unilateral or lobar radiolucency, such as proximal interruption of a pulmonary artery, hypogenetic lung syndrome, and obstruction of a main pulmonary artery or one of its branches by thromboemboli, are readily differentiated by the absence of air trapping during expiration and by other radiographic signs that characterize these conditions.

In one study, the data obtained from a series of 40 consecutive patients who had chronic unilateral hyperlucent lung were analyzed to determine the etiology;[156] cases of

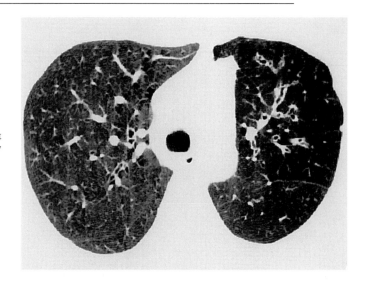

**Figure 58–20. Swyer-James Syndrome.** An HRCT scan in a patient with Swyer-James syndrome demonstrates decreased size and vascularity of the left lung and left upper lobe bronchiectasis.

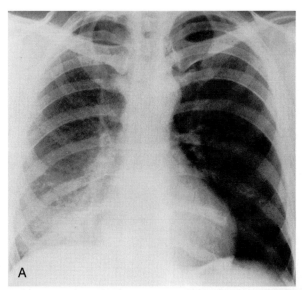

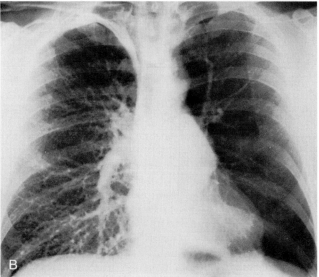

**Figure 58–21. Swyer-James Syndrome: Angiographic and Bronchographic Manifestations.** A posteroanterior radiograph *(A)* reveals the typical appearance of unilateral hyperlucent lung. A pulmonary angiogram *(B)* shows the marked disparity in perfusion of the two lungs, vessels on the left being narrow and attenuated.

*Illustration continued on following page*

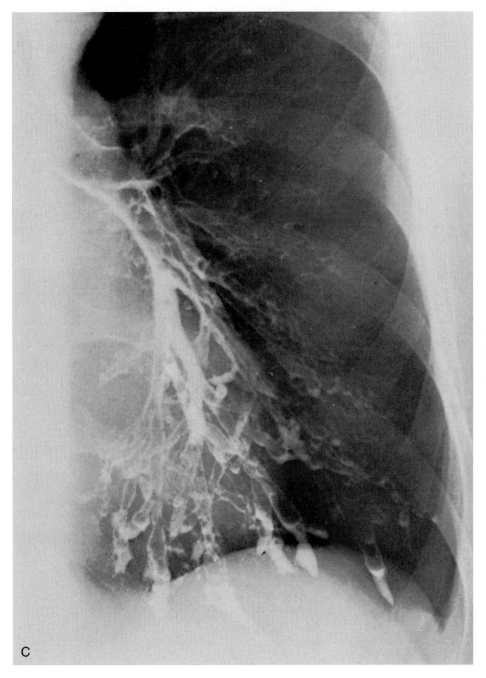

C

**Figure 58–21** *Continued.* A left bronchogram *(C)* demonstrates irregular dilation of all visualized segmental bronchi in the form of "varicose" bronchiectasis; all bronchi terminate in squared or tapered endings, and there is a notable absence of filling of peripheral bronchiolar radicles. This 34-year-old man complained of paroxysmal attacks of dyspnea over a period of several years.

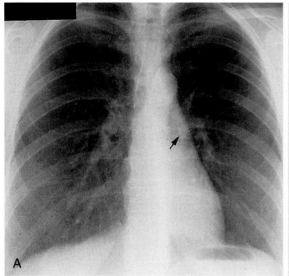

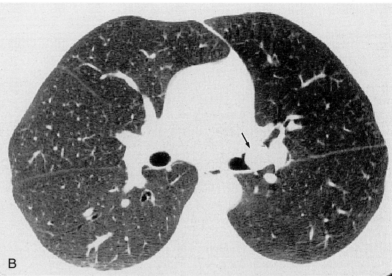

**Figure 58–22. Unilateral Radiolucency Caused by a Partly Obstructing Endobronchial Mass.** A posteroanterior chest radiograph *(A)* in a 35-year-old woman shows increased radiolucency and decreased vascularity and size of the left lung. An endobronchial tumor *(arrow)* is present in the distal left main bronchus. An HRCT scan at end inspiration *(B)* demonstrates the tumor *(arrow)*, decreased vascularity of the left lung, and a slight decrease in attenuation. Note the decrease in size of the left lung with shift of the mediastinum and anterior junction line to the left. An HRCT scan at end expiration *(C)* demonstrates air trapping distal to the endobronchial tumor with shift of the mediastinum and anterior junction line to the right.

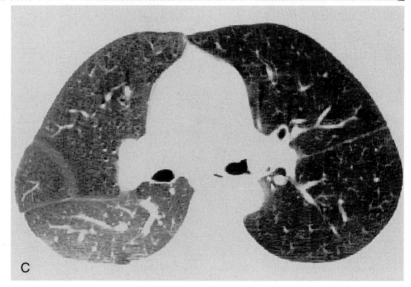

acute thromboembolism were excluded. Etiologies included the Swyer-James syndrome in 18 patients (45%), unilateral bullae in 8 (20%), congenital hypoplastic pulmonary artery in 4 (10%), previous massive pulmonary thromboembolism in 4 (10%), a partly obstructing pulmonary carcinoma in 3 (7.5%), the late sequelae of radiation therapy in 2 (5%), and a benign intrabronchial neoplasm in 1 (2.5%). On the basis of a scoring system for reduction in pulmonary vasculature, patients who had the Swyer-James syndrome were found to have the most significant oligemia, whereas those with carcinoma had the least.

### Clinical Manifestations

The clinical presentation is highly variable. Some patients have no symptoms,[137, 157] and some complain of dyspnea on exertion;[135, 145, 158] still others present with a history of repeated lower respiratory tract infections.[130, 145] Physical examination reveals restriction of chest expansion on the affected side, associated with diminished breath sounds,

relative hyper-resonance, and (sometimes) scattered crackles.[130, 159] In one patient who also developed Goodpasture's syndrome, pulmonary hemorrhage occurred exclusively on the side of the normal lung.[160]

Pulmonary function test results vary with the amount of affected lung. In cases in which an entire lung is involved, there is reduction in vital capacity and expiratory flow. Diffusing capacity measured by the steady-state method usually is reduced; however, it may be normal with the single-breath method because breath-holding permits time for more uniform gas distribution. Blood gas concentrations are usually normal but may decrease during exercise. When bronchospirometry was done, the results revealed reduction in ventilation by as much as 90% on the affected side; oxygen uptake was reduced to as low as 5% of normal.[158, 161] Cases of unilateral hyperlucent lung associated with hypoxemia, polycythemia, pulmonary hypertension, and cor pulmonale probably are the result of the subsequent development of air-flow obstruction (with or without emphysema) in the contralateral lung.[162]

### Bronchiolitis Obliterans Organizing Pneumonia

#### Etiology and Pathogenesis

Although *organizing pneumonia* has been used as a descriptive term histologically in a variety of conditions, the idea that it could represent a distinct clinicopathologic entity was first recognized only in 1982.[13, 14] The first report included eight patients who presented with a short history of severe dyspnea, cough, malaise, and weight loss, bilateral radiographic shadowing, and a raised erythrocyte sedimentation rate;[13] pathologic examination showed an organizing inflammatory exudate in the lumens of transitional airways and alveolar air spaces and no evidence of an infectious or other etiologic agent. Although there was a dramatic clinical and radiologic response to prednisolone, relapse occurred quickly as the dose was reduced. To avoid confusion with postinfective organizing pneumonia, the authors suggested the term cryptogenic organizing pneumonia.

In 1985, another group described an identical clinicopathologic disorder that they termed bronchiolitis obliterans organizing pneumonia.[12] This report was based on a retrospective analysis of 2,500 open-lung biopsy specimens obtained for the diagnosis of diffuse lung disease. Sixty-seven cases were identified in which bronchiolitis obliterans was a prominent histologic feature; in 57 (85%) of these, the bronchiolitis was associated with organizing pneumonia, and in 50 of these, there was no apparent cause or underlying disorder. As discussed previously, we prefer the term cryptogenic organizing pneumonia to describe this condition; nevertheless, because BOOP is well established in the literature, we continue to use it here. It is important to remember that the histologic reaction pattern of BOOP can be seen in association with a number of etiologies, including connective tissue disease, drugs, infection, and aspiration; the following discussion refers mainly to those cases in which an etiology is not identified (idiopathic BOOP). It is also important to note that the radiographic appearance occasionally suggests interstitial disease and pulmonary function studies reveal a restrictive rather than an obstructive derangement, in which situation BOOP can be confused with idiopathic pulmonary fibrosis or other forms of interstitial lung disease.[11]

#### Pathologic Characteristics

Pathologically, BOOP is typically distributed in a patchy fashion throughout the lung, both grossly (Fig. 58–23) and microscopically within secondary lobules. Characteristically, plugs of loose fibroblastic connective tissue can be identified within respiratory bronchioles and alveolar ducts (Fig. 58–24). These are associated with the deposition of a variety of connective tissue proteins and adhesion molecules, including type III collagen, fibronectin, versican, and hylaronan.[163] The parenchyma adjacent to the affected bronchioles shows filling of alveolar air spaces by similar fibroblastic tissue; occasionally, a proteinaceous exudate can be identified in the central portion of the fibroblastic tissue, representing a more direct manifestation of prior epithelial or endothelial injury. A variable degree of nonspecific chronic inflammation and interstitial fibrosis is also evident. Eosinophils may be seen in some cases.[164]

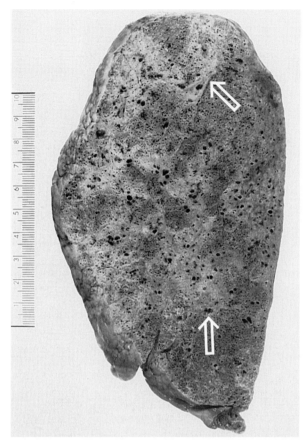

**Figure 58–23. Bronchiolitis Obliterans Organizing Pneumonia.** A slice of an upper lobe shows patchy, irregularly shaped foci of parenchymal consolidation *(arrows)*, shown on histologic examination to be organizing pneumonia. The patient was a 55-year-old man with typical radiologic features of bronchiolitis obliterans organizing pneumonia who died unexpectedly of an acute myocardial infarct; the etiology of the pulmonary disease was undetermined.

#### Radiologic Manifestations

BOOP can be associated with four rather distinctive radiographic and CT patterns: (1) multiple, usually bilateral, symmetric, patchy air-space opacities; (2) diffuse, bilateral interstitial opacities, which may be reticular, nodular, or reticulonodular; (3) focal consolidation; and (4) multiple large nodules or masses.[165–167] A mixed pattern of combined air-space and interstitial opacities has also been described.

Patchy air-space consolidation is the most characteristic and the most common of these patterns (Fig. 58–25): of 124 patients reported in five studies, 89 (72%) had this manifestation of disease.[12, 168–171] The opacities are most often peripheral and pleural based (*see* Fig. 58–8, page 2330). They may decrease in size in one area and appear in previously unaffected regions.[172] An unusual case of "levitating" lesions has been described, the bilateral areas of consolidation migrating cephalad over a period of months and gradually disappearing after reaching the lung apices.[173] The size of the individual opacities ranges from about 3 cm to nearly complete lobar consolidation. The margins of the individual opacities are indistinct, and they may contain air bronchograms. The lung volume may appear preserved or decreased. Concomitant pleural disease is not infrequent; in

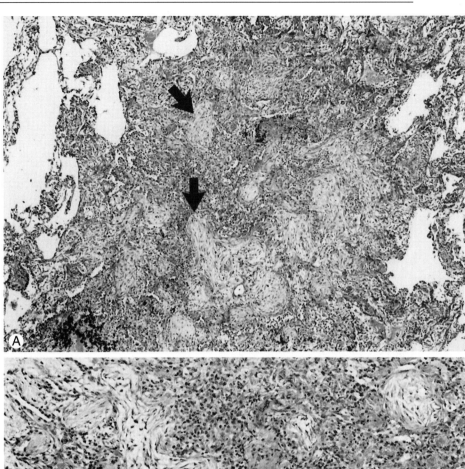

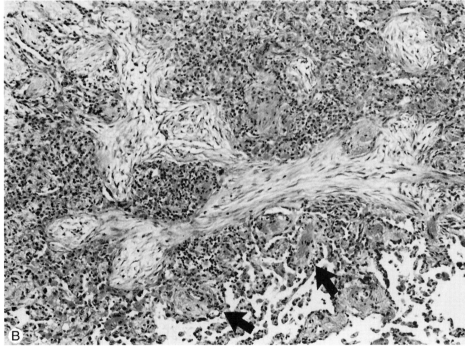

**Figure 58–24. Bronchiolitis Obliterans Organizing Pneumonia.** A histologic section of lung parenchyma *(A)* shows a poorly defined focus of chronic inflammation associated with numerous small foci of loose connective tissue *(arrows)*. A magnified view of similar disease from another area *(B)* shows branching of the connective tissue plugs, implying that they are present in the lumens of alveolar ducts and respiratory bronchioles. The interstitial nature of the chronic inflammatory infiltrate is apparent at the junction with normal lung *(arrow)*. *(A, ×40; B, ×100.)*

one study of 24 patients, it was seen in 5 (21%).[168] In another study of 14 patients, small pleural effusions were detected in 4 (29%).[169] Although the bilateral air-space pattern of BOOP is reasonably characteristic, it is by no means specific, and the differential diagnosis includes chronic eosinophilic pneumonia, bronchioalveolar carcinoma, lymphoma, pulmonary alveolar proteinosis, and alveolar hemorrhage.[165]

A pattern of reticular or reticulonodular opacities may be seen in association with air-space opacities or, occasionally, as an isolated finding. In two series of 24 and 14 patients, it was reported in 42%[168] and 18%,[169] respectively. A less common radiologic presentation is as a focal area of consolidation. The differential diagnosis includes pulmonary carcinoma, a suspicion that may be enhanced by the presence of fever, weight loss, and hemoptysis; the diagnosis is most often established by resection of the lesion, which tends not to recur.[170] The last and least common manifestation is as multiple large nodules or masses, which may simulate metastatic disease.[167]

On HRCT, most patients show areas of air-space consolidation *(see* Fig. 58–14), small nodules, or both [40, 41, 43, 174] (Fig. 58–26); peripheral reticular areas of increased attenuation and ground-glass opacities are seen less often[40, 174] (Fig. 58–27). In one study of 43 patients (of whom 32 were immunocompetent and 11 were immunocompromised secondary to a variety of conditions), consolidation was more

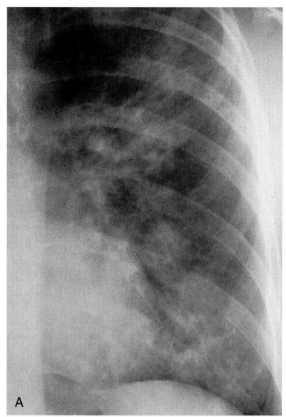

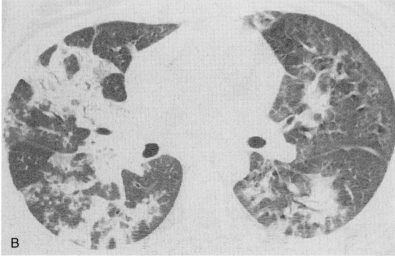

**Figure 58–25. Idiopathic Bronchiolitis Obliterans Organizing Pneumonia.** A view of the left lung from a posteroanterior chest radiograph *(A)* in a 20-year-old woman demonstrates patchy areas of consolidation. An HRCT scan *(B)* shows a predominantly peribronchial and subpleural distribution of the consolidation. Air bronchograms, focal areas of ground-glass attenuation, and a few centrilobular nodules are also evident.

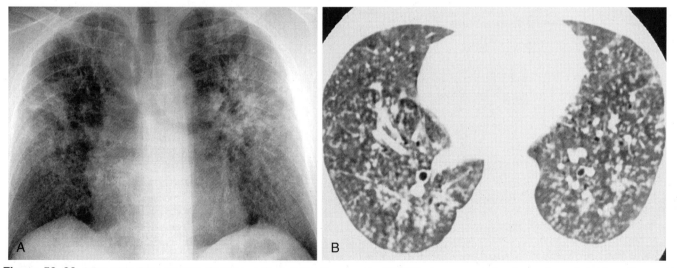

**Figure 58–26. Idiopathic Bronchiolitis Obliterans Organizing Pneumonia (BOOP).** A posteroanterior chest radiograph *(A)* in a 47-year-old man shows an extensive bilateral reticulonodular pattern. A CT scan *(B)* demonstrates numerous bilateral small nodules in a predominantly centrilobular distribution. The diagnosis of idiopathic BOOP was confirmed by open biopsy.

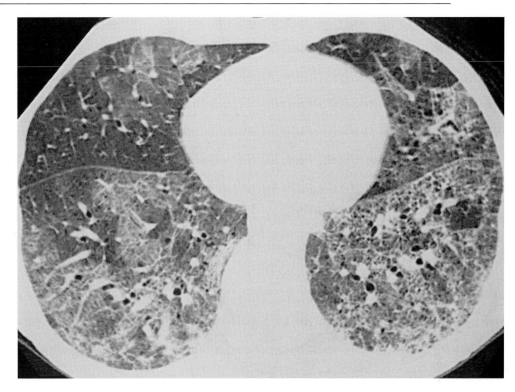

**Figure 58–27. Idiopathic Bronchiolitis Obliterans Organizing Pneumonia (BOOP).** An HRCT scan in a 58-year-old man shows extensive bilateral areas of ground-glass attenuation. Also noted are small linear opacities giving a linear pattern, particularly in the left lower lobe. The diagnosis of idiopathic BOOP was made at transbronchial biopsy.

common in immunocompetent (91%) than in immunocompromised (45%) patients;[41] in the former group, such consolidation was most frequently subpleural or peribronchial in distribution. Ground-glass attenuation and nodules were more common in immunocompromised patients (73% and 55%, respectively) than in immunocompetent patients (56% and 23%, respectively). Occasionally, patients in whom BOOP is confirmed by biopsy have a CT pattern of small centrilobular nodules and branching shadows that is more characteristic of acute infectious bronchiolitis or DPB.[22]

### Clinical Manifestations and Pulmonary Function

BOOP usually appears as a subacute illness whose duration of symptoms before diagnosis is about 2 to 6 months.[12, 175, 176] The most common symptoms are cough (90%), dyspnea (80%), fever (60%), sputum expectoration, malaise, and weight loss (50%). Crackles are audible on auscultation in 75% of cases, but clubbing is not observed.

Most patients who have diffuse BOOP show restrictive disease and gas exchange impairment.[22, 175] The presence of such marked bronchiolar pathology without air-flow obstruction is confusing. A possible explanation for the apparent paradox is that the areas of lung parenchyma subtended by the diseased airways are completely nonfunctional because of the airway obstruction and distal pneumonitis; these areas of parenchyma, therefore, do not contribute to lung emptying, whereas noninvolved areas of parenchyma are subtended by airways that are not obstructed.[175]

### Prognosis and Natural History

In many patients, the clinical and radiographic signs of disease remit completely after systemic corticosteroid therapy.[22, 175, 176] However, there is a subset of patients who

have a much more rapid course and worse prognosis; although some of these patients are still found to have idiopathic disease after careful investigation,[177] rapid progression is more likely to be associated with an underlying condition, such as connective tissue disease or drug therapy.[178] For example, in one study of 74 patients whose lung biopsies showed predominant organizing pneumonia, three groups were analyzed:[179] symptomatic BOOP (37 patients [50%]), symptomatic secondary organizing pneumonia (27 patients [36%]), and asymptomatic organizing pneumonia presenting as a focal nodule (10 patients [14%]). No difference was found between the first two groups with respect to the type or severity of symptoms, signs, laboratory and pulmonary function test results, or radiologic or pathologic findings. Spontaneous or steroid-induced resolution of symptoms was more frequent in patients with BOOP than in those with secondary organizing pneumonia; however, relapse was infrequent in both groups. The 5-year survival rate was higher in patients who had BOOP (73%) than in those who had secondary disease (44%). Organizing pneumonia that manifested as an asymptomatic focal opacity was most often detected on chest radiograph and diagnosed on lung biopsy performed because of a suspicion of carcinoma. Patients who had this form of organizing pneumonia required no treatment and had no relapse or respiratory-related deaths.

The radiologic pattern is also related to prognosis. In one study in which patients who had idiopathic BOOP were divided into three groups based on their radiologic presentation, those who had a pattern of bilateral air-space opacities demonstrated a good response to steroid therapy (although their disease tended to relapse when steroids were discontinued);[170] by contrast, patients who had a localized masslike lesion or widespread interstitial opacities had less consistent responses to therapy. Similar results were reported in another study of six patients who had an interstitial pattern on chest radiography;[180] all had persistent abnormalities, and two died of progressive disease.

### Respiratory Bronchiolitis

The term *respiratory bronchiolitis* has been used to describe a variety of histologic abnormalities, including accumulation of pigment-laden macrophages in the respiratory bronchioles and adjacent alveoli[181] and thickening of the respiratory bronchial walls by inflammatory cells and fibrous tissue.[182] The lesion is invariably associated with cigarette smoking[183] and, in fact, has been considered to be one of the earliest pathologic reactions to this agent.

In its mildest form, respiratory bronchiolitis is associated with few if any symptoms and minimal abnormalities of lung function. In this situation, it is typically discovered as an incidental finding on histologic examination of lungs removed at autopsy or for transplantation. Rarely, a patient presents with cough, dyspnea, crackles, and a combined restrictive and obstructive pattern on lung function testing. When associated with typical radiologic and pathologic findings (*see* farther on), this clinicopathologic syndrome has been called *respiratory bronchiolitis–associated interstitial lung disease*.[183–185] Patients with this syndrome may constitute no more than a subset of individuals who have a more severe form of cigarette smoke–induced respiratory bronchiolitis. However, the lesion has also been considered to represent part of a histologic spectrum of disease that includes desquamative interstitial pneumonitis (DIP) (*see* page 1611).[186]

Histologic abnormalities are seen in both membranous and respiratory bronchioles and consist of a mononuclear inflammatory cell infiltrate (predominantly lymphocytes) and fibrosis in the airway wall[183, 187] (Fig. 58–28); extension of the fibrous tissue into the adjacent alveolar septa is not uncommon. Characteristically, numerous tan-colored macrophages are present within the airway lumen and the alveolar air spaces surrounding the affected bronchiole. Goblet cell hyperplasia and mucous plugging may also be seen in some cases. The abnormality has been confused histologically with other forms of diffuse lung disease, particularly idiopathic pulmonary fibrosis.[183, 187] However, the prominent bronchiolar localization of disease usually enables easy distinction from this condition.

The radiologic features of respiratory bronchiolitis consist of poorly defined centrilobular nodules or ground-glass opacities[22, 29, 30] (*see* Fig. 58–11). These may be diffuse but often involve predominantly or exclusively the upper lobes. The findings in respiratory bronchiolitis–associated interstitial lung disease are similar to those of DIP and consist of ground-glass opacities with or without associated fine reticular or reticulonodular interstitial opacities; in contrast to DIP, lung volumes are usually normal.[22, 184, 187] On HRCT, the abnormalities consist of diffuse or patchy areas of ground-

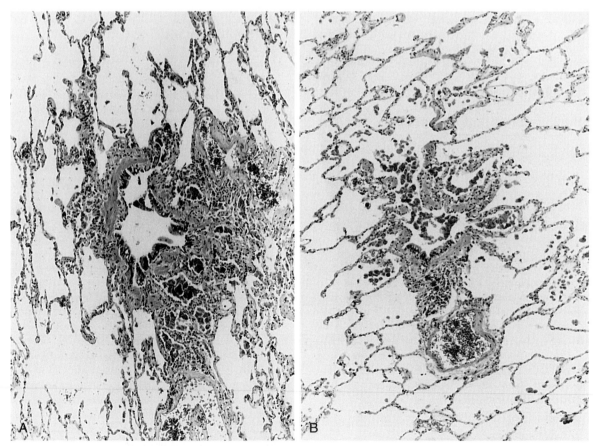

**Figure 58–28. Respiratory Bronchiolitis.** Sections show membranous *(A)* and proximal respiratory *(B)* bronchioles, each with mild to moderate thickening of their walls by fibrous tissue and a lymphocytic infiltrate. Aggregates of alveolar macrophages are present in the lumen of the respiratory bronchiole and the alveolar air spaces adjacent to each airway. The patient was a 30-year-old man who died in a motor vehicle accident; his smoking history was unknown.

glass attenuation with or without fine reticular or poorly defined nodular opacities.[21, 22, 42]

Although the natural history of the condition is uncertain, it responds dramatically to smoking cessation and corticosteroid therapy.[184]

### Follicular Bronchiolitis

The term *follicular bronchiolitis* refers to a form of bronchiolar disease characterized histologically by the presence of abundant lymphoid tissue, frequently with prominent germinal centers, situated in the walls of bronchioles and, to some extent, bronchi[188, 189] (Fig. 58–29). Although the alveolar interstitium may contain a similar lymphocytic infiltrate, this is typically minimal. The most common clinical finding is progressive shortness of breath;[188–190] cough, fever, and recurrent pneumonia are occasionally present. Pulmonary function studies reveal evidence of airway obstruction,[189] restriction, or both.

The lesion is not specific and can be found in association with connective tissue diseases (particularly adult and juvenile rheumatoid disease and Sjögren's syndrome), immunodeficiency diseases, systemic hypersensitivity reactions, and infection by *M. pneumoniae* or viruses.[188, 189] The last-named has been seen particularly in children as a sequela of viral infection and in patients who are infected by Epstein-

Barr virus or human immunodeficiency virus.[191] In some instances, the condition is an isolated finding. For example, in one study of five children who had biopsy-confirmed follicular bronchiolitis and who were followed for 2 to 15 years, none had a connective tissue or other autoimmune disorder, and no pathogenetic organisms were isolated from the sputum or biopsy specimen.[192] The children presented with cough and tachypnea before 6 weeks of age and improved between 2 and 4 years of age; however, mild residual obstruction persisted in some patients. A familial form of the condition associated with elevated serum immunoglobulin and antinuclear antibodies has also been described.[193]

The chest radiograph characteristically shows a diffuse reticulonodular pattern.[188, 189] HRCT may demonstrate nodular opacities mainly in a peribronchovascular or subpleural distribution, consistent with the presence of lymphoid aggregates; these opacities are usually small (1 to 3 mm diameter),[194, 195, 195a] but occasionally are as large as 1 to 2 cm in diameter (Fig. 58–30). Other findings include centrilobular branching structures, bronchial wall thickening, and (occasionally) patchy areas of low attenuation.[195a]

Although it is possible that the lymphocytic infiltrate is a manifestation of active inflammation of the bronchioles in some cases (i.e., a true bronchiolitis), in others, it is probable that it represents hyperplasia of the lymphoid tissue that normally occurs in this region. The presence of lymphoid aggregates in the pleura and interlobular septa,[188, 196] sites of normal lymphatic drainage, supports the latter interpretation. Lymphocytic infiltration without follicle formation is a feature of some cases of bronchiolitis, especially in association with Sjögren's syndrome.[197]

### Diffuse Panbronchiolitis

DPB is a disease of unknown etiology and pathogenesis associated with chronic inflammation of the paranasal sinuses and respiratory bronchioles, the latter characterized histologically by luminal obliteration and a striking accumulation of foamy macrophages.[198, 199]

The disease has been recognized almost exclusively in Japan; a survey in that nation between 1978 and 1980 identified more than 1,000 probable cases, of which 82 were confirmed pathologically.[200] The condition has also been reported in Korea,[201] China,[202] Europe,[203, 204] and North America.[205, 206] Although some affected patients in the last two regions have been Asian,[203, 203a] others have been white. The disease has also been reported occasionally in whites who have traveled in Asia.[207] Most patients are between 30 and 60 years of age; the male-to-female ratio is about 2:1.[200]

#### Etiology and Pathogenesis

The rather limited racial and geographic distribution of DPB suggests the presence of specific factors in its etiology and pathogenesis. The two most likely to be involved are infection by a microorganism prevalent in the Far East and the presence of genetic susceptibility in individuals who reside therein.[208] DPB has been shown to occur with increased frequency in family members; this may be related to a strong association with a specific HLA class II antigen, Bw54.[209] The relative risk for DPB associated with this genotype has been found to be between 3 and 13;[209, 210, 210a]

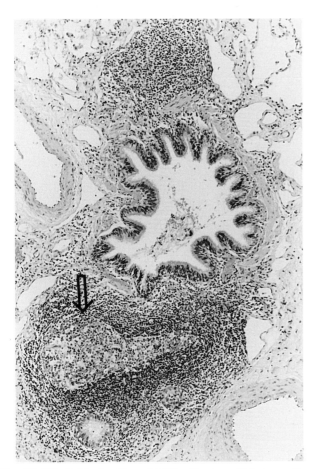

**Fig. 58–29. Follicular Bronchiolitis.** The interstitial tissue adjacent to a membranous bronchiole is expanded by an infiltrate of lymphoid cells, focally with germinal center formation *(arrow).* Similar disease was present in relation to many other bronchioles. The patient had rheumatoid disease.

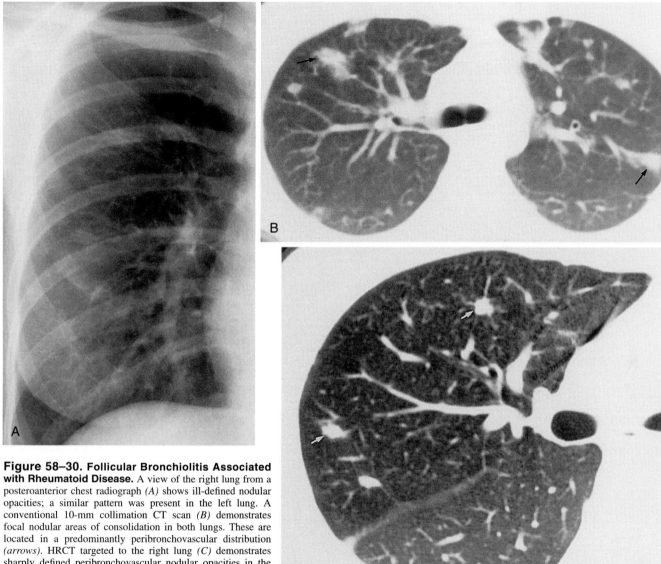

**Figure 58–30. Follicular Bronchiolitis Associated with Rheumatoid Disease.** A view of the right lung from a posteroanterior chest radiograph *(A)* shows ill-defined nodular opacities; a similar pattern was present in the left lung. A conventional 10-mm collimation CT scan *(B)* demonstrates focal nodular areas of consolidation in both lungs. These are located in a predominantly peribronchovascular distribution *(arrows)*. HRCT targeted to the right lung *(C)* demonstrates sharply defined peribronchovascular nodular opacities in the right upper lobe *(arrows)*. The patient was a 24-year-old woman who had rheumatoid disease and biopsy-confirmed follicular bronchiolitis.

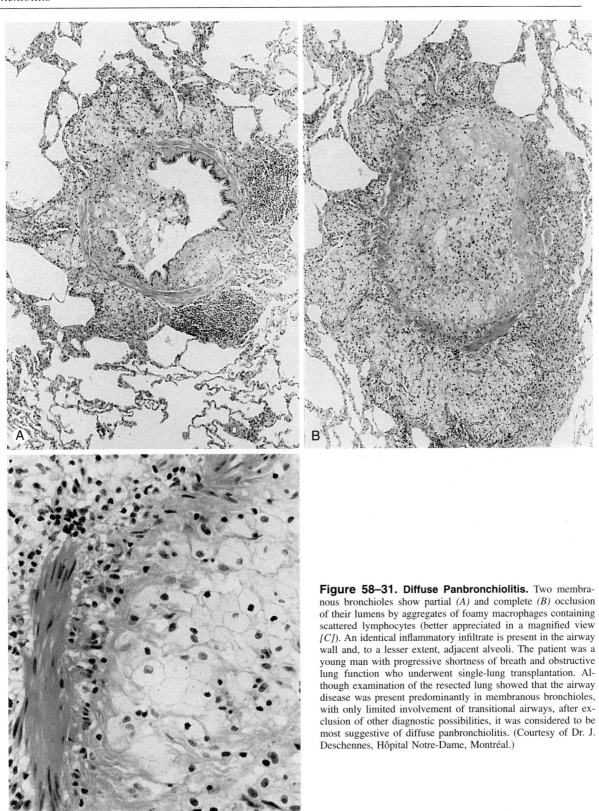

**Figure 58–31. Diffuse Panbronchiolitis.** Two membranous bronchioles show partial *(A)* and complete *(B)* occlusion of their lumens by aggregates of foamy macrophages containing scattered lymphocytes (better appreciated in a magnified view *[C]*). An identical inflammatory infiltrate is present in the airway wall and, to a lesser extent, adjacent alveoli. The patient was a young man with progressive shortness of breath and obstructive lung function who underwent single-lung transplantation. Although examination of the resected lung showed that the airway disease was present predominantly in membranous bronchioles, with only limited involvement of transitional airways, after exclusion of other diagnostic possibilities, it was considered to be most suggestive of diffuse panbronchiolitis. (Courtesy of Dr. J. Deschennes, Hôpital Notre-Dame, Montréal.)

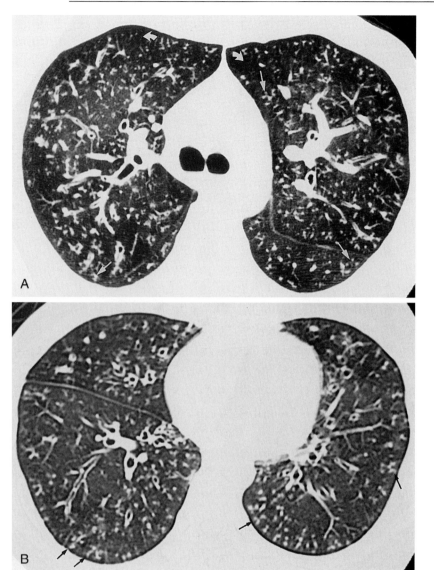

**Figure 58–32. Diffuse Panbronchiolitis.** An HRCT scan in a 32-year-old man with panbronchiolitis *(A)* demonstrates centrilobular nodules *(straight arrows)*, marked bronchial wall thickening, bronchiectasis, and localized areas of decreased attenuation and perfusion *(curved arrows)*. An HRCT scan in another patient *(B)* shows centrilobular nodules and branching lines, giving a characteristic tree-in-bud appearance *(arrows)*. Extensive bronchial wall thickening and bronchiectasis are also evident. (Courtesy of Dr. Kyung Soo Lee, Samsung Medical Center, Seoul, Korea.)

because this allele exists only in Japanese, Chinese, and Korean populations, this may explain the racial distribution of the condition.

Investigation for a causative organism has not yielded consistent results. The typical features of DPB have been described in single patients infected with *C. pneumoniae*[211] and with human T-cell lymphotropic virus type 1.[212] Patients who have DPB are frequently infected with *Pseudomonas aeruginosa* and *Haemophilus influenzae*; however, this is thought to represent opportunistic infection in damaged airways rather than a cause of the disorder.[213]

Analysis of BAL fluid from patients who have DPB demonstrates evidence of an intense inflammatory reaction. In addition to increased numbers of neutrophils and CD8[+] T lymphocytes,[214] the fluid contains high concentrations of elastase[215] and the potent chemoattractants leukotriene B4[216] and interleukin-8.[217] In one African American patient who underwent double-lung transplantation for DPB, the disease recurred in the transplanted lungs within 10 weeks of transplantation but then responded to erythromycin therapy; the investigators suggested that this occurrence argues for a systemic factor in the pathogenesis.[218] Although some pa-

tients have been reported in whom DPB has accompanied rheumatoid arthritis[219] or adult T-cell leukemia,[220] evidence for abnormal immune function has not been found in most patients.

### Pathologic Characteristics

Grossly, DPB is manifested by multiple, fairly discrete gray or yellow nodules 1 to 3 mm in diameter; although some of these are clearly associated with airways, in many, this relationship can only be surmised by noting their central location in a secondary lobule. Histologically, the condition is characterized by an accumulation of mononuclear inflammatory cells (predominantly lymphocytes, plasma cells, and foamy histiocytes) in the walls of respiratory bronchioles, alveolar ducts and, to a lesser extent, adjacent alveoli.[200, 206, 221] Mucus and aggregates of neutrophils may be seen within the airway lumen;[206] occasionally, intraluminal fibrosis is present.[221] The distal lung parenchyma may be normal or may show features of airway obstruction (such as an increase in alveolar macrophages and a mild degree of interstitial inflammation).

The histologic pattern of bronchiolar inflammation accompanied by foamy histiocytes is not by itself diagnostic, because a DPB-like lesion can be seen in a variety of other conditions, including bronchiectasis, cystic fibrosis, aspiration pneumonia, extrinsic allergic alveolitis, Wegener's granulomatosis, and lymphoma.[199] In some of these conditions, the inflammatory infiltrate appears to be centered on more proximal airways (membranous bronchioles and small bronchi) (Fig. 58–31) than in DPB;[199] in fact, localization of the inflammation to respiratory bronchioles and alveolar ducts (the so-called unit lesion[222]) has been considered to be a distinctive feature of DPB.[199] Three-dimensional morphometric study of the airways has also shown the site of airway obstruction in DPB to differ from that of obliterative bronchiolitis.[223]

### Radiologic Manifestations

Radiographic abnormalities consist of diffuse nodules smaller than 5 mm in diameter and mild to moderate hyperinflation.[200, 224] The findings on HRCT are characteristic and include small centrilobular nodules and branching linear opacities, bronchiolectasis, bronchiectasis, and mosaic areas of decreased parenchymal attenuation (Fig. 58–32).[24–26] The presence of these findings is related to the stage of the disease:[26] the earliest manifestation consists of centrilobular nodular opacities, followed by branching linear opacities that connect to the nodules, followed by bronchiolectasis and, eventually, bronchiectasis.[26] Large cystic spaces or bullae may be seen in the late stage.

In addition to diagnosis, HRCT has been useful in following the evolution of disease.[225] For example, in one study of 17 patients, centrilobular and branched linear areas of soft tissue attenuation progressed to dilation of proximal airways in 5 untreated patients, whereas these lesions decreased in number and size after erythromycin therapy in 12 patients.[226]

### Clinical Manifestations

The chief clinical manifestations are dyspnea on exertion and cough, often with sputum production. Sinusitis is common.[200, 221] Progressive disease is common and is sometimes accompanied by respiratory failure. Colonization with *P. aeruginosa* frequently complicates the late stages of the disease and appears to be associated with a worse prognosis; in one study, the 10-year survival rate for those infected with the organism was only 12%, compared with 73% for those who remained uninfected.[213] Pulmonary function tests show marked obstructive and mild restrictive impairment. Arterial hypoxemia is common.[221]

The beneficial effect of chronic therapy with erythromycin in the treatment of DPB was first reported in 1987[227] and has been supported by the results of subsequent studies.[228] The mechanism by which the drug exerts its beneficial effect is unclear. It is possible that its action may not be as an antimicrobial; in one study of 28 patients who had DPB, 16 with and 12 without chronic infection with *P. aeruginosa*, improvement occurred after erythromycin irrespective of their bacteriologic status or whether the organism was cleared from the sputum.[229] Erythromycin has also been reported to decrease the neutrophil chemotactic activity in BAL fluid,[230, 231] reduce the airway concentration of interleukin-8[232] and neutrophil elastase,[233] and decrease neutrophil superoxide formation.[234]

# REFERENCES

1. Adekunle MA, Vallyathan V, McQuillen EN, et al: Bronchiolar inflammation and fibrosis associated with smoking. Am Rev Respir Dis 143:144, 1991.
2. Yousem SA: Lymphocytic bronchitis/bronchiolitis in lung allograft recipients. Am J Surg Pathol 17:491, 1993.
3. Matsuse T, Oka T, Kida K, et al: Importance of diffuse aspiration bronchiolitis caused by chronic occult aspiration in the elderly. Chest 110:1289, 1996.
4. Wright JL, Churg A: Morphology of small-airway lesions in patients with asbestos exposure. Hum Pathol 15:68, 1984.
5. Churg A, Wright JL: Small-airway lesions in patients exposed to non-asbestos mineral dusts. Hum Pathol 14:688, 1983.
6. Kraft M, Mortenson RL, Colby TV, et al: Cryptogenic constrictive bronchiolitis: clinicopathologic study. Am Rev Respir Dis 148:1093, 1993.
7. Macklem PT, Thurlbeck WM, Fraser RG: Chronic obstructive disease of small airways. Ann Intern Med 74:167, 1971.
8. Kindt CG, Weiland JE, Davis WB, et al: Bronchiolitis in adults. A reversible cause of airway obstruction associated with airway neutrophils and neutrophil products. Am Rev Respir Dis 140:483, 1989.
9. Edwards C, Cayton R, Bryan R: Chronic transmural bronchiolitis: A non-specific lesion of small airways. J Clin Pathol 45:993, 1992.
10. Bai T, Eidelman DH, Hogg JC, et al: Proposed nomenclature for quantifying subdivisions of the bronchial wall. J Appl Physiol 77:1011, 1994.
11. Epler GR, Colby TV: The spectrum of bronchiolitis obliterans. Chest 83:161, 1983.
12. Epler GR, Colby TV, McLoud TC, et al: Bronchiolitis obliterans organizing pneumonia. N Engl J Med 312:152, 1985.
13. Davison AG, Heard BE, McAllister WAC, et al: Steroid-responsive relapsing cryptogenic organising pneumonitis. Thorax 37:785, 1982.
14. Davison AG, Heard BE, McAllister WAC, et al: Cryptogenic organizing pneumonia. Q J Med 52:382, 1983.
15. du Bois RM, Geddes DM: Obliterative bronchiolitis, cryptogenic organizing pneumonia and bronchiolitis obliterans organizing pneumonia: Three names for two different conditions. Eur Respir J 4:774, 1991.
16. McLoud T, Epler G, Colby T, et al: Bronchiolitis obliterans. Radiology 159:1, 1986.
17. Sweatman M, Millar A, Strickland B, et al: Computed tomography in adult obliterative bronchiolitis. Clin Radiol 41:116, 1990.
18. Davies HD, Wang EE, Manson D, et al: Reliability of the chest radiograph in the diagnosis of lower respiratory infections in young children. Pediatr Infect Dis J 15:600, 1996.
19. Babcook CJ, Norman GR, Coblentz CL: Effect of clinical history on the interpretation of chest radiographs in childhood bronchiolitis. Invest Radiol 28:214, 1993.
20. Dawson KP, Long A, Kennedy J, et al: The chest radiograph in acute bronchiolitis. J Paediatr Child Health 26:209, 1990.
21. Lynch DA: Imaging of small airways diseases. Clin Chest Med 14:623, 1993.
22. Müller NL, Miller RR: Diseases of the bronchioles: CT and histopathologic findings. Radiology 196:3, 1995.
22a. Worthy SA, Flint JD, Müller NL: Pulmonary complications after bone marrow transplantation: High-resolution CT and pathologic findings. Radiographics 17:1359, 1997.
23. Logan PM, Primack SL, Miller RR, et al: Invasive aspergillosis of the airways: Radiographic, CT and pathologic findings. Radiology 193:383, 1994.
23a. Im J-G, Itoh H, Shim Y-S, et al: Pulmonary tuberculosis: CT findings—early active disease and sequential change with antituberculous therapy. Radiology 186:653, 1993.
24. Nishimura K, Kitaichi M, Izumi T, et al: Diffuse panbronchiolitis: Correlation of high-resolution CT and pathologic findings. Radiology 184:779, 1992.
25. Akira M, Higashihara T, Sakatani M, et al: Diffuse panbronchiolitis: Follow-up CT examination. Radiology 189:559, 1993.
26. Akira M, Kitatani F, Yong-Sik L, et al: Diffuse panbronchiolitis: Evaluation with high-resolution CT1. Radiology 168:433, 1988.
27. Kang EY, Miller RR, Müller NL: Bronchiectasis: Comparison of preoperative thin-section CT and pathologic findings in resected specimens. Radiology 195:649, 1995.
28. Gruden JF, Webb WR, Warnock M: Centrilobular opacities in the lung on high-resolution CT: Diagnostic considerations and pathologic correlation. Am J Roentgenol 162:569, 1994.
29. Remy-Jardin M, Remy J, Gosselin B, et al: Lung parenchymal changes secondary to cigarette smoking: pathologic-CT correlations. Radiology 186:643, 1993.
30. Gruden JF, Webb WR: CT findings in a proved case of respiratory bronchiolitis. Am J Roentgenol 161:44, 1993.
31. Padley SPG, Adler BD, Hansell DM, et al: Bronchiolitis obliterans: High resolution CT findings and correlation with pulmonary function tests. Clin Radiol 47:236, 1993.
32. Worthy SA, Park CS, Kim JS, et al: Bronchiolitis obliterans after lung transplantation: High-resolution CT findings in 15 patients. Am J Roentgenol 169:673, 1997.
32a. Leung AN, Fisher K, Valentine V, et al: Bronchiolitis obliterans after lung transplantation: Detection using expiratory HRCT. Chest 113:365, 1998.
33. Garg K, Lynch DA, Newell JD, et al: Proliferative and constrictive bronchiolitis: Classification and radiologic features. Am J Roentgenol 162:803, 1994.
34. Stern EJ, Frank MS: Small airway diseases of the lungs: Findings at expiratory CT. Am J Roentgenol 163:37, 1994.
34a. Desai SR, Hansell DM: Small airways disease: Expiratory computed tomography comes of age. Clin Radiol 52:332, 1997.
35. Webb WR, Stern EJ, Nanth N, et al: Dynamic pulmonary CT: Findings in healthy adult men. Radiology 186:117, 1993.
36. Park CS, Müller NL, Worthy SA, et al: Airway obstruction in asthmatic and healthy individuals: Inspiratory and expiratory thin-section CT findings. Radiology 203:361, 1997.
37. Brown MJ, English J, Müller NL: Bronchiolitis obliterans due to neuroendocrine hyperplasia: High-resolution CT-pathologic correlation. Am J Roentgenol 168:1561, 1997.
38. Hansell DM, Wells AU, Padley SP, et al: Hypersensitivity pneumonitis: Correlation of individual CT patterns with functional abnormalities. Radiology 199:123, 1996.
39. Small JH, Flower CDR, Traill ZC, et al: Air-trapping in extrinsic allergic alveolitis on computed tomography. Clin Radiol 51:684, 1996.
39a. Lynch DA, Newell JD, Tschomper BA, et al: Uncomplicated asthma in adults: Comparison of CT appearance of the lungs in asthmatic and healthy subjects. Radiology 188:829, 1993.
39b. King GG, Müller NL, Paré PD: Pulmonary perspective: Evaluation of airways in obstructive lung disease using high-resolution CT. Am J Respir Crit Care Med 1999: in press.
39c. Arakawa H, Webb WR, McCowin M, et al: Inhomogeneous lung attenuation at thin-section CT: Diagnostic value of expiratory scans. Radiology 206:89, 1998.
39d. Worthy SA, Müller NL, Hartman TE, et al: Mosaic attenuation pattern on thin-section CT scans of the lung: Differentiation among infiltrative lung, airway, and vascular diseases as a cause. Radiology 205:465, 1997.
40. Müller NL, Staples CA, Miller RR: Bronchiolitis obliterans organizing pneumonia: CT features in 14 patients. Am J Roentgenol 154:983, 1990.
41. Lee KS, Kullnig P, Hartman TE, et al: Cryptogenic organizing pneumonia: CT findings in 43 patients. Am J Roentgenol 162:543, 1994.
42. Holt RM, Schmidt RA, Godwin JD, et al: High resolution CT in respiratory bronchiolitis-associated interstitial lung disease. J Comput Assist Tomogr 17:46, 1993.
43. Nishimura K, Itoh H: High-resolution computed tomographic features of bronchiolitis obliterans organizing pneumonia. Chest 102:26S, 1992.
44. Epler GR, Colby TV: The spectrum of bronchiolitis obliterans. Chest 83:161, 1983.
45. Seggev JS, Mason UG, Worthen S, et al: Bronchiolitis obliterans: Report of three cases with detailed physiologic studies. Chest 83:169, 1983.
46. Wohl M, Chernick V: State of the art: Bronchiolitis. Am Rev Respir Dis 118:759, 1978.
47. Panitch HB, Callahan CW, Schidlow DV: Bronchiolitis in children. Clin Chest Med 14:715, 1993.
48. Holberg CJ, Wright AL, Martinez FD, et al: Risk factors for respiratory syncytial virus-associated lower respiratory illness in the first year of life. Am J Epidemiol 133:1135, 1991.
49. Welliver JR, Welliver RC: Bronchiolitis. Pediatr Rev 14:134, 1993.
50. Denny FW, Clyde WA: Acute lower respiratory tract infections in nonhospitalized children. J Pediatr 108:635, 1986.
51. Young S, O'Keefe PT, Arnott J, et al: Lung function, airway responsiveness, and respiratory symptoms before and after bronchiolitis. Arch Dis Child 72:16, 1995.
52. Khan MA, Potter CW: The nPCR detection of *Chlamydia pneumoniae* and *Chlamydia trachomatis* in children hospitalized for bronchiolitis. J Infect 33:173, 1996.
53. Heycock JB, Noble TC: 1,230 Cases of acute bronchiolitis in infancy. Br Med J 2:879, 1962.
54. Thompson MEM, Nelson JK, McMastre C, et al: Risk factors for bronchiolitis: Presentation of an on-going perspective clinical study. Inflamm Res 46:S85, 1997.
55. Tsutsumi H, Sone S, Yoto Y, et al: Respiratory syncytial virus bronchiolitis in a girl undergoing chemotherapy for acute lymphoblastic leukemia: An immunologic study of local secretion. Pediatr Infect Dis J 15:635, 1996.
56. Piscacane Z, Graziano L, Zona G, et al: Breast feeding and acute lower respiratory infection. Acta Paediatr 83:714, 1983.
57. Holberg CJ, Wright AL, Martinez FD, et al: Risk factors for respiratory syncytial virus-associated lower respiratory illnesses in the first year of life. Am J Epidemiol 133:1135, 1991.
58. Dezateux C, Fletcher ME, Dundas I, et al: Infant respiratory function after RSV-proven bronchiolitis. Am J Respir Crit Care Med 155:1349, 1997.
59. Spencer N, Logan S, Scholey S, et al: Deprivation and bronchiolitis. Arch Dis Child 74:50, 1996.
60. Buckley CE III, Tucker DH, Thorne NA, et al: Bronchiolectasis: The clinical syndrome and its relationship to chronic lung disease. Am J Med 38:190, 1965.
61. Sturtevant HN, Knudson HW: Bronchiolar ectasia: A report of twelve cases. Am J Roentgenol 83:279, 1960.
62. Sterner G, Wolontis S, Bloth B, et al: Respiratory syncytial virus: An outbreak of acute respiratory illness in a home for infants. Acta Paediatr Scand 1966;55,273.
63. Simpson W, Hacking PM, Court SDM, et al: The radiological findings in respiratory syncytial virus infection in children. Pediatr Radiol 1974;2,155.

64. Gold R, Wilt JC, Adhikari PK, et al: Adenoviral pneumonia and its complications in infancy and childhood. J Can Assoc Radiol 20:218, 1969.

65. Wahlgren H, Mortensson W, Eriksson M, et al: Radiographic patterns and viral studies in childhood pneumonia at various ages. Pediatr Radiol 25:627, 1995.

66. Sawazaki H, Watabe S, Onoki S, et al: Two cases of bronchiolitis obliterans. Jap J Chest Dis 21:635, 1962.

67. Osborne D: Radiologic appearance of viral disease of the lower respiratory tract in infants and children. Am J Roentgenol 130:29, 1978.

68. Rosmus HH, Paré JAP, Masson AM, et al: Roentgenographic patterns of acute mycoplasma and viral pneumonitis. J Can Assoc Radiol 19:74, 1968.

69. Cameron DC, Borthwick RN, Philp T, et al: The radiographic patterns of acute mycoplasma pneumonitis. Clin Radiol 28:173, 1977.

70. Lemen RJ: Respiratory syncytial virus and bronchiolitis. Acta Paediatr Sin 36:78, 1995.

71. Seidenberg J, Masters IB, Hudson I, et al: Disturbance in respiratory mechanics in infants with bronchiolitis. Thorax 44:660, 1989.

72. Mulholland EK, Olinsky A, Shann FA: Clinical findings and severity of acute bronchiolitis. Lancet 335:1259, 1990.

73. Klassen TP: Recent advances in the treatment of bronchiolitis and laryngitis. Pediatr Clin North Am 44:249, 1997.

74. Kellner JD, Ohlsson A, Gadomski AM, et al: Efficacy of bronchodilator therapy in bronchiolitis: A meta-analysis. Arch Pediatr Adolesc Med 150:1166, 1996.

75. Menon K, Sutcliffe T, Klassen TP: A randomized trial comparing the efficacy of epinephrine with salbutamol in the treatment of acute bronchiolitis. J Pediatr 126:1004, 1995.

76. Ham JC: Acute infectious obstructing bronchiolitis: A potentially fatal disease in the adult. Ann Intern Med 60:47, 1964.

77. Hogg JC, Williams J, Richardson JB, et al: Age as a factor in the distribution of lower-airway conductance and in the pathologic anatomy of obstructive lung disease. N Engl J Med 282:1283, 1970.

78. Wright JL: Inhalational lung injury causing bronchiolitis. Clin Chest Med 14:635, 1993.

79. Kirkpatrick B, Bass JB: Severe obstructive lung disease after smoke inhalation. Chest 76:108, 1979.

80. Ramirez RJ: The first death from nitrogen dioxide fumes: The story of a man and his dog. JAMA 229:1181, 1974.

81. Ramirez RJ, Dowell AR: Silo-filler's disease: Nitrogen dioxide-induced lung injury. Long term follow-up and review of the literature. Ann Intern Med 74:569, 1971.

82. Tse RL, Bockman AA: Nitrogen dioxide toxicity: Report of four cases in firemen. JAMA 212:1341, 1970.

83. Jones GR, Proudfoot AT, Hall JI: Pulmonary effects of acute exposure to nitrous fumes. Thorax 28:61, 1973.

84. Wright JL, Cagle P, Churg A, et al: Diseases of the small airways. Am Rev Respir Dis 146:240, 1992.

85. Sparrow D, Bosse R, Rosner B, et al: The effect of occupational exposure on pulmonary function. Am Rev Respir Dis 125:319, 1982.

86. Perez-Padilla R, Gaxiola M, Salas J, et al: Bronchiolitis in chronic pigeon breeder's disease: Morphologic evidence of a spectrum of small airway lesions in hypersensitivity pneumonitis induced by avian antigens. Chest 110:371, 1996.

87. Selman-Lama M, Perez-Padilla R: Airflow obstruction and airway lesions in hypersensitivity pneumonitis. Clin Chest Med 14:699, 1993.

88. Chan-Yeung M, Enarson DA, Kennedy SM: The impact of grain dust on respiratory health. Am Rev Respir Dis 145:476, 1992.

89. Malmberg P, Rask-Andersen A, Hoglund S, et al: Incidence of organic dust toxic syndrome and allergic alveolitis in Swedish farmers. Int Arch Allergy Appl Immunol 87:47, 1988.

90. Emanuel DA, Wenzel FJ, Lawton BR: Pulmonary mycotoxicosis. Chest 67:293, 1975.

91. May JJ, Stallones L, Darrow D, et al: Organic dust toxicity (pulmonary mycotoxicosis) associated with silo unloading. Thorax 41:919, 1986.

92. Cormier Y, Boulet LP, Bedard G, et al: Respiratory health of workers exposed to swine confinement buildings only or to both swine confinement buildings and dairy barns. Scand J Work Environ Health 17:269, 1992.

93. Schwartz DA, Landas SK, Lassie DL, et al: Airway injury in swine confinement workers. Ann Intern Med 116:630, 1992.

94. Mulhausen JR, McJilton CE, Redig PT, et al: Aspergillus and other human respiratory disease agents in turkey confinement homes. Am Ind Hyg Assoc J 48:894, 1987.

95. Heederik D, Brouwer R, Biersteker K, et al: Relationship of airborne endotoxin and bacteria levels in pig farms with the lung function and respiratory symptoms of farmers. Int Arch Occup Environ Health 6:595, 1991.

96. Geddes DM, Corrin B, Brewerton DA, et al: Progressive airway obliteration in adults and its association with rheumatoid disease. Q J Med 46:427, 1977.

97. Epler GR, Snider GL, Gaensler EA, et al: Bronchiolitis and bronchitis in connective tissue disease, a possible relationship to the use of penicillamine. JAMA 242:528, 1979.

98. Chebat J, Seigneur F, Lechien J, et al: Severe bronchiolitis in three cases of rheumatoid polyarthritis treated with D-penicillamine. Rev Fr Mal Respir 9:147, 1981.

99. Herzog CA, Miller RR, Hoidal JR, et al: Bronchiolitis and rheumatoid arthritis. Am Rev Respir Dis 124:636, 1981.

100. Murphy KC, Atkins CJ, Offer RC, et al: Obliterative bronchitis in two rheumatoid arthritis patients treated with penicillamine. Arthritis Rheum 24:557, 1981.

101. Jacobs P, Bonnyns M, Depierreux M, et al: Rapidly fatal bronchiolitis obliterans with circulating antinuclear and rheumatoid factors. Eur J Respir Dis 65:384, 1984.

102. Gibson JM, O'Hara MD, Beare JM, et al: Bronchial obstruction in a patient with Behçet's disease. Eur J Respir Dis 63:356, 1982.

103. Wells AU, du Bois RM: Bronchiolitis in association with connective tissue disorders. Clin Chest Med 14:655, 1993.

104. Kinoshita M, Higashi T, Tanaka C, et al: Follicular bronchiolitis associated with rheumatoid arthritis. Int Med 31:674, 1992.

105. Hayakawa H, Sato A, Imokawa S, et al: Bronchiolar disease in rheumatoid arthritis. Am J Respir Crit Care Med 154:1531, 1996.

106. Sugiyama Y, Ohno S, Kano S, et al: Diffuse panbronchiolitis and rheumatoid arthritis: A possible correlation with HLA-B54. Int Med 33:612, 1994.

107. Wolfe F, Schurle DR, Lin JJ, et al: Upper and lower airway disease in penicillamine-treated patients with rheumatoid arthritis. J Rheumatol 10:406, 1983.

108. Tomioka R, King TE Jr: Gold-induced pulmonary disease: Clinical features, outcome and differentiation from rheumatoid lung disease. Am J Respir Crit Care Med 155:1011, 1997.

109. Yousem SA, Colby TV, Carrington CB: Lung biopsy in rheumatoid arthritis. Am Rev Respir Dis 131:770, 1985.

110. Turton CW, Williams G, Green M, et al: Cryptogenic obliterative bronchiolitis in adults. Thorax 36:805, 1981.

111. Green M, Turton CW: Bronchiolitis and its manifestations. Eur J Respir Dis 63:36, 1982.

112. Reichenspurner H, Girgis RE, Robbins RC, et al: Stanford experience with obliterative bronchiolitis after lung and heart-lung transplantation. Ann Thorac Surg 62:1467, 1996.

113. Sweet SC, Spray TL, Huddleston CB, et al: Pediatric lung transplantation at St. Louis Children's Hospital, 1990–1995. Am J Respir Crit Care Med 155:1027, 1997.

114. Philit F, Wiesendanger T, Archimbaud E, et al: Post-transplant obstructive lung disease ("bronchiolitis obliterans"): A clinical comparative study of bone marrow and lung transplant patients. Eur Respir J 8:551, 1995.

115. Trulock EP: Management of lung transplant rejection. Chest 103:1566, 1993.

116. Dauber JH: Posttransplant bronchiolitis obliterans syndrome: Where have we been and where are we going? Chest 109:857, 1996.

117. Keller CA, Cagle PT, Brown RW, et al: Bronchiolitis obliterans in recipients of single, double and heart-lung transplantation. Chest 107:973, 1995.

118. Sundaresan S, Trulock EP, Mohanakumar T, et al: Prevalence and outcome of bronchiolitis obliterans syndrome after lung transplantation. Washington University Lung Transplant Group. Ann Thorac Surg 60:1341, 1995.

119. Judson MA: Clinical aspects of lung transplantation. Clin Chest Med 14:335, 1993.

120. Nathan SD, Ross DJ, Belman MJ, et al: Bronchiolitis obliterans in single-lung transplant recipients. Chest 107:967, 1995.

121. Sharples LD, Tamm M, McNeil K, et al: Development of bronchiolitis obliterans syndrome in recipients of heart-lung transplantation: Early risk factors. Transplant 61:560, 1996.

122. Burke GJ, Malouf MA, Glanville AR: Opportunistic lung infection with *Corynebacterium pseudodiphtheriticum* after lung and heart transplantation. Med J Aust 166:362, 1997.

123. Soghikian MV, Valentine VG, Berry GJ, et al: Impact of ganciclovir prophylaxis on heart-lung and lung transplant recipients. J Heart Lung Transplant 15:881, 1996.

124. Urbanski SJ, Kossakowska JC, Chan CK, et al: Idiopathic small airways pathology in patients with graft-versus-host disease following allogeneic bone marrow transplantation. Am J Surg Pathol 11:965, 1987.

125. Chan CK, Hyland RH, Hutcheon MA, et al: Small-airways disease in recipients of allogeneic bone marrow transplants: An analysis of 11 cases and a review of the literature. Medicine 66:327, 1987.

126. Clark JG, Schwartz DA, Flourtnoy N, et al: Risk factors for airflow obstruction in recipients of bone marrow transplants. Ann Intern Med 107:648, 1987.

127. Rosenberg ME, Vercellotti GM, Snover DC, et al: Bronchiolitis obliterans after bone marrow transplantation. Am J Hematol 18:325, 1985.

128. St. John RC, Gadek JE, Tutschka PJ: Analysis of airflow obstruction by bronchoalveolar lavage following bone marrow transplantation. Chest 98:600, 1990.

129. Clark JG, Crawford SW, Madtes DK, et al: Obstructive lung disease after allogeneic marrow transplantation. Ann Intern Med 111:368, 1989.

130. Swyer PR, James GCW: A case of unilateral pulmonary emphysema. Thorax 8:133, 1953.

131. MacLeod WM: Abnormal transradiancy of one lung. Thorax 9:147, 1954.

132. Ohri SK, Rutty G, Foundation SW: Acquired segmental emphysema: The enlarging spectrum of Swyer-James/Macleod's syndrome. Ann Thorac Surg 56:120, 1993.

133. Warrell DA, Hughes JMB, Rosenzweig DY: Cardiopulmonary performance at rest and during exercise in seven patients with increased transradiancy of one lung (Macleod's syndrome). Thorax 25:587, 1970.

134. Reid LM, Millard FJC: Correlation between radiological diagnosis and structural lung changes in emphysema. Clin Radiol 15:307, 1964.

135. Fouché RF, Spears JR, Ogilvie C: Unilateral emphysema. Br Med J 1:1312, 1960.

136. Houk VN, Kent DC, Fosburg RG: Unilateral hyperlucent lung: A study in pathophysiology and etiology. Am J Med Sci 253:406, 1967.

137. Leahy DJ: Increased transradiancy of one lung. Br J Dis Chest 55:72, 1961.

138. Peters ME, Dickie HA, Crummy AB, et al: Swyer-James-Macleod syndrome: A case with a baseline normal chest radiograph. Pediatr Radiol 12:211, 1982.

139. Gold RE, Wilt JC, Adhikari TK, et al: Adenoviral pneumonia and its complications in infancy and childhood. J Can Assoc Radiol 20:218, 1969.

140. Culiner MM: The hyperlucent lung, a problem in differential diagnosis. Dis Chest 49:578, 1966.

141. Bernardi F, Cazzato S, Poletti V, et al: Swyer-James syndrome: bronchoalveolar lavage findings in two patients. Eur Respir J 8:654, 1995.

142. Reid L, Simon G: Unilateral lung transradiancy. Thorax 17:230, 1962.

143. Reid L, Simon G: The role of alveolar hypoplasia in some types of emphysema. Br J Dis Chest 58:158, 1964.

144. Rakower J, Morgan E: Unilateral hyperlucent lung (Swyer-James syndrome). Am J Med 33:864, 1962.

145. Margolin HN, Rosenberg LS, Felson B, et al: Idiopathic unilateral hyperlucent lung: A roentgenographic syndrome. Am J Roentgenol 82:63, 1959.

146. Stern EJ, Samples TL: Dynamic ultrafast high resolution CT findings in a case of Swyer-James syndrome. Pediatr Radiol 22:350, 1992.

147. Ghossain MA, Achkar A, Buy JN, et al: Swyer-James syndrome documented by spiral CT angiography and high resolution inspiratory and expiratory CT: An accurate single modality exploration. J Comput Assist Tomogr 21:616, 1997.

148. Marti-Bonmati L, Perales FR, Catala F, et al: CT findings in Swyer-James syndrome. Radiology 172:477, 1989.

149. Moore ADA, Godwin JD, Dietrich PA, et al: Swyer-James syndrome: CT findings in eight patients. Am J Roentgenol 158:1211, 1992.

150. McKenzie SA, Allison DJ, Singh MP, et al: Unilateral hyperlucent lung: The case for investigation. Thorax 35:745, 1980.

151. Salmanzadeh A, Pomeranz SJ, Ramsingh PS: Ventilation-perfusion scintigraphic correlation with multimodality imaging in a proven case of Swyer-James (Macleod's) syndrome. Clin Nucl Med 22:115, 1997.

152. Daniel TL, Woodring JH, Vandiviere HM, et al: Swyer-James syndrome: Unilateral hyperlucent lung syndrome. A case report and review. Clin Geriatr 23:393, 1984.

153. O'Dell CW Jr, Taylor A, Higgins CB, et al: Ventilation-perfusion lung images in the Swyer-James syndrome. Radiology 121:423, 1976.

154. Gottlieb LS, Turner AF: Swyer-James (MacLeod's) syndrome: Variations in pulmonary-bronchial arterial blood flow. Chest 69:62, 1976.

155. Piovan M, Vallis G, Sanson A, Milani L: Echocardiographic findings in one case of Swyer-James syndrome. Clin Cardiol 4:352, 1991.

156. Hekali P, Halttunen P, Korhola O, et al: Chronic unilateral hyperlucent lung: A consecutive series of 40 patients. Fortschr Rontgenstr 136:41, 1982.

157. Prowse OM, Fuchs JE, Kaufman SA, et al: Chronic obstructive pseudoemphysema: A rare cause of unilateral hyperlucent lung. N Engl J Med 271:127, 1964.

158. Nairn JR, Prime FJ: A physiological study of Macleod's syndrome. Thorax 22:148, 1967.

159. Dornhorst AC, Heaf PJ, Semple SJG: Unilateral "emphysema." Lancet 2:873, 1957.

160. Mont JL, Botey A, Subias R, et al: Unilateral pulmonary hemorrhage in a patient with Goodpasture's and Swyer-James' syndrome. Eur J Respir Dis 67:145, 1985.

161. Bates DV, Macklem PT, Christie RV: Respiratory Function in Disease: An Introduction to the Integrated Study of the Lung. 2nd ed. Philadelphia, WB Saunders, 1971.

162. Llamas R, Schwartz A, Gupta SK, et al: Unilateral hyperlucent lung with polycythemia and cor pulmonale. Chest 59:690, 1971.

163. Bensadoun ES, Burke AK, Hogg JC, et al: Proteoglycan deposition in pulmonary fibrosis. Am J Respir Crit Care Med 154:1819, 1996.

164. Olopade CO, Crotty TB, Douglas WW, et al: Chronic eosinophilic pneumonia and idiopathic bronchiolitis obliterans organizing pneumonia: Comparison of eosinophil number and degranulation by immunofluorescence staining for eosinophil-derived major basic protein. Mayo Clin Proc 70:137, 1995.

165. Cordier JF: Cryptogenic organizing pneumonia. Clin Chest Med 14:677, 1993.

166. Yamamoto M, Ina Y, Kitaichi M, et al: Clinical features of BOOP in Japan. Chest 102:21S, 1992.

167. Akira M, Yamamoto S, Sakatani M: Bronchiolitis obliterans organizing pneumonia manifesting as multiple large nodules or masses. Am J Roentgenol 170:291, 1998.

168. Chandler P, Shin M, Friedman S, et al: Radiographic manifestations of bronchiolitis obliterans with organizing pneumonia vs usual interstitial pneumonia. Am J Roentgenol 147:899, 1986.

169. Müller N, Guerry-Force ML, Staples C, et al: Differential diagnosis of bronchiolitis obliterans with organizing pneumonia and usual interstitial pneumonia: Clinical, functional, and radiologic findings. Radiology 162:151, 1987.

170. Cordier J, Loire R, Brune J: Idiopathic bronchiolitis obliterans organizing pneumonia. Chest 96:999, 1989.

171. Izumi T, Kitaichi M, Nishimura K, et al: Bronchiolitis obliterans organizing pneumonia: Clinical features and differential diagnosis. Chest 102:715, 1992.

172. Spiteri M, Klenerman P, Sheppard M, et al: Seasonal cryptogenic organizing pneumonia with biochemical cholestasis: A new clinical entity. Lancet 340:281, 1992.

173. Reich J, Scott D: Levitating lung lesions due to bronchiolitis obliterans organizing pneumonia. Chest 103:623, 1993.

174. Bouchardy LM, Kuhlman JE, Ball WC, et al: CT findings in bronchiolitis obliterans organizing pneumonia (BOOP) with radiographic, clinical and histologic correlation. J Comput Assist Tomogr 17:352, 1993.

175. Guerry-Force ML, Müller NL, Wright JL, et al: A comparison of bronchiolitis obliterans with organizing pneumonia, usual interstitial pneumonia, and small airway disease. Am Rev Respir Dis 135:705, 1987.

176. King TE Jr, Mortenson RL: Cryptogenic organizing pneumonia: The North American experience. Chest 102(1 Suppl):8S, 1992.

177. Nizami IY, Kissner DG, Visscher DW, et al: Idiopathic bronchiolitis obliterans with organizing pneumonia: An acute and life-threatening syndrome. Chest 108:271, 1995.

178. Cohen AJ, King TE Jr, Downey GP: Rapidly progressive bronchiolitis obliterans organizing pneumonia. Am J Respir Crit Care Med 149:1670, 1994.

179. Lohr RH, Boland BJ, Douglas WW, et al: Organizing pneumonia: Features and prognosis of cryptogenic, secondary, and focal variants. Arch Intern Med 157:1323, 1997.

180. Katzenstein A, Myers J, Prophet D, et al: Bronchiolitis obliterans and usual interstitial pneumonia: A comparative clinicopathologic study. Am J Surg Pathol 10:373, 1986.

181. Cosio MG, Hale KA, Niewoehner DE: Morphologic and morphometric effects of prolonged smoking on the small airways. Am Rev Respir Dis 122:265, 1980.

182. Wright JL, Lawson LM, Paré PD, et al: Morphology of peripheral airways in current and ex-smokers. Am Rev Respir Dis 127:474, 1983.

183. Yousem SA, Colby TV, Gaensler EA: Respiratory bronchiolitis-associated interstitial lung disease and its relationship to desquamative interstitial pneumonitis. Mayo Clin Proc 64:1373, 1989.

184. King TE: Respiratory bronchiolitis-associated interstitial lung disease. Clin Chest Med 14:693, 1993.

185. Bosi F, Oggionni T, Vaiana E, et al: Respiratory bronchiolitis-associated interstitial lung disease: A case report with bronchoalveolar lavage findings. Monaldi Arch Chest Dis 50:448, 1995.

186. Katzenstein AA, Myers JL: Idiopathic pulmonary fibrosis: Clinical relevance of pathologic classification. Am J Respir Crit Care Med 157:1301, 1998.

187. Myers JL, Veal CF, Shin MS, et al: Respiratory bronchiolitis causing interstitial lung disease: A clinico-pathologic study. Am Rev Respir Dis 135:880, 1987.

188. Yousem SA, Colby TV, Carrington CB: Follicular bronchitis/bronchiolitis. Hum Pathol 16:700, 1985.

189. Fortoul TL, Cano-Valle F, Oliva E, et al: Follicular bronchiolitis in association with connective tissue diseases. Lung 163:305, 1985.

190. Kinoshita M, Higashi T, Tanaka C, et al: Follicular bronchiolitis associated with rheumatoid arthritis. Intern Med 31:674, 1992.

191. Scully RE, Mark EJ, McNeely WF, et al: Case records of the Massachusetts General Hospital. Case 23-1993. N Engl J Med 328:1696, 1993.

192. Kinane BT, Mansell AL, Zwerdling RG, et al: Follicular bronchitis in the pediatric population. Chest 104:1183, 1993.

193. Franchi LM, Chin TW, Nussbaum E, et al: Familial pulmonary nodular lymphoid hyperplasia. J Pediatr 121:89, 1992.

194. Remy-Jardin M, Remy J, Wallaert B, et al: Pulmonary involvement in progressive systemic sclerosis: Sequential evaluation with CT, pulmonary function tests, and bronchoalveolar lavage. Radiology 188:499, 1993.

195. Remy-Jardin M, Remy J, Cortet B, et al: Lung changes in rheumatoid arthritis: CT findings. Radiology 193:375, 1994.

195a. Hayakawa H, Sato A, Imokawa S, et al: Bronchiolar disease in rheumatoid arthritis. Am J Respir Crit Care Med 154:1531, 1996.

196. Yousem SA, Colby TV, Carrington CB: Lung biopsy in rheumatoid arthritis. Am Rev Respir Dis 131:770, 1985.

197. Newball HH, Brahim SA: Chronic obstructive airway disease in patients with Sjögren's syndrome. Am Rev Respir Dis 115:295, 1977.

198. Sugiyama Y: Diffuse panbronchiolitis. Clin Chest Med 14:765, 1993.

199. Iwata M, Colby TV, Kitaichi M: Diffuse panbronchiolitis: Diagnosis and distinction from various pulmonary diseases with centrilobular interstitial foam cell accumulations. Hum Pathol 25:357, 1994.

200. Homma H, Yamanaka A, Tanimoto S, et al: Diffuse panbronchiolitis: A disease of the transitional zone of the lung. Chest 83:63, 1983.

201. Kim YW, Han SK, Shim YS, et al: The first report of diffuse panbronchiolitis in Korea: Five case reports. Intern Med 31:695, 1992.

202. Tsang KWT, Ooi CGC, Ip MSM, et al: Clinical profiles of Chinese patients with diffuse panbronchiolitis. Thorax 53:274, 1998.

203. Brugiere O, Milleron B, Antoine M, et al: Diffuse panbronchiolitis in an Asian immigrant. Thorax 51:1065, 1996.

203a. Fisher MS Jr, Rush WL, Rosado-de-Christenson ML, et al: Diffuse panbronchiolitis. Histologic diagnosis in unsuspected cases involving North American residents of Asian descent. Arch Pathol Lab Med 122:156, 1997.

204. Poletti V, Patelli M, Poletti G, et al: Diffuse panbronchiolitis observed in an Italian male. Sarcoidosis 9:67, 1992.

205. Fitzgerald JE, King TE Jr, Lynch DA, et al: Diffuse panbronchiolitis in the United States. Am J Respir Crit Care Med 154:497, 1996.

206. Randhawa P, Hoagland MH, Yousem SA: Diffuse panbronchiolitis in North America: Report of three cases and review of the literature. Am J Surg Pathol 15:43, 1991.

207. Homer RJ, Khoo L, Smith GJ: Diffuse panbronchiolitis in a Hispanic man with travel history to Japan. Chest 107:1176, 1995.

208. Corne J: Diffuse panbronchiolitis: A new Japanese export? Lancet 348:1465, 1996.

209. Sugiyama Y, Kudoh S, Maeda H, et al: Analysis of HLA antigens in patients with diffuse panbronchiolitis. Am Rev Respir Dis 141:1459, 1990.

210. Tomita Y, Hashimoto S, Shimizu T, et al: Restriction fragment length polymorphism analysis in the HLA class III genes of patients with diffuse panbronchiolitis. Intern Med 35:693, 1996.

210a. Keicho N, Tokunaga K, Nakata K, et al: Contribution of HLA genes to genetic predisposition in diffuse panbronchiolitis. Am J Respir Crit Care Med 158:846, 1998.

211. Miyashita N, Matsumoto A, Kubota Y, et al: Continuous isolation and character-

ization of *Chlamydia pneumoniae* from a patient with diffuse panbronchiolitis. Microbiol Immunol 40:547, 1996.

212. Kikuchi T, Saijo Y, Sakai T, et al: Human T-cell lymphotropic virus type 1 (HTLV-1) carrier with clinical manifestations characteristic of diffuse panbronchiolitis. Intern Med 35:305, 1996.

213. Hoiby N: Diffuse panbronchiolitis and cystic fibrosis: East meets West. Thorax 49:531, 1994.

214. Mukae H, Kadota J, Kohno S, et al: Increase in activated CD8 + cells in bronchoalveolar lavage fluid in patients with diffuse panbronchiolitis. Am J Respir Crit Care Med 152:613, 1995.

215. Yasuoka S, Fujisawa K, Ueta Y, et al: Cell profile and elastase activity in diffuse panbronchiolitis investigated by bronchoalveolar and bronchial lavage. Intern Med 31:599, 1992.

216. Oda H, Kadota J, Kohno S, et al: Leukotriene B4 in bronchoalveolar lavage fluid of patients with diffuse panbronchiolitis. Chest 108:116, 1995.

217. Koga T: Neutrophilia and high level of interleukin 8 in the bronchoalveolar lavage fluid of diffuse panbronchiolitis. Kurume Med J 40:139, 1993.

218. Baz MA, Kussin PS, Van Trigt P, et al: Recurrence of diffuse panbronchiolitis after lung transplantation. Am J Respir Crit Care Med 151:895, 1995.

219. Sugiyama Y, Saitoh K, Kano S, et al: An autopsy case of diffuse panbronchiolitis accompanying rheumatoid arthritis. Respir Med 90:175, 1996.

220. Ono K, Shimamoto Y, Matsuzaki M, et al: Diffuse panbronchiolitis as a pulmonary complication in patients with adult T-cell leukemia. Am J Hematol 30:86, 1989.

221. Maeda M, Saiki S, Yamanaka A: Serial section analysis of the lesions in diffuse panbronchiolitis. Acta Pathol Jpn 37:693, 1987.

222. Kitaichi M, Nishimura K, Izumi T: Diffuse panbronchiolitis. In: Sharma OP (ed): Lung Disease in the Tropics. New York, Marcel Dekker, 1991, pp 479.

223. Yaegashi H, Takahashi T: The site, severity, and distribution of bronchiolar obstruction in lungs with chronic obstructive pulmonary disease: Morphometry and computer-assisted three-dimensional reconstruction of airways. Arch Pathol Lab Med 118:975, 1994.

224. Nakata K, Tanimoto H: Diffuse panbronchiolitis. Jpn J Clin Radiol 26:1133, 1981.

225. Ichikawa Y, Hotta M, Sumita S, et al: Reversible airway lesions in diffuse panbronchiolitis: Detection by high-resolution computed tomography. Chest 107:120, 1995.

226. Akira M, Higashihara T, Sakatani M, et al: Diffuse panbronchiolitis: Follow-up CT examination. Radiology 189:559, 1993.

227. Kudoh S, Uetake T, Hagiwara K, et al: Clinical effects of low-dose long-term erythromycin chemotherapy on diffuse panbronchiolitis. Jpn J Thorac Dis 25:632, 1987.

228. Kudoh S, Azuma A, Yamamoto M, et al: Improvement of survival in patients with diffuse panbronchiolitis treated with low-dose erythromycin. Am J Respir Crit Care Med 157:1829, 1998.

229. Fujii T, Kadota J, Kawakami K, et al: Long-term effect of erythromycin therapy in patients with chronic *Pseudomonas aeruginosa* infection. Thorax 50:1246, 1995.

230. Oda H, Kadota J, Kohno S, et al: Erythromycin inhibits neutrophil chemotaxis in bronchoalveoli of diffuse panbronchiolitis. Chest 106:1116, 1994.

231. Kadota J, Sakito O, Kohno S, et al: A mechanism of erythromycin treatment in patients with diffuse panbronchiolitis. Am Rev Respir Dis 147:153, 1993.

232. Sakito O, Kadota J, Kohno S, et al: Interleukin 1 beta, tumor necrosis factor alpha, and interleukin 8 in bronchoalveolar lavage fluid of patients with diffuse panbronchiolitis: A potential mechanism of macrolide therapy. Respiration 63:42, 1996.

233. Ichikawa Y, Ninomiya H, Koga H, et al: Erythromycin reduces neutrophils and neutrophil-derived elastolytic-like activity in the lower respiratory tract of bronchiolitis patients. Am Rev Respir Dis 146:196, 1992.

234. Umeki S: Anti-inflammatory action of erythromycin: Its inhibitory effect on neutrophil NADPH oxidase activity. Chest 104:1191, 1993.

235. Diaz F, Collazos J, Martinez E, et al: Bronchiolitis obliterans in a patient with HIV infection. Respir Med 91:171, 1997.

236. Schwartz DA, Visvesvara GS, Leitch GJ, et al: Pathology of symptomatic microsporidial *(Encephalitozoon hellum)* bronchiolitis in the acquired immunodeficiency syndrome: A new respiratory pathogen diagnosed from lung biopsy, bronchoalveolar lavage, sputum, and tissue culture. Hum Pathol 24:937, 1993.

237. Sieber SC, Cole SR, McNab JM, et al: Bronchiolitis associated with the finding of the fungus aspergillus. Conn Med 58:13, 1994.

238. Ogawa H, Fujimura M, Matsuda T, et al: Transient wheeze: Eosinophilic bronchiolitis in acute eosinophilic pneumonia. Chest 104:493, 1993.

239. Wilcox P, Miller R, Miller G, et al: Airway involvement in ulcerative colitis. Chest 92:18, 1987.

240. Chatte G, Streichenberger N, Boillot O, et al: Lymphocytic bronchitis/bronchiolitis in a patient with primary biliary cirrhosis. Eur Respir J 8:176, 1995.

241. Miller RR, Müller NL: Neuroendocrine cell hyperplasia and obliterative bronchiolitis in patients with peripheral carcinoid tumors. Am J Surg Pathol 19:653, 1995.

242. Chang H, Wang J-S, Tseng H-H, et al: Histopathologic study of *Sauropus androgynus*-associated constrictive bronchiolitis obliterans. A new cause of constrictive bronchiolitis obliterans. Am J Surg Pathol 21:35, 1997.

# Index

Note: Page numbers in *italics* refer to illustrations; numbers followed by t indicate tables; numbers followed by n indicate notes.

Abdomen, pleural effusion related to disease within, 2763–2766
  sarcoidosis involving, 1563, 1565
  surgery on, pleural effusion after, 2763–2765, 2766
    pulmonary complications in, 2672, 2674
  upper, mechanoreceptors in, in ventilatory control, 238
Abdominal drainage tubes, complications of, 2677
Abdominal muscles, in ventilation, 247, 255, 256, 3056
  recruitment of, in diaphragmatic paralysis, 3059, *3060*
Abscess, cavity vs., 462
  hepatic, in amebiasis, 1034, 1035, *1035,* 2753
  intrabdominal, pleural effusion due to, 2765
  lung. See *Lung abscess.*
  mediastinal, radiologic features of, 2852, *2854, 2855*
    retropharyngeal abscess with, upper airway obstruction due to, 2022, *2023*
    retropharyngeal, acute, upper airway obstruction due to, 2021, 2022, *2023*
    mediastinitis due to, *2852*
  retrosternal, after sternotomy, 2660, *2660, 3019, 3019*
  subphrenic, in amebiasis, 1034
    pleural effusion with, 2766
    postoperative, 2672–2674
  with skeletal tuberculosis, 837–838, *838*
Acanthosis nigricans, in pulmonary carcinoma, 1174
Acariasis, 1061
Accessory cardiac bronchus, 626–627, *627*
Accessory diaphragm, 3006
Accessory fissures, imaging of, 160–165, *163–166*
Accessory lobe, inferior, 164–165, *165*
Accessory lung, 628
  bronchopulmonary sequestration vs., 601
Acetaldehyde, defect in metabolism of, alcohol-induced asthma and, 2116
Acetylation, slow, drug-induced lupus and, 1424–1425
Acetylcholine, endothelial response to, 148
  pulmonary vascular response to, 106
Acetylcysteine, mucus viscosity and, 63
Acetylsalicylic acid. See also *Salicylates.*
  asthma provoked by, 2112–2113
  leukotrienes in, 2091, 2113
  mucociliary clearance and, 129
  thoracic disease due to, 2539t, 2565

Achalasia, 2967, *2967, 3183*
  esophageal involvement in progressive systemic sclerosis vs., 1457
Acid, daily production of, 115
Acid maltase deficiency, 2727, 3064
Acid-base balance, 115–119
  disorders of. See also *Acidosis; Alkalosis.*
    classification of, 115
    compensatory mechanisms in, 115–116
    mixed, 115
    nomogram for, 119, *120*
    renal response to, 116
    in COPD, 2228
Acidemia, acidosis vs., 115n
Acidosis, carotid body response to, 235–237
  defined, 115n
  metabolic, 117–118, 118t
    central ventilatory response to, 237
    hyperventilation in, 3067
    in asthma, 2139
    pulmonary vascular response to, 106
    pleural fluid, 2743
  respiratory, 116–117
    in COPD, 2228
Acinar adenocarcinoma, pulmonary, 1101, *1102.* See also *Adenocarcinoma, pulmonary.*
Acinar nodule, 438
*Acinetobacter* infection, 764
Acinic cell carcinoma, tracheobronchial gland, 1258
Acino-nodose lesions, in tuberculosis, problems with term, 828
Acinus(i), 26–31, *31, 32, 2190*
  channels of airway communication with, 31–33, *32*
  development and growth of, 137, *139*
    postnatal, 138–139
  gas composition in, 53, *54*
  gas diffusion in, 107
  perfusion of, 104
    matching acinar ventilation to, 108–111, *109.* See also *Ventilation/perfusion* entries.
  ventilation of, 53–60
    matching capillary blood flow to, 108–111, *109.* See also *Ventilation/perfusion* entries.
Acquired immunodeficiency syndrome (AIDS). See also *Human immunodeficiency virus (HIV) infection.*
  bronchoalveolar lavage in infection diagnosis in, 343
  epidemiology of, 1641–1643, *1642*

Acquired immunodeficiency syndrome (AIDS) *(Continued)*
  Kaposi's sarcoma in. See *Kaposi's sarcoma, in HIV infection.*
  *Mycobacterium avium* complex infection in, 1654–1655, *1654–1656*
    histologic features of, 853, *854*
  *Pneumocystis carinii* pneumonia in. See Pneumocystis carinii *pneumonia, in HIV infection.*
  spontaneous pneumothorax in, 2787
Acrocyanosis, 398
Acrodermatitis enteropathica, 726
Acromegaly, 2729
  with carcinoid tumor, 1241, 1242
Acrylate glue embolism, 1865, *1867*
ACTH, intraoperative measurement of, during carcinoid tumor excision, 1242
*Actinobacillus actinomycetemcomitans* infection, 776
Actinomycosis, 952–957
  cavities or cysts in, 3102t
  clinical features of, 956–957
  endobronchial, 957
  epidemiology of, 953
  homogeneous nonsegmental opacity in, 3080t
  pathogenesis of, 953–954
  pathologic features of, 954, *954*
  pleural boundary crossing by, 460
  pleural effusion in, 2751
  radiologic features of, 954–956, *955, 956*
Acute lung injury. See also *Adult respiratory distress syndrome (ARDS); Pulmonary edema, permeability.*
  diagnostic criteria for, 1995, 1995t
Acute respiratory disease syndrome, adenovirus infection and, 995
Acute-phase reactants, in tuberculosis, 847
Acyclovir, thoracic disease due to, 2572
Addison's disease, due to tuberculosis, 840
Adenocarcinoid tumor, 1232
Adenocarcinoma. See also *Carcinoma.*
  cervical, metastatic to lung, 1408
  colorectal, metastatic to lung, *1385, 1387, 1396, 1400*
  endometrial, metastatic to lung, 1407
  mesothelioma vs., 1165, *1165,* 2818–2820, *2819,* 2826
  metastatic to lung, calcification in, 467
    from cervical primary, 1408
    from colorectal primary, *1385, 1387, 1396, 1400*
    from endometrial primary, 1407

Vol. 3 ISBN 0-7216-6197-1

9 780721 661971

90071